D1310132

NEURORADIOLOGY

Third Edition

NEURORADIOLOGY

Third Edition

Juan M. Taveras, M.D.

Professor of Radiology (Emeritus)
Harvard Medical School
Radiologist
Former Radiologist-in-Chief
Massachusetts General Hospital
Boston, Massachusetts

with a chapter on
Endovascular
Therapeutic
Neuroradiology
by

John Pile-Spellman, M.D.

Associate Professor of Radiology and Neurosurgery
Columbia University College of Physicians and Surgeons
Director of Interventional Neuroradiology
Columbia Presbyterian Medical Center
New York, New York

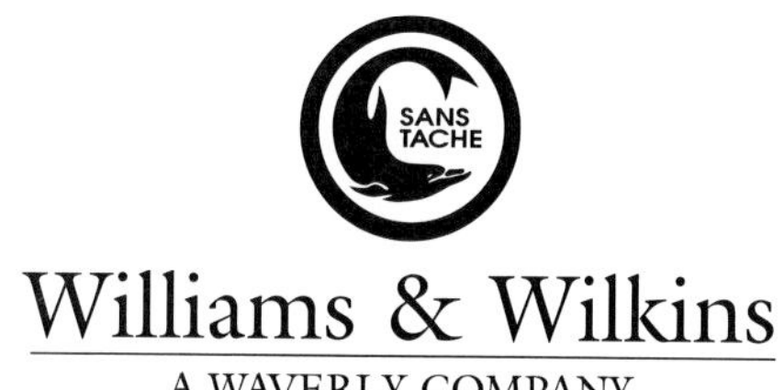

Williams & Wilkins
A WAVERLY COMPANY

BALTIMORE • PHILADELPHIA • LONDON • PARIS • BANGKOK
BUENOS AIRES • HONG KONG • MUNICH • SYDNEY • TOKYO • WROCLAW

Editor: Charley Mitchell
Managing Editor: Margie Keating
Production Coordinator: Linda Carlson
Production Service: Editorial Services of New England, Inc.
Project Managers: John Svatek and Rojean Wagner
Copyeditor: Beverly Miller
Illustration Planner: Linda Dana-Willis
Cover Designer: Tom Scheuerman
Typesetter: Maryland Composition
Printer: R. R. Donnelley, Crawfordsville, IN

351 West Camden Street
Baltimore, Maryland 21201-2436 USA

Rose Tree Corporate Center
1400 North Providence Road
Building II, Suite 5025
Media, Pennsylvania 19063-2043 USA

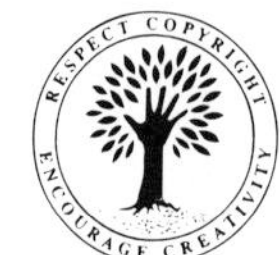

Visit Williams & Wilkins on the Internet: http://www.wwilkins.com

Accurate indications, adverse reactions, and dosage schedules for drugs are provided in this book, but it is possible that they may change. The reader is urged to review the package information data of the manufacturers of the medications mentioned.

Printed in the United States of America

Third Edition

Library of Congress Cataloging in Publication Data

Taveras, Juan M., 1919–
Neuroradiology / Juan M. Taveras. — 3rd ed.
p. cm.
Rev. ed. of: Diagnostic neuroradiology / Juan M. Taveras, Ernest H. Wood. 2nd ed., c1976.
Includes bibliographical references and index.
ISBN 0-683-08112-8
1. Nervous system—Radiography. I. Taveras, Juan M., 1919– . Diagnostic neuroradiology. II. Title.
[DNLM: 1. Central Nervous System Diseases—radiography. 2. Neuroradiography. WL 141 T233n 1996]
RC349.D52T38 1996
616.8′047572—dc20
DNLM/DLC
for Library of Congress 95-33623
CIP

The Publishers have made every effort to trace the copyright holders for borrowed material. If they have inadvertently overlooked any, they will be pleased to make the necessary arrangements at the first opportunity.

96 97 98 99 00
1 2 3 4 5 6 7 8 9 10

Reprints of chapters may be purchased from Williams & Wilkins in quantities of 100 or more. Call our Special Sales Department, (800) 358-3583.

ISBN 0-683-08112-8

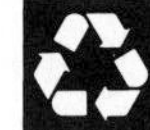

To my wife, Margot, for her understanding and encouragement
To my children, Louisa and Jeffrey, and my grandchildren, Tiffany and Olivia

Contents

Preface

This work represents the third edition of *Diagnostic Neuroradiology*. The first edition appeared in 1964 and the second in 1976 and were authored with Dr. Ernest H. Wood. Dr. Wood passed away over two decades ago and this edition has been done by myself with the exception of one important chapter on endovascular therapeutic neuroradiology, authored by John Pile-Spellman with some assistance from three collaborators, Dr. William L. Young, Dr. Lotfi Hacein-Bey, and Dr. E. Sander Connolly, Jr. Since the second edition of *Diagnostic Neuroradiology*, revolutionary changes have taken place in all of radiology but particularly in the radiology of the nervous system. In addition to the developments and improvements in computed tomography, magnetic resonance was introduced for clinical applications in the early 1980s, and these technical advances totally changed our approach to diagnosis of diseases of the central nervous system. The advances in neuroradiology have created the need for a change in the title of the book as well as in the emphasis. The changes have been so radical that only a small portion, about 15 or 20% of the second edition could be used here. For instance, the chapter on skull radiography was deleted because radiography of the skull has been relegated to a secondary position. It is performed only when needed, after computed tomography.

The work is organized in 18 chapters. In the first two editions, the subdivision of the material was based on the radiologic examination. In this edition, the presentation of the material is focused on the pathologic condition being described and on what imaging methods of examination can be utilized to arrive at a diagnosis. The only exception to this is the first three chapters: an introduction, technical considerations, in which the cross-imaging procedures are described in some detail, and the anatomy of the central nervous system. In addition, a large chapter on endovascular therapeutic neuroradiology is integrated into the work (Chapter 18). A discussion of angiographic technique and anatomy (Chapter 17) precedes the chapter on endovascular therapeutic neuroradiology. That chapter represents the angiographic section of the second edition, which has been revised, with some assistance from Dr. Pile-Spellman, and reduced in size to conform to current practice. In the anatomy and technical considerations of angiography, some pathologic aspects are mentioned and illustrated, although they are not usually utilized for diagnosis. However, the abnormalities are observed and it is important to be able to interpret them in the angiograms. Also, the interventional neuroradiologist needs to be able to interpret the findings.

The present work deals only with neuroradiology and does not include the radiology of the head and neck. For this reason, the orbit is only dealt with in passing and there are no descriptions of the paranasal sinuses, the facial bones, or the other structures. The endovascular therapeutic chapter includes a small section dealing with craniofacial pathology because of the intimate relationship that exists between the extra and intracranial circulations and because they are likely to be cared for by the neuroradiologists.

In addition to the evolutionary changes in diagnosis, spectacular developments have taken place in the area of percutaneous therapeutic procedures, which have come to be known as interventional neuroradiology. While the concept of interventional neuroradiology could be broadened to include such procedures as brain biopsies or percutaneous discectomy, only the endovascular procedures are described here, because I believe that the others are likely to be performed by neurosurgeons or orthopedic surgeons.

As with the first edition of *Diagnostic Neuroradiology*, it is my purpose to present here what I believe to be the present status of neuroradiology. I adhere to the concept that the diagnostic and therapeutic aspects of neuroradiology are inseparable and that the two portions represent the subspecialty as it is today. It is expected that from now on training programs will include both aspects.

This book was prepared for the student as well as for the specialist, for the radiologist as well as for the neurologist and the neurosurgeon, and it is my hope that they find it useful in many aspects of their clinical and scientific activities.

I am most grateful to many who helped me during the last five years of preparation of this work. Life has its difficult moments and the passing away of my wife Berenice caused a long delay in the first two years of working on this revision, but fortunately this passed. Margot has now successfully filled the void, and happiness has returned. I thank her for her understanding and for adapting to the difficult schedule and also for contributing a number of anatomical drawings and diagrams throughout the text.

My thanks also goes to several of my colleagues, nationally and internationally, who contributed cases for illustrations. These include: Dr. Cosma Andreula of Bari, Italy; Dr. Luiz Bacheschi of Sao Paulo, Brasil; Dr. William Bradley, Los Angeles, CA; Dr. R. K. Breger, Madison, WI; Dr. Jan Brismar of King Faisal Specialist Hospital in Saudi Arabia; Dr. F. Ebner of Vienna, Austria; Dr. Allen D. Elster, Winston-Salem, NC; Dr. Richard E. Fernandez,

Tom's River, NJ; Dr. Ramon Figueroa, Augusta, GA; Dr. Massimo Gallucci, L'Aquila, Italy; Dr. R. K. Gupta, New Delhi, India; Dr. John Hesselink, San Diego, CA; Dr. J. Randy Jinkins, San Antonio, TX; Dr. Alvaro Magalhaes, Sao Paulo, Brazil; Dr. Alexander Mamourian, Lebanon, NH; Dr. Kenneth Maravilla, Seattle, WA; Dr. Michael Mikhael, Chicago, IL; Dr. Sergio Moguillansky, Cipolletti, Argentina; Dr. Robert Peyster, Stony Brook, NY; Dr. James Provenzale, Durham, NC; Dr. Joseph Sackett, Madison, WI; Dr. Stephen Sweriduk, Boston, MA; Dr. Robert Tien, Durham, NC; Dr. Charles Truwit, Minneapolis, MN; Drs. J. Valk and M. van der Knaap, Amsterdam, the Netherlands; Dr. Daniel Williams, Winston-Salem, NC.

In the Department of Radiology at Massachusetts General Hospital, I am most grateful to the entire neuroradiology staff and fellows for their help and understanding. Drs. Bradley Buchbinder, Richard Robertson, Greg Sorenson, and Gilberto Gonzalez deserve special thanks. Dr. James Thrall, the department chairman, was most gracious to me throughout the preparation of this manuscript. My deepest appreciation also goes to many others. Practically all the photography was carried out by Nancy J. Speroni, M.Ed., Laurie Lizotte, Catherine Otis, and Kristin Toohey in the Photographic Laboratory of the Department of Radiology. Many of the anatomical drawings were performed by a former Research Fellow in our Department, Dr. Martha Sideregts of Venezuela. Ms. Betty Emanuel and, particularly, Maureen Stimpson typed and retyped the entire manuscript. I also wish to thank Dr. James Provenzale for assisting me in the preparation of many of the tables throughout the text.

The Williams and Wilkins staff have always been helpful and very patient as they waited for the manuscript. I would like to thank Mr. Charles Mitchell for speeding up the review and the copyediting of the manuscript once it was complete and Margie Keating for her handling of it. The chosen group of copyeditors in Boston was outstanding and very helpful.

JUAN M. TAVERAS

1

Introduction and Examination Approach

For a number of decades we have been living through what might be called the diagnostic era of medicine. We are no longer content with simply making an approximate diagnosis of a lesion; rather, we strive to get considerably more information before deciding to treat the lesion, if one is found, and selecting the method of treatment that is best suited to the diagnosis. Before the discovery of x-rays, it was only possible to suspect the presence of an organic lesion and to approximate its location through neurologic examination. Following the discovery of x-rays, we were able to diagnose some lesions that produced calcification within the cranial cavity, which produced changes in the skull bones that could be detected by radiography. In addition, we were able to see enlargement and erosion of the sella turcica, and thus suspect the presence of pituitary tumors; the same was true of other lesions around the base of the skull and in the vault that led to bone destruction (1).

Following the introduction of contrast media, nearly 25 years after Roentgen's discovery, the localization of space-occupying lesions and of certain vascular problems improved dramatically. The first contrast examination was described by Walter Dandy, who, in 1918, introduced air ventriculography by injecting air directly into the ventricles (2); in 1919, Dandy introduced pneumoencephalography, which could be performed after the injection of air following a lumbar spinal puncture (3). Dandy also spoke about the possibility of diagnosing intraspinal space-occupying lesions by showing the arrest of the injected air in the spinal canal, but it was Sicard who, in 1921, described a radiopaque oily contrast substance that could be injected into the spinal canal and used to diagnose intraspinal lesions (4,5). Egas Moniz, in 1927, described cerebral angiography (6). These developments represented considerable progress in the diagnosis of lesions of the central nervous system. Once these three invasive approaches could be utilized, it was possible to diagnose space-occupying lesions within the brain and within the spinal canal, and also to diagnose lesions of the blood vessels of the brain.

In 1948, George Moore described the use of radioactive isotopes to diagnose the location of tumors of the brain (7). This was an important noninvasive approach to diagnosing brain neoplasms and other conditions. Although Dussik and Dussik of Vienna had described the possibility of using ultrasound in diagnosing lesions of the brain (8), it was not until 1956, when Leksell published a paper on the use of ultrasound to detect brain abnormalities following head trauma (9), that ultrasound began to be used more extensively to diagnose brain lesions. He termed this examination *echoencephalography*, and it involved mostly the detection of displacement of the midline structures, which would take place in the presence of intracerebral hemorrhage, or a subdural or epidural hematoma as a result of head trauma.

With the exception of plain films of the skull, there were no other noninvasive approaches to diagnose brain tumors when I started in neuroradiology; it was not until the late 1950s and early 1960s that we began to utilize radionuclide encephalography and echoencephalography.

In the 1960s the diagnostic procedures, particularly angiography, continued to improve and were getting progressively more invasive as we strove to make more complete diagnoses through the use of selective and superselective angiographic approaches; the same was true of pneumographic and cisternographic procedures.

The discovery of computed tomography (CT) by Godfrey Hounsfield, in 1972, opened a new era in noninvasive diagnosis of brain lesions (10). Shortly after, in 1973, the possibility of utilizing nuclear magnetic resonance to produce images was suggested by Paul Lauterbur (11), but it took several years before we could produce satisfactory images of the brain and the spine utilizing magnetic resonance.

Today we have a good number of noninvasive procedures that are very effective in arriving at a diagnosis of pathologic processes in the brain and spine. For this reason, we should start with the least invasive approaches to diagnose the presence, the type, the location, and the probable histology of the lesion before proceeding with a more invasive approach. The result was that *pneumoencephalography* disappeared as a diagnostic procedure, and *angiography* is carried out only to obtain some specific information. For instance, it is needed to diagnose saccular aneurysm of the cerebral vessels and to demonstrate the configuration of arteriovenous malformations, which are usually already diagnosed by CT or magnetic resonance imaging (MRI). Angiography is also used to visualize the vascularity of certain tumors such as meningiomas, and when a closed biopsy is going to be performed because it is important to know how vascular the lesion is prior to putting a probe into it without a craniotomy. Angiography is also used in the study of vascular occlusive disease, but much less frequently than previously.

For these reasons, today we carry out the diagnostic approach to a patient with a suspected brain or spinal cord lesion as follows:

In a nonurgent condition we would start with CT without and with intravenous iodide contrast media and, if needed, MRI without and with gadolinium injection. The diagnosis would usually be strongly suspected or clearly made after these two procedures. *Plain-film examinations of the skull* are no longer done routinely unless there is a condition that may show skull abnormalities. In general, following either CT or MRI, no further examinations are carried out unless there is doubt that the findings obtained by either of these two procedures are accurate or complete. We no longer do *radionuclide encephalography* because in this group of nonurgent diagnostic problems, it does not add any information over and above that which can be shown by CT or MRI. Angiography is carried out only if there is a perceived need, as explained earlier. In the spine, *myelography* may be needed; we still use it to diagnose more accurately the intervertebral discs in the lumbar and cervical regions. We rarely use myelography to study intraspinal neoplasms, because MRI without and with contrast enhancement is usually sufficient to diagnose the presence of the lesion and the relationship of the lesion to the spinal cord to differentiate intramedullary from extramedullary lesions, whether intradural or extradural. If MRI is unavailable or contraindicated, CT myelography is recommended.

In acute conditions, such as in a patient with head trauma, a suspected stroke, or subarachnoid hemorrhage, the approach would be similar, except that CT is preferable in this type of procedure, whereas in the nonurgent situation, MRI is becoming the ideal procedure to start with as equipment becomes more widely distributed.

In acute conditions, owing to the fact that the patient may be uncooperative, may present intracranial bleeding, or, as in the case of trauma, may also present fractures and depressions of the skull bones, CT is superior to MRI because of the shorter exposure required (1 to 3 sec for CT, while still obtaining optimum resolution, and several minutes for MRI to obtain optimum resolution) and also because it is much easier to diagnose acute bleeding with CT than with MRI. Subarachnoid hemorrhage may be entirely overlooked by MRI. Also, there are no contraindications to CT imaging.

In acute conditions involving the spine or spinal cord, however, MRI is superior because it will show the direct effect on the spinal cord itself; it also allows the taking of sagittal views, showing the deformity of the vertebral bodies as well as the presence or absence of compression of the spinal cord. This applies not only to a patient who has a rapidly progressing paraparesis or paraplegia but also to a patient who has had spinal injury, if there are signs suggesting the possibility of cord compression. In the absence of any signs that would indicate cord compression, plain films of the spine are usually considered sufficient.

The organization of this book will follow the approaches just described. That is, the noninvasive diagnostic procedures will be discussed first, followed by discussion of the more invasive procedures such as cerebral angiography. A similar approach will be followed when describing the examination of the spine and spinal cord. Owing to the profound changes in our ability to diagnose lesions by cross-sectional imaging, the chapter dealing with plain-film examination of the skull has been moved to last in this edition.

REFERENCES

1. Taveras JM: Neuroradiology: Past, present, future. The Diamond Jubilee Lecture. Radiology 1990;175:593–602.
2. Dandy WE: Ventriculography following the injection of air into the cerebral ventricles. Ann Surg 1918;68:4–11.
3. Dandy WE: Roentgenography of the brain after the injection of air into the spinal canal. Ann Surg 1919;70:397–403.
4. Sicard JA, Forestier J: Méthode générale d'exploration radiologique par l'huile iode (Lipiodol). Bull Mem Soc Med Hop 1922;46: 463–469.
5. Sicard JA, Forestier J, LaPlane: Radio-diagnostic lipiodole au cours des compressions rachidiennes. Rev Neurol 1923;31:676.
6. Moniz E: Arterial encephalography: Its importance in the location of cerebral tumors. Rev Neurol 1927;1:48–72.
7. Moore G: Use of radioactive diiodofluorescein in diagnosis and localization of brain tumors. Science 1948;107:569–571.
8. Dussik KT, Dussik F, Nyt L: Aub dem weg! zur hyperphonogrpahie des gehirnes. Wien Med Wochenschr 1947;97:425.
9. Leksell L: Echoencephalography: Detection of intracranial complications following head injury. Acta Chir Scand 1956;110:301–305.
10. Hounsfield G: Computerized transverse axial scanning (tomography): I. Description of system. Br J Radiol 1973;46:1016–1022.
11. Lauterbur P: Image formation by induced local interactions: Examples employing nuclear magnetic resonance. Nature 1973;242: 190–191.

SELECTED READING

Ambrose J: Computerized transverse axial scanning (tomography): II. Clinical application. Br J Radiol 1973;46:1023–1047.

2

Technical Considerations

COMPUTED TOMOGRAPHY

Computed tomography (CT) is based on the principle that the different tissues of the body absorb x-rays in different proportions depending on their molecular weight. CT therefore is based on the same single principle upon which ordinary radiography is based. However, CT scanning is considerably more sensitive than ordinary radiography in recording the absorption differences. Why is this so? It is because ordinary radiography exposes the entire area to be radiographed to a single exposure; this causes a considerable amount of scattering of the x-ray beam from areas adjacent to and remote from a given point, which works to decrease the contrast that might otherwise be possible if there were not so much scattering. In addition, in ordinary radiography one superimposes all of the tissues throughout the area of the body being radiographed. These two factors decrease considerably the ability of an ordinary radiographic film to show the anatomy and the pathology. In CT, on the other hand, scatter is eliminated by the use of a very narrow x-ray beam, and only a single slice of the body is being radiographed. In addition, the effects of superimposition are eliminated by viewing any given point from all possible aspects, up to 360°. In the initial CT scanner, marketed by the EMI Company, each point was viewed from at least 180° (1). This first-generation scanner took from 2 to 5 min to generate an image. In the second generation, the approach was essentially the same, utilizing up to 200 or 220° instead of 180°, but the exposure could be completed in about 20 to 30 sec. In the so-called third generation, both x-ray tube and detector rotate together 360° around the patient. In the fourth generation, the detector is fixed in a wide, complete circle around the patient, and the x-ray tube rotates 360° around the patient. A fifth-generation x-ray scanner is now available that consists of an x-ray tube that is shaped so that it is wrapped around the patient two-thirds of the way, and the x-ray focal spot is curved round the patient so that only the electron beam needs to be moved electronically. In this method there are no moving parts, and exposures can be made as short as 1/20 sec. This may well be the CT scanner of the future, but at present it still has sufficient problems so that it cannot be considered competitive with the third- and fourth-generation scanners. Also, the gantry cannot be angled; if angulation is desired, the couch on which the patient lies must be tilted.

Finally, it may be stated that the ideal CT scanner may be one that uses a monochromatic beam of radiation and presents a uniform concentration of equal wavelength photons throughout the thickness of the slice. This, however, is very difficult to achieve and has been attempted only at the National Synchrotron Light Source installation in Brookhaven National Laboratories. Unfortunately, in this installation the patient must be rotated, which may introduce motion artifacts. Monochromatic CT might be a great tool for research, for it may be possible to detect the concentration in tissues of certain intermediate atomic weight elements such as phosphorus, potassium, sulfur, and calcium by utilizing a dual-photon absorptiometry technique between 30 and 100 keV. Also, the iodine enhancement after intravenous (IV) injection could be multiplied severalfold by utilizing two monochromatic beams of different kiloelectron volt values, one at the optimal level for iodine. This would allow for subtraction and considerable enhancement of the iodine component of the image. CT angiography similar to magnetic resonance imaging (MRI) angiography may be possible.

Another method for producing near-monochromatic x-ray beams is by the free electron laser and Compton backscatter. This approach is more likely to be available than the very special and unique installation at Brookhaven. In this approach, "the intense photon output of a free electron laser may be made to collide with its own high energy electron beam to create nearly monochromatic x-rays using Compton backscatter techniques" (2).

All manufacturers strive to decrease the tremendous range of wavelength values present in the output of an x-ray tube. This is accomplished by utilizing a higher kilovolt peak to produce the x-rays and by adding a fair amount of filtration, usually 3 or 4 mm of aluminum. However, the beam is still quite heterogeneous, and much of the radiation is still composed of longer wavelength photons that are absorbed by the skull, producing what is termed *beam hardening.* Beam hardening is the source of many artifacts (see under "Artifacts in CT Scans").

More recently, a manufacturing improvement—the *spiral CT*—has been introduced. It allows for continuous rotation of the tube that can spiral down for an unlimited number of slices. This provides the possibility of obtaining continuous slices over an area and yields CT angiography through reconstruction of the images in three dimensions, which can later be reformatted in coronal and sagittal projections. In fact Aoki et al. have demonstrated intracranial aneurysms with a three-dimensional reconstruction technique utilizing a modern scanner, A GE9800 HR (not specially equipped for spiral angiography) (3). In a study of 15 patients the aneurysms were demonstrated in all cases.

Positioning of the Patient

AXIAL IMAGES

In the early days of CT it was decided that the best angle to examine the brain would be one that would show the intracranial contents without much superimposition of the surrounding structures. For that reason, it was felt that the best angle was one that would start at the upper margin of the orbit and pass through the external auditory meatus. This was a plane 20 to 25° above Reid's base line, and the thickness of the slice was usually around 10 mm. This approach was used for about 10 years, after which a tendency developed to abandon this angulation and instead to use planes that are parallel to Reid's base line. In this way, the cerebellum is more thoroughly studied; at the same time, it is possible to visualize the base of the skull and the paranasal sinuses and orbit more completely (Fig. 2.1). In addition, this angulation is more advantageous to study the temporal lobes of the brain. The anatomy looks slightly different from that demonstrated with the 20 or 25° angulation views, but it is easy to become accustomed to the difference. The same angle is being employed in MRI. When it is necessary to visualize the temporal lobes, it has been suggested that taking axial views following Reid's base line or 5 to 10° negative (below) the lower orbital margin would improve visualization of the temporal horn and surrounding structures. El Gammal et al. recommend sections following a plane passing through the top of the dorsum sellae and 3 mm below the tuberculum sellae as determined on a digital lateral view taken during the CT examination (4).

Preferably, the patient should be immobilized as effectively as possible to prevent any motion during the exposures. Children under a certain age may need to be sedated and sometimes anesthetized. Sedation can be accomplished by an enema of chloral hydrate solution, but in some children stronger sedatives are required.

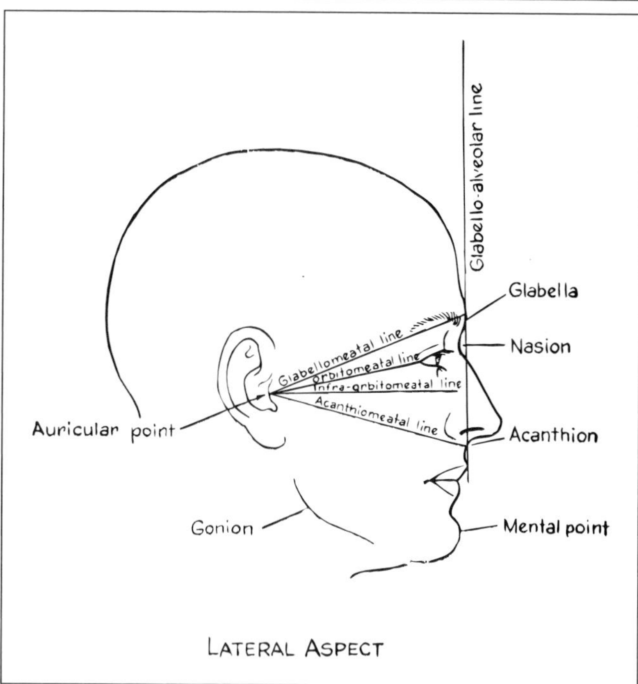

Figure 2.1. Lines and points used for positioning. The recommended line is the infraorbitomeatal line.

CORONAL IMAGES

Reformatted coronal images can be made out of the axial images. However, unless the slices are thin enough, the resolution of the reformatted images is suboptimal. For best results, slices 1.0, 1.5, or 2.0 mm in thickness would be necessary. In order to save on time and patient exposure, only the area in question needs to be imaged in detail.

Glenn et al. recommend overlapping images by 1 mm (5). In this way, slightly thicker slices (e.g., 3 mm) may produce good results.

Direct coronal views require that the patient lie in the supine position and be capable of extending the head sufficiently so that the orbital meatal line is parallel to the table surface. Lacking this, it is possible to angle the gantry to compensate for whatever is necessary to obtain coronal images. One of the more important problems is avoiding overlap of the teeth, which will produce considerable artifacts, particularly if there are metallic fillings. It is also important to prepare everything so that the images can be obtained as rapidly as possible in order to prevent motion as the patient becomes fatigued from the uncomfortable position.

It is also possible to put the patient in the prone position, and to extend the head with the patient's chin on the table or elevated, as needed, and to add to this the tilting of the gantry to obtain a satisfactory coronal projection. For some patients the prone position is easier to maintain, but, in general, if the patient is not able to extend the head sufficiently in the supine position, the same may well apply to the prone position.

SAGITTAL VIEWS

Again, these may be obtained through image reconstruction or reformatting if the original slices were thin enough; this method is utilized in the great majority of cases. However, particularly in infants and young children, it may be possible to obtain direct sagittal views (6). These are difficult to obtain because of the awkward positioning, but they are possible even in many adults (7,8). While the images obtained may not be truly lateral, the resolution is excellent and may be worth the extra effort and time. The effort may be particularly worthwhile in installations where MRI is not available.

Thickness of the Slices

It is important to be acquainted with some physical aspects of image production with CT scanning. In a 10-mm slice, the resolution near the upper or lower surface of the slice may not be as optimal as that in the middle, and if one has a small structure that falls between two adjacent images, it may be overlooked because it does not cast enough of a contrast difference to be visualized. For this reason, theoretically, perhaps images should be overlapped slightly (1 or 2 mm if a 10-mm slice is to be used). Also, there is the question of the partial volume effect, which is more pronounced in the thicker slices than in thinner slices. For this reason, we recommend 5-mm slices for the posterior fossa and 10-mm slices for the supratentorial space, but possibly overlapping 1 or 2 mm. Recently, we have changed to 3-mm slices for the posterior fossa and 5-mm slices for the supratentorial space. This decreases the possibility of overlooking small pathologic processes and allows for reformatting of the images in sagittal or coronal planes if it is considered desirable (see text following). I believe the most practical approach is to take 5-mm slices throughout, which tends to speed up the examination while decreasing the chances of overlooking a small lesion. The 3-mm section can be made in any case where it is considered necessary. Sometimes 1.0- or 1.5-mm slices are indicated, such as in the examination of the pituitary.

Photographic Recording

In spite of the fact that images can be analyzed more thoroughly on the viewing screen of the CT instrument, we continue to photograph the images as a permanent record. In general, images are photographed with the correct windows (window level and window width) to show the soft tissues optimally. In addition, a second picture is made with the window setting to show the bones (the so-called bone window). For the brain soft tissues, a window level of 30 to 40 and a window width of 80 to 100 are usually satisfactory. For the posterior fossa structures, near the base of the skull, a window level of about 50 and a window width of 150 to 250 may be required, and through the middle of the cerebellum, a window level of 40 or 50 and a window width of 150 would be advantageous. Again, as one approaches the top of the skull, it may be necessary to raise the window width by 20 to 50 points for best results.

If the orbits are to be demonstrated optimally, a window level of 50 and a window width of 300 to 500 may be used for best results. In order to visualize the bones, a bone window should be utilized using a window level of 300 to 500 and a window width of 2000 to 4000, depending on the manufacturer of the unit. It has been our custom to take bone windows for every level where we also have soft tissue windows. This utilizes more films, but we find it useful in a busy department. In order to save on films, it is possible to photograph the images in the bone window settings in smaller sizes than in the soft tissue windows. Also, in nontrauma cases and in cases where metastases are not being sought, the bone windows can be eliminated, for the paranasal sinuses, which can be seen better in bone window settings, can be seen well enough on ordinary soft tissue settings.

Image Reformatting

As mentioned previously, from the axial views it is possible to produce images in coronal, sagittal, or any degree of obliquity. For best results this requires that the original slices be as thin as possible. Slices 1 to 2 mm are best, although, as explained earlier, in the spine, slices of 5-mm thickness with an overlap of 2 mm yield excellent results, as suggested by Glenn et al. (5). The newer CT scanners are capable of producing reformatted images very rapidly.

In addition, it is possible to produce three-dimensional images of the surface, or of deeper areas utilizing soft tissue or bone windows. The images can be rotated on the viewing screen. This approach is particularly useful for plastic and reconstructive surgery, in cases where there has been a fracture of the facial bones with deformity, and also in children with premature suture synostosis and plagiocephaly.

Absorption Coefficient of Tissues

The entire technology of CT is based on the differential absorption of tissues. Initially, the attenuation values for blood, fat, air, bone, and so forth were set up by Hounsfield, utilizing numbers 500 above 0 and 500 below 0. The 0 value represents water. These came to be called *EMI numbers* (after EMI, the company that sponsored the development of the original instrument). Later this scale was doubled to offer somewhat more flexibility; it now goes from 1000 above to 1000 below 0. Each subdivision within the scale is now called the *Hounsfield (H) number*. Figure 2.2 explains the average numbers for circulating blood, clotted blood, gray and white matter, fat, air, and bone. Zero refers to pure water, and the value of cerebrospinal fluid is slightly above that of water.

The absorption coefficient of tissues is also related to the amount of protein. A greater percentage of protein increases the H number. This is the case, for instance, with

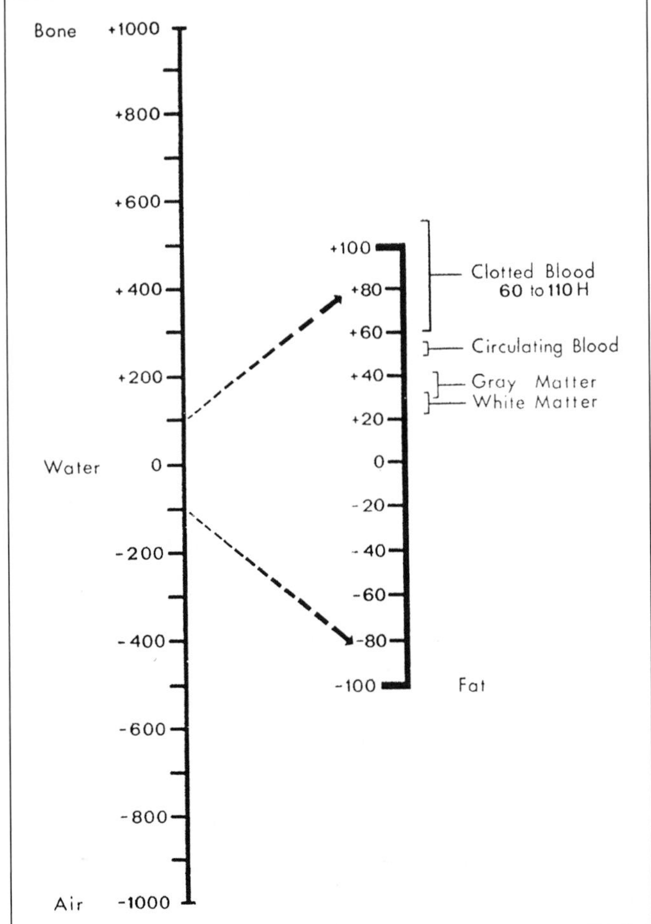

Figure 2.2. Hounsfield number scale as seen on CT scan images. See text.

neoplasms. The tumors that are more cellular will be higher in density (see Chapter 11). In the case of blood, the H number is related to the hematocrit value: the higher the hematocrit, the higher the H number. The presence of calcium in the tissues elevates the H numbers. If the calcium is present in concentrated areas, it would be obvious; however, it may be more or less uniformly distributed, as may occur in a meningioma full of psammoma bodies, in which case the H numbers will be higher.

It is also possible to move a region of interest (point or square) around the organ being examined and to read out the actual number involved with the appropriate standard deviation. The reading could be inaccurate because a segment of the tissue could be adjacent to another tissue with a different number (the partial volume effect). The thinner the slice, the smaller the partial volume effect. The smaller the region of interest, the more accurate the number is likely to be. However, there are limitations to this; when the slices are too thin, there is increased quantum noise because of a reduction in the number of photons, which reduces the total beam flux. Thus, the readings should always be obtained with the accompanying standard deviations; they are, in general, very useful. For instance, when it is necessary to differentiate between a density that could be hemorrhage in the brain or a partially calcified area, the blood would be somewhere between the 50 and 100 range, whereas if it were calcium, it probably would have a value higher than 120. By the same token, sometimes it is necessary to differentiate cerebrospinal fluid (CSF) from fat. The CSF should have a number around 0, or slightly above, whereas fat would definitely have a number lower than 0, in the −10 to −50 or lower range, depending upon how pure the fat is. CSF is usually found to be between 0 and 14 H. This fluctuation is probably related to the partial volume effect, because CSF-containing cavities always have some soft tissue near them unless the slice passes through the ventricles when they are dilated.

Spatial Resolution

Modern CT scanners are capable of excellent resolution, slightly under 1 mm. Increasing the resolution usually requires a higher radiation dose. In general, it is not necessary to increase the resolution beyond 0.8 mm because the slice is usually several millimeters in thickness. What we deal with, in general, assuming a resolution of 1 mm, would be a square column 1 to 10 mm high (voxel). The size of the matrix actually determines the degree of resolution possible. Scanners can use a matrix that is 512 × 512 pixels. A 256 × 256 matrix yields satisfactory results, but the 512 × 512 matrix will show greater detail and smoothness in the images. The actual size of the pixel depends on the size of the reconstructed circle. For instance, if the reconstructed circle has a diameter of 40 cm, the size of the pixel is 1.56 × 1.56 mm. However, if the size of the reconstructed circle is cut in half, to 20 cm, the pixel size drops to half, or 0.78 mm. This will increase the resolution, and for this reason the head should be examined with the smallest possible circle. In the body, a smaller circle should be used to examine the spine. When the circle of interest is smaller than the body part being examined, artifacts are produced by irradiated tissue outside the circle of interest, but these can be handled by appropriate computer algorithms. The amount of data necessary for a 512 × 512 reconstruction is four times greater than that required for a 256 × 256 matrix reconstruction; thus, the computer capacity will have to be much greater so that the reconstruction can take place in a relatively short period of time. Matrices of 1024 × 1024 have been tried, but in general have not been found to be practical, mostly because of cost. It would require a very powerful computer reconstruction system, special viewing screens, and special photographic arrangements, all of which add considerably to the cost without increasing the resolution sufficiently. The output of the x-ray tube also needs to be higher if a higher spatial rsolution matrix is to be utilized. As stated earlier, the density or contrast resolution turns out to be more important than spatial resolution once a certain degree of spatial resolution has been achieved.

Density resolution is also dependent on the contrast of the object being scanned. For instance, if the object contrast is high, the spatial resolution is of the order of 1 mm or less, but if the object contrast is low, the resolution will decrease to 4 to 5 mm. The latter is typical for tissue resolution, which normally has low contrast.

There is an important relationship between resolution and the dose of x-ray applied to obtain the image. In modern CT scanners, the radiation dose has been raised to the optimal level to obtain sufficient spatial and contrast resolution while keeping the radiation dose to the patient as low as practical (9). (See text following for further details.)

Artifacts in CT Scans

Artifacts usually result from factors that cause a specific voxel (the volume represented by each pixel) to have a different absorption coefficient when viewed from opposing angles. The great majority of CT scanners today utilize a 360° rotation. The absorption coefficient of a given voxel should be identical when its absorption is calculated as the x-ray beam goes from 1 to 180° as from 181 to 360°. If this is not the case, artifacts will result.

Most frequently, artifacts show up as either dark or light *straight streaks*. Perhaps the most important single factor that helps in diagnosing an artifact from a pathologic condition is the fact that the lighter or darker artifact almost always is bandlike. Often, the artifact is not obvious, and only careful examination will allow us to conclude that we are dealing with an artifact because of the bandlike or streaky configuration.

MOTION

Motion is one of the most common causes of artifacts and perhaps the easiest to evaluate. It is also the easiest to understand because, obviously, the absorption coefficient of a given voxel will be different as it is viewed from the opposing angles. Motion causes not only streaking but also degradation of detail resolution, which at times may be difficult to evaluate as one views the images, if there are no obvious linear artifacts (Fig. 2.3). The newer scanners, which utilize an exposure time of 1 to 3 sec, have decreased the incidence of motion artifacts, but these will probably not disappear until the exposure time can be reduced further, possibly to as little as 1/20 sec, as discussed earlier.

BEAM-HARDENING EFFECTS

The x-ray beam is always polychromatic, that is, made up of photons with many different wavelengths. The longer-wavelength photons are absorbed in greater percentage; thus, as the x-ray beam penetrates farther, it becomes "harder" because the softer photons have been filtered out. For instance, in the skull, the brain cortex on the left side of the patient is imaged by a softer ray when the beam enters from the left than when it enters from the right, which is the case with every CT image. The beam-hardening artifact was responsible for the erroneous assumption

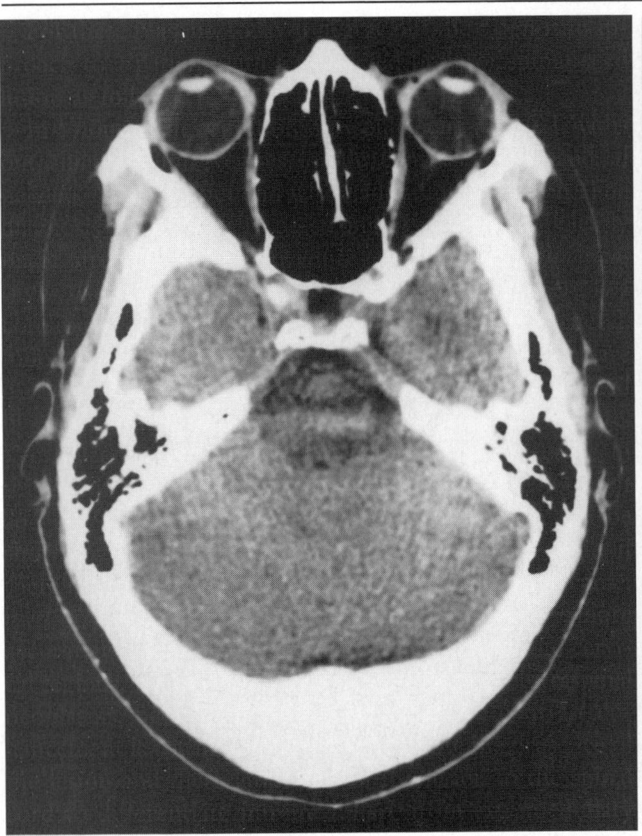
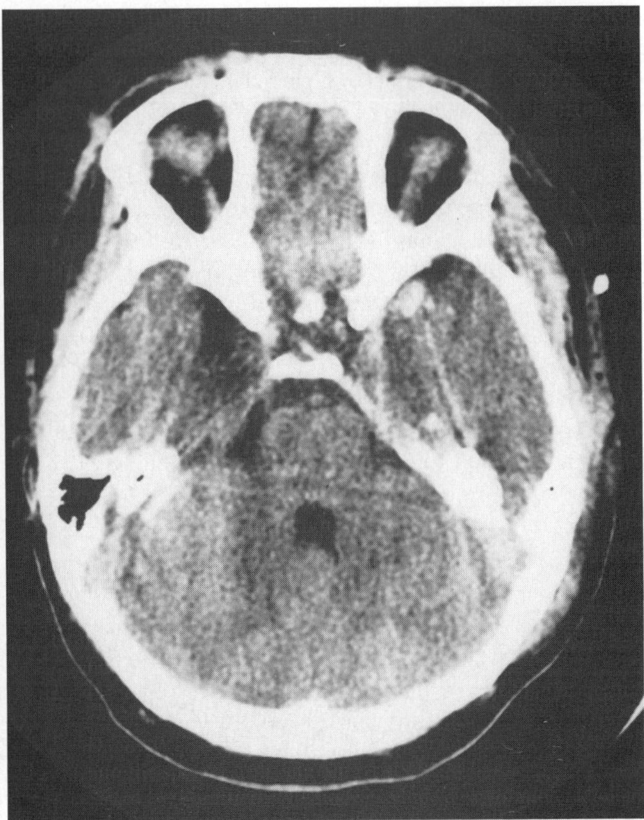

A B

Figure 2.3. Interpetrous artifact (Hounsfield artifact) and linear artifacts arising from motion. **A.** The transverse light and dark bands overlying the brainstem are typical. This interferes with visualization of the brainstem. Thinner slices help in decreasing the severity of the artifact but do not eliminate it entirely. See text. **B.** In another patient, after trauma, there are a number of dark and light bands in the middle fossa and to a lesser extent in the posterior fossa due to some patient motion because the patient was not fully cooperative. Similar artifacts result from large paranasal sinuses, which is not the case here.

of Ambrose in his initial publication in 1973 (10), which led him to state that the lighter zone under the inner table of the skull represented the brain cortex.

STAR ARTIFACTS

These are usually produced by the presence of dense bone or a heavy calcified or metallic object. Dense radiation streaks are usually the result.

INTERPETROUS ARTIFACTS

These are irregular dark bands between the two petrous pyramids. They were more prominent in the earlier scanners and have been reduced through special algorithms, but unfortunately they are still very common and interfere with visualization of the pons (Fig. 2.3).

It has been suggested that taking thinner slices (1.5 or 2.0 mm) and "adding" the images significantly reduces the artifacts at the same area as compared with a thicker slice—for instance, a 6.0-mm slice as against four "added" 1.5-mm slices (11).

BONE AND AIR ARTIFACTS

These are frequently seen when the paranasal sinuses and surrounding dense cortical bones have nonspecific configurations that lead to uneven attenuation coefficient of adjacent voxels. The uneven attenuation is exaggerated by minimal motion of the patient (Fig. 2.4). These are frequently seen behind the frontal sinuses, particularly if these are large.

The posterior fossa is surrounded by heavy bone, particularly the petrous pyramids, and also contains pneumatized sinuses in the mastoids. Artifacts are most abundant in the posterior fossa, and the result is that CT scanning is significantly less accurate in the posterior fossa than MRI, which is free of artifacts of this type, although motion artifacts are more common because of the longer exposure time required for MRI.

OTHER CAUSES OF ARTIFACTS

In addition to motion, heavy bone and air combinations, and beam hardening, artifacts may be produced by equip-

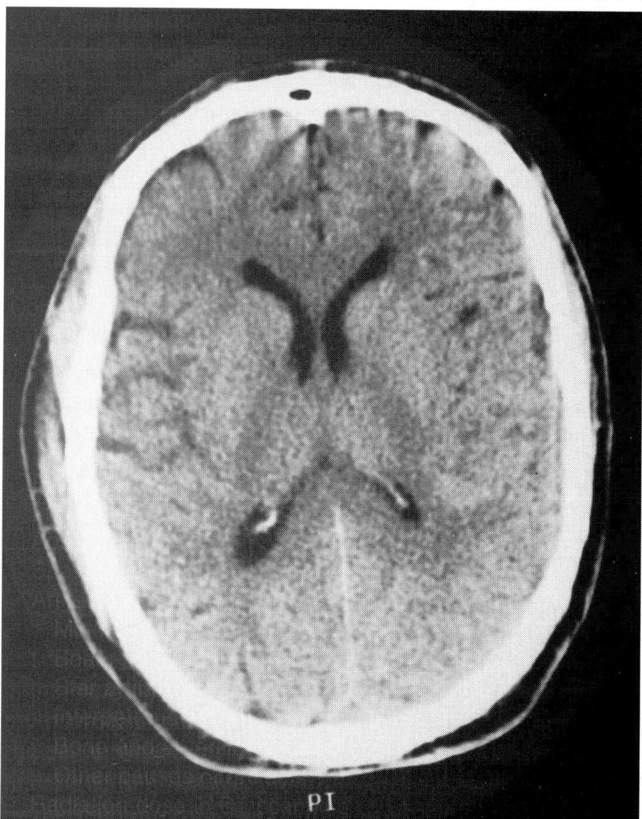

Figure 2.4. Artifacts in the frontal region partly related to the frontal sinuses, which in this case are small. The midline frontal crest often produces a star artifact, which in this example is responsible for the dark band running obliquely to the right. The light and dark streaks are also due to slight motion, for the patient came after head trauma and probably was not fully cooperative.

ment misalignment between the x-ray tube focal spot and the radiation detectors, or by faulty x-ray source, which may be caused by variations in electrical current or voltage in the incoming lines. Some of these are partly corrected by reference detection outside the field of view, but artifacts usually result in spite of this.

A characteristic of CT slices is that the two surfaces of the slice are not parallel to each other. Rather, they are slightly concave owing to the fact that the collimator allows a flat beam of x-rays to enter the object, but the beam diverges and is significantly wider at its exit from the object being examined than at its entrance. The detectors see a wider beam on the exit side, and this is the volume of tissue that is "seen" by the computer. However, the collimator on the entrance side should be made as narrow as possible both to lower radiation to the patient and to decrease scattering. The end result is the so-called dishing artifact; that is, the slice of tissue is in fact thinner in and around the center than at the periphery. For this reason, slices should be made without any space between them; in fact, slight overlapping would totally eliminate the problem. The artifact is potentially greater if thicker slices are made. The effect of "dishing" is exaggerated by the partial volume effect discussed earlier.

Radiation Dose in CT Scanning

In order to obtain optimal resolution, it is necessary to generate sufficient x-rays with sufficient penetrating power so that enough photons can be detected by the detectors on the exit side. Insufficient numbers of photons cause noise and yield a grainy image. Increasing the strength of the x-ray beam increases the patient dose. Manufacturers have turned to higher kilovolt values (around 140 kV) and to higher filtration (3 to 4 mm of aluminum equivalent in copper) to harden the x-ray beam and thus decrease the radiation dose to the tissues on the entrance side. More efficient detectors decrease the needed radiation dose.

The actual radiation dose to the tissues varies somewhat between manufacturers. Also, the dose is greater at the skin than in the deeper tissues. In general the dose is about 2 to 3 cGy (2 rads) per slice and higher when adjacent slices are considered. The dose would be higher if adjacent slices are overlapped. Thinner multiple slices will increase the total dose. Certain organs such as the eye lens receive a higher dose than the tissue average; this is unavoidable because the skin dose is higher than the average tissue dose. Scattered radiation outside the field being scanned is progressively lower as the distance increases from the area being scanned. For instance, the dose to the ovaries when scanning the head is on the order of one-half of one millirad per scan. To lower the dose to the eye, an angled view (15° above the orbitomeatal line) may be used. As explained earlier, we no longer use this angle unless it is desired to reduce the dose to the lens in a patient undergoing multiple CT examinations.

Contrast Enhancement

Soon after Ambrose pointed out in his initial report that the IV injection of the iodide contrast media ordinarily used for urography would enhance the contrast in certain tumors and other pathologic entities, it became obvious to the early workers in the field that contrast enhancement was an extremely valuable technical improvement. A large proportion of all CT examinations currently are performed with contrast enhancement. In some centers the examination is carried out without contrast, followed by repeat examination after contrast. This is time-consuming and therefore more expensive. In other centers the contrast is given before the examination and only one series of scans is performed unless there is a contraindication to the use of contrast; a specific request has been made to perform the examination without contrast; or the patient was referred for a condition, such as suspected intracranial bleeding, acute head trauma, and others, that ordinarily calls for noncontrast CT examination. The creatinine level is the laboratory value we use at the Massachusetts General Hospital. A creatinine value above 2.0 mg/100 ml is a contraindication to the use of iodine contrast media; a value between 1.5 and 2.0 mg/100 ml may represent a relative contraindication, which would require a judgment decision as to the need for contrast imaging in a given patient.

The dose of contrast varies somewhat between institutions, but in the last 10 years it has become more or less standard after having increased from the earlier lower quantity. A single dose of contrast might be described as 50 or 60 ml of a 60 percent concentration of the contrast injected as a bolus. A double dose might be described as a 100- to 150-ml IV injection of 60 percent contrast. When using these quantities, it is more practical to use a 30 percent concentration and to administer it as an IV drip. Again, it may be possible to administer the equivalent of 50 ml of 60 percent concentration as a bolus and an additional 100 to 200 ml of 30 percent concentration as an IV drip. The latter technique may be used, for instance, to rapidly elevate and then maintain the concentration of contrast in the blood. While images are being generated, it is used to visualize the pituitary gland, aneurysms, and arteriovenous malformations to better advantage and may be helpful when trying to differentiate scarring from a recurrent herniated lumbar intervertebral disc. Manufacturers provide contrast in sacs of 300 ml of a 30 percent concentration for IV drip infusion; and this is the method and the quantities most frequently used in our department at the Massachusetts General Hospital. Exposures are usually started when about two-thirds of the injection has been completed. The injection rate is rather rapid, but it takes 7 to 10 min to complete because of the relatively large amount of fluid.

No special preparation of the patient is recommended in our practice. The examinations are carried out when the patient arrives regardless of whether the patient has eaten a meal. It is surprising how uncommon it is to see a significant reaction. It is our impression that untoward reactions are less common in our CT practice than in IV urography, possibly because for the latter the patient is prepared with a physic and/or enemas to clean the bowel and may be asked to fast at least partially, all of which may lead to some degree of dehydration and apprehension, which is not the case with CT of the head.

There is controversy, at the time of this writing, regarding the use of the conventional hypertonic or hyperosmolar iodine contrast media as against the newer lower osmolar compounds. At the Massachusetts General Hospital, we continue to use the conventional contrast media because the observed occurrence of untoward reactions is extremely low and the results have been uniformly satisfactory. The low osmolar compounds are used when there is a history of significant cardiac coronary disease or when a history of an "allergic" reaction to a previous injection exists. Hypersensitivity reactions do occur with the low osmolar compounds as well, but the molecules are different, and thus an individual who had a reaction to the conventional contrast media may not have any with the new compounds. In the past, a history of a severe previous reaction made us prepare the patient with steroids for a day (20 mg of prednisone 24 and 12 h) before injecting the contrast when contrast enhancement was considered necessary in that particular patient. This patient preparation would be followed even if a nonionic contrast agent was going to be used if the reaction to the contrast was classified as severe. Today, however, we would most likely recommend an MRI examination without and with contrast because hypersensitivity reactions are much less common with the gadolinium-DTPA–type compounds.

MAGNETIC RESONANCE

Human tissues first became visible following the discovery of x-rays by Konrad Roentgen in 1895. Biological tissues are transparent to short-wave electromagnetic radiation represented by x-rays but are opaque to other variations of the light spectrum such as visible light or infrared radiation. However, the tissues again become transparent to waves such as ultrasound or radio waves. It is the latter possibility that allows us to utilize the nuclear magnetic resonance.

Cross-sectional imaging of the human body represents a real revolution in diagnosis. Tomographic imaging with x-rays was first suggested about 30 years following the discovery of x-rays and was actually implemented relatively shortly thereafter by Vallebona (12) and others. The principle of tomography is also utilized in ultrasound, where essentially all the images produced are cross-sectional. However, the concept was not really developed until the discovery of CT in 1972. MRI had been well known and had been developed rather extensively by chemists since its discovery by Purcell of Harvard in 1946 (13) and by Bloch of Stanford, working independently, the same year (14). They received the Nobel Prize in chemistry jointly in 1953. It was not until 1973 that Paul Lauterbur of the State University of New York in Stonybrook published a paper on the first spatially differentiated NMR measurements or NMR images (15). He suggested the use of magnetic field gradients to encode position-dependent imaging information. Up to that time, only spectroscopic tracings had been obtained. It is interesting that publication of the possibility of creating cross-sectional images with magnetic resonance occurred very shortly after the announcement of the development of CT, made by Hounsfield and Ambrose (1,10).

The article by Lauterbur aroused much attention, particularly in England, and it is for this reason that some of the early publications involved mostly authors in Great Britain. One of the most influential papers was that of Waldo Hinshaw (an American working in England) and coauthors (1977) from Nottingham University demonstrating excellent anatomic resolution of the human wrist and forearm (16). These images attracted attention all over the world. I became interested in the potential of MRI at that time and, by 1978, had established a laboratory at the Massachusetts General Hospital, directed by Waldo Hinshaw. The field moved very rapidly following these developments, and a number of publications by the Thorn-EMI group, the Nottingham University group, the Aberdeen group, and the group at Hammersmith Hospital, all in England, began to appear in 1980, followed shortly thereafter by others.

Magnetic resonance is based on the fact that the nucleus of the atoms, made up of protons and neutrons, contains most of the elemental mass of the atoms. The nuclei in some elements, those that have one unpaired proton or neutron, possess angular momentum or spin. Because the nuclei have an electric charge, the spinning produces a magnetic field around them. One could assimilate the nuclei with a tiny bar magnet that has a north and a south pole. In nature the tiny bar magnets are randomly oriented in space and therefore do not create a magnetic field because they cancel each other out. However, if placed inside a strong magnetic field, the bar magnets representing the atoms tend to align with it (Fig. 2.5).

The stronger the external field, the larger the percentage of atoms that align with the field. It must be said that in a field of 1000 gauss (G) only about one atom per million is aligned, which is a rather small figure. The alignment could take place in the same direction as the external field (paramagnetic atoms) or in the opposite direction (diamagnetic atoms). The ferromagnetic materials are very strong paramagnetic substances, and their response is proportionately much greater. Each atom creates its own magnetic field around it, created by the spinning nucleus and the spinning and rotating electrons. The field created by the spinning and orbiting electrons turns out to be the strongest. However, it is the nuclear spin field that is used in MRI. The nuclear fields that are aligned with the external field are made to rotate 90 or 180° by applying a radio frequency (RF) pulse of appropriate duration and at the appropriate megahertz (MHz) frequency for the element in question, and are observed as they return to be realigned (to a relaxed state). The *rate* of this realignment is modified by the electron fields surrounding the nuclei; this modification, in turn, is dependent on the chemical composition of the tissue. Even slight differences in tissue composition may cause sufficient change in relaxation time, and it is this fundamental quality that makes MRI such a powerful method.

The nuclei are constantly spinning around their own axes. As they try to align with the applied external field, their axes will not be exactly parallel to the external field; instead, they will precess around this axis at a speed that is proportional to the strength of the external field. The stronger the field, the faster the precession. For instance, protons (the nuclei of hydrogen) precess exactly at 42.58 MHz per second if placed in an external magnetic field of 10,000 G (1.0 T). If the external field is increased by 100 G, the nuclear precession, or Larmor frequency, will increase slightly, to 43.0058 MHz, and this can be measured. This sensitivity to the strength of the magnetic field is the fundamental quality on which MRI is based. (See text following.)

While the Larmor precession frequency for hydrogen is 42.58 MHz/T, that of carbon 13 is 10.70; fluorine 19 is 40.05; sodium 23 is 11.26; and phosphorus 31 is 17.32 MHz/T. Each element has a constant relationship, between the external magnetic field and its Larmor frequency, which is called the *gyromagnetic ratio*. At 1.5 T the Larmor frequency of hydrogen is 63.87 MHz (or about 64 MHz).

Precession is a rotating movement that a spinning object, such as a top or gyroscope, describes around an axis. The precession is in addition to the spinning, and in the case of the nuclei is conceived as being clockwise when looked at from above the *xy* axis (Fig. 2.6).

As mentioned previously, the percentage of nuclei that align with the external field is very small: only about 1 in 100,000 in a field of 1.0 T. However, even this small fraction is a rather large number in the case of hydrogen when one considers that the body tissues are made up of about 90 percent water and that each water molecule contains two hydrogen nuclei, yielding a total of about 10 to the 19th power protons per gram of tissue, aligned or precessing around the axis of the external magnetic field. This makes hydrogen the most widely used element for MRI. The percentage is proportional to the strength of the external field and inversely proportional to the temperature. The closer to zero temperature, the greater the percentage of aligned nuclei. The latter quality works against us, for there is a decrease in the number of aligned nuclei at body temperature.

Image Formation

If an object is placed in a uniform strong magnetic field, any changes generated in the orientation of the nuclear fields take place rapidly and from then on the change is relatively stable. The nuclear dipoles are not totally aligned or parallel; rather, they tend to align but instead precess

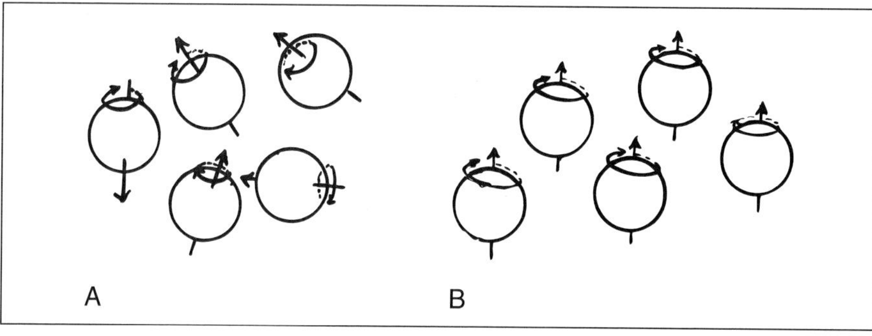

Figure 2.5. Effect of a magnetic field on nuclear dipoles. **A.** The nuclear dipoles are pointing in all directions. **B.** The dipoles are lined up with the applied magnetic field and rotate at the speed corresponding to the strength of the magnetic field.

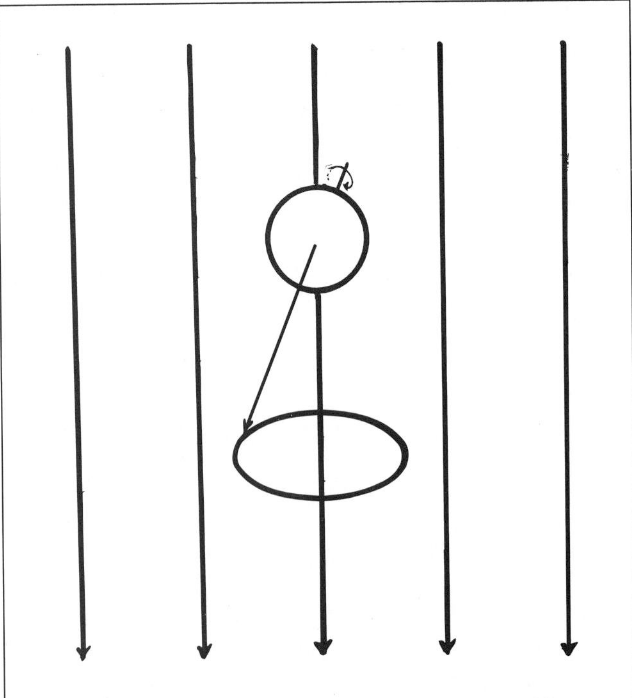

Figure 2.6. Nuclear alignment and precession. The nuclei are aligned in relation to the lines of force of the magnetic field. In addition to rotating around their own axis, the nuclei precess around the lines of force of the magnetic field, like a top or gyroscope.

around the axis of the external field (Fig. 2.6). The relatively stable situation created by the application of the external field is not sufficient to create images or spectroscopy. What is done is to apply an RF pulse at the Larmor frequency, which creates a torque on the net magnetic moment of the entire sample, making the nuclear dipoles tip away from the axis of the external field usually 90 or 180°. The amount of the tilt away from the axis depends on the strength and the duration of the RF pulse. If a 90° or less than 90° pulse is used, the precession, now in the *xy* axis (Fig. 2.7), creates a magnetization that can be detected, whereas before the RF pulse it could not because it was aligned with the axis of the external magnetic field. The magnetization along the *xy* axis oscillates, creating an oscillating voltage detectable by a phase-sensitive detector. The oscillating voltage is also at Larmor frequency.

SLICE SELECTION: TWO-DIMENSIONAL

In order to concentrate our attention on one slice, it is necessary to add a magnetic field gradient, that is, a magnetic field slightly higher on one side than on the other. This is a weak magnetic field, around 2000 times weaker than the applied external field, usually arranged perpendicular to the direction of the desired slice. For instance, for a sagittal slice, the gradient field would be arranged from right to left with the patient lying supine (Fig. 2.7). For an

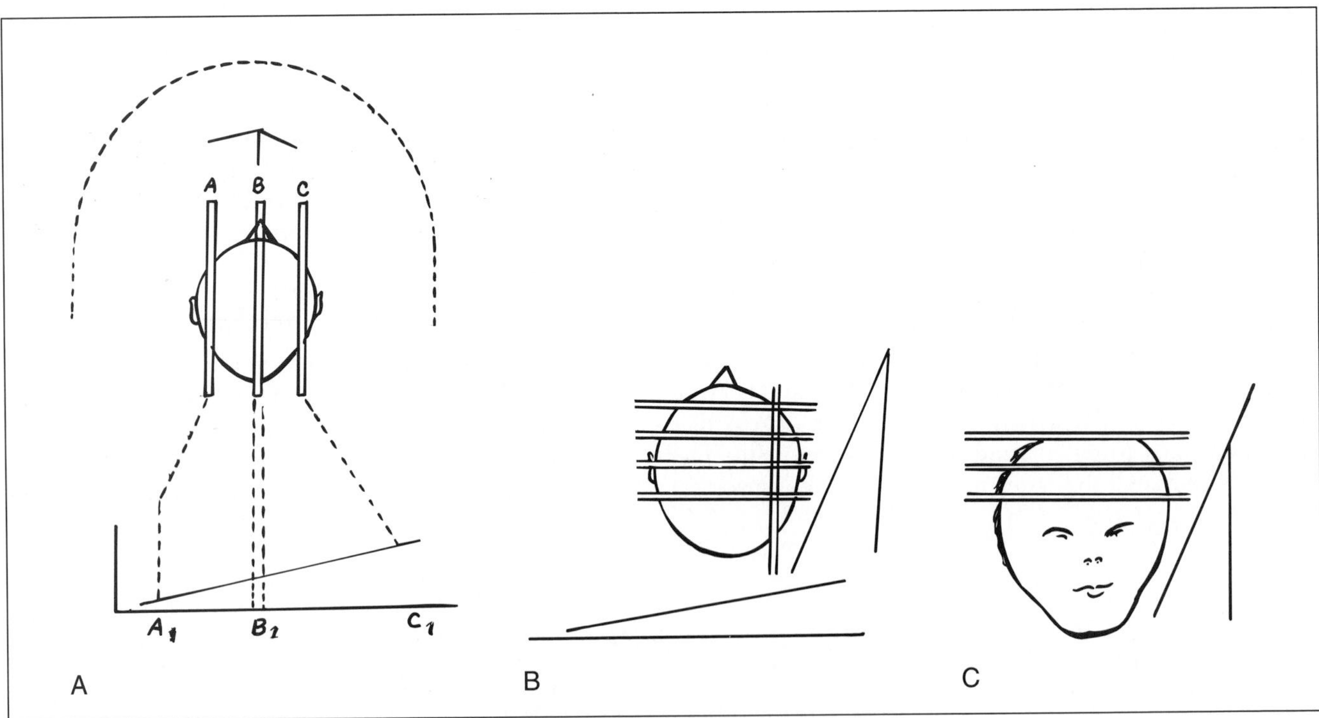

Figure 2.7. Slice selection by MRI. **A.** Diagram representing the use of a gradient magnetic field superimposed on the uniform outside field to select the desired section, as explained in the text. The position in relation to the gradient will generate sagittal slices. **B.** The position of this gradient will generate coronal sections. **C.** The position of this gradient will generate axial sections. The gradient is indicated by the inclined plane; the total magnetic field in A is slightly higher in C_1 than in B_1 or A_1; thus the spin frequency in C is higher. In order to excite one of the three slices, an RF pulse of appropriate frequency is chosen.

axial slice the gradient field is arranged from cephalad to caudad, and for a coronal slice the gradient field is arranged from front to back; that is, in the latter case, the field would be stronger in the front than in the back of the head or vice versa.

If an RF pulse with a bandwidth broad enough to cover the expected range of Larmor frequencies (slightly lower at the weaker side and slightly higher at the stronger side of the gradient) were to be applied, it would be possible to set the phase-sensitive detectors to receive, at any one time, only a very narrow range of frequencies that would be concentrated in a given slice. The narrower the range of frequencies, the narrower the slice. The thickness of the slice is dependent either on the grouping of Larmor frequencies (or bandwidth set in the receiver to "listen" to the nuclear resonance) or on how steep the magnetic gradient is. If the bandwidth is narrow, the slice is thinner and vice versa. Also, if the gradient is steeper, the slice can be thinner. The applied RF pulse could have a bandwidth sufficiently broad to encompass all the frequencies expected in the field of view (FOV). For instance, in the example given previously, if the 1.0 T magnet is used and the gradient applied goes from 0 to 100 G, the Larmor frequencies would range from 42.58 to 43.0058 MHz, or 425.8 kHz. In practice, smaller gradients may be used, depending on the desired width of the slices.

As can be easily understood, there is likely to be cross talk between adjacent slices, separated only by the Larmor frequency. In order to accomplish a better separation a "dead space," usually around 1 or 2 mm, is left unimaged between any two slices. If no dead space is desired, it is necessary to offset the patient by a few millimeters and repeat the study; this also can be accomplished electronically, but in either case it adds time to the examination.

It is also possible to record the data on all the slices in rapid sequence so that signals can be received sequentially from all the slices. The phase-sensitive detector is then set to receive signals of increasing or decreasing Larmor frequencies in very rapid sequence, within a few milliseconds, each narrow group of frequencies representing a different slice. In this way it is possible to produce all slices simultaneously.

Three gradient coils are required to allow for selection of the slice and to provide the required encoding to produce an image. One gradient coil is used to select the slice, one to frequency encode, and the other to phase encode the signals (Fig. 2.7). There are a number of factors that complicate slice selection, related to the flip angles and other parameters that cannot be discussed here.

FREQUENCY ENCODING

A magnetic gradient is applied in a different, orthogonal, plane, from that used in slice selection, such as shown in Figure 2.7. This would allow the generation of successive very thin slices, or lines of the selected slice to be separated by their frequency, typically 256 lines, usually in the x direction. In this way it becomes possible to localize in space one line at the time. The entire line will have the same RF, but the frequency will increase (or decrease) as we move successively to adjacent lines. We might call this the first component of the matrix, which will be completed by the phase-encoding gradient. The signal or voltage received by the detector is converted into a digital signal by using the Fourier transformation approach, which is the method employed to convert an analog into a digital signal that can be handled by the computer.

PHASE ENCODING

We now need to consider how it is possible to obtain data in a direction at right angles (y direction) to the frequency encoding just discussed. It turns out that it is possible to encode the phase angle of the spins. This is accomplished as follows: following the application of the 90° excitation pulse for a spin-echo (SE) sequence, the spins are at the same phase angle (line A, Fig. 2.8). A brief application of a gradient field causes the spins to accelerate on the stronger side of the gradient in relation to those on the

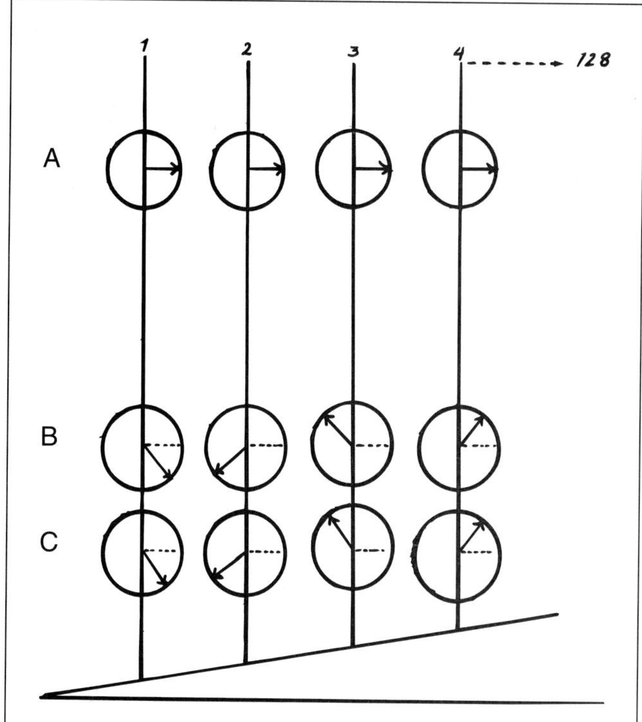

Figure 2.8. Phase encoding. **A.** At gradient 0 (the gradient has not been applied yet), all spins are at the same phase following the application of a 90° RF pulse. **B** and **C.** The magnetic field gradient is now applied for a very brief period, causing spins at line 4 to precess faster (stronger magnetic field) than at line 3, and these in turn rotate a little faster than those at lines 2 and 1. The result is that in the steady state they return to precess at the same speed corresponding to the surrounding uniform magnetic field, but still maintain the same changed phase angle as shown in lines 1, 2, 3, and 4. In other words, they "remember" the phase angle (row C). It is then possible to encode the vertical lines (as shown) in the phase of the MR signal.

weaker side (line B, Fig. 2.8). This causes a change in the phase angle of the spins. When the gradient is turned off, all the spins return to the original speed, in accordance with the surrounding uniform magnetic field, but remain at the same changed phase angle, which can be recorded. Usually 128 lines are recorded in the *y* direction; more lines could be used, if desired, but it would take longer to complete the scan.

Imaging Parameters

The six intrinsic properties of tissue related to MRI and contrast are T1 relaxation time, T2 relaxation time, proton density (N), magnetic susceptibility (X), chemical shift (S), and flow. The importance of examining the appropriate inherent properties can be highlighted by a historical note. During the early days of clinical investigation of MRI, the T1-weighted images, particularly those generated with the inversion recovery sequence, yielded beautiful anatomic images with high spatial resolution. However, the T1-weighted images failed reliably to identify pathologic lesions and required the addition of T2-weighted images. The introduction of SE imaging sequences, which permitted the acquisition of T1-weighted, intermediate (proton density), and T2-weighted images, was an important contribution.

SE images represent the basic imaging sequences used in medical diagnosis. Modifications are introduced from time to time, but the interpretation of images and the long experience acquired with their use tend to minimize any changes, for a long period of usage is required to ascertain that lesions are not missed or misinterpreted because of the change. A recent development is the *fast spin echo* (FSE), a variation that requires 30 percent less time in data acquisition but does produce some minor alterations in the intensity of the various normal and pathologic tissues. The tissue changes that are obvious are of no concern; it is the minor changes that are more difficult to interpret and that can be easily misinterpreted.

RELAXATION TIMES

Following the application of an RF pulse, the precessing axis of the nuclear dipoles is tilted, for instance, at 90° from the *z* axis (or Bo), the axis of the external magnet. The precession will now be in the *xy* plane, perpendicular to the *z* axis (Figs. 2.9 and 2.10). If left alone, the angles of the dipoles will gradually decrease while continuing to precess until they reach the relaxed position. There are two time constants related to this phenomenon: the longitudinal or spin-lattice relaxation time (T1), and the transverse or spin-spin relaxation time (T2).

The energy imparted by the RF pulse is gradually passed to the surrounding lattice and thus the expression of spin-lattice relaxation time applied to T1. Liquids have a longer T1 and T2. In the case of water, they both approach 2 sec. As the tissue becomes more solid, the T2 becomes much

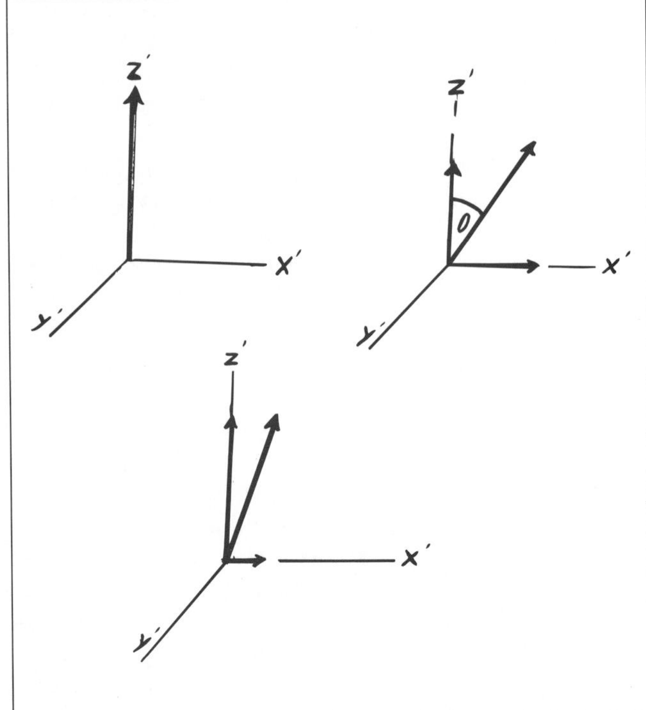

Figure 2.9. T1 or spin-lattice relaxation time. Starting at the left top, a 90° radiofrequency pulse is given, and some milliseconds later the imparted energy decreases until it reaches equilibrium along the *Z′* axis.

shorter than T1. The detection of T2 signals turns out to be considerably more useful than T1 in clinical MRI. This is because T2 is an expression of the loss of coherent precession of the nuclei following the RF pulse. That is, immediately after turning off the RF pulse, all the nuclei are precessing together and a signal is produced. However, some milliseconds later, owing to the fact that the nuclei are components of different molecules and the fact that there are some local inhomogeneities within the tissues as well as in the external magnetic field, some of the nuclei precess slightly more slowly than others. Some milliseconds later the spread between the spinning nuclei becomes broad enough that the signal disappears. That is T2. Because the inhomogeneities that cause the loss of coherent motion are dependent on chemical composition as well as on other factors, MR images based on T2 are more sensitive to tissue changes than those based on T1 and therefore more useful in the clinical situation. Free water has a longer T2 (it is brighter) than bound water in the tissues. This is the usual explanation as to why edema in the brain or in neoplasms has a longer T2 than the surrounding normal brain, where water is a component of the cell molecular structure. T1 is also longer and yields a lower-intensity image.

The T1 relaxation time becomes proportionately longer if the strength of the magnetic field is increased. A doubling of the field strength causes a 25 to 40 percent increase in

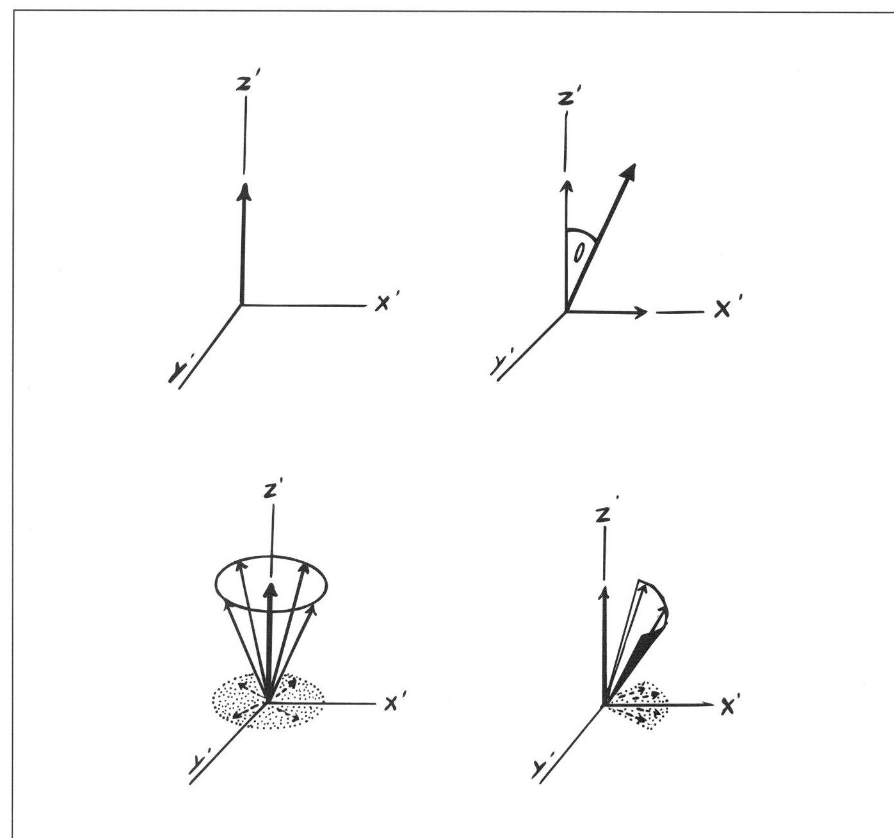

Figure 2.10. T2 or spin-spin relaxation time. Starting at the left top sketch, assuming a 90° radiofrequency pulse is applied, the transverse magnetization acquired begins to change rapidly. The precession is assumed to be coherent or in unison immediately after the pulse, but milliseconds later, because of inhomogeneity in the magnetic field and in the tissues, the spins are not equal in speed and thus become separated; when they become sufficiently separated, the signal is lost, as in the last, bottom left image, moving clockwise. T2 is always shorter than T1. Actually, as shown on the diagram, the vector has not returned to the *Z'* axis, meaning that T1 relaxation (occurring at the same time) is not yet complete.

T1. While free water has a T1 of 2.0 sec or longer in a 1.5-T magnet, water in the tissues has a much shorter T1. Thus, CSF has a T1 of 2 to 3 sec and a T2 of several hundred milliseconds, whereas water in brain tissue has a T1 of 600 to 800 ms for white matter and 800 to 1000 ms for gray matter at 1.5 T. T2 of brain is approximately 90 ms for white matter and 100 ms for gray matter. The T2 relaxation time is relatively independent of the strength of the external magnetic field; it is always shorter than T1 and, in tissues, much shorter (Table 2.1).

Table 2.1.
T1 and T2 in Various Mammalian Tissues at 1.5 T

	Milliseconds	
	T1	*T2*
Muscle:		
Skeletal	870	47
Heart	870	57
Liver	490	43
Kidney	560	58
Spleen	780	62
Adipose	260	84
Brain:		
Gray matter	920	101
White matter	790	92

CONTRAST IN MR IMAGES

Contrast is defined as the intensity difference between adjacent points or areas in the image. It is a fundamental parameter because it enables us to distinguish between adjacent anatomic structures. Since there is no color in the MRI, we depend on difference in shades of gray from white to black. In MRI, the whiter or brighter the area, the higher the signal intensity, and vice versa, in that particular area. In CT a light area means greater absorption of photons, and a darker area means lesser absorption of photons. In MRI this is totally different.

Three factors influence contrast in MR images: proton density (the number of hydrogen atoms) and T1 and T2 relaxation times. In brain tissue proton density does not vary greatly; it is slightly higher in gray than in white matter (about 12 to 15 percent) and higher in CSF. Relaxation times vary considerably more: T1 of CSF is four or five times longer than that of white or gray matter, and T2 of CSF is also several times longer than that of white and gray matter. The T2 of gray matter is about 10 to 15 percent longer than that of white matter (see Table 2.1).

Practically all the signals come from protons in tissue water and in lipids. The protons in heavy proteins (such as DNA) and in bone do not ordinarily contribute to the MR signals that generate the images in clinical MRI systems. Nevertheless, the intracellular water interacts with the macromolecules, and this modifies the proton relaxation times, which accounts for the differences in relaxation times between different tissues as well as between CSF and brain tissue discussed earlier. Freely mobile protons, such as those in liquids, have a longer relaxation time and a rapid tumbling rate. The protons in protein macromolecules have little motion because of the slow tumbling rate of these large molecules. Their relaxation time is so short as to be undetectable in the clinical MRI systems. The same is true, perhaps even more so, in bone, where the protons are relatively immobile.

A smaller object requires a higher degree of contrast between it and adjacent tissues in order to be sure that a slight contrast change does not represent random noise. The presence of noise in all the images tends to degrade them. Our aim is always to try to decrease the noise so as to make the images clearer. That is one reason to utilize higher Tesla values because, as mentioned previously, the number of precessing protons aligned with the magnetic field increases as the power of the magnetic field increases, and thus the signals are likely to be stronger. This improves the signal-to-noise ratio. A method that is ordinarily employed in MRI is to repeat the pulses two to four times at each slice level. This doubles or triples the imaging time and is one reason that the imaging time must be longer with the lower-field magnets, for they require more repetitions to improve the signal-to-noise ratio.

IMAGING SEQUENCES

The relaxation times and the chosen times at which the echoes are received have a profound effect on the appearance of the images. The resolution of MRI systems is around 1 to 2 mm. A number of pulse sequences are used in the production of images. The most common are the SE and the gradient-echo (GRE) pulse sequences, of which there are a number of variants. A third, less frequently used sequence is the *inversion recovery pulse sequence*, which is a variant of the SE sequence. The SE pulse sequences utilize RF pulses that generate flip angles of 90 and 180°, whereas the GRE pulse sequences utilize flip angles of less than 90°.

In the typical SE pulse sequence a 90° pulse is applied followed by a 180° refocusing pulse, after which the echo is received at a variable time (echo time, TE), a number of milliseconds later, depending on the desired effect. If it is desired to emphasize T1, the echo is received at about 10 to 30 ms. However, in this case it is also important to use a short repetition time (TR), that is, the time at which the entire sequence is repeated. To emphasize T1, the TR should be less than 1 sec. This is usually referred to as a *short TR–short TE sequence*, which emphasizes T1. The phase-encoding gradient is applied between the two pulses, and the frequency-encoding gradient is applied at the time the echo is received. If it is desired to emphasize T2, it is necessary to use a long TR of 2 sec or longer. In addition, the TE should be longer, 80 to 120 ms, depending on the strength of the magnetic field. In a 0.5-T magnet, 120 ms may be needed, whereas in a 1.5-T magnet, 80 ms is sufficient.

In addition, when obtaining T2-weighted images, it is customary to obtain two echoes, one at 30 to 40 ms, which is called the *first echo* or the *proton density* or *spin density image*, and the other at 80 to 120 ms, which yields a T2-weighted image. While the first echo (also referred to as *long TR–short TE*) is usually called a proton density image, it is not entirely so; perhaps it is more appropriate to call it the *first echo* in the T2 sequence. The other would then be referred to as the *second echo*, which yields the more heavily T2-weighted images.

T1-WEIGHTED IMAGES

In order to obtain a T1-weighted image, it is necessary to use a short TR, around 400 to 800 ms. The longer time is required in order to obtain more slices and for no other reason, for it adds to the total imaging time. If it is desired to obtain 10 images at a TE of 30 ms, a shorter TR would be needed than if 15 slices are desired. Obtaining a T1-weighted image also requires a short TE.

In a T1-weighted image, a tissue with a short T1 appears bright, and a long T1 appears dark. In between the two extremes the image will show various shades of gray. Fat is bright, almost white, on T1 images both as fat and as a bone marrow component. Water is dark, almost black. Increased water in tissue, such as edema fluid, yields shades of gray darker than the surrounding normal tissue. Water has a long T1 relaxation time of 2 sec or longer. If the TR is much shorter, such as is used in T1 SE pulse sequences, the water protons are far from reaching a relaxed state and thus yield a low signal. On the other hand, if the T1 is short, such as that of protons in fat, the short TR catches them when they are almost fully relaxed and thus yield a stronger signal.

In a T1-weighted image the CSF is always dark, and the surface sulci are also dark. The white matter is lighter than the gray matter. The white matter has a shorter T1 relaxation time than the gray matter, and for that reason it is brighter on the T1 images. It was assumed that the white matter has a shorter T1 than the gray matter because it contains myelin, which is made up of lipoprotein, but this apparently is not the case. It is partly related to the fact that white matter has less water than gray matter and possibly it is also related to the presence of cholesterol in the cell membrane.

Aside from fat, very few tissues have a short T1. Perhaps the most important to mention here is blood in the methemoglobin stage following hemorrhage, a common condition in the intracranial space. Protein in tissue or in a cyst may be bright if it reaches a high enough concentration (e.g., 9 g/1000 g or more). The presence of a dark area on a T1-weighted image does not necessarily indicate CSF or other fluid; it could be bone, calcification, a flow void produced by an artery or a vein, or extremely thick high-protein fluid, because macromolecules possess poorly "mobile" protons. Hemosiderin, the result of old hemorrhage, may also be very dark on T1-weighted images, but this is much more conspicuous on T2-weighted images. Membranes such as dura mater and ligaments are T1-dark, possibly because they are rich in collagen.

The T1-weighted image obtained with the SE sequence is not a pure T1 image; the T2 relaxation time is also expressed in these images. The T1-weighted image generated with the inversion recovery sequence is closer to being a true T1-weighted image but still not entirely so.

T2-WEIGHTED IMAGES

In the SE sequences these images are obtained by using a long TR (800 to 3000 ms) and a long TE (70 to 120 ms or longer). However, as described earlier, with the same long TR it is possible to obtain two images, one at a TE of 10 to 40 ms and another at the higher TE value. The second image is more heavily T2-weighted. As mentioned earlier, the first echo image is often referred to as the proton density or spin density image because it is somewhat related to the number of protons in tissue. In the T2-weighted images (the second echo), water has a high signal and is very bright, white on the image, because it possesses a long T2. The long TR emphasizes any fluid or tissue that has a long T2.

In both the first and second echoes the gray matter is brighter than the white matter; the basal ganglia (caudate nucleus, globus pallidus, putamen) are brighter, similar to gray matter. In the first echo, the CSF is usually gray and more or less isointense with the surrounding white or gray matter. In the second echo, the CSF is white.

A "dark" image on T2-weighted images most commonly may be a flow void produced by flowing blood in arteries or veins and sometimes flowing CSF, for instance, near the foramen of Monro, the aqueduct, or in the neighborhood of a pulsating artery such as the basilar artery in the interpeduncular fossa. The globus pallidus and to a lesser extent the putamen are usually dark on T2 images due to a susceptibility effect produced by an increase in iron content, which increases with age in these structures (17). In addition, the red nucleus, the substantia nigra, and the dentate nucleus of the cerebellum contain iron, which increases with age, giving these structures a darker appearance on T2 images. This susceptibility effect is more marked in the higher-field magnets.

"Dark T2" images are also produced by calcium, hemosiderin, and others (see text following). In general, pathologic processes of all types tend to be hyperintense on first and second echo T2-weighted images, usually because of edema or increased fluid in the lesion, be it inflammatory, neoplastic, or degenerative.

There are relatively few types of lesions that are dark on T2 images. These include old hemorrhage because of hemosiderin, some meningiomas because of diffuse psammoma bodies, calcified lesions, some sarcoid granulomas possibly because of increased collagen, nonthrombosed aneurysms due to a flow void, blood in the deoxyhemoglobin stage, or a cyst containing very high protein fluid such as some colloid cysts and some mucoceles. Other T2 hypointense lesions include neoplasms in the primitive neuroectodermal group (PNET) (medulloblastoma, pineoblastoma, esthesioneuroblastoma), and also some lymphomas, plasmacytomas, and melanomas. The dura mater and the ligaments are usually T2-dark.

On SE T2-weighted images, fat is much less bright than on T1 images. However, in FSE images, fat tends to be bright related to the use of short echo in the images. On GRE images emphasizing T2, fat is actually dark, whereas fluid remains bright (see text following).

GRADIENT ECHO

The GRE is an imaging sequence in which a refocusing 180° RF pulse, used in the SE imaging sequence, is not employed. Instead, any flip angle of less than 90° may be used, depending on the desired effects, combined with various TRs and TEs. For instance, to obtain a T2 effect, a relatively longer TR (over 2000 ms) and longer TE (over 15 ms) combined with a low flip angle (less than 20°) may yield the desired result. A T1 effect would be produced by a longer TR, a short TE (less than 15 ms), and a higher flip angle (over 20°). In the GRE sequences the predominance is in longitudinal magnetization, while only minimal residual transverse magnetization remains. This residual transverse magnetization is eliminated in the General Electric gradient variant called *spoiled* GRASS (SPGR) or other GRE variants from different manufacturers (see text following).

The T2 effect in GRASS is referred to as T2* (T-2 star) to indicate the signal loss due to T2 effects plus that related to static field inhomogeneites that are not compensated for due to the lack of a 180° refocusing pulse in GRE sequences. GRE images exaggerate magnetic field inhomogeneities both intrinsic to the magnet and resulting from induced local magnetic fields (for example, the presence of iron in old hemorrhage). For this reason this sequence is preferred when looking for signs of old hemorrhage, usually referred to as a *magnetic susceptibility image* or sequence.

MAGNETIC SUSCEPTIBILITY

Magnetic susceptibility is the ability of a substance to become magnetized when placed in an applied magnetic field. A substance can be diamagnetic, paramagnetic, or ferromagnetic, depending on whether the induced local field opposes, weakly augments, or strongly increases the applied field. GREs are extremely sensitive to the presence of small amounts of paramagnetic and ferromagnetic substances because of the induced local magnetic fields. These local magnetic fields cause visible signal loss on GRE T2-weighted images because of T2*. This signal loss can be emphasized in GRE by decreasing the flip angle, and/or prolonging the TE. The greatest value of investigating magnetic susceptibility is in identifying diamagnetic substances (calcifications) and paramagnetic substances (physiologic and pathologic areas of iron deposition).

While advantages of GRE T2-weighted images over SE T2-weighted images include their short acquisition time and their ability to maintain signal in fluids or substances with long T2* (e.g., CSF and intervertebral discs), a weakness is the greater signal loss from T2*, which can overshadow signal loss from spin-spin relaxation (T2 relaxation), thereby hiding lesions. Large differences of local magnetic fields at interfaces cannot support the same magnetic flux density, thereby creating a signal loss at interfaces. This is most noticeable at the sinus-brain interface and the CSF-osteophyte interface.

GRE allows rapid chemical shift evaluation by choosing the appropriate TE. Water protons precess at a faster rate than fat protons (3.5 ppm). After being perturbed by an RF pulse and placed on the transverse plane, the protons of water and fat dephase. There is a cyclic increased and decreased signal depending on whether the water and fat protons are in or out of phase. If the water and fat protons are in phase, their signals are additive. If they are 180° out of phase, their signals are canceled. The choice of the TE determines whether protons have cycled to a position in or out of phase. At 0.6-T field strength, the water and fat protons are out of phase at 18, 29, 40, and 51 ms. Chemical shift becomes important in evaluating the spine for metastasis or a subtle fracture. Nulling the normal signal from the marrow increases the conspicuity of water-dominant tumors and trauma.

Because of the rapid acquisition of single-slice GRE T1-weighted images, flowing blood can be made bright using the "entry slice phenomenon." Blood flowing into the imaging slice has not received a pulse and is fully magnetized. The stationary tissue within the slice is partially saturated by the repeated pulses, not having recovered full magnetization. Therefore, the strong signal elicited from unsaturated blood reflects full magnetization. The entry slice phenomenon has been used to create a bright signal in arteriovenous malformations with rapid flow, while thrombosed arteriovenous malformations would have a null signal. Arteriovenous malformations containing blood clots with methemoglobin, however, will be bright using flow techniques based on in-flow. In this case, phase imaging would be preferred.

Contrast in GRE images is controlled by the flip angle and the TE. GRE should be used as a supplemental pulse sequence to investigate lesions seen on SE pulse sequences. This rapid acquisition and the ability to choose only the appropriate sequence to study an intrinsic tissue parameter are extremely advantageous (18,19). GRE T2-weighted images, however, should not be primary imaging sequences because they are hampered by their magnetic susceptibility at interfaces, and lesions having subtle spin-spin relaxation changes may be obscured by the T2* effects. Also, GREs are more susceptible to artifacts produced by paramagnetic material, such as that found in CSF shunt valves.

There is a great variety of approaches and variations of GRE images, and this has led to a growing variety of designations used by the various manufacturers and by individuals who have developed and employed them. In order to simplify communication, the terms have been replaced by acronyms. Some of the better-known and more frequently used terms and acronyms are listed here, but the list is not intended to be complete. A more complete listing may be found in the literature (19,20). They can be divided into the following four groups:

1. Basic GREs

   MPGR = Multiplanar GRASS (GE Medical Systems)

   FE = Field echo (Picker, Phillips, Toshiba, Otsuka)

   FESUM = Field echo with echo time (ET) set for water and fat in phase (Picker)

   FEDIF = Field echo with echo time set for water and fat in opposition (Picker)

   GRECHO = Gradient-recalled echo (Resonex)

   GFE = Gradient field echo (Hitachi)

   PFI = Partial flip angle (Toshiba)

   STIR = Short time inversion recovery

2. Steady state

   Steady state with FID (free induction decay) sampling
   - FFE = Fast field echo (Philips)
   - FAST = Fourier-acquired steady state (Picker)
   - GRASS = Gradient-recalled acquisition in the steady state (GE Medical Systems)
   - FISP = Fast imaging with steady-state precession (Siemens)
   - SSFP = Steady-state free precession (GE, Shimadzu, Toshiba)

   Steady state with stimulated echo
   - E-SHORT = Steady-state GRE with stimulated echo sampling (Elscint)
   - SSFP = Steady-state free precession (GE, Shimadzu, Toshiba)
   - PSIF = Reversed FISP (Siemens)

3. Non-steady-state

   FLASH = Fast low-angle shot (Siemens)
   CE-FFE-T1 = Contrast-enhanced fast field echo with T1 weighting (Philips)
   CE-FFE-T2 = Contrast-enhanced fast field echo with T2 weighting (Philips).
   RF-FAST = RF-spoiled FAST (Picker)

   SPGR = Spoiled GRASS (GE)

4. Rapid (prepared) GRE sequences

   FSPGR = Fast spoiled GRASS (GE)

   RAM-FAST = Rapidly acquired magnetization-prepared FAST (Picker)

   Turbo FLASH = Turbo FLASH (Siemens)

   MP-RAGE (3-D) = Magnetization-prepared rapid GRE (Siemens)

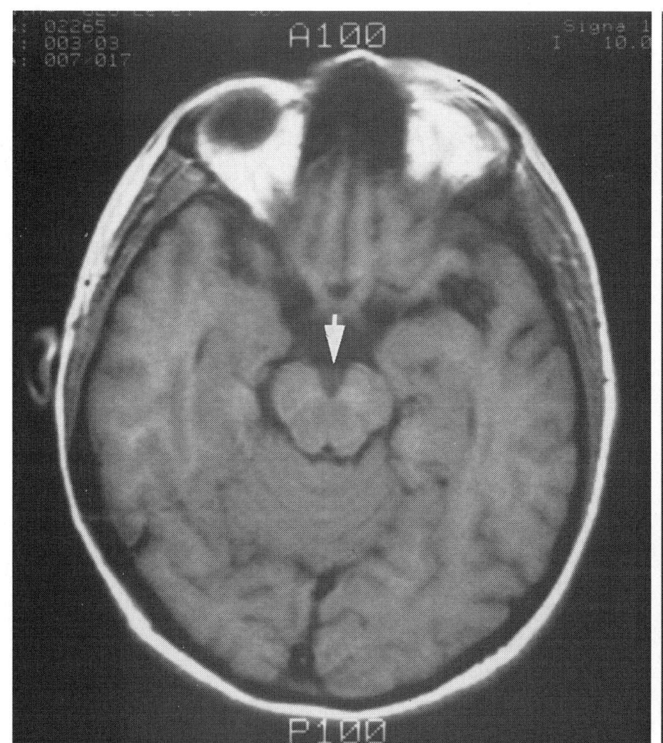

A

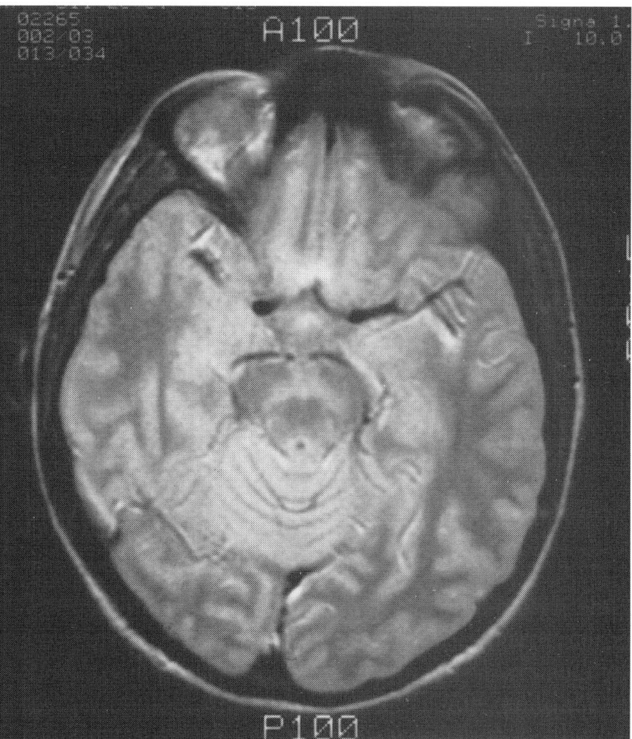

B

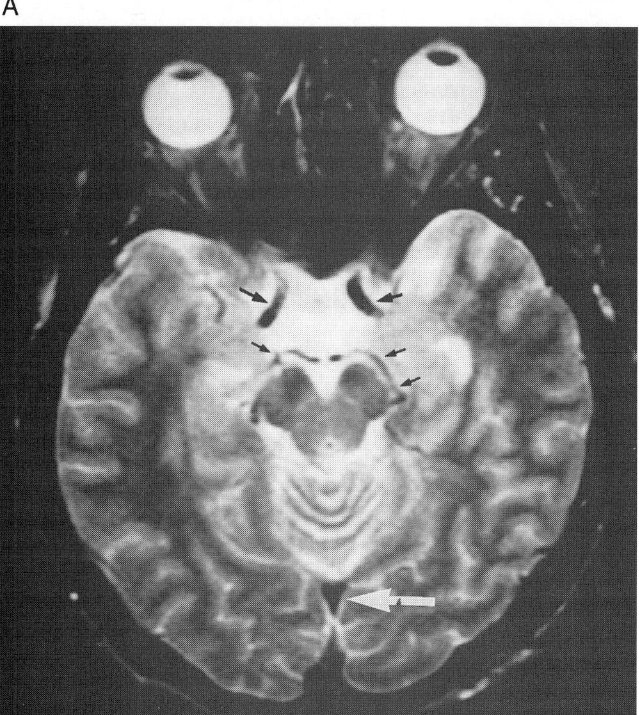

C

Figure 2.11. A. T1-weighted axial image. The CSF is dark, and the gray matter is darker than the white matter. The anatomy is very clearly demonstrated (TR 700 ms; TE 11 ms). **B.** First-echo T2-weighted axial image (proton density). The CSF is isodense with the white matter, and the gray matter is brighter than the white matter. The interpeduncular fossa cannot be discerned because of the isodense CSF (compare with A). The dark shadows represent flow voids of the anterior and middle cerebral artery, of the posterior cerebral arteries around the midbrain, and of the straight sinus posteriorly, as well as bone in the right orbital wall and calvarium. The aqueduct is seen partly because it is surrounded by periaqueductal gray matter, which is brighter, and partly because of CSF flow in it, which may produce a variable flow void. **C.** T2-weighted axial image on another subject (TR 2000 ms; TE 80 ms). The CSF is white, and the gray matter is brighter than the white matter. Posteriorly, the image shows a flow void in the straight sinus (arrow), and in the torcular behind; laterally, it shows flow voids in the posterior cerebral arteries (small arrows) around the midbrain; anteriorly, flow voids are in the internal carotid. In A the interpeduncular fossa is dark (T1) (arrow); in B the fossa is not seen because the CSF is isodense (proton density, first-echo (proton density) T2-weighted image); in C the interpeduncular fossa is bright. In A the optic chiasm and nerves (just anterior to the white arrow) are well seen because they are surrounded by dark CSF; but in B and C they are not visible, since the isointense CSF in B and the hyperintense CSF in C obscure the anatomy. In A, the orbital fat is bright and the eye is dark, and in C it is the reverse.

Effects of Flow on MR Images

It is necessary to become acquainted with the various manifestations of flow in MRI. In the head, two liquids must be considered: blood and CSF. The flow of blood is mostly rapid, but some blood moves more slowly, particularly in the veins. Here we will deal only with larger and medium-sized vessels. Flow through the arteriolar capillary bed is not ordinarily imaged by MRI, although blood volume can be estimated with special techniques. CSF flow is mostly very slow but can be more rapid, such as through the aqueduct and in the region of the foramen of Monro.

The blood flow through vessels the size of those in the human brain is ordinarily laminar flow. Turbulent flow develops if the speed of flow increases, whereas in larger vessels turbulence develops at lower speeds.

Some of the phenomena related to flow which one must understand are as follows:

FLOW VOIDS IN SPIN-ECHO SEQUENCES

A flow void is produced when moving fluid leaves a slice where it has received the 90° and the 180° RF pulses and is replaced by fluid that has been only partially saturated. This washout effect is termed *flow void* to indicate that a signal loss has occurred. The effect is magnified by using thin slices and longer TEs. Faster flow increases the flow void effect. For these reasons flow voids are much more

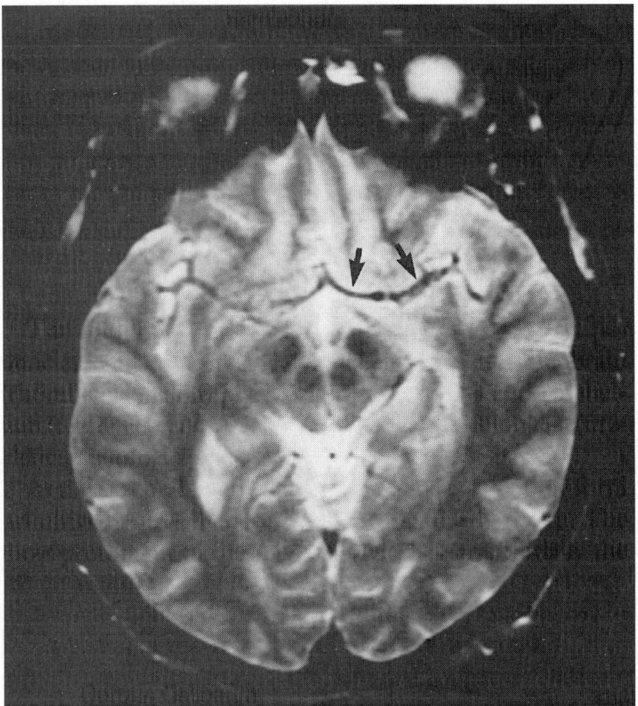

Figure 2.12. Flow voids produced by the middle and anterior cerebral arteries on both sides (arrows). The direction of the flow does not matter (the anterior cerebral arteries are flowing toward the midline and the middle cerebral arteries are flowing away from the midline); only the speed of flow matters, which is likely to be high in arteries as opposed to veins.

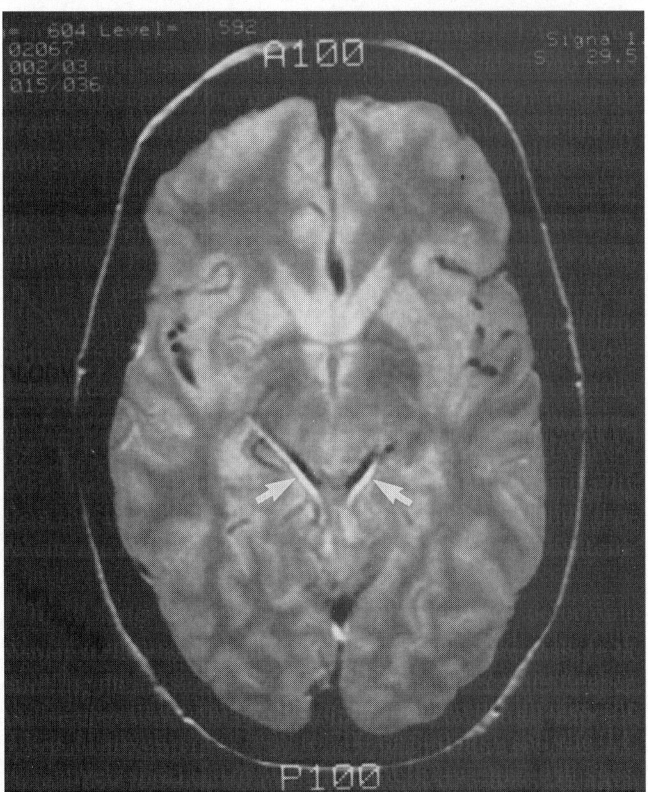

Figure 2.13. Misregistration of slow flow oblique to the phase-encoding axis. The two basal veins are frequently a source of this artifact because they usually run oblique to the plane of the phase-encoding axis in axial views (arrows). The basal veins are bright and are parallel to a dark band representing the true position of the veins.

pronounced in T2-weighted images, which utilize fairly thin slices and a long TE (Figs. 2.11 and 2.12). Arteries produce a clearer flow void, whereas veins may or may not.

Flow oblique to the direction of the phase-encoding axis may place the flow void or the intensity of a slowly flowing vessel in the wrong position due to misregistration between the time that gradient pulse is applied and the echo is received. In other words, the fluid has moved at every level, which causes it to be placed farther away or closer depending on the direction of the flow (Fig. 2.13).

FLOW-RELATED ENHANCEMENT

The blood flowing into an area that has received a saturating pulse is fully magnetized but unsaturated. As it enters the field being imaged, it may present a bright image. This occurs if the flow is not too rapid, and the image is brightest if the flow is at the same speed as the slice thickness being imaged, for instance, if the flow is 1 cm per second and the slice thickness is 1 cm. This is rather slow flow, which may be seen in some veins but also may be seen over a longer distance if the plane of the vessel is not perpendicular but inclined in relation to the imaging plane. This flow-related enhancement is seen usually in the first slices of a multislice imaging train and may extend to the first two or three slices (Fig. 2.14); it sometimes may be seen in several

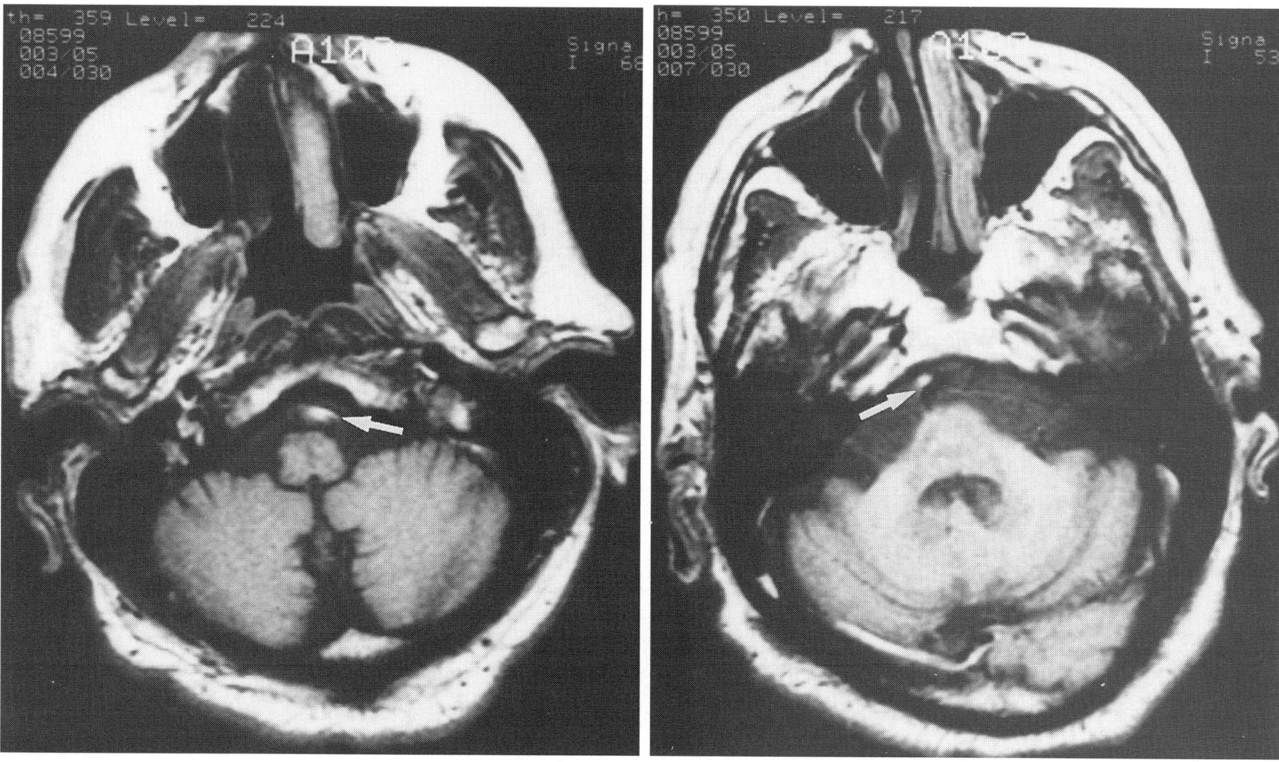

A B

Figure 2.14. A. Flow-related enhancement of vertebral artery in the first slice of a T1-weighted sequence (arrow). **B.** Twelve millimeters higher up there is partial brightness of the basilar artery combined with a flow void (arrow) due to flow-related enhancement.

slices but only in the center of the vessel (21). Flow-related enhancement of the first slice may be seen on T1-weighted images as well as on T2-weighted images. Flow-related enhancement can be a source of artifacts that at times are difficult to interpret; this is particularly true when performing magnetic resonance angiography. However, because flow-related enhancement occurs when fully magnetized but unsaturated protons flow into the imaging area, it may be eliminated by presaturating the adjacent tissues from which blood is flowing.

STAGNANT FLOW

Very slow flow may yield a brighter image. This sometimes may be seen in the jugular vein if the head is overflexed, and would be seen on T2-weighted images.

EVEN ECHO REPHASING

This applies to the use of the first and second echo T2 images where if the second echo is twice the echo time of the first echo (e.g., 40 and 80 ms, respectively), there may be enhancement of signal owing to rephasing of the spins taking place at the time of the second echo. This would yield a much stronger signal on the par-numbered echo compared with the preceding and following odd-numbered echoes. It could also occur if the echoes were 20 and 80 ms. This phenomenon can be used clinically—for instance, to demonstrate patency of a dural sinus. The first echo may show a signal loss, whereas the second echo may show brightness if the vessel is patent and flowing.

DIASTOLIC PSEUDOGATING

The high signal of stagnant flow may be seen during diastole. For instance, increased intensity is often seen in the aorta in gated acquisitions.

MR ANGIOGRAPHY

See Chapter 10.

CSF FLOW

A flow void is produced by flowing CSF, usually in the region of the foramen of Monro, in the third ventricle, or in the aqueduct. The last is the most common and is likely to show up during systole and to disappear during diastole if cardiac gating is used during image data acquisition (Fig. 2.15*A*). CSF flow voids may also be seen around pulsating arteries, particularly in the interpeduncular fossa, owing to pulsations of the basilar artery bifurcation. This can be confused with an aneurysm (Fig. 2.15*B* and *C*).

DIFFUSION IMAGING

Water molecules within the tissues move at random. Blood moves through vessels in a defined way, but water leaves

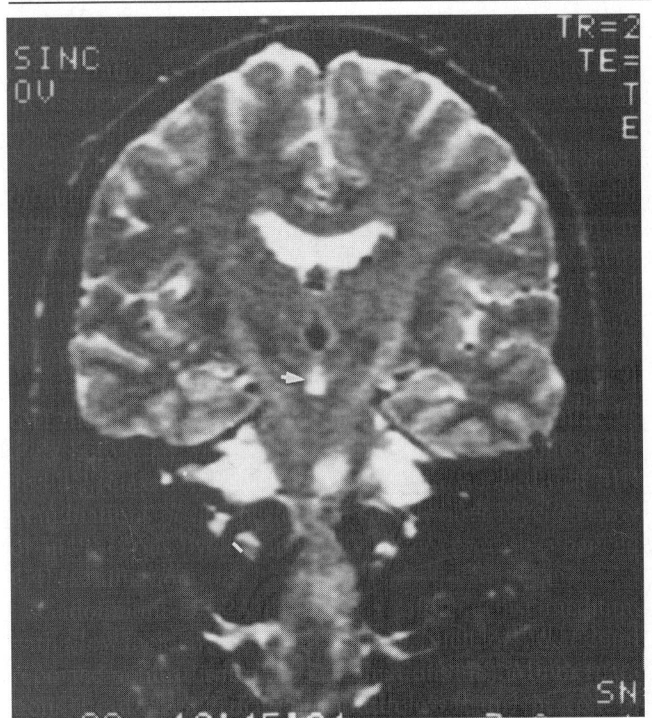

A

Figure 2.15. Flow void in third ventricle and in aqueduct. Flow void in interpeduncular fossa. **A.** T2-weighted coronal image shows that the lateral ventricles are bright, and the CSF in the region just below the foramen of Monro and in the rest of the third ventricle is dark because of movement of the CSF. The bright midline shadow below the third ventricle (arrow) represents CSF in the interpeduncular fossa. This patient has bilateral eighth-nerve schwannomas, seen in the lower part of the figure. **B.** Axial proton density image in another patient. The aqueduct shows a flow void. The interpeduncular fossa presents a round flow void due to pulsations related to the basilar artery (arrow). **C.** T2-weighted image reveals disappearance of the pseudoaneurysm. Only the basilar artery produces a flow void (arrow).

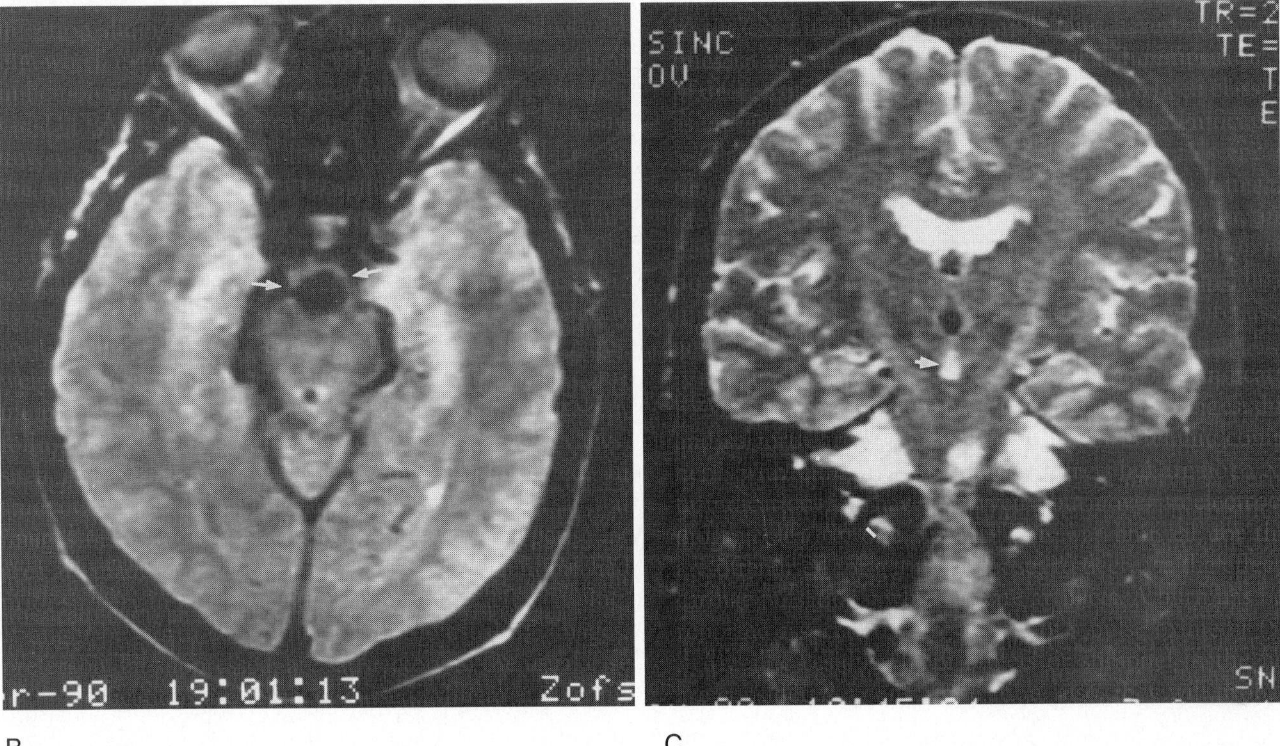

B

C

the blood vessels and moves freely outside the blood vessels. The extravascular water movement is very slow in relation to intravascular flow: possibly 50 micrometers per second, much less than the dimension of a voxel. Nevertheless, this motion generates some signal loss in MRI. The rate of diffusion may increase or decrease with pathologic conditions, and increased diffusion is probably more common than the opposite. A diffusion-weighted image can be obtained by using a long TR and a double echo separated by a relatively long time (e.g., 100 ms between the two echoes), using a different gradient before each echo. Clinical applications of the technique have developed very slowly. It was thought that ischemic strokes could be diagnosed earlier using diffusion imaging (22); the usefulness promised by preliminary findings in animals is just beginning to reach clinical practice. This is believed to be due to lack of proper instrumentation. The current evidence suggests that the introduction of newer MRI techniques such as echoplanar and other fast imaging variations may increase clinical applications of diffusion-weighted imaging to study early ischemic lesions in the brain as well as other pathologic conditions. Rapid imaging is essential to decrease the artifacts produced by motion in this motion-sensitive technique. Sevick et al. concluded, after some experimental evidence in rats, that diffusion-weighted MRI may be useful to reach a quantitative evaluation of cytotoxic edema (23).

Doran et al. emphasized the influence of the direction of fibers in fiber tracts on diffusion (24). Diffusion imaging parallel to the direction of fiber tracts demonstrated the tracts, but not if the gradient was perpendicular to the direction of the fibers.

Two terms frequently used are *intravoxel incoherent motion* (IVIM), which refers to other kinds of motion such as capillary flow, and *apparent diffusion coefficient* (ADC). The latter term has been suggested to describe quantitatively the results of diffusion imaging experiments in vivo (25). The ADC has been measured in many conditions, such as multiple sclerosis plaques, inflammatory conditions, and neoplasms (26). Brunberg et al. reported on the use of ADC and average ADC in combination with determination of an index of diffusion anisotropy (IDA) in brain tumors of the astrocytoma and malignant astrocytoma type (27). They found higher IDAs at the margin of the tumor than in the central portions, which they thought were consistent with disruption of myelin membranes, which normally restrict diffusion. However, the higher marginal diffusion could also be due to IVIM due to a heavy hypervascular capillary bed in the periphery of the tumor.

CSF Flow Velocity

This is a specialized form of phase contrast that allows imaging of CSF flows. When spins move through a gradient, their acquired phase is proportional to velocity. Thus, it is possible to subtract the stationary background and image only the moving parts. It is possible to image midline structures such as the aqueduct or the fourth ventricle to determine the direction of CSF flow. Cardiac pulsations generate a to-and-fro motion through the aqueduct, which may be exaggerated in hydrocephalus of the communicating type (see Chapter 4). The outlet of the fourth ventricle and the midline of the foramen magnum region may also be imaged in some cases where there is pathology in this region and knowledge of CSF flow may be useful.

Magnetization Transfer Imaging

Magnetization transfer imaging (MTI) is a technique that examines the effect of large-protein-molecule-bound protons on free unbound water protons. Yousem et al. carried out a series of studies to determine the influences of high signal secretions in the paranasal sinuses as seen on T1-weighted images (which is an indication of higher protein content) on the magnetization transfer ratio (MTR) and found a higher MTR in these cases (28). Tumor versus edema may well show the same relationship. According to Mehta et al. it is possible to improve the detection of tumors by utilizing MTI techniques in combination with gadolinium enhancement (29). MTI can be carried out by using a gradient-echo sequence of TR 500 ms, TE 12 ms, and a 20° flip angle with and without the MTI suppressor pulse applied. The MTI suppressor pulse is placed at a certain frequency—e.g., 2000 Hz off the resonance of water and applied for 19 ms at an amplitude about 10 times that of the 90° flip angle pulse according to Yousem et al., who found improved contrast between lesion and surrounding background (30). The same was also reported in brain lesions by Nguyen et al. (31). Improved visualization of ischemic lesions is another possibility, as is the characterization of water versus demyelination (32).

MR Functional Imaging

See Chapter 14.

Artifacts in MRI

MOTION

This is the most common technical problem in MRI owing to the fact that data acquisition takes several minutes. Any subject motion is likely to degrade the images; thus, all efforts should be made to eliminate motion. These artifacts are usually recognized because they produce blurring of all detail in the images; this would be the case in all views. Contrary to CT, where motion may be seen in some sections but not in others, in MRI all the images of a particular sequence would show loss of sharpness because they are generated simultaneously. In the abdomen, motion artifacts are usually associated with respiratory motion. Periodic motion leads to the production of ghost images and general degradation of the resolution. Ghost images occur along the phase-encoding direction regardless of the direction of motion.

Motion artifacts occurring along the phase-encoding axis due to arterial pulsations are very common. They also occur, particularly after contrast enhancement, across from the basilar artery or the lateral sinuses in the posterior fossa in axial or coronal views; or arising from the anterior cerebral arteries and the superior sagittal sinus in sagittal views (Fig. 2.16). This artifact can be eliminated (or made to change to other locations) by shifting the phase-encoding axis 90° and doing the same with the frequency-encoding axis.

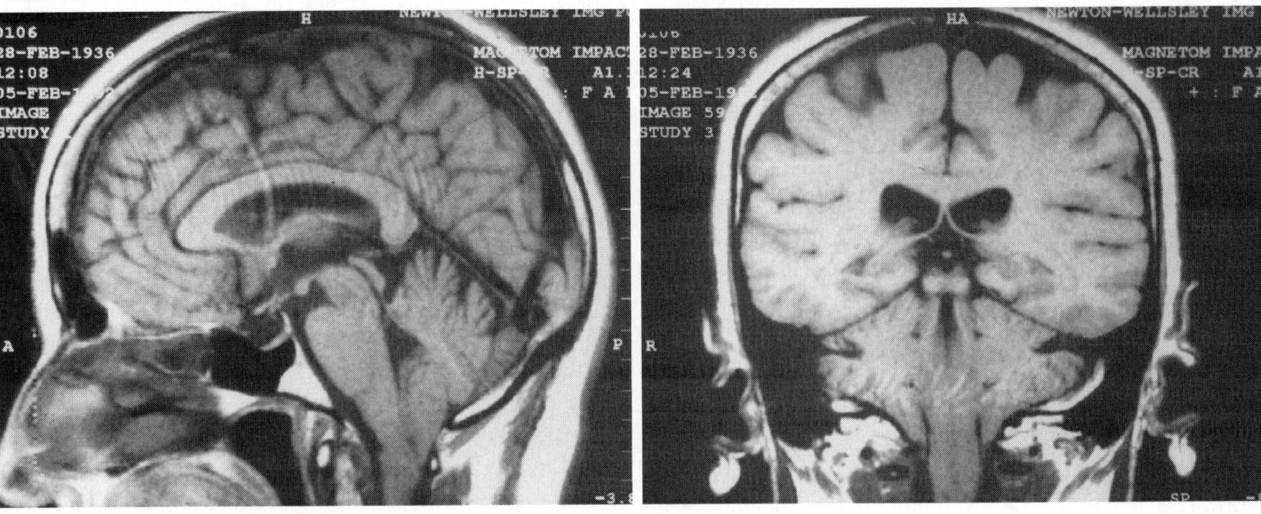

A B

Figure 2.16. Phase-encoding artifacts due to pulsations. **A.** Artifacts arising in the midline sagittal view from pulsations from the anterior cerebral arteries or flow effects in the sagittal sinus. **B.** Phase artifacts in the posterior fossa between the lateral sinuses. The pulsating fourth ventricle, the choroid plexus, and the basilar artery all contribute to these frequently encountered artifacts, which appear as straight bands composed of a combination of bright and gray curved lines. They are sometimes difficult to interpret but must always be kept in mind if a combination of unexplained brighter and gray images is seen in this region, particularly on T1-weighted images. After contrast enhancement this artifact becomes worse and is seen in nearly all cases, in both axial and coronal views. Other pulsation artifacts elsewhere become more prominent after contrast injection. This patient has an unrelated Chiari I malformation and also an empty sella.

METALLIC ARTIFACTS

These usually can be identified because they produce a signal void in the area sometimes associated with geometric distortion and arcs of high signal intensity. Ferromagnetic materials as well as nonferromagnetic materials cause localized artifacts because they cause nonuniformity of the magnetic field. The amount of material required to produce an artifact is surprisingly small and may not be visible on radiography. Eye makeup is a frequent source of artifacts around the orbits.

CHEMICAL SHIFT ARTIFACTS

These usually occur at the interfaces between fat and a body organ, such as the orbital fat surrounding the optic nerve or adjacent to the orbital muscles. Typically a dark line or band is seen, followed by a bright band. The artifact results from the difference in Larmor frequency of hydrogen nuclei in aliphatic carbon chains in lipids and hydrogen nuclei that are part of water molecules. When the frequency gradient is applied, the protons in fat precess slightly more slowly than those in water molecules and thus will be frequency encoded in a wrong location. The misregistration always occurs in the frequency-encoding direction, and the dark and bright bands will be perpendicular to the encoding direction (Fig. 2.17). In some cases a chemical shift can suggest the presence of dissection of the internal carotid artery in the neck when the artery is partly surrounded by fat. Fat suppression techniques would eliminate this artifact (33).

TRUNCATION ARTIFACTS (GIBB PHENOMENON, RINGING ARTIFACTS)

These consist of parallel bands occurring along both the frequency- and the phase-encoding axis, where there is a fairly sharp boundary between high- and low-signal intensities. A classic truncation artifact is the low-intensity line along the middle of the spinal cord, suggesting the central canal of the cord on T1-weighted sagittal images, or the bright central line on T2-weighted images (34). The truncation artifacts are produced by the use of Fourier transformations to generate the MR images and are worse when using a matrix with fewer lines; for instance, in a 128 $\times$ 256 pixel matrix the artifact would be worse along the 128 direction (usually the phase-encoding axis). In this example, the truncation artifacts would decrease by changing to a 256 $\times$ 256 matrix. However, this decreases but does not eliminate the artifacts. Daniels et al. have also demonstrated these artifacts in the internal acoustic canal (35).

Fourier transformations are best when imaging gradual transitions from bright to black passing through grades of gray, but they do poorly when imaging any abrupt transitions from bright to dark and vice versa. Such is the case when moving from CSF to spinal cord and from cord to CSF, but examples are common in other locations; this fact

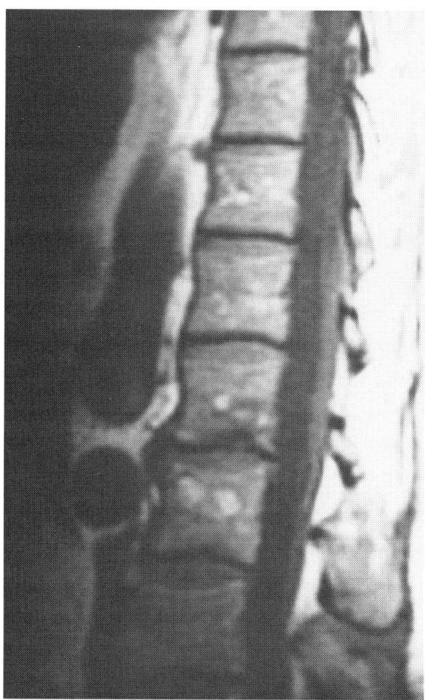

Figure 2.17. Chemical shift artifact. A dark band is seen under each vertebral body at the interface between the fat-containing bone marrow in the vertebral body and the water-containing intervertebral disc. This is seen at all levels and occurs in the frequency-encoding direction.

should be kept in mind to explain some of the many artifacts observed in MRI.

ALIASING ARTIFACTS

These artifacts occur when the dimension of the object exceeds the image FOV, causing signals generated outside the FOV to be superimposed on the opposite side of the field (wraparound artifacts). This problem places limits on the image parameters such as the size of the FOV and also on the choice of frequency-encoding and phase-encoding axes. Manufacturers have solved the problems in the frequency-encoding axes but not in the phase-encoding direction. An aliasing artifact may occur when the nose falls outside the FOV: the nose is imaged in the occipital region.

SURFACE COIL SIGNAL LOSS

The signal is strongest closer to the surface coil, and the intensity of the signal decreases as it moves away from the coil. This is particularly noticeable in the spine. The subcutaneous tissue and the paraspinal muscles have the highest intensity and appear white on the images. The brightness gradually decreases as one moves away from the back.

FAT-SUPPRESSION TECHNIQUES

The high intensity of fat in T1-weighted images obscures some of the anatomy as well as some pathologic lesions. This is particularly significant in the orbit and in the pituitary but also applies to lesions located near or at the base of the skull. Some of the lesions are small, and the presence of fat in the bone marrow and sometimes in the cavernous sinus may make interpretation more difficult.

Fat-saturation techniques consist basically of covering the tissues to be imaged with a preparatory pulse to saturate the fat, followed by in-phase and out-of-phase chopper components. In general, because of frequent artifacts related to air-containing structures, we no longer use fat-suppression techniques when examining the pituitary with gadolinium unless the patient has had surgery. Fat suppression is useful when studying a lesion near the base of the skull, such as detection of perineural infiltration by tumor, and also when a fat-containing intracerebral lesion is suspected (lipoma, teratoma). In the spine, this technique is used in all cases where contrast enhancement is carried out.

Fat suppression may also be useful in T2-weighted images because it increases the sharpness of some structures and of lesions partly surrounded by fat. This is particularly important in the head and neck (36).

It may be worth mentioning here that fat-suppression techniques may introduce artifacts, particularly in the lower aspect of the orbits and in the high nasopharynx, due to the proximity of air-containing cavities (37).

Practical Considerations in MRI in Clinical Practice

HEAD EXAMINATIONS

The axial images are the most important and most useful on a routine basis. However, sagittal and, particularly, coronal views are important to reach a complete understanding of the morphology of a lesion and its relationship to the surrounding structures. A routine examination of the head consists of a T1-weighted set of sagittal images and a T2-weighted set of axial images, consisting of first echo (proton density or spin density) and second echo, where the second echo images are the truly T2-weighted images.

The SE sequence is used routinely. However, the development of the FSE technique has led many investigators to try it in many types of cases, for instance, in pediatric examinations to reduce movement artifacts and to save time (38). Because time is an important factor in MR examinations, FSE is being used more and more in routine examination of the head and spine (39,40,41).

However, FSE presents some disadvantages in the demonstration of certain lesions. For instance, Norbash et al. found that FSE was equivalent to spin echo in the detection of high-intensity lesions but was inferior to spin echo in the demonstration of small, low-signal-intensity lesions (42). Thus it is important to keep these factors in mind, for we would not wish to expose ourselves to the possibility of overlooking a lesion. Also, FSE is somewhat insensitive to magnetic susceptibility, meaning that one can miss old hemorrhagic lesions, a most important consideration. For this reason, if there is any suspicion of old hemorrhage of any type, it is important to supplement the examination with a GRE sequence, particularly if the FSE technique is being used routinely, which is the case in many installations at present. FSE has been specifically recommended to reduce metallic artifacts in postoperative patients, precisely because of the insensitivity to magnetic susceptibility noted earlier.

REDUCTION OF IMAGING TIME

Methods to decrease imaging time are under operator control and are determined by the products of the repetition time (TR), matrix size (M), and number (N) of acquisitions. Total time T = TR × M × N. One or all three can be changed to decrease imaging time (20).

TR reduction is used in gradient echoes (e.g., 2000 ms TR for conventional spin echo and 100 to 200 ms for GRE). The matrix (M) can be manipulated via lowering resolution (e.g., 128 × 256), but other approaches are preferable to lowering resolution. The phase steps can be decreased by partial Fourier transformation or by rectangular FOV. Half-Fourier transformation maintains contrast, but the signal is reduced because the number of samples is reduced (only half of the phase steps are obtained, and the other half are created by mathematical conjugation). Also, phase steps can be scanned more quickly, which is the technique used in FSE and echoplanar imaging. The number of acquisitions (N) can be reduced; this works particularly well with the use of surface coils, which improves the signal-to-noise ratio. High-field magnets allow for a reduction of N without loss of resolution, as against the low-field magnets, which require a higher number of acquisitions and therefore longer imaging time.

The most important time reduction, at present, is obtained through the use of FSE. It allows for faster scanning with retained image resolution and contrast. The speed of FSE is gained from faster acquisition of phase steps.

In FSE for each 90° RF pulse, 4 to 16 echoes can be obtained, whereas in conventional SE only a single echo is obtained. The different echo times obtained during one repetition time (TR) are called echo train length (ETL).

Increasing the ETL decreases imaging time. Because the echo in FSE is the combination of several echoes, the echo is called the effective TE (TE eff.). Image contrast is retained because the echoes are formed by 180° RF pulses, similar to conventional SE.

Other weaknesses to FSE, in addition to the lower magnetic susceptibility discussed earlier, include slight blurring of the proton density T2 images and the persistent bright signal of fat on second echo T2; however, a higher matrix (e.g., 512 × 256) for brain examination images may be used, which increases image resolution.

The reduced magnetic susceptibility in FSE is related to the rapid rephasing of the protons by the repetitive 180° refocusing pulses, which limits the effects of water diffusion produced by the local variations in the magnetic field at the microscopic level, engendered by the paramagnetic iron deposits (either from hemosiderin or other, such as found in the basal ganglia, substantia nigra, etc.).

The sagittal T1-weighted image is useful to demonstrate the anatomy in this projection, and because it is T1-weighted, any pathology present is often difficult to see or is not seen at all. The rationale for obtaining a T1-weighted sagittal image as against a T1-weighted axial image is to have a different projection, and it represents a trade-off in order to save time. A T1-weighted axial image would be more useful but would present the same anatomy as the T2-weighted images. Because of the extra time required (in a very expensive installation), however, the axial T1 is eliminated in favor of the sagittal image, whereas both should be obtained, for there are many instances where the T1-weighted image is needed for complete interpretation. This is frequently the case with calcifications, blood products, and, often, simple anatomic structures, which usually show up more clearly on T1-weighted images. Nevertheless, it is well known that the T2-weighted images show even minor pathologic changes with much greater clarity than the T1-weighted images, and for this reason they represent the basic images for detection of pathologic alterations.

In looking at images, it is usually easy to determine whether an image of the brain is T1-weighted. The CSF is dark, and the gray matter is darker than the white matter (Fig. 2.11). In looking at the inscription on the images, the TR is relatively short (400 to 700 or 800 ms), and the TE is relatively short (10 to 30 ms). In the T2-weighted images, the first echo (proton density), the CSF is either isointense with white matter or it is slightly darker or brighter; the gray matter is brighter than the white matter (Fig. 2.11). In the second echo, the CSF is white and the gray matter is brighter than the white matter.

Any dark image on the T2-weighted sequence is likely to be a flow void; flowing blood or flowing CSF (Figs. 2.11 and 2.15); blood products (hemosiderin or acute blood in the deoxyhemoglobin or early intracellelar methemoglobin state); iron in tissues such as basal ganglia; calcification; or occasionally a high-protein-containing cyst or granuloma (see Figs. 6.29, 6.30, and 11.37).

Modification of Imaging Sequences

The basic imaging sequences must be modified to meet the different circumstances posed by the patient's problem.

INFANT

When an infant is being examined and it is desired to see the anatomy clearly to determine the presence or absence of anomalies, T1-weighted axials are needed in addition to T1-weighted sagittals, and the T2-weighted images because the T1-weighted images demonstrate the anatomy more clearly. Because in all infants it is desirable to ascertain the state of myelination, the T1-weighted axials are also needed, particularly during the first year of life. The inversion recovery (T1-weighted) images are preferable for this purpose but, unfortunately, they take a longer time to complete, and for this reason other alternatives are preferred. After the first year the routine images are sufficient to evaluate myelination (see Chaps. 4 and 5).

CHILD OR ADULT

In a child or adult with a convulsive disorder, one should perform routine imaging plus coronal, T2-weighted images to see the medial temporal lobe region bilaterally. In a child, if no abnormalities are seen, it is questionable as to whether a postcontrast sequence is needed. In the adult, on the other hand, a postcontrast sequence in both axial and coronal projections should be made to rule out a vascular process that might not be seen without contrast. A neoplasm is likely to show up in the T2-weighted sequences, and contrast would be used to characterize the lesion.

TUMOR

If the patient is suspected of harboring a tumor, routine series plus contrast is performed.

POSTTRAUMATIC CONDITIONS

In the acute stage CT is usually done. In the subacute or chronic stage, routine MRI plus GRE susceptibility study is done to analyze the presence of blood products in the brain. Also extracerebral collections show up better on MRI.

STROKE

CT is usually done first to rule out acute hemorrhage and also because, more often than not, the patient is somewhat uncooperative. Subsequently, in the acute or subacute stage, MR routine imaging is usually carried out. If a hemorrhagic infarction (recent or old) is suspected a GRE susceptibility study is useful.

A magnetic resonance angiogram may be performed, visualizing both the cervical portion and the intracranial portion of the carotid and vertebrobasilar arterial systems. Additional imaging sequences might include GRE flow imaging sequence (for further details see Chapter 10). If the CT carried out in the acute stage is negative, MR examination should be done next because MRI is more likely than CT to show early ischemic findings.

Contrast examination in hemorrhagic or ischemic lesions is not usually carried out except in special circumstances.

INFLAMMATORY CONDITIONS

Routine imaging plus postcontrast examination should be performed. This would be required if the suspected diagnosis is meningitis, abscess, or some other inflammatory process. A contrast study is nearly always indicated in an inflammatory condition, for both the enhancement and the lack of enhancement of a lesion have important differential diagnostic implications.

Contrast Media in Brain MRI

In the CNS, the contrast media remain in the intravascular space because of the presence of the blood-brain barrier, resulting from the tight junction between the endothelial cells of the walls of the brain capillaries, which does not allow the passage of any relatively large molecule through the intercellular space. Thus, it is necessary to have a breakdown of the blood-brain barrier to observe passage of contrast outside the vessels.

To be sure, in the brain, it is possible to detect the rapid passage of an intravascular MR contrast agent such as gadolinium-DTPA without extravasation, but this effect is very rapid (3 to 6 sec), and the effects require special instrumentation to be observed. It is a very rapid imaging, and instead of enhancement, what is seen is a susceptibility effect (a decrease in intensity) (43). Yousem et al. reported seven cases in which there was a decrease in intensity compared with the initial T1-weighted images in patients with lesions suspected of being associated with blood-brain barrier breakdown (44). All lesions were hyperintense on short TR–short TE images, and in four cases the lesions were T2-dark. The explanation for this paradoxical result is not known at this point; possibly the T2 shortening effect was too strong and affected the T1 response. Four of the lesions were hemorrhagic, and one was melanoma.

When there is a defect in the blood-brain barrier, such as may exist in the presence of a neoplasm, an inflammatory process, a posttraumatic condition, or a cerebral infarction, the contrast enters the intercellular space, where it produces changes in proton relaxation. Gadolinium-based compounds induce a shortening of the T1 relaxation time, which increases the signal intensity of the tissues. There is also a T2 relaxation effect, but this is minor and does not really affect the imaging characteristics. That is, T2-weighted images can be taken after gadolinium administration, and usually no significant changes in the images are observed. Nevertheless, it is preferable to carry out the routine imaging sequences prior to doing the postcontrast sequences.

In general, a dose of 0.1 mmol of gadolinium-DTPA per kilogram of body weight is employed; greater enhancement could possibly be obtained with up to twice this dose. However, the enhancement of pathologic processes appears to be sufficient for diagnostic purposes with the lower dose, and, in accordance with the principle of using the lowest dose that produces the desired effect, there is no reason to go higher. If it is feared that a lesion is being missed because of insufficient dose, the use of a higher dose would be justified and can be accomplished by injecting a second dose of contrast (45).

The effect of gadolinium begins within a few minutes following injection and reaches a peak in about 15 to 25 min, after which it decreases. Thus, imaging should be carried out starting soon after the injection is completed to allow for axial as well as coronal and sagittal views if the latter are considered desirable. Although the peak concentration in the tumor decreases after 30 to 35 min, there is still sufficient contrast so that enhanced imaging can be done if necessary. In the necrotic portion of a tumor, the concentration of gadolinium is low in the early period and increases with time so that at 45 to 60 min, the concentration is higher (46).

Gadolinium-DTPA is excreted by tubular filtration through the kidneys, and in 3 h over 90 percent has been eliminated. In terms of its biodistribution, it is quite similar to that of iodide contrast media. It is first intravascular, and, fairly rapidly, it begins to leave the vascular space and to enter the interstitial (extravascular) space in tissue outside the CNS.

It is worth mentioning here that Jinkins et al. reported that the administration of iodide contrast media immediately before an MRI examination may cause reduced T1 and T2 relaxation times (47). It is recommended that MR examinations not be performed shortly after myelography or intravenous pyelography or after a contrast-enhanced CT examination.

Gadolinium-DTPA has been a safe contrast medium, with a low incidence of complications. Niendorf and Ezumi reported no deaths in 7000 examinations (48). Minor reactions (headaches, urticaria) occur in less than 1 percent of patients. Extravasation at the time of injection can be painful. Gadolinium-DTPA is a hypertonic agent, and rapid injection should be avoided to prevent nausea and vomiting, which may occur in some patients. It is contraindicated in hemolytic anemias and in pregnancy. In young children Gd-DTPA has been used sparingly. We have not seen any untoward reactions when it has been used in children at the Massachusetts General Hospital.

When contrast is used, it is the protocol at the Massachusetts General Hospital to take precontrast sagittal T1-weighted images, first and second echo T2-weighted images, and T1-weighted axial images and then to give contrast using a relatively slow injection (0.1 mm/kg body weight). Imaging is started shortly after injection is completed. Postcontrast axial T1-weighted images are taken, followed by coronal T1-weighted images. Other views, such as sagittal postcontrast, are made if indicated. In studying the pituitary gland, magnified coronal and sagittal images before and after contrast limited to the perisellar area are made, usually fat suppressed if the patient has had prior surgery in which the surgeon may have left a fat plug. It might be worth commenting that the usual SE images, preferably fat suppressed, are satisfactory in the usual case and modifications are rarely discussed. Mihara et al. compared SE with STIR (short T1 inversion recovery) and found that when the signal intensity of a lesion is 80 percent of adjacent fatty tissue, STIR images provide better delineation of the lesion (49). This might be useful in some head and neck lesions.

Some brain structures (the pineal gland, the pituitary stalk, the area postrema, the dura mater) have no blood-brain barrier and thus are seen as enhanced areas, points, or lines on all postcontrast T1-weighted images.

Other compounds of gadolinium will be marketed as contrast agents for MRI, and other metals are being investigated for the same purpose. The future may see special contrast agents that are more specific for certain anatomic locations and for certain disease processes, but this may well apply to MRI of other organs more than to the central nervous system.

For instance, much work has been done to develop and clinically assess iron compounds (50). Compounds such as superparamagnetic iron oxide, sometimes covered with dextran, are made up of tiny particles that are fixed by the reticuloendothelial system of the body, such as the liver, spleen, bone marrow, and lymph nodes. The iron particles generate a susceptibility effect. Again, the compound remains within the brain vascular system and could generate a low signal as it passes through the brain, lasting 15 to 20 sec. Much finer iron particle compounds can be produced in which the contrast remains in the bloodstream for a considerably longer period before being picked up by the reticuloendothelial system (51,52). Other metals such as manganese and dysprosium are also being investigated.

Risks of MRI of the Brain and Spine

Except for risks associated with metal objects within the patient or on the patient, there are no real risks attributable to the examination itself. Many studies have been carried out that indicated minor elevations of skin temperature or of deeper tissue temperature, but these have been classified as either inconsequential or not statistically significant.

Claustrophobia continues to be a problem in some patients. In these patients it is necessary to use CT instead, or, if the MRI is necessary, sedation is helpful; sometimes heavy sedation is needed. Unfortunately, simple sleep may not be sufficient, for the loud noise within the unit during imaging wakes up the patient. Good earplugs are useful and should be used routinely.

Aneurysm clips have been considered a contraindication to MRI brain examinations. Clips over the meninges, dura, and so forth are not a contraindication. Metallic components with shunt valves produce artifacts but are not a contraindication. We have observed a burn over an electrocardiogram lead in one patient. This was unusual, for these are often used for gating purposes to decrease the effect of cardiac pulsations, which create artifacts. A burn has been reported associated with the use of a pulse oximeter (53).

Metallic residues from bullets or shrapnel in the head are considered a contraindication; also, they will probably produce severe artifacts. It is important to obtain a complete history about metallic foreign bodies before an MRI examination; if any suspicion exists, a lateral and frontal skull x-ray examination is recommended. Orbital foreign bodies are particularly important. One case of blindness, produced by a ferromagnetic foreign body in the orbit, has been reported (54).

Implanted pacemakers are a contraindication. Large prosthesis in hips and extremities are not considered a contraindication for MRI examinations, but they may produce artifacts.

REFERENCES

1. Hounsfield G: Computerized transverse axial scanning (tomography). Part I. Description of system. Br J Radiol 1973;46:1016–1022.
2. Carroll FE, Waters JW, Price RR, et al: Near-monochromatic x-ray beams produced by the free electron laser and Compton backscatter. Invest Radiol 1990;25:465–471.
3. Aoki S, Sasaki Y, Machida T, et al: Cerebral aneurysms: Detection and delineation using 3-D-CT angiography. AJNR 1992;13: 1115–1120.
4. El Gammal T, Adams RJ, King DW, et al: Techniques in the evaluation of temporal lobe epilepsy prior to lobectomy. AJNR 1987;8: 131–134.
5. Glenn WV, Rhodes ML, Altschuler EM, et al: Multiplanar display of computerized body tomography. Applications in lumbar spine. Spine 1979;4(4):282–352.
6. Altman M, Harwood-Nash D, Fitz CR, et al: Evaluation of infant spine by direct sagittal computed tomography. AJNR 1985;6:65–69.
7. Osborn AG, Anderson RE: Direct sagittal computed tomographic scans of the face and paranasal sinuses. Radiology 1978;129:81–87.
8. Bluemn P: Direct sagittal (positional) computed tomography of the head. Neuroradiology 1982;22:199–201.
9. Trefler M, Haughton VM: Patient dose and image quality in computed tomography. AJR 1981;137:25–27.
10. Ambrose J. Computerized transverse axial scanning (tomography). Part 2. Clinical applications. Br J Radiol 1973;46:1023–1047.
11. Levy JM, Hupke R: Composite addition technique: A new method in CT scanning of the posterior fossa. AJNR 1991;12:686–688.
12. Vallebona A: Una modalità di tecnica perla dissociazione radiografica delle ombre applicata allo studio del cranio. Radiol Med 1930; 17:1090.
13. Purcell EM, Torrey HC, Pound RF: Resonance absorption by nuclear magnetic moments in a solid. Physiol Rev 1946;69:37–38.
14. Bloch F: Nuclear induction. Physiol Rev 1946;70:460–473.
15. Lauterbur P: Image formation by induced local interactions: Examples employing nuclear magnetic resonance. Nature 1973;242: 190–191.
16. Hinshaw WS, Bottomley PA, Holland GN: Radiographic thin-sectioned image of the human wrist by nuclear magnetic resonance. Nature 1977;270:722–723.
17. Drayer B, Burger P, Darwin R, et al: Magnetic resonance imaging of brain iron. AJNR 1986;7:373–380.
18. Norfray JF, Rosen B, Taveras JM: Newer pulse sequences in magnetic resonance imaging: Their uses and acronyms. In JM Taveras, JT Ferrucci (eds), Radiology: Diagnosis, Imaging, Intervention. Vol. 3. Philadelphia: Lippincott, 1994.
19. Elster AD: Gradient-echo MR imaging: Techniques and acronyms. Radiology 1993;186:1–8.
20. Wehrli FW: Fast Scan Magnetic Resonance: Principles and Applications. New York: Raven, 1991, pp 1–138.
21. Bradley WG, Walluch V: Blood flow: Magnetic resonance imaging. Radiology 1985;154:443–450.
22. Mosely ME, Kucharczyk J, Mintoravitch J, et al: Diffusion-weighted MR imaging of acute stroke: Correlation with T2-weighted and magnetic susceptibility-enhanced MR imaging in cats. AJNR 1990; 11:423–429.
23. Sevick RJ, Kanda F, Mintorovitch J, et al: Cytotoxic brain edema: Assessment with diffusion-weighted MR imaging. Radiology 1992; 185:687–690.
24. Doran M, Hajnal JV, von Bruggen N, et al: Normal and abnormal white matter tracts shown by MR imaging using directional diffusion weighted sequences. J Comput Assist Tomogr 1990;14:865–873.
25. Le Bihan D, Breton E, Lallemand D, et al: Separation of diffusion and perfusion in intravoxel incoherent motion (IVIM) MR imaging. Radiology 1988;168:497–505.
26. Le Bihan D, Turner R: Diffusion and perfusion. In DD Starle and WG Bradley (eds), Magnetic Resonance Imaging, ed 2. St. Louis: Mosby, 1992.
27. Brunberg JA, Chenevert TL, Ross DA, et al: In vivo MR determination of water diffusion coefficients and diffusion correlation with alteration in astrocytomas of the cerebral hemispheres already tested. Presented at the annual meeting of the American Society of Neuroradiology, Vancouver, 1993.
28. Yousem DM, Jarvik J, Tae Sub Chung: Magnetization transfer imaging sinonasal secretions and tumors. Presented at the annual meeting of the American Society of Neuroradiology, Vancouver, 1993.
29. Mehta RC, Pike GB, Enzman DR, et al: Gadolinium enhanced MR (magnetization transfer) MR imaging: Improved detection of CNS tumors, infections and infarctions. Presented at the annual meeting of the American Society of Neuroradiology, Vancouver, 1993.
30. Yousem DM, Weinstein G, Hayden R, et al: Magnetization transfer imaging of the head and neck cancers. Presented at the annual meeting of the American Society of Neuroradiology, Vancouver, 1993.
31. Nguyen HD, Yuh WTC, Fisher DJ, et al: Comparative effect of MTC and gadolinium dosage on lesion contrast. Presented at the annual meeting of the American Society of Neuroradiology, Vancouver, 1993.
32. Wong KT, Grossman RI, Boorstein JM, et al: Magnetization transfer imaging of periventricular hyperintense white matter in the elderly. AJNR 1995;16:253–258.
33. Pacini R, Simon J, Ketomen L, et al: Chemical-shift-imaging of a spontaneous internal carotid artery dissection: Case report. AJNR 1991;12:360–362.
34. Czervionke LF, Czervionke JM, Daniels DL, Haughton VM: Characteristic features of MR truncation artifacts. AJNR 1988;9: 815–824.
35. Daniels DL, Czervionke LF, Breger RK, et al: "Truncation" artifact in MR images of the internal auditory canal. AJNR 1987;8:793–794.
36. Tien RD, Hesselink JR, Chu PK, et al: Informed detection and delineation of head and neck lesions with fat suppression skin-echo MR imaging. AJNR 1991;12:19–24.
37. Anzai Y, Lufkin RB, Jabour BA, Hanafee WN: Fat-suppression failure artifacts simulating pathology on frequency-selective fat-suppression. MR images of the head and neck. AJNR 1992;13: 879–884.
38. Ahn SS, Mantello MT, Jones KM, et al: Rapid MR imaging of the pediatric brain using the fast spin-echo technique. AJNR 1992;13: 1169–1177.
39. Jolesz FA, Jones KM: Fast spin echo imaging of the brain. Magn Reson Imaging 1993;5:1–13.
40. Sze G, Merriam M, Oshio K, et al: Fast spin-echo imaging in the evaluation of intradural disease of the spine. AJNR 1992;13:1383.
41. Sze G, Kawamuray, Negishi C, et al: Fast spin-echo MR imaging of the cervical spine: Influence of echo train length and echo spacing on image contrast and quality. AJNR 1993;14:1203–1213.
42. Norbash AM, Glover GH, Enzman DR: Intracerebral lesion contrast with spin-echo and fast spin-echo pulse sequences. Radiology 1992;185:661–665.
43. Rosen BR, Belliveau JW, Vevea JM, Brady TJ: Perfusion imaging with NMR contrast agents. Magn Reson Med 1990;14:249–265.
44. Yousem DM, Ihmeidan I, Quencer RI, et al: Paradoxically decreased signal intensity of postcontrast short-TR MR images. AJNR 1991; 12:875–880.
45. Yuh WTC, Engelken JD, Muhonen MG, et al: Experience with high-dose gadolinium MR imaging in the evaluation of brain metastases. AJNR 1992;13:335–345.
46. Laniado M, Clausen C, Weinman HJ, Schörner W: Paramagnetic contrast media in magnetic resonance imaging of the brain. In JM Taveras and JT Ferrucci (eds), Radiology: Diagnosis, Imaging, Intervention, Vol. 3, Chapter 59. Philadelphia: Lippincott, 1989.

47. Jinkins JR, Robinson JW, Sisk L, et al: Proton relaxation enhancement associated with iodinated contrast agents in MR imaging of the CNS. AJNR 1992;13:19–27.
48. Niendorf HP, Ezumi K: Magnevist (Gd DTPA): Tolerance and safety after four years of clinical trials in more than 7000 patients. In Abstracts of the 2nd European Congress of NMR in Medicine and Biology, Berlin, 1988.
49. Mihara F, Gupta, KL: Gd-DTPA-enhanced short repetition time and short inversion time inversion recovery magnetic resonance imaging: Experimental and clinical assessment. Invest Radiol 1991;26: 734–741.
50. Saini S, Stark DD, Hahn PF, et al: Ferrite particles: A superparamagnetic MR contrast agent for the reticuloendothelial system. Radiology 1987;162:217–222.
51. Raynaud M, Chambon C, Caille JM: MR perfusion imaging using AM1227 as a contrast agent in rabbit brain with a cold induced edema. Presented at the annual meeting of the American Society of Neuroradiology, Vancouver, 1993.
52. Weissleder R, Elizondo G, Wittenberg J, et al: Ultrasmall superparamagnetic iron oxide: Characterization of a new class of contrast agents for MR imaging. Radiology 1990;175:489.
53. Shellock FG, Slimp G: Severe burn of the finger caused by using a pulse oximeter during MRI. AJR 1989;153:1105.
54. Kelly WM, Paglen PG, Pearson JA, et al: Ferromagnetism of intraocular foreign body causes unilateral blindness after MR study. AJNR 1986;7:243–245.

SUGGESTED READINGS

Berns D, Blaser S, Ross JS, et al: MR imaging with Gd-DTPA in leptomeningeal spread of lymphoma. J Comput Assist Tomogr 1988;12:499.

Gallen CC, Sobel DF, Lewine JD, et al: Neuromagnetic mapping of brain function. Radiology 1993;187:863–867.

Goldstein HA, Kashanian FK, Blumetti RF, et al: Safety assessment of gadopentetate dimeglumine in United States clinical trials. Radiology 1990;174:17–23.

Harada K, Fujita N, Sakurais, et al: Diffusion imaging of the human brain: A new pulse sequence application for a 1.5-T standard MR system. AJNR 1991;12:1143–1148.

Kieffer SA: Gadopentetate dimeglumine: Reassessment of the clinical research process. AJNR 1990;11:1168–1169.

Klucznik RP, Carrier DA, Pyka R, Haid RW: Placement of a ferromagnetic intracerebral aneurysm clip in a magnetic field with a fatal outcome. Radiology 1993;187:855–856.

Le Bihan D, Turner R, Doucek B, et al: Diffusion MR imaging: Clinical application. AJR 1992;159:591–599.

Lenz GW, Haacke EM, Masaryk TJ, et al: In-plane vascular imaging: Pulse sequence design and strategy. Radiology 1988;166:875–882.

Lufkin RB, Pusey E, Start DD, et al: Boundary artifact due to truncation errors in MR imaging. AJR 1986;147:1283–1287.

McCullough EC, Payne JT, Baker HL: Performance evolution and quality assurance of computed tomography scanners with illustrations from the EMI, beta and delta scanners. Radiology 1976;120:173–188.

New PFJ, Aronaw S: Attenuation measurements of whole blood fractions in computed tomography. Radiology 1976;121:635.

Njuyen HD, Yuh WTC, Fisher DJ, et al: Comparative effect of MTC and gadolinium dosage on lesion contrast. Presented at the annual meeting of the American Society of Neuroradiology, Vancouver, 1993.

Tien RD, Mac Fall JM, Heinz R: Evaluation of complex cystic masses of the brain: Value of steady-state-free-precession MR imaging. AJR 1992; 159:1049–1055.

Tishler S, Hoffman JC: Anaphylactoid reaction to IV gadopentetate dimeglumine treated with benadryl, epinephrin, and cortisone. AJNR 1990;11:1167.

3

Anatomy

A careful study of brain anatomy has always been very important in neuroradiology. In the past, however, the only aspects of this anatomy that could be seen in vivo were the ventricular system, the subarachnoid space, and the subarachnoid cisterns; that is, the area that became visible on the brain surface and on the surface of the lateral ventricles as well as on the third and fourth ventricles through the injection of air. In addition, a detailed study of the anatomy of the arterial and venous systems of the brain was most important for the interpretation of cerebral angiograms.

The introduction of computed tomography (CT) and magnetic resonance imaging (MRI) has added another requirement to the study of anatomy in neuroradiology: the identification of actual structures of the brain—the gray and white matter, the basal ganglia, and the brainstem and its pathways—as well as the degree of myelination. Even ultrasound has reached such a degree of resolution that one needs a good knowledge of structural brain anatomy to interpret ultrasound cross-sectional images in the infant.

BRAIN DEVELOPMENT

After the neural tube closes, the brain develops from the expanded anterior part. Within days, this anterior part of the closed neural tube develops into three expanded areas, usually termed the *forebrain* (prosencephalon), the *midbrain* (mesencephalon), and the *hindbrain* (rhombencephalon). These areas are already well developed at the fourth and fifth weeks after gestation (Fig. 3.1).

The forebrain develops into two important portions: the diencephalon, which generates the thalamus, hypothalamus, and globus pallidus, and the telencephalon. The telencephalon will generate the cerebral hemispheres, the caudate nucleus, and the putamen, as well as the rhinencephalon. The rhinencephalon is the "oldest" part of the telencephalon in evolutionary terms; it is highly developed in animals but is much less so in man (Fig. 3.2). It comprises the olfactory lobe, the anterior perforated substance, the septum pellucidum, the subcallosal, supracallosal, and dentate gyri, the fornix, the hippocampus, and the uncus. This formation constitutes mostly what is termed the *limbic system*, which has acquired more importance in the last decades as its functions have become better understood. The limbic system also includes the cingulate gyri.

Cells that will later form the various components of the diencephalon arise from the germinal matrix in the wall of the third ventricle (which has not yet formed). Cells that will later compose the telencephalon, which represents the most bulky portion of the brain, arise from the germinal matrix in the walls of the lateral ventricles.

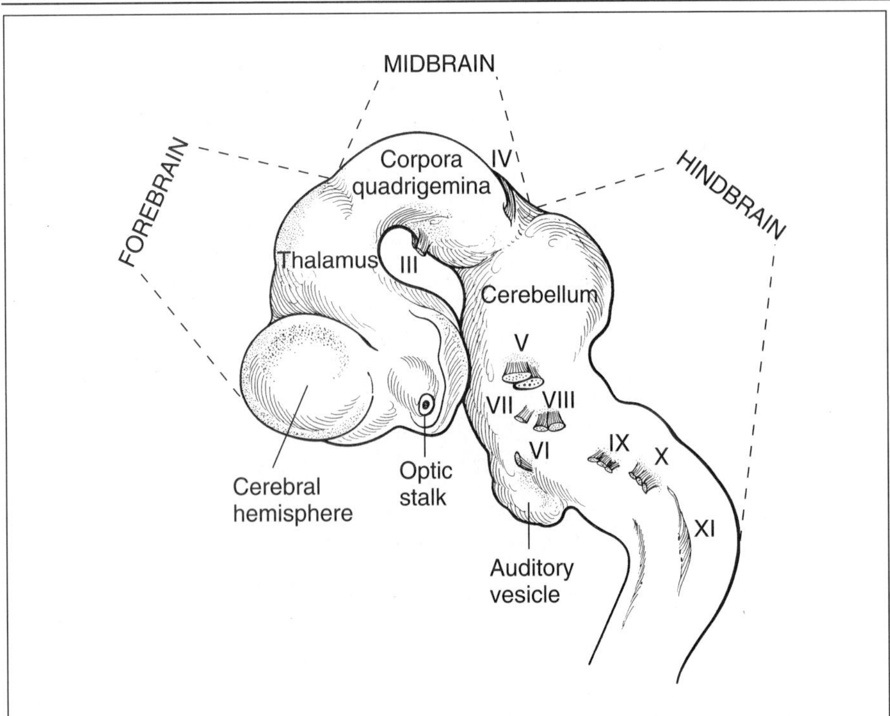

Figure 3.1. Brain of human embryo at 4½ weeks according to His.

The midbrain (mesencephalon) forms the cerebral peduncles and the quadrigeminal plate. The hindbrain (rhombencephalon) gives origin to the pons and cerebellum (metencephalon) as well as the medulla oblongata (myelencephalon).

As the cerebral hemispheres grow and expand, they form primitive fissures that are visible by the fourth month. The most prominent of these is the sylvian fissure. Initially the insular surface is almost totally flat, but with the passage of time the depression of the insular surface becomes deeper and deeper as the orbital, frontal, parietal, and temporal opercula develop (Fig. 3.3). The sylvian fissure is not completely developed until near the end of the first year after birth. The orbital and frontal opercula are the last to develop.

At about 2½ months, fibers from both hemispheres begin to grow into the midline in the region of the primi-

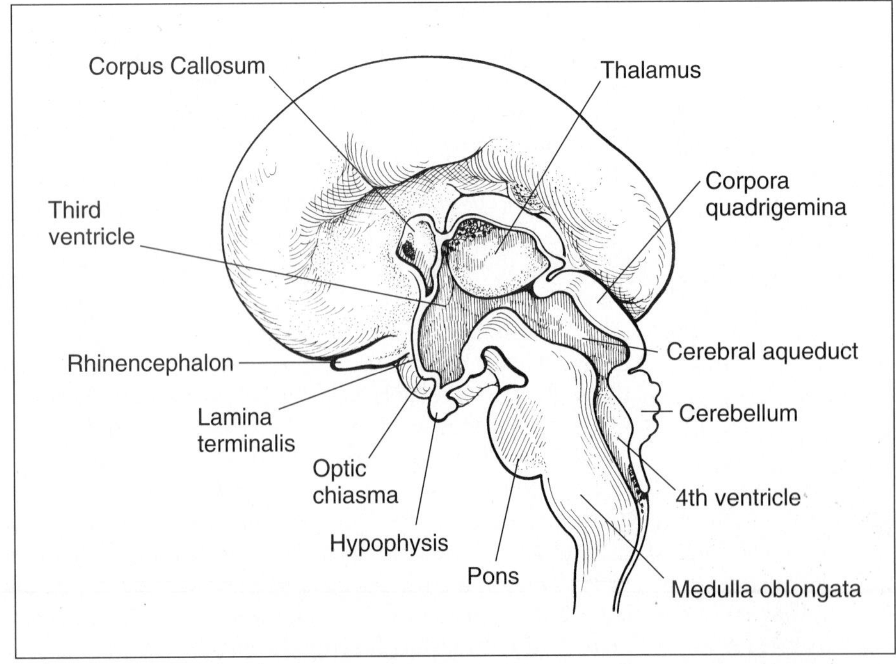

Figure 3.2. Median sagittal section of human embryo at 4 months.

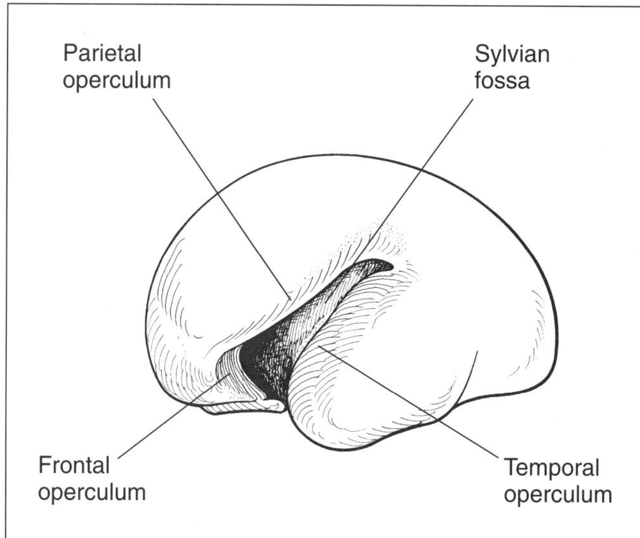

Figure 3.3. Lateral surface of human embryo at about 5 months showing the gaping sylvian fissure and the absence of gyri and sulci.

tive lamina terminalis, which will later differentiate into the three main commissures: the anterior commissure, the hippocampal commissure (fornix), and the corpus callosum. The corpus callosum itself develops progressively from the anterior aspect, the genu, to the splenium (that is, from front to back). But the rostrum of the corpus callosum, which is anterior and below the genu, ending down into the permanent lamina terminalis, develops after the splenium. Anomalies of the corpus callosum would normally follow the sequence of embryologic development, which is further explained under congenital anomalies (Chapter 5).

TOPOGRAPHIC ANATOMY OF THE CEREBRAL HEMISPHERES

Lateral Surface

The cerebral hemispheres present two types of furrows on their surfaces. The first type is the fissures, which are rather deep; the second is the sulci, which are less deep. The fissures are fairly constant in their relationships, whereas the sulci show considerable individual variation. The interhemispheric fissure incompletely divides the two hemispheres into right and left; the sylvian or lateral fissure, which is quite deep, divides the frontal and parietal lobes from the temporal lobes. The central fissure (rolandic fissure) is most important and separates the frontal lobe from the parietal lobe. The fissures may produce some indentation on the ventricular surface. For instance, the calcarine fissure, involved with vision, produces the calcar avis on the medial surface of the occipital horn. This indentation can be deep enough to almost cut off the occipital horn and accounts for the frequent asymmetry of the occipital horns. The parieto-occipital fissure separates the precuneus from the cuneus on the medial surface of the posterior aspects of the hemisphere.

On the outer surface of the hemisphere, the shallower sulci separate the various convolutions (Fig. 3.4). There is considerable individual variation in the actual configuration of sulci and gyri. In the frontal lobe, the precentral gyrus is located at the posterior limit, just in front of the central fissure. This important gyrus contains all of the motor area with the body essentially represented upside down (that is, the facial area is at the lower part and the leg is at the top). On the inner surface of the upper margin of the hemisphere is the paracentral lobule (Fig. 3.5). In front of the precentral gyrus are the superior, middle, and inferior frontal gyri. The inferior frontal gyrus in its pars triangularis contains Broca's area, which has to do with the motor mechanisms of speech (1). The inferior aspect of the frontal lobe is shown in Figure 3.6.

The *parietal lobe* on its outer surface presents the postcentral gyrus, which represents the somatosensory, tactile thermal, and kinesthetic areas. Again, the representation is upside down (that is, the lower parts of the gyrus represent the face and adjacent areas, and the leg is in the upper portion of the gyrus going over the upper margin to the medial surface). The inferior parietal lobule contains the supramarginal and angular gyri at the back end of the sylvian fissure. These structures are part of the inferior parietal lobule and are very important in the dominant hemisphere, for they control the individual's ability to read, calculate, identify body parts, and distinguish right from left. The region of the angular gyrus is termed *Wernicke's area*, an area very important in language comprehension.

The *temporal lobe* contains the superior, middle, and inferior temporal gyri. Along its superior margin the superior temporal gyrus is continuous with the gyri in the floor of the posterior aspect of the sylvian fissure. These are three or four in number and are called the *transverse temporal gyri of Heschl*, structures that contain the primary auditory cortical areas on both sides. They are continuous with the sulci on the insula.

The *occipital lobe* comprises the posterior pole of the brain starting at the parieto-occipital fissure and extending inferiorly to the preoccipital notch in the inferior aspect of the temporal lobe. The division here is somewhat arbitrary on the outer surface. The preoccipital notch is difficult to identify in its usual position about 4 cm in front of the occipital pole. The lateral occipital gyri are associated with visual function.

The *insula* is buried inside the sylvian fissure; to see it, the frontoparietal and temporal opercula must be separated. So that it can be visualized fully, the frontoparietal and temporal opercula are customarily resected, as shown in Figure 3.7.

Medial Surface

The most permanent feature in the medial surface is the *corpus callosum*, the important commissure that connects the two hemispheres (Figs. 3.5*A* and 3.11). In the rostral portion of the corpus callusom, located below the genu, is

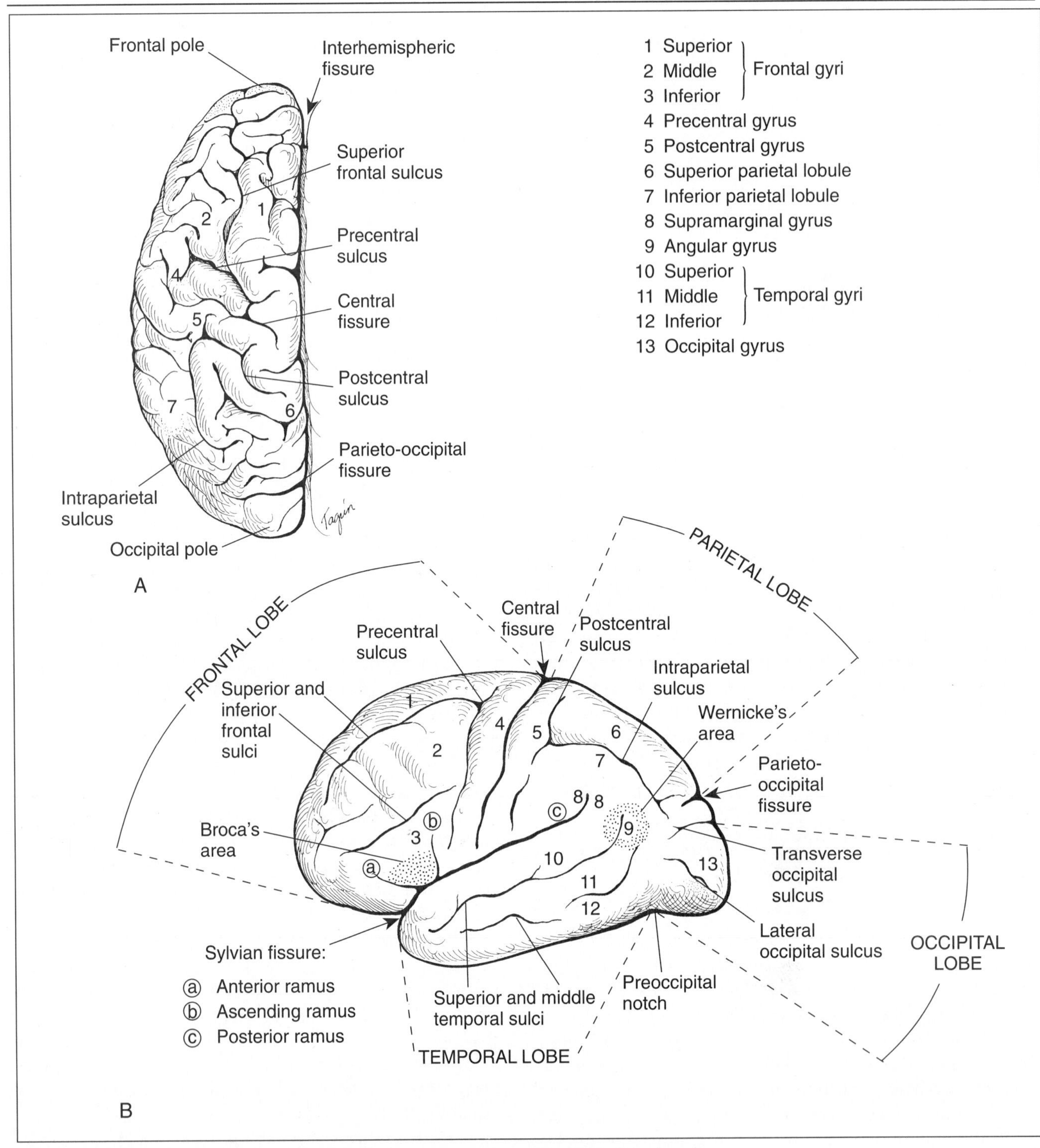

Figure 3.4. Brain surface. **A.** Seen from above. **B.** Seen from the left side. The inferior frontal gyrus (3) contains the pars triangularis, situated between the anterior and the ascending sulci (where Broca's area is situated), and behind the ascending ramus is the pars opercularis. These areas can usually be identified on sagittal MRI (see Fig. 3.46).

the *anterior commissure*, just slightly ventral to the rostrum. This commissure connects certain portions of middle and inferior temporal gyri.

The *fornix* is situated immediately below the corpus callosum in its posterior aspect. First, the columns of the fornix are separated by the commissure of the fornix, and about in the center of the corpus callosum, the two columns of the fornix come together (body of the fornix) but remain separate. They continue forward and swing down toward the anterior commissure, passing anterior to the foramen

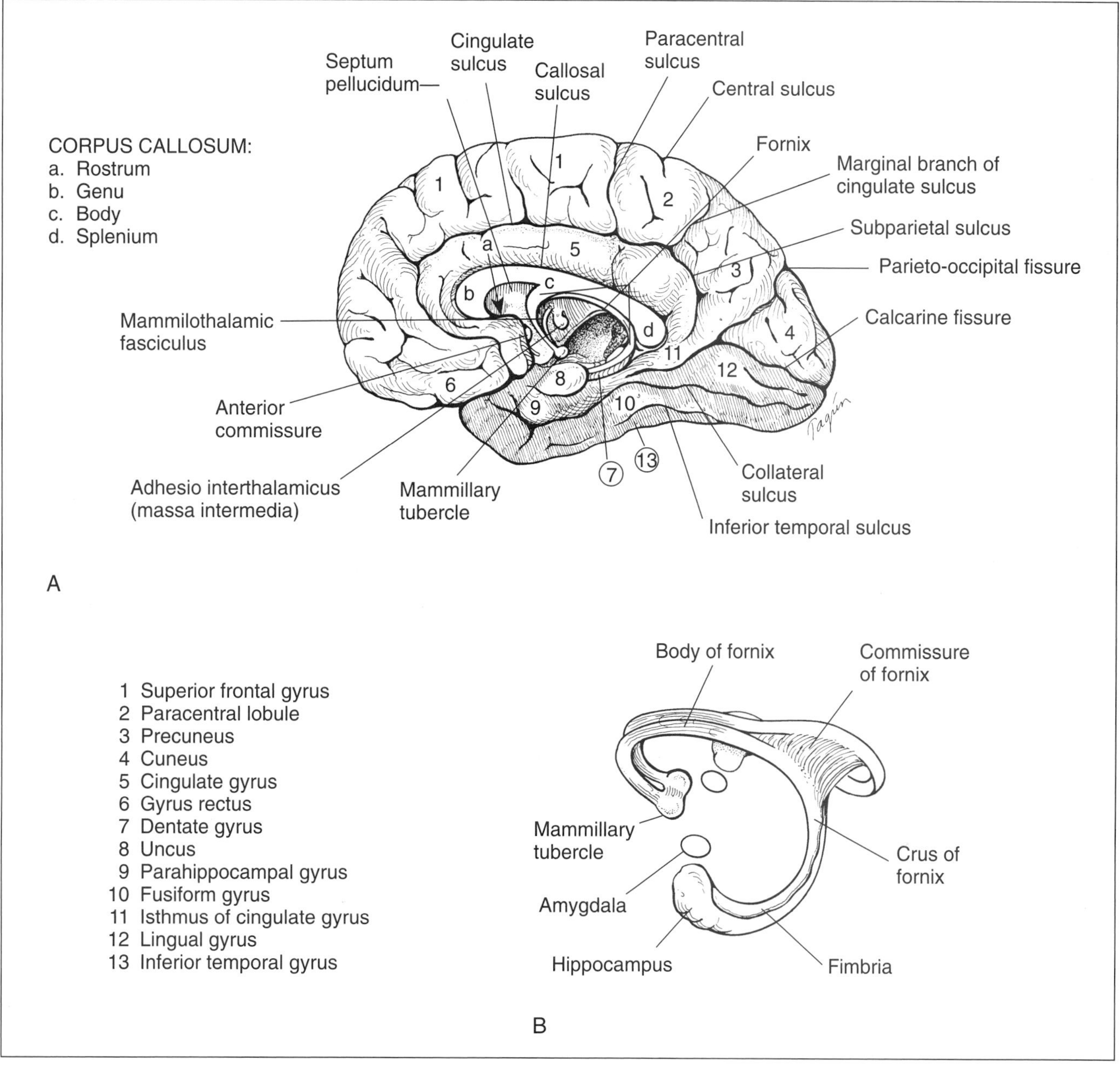

Figure 3.5. A. Medial surface of the brain. **B.** Configuration of the fornix.

of Monro. The two components of the body of the fornix do not join the anterior commissure but pass on each side of the midline slightly posteriorly to continue down before swinging backward to end at the mammillary tubercle on each side of the hypothalamus (Fig. 3.5*B*). Between the fornix and the posterior aspect of the genu and the anterior aspect of the body of the corpus callosum is the *septum pellucidum* (Figs. 3.5*A* and 3.11). Posteriorly, the fornix swings downward and forward following the medial aspect of the temporal horn parallel to the hippocampal formation, where it is called the *fimbria*, and ends near the anterior end of the hippocampus in the region of the uncus (Fig. 3.5*B*).

Above the corpus callosum is the callosal sulcus, and immediately above this sulcus is the *cingulate gyrus*, which in its posterior aspect swings upward and circumscribes the *paracentral lobule* posteriorly. However, the cingulate gyrus is felt to pass behind the splenium of the corpus callosum as shown in Figure 3.5, forming part of the limbic lobe.

The parieto-occipital fissure separates the precuneus from the cuneus, and in turn the cuneus is separated from the lingual gyrus by the calcarine fissure. The slanted medial-inferior aspect of the temporal lobe is seen on the medial surface, and one can see the uncus of the hippocampus, the parahippocampal gyrus, and the fusiform gyrus. The posterior aspect of the cingulate gyrus swings down behind

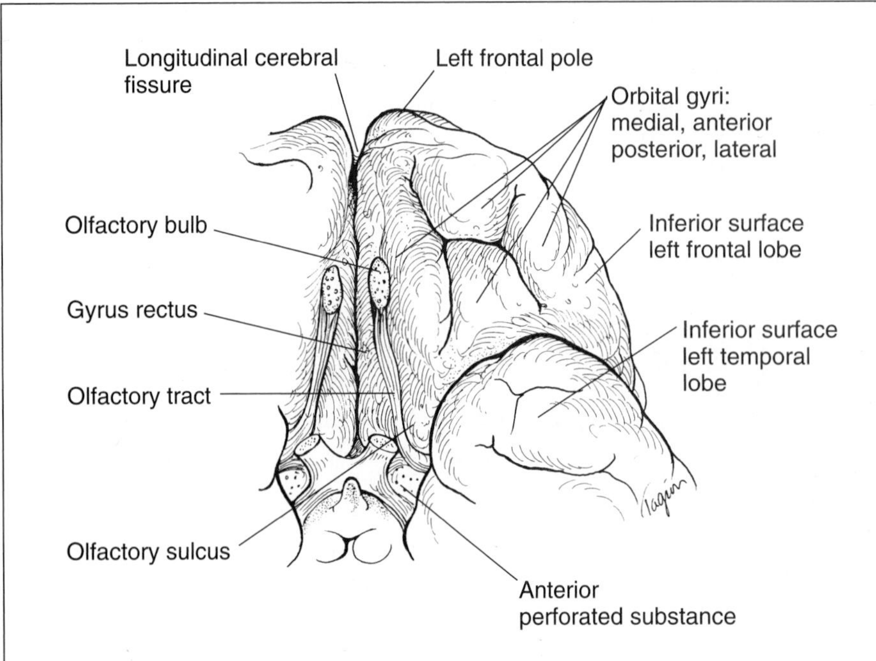

Figure 3.6. Inferior surface of brain, anterior aspect.

the corpus callosum, forming the portion called the *isthmus of the cingulate gyrus* (Fig. 3.5).

Below the fornix is the tela choroidea and the choroid plexus of the third ventricle. Between the fornix and the roof of the third ventricle are the two layers of the velum interpositum, and between its two layers is the cistern of the velum interpositum, which can receive cerebrospinal fluid. In fact, the velum interpositum cistern has a triangular configuration, like the commissure of the fornix, and connects with the subarachnoid space on its wider, dorsal aspect (Figs. 3.5*A* and 3.11). The thalamus forms the wall of the third ventricle and, anteriorly, crossing the third ventricle, is the massa intermedia or interthalamic adhesion (Fig. 3.11).

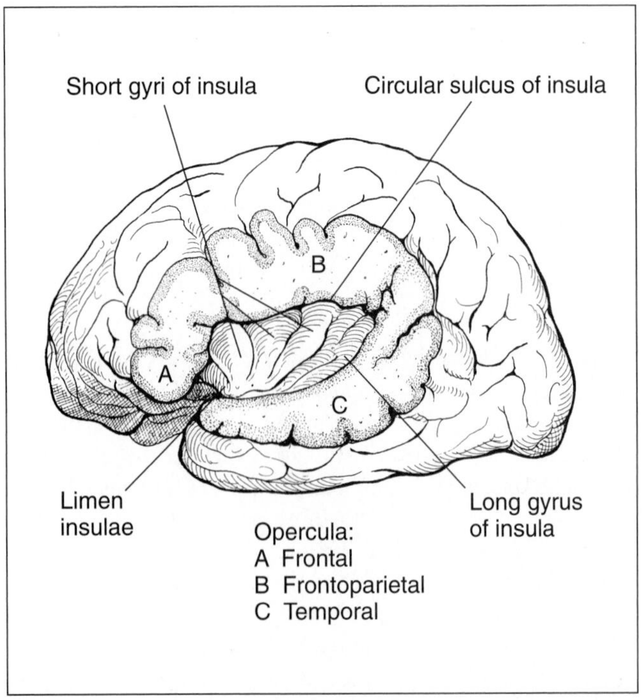

Inferior Surface

The inferior surface is not usually clearly visible on axial or in coronal or sagittal views. Nevertheless, some segments of it can be identified (Fig. 3.6). In coronal sections, the gyrus rectus is visible on each side of the midline, and lateral to it is the olfactory sulcus.

SOME FUNCTIONAL CONSIDERATIONS

The *motor* function of the brain is mainly represented by the cortical spinal tract. The cells are mainly located in the precentral gyrus, and the fibers pass through the centrum semiovale, the corona radiata, and the internal capsule, continuing down to the cerebral peduncle, the basis pontis, and down through the medulla, where they form the paramedian pyramids (Fig. 3.8). The pyramids seem to disappear at about the level just below the foramen magnum where decussation of pyramidal tract takes place. In this area the median sulcus tends to be erased. The pyramidal tracts continue to the various levels of the spinal cord and run on the lateral aspect of the spinal cord just in front of a plane bisecting the spinal cord in the coronal plane.

Figure 3.7. Diagram demonstrating the insula after the frontal, frontoparietal, and temporal opercula are resected.

The centrum semiovale and the corona radiata carry all of the fibers that are formed by the cortical cells and that radiate down to the internal capsule and the brainstem.

In addition to the fibers described as a corona radiata, there are the arcuate fibers or U fibers, which start in a given gyrus and swing again toward the adjacent gyrus, thus acquiring the term *U fibers*. In fact, the motor cortex occupies a broader area than just the precentral gyrus and includes some adjacent postcentral gyrus and the adjacent frontal lobe.

The sensory system is considerably more complex. In addition to the postcentral gyrus, the thalamus is involved in some aspects of pain, touch, and temperature as well as in the sense of movement, weight, and position. The visual pathways follow the optic chiasm, the optic tracts around the cerebral peduncles, to terminate in the lateral geniculate bodies. From there, the geniculate calcarine tract swings around the temporal horn and passes along the lateral aspect of the atrium of the ventricle to terminate in the medial aspect of the occipital lobe at the calcarine fissure. Actually, the fibers that terminate in the superior aspect of the calcarine fissure carry visual impulses from the upper quadrants of the eye, whereas those carrying visual impulses from the lower quadrants terminate in the inferior aspect of the calcarine fissure.

The auditory pathways are even more complex. The auditory cortex is located in the region of the insula and the superior aspect of the temporal lobe bilaterally. Imaging methods are not usually used to try to locate auditory difficulties, except when the auditory nerves are involved.

The *extrapyramidal system* is an old term for a system that complements the pyramidal motor system and which contains motor neurons and pathways related to the basal ganglia. The basal ganglia are composed of the caudate

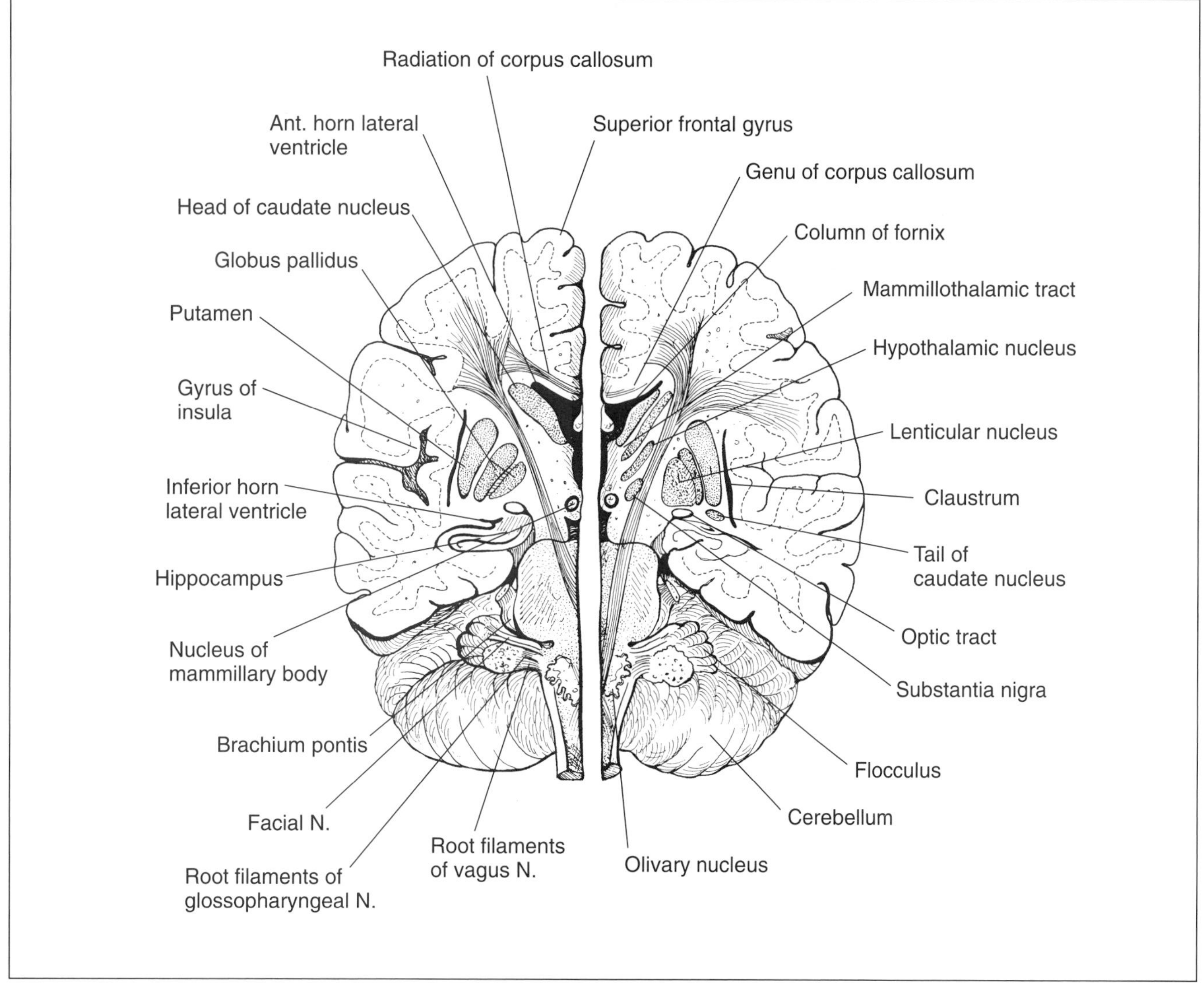

Figure 3.8. Vertical cross section of the brain. The drawing to the right was cut about 1 cm behind the one to the left. The corticospinal tracts are shown in their relationship to the various structures.

nucleus, the putamen, and the globus pallidus, the components of the corpus striatum. However, additional components of what might be called the extrapyramidal system include a number of other gray matter structures and nuclei that are functionally related. These are the subthalamic nucleus, the claustrum, the substantia nigra, the red nucleus, the ventral basal thalamus, and the reticular formation in an area anterolateral to the aqueduct. The aqueduct is surrounded by the periaqueductal gray matter (Fig. 3.19*B*).

DEEP STRUCTURES OF THE BRAIN

Basal Ganglia

The basal ganglia are partially components of the brainstem, but for practical reasons they should be described and illustrated separately (Figs. 3.8 to 3.10). The basal ganglia are composed of the caudate nucleus, putamen, globus pallidus, and amygdaloid nucleus. The putamen, globus pallidus, and caudate nucleus form what is generally termed the *corpus striatum*. Initially, these three gray matter masses develop together, but later they become separated as the fibers of the internal capsule pass between the caudate nucleus on the upper aspect and the putamen and globus pallidus on the lower, lateral aspect. Many thin, gray bridges remain between the caudate nucleus and the putamen and the globus pallidus. The last two together are usually labeled the *lenticular nucleus* because of their shape. The presence of these connections generated the term *corpus striatum*.

The *caudate nucleus* contains the head, which is situated on the lateral and inferior aspect of the frontal horn of the lateral ventricle. The tail, which continues along the lateral aspect of the lateral ventricle, rests on the dorsolateral area of the thalamus, from which it is separated by the stria terminalis and the thalamostriate vein. The tail turns downward behind the thalamus, continues along the ventricular contour on the superior aspect of the temporal horn, and ends in the amygdaloid nucleus (Fig. 3.9).

The *amygdaloid nucleus* is situated above and anterior to the tip of the temporal horn. The nucleus is a complex of gray masses covered by a thick layer of brain cortex medially and continuous with the uncus of the hippocampus.

The *putamen*, the lateral component of the lenticular nucleus, is larger than the globus pallidus. Anteriorly it connects directly with the head of the caudate nucleus. Toward the back the putamen is separated from the caudate nucleus, although still connected with it through the gray bridges previously mentioned. Lateral and anterior to the thalamus (Fig. 3.9) the putamen is separated from the globus pallidus by a thin lateral medullary lamina containing many myelinated fibers going transversely through the globus pallidus (Figs. 3.8 to 3.10).

The *globus pallidus* is medial to the putamen and separated from the thalamus and caudate nucleus by the capsule. The two parts of the globus pallidus, the lateral and the medial portions, are separated by a thin medial medullary lamina. The globus pallidus derives its name from its color, which is lighter than that of the putamen because it contains many myelinated and unmyelinated fibers (Figs. 3.8, 3.10, and 3.13).

The *claustrum* is a thin layer of gray matter situated between the lateral aspect of the putamen and the medial aspect of the insula. The claustrum is separated from the putamen by the external capsule and from the insular surface by the extreme capsule (Figs. 3.8, 3.10, and 3.13).

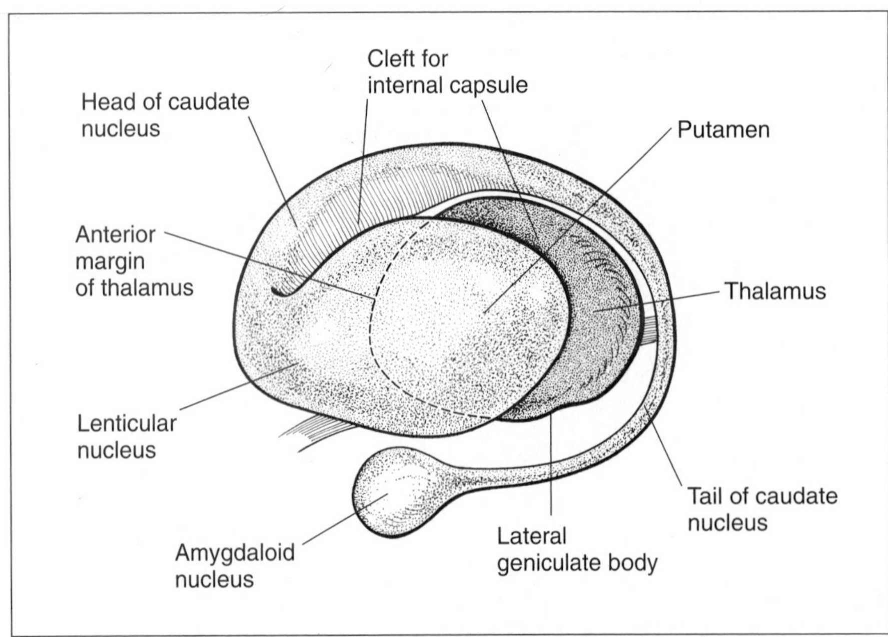

Figure 3.9. Corpus striatum seen from the left side. Note that the putamen portion of the lenticular nucleus merges with the head of the caudate nucleus anteriorly. This can be seen on sagittal and coronal MRI. The anterior limb of the internal capsule passes between the caudate nucleus and lenticular nucleus.

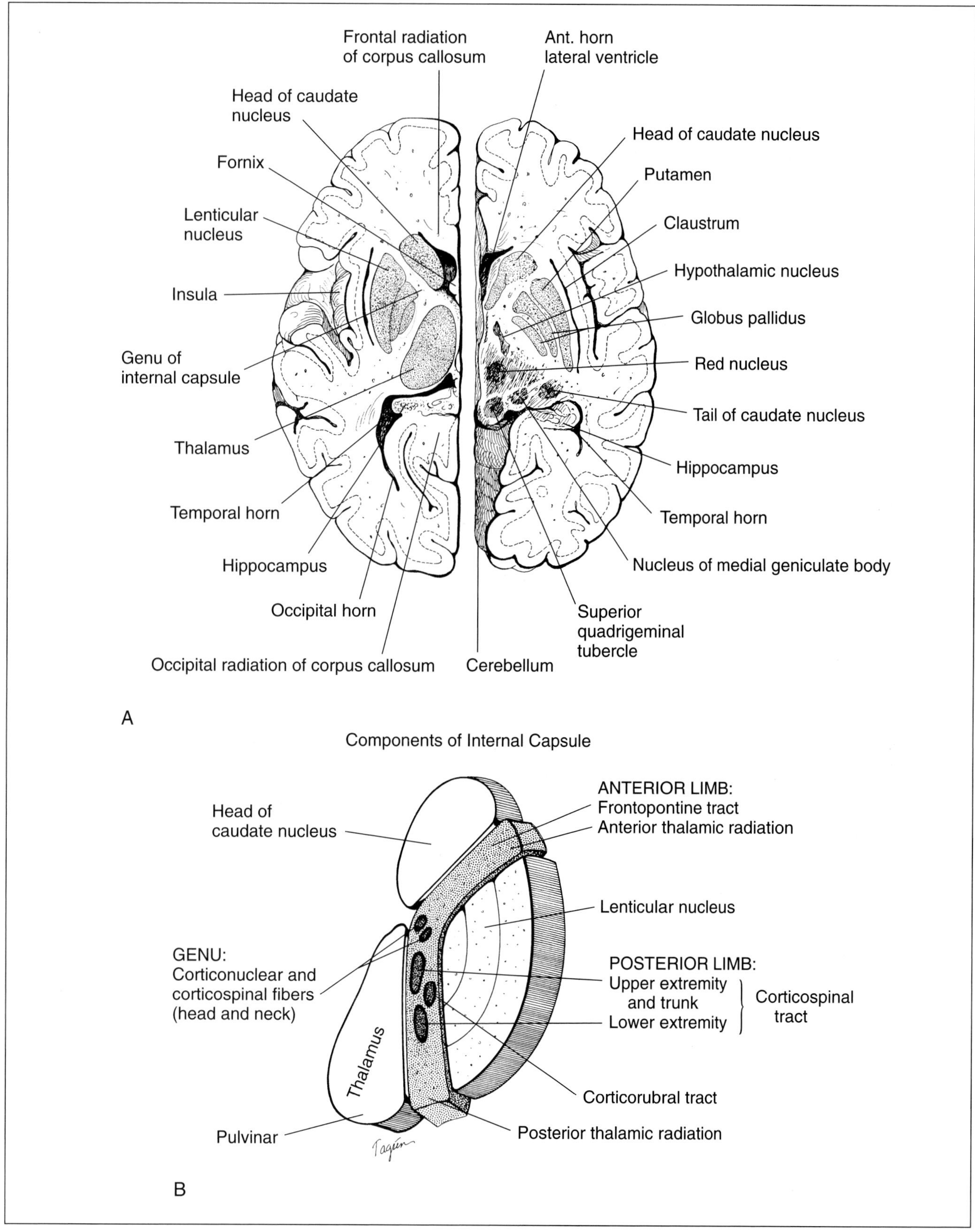

Figure 3.10. A. Horizontal cross section of the brain. The right side of the drawing on the reader's side is about 1 cm caudal to the one on the left. **B.** The internal capsule in cross section as seen on cross-sectional images on CT and MRI.

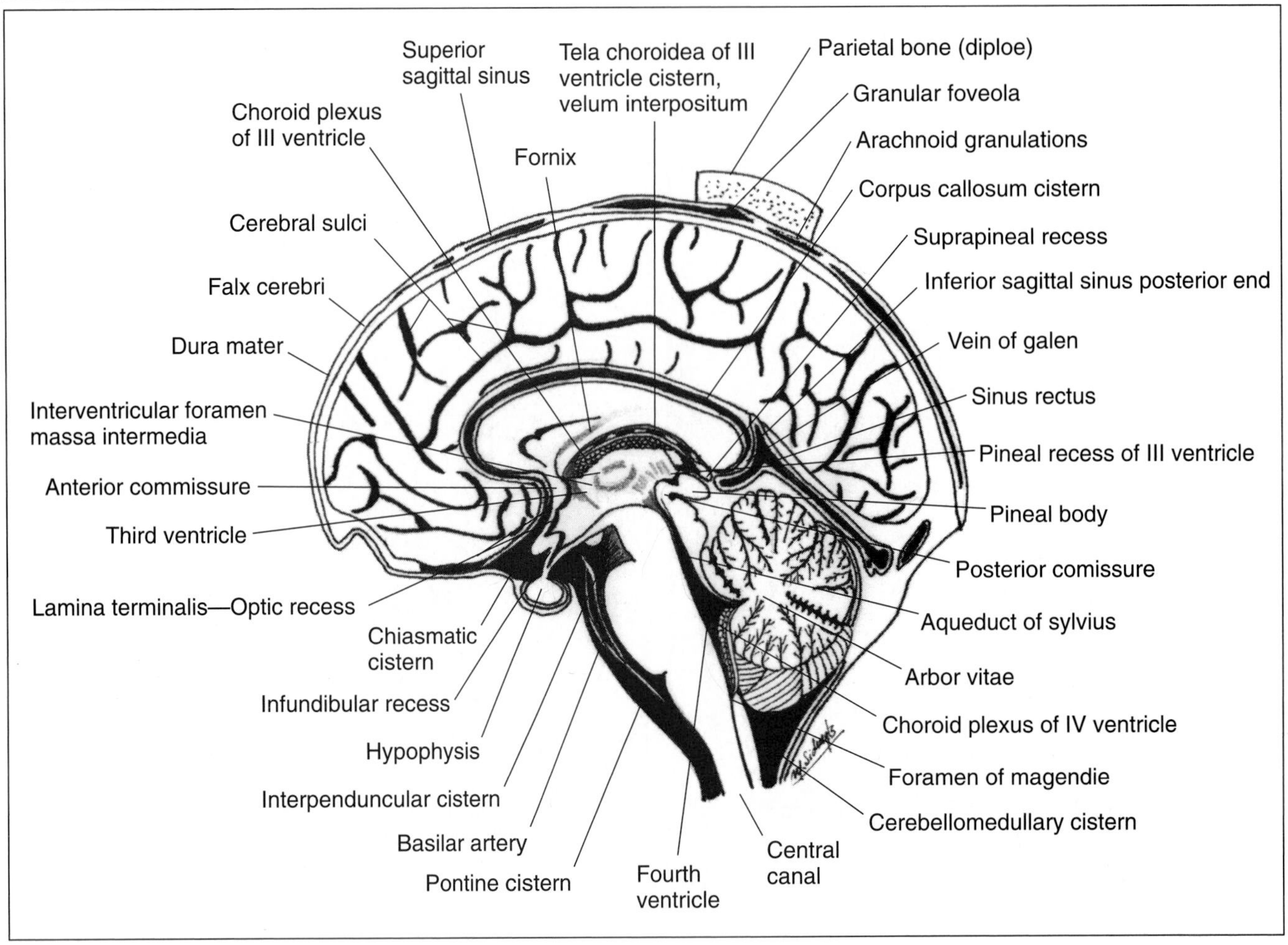

Figure 3.11. Medial surface of hemisphere, including the midline structures, brainstem, and cerebellum.

Limbic System

The concept of the limbic system started with the original description of Broca (1878), who referred to the *grand lobe limbique* (2). The limbic lobe included the subcallosal, cingulate, and parahippocampal gyri and the hippocampus. Today this concept has been expanded, and physiologically the limbic system is presumed to have much to do with emotions. In lower species, the olfactory system is the major part of the limbic lobe or system, but in man the olfactory component is significantly smaller. Today the limbic system comprises the cingulate gyrus, the subcallosal gyrus, the parahippocampal gyrus, the hippocampal formation, the dentate gyrus, the amygdaloid nucleus, the olfactory nerves, and the olfactory nucleus and striae; the olfactory trigone and anterior perforated substance; the septal areas, septum pellucidum, fornix, hypothalamus, medial part of the thalamus, and anterior commissure; and other smaller components.

THALAMUS

The thalamus on each side of the third ventricle is a gray matter mass about 4 cm long that reaches caudally below

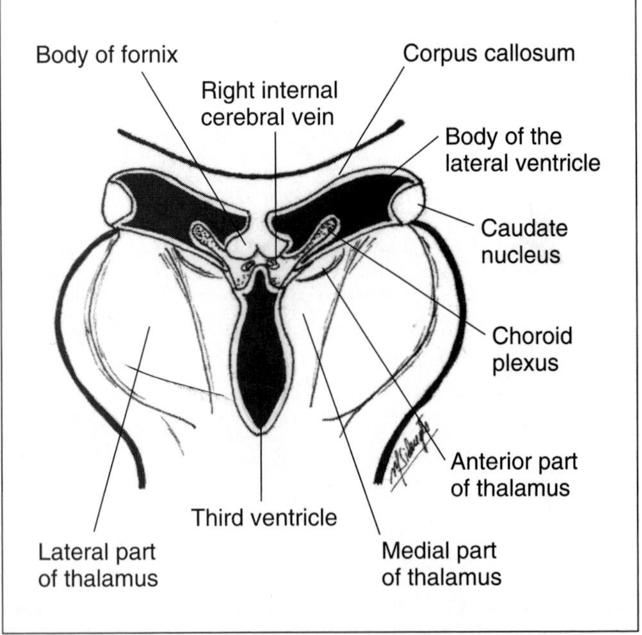

Figure 3.12. Diagram of lateral and third ventricles. Coronal cross section passing through the thalamus.

the third ventricle (Figs. 3.9 to 3.13). *Anteriorly* the thalamus reaches to the posterior aspect of the foramen of Monro and overhangs the quadrigeminal plate. The anterior end is narrow and the *posterior* end, or *pulvinar*, is broader. Immediately below the thalamus is the lateral geniculate body, and medially the inferior surface is separated from the medial geniculate body by the brachium of the superior colliculus.

Superiorly the thalamus is covered by a layer of white matter and is separated from the caudate nucleus, which lies over it, by a white band, the *stria terminalis*, and by the *thalamostriate vein*. The lateral aspect of the superior surface of the thalamus forms a small part of the floor of the lateral ventricle. This portion of the superior surface is covered by the tela choroidea of the third ventricle, which separates the thalamus from the fornix. The tela choroidea invaginates into the medial inferior aspect of the lateral ventricles to form the choroid plexus. The space through which the tela choroidea passes is part of the choroidal fissure, which in this area is located between the lateral aspect of the fornix superiorly and the upper surface of the thalamus inferiorly. The medial surface of the thalamus forms the lateral wall of the third ventricle, and the two thalami are joined by the interthalamic mass, which contains some nerve cells and nerve fibers.

The *medial surface* is limited inferiorly by a curved groove called the *hypothalamic sulcus*, often ill defined, which extends from the upper end of the aqueduct of Sylvius to the lower aspect of the interventricular foramen. The *inferior surface* rests anteriorly on the hypothalamus and more posteriorly on the midbrain.

Although the thalamus is mostly composed of gray matter, the superior and lateral aspects are covered by white matter containing white fiber tracts. Many gray nuclei have been identified within the thalamus, but the function of many of these is not known. The three-dimensional configuration and position of these nuclei are rather complex. No effort is made here to illustrate these structures except in the simplest manner because they are not identified on MRI or CT and are rather complex (see Figs. 3.13*C* and *D* and 3.33*C* and *D*).

The three major subdivisions are the anterior nuclear group, the medial nuclear group, and the lateral nuclear group; the posterior portion of the thalamus is the pulvinar. The three groups are separated by the internal medullary lamina, which has a Y shape (Figs. 3.13*C* and 3.33*C* and *D*). Below the thalamus laterally is the subthalamic nucleus, and below it medially is the red nucleus (Fig. 3.13*C*). Immediately below the red nucleus, in a coronal cross section, is the substantia nigra (Fig. 3.13*C*).

HYPOTHALAMUS

The hypothalamus is the portion of the brain situated below the basal ganglia and the thalamus and surrounding the lower aspect of the third ventricle below the hypothalamic sulcus. It contains the mammillary bodies just anterior to the interpeduncular fossa, the tuber cinereum (an elevation situated behind the infundibulum), the infundibulum and pituitary stalk, the lamina terminalis, and the optic chiasm up to the anterior commissure (Figs. 3.11, 3.13*B*, 3.15, and 3.18). On each side of the third ventricle are a number of important hypothalamic nuclei that usually cannot be individually recognized on sagittal or coronal MRI sections (Fig. 3.14).

ANTERIOR COMMISSURE

See text following for a discussion of the anterior commissure.

Posterior Fossa: Brainstem and Cerebellum

The anatomy of the posterior fossa is poorly shown by CT because of many artifacts from the heavy bone in the petrous pyramids anterolateral to the brainstem (interpetrous artifacts) and because of structures like the internal occipital protuberance, which often produces star artifacts. In the brainstem, artifacts are often related to pneumatization of the sinuses, which vary in size, and to the anterior clinoid processes, which line up and may produce enough compact bone to cause streak artifacts.

MRI is significantly superior to CT in that dense bone does not in any way interfere with the production of images. The only things that may produce MRI artifacts are motion—sometimes pulsatile motion because of the arteries and the movement of cerebral spinal fluid—and paramagnetic metal, no matter how small. Moreover, MRI can be used to study structures in axial, coronal, sagittal, and any oblique plane that one wishes to generate. For these reasons, it is useful to describe and illustrate the anatomy of the posterior fossa structures, cerebellum, and brainstem in somewhat more detail than was previously necessary.

A large number of anatomic formations cannot be adequately shown on MRI because of the lack of contrast between them, but if one knows where to look for the various structures, one is more likely to identify them. Pathologic conditions in the brainstem can be quite small, and familiarity with normal anatomy is helpful in determining whether what is seen is in fact pathologic or normal. Fortunately, nature has helped by providing symmetrical structures so that one can compare one side with the other; if pathology is present, the appearance is likely to be asymmetrical.

The brainstem comprises the medulla, pons, midbrain, two thalami, putamen and globus pallidus (on each side), and the pineal body, posterior commissure, habenula, and stria medullaris. The thalami and the basal ganglia are described elsewhere; here only the brainstem per se is assessed. The discussion is brief because the morphology and cross-sectional images are more important to diagnostic imaging than a description of various tracts and connections.

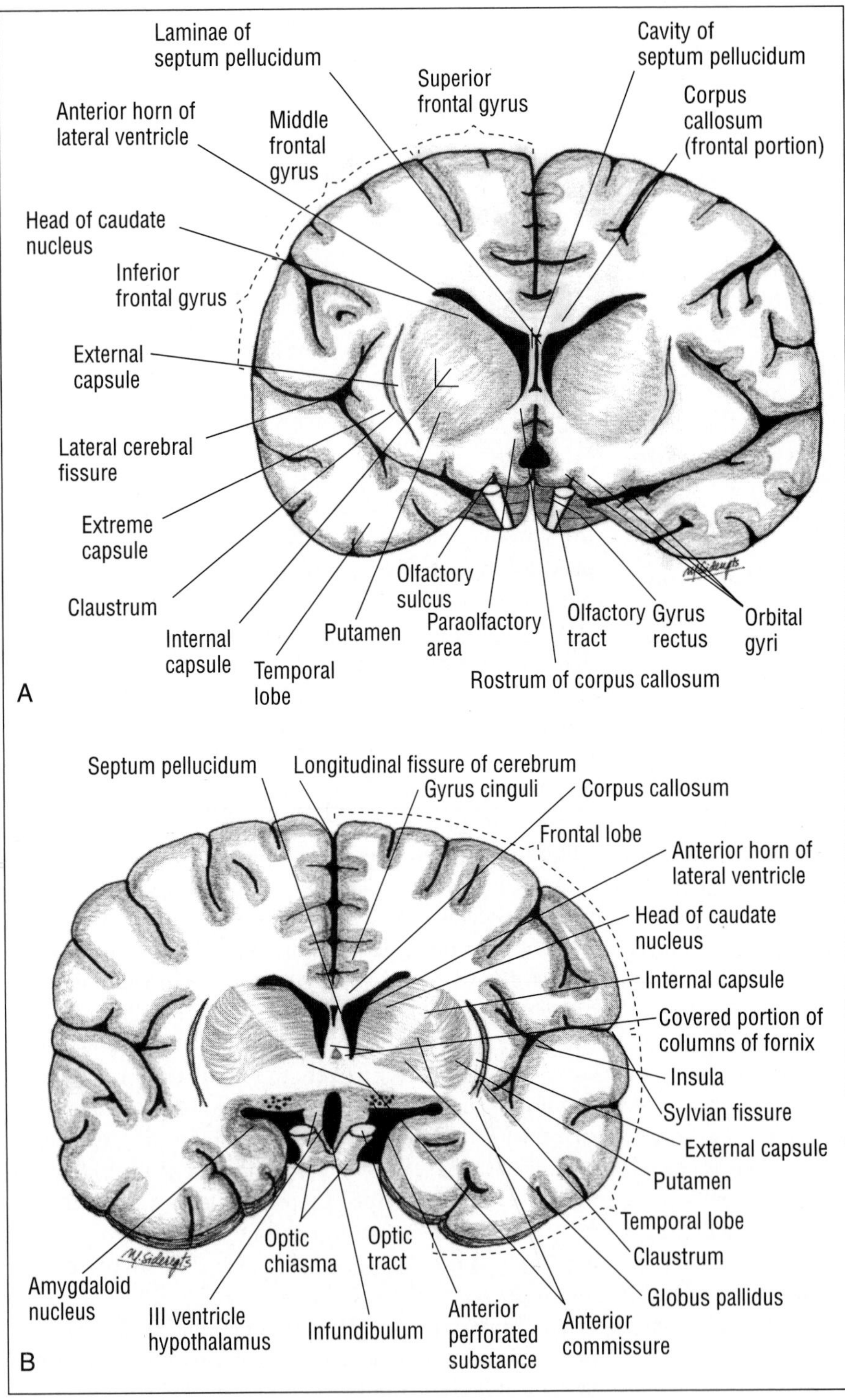

Figure 3.13. Coronal sections of brain. **A.** Passing anteriorly just behind the junction of the caudate nucleus and putamen. **B.** Passing about 1 cm behind A, anterior to the foramen of Monro. **C.** Passing about 1.3 cm behind B. **D.** Diagram of coronal section behind C passing through the thalamus to depict some of the thalamic components.

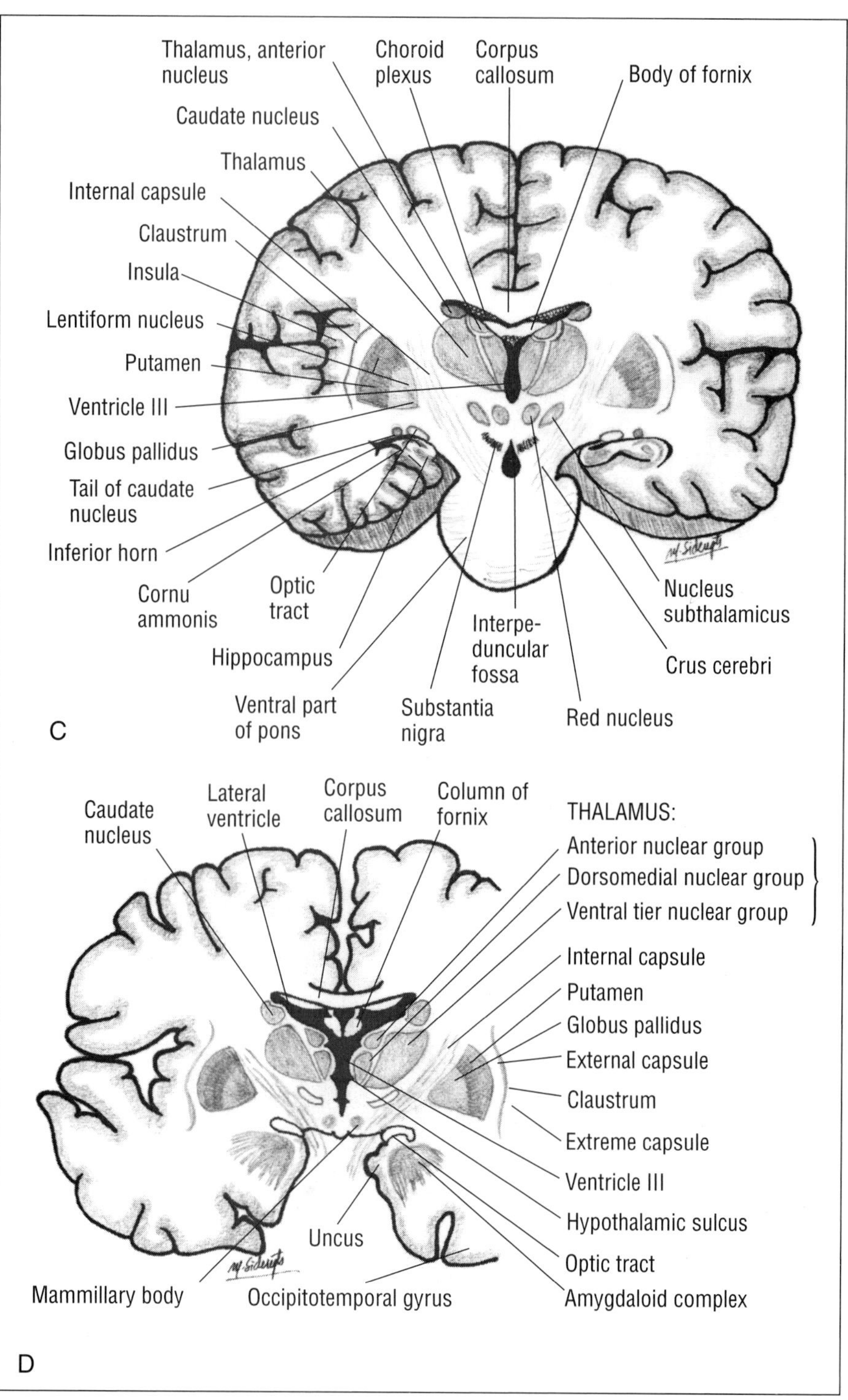

Figure 3.13. *(continued)*

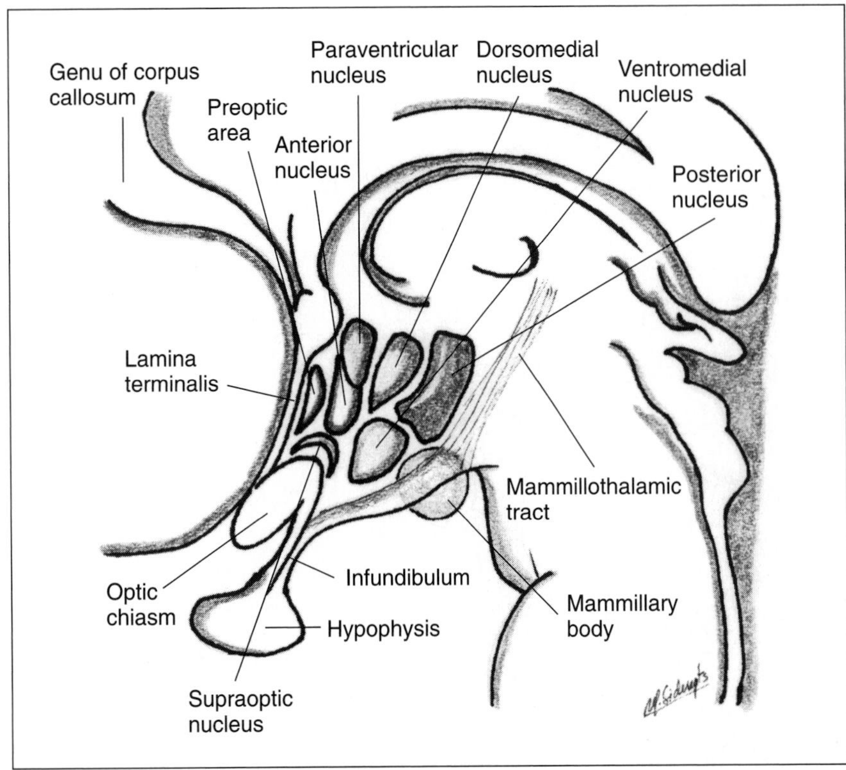

Figure 3.14. Semischematic diagram of the medial hypothalamic nuclei. These cannot be distinguished on MRI.

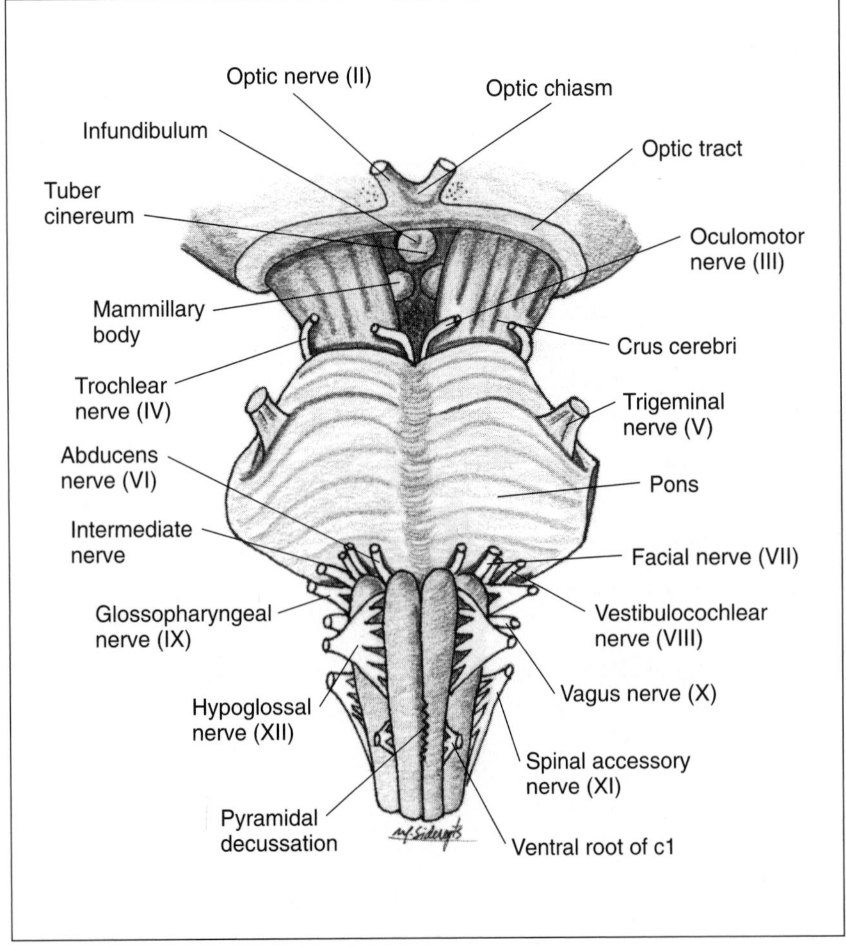

Figure 3.15. Frontal view of brainstem.

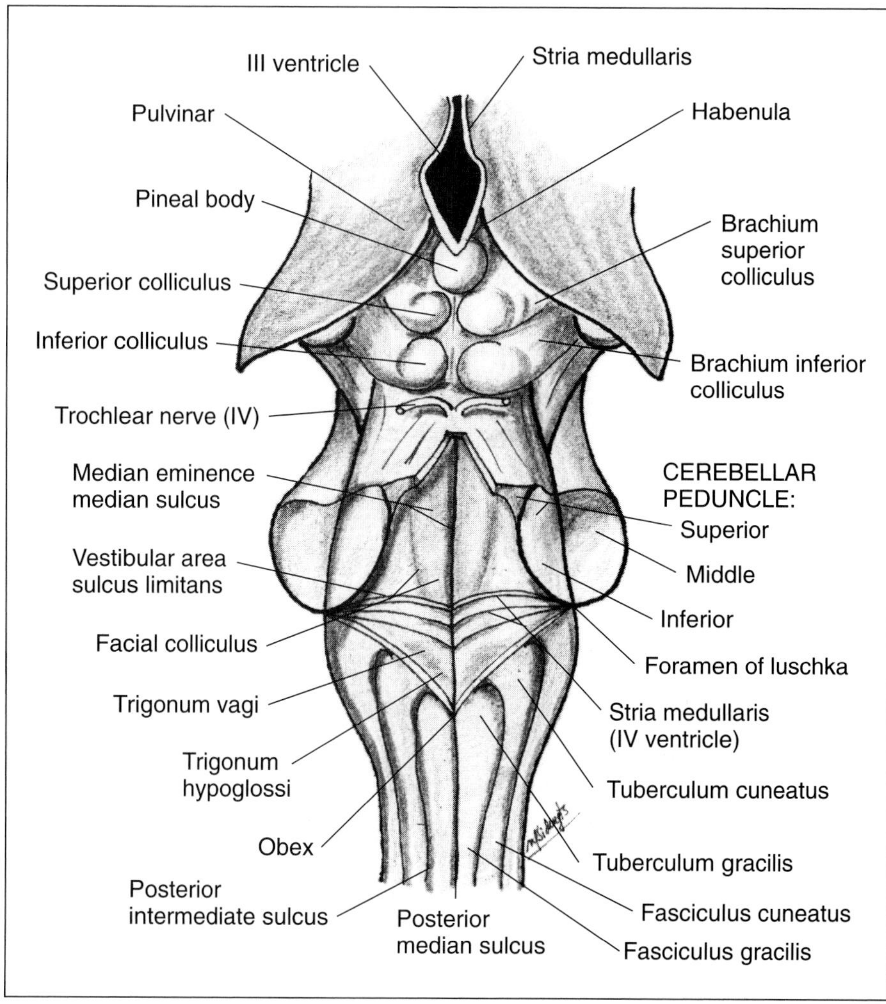

Figure 3.16. Dorsal view of brainstem. The cerebellum has been removed.

MIDBRAIN

The midbrain is only about 2 cm in length. On the dorsal side, behind the aqueduct, is the quadrigeminal plate, usually termed the *tectum*. The plate contains the two pairs of eminences called the superior and inferior collicula or superior and inferior quadrigeminal tubercles (Fig. 3.16). In front of the aqueduct and tegmentum are the cerebral peduncles, two heavy bundles of fibers diverging upward from below on the rostral side, usually called the crura (Fig. 3.15), and limited dorsally by the substantia nigra. Behind the substantia nigra is the tegmentum, which is the portion between the substantia nigra anteriorly and the aqueduct posteriorly.

Between the crura is the interpeduncular fossa. In the depth of the interpeduncular fossa is the posterior perforated substance, through which pass perforating blood vessels. The interpeduncular fossa is limited anteriorly by the mammillary bodies (Figs. 3.15 and 3.18). See the cross-sectional images for further detail concerning the internal structure of the midbrain (Figs. 3.8, 3.13, and 3.19).

PONS

Viewed anteriorly, the pons is a bulging mass of brain tissue, about 20 to 30 mm in length, situated in front of the cerebellum and separated from it by the fourth ventricle. The pons is united to the cerebellum by the middle cerebellar peduncle or brachium pontis, and it is superficially delineated from the medulla by the inferior pontine sulcus and from the midbrain by the superior pontine sulcus (Figs. 3.15, 3.17, and 3.18). See Figure 3.20 for further detail on internal structure.

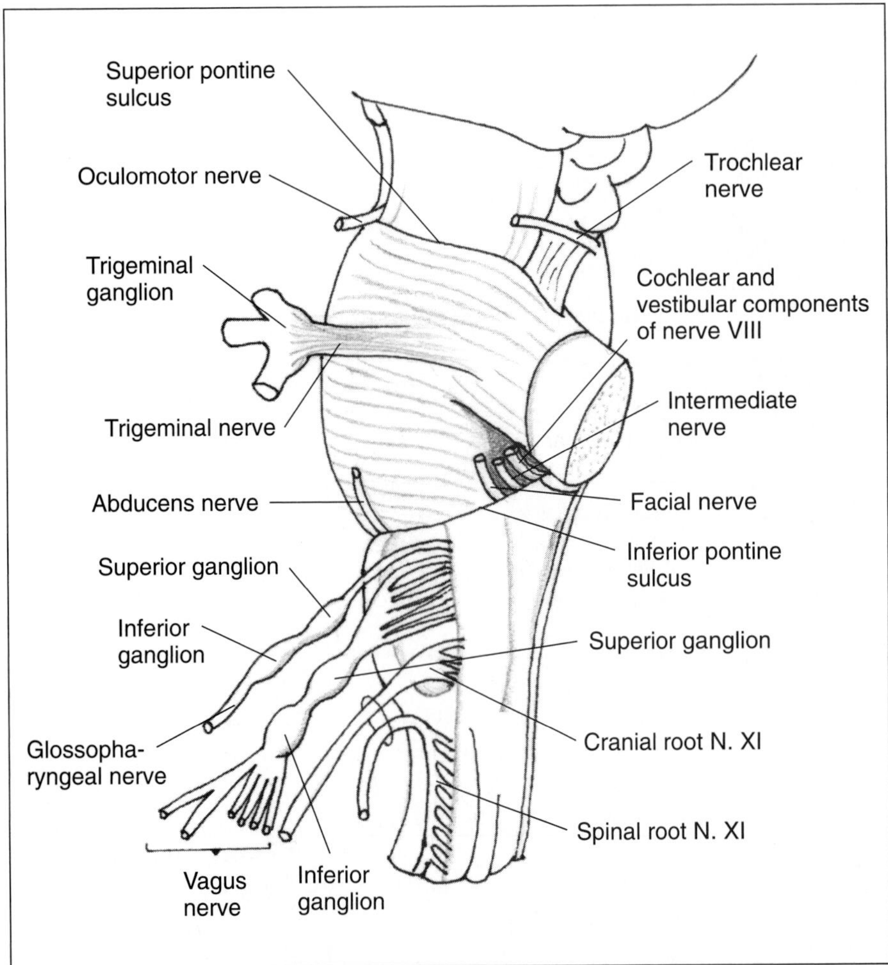

Figure 3.17. Lateral view of brainstem showing the emergence of some of the cranial nerves.

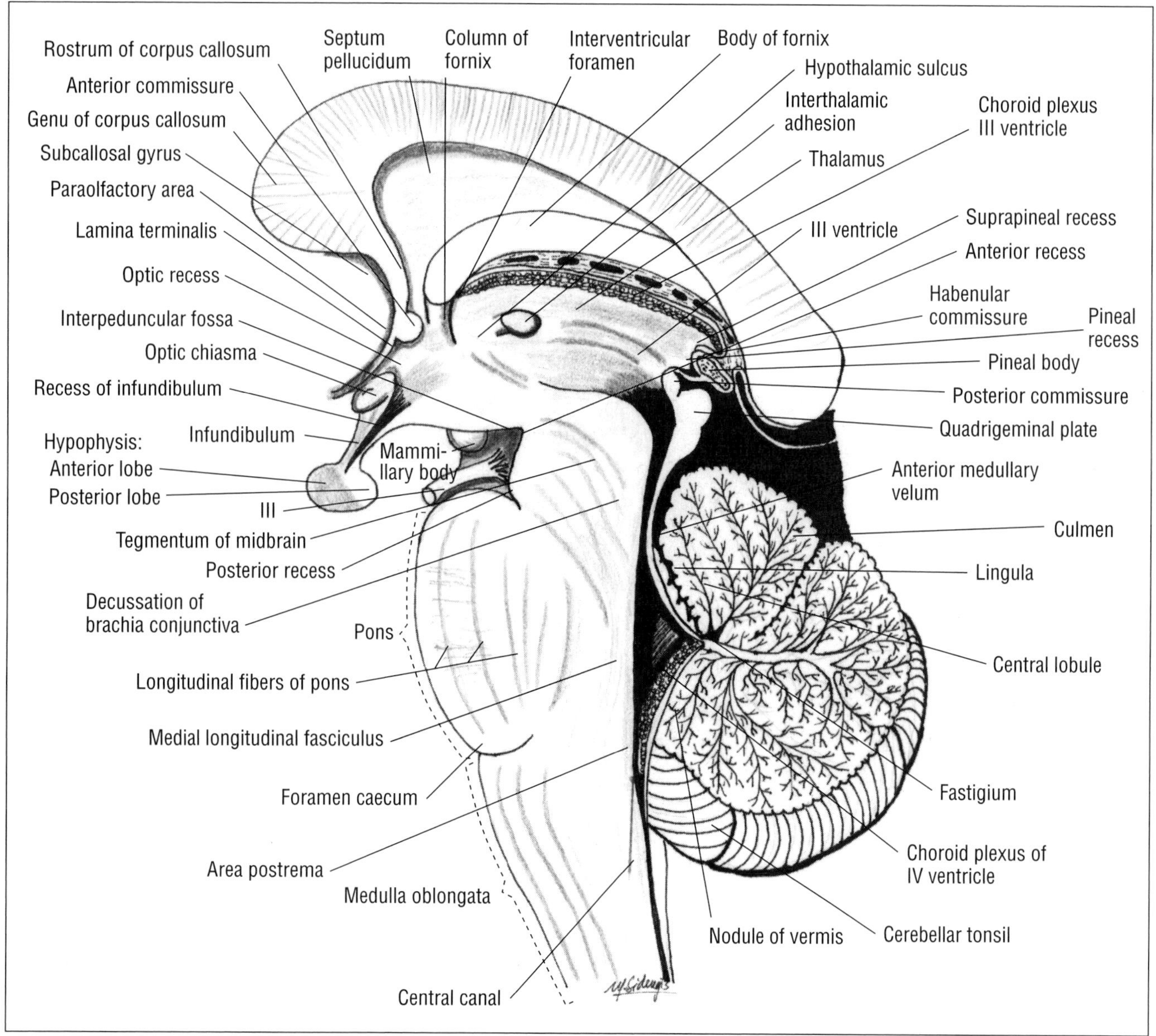

Figure 3.18. Midline sagittal section of brainstem and cerebellum including the corpus callosum and third ventricle.

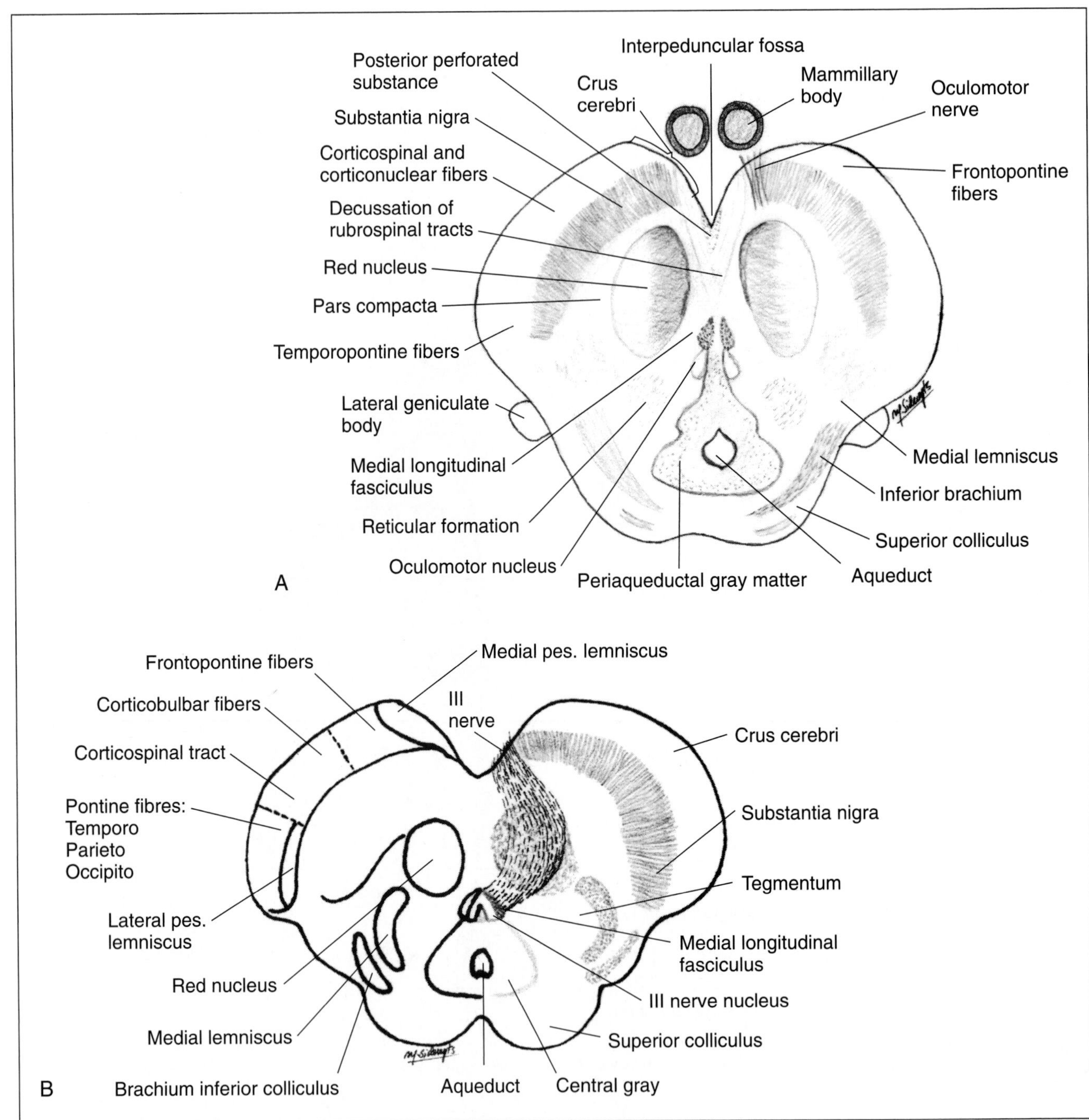

Figure 3.19. A. Transverse section of midbrain in its upper portion passing through the red nucleus and mammillary tubercles. **B.** Transverse section passing through the superior colliculus. **C.** Transverse section passing through the inferior colliculus. The tectum of the midbrain is the portion behind the cerebral aqueduct. The tegmentum is the portion between the aqueduct posteriorly and the substantia nigra anteriorly.

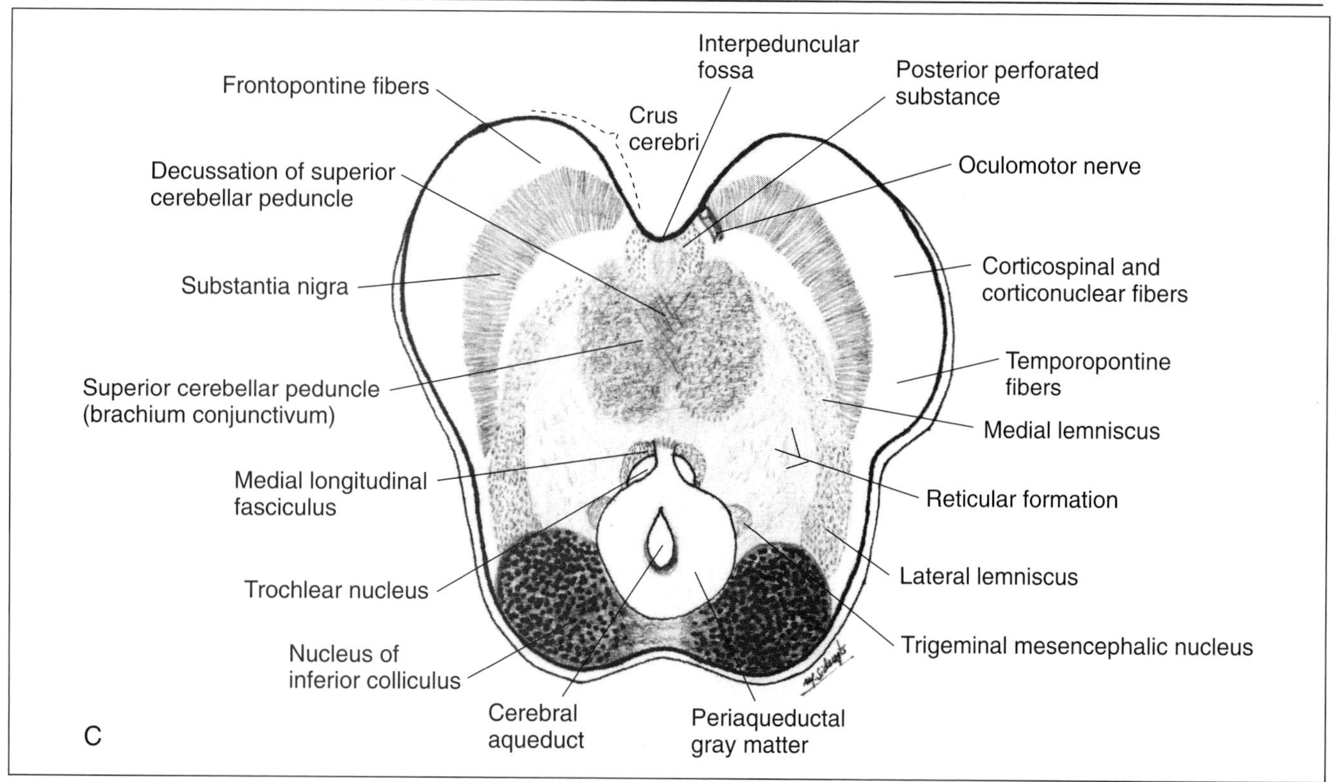

Figure 3.19. *(continued)*

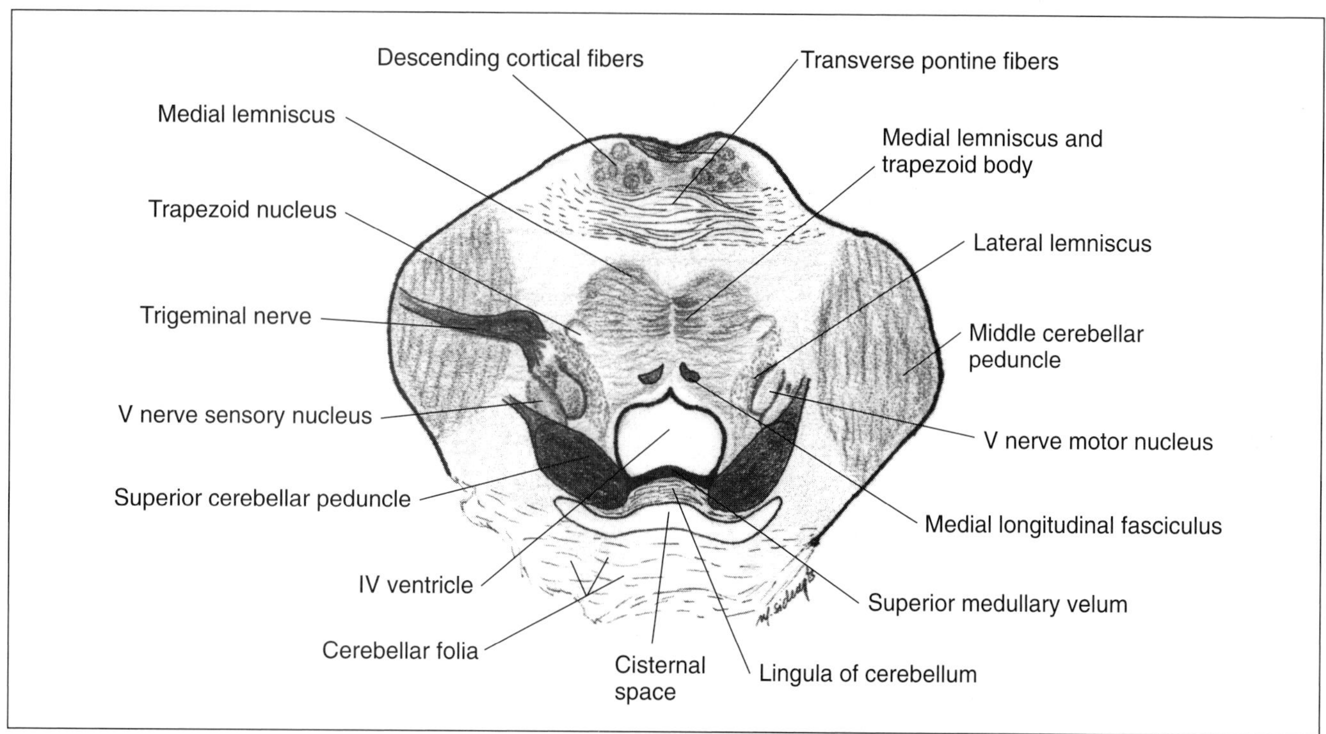

Figure 3.20. Transverse section passing through the pons at the level of the fifth (trigeminal) nerve.

MEDULLA

The medulla is the lower part of the brainstem and continues caudally with the spinal cord. Externally, the medulla presents a number of sulci and elevations that ascend from the spinal cord but are more prominent. These are the anterior median sulcus (which disappears where the decussation of the pyramidal tract takes place at the lower medulla) and the anterolateral (preolivary) sulcus, through which emerge the twelfth nerve (hypoglossal) and the ventral root of the first cervical nerve. The eminence between the anterior median sulcus and the anterolateral sulcus is the pyramid, under which passes the pyramidal tract before decussating. The anterolateral sulcus separates the pyramid from the olive. The root fibers of the eleventh nerve or spinal accessory nerve emerge behind (or lateral) to the olive along most of the length of the medulla. The ninth

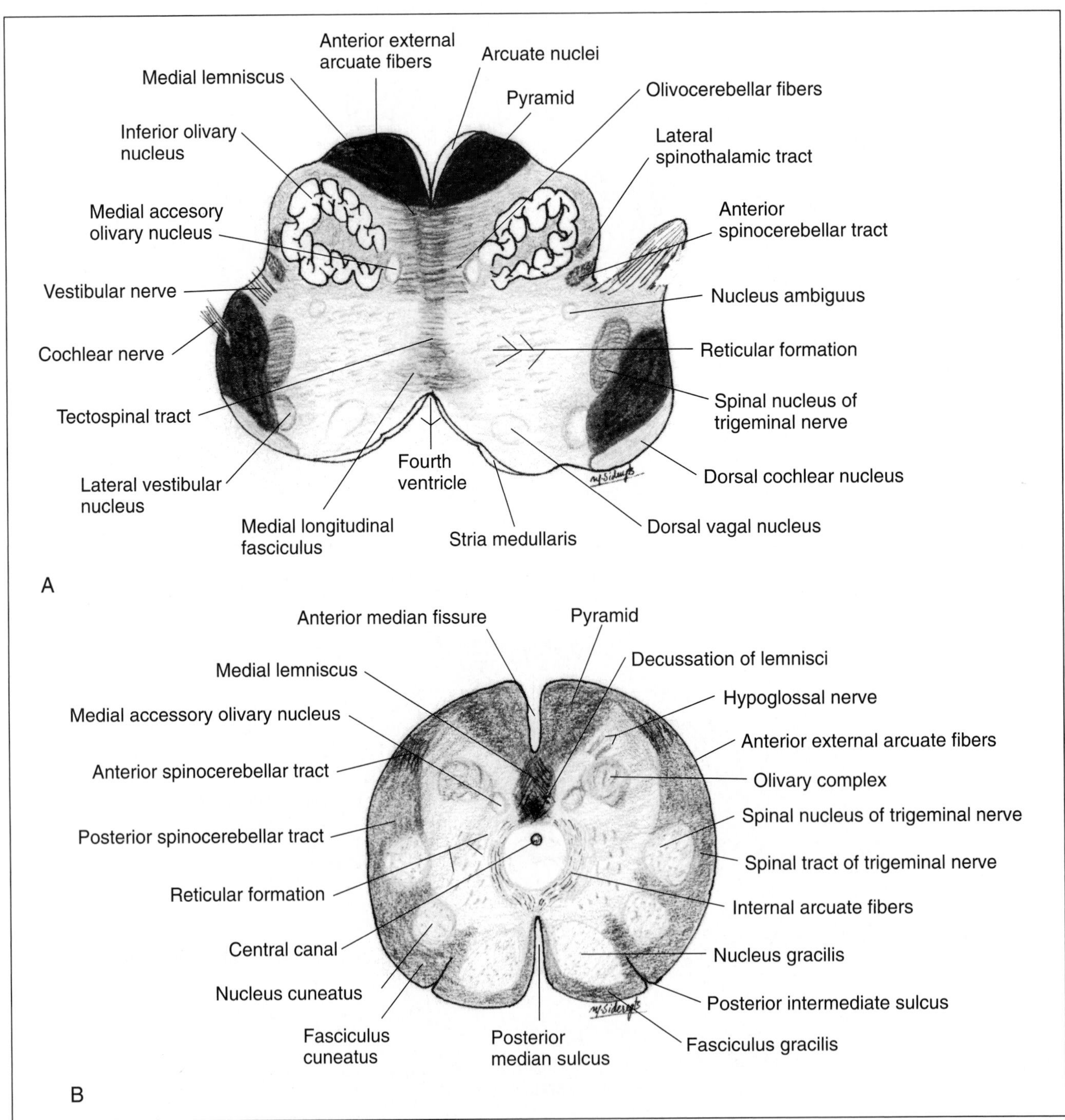

Figure 3.21. A. Transverse section through the upper half of the medulla oblongata. **B.** Transverse section through the medulla just above the decussation of the pyramidal tracts.

(glossopharyngeus) and the tenth (vagus) nerves also arise lateral to the olive in the upper part, closer to the pons (Figs. 3.15 and 3.17).

Posteriorly, in the upper part, is the lower aspect of the fourth ventricle, which terminates at the obex. Below it are the posterior median sulcus, the posterior intermediate sulcus, and the posterolateral sulcus. Between the midline and intermediate sulci is the gracilis tubercle, and between the intermediate and posterolateral sulci is the cuneate tubercle, above which and continuing along the same elevation is the inferior cerebellar peduncle or restiform body (Figs. 3.15 and 3.16).

These elevations and sulci are visible on high-quality T1-weighted images. See cross-sectional images for further detail on internal structure (Fig. 3.21). The position of some of the cranial nerve nuclei in the brainstem is shown in Figure 3.22.

THE FOURTH VENTRICLE

The fourth ventricle, situated between the upper medulla and pons anteriorly and the cerebellum dorsally, is an important structure because it is conspicuous in all examinations of the posterior fossa by CT or MRI. As seen from the front or back it has a rhomboidal shape. Its upper angle is on a level with the upper margin of the pons and is continuous with the aqueduct. Its inferior angle is at the level of the inferior border of the olive of the medulla. It opens out into the cisterna magna through the midline foramen of Magendie, but it also opens into the central canal of the spinal cord.

The anterior wall of the fourth ventricle presents the median sulcus in the midline; on each side is the median eminence, and lateral to it is the sulcus limitans. The median eminence is also called the *colliculus facialis* because under it are the nuclei of the sixth and part of the seventh nerves (Fig. 3.16 and 3.31*A*). Two-thirds of the way down is a formation, the *striae medullares*, consisting of white strands starting in the midline and extending to either side to enter the opening of the lateral recesses on either side (Fig. 3.16). At the upper part of the sulcus limitans as it joins the lateral boundary of the fourth ventricle is located the *locus ceruleus*, an underlying patch (on each side) of deeply pigmented nerve cells that give the small area a bluish color, from which the name comes.

The lateral recesses (foramina of Luschka) are situated three-fifths of the way down from the top; they extend laterally, passing under the inferior cerebellar pendungle to open laterally to the medulla on each side (Fig. 3.16).

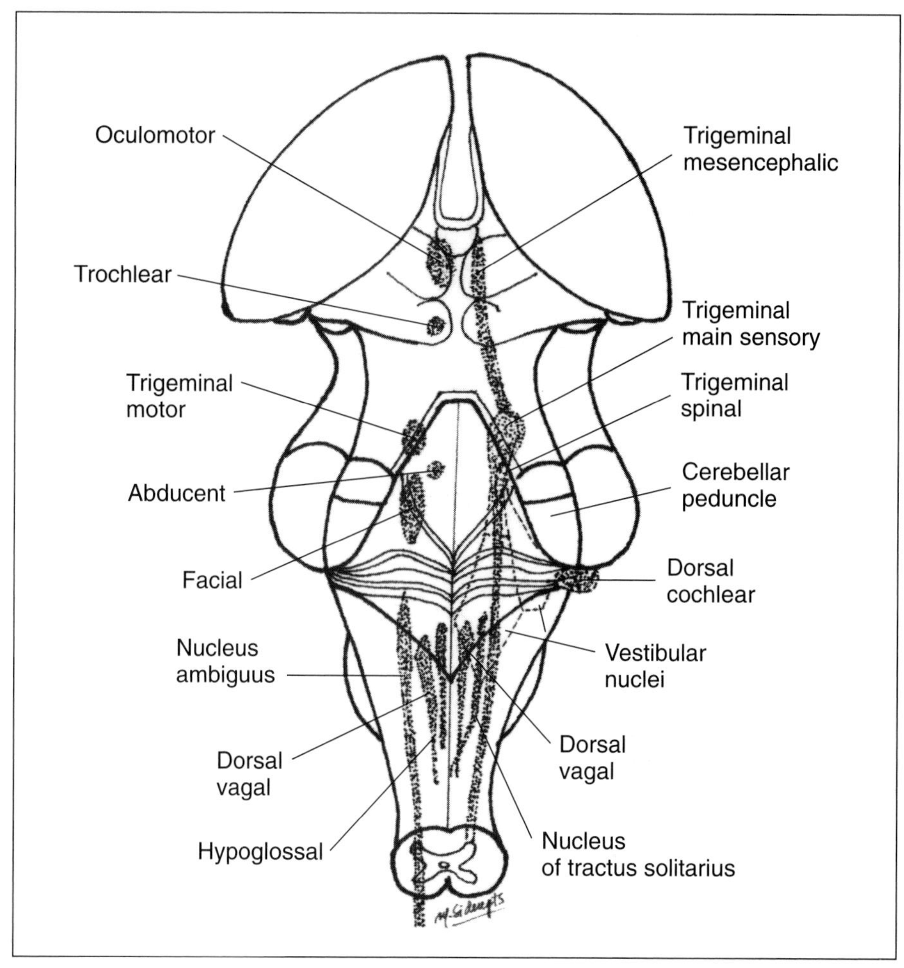

Figure 3.22. Relative positions of the nuclei of the cranial nerves in the brainstem, excluding the olfactory and optic centers.

The posterior wall of the fourth ventricle is bounded by the anterior (or superior) medullary velum, the upper posterior boundary. Its configuration is best appreciated in a sagittal cross section (Figs. 3.18 and 3.29). It arches down and back to the *fastigium*, a sharp angle that is almost always well outlined (Fig. 3.29). On each side and immediately below the level of the fastigium are the superior posterior recesses, which are seen in good detail in sagittal sections (Fig. 3.29) but are best demonstrated in coronal cross sections (3).

Below the fastigium, in the posterior wall, is the choroid plexus, which has a midline component and two lateral components that extend out through the lateral recesses to reach the posterior lateral aspect of the medulla. The *nodulus* of the cerebellar vermis forms the rounded configuration of the lower aspect of the posterior wall. There is a

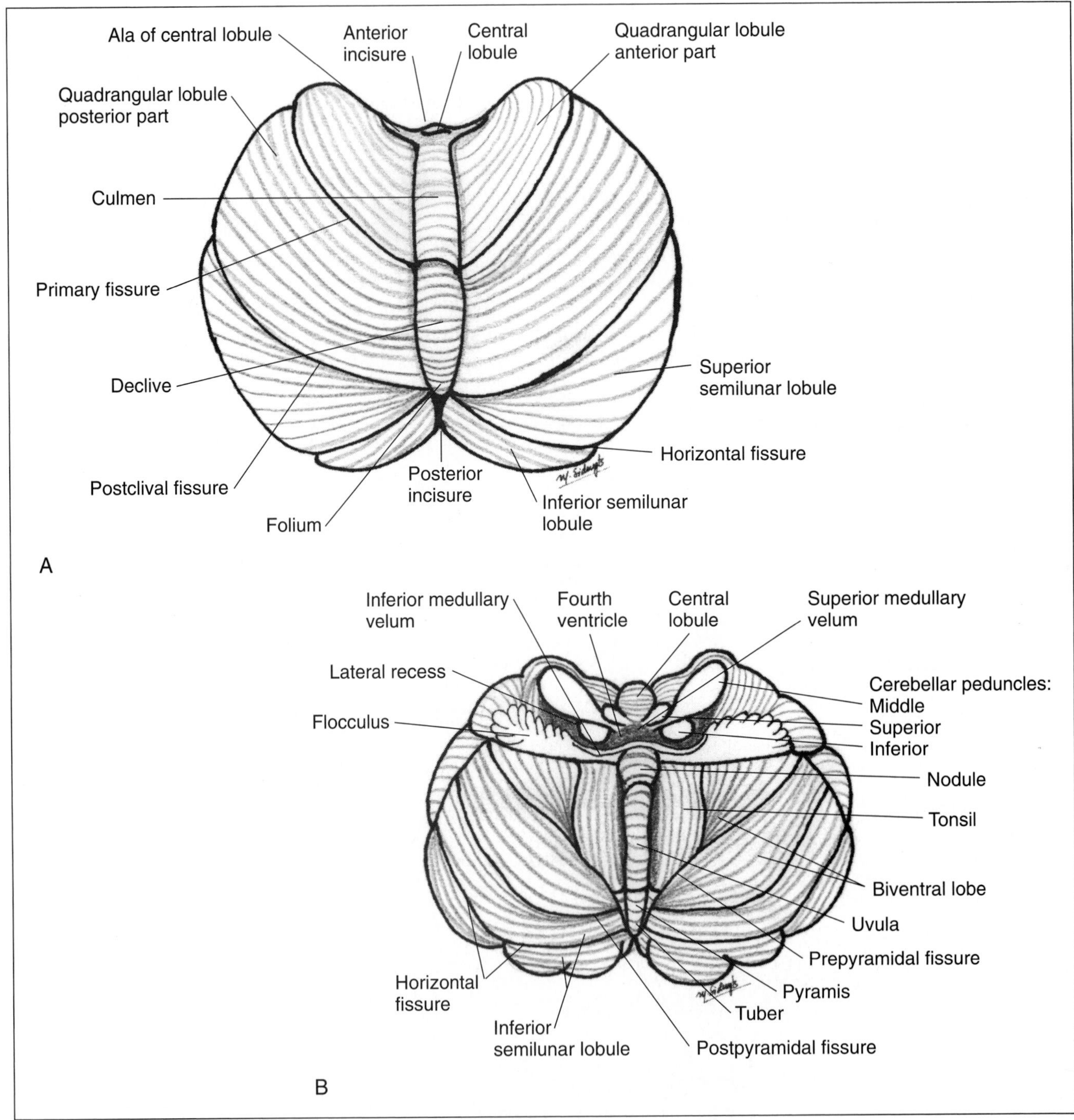

Figure 3.23. Diagram of the cerebellum. **A.** Superior surface. **B.** Inferior surface. **C.** Sagittal section passing through vermis (Courtesy of GA Press, et al: AJNR 1989;10:667–676, with permission.)

posterior (or inferior) *medullary velum* in the midline that has the foramen of Magendie, but this is never seen on CT or MRI examinations.

THE CEREBELLUM

The cerebellum consists of two hemispheres joined by the vermis. This area is separated from the occipital and temporal lobes by the tentorium cerebelli, except in its anterior superior surface, where the free margin of the tentorium forms the tentorial notch.

In the superior surface, the vermis is poorly separated from the hemispheres; only a shallow midline depression is seen here, whereas the inferior aspect of the vermis is separated from the cerebellar hemispheres by a deep sulcus on each side (Figs. 3.23 and 3.24). The vermis contains a number of segments that have been named anatomically but which have no particular practical importance except for purposes of description (Fig. 3.23*C*). The lingula, anterior superiorly, is against the superior medullary velum, the superior and rostrally directed membrane delimiting the fourth ventricle; the nodule is against the inferior medullary velum, which borders the fourth ventricle inferiorly (Fig. 3.23*C*). On each side of the inferior vermis are the two cerebellar tonsils, and between them is a space that is part of the cisterna magna, the vallecula (little valley).

The cerebellar hemispheres as well as the vermis are covered by a mantle of gray matter, the cerebellar cortex, covering a mass of white matter, the corpus medullare. The hemispheres present numerous small gyri or folia and several fissures (Fig. 3.23). Some of the fissures are deep enough so that they almost reach the surface of the fourth ventricle. The only fissure that is important to recognize is the horizontal fissure, which almost divides the cerebellum into a superior and an inferior portion. Portions of the horizontal fissure are often seen on axial images on CT or MRI and may be mistaken for an ischemic infarct, particularly if the fissure happens to be seen on one side only (Fig. 10.23). The horizontal fissure is more prominent in older individuals.

Within the cerebellum, four pairs of nuclear masses are situated in the center of the white matter at about the level of the fastigium around and close to the posterior aspect of the fourth ventricle. These are the fastigial, the globose, the emboliform, and the dentate nuclei (Fig. 3.25). Of these, the most important from the imaging point of view is the dentate nucleus, which is frequently seen on CT and particularly on MRI.

The flocculus is a distinct formation of the cerebellum situated just inferior and lateral to the middle cerebellar peduncle. Because it is on the surface, it may sometimes simulate a small tumor mass in the region of the cerebellopontine angle. The flocculus is usually symmetrical but may be seen better on one side (Figs. 3.24 and 3.31*B*) (4).

The cerebellum is attached to the brainstem by three bridges on each side, called the *cerebellar peduncles.* Of these, the largest and most easily identified is the *middle cerebellar*

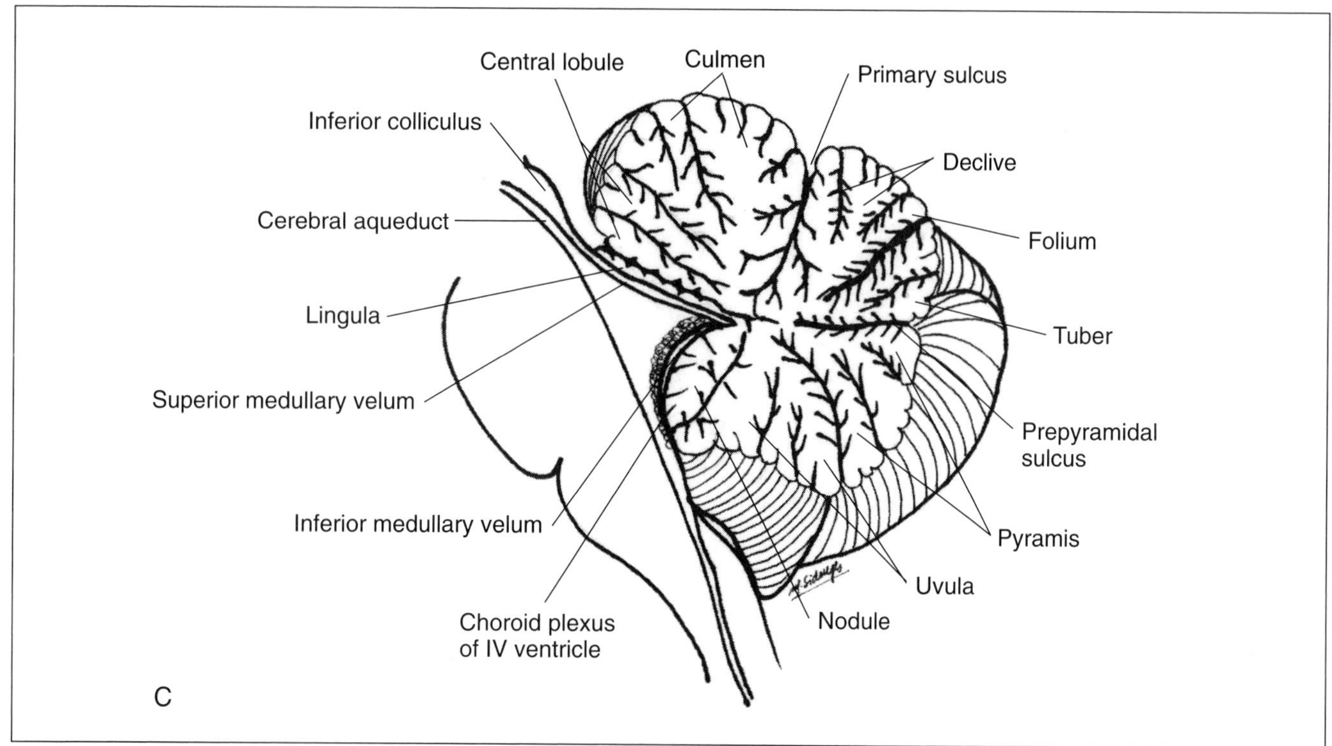

Figure 3.23. *(continued)*

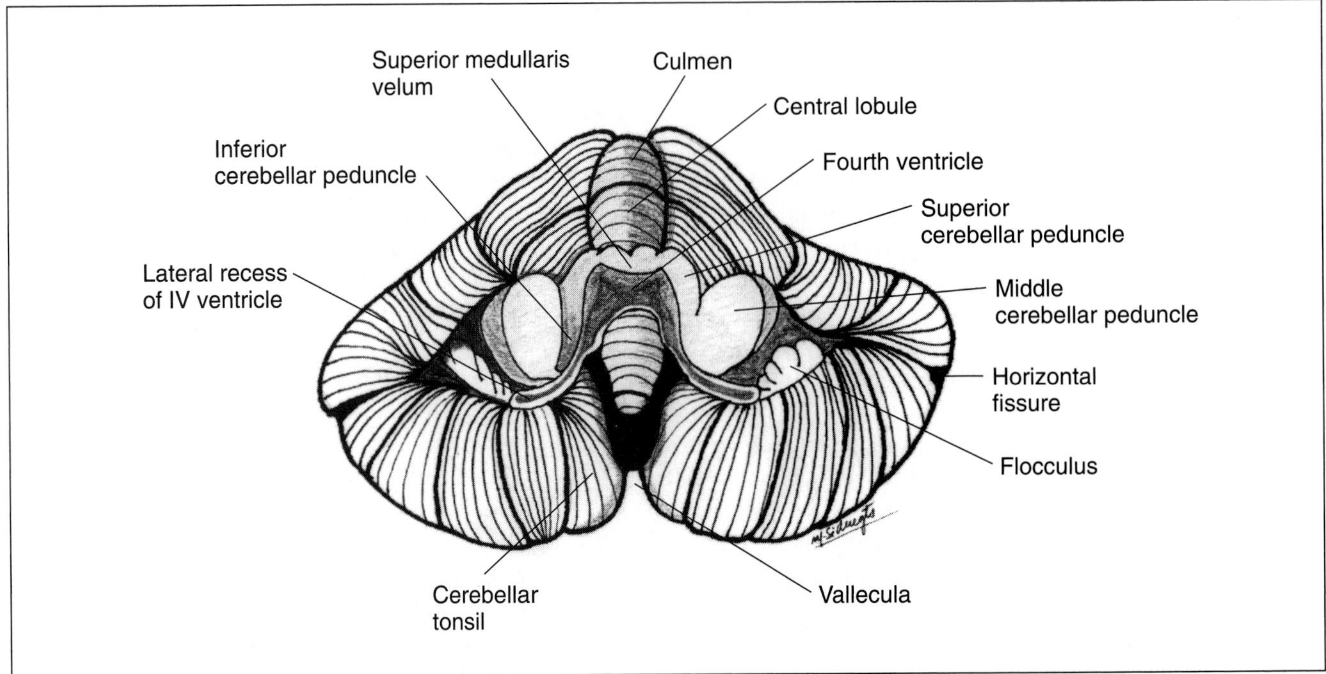

Figure 3.24. Diagram of the anterior surface of cerebellum after severing it from its attachments to the brainstem.

peduncle or *brachium pontis*, which comes out of the pons into the cerebellum, where it fans posteriorly and slightly caudally. This structure carries fibers to and from the cerebellum (Figs. 3.20 and 3.31*A*).

The *superior cerebellar peduncles* (brachium conjunctivum) are on each side of the upper part of the fourth ventricle and are connected with each other by the superior medullary velum. They ascend, coming closer together and then disappearing just caudal to the inferior colliculus. Within the midbrain, the majority of the fibers decussate, and most end at the red nucleus of the opposite side (Fig. 3.19*C*). The superior cerebellar penduncles and their decussation can be seen most often on MR axial images and sometimes on CT images (Fig. 3.32*A*).

The inferior cerebellar peduncle (restiform body) contains fibers originating in the medulla and spinal cord and terminating in the medial side of the cerebellar hemispheres as well as fibers originating in the cerebellum and entering the medulla. The inferior cerebellar peduncles are formed on the dorsolateral aspect of the upper medulla oblongata. They ascend and diverge, but upon entering the cerebellum, bend medially and posteriorly (Fig. 3.16).

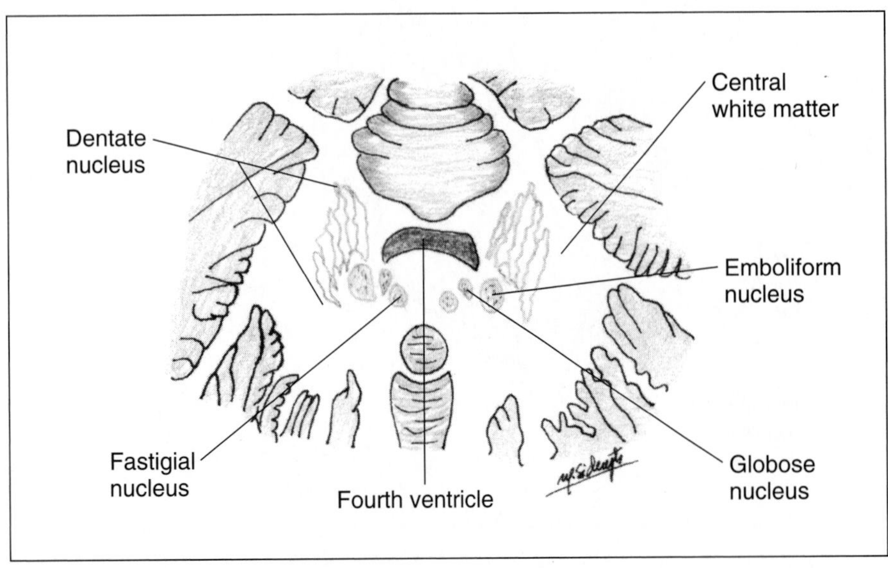

Figure 3.25. Transverse section of cerebellum passing through the fastigium of the fourth ventricle to show the relationship of the cerebellar nuclei.

SPECIAL FORMATIONS

Some special formations in the brain are described below.

Hippocampal Formation

The term *hippocampus* originated because the shape of the structure resembles a sea horse when viewed in coronal section. Starting at the collateral sulcus and extending medially is the parahippocampal gyrus, which is situated at the border between the inferior and medial surface of the hemisphere. On the medial surface the parahippocampal gyrus is limited superiorly by the hippocampal fissure. The upper portion of the medial surface continuing into the hippocampal fissure is called the *subiculum* (Figs. 3.26 and 11.130). Bordering the hippocampal fissure above is the dentate gyrus, and immediately above is the fimbria, which is the inferior aspect of the fornix.

Immediately above the fimbria is the choroidal fissure, through which enters the choroid plexus of the inferior (temporal) horn of the lateral ventricle (Fig. 3.26). This arrangement applies from the dorsal to the rostral portion of the temporal horn. Anteriorly, the hippocampus bends up and back, creating what is called the *uncus* (Fig. 3.44 and 3.45). The entire hippocampus, including the upper aspect of the uncus, projects into the temporal horn. The temporal horn tip is wrapped around the anterior aspect of the hippocampus. On its expanded anterior extremity, the hippocampus presents a few depressions and slight elevations that resemble a paw, which have received the name of *pes hippocampi.* These slight irregularities were visible on pneumoencephalography but may be seen sometimes on CT or MRI studies (Fig. 3.45).

The ventricular surface of the hippocampus is covered by ependyma, but immediately beneath it is a white layer, the alveus. Fibers of the alveus converge to form the fimbria of the fornix (Fig. 3.26). The dentate gyrus is cortical tissue. The subiculum has a thinner covering of gray matter than the parahippocampal gyrus. The parahippocampal gyrus has a six-layer cellular organization that gradually decreases to a three-layer cell organization in the upper part of the subiculum and in the hippocampus and dentate gyrus (5).

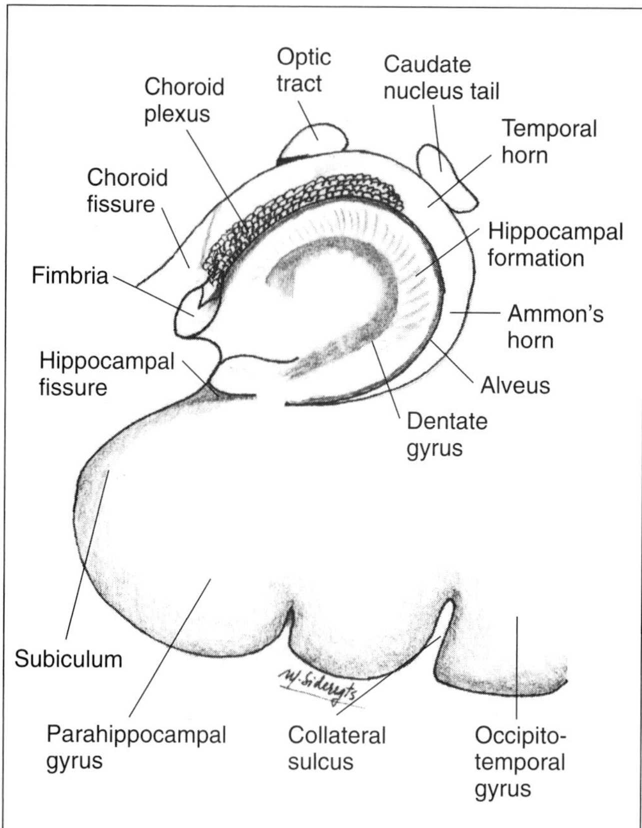

Figure 3.26. Hippocampal formation. Diagram of coronal cross section of the hippocampus.

Fiber Tracts of the Brain

A number of nerve fibers that accumulate in the cerebral hemispheres deserve special description. An axial cross section of the brain about 1 to 2 cm above the corpus callosum shows a mass of white matter on each hemisphere that is usually referred to as the *centrum semiovale.* The fibers that arise from the brain cortex and converge to the internal capsule and those that arise below the basal ganglia region and ascend toward the centrum semiovale form the *corona radiata.* The corona radiata occupies a relatively narrow space on each side of the bodies of the lateral ventricles.

CORPUS CALLOSUM

The corpus callosum is the largest commissure connecting the cerebral hemispheres. The structure has a central portion, the body or trunk; an anterior portion, the genu; and a posterior portion, the splenium. The genu bends downward and dorsad around the frontal horns of the lateral ventricles (Fig. 3.18). This portion, called the rostrum, becomes thinner and continues caudally below the foramen of Monro until it reaches the optic chiasm. This lower, thinner portion is called the lamina terminalis (Figs. 3.11 and 3.18).

The fibers of the genu curve forward in front of and lateral to the diverging frontal horns, a portion of the corpus callosum known as the *forceps minor.* The corpus callosum forms the roof of the lateral ventricles, and its crossing myelinated fibers reach all aspects of the cerebral hemisphere cortex. The large number of fibers of the posterior part of the trunk and the *splenium* that cover the roof of the ventricles and extend to cover the lateral aspect of the temporal horn on each side are the *tapetum.* The most posterior fibers of the splenium curve backwards into the occipital lobes and are called the *forceps major.* The splenium makes a broad indentation on the superior medial aspect of the posterior horn of the lateral ventricle (Fig. 3.33).

Above the corpus callosum is the callosal sulcus, separating the corpus callosum from the cingulate gyrus (Fig. 3.5).

ANTERIOR COMMISSURE

The anterior commissure is a tight bundle of myelinated fibers about 3.0 mm thick situated just anterior to the foramen of Monro and the columns of the fornix (Fig. 3.11). It is imbedded in the lamina terminalis and extends horizontally (Fig. 3.13*B*). The majority of the fibers form a posterior bundle that extends and fans into the medial aspect of the temporal lobe. Passing laterally, this posterior bundle produces a groove on the anterior inferior aspect of the lentiform nucleus. The anterior bundle curves forward into the olfactory tract and anterior perforated substance. The anterior commissure can be seen almost regularly on sagittal axial and coronal images (Figs. 3.28 and 3.33*B*).

In addition, the white matter of the hemispheres contains some compact white matter tracts and interconnections that are worth describing briefly. Curnes et al. reported on the MRI demonstration of some of these white matter tracts (6).

SUPERIOR LONGITUDINAL FASCICULUS

This structure extends from the frontal to the parieto-occipital lobes and is situated just lateral to the corona radiata. It is sometimes seen on proton density and T2-weighted images as a dark band medial to the brain sulci above the level of the insula.

FRONTO-OCCIPITAL FASCICULUS

This structure extends from the frontal pole to the occipital lobe and is situated medial to the corona radiata and lateral to the caudate nucleus. It is seen very frequently on axial T2-weighted images as a dark band parallel to the lateral ventricle. It is visible also in coronal views, just lateral to the ventricle and the caudate nucleus. It is best seen in the anterior aspect of the hemisphere.

SHORT ARCUATE FIBERS (U FIBERS)

These connect adjacent gyri. Some longer connecting fiber groups are also present (Fig. 3.27) but are not usually visible on MRI.

INFERIOR LONGITUDINAL FASCICULUS

This structure begins in the occipital pole and extends to the temporal lobe, passing laterally to the lateral ventricle and the tapetum. This structure is not usually identified on MRI.

UNCINATE FASCICULUS

This structure connects the gyri on the orbital surface of the frontal lobe and the speech area with the cortex of the temporal lobe pole. Its sharply angulated course (Fig. 3.27) is visible on axial T2-weighted images, starting at the same level where the anterior commissure fibers reach the temporal lobe. It is also visible in coronal views below the claustrum and the external and extreme capsules.

CINGULUM

This is a tight band of myelinated fibers that is contained in the cingulate gyrus and is shaped like it. Posteriorly it rounds the corpus callosum, and inferiorly it enters the parahippocampal gyrus. It is seen in coronal T2-weighted images and on axial images above the corpus callosum near the medial surface of the hemisphere.

OPTIC RADIATION

These fibers arise from the lateral geniculate body, pass in the retrolenticular portion of the internal capsule, swing around the temporal horn (Meyer loop), and turn posteriorly adjacent to the lateral surface of the atrium and occipital horn of the ventricle, where they swing medially to reach the visual cortex (calcarine fissure area) (Figs. 3.27*B* and 3.33*B*).

FORNIX AND INTERNAL CAPSULE

These have been described in the text preceding.

MAMMILLOTHALAMIC TRACT

This tract extends from the mammillary body across the medial thalamus to end in the anterior thalamic nucleus. It is adjacent to the third-ventricular wall in the hypothalamus. In axial T2-weighted images it is visible as a dark round area adjacent to the bright cerebrospinal fluid (CSF)–containing third ventricle behind the pillars of the fornix.

POSTERIOR COMMISSURE

This structure is situated on the dorsal aspect where the cerebral aqueduct enters the third ventricle. It is a constant structure and of fairly good size, and is used as a most important point of reference in stereotactic surgical interventions. Laterally it does not extend much away from the midline. It is related to the habenular commissure, which is situated just above it in front of the pineal body (Figs. 3.11 and 3.18). The habenular commissure calcifies somewhat less frequently than the pineal body and can be seen on plain skull films as well as on CT axial images.

HABENULAR COMMISSURE

Two small habenular nuclei are situated on the dorsomedial aspect of the thalamus. They connect with each other through the habenular commissure (Fig. 3.18).

LEFT-RIGHT BRAIN DYSSYMMETRY

This term has been used by LeMay to describe the asymmetry often seen in axial tomograms, CT or MRI, of the head (7). In the right-handed individual the best-developed asymmetry involves the occipital region; the left occipital lobe extends slightly farther back than the right, causing some thinning of the bone in the left occipital area, and sometimes slight bulging (usually called petalia). The left occipital horn of the lateral ventricle is usually longer than the right (five times more frequently than the right, according to McRae, Brauch, & Milner [8]). The lateral venous sinus on the right (usually the dominant draining sinus) is higher than the left in slightly over half of the individuals seen with angiography. Other asymmetries reported by LeMay have included racial differences (7). Arteriographic differences in the cerebral hemispheres have also been reported (9).

ILLUSTRATION OF BRAIN ANATOMY BY MRI

Detailed illustrations with legends are shown in Figures 3.28 through 3.49.

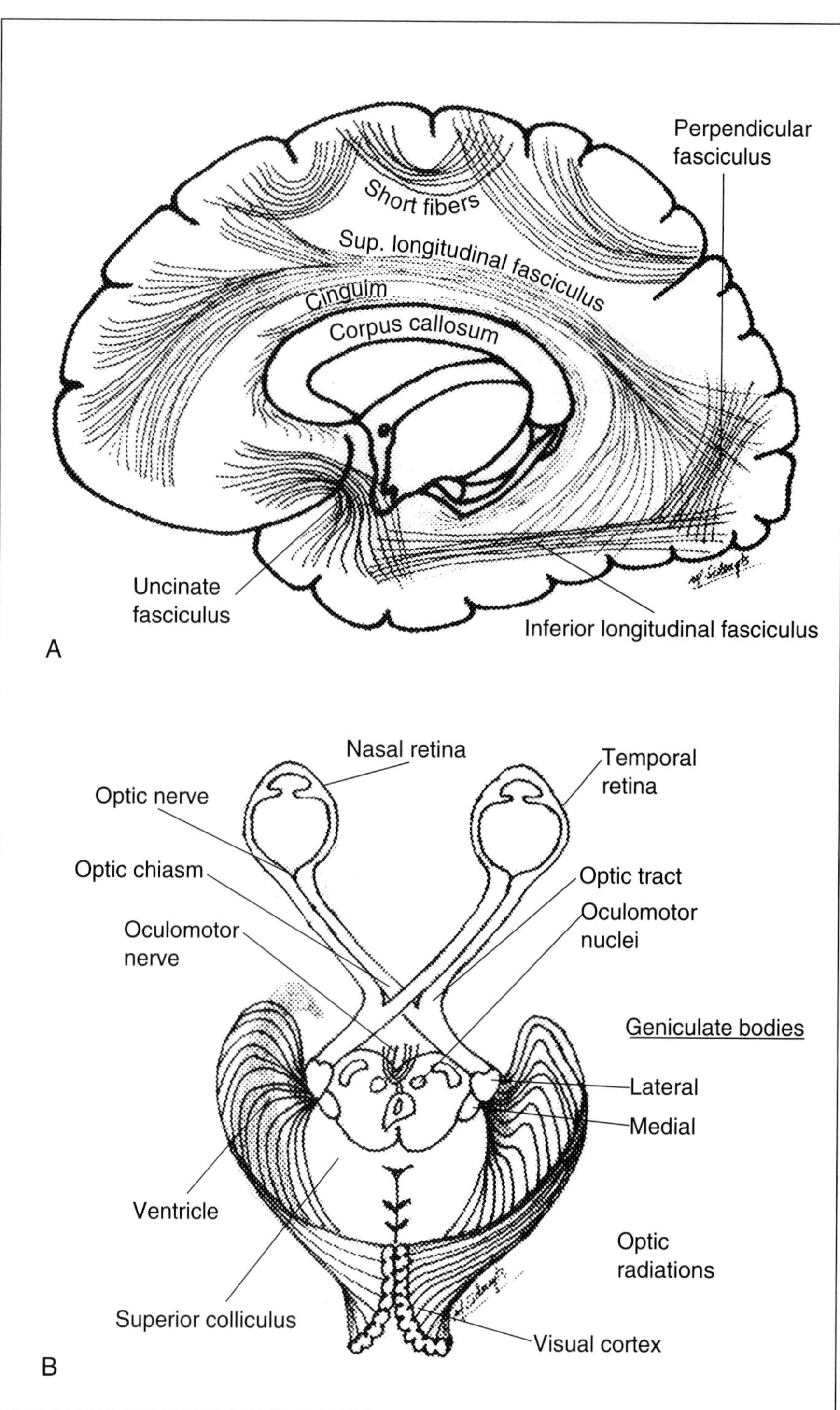

Figure 3.27. A. Diagram of some fiber tracts within the brain. Some are visible on MRI. **B.** Diagram of optic pathways.

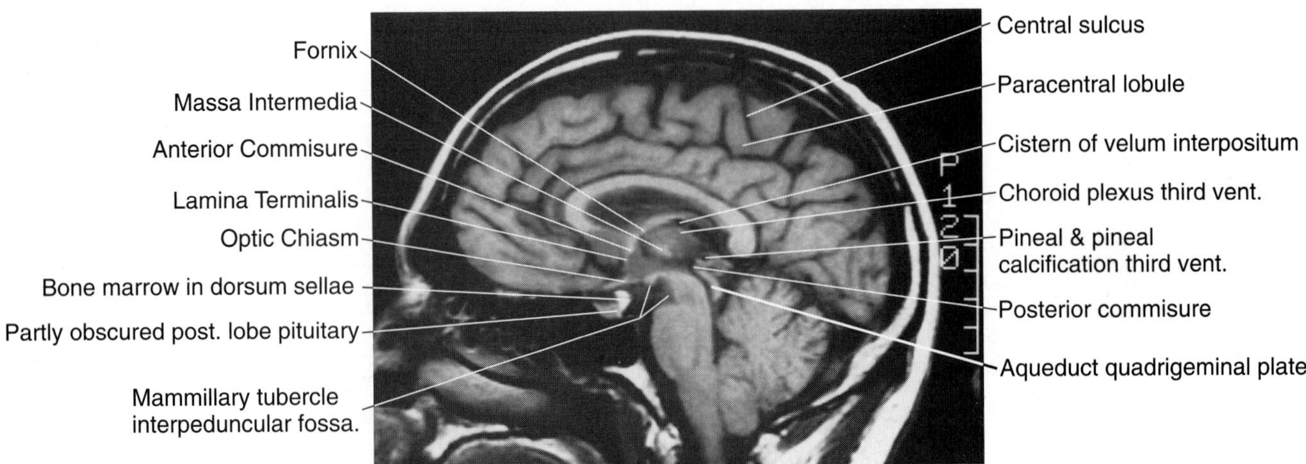

Figure 3.28. Mildline sagittal view, MRI T1 weighted.

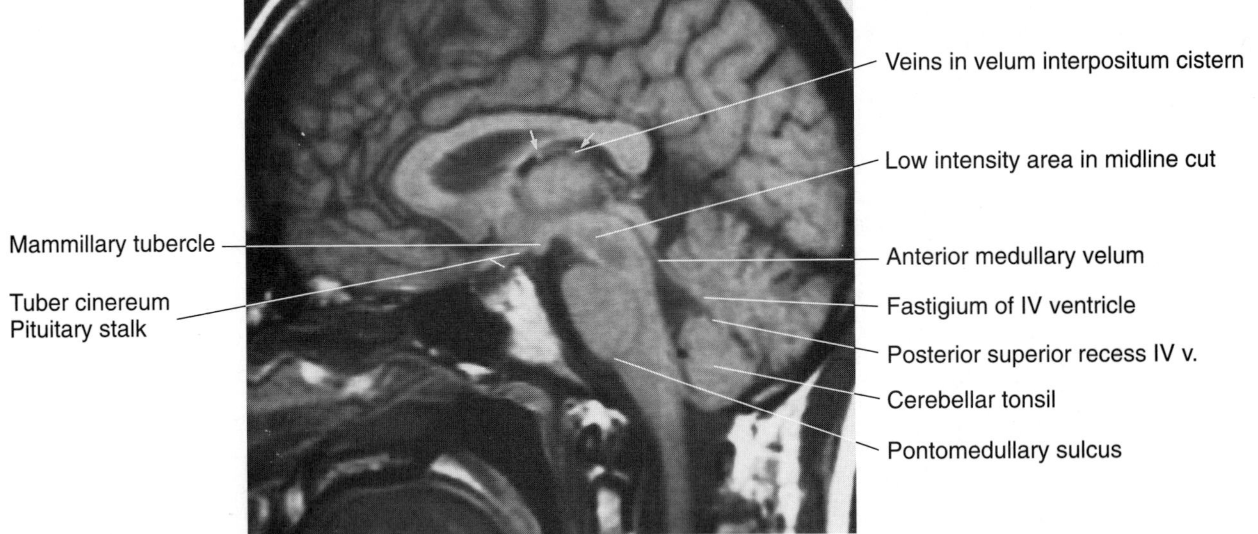

Figure 3.29. Midline T1-weighted sagittal view. The low-attenuation area in the midbrain is a frequent finding; it is seen in the midline section and thus in the tegmentum of the midbrain. It is probably produced by periaqueductal gray matter and nuclei of the oculomotor nerves, and possibly by partial volume of the red nuclei. The decussation of the superior cerebellar peduncles is in the same area, and one would expect them to be like myelinated fibers and therefore brighter on T1-weighted images. However, they may be low intensity in both T1- and T2-weighted images (see Fig. 3.32*B*). The small arrows point at slowly flowing veins in the region of the velum interpositum.

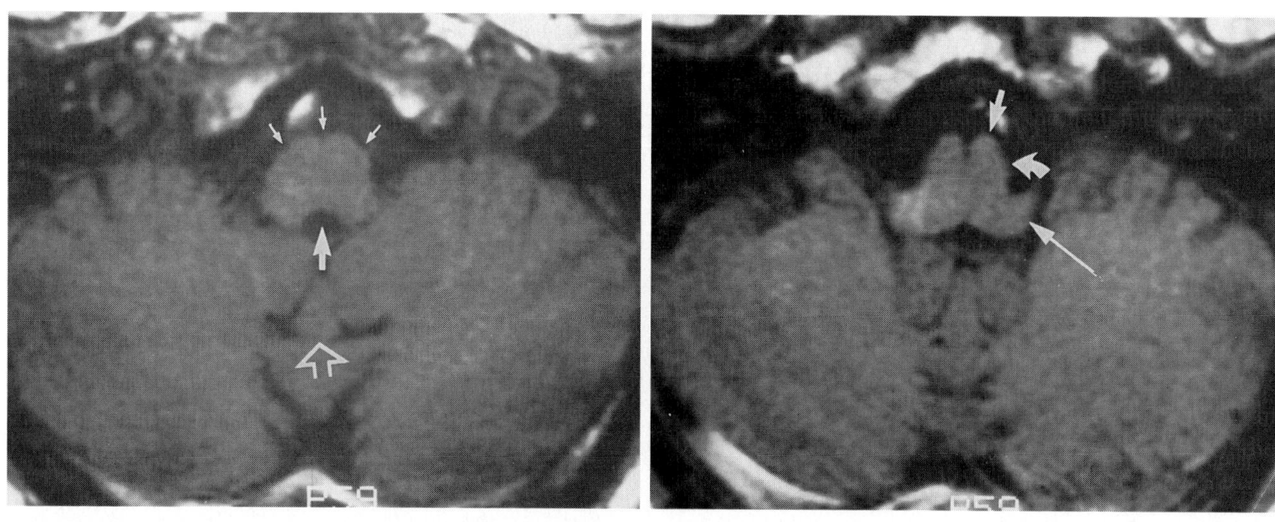

A B

Figure 3.30. Cross section (T1-weighted) through medulla. **A.** The anterior median fissure (small white arrow) is shallow because the section passes through the upper part of the pyramidal decussation. The posterior median fissure is widening (white dorsal arrow) as it reaches the lower aspect of the fourth ventricle. No structures can be discerned in the MRI cross sections of the medulla, and only pathological changes can produce variations in the signal intensity. In the isolated specimens much more detail can be seen (Solsberg, Fournier, Potts, 1990). The anterolateral sulcus on each side of the midline (small white arrows) is faintly outlined. Through it emerge the component fibers of the hypoglossal nerve and more caudally the anterior rootlets of the spinal nerves. Likewise, there is a posterolateral sulcus through which emerge the fibers of the glossopharyngeal, vagus, and spinal accessory nerves and further down the posterior rootlets of the spinal nerves. The corticospinal tract (pyramids) runs on each side of the anterior median sulcus. The open arrow points at the uvula of the vermis, and the arrow is sitting on the pyramid of the cerebellum. On each side are the cerebellar tonsils. **B.** Cross section 8 mm above A. The pyramidal tract is between the median and shallow anterolateral sulcus (white arrow). The olive (inferior olivary nucleus) is shown by the curved arrow, and the inferior cerebellar peduncle (restiform body) by the long-stem arrow. Just behind it is the inferior lateral recess of the fourth ventricle (foramen of Luschka).

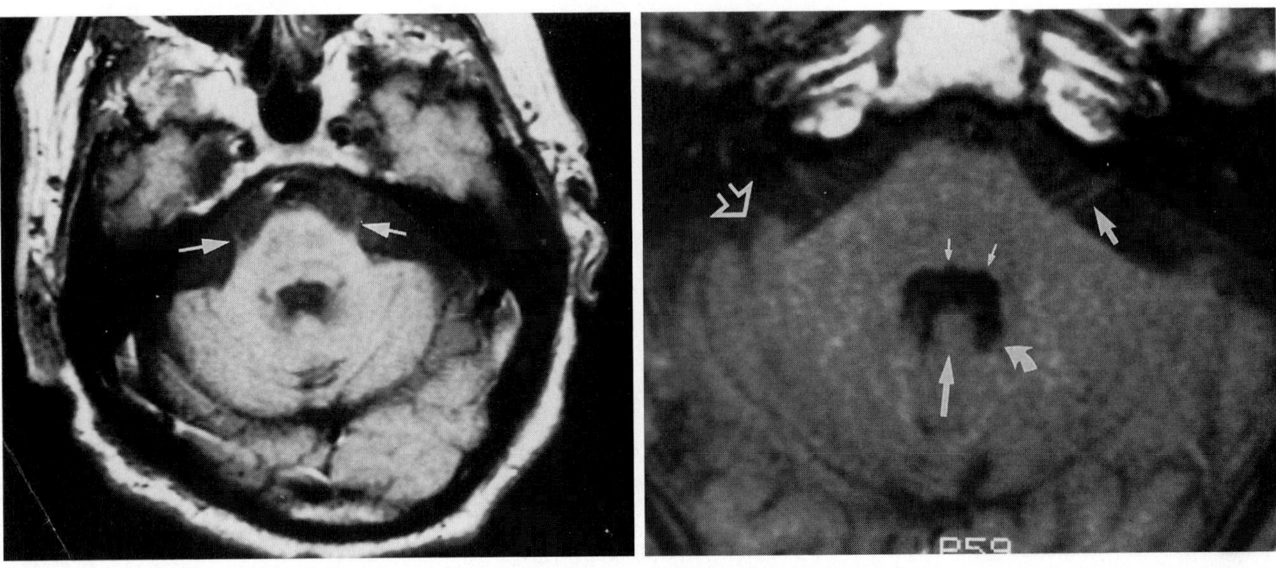

A B

Figure 3.31. A. T1-weighted cross section through the pons reveals the fourth ventricle and its anatomical components as described in B and C. The fifth nerves are seen to arise from the lateral aspect of the pons and to move anteriorly through the cisterna pontis to reach Meckel's cave (arrows). **B.** Cross section through the pons, T1-weighted image. The section is at the level of the seventh and eighth nerves, which can be seen crossing the cerebellopontine cistern on each side (arrow). The fourth ventricle reveals the median sulcus (small arrows); on each side is the median eminence, delineated laterally by the sulcus limitans (small arrow to right). Under the median eminence are the nuclei of the sixth and seventh nerves, which give the median eminence the name *colliculus facialis.* The posterior extensions of the fourth ventricle represent the posterior superior recesses (curved arrow). Between them is the nodule (long-stem arrow). On each side of the fourth ventricle, anterolaterally, is the middle cerebellar peduncle (brachium pontis). The anterior margin of the pons is slightly irregular because the cut was near the pontomedullary junction. The open arrowhead points at the flocculus (10,11).

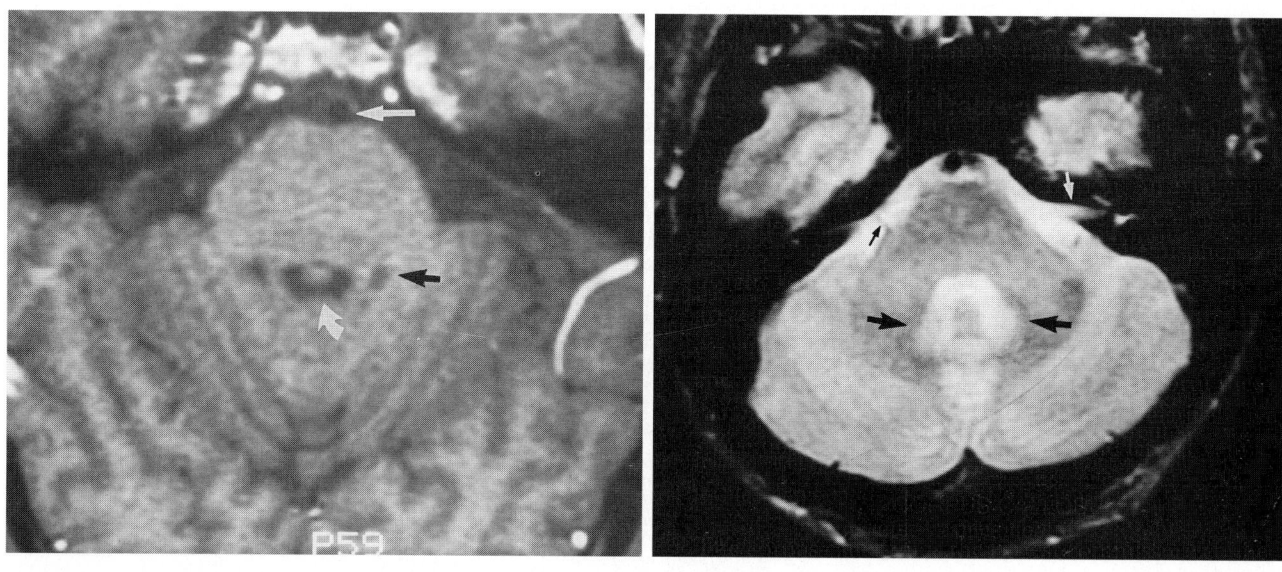

C D

Figure 3.31. *(continued)* **C.** Section 4 mm above B, T1-weighted image. The section is above the fastigium of the fourth ventricle. The basilar artery shows a normal flow void (arrow). The anterior (superior) medullary velum is shown at the curved white arrow. Inside the fourth ventricle is soft tissue, which may represent some redundant choroid plexus. On each side of the fourth ventricle is a CSF-containing symmetrical space that is seen on axial images in many MRI and CT examinations (also seen in A). It represents a subarachnoid space around the fourth ventricle (arrow); see also Figure 3.20. The occipital lobes are surrounding the cerebellum as the latter becomes smaller. **D.** T2-weighted image passing at the same level as B. The posterior superior recesses are seen (arrows), and between tem is the nodule. The cerebellopontine cistern is now bright; the anterior-inferior cerebellar artery is seen on the right (small black arrow). The internal acoustic canal is now bright (CSF-containing), and the inner ear structures are seen lateral to it.

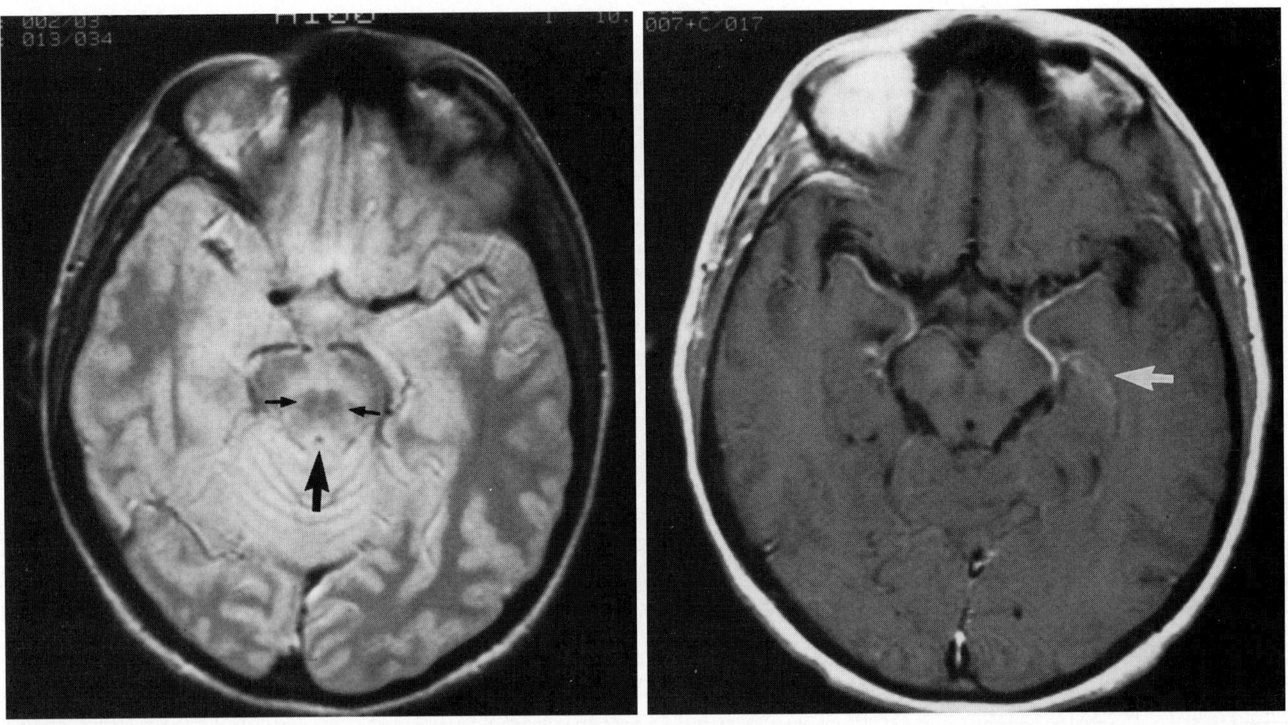

A B

Figure 3.32. MR cross-sectional images through midbrain. **A.** Inferior aspect. The aqueduct surrounded by periaqueductal gray matter is well seen (vertical arrow) on a first-echo T2-weighted image. The decussation of the superior cerebellar peduncles is well seen (horizontal small arrows). Immediately in front is the substantia nigra, which on first-echo T2-weighted image does not show the magnetic susceptibility from iron accumulation. The interpeduncular fossa is not clearly seen in the midline because the CSF is isointense. Anterior to the peduncles is the flow void of the posterior cerebral (and superior cerebellar?) arteries on each side. **B.** T1-weighted image, after contrast, at the same level shows the same structures. The interpeduncular fossa is now well seen. The basal vein on each side is well shown originating in the deep temporal region and coming around the uncus of the hippocampus and around the midbrain as it proceeds backward and upward (going off this slice) to join the vein of Galen. Lateral to the crus cerebri on each side is the temporal horn containing the contrast-enhanced choroid plexus (arrow).

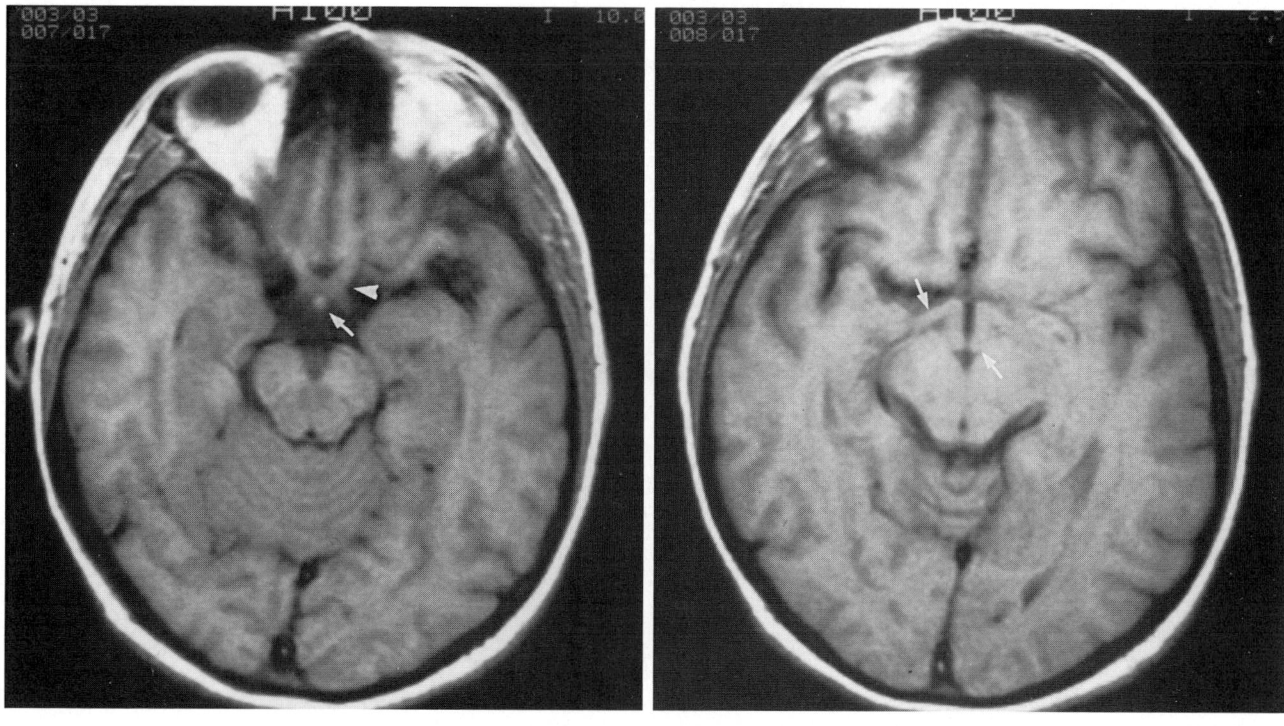

C D

Figure 3.32. *(continued)* **C.** T1-weighted image, same level, before contrast. The pituitary stalk (arrow) and the optic chiasm are shown in front of the midbrain (arrowhead). **D.** A higher cross section, T1-weighted, shows the interpeduncular fossa, within which are seen the mammillary tubercles (small arrow) and the hypothalamus on each side of the third ventricle. From the hypothalamus are seen to spring the optic tracts (small arrow on right). Since the patient's head was canted toward the right, the section is slightly higher on the left than on the right. Thus, the outline of the left peduncle (crus) is not seen as it merges with the thalamus.

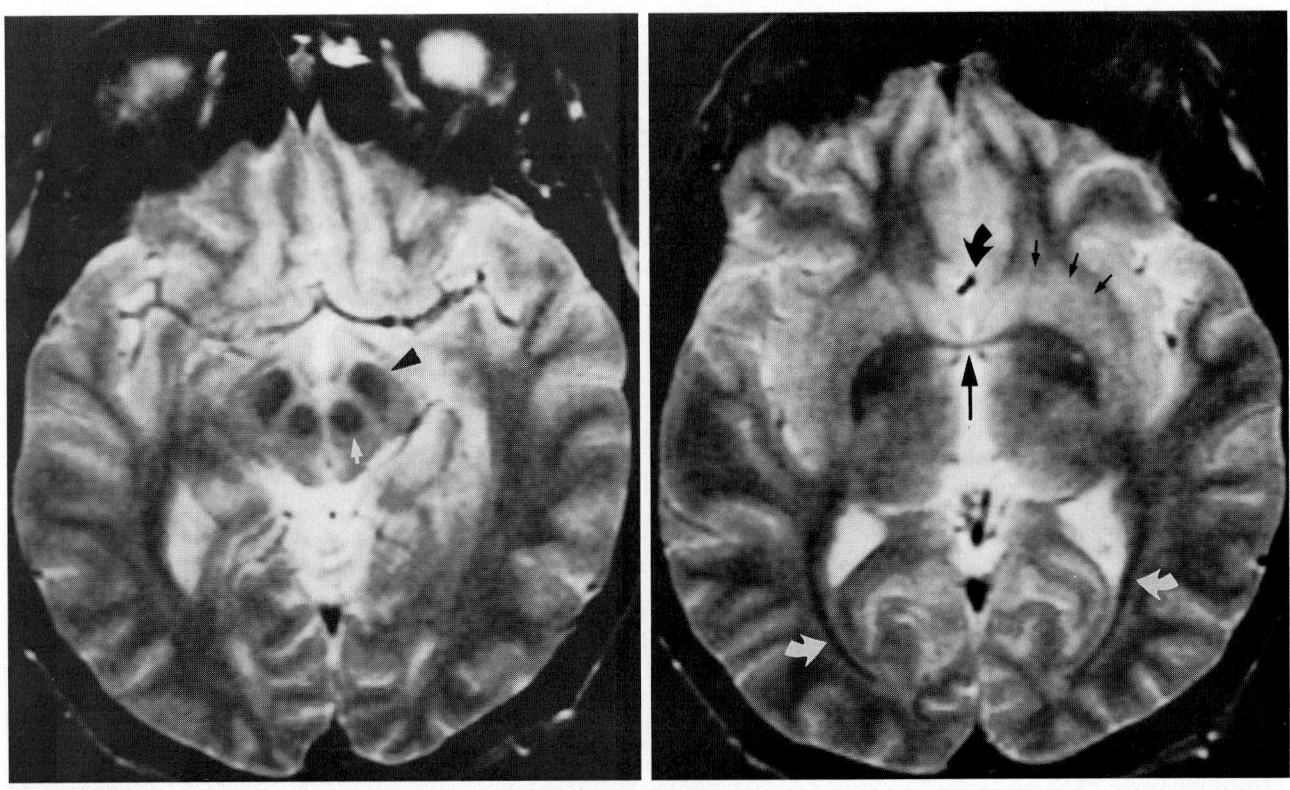

Figure 3.33. A to **C.** Normal brainstem and basal ganglia containing iron in a 27-year-old man. **A.** T2-weighted image shows rather low intensity over the red nucleus (small white arrow) and substantia nigra (arrowhead) on both sides as the result of normal iron accumulation. This susceptibility effect is much more pronounced in images made with a higher-strength magnet (1.5 T), than with a lower-strength one. **B.** A higher section passing through the lower aspect of the basal ganglia shows iron (magnetic susceptibility) in the globus pallidus. The putamen does not show evidence of susceptibility effect from iron accumulation. Note that in this lower section through the basal ganglia the putamen is practically merged with the head of the caudate nucleus (small arrows). The black vertical arrow is over the third ventricle and points at the anterior commissure, a dark, thin band extending across, presenting the shape of a bicycle handlebar. On each side of the arrowhead is a low-intensity image produced by the columns of the fornix. Anterior to the commissure are two faint, low-intensity areas on each side of the midline, probably representing a flow effect of CSF on each side of the Y-shaped foramen of Monro. About 1 cm anterior to the commissure is an elongated, very dark, somewhat oblique dash representing a flow void of the two anterior cerebral arteries (curved black arrow). The two white arrows posteriorly represent the optic radiation passing lateral to the atrium of the lateral ventricles and curving toward the calcarine fissure in the medial occipital lobe.

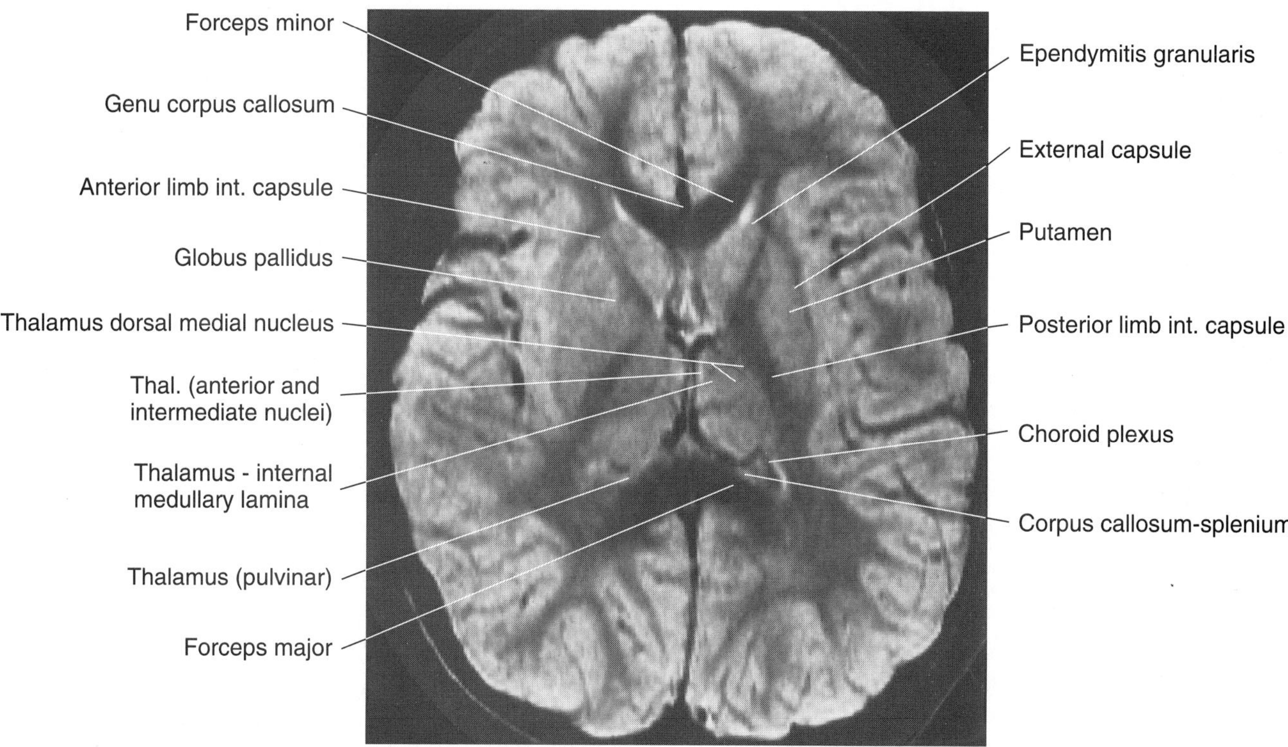

C

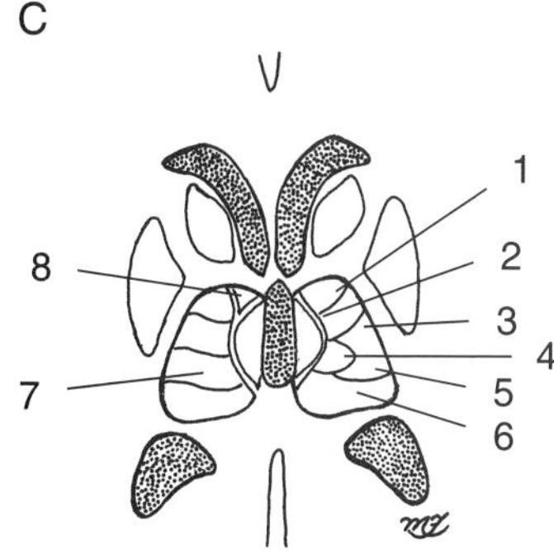

D

Figure 3.33. *(continued)* **C.** Proton density axial view passing through the basal ganglia region. **D.** Diagram of thalamic region in axial projection to show position of thalamic nuclei. 1, anterior ventral nucleus; 2, dorsal medial nucleus; 3, intermediate ventral nucleus; 4, centromedial nucleus; 5, posterolateral ventral nucleus; 6, pulvinar; 7, posterior lateral nucleus; 8, anterior nucleus. (Courtesy of TM Koci, et al: AJNR 1990;11:1229–1233, with permission.)

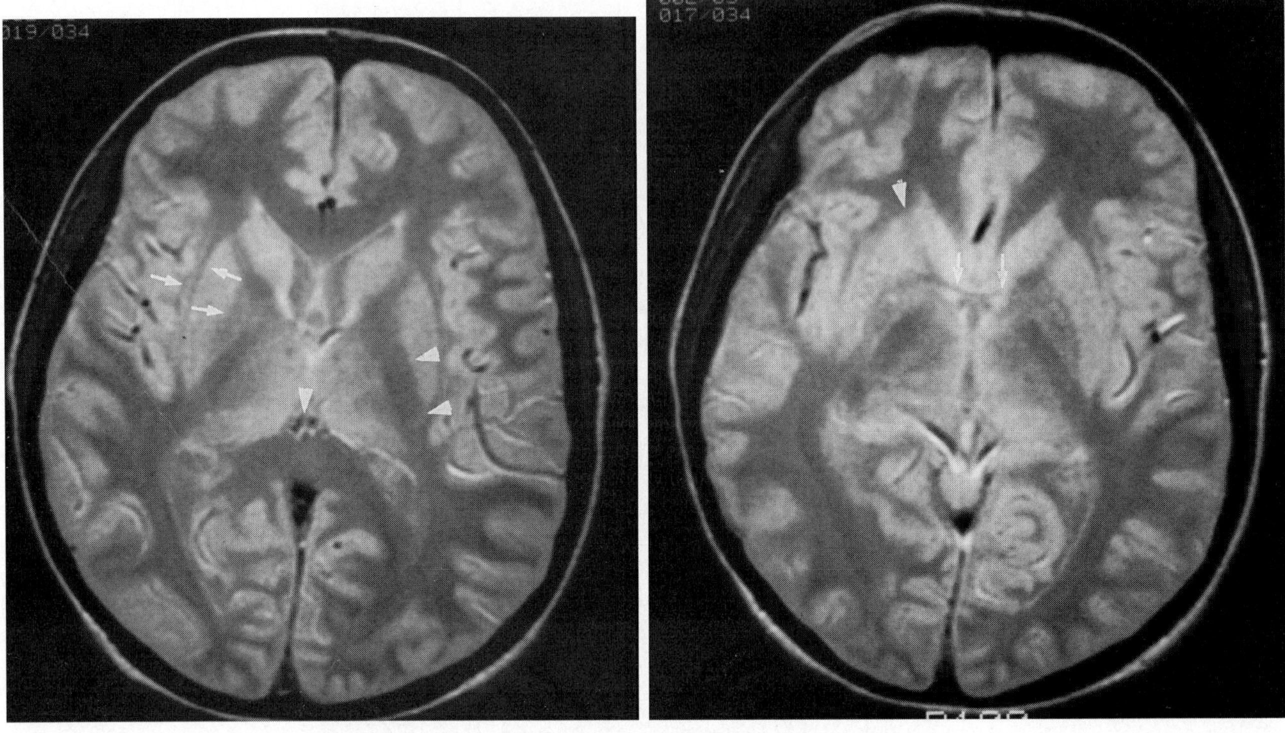

A B

Figure 3.34. Normal axial views of the brain. **A.** Axial view passing through the inferior aspect of the lateral ventricles. Because the head is slightly canted toward the right, the globus pallidus is well seen on the patient's right side (right small arrow) but passes just below it on the left. For that reason, the posterior limb of the internal capsule is better seen on the left than on the right (arrowheads). Because this is a first-echo T2-weighted image (proton density), the CSF within the ventricle is almost isointense with the white matter. The frontal horn tips have a hyperintense appearance, probably due to ependymitis granularis, a normal finding in this 27-year-old man. Lateral to the putamen is the external capsule (white matter, small arrow pointing laterally), and immediately lateral to it is the claustrum, a thin shell of gray matter (small arrow pointing medially). Both can be seen in this image. The claustrum is just medial to the insular cortex. Lateral to the insula is the sylvian fissure. The two internal cerebral veins are seen in cross section (arrowhead) in front of the splenium of the corpus callosum. **B.** Proton density axial image passing lower than A. At this level the putamen and the caudate nuclei are almost fused; the anterior limb of the internal capsule is very thin (arrowhead). The putamen is brighter than the globus pallidus. The posterior limb of the internal capsule between the globus pallidus and the thalamus is not clearly seen; the thalamus is joining the cerebral peduncles. The anterior commissure is well seen (arrows) extending out toward the temporal lobes. The basal veins show a flow void. However, there is a parallel bright band behind them that represents an artifact caused by a misregistration of the phase encoding secondary to the oblique flow.

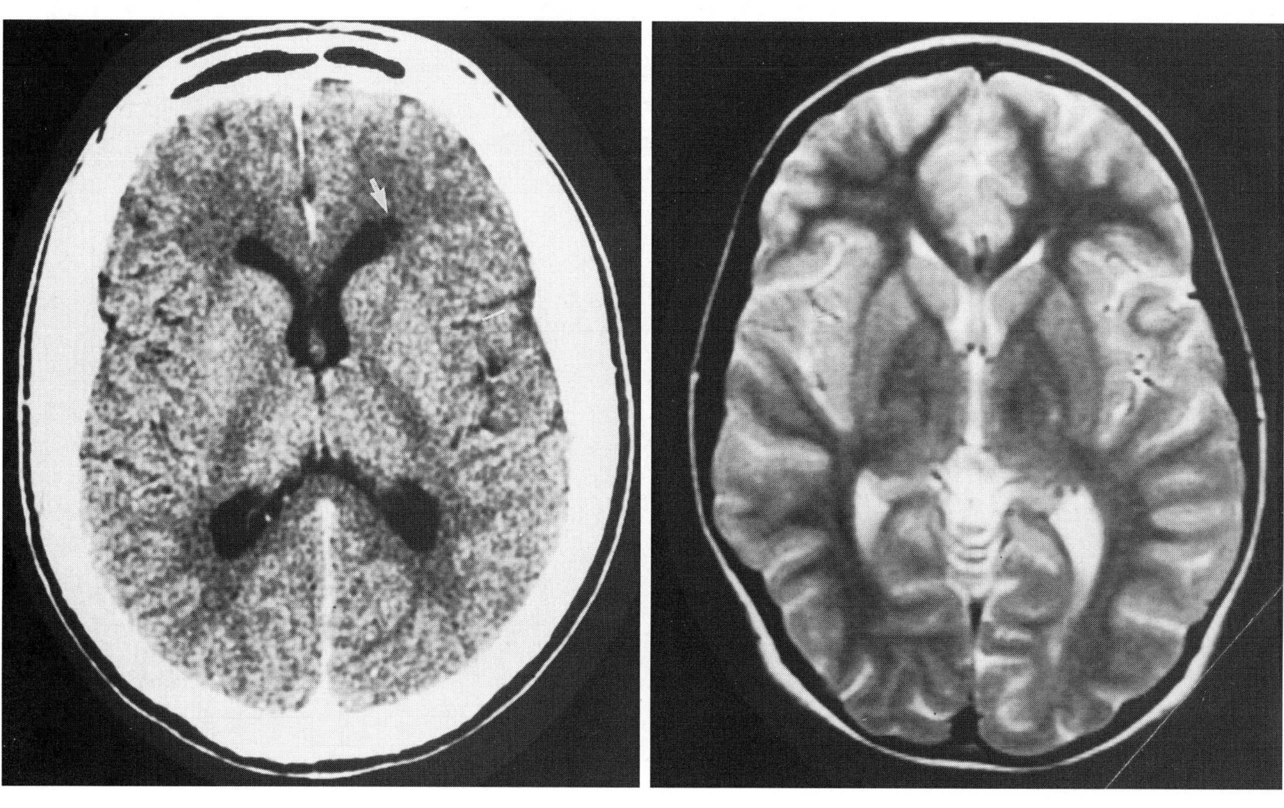

Figure 3.34. *(continued)* **C.** Axial CT image passing through the same area. The internal capsules are well seen on both sides, as well as the basal ganglia and thalami. The arrow points at a small diverticulum of the left frontal horn of the lateral ventricle, which is a normal variant. **D.** T2-weighted image in another subject. The anatomy is similar. The ventricles are now white, as are the surface sulci.

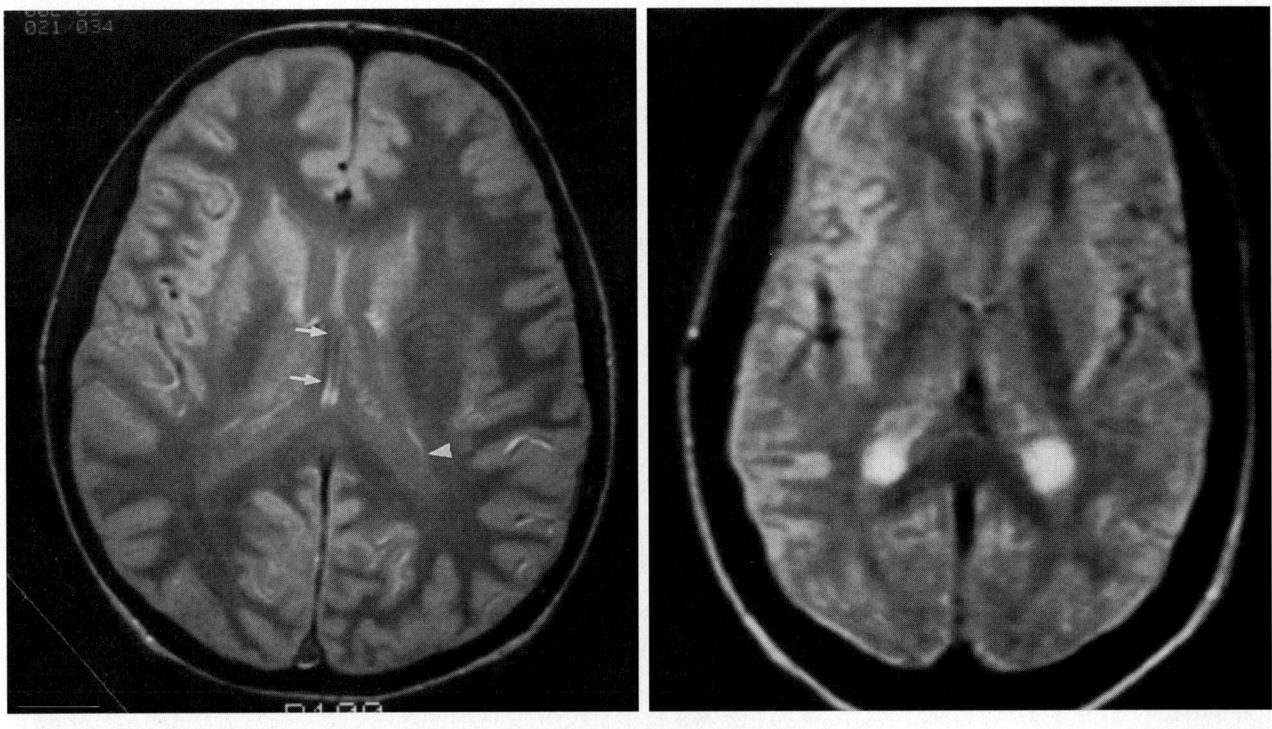

A B

Figure 3.35. Normal axial view 7 mm higher than 3.34*A,* same subject. **A.** View passing higher through the lateral ventricles. The putamen is still visible on the right but not on the left because the head is tilted. Lateral to the putamen is the external capsule, and immediately lateral to it is the insular cortex, followed by the sylvian fissure, which contains some flow voids caused by the arteries within it, and two layers of gray matter, the medial cortex of the operculum and the lateral insular surface. The internal capsule is wider in this higher slice than in Figure 3.34. The two internal cerebral veins show up bright, probably because of slow flow. This is a postcontrast scan, but it is a proton density image. There are also a few fragments of cortical veins, which are bright. The glomus of the choroid plexus is slightly hypointense in relation to the CSF (arrowhead); compare with B. **B.** Proton density axial image in a patient with xanthomatous degeneration of the choroid glomus.

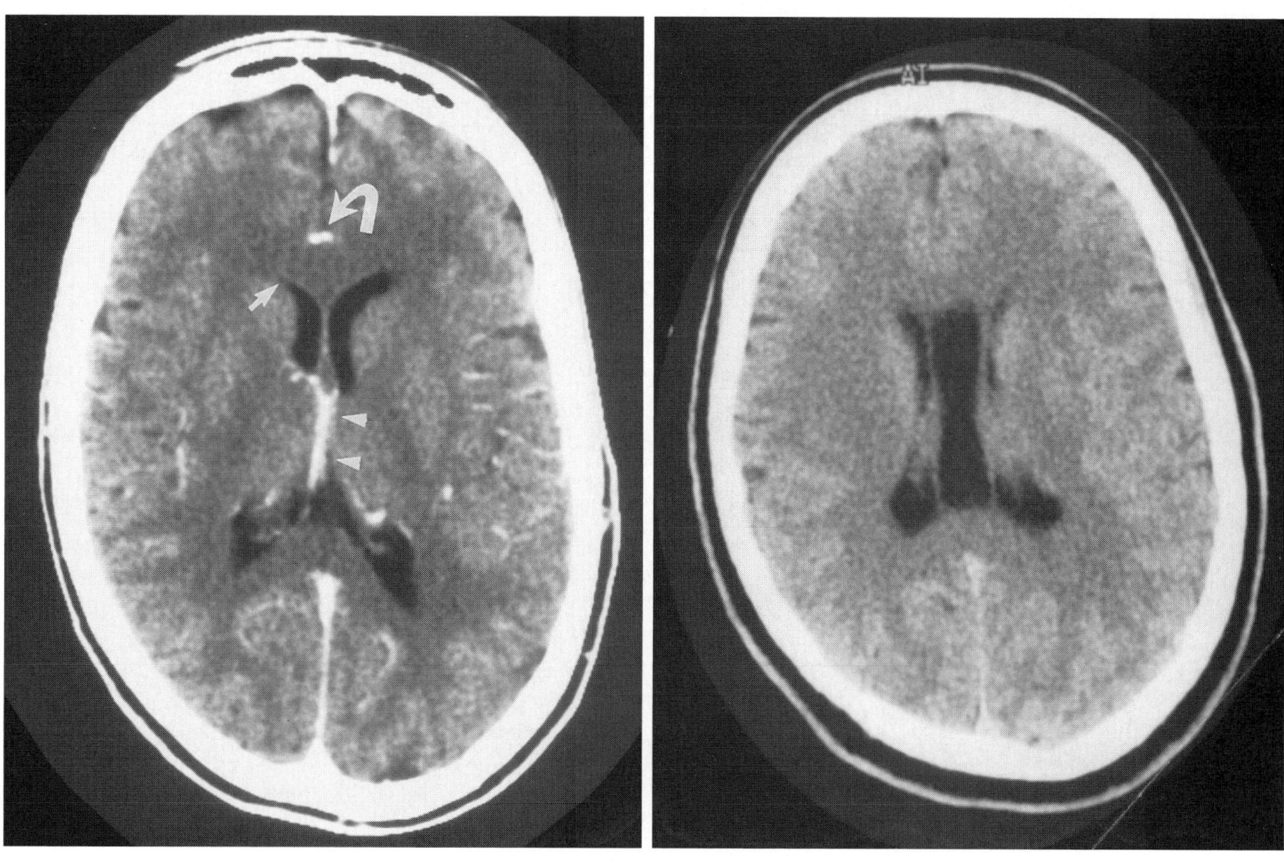

A B

Figure 3.36. Normal axial views. **A.** CT image after contrast shows that the right frontal horn of the lateral ventricle ends in a sharp point as compared to the left (arrow). This is caused by coarctation of the lateral angle of the ventricle, a normal finding that should not be confused with ventricular compression or periventricular edema. The two anterior cerebral arteries are seen anterior to the genu of the corpus callosum (curved arrow), and the internal cerebral veins are also well opacified (arrowheads). **B.** The axial CT image at the level of the ventricles shows a large "cystic" elongated space between the lateral ventricles representing the cavum septum pellucidum and cavum vergae. This is a normal variant. It is frequently seen in young infants but usually disappears as the child grows older.

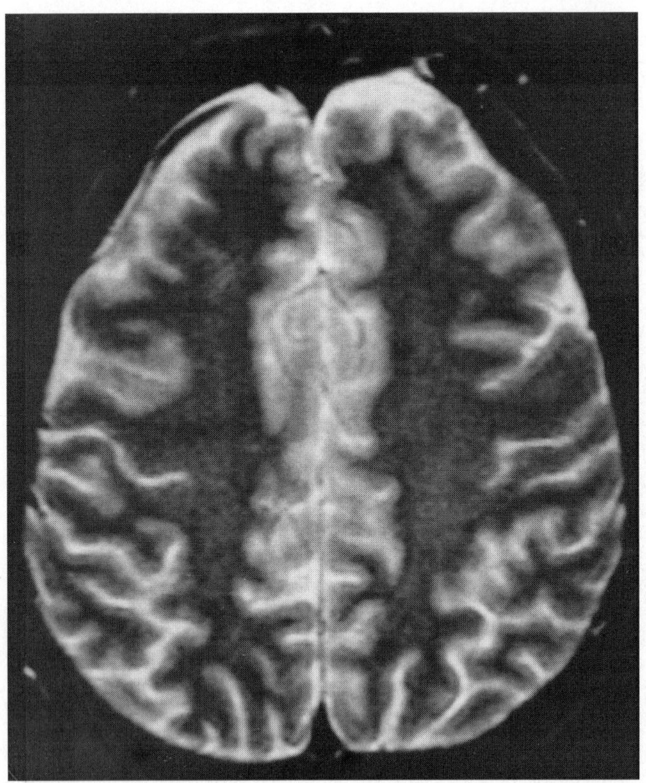

Figure 3.37. Centrum semiovale seen in a T2-weighted axial view. The myelinated white matter is dark. The term *semiovale* refers to the half-moon shape of the white matter in each hemisphere. The size of the white matter space between the lateral and medial cortex is somewhat variable. It is usually well developed, as in this subject. At other times there appears to be a narrower centrum semiovale with the cortical convolutions crowding the center in normal young adults, and particularly in children of 5 to 15 years. In the latter group this may be part of the growth process. The brain is fully myelinated by the age of 9, but the thickness of the myelin sheaths continues to increase for some years.

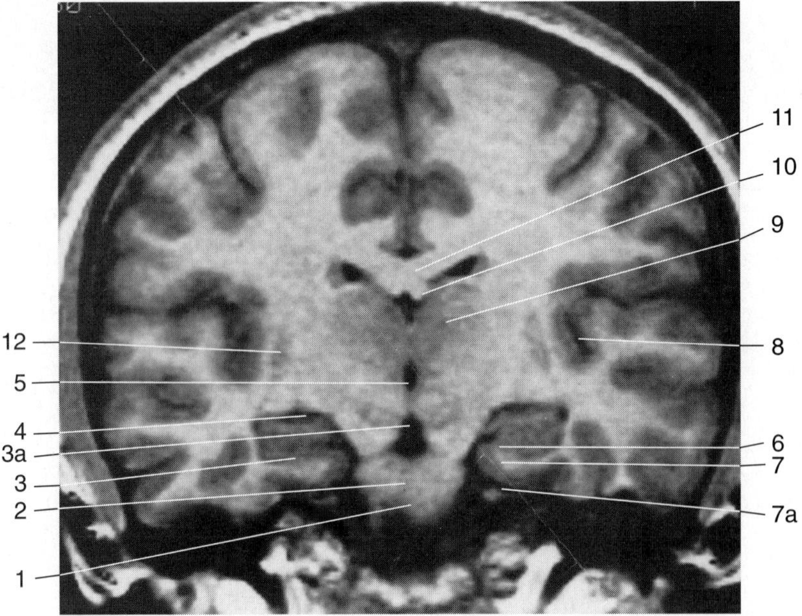

Figure 3.38. Coronal section of brain passing through the anterior portion of the temporal horn, T1-weighted image. 1, belly of the pons; 2, interpeduncular fossa; 3, hippocampus; 3a, substantia nigra; 4, temporal horn; 5, third ventricle; 6, hippocampal fissure; 7, subiculum; 7a, fifth cranial nerve; 8, sylvian fissure; 9, thalamus; 10, fornix; 11, corpus callosum; 12, claustrum, anterior aspect.

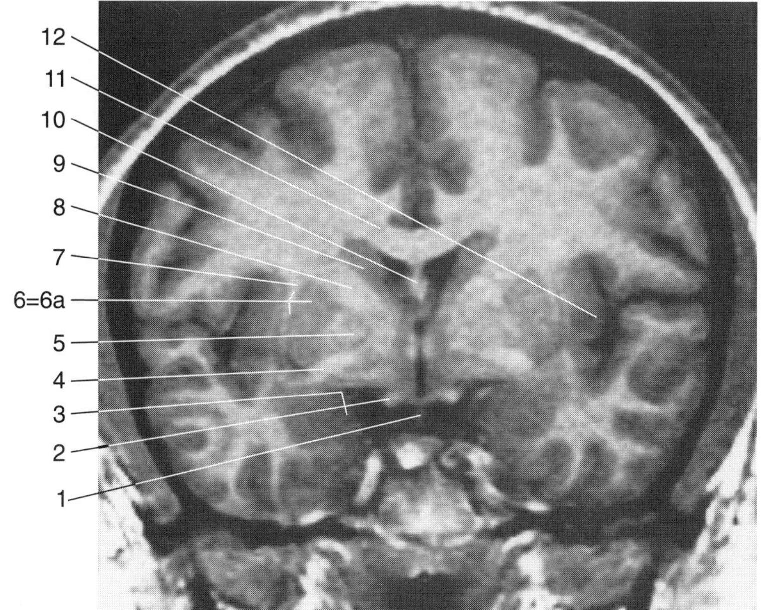

Figure 3.39. Coronal T1-weighted image passing 1.0 cm in front of image in Figure 3.38: 1, pituitary stalk; 2, optic tract; 3, hippocampus; 4, anterior commissure, lateral extension; 5, globus pallidus; 6, putamen; 6a, claustrum; 7, external capsule; 8, internal capsule; 9, caudate nucleus; 10, fornix; 11, corpus callosum; 12, insular surface of gray matter.

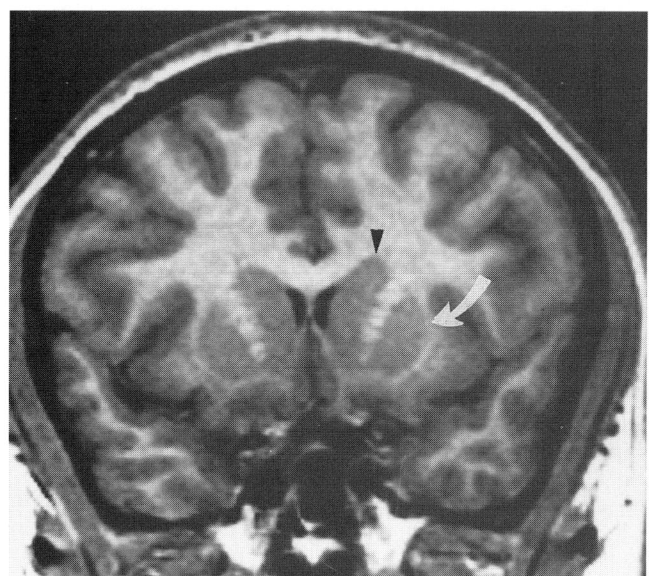

Figure 3.40. Coronal section about 1.0 cm anterior to section in Figure 3.39, T1-weighted image. On each side, the caudate nucleus (upper arrow) and the lenticular nucleus (curved arrow) are coming closer together and are now clearly connected by the striations that give the corpus striatum its name. The temporal lobes are now completely separated from the frontal lobes.

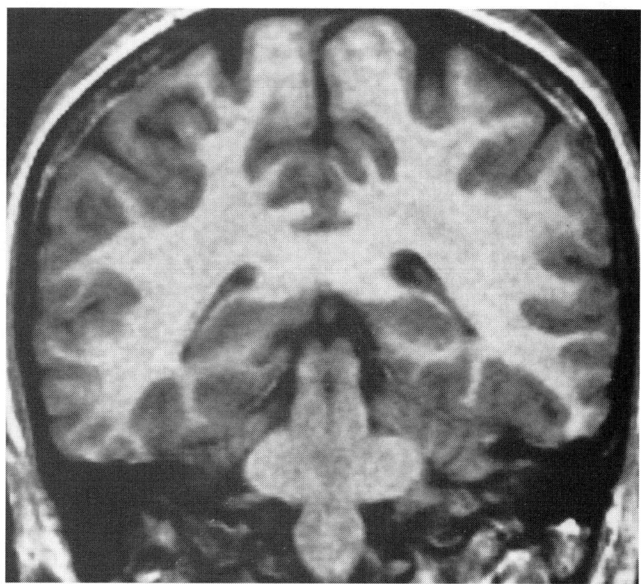

Figure 3.41. Coronal T1-weighted image passing through the atrium of the lateral ventricles. The atrium of the lateral ventricles is shown on each side, diverging downward and laterally (arrows). Medial to the atrium is the hippocampal formation. Above and lateral to the atria are the corpus callosum and the tapetum.

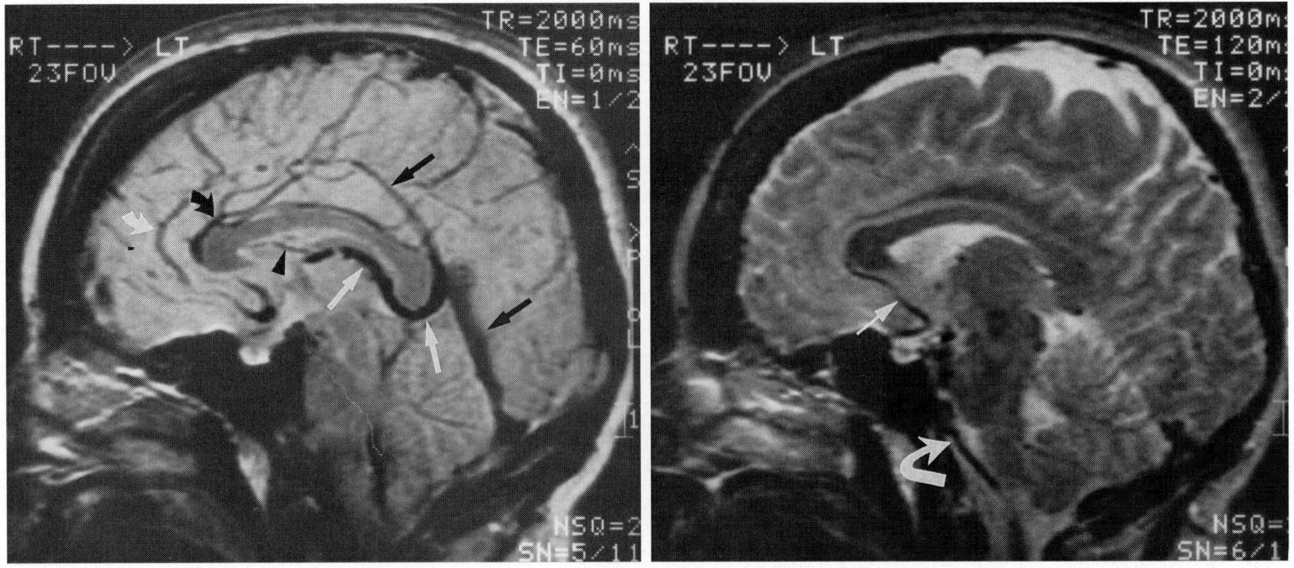

A B

Figure 3.42. Sagittal images near midline. **A.** Proton density (first-echo, T2-weighted) image. Image is slightly off the midline, showing flow voids corresponding to venous and arterial flow. The venous flow is particularly prominent; visible are the inferior sagittal sinus and straight sinus (black arrows); the internal cerebral veins and the vein of Galen (white arrows); the septal vein (black arrowhead); and the pericallosal (curved black arrow) and cellosomarginal arteries (curved white arrow). Ascending veins on the medial surface of the hemisphere are seen as flow voids. **B.** T2-weighted midline sagittal views. Only the basilar artery posteriorly (curved arrow) and the anterior cerebral artery (white arrow) are seen because this is closer to being a midline section.

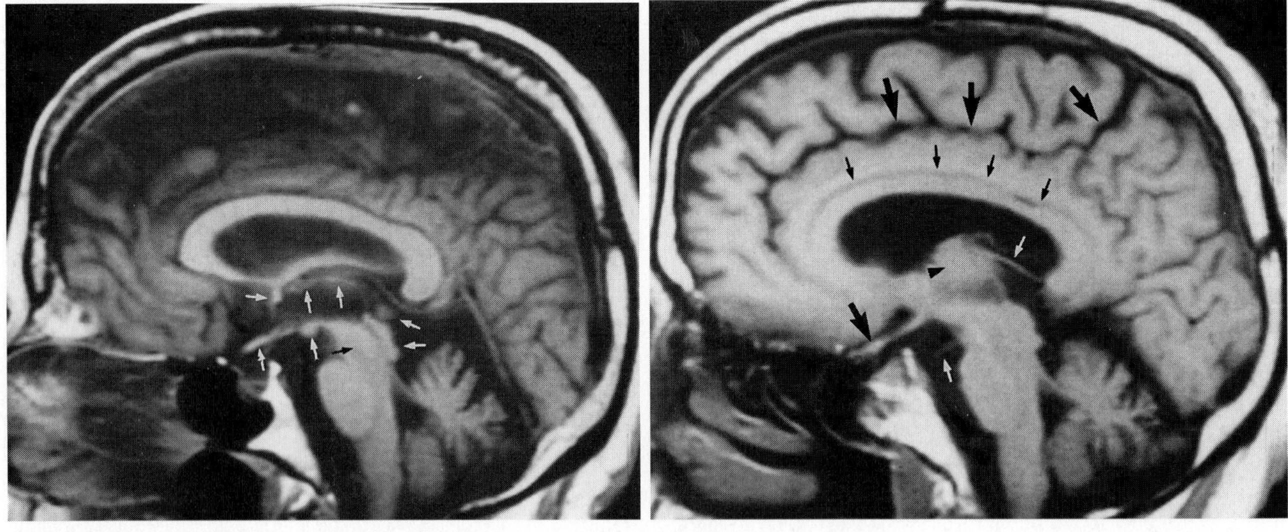

A B

Figure 3.43. Sagittal images. **A.** Midline section. It shows well, from front to back (arrows), the anterior commissure, the choroid plexus of the third ventricle below the fornix, the pineal gland (above it is the internal cerebral vein and the vein of Galen), and the quadrigeminal plate. The lower arrows show the optic chiasm, the mammillary tubercle, the interpeduncular fossa, and the tegmentum of the midbrain (black arrow). **B.** Section 7.5 mm lateral to the midline. The thalamus is now seen (arrowhead), as well as the internal cerebral vein (upper white arrow), the optic nerves and tract (lower anterior arrow), the third nerve (lower arrow) crossing the premesencephalic CSF space, and the cingulate gyrus, separated from the corpus callosum by the pericallosal sulcus (small arrows). The cingulate sulcus continues back and up behind the paracentral lobule (three arrows).

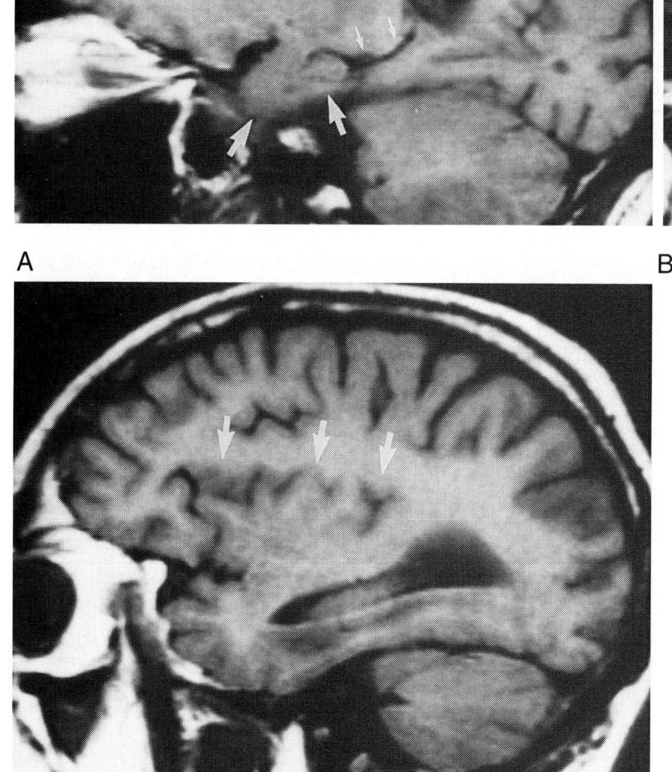

A

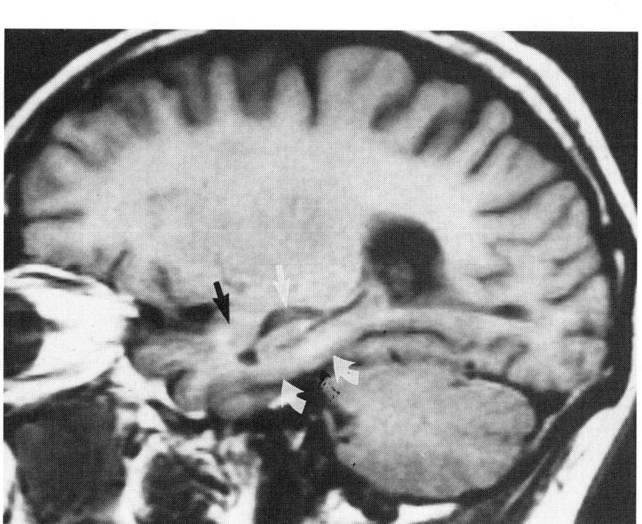

B

C

Figure 3.44. Sagittal MR T1-weighted image passing through temporal lobe. **A.** Hippocampus (white arrow); choroidal fissure swings under and behind thalamus (small white arrows). **B.** Section passing 5 mm more laterally than A. Temporal horn (white vertical arrow); amygdaloid nucleus (black arrow); parahippocampal gyrus (curved white arrows). **C.** Section passing 5 mm more laterally than B. The temporal horn is cut in its entire length and followed as it joins the atrium. The upper margin of the insula between its surface and the medial aspect of the frontoparietal operculum is well seen at this level (three white arrows).

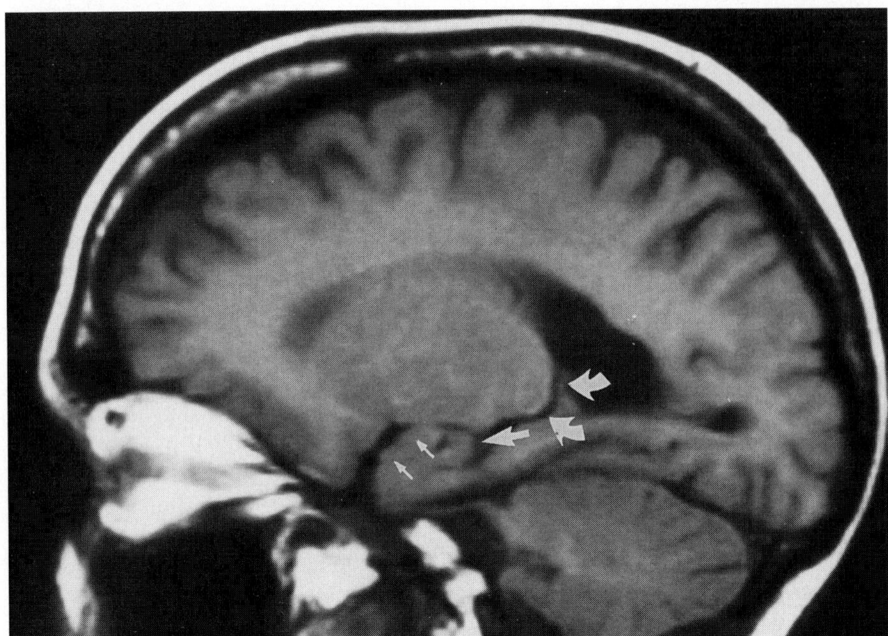

Figure 3.45. Hippocampus. Uncus of hippocampus (white arrow); pes hippocampi (small white arrows); choroid fissure and pulvinar of thalamus (curved white arrows).

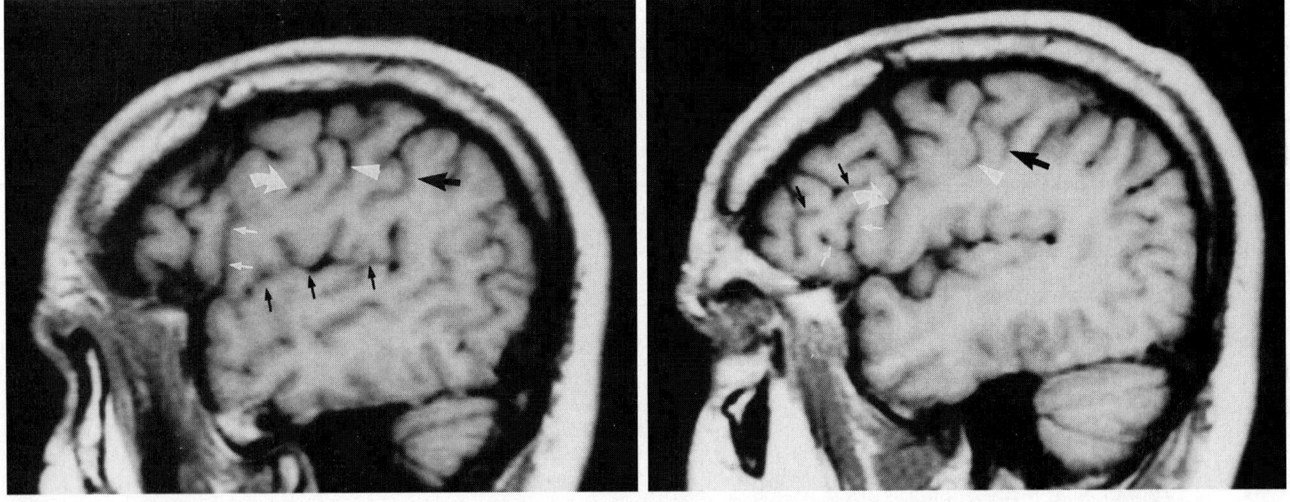

A B

Figure 3.46. Lateral aspect of hemisphere. **A.** Sagittal T1-weighted image approximately 45 mm from the midline shows the sylvian fissure running nearly horizontally (small black arrows) (compare with Fig. 3.4). The anterior ascending ramus extending from the sylvian fissure (small white arrows) separates the pars triangularis, in front, from the pars opercularis behind it. The precentral sulcus does not reach the sylvian fissure in this case (curved white arrow). The inferior frontal sulcus is not well seen in this image and at this depth from the surface. The central sulcus (white arrowhead) and the postcentral sulcus (black arrow) are visible. The central sulcus *does not* reach the sylvian fissure in about 90% of cases. **B.** At 40 mm from the midline the inferior aspect of the precentral sulcus is more defined (curved white arrow). The ascending ramus (small white arrow) and the anterior horizontal ramus (anterior small white arrow) are well seen. The central sulcus (white arrowhead) and the postcentral sulcus (black arrow) are again seen. The inferior frontal sulcus is seen more clearly (small black arrows).

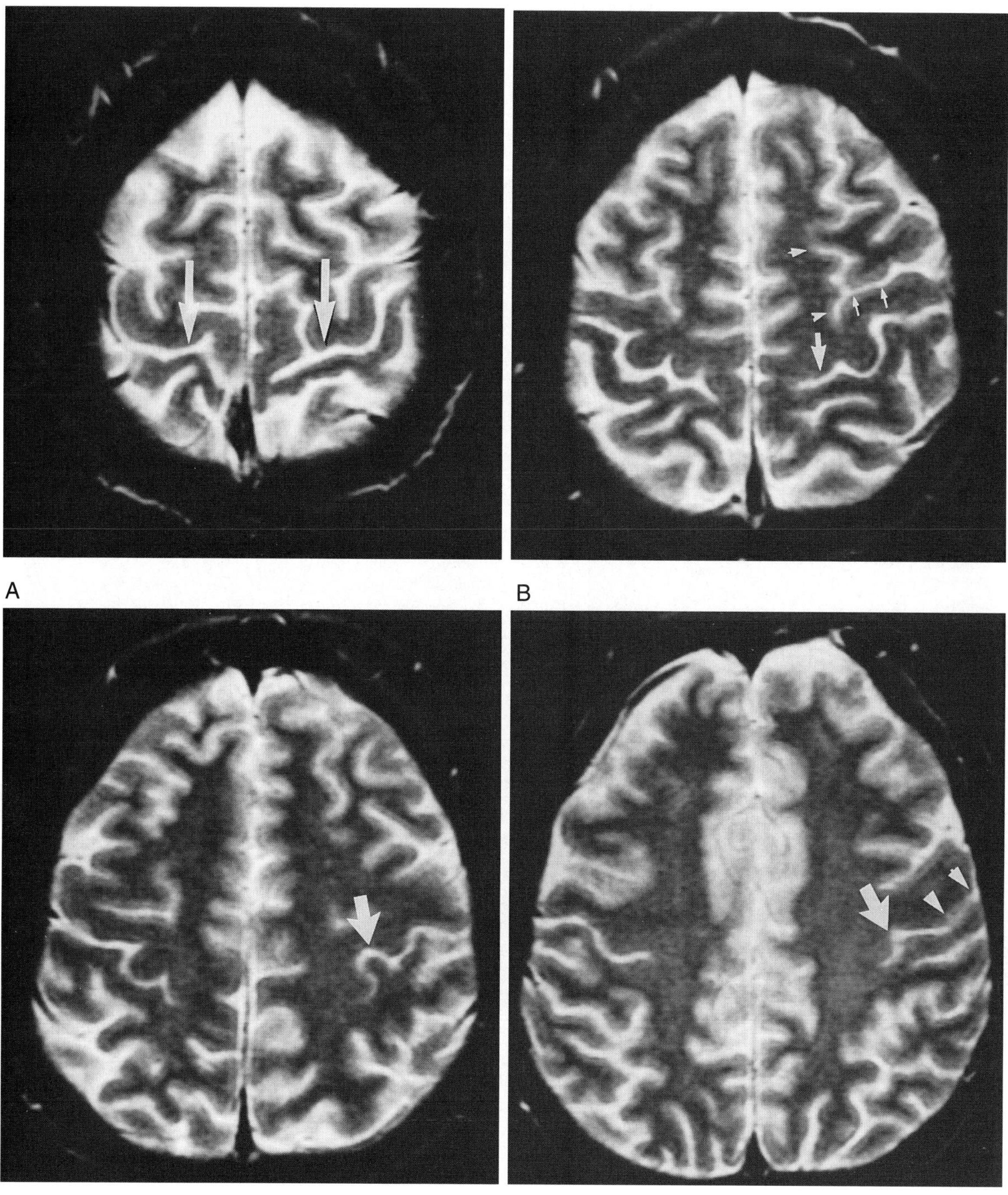

Figure 3.47. Normal brain, T2-weighted axial images. The central sulcus can be identified in sections through the superior aspect of the hemispheres with greater accuracy. With the usual head position, the slices are approximately parallel to the infraorbitomeatal line (Reid's base line); the central sulcus is closer to the center in the sections above the sylvian fissure and moves back closer to the dorsal edge of the brain image as the section approaches the top. Thus it is best to start with the highest slices, in which the longest sulcus, almost reaching the dorsally located midline, is usually the central sulcus (arrows in A, B, C, D). Note that in D, the lowest section (2.3 cm below A), the central sulcus is in the middle of the brain as it reaches the lateral brain surface (arrowheads). In front of it is the precentral gyrus, which has to do with motor function, and behind it is the postcentral gyrus, which is involved in sensory function. The superior frontal gyrus, extending from front to back, ends in the precentral sulcus, and this gyrus can be used to identify the central sulcus. The arrows in A are over the superior frontal gyrus (it shows an anatomical variant), and the arrow in B is also over the superior frontal gyrus. In B the precentral sulcus is marked by the small white arrows; the superior frontal sulcus is marked by the white arrowheads (12,13,14). The precentral sulcus can usually be recognized because it is interrupted by the superior frontal sulcus, as shown in B.

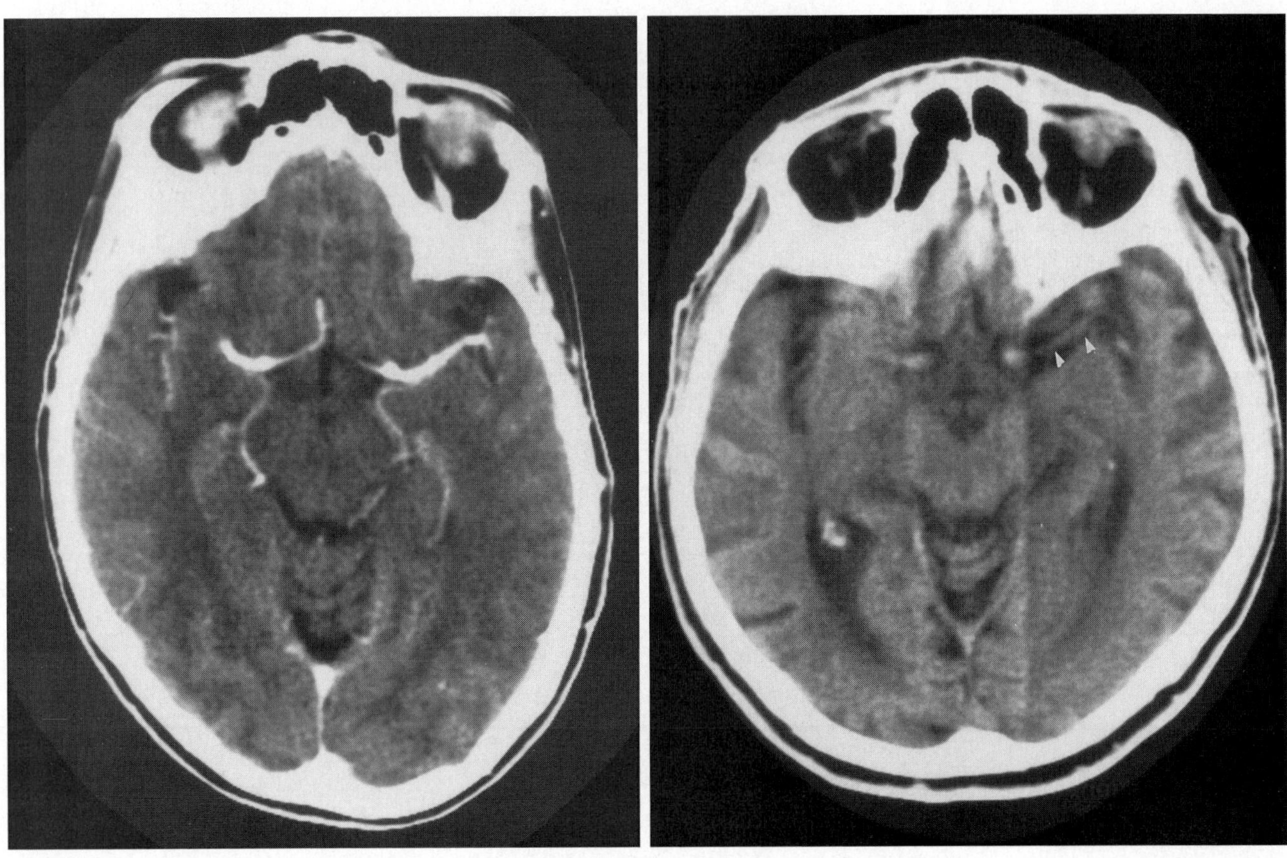

Figure 3.48. Arteries with and without contrast seen on CT images. **A.** With contrast, most of the components of the circle of Willis are visible. However, the first segments of the posterior cerebral arteries are not seen, probably because they are just below the slice, along with the top of the basilar artery. The right anterior cerebral artery is slightly larger than the left. **B.** A noncontrast CT scan in another patient. The top of the internal carotid arteries and the middle cerebral arteries are seen within the sylvian cistern (arrowheads) because this patient has some cerebral atrophy. It is frequent to see this segment of the middle cerebral artery even in young patients, and it should not be taken to represent pathology such as thrombosis. Only rarely does one see a dense middle cerebral artery in a patient with a stroke on the same side.

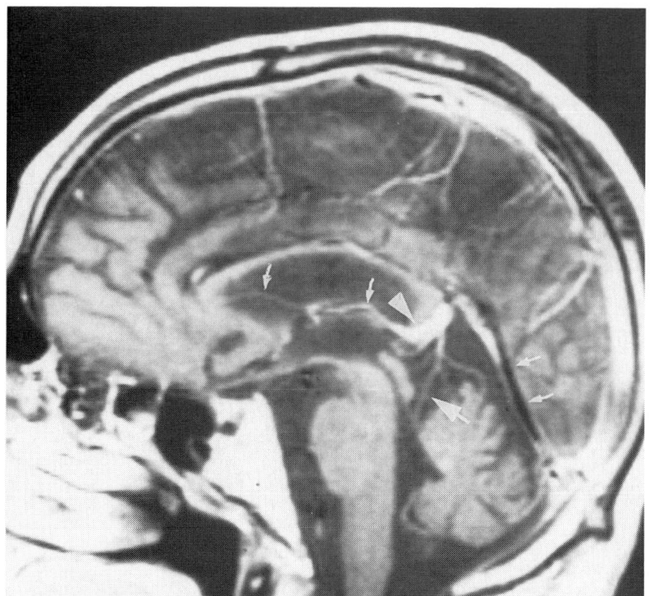

Figure 3.49. Postcontrast T1-weighted midline sagittal image. The contrast has enhanced any veins that present a relatively low speed of flow. The arteries are not usually so visible with contrast because the speed of flow is higher. In this instance, the straight sinus presents a flow void (small arrows), indicating a higher flow velocity. The surface midline veins are seen to join the superior sagittal sinus. The septal vein and internal cerebral veins are well seen (arrows) as they join the vein of Galen (arrowhead). Also note the precentral cerebellar vein (lower arrow) joining other superior cerebellar draining veins to end apparently in the vein of Galen, but they may have first joined the basal vein, which is not clearly shown here.

REFERENCES

1. Broca P: Remarques sur la siège de la faculté du langage articulé, suivies d'une observation d'abhemie (père de là parole). Bull Soc Anat (Paris) 1861;6:330.
2. Broca P: Anatomie comparée circonvolutions cérébrales. Le grand lobe limbique et la scissure limbique dans la série des mammifères. Rev Anthropol 1878;Ser. 2, 1:384–498.
3. Corrales M, Greitz T: Fourth ventricle: 1. A morphologic and radiologic investigation of the normal anatomy. Acta Radiol (Diagn) 1972; 12:113–133.
4. Daniels DL, Haughton MM, Williams AL, Berns TF: The flocculus in computed tomography. AJNR 1981;2:227–229.
5. Loes DJ, Barloon TJ, Yuh WTC, DeLaPaz RL, Sato Y: MR anatomy and pathology of the hypothalamus. AJR 1991;156:579–585.
6. Curnes JT, Burger PC, Djang WT, Boyko OB: MR imaging of compact white matter pathways. AJNR 1988;9:1061–1068.
7. LeMay M: Left-right dyssymmetry—handedness. AJNR 1992;13: 493–504.
8. McRae DL, Branch CL, Milner B: The occipital horns and cerebral dominance. Neurology 1968;18:433–438.
9. Hochberg FH, LeMay M: Arteriographic correlates of handedness. Neurology 1975;25:218–222.
10. Flannigan BD, Bradley WG, Mazziotta JC, et al: Magnetic resonance imaging of the brainstem: Normal structure and basic functional anatomy. Radiology 1985;154:375–383.
11. Hirsch WL, Kemp SS, Martinez AJ, et al: Anatomy of the brainstem: Correlation of in vitro MR images with histologic sections. AJNR 1989;10:923–928.
12. Eberlin U, Steinmetz H, Huang Y, Kahn T: Topography and identification of precentral sulcus in MR imaging. AJNR 1989;10: 937–942.
13. Febeling U, Steinmetz H, Huang Y, Kahn T: Topography and identification of the inferior precentral sulcus in MR imaging. AJNR 1989;10:937–942.
14. Vannier MW, Brunsden BS, Hildebolt CF, et al: Brain surface cortical sulcal lengths: Quantification with three-dimensional MR imaging. Radiology 1991;180:479–484.

SELECTED READINGS

Courchesne E, Press GA, Murakami J, Berthoty D: The cerebellum in sagittal plane-anatomic-MR correlation: I. The vermis. AJNR 1989; 10:659–665.

Heier LS, Bauer CJ, Schwartz L, et al: Large Virchow-Robin spaces: MR-clinical correlation. AJNR 1989;10:929–936.

Jack CR, Bentley MD, Twomey CK, Zinsmeister AR: MR imaging–based volume measurements of the hippocampal formation and anterior temporal lobe: Validation studies. Radiology 1990;176:205–209.

Koci TM, Chiang F, Chow P, et al: Thalamic extrapontine lesions in central pontine myelinolysis. AJNR 1990;11:1229–1233.

Lee BCP, Kneeland B, Knowles RJR, Chaill PT: Quantification of gray/ white matter in neonates and adults. AJNR 1983;4:692–695.

Press GA, et al: The cerebellum in sagittal plane—anatomic-MR correlation: 2. The cerebellar hemispheres. AJNR 1989;10:667–676.

Sedat J, Duvernoy H: Anatomical study of the temporal lobe. J Neuroradiol 1990;17:26–49.

Solsberg MD, Fournier D, Potts DG: MR imaging of the excised human brainstem: A correlative neuroanatomic study. AJNR 1990;11: 1003–1013.

Suzuki M, Takahima T, Kadoya M, et al: MR imaging of olfactory bulb and tract. AJNR 1989;10:955–957.

4

General Pathologic Conditions

This chapter considers four conditions that may be a component of many diseases of the nervous system and that are important to recognize as the images are analyzed. Some are important from the patient management point of view, and others have significance because they influence the differential diagnostic considerations. The four conditions are (a) brain calcification, (*b*) cerebral edema, (*c*) intracranial pressure and hydrocephalus, and (*d*) myelin and demyelination.

BRAIN CALCIFICATIONS

Deposition of calcium salts in tissues other than bone is a pathologic process known as *calcification*. In calcification the same salts concerned with ossification are deposited in tissue that is either dying or dead and from which cell structure has disappeared. In the presence of hypercalcemia, degeneration on the part of the tissues is not involved, and lime salts are deposited in living cells. More commonly, however, calcium is laid down in dead tissue without reference to blood calcium.

Necrosis and hyalin changes are the two chief antecedents of calcification. Physical rather than chemical structure appears to be the important factor in determining the deposition of calcium. Tissue inactivity results in a low carbon dioxide tension, and by diffusion the phosphate and carbonate calcium salts are absorbed by the hyalinized substance from the accessible body fluids of surrounding living tissue.

Another process of calcification, thought to occur less frequently, takes place through fatty degeneration.

Table 4.1.
Common Causes of Intracranial Calcification

A. Surface (extracerebral)
  1. Membranous
    a. Physiologic
      (1) Falx cerebri and superior longitudinal sinus
      (2) Falx cerebelli
      (3) Tentorium and petroclinoid ligaments
      (4) Diaphragma sellae, bridged clinoids
      (5) Dural plaques
      (6) Basal cell nevus syndrome
      (7) Arachnoid granulations
    b. Pathologic
      (1) Subdural hematoma
      (2) Psammomatous meningioma
      (3) Tuberculous meningitis
  2. Intrasellar and juxtasellar
    a. Craniopharyngioma
    b. Pituitary adenoma
    c. Cranial tumors of the basisphenoid
      (1) Chordoma
      (2) Osteochondroma
    d. Vascular
      (1) Arterial calcification
        i. Arteriosclerosis
        ii. Arterial aneurysm
        iii. Metastatic
      (2) Angiomatous malformations
        i. Venous angioma (Sturge-Weber)
        ii. Arteriovenous malformation
B. Deep (intracerebral)
  1. Localized
    a. Physiologic
      (1) Pineal
      (2) Habenular
      (3) Choroid
    b. Pathologic
      (1) Sturge-Weber syndrome
      (2) Neurofibromatosis
      (3) Cockayne syndrome
      (4) Fahr disease
      (5) Lipoid proteinosis
      (6) Wilson disease
      (7) Brain abscess
      (8) Granuloma (tuberculoma, etc.)
      (9) Hematoma
      (10) Dystrophy (from hemorrhage and/or necrosis)
      (11) Teratoma (dermoid and epidermoid)
      (12) Angioma
      (13) Arteriovenous malformation
      (14) Choroid plexus papilloma
      (15) Agyria
      (16) Other focal calcifications
      (17) Meningioma
      (18) Glioma (astrocytoma, oligodendrocytoma, retinoblastoma)
      (19) Xanthogranuloma
      (20) Postthyroidectomy
  2. Multiple scattered
    a. Tuberous sclerosis
    b. Encephalitis
      (1) Toxic
      (2) Viral
        (a) Cytomegalic inclusion disease
        (b) Rubella
        (c) Herpes simplex, etc.
      (3) Parasitic
        (a) Toxoplasmosis
        (b) Cysticercosis, paragonimiasis, sparganosis, etc.
    c. Metastatic neoplasm
    d. Endarteritis calcificans
    e. Miscellaneous
    f. Coccidioidomycosis
  3. Multiple symmetric
    a. Neoplastic (lipoma)
    b. Basal ganglia
      (1) Hypoparathyroidism
      (2) Pseudohypoparathyroidism
      (3) Fahr disease
      (4) Wilson disease
      (5) MELAS syndrome
    c. Dentate nucleus
    d. Red nucleus
    e. Hippocampus
    f. Cortical

Through hydrolysis of fat, a fatty acid is liberated when calcium is first deposited through union with the acid to form a calcium soap. Carbonate and phosphate later replace the fatty acid radical. Such a process probably occurs in fat necrosis and may be seen in a degenerating lipoma.

It is of interest that the calcification with which physicians ordinarily concern themselves in clinical work does not occur in neural tissue. Some calcium salts may be deposited in dead ganglion cells of the brain and in the corpora amylacea of glial origin, and perhaps under other circumstances at the cellular aggregate level. The calcifications in which we are interested, however, are large enough to be visible to the unaided eye and are sufficiently large to be seen on plain films or particularly by computed tomography (CT). Essentially, all such calcifications develop through degenerative changes in fibrous tissue.

The diagnosis of intracranial calcification may be divided into two parts: detection of calcification in the cranial cavity of the living subject by imaging methods, and once detected, identification of the pathologic process involved. Table 4.1 lists the causes of intracranial calcification. They are divided into two major groups: the surface or extracerebral calcifications, and the deep or intracerebral calcifications.

A deposit of calcium has to be fairly heavy before it can be shown by plain film radiography. Today, with the frequent use of CT, even minor degrees of calcification can be detected. It is surprising, for instance, to see how frequently calcification in the globus pallidus on one or both sides, most often bilaterally, is encountered, particularly in the older age group. Slight calcification in this area is encountered in many patients over 60 years of age.

The radiologist interpreting radiographs and cross-sectional images must be familiar with the location of the normal calcifications that are frequently found and with the various appearances of calcification in magnetic resonance imaging (MRI), which presents a variety of appearances but which at times is baffling. In CT it is easy to understand that calcium absorbs more x-rays than surrounding tissues and therefore may appear as a lighter area in the images. Calcium ions do not contain mobile protons and thus would yield an absent signal on MRI. It is thus expected that calcium would produce a dark image on both T1- and T2-weighted images. This appearance is usually seen only in very heavy deposits of calcium, however, and even in fairly heavy deposits the absence of the signal is not as expected (see Fig. 4.12*B* to *D*). A calcification is probably more likely to appear dark on a T2-weighted image. Sometimes the calcification may be dark on T1-weighted images and brighter, or somewhat isodense, on T2-weighted images, and it might even vary between the first and the second echoes. In addition, spotty calcifications may be obscured by partial volume or averaging from higher-intensity surrounding areas. This is often the case in lesions such as oligodendrogliomas (see Fig. 11.26). The presence of a calcified or calcifying area of the brain that is hyperintense on T2-weighted images is easier to understand than when it is hyperintense on T1-weighted images. The explanation is not clear at the moment as to why the latter may occur, but it is attributed to some metabolic process in which the calcium is fixed to a protein (1). Dell et al. reported on a case of pseudohypoparathyroidism with extensive calcification in the basal ganglia on CT but with a hyperintense signal on T1-weighted images (2). They reported similar signal characteristics in an experimental model using a calcium phosphate suspension in water.

In general, calcification is often not seen on spin-echo images, and Atlas et al. have described how a gradient-echo technique may demonstrate marked hypointensity in the area of calcification (3). However, this is somewhat nonspecific, for there are other reasons for marked hypointensity on gradient-echo images. Zimmerman et al. reported on 15 meningiomas in which calcifications were detected on CT images; only in 3 were they seen on MRI (4). Thus, if one is looking for calcification, rather than carrying out multiple sequences to clarify the images on MRI, it would be better to simply carry out a CT examination (5).

Membranous Calcifications

Most of the membranous calcifications lie in the processes of the cranial dura mater, which project into the cavity of the skull. The dura is composed of two layers, an outer or endosteal layer, constituting the periosteum of the inner surface of the cranial bones, and an inner or meningeal layer. Processes are formed by duplication of the inner layer of the membrane and are four in number: the falx cerebri, the falx cerebelli, the tentorium cerebelli, and the diaphagma sellae.

The dura mater is composed of white fibrous tissue and elastic fibers, and like all collagenous connective tissue, it often undergoes hyaline degeneration and calcification. Just why calcification occurs so frequently in this cerebral membrane is not clear. Although it supports an abundant vascular supply for other structures, it is not particularly vascular itself, and this may be the principal cause. Trauma, particularly birth injury, has often been suggested as an explanation for the extensive calcifications sometimes found, but the correlation of a history of very remote trauma and the discovery of extensive dural calcification is difficult to establish.

Some form of membranous calcification occurs in approximately 10 percent of normal persons, as seen on plain films. However, on CT examination of the skull, membranous calcifications are probably more commonly seen if looked for.

The petroclinoid reflection of the tentorium is particularly subject to the development of calcification, although it may occur in the tentorial apex or in any one of its reflections. The extent of petroclinoid calcification is quite variable and may be heavy. The shadows are linear and are disposed in an oblique plane as seen in a lateral view of the skull, forming an angle with the clivus. Calcification is more often seen at the clinoid end of the dura reflection, and it extends backward and downward toward the internal acoustic canal. In general this is easy to recognize, and it can rarely be confused with calcification in the basilar artery (Fig. 4.1).

Falx calcification is the most common. On MRI, very occasionally the calcification, which sometimes extends toward one side or the other, away from the surface of the falx for several millimeters, may show that there is ossification with development of bone marrow, which on T1-weighted images would be hyperintense (Fig. 4.2*A* and *B*). Heavy calcification in the falx and tentorium is seen in basal cell nevus syndrome (Gorlin syndrome), discussed in following text (Fig. 4.2*C*), as well as in congenital myotonic dystrophy (6).

Subdural and epidural hematomas rarely calcify, and when they do, they have the fairly characteristic appearance seen in Figure 4.3.

Meningiomas are sometimes hyperdense because of the presence of calcareous deposits, usually termed *psammoma bodies*. In addition, they may stimulate osteoblastic activity, which produces a diffuse increase in the density of the bone and also hyperostosis. These findings are easily visible on plain films and may also be shown on CT scanning but will not be shown on MRI. The great majority of meningiomas in the convexity of the brain and skull do not calcify and generally do not develop visible changes in the bone on plain films or CT. In the suprasellar and parasellar regions a high proportion will show calcification or changes in the bone (Fig. 4.4).

Following meningitis, particularly tuberculous meningitis, calcification may occur, even in the basal meninges. The lime salts are deposited in the organized exudate and in the base of the brain, most commonly in the sella turcica.

Intrasellar and Juxtasellar Calcifications

These include the craniopharyngiomas, saccular aneurysms, and occasional suprasellar gliomas in the region of the hypothalamus or in the optic chiasm, and sometimes a tumor of the pituitary. This may happen following hemorrhage into a tumor. In the case of an adenoma, calcification may occur in the capsule of the tumor as well, in which case it will probably be situated above the sella as a result

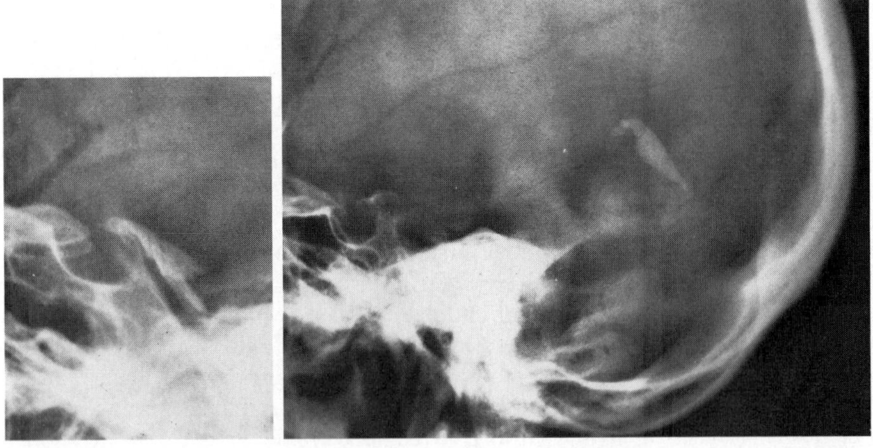

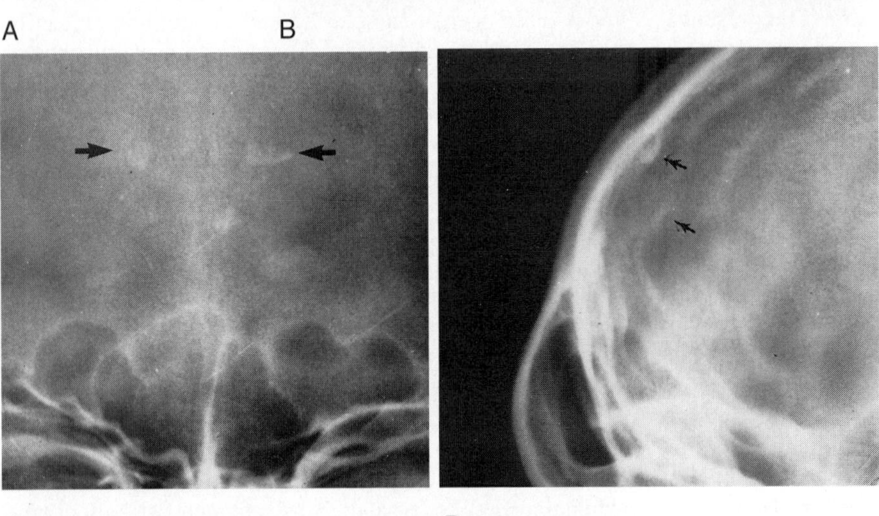

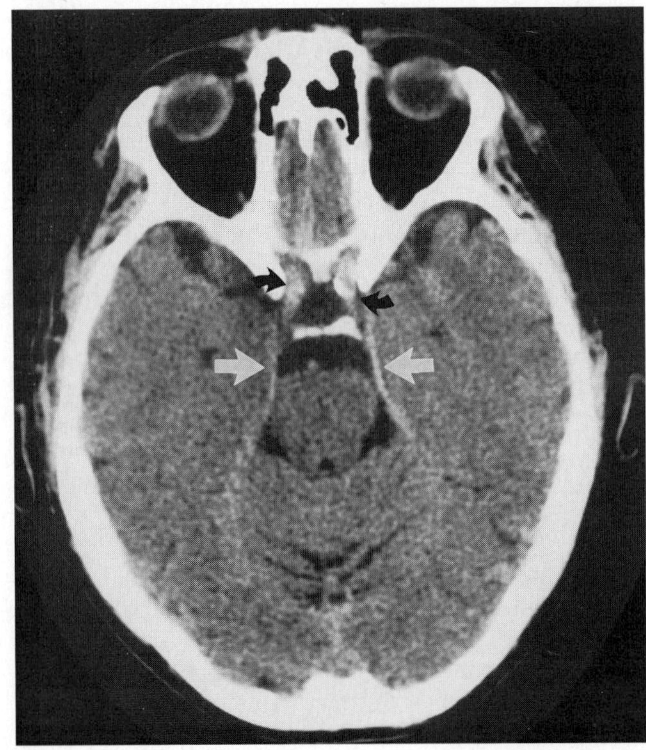

Figure 4.1. Membranous calcifications. **A.** Petroclinoid ligament calcification. This is rather commonly seen in skull examinations in lateral views but less frequently recognized in CT axial examinations. **B.** Dural calcification at the apex of the tentorium. These calcifications, as well as those in the falx, may be ossified and sometimes contain bone marrow. **C** and **D.** Calcification in arachnoid granulations. These are usually found in a parasagittal location (arrows). **E.** Petroclinoid ligament calcification seen in noncontrast CT (arrows). There is also calcification in the internal carotid arteries (small arrows).

of suprasellar extension of the tumor. In the region of the sella we must also consider chordomas and chondromas.

Vascular Calcifications

Vascular calcifications, particularly in the *internal carotid arteries* in the intracavernous segment, are common in the older age group and indicate atherosclerosis of varying degrees (Fig. 4.5).

Saccular aneurysms may calcify. The calcification is usually in the wall of the aneurysm. Atherosclerosis develops frequently in the intima of the aneurysmal sac, and it is through this process that the wall calcification develops (Figs. 4.6 and 4.7). CT scanning may show the calcium deposits before they become visible on plain films of the skull.

Whereas arterial calcifications occur quite commonly in the internal carotid and the basilar and vertebral arteries, calcifications in smaller arteries (middle, anterior, posterior cerebral) are sometimes seen on CT examination but are rare.

Arteriovenous malformations also may calcify, sometimes appearing as curvilinear or ringlike calcifications. Sometimes the shell-like calcification is associated with stippled deposits (Fig. 4.8). Occult vascular malformations or angiomas may also calcify.

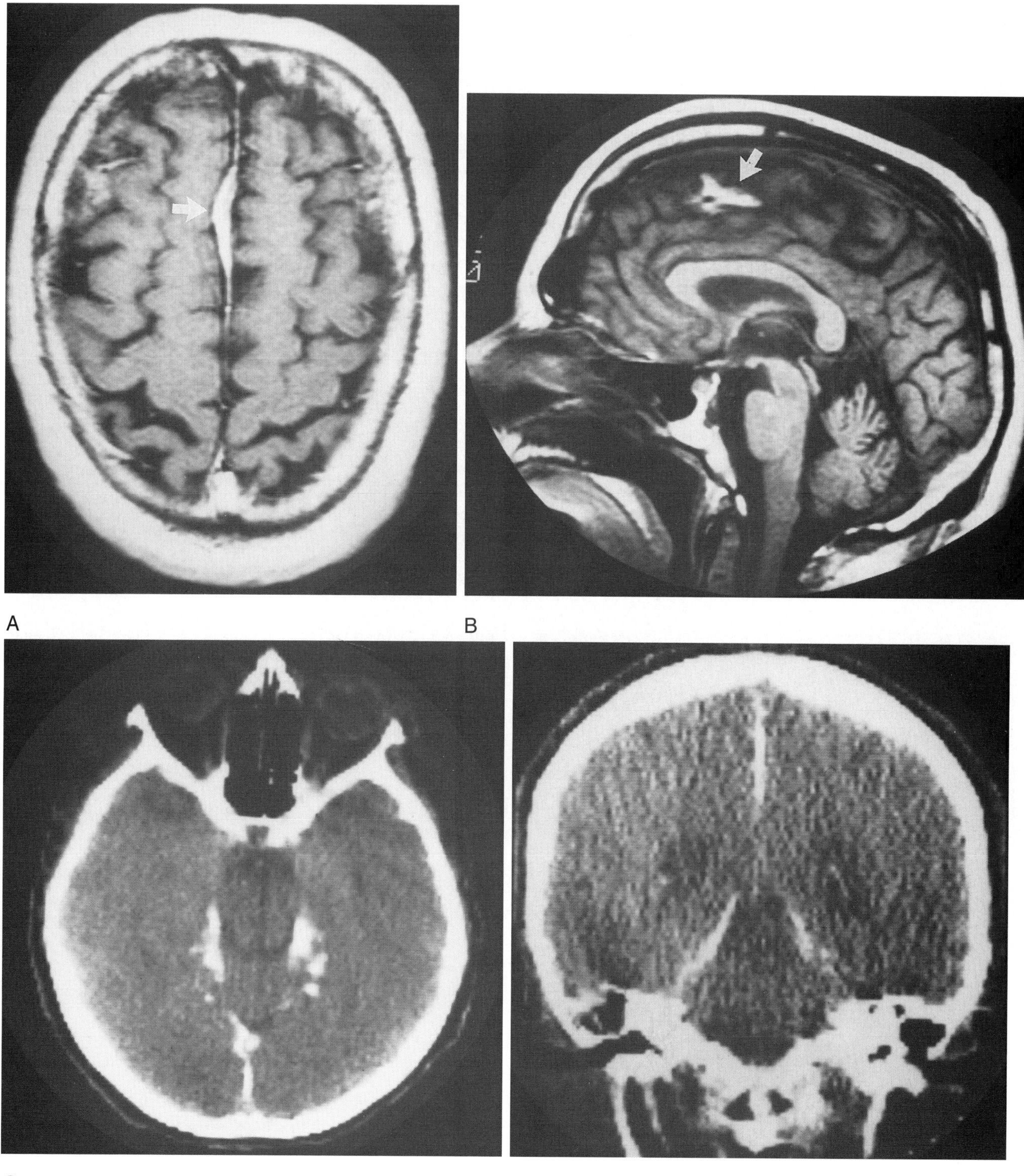

Figure 4.2. Falx cerebri calcification showing brightness on T1-weighted images. **A** and **B.** Sagittal and axial T1-weighted images reveal brightness in the frontal region representing bone marrow within the calcified falx (arrow). **C.** Extensive calcification in dura in patient affected by basal cell nevus syndrome (Gorlin syndrome). The patient was a 60-year-old woman who had had many basal cell carcinomas removed from the face since before age 20.

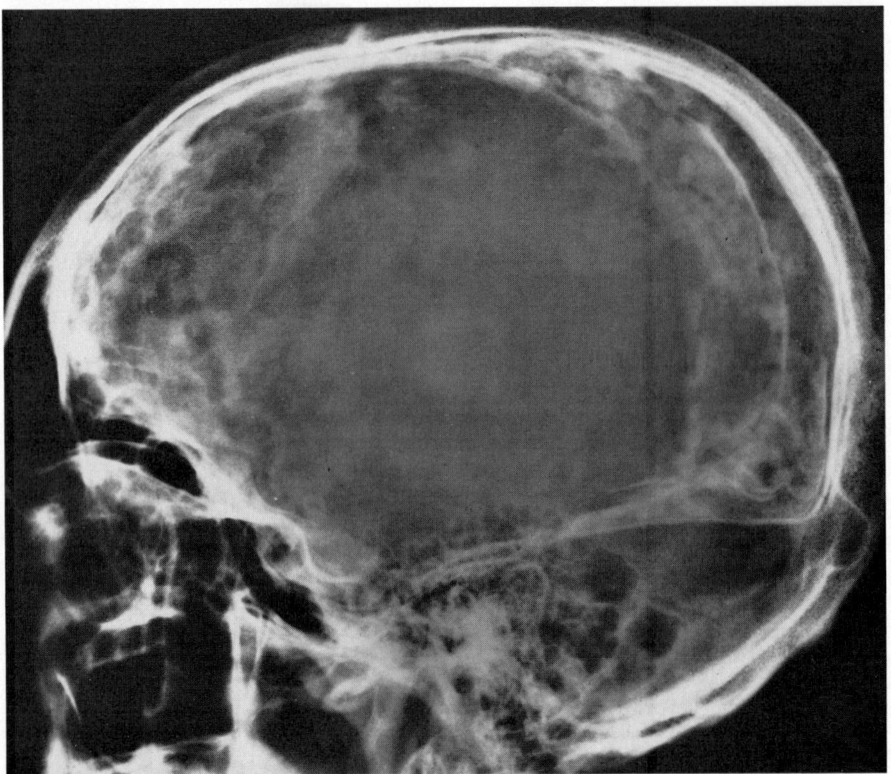

A

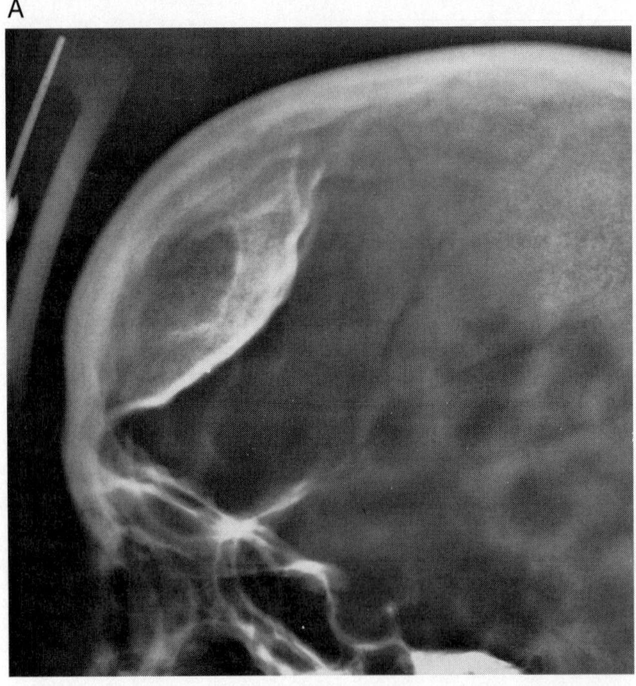

B

Figure 4.3. Calcified subdural and epidural hematoma. **A.** Subdural hematoma. There may be calcification in the membrane. Irregular calcification is present throughout the organized hematoma. **B.** Epidural hematoma seen 2 years after decompression and shunting in a young patient with hydrocephalus. Presumably the decompression led to epidural hemorrhage that was not recognized at the time.

Calcifications of Sturge-Weber syndrome are characteristic in that they present a series of parallel, straight lines or curvilinear densities most frequently in the parieto-occipital region, described in text following (see Fig. 5.44). The calcifications in Sturge-Weber syndrome are not primarily in the blood vessels.

Intracerebral Calcifications

LOCALIZED CALCIFICATIONS

Localized calcifications are lime salts that have been deposited in one area or structure of the brain. Since calcification occurs below the cellular level, it is obvious that multiple

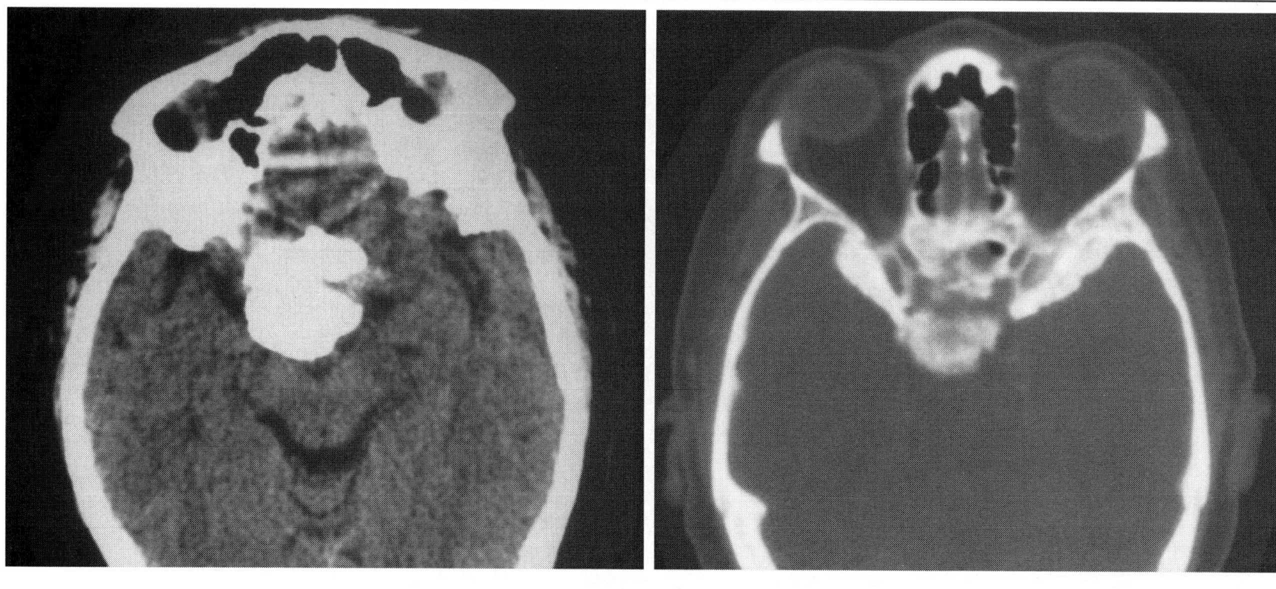

Figure 4.4. Calcified suprasellar meningioma. **A.** There is a calcified mass in the suprasellar region, slightly off center to the right. The bone window (**B**) shows the exact position of the calcium deposits and their relationship to the sella and the sphenoid ridge. There is sclerosis of the right anterior clinoid and adjacent lesser wing of the sphenoid, more so on the right than on the left. The calcification is fairly homogeneous and may be composed of myriad of the calcified psammoma bodies seen in meningiomas. The lesion is large enough to produce slight compression of the right midbrain peduncle.

foci must form an aggregate before they can be seen. Whether fused or separated by noncalcified elements, the deposits are at a single morphologic site or in a lesion with continuity; the change indicates focal degeneration in tissue in a restricted part of the brain.

Physiologic Calcifications

The pineal gland is the most common structure to calcify sufficiently to be visible on plain radiographs, and particularly on CT examinations. The pineal is located just behind the posterior margin of the third ventricle. It is a midline structure. In the past, when dealing with skull films as the only noninvasive examination, it was necessary to determine the midline position of the calcified pineal. Today, with the frequent use of CT and MRI, this is not usually necessary, and in most instances plain films of the skull have been eliminated and are taken only if they become necessary.

Calcification in the pineal can be very heavy at times. Cystic degeneration of the pineal may occur at the same time, and the size of the cyst can at times be fairly large. In general, if the partially calcified, cystic pineal measures up to 14 mm in diameter, it is considered to be a cystic pineal. A larger measurement should be considered as possibly pathologic, and follow-up is recommended if there are no clinical manifestations. An occasional patient has been reported who required surgical intervention, but in general, this should be considered an unnecessary procedure (Fig. 4.9).

Habenular calcification occurs almost as frequently as calcification in the pineal body. The habenula is situated immediately anterior to the pineal. On lateral radiographs, the calcified habenula has a curvilinear shape that is concave backward. Sometimes the habenular commissure is calcified when the pineal is not visible on plain radiographs. CT usually demonstrates it, however, and usually shows calcification in the pineal as well.

Choroid plexus calcification is also very common. Usually the glomus of the choroid plexus, situated in the atrium of the lateral ventricle, is the one that most frequently calcifies. It should be remembered that the glomus can be quite large and that sometimes it is slightly pedunculated; in these cases it can change positions when the patient's head changes. The relationship of the calcified glomera and pineal is quite typical and is usually well seen on axial views (Fig. 4.9). The glomus of the choroid plexus can be displaced by masses when the atrium of the ventricle is also displaced. Calcification in the choroid plexus may occur at other points. These aberrant calcium shadows may be seen anywhere along the course of the choroid plexus in the lateral ventricles, but they are most common near the foramen of Monro (7). (Fig. 4.10*A* to *C*). Calcification may occur in the tela choroidea of the third ventricle or in the choroid plexus in the roof of the fourth ventricle. It is common to find calcifications extending along the foramina of Luschka on both sides. Sometimes this is unilateral, and in such cases it could be confusing. Ordinarily, however, it is bilateral and easier to interpret because of the symmetry (Fig. 4.10*D*).

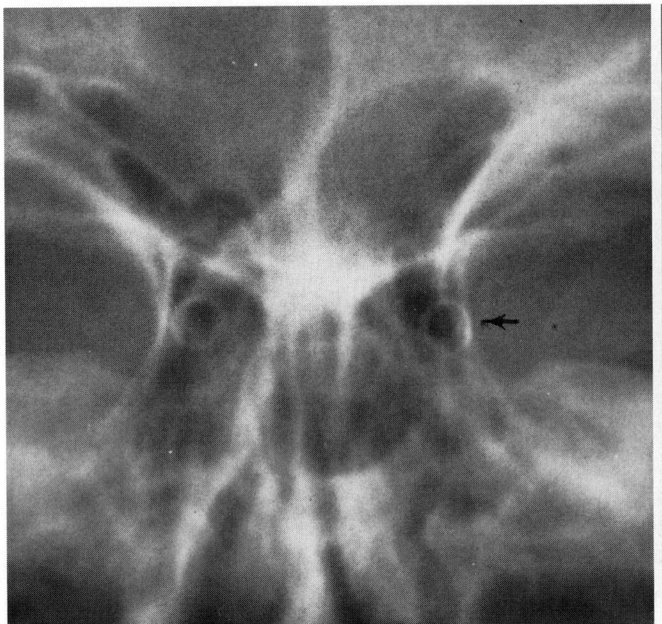

A

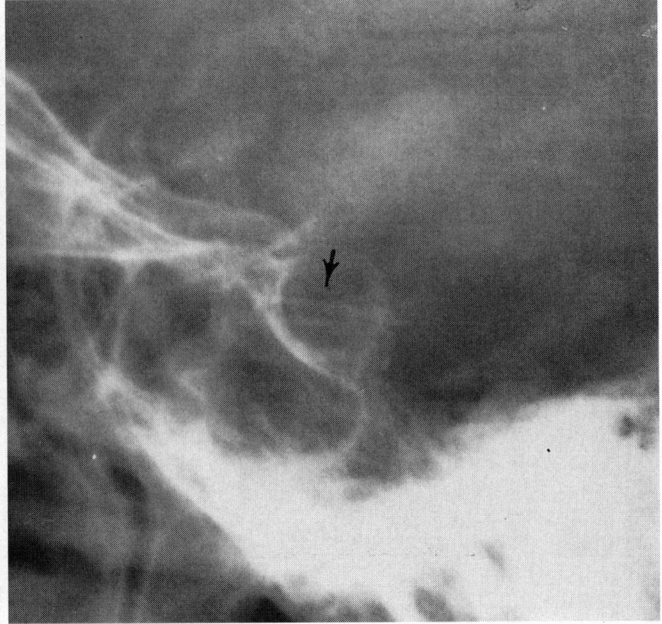

B

C

Figure 4.5. Calcification in the internal carotid artery. **A.** Frontal (arrow). **B.** Lateral skull (arrow). **C.** Lateral view showing calcification in the carotid siphon and in the supraclinoid portion of the artery.

Inflammatory Calcifications

Brain abscesses may calcify, but probably do so rarely. Certainly the majority of abscesses that we see do not seem to be followed by calcification. *Tuberculomas* are apparently the granulomatous type of lesion that most frequently calcifies. However, tuberculomas are very rare in the United States, and when we encounter a calcification we list a tuberculoma as a statistically less likely lesion. In other countries, however, particularly in South America and Asia, tuberculomas are considerably more common and would be the first possibility to consider (see Fig. 4.16*C*). Other granulomatous lesions are actinomycosis, coccidioidomycosis, cryptococcosis, mucormycosis, and other fungal diseases.

Hemorrhagic Calcifications

Unidentified solitary intracerebral calcifications are often labeled as being the result of intracerebral hemorrhage. The exact nature of some lime deposits can never be determined even at the time of microscopic examination, since they are amorphous masses that have no distinguishing features. Study of the pathologic processes occurring with intracerebral bleeding suggests that calcification should not occur frequently. A gross intracerebral hemorrhage in which the patient survives ultimately comes to resolution, and with its disappearance the cavity becomes smaller through the restoration of marginal brain architecture, the disappearance of edema, and ventricular enlargement. A capsule does not usually develop around an intracerebral hematoma, and for this reason a connective tissue scar is not the common end result of the lesion, as is the case with an abscess or a granuloma. Nevertheless, it is quite possible that intracerebral calcification may, in some instances, be the result of an old hemorrhage. Calcification sometimes develops in the needle tract following puncture of the lateral ventricles for ventriculostomy. Interestingly enough,

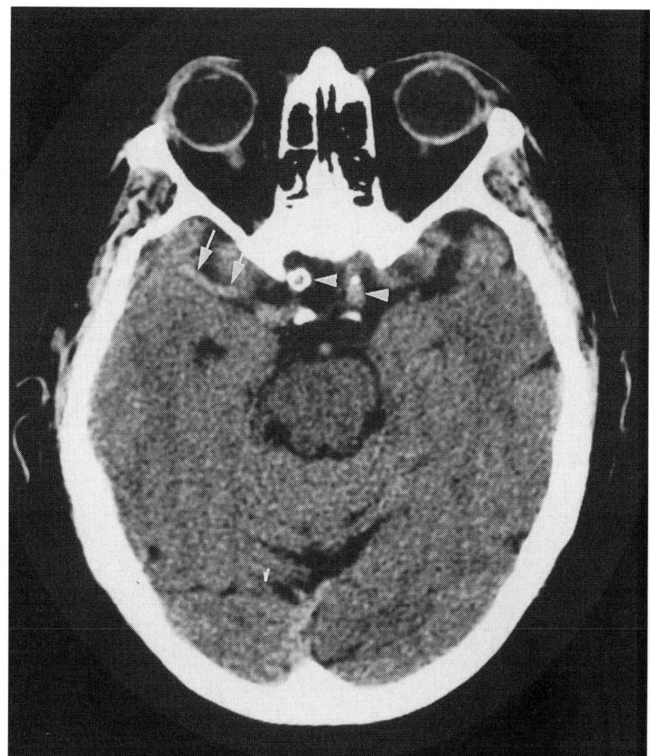

A

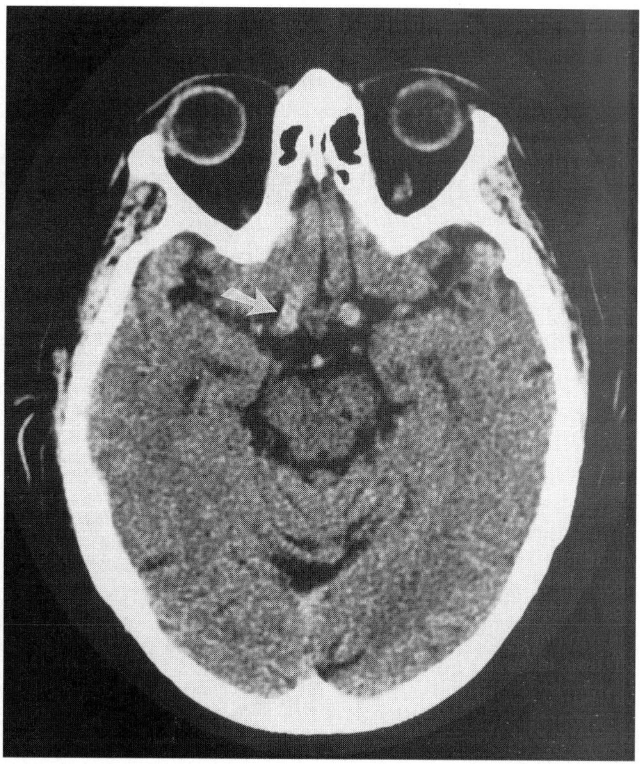

B

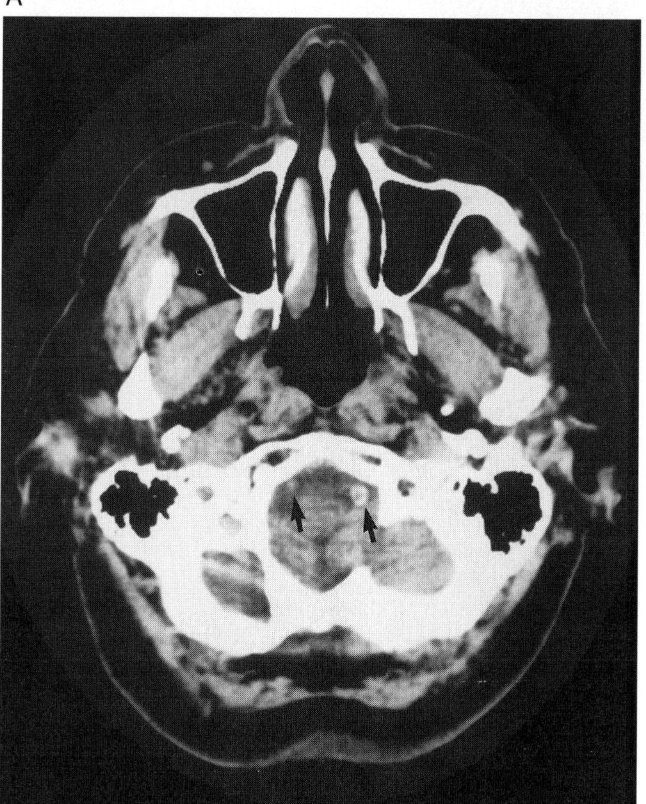

C

Figure 4.6. Vascular calcifications shown by CT in a 73-year-old woman. **A.** Axial view showing bilateral carotid calcifications (arrowheads). There is also calcification in a branch of the middle cerebral artery (arrows). **B.** View 5.0 mm higher showing calcification in the supraclinoid portion of the carotid artery (arrow). **C.** Vertebral artery calcification (arrows); the right vertebral artery is probably hypoplastic.

however, we rarely see calcification in the brain—even with CT, which is very sensitive to the presence of calcium—following shunting for the treatment of hydrocephalus, either acute or chronic. Perhaps the type of instrumentation previously used for ventriculography, which was often performed for diagnosis, may have improved in recent years. Obviously, if a hemorrhagic event is later followed by the presence of calcification in the same area, it is difficult to conclude that the calcification was not the result of the hematoma.

Neoplastic Calcifications

The tumors of the brain that most frequently calcify are the gliomas. Statistically the astrocytomas are so much more common than the others that the majority of calcified intracerebral tumors turn out to be astrocytomas. However, oligodendrogliomas calcify more frequently than astrocytomas, though they are far less common (Figs. 4.11 and 4.12). The calcification of astrocytomas is more subtle than that of oligodendrogliomas, which tend to have heavier and more conglomerate calcium deposits. Glioblastomas do not usually calcify, but when they do, the calcification may increase following radiation therapy. Ependymomas also frequently calcify. They tend to be intraventricular and may be found in the lateral ventricles or, more frequently, in the region of the fourth ventricle. Calcification in a tumor either totally inside the fourth ventricle or partially outside it is typical of ependymoma. Another intraventricular tumor that may present calcium deposits is a choroid plexus papilloma and xanthogranulomas of the choroid plexus. Tumors of pineal origin may also calcify. They may be pineal teratomas, gliomas, or germinomas. CT scanning usually clarifies the diagnosis in the majority of these neoplasms.

MULTIPLE SCATTERED CALCIFICATIONS

Tuberous Sclerosis

These multiple calcifications are usually intraventricular, in the wall of the ventricles. This lesion is described and illustrated in Chapter 5 (see Figs. 5.45 and 5.46).

Encephalitis

The most common of these multiple calcifications are toxoplasmosis and cytomegalovirus infections. These are often prenatal infections, and the calcification is present shortly after birth or may develop sometime later. The calcifications tend to be periventricular and may become scattered

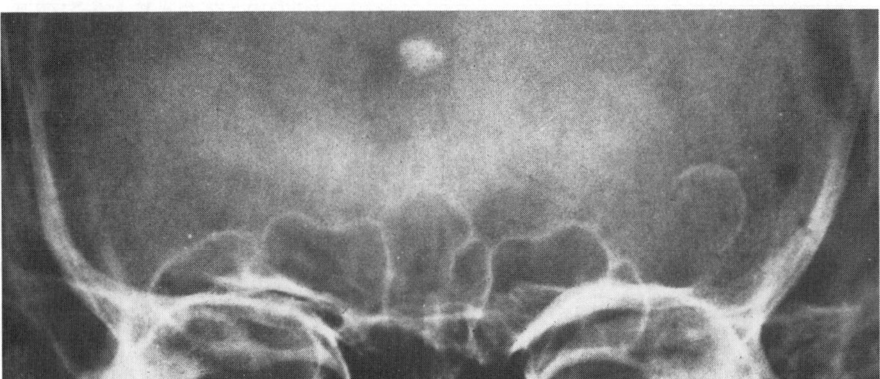

A

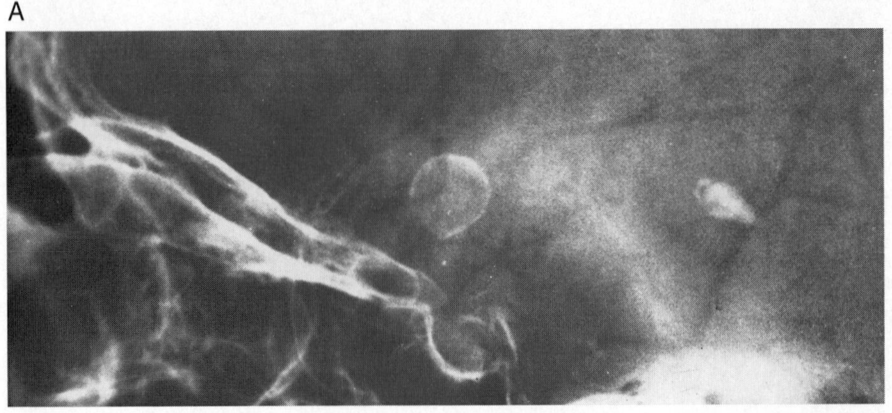

B

Figure 4.7. Calcified aneurysm of the middle cerebral artery seen on frontal (**A**) and lateral (**B**) radiographs. Calcifications in aneurysms are much more frequently encountered on CT images because the calcium may be seen even if the deposits are small.

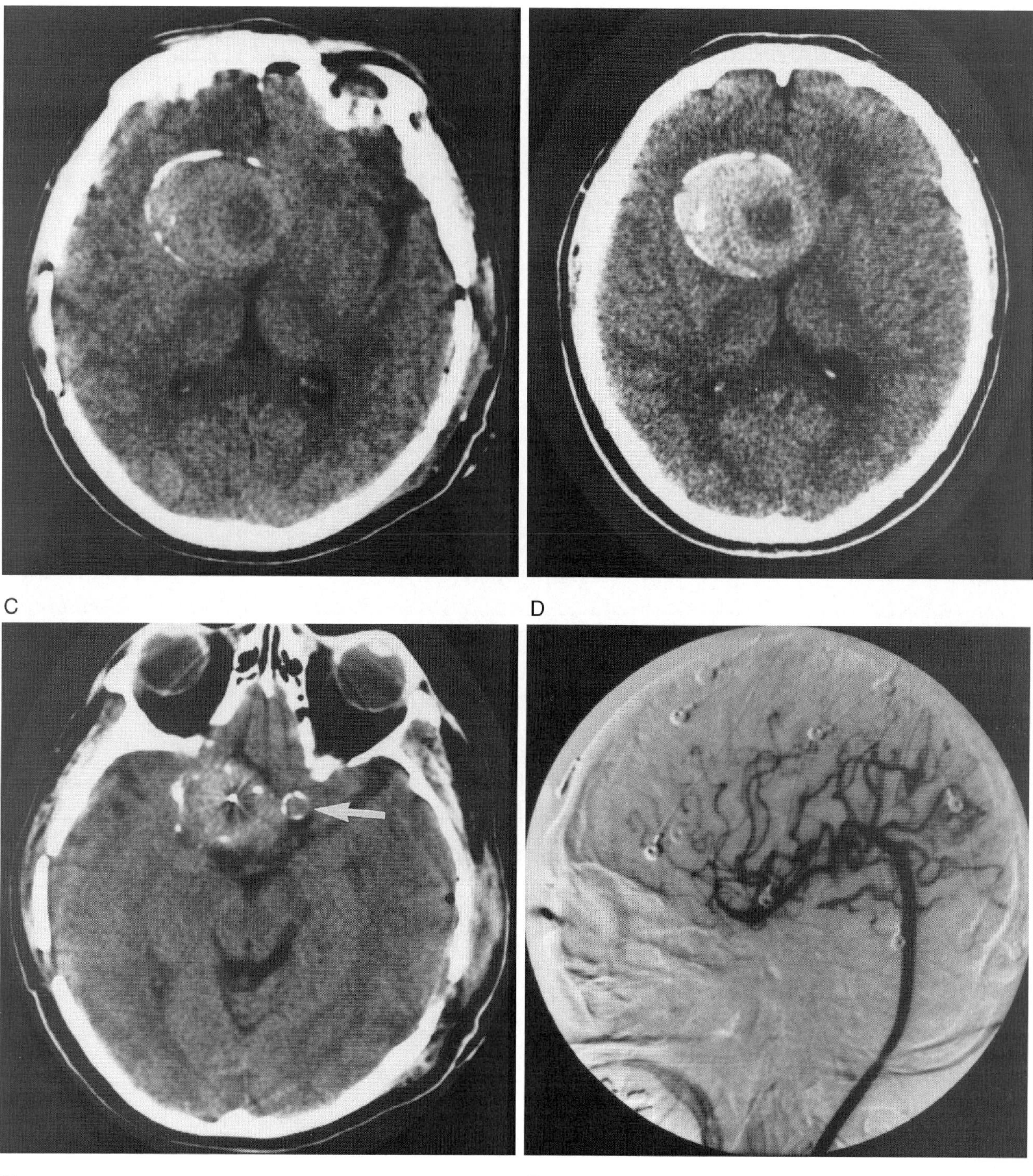

Figure 4.7. *(continued)* **C.** CT scan showing calcified aneurysm. Within the ringlike calcification there is a rounded, low-attenuation area representing a balloon from a previous transluminal interventional procedure. **D.** Following contrast enhancement the aneurysm enhances but the lumen is not open. It is felt that the tissue filling the old aneurysmal sac enhances. **E.** A section caudal to the previous image shows another calcified small aneurysm on the opposite carotid artery (arrow). Bilateral carotid occlusion was carried out for treatment and the patient tolerated it well. Preocclusion external-internal carotid anastomosis (ECIC) was carried out. **F.** Post-ECIC bypass angiogram showing excellent blood supply to the middle cerebral artery territory.

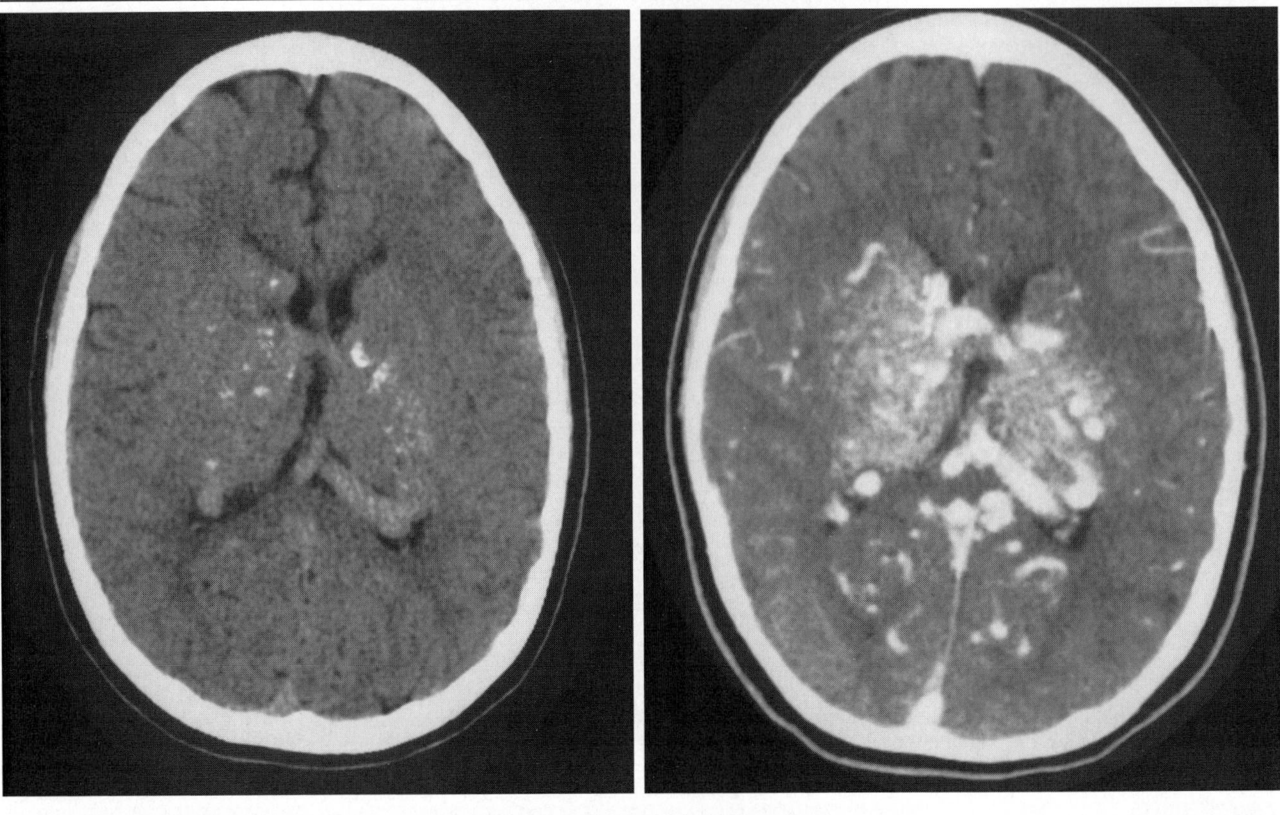

Figure 4.8. Calcification in arteriovenous malformation. **A.** CT without contrast shows bilateral calcifications in the region of the basal ganglia and thalamus. A slightly hyperdense tubular structure is seen in the atrial region of the left ventricle and a round, slightly hyperdense structure in the right atrium (noncalcified). These turned out to be venous structures, which enhanced with intravenous contrast media (**B**). Several other enhancing large vessels, probably veins, are seen anterior and posterior to the main vascular malformation. There is also diffuse increase in density.

as the lateral ventricles dilate because of brain atrophy. They may sometimes be associated with aqueductal stenosis secondary to the same encephalitic process. Calcifications are also found in the basal ganglia region, and indeed anywhere in the brain. Plain film diagnosis is possible if the calcifications are heavy enough (Figs. 4.13 and 4.14). CT can demonstrate the calcium deposits when they are much more subtle. MRI is not very accurate in diagnosing these finer calcifications; CT is recommended as the first study in any infant in whom the possibility of a prenatal infection is clinically suspected (Fig. 4.15).

Cysticercosis

Involvement of the nervous system by infestation with the pork tapeworm (*Taenia solium*) is an important problem in many countries around the world, particularly in Latin America but also in Asia. In the United States it is only seen in immigrants or in the southern part near the frontier with Mexico. The individual acquires the infection by ingesting *Taenia solium* eggs. When the egg enters the acid and enzymatic conditions of the stomach, dissolution of the embryophore takes place and the oncosphere is activated and liberated after dissolving the oncospherial membrane. The embryo invades the intestinal wall, enters the circulation, and finally establishes itself in various organs. The embryo then develops into a cysticercus, a cystic organism composed of a complex wall surrounding a cavity containing a vesicular fluid and a scolex. The cysticercus will die or remain as such until it is eventually ingested by the definitive host. Once again, the parasite meets adequate conditions in the digestive tract, where it stays to develop into an adult tapeworm, which is again capable of producing new eggs.

The diagnosis of cysticercosis is discussed elsewhere. The cysts can easily be seen by CT or MRI. Calcifications, which take place after the death of the parasite, can be seen by CT and sometimes on plain films of the skull (Fig. 4.16). Typically, the calcifications are round, and they may present, at least during some stages, as a small dot within a dense circle; the dot represents the scolex or small parasite, which initially was contained within a vesicle. This configuration is typical of cysticercosis. Serological testing is usually necessary to confirm the diagnosis. One of the problems with the eradication of cysticercosis is that man is a definitive host for *Taenia solium*.

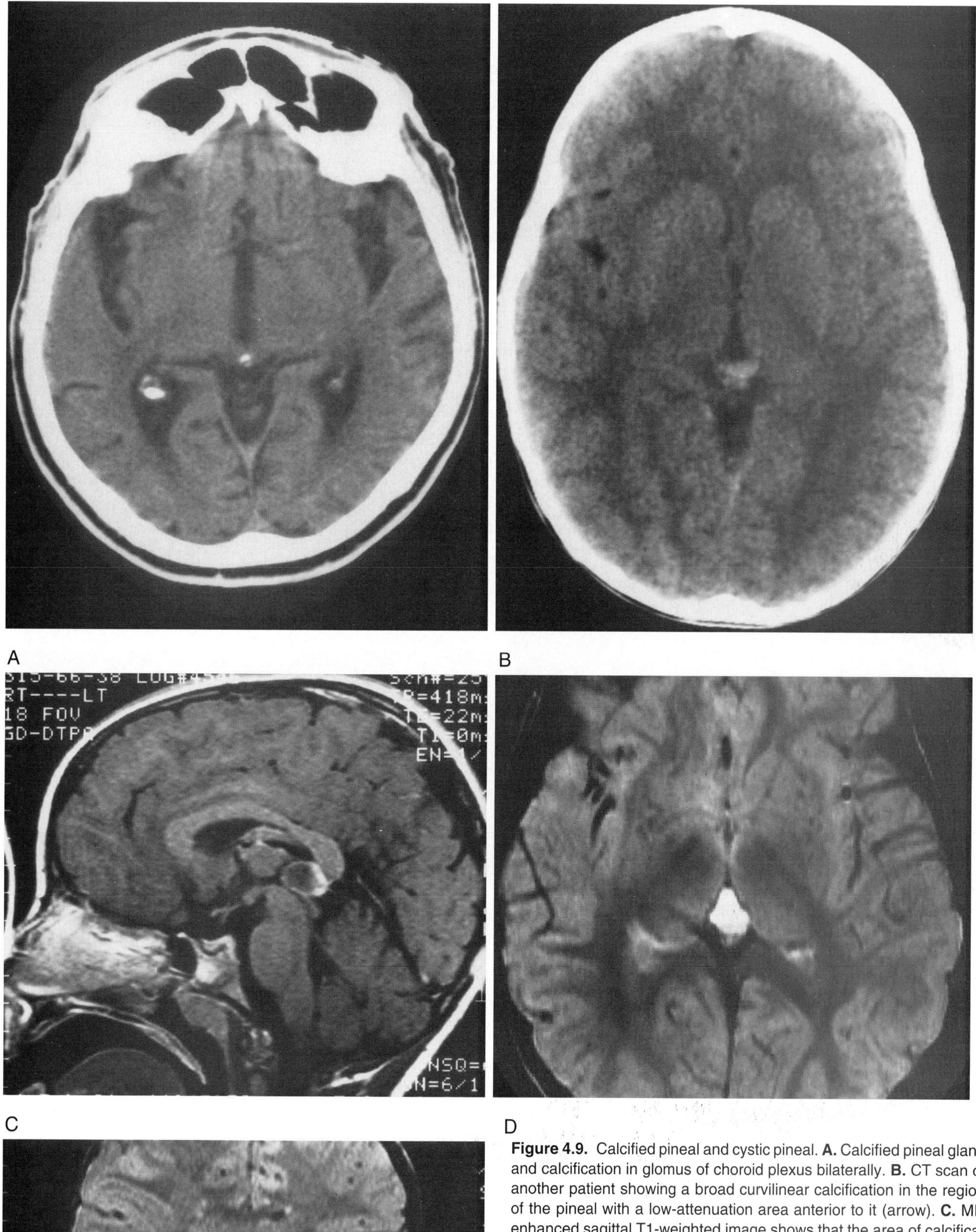

Figure 4.9. Calcified pineal and cystic pineal. **A.** Calcified pineal gland and calcification in glomus of choroid plexus bilaterally. **B.** CT scan of another patient showing a broad curvilinear calcification in the region of the pineal with a low-attenuation area anterior to it (arrow). **C.** MR enhanced sagittal T1-weighted image shows that the area of calcification is hyperintense and that there is a rounded cystic space anteriorly. **D** and **E.** The cystic space is hyperintense on first-echo T2-weighted images, indicating that it does not contain CSF-like fluid (which would be isointense). This cystic pineal actually measured 1.7 cm in diameter, which is 3 mm longer than the author usually considers a normal variant. Under these circumstances it is probably wise to recommend a follow-up in 6 to 12 months to make sure the cystic pineal is not growing.

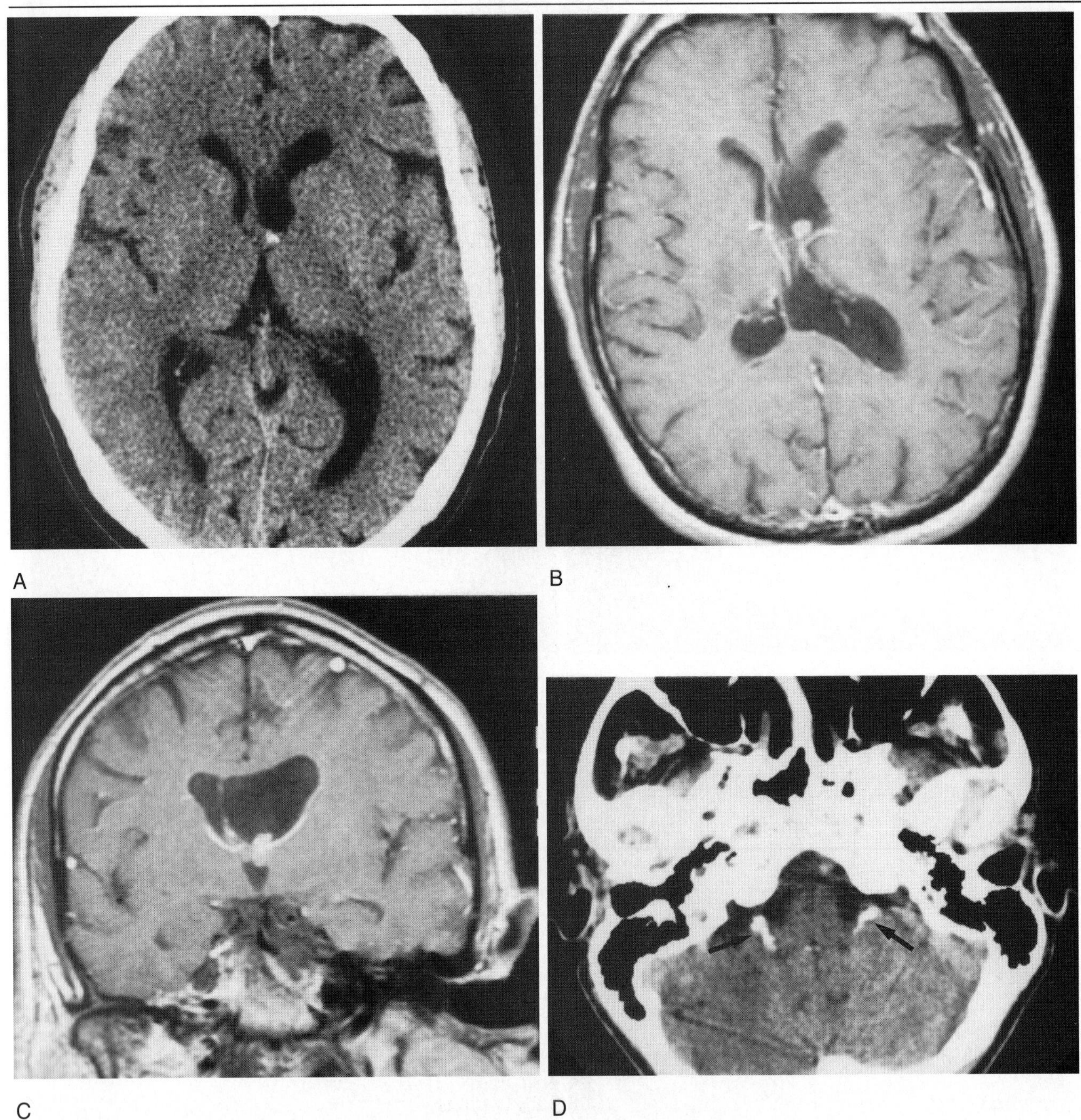

Figure 4.10. Aberrant glomus of the choroid plexus in the upper aspect of the foramen of Monro causing slight, stable ventricular dilatation on one side in a 66-year-old man. **A.** CT axial view shows the calcified aberrant glomus and slight ventricular enlargement on the right side. **B.** Axial MR, postcontrast, T1-weighted image shows the small calcified mass, which is bright on T1. **C.** Coronal view after contrast. The ventricular enlargement is well shown. Reexamination 3 months later showed no change in the size of the left ventricle. **D.** In another patient, calcification in the choroid plexus is shown along the foramina of Luschka (arrow).

Echinococcosis (Hydatid Disease)

This disease is prevalent in South America, particularly in Argentina and Chile. The definitive host for the adult form is usually the dog, where the tapeworm lives in large numbers in the intestines. Eggs are passed in the excreta, from which they are commonly picked up by sheep, although other mammals, including man, may serve as intermediate hosts. The usual cycle is completed by the dog's eating mutton containing the larval cysts. Shepherds are commonly affected, as are children. Only about 2 percent of patients with echinococcosis develop hydatid cysts of the

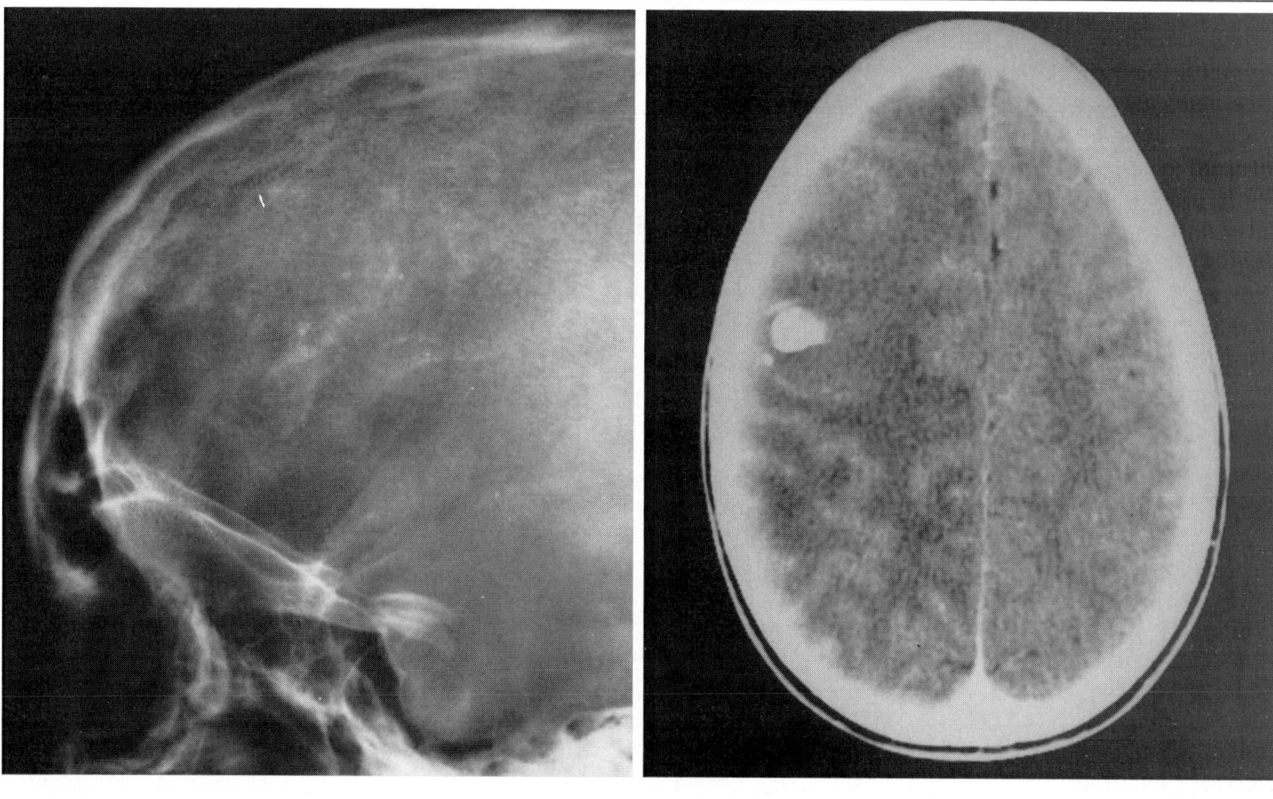

Figure 4.11. Calcified astrocytoma. **A.** Granular, nodular, and linear calcifications, a combination seen in astrocytoma. Compare with the oligodendroglioma in Figure 4.12. The tumor caused total deossification of the walls of the sella turcica that was associated with chronic increased intracranial pressure. **B.** Calcification in astrocytoma in the right frontal region. There is evidence of edema in the surrounding brain; the edema involves a good portion of the hemisphere, causing separation of the surface gyri and a decrease in density of the white matter.

brain; the majority of the larvae are filtered out in the liver and lungs. For this reason hydatid cysts in these organs are much more common. As with cysticercosis, calcification may occur after the death of the parasite. By that time the hydatid cyst may have reached several centimeters in diameter, even in the brain. In contrast to cysticercosis, the hydatid cyst is more often solitary in the brain. When calcification occurs, it is mainly about the perimeter of the cyst, but sometimes there is a reticular or "ground glass" calcification within the cyst cavity, suggesting that it may have been infected or otherwise damaged before the death of the larva.

Other Parasitic Diseases

Trichinosis and paragonimiasis are among the other less common parasitic diseases that produce intracranial calcifications. Trichinosis, however, is rarely considered in the differential diagnosis of intracranial calcifications. Although it may occur, it must be very rare, in spite of the fact that it is not an uncommon infestation in the United States. The cysts are tiny, about a millimeter or so.

Paragonimiasis, which is common in the Orient, is much more common than trichinosis as a cause of calcification in the brain. The lungs are chiefly affected. In the case of the lung fluke (*Paragonimus westermani*), human infestation is by ingestion of poorly prepared shellfish, one of the intermediate hosts, which contains encysted cercariae. Meningoencephalitis occurs in approximately 25 percent of patients infested with the lung fluke, and cystic lesions and granulomas may be formed. Large numbers of shell-like calcifications of varying size may be seen in some patients, and at other times the calcium is punctate and nodular. Calcification is said to occur in almost one-half of the patients with cerebral paragonimiasis (Fig. 4.17). Oh described the calcification that occurs in some cases as resembling soap bubbles (8).

Mycotic Infections

Mycotic infections producing meningoencephalitis may result in intracranial calcium deposits in some cases. The invisible microorganisms, *Cryptococcus neoformans*, *Blastomyces dermatitidis*, and *Coccidioides immitis*, are among the more common causative agents in this group. Cryptococcosis often affects infants and children, producing wide-

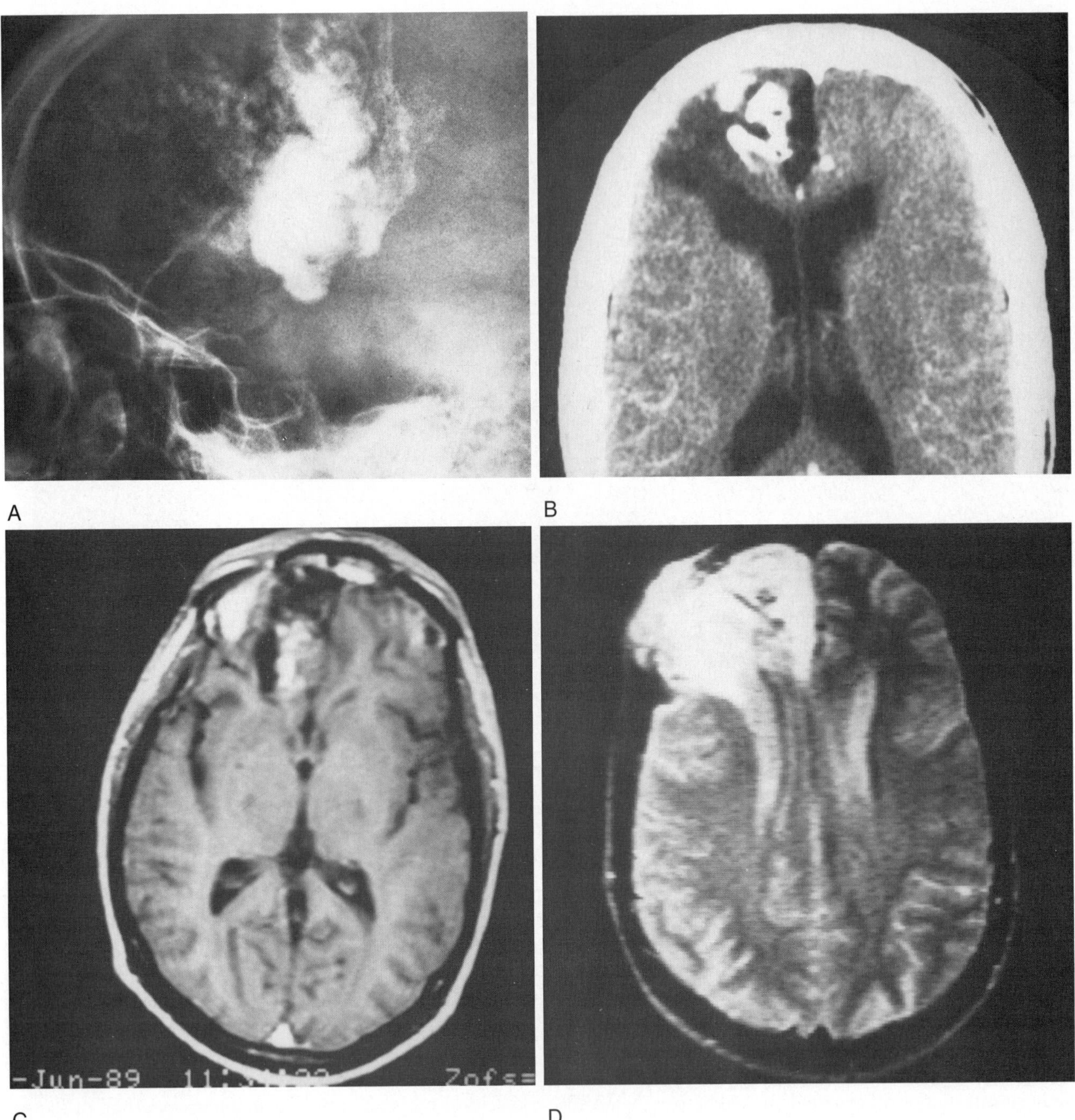

Figure 4.12. Calcified oligodendroglioma. **A.** Lateral skull image showing heavy nodular and spotty calcification. The heavy deposits suggest the proper histology, which is not usually encountered in other types of intracerebral tumors. **B.** CT scan of another case showing heavy calcification in the neoplasm. **C.** MRI examination shows that on a T1-weighted image there is hyperintensity over part of the calcified area. The low-intensity areas are edema or cystic spaces (the patient had prior surgery). **D.** A T2-weighted image shows the edema and cystic spaces as well as the postoperative change, but the calcification can only be suspected because of the low-intensity areas, which, in the absence of a CT examination, may be taken to represent old hemorrhage following the surgical procedure.

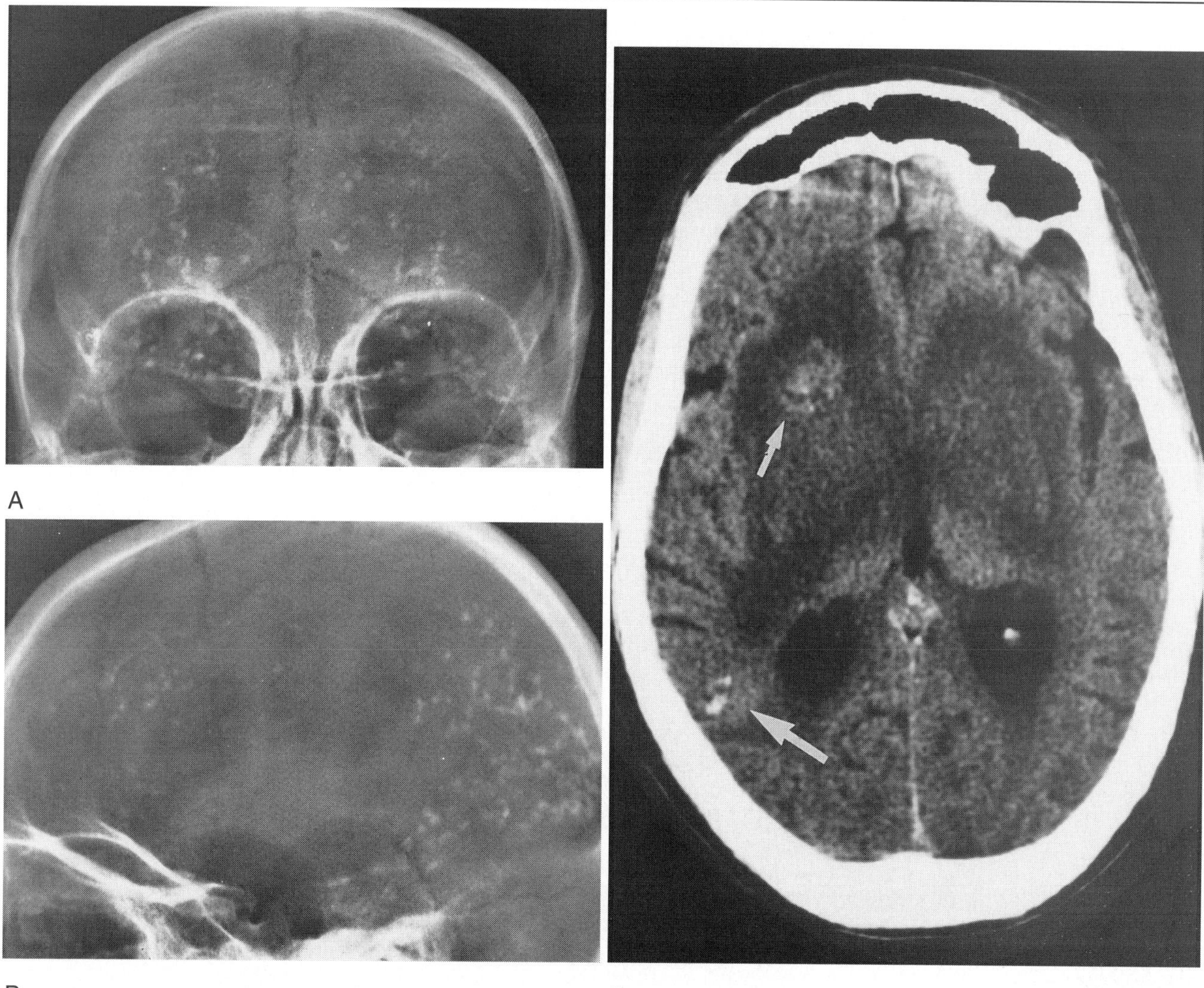

Figure 4.13. Toxoplasmosis with calcification. A young child with hydrocephalus shows extensive punctate scattered calcifications, bilaterally and following the contour of dilated ventricles. (**A,** frontal view; **B,** lateral view.) **C.** Calcification in lesions of toxoplasmosis in an adult patient with AIDS. Two calcified areas are seen in this section; one is ringlike and the other is more punctate (arrows). The patient also had more recent active lesions with much edema.

spread granulomatous lesions within the brain, on the brain surface, and in the spinal cord. As with other granulomas, lime salts may be deposited in the lesions and in adjacent necrotic brain tissue. Calcific deposits in cryptococcosis are punctate or small nodular lesions with a tendency to coalesce. Many are seen in subependymal locations, where they may appear as grossly curvilinear, aligning roughly with the configuration of enlarged ventricles. Others may be found scattered through the brain. Calcium deposits may also be found in the granulomatous residues in the basal meninges, resembling those deposits seen in tuberculous meningitis. Coccidioidomycosis also produces a basilar meningitis with a heavy exudate that becomes organized and that may contain calcific plaques after fibrosis and healing. In both cryptococcosis and coccidioidomycosis, the posterior fossa is prominently affected, and calcifications found here may be a clue to the cause of obstructive hydrocephalus. Mucormycosis is a rapidly progressive infection usually occurring in diabetics or in immunocompromised patients. It often leads to death but may be controlled if treated early (Fig. 4.18).

Metastatic Tumors

Metastatic tumors would not be expected to calcify in an appreciable number of instances. Calcium deposits are not infrequently seen, however, at pathologic examination, and lime deposits were identified in 7 percent of specimens by Potts and Svare (9). The same investigators found that in 1 to 2 percent of the group of cases studied, calcium shadows could be identified on the plain skull films. More than one-half of the metastases showing calcification were from the lung; in another case a breast metastasis to the midbrain

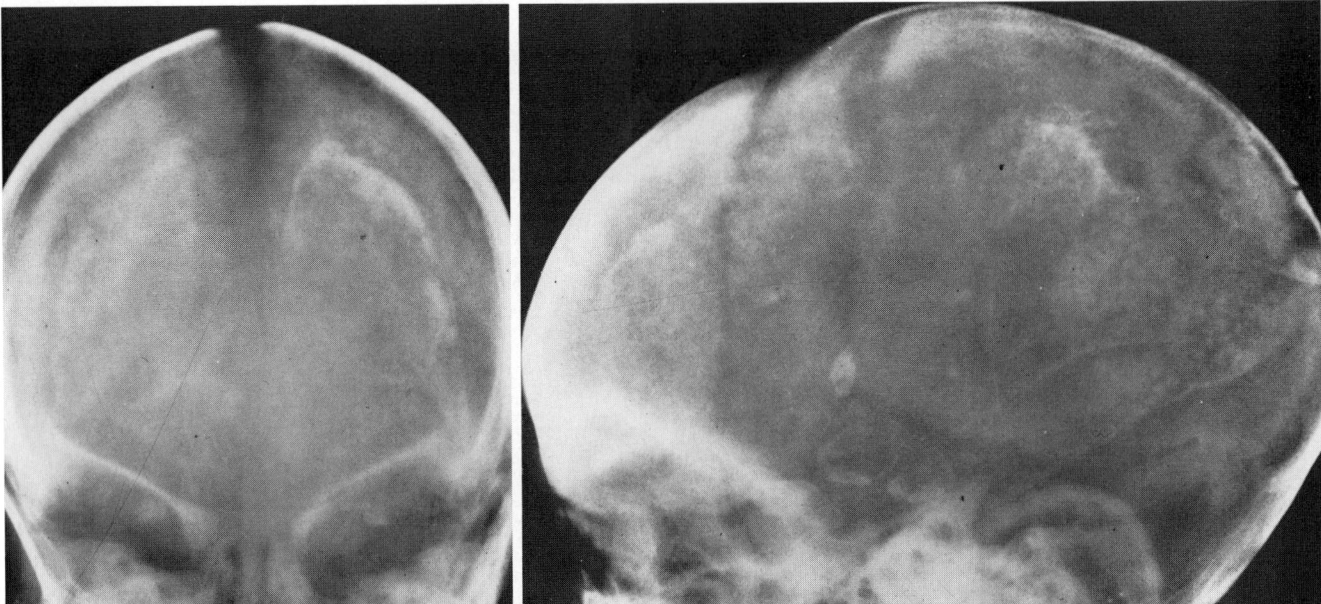

Figure 4.14. Cytomegalovirus infection in a newborn infant. The calcification is mostly periventricular and demonstrates the symmetrical ventricular enlargement. Differentiation of cytomegalovirus from congenital toxoplasmosis cannot really be made on the basis of the distribution of calcifications. Possibly in toxoplasmosis the calcifications tend to be more scattered in the brain as well as periventricular in location.

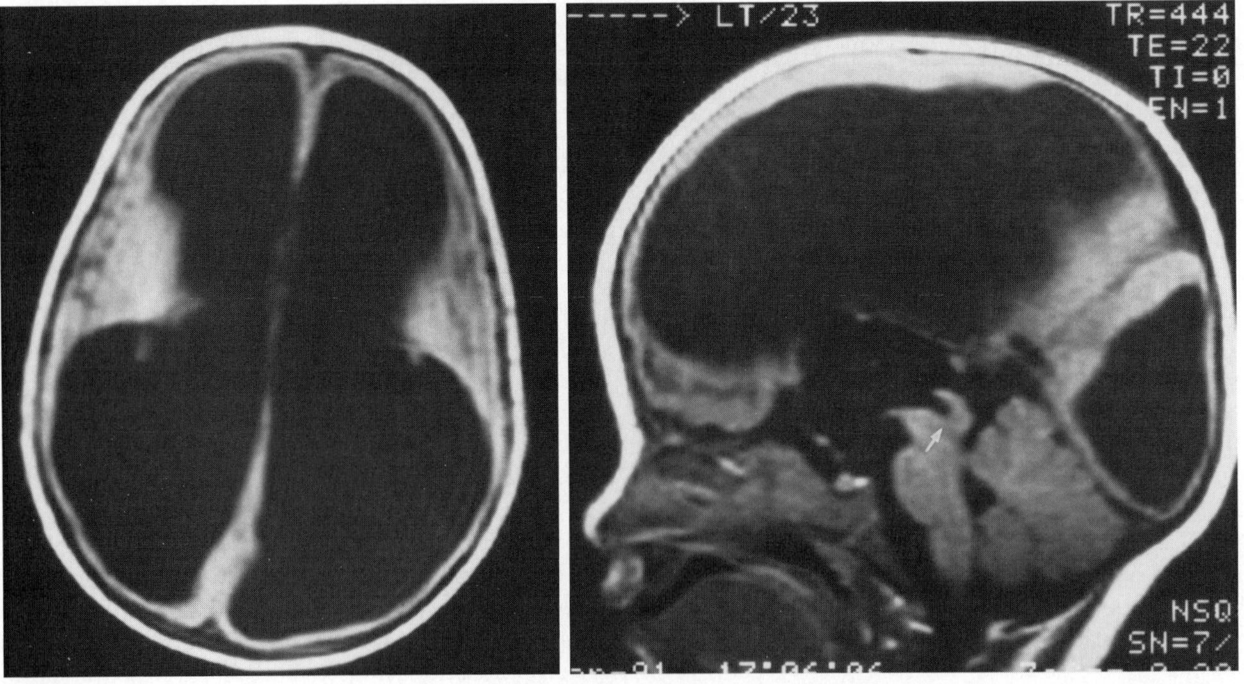

A B

Figure 4.15. "Hydrocephalus" at birth secondary to infection with brain calcifications. **A** and **B.** An MRI examination was carried out first and demonstrated marked ventricular dilatation. The sagittal image shows aqueductal obstruction (arrow). The diagnosis was congenital hydrocephalus on the basis of the MRI, but CT was recommended to rule out calcified lesions.

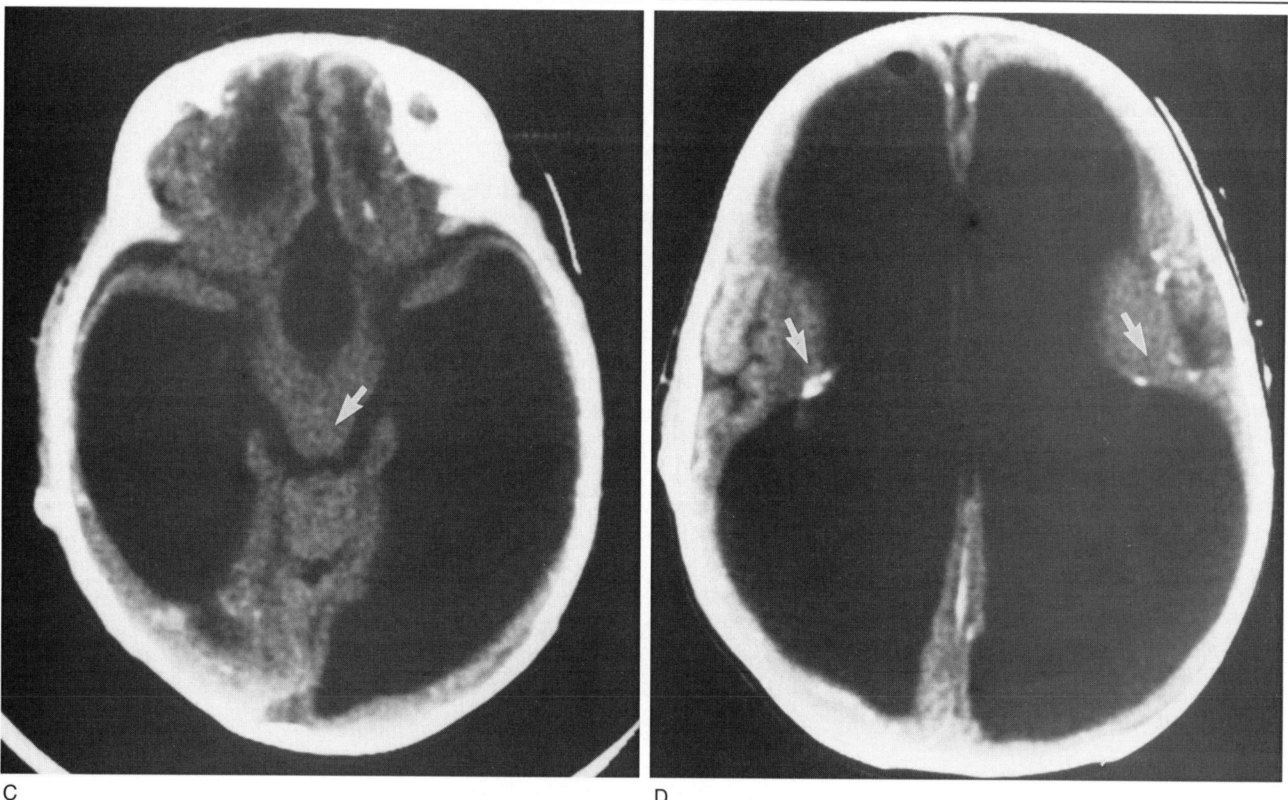

C D

Figure 4.15. *(continued)* **C** and **D.** Axial CT images demonstrate numerous calcifications in the brain (arrows) consistent with prenatal infection with toxoplasmosis or cytomegalovirus. The absence of the aqueduct in C (arrowhead) indicates aqueductal obstruction. The presence of calcifications was not suspected on MRI.

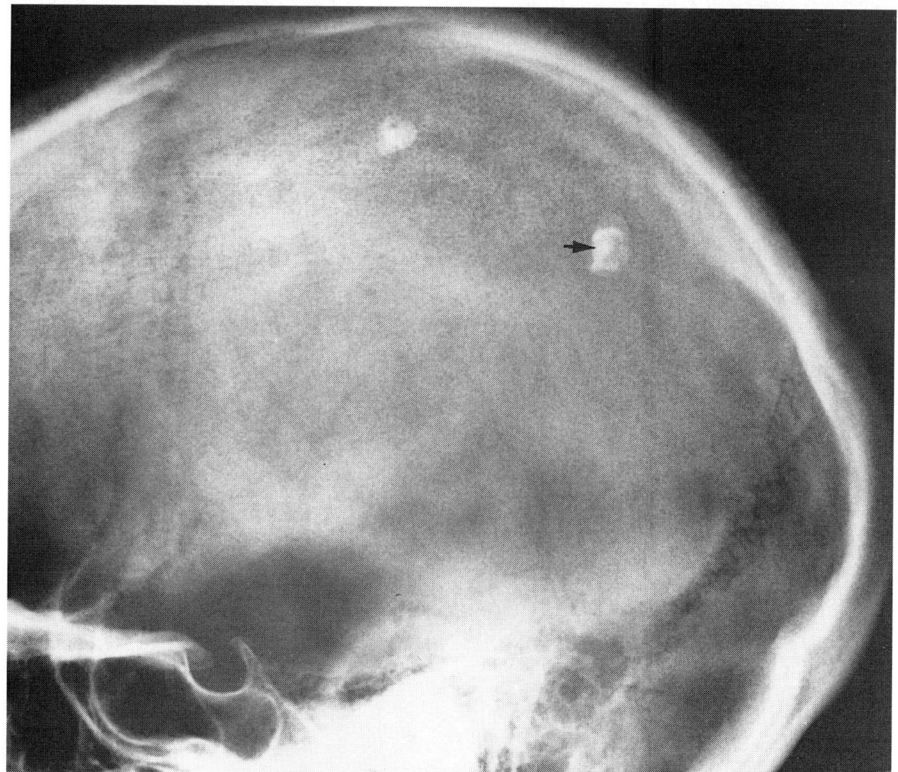

A

Figure 4.16. A. Calcified lesions of cysticercosis. Two dense calcifications are seen. One (arrows) shows the calcified parasite on one side of the calcified cyst; in the one on the other side, the calcified scolex is probably projected over the center of the calcified lesion. See discussion under "Infectious Diseases," Chapter 6.

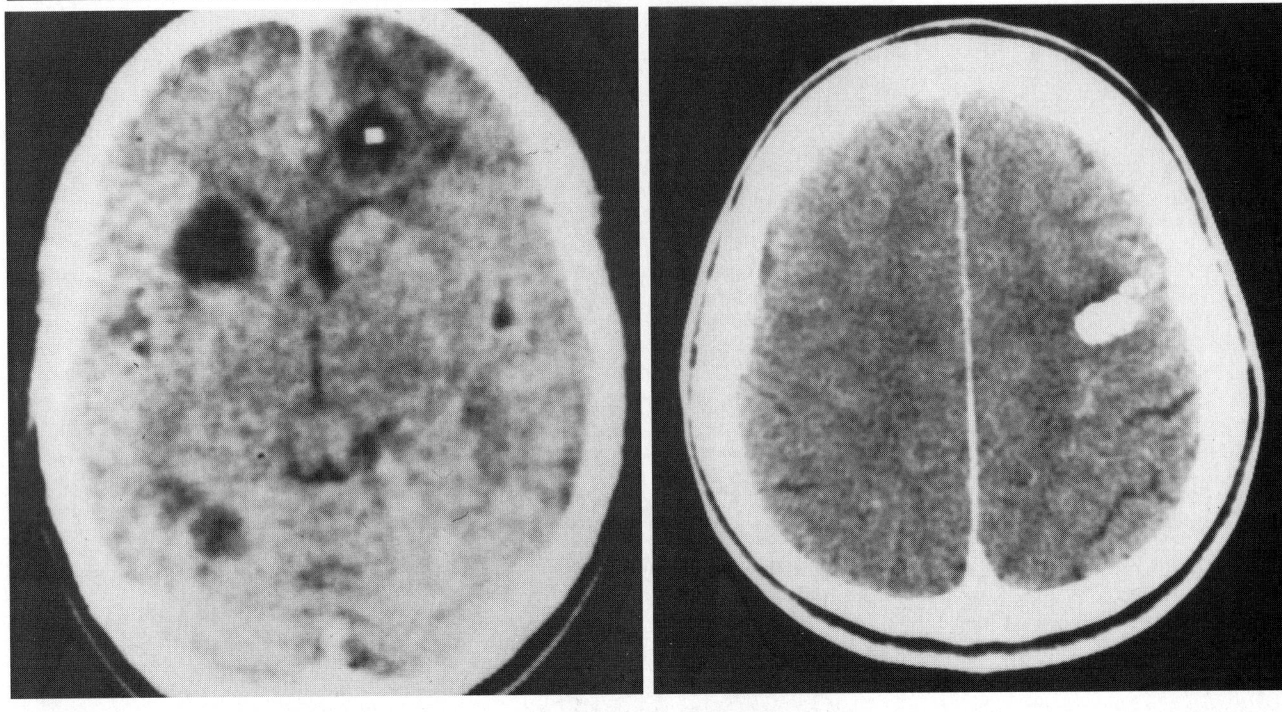

B C

Figure 4.16. *(continued)* **B.** CT showing a cystic lesion with a calcification typical of cysticercosis. There is a cyst on the other side. **C.** Calcified nodule in the upper posterior frontal region believed to be typical of tuberculoma from the point of view of size and location. There is an area of diminished attenuation anterior to it, probably representing an area of gliosis from prior inflammation.

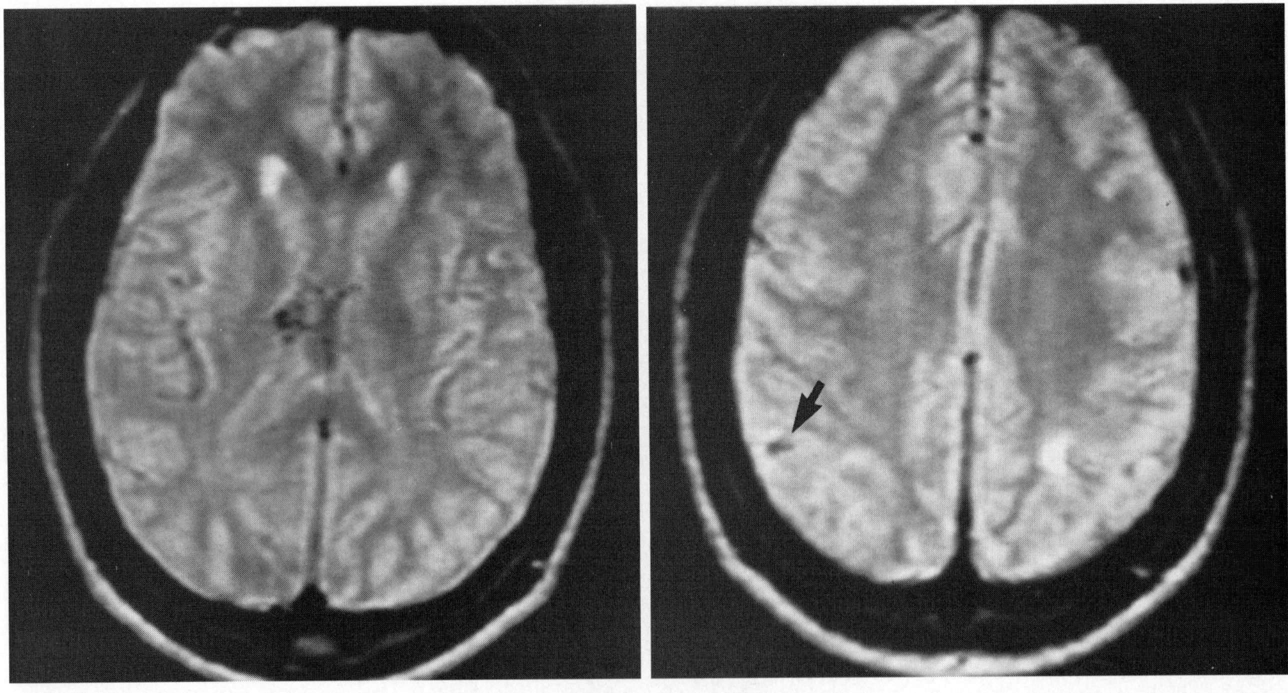

A B

Figure 4.17. Multiple calcifications, possibly paragonimiasis or sparganosis in a 57-year-old American soldier who spent time in South Korea. **A** and **B.** MRI showed a low-intensity area and an area of high intensity on a first-echo T2-weighted image. A third area near the right cortex is low intensity (arrow). On a T1-weighted image the three lesions were low intensity.

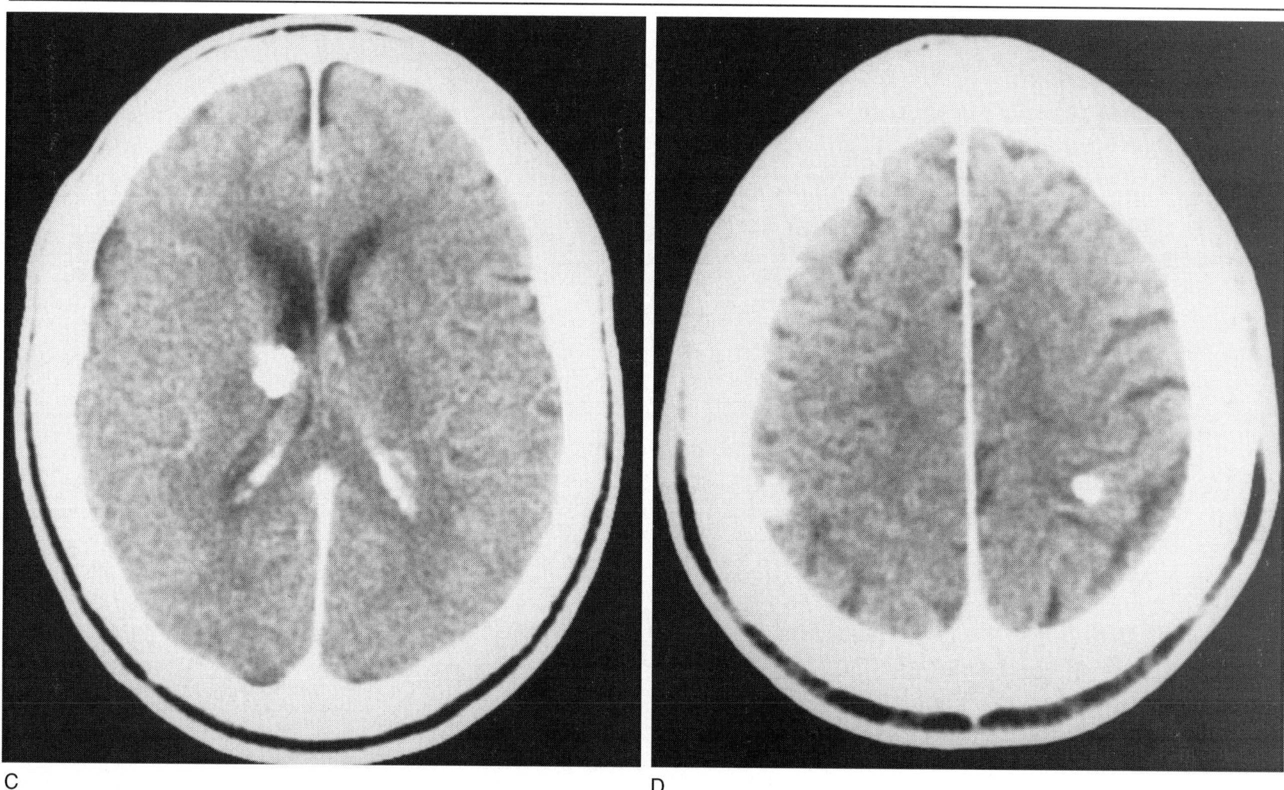

C D

Figure 4.17. *(continued)* **C** and **D.** CT demonstrated heavy calcifications in all three areas. Reexamination 4 years later revealed no change in CT appearance.

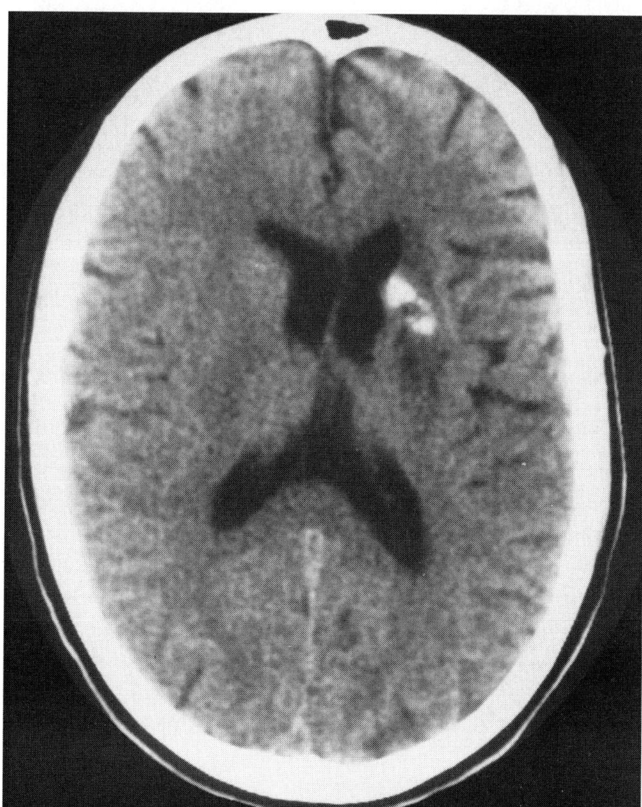

Figure 4.18. Calcified mucormycosis lesion 7 months after initial acute infection in patient with HIV. See Figure 6.35 for other images of same patient.

contained gross calcium. Several metastases from gastrointestinal tumors are occasionally seen to contain calcium on plain film examination. In all of the cases, the lime salts had been deposited in areas of necrosis in the larger tumor nodules. In most of the cases observed by the authors and described by others, the calcium deposits were small and granular, at times coalescing to form a miliary or small nodular pattern. Calcium shadows are sometimes of very light density and amorphous, and, on plain skull films, careful stereoscopic film examination is required to detect their presence. However, CT scanning can easily pick up these calcium deposits. Obviously, unless they are in multiple locations, the diagnosis of metastatic tumor as against a glioma cannot usually be made.

Various causes for scattered intracranial calcifications have been recognized. Calcifications sometimes occur in necrotic portions of tumors after radiation therapy and occasionally in nonneoplastic tissue in the field of treatment. In rare instances calcification is seen in patients with an aneurysm of the vein of Galen, both as linear deposits in the wall of the Galenic lesion and in the area of the primary arteriovenous malformation; the nature of these latter calcifications was described previously. Calcification in infantile hemiplegia may occur at multiple sites, especially along the course of the terminal branches of the anterior and middle cerebral arteries, in addition to presenting as a single calcification in some instances. Idiopathic cerebral calcifications are found in some familial diseases. So-called

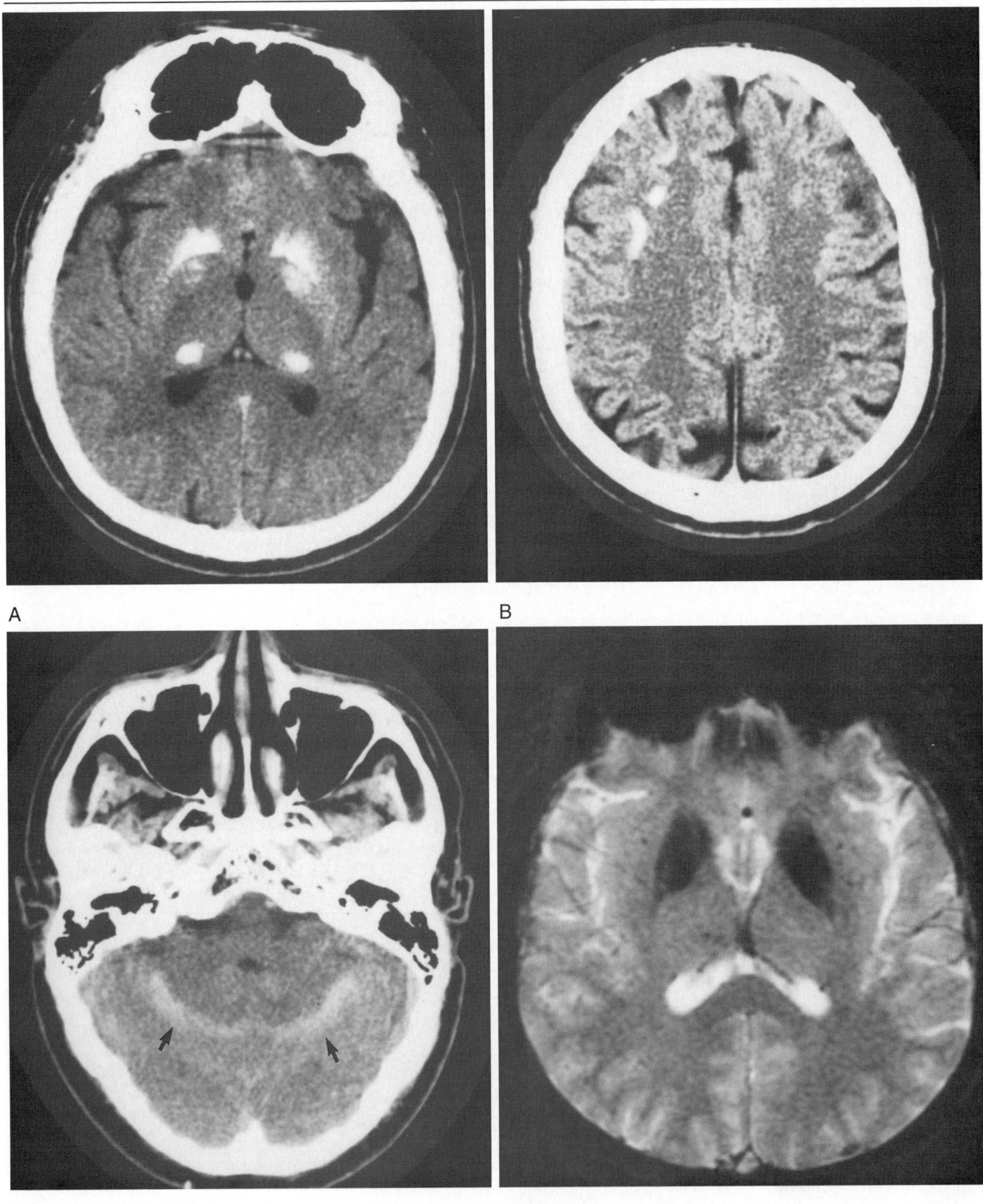

Figure 4.19. Hypoparathyroidism. **A.** CT scan showing bilateral calcification in the basal ganglia and in the pulvinar of the thalamus. **B.** Some subcortical calcifications are seen involving the cerebral corticomedullary junction. **C.** There is also calcification in the dentate nucleus of the cerebellum bilaterally (arrows). **D.** Axial MR susceptibility image shows very low intensity in basal ganglia bilaterally that cannot be differentiated from iron deposits.

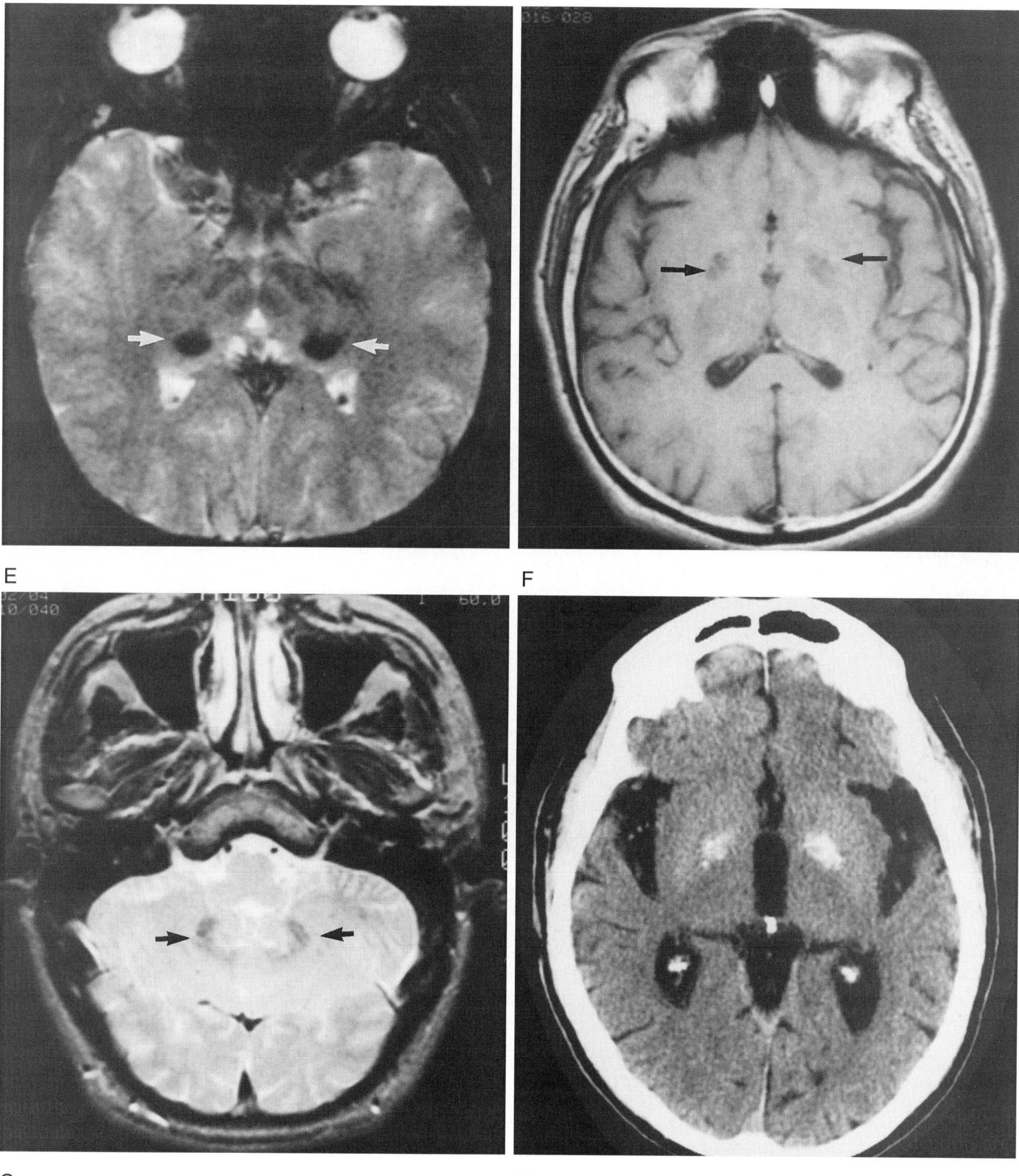

E F G H

Figure 4.19. *(continued)* **E.** An MR susceptibility section lower than D reveals the posterior thalamic calcifications as very-low-intensity areas consistent with calcifications (arrows). **F.** T1-weighted image shows that the calcific areas in the basal ganglia and thalami are only faintly visualized. **G.** The same is true in the dentate nuclei of the cerebellum (arrows). **H.** Bilateral calcification in globus pallidus in 70-year-old woman complaining of memory loss. As explained in the text, this is an extremely common finding in the older age group and is of no clinical significance. It usually exists alone; if it is accompanied by other calcifications, a pathologic condition is suspected.

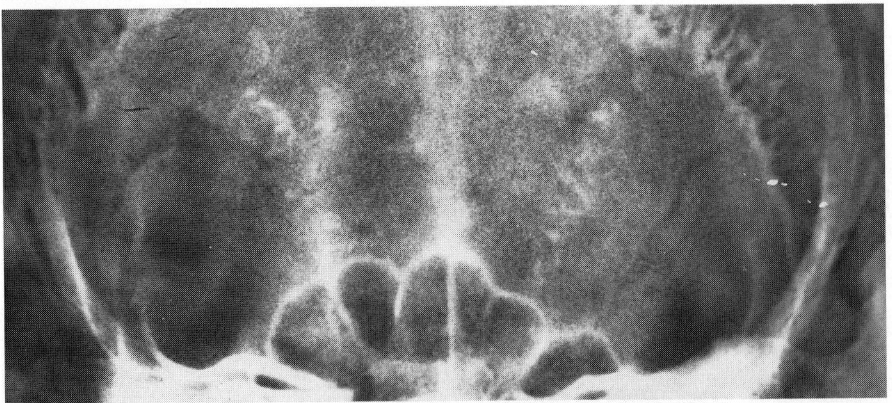

A

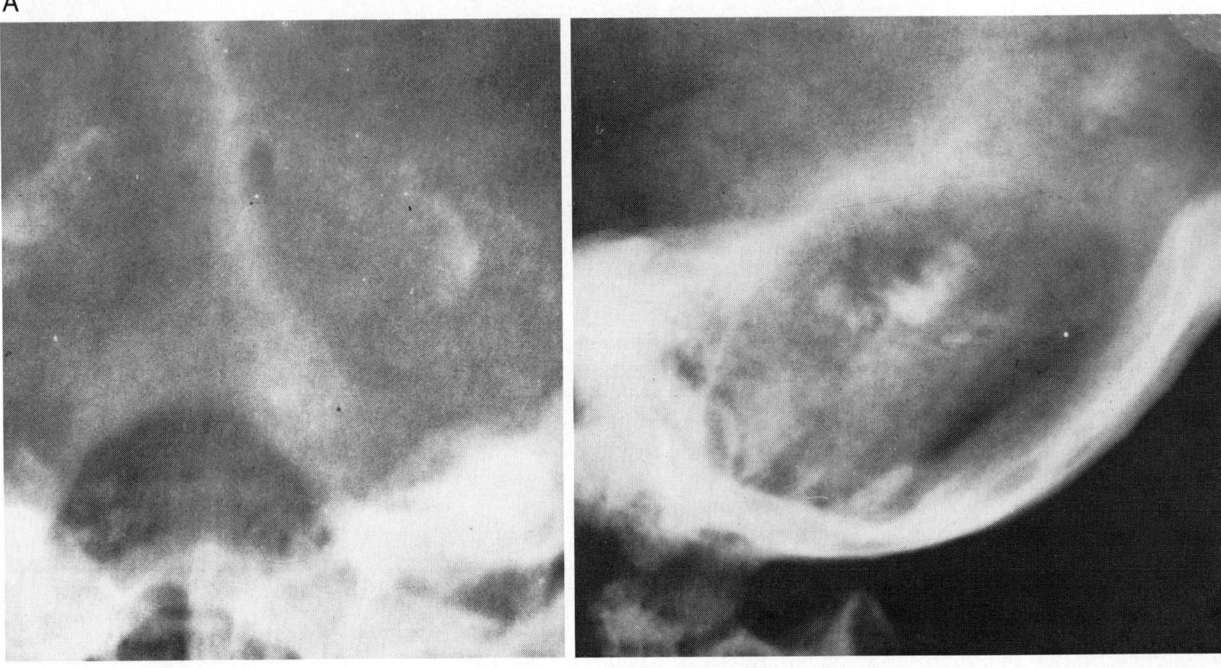

B C

Figure 4.20. A to **C.** Hypoparathyroidism with calcification in both basal ganglia and in the dentate nucleus of the cerebellum bilaterally seen on plain skull films. The same appearance may be seen in pseudohypoparathyroidism. The calcification in hypoparathyroidism is similar to that found in other conditions, such as Fahr disease. The distribution is similar. The calcifications look much heavier on CT than on plain films (see Fig. 5.68).

brainstones occasionally are found for which no particular pathology can be ascertained.

MULTIPLE SYMMETRIC CALCIFICATIONS

The most common form of symmetrical intracranial calcification is that which occurs in the choroid plexus, mentioned previously.

Basal Ganglia Calcifications

Perhaps the next most common symmetric calcifications are those found in the basal ganglia, particularly in the globus pallidus, on CT scans in older patients (Fig. 4.19*H*). The calcifications are usually punctate and can be very slight on both sides. They are sometimes moderately heavy and sometimes quite heavy, but still localized in the globus pallidus. When the putamen is also involved, we must think about the possibility of another condition, such as hypoparathyroidism or pseudohypoparathyroidism (Figs. 4.19 and 4.20). The dentate nuclei of the cerebellum may also be involved in these cases. The occurrence of colloid material is so common in the anterior half of the globus pallidus and in the dentate nucleus of the cerebellum that its presence is considered essentially normal. The colloid deposits develop in and about the finer cerebral blood vessels, and subsequent calcification takes place, apparently the result of some abnormality of the interstitial fluids that nourish

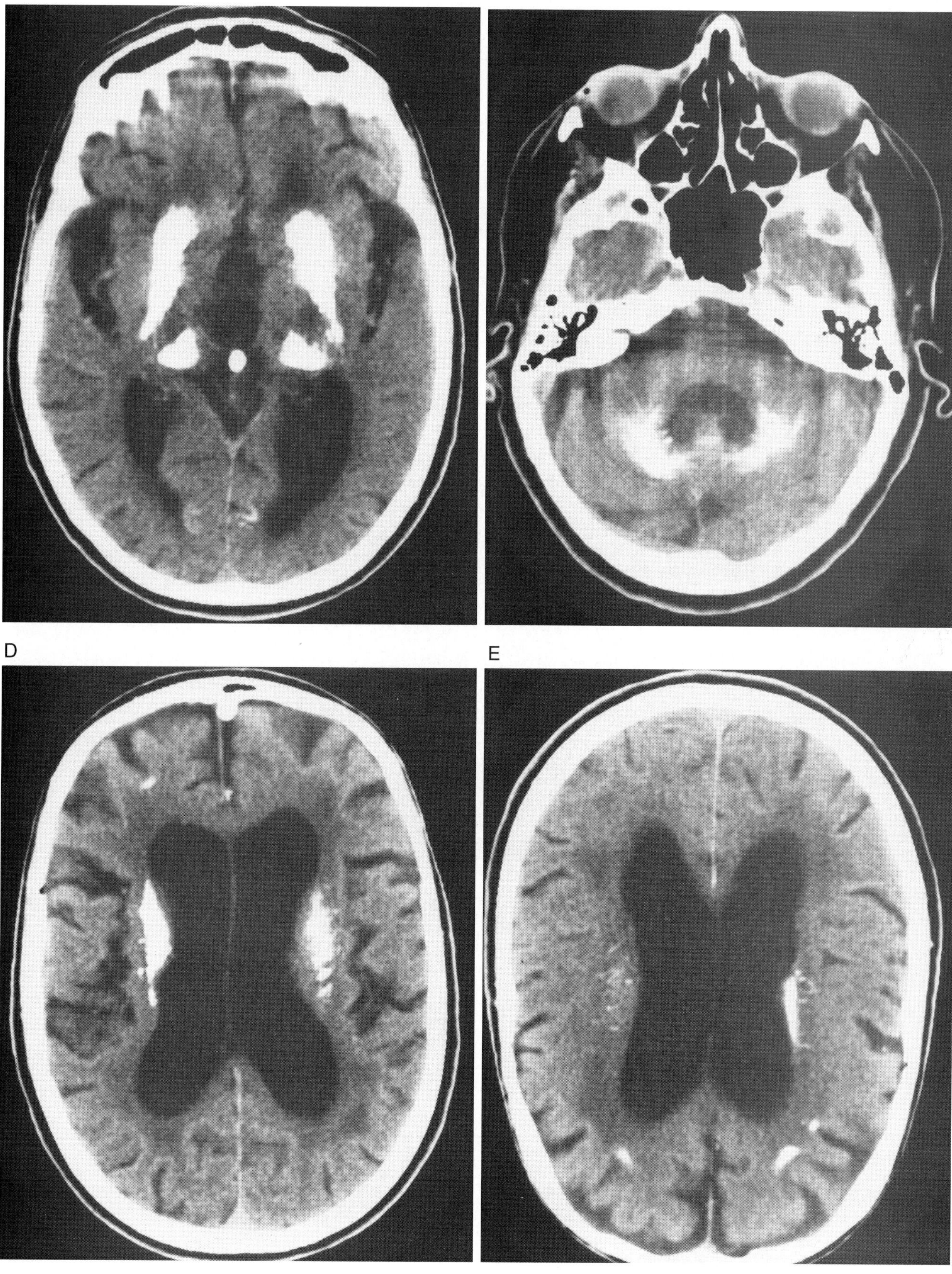

Figure 4.20. *(continued)* **D** and **E.** CT scan on another patient with Fahr disease showing calcification in the same areas. **F** and **G.** In addition, this patient had calcifications in the caudate nuclei and a few calcifications in the brain at the gray/white matter junction as well as ventricular dilatation.

the blood vessels. Albright and Reifenstein have thrown some light on the mechanism by explaining that in hypoparathyroidism there is an excess of ionic calcium in the interstitial tissues, whereas the circulating calcium values are low (10). The same distribution of calcification (globus pallidus, putamen, dentate nuclei of cerebellum, and some brain calcification) is found in some postoperative thyroidectomy patients (11).

In Fahr disease, the deposition of calcium and iron takes place in essentially the same areas, mainly the lenticular and dentate nuclei and to a lesser extent in the brain's subcortical areas. In Cockayne syndrome the calcifications are also in essentially the same locations, and occasionally cortical calcifications are found. Calcification in the basal ganglia also occurs in some of the mitochondrial cytopathies, such as Kearns-Sayre, MELAS, and MERRF (see under "Metabolic Anomalies," Chapter 5). A case of osteopetrosis was described by Demirci and Sze in which extensive calcification in the basal ganglia, thalamus, and brain white matter was found, similar in configuration to Fahr disease (12).

The lipoma of the corpus callosum sometimes calcifies symmetrically with a shell-like calcification on each side (Fig. 4.21). This is particularly well seen on frontal radiographs of the skull. However, CT scanning, with axial projections, is likely to show these calcifications particularly well.

Hippocampal Calcifications

These calcifications are an important feature of *lipoid proteinosis*, a hereditary disorder following an autosomal recessive pattern. In a well-documented case, it was found at necropsy that the calcifications were perivascular in location, being chiefly around the capillaries in the hippocampal gyri (13). The appearance on plain films or on CT scans is that of fairly dense, paired conglomerates that produce a comma-shaped shadow. The deposits are placed symmetrically in the anterior and medial walls of the temporal horns and are generally vertical in disposition on frontal or coronal views. Calcifications in the choroid plexus of the temporal horns are frequently seen on CT axial views. In this case the calcification is inside the ventricles and toward the medial edge.

Cerebral Cortical Calcifications

These are sometimes seen where no particular explanation can be found. A case of symmetrical cortical calcifications was reported by Williams and Fowler in a child who had a normal birth but had a severe illness at 3 weeks of age with a diagnosis of encephalitis (14). At 7 months of age, gyriform calcifications were demonstrated bilaterally in the occipital, parietal, and frontal regions similar to those of Sturge-Weber syndrome. Cerebral atrophy also developed.

OTHER CALCIFICATIONS

Other rare causes of symmetrical calcifications include Möbius syndrome, in which calcifications in the brainstem and in the region of the fourth-nerve nuclei have been

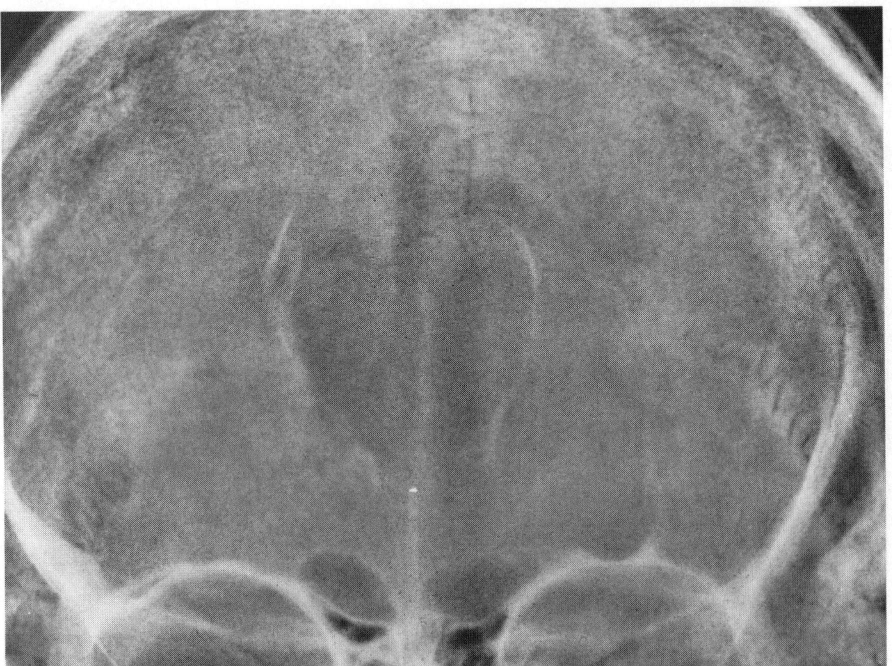

Figure 4.21. Calcified corpus callosum lipoma. The calcification as seen in the frontal view is typical of corpus callosum lipoma. The lateral view (not shown) shows nothing characteristic. In addition, there is a slightly diminished attenuation between the comma-like shells of calcium due to the adult-type fat in the lipoma. See discussion of agenesis of the corpus callosum under "Congenital Malformations" (Chapter 5), for additional details see also Fig. 5.34.

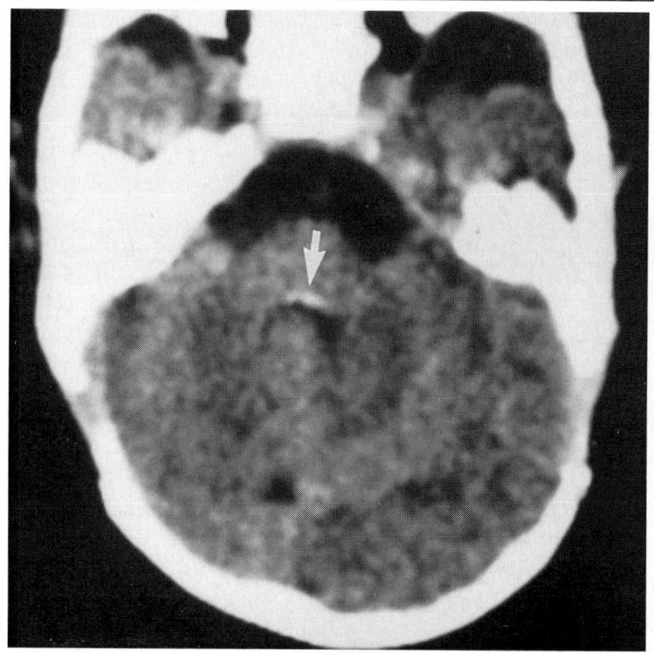

A

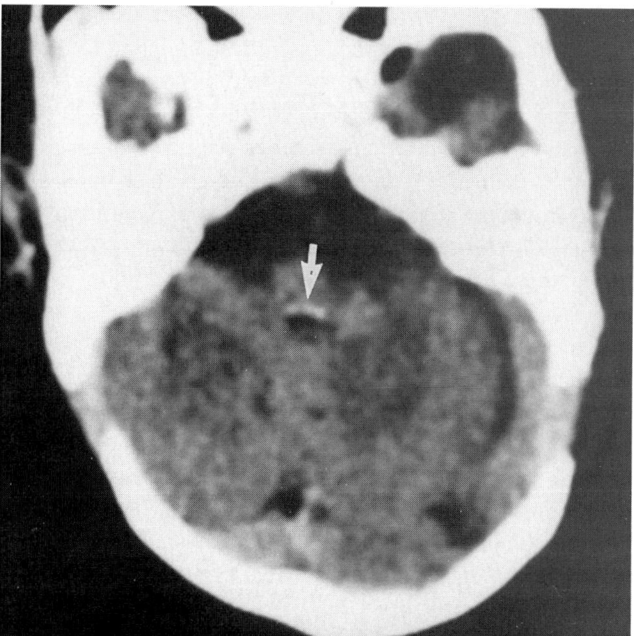

B

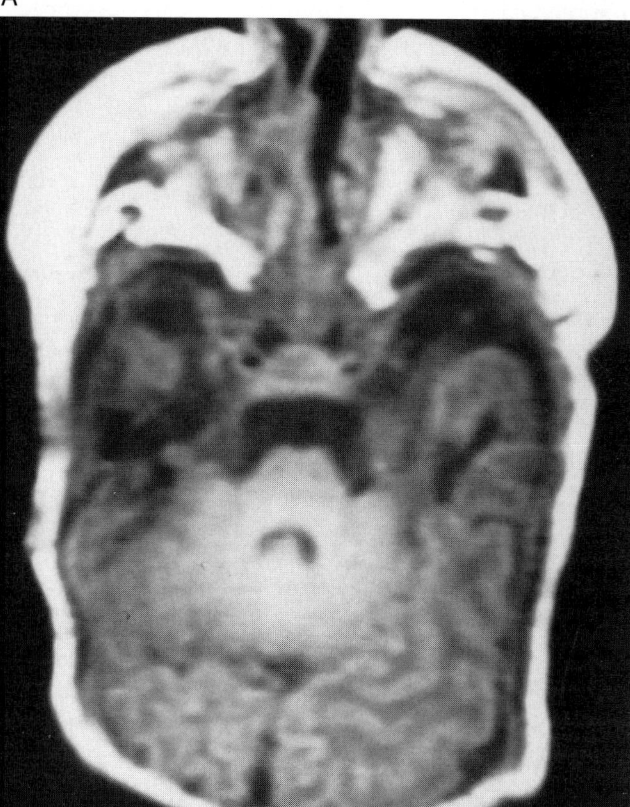

C

Figure 4.22. Möbius syndrome. **A** and **B.** CT scan without contrast in a 6-day-old infant showing extraocular muscle abnormalities (abducens palsy). Calcification in the anterior wall of the fourth ventricle is seen at two levels (arrows). **C.** MRI examination was negative and revealed normal myelination in the pons and cerebellar periventricular area. The image is a T1-weighted horizontal cross section.

described (15). Möbius syndrome is a congenital neuromuscular disorder in which there may be inability to abduct the eyes, and facial weakness. In most instances there is involvement of the eye muscles and the facial nerves or nuclei, although the lesions could all be outside the central nervous system (Fig. 4.22).

In osteopetrosis, symmetrical calcification in the basal ganglia and also in the brain white matter is quite similar to that found in Fahr's disease and in hypoparathyroidism. The appearance is so similar that one wonders whether there is a connection between the conditions. On the other hand, it is known that deposition of lime salts in the basal ganglia and in the dentate nuclei of the cerebellum occurs as a result of many conditions affecting these structures. The development of hypodensity on CT and of high signal on MRI T2-weighted images occurs frequently in asphyxia, whether due to circulatory arrest or to carbon monoxide poisoning. Presumably, focal necrosis could occur leading to calcification (16, 17, 18, 19, 20).

In chronic lead poisoning multiple calcifications have been described in the basal ganglia, subcortical white matter, vermis, and cerebellum (17). The blood lead values may reach high levels (54–72 μg as against 0–30 μg). Clinically the patients may present dementia, decreased visual acuity, peripheral neuropathy, dizziness, nystagmus, and a history of work in lead smelting plants. Brain calcifications are summarized in Table 4.1.

CEREBRAL EDEMA

Cerebral edema is an increase in brain volume due to increased tissue-water content and is a well-known reaction of brain tissue to various injuries.

Under normal circumstances the water content of the gray matter of the brain is 80 percent and that of the white matter 68 percent. The subcortical arcuate fibers have a water content that is quite similar to that of the adjacent gray matter. The extracellular space in gray matter is 13 percent of the tissue volume, whereas in white matter it is 18 percent, although a considerable amount of discussion is found in the literature with respect to the cerebral extracellular space (21). At one time the extracellular space was thought to be so small as to be virtually nonexistent.

Cerebral edema is always greatest in the white matter, quite possibly because there is less water in the white matter and slightly more extracellular space. This has been clarified to a large extent in vivo by CT and MRI. Edema appears on CT images as a radiolucent shadow surrounding the area of pathology, and on MRI it is a hyperintense area in the T2-weighted images or a hypointense area in the T1-weighted images. Sometimes the edema may extend for a considerable distance away from the lesion and follow tracts within the white matter. Edema does tend to spare the long tracts, such as the internal capsule and the optic radiations, but it is frequently seen to follow the external capsule and other tracts within the white matter of the brain. It usually spares the corpus callosum. Undoubtedly, some edema also occurs in the gray matter, but it is much more difficult to observe because of its lesser extent as compared to the white matter. Edema usually also spares or is less pronounced in the subcortical arcuate fibers. Because it usually spares the corpus callosum, it does not ordinarily pass from one hemisphere to another.

In general, the margins of edema are diffuse; the image of edema fades into the normal area rather than presenting a sharp edge.

Edema acts as a space-occupying lesion. It flattens the gyri, displaces and deforms the ventricles, and produces or increases a shift of the midline structures toward the opposite side (see Fig. 4.36).

Long-standing edema produces some gradual destruction of axons and myelin sheaths and moderate astrocytic gliosis. It does not affect the oligodendroglia. Long-standing edema may cause some slight changes in the gray matter, such as swelling of nerve cells. The edema fluid contains water, sodium, chloride, and potassium, similar to a serum filtrate, as well as increased albumin. The composition is that of interstitial fluid and not the result of breakdown of cells.

In general, two major types of edema are described: (1) *vasogenic edema* and (2) *cytotoxic edema*. Cytotoxic edema may be due to an energy failure, such as may be found in a cerebral infarct, and may involve the gray matter more than the white matter. Cytotoxic edema may be due to poisoning. Experimental cytotoxic edema may be produced by a toxic substance such as triethyl tin. Miller and Adams also include hydrostatic edema (a form of interstitial edema) and hypo-osmotic edema (22).

Because the edema fluid comes from the blood vessels, it is most severe near the lesion, probably because of leakage from vessels in the lesion or at the edge of the lesion. The cause of the edema under these circumstances could be venous compression (as may be the case in a tumor such as meningioma); thrombosis of arteries or veins (as may be the case in malignant glioma); damage of the blood vessels by toxic metabolites (as might be the case in an abscess); or secondary to anoxia (as would be the case in an infarct or a massive hemorrhage).

An important concept is that *vasogenic edema* does not develop immediately in the great majority of instances: it takes some time to develop. Thus it appears that passage of fluids from the vascular system into the tissues is not necessarily due to a break in the blood-brain barrier. Rather, it may be due to an increase in pinocytotic activity, which is responsible for at least the passage of protein across the vessel wall and into the intercellular space (Fig. 4.23). Contrast media, such as iodide contrast medium or gadolinium, *do not enhance edema*. This would tend to suggest that the accumulation of fluid is not due to a break in the blood-brain barrier (Fig. 4.24), since contrast enhancement in the brain is due to an abnormality of the vessels usually attributed to a break in the blood-brain barrier, which permits the passage of fluid outside of the blood vessels and into the tissues.

In vasogenic edema, the astrocytes may become larger as a result of the swelling, but in general this is not an important feature. The oligodendrocytes usually remain unchanged. Cytotoxic edema, on the other hand, is usually

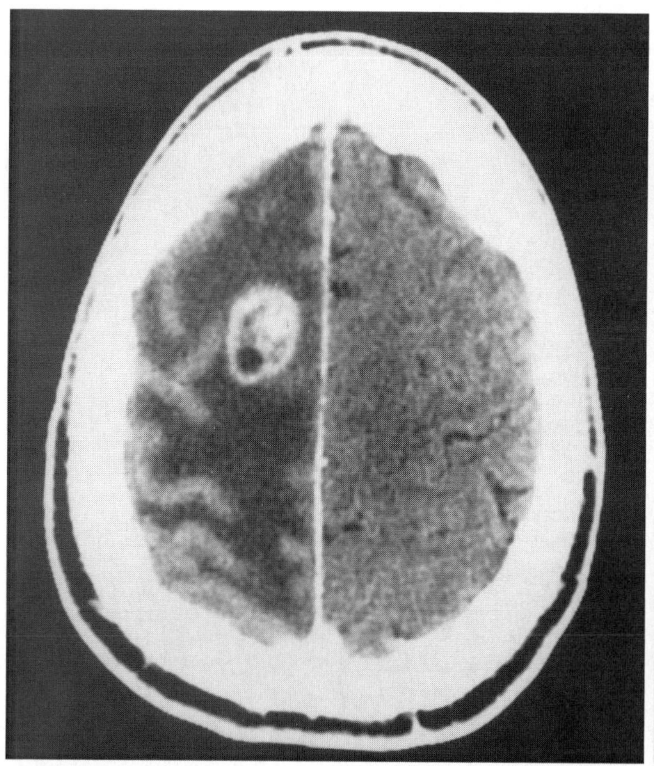

A

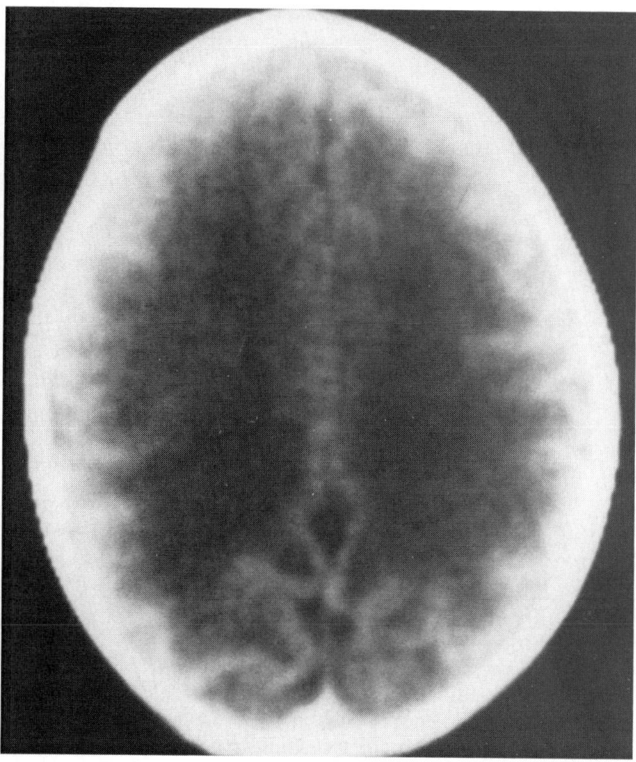

B

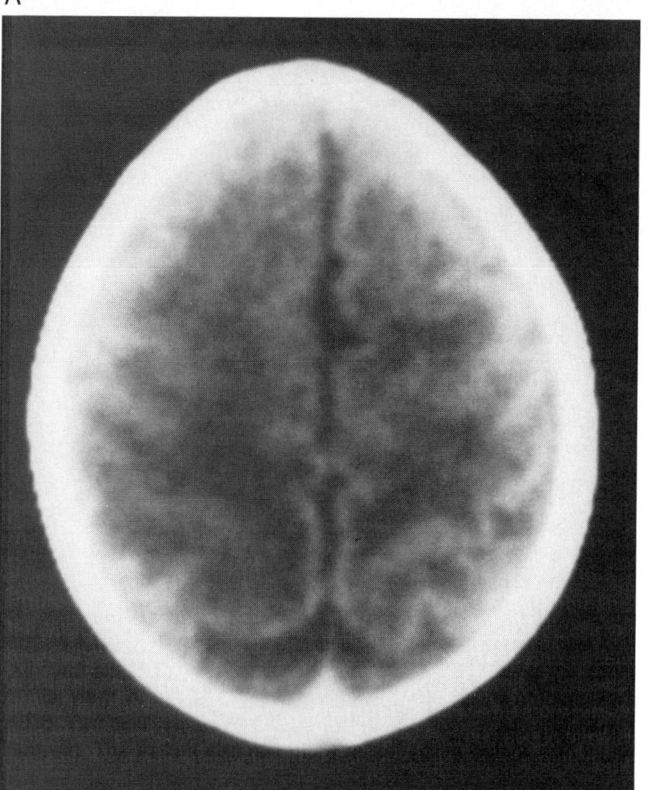

C

Figure 4.23. Vasogenic edema associated with a glioblastoma. **A.** There is a relatively small tumor but a considerable degree of low attenuation secondary to increased edema fluid. The presence and amount of edema vary considerably with the histology. Malignant tumors are likely to present more edema than benign ones, but this response is unpredictable, having to do with the tolerance of the brain tissue to the presence and histology of the tumor. Metastatic tumors usually present proportionately more edema than gliomas, but there are exceptions. The edema presumably develops slowly over a period of weeks or months (see text). **B** and **C.** Cytotoxic edema secondary to prolonged hypoxia in a young infant. There is diffuse decrease in density with apparent enlargement of the white matter in proportion to the gray matter. The gyri seem to be pushed away from the center of each hemisphere.

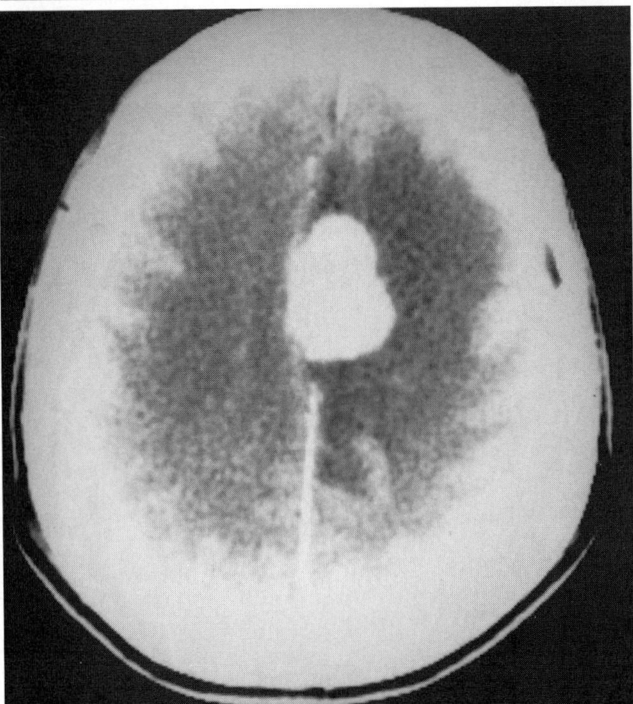

Figure 4.24. Large amount of edema associated with a lymphoma of the brain seen on an enhanced CT image. Edema does not show a blood-brain barrier breakdown and thus does not enhance after intravenous contrast. This is an important characteristic of all edema that is used in differential diagnosis.

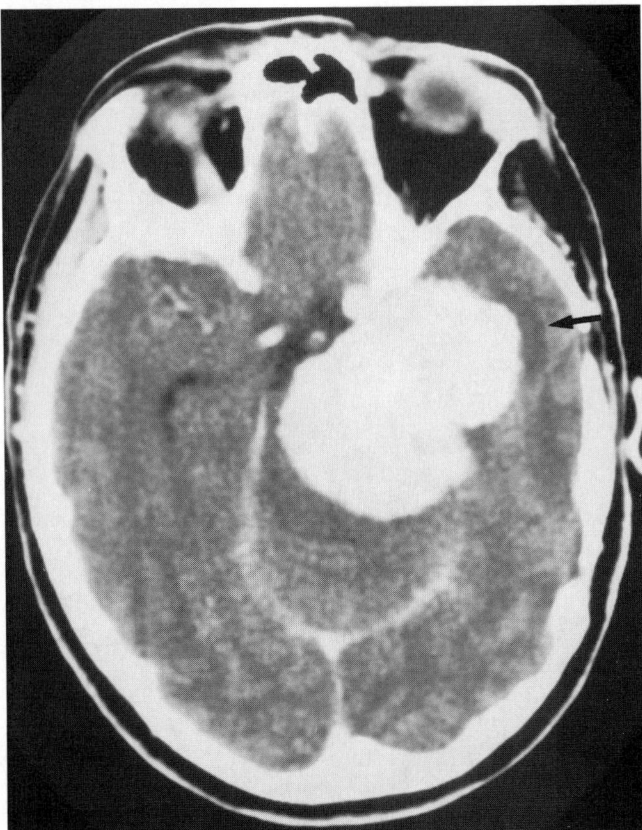

Figure 4.26. Large incisural meningioma showing no perineoplastic edema; contrast-enhanced CT. In spite of the large tumor and the strategic location, there is no discernible edema present. The low-intensity area in the left lateral temporal lobe region is produced by the laterally displaced temporal horn, which is also dilated (arrow).

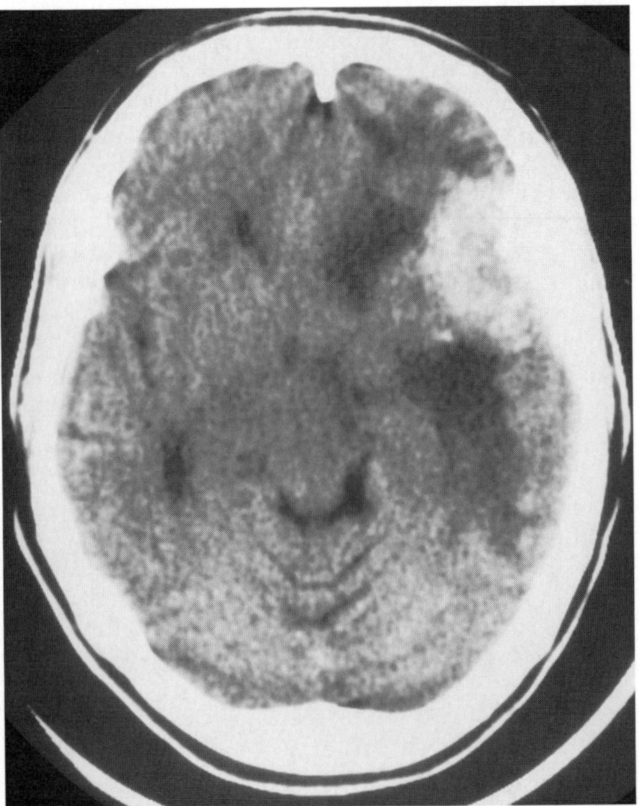

Figure 4.25. Pterional meningiomas associated with much vasogenic edema; contrast-enhanced CT. The tumor enhances with contrast and is surrounded by marked edema in all areas surrounding the lesion and extending at a distance from the tumor. There is a mass effect that is mostly due to the edema and there is displacement of the temporal lobe, which displaces the midbrain. There may be a threatened hippocampal tentorial herniation.

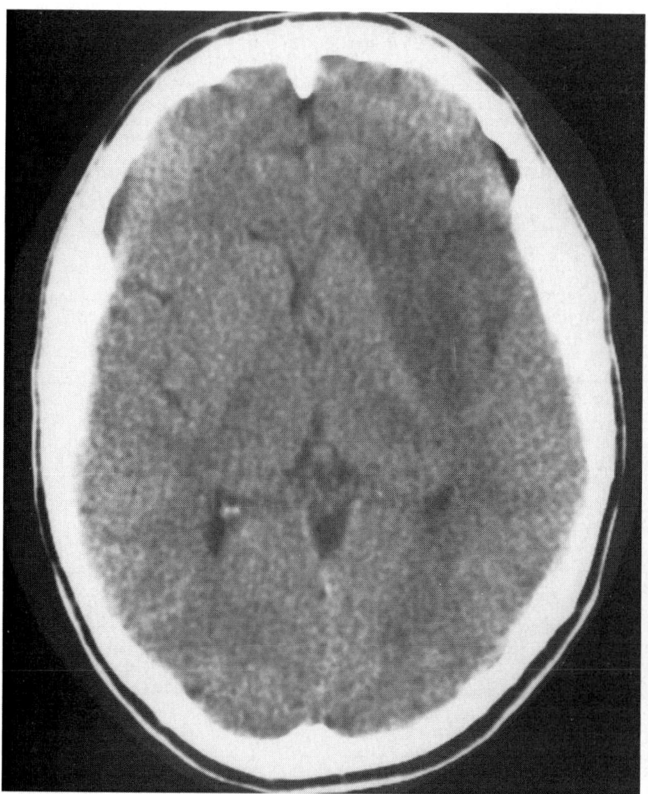

A

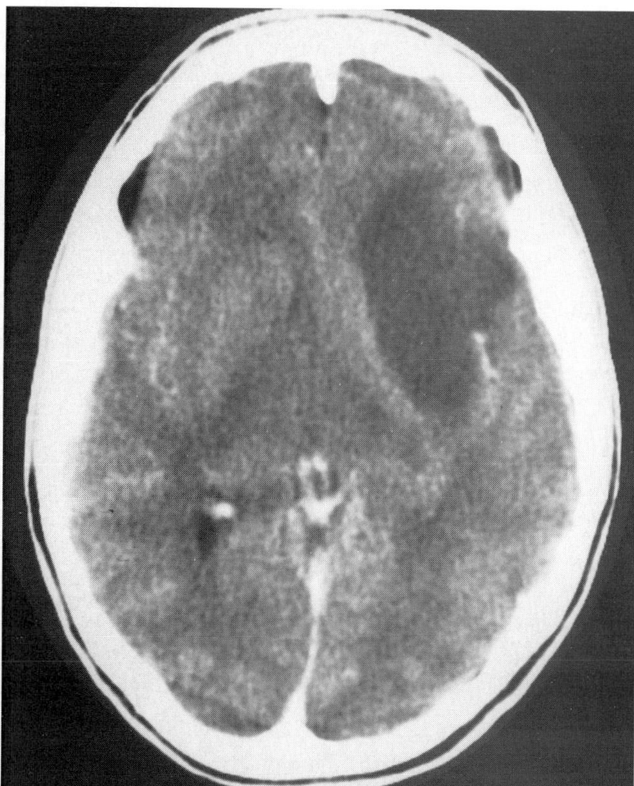

B

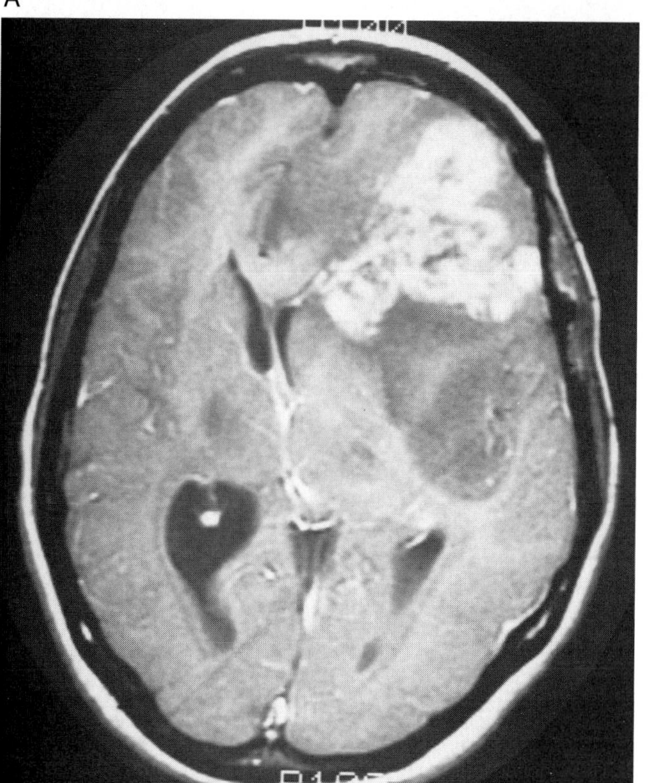

C

Figure 4.27. Slowly growing glioma showing no contrast enhancement with malignant degeneration 5 years later. **A.** CT scan showing hypodense oval area in left frontal region with slight mass effect. **B.** There was no enhancement with contrast. **C.** Five years later the tumor degenerated to glioblastoma and at that time showed considerable edema with subfalcial herniation producing considerable midline shift, as seen in this postcontrast T1-weighted axial view.

accompanied by enlargement and disruption of cell architecture, both in the neural cells and in the glial cells.

The reaction of the brain to a lesion, such as a neoplasm, varies considerably. Some meningiomas present no visible edema on CT or MRI, whereas others produce a considerable degree of swelling of the surrounding brain (Fig. 4.25). The etiology of the edematous reaction is not known. The histology of meningiomas that are accompanied by edema is no different in general from that of those that do not produce brain swelling. The more rapidly growing and recurring meningiomas do not produce more edema than others. However, the very slowly growing meningiomas tend to produce less edema (Fig. 4.26). Slowly growing gliomas produce significantly less edema than more rapidly growing ones. For that reason, it is quite possible to miss a slowly growing glioma on CT scans because there is no significant increase in the amount of water present and thus

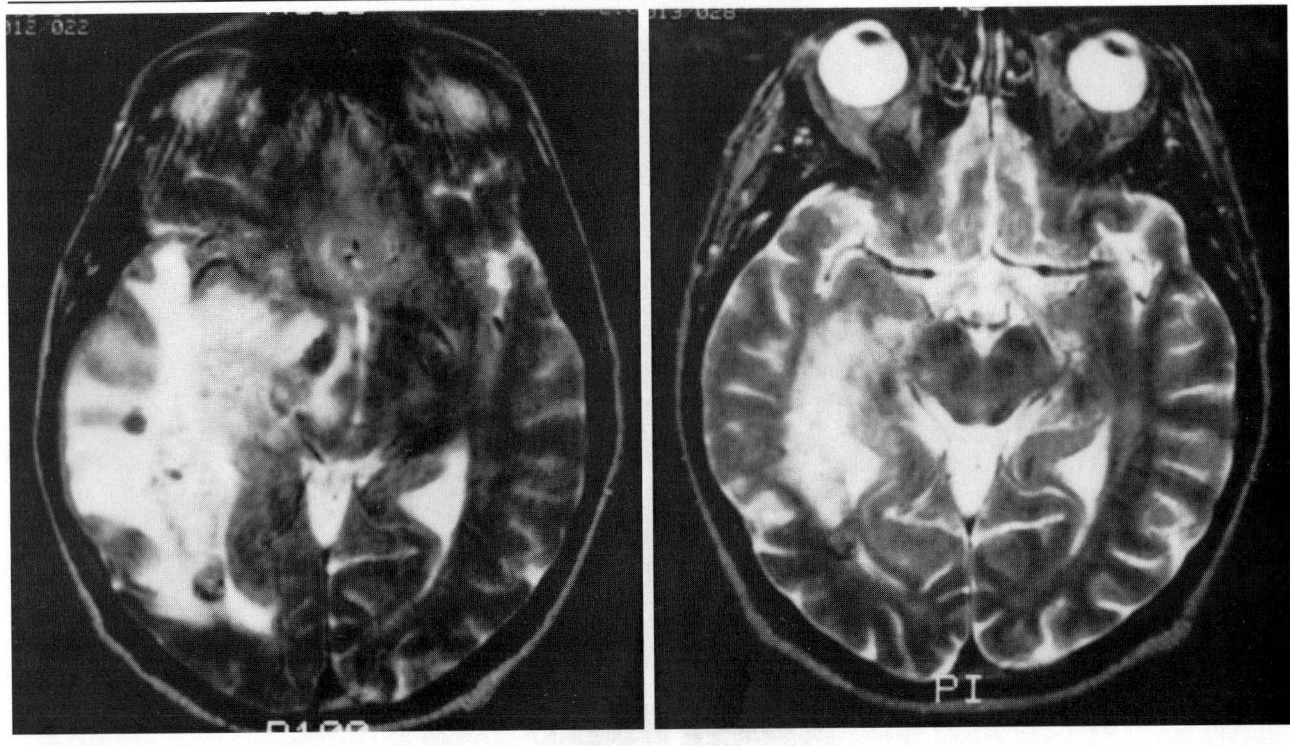

A B

Figure 4.28. Decreased edema in temporal lobe tumor following treatment. There is marked edema (**A**) that improved 2 months following radiation therapy (**B**), although the tumor is still present.

the usual radiolucency of these neoplasms does not show up. MRI, on the other hand, will demonstrate these lesions because a change in the water molecules affects the proton relaxation time sufficiently for them to be seen.

Malignant gliomas are always accompanied by edema, which sometimes is very pronounced (Fig. 4.27). It may be interesting to mention here that during the period of active growth, a malignant glioma is accompanied by considerable edema. Following treatment, it is common to see minor diminution in the size of the enhancing mass but a considerable decrease in the amount of accompanying edema. One cannot help but speculate that the quiescent cells, during the period of remission, do not have the element that leads to the vascular abnormality generating the edema (Fig. 4.28).

Types of Edema

HYDROSTATIC EDEMA

This type of edema is presumably due to a rapid increase of intracranial pressure. This generates increased arterial pressure that overcomes the cerebral vascular resistance. This type of edema might also be produced following a sudden decompression of the brain such as may occur following the removal of a large tumor or sometimes following the removal of a large extracerebral hematoma, such as an epidural or subdural hematoma. This is the type of edema that neurosurgeons are well acquainted with and which they guard against.

INTERSTITIAL EDEMA

Fishman described this edema as associated with hydrocephalus (23). Fluid is forced through damaged ependyma and into the surrounding periventricular tissues and surrounding white matter. It may be responsible for the signal hyperintensity seen on T2-weighted images and for the radiolucency in the periventricular area seen on CT (Fig. 4.29).

HYPEROSMOTIC EDEMA

This condition is caused by overhydration. It could be produced by too much intravenous fluid or inappropriate secretion of antidiuretic hormone.

Vasodilatation increases the amount of cerebral edema, whereas vasoconstriction decreases edema. Thus factors that tend to increase capillary pressure favor the formation and spread of edema, as do factors that decrease plasma osmotic pressure.

CONGESTIVE BRAIN SWELLING

In congestive brain swelling the brain rapidly expands, particularly if the arterial pressure is high. This rapid expansion, caused by rapid accumulation of extravascular water,

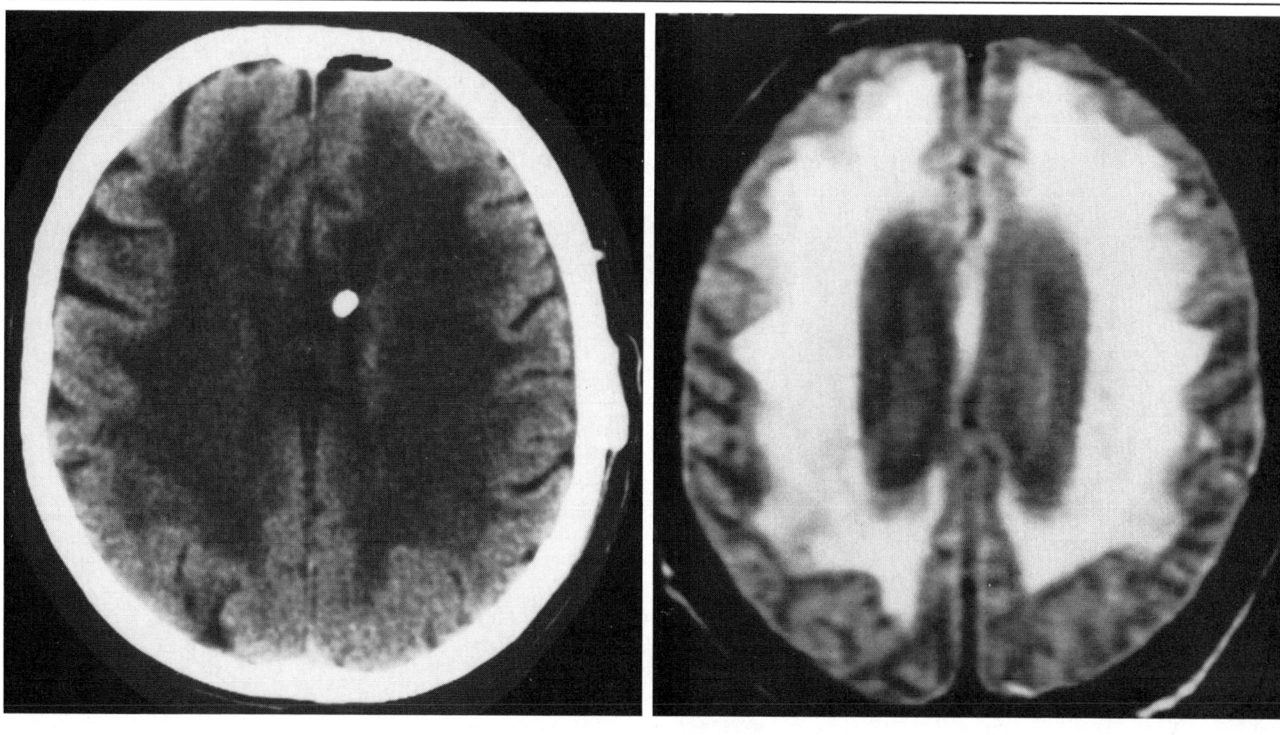

Figure 4.29. Transependymal passage of fluid in patient with partial obstruction of CSF flow in basal cisterns. There is low attenuation on CT (**A**) and marked hyperintensity on T2-weighted MRI (**B**) in the patient, who developed diffuse meningeal mestastases from cancer of the breast. The meningeal involvement was particularly heavy in the posterior fossa, causing obstruction of CSF pathways that resulted in increased intraventricular pressure.

causes a decrease in the cerebrospinal fluid (CSF) space and constriction of the ventricles. At this point, intracranial pressure increases in waves and may reach very high levels, up to the systolic blood pressure. This type of irreversible edema can occur as a result of severe head trauma. As vasomotor paralysis occurs, the arterioles and capillaries remain dilated and edema increases to the point where the intracranial pressure reaches the systolic blood pressure. At this point, an irreversible state is reached that leads to brain death (24, 25, 26).

An important concept is that edema does not necessarily interfere with brain function. It decreases cerebral blood flow, and if it is severe enough, it reduces cerebral blood flow to a point where it may become critical. Increased intracranial pressure may reduce cerebral blood flow. Autoregulation (the ability of the brain blood vessels to adapt to changes in blood pressure) is also impaired locally if there is tissue damage. It is questionable whether the local tissue pressure may be high enough to decrease local cerebral blood flow. External methods of blood flow measurement frequently show a decrease in cerebral blood flow in the area of the lesion, but only if it is a lesion with low vascularity.

The effects of cerebral edema are important. The edema tends to increase the mass effect, sometimes to a very large extent. For instance, the volume of a tumor may be 25 or 30 cc, but the edema that surrounds the lesion could easily be 10 times that much or even more. Under those circumstances, edema causes a considerable increase in the mass effect. Metastatic tumors tend to produce more edema than primary brain neoplasms (Fig. 4.30). As is well known, steroid therapy decreases the edema of the surrounding brain and improves the patient's condition. The steroids probably close or narrow the junctions between the endothelial cells of the capillary walls and thus cause a diminution in the extravasation of fluid.

Herniations

The presence of the mass and the accompanying edema causes displacement of the adjacent brain structures (Table 4.2). Thus there is usually compression of the lateral and third ventricles, displacement of the midline structures to the opposite side, and possibly displacement of brain structures through the tentorial incisura. Subfalcial herniation or midline shift is not usually a severe complication unless it is very marked, in which case it may produce necrosis of the cingulate gyrus where the edge of the falx presses against it. On the other hand, transtentorial herniation is likely to be much more important. The reason is that the tissue that herniates downward (the medial portion of the temporal lobe or parahippocampal gyrus) compresses the

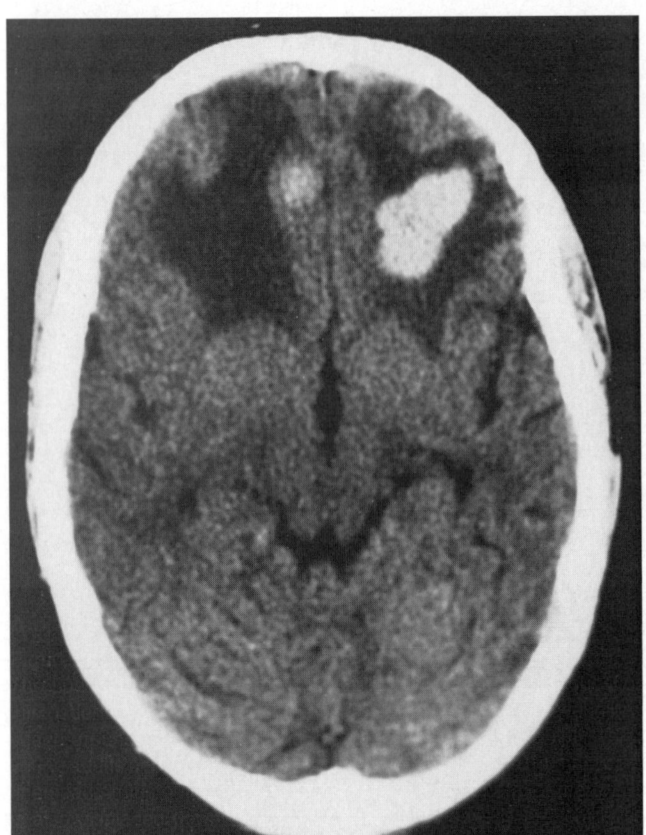

A

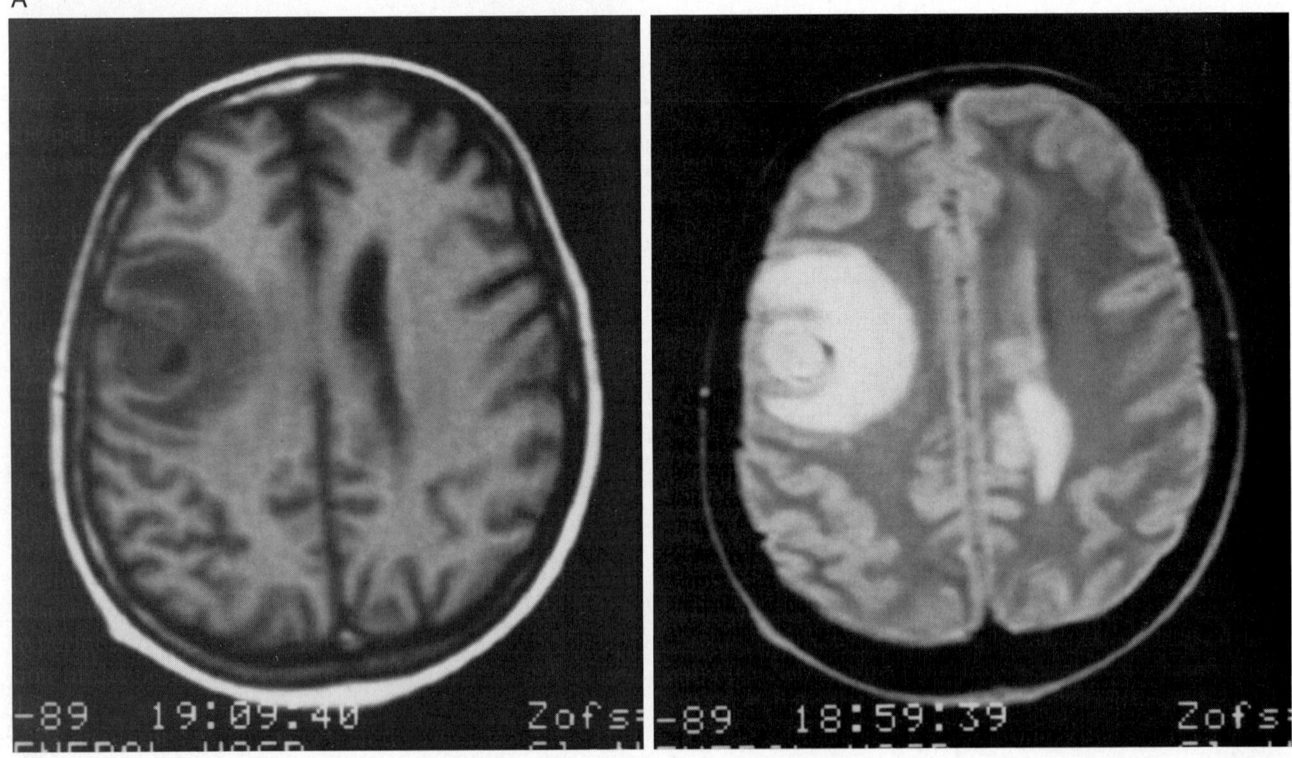

B C

Figure 4.30. Metastatic nodules associated with marked edema. **A.** The nodules in the right frontal area are small but the edema is as much as on the other side. **B** and **C.** Another example showing the typical appearance of edema on T1-weighted (B) and T2-weighted (C) images: dark on T1 and bright on T2.

Table 4.2.
Types of Brain Herniation

I. Subfalcine: contralateral shift of midline and paramidline structures under falx cerebri
II. Transtentorial
  A. Upward: cephalad displacement of cerebellum through tentorial incisura
  B. Downward
    1. Anterior: uncal herniation by lesions in anterior half of brain
    2. Posterior: herniation of posterior portion of parahippocampal gyrus
    3. Total: herniation of uncus and parahippocampal gyrus
III. Retroalar: posterior herniation of frontal lobe across edge of sphenoid ridge
IV. Trans–foramen magnum: downward displacement of inferior mesial portions of one or both cerebellar hemispheres

midbrain. The shifting structures usually also displace and stretch the third cranial nerve, which leads to dilatation of the pupil, an important clinical sign of impending or actual transtentorial herniation.

UPWARD TRANSTENTORIAL

Transtentorial herniation may be downward, as just explained, or upward, in which case the cerebellum is pushed up through the tentorial incisura posteriorly as the result of a mass in the cerebellum itself or a mass that displaces the cerebellum upward. This mass could be produced by sudden hemorrhage in the cerebellum or by a tumor. In the case of tumor, the upward transtentorial herniation

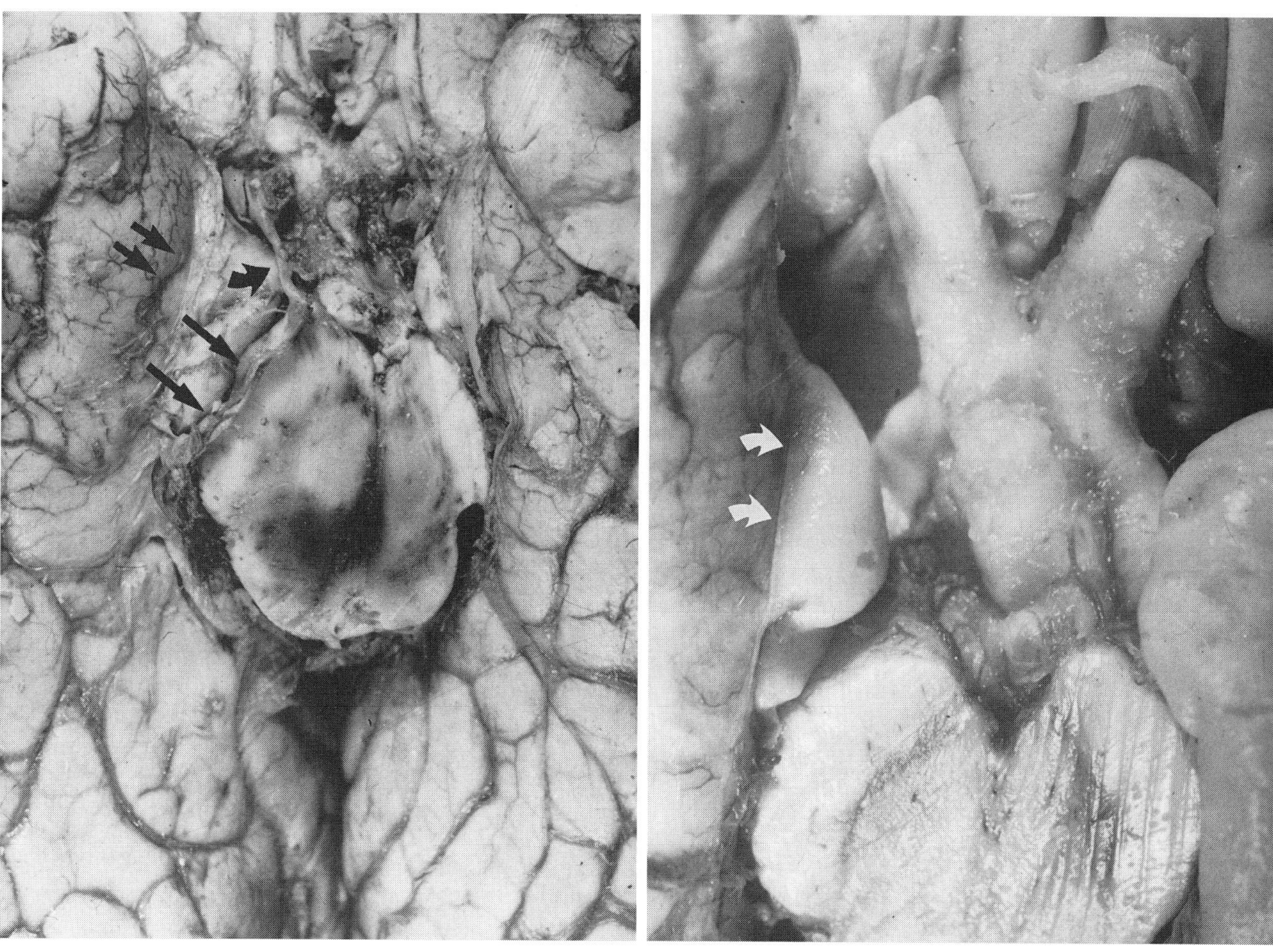

Figure 4.31. A. Anterior transtentorial herniation. There is medial displacement of the uncus of the hippocampus; a groove is seen in the position where the edge of the tentorium would be (arrows). The midbrain is displaced toward the opposite side, against the edge of the tentorium. The cerebral peduncle is flattened (longer tail arrows), and the interpeduncular fossa is almost totally compressed. The oval small mass is the right mammillary body. The posterior communicating artery is displaced medially (curved arrow), and the posterior cerebral artery is displaced medially and backward. There is hemorrhagic congestion of the midbrain due to elongation and rupture of the veins as the anteroposterior diameter of the structure is increased. **B.** Small anterior transtentorial hernia in another autopsy case (arrows). There is minimal evidence of compression of the cerebral peduncle and no evidence of hemorrhage.

takes place more slowly, whereas in the case of spontaneous hemorrhage it develops more rapidly. The same might be the case if bleeding were to develop within a neoplasm. Under these circumstances, the patient may rapidly deteriorate clinically.

DOWNWARD TRANSTENTORIAL

Downward transtentorial herniation can be classified as anterior, posterior, or total. In *anterior herniation,* the most common type, the anterior portion of the hippocampus (the uncus) herniates downward, compressing and displacing the cerebral peduncle posteriorly and toward the other side. At the same time, it may stretch or compress the third cranial nerve. This condition is produced by lesions situated in the anterior half of the brain, possibly in the frontal or temporal lobe (Fig. 4.31).

Lateral and *posterior herniation* involves, respectively, the lateral and posterior aspects of the parahippocampal gyrus. It compresses the lateral and posterior aspect of the midbrain and displaces it toward the opposite side, together with the aqueduct. Such movement can lead to ventricular dilatation. If the compression is sudden, the ventricular dilatation is acute and can lead to sudden worsening of the patient's condition, with loss of consciousness (Fig. 4.32).

In *total herniation* the entire hippocampus is displaced downward through the tentorial incisura, and the degree of displacement and flattening of the midbrain is greater. Elongation of the anteroposterior diameter of the midbrain leads to elongation of the veins and rupture of some of these veins, which causes hemorrhage within the midbrain. Posterior herniation is caused by a tumor situated in the posterior half of the brain, whereas total herniation may be caused by a very large tumor or by a large subdural or epidural hematoma (Figs. 4.33 and 4.34) (27, 28).

When the brainstem is compressed and flattened by a lateral or total unilateral herniation, the midbrain is also displaced toward the opposite side and may, in addition, be compressed on the other side as it is pressed against the tentorial edge. The edge of the tentorium is sharper than the herniated hippocampus, and the contralateral compression may lead to clinical signs referable to the opposite hemisphere. Thus a large subdural hematoma on the right side may produce a right dilated pupil due to hippocampal herniation and a right hemiparesis due to compression of the midbrain against the left tentorial edge.

Bilateral transtentorial herniation may also occur, such as in bilateral extracerebral collections (subdural or epidural hematomas) or in severe generalized supratentorial brain edema (Fig. 4.34).

RETROALAR

In addition to downward transtentorial herniation, the inferior aspect of the frontal lobe can herniate behind the edge of the sphenoid ridge. This is called a *retroalar herniation* and is caused by lesions situated in the anterior aspect of the frontal lobe. From the clinical point of view, this movement is not as important as the transtentorial herniation but may lead to some ischemic changes in the inferior frontal lobe (Fig. 4.35).

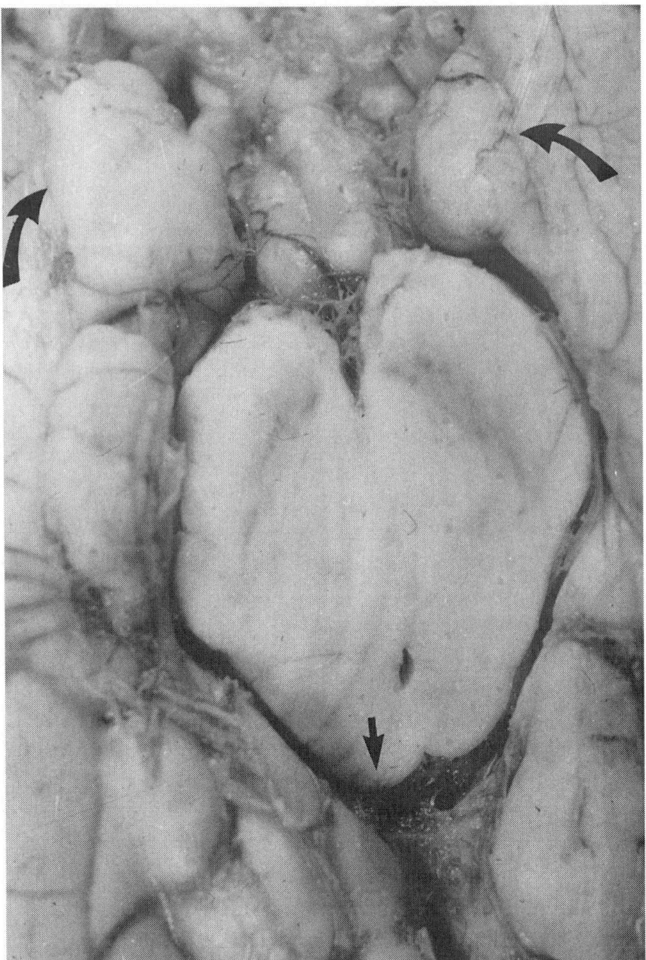

Figure 4.32. Lateral transtentorial hippocampal herniation. The deformity is obvious. As yet there is no evidence of hemorrhage in the midbrain. There is also evidence of anterior hippocampal hernation bilaterally, larger on the right (curved arrows). Lateral transtentorial herniation is usually seen when there is also anterior and/or posterior herniation. The right side of the quadrigeminal plate is dorsally displaced (arrow), and the aqueduct is narrowed and elongated.

It should be remembered that in the presence of impending or actual transtentorial herniation, a spinal puncture with removal of CSF could be very dangerous and is usually considered contraindicated. The same applies to the presence of a posterior fossa tumor where the lower part of the cerebellum could herniate through the foramen magnum. In general, the cerebellar tonsils and adjacent portion of the biventral lobule of the cerebellum are low and just above the foramen magnum; lowering the pressure in the spinal canal by removing CSF could provoke a complete herniation and blockage of the outlets of the fourth ventricle.

CT AND MRI DIAGNOSIS

CT scanning and MRI are excellent for diagnosing *subfalcial herniations* (midline shift) and transtentorial hernia-

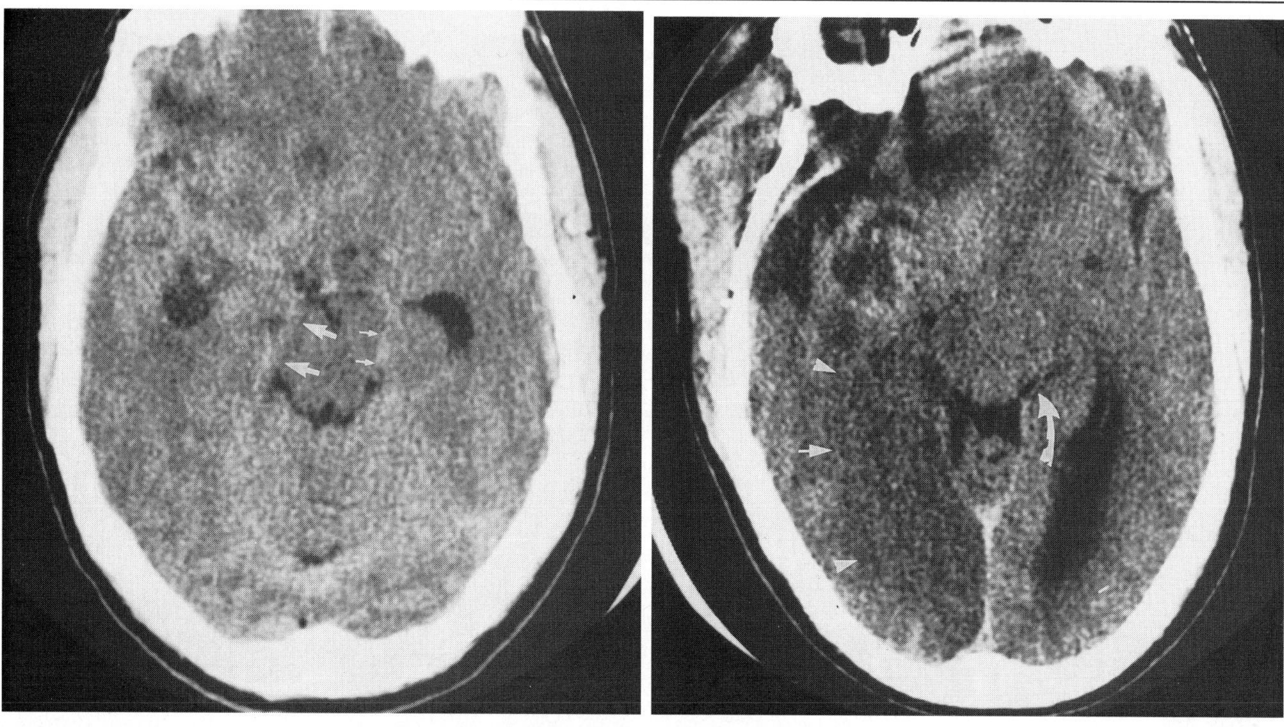

Figure 4.33. Hippocampal herniation causing compression of posterior cerebral artery and occipital infarction. **A.** CT image of a 41-year-old man with a malignant right frontal glioma causing hippocampal herniation (arrows). There is also some medial displacement of the left hippocampus (small arrows) causing some further compression of the midbrain. **B.** Following surgery there was some change in the position of the brain; the previous right transtentorial hernia caused compression of the right posterior cerebral artery and an occipital infarct visible as a large low-density area (arrows). However, because of the generalized brain edema and ventricular dilatation, the patient also developed a posterior transtentorial herniation on the left side (curved arrow).

tions. The degree of midline shift can be estimated by measuring the distance from the inner table of the skull to the lower portion of the septum pellucidum and from that to the opposite inner table. If one then determines where the midline should be, it is easy to estimate the degree of displacement of the midline structures by comparing it with the minification factor, which is always photographed on the films. The third ventricle can also be used for this purpose, but it is often not clearly seen because of the compression produced by the pathology (Fig. 4.36).

It is more difficult to diagnose *downward transtentorial herniation.* In an anterior hippocampal herniation, the herniated uncus moves medially over the anterior edge of the tentorial incisura and compresses the peduncle of the midbrain, producing flattening. If the herniation is large enough, it will rotate the midbrain slightly (see Fig. 4.31). In a lateral or total transtentorial herniation, the CSF space around the lateral aspect of the brain decreases or disappears, the midbrain is displaced against the opposite edge of the tentorium, and the CSF space on this side may also disappear. The midbrain may become flattened and elongated in the anterior posterior diameter. In total herniation the posterior aspects of the CSF spaces also disappear or become considerably decreased in size. The quadrigeminal cistern is deformed and narrowed and may disappear altogether. If the compression is severe, there are signs of hemorrhage in the midbrain (Figs. 4.32 and 4.34). In posterior herniation, only the posterolateral aspect of the midbrain is compressed and displaced.

On CT, all of these changes must be observed on axial views. When MRI is available, the transtentorial herniations may be observed on axial, sagittal, and coronal views. Often the coronal views show transtentorial herniations most clearly. *Upward transtentorial herniation* brings the upper aspect of the vermis and the cerebellum upward behind the midbrain. The inferior aspect of the quadrigeminal cistern is compressed and disappears, and the midbrain is flattened from behind. The superior cerebellar cistern also disappears or becomes very small (Fig. 4.37).

Generalized Edema

Generalized edema of the brain is another condition that is important to recognize. It occurs most frequently following head injuries and may or may not be associated with extracerebral hematomas. It may also be seen as a result of cardiorespiratory arrest or of any cause of total arrest of brain

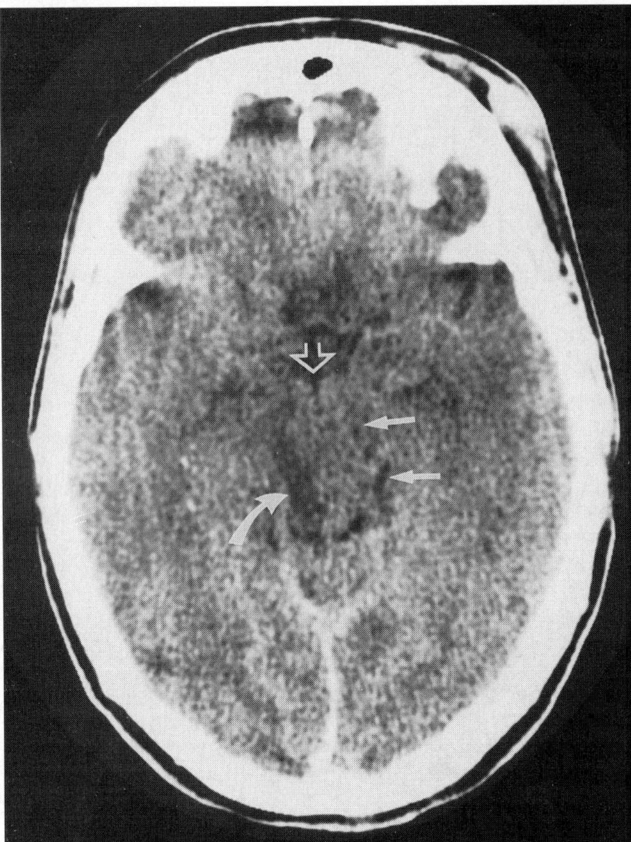

Figure 4.34. Total downward transtentorial herniation in a patient with acute severe head injury. The edge between the herniated medial temporal lobe and the compressed midbrain is outlined by an irregular thin dark edge (two white arrows). There is edema and flattening of the midbrain also on the right side (curved arrow). The interpeduncular fossa is markedly compressed (open arrow).

circulation. In general, the first signs that can be observed are diminution in the size of the lateral ventricles and decrease in the size of the subarachnoid CSF spaces. This may be more difficult to appreciate when the changes are only slight or moderate.

In young subjects, the sylvian fissures and the subarachnoid sulci over the surface of the brain may be quite small under normal circumstances, but some subarachnoid space is always present if looked for. Perhaps the most important finding is the decrease in size of the cisternal spaces at the base of the brain. This includes, in the early stage, the disappearance of the perimesencephalic CSF space and the slight downward displacement of the midbrain and pons, which causes a diminution in size of the prepontine CSF space situated below the tentorium (Fig. 4.38). One should be careful in interpreting small but present perimesencephalic and quadrigeminal cistern CSF spaces in young individuals because often the spaces are normally small. If they have disappeared completely, then that should be a clear indication of generalized edema of the brain (Fig. 4.39). Brain edema would also cause a depression of the brainstem caudally, producing a forward movement of the belli of the

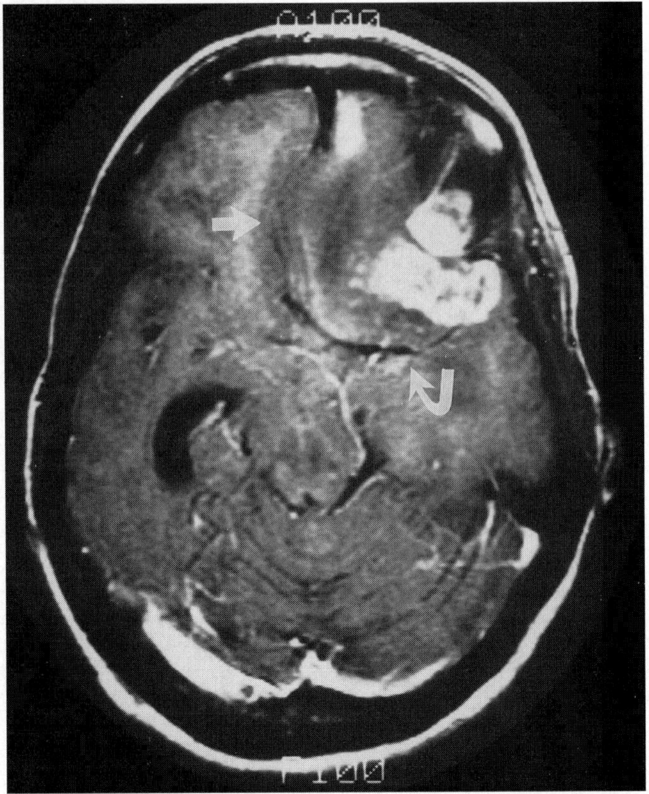

A

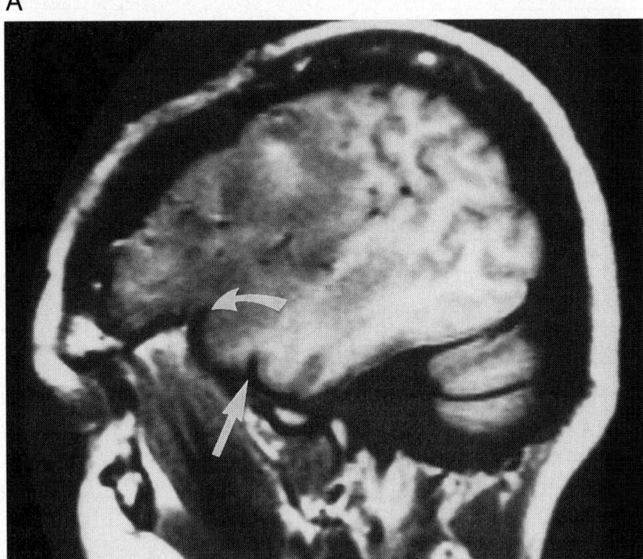

B

Figure 4.35. Retroalar herniation in patient with left frontal glioblastoma. **A.** Axial T1-weighted postcontrast image shows hyperintensity in the tumor surrounded by considerable edema; the frontal lobe is displaced to the opposite side (single arrow), and the edematous frontal lobe bulges dorsally, displacing the temporal lobe (curved arrow). **B.** Sagittal view shows the notch between the inferior frontal and the temporal lobes displaced backwards (arrow). The inferior aspect of the frontal lobe is deeply notched by the sphenoid ridge (curved arrow).

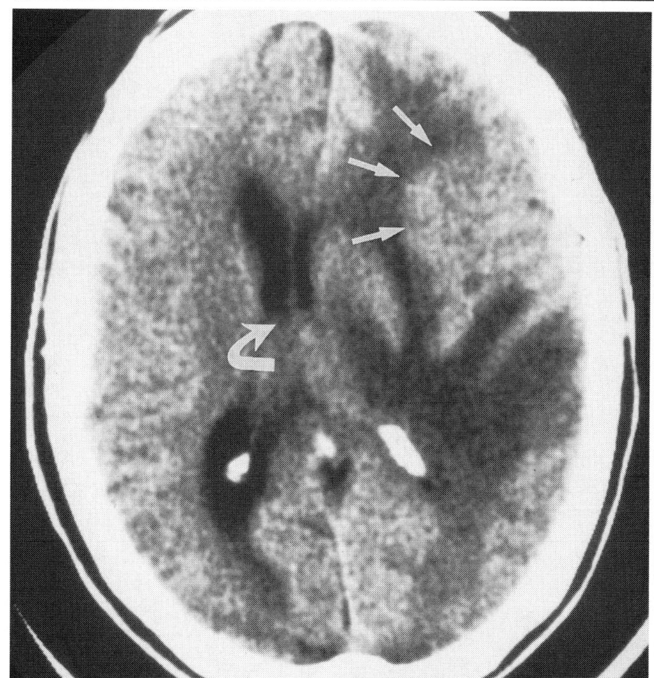

A

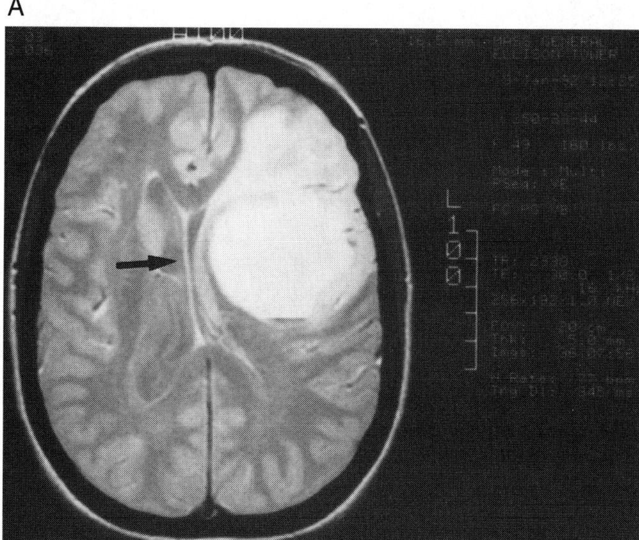

B

Figure 4.36. Midline shift mostly due to brain edema. **A.** The tumor was not large (arrows). The edema extends through the usual white matter pathways (external capsule, posterior limb of internal capsule, intergyral white matter). The septum and third ventricle are displaced across the midline to the opposite side. The shift is more pronounced anteriorly, partly because the tumor is anterior and partly because the anterior half of the brain shifts across the midline more easily due to the wider configuration of the falx posteriorly. **B.** Another example: T2-weighted MR image. The cystic tumor and the edema cause a midline shift that is less than that noted on A because there is less edema present, although the tumor mass is larger. To estimate the degree of midline shift for comparison with other examinations, the best point to measure is the septum pellucidum at the foramen of Monro (curved arrow in A, straight black arrow in B).

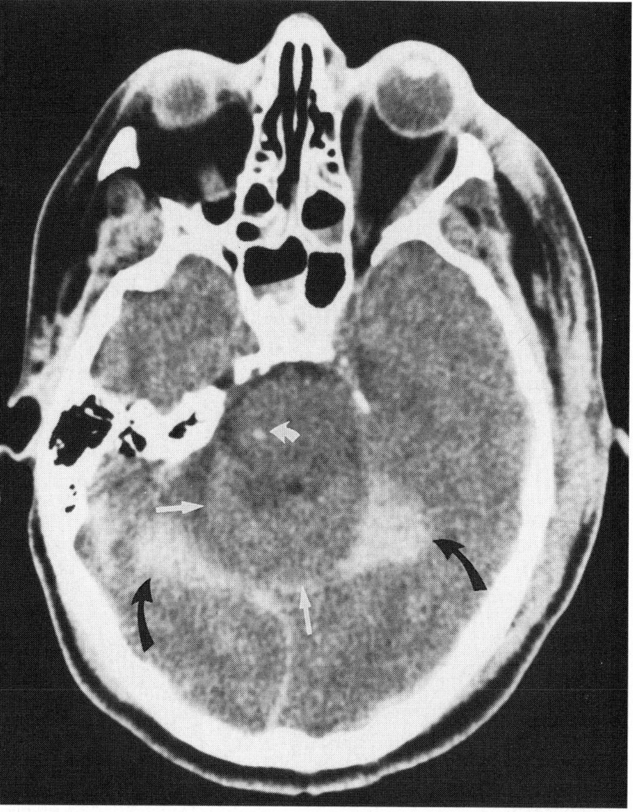

Figure 4.37. Upward transtentorial herniation of the cerebellum due to subtentorial subdural hematoma compressing the cerebellum (curved black arrows). The posterior aspect of the incisura is widened (white arrows), and the brainstem is displaced forward against the clivus. The bright spot over the right side of the brainstem is due to hemorrhage (curved white arrow).

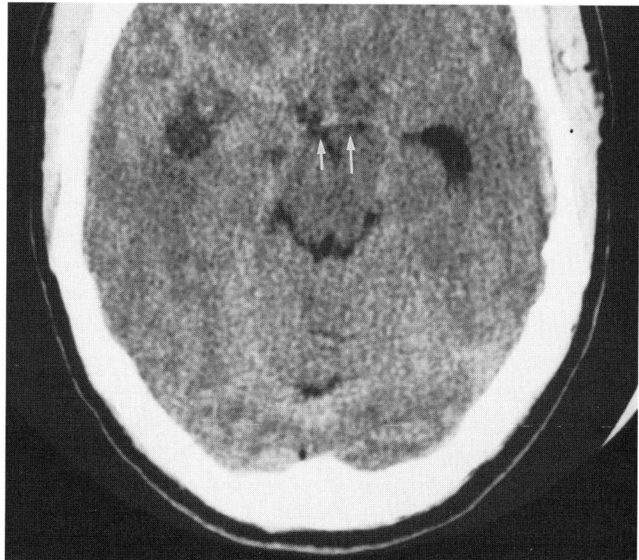

Figure 4.38. Decreased perimesencephalic space in a patient with tumor and bilateral edema. There is a decrease in CSF space anterior to the brainstem (arrows) as well as hippocampal herniation, larger on right side (same case as Fig. 4.33).

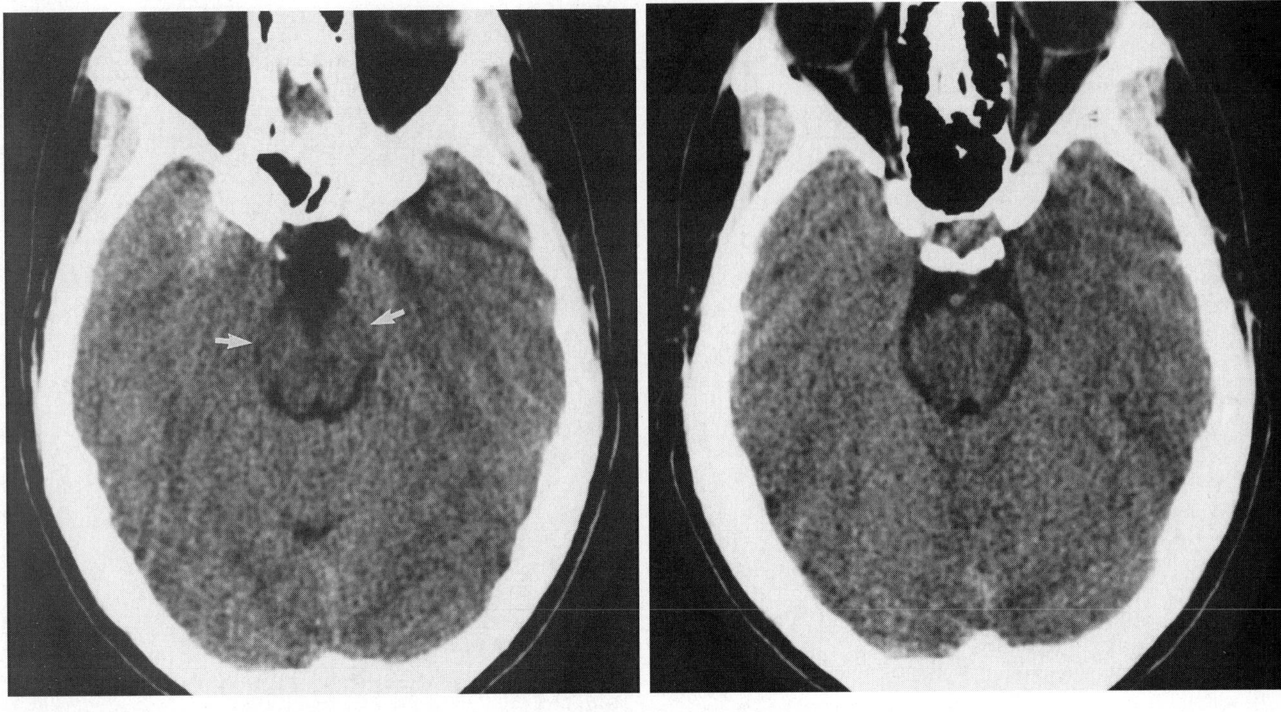

A B

Figure 4.39. **A** and **B.** Decreased normal perimesencephalic CSF space in 19-year-old girl. **A.** The space around the midbrain is small and could raise the question of diffuse brain edema in this patient, who was brought in because of a question of head injury following an accident. The space around the quadrigeminal plate is also somewhat small. This is a normal appearance in young adults and is sometimes difficult to interpret. **B.** The normal appearance of the upper prepontine space rules out bitemporal brain swelling. In general, if there is brain edema, the brainstem is also displaced downward, in which case the pons is brought in contact with the clivus, or at least there is a significant decrease in the distance between the upper pons and the clivus, such as is shown in Figures 4.34 and 4.38.

pons against the clivus that diminishes the space between the pons and the clivus.

Another sign of edema is disruption of the gray/white matter relationships. In the CT or MRI examination, the gray and white matter are clearly separated. On the CT scan, the examination that is almost always carried out first in patients with head injuries, the white matter is more radiolucent than the gray matter and there is a distinct, even separation. In the presence of edema, this separation becomes blurred, and large areas of decreased density may lie adjacent to areas of relatively normal density. This appearance may indicate a severe type of condition due to generalized edema (Fig. 4.40). Edema of the brainstem may also be observed as a generalized decrease in density of the brainstem in relation to the surrounding brain structures (thalamus, hippocampal cortex). On MRI, the same general observations may be made. Although the brain may not be hyperintense on T2-weighted images, there may be disruption of the normal gray/white matter relationships (Table 4.3).

As mentioned earlier, edema in the white matter usually extends following some fiber tracts or bundles. Thus edema in the temporoparietal region may extend forward along the fiber bundles, such as the inferior fronto-occipital fasciculus and inferior longitudinal fasciculus. It may also extend forward along the external capsule and involve the posterior limb of the internal capsule. The anterior limb of the internal capsule is rarely involved in edema as seen by CT or MRI (Figs. 4.36 and 4.41). Edema in the subarcuate fibers is often demonstrated by CT or MRI when it may not be appreciated pathologically on brain specimens. We know, however, that it is difficult to ascertain the presence of edema in pathologic specimens and that examinations by cross-sectional imaging in vivo are much more accurate. The earliest cross-sectional imaging analysis and discussion of these findings was reported by Crowley (29). It should be mentioned here that the CT and MRI appearance of edema sometimes needs to be differentiated from diffuse gliosis, but in general, the cause of the gliosis is evident, such as postoperative changes, a focal scar following trauma, or infection. In the case of other, more diffuse static conditions (such as radiation cerebritis), the cause of the appearance is mostly chronic edema, although there are other histological changes such as gliosis (Fig. 9.7).

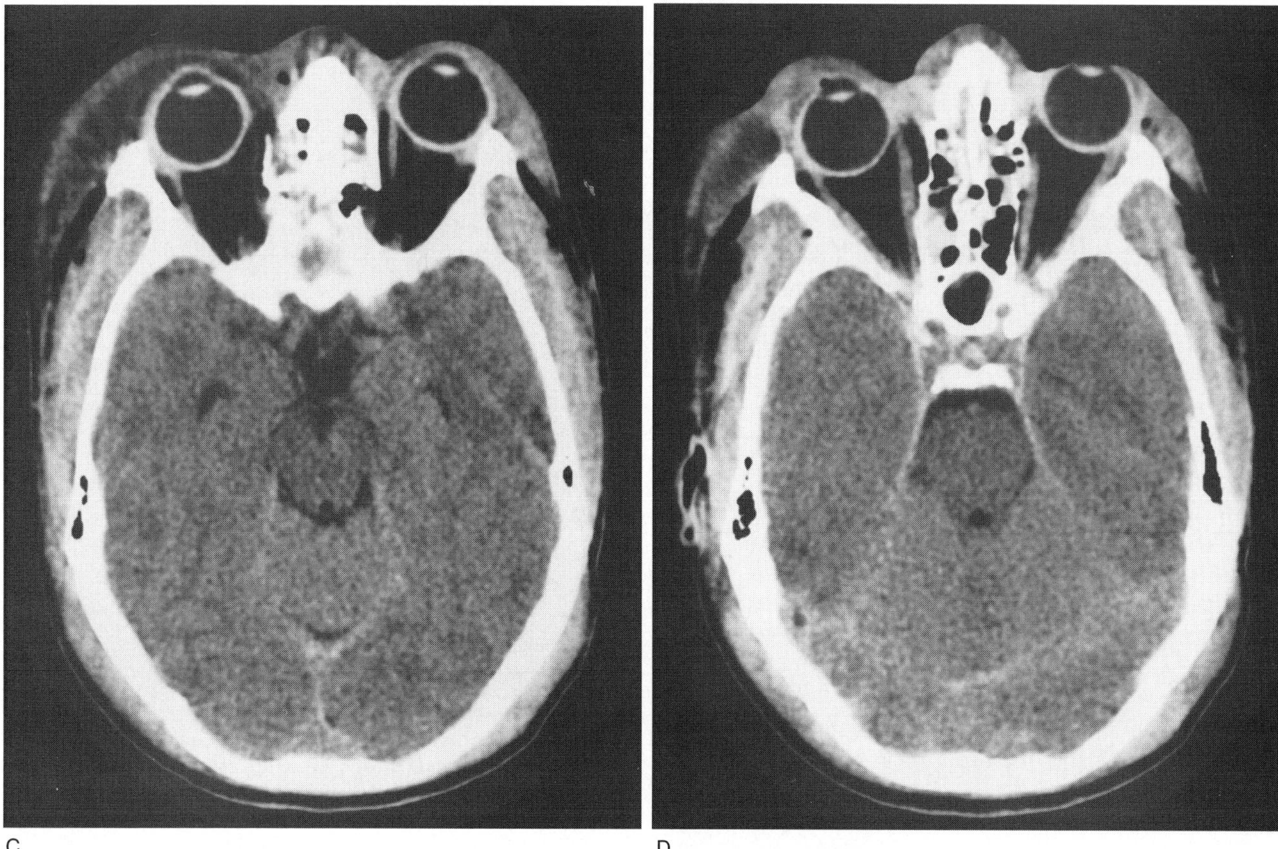

Figure 4.39. *(continued)* **C.** Head trauma patient with a depressed frontal fracture. The perimesencephalic space is small but normal for this 15-year-old boy; however, there is slight enlargement of the right temporal horn. **D.** Scan of same patient showing a normal prepontine space. The appearance was considered normal for this young patient, who recovered rapidly. The enlargement of the temporal horn raised the question of a degree of ventricular obstruction, but the aqueduct was widely patent and did not give the impression of being compressed or deformed. In addition, the temporal horn enlargement was unilateral.

The extension of edema along fiber tracts is a manifestation of local edema. Diffuse edema, such as may be seen in a diffuse encephalitic process, does not ordinarily show this appearance.

Pseudotumor Cerebri

In this condition an increase in brain mass leads to papilledema due to increased intracranial pressure. The reason for the increased intracranial pressure is not known. Undoubtedly there must be some generalized "brain edema," but this is not visible on CT or MRI. Venous or sinus obstruction is postulated as a possible etiology, and it should be looked for by MRI flow studies or, if necessary, by cerebral angiography before a diagnosis of idiopathic pseudotumor is made. Spinal tap always demonstrates increased CSF pressure. The increased intracranial pressure may also be due to "too much CSF." However, if this were the case one would have to postulate a disturbance in the absorption of CSF. Moreover, hydrocephalus does not usually develop. The ventricles do not enlarge; rather, they become smaller (compressed) or remain normal in size. Occasionally some slight ventricular enlargement may be encountered on CT or MRI.

Table 4.3.
CT/MRI Findings in Diffuse Cerebral Edema

Narrowing or obliteration of basal cisternal spaces
Caudal and forward brainstem displacement
Blurring of gray/white matter junction
Obliteration of cortical sulci and sylvian fissures

The most important problem is the papilledema, which can become severe enough to produce visual impairment. Treatment is usually directed to avoid this complication. The patient usually presents with persistent headaches. Spinal taps with CSF removal improve the symptoms.

Pseudotumor cerebri may occur in the presence of a variety of conditions, and it usually affects young, obese women. Oral contraceptive use has been in the background. Other conditions are hypo- and hyperthyroidism, hypoparathyroidism, and adrenal insufficiency. Supplemental vitamin A, tetracycline, lithium, indomethacin, and phenytoin have been implicated.

The clinical manifestations of cerebral edema are related to increased intracranial pressure. In addition to headache, nausea, and vomiting, papilledema may be seen by ophthalmoscopy. Papilledema can be demonstrated by MRI on T2-weighted images; the "swollen" optic nerve head is less bright than the adjacent vitreus, which, according to Jinkins et al. (30), probably means that other factors in addition to plain edema of the optic nerve head may be involved.

CT and MRI images are usually normal. The ventricles may be of normal size or slightly smaller. They may also be slightly enlarged, but the enlargement is minimal. No alteration in the gray/white matter relationship is seen.

Emphasis has been placed on the possible association of pseudotumor and venous sinus thrombosis. It is important to investigate all suspected patients with appropriate imaging techniques to exclude this possibility.

Severe systemic hypertension may cause some degree of brain edema, but only if it occurs suddenly, and only if it rises above a certain level, possibly over systolic 220/140 diastolic mmHg, beyond the point where autoregulation protects the brain. In certain conditions, such as eclampsia, brain edema occurs rapidly, usually beginning in the bioccipital areas. The location in this area is attributed to the difference in the sympathetic innervation between the vertebrobasilar and the carotid system. The brain edema may worsen and cause death. If the eclampsia is controlled, the edema disappears (31) (see Fig. 13.11).

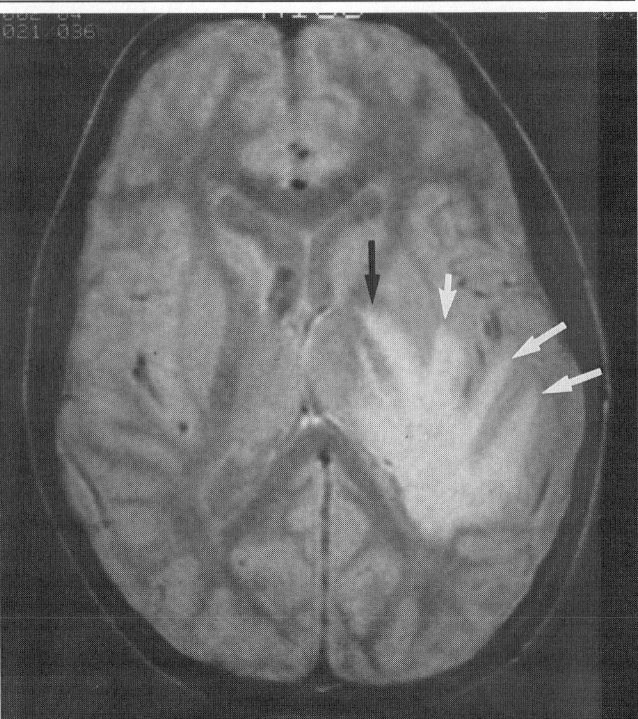

Figure 4.41. Edema in periatrial region. The edema extends along the posterior limb of the internal capsule (upper black arrow), along the external capsule (upper white arrow), and along the intergyral white matter (lateral arrows). The anterior limb of the internal capsule serves less frequently as a path for edema extension.

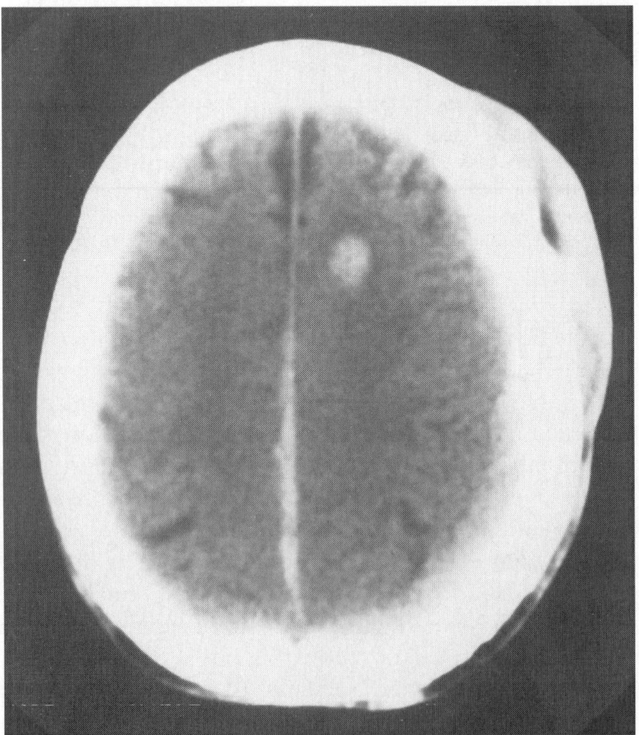

Figure 4.40. Generalized posttraumatic edema causing loss of gray/white matter discrimination on CT. There is a hemorrhagic focus in the left frontal area, probably due to shear injury, as well as a thin subdural collection around the falx. The diminution or disappearance of gray/white matter discrimination is due to diffuse edema of the white and gray matter associated with blood volume changes (hyperemia). It may also be associated with numerous petechial hemorrhages diffusely distributed in the tissues. It is seen in severe head injuries.

INTRACRANIAL PRESSURE AND HYDROCEPHALUS

The concept of increased intracranial pressure is very important. The brain is surrounded by and filled with CSF. Pressure within the rigid cranial cavity is maintained within certain limits. Normal, temporary increases in intracranial pressure are generated mostly by increased venous pressure in the presence of strain or severe coughing and by dilatation of arterial channels of the brain caused by an increased carbon dioxide concentration in the blood.

Intracranial pressure may rise slowly in the case of a growing neoplasm or rapidly in the case of an intracerebral hematoma due to arterial bleeding or following trauma, in which case the hematoma is probably located outside the brain. The brain can tolerate slowly increasing intracranial pressure caused by a combination of a brain tumor or an abscess accompanied by edema, but rapid increases of intracranial pressure are usually followed by loss of consciousness and other more severe interference with brain function. An increase in intracranial pressure is usually manifested by papilledema on clinical examination. Symptoms may vary, but nausea and projectile vomiting or headache are also common manifestations.

Increased intracranial pressure cannot be measured by imaging methods but can be suspected from the presence of very small ventricles and the disappearance of some CSF spaces at the basal cisterns, as well as by flattening of the gyri of the brain, diminution of the surface sulci, and even disappearance of the sulci. These changes are also a manifestation of brain edema in the presence of a space-occupying mass, as described in the preceding section. However, these are all signs of a decrease in the available space for the brain within the cranial cavity and do not indicate necessarily that there is increased intracranial pressure.

Increased intracranial pressure can only be estimated by the presence of papilledema and by placing a measuring instrument in the cranial cavity, usually in the subdural space. It may also be measured during a spinal puncture. Any pressure over 300 mmH_2O or 30 mmHg is considered high. However, the measurements in the spinal canal may not be accurate because a partial effect in the tentorial incisura or in the foramen magnum may be acting somewhat like a cork, giving a false low reading. In addition, it may be dangerous to carry out the spinal tap. A decision concerning a contraindication for a spinal tap is currently made by CT or MRI. If these images show the absence of any intracranial mass and nothing to suggest cerebral edema or impending tentorial or foramen magnum herniation, a spinal tap is considered safe.

The brain circulation has much to do with how increases in intracranial pressure are tolerated. Lundberg describes two types of increases in intracranial pressure: the *A wave* and the *B wave* (32). The A wave is seen in patients with intracranial tumors or masses; the pressure may rise fairly rapidly from a baseline up to a point, for instance, of 50 mmHg, and stay at that level for some time, after which it may again decrease rather rapidly. Dilatation of brain blood vessels is felt to be involved in the behavior of intracranial pressure. The B wave is more frequently encountered and consists of sharp increases in intracranial pressure from the baseline with an equally sharp decrease to the previous level. These waves occur at short intervals. Miller attributes the fluctuations to changes in cerebral vascular tone and cerebral blood volume (33).

As mentioned earlier, increases in intracranial pressure may result in a decrease in cerebral blood flow, but this does not occur until the intracranial pressure has reached about 60 mmHg. A continuous rise in intracranial pressure eventually results in a total arrest of cerebral circulation when the intracranial pressure reaches the level of the systolic blood pressure. This is a state of brain death and can be proved beyond doubt by carrying out a cerebral angiogram. However, it has been suggested that this state can be ascertained by a more noninvasive method, such as a radionuclide angiogram or, more recently, a MR angiogram. Electroencephalography is most frequently used as the first procedure because it shows a disappearance of brain electrical activity (34).

Cerebrospinal Fluid

PRODUCTION AND ABSORPTION

The CSF is a most important component of the intracranial contents. There is a total of about 140 ml of CSF, and about 20 ml/h are produced and presumably absorbed. The majority of CSF is produced by the choroid plexus situated in the lateral, third, and fourth ventricles. Although statements have been made concerning the production of CSF elsewhere in the brain, the amount produced outside the choroid plexus is difficult to determine. CSF is produced by the choroid plexus by a filtration mechanism through fenestrated capillaries and also by active secretion by the epithelium through both pinocytosis and vesicular transport. The rate of CSF formation appears to be fairly constant and does not seem to be decreased by increased intracranial pressure.

Absorption of CSF depends upon a pressure gradient between the venous pressure and the CSF pressure. The venous pressure is normally higher than the CSF pressure; if it were not, the veins would collapse. Absorption of the CSF takes place at the level of the arachnoid granulations, which are in contact with the veins of the dural sinuses and also penetrate the dura of the spinal roots into small spinal veins (35). Protein in the CSF seems to be absorbed only at the arachnoid granulations connected with the superior sagittal sinus. For this reason, when trying to image the circulation of CSF by radionuclide methods, an indicator with a protein, usually albumin, is used because it will rise to the upper brain surface, where it is absorbed. If no protein is included in the radionuclide spinal injection, the material will be absorbed before reaching the upper surface of the brain (24).

As explained earlier, the volume of CSF tends to decrease to compensate for a tumor mass or edema, up to a point. In addition, the blood vessels of the brain (capillaries, venules, and veins) do increase or decrease in size and affect the adjustment or maladjustment of intracranial volume and pressure.

If a balloon is placed intracranially in a dog and inflated slowly, the intracranial pressure rises slowly to a point as the inflation of the balloon proceeds. After reaching a certain level, each volume increase in the balloon produces a sharp rise in intracranial pressure. The same might be occurring in patients who deteriorate rapidly when they harbor a neoplasm or another intracranial mass. This sudden deterioration is most often due to increased vasodilatation, venous obstruction, or edema rather than to a hemorrhage, although sometimes it may be caused by hemorrhage. Today, when a patient deteriorates fairly rapidly, a CT examination is carried out to determine if there is intracranial hemorrhage.

CIRCULATION

As explained earlier, CSF is produced in the lateral, third, and fourth ventricles. In the first place, the liquid must pass

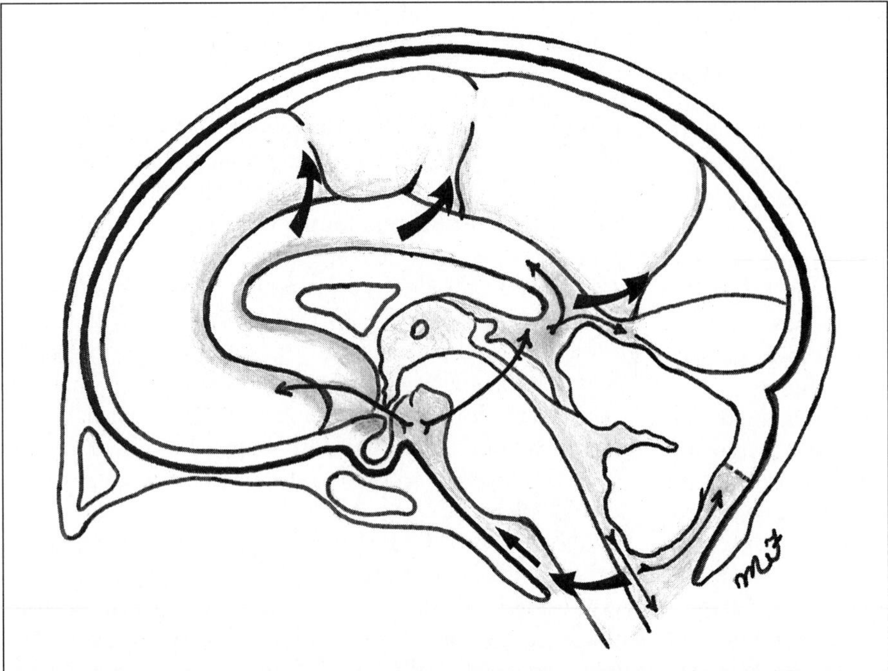

Figure 4.42. Flow of CSF after exit from fourth ventricle as seen in sagittal view. The main cerebrospinal fluid pathways are shaded. From the cisterna magna (cerebellomedullaris), the main course is rostral and upward through the pontine and interpeduncular cisterns. Fluid then flows in one of two main directions: it may continue forward, or it may be funneled in a broad, thin band from the lateral extensions of the basal cisterns through the lateral communicating channels around the brainstem (long arrow) into the quadrigeminal cistern. The forward passage goes through the postchiasmatic and prechiasmatic portions of the suprasellar cistern. The thin cisterna lamina terminalis is shown diagrammatically as the main forward channel providing communication to the callosal sulcus through the subarachnoid space around the rostrum and genu. A corresponding communication is through the subarachnoid space around the splenium. A number of important subarachnoid extensions visible in lateral view are not indicated in the diagram in this figure and Figure 4.43.

through the foramen of Monro into the third ventricle and from here through the aqueduct into the fourth ventricle. The CSF leaves the fourth ventricle via the foramen of Magendie and the lateral foramina of Luschka into the cisterna magna. From here, some of the CSF does go down the spinal subarachnoid space surrounding the spinal cord. However, most of it turns up around the medulla in front of the pons, between the pons and the clivus, up to the region of the interpeduncular cistern, and from there into the suprasellar cistern. From the suprasellar cistern, the CSF current divides into three streams before emerging to the surface of the brain: one midline interhemispheric stream and two streams on each side following the anterior and superior aspects of the temporal lobes into the sylvian fissure region. The CSF will continue to rise up to the upper brain surface, where it is absorbed (Figs. 4.42 and 4.43). As the CSF emerges from the fourth ventricle, it goes into the cisterna magna. The cisterna magna is limited on its upper aspect, so the CSF does not continue to rise over the top of the cerebellum via this route. It reaches the upper part of the cerebellum by way of the perimesencephalic cisterns to the superior cerebellar cistern, which connects with the quadrigeminal cistern and also with the thin cisternal space behind the thalamus on each side and on the roof of the third ventricle in what is called the *cistern of the velum interpositum*, which can be fairly large in children but which is rather small in adults (see Figs. 4.42 and 4.43).

The latter group of cisterns communicate with the CSF space behind the splenium of the corpus callosum and through this with the rest of the interhemispheric subarachnoid space. These pathways were commonly demonstrated with pneumoencephalography by recording the movement of air. CSF movement cannot be observed with CT or MRI.

Hydrocephalus

Enlargement of the lateral ventricles is common and is often determined by simple visual inspection. It is usually not necessary to determine the presence of enlargement by measurement; however, if the change is minor, measurement may be necessary to determine whether there is an increase or decrease in the size of the ventricles in comparison with a prior examination. In general, this could be done

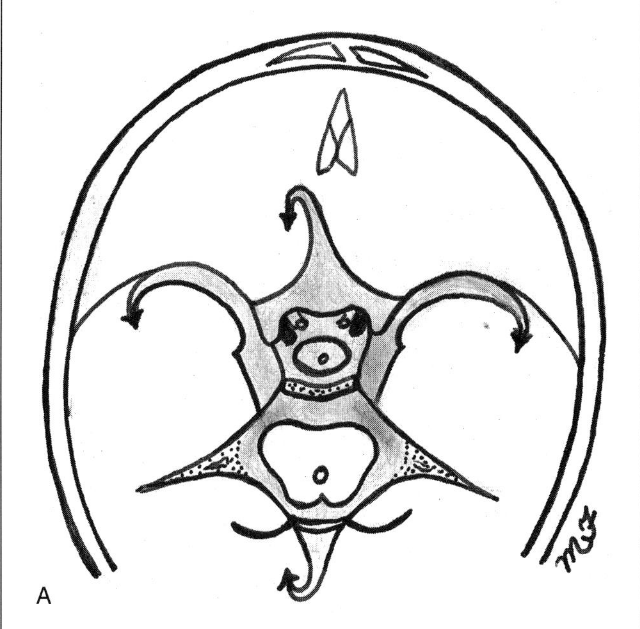

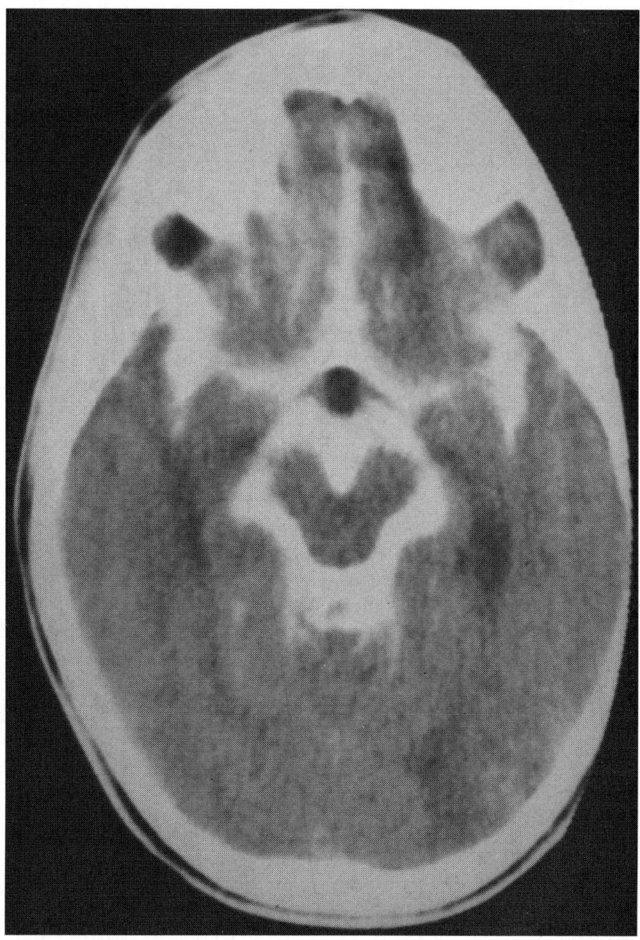

Figure 4.43. Circulation of cerebrospinal fluid diagrammed in axial view. **A.** The CSF flow from the central and lateral cisterns is shown diagrammatically. After the CSF leaves the fourth ventricle and ascends in front of the pons, it reaches the suprasellar cistern, from where it divides into three main streams: the midline, as shown in Figure 4.42, and the two lateral streams (the two large lateral communicating channels, the sylvian cisterns behind the sphenoid ridge resembling the long horn of a steer). The stream reaches the sylvian fissure, and from there the CSF ascends on the outer surface of the hemisphere to reach the superior surface, where fluid is absorbed around the pacchionian granulations and superior sagittal sinus. From the interpeduncular cistern in the midline behind the dorsum sella, the CSF flows around the midbrain to reach the quadrigeminal cistern, as shown in Figure 4.42. This is not as important a channel for flow as the midline and sylvian cisterns anteriorly. **B.** The three anterior streams are well shown in a cisternogram performed with water-soluble contrast.

by measuring the bifrontal diameter, between the lateral aspects of the two frontal horns. The bicaudate diameter is also used for this purpose, and it is also possible to measure the distance between the lateral aspects of the bodies of the lateral ventricles. Currently these measurements are always made on cross-sectional images, and it is often difficult, because of partial volume effects, to be sure that one is measuring the maximum diameter. However, this can be approximated well enough to make a comparison between two examinations. The transverse diameter of the lateral ventricles measured at their maximum diameter between the outer edges of the bodies is 3.5 to 4 cm. All measurements must be adjusted to the minification factor that appears on all of the images. The width of the temporal horns is 3 to 5 mm, and anything over 5 mm is considered enlarged. The width of the third ventricle is 4 to 8 mm, and anything over 8 mm is considered abnormal.

Enlargement of the lateral ventricles is so common in everyday practice that reports usually mention it without attempting to determine the cause. Symmetrical enlargement occurs with increasing age. Any individual over 50 years of age is likely to have ventricles that begin to enlarge and which continue to enlarge slightly with advancing age. The third ventricle usually follows the enlargement of the lateral ventricles, indicating some loss of brain mass. When slight ventricular enlargement is found in children, we must assume there was a cause that may be related to trauma, some minor degree of brain hypoplasia, or some vascular, hypoxic, or inflammatory condition occurring before or after birth. However, the question usually remains unanswered if the child is otherwise normal.

Unilateral ventricular dilatation in a relatively young subject is probably secondary to head trauma occurring sometime during childhood or later. The specific cause may not be ascertained by history for several reasons: not enough importance may have been paid to the trauma or it may have occurred during childhood and the individual does not know about it. We know that head trauma usually results in enlargement of the ventricle on one or both sides within 4 to 8 weeks after a trauma (Fig. 4.44). The enlarge-

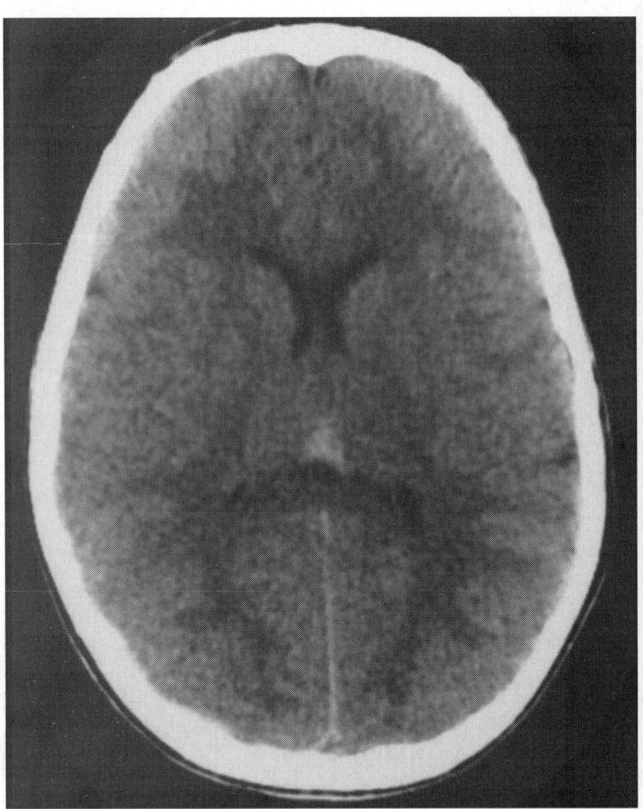

A

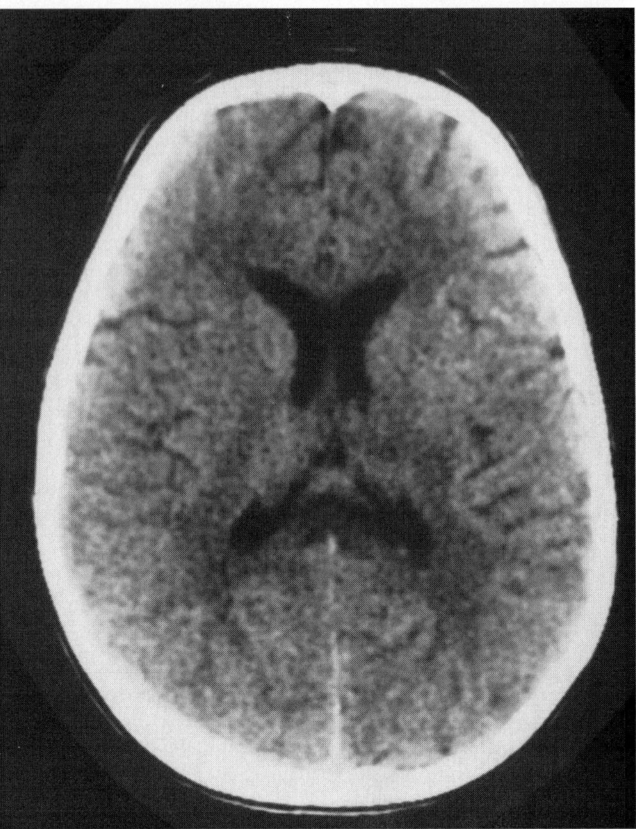

B

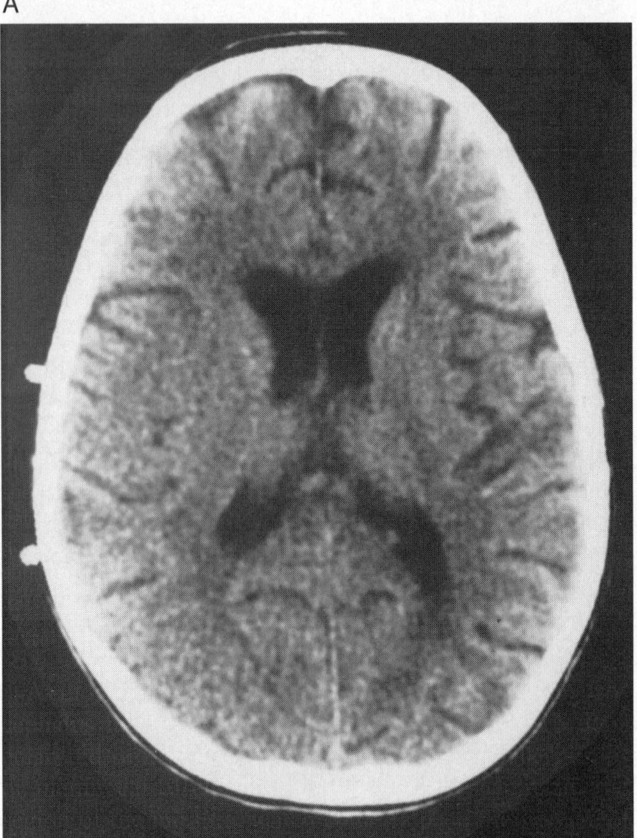

C

Figure 4.44. Posttraumatic ventricular enlargement in a period of 3 weeks after trauma. The 3-year-old boy was involved in a moving vehicle accident. **A.** CT showed hemorrhage in the velum interpositum (arrow) and revealed no other brain abnormalities. The boy recovered fairly rapidly but was kept under observation because of the hemorrhage. CT examination repeated 10 days later (**B**) and 3 weeks after onset (**C**) demonstrated progressive ventricular enlargement felt to be due to posttraumatic tissue loss or atrophy. This is common after trauma and can be unilateral or bilateral. Because the ventricles do not continue to enlarge and the patients are usually normal after the acute head trauma, it is difficult to attribute the change to other mechanisms than posttraumatic brain shaking with the production of numerous minor tissue changes. In this instance there was a small hemorrhage, but usually no CT findings can be demonstrated. The brain reacts to injury of any type (traumatic, inflammatory, vascular, toxic) by loss of tissue mass that is seen as ventricular enlargement or sulcal widening, but ventricular enlargement is by far the more common appearance, perhaps because it is easier to appraise. **D** and **E.** Posttraumatic bifrontal atrophy in a 62-year-old alcoholic who had sustained a number of head trauma episodes. D shows the posttraumatic ventricular dilatation, particularly in the frontal horns. E reveals the bilateral sulcal widening due to tissue loss.

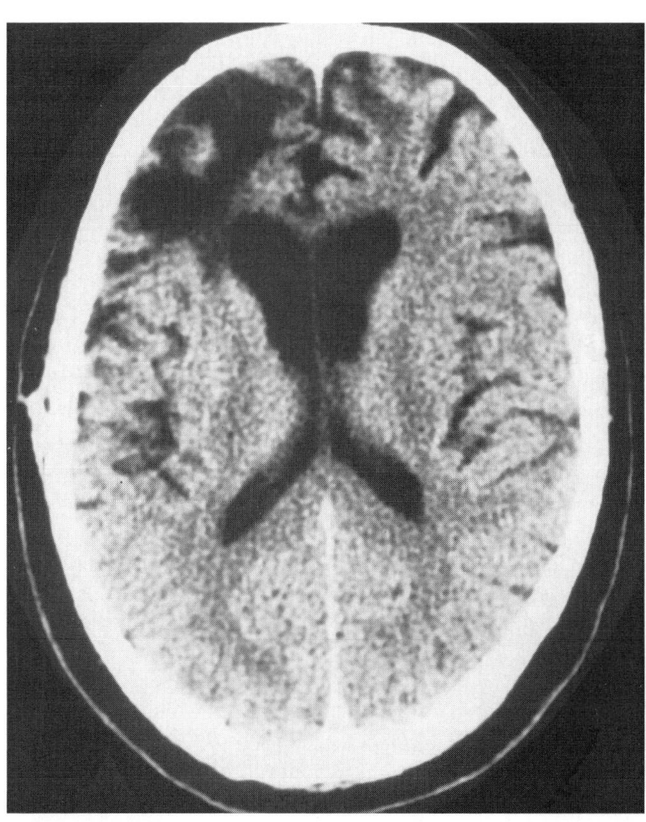

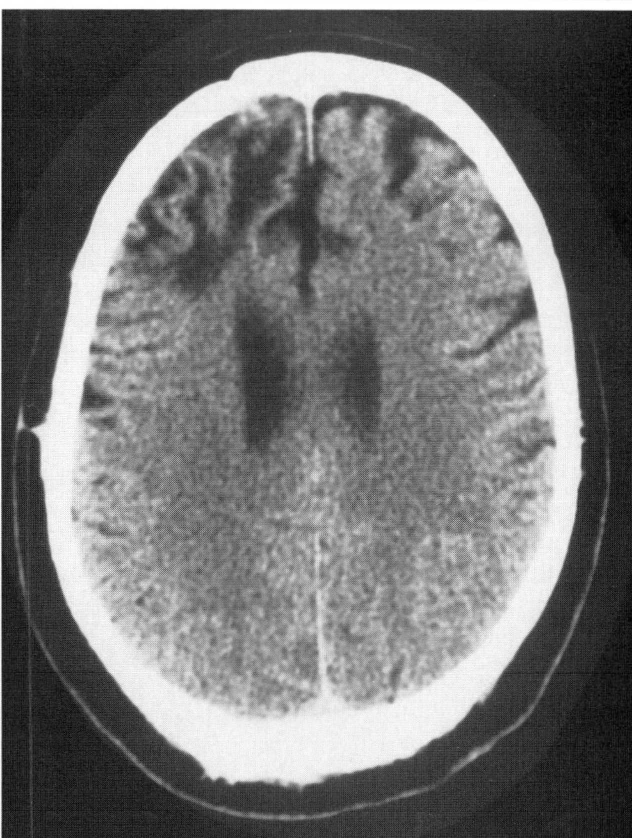

D E

Figure 4.44. *(continued)*

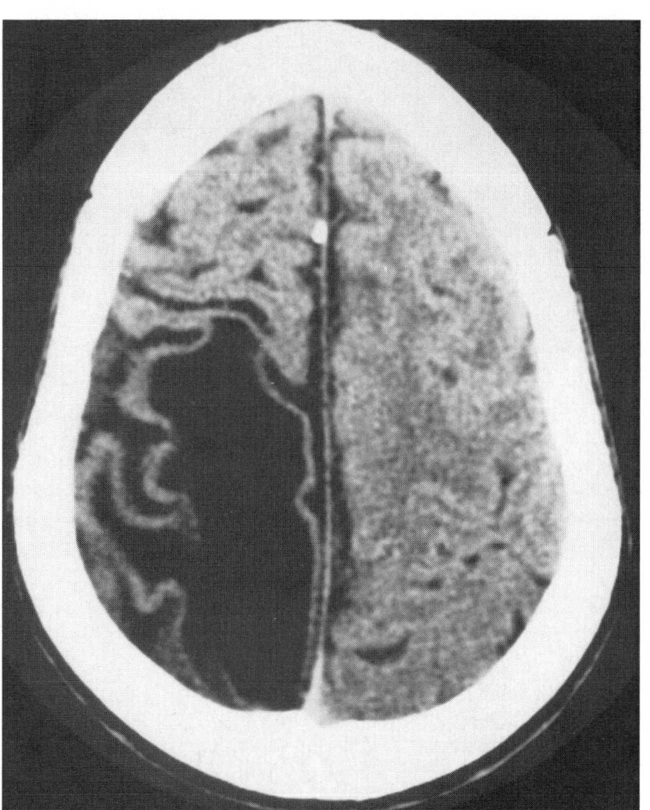

Figure 4.45. Porencephaly in a 7-year-old boy who had a large hemispheric infarction associated with basal arachnoiditis. The large ventricular extension is seen in spite of adequate shunting because it is due to focal brain tissue loss.

ment is probably secondary to changes in the brain tissue after the sudden shaking provoked by the trauma. The movement may generate millions of tiny petechial hemorrhages or some other change leading to a slight decrease in brain mass. Cortical atrophy does not usually accompany this slight shrinkage of brain tissue. Unilateral atrophy may also be produced by a vascular occlusive lesion or by an inflammatory process.

Slight ventricular asymmetry is frequently observed on CT or MRI examinations and could be congenital if the larger of the ventricles is still normal in size. However, if it is larger than normal, we must conclude there was a cause, as previously described.

Focal ventricular enlargement may be mild or pronounced. If pronounced, it is called *porencephaly* (Fig. 4.45). Unless it is congenital, the cause of porencephaly is usually known (trauma, infection, vascular, surgical).

The term *hydrocephalus* is not usually applied unless the ventricles are significantly enlarged. At this point we try to determine whether we are dealing with an obstructive or a communicating type of hydrocephalus.

OBSTRUCTIVE (HYPERTENSIVE) HYDROCEPHALUS

The majority of spinal fluid is produced in the lateral ventricles and in the fourth ventricle. A lesser amount is produced in the third ventricle. If the foramen of Monro is obstructed, both lateral ventricles are dilated, but not the third ventricle. If the obstruction is on one side of the Y-shaped foramen of Monro, only one ventricle will be dilated. Partial obstruction of one side of the foramen of Monro is common in the presence of masses occupying one side of the brain and distorting the region of the interventricular foramen, which would usually be displaced toward the opposite side. The dilatation in this case would be of the ventricle on the side opposite that of the tumor or mass.

If the obstruction is in the region of the posterior aspect of the third ventricle or in the aqueduct, both lateral ventricles and the anterior aspect of the third ventricle or the whole ventricle will be dilated, depending on the location of the obstruction. Dilatation of the ventricles makes it easy to determine the site of obstruction even though the actual cause of the obstruction may not be visible on CT or MRI. If the obstruction is at the outlet of the fourth ventricle, then the lateral, third, and fourth ventricles and the aqueduct become dilated.

In general, obstruction may not be complete and may develop rapidly or somewhat more slowly. When complete obstruction develops rapidly, the patient deteriorates clinically and loses consciousness. This may be produced, for instance, by intraventricular bleeding, by a cerebellar hemorrhage, or by a blood clot in the aqueduct.

The result of obstruction of the CSF pathways is dilatation of the ventricles. The dilatation occurs rather rapidly in the presence of a high degree of obstruction and more slowly if the obstruction is incomplete. Expansion of the ventricle is at the expense of the white matter of the brain, which becomes progressively thinner as the ventricles become larger. It is interesting to note, however, that in addition to the decreased thickness, the white matter also contains an increased amount of water, presumably because of passage of CSF across the damaged ependymal membrane and into the white matter. Histological examination of enlarged ventricles, in the early stages of hydrocephalus,

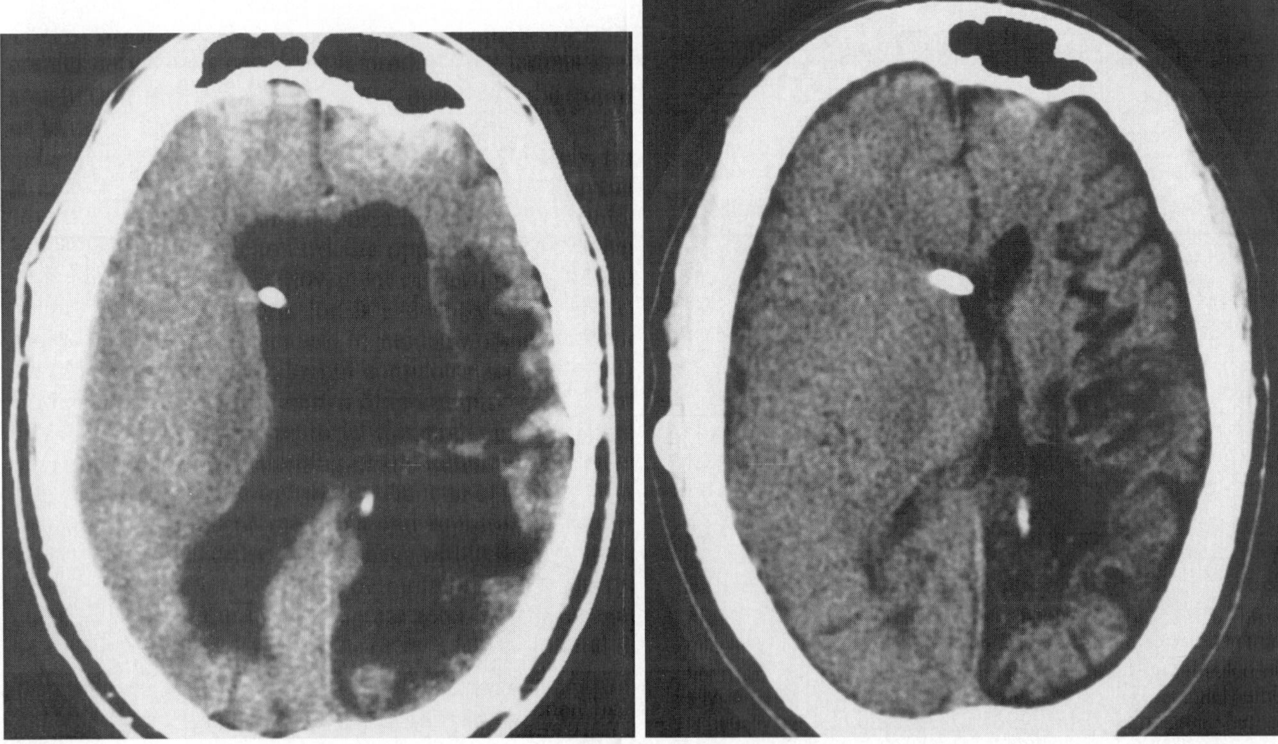

Figure 4.46. Porencephaly and transependymal CSF passage in a 31-year-old man who had had a brain abscess and later developed ventriculitis. **A.** Shunt malfunction in the two required shunts, because of intraventricular adhesions, led to bulging of the isolated porencephalic cavity and considerable extravasation of CSF across the ependyma. **B.** Following shunt revision, the ventricles returned to normal size, the porencephalic cavity became smaller, and the CSF transependymal passage (giving the dilated ventricular surface a scalloped appearance on both sides, particularly noticeable in the occipital area) disappeared. There is also a dilatation in the sylvian fissure area in A representing CSF extravasation.

shows disruption of the ependymal layer. As the hydrocephalus becomes chronic, the ependymal layer of cells becomes continuous but flattened.

Periventricular edema can be demonstrated by CT or MRI (Figs. 4.46 and 4.47). In the presence of obstruction, ventricular dilatation can be demonstrated within 24 h or less (Fig. 4.48). Extreme degrees of ventricular enlargement can be reached in infants and young children. A diverticulum of the medial atrial aspect of the lateral ventricle may occur because of the increased intraventricular pressure. In these cases, the diverticulum may herniate downward through the tentorial incisura, sometimes producing confusing CT images because of the lucent image outlining the tentorium and bulging into the upper aspect of the posterior fossa. A contrast ventriculogram using water-soluble contrast and CT will sometimes be required for diagnosis (36). The direct connection with the medial atrial portion of the ventricle is often difficult to demonstrate.

Presumably, in these cases, the obstruction, usually in the aqueduct, may have occurred in utero or shortly after birth (Figs. 4.15 and 4.47). It is surprising to see the compliance of brain tissue in infants. Cross-sectional imaging may show only a thin brain mantle as the result of an extreme degree of hydrocephalus. However, following an appropriate shunting procedure, the thickness of the brain tissue increases fairly rapidly and reaches a nearly normal appearance. In these cases the shunting makes for a virtual collapse of the lateral ventricles, which become small. One wonders how the brain could have withstood so much compression and could return to what apparently is a normal thickness so rapidly. Infants treated for hydrocephalus do not necessarily develop a normal intelligence, although some do.

Aqueductal Stenosis

This form of obstructive hydrocephalus may be congenital or acquired. In the congenital type the aqueduct may be malformed or atretic in a manner similar to congenital atresia in the gastrointestinal tract. The columns of ependymal cells, which ordinarily are well aligned to form the wall of the lumen of the aqueduct, do not proliferate properly or join in the usual manner. Often multiple blind pockets or isolated microscopic cavities are present (forking of the aqueduct) along the normal course of the aqueduct, rather than a point of true focal narrowing of an otherwise normal lumen. The grade of obstruction in the iter depends on the extent of the blind ending of the malformed channels and the number that join, even though abnormally, to allow the transmission of CSF. In some cases there is only a low-grade obstruction and clinical manifestations do not occur until adolescence or adult life (37). Total obstruction rarely exists, even though this fact may not be demonstrable by the injection of contrast material or air.

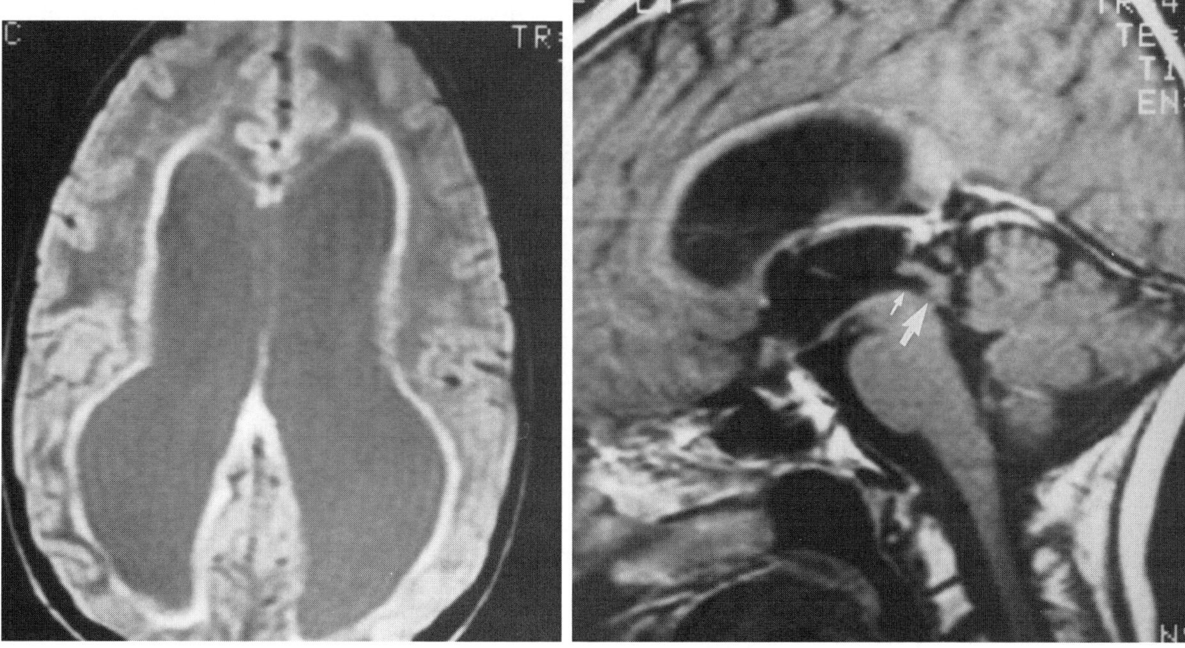

A B

Figure 4.47. Focal aqueduct stenosis in a 10-year-old boy with type I neurofibromatosis. **A.** Proton density image showing marked ventricular dilatation and sharp, uniform, increased periventricular hyperintensity attributed to transependymal passage of CSF. **B.** The sagittal image reveals focal aqueductal obstruction with dilatation of the proximal aqueduct (arrows). The size of the ventricles is not as great as is usually seen in untreated congenital aqueductal obstruction, showing that the condition was acquired sometime later. Probably the aqueduct is not completely obstructed.

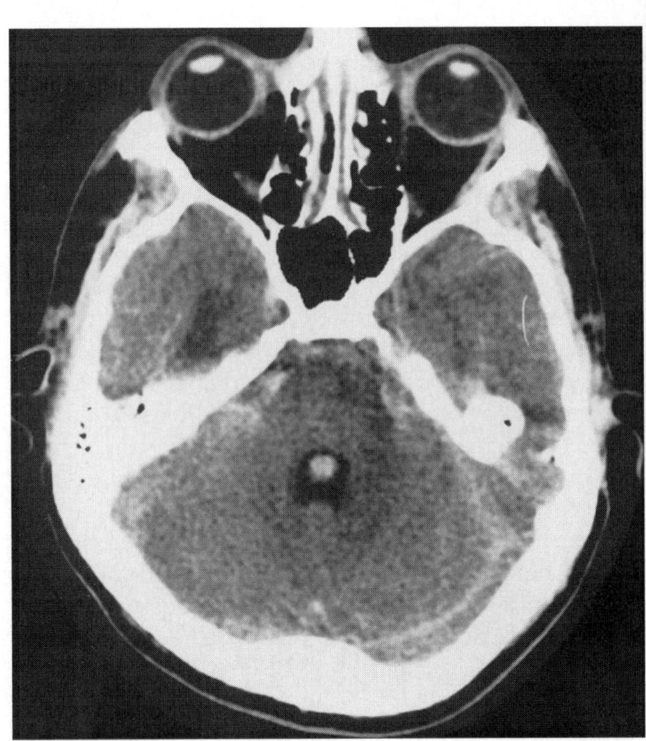

A

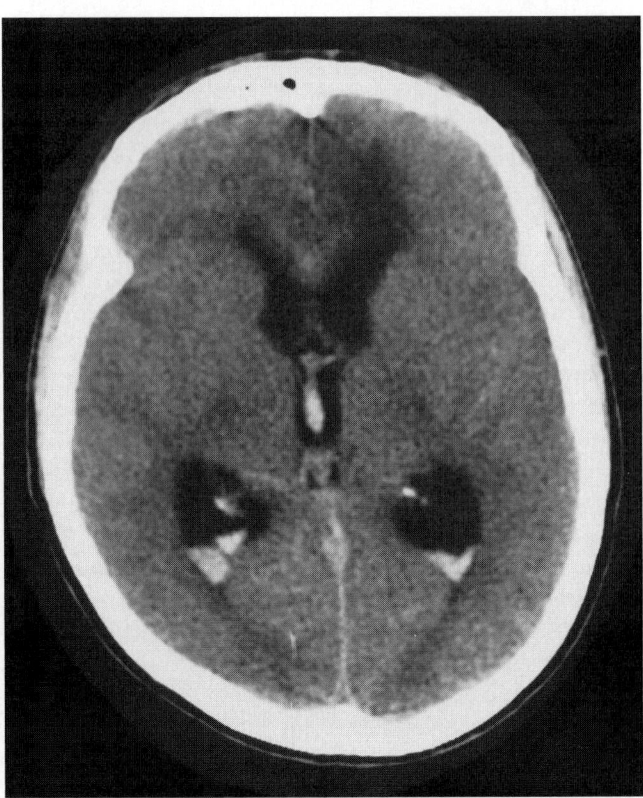

B

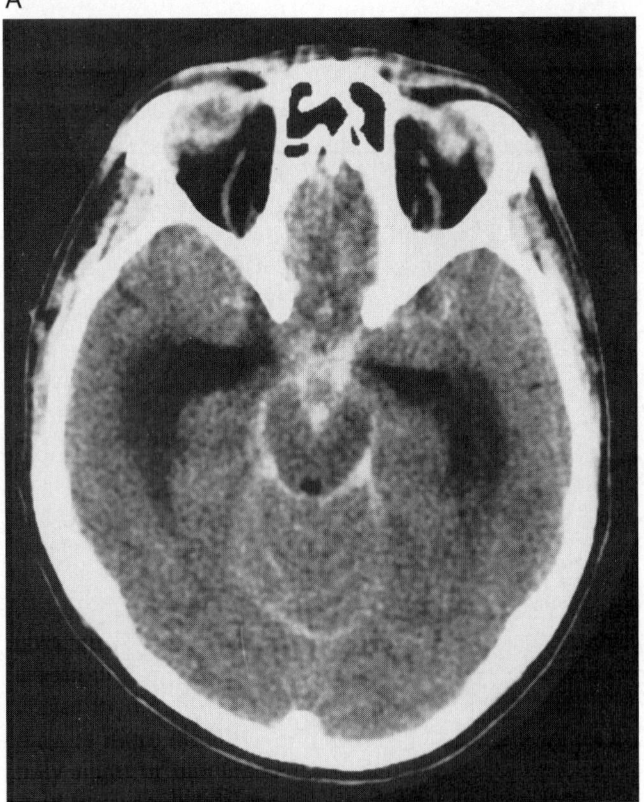

C

Figure 4.48. Rapid ventricular dilatation occurring within 24 to 48 hours after ruptured aneurysm and subarachnoid and intraventricular hemorrhage. **A.** The intraventricular bleed with partial blocking of the aqueduct causes more rapid ventricular enlargement. **B** and **C.** The enlargement of the temporal horns is greater than that of the rest of the lateral ventricles, indicating active hydrocephalus.

The diagnosis can be made by MRI, particularly in sagittal midline images, or by CT utilizing reformatted sagittal images. Radiographic contrast can be easily injected into the dilated ventricles through the anterior fontanelle and the contrast maneuvered into the third ventricle.

Acquired aqueductal stenosis may occur as the result of inflammation, although a clear-cut history is often lacking. It may also result from severe trauma, although probably infrequently. Pathologically there may be thickening of the ependymal lining, but the most prominent microscopic change is subependymal, where scarring caused by proliferation of astrocytes and other glial elements is found. The reaction is inflammatory, although frequently not postinfectious. The aqueductal obstruction may begin proximally, at the level of the superior colliculi or at the level of the intercollicular sulcus (38). Occasionally, instead of a long stenosis, a web may be the cause of obstruction, and in these cases the degree of ventricular dilatation may be less marked. The diagnosis can be made by sagittal MRI.

The most common cause of acquired aqueductal stenosis is neoplasm, which may be periaqueductal or may be in the midbrain tectum or in any portion of the upper brainstem compressing or invading the aqueduct (Fig. 4.49*C*). Any mass that is large enough or strategically situated in relation to the aqueduct may cause sufficient interference with the passage of CSF through the aqueduct to cause obstructive hydrocephalus.

Extraventricular Hydrocephalus

If the obstruction is beyond the outlets of the fourth ventricle, it may be situated in the posterior fossa basal cisterns, in the suprasellar and perimesencephalic regions. As explained under "Circulation," the majority of the CSF will pass through the suprasellar region in order to reach the upper surface of the brain, where absorption takes place. A strategically located adhesive process will not allow the CSF to pass through this area and distribute itself into the three normal streams previously described. If the adhesive process also involves the perimesencephalic cisterns, the CSF cannot circulate around to reach the posterior surface of the brainstem to the quadrigeminal cistern and from there to pass behind the splenium of the corpus callosum to reach the interhemispheric fissure. Although the pathologic process just described might be called *communicating hydrocephalus*, in fact the hydrocephalus is obstructive, but the obstruction is beyond the outlets of the fourth ventricle.

An adhesive process beyond the suprasellar and perimesencephalic cisterns is less common and probably does not lead to progressive hydrocephalus because it is not likely to be strategically located to impede normal circulation of the CSF. It may result from meningitis over the brain surface or some other process, such as subarachnoid bleeding or extensive meningeal carcinomatosis.

The diagnosis of hydrocephalus depends entirely on obtaining an image. Previously it was based on pneumoencephalography or ventriculography, and later on cerebral angiography. After the development of CT and MRI, the diagnosis became entirely dependent on these cross-sectional imaging procedures. Normally, the aqueduct is always visible on CT or MRI, and if it is not seen, one must conclude that the hydrocephalus is related to aqueductal insufficiency or occlusion. Quencer et al. (39) and Quencer (40) have indicated that cine-MRI is valuable in arriving at a valid conclusion regarding the pathophysiology of CSF flow under abnormal conditions, in both children and adults.

COMMUNICATING HYDROCEPHALUS

The term *communicating hydrocephalus* is used to indicate that there is no obstruction in the ventricular system. The pathogenesis of communicating hydrocephalus is presumably an imbalance between production and absorption of CSF. Too much CSF is produced in relation to the available capacity for absorption of the liquid. Overproduction of CSF has been suggested in patients with papilloma of the choroid plexus, but even in these cases blockage of the arachnoid granulations may be produced by repeated small hemorrhages, commonly caused by choroid papillomas.

As just explained, an obstruction in the suprasellar and perimesencephalic cisterns is sometimes described as communicating hydrocephalus when in fact it is due to obstruction, an incisural block. Beyond this point, however, an organized obstruction cannot usually be produced without an extensive generalized meningitic process. The obstruction can be located where CSF is normally absorbed, at the level of the pacchionian (arachnoid) granulations at the top of the brain where the granulations penetrate the superior sagittal sinus. Although this might be considered a true communicating hydrocephalus, nevertheless it is obstructive because there is an obstruction, which could be partial or fairly complete, of the arachnoid granulations. The obstruction of the arachnoid granulations could be produced by an inflammatory process or by blood in the CSF, a subarachnoid hemorrhage. A moderately severe or large subarachnoid hemorrhage often produces sufficient obstruction of the arachnoid granulations that ventricular dilatation develops and requires ventricular shunting. The obstruction may be seen in the acute stage and may improve later so that the ventricular drainage catheter can be removed, or it may involve such a high percentage of the arachnoid granulations that ventricular shunting must be permanent.

The diagnosis of hydrocephalus should not be made only because there is enlargement of the ventricular system. The ventricles may also become enlarged because of cerebral atrophy or hypoplasia, sometimes called *hydrocephalus ex vacuo*. Because the latter term is somewhat confusing, this appearance is generally described as *ventricular enlargement due to atrophy* or *hypoplasia* (the latter term is used if it may be congenital).

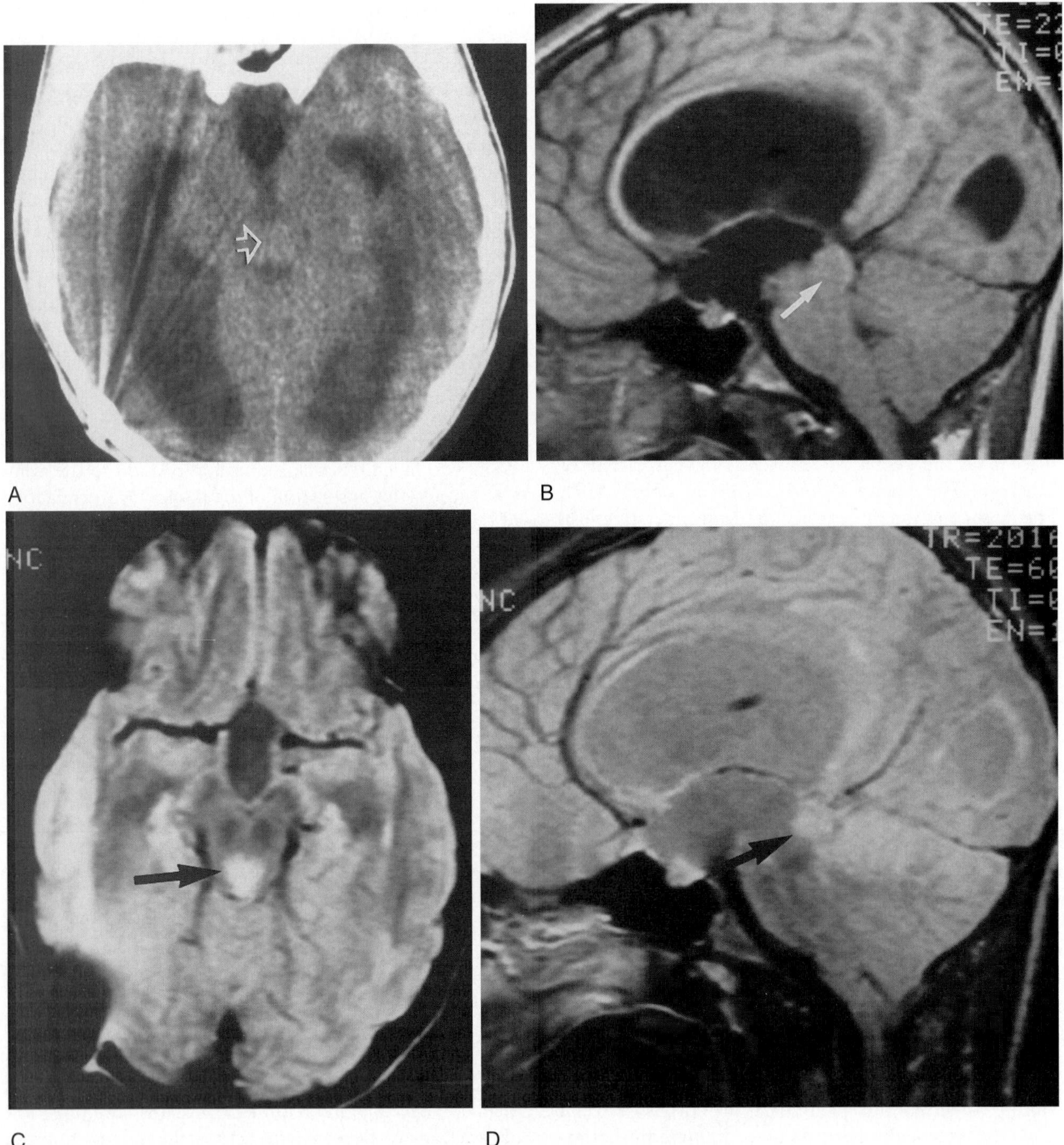

Figure 4.49. Periaqueductal glioma diagnosed previously as aqueductal stenosis on CT. **A.** CT showed absence of the aqueductal image (arrow). The diagnosis of stenosis was made and the patient was shunted. **B.** Two years later, reexamination by MRI revealed an enlargement of the quadrigeminal plate (arrow) and absence of the aqueduct. **C** and **D.** Proton density axial and sagittal images revealed abnormal signal in the area, indicating that the tissue was pathologic (arrows).

As indicated earlier, the cause of communicating hydrocephalus may be adhesions in the region of the interpeduncular and suprasellar cisterns or a large suprasellar tumor or meningeal carcinomatosis with diffuse seeding in the region of the incisura, which could impede the passage of CSF into the supratentorial area. This would be a communicating hydrocephalus but with a true obstruction demonstrable in the perisellar region.

Perhaps the most frequent and important type of communicating hydrocephalus is that in which there is no demonstrable obstruction anywhere but there is interference with normal absorption of CSF by arachnoid granulations at the top of the brain. This may result, for instance, from a severe subarachnoid hemorrhage that plugs normal arachnoid granulations. It may also result from any cause that would produce subarachnoid blood, such as trauma. Bleeding aneurysms are a frequent cause of temporary obstruction that requires a shunting procedure or ventricular drainage for a limited period of time. Later, an equilibrium between production and absorption is reached and the shunting procedure may no longer be necessary.

The diagnosis would depend on examination by CT or MRI demonstrating the absence of obstruction. Clinically, patients show signs of developing hydrocephalus, such as headaches and obtundedness. A demonstration on CT or MRI of dilating ventricles in comparison with the previous recent examination would then be an indication of developing hydrocephalus.

If the condition is allowed to proceed without any attempts at a shunting procedure, the ventricles will probably continue to dilate until equilibrium is reached between production and absorption of CSF. Usually an increased amount of CSF leaves the lateral ventricles through the ependymal surface and passes into the periventricular white matter, demonstrable by CT or MRI (Fig. 4.47).

Normotensive Hydrocephalus (Hakim Syndrome)

This form of communicating hydrocephalus was first described by Hakim (41) and by Adams et al. (42). It usually has an unknown etiology. Sometimes an old head trauma or subarachnoid hemorrhage may be in the history, but in general no cause can be detected by history or otherwise (43). As originally described, the pressure within the ventricles as measured directly in the ventricles or by a spinal tap is normal or at the normal upper limits. The condition occurs in older individuals and is clinically characterized by difficulty in walking, sleepiness, urinary incontinence, and some intellectual deterioration, all of which can improve if a successful shunting procedure is carried out. The diagnosis can be made by a combination of cross-sectional imaging and by carrying out spinal puncture and removal of a fair amount of CSF. The latter procedure will improve the patient's condition for a few days.

From the point of view of cross-sectional imaging, the diagnosis is made because of enlargement of the lateral ventricles, including the temporal horns, and of the third ventricle. Interestingly enough, the aqueduct of Sylvius may also be somewhat large and may show a flow void on MRI due to back-and-forth motion of CSF, as described by Bradley et al. (44). Bradley et al. propose that the dilated ventricles produce a reactive diminution of space in the cranial cavity for the brain. As proof of this, they emphasize the flattening of the gyri against the inner skull surface. Since the brain cannot pulsate normally, more of the pulsating movement is transmitted to the ventricular wall, which in turn displaces the CSF through the third ventricle and aqueduct, producing a rapid back-and-forth movement. A flow void may be observed in the posterior third ventricle and in the aqueduct on MRI (Figs. 4.50 and 4.52).

The surface sulci of the brain and the sylvian fissure are not enlarged and in fact may be disproportionately smaller than the size of the ventricles. The gyri are flattened against the inner table of the skull. This is visible on axial cross-sectional images but may also be shown on MRI coronal images. The corpus callosum has a rounded (humped) configuration as seen on sagittal MR images because of elevation by the enlarged ventricles (Fig. 4.51).

Jinkins suggests that the elevation of the posterior aspect of the corpus callosum raises this structure to impinge on the rigid inferior aspect of the falx, producing symptoms that may accompany hydrocephalus (gait disturbance, imbalance, incontinence, short-term memory deficits, and global dementia) (45). The edge of the falx produced focal flattening of the posterior corpus callosum in 21 of his 24 patients with this complex of symptoms, whereas in 16 patients similarly hydrocephalic but without flattening of the corpus callosum against the falx, these symptoms were absent with one possible exception. The cases described by Jinkins were not selected. The falx cerebri varies in configuration between subjects but is always wider in vertical diameter posteriorly than it is anteriorly. For this reason impingement of the elevated corpus callosum in hydrocephalus is always posterior (Fig. 4.51).

Enlargement of the sylvian fissure on both sides has been described in documented cases (46). In such cases, the surface sulci still are closer to normal.

The diagnosis of normotensive hydrocephalus is difficult (47). Perhaps the main difficulty lies in differentiating it from atrophy. Although we assume that atrophy is usually accompanied by enlarged sulci in the brain cortex, this abnormality may also be found in cases of normotensive hydrocephalus. El Gammal et al. have suggested four items to be sought on MRI examinations (48): (a) the *mammillo-pontine distance* (distance from the mammillary body to the belli of the pons as measured on sagittal T1-weighted images), normally 1.2 cm, is reduced to 7 to 8 mm in hydrocephalus but not in atrophy; (b) the anterior third ventricle is dilated in hydrocephalus; (c) the corpus callosum is elevated in hydrocephalus but not in atrophy; (d) the average thickness of the corpus callosum at the level of the foramen of Monro is under 6 mm in hydrocephalus. Because of the atrophy, however, this measurement may also be decreased in patients with cerebral atrophy. When a clinical diagnosis cannot be made by available methods, sometimes a shunting procedure is necessary to test whether the patient will improve. If the patient has the pathologic condition being described, he or she is likely to improve dramatically. On the other hand, if the diagnosis is not correct, the shunting procedure will probably produce very little or no improvement.

Concerning the CT or MRI diagnosis of normotensive hydrocephalus, Jinkins et al. have recently analyzed all the

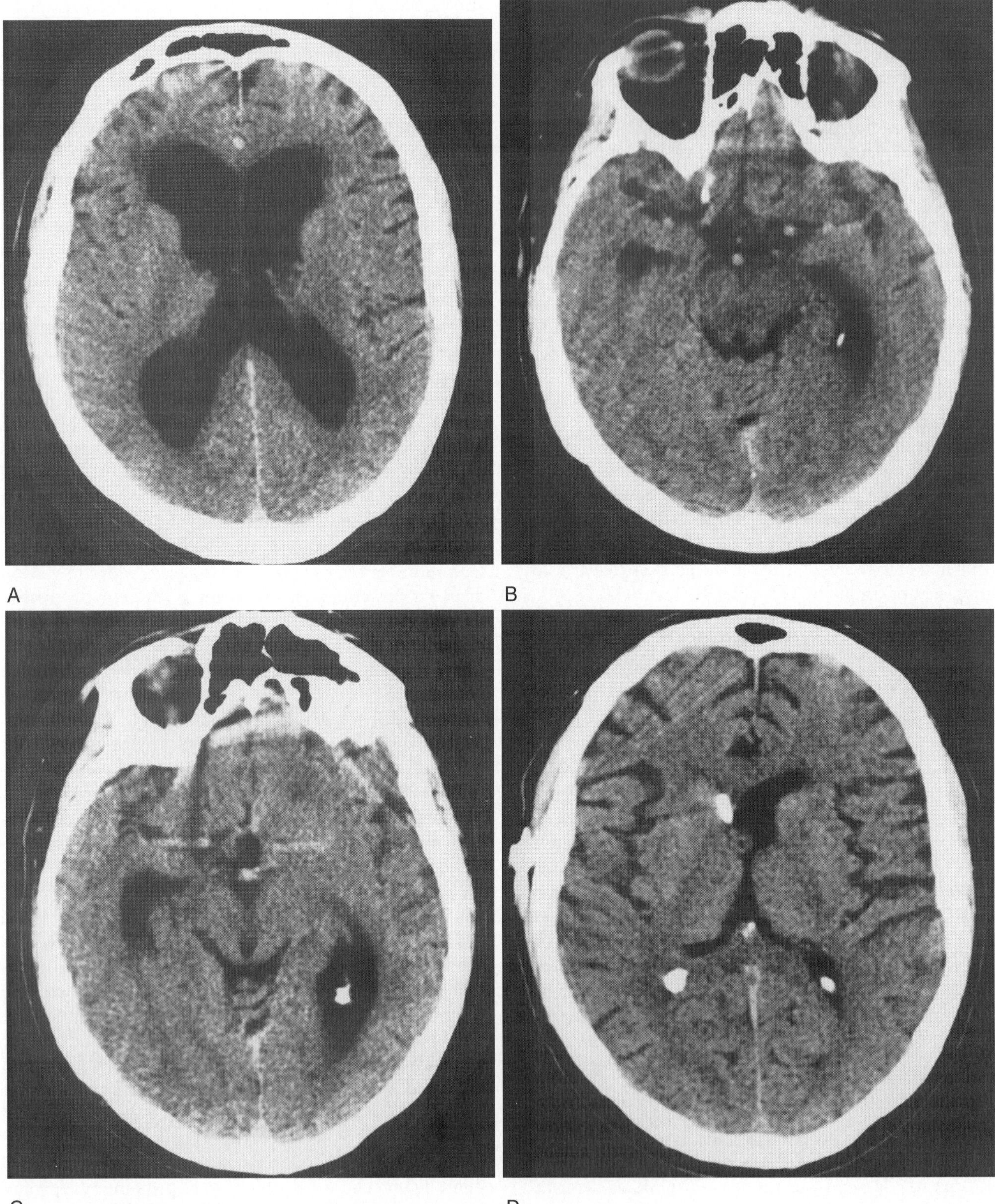

Figure 4.50. Normotensive hydrocephalus showing improvement after shunting. **A.** Image shows considerable ventricular dilatation without evidence of enlargement (actually compression) of the surface sulci or sylvian fissures. The patient was a 66-year-old man who had difficulties walking and was confined to a wheelchair. **B** and **C.** The temporal horns are dilated; the aqueduct is large, which is a feature of this condition. **D.** Reexamination 9 months after shunting revealed that the ventricles had returned to normal and the sylvian fissures and surface sulci were not compressed by the dilated ventricles. The patient was now walking normally.

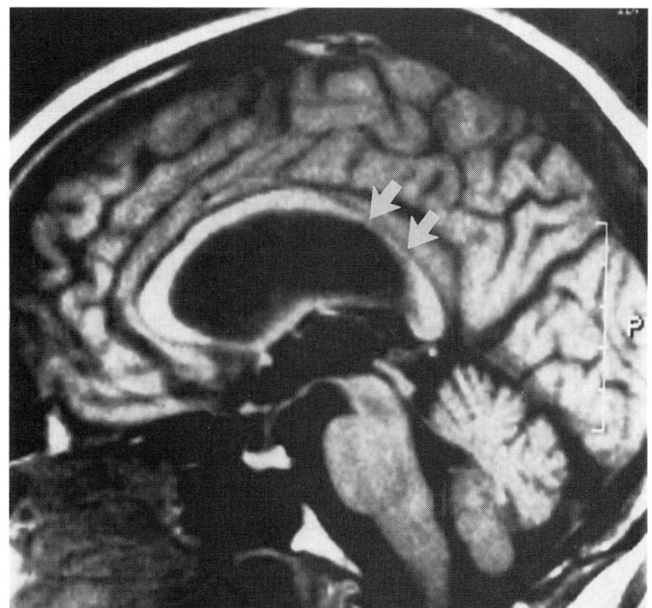

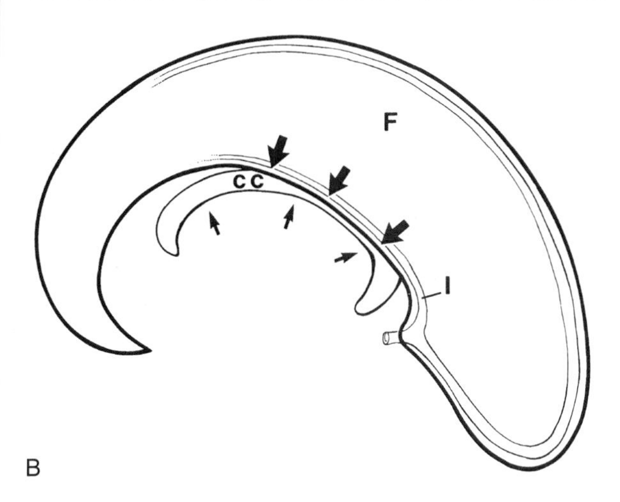

A

Figure 4.51. Impingement of the corpus callosum on the edge of falx in a patient with normotensive hydrocephalus. **A.** Sagittal T1-weighted image. The lateral ventricles are dilated and elevate the corpus callosum, which assumes a more curved configuration. This elevation brings the corpus callosum against the falx in its wider portion, posteriorly (arrows). **B.** Diagram demonstrating the pathogenesis. There is elevation of the corpus callosum (cc, small arrows) and an associated curvilinear flattening and thinning of the caudal aspect of the dorsal surface of the corpus callosum (large arrows) caused by impinging falx cerebri (F). (I = interior sagittal sinus.) (Courtesy of Dr. J. Randy Jinkins, University of Texas, Health Services Center, San Antonio [AJNR 1991;12: 331–340], with permission.)

findings, and have concluded that the only finding that seems to be encountered in all of these patients as against those with deep cerebral atrophy is enlargement of the temporal horns (49). The other findings (flattening of the gyri against the inner table of the skull, ballooning of the frontal horns and the atrium of the lateral ventricles, thinning of the corpus callosum, and enlargement of the third and fourth ventricles) can be found in both groups, although they occur much more frequently in normotensive hydrocephalus than in cerebral atrophy. If enlargement of the temporal horns is not present, the diagnosis of normotensive hydrocephalus is doubtful.

In fact, no reliable method exists today to determine whether shunting will produce improvement. Greitz et al. (50) and Meyer et al. (51) state that cerebral blood flow (CBF) decreases in normotensive hydrocephalus (maximal in frontal and temporal lobes) and that, in the cases where the shunting was properly indicated, there is an increase in CBF following the procedure. Meyer et al. also suggest that it may be possible to use the CBF test before and after spinal puncture with removal of CSF to determine the probable response to shunting. They also indicate that the local partition coefficient of xenon diminishes, particularly in the white matter, in normotensive hydrocephalus because of increased water in the brain tissue, and that abnormal partition coefficients are never seen in Alzheimer's disease and other degenerative dementias associated with brain atrophy. They suggest that this could be used to differentiate between the two conditions. However, the xenon CBT test is used in relatively few institutions. A reduction in CBF may also be found in Alzheimerlike dementias.

In a recent study, Bradley et al. (44, 52, 53) reported on the use of a high-resolution phase contrast MRI technique to measure the CSF stroke volume through the aqueduct of Sylvius in patients suspected of having normotensive hydrocephalus. If the stroke volume (SV) was greater than 40 μl, the diagnosis was considered more secure and shunting would probably achieve desired results. The higher the figures above 40 μl the more likely the good results after shunting. However, the higher stroke volumes did not necessarily yield clear flow voids in the aqueduct on routine spin-echo images. If the stroke volume is below 40 μl, the chances are that a ventriculoperitoneal shunt will not lead to improvement, although exceptions may well occur.

Following shunting it is possible to measure the flow through the tube by a spin-echo phase contrast MRI technique (54).

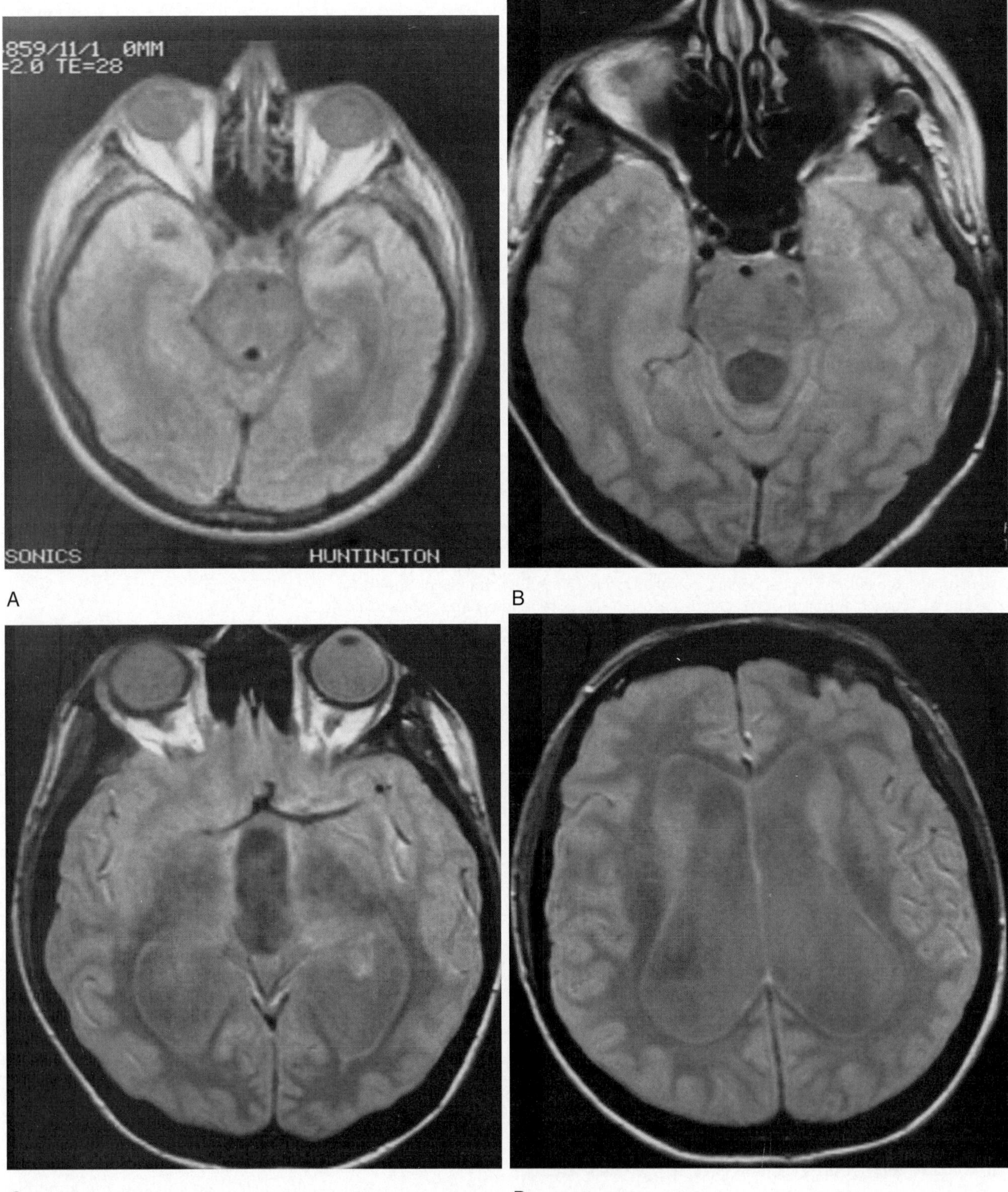

Figure 4.52. Normotensive hydrocephalus showing marked flow void in aqueduct and flattening of gyri against inner table of skull. **A.** Proton density image demonstrates an enlarged aqueduct with low intensity, indicating a flow void from increased pulsations. **B** to **D.** MRI of another case shows marked ventricular enlargement including the third and fourth ventricles and only slight periventricular hyperintensity, indicating normotensive as against hypertensive hydrocephalus, in which we may expect greater transependymal passage of CSF. The surface sulci are relatively small because of brain compression against the inner table of the skull. (Courtesy of Dr. William G. Bradley, Jr., Medical MRI Center, Long Beach Memorial Medical Center, Calif., with permission.)

Focal Hydrocephalus

A portion of the ventricle or an isolated ventricle can become dilated if there is an obstruction. A unilateral obstruction of the foramen of Monro causes dilatation of one lateral ventricle. When an obstruction is in the atrium of the ventricle, such as may be produced by a neoplasm or by an adhesive process, the temporal horn becomes dilated because the choroid plexus in the temporal horn continues to produce CSF. This is ordinarily called *trapping* of the ventricle (Fig. 4.53). The fourth ventricle may become dilated if its outlets are obstructed and at the same time a shunting procedure of the lateral ventricle is carried out. The isolated fourth ventricle may become dilated, as in the presence of a Chiari II malformation with shunting or in basal arachnoiditis. In the presence of aqueductal obstruction, the fourth ventricle does not become dilated because the CSF produced within it passes out into the basal cisterns and is absorbed by the usual mechanisms. For this reason, in cases of aqueductal obstruction, the fourth ventricle is normal or somewhat smaller in size.

ETIOLOGY OF HYDROCEPHALUS

There are many causes for hydrocephalus (Table 4.4). In general, the cause will be congenital, inflammatory, traumatic, neoplastic, or vascular (either directly or usually due to hemorrhage). Sometimes the cause may be unknown. At other times overproduction of CSF may be a cause, such as may be seen in patients with choroid plexus papilloma, although this connection has not been proved. In each location, as shown in Table 4.4, the etiology may vary somewhat.

The diagnosis of hydrocephalus in infants is usually made by ultrasound followed by a CT or MRI examination to ascertain the probable etiology. The diagnosis can be made in utero by sonography. This allows the parents to elect interruption of pregnancy, which is an important contribution to management, for these children have a probability of being mentally retarded even if adequate surgical treatment is applied early.

TREATMENT OF HYDROCEPHALUS

The basic treatment of hydrocephalus is shunting of the CSF to another location where the fluid can be absorbed. Although choroid plexectomy of the lateral ventricles was used by Scarff (56) and others for a number of years, it was given up because the procedure was surgically more difficult, had more complications, and could be properly used only in communicating hydrocephalus. Puncture of the dilated third ventricle in the suprasellar region was also tried, originally with poor results, but recently stereotactic third ventriculostomy is being advocated using CT scanning guidance. The cannula is inserted through the foramen of Monro and the opening is made in the hypothalamus. A flow void may be seen when the ventriculostomy is functioning (57). One of the earlier shunting procedures was the Torkildsen procedure, which consisted of shunting the lateral ventricles into the cisterna magna. This worked well in some patients, but again, the surgical procedure is more difficult and could not work in the long term in the growing infant. For this reason it was mostly reserved for older children or adults with aqueductal obstruction.

Then came other shunting procedures, such as ventriculospinal, ventriculoureteral, ventriculofallopian (in girls), ventriculopleural, ventriculoatrial, and ventriculoperitoneal. The two most extensively utilized procedures were the ventriculoatrial and the ventriculoperitoneal shunts. In the ventriculoatrial, the shunt tube was inserted into the occipital or frontal horn of the lateral ventricle at the upper end and into the jugular vein down to the right atrium of the heart. It was relatively easy to perform. Because of possible, and actual, complications (clotting, bloodstream infection), the procedure is used much less frequently now. It has been replaced by the ventriculoperitoneal shunt, which is initially more difficult to perform but has a better chance of satisfactory long-term function, particularly since the development of the slit valve.

Concomitant with the development of shunting procedures was that of pressure valves to maintain optimal CSF pressure. The valves have to remain patent for a long period and ideally should maintain the CSF pressure within a narrow range for optimum results. The Holter valve was one of the earliest; the Hakim valve is carefully engineered; the slit valve has the advantage of simplicity and lack of invasion by surrounding tissue such as the peritoneum. The choroid plexus may grow in size to surround or invade an intraventricular shunt tube, which requires multiple holes to remain open. Shunt revisions were very frequent in the early period, but this problem has improved greatly.

Chronic, long-term shunting may produce thickening of the dura that may be quite pronounced at times (58). The meningeal fibrosis may be so marked that it needs to be differentiated from a subdural collection. Enhanced CT or MRI will show enhancement of the entire thickened dura, usually also around the tentorium and falx (Fig. 4.54).

Complications of shunting include infection and hemorrhage, which usually require reinsertion in another location. In ventriculoatrial shunts, infection may lead to endocarditis.

Malfunction is common and may be due to a variety of causes, including obstruction by the choroid plexus or by gliosis. If the ventricles become too small (slit ventricles), malfunction due to obstruction may lead to intermittent symptoms. The pressure adjustment in the shunt valve may be important in such cases.

Rapid decompression of the ventricles may result in accumulation of a subdural hematoma or hygroma, which will impede expansion of the brain in an infant with severe hydrocephalus. It is common after shunting of normotensive hydrocephalus in the elderly, possibly because of failure of the brain tissue to expand to fill in the space made available by ventricular shunting. For this reason it

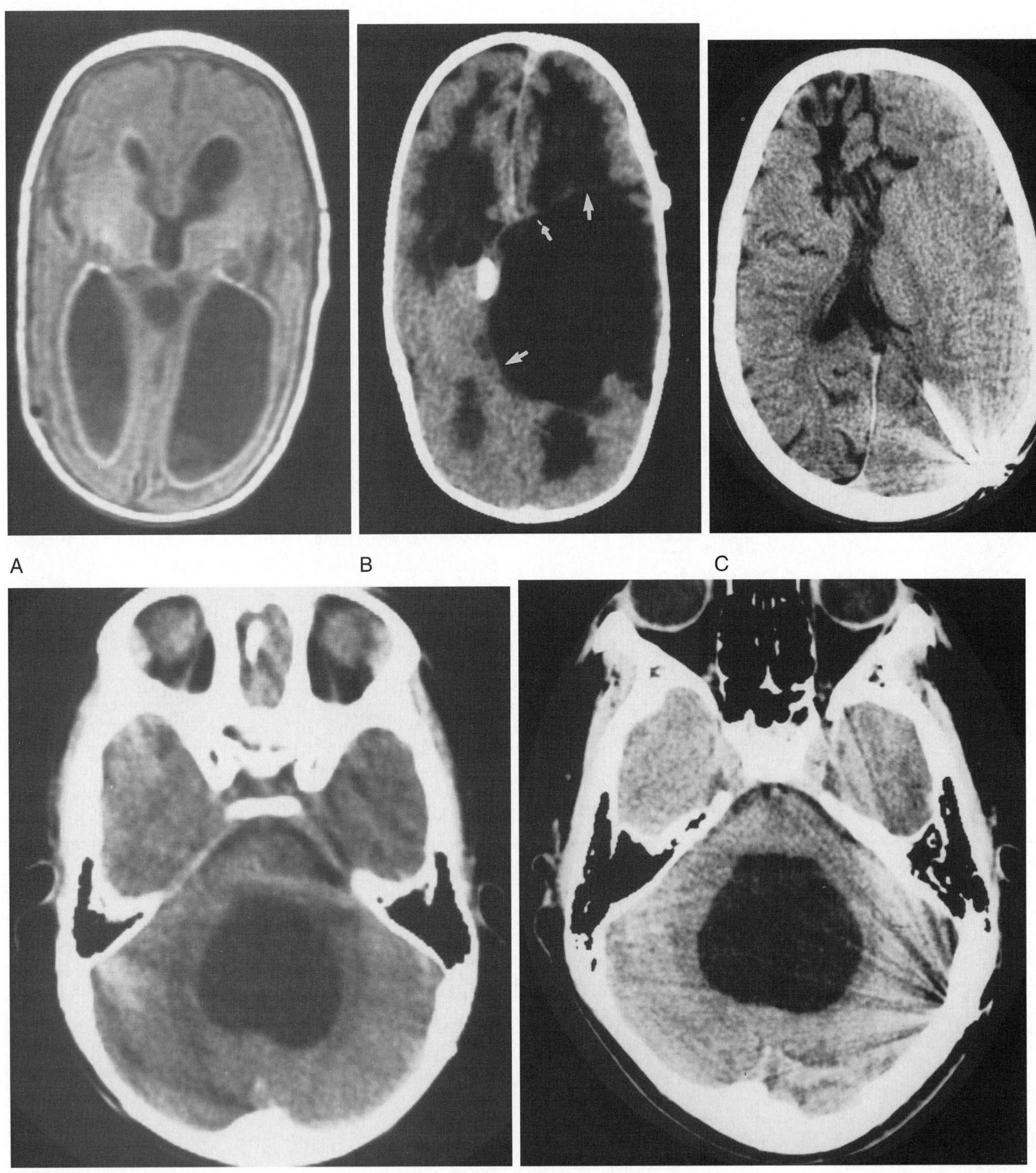

Figure 4.53. Trapping of temporal horn in a 5-month-old child with meningitis and ependymitis requiring a shunting procedure. **A.** Hydrocephalus due to meningitis and ependymitis. This T1-weighted image without contrast shows hyperintensity in the ependymal lining. **B.** CT image. Shunt malfunction resulted in considerable dilatation of the left temporal horn, which is acting like a cyst and producing a mass effect (arrows). The CSF produced in the temporal horn cannot join the rest of the ventricle because of intraventricular adhesions secondary to ependymitis. In addition, there is ventricular obstruction and a marked irregular outline of the lateral ventricles due to transependymal passage of fluid. **C.** The shunt is functioning and maintaining normal ventricular size. There is a shift of midline structures to the right because of a large hemispheric infarct. **D to E.** Trapping of the fourth ventricle in a 7-year-old boy with a history of basal arachnoiditis and shunting. **D.** The fourth ventricle is markedly enlarged as the result of basal arachnoiditis and associated aqueductal stenosis, probably from old ependymitis. **E.** Examination 5 years after D shows that the fourth ventricle is slightly larger but that equilibrium must have taken place, and no specific treatment was applied.

Table 4.4.
Obstructive Hydrocephalus by Etiology of Obstruction

At Foramen of Monro
- Congenital: Tuberous sclerosis
- Inflammatory: Ependymitis
- Traumatic: Disruption of structures, ependymal adhesions
- Neoplastic: Colloid cyst; ependymoma; glioma arising from septum pellucidum, rostrum of corpus callosum, or third ventricle tumor (germinoma, intraventricular craniopharyngioma, ependymoma, astrocytoma)
  - Suprasellar tumor (pituitary adenoma, craniopharyngioma, suprasellar arachnoid cyst, other)

At posterior third ventricle and aqueduct
- Aneurysm of vein of Galen
- Pineal-origin tumor (germinoma, glioma, teratoma)
- Aqueduct stenosis (congenital, acquired due to ependymitis), periaqueductal glioma, tumors pressing on aqueduct (gliomas arising from quadrigeminal plate, meningiomas arising from tentorium, superior cerebellar tumors)

At aqueduct
- Congenital: aqueduct stenosis, forking, gliosis or septum
- Inflammatory: ependymitis
- Traumatic: hemorrhage, gliosis, ependymitis, and adhesive process
- Neoplastic: periaqueductal glioma, other neoplasms arising in quadrigeminal plate or brainstem. Tumor pressing on aqueduct (tentorial meningiomas, cerebellar tumors, arachnoid cysts, other)

At the fourth ventricle
- Intraventricular tumor (ependymoma, choroid plexus papilloma, meningioma)
- Cerebellar masses (hemorrhage, abscess, neoplasms)
- Brainstem tumor: gliomas
- Extra-axial posterior fossa lesions (basal arachnoiditis, cysticercosis, cerebellopontine-angle tumors, large basilar artery aneurysm)

Metaventricular causes
- Incisural and suprasellar (arachnoiditis, neoplasms)
- Diffuse arachnoidal (postmeningitic, subarachnoid hemorrhage, meningeal carcinomatosis)
- Suprahemispheric (blockage of arachnoid granulations by hemorrhage, inflammation, other)

is important to effect the decompression gradually. Hakim also emphasizes the need to maintain a reduced but not too low intraventricular pressure to prevent rapid ventricular size reduction. Follow-up of a number of older patients with bilateral subdural hygromas at the Massachusetts General Hospital has shown a stable improved clinical status, which suggests that there is no need to remove the extracerebral fluid.

Malfunction may be related to disconnection of the shunt tube, such as when the child grows. Shunt tubes can usually be tested without having to inject contrast material and using radiography.

The diagnosis of shunt malfunction is made by the presence of ventricular enlargement in comparison with previous examinations. The injection of contrast intraventricularly is not necessary unless an ependymal adhesive process leading to multiple compartments is suspected. Lemann et al. described a white matter complication in patients with a shunt when an Ommaya reservoir had been used, which is usually used for treatment of a neoplastic or inflammatory condition (59). The white matter (usually in the frontal region where the catheter is inserted) becomes edematous in a wide area, and contrast enhancement will usually be observed around the catheter. When this is recognized, the catheter should be removed and checked for possible infection.

It is interesting to note that nature has not provided for a limitation or arrest of CSF production in the presence of obstruction. For instance, an isolated fourth ventricle that is obstructed by outlet adhesions or other causes will continue to grow and compress the brainstem until some adjustment is reached between CSF production and passage of fluid transependymally, but not before symptoms of cerebellar and/or brainstem dysfunction may have occurred. The same is true of other obstructive cavities where CSF production is taking place (Fig. 4.53). (See "Arachnoid Cysts," for further discussion.)

Rare causes of hydrocephalus include spinal tumor. This has been described in patients with meningioma and also in ependymoma of the filum terminale. The cause is obscure but may be related to long-standing elevation of CSF protein, which may interfere with its absorption at the arachnoid granulations. As explained earlier, the fluid component of CSF can be absorbed in the spinal root meninges, but the protein is not. The hydrocephalus usually improves following tumor removal (60, 61).

COLPOCEPHALY

The term *colpocephaly* is often used to refer to dilatation of the atrial and occipital portions of the lateral ventricles. In the past it was believed to represent some special condition, but it appears that greater dilatation of the posterior aspects of the lateral ventricles is commonly seen in both obstructive hydrocephalus in the newborn and in the infant and child with brain hypoplasia or atrophy accompanied by ventricular enlargement. The latter group of children usually present mental retardation, motor deficits, seizures, and sometimes visual difficulties. The term *colpocephaly* is usually applied to this group. As mentioned above, however, greater atrial and occipital horn dilatation is also seen in the hydrocephalic infant. This can be attributed to greater ease of enlargement of the ventricles posteriorly because of the presence of several sutures, whereas in the frontal region there are no sutures to allow the skull to widen secondary to increased ventricular pressure. Unless there is an extreme degree of occipital horn enlargement, the term *colpocephaly* has no significance. In some cases, such as those described by Herskowitz et al. (55), one might be justified in using it, but simply to describe the ventricular configuration, not to imply a unifying etiology.

EXTERNAL HYDROCEPHALUS

It is questionable whether such an entity exists. If one accepts the well-established fact that practically all of the CSF is produced within the ventricles, one cannot easily accept the premise that CSF will accumulate in the extracerebral space without significant ventricular enlargement and without adhesions in the subarachnoid space such as may result from meningitis. Nevertheless, the term has been

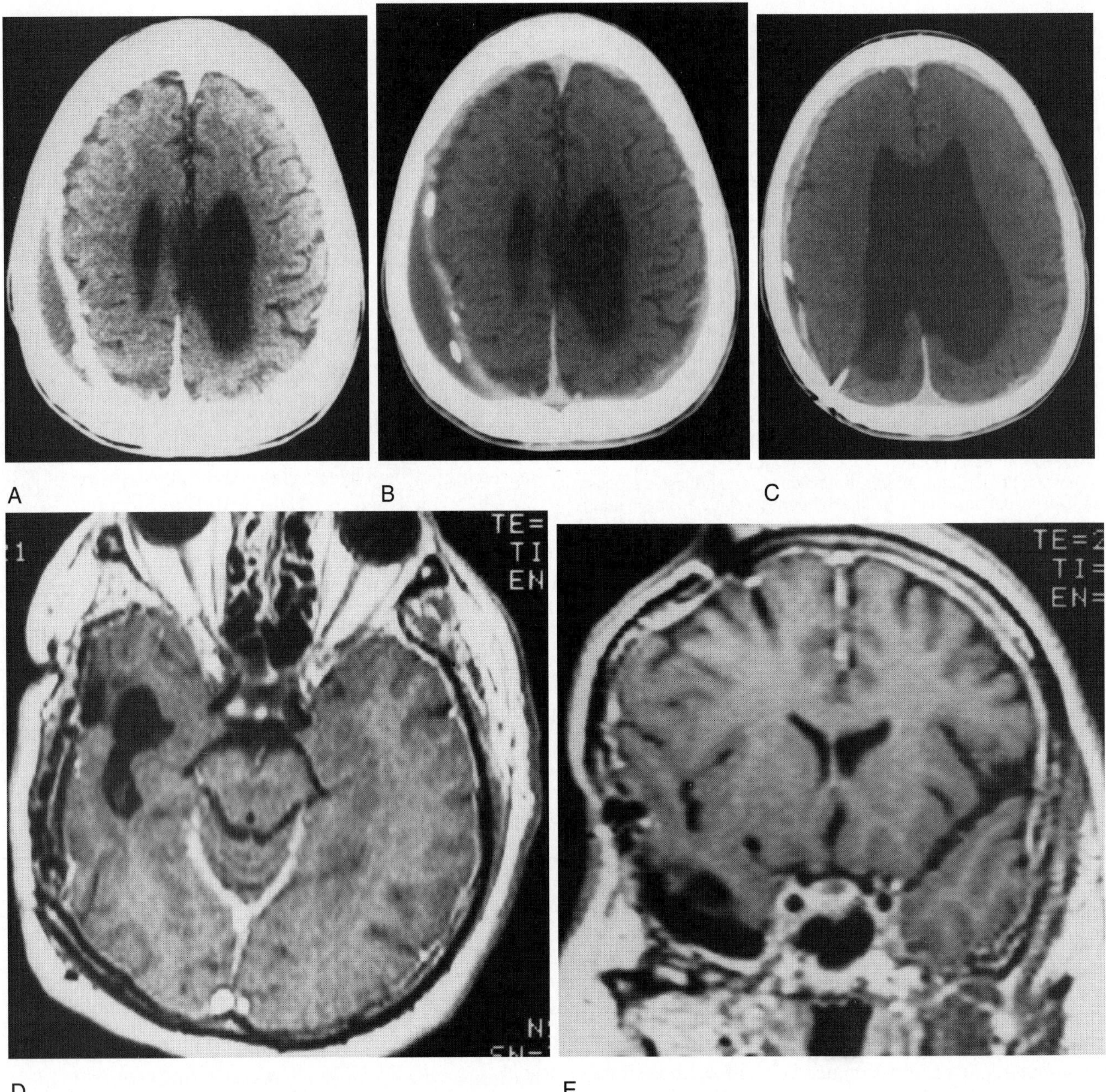

Figure 4.54. Marked dural thickening and fibrosis in a patient with a long-standing ventricular shunt (24 years). **A.** Contrast-enhanced CT shows marked enhancement of dural bridging over an epidural CSF collection at the site of entrance of the shunting tube. The falx is also markedly enhanced. **B** and **C.** The postcontrast CT images show thickened dura all around the brain. Note that the septum pellucidum is not seen, probably because of the rupture and reabsorption that occurs in early severe hydrocephalus. The dura can acquire a thickness approaching 1.0 cm in these cases. **D** and **E.** Meningeal enhancement in postoperative patient. The postcontrast T1 images show diffuse meningeal enhancement, not only near the area of surgery (5 years after removal of acoustic neuroma), but also around all meningeal surfaces.

used to describe infants with growth of the head beyond the normal, minimal enlargement of the ventricles, and with enlargement of the extracerebral fluid space. In the children with megalencephaly described by Maytal et al. (62), the fluid was bifrontal in location, the frontal interhemispheric space was widened, and the ventricles were slightly enlarged (Fig. 4.55). Follow-up usually shows disappearance of the abnormality by about 2 years of age. Some infants have a family history of benign familial macrocephaly.

The CSF accumulation in the frontal region may relate to the supine position in which the examinations are per-

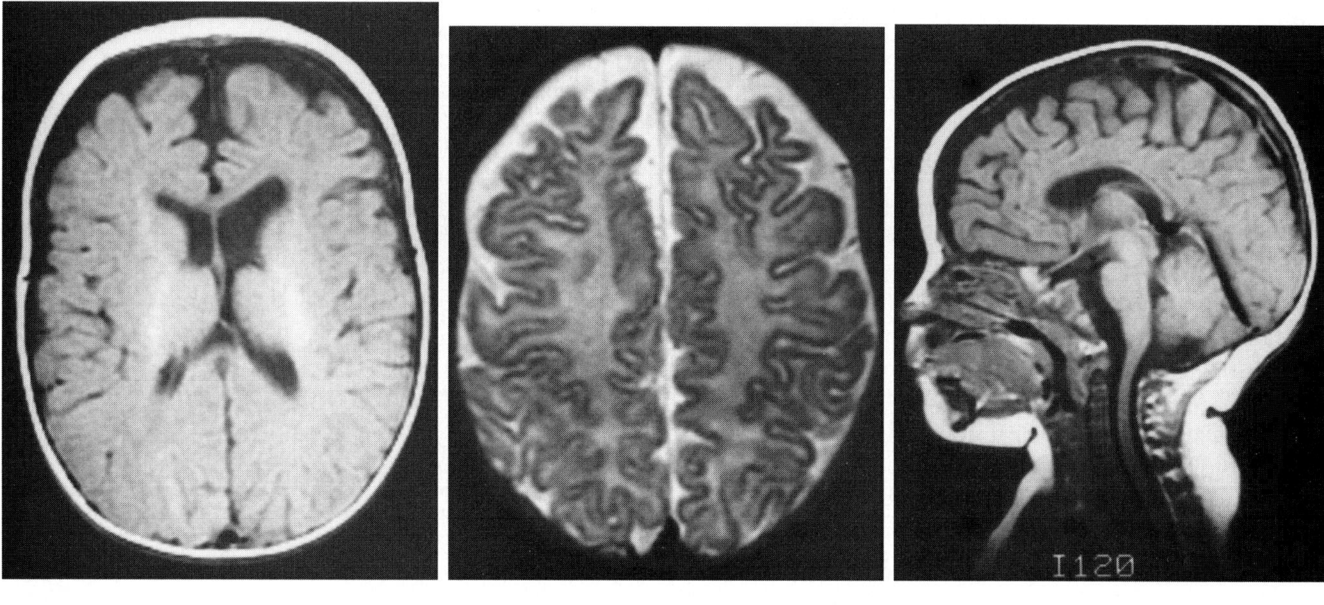

A B C

Figure 4.55. External hydrocephalus in a 3-month-old female infant who was brought in because of a large head. **A.** T1-weighted axial image shows a large extracerebral fluid space with normal gyri bilaterally. The frontal location is due to gravity; the brain is slightly heavier than the CSF. The ventricles are slightly to moderately enlarged. Myelination is normal; there is evidence of it in the basal ganglia and the internal capsule. **B.** A higher T2-weighted axial image confirms the large extracerebral space, also in the interhemispheric fissure. **C.** Sagittal T1-weighted image demonstrates a normal appearance of the brain. The corpus callosum shows mild early myelination. The term *benign enlargement of the subarachnoid spaces* may well be applied to this condition (see text).

formed. Examination in the prone position probably would decrease the appearance or show more CSF in the occipital region.

Atrophy or brain hypoplasia may produce a similar picture, but Maytal et al. indicate that in these patients the cerebral sulci are usually more prominent (62). Some infants with CT and MRI signs of external hydrocephalus may have a congenital metabolic anomaly. The term *benign enlargement of the subarachnoid spaces* has been proposed by Nickel et al. (63), and it appears to be a preferable and less confusing term than *external hydrocephalus.* Wilms et al. emphasize the importance of MRI examination to differentiate between this entity and subdural collections, with which it may be confused and which are less specific with CT (64). The subdural collections usually show some signal changes in the fluid and slight hyperintensity on T1 weighted images, and the double collections (subdural and subarachnoid) are clearly seen, but not so clearly differentiated on CT images.

Spontaneous Intracranial Hypotension

The post–lumbar puncture headache is well known and is attributed to low intracranial pressure caused by removal of CSF and leakage of CSF outside the subarachnoid space. A similar condition is seen postoperatively in many patients, although it may be masked by the postoperative condition of the patient. Although perhaps rare, a condition exists in which there is decreased intracranial pressure in a patient who has not had any prior history of surgery or spinal puncture or trauma. The clinical manifestation is a headache that is completely relieved by lying supine. In a recent report, Baum et al. found that 3 of 3 patients had diffuse dural enhancement and what they called distention of the dural sinuses. Two had bilateral thin subdural collection (65). The patients also showed a decrease in the size of the suprasellar cisterns and of the cisterns of the posterior fossa, which was attributed to sagging of the brain.

The clinical history should raise the question of a CSF leak, and a careful search for such should be made (radionuclide cisternography, myelography). Baum et al. indicate that the subdural collections are not the cause of the headaches, but a result of the intracranial hypotension (65).

MYELIN AND DEMYELINATION

Myelin, which might be considered an insulator for axons, is a very important component of the nervous system. The fibers that conduct impulses within the nervous system are covered by myelin, and the absence of myelin, either because it has not formed or because it has been destroyed, will make the nerve fibers incapable of cleanly conducting electrical nerve impulses. Myelinated fibers characteristically have a larger diameter than unmyelinated fibers. Myelin is a proteophospholipid, and in the peripheral nerves the myelin sheath is composed of a multilayered spiral derived from the apposed and compacted membranes of a greatly elaborated Schwann cell (66).

Normal myelin has a complicated molecular structure, and in the brain it is formed by modification of the oligodendrocytic cell membrane. This is different in the brain than it is in the peripheral nerves, where the Schwannn cells are the major participants. Each oligodendrocyte has cell processes, each of which forms a segment of the myelin sheath of an axon (67). An oligodendrocyte may lend its processes to more than one axon to produce segments of myelination.

Myelination in the central nervous system starts early, and some is already present at birth in the brainstem, the cerebellum, and the internal capsule, particularly in its posterior limb. Myelin deposition progresses rapidly after birth and can be well demonstrated by MRI. The T1-weighted image, particularly the inversion recovery sequence, images myelin best in the first 6 to 8 months of life. Thereafter, the T2-weighted images are satisfactory. MRI has shown that by 2 to 3 years myelination is very advanced, quite similar to the grown brain, and for all practical purposes myelination is complete by 4 to 5 years of age. However, histologically, complete myelination is not reached until 8 to 9 years of age, when growth of the brain is considered complete. The progress of myelination is described and illustrated in Chapter 5, "The Developing Brain in the Infant and Child."

An important point to keep in mind is that on T1-weighted images myelin is hyperintense in relation to surrounding brain tissue and on T2-weighted images it is darker than gray matter. The reason is that myelin contains significantly less water than the surrounding brain tissue. Its brightness on T1-weighted images is not due to the fact that it is a phospholipid but to the fact that it contains fewer water molecules. The usual fat-suppression technique does not change the image of myelinated brain tissue. Although by around 2 years the brain presents an MRI pattern similar to that of the adult brain, there may be areas of incomplete myelination around the poles of the ventricles, particularly near the occipital region in the periatrial portion of the lateral ventricles (68). See Table 4.5.

Table 4.5.
Myelin and Demyelination

Myelination process (discussed in Chapter 5)
Demyelination and dysmyelination
- a) Inborn errors of metabolism (discussed in Chapter 5)
- b) Multiple sclerosis
  - 1- Classic type
  - 2- Acute (Marburg type)
  - 3- Diffuse cerebral sclerosis (Schilder type)
  - 4- Concentric sclerosis (Baló type)
  - 5- Neuromyelitis optica
- c) Acute disseminated (perivenous) encephalomyelitis
  - 1- Classic (parainfectious)
  - 2- Postimmunization (idiopathic)
  - 3- Hyperacute (acute hemorrhagic leukoencephalitis) (discussed under Infectious Diseases, Chapter 6)
- d)
  - 1- Central pontine myelinolysis
  - 2- Marchiafava-Bignami disease
  - 3- Progressive multifocal leukoencephalopathy (discussed under Infectious Diseases, Chapter 6)

Classification of Demyelinating Diseases

Demyelination is a very important chapter in neurology. The demyelinating diseases are usually of unknown etiology. They have different clinical, epidemiologic, and pathologic features but have one common pathologic feature, *periaxial demyelination*, which means that the myelin sheath is destroyed but that the axon is preserved, completely or at least partially.

Another term that is important to understand is that of *dysmyelination*, which is usually applied to congenital defects leading to defective formation or lack of myelin deposition along the fibers, as described in Chapter 5. Other conditions causing breakdown of the myelin (such as wallerian degeneration) are secondary to neuronal destruction. However, there are other conditions in which periaxial demyelination occurs, such as viral infections or intoxications. Allen indicates they are not usually included among the demyelinating diseases because they have other features in addition to pure demyelination (67).

Allen lists three classes of demyelinating diseases:

1. Multiple sclerosis (disseminated sclerosis). This includes the classic Charcot type, acute (Marburg) type, diffuse cerebral (Schilder) type, concentric (Baló) type, and neuromyelitis optica (Devic) type.
2. Acute disseminated (perivenous) encephalomyelitis (acute perivascular myelinolysis). This includes classic (parainfectious), postimmunization (idiopathic), and hyperacute (acute hemorrhagic leukoencephalitis).
3. Demyelinating disorders associated with systemic disease. This is a rare type. It includes central pontine myelinolysis, Marchiafava-Bignami disease, and progressive multifocal leukoencephalopathy.

The mechanism by which demyelination is produced is not known, but it can be produced by damage to the oligodendrocyte, by direct damage to the myelin sheath, or by damage to both simultaneously. As explained earlier, myelin is composed of a protein and a lipid from sphingolipid phospholipid, glycolipid, and cholesterol. The breakdown of the myelin then leads to loss of the protein, the presence of glycerol and fatty acids, and free cholesterol. The latter three would free triglycerides from cholesterol esters and neutral fats.

Another important concept is that proposed by Blakemore, who said that disintegration of the myelin sheath may not be complete under all circumstances and that partial demyelination may be produced by sublethal damage to the parent oligodendrocyte (69).

Multiple Sclerosis

The advent of MRI, which permits the visualization of multiple sclerosis (MS) plaques in vivo, has allowed us to visualize many more types of lesions that can occur in multiple sclerosis. Perhaps the most frequent general location is the periventricular area near the lateral angles of the lateral ventricles. The lesions near the floor of the fourth ventricle and aqueduct, described pathologically in autopsy material, are not as commonly discovered on MRI examinations. The cases seen at autopsy are likely to be much more advanced and chronic than those that are commonly subject to diagnostic imaging examinations. The same is true of the frequency with which optic nerve changes may be found at autopsy, for these are difficult to detect by MRI.

Involvement of the corpus callosum is common and is an important feature in the differential diagnosis, for the presence of lesions in the corpus callosum is almost surely related to MS (70).

IMAGING DIAGNOSIS

CT scanning often shows multiple areas of decreased attenuation in the periventricular white matter and sometimes in the cerebellum and in the middle cerebellar peduncles as well as in the brainstem. However, sometimes no lesions are seen or very few lesions can be visualized even after the intravenous injection of iodine contrast material. Thus the absence of lesions as seen by CT scanning cannot be relied upon to exclude the diagnosis of MS: Such was the case in an instance of acute and subacute MS occurring primarily

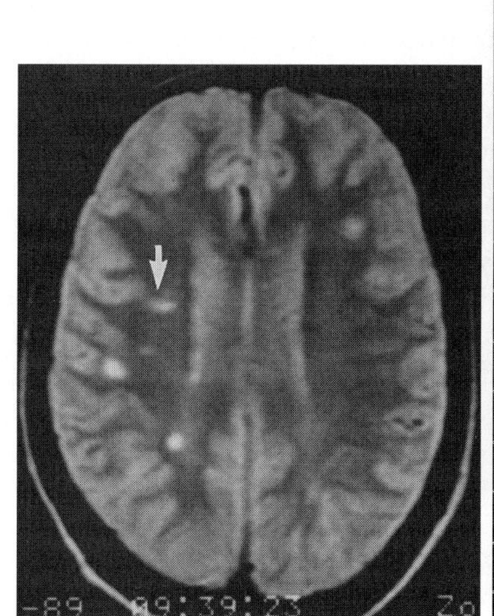

A

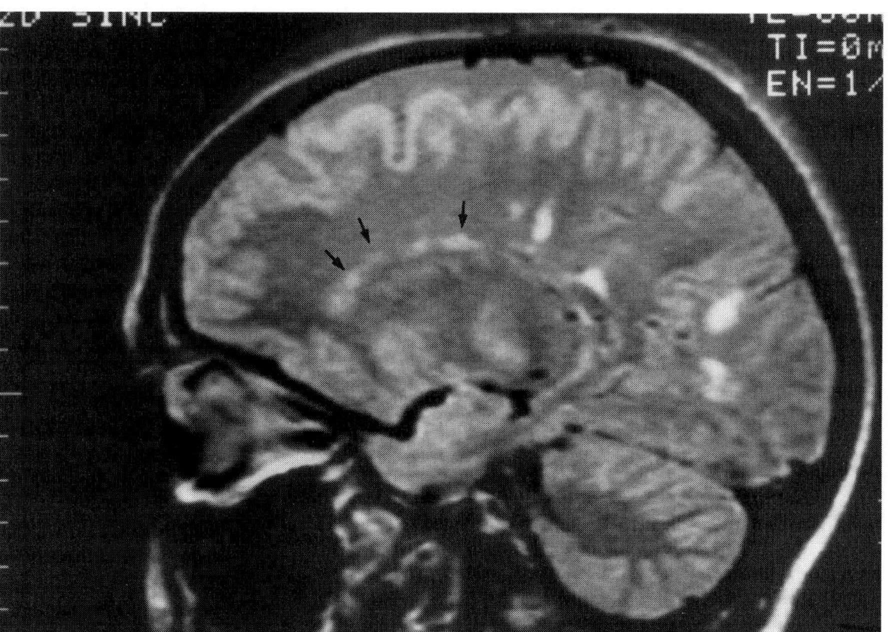

B

C

Figure 4.56. Multiple sclerosis. **A.** Proton density axial image shows scattered bright lesions. Some are elongated and oval, perpendicular to the ventricular wall (white arrow). Some are round. **B.** The sagittal proton density image reveals the elongated lesions (Dawson fingers); they are directed toward the ventricular wall because they tend to follow the deep vascular pattern. There is irregularity of the corpus callosum, which has a number of MS plaques. **C.** MS lesions in cerebellum and pons.

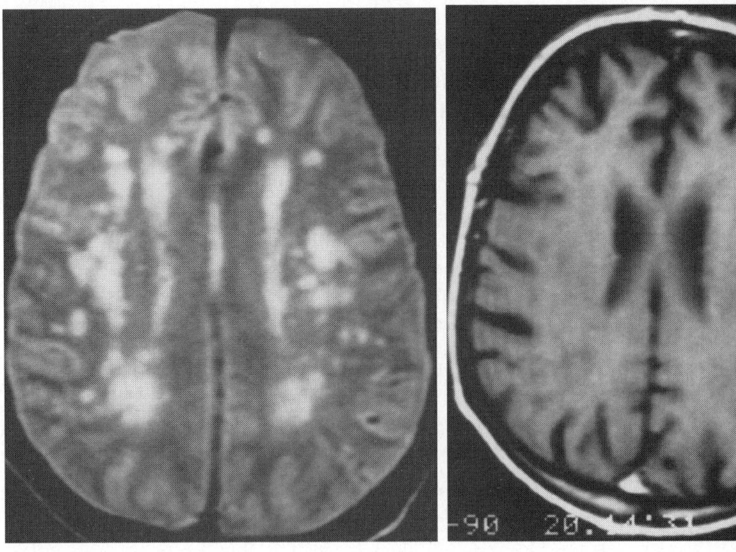

Figure 4.57. Extensive white matter hyperintense foci (leukoariosis) simulating multiple sclerosis (77). **A.** Proton density axial image. **B.** T1-weighted image. Some irregularities are barely seen. This is typical of idiopathic white matter hyperintense foci. Because of the patient's age (70 years) and the absence of an MS history, the diagnosis is easy. However, from imaging alone it would be difficult to make a conclusive diagnosis. These idiopathic "lesions" do not usually involve the corpus callosum, which is a good differential point in doubtful cases. Periventricular bright foci on T2-weighted images are seen, and sometimes uniform periventricular hyperintensity is present, but the lesions are not in the corpus callosum. CT may be entirely negative in these cases.

in the brainstem, cerebellum, and spinal cord reported in the Massachusetts General Hospital case records (71).

On the other hand, MRI is capable of showing lesions of multiple sclerosis at any stage, the acute stage or the intermediate or chronic stage, with a high degree of accuracy. The absence of any lesions in the brain, brainstem, or spinal cord as seen by MRI is evidence against the diagnosis of multiple sclerosis. When lesions are visualized by MRI, the specificity of the diagnosis is rather high, estimated to be 95 to 99 percent by Yetkin et al. (72).

MS lesions tend to have an oval configuration in most instances; the long axis may follow a line perpendicular to the wall of the lateral ventricles as seen in axial projections, or may follow the direction of the blood vessels in coronal views (Fig. 4.56). The long axis of the lesions may well follow the direction of the medullary veins of the white matter of the brain, which do have a radial configuration or position in relation to the ventricular wall, and the presumption is that these lesions tend to develop around small blood vessels. Horowitz et al. (73) were the first to point out the frequency of this configuration as seen on MRI, but it is well known pathologically that MS lesions do tend to occur around blood vessels (Dawson fingers). However, spherical lesions of various sizes are seen, and lesions around the frontal and occipital poles of the ventricles are likely to be of any shape (Fig. 4.56*B*). Some lesions of MS are very large, measuring 3 cm or more in diameter, in which case they are usually fewer in number (Fig. 4.58). Most MS lesions tend to be fairly well circumscribed, but some, particularly when they are large, tend to be more diffuse in their margins. The lesions are usually bright on T2-weighted images and may not be visible on T1-weighted images. However, many are visible, and this would tend to differentiate them from those that are seen as idiopathic bright foci only on long TR images in the older age group and sometimes in younger individuals (Fig. 4.57). In general, standard imaging with axial first- and second-echo T2-weighted images is sufficient to visualize the lesions without any special sequences. When the lesions are few, T1-weighted images are useful, because if lesions are seen this will provide a differential diagnosis between an MS plaque (or a small infarct) and an incidental bright T2 focus, not usually seen on T1-weighted images.

It is important always to look for involvement of the corpus callosum, for, as previously stated, the presence of corpus callosum lesions is almost specific for MS. Sometimes only irregularity or scalloping of the ventricular margin is seen, particularly in the sagittal views (Fig. 4.59). The scalloping is therefore on the upper margin of the ventricle, formed by the corpus callosum. The lesions may also be visible in the rostrum or splenium of the corpus callosum in axial views (Fig. 4.59) (70, 74, 75). The lack of involvement of the corpus callosum is typical of the T2 hyperintense white matter foci known as leukoariosis (76, 77).

A common radiologic feature in MS is the lack of mass effect or edema in the surrounding white matter, even in large lesions. Many lesions of MS enhance with gadolinium, indicating a local break in the blood-brain barrier. Nesbit et al. described three predominant enhancing patterns on radiologic imaging: a relatively small homogeneous lesion with no or minimal diffuse enhancement after intravenous contrast; a lesion that enhances and is surrounded by an isointense ring; and lesions somewhat less well circumscribed and with scattered enhancement with intravenous contrast agent (75). In their cases, the lesions were somewhat atypical or acute and required a biopsy for diagnosis. Thus the lesions that they reported do not represent the usual cases and probably apply more to acute or subacute lesions, usually solitary, where differentiation

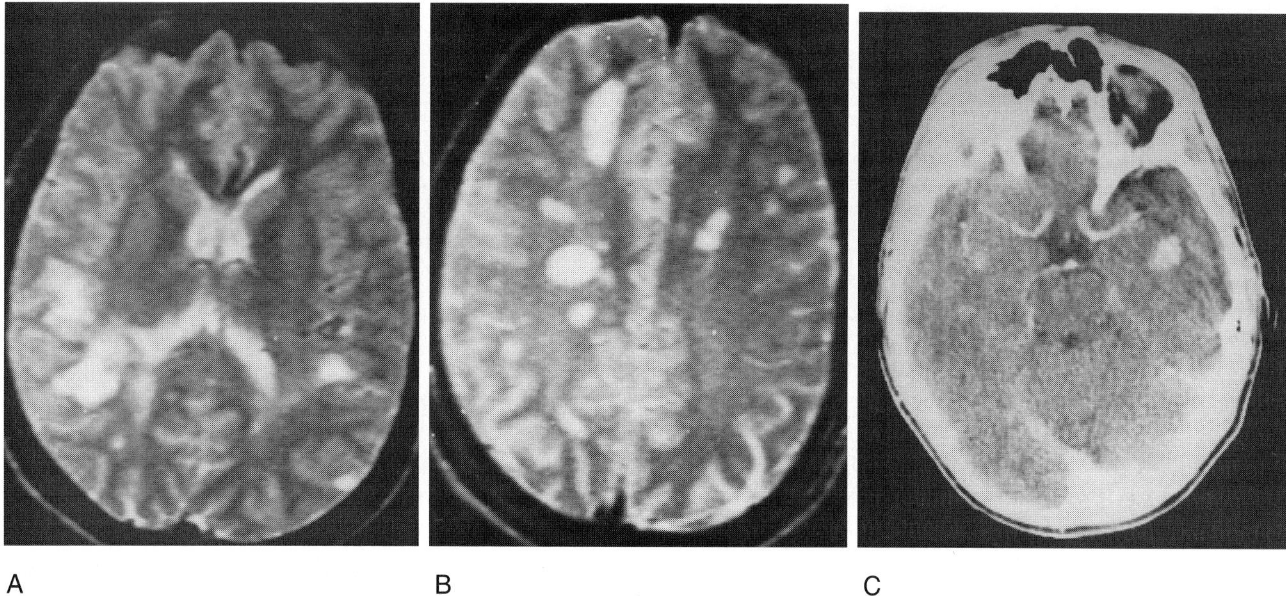

A B C

Figure 4.58. Multiple sclerosis, large lesions. **A.** On proton density images there are large lesions in the right frontal and parietal white matter. **B.** Other larger-than-usual lesions are seen higher up in the centrum semiovale. **C.** CT with contrast enhancement shows enhancing lesions in both temporal lobes. This may indicate that these lesions are active or more recent, but contrast uptake may not have the same meaning in all cases. The only statement that can be made is that there is a loss of the blood-brain barrier in the lesion, and this is usually temporary.

between focal and inflammatory causes and MS cannot be made by imaging alone.

The question of enhancement of an acute or subacute lesion as opposed to a chronic lesion is important to discuss here because it is not always possible to conclude that a breakdown of the blood-brain barrier is in fact due to an acute active lesion (Fig. 4.60). The enhancement could be rather ephemeral or may never occur, and thus it cannot be concluded that a lesion that does not enhance is not acute or subacute. Diffusion imaging techniques might help in differentiating subacute from older lesions, but at this writing this has not been proven.

The enhancement of a lesion could involve the entire lesion or only part of it. It could also have a ring shape (Fig. 4.60*E* and *F*).

Gean-Marton et al. emphasized the fact that in detecting corpus callosum involvement the sagittal proton density image (long repetition time, short echo time) is particularly

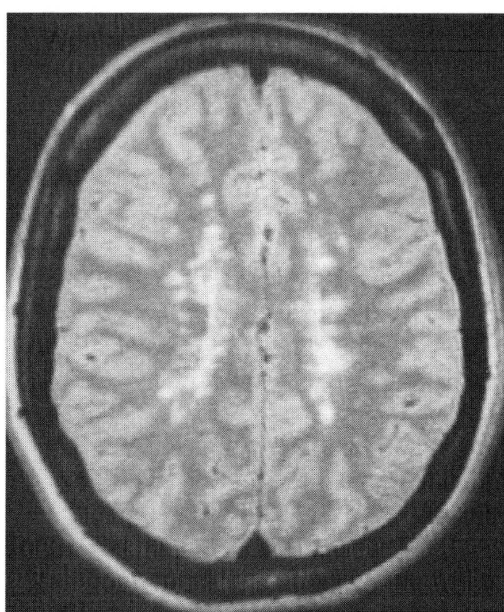

A

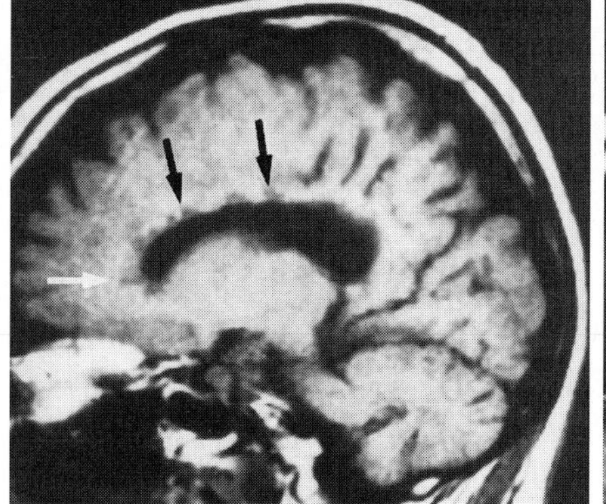

B

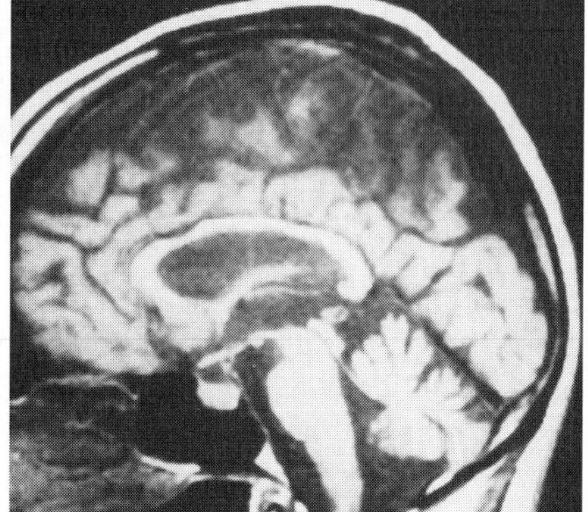

C

Figure 4.59. Multiple sclerosis with extensive involvement of the corpus callosum. **A.** Axial proton density image shows extensive coverage of the corpus callosum by lesions on both sides. **B.** Sagittal, off-midline, T1-weighted image shows irregular scalloping of ventricular surface, which is considered typical of MS (arrows). **C.** A midline T1-weighted image shows the absence of irregularity of the corpus callosum that is clearly shown on A. The irregularity of the ventricular surface is also present in the rostrum of the corpus callosum in B (white arrow).

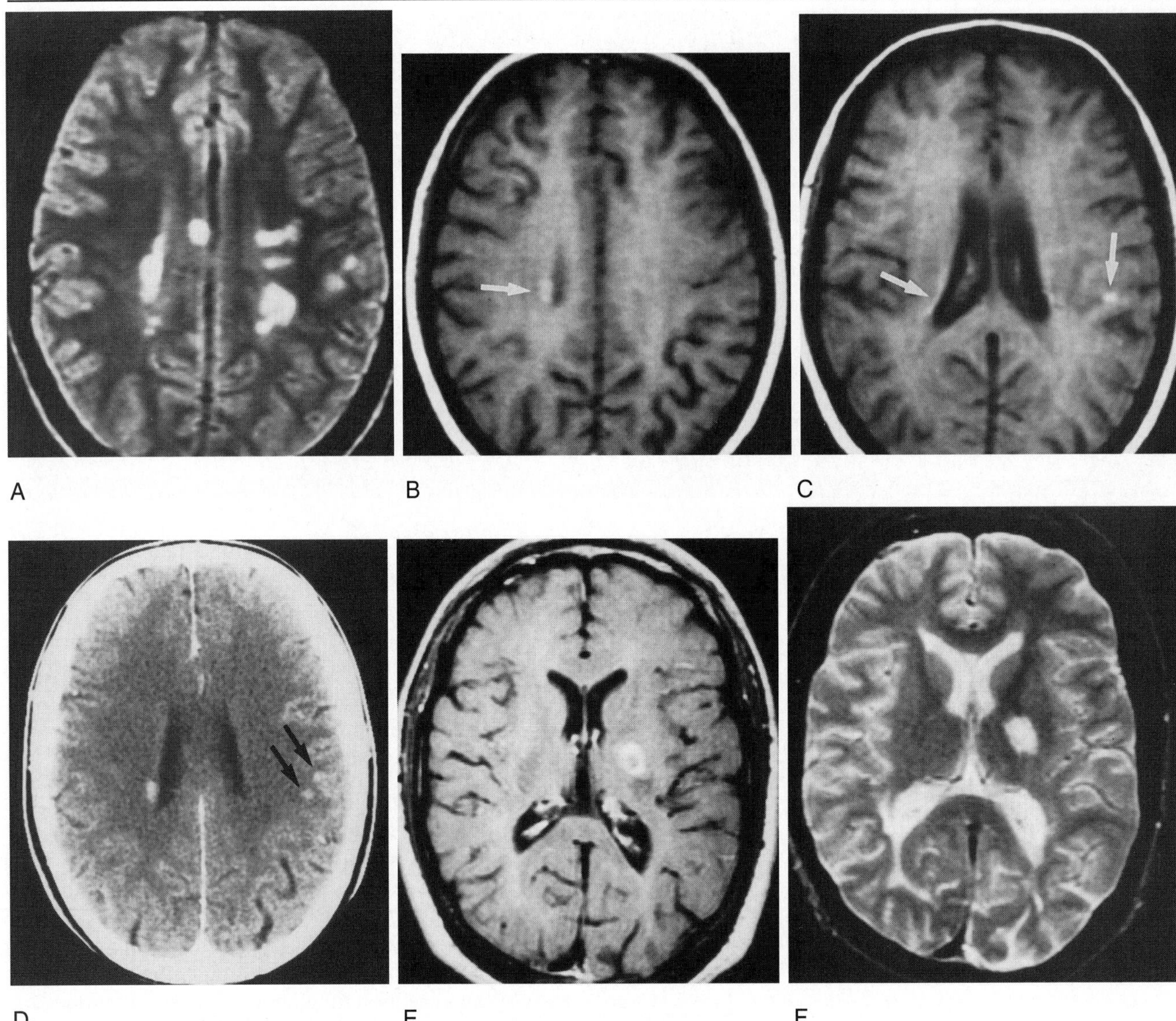

Figure 4.60. Multiple sclerosis lesions enhanced with contrast on MRI and CT. **A.** Proton density image. **B** and **C.** T1-weighted image after contrast shows enhancement of some lesions and only parts of others (arrows). **D.** CT with contrast shows enhancement of the same lesions that enhanced on MRI (arrows). **E.** Another case. Ring enhancement can occur. In this case, and because of the location in the basal ganglia-thalamic region, MS must be differentiated from toxoplasmosis, which can yield a similar appearance and be in the same location. **F.** T2-weighted image.

useful in detecting involvement of the corpus callosum in MS (70). In a group of 42 patients with MS and 127 control patients with other periventricular white matter disease who showed corpus callosum involvement optimally demonstrated on sagittal views, the involvement was not seen on axial views in 45 percent of the cases. Only in 2.4 percent of the control patients were lesions of the corpus callosum seen. The authors emphasized that the lesions were seen particularly well on sagittal views at the callosal-septal interface. The axial proton density images usually showed an asymmetry of the normally triangular callosal-septal interface. This interface, originally described by Gean-Marton et al. (78), consists of the interface between the septum pellucidum and the corpus callosum. It is triangular in shape on coronal cuts or on axial cuts at the rostrum of the corpus callosum. On midline sagittal views, the interface is bright on first- and second-echo T2 images and is uniform and smooth; this is most clearly seen in older individuals. In MS patients, it is irregular as a result of the involvement as previously described (Fig. 4.61*F*, *G*). Corpus callosum atrophy was present in chronic MS cases (Fig. 4.61).

Some acute MS lesions can be quite large and can produce a mass effect. In these cases it is necessary to carry out

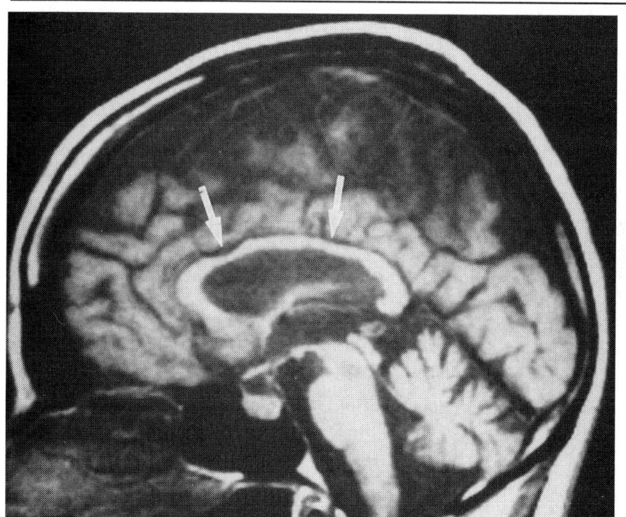

A

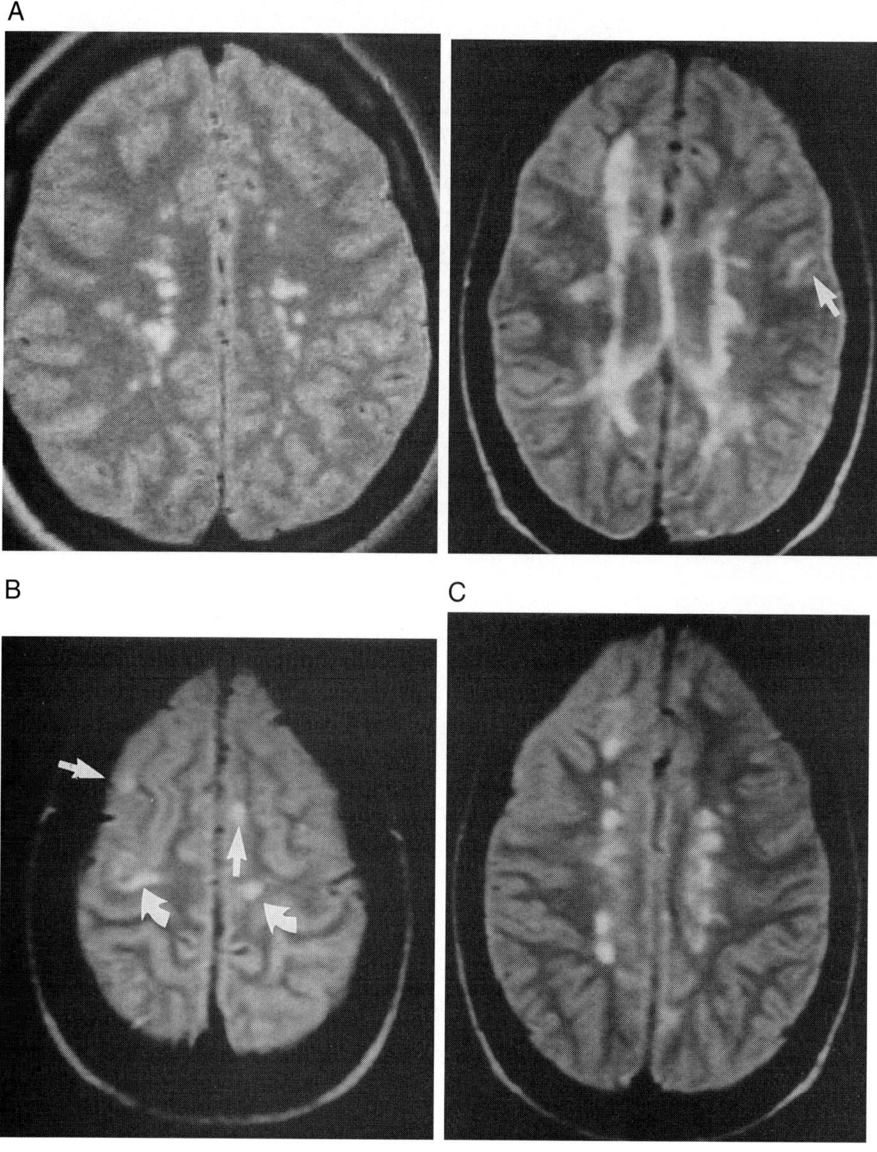

B C D E

Figure 4.61. **A** and **B.** Corpus callosum atrophy in patient with chronic multiple sclerosis. **A.** The corpus callosum shows irregularity and thinning due to chronic disease (arrows). **B.** There is extensive disease involving the corpus callosum and adjacent white matter. **C** and **D.** MS lesions in gray matter (arrows) and in subcortical U fibers (curved white arrows). **E.** Typical lateral corpus callosum lesions in same patient as C and D.

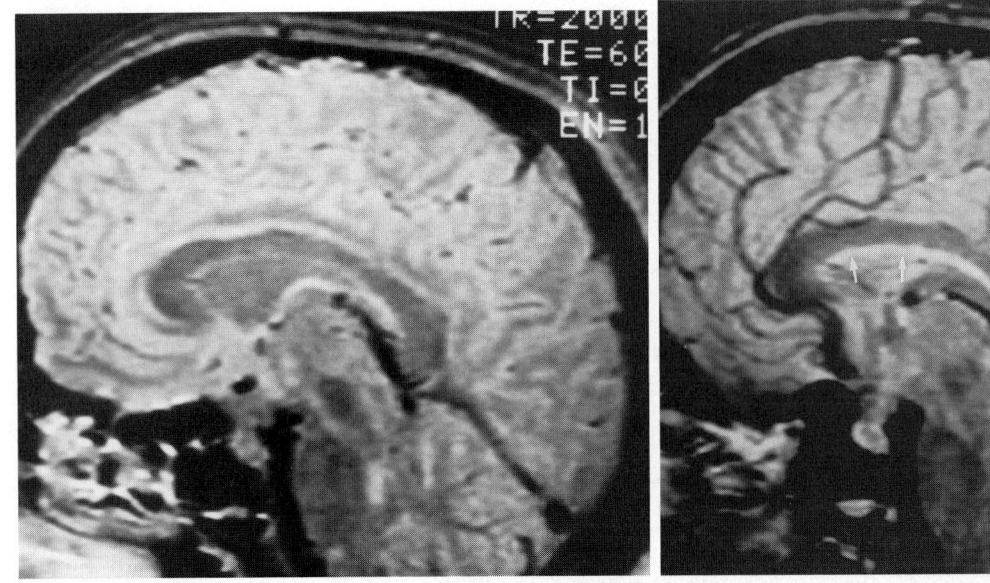

F

G

Figure 4.61. *(continued)* **F** and **G.** Proton density weighted image. Normal callosal-septal interphase in sagittal view. The contour is smooth (arrow). **H.** Callosal-septal interphase in patient with MS and corpus callosum involvement (small vertical arrows).

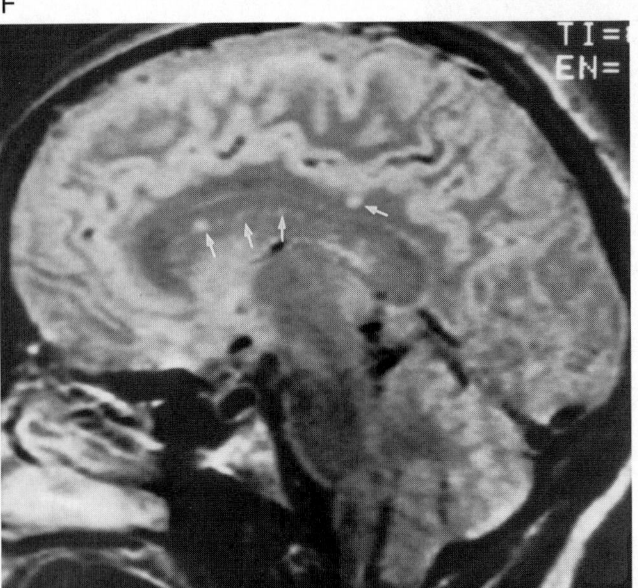

H

a complete examination, including contrast enhancement, with both MRI and CT. A biopsy may be required because it is not possible to differentiate these lesions from a tumor (Fig. 4.62) (79).

The temporal evolution of MS lesions is of interest. Few serial studies have been carried out now that MRI is available. The clinical relapses are not necessarily related to the appearance of new lesions by MRI. It may be that some old lesions reactivate or that new MRI-visible lesions will become apparent somewhat later, possibly 4 to 6 weeks later (80). Willoughby et al. reported that new lesions reached a maximum size in about 4 weeks and then decreased to leave a smaller lesion presenting an appearance indistinguishable from a chronic lesion (81). It is difficult at present to know whether the total lesion burden increases or decreases with exacerbations and remissions. The number of lesions may vary in a given patient if 10-mm as against 5-mm sections are obtained (82, 83).

Cases of acute disseminated encephalomyelitis (ADEM) may have similar MRI characteristics as acute MS. However, the lesions are usually larger, and ADEM is a monophasic disease that usually clears without significant sequelae and does not recur in most cases (84, 85, 86).

Barkhof et al. reported a patient with typical MS in whom meningeal enhancement after gadolinium was demonstrated and in whom the enhancement disappeared sometime after steroid therapy (87). Although leptomeningeal infiltration is sometimes found pathologically in MS

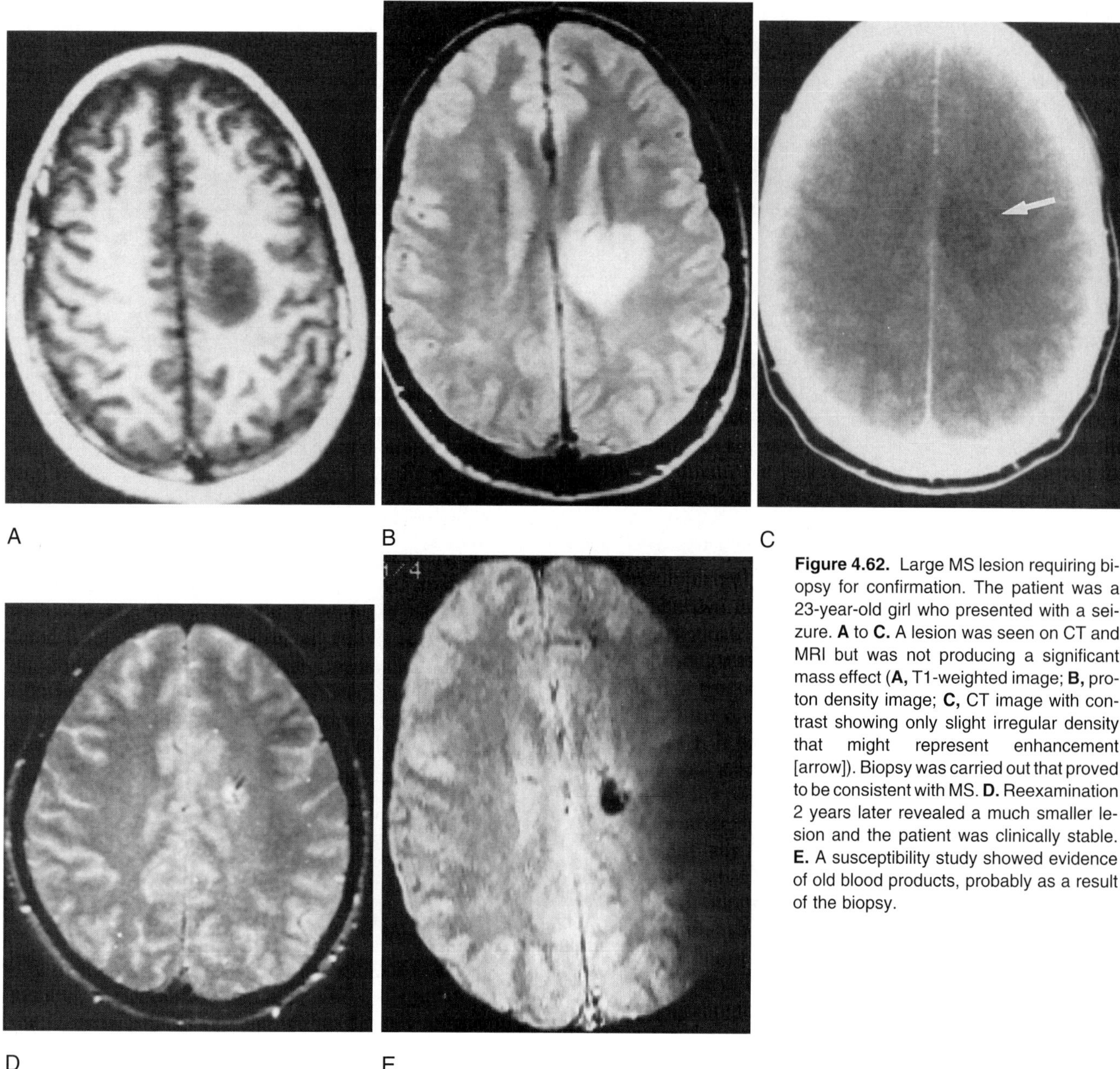

Figure 4.62. Large MS lesion requiring biopsy for confirmation. The patient was a 23-year-old girl who presented with a seizure. **A** to **C.** A lesion was seen on CT and MRI but was not producing a significant mass effect (**A,** T1-weighted image; **B,** proton density image; **C,** CT image with contrast showing only slight irregular density that might represent enhancement [arrow]). Biopsy was carried out that proved to be consistent with MS. **D.** Reexamination 2 years later revealed a much smaller lesion and the patient was clinically stable. **E.** A susceptibility study showed evidence of old blood products, probably as a result of the biopsy.

(88), the report of meningeal enhancement on MRI needs further confirmation (89).

Contrast enhancement is useful in demonstrating lesions in the optic nerves and chiasm. If the examination is carried out during an acute or subacute episode of optic neuritis, gadolinium enhancement may well demonstrate the lesion. In the cases reported by Merandi et al., enhancing lesions were demonstrated in the optic nerve in 7 of 14 cases; in 2 of 14 cases the lesion was in the optic chiasm, and in 6 of the 14 cases enhancing lesions were demonstrated in the brain (90). In 1 of the cases there was an enhancing lesion in the optic nerve but no brain lesions were demonstrated. The absence of brain lesions in that instance is not surprising, for it is well known that optic neuritis may be the first manifestation of MS. A few of the patients had enlargement of the optic nerve or chiasm on the involved side, and the enlarged portion in these cases enhanced. A fat-suppression technique is advisable, particularly to visualize the intraorbital optic nerves (Fig. 4.63).

Although lesions are most frequently seen in the cerebral hemispheres, chiefly in the periventricular white matter but also in the centrum semiovale, they may also be found occasionally in the gray matter and in the gray matter nuclei (Figs. 4.60*E*, *F* and 4.61). Lesions in subcortical U fibers are much more common. Lesions in the brainstem are common, and they may be scattered from the midbrain down to the medulla and upper cervical spinal cord. Cerebellar lesions are also quite common, and in this area pa-

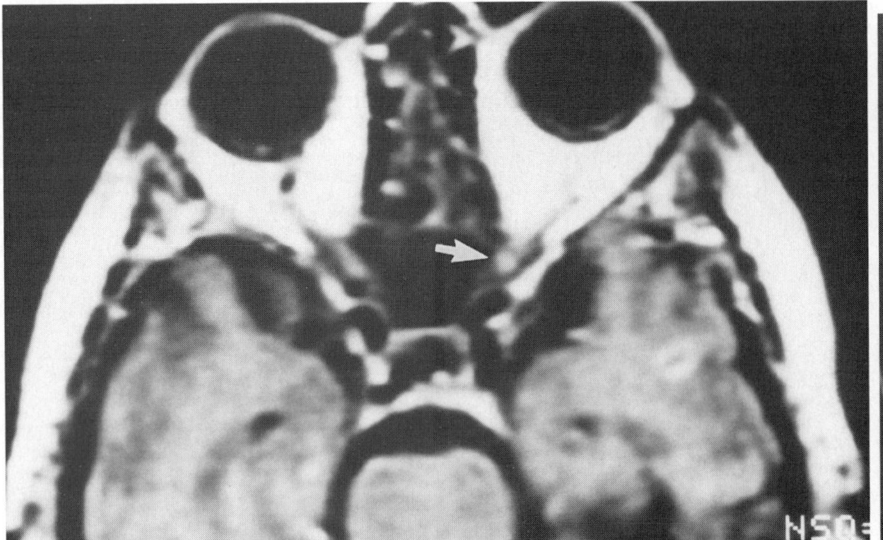

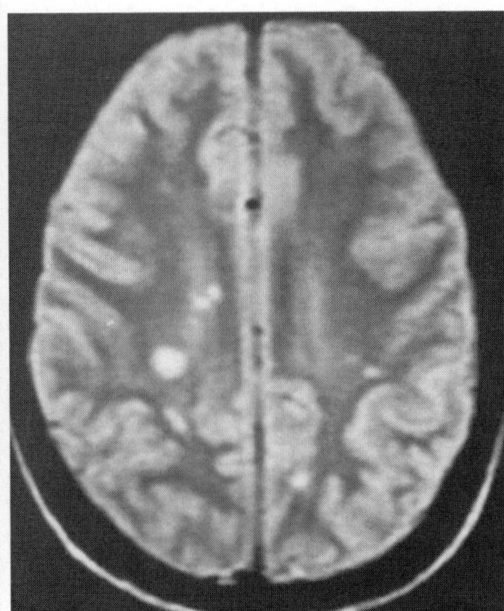

A B

Figure 4.63. Optic neuritis in patient with multiple sclerosis. **A.** A non-fat-suppressed, contrast-enhanced axial image shows an area of increased intensity in the left optic nerve (arrow). This was the first symptom for this 37-year-old woman. However, the brain demonstrated a number of typical lesions consistent with MS (shown in **B**). Fat-suppression techniques should be used to improve visualization of optic nerve MS lesions. However, the majority are not seen either with or without contrast, probably because the lesions are too small and the nerve is surrounded by various structures that interfere with clear visualization.

thologists emphasize the periventricular distribution around the fourth ventricle and lower aqueduct (Fig. 4.56).

In the spinal cord, lesions are often not demonstrated on MRI even though the history and clinical findings are strongly indicative of a spinal cord lesion. Of course, in some of these cases, the diagnosis may well be other than MS, and the examination is ordered by the neurologist to rule out MS. In other cases, however, the examination of the spinal cord is negative without and with gadolinium enhancement, and yet the examination of the brain will show lesions that would have to be described as silent lesions in patients in whom all the clinical manifestations are localized to the spinal cord. In a group of 10 patients reported by Edwards et al. with isolated spinal cord manifestations diagnosed clinically as possible MS, typical lesions of MS were found on cranial MRI in 6 patients (91). Thus it is essential to recommend MRI examination of the head in any patient with spinal cord symptoms that might suggest the possibility of MS (Fig. 4.64; Table 4.6).

Advanced cases of MS usually present varying degrees of cerebral atrophy, as is the case with most chronic brain diseases.

MS occurs in children as well as adults, usually in the second decade, and the MRI manifestations are similar to those found in adults, but some of the cases shown in teenagers are likely to demonstrate larger lesions with edema (92). In the cases reported by Ebner et al. (93), the average age of onset was 12 years and the female-male ratio was 5:1. Interestingly, the first MRI examination showed an average of 16 lesions per patient (range, 3 to 50); a follow-up MRI about 2 months later showed an average of 21 lesions per patient; and a third examination approximately 5 months later showed an average of 27 lesions per patient. Many of the lesions were silent in that the patients had not

Table 4.6.
Multiple Sclerosis

I. Lesion number
  A. Often large number (>6).
  B. Lesions often not associated with clinical symptoms or signs.
  C. Lesion number often increases during course of disease even in the absence of clinical progression.
II. Lesion size
  A. Usually less than 1.5 cm.
  B. Occasionally larger than 3 cm, and may mimic a mass lesion.
III. Favored lesion distribution
  A. Periventricular.
  B. Corpus callosum.
  C. Pons.
  D. Brachium pontis.
  E. Internal capsule.
  F. Spinal cord.
  G. Optic nerve/chiasm.
IV. Appearances suggestive of MS diagnosis
  A. Location in corpus callosum or brachium pontis.
  B. Oval-shaped lesion with long axis perpendicular to lateral ventricle (Dawson fingers).
  C. Location in both brain and spinal cord.
V. Atypical lesion appearance
  A. Location in gray matter.
  B. Ill-defined lesion margin.
  C. Mass effect/edema.

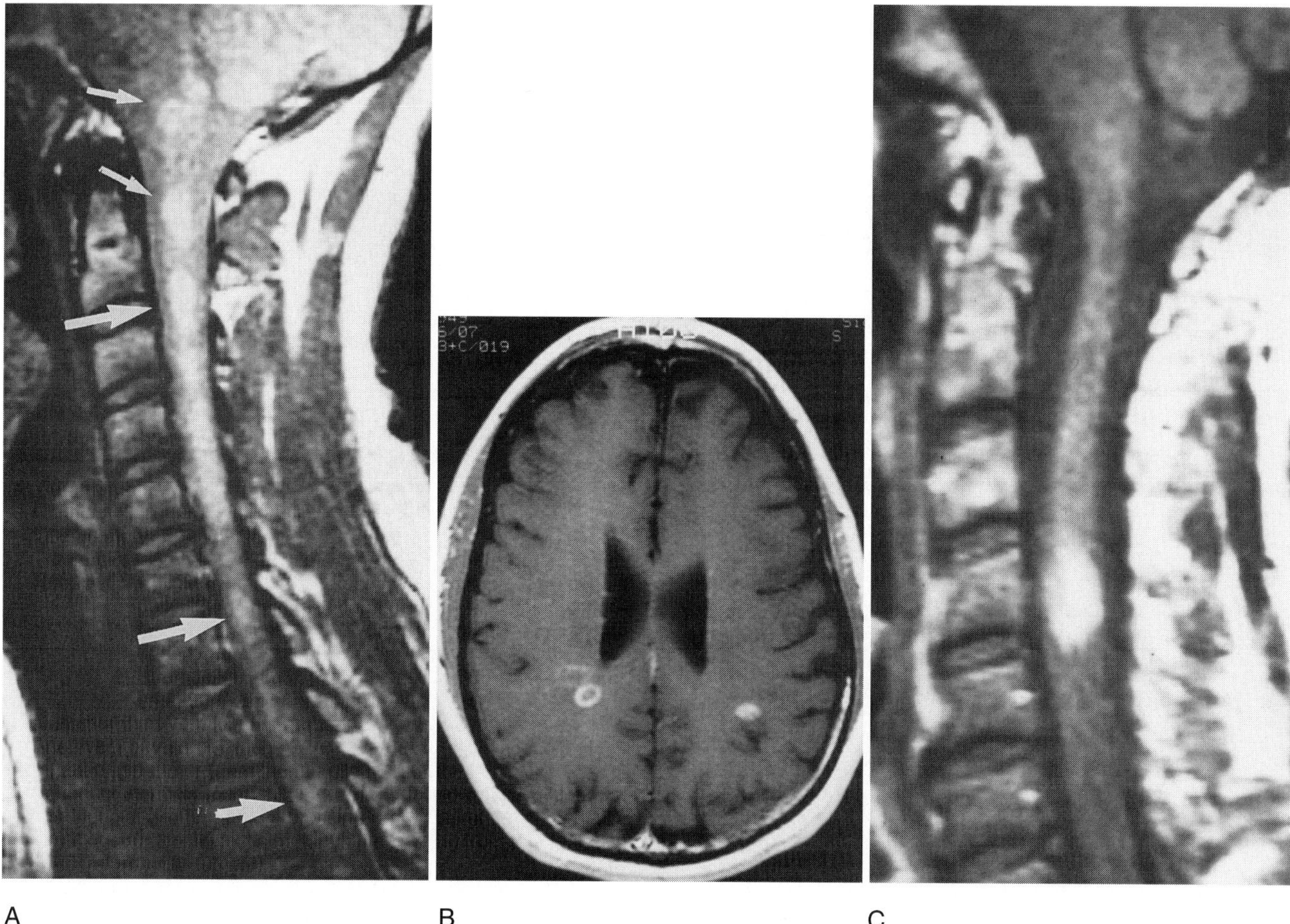

A B C

Figure 4.64. Multiple sclerosis spinal cord lesions; two cases. **A.** Several lesions extending from the medulla to the second thoracic vertebra are well shown in this proton density image (arrows). **B.** The same patient also had enhancing lesions in the brain, one of which shows ring enhancement. **C.** A single lesion in the cervical cord that enhances.

complained of any recurrence of symptoms or new symptoms in the interval. The lesions may simulate those seen in acute disseminated encephalomyelitis (85).

SPECIFIC TYPES

Concentric sclerosis (Baló Type)

This probably cannot be diagnosed by MRI without a biopsy. However, a recent case I saw showed large lesions with central areas that were different from the periphery and on biopsy were found to be consistent with MS.

Neuromyelitis Optica

This is a clinical classification and does not necessarily demonstrate any imaging characteristics. The eye and spinal cord involvement may be seen in other conditions, such as lupus erythematosus (94). It implies the development of eye symptoms up to blindness accompanied by paraplegia. At autopsy, optic nerve and spinal cord demyelination is found, but it is not clear whether the syndrome is a variant of MS or whether it may occur in more than one entity.

Schilder Disease

Schilder disease is a condition in which widespread demyelination occurs with axonal damage in both cerebral hemispheres and often in the brainstem and cerebellum as well. The lesions are not symmetrical but do involve both hemispheres in a variable way and usually do not involve the subcortical U fibers. The findings are much more severe than those that are found in juvenile MS, although transitional cases with multiple small plaques have been described. It is questionable whether a true entity called Schilder disease does in fact exist or whether it is a very severe form of MS (95). As Osborn et al. have reported, adolescent patients affected by MS tend to have more severe disease characteristics as well as more frequent infratentorial involvement (92). The MR findings are likely to be more diffuse in this group.

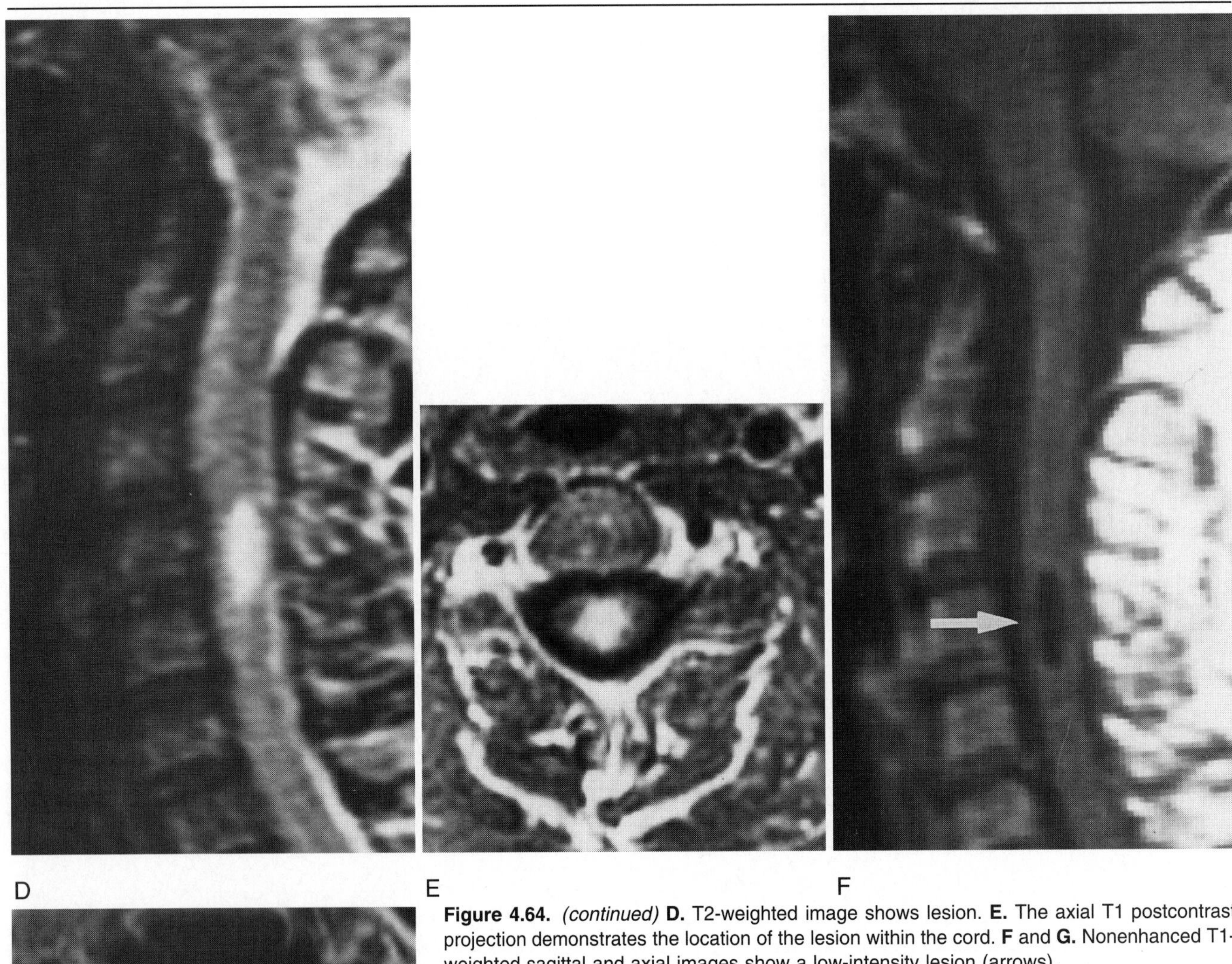

Figure 4.64. *(continued)* **D.** T2-weighted image shows lesion. **E.** The axial T1 postcontrast projection demonstrates the location of the lesion within the cord. **F** and **G.** Nonenhanced T1-weighted sagittal and axial images show a low-intensity lesion (arrows).

Central Pontine Myelinolysis (CPM)

Central pontine myelinolysis, first described in 1959 by Adams et al. (96), is characterized by regions of demyelination involving particularly the pons but sometimes also other areas of the brain. The lesions usually occur in alcoholics or in association with acute or prolonged alcoholic exposure. However, not all patients are alcoholics, and the condition has been found in children and in other patients with electrolyte abnormalities, mostly hyponatremia. The symptoms may appear quite acutely and include quadriparesis, pseudobulbar palsy, and acute changes in mental status that may lead to loss of consciousness, coma, or death. It is important to remember that rapid correction of the hyponatremia seems to be associated with the occurrence of

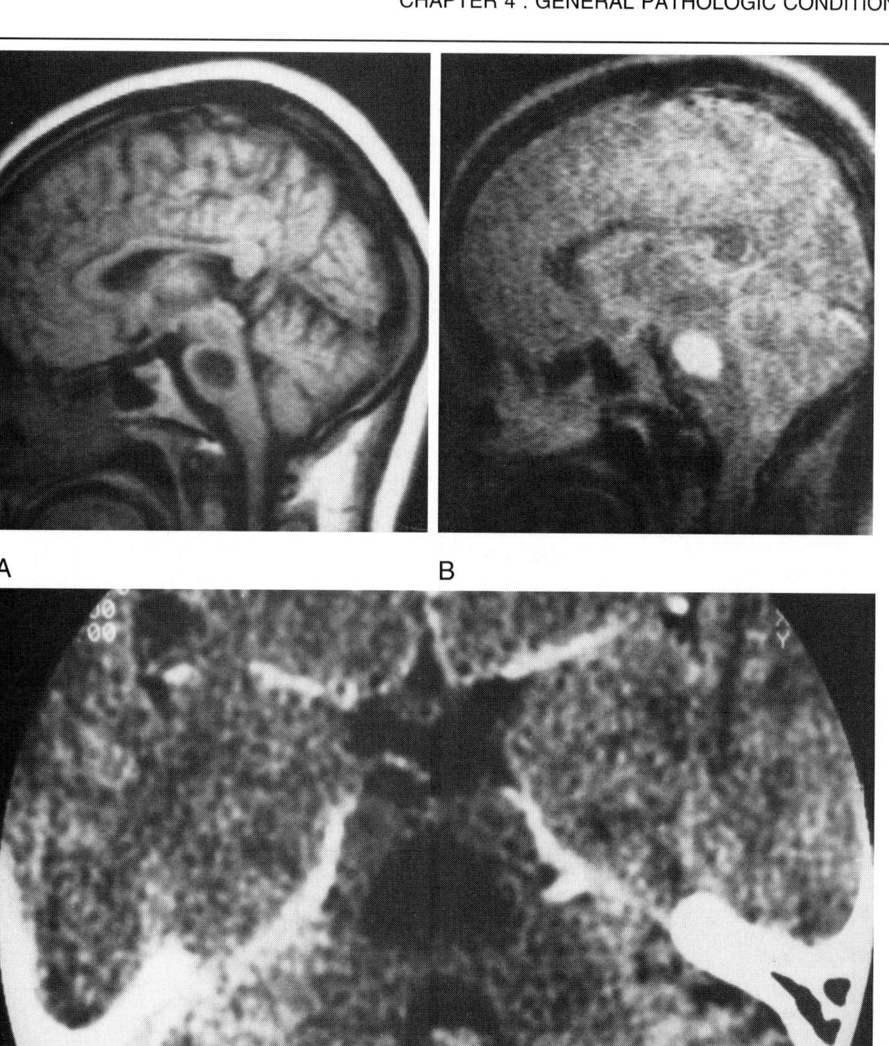

Figure 4.65. Central pontine myelinolysis in a young woman following an extended acute alcoholic exposure. **A.** T1-weighted sagittal image shows typical oval, low-intensity area in the pons. **B.** T2-weighted image reveals hyperintensity in the same area. **C.** Postcontrast CT reveals a large area of decreased attenuation in the center of the pons. Extrapontine manifestations are also seen in this entity.

central pontine myelinolysis, and that the hyponatremia should always be corrected slowly. Originally it was thought that this condition was fatal; however, following the recognition of the hyponatremia and the fact that this can be corrected, many of the patients recover, sometimes completely and sometimes with continuing neurologic deficits.

The diagnosis can be made by cross-sectional imaging, either CT or MRI, because of the typical broad area of low attenuation on CT and an area of low intensity on T1-weighted images and of high intensity on T2-weighted images occupying the pons (Fig. 4.65). However, the CT image may be negative, and for this reason MRI is preferred. Miller et al. point out that pontine lesions that look somewhat like those found in central pontine myelinolysis may be seen due to infarct, metastases, glioma, MS, encephalitis, and radiation or chemotherapy (26). However, when one puts the CT or MRI findings together with the clinical picture in the setting of hyponatremia, the diagnosis becomes certain. Koci et al. emphasize the presence of extrapontine lesions in central pontine myelinolysis; they presented three cases in which symmetric thalamic lesions were demonstrated by MRI (97). However, extrapontine lesions have also been frequently found in the cerebellum, lateral geniculate body, cerebral cortex, putamen, and subcortical areas. One case of Koci et al. also showed lesions in the caudate nucleus. A trident-shaped pontine lesion is supposed to be characteristic of central pontine myelinolysis, but it is probably more accurate to state that the shape of the lesion is variable but usually is fairly broad. Brunberg et al. reported on the occurrence of central pontine myelinolysis in patients with liver failure (98).

Korogi et al. reported two cases in which a mild pontine myelinolysis picture by MRI was found, limited to the pons and seen only on T2-weighted images (99). Both patients were diabetics, one with chronic renal failure on dialysis, and the other an alcoholic. Both patients presented dysarthria that cleared completely, accompanied by other mild neurological symptoms. Both had mild hyponatremia.

Marchiafava-Bignami Disease

This is also a syndrome associated with alcohol, first described in heavy drinkers of Italian red wine but later described outside of Italy (France, Americas). The typical lesion is corpus callosum atrophy. Histologically, demyelination occurs in regions of the corpus callosum, the anterior commissure, and sometimes the middle cerebellar peduncles. I have not seen a case of this condition, but the findings on MRI can be expected to be those described pathologically, particularly on T2-weighted images (atrophy of the corpus callosum, hyperintense areas in the brachium pontis).

References

1. Henkelman R, Watts J, Kuchrazyk W: High signal intensity on MR images of calcified brain tissue. Radiology 1991;179:199.
2. Dell LA, Brown MS, Orrison WW, et al: Physiologic intracranial calcification with hyperintensity on MR imaging: Case report and experimental model. AJNA 1988;9:1145–1148.
3. Atlas SW, Grossman RI, Hackney DB, et al: Calcified intracranial lesions: Detection with gradient-echo-acquisition rapid imaging. AJNR 1988;9:253–259.
4. Zimmerman RD, Fleming CA, Saint-Louis LA, et al: Magnetic resonance imaging of meningiomas. AJNR 1985;6:149–157.
5. Oot RF, New PF, Pile-Spellman J, et al: The detection of intracranial calcification by MR. AJNR 1986;7:801–809.
6. Uggetti C, Sibilla L, Zappoli F, Martelli A: La risonanza magnetica del'encefalo nella distrofia miotonica. Riv Neuroradiol 1991;4: 53–60.
7. Wood EH: Some roentgenological and pathological aspects of calcification of the choroid plexus. Am J Roentgenol 1944;52:388.
8. Oh SJ: Roentgen findings in cerebral paragonimiasis. Radiology 1968;90:292.
9. Potts GD, Svare GT: Calcification in intracranial metastases. Am J Roentgenol 1964;92:1249.
10. Albright F, Reifenstein ED Jr: The Parathyroid Glands and Metabolic Bone Disease. Baltimore: Williams and Wilkins, 1948.
11. Bhimani S, Sarwar M, Virapongse C, et al: Computed tomography of cerebrovascular calcification in post surgical hypoparathyroidism. J Comput Assist Tomogr 1985;9:121–124.
12. Demirci A, Sze G: Cranial osteopetrosis: MR findings. AJNR 1991; 12:781–782.
13. Holtz KH: Uber Gehirn-und Augeveranderungen bei Hyalinosis cutis et mucosae (lipoid proteinosis) mit Autopsiebefund. Arch Klin Exp Dermatol 1962;214:289.
14. Williams JP, Fowler GW: Gyriform calcifications following encephalitis: Case report. Neuroradiology 1972;4:57.
15. Kuhn MJ, Clark HB, Morales A, Shekar PC: Group III Möbius syndrome: CT and MR findings. AJNR 1990;11:903–904.
16. Sarwar M, Ford K: Rapid development of basal ganglia calcification. AJNR 1981;2:103–104.
17. Reyes PF, Gonzalez CF, Zalewska MK, Berarato A: Intracranial calcification in adults with chronic lead poisoning. AJNR 1985;6: 905–908.
18. Brennan TS, Burger AA, Chaudhary MY: Basal ganglia calcifications visualized on CT scan. J Neurol Neurosurg Psychiatry 1980;43: 403–406.
19. Burt TB, Boise ID, Yang PJ, et al: Calcified brain metastases from ovarian cancer. AJNR 1988;9:613.
20. Sly WS, Whyte MP, Sundaram V, et al: Carbonic anhydrase II deficiency in 12 families with the autosomal recessive syndrome of osteopetrosis with renal tubular acidosis and cerebral calcification. N Engl J Med 1985;313:139–145.
21. Adachi M, Feigin I: Cerebral edema and the water content of normal white matter. J Neurol Neurosurg Psychiatry 1966;29:446–450.
22. Miller JD, Adams JH: The pathophysiology of raised intracranial pressure. In JH Adams, JAN Corsellis, LW Duehen (eds), Greenfield's Neuropathology, ed 4. New York: Wiley, 1984.
23. Fishman RA: Brain edema. N Engl J Med 1975;293:706–711.
24. Taveras JM: Low pressure hydrocephalus. Neuro-ophthalmology 1968;4:293.
25. Leech JM, Miller JD: Intracranial volume/pressure relationships during experimental brain conditions in primates: I. Pressure responses to changes in ventricular volume. J Neurol Neurosurg Psychiatry 1974;37:1093–1098.
26. Miller GM, Baker HL, Okazaki H, Whismant SP: Central pontine myelinolysis and its imitators: MR findings. Radiology 1988;168: 795–802.
27. Azambuja N, Lindgren E, Sjögren SE: Tentorial herniations: I. Anatomy. Acta Radiol 1956;46:215.
28. Azambuja N, Lindgren E, Sjögren SE: Tentorial herniations: III. Angiography. Acta Radiol 1956;46:232.
29. Crowley AR: Influence of fiber tracts on the CT appearance of cerebral edema: Anatomic-pathologic correlation. AJNR 1983;4: 915–925.
30. Jinkins JR, Athale S, Xiong L, et al: MR characteristics of optic papilla protrusion in conditions associated with raised intracranial pressure. Paper presented at the annual meeting of the American Society of Neuroradiology, Vancouver, 1993.
31. Schwartz RB, Jones KM, Kalina P, et al: Hypertensive encephalopathy: Findings on CT, MR imaging, and SPECT imaging in 14 cases. AJR 1992;159:379–383.
32. Lundberg N: Continuous recording and control of ventricular fluid pressure in neurosurgical practice. Acta Psychiatr Neurol Scand 1960;36, Suppl 149.
33. Miller JD: Volume and pressure in the craniospinal axis. Clin Neurosurg 1975;22:76–105.
34. Langfitt TW, Weinstein JD, Kassell NF: Cerebral vasomotor paralysis produced by intracranial hypertension. Neurology 1965;15: 622–641.
35. Fishman RA: Cerebrospinal Fluid in Diseases of the Nervous System. Philadelphia: Saunders, 1980.
36. Naidich TP, McLone DG, Hahn YS, Hanaway J: Atrial diverticula in severe hydrocephalus. AJNR 1982;3:257–266.
37. Schechter MM, Zingesser LH: The radiology of aqueduct stenosis. Radiology 1967;88:905.
38. Barkovich AJ, Newton TH: MR of aqueduct stenosis: Evidence of broad spectrum of testal distortion. AJNR 1989;10:471–476.
39. Quencer RM, Post MJD, Hinks RS: Cine-MR in the evaluation of normal and abnormal CSF-MR in the evaluation of normal and abnormal CSF flow: Intracranial and intraspinal studies. Neuroradiology 1990;32:371–391.
40. Quencer RM: Intracranial CSF flow in pediatric hydrocephalus: Evaluation with cine-MR imaging. AJNR 1992;13:601–608.
41. Hakim S, Adams RD: Clinical problem of symptomatic hydrocephalus with normal cerebrospinal fluid pressure: Observations on cerebrospinal fluid hydrodynamics. J Neurol Sci 1965;2:307–327.

42. Adams RD, Fisher CM, Hakim S, et al: Symptomatic occult hydrocephalus with "normal" cerebrospinal fluid pressure: A treatable syndrome. N Engl J Med 1965;273:117–126.
43. Koto A, Rosenberg G, Zingesser LH, et al: Syndrome of normal pressure hydrocephalus: Possible relation to hypertensive and arteriosclerotic vasculopathy. J Neurol Neurosurg Psychiatry 1974;40: 73–79.
44. Bradley WG, Mullin WJ, Wong P, et al: Use of quantitative CSF velocity imaging in the evaluation of shunt-responsive NPH. Paper presented at the annual meeting of the American Society of Neuroradiology, Vancouver, 1993.
45. Jinkins JR: Clinical manifestations of hydrocephalus caused by impingement of the corpus callosum on the falx: An MR study in 40 patients. AJNR 1991;12:331–340.
46. Shier CK, George AE, DeLeon MJ, et al: CT and MR features of hydrocephalus: Paradoxical sylvian fissure enlargement and significance of the hippocampal lucency. AJNR 1989;10:904.
47. Roman GC: White matter lesions and normal-pressure hydrocephalus: Binswanger disease or Halsim syndrome? AJNR 1991;12:40–41.
48. El Gammal T, Allen MB Jr, Brooks BS, Mark EK: MR evaluation of hydrocephalus. AJNR 1987;8:591–597.
49. Jinkins JR, Ripeckyj GT, Rauch RA, Xiong L: A reappraisal of the imaging criteria of hydrocephalus versus deep cerebral atrophy: A retrospective MR study of 44 cases. Paper presented at the annual meeting of the American Society of Neuroradiology, Vancouver, 1993.
50. Greitz TVB, Grepe AOL, Kalmer MSF, Lopez J: Pre- and postoperative evaluation of cerebral blood flow in low-pressure hydrocephalus. J Neurosurg 1969;31:644–651.
51. Meyer JS, Yasuhisa K, Tanhashi N, et al: Pathogenesis of normal pressure hydrocephalus: Preliminary observations. Surg Neurol 1985;23:121–133.
52. Bradley WG, Whitemore AR, Kortman KE, et al: Marked cerebrospinal fluid void: Indicator of successful shunt in patients with suspected normal-pressure hydrocephalus. Radiology 1991;178: 459–466.
53. Bradley WG, Whitemore AR, Watanabe AS, et al: Association of deep white matter infarction with chronic communicating hydrocephalus: Implications regarding the possible origin of normal-pressure hydrocephalus. AJNR 1991;12:31–39.
54. Norbash AM, Pelc NJ, Shimakawa A, Enzman DR: Accuracy of shunt flow measurement and evaluation of valve oscillation with spin-echo phase contrast MR imaging. Paper presented at the annual meeting of the American Society of Neuroradiology, Vancouver, 1993.
55. Herskowitz J, Rosman NP, Wheeler CB: Colpocephaly: Clinical, radiologic, and pathologic aspects. Neurology 1985;35:1594–1598.
56. Scarff J: The treatment of nonobstructive (communicating) hydrocephalus by endoscopic cauterization of the choroid plexuses. J Neurosurg 1970;33:1.
57. Jack CR Jr, Kelly PJ: Stereotactic third ventriculostomy: Assessment of patients with MR imaging. AJNR 1989;10:515–522.
58. Destian S, Heier LA, Zimmerman RD, et al: Differentiation between meningeal fibrosis and chronic subdural hematoma after ventricular shunting: Value of enhanced CT and MR. AJNR 1989;10: 1021–1026.
59. Lemann W, Wiley RG, Posner JB: Leukoencephalopathy complicating intraventricular catheters: Clinical, radiographic and pathologic study of 10 cases. J Neurooncol 1988;6:67–74.
60. Wang AM, Haykae HA: Thoracic spinal meningioma associated with hydrocephalic dementia. AJNR 1990;11:383–384.
61. Gibbard FB, Ngan H, Swann GF: Hydrocephalus, subarachnoid hemorrhage and ependymomas of the cauda equina. Clin Radiol 1972;23:422–429.
62. Maytal J, Alvarez LA, Elkin CM, Shinnar S: External hydrocephalus: Radiologic spectrum and differentiation from cerebral atrophy. AJNR 1987;8:271–278.
63. Nickel RE, Gallenstein JS: Developmental prognosis for infants with benign enlargement of the subarachnoid spaces. Dev Med Child Neurol 1987;29:181–186.
64. Wilms G, Vanderschueren G, Demaerel PH, et al: CT and MR in infants with pericerebral collections and macrocephaly: Benign enlargement of the subarachnoid spaces versus subdural collections. AJNR 1993;14:855–860.
65. Baum PA, Dillon WP, Fishman RA: Imaging features and diagnostic evaluation of spontaneous intracranial hypotension. Paper presented at the annual meeting of the American Society of Neuroradiology, Vancouver, 1993.
66. Geren BB: The formation from the Schwann cell surface of myelin. Exp Cell Res 1954;7:558–562.
67. Allen IV: Demyelinating diseases. In JH Adams, JAN Corsellis, LW Duchen (eds), Greenfield's Neuropathology. New York: Wiley, 1984.
68. Barkovich AJ, Kjos BO: Normal maturation of the neonatal and infant brain: MR imaging at 1.5 T. Radiology 1988;166:173–180.
69. Blakemore NF: Myelination, demyelination and remyelination in the CNS. In WJ Smith, JB Cavanagh (eds), Recent Advances in Neuropathology. London: Churchill Livingston, 1982, p 53.
70. Gean-Marton AD, Vozina LG, Marton KI, et al: Abnormal corpus callosum: A sensitive and specific indicator of multiple sclerosis. Radiology 1991;180:215–222.
71. Case records of the Massachusetts General Hospital. N Engl J Med 1990;323:1123–1135.
72. Yetkin FZ, Haughton VM, Papke RA, et al: Multiple sclerosis: Specificity of MR for diagnosis. Radiology 1991;178:447–451.
73. Horowitz AL, Kaplan RD, Grewe G, et al: The ovoid lesion: A new MR observation in patients with multiple sclerosis. AJNR 1989;10: 303–305.
74. Runge VM, Price AC, Kirshner HS, et al: Magnetic resonance imaging of multiple sclerosis: A study of pulse technique efficiency. AJNR 1984;5:691–702.
75. Nesbit GM, Forbes GS, Scheithauer BW, et al: Multiple sclerosis: Histopathologic and MR and/or CT correlation in 37 cases at biopsy and three cases at autopsy. Radiology 1991;180:467–474.
76. Kobari M, Meyer JS, Ichijo M, Oravez WT: Leukoaraiosis: Correlation of MR and CT findings with blood flow, atrophy, and cognition. AJNR 1990;11:273–281.
77. Hashinski VC, Potter P, Meskey H: Leukoaraiosis. Arch Neurol 1987;44:21–23.
78. Gean-Marton AD, Vezina LG, Engel E, et al: The callosal-septal interface: MR imaging, neuroanatomy, and neuropathological manifestations. AJNR 1990;10:893.
79. Longo M, Maiorana A, Meduri M, et al: Acute multiple sclerosis simulating a cerebral tumor: A case report. Rays (Milano) 1987;12: 45–48.
80. Uhlenbrock D, Seidel D, Gehlen W, et al: MR imaging in multiple sclerosis: Comparison with clinical, CSF, and visual evoked potential findings. AJNR 1988;9:59–67.
81. Willoughby EW, Grochowski E, Li DKB, et al: Serial magnetic resonance scanning in multiple sclerosis: A second preoperative study in relapsing patients. Ann Neurol 1989;25:43–49.
82. Grossman RI, Braffman BH, Bronson JR, et al. Multiple sclerosis: Serial study of gadolinium-enhanced MR imaging. Radiology 1988; 169:117–122.
83. Heinz ER, Drayer BD, Haenggeli CA, et al: CT in white matter disease. Radiology 1979;130:370–378.
84. Atlas SW, Grossman RI, Goldberg I, et al: MR diagnosis of acute disseminated encephalomyelitis. J Comput Assist Tomogr 1986;10: 798–801.
85. Dunn V, Bale JF, Zimmerman RA, et al: MRI in children with postinfectious disseminated encephalomyelitis. Magn Reson Imaging 1986;4:25.
86. Kesselring J, Miller DH, Robb SA, et al: Acute disseminated encephalomyelitis: MRI findings and the distinction from multiple sclerosis. Brain 1990;113:291.

87. Barkhof F, Valk J, Hommes OR, Scheltens P: Meningeal 9d-DTPA enhancement in multiple sclerosis. AJNR 1992;13:397–400.
88. Guseo A, Jellinger K: The significance of perivascular infiltration in multiple sclerosis. J Neurol 1975;211:51–60.
89. Grossman RI: Meningeal enhancement in multiple sclerosis truth or coincidence? AJNR 1992;13:401–402.
90. Merandi SF, Kudryk BT, Murtagh FR, Arrington JA: Contrast-enhanced MR imaging of optic nerve lesions in patients with acute optic neuritis. AJNR 1991;12:923–926.
91. Edwards MK, Farlow MR, Stevens JC: Cranial MR in spinal cord MS: Diagnosing patients with isolated spinal cord symptoms. AJNR 1986;7:1003–1005.
92. Osborn AG, Harnsberger HR, Smoker WRK, Boxer RS: Multiple sclerosis in adolescents: CT and MR findings. AJNR 1990;11: 489–494.
93. Ebner F, Millner MM, Justich E: Multiple sclerosis in children: Value of serial MR studies to monitor patients. AJNR 1990;11: 1023–1027.
94. Allen IV, Millar JHD, Kirk J, et al: Systemic lupus erythematosus clinically resembling multiple sclerosis and with unusual pathological and ultrastructural features. J Neurol Neurosurg Psychiatry 1979;42:392–401.
95. Mehler MF, Rabinowich L: Inflammatory myelinoclastic diffuse sclerosis (Schilder disease): Neurologic findings. AJNR 1989;10: 176–180.
96. Adams RD, Victor M, Mancall EL: Central pontine myelinolysis: A hitherto undescribed disease occurring in alcoholic and malnourished patients. Arch Neurol Psychiatry 1959;81:154–172.
97. Koci TM, Chiang F, Chow P, et al: Thalamic extrapontine lesions in central pontine myelinolysis. AJNR 1990;11:1229–1233.
98. Brunberg JA, Kanal E, Hirsch W, Van Thiel DH: Chronic acquired hepatic failure: MR imaging of the brain at 1.5 T. AJNR 1991;12: 909–914.
99. Korogi Y, Takahashi M, Shinzato J, et al: MR findings in two presumed cases of mild central pontine myelinolysis. AJNR 1993;14: 651–654.

5

Brain Congenital Anomalies

- The developing brain in the infant and child
  - Migration
  - Myelination
  - Additional developmental features
- Congenital anatomic abnormalities
  - Classification of brain malformations
  - Disorders of dorsal induction
    - Anencephaly
    - Encephalocele, meningoencephalocele
    - Frontonasal meningoceles
    - Nasopharyngeal meningoceles
    - Chiari malformation
    - Other cerebellar anomalies
  - Anomalies occurring between 5 and 10 Weeks of gestation
    - Holoprosencephaly
    - Septo-Optic dysplasia (de Morsier syndrome)
    - Absence of septum pellucidum
    - Diencephalic cysts
    - Other anomalies
    - Dandy-Walker syndrome
    - Premature craniosynostosis
  - Anomalies occurring between 2 and 5 Months of gestation
    - Disorders of cell migration
    - Corpus callosum anomalies
    - Neuronal proliferation, differentiation, and histogenesis (2 to 5 Months' Gestation)
- Congenital metabolic anomalies
  - Metabolic conditions affecting the white matter
    - Alexander's disease
    - Canavan's disease
    - Pelizaeus-Merzbacher disease
    - X-Linked adrenal leukodystrophy
    - Refsum disease
    - Neonatal adrenal leukodystrophy
    - Zellweger syndrome
    - Rhizomelic chondrodysplasia calcificans punctata
    - Metachromatic leukodystrophy
    - Krabbe's disease
    - Maple syrup urine disease
    - Phenylketonuria
    - Malignant hyperphenylalaninemia
    - Nonketotic hyperglycinemia
    - Homocystinuria
    - Oculocerebrorenal syndrome (Lowe's syndrome)
    - Glutaric acidemia, type 1
  - Peroxysomal disorders
    - Single enzyme deficiency
    - Multiple enzyme deficiency
  - Lysosomal diseases
    - Mucopolysaccharidoses
    - Lipid storage diseases (sphyngolipidoses)
  - Mitochondrial cytopathies
    - Leigh's disease (subacute necrotizing encephalomyelopathy)
    - Menkes' disease (kinky hair disease)
    - Zellweger syndrome
    - Kearns-Sayre syndrome
    - MELAS syndrome (mitochondrial myopathy, encephalopathy, lactic acidosis, and stroke)
    - MERRF (myoclonic epilepsy with ragged red fibers)
    - Cerebrotendinous xanthomatosis
    - Cytoplasmically inherited striatal degeneration
  - Disorders of amino acid metabolism
    - Maple syrup urine disease
    - Phenylketonuria
    - Malignant hyperphenylalaninemia
    - Nonketotic hyperglycinemia
    - Homocystinuria
    - Methylmalonic acidemia
    - Glutaric acidemia
    - Oculocerebrorenal syndrome
    - Leucine metabolism
  - Gray matter diseases
    - Neuronal ceroid lipofuscinosis
    - Other diseases affecting gray matter
  - Miscellaneous conditions
    - Navajo neuropathy
    - Partial albinism
    - Congenital x-linked agammaglobulinemia
    - Mobius syndrome
    - Congenital bilateral perisylvian syndrome
  - Diseases affecting the basal ganglia
    - Wilson's disease (hepatolenticular degeneration)
    - Huntington's disease
    - Fahr's disease
    - Hallervorden-Spatz disease
    - Methylmalonic acidemia

THE DEVELOPING BRAIN IN THE INFANT AND CHILD

Evaluation of a preterm infant's brain is often difficult because of our inability to determine with accuracy the time of conception. For this reason and in view of the very rapid progression of brain development, where a significant change in the externally visible brain takes place on a weekly basis, we can only speak of an approximate number of weeks. According to Fitz, absolutely reliable age data in vivo and even post mortem is difficult to obtain, and one must rely on experience based on observations (1) made on computed tomography (CT) and magnetic resonance imaging (MRI).

The time of appearance of cerebral convolutions in the fetus is the only parameter we can rely on after birth to estimate the age of the fetal brain by CT or MRI (Fig. 5.1). Before 28 weeks, the brain presents no recognizable gyri or fissures except for the sylvian and interhemispheric fissures on CT and MRI. Autopsy specimens show more sulci and gyri (2), also shown in Figure 5.1. The subarachnoid space is large, particularly in the occipital region and in the midline; and the ventricles are relatively large. The gray matter is rather thin and difficult to see peripherally on CT, but on MRI the gray matter is clearer. The germinal matrix is likely to be denser than the gray matter and extends along the length of the lateral ventricle. In some areas the matrix may simulate hemorrhage because of its relatively high density on CT. The glomus of the choroid plexus is usually large, particularly on ultrasound, and may be confused with a hemorrhage of the choroid plexus.

As shown in Figure 5.1, 2 weeks later (28 to 30 weeks' gestation), the brain rapidly presents gyral-sulcal development. The central fissure may be discernible. The gray matter is still thin, the basal ganglia are slightly denser than the surrounding white matter, and the germinal matrix is less distinguishable (only anteriorly is it well seen). The sylvian fissures are large, and the amount of cerebrospinal

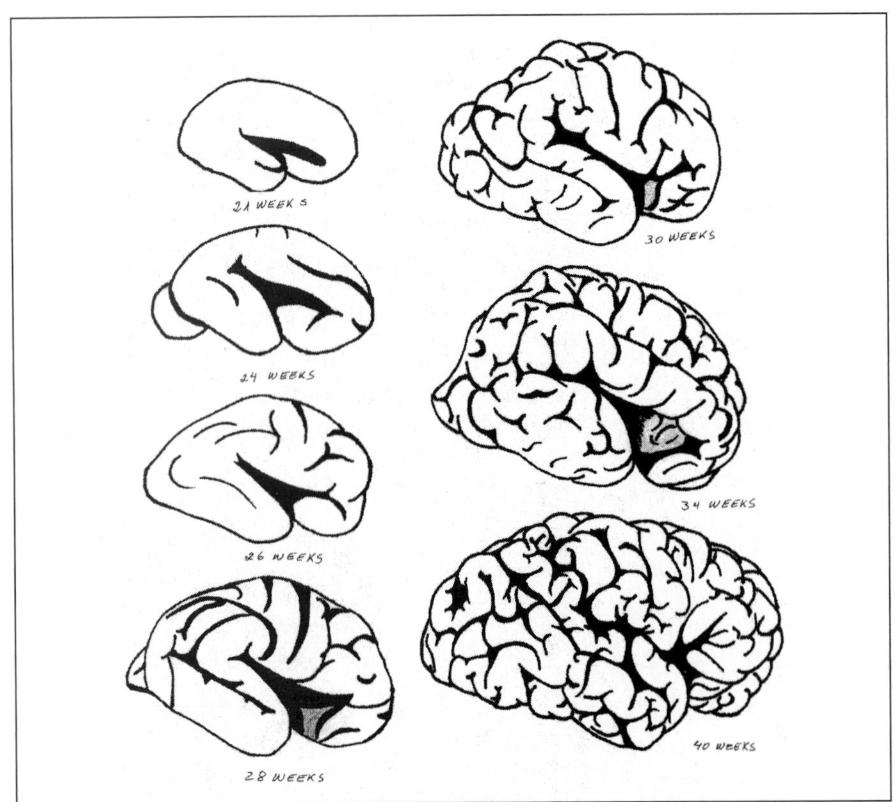

Figure 5.1. Drawing based on photographic images to show the development of the cerebral convolutions. As can be seen, convolutions begin to develop after the twenty-fourth week of gestation. (Adapted from Warwick R and Williams PL [eds], Gray's Anatomy, ed 35. London: Saunders, 1973.)

fluid (CSF) space over the interhemispheric fissure is prominent. The cavum septum pellucidum and cavum vergae are usually prominent. The gray matter gradually becomes thicker in subsequent weeks, and on MRI it may be seen going around the brain sulci (3).

The cisterna magna tends to be much larger until near term. The ventricles, which are larger early on, become gradually smaller, reaching the normal, smaller, size at term (38 to 40 weeks), although the occipital horns and atria may be slightly larger. At 28 to 30 weeks of gestation, the cerebellum is likely to be a fairly good size and the fourth ventricle has become visible. The sylvian fissures remain wide until birth and do not close until about the end of the first year.

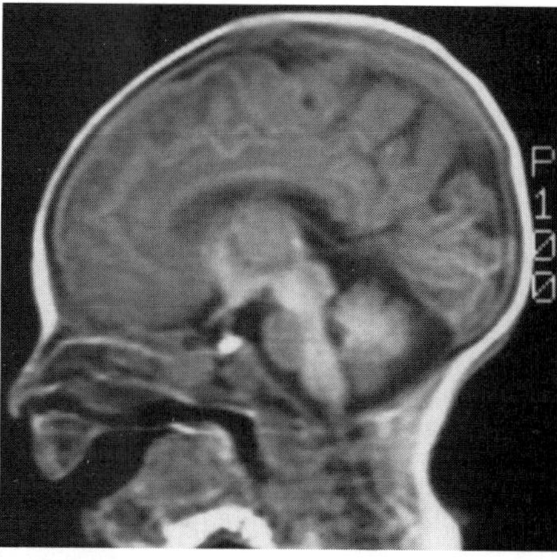

Figure 5.2. "Normal" infant—first week of life. T1-weighted midline sagittal image shows some myelination in brainstem (medulla, posterior aspect of pons and midbrain) and cerebellum (brighter than the rest of tissue). The corpus callosum is seen but not conspicuous; it has minimal myelination.

Migration

Migration of cells from the germinal matrix is the result of movement of neuroblasts, which make up the germinal matrix, across the white matter to form the gray matter of the brain cortex as well as the basal ganglia nuclei. This highly complex development is spread over a fairly long period, starting around the eighth or ninth week to the twentieth week of gestation, thereby increasing the possibility of being affected by unfavorable factors. At about the twenty-sixth week of gestation, the germinal matrix is still rather prominent around the lateral ventricles on CT but becomes less prominent within 2 to 4 weeks. This change can only be interpreted as continuous migration of cells. The active process in this area accounts for the frequency of germinal matrix hemorrhages occurring in premature infants.

Myelination

Some myelination already exists at birth, having started several weeks before birth. It is not possible to get an idea about myelination with CT. MRI allows us to study myelination and to observe the progress of the myelinating process to determine whether it is occurring at a normal rate.

Myelination in the early postnatal stages can be studied better with T1-weighted images, particularly utilizing the inversion recovery technique. After 6 months, the T2-weighted images are satisfactory. The infant brain has a higher proportion of water (over 90 percent), which decreases gradually to maturity. In the adult, the proportion of water is 80 percent in gray matter and 68 percent in white matter. The T1 brightness of myelinated brain is not due to the myelin's being a fatty substance; rather, there is very little water in myelin, and it is for this reason that it is brighter on T1 (Figs 5.2 through 5.5). As the myelination process is accomplished, a local loss of water occurs, which, in the early period, is more clearly demonstrated with a T1 image.

At birth mature myelination is evident in the dorsal aspect of the pons, in portions of the superior and inferior cerebellar peduncles, in the posterior aspect of the internal capsule, and in the adjacent thalamus. Some myelin evidence is also visible around the basal ganglia, which on T2 images are darker than surrounding areas. During this period the entire white matter of the brain in the cerebral hemispheres is bright on T2 images and relatively isodense with the gray matter on T1 images (2,4,5) (Figs. 5.5 and 5.6).

By 1 month of age the optic radiations clearly extend from the region of the temporal lobes, as seen on MR axial images, and back along the lateral aspect of the atrium to the occipital horn of the lateral ventricles. Some myelination of the corona radiata can be seen extending upward from the internal capsule. The brainstem shows a fair amount of myelination soon after birth, and some aspects of white matter of the cerebellum show myelination on T1-weighted images, particularly utilizing inversion recovery.

The degree of myelination may vary somewhat from one infant to another, but in general the normal progression is such that one can state that the brainstem has myelination at birth, which is mature at 6 months, and the same is true of the cerebellar peduncles; the superior and inferior cerebellar peduncles myelinate before the middle cerebellar ones. Cerebellar white matter, which presents some myelin at birth, matures by around 6 months to 1 year. The optic radiations, which are already seen by around the first month of a term infant, are mature by 6 months. Myelination of the posterior limb of the internal capsule, which is present at birth, matures early, whereas the anterior limb is present by around 4 months of age and the anterior and posterior limbs are about equal by around 8 months.

Corpus callosum myelination begins in the splenium by around 4 to 6 months, which is somewhat earlier than the rest of the structure, and then moves in a rostral direction into the trunk, the genu, and the rostrum, to reach full

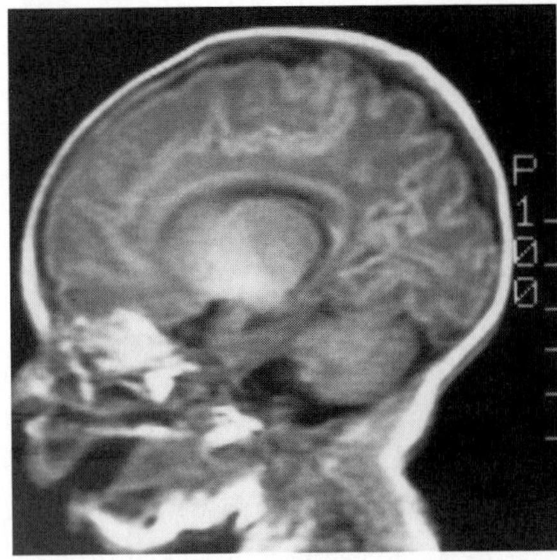

A

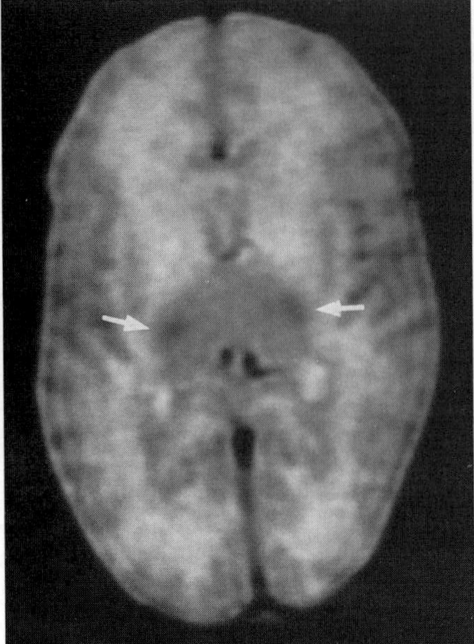

B

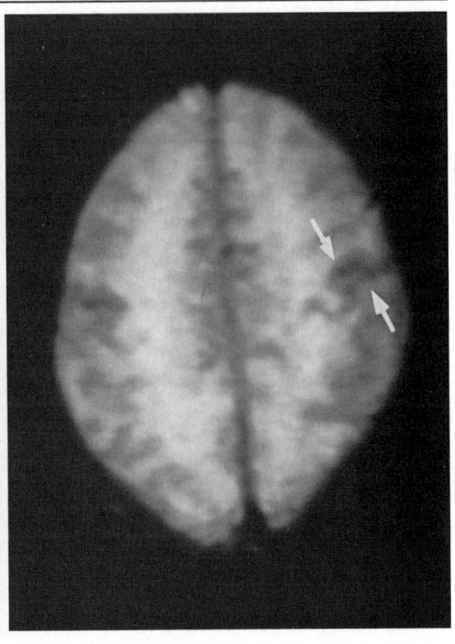

C

Figure 5.3. Normal myelination, first week of life. **A.** Sagittal off center, T1-weighted, shows brightness at level of basal ganglia—internal capsule indicative of myelination. **B.** T2-weighted axial shows darkness in region of posterior limb of internal capsule (small arrows). **C.** T2-weighted axial shows low intensity in region of central fissure indicative of myelination (small arrows). The white matter in the newborn is brighter than the gray matter on T2-weighted images because it has a higher water concentration.

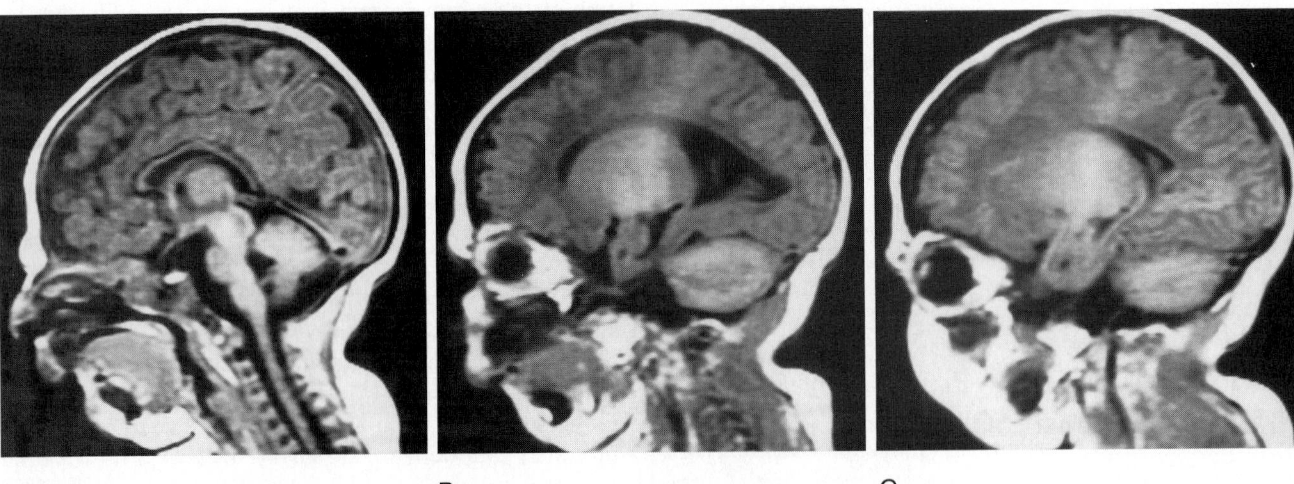

A B C

Figure 5.4. Normal myelination in first 4 weeks of life. **A.** Midline sagittal T1-weighted image shows the normal myelination (emphasis on T1) of upper brainstem and cerebellum (compare cerebellum with Fig. 5.2). There is myelination also in medulla. The corpus callosum shows slight brightness throughout. **B** and **C.** Sagittal T1-weighted images on each side of the midline passing through internal capsules and corona radiata reveal a band of hyperintensity symmetrically arranged and moving toward the central fissure, indicative of progression of myelination. The gray matter is still hyperintense in relation to the white matter because of greater water content of the latter.

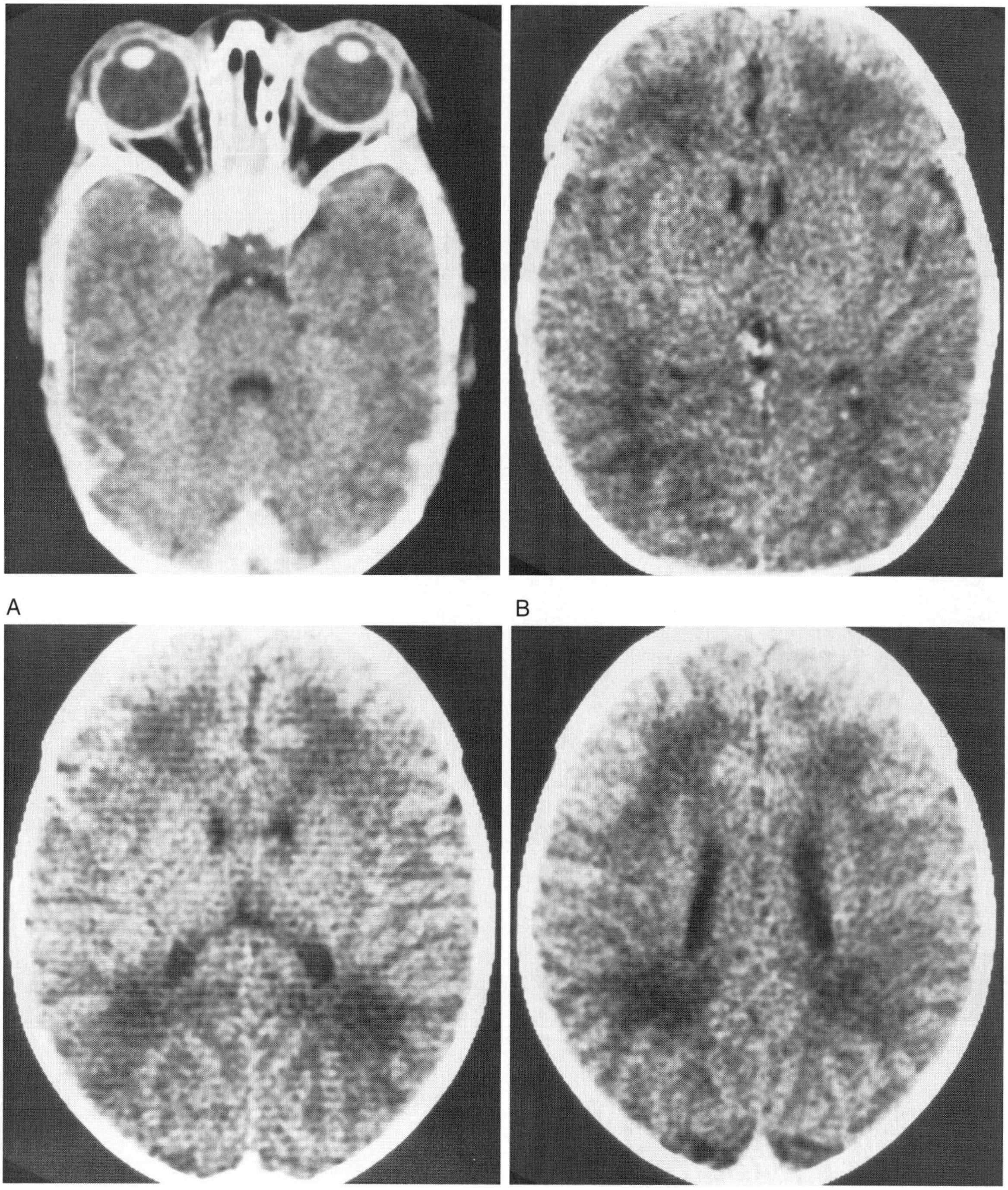

A

B

C

D

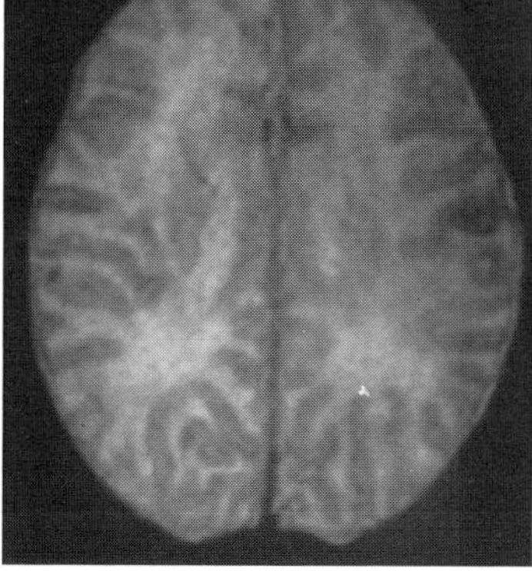

E

Figure 5.5. Normal infant, first 4 weeks of life. **A** to **D.** CT axial views of 2-week-old infant at level of upper pons, basal ganglia, upper basal ganglia, upper ventricular level. The gray-white matter separation is sharp because the white matter has increased water content at this age prior to myelination. The internal capsule cannot be separated from the basal nuclei (compare Fig. 5.5D with Fig. 5.6E, a T2-weighted MR image of same infant). The appearance is similar to the CT image. Note in C the relative increased density of the confluence of the venous sinuses. **E.** A T2-weighted MRI to show the similarity with the CT image at the same level (D).

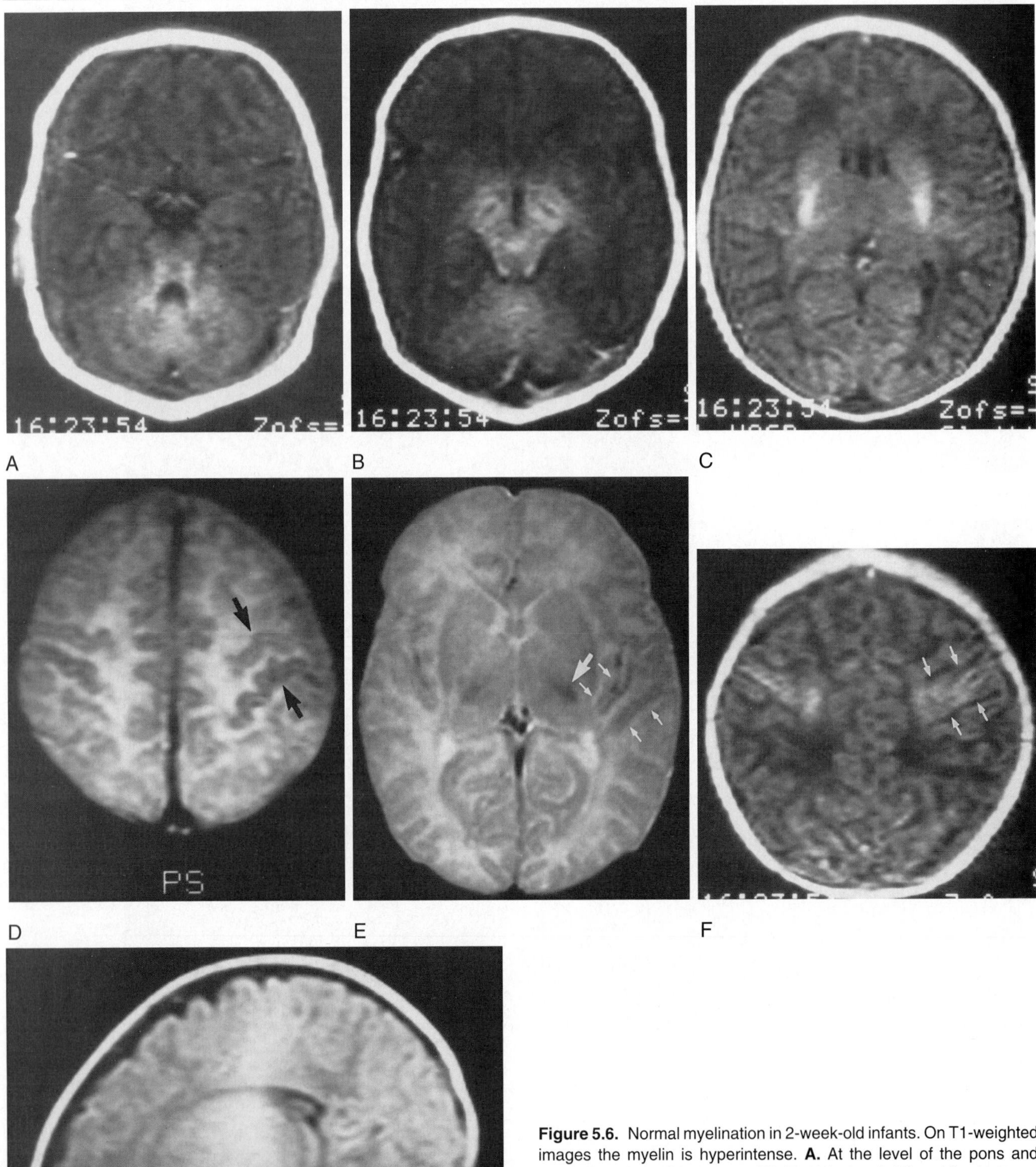

Figure 5.6. Normal myelination in 2-week-old infants. On T1-weighted images the myelin is hyperintense. **A.** At the level of the pons and cerebellum. Inversion recovery T1. **B.** At the level of the midbrain. Inversion recovery. **C.** At the corona radiata. Inversion recovery. **D.** Around the central sulcus on another child. On T2-weighted images, myelin is hypointense in relation to gray matter. **E.** At the level of the internal capsule. Posterior limb is hypointense on T2-weighted image. There is myelination around the central sulcus area (dark on T2) (arrows). **F.** Hyperintensity around the central sulcus is due to myelination. This area is bright on T1-weighted images (inversion recovery). **G.** Sagittal T1-weighted spin-echo view shows the wide path of myelination extending from the basal ganglia–internal capsule region through the corona radiata to the cortex in the central area (cut 1 cm from midline). The image was identical at 1 cm on the opposite side of the midline.

myelination by 1 year of age. The precentral gyrus presents myelination that begins during the first month, and the postcentral gyrus is present at birth. Myelination of the subcortical white matter is mature by 21 to 25 months. The occipital pole, the calcarine cortex, and the precentral gyrus are usually mature by 7 to 15 months (Figs. 5.7 and 5.8) (Table 5.1).

As the infant's brain develops, CT and MRI show the evolving anatomy. In the first 6 months, on the T2-weighted images, the cerebral hemispheres present a fairly bright white matter and a gray matter that is gray; on T1-weighted images the appearance tends to be more uniform between the gray and the white matter. In the second half of the first year, the gray and white matter become relatively isointense on T2-weighted images of the cerebral hemispheres because the water content of the partially myelinated white matter and the gray matter is fairly similar. After the first year myelination has progressed sufficiently that the white matter of the brain hemispheres tends to be darker than the gray matter on T2-weighted images. Throughout the first year, the early myelinated structures show the usual characteristics of myelination: darker than the gray matter on T2-weighted images and lighter than the gray matter on T1-weighted images (Figs. 5.6 through 5.8).

Additional Developmental Features

The myelination process is the most striking change to be noted on sequential MRIs of infants. As mentioned previously, however, the ventricles can vary in size because they usually become slightly smaller after birth and tend to remain so for several days, which Fitz attributes to mild postnatal swelling (1). When the mild edema subsides, the ventricles become slightly larger and then gradually become smaller with the passage of time. The cavum septum pellucidum is often visible at birth but disappears in the majority of instances, although sometimes it remains large. The cavum vergae may also be visible at birth and tends to disappear later.

Surface sulci are slightly more prominent in the early months and get smaller gradually as the brain convolutions gain in size by growth of the gray matter. The pituitary gland is hyperintense at birth on T1 images, and several months later it acquires its normal mature appearance: an isointense (with the gray matter) anterior lobe and hyperintense posterior lobe on T1 images. The hyperintensity was once attributed to fatty substances, but fat suppression images have since shown no difference in the bright posterior lobe of the pituitary gland from the usual T1 images.

Perhaps the most important aspect to note here is the accumulation of ferric iron in certain locations in the brain, which is almost nil at birth and gradually increases with age. It is not very noticeable in children and it becomes more and more so in adults and in the elderly. Since the initial publication of Drayer et al. (6), it has become well known that the globus pallidus, the reticular portion of the substantia nigra, the red nucleus, the dentate nucleus of the cerebellum, and the putamen are involved most frequently. With the passage of time, nearly every tissue in the brain accumulates a certain amount of ferric iron. The amount of iron in the basal ganglia structures, brainstem, and cerebellum tends to increase until about 20 years of age. At that time, the iron content becomes stationary until about age 60, at which time the accumulation of ferric iron again spurts.

The imaging of this physiologic phenomenon is easy because iron has a strong susceptibility effect, which is shown extremely well on T2- but not on T1-weighted images. In the rest of the brain, the U fibers in the subcortical area of the brain have a greater iron content than the gray or white matter. More iron gathers in the frontal than in the occipital white matter, and almost no ferric iron is deposited in the posterior aspect of the posterior limb of the internal capsules and in the optic radiations. In infants, iron stains first become positive at approximately 6 months of age in the globus pallidus and at 9 to 12 months in the reticular portion of the substantia nigra. The red nucleus becomes visible at 18 to 24 months and the dentate nucleus at 3 to 7 years, according to Diezel (7).

Perls' stain is more sensitive than T2 images, although the ability to demonstrate a susceptibility effect goes up exponentially with the strength of the magnetic field. Thus,

Table 5.1.
Important Stages in MR Visualization of Myelination

T-1-weighted images	
Birth	Medulla
	Dorsal midbrain
	Inferior and superior cerebellar peduncles
	Posterior limb of internal capsule
	Ventrolateral portion of thalamus
1 Month	Optic tract and optic radiations
	Cerebral peduncles
	Central portion of centrum semiovale
	White matter of precentral and postcentral gyri
3 Months	Anterior limb of internal capsule
	Occipital white matter
4–5 Months	Splenium of corpus callosum
6 Months	Genu of corpus callosum
	Centrum semiovale
8–11 Months	Peripheral white matter
T-2-weighted images	
Birth	Superior and inferior cerebellar peduncles
	Dorsal pons
	Ventrolateral thalamus
1 Month	Pre- and Postcentral gyri
	Optic tracts
2 Months	Portions of the centrum semiovale
4 Months	Calcarine fissure
6 Months	Splenium of corpus callosum
8 Months	Genu of corpus callosum
9–12 Months	Posterior centrum semiovale
11–14 Months	Anterior centrum semiovale

Adapted from Barkovich et al. Radiology 1988;166:173–180.

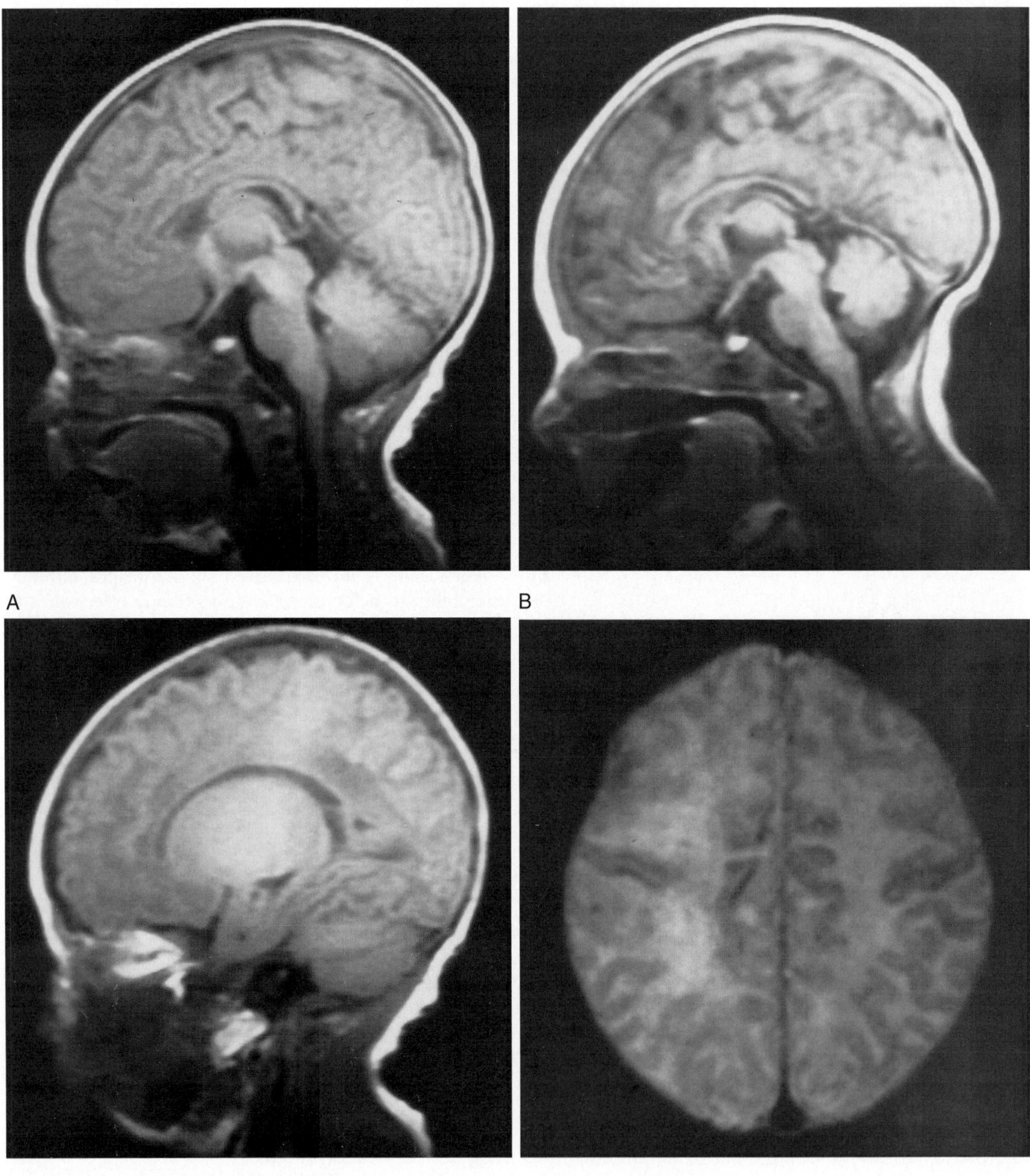

Figure 5.7. Progress of myelination at 4 weeks. **A.** At 2 weeks the corpus callosum is poorly outlined although visible, but (**B**) at 4 weeks it is more visible. **C.** T1-weighted sagittal view shows a wider bright band of meylination. **D.** T2-weighted axial view. The myelinated area around the central fissure is better defined.

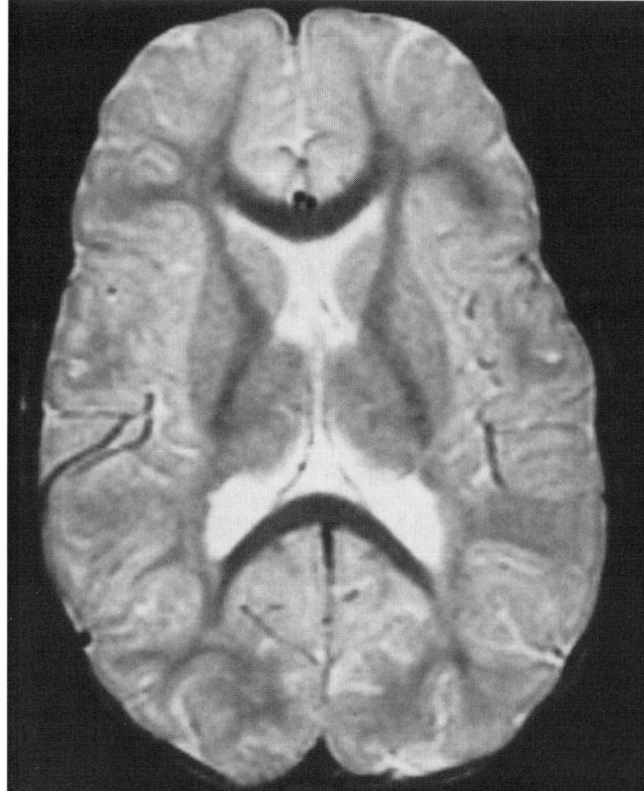

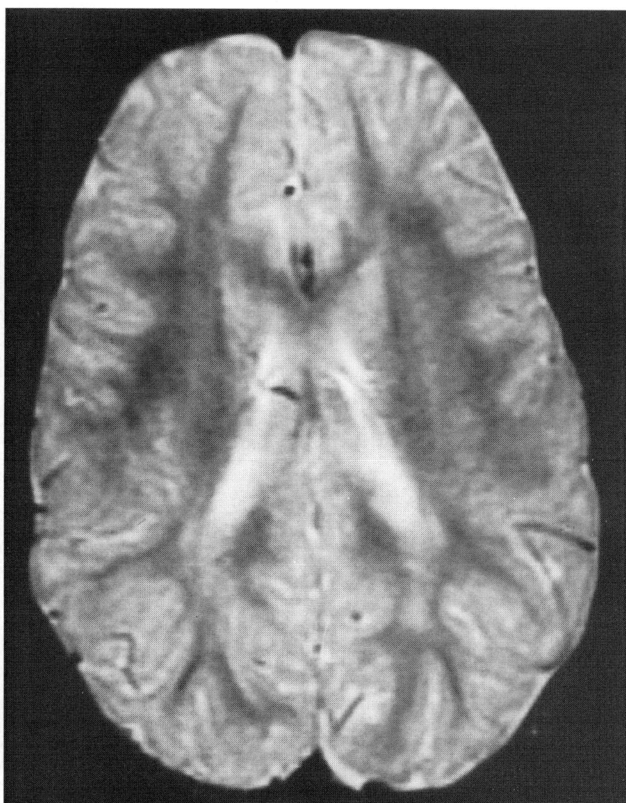

A B

Figure 5.8. Normal myelination at 15 months. **A.** Axial T2-weighted image shows the dark, normal myelination in the corpus callosum, internal capsules, and white matter in the frontal and occipital areas. **B.** Higher section shows that the centrum semiovale, bilaterally, shows some irregular brightness, suggesting incomplete myelination. This is a difficult condition to interpret, for minor variants of this normal appearance are found in adults and in that group it should be considered abnormal.

this effect is seen much more strongly on 1.5-T images than in those images made with lower magnet strength (Figs. 5.9 and 5.10).

On CT examinations the region of the straight sinus and the torcular Herophili as well as the transverse sinuses tend to be denser in infants than in older children or adults, probably because the blood pool is relatively denser than the brain due to the higher content of water in the infant brain. In some infants, the sinuses, including the superior sagittal sinus in its posterior aspect, are so relatively dense that we may suspect thrombosis, particularly if confusing clinical signs could relate to sinus thrombosis. MRI may clarify the problem in these instances (Fig. 5.11).

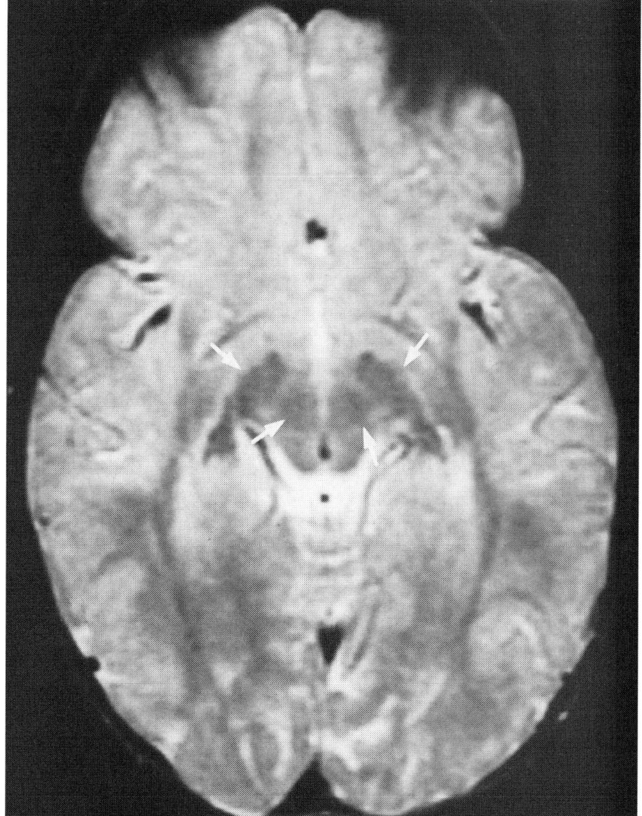

Figure 5.9. T2-weighted axial image in a 15-month-old child. Taken with a 1.5-T MRI unit. There is evidence of hypointensity in the red nucleus (posterior arrow) and substantia nigra (anterior arrow) bilaterally due to normal early accumulation of ferric iron.

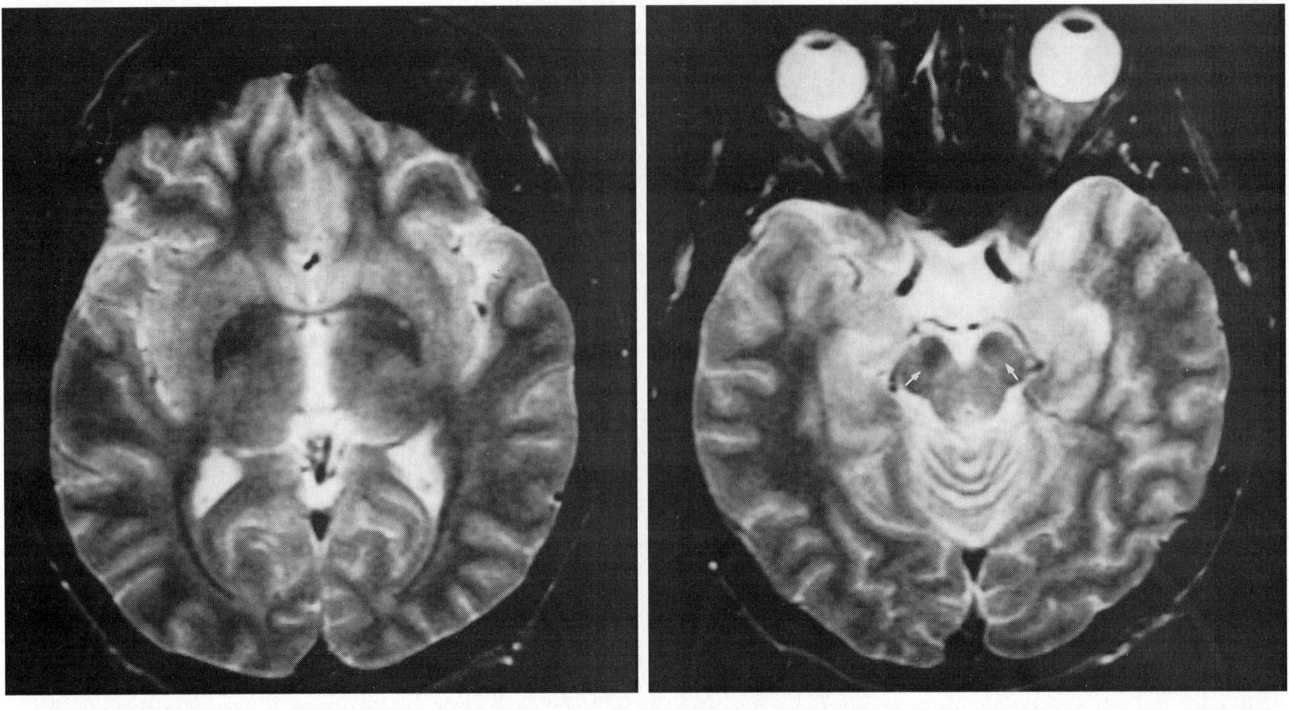

A B

Figure 5.10. Ferric iron accumulation in globus pallidus in a 50-year-old man. **A.** Hypointensity in the globus pallidus bilaterally in this T2-weighted axial; also in the substantia nigra in (**B**) (arrow). It has been said that in children who suffer a vascular insult, increased iron concentration for age may be found in the lenticular nucleus.

CONGENITAL ANATOMIC ABNORMALITIES

The congenital anomalies of the central nervous system (CNS) and its surroundings, the skull and spine, are the most frequently encountered malformations. Also, they have far greater consequences, for, in addition to causing the death of the infant (the most frequent cause of stillbirths), they may cause death at an early age or may cause significant mental and physical retardation of normal development and performance, a most important problem. This applies to both the anatomic anomalies, usually termed *malformations*, and to the biochemical and metabolic anomalies, a group that continues to grow as more of these derangements are recognized.

Congenital anatomic anomalies are malformations of the entire organ or portions of the organ. The term *anatomic variant* applies to a separation from the normal that does not in itself lead to any pathologic manifestations or malfunction.

Classification of Brain Malformations

The discovery of CT was a great advance in our ability to recognize malformations of the various components of the brain. Prior to that, we made many diagnoses because the ventricular system and the subarachnoid cisterns could be well seen by pneumoencephalography and the blood vessels of the brain could be studied by cerebral angiography. These capabilities, in addition to plain-film examination of the skull, provided a means of identifying the probable malformation. However, CT provided us with a method to actually see brain anatomy without performing an invasive study, except for the injection of intravenous (IV) contrast material when needed. Only axial views could be made easily, but it was possible to carry out sagittal or coronal reformatting of the axial image data. The introduction of MRI has added yet another method with which to see brain anatomy in any plane. In addition, MRI provides images without any artifacts, particularly in the posterior fossa, where CT is frequently suboptimal because of bone artifacts.

Causes of malformations of the brain can be varied and are mostly unknown. Use of narcotics such as cocaine and others has been associated with certain nervous system malformations, and the same is true of some pharmaceutical drugs. Some malformations have been related to the ingestion of alcohol in excess during early pregnancy and even to heavy smoking. But in the majority of instances, anatomic malformations of the brain and spine are considered to be idiopathic. Most of them are not hereditary or familial.

None of the various ways of classifying these malformations can be considered perfect. The time at which the injury or the aberration of normal development occurred in utero in relation to gestation has much to do with the type of malformation that will occur. The more severe ones

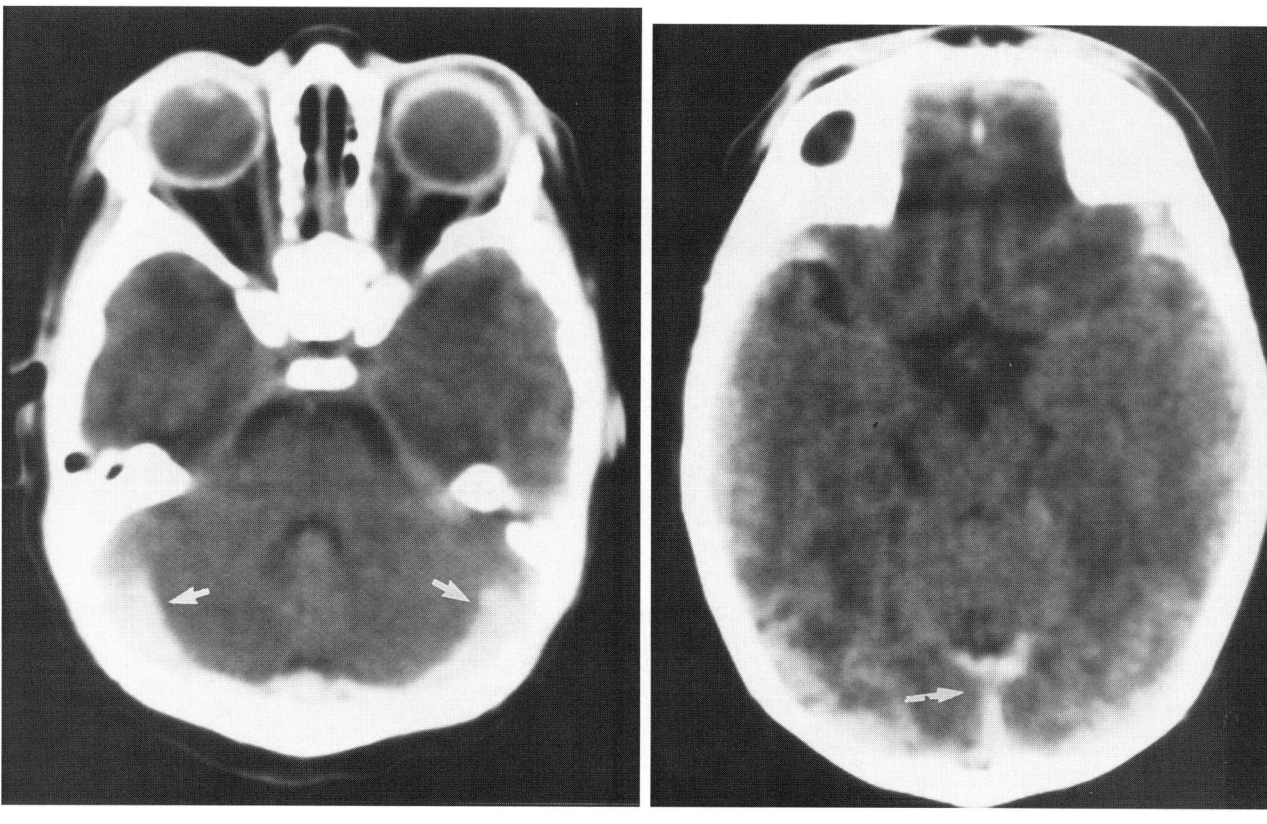

Figure 5.11. A and **B.** Dense torcular herophilii and lateral venous sinuses in a 1-day-old infant (arrows). The relative increased density on CT is owing to the high water content of the infant brain in relation to the blood in the venous sinuses.

occur early, and usually, the later they occur during gestation, the more they are likely to be compatible with a handicapped but acceptable level of development. This has led Volpe (8) and later van der Knaap and Valk (4) to use timing as a basis for the classification of the anomalies. A modified form of this system is utilized here, but when needed, the malformations are grouped according to the segment of the organ that is involved as seen by CT or MRI.

In this section only congenital anomalies of the brain are considered. Disorders of the spine and spinal cord are addressed in the chapters dealing with these structures.

Disorders of Dorsal Induction

These disorders of closure or cranial dysraphic states tend to occur in the first 4 weeks of gestation and are related to derangements of closure of the neural tube. Because the neural tube as well as adjacent mesoderm are involved, the dura, arachnoid, pia, vertebrae, and skull participate in the malformations.

ANENCEPHALY

The term applies to congenital absence of the cranial vault when cerebral hemispheres are missing or are very hypoplastic. Usually the posterior fossa structures are present. The diagnosis is made by clinical observation.

ENCEPHALOCELE, MENINGOENCEPHALOCELE

Encephaloceles usually do not exist alone. Ordinarily the aberration is a meningoencephalocele because the meninges are developed and accompany the brain as it herniates through the cranial opening. Many of these infants are stillborn or die a short time after birth. In the United States and Western Europe, the majority of these anomalies occur in the occipital region. In the series of 265 cases published by Matson, there were 196 occipital, 34 parietal, 17 frontal, 14 nasal, and 4 nasopharyngeal encephaloceles (9). The diagnosis is usually apparent by inspection; cross-sectional imaging by CT or MRI is utilized to determine the type of tissue that is present in the meningocele sac. It may all be filled with fluid or it may contain variable amounts of brain tissue. This is easy to appreciate by CT or, particularly, by MRI (Fig. 5.12).

FRONTONASAL MENINGOCELES

These are common in Asian countries but relatively rare in the Western world. The congenital absence of the

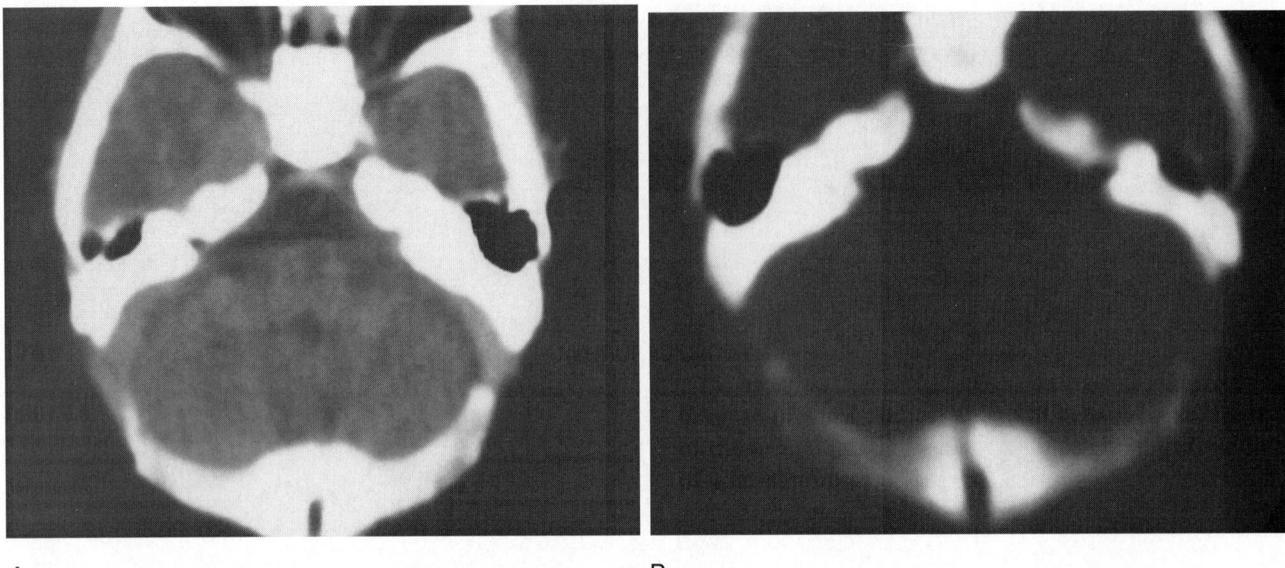

A B

Figure 5.12. Occipital encephalocele. **A.** There is a soft tissue mass in the occipital region. **B.** A bone window reveals the cleft in the bone associated with meningoencephalocele.

greater wing of the sphenoid, which is seen in association with neurofibromatosis, may or may not be associated with a meningocele in the temporal region causing exophthalmus.

Barkovich et al. analyzed the congenital nasal masses and found that CT and MRI are both satisfactory for diagnosis (10). MRI has the advantage of multiple high-resolution images in all planes. The lesions occurring in this area are nasofrontal encephaloceles resulting from failure to close the small frontonasal fontanelle (the fonticulus frontalis). The fonticulus frontalis normally closes before retraction of the dural extension through the foramen cecum. If the dura does not retract, a nasal glioma may form (connecting with the brain by a thin stalk) or a dermal sinus may result. The latter may involute partially, and a dermoid or epidermoid tumor may form by the usual mechanism of desquamation of the cells lining the sinus tract (Fig. 5.13*A*). Some cases may go undiagnosed until later if there is no visible lump outside and there is no evidence of nasal obstruction (Fig. 5.13*B*).

NASOPHARYNGEAL MENINGOCELES

These may exist alone (Fig. 5.14) or may be associated with other anomalies such as partial or complete agenesis of the corpus callosum. They may present as a mass in the nasopharynx, which will interfere with breathing. Sagittal MRI will usually give a clear image of the anatomy. The meningeal opening may go through the sphenoid bone in the region of the sella turcica (Fig. 5.14), or the bone defect in the skull base could be farther forward in the ethmoidal area.

The connection between the brain tissue in the nasopharynx and the intracranial contents may not be apparent on MRI or otherwise. In this case the isolated brain tissue may be called *aberrant* or *heterotopic.* Braun et al. reported on two cases of brain tissue heterotopia in the nasopharynx; in one case there was a patent craniopharyngeal canal and in the other there was none, but the infant had a cleft palate (11). No brain anomalies were observed. The pituitary gland may be ectopic or unrecognizable on surgical intervention in cases of nasopharyngeal meningoencephaloceles and thus could be either damaged or inadvertently removed (12).

CHIARI MALFORMATION

This disorder, as well as anencephaly, encephaloceles, and encephalomeningoceles, occurs with aberrations taking place during the first 4 weeks of gestation. There are three types of Chiari malformation that are usually described (13).

In *Chiari type I malformation*, the cerebellar tonsils are below the foramen magnum (Fig. 5.15). Normally, the lower margin of the cerebellar tonsils is slightly above the foramen magnum level as measured from the tip (lower margin) of the clivus to the posterior aspect of the foramen magnum. However, the lower margin of the cerebellar tonsils in some normal individuals may extend slightly below the foramen magnum. In their review of 200 cases, Barkovich et al. found that 14 percent of normal patients had tonsils extending slightly below the foramen magnum (14). They concluded that up to 2 mm below the foramen magnum can be considered as normal and probably has no clinical significance unless associated with other anomalies such as hydromyelia.

However, Mikulis et al. indicate that the cerebellar tonsils ascend with age; they state, based on an investigation of 221 subjects, that any measurement must be considered according to the age of the patient (15). The maximum normal level of the tonsils below the foramen magnum is first decade, 6 mm; second and third decades, 5 mm; fourth to eighth decade, 4 mm; and ninth decade, 3 mm. Some would call the Chiari I malformation *tonsillar ectopia*, and indeed, in some of these cases the tonsils are down but no other anomalies or neurologic signs are evident. Because of the frequent association between a Chiari type I or type II malformation with hydromyelia and possibly spinal meningoceles, these anomalies evidently tend to occur at the same time during gestation. Hydromyelia and spinal meningoceles are not considered in this chapter but are described under congenital anomalies of the spine in chapter 16.

Chiari type I anomalies are best seen on sagittal MRI views, which usually show the level of the foramen magnum even though the actual tip of the posterior aspect of the foramen magnum cannot be seen clearly because it does not contain bone marrow. Some bone marrow development usually approaches the posterior margin of the foramen magnum, however, and provides a marker that allows the tracing of a line between the bottom of the clivus and the posterior margin (Fig. 5.15). The tonsillar herniation is easily visible in a coronal plane on MRI. CT may suggest Chiari type I malformation because the tonsils are shown to be at the level of the foramen magnum with less than the usual amount of CSF and might be seen in the cross section just below the foramen magnum. In addition, the cisterna magna is usually small or absent. Asymmetry of the cerebellar tonsils is common; one side may be larger and lower in position than the other. This may be the case in normal subjects as well as those presenting tonsillar ectopia.

The fourth ventricle may be in normal position or slightly lower and perhaps minimally elongated. There is no evidence of displacement of the brainstem downward into the upper spinal canal, and the foramen magnum may be either slightly enlarged or normal. Usually no anomalies affect the cerebellum, the brainstem, or the region of the third ventricle with Chiari type I malformation. Anomalies of the bone may include basilar impression, atlanto-occipital fusion, and spina bifida of C1; the last is a relatively common normal variant. The cervical spine may show Klippel-Feil syndrome (reduction in the number of vertebrae or fusion of two or more vertebrae with hemivertebrae and a low hairline).

The anomaly may be asymptomatic for years and may manifest itself during adolescence or young adulthood. When symptoms arise, surgical decompression of the foramen magnum usually produces good and lasting results, particularly in those patients who presented with some variable intracranial hypertension or cerebellar dysfunction. Thus, it is important to make a clinical diagnosis, usually with MRI or CT. Unfortunately, about 19 percent of patients may show initial improvement but later they regress.

According to Saez et al. the patients who have signs of central cord involvement are most likely to do poorly in the long term (16).

Contrary to the Chiari type I malformation, the *Chiari type II malformation* is usually associated with other anomalies, most commonly with a myelomeningocele. Hydrocephalus is also common due to aqueductal stenosis or to compression of the outlet of the fourth ventricle at the foramen magnum. Other anomalies are detailed later in the text.

In the Chiari type II malformation the cerebellum, medulla, and pons are displaced downward through an enlarged foramen magnum (Fig. 5.16). A careful and complete study of the pathologic anatomy and the CT as well as plain-film findings in this anomaly have been described by Naidich et al. (17–20). The fourth ventricle may be massively enlarged or relatively small, but it is usually elongated and displaced caudally. The posterior fossa is small and the foramen magnum is widened.

Although CT is an excellent method to diagnose the Chiari malformation, MRI offers a more complete evaluation of any associated anomalies (21). MRI allows us to get excellent images in all projections, of which the sagittal view is one of the most useful, and to study the altered anatomy (Fig. 5.17).

In addition to the downward displacement of the lower part of the cerebellum and cerebellar tonsils, the upper aspect of the cerebellum may be herniated through the tentorium, probably secondary to the small posterior fossa, which cannot contain the volume of the brainstem and cerebellum (Fig. 5.17). In addition, the cerebellum may wrap around the lateral aspects of the pons on each side. The cerebellum may become impacted inferiorly through the foramen magnum, and necrosis of some aspects of the lower cerebellum can take place. The cerebellar tonsils may extend down for several cervical vertebral segments to C4, C5, or lower (22). Considerable hypoplasia of the cerebellum may occur. In these cases the occipital lobes seem to occupy most of the posterior fossa.

The ventricles are usually dilated in the Chiari type II malformation. The anterior horns of the lateral ventricles have a pointed anteroinferior configuration that is visible in most instances (11 of the 12 patients in the Wolpert et al. [21] series). Coronal scans are needed to see this configuration more clearly. There is usually flattening of the lateral angles of the lateral ventricles, particularly in the frontal horns. The third ventricle is usually relatively small and may have a large massa intermedia or interthalamic adhesion. The septum pellucidum is often absent. The fourth ventricle, as indicated previously, is sometimes very

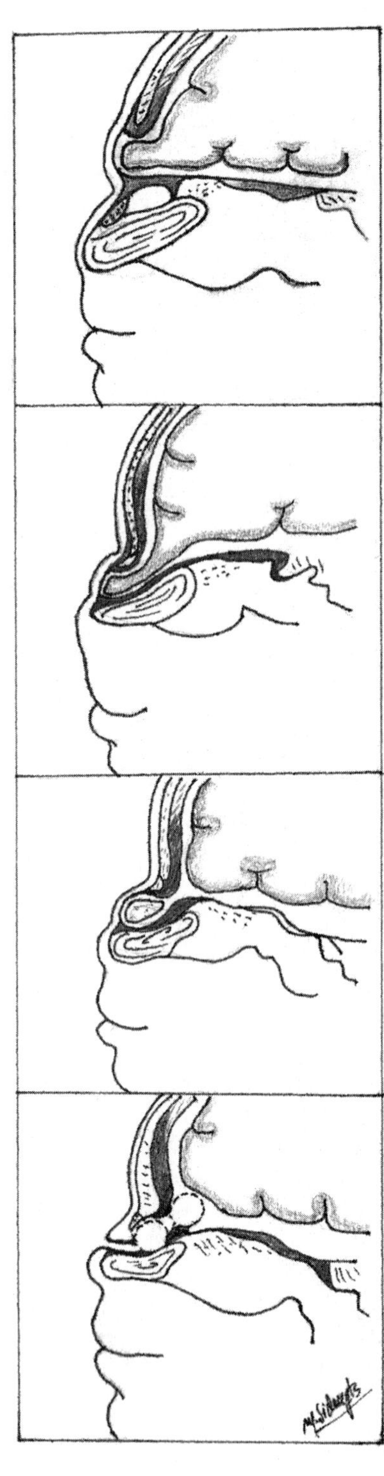

A

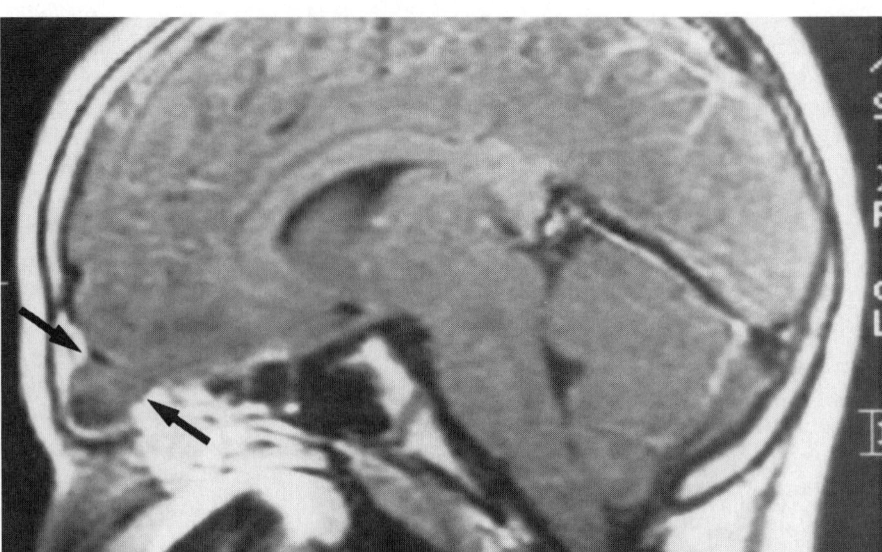

B

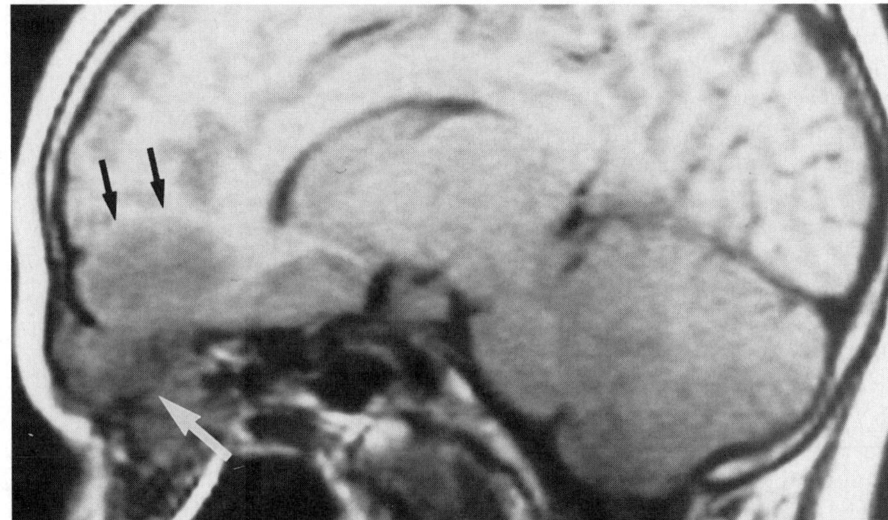

C

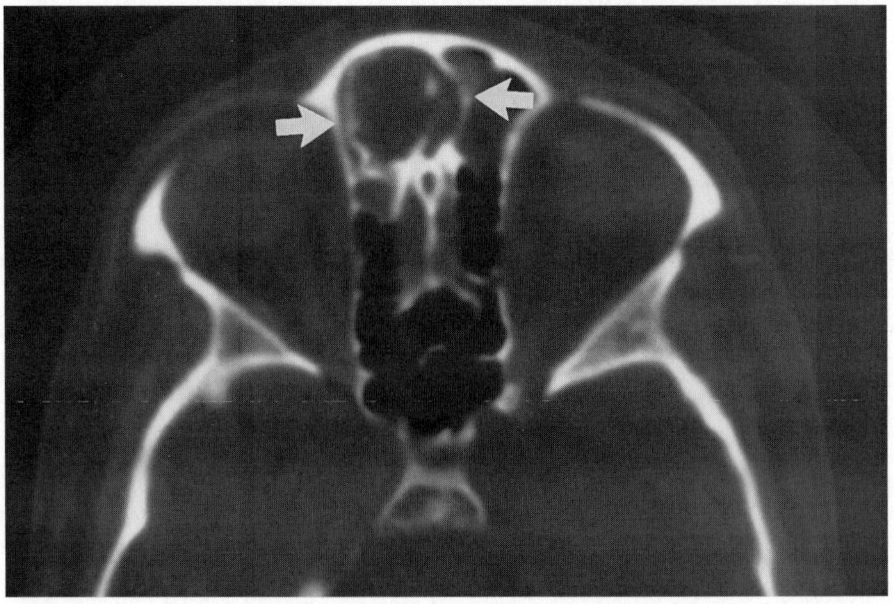

D

Figure 5.13. A. Drawing according to Barkovich et al. (10). For explanation on drawing, see text. **B** to **F.** Frontonasal meningocele in a 15-year-old boy who presented with a sinus infection and signs of meningitis. **B.** Sagittal view near the midline showing the direct extension into the frontonasal area, on gadolinium-enhanced T1 image (arrows). **C.** More laterally, there is low intensity and presence of edema in the brain secondary to infection. No enhancement is seen (arrows). **D.** Axial CT shows the bone erosion in the frontonasal area (arrows). **E.** Reformatted CT sagittal view shows the bone defect in the frontal region. **F** and **G.** Frontonasal encephalocele associated with schizencephaly. **F.** CT axial with contrast. There is a large meningoencephalocele with hypertelorism. A CSF space is present in the left frontotemporal area. **G.** A higher section reveals that a CSF collection projects medially through a wide cleft apparently lined by gray matter consistent with open lip schizencephaly.

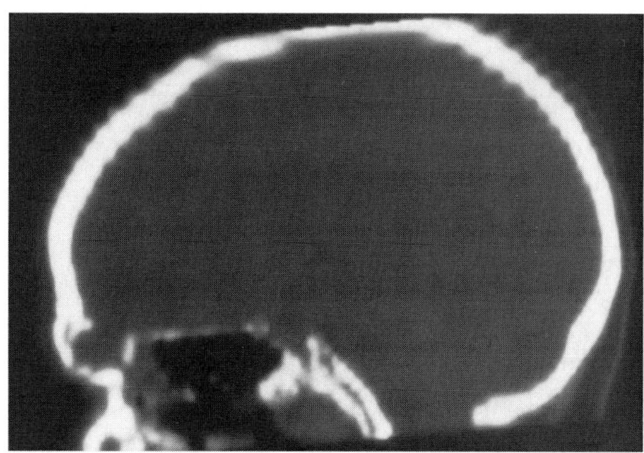

E

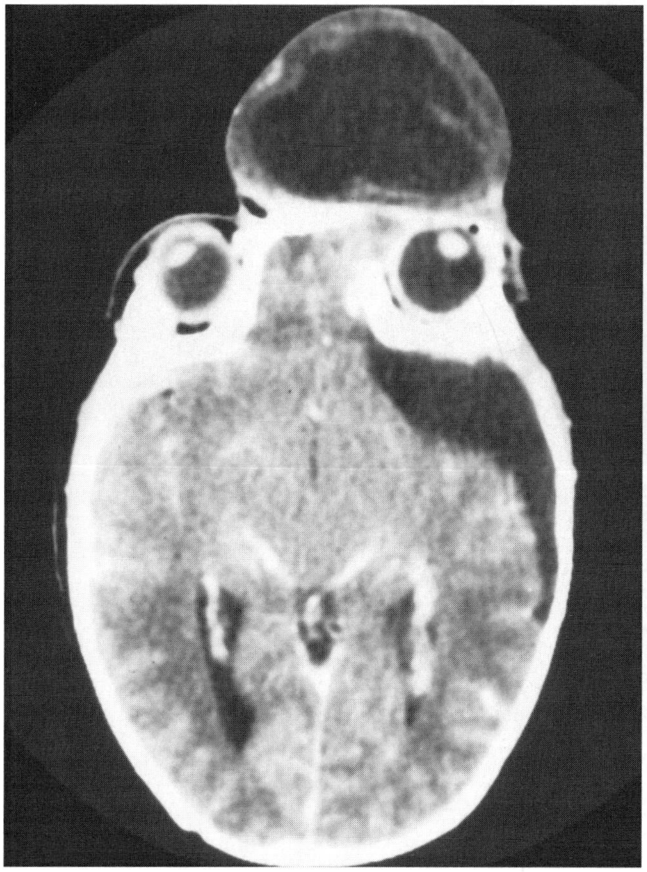

F

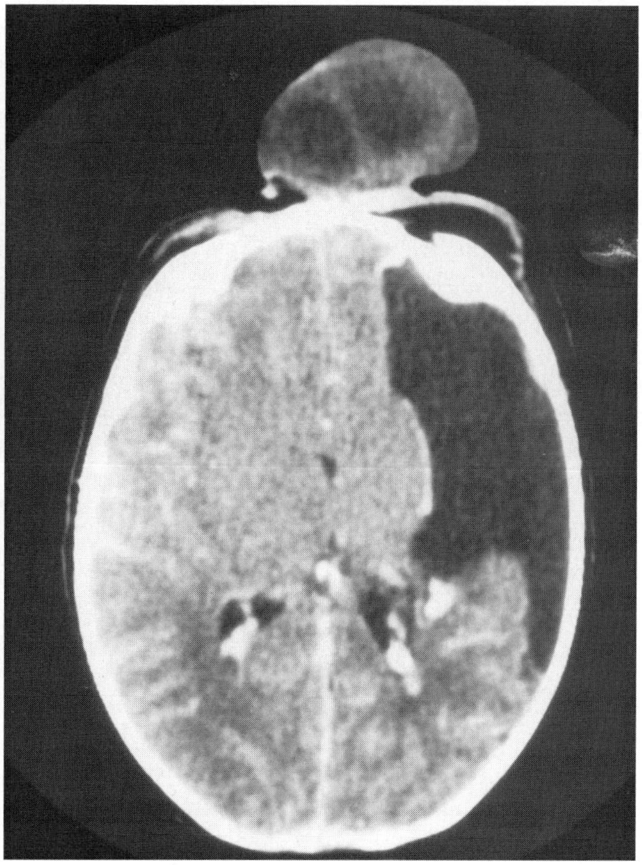

G

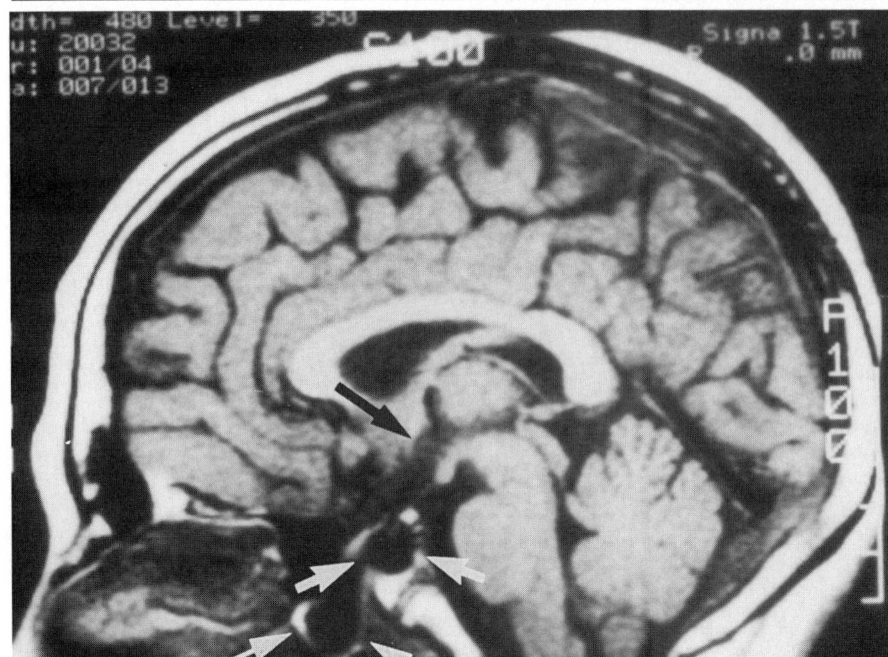

A

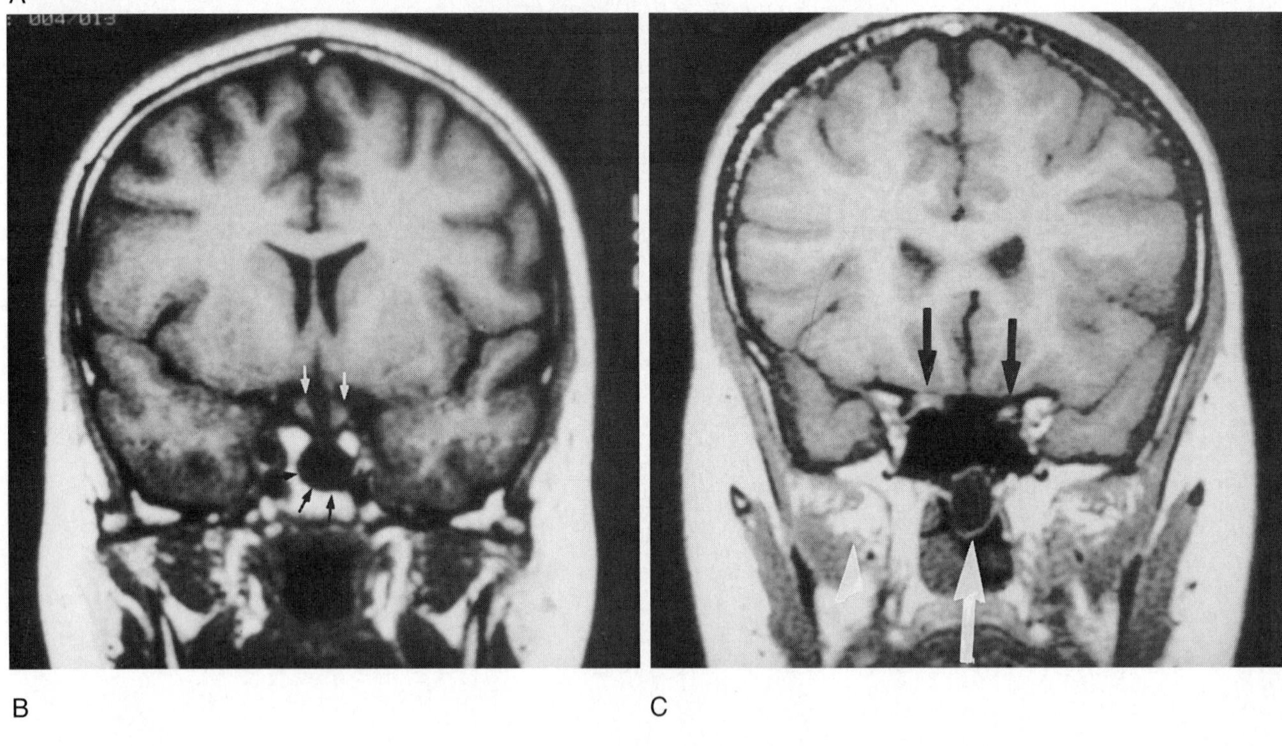

B C

Figure 5.14. Transphenoidal meningocele in a 19-year-old woman who complained of blindness in one eye, probably since birth. **A.** Sagittal T1-weighted image (midline) shows that the third ventricle is not closed caudally (black arrow). A pouch is seen in the nasopharynx (white arrows). **B.** Coronal T1-weighted image shows separation of the optic nerves near the chiasm (small arrows). A complete chiasm was not seen. The pouch is seen below (small black arrows). **C.** More anteriorly, the two nerves are asymmetrical (upper arrows), and the bottom of the pouch can be seen in the nasopharynx (lower arrow). (Courtesy of Dr. B. Swearingen, Boston, Massachusetts.)

Figure 5.15. Chiari I malformation (tonsillar ectopia). **A.** T1-weighted sagittal view close to the midline demonstrates the cerebellar tonsil to be over 1 cm below the edge of the foramen magnum shown by the arrow. There is no evidence of syringomyelia. It is possible the patient has platybasia (basal angle 145 to 150°), but there is no evidence of basilar invagination. The fourth ventricle is in the normal position. **B.** Another patient, a young woman, complained of neck pain, headaches, and vertigo. Sagittal view just off the midline shows tonsillar herniation. The fourth ventricle may be slightly lower in position. There is no platybasia (compare with A). **C.** Coronal view. The tonsils are squeezed together as they go through the foramen magnum. **D.** A section slightly more anterior than C shows that the tonsils are not only dorsally but also laterally placed around the spinal cord. No syringomyelia was detected. The second patient (B, C, D) had symptoms and findings suggesting that surgical decompression might be indicated. In the patient shown in A, the tonsillar ectopia may have been an incidental finding. **E.** Chiari I malformation in another patient, a 27-year-old woman who complained of headaches. The axial CT demonstrates the low cerebellar tonsils at the foramen magnum (arrows). **F.** A higher slice demonstrates the absence of the cisterna magna.

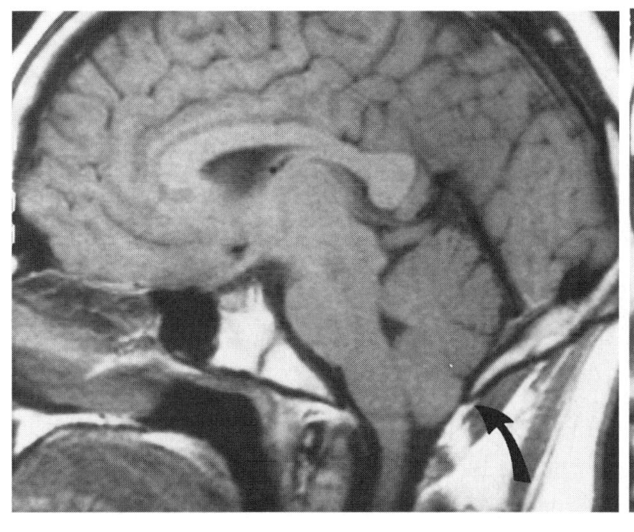

A

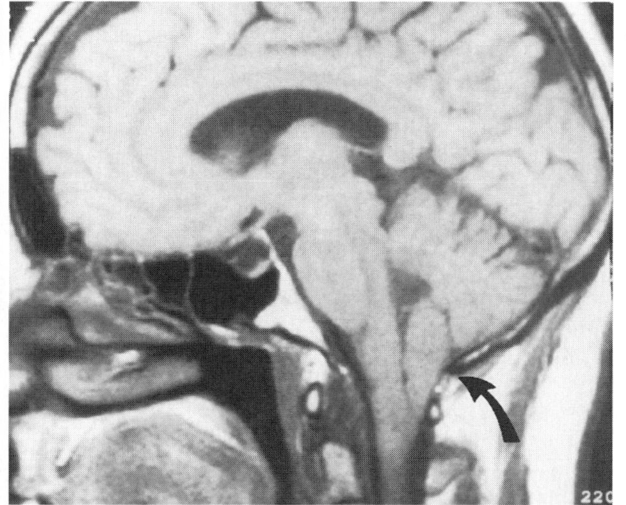

B

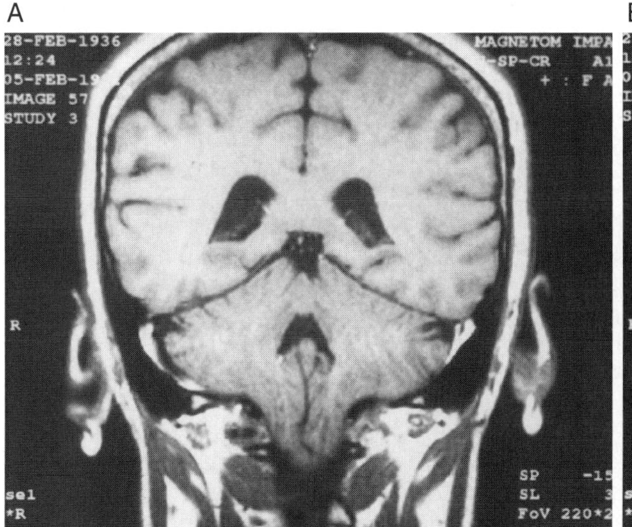

28-FEB-1936
12:24
IMAGE 57
STUDY 3
R
sel
*R

C

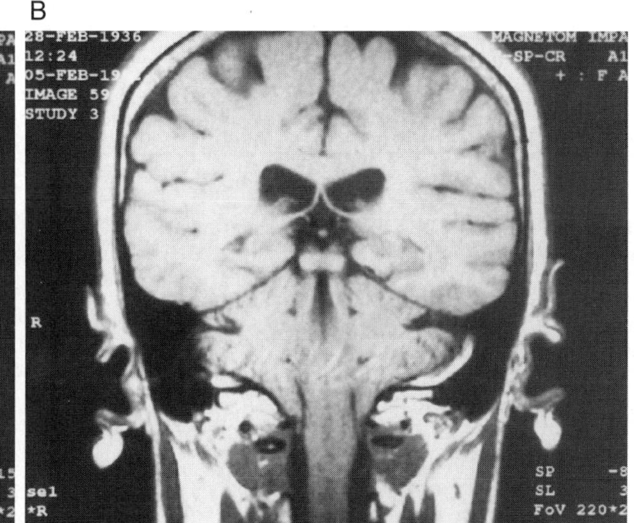

28-FEB-1936
12:24
IMAGE 59
STUDY 3
R
sel
*R

D

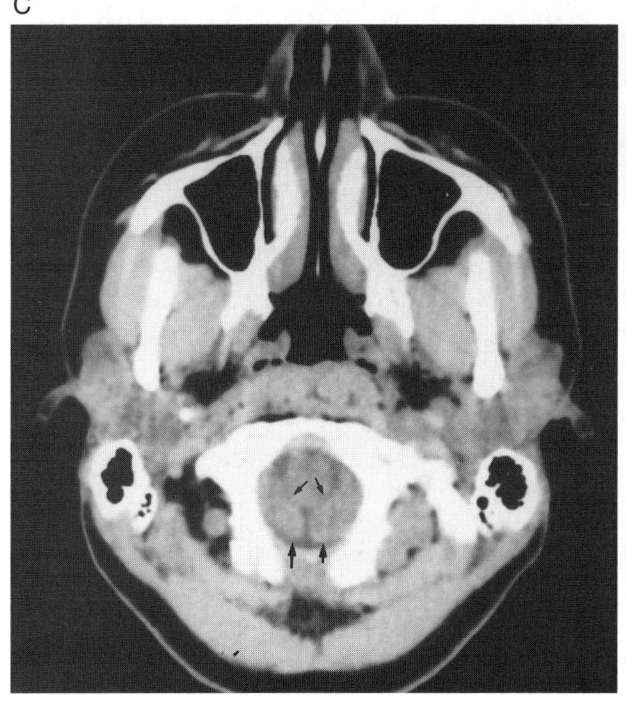

E

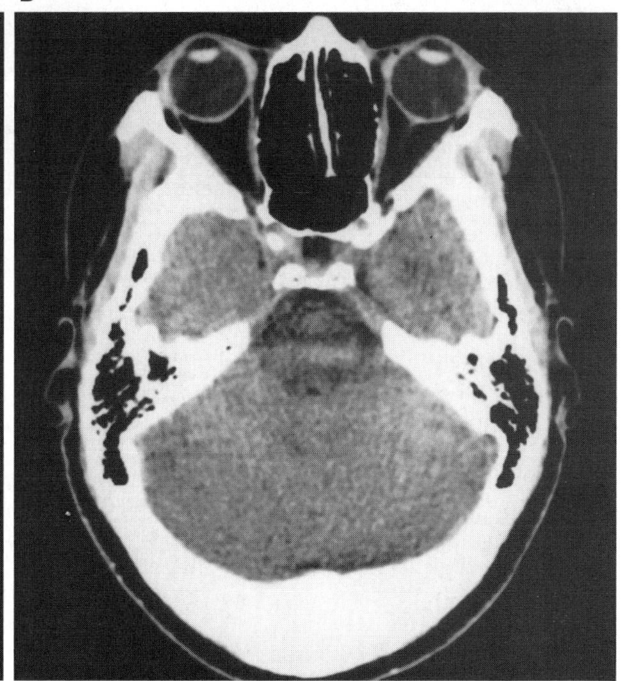

F

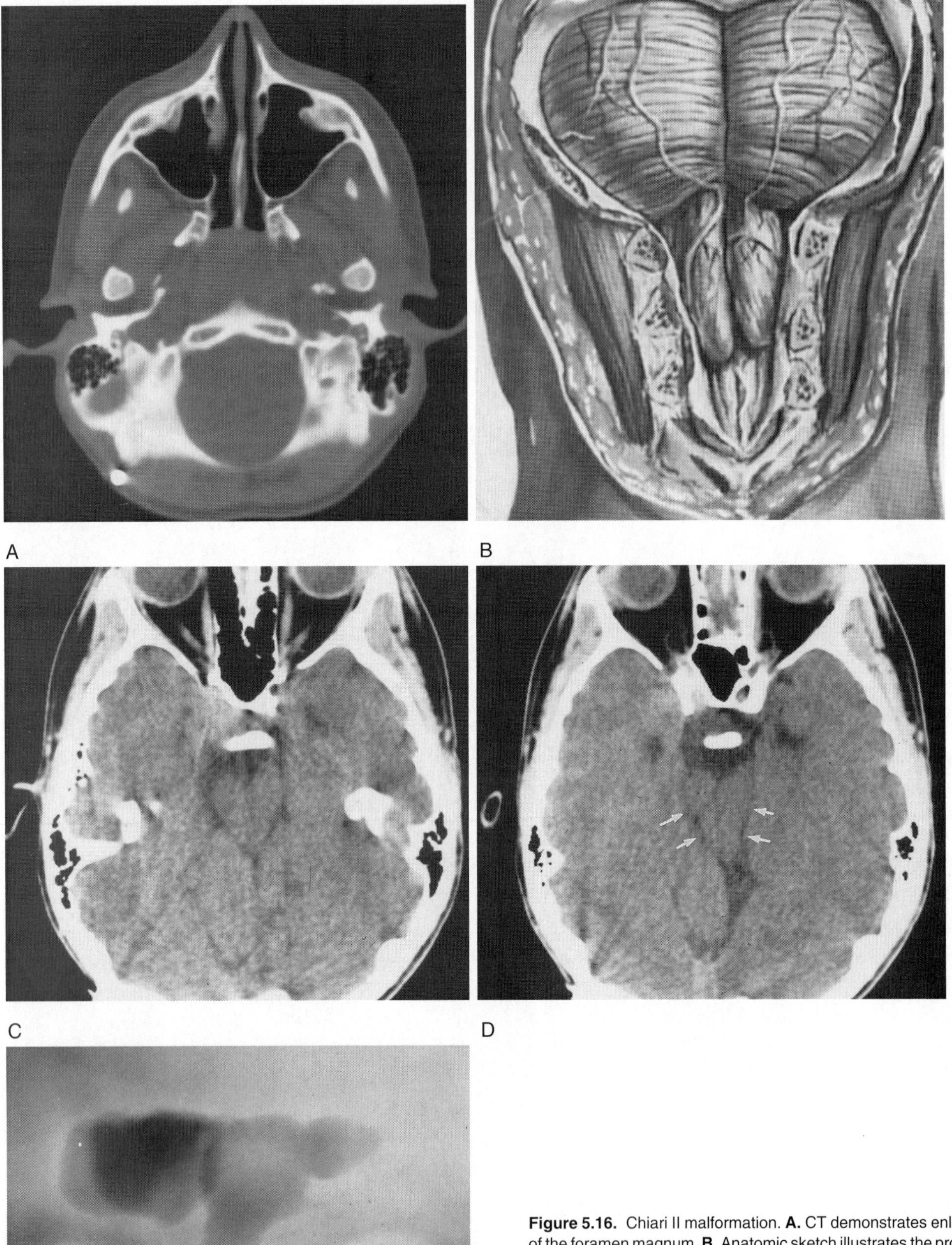

Figure 5.16. Chiari II malformation. **A.** CT demonstrates enlargement of the foramen magnum. **B.** Anatomic sketch illustrates the pronounced tonsillar herniation and elongation into the vertebral canal. (Courtesy of Dr. F. H. Netter and Ciba, New York.) **C.** Inverted flame shape of midbrain due to forward extension of upper cerebellum on both sides of the brainstem. **D.** CT slice at a higher level shows even greater deformity of the midbrain. **E.** Sagittal view from a pneumoencephalogram shows diverticula arising from the third ventricle anteriorly posteriorly above the infundibular and optic recesses of the third ventricle. These diverticula are usually not seen on CT or MR images of Chiari II malformation.

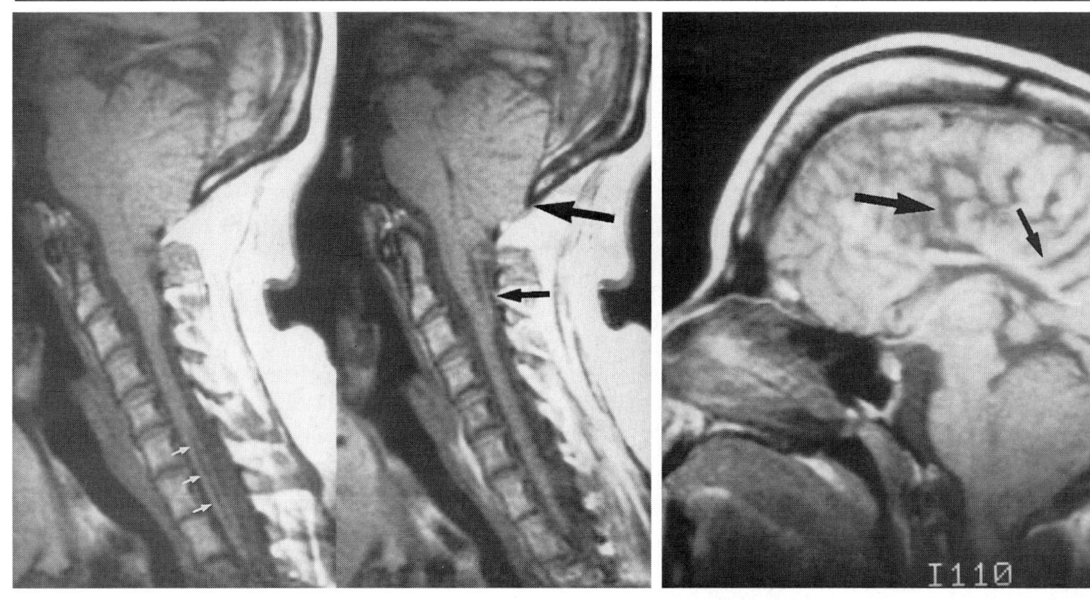

A B

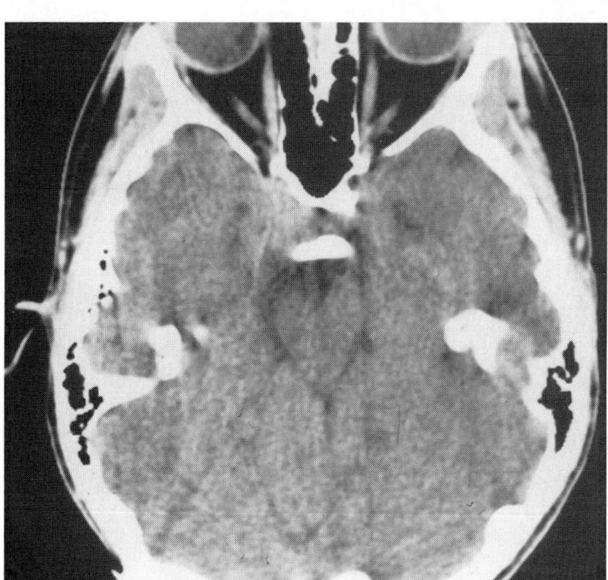

C

Figure 5.17. Chiari II malformation in 18-year-old girl. **A.** The sagittal view of the upper spine and posterior fossa shows that about one-fourth of the cerebellum extends through a wide foramen magnum and lies in the spinal canal (arrows). The fourth ventricle is low and elongated. Its outlet extends down to C2 (arrows on right image). On the left image there is evidence of a syringomyelia (small white arrows). **B.** A midline sagittal view of the head reveals that the corpus callosum is absent. Note that gyri and sulci on the medial hemisphere surface come down to the flat roof of the third ventricle (arrows). The posterior fossa is too small, and the cerebellum also protrudes upward. **C.** Axial view through the midbrain reveals that the cerebellum is wrapped around the brainstem (arrows) on both sides. This is not seen in B because it is a midsagittal section.

large, but more commonly it is small and sometimes not visible. The third ventricle may present diverticula, but these are not observed commonly on CT or MRI. Such changes were commonly observed when air studies (pneumoencephalography) were carried out.

In addition to the cerebellar changes, changes in the posterior fossa include partial or complete fusion of the quadrigeminal tubercles. The tentorium shows a wide incisura through which the upper portion of the cerebellum bulges upward above the tentorium. In addition, the falx is hypoplastic or shows some fenestrations or both.

Agenesis of the corpus callosum is fairly common in association with Chiari type II malformation. Partial or complete agenesis was present in 33 percent of the patients reported by Wolpert et al. (21).

Wolpert et al. also reported the presence of many thin gyri over the surface of the hemispheres, particularly in the medial side (21). They termed this finding *stenogyria*, indicating narrowing of the gyri of the brain. This name distinguishes the aberration from polymicrogyria, which, in addition to the multiple thin gyri, presents abnormal histology of the cerebral cortex. In the Chiari type II malformation, the cerebral cortex has a normal histology.

Naidich et al. also described an enlargement of the superior cerebellar cistern and of the subarachnoid space surrounding the upwardly displaced cerebellum (17–20). The same finding was observed frequently by Wolpert et al. (about 40 percent of their cases) (21).

The cause of the hydrocephalus is controversial. Some believe it is due to compression of the posterior brainstem

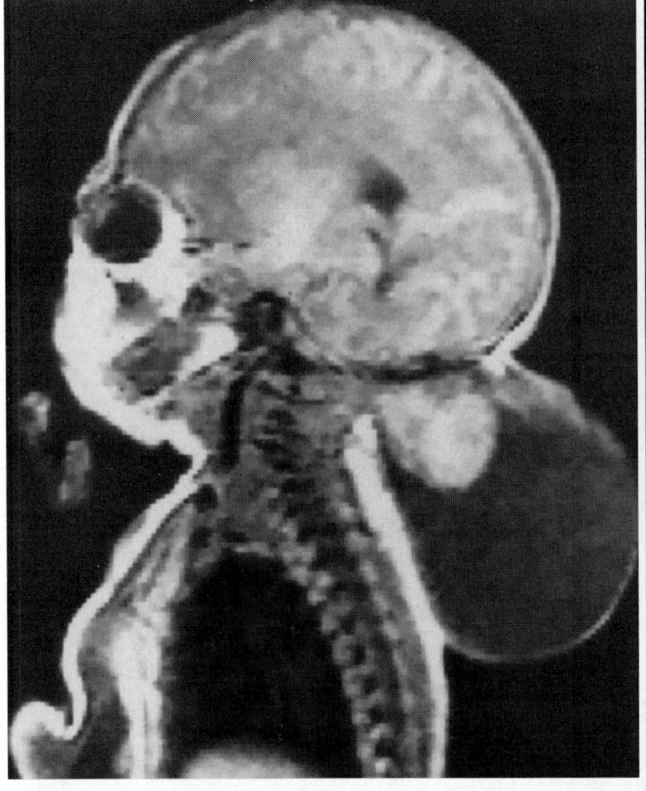

A

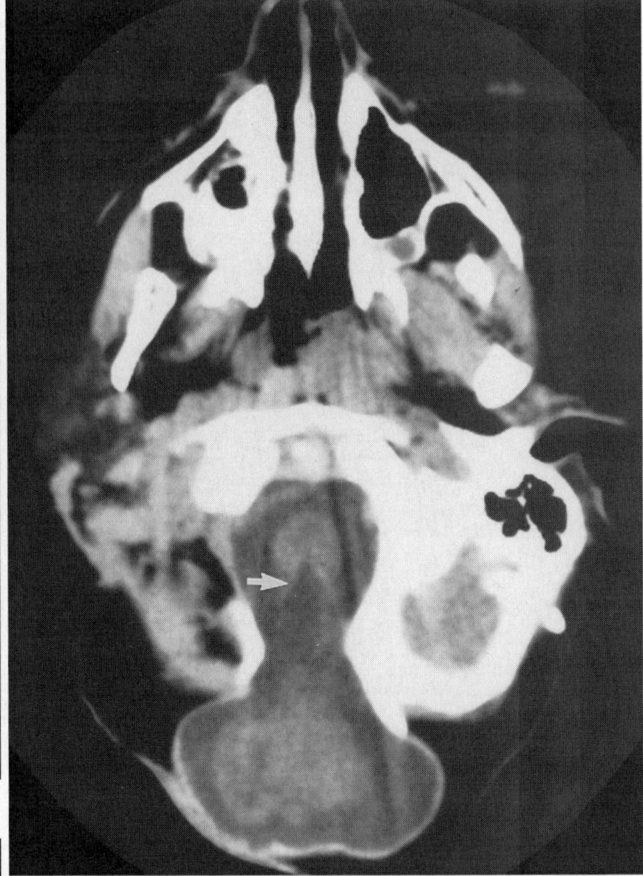

B

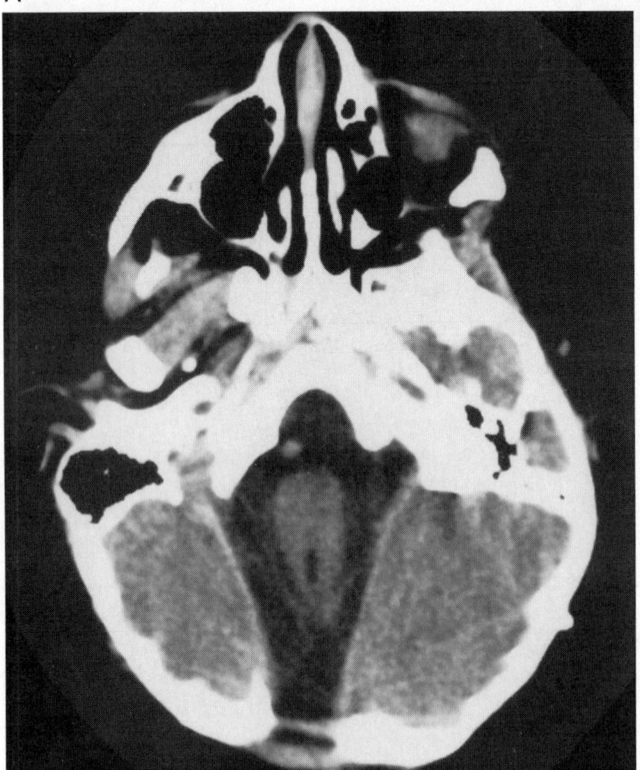

C

Figure 5.18. Chiari III malformation. **A.** Sagittal T1-weighted MR image shows an encephalomeningocele in the lower occipital area. The spinal cord in not shown, but there was evidence of syringohydromyelia. **B.** Axial T1-weighted image shows the cerebellum extending into the sac. The posterior aspect of the upper medulla presents an appearance suggestive of a large fourth ventricle (arrow). **C.** A higher cut shows the upper part of the fourth ventricle extending into the lower aspect of the midbrain, which is elongated as is common in the Chiari II malformation.

and aqueductal region by the various anomalies and narrowing of the posterior fossa. Others think the aqueduct is very small and usually short. The passage is open, however, and Yamada et al. found that the aqueduct was patent in all 65 patients studied with intraventricular water-soluble contrast agents (23).

The *Chiari type III malformation* is similar in many respects to the Chiari II malformation, but, in addition, the hindbrain herniates into a meningocele sac located posteriorly in the lower occipital–upper cervical spine region (Fig. 5.18). The brainstem may be buckled as if it were pulled by the other structures herniated into the encephalocele sac. This malformation is far less common than the Chiari type II malformation (Table 5.2).

OTHER CEREBELLAR ANOMALIES

In addition to the Chiari malformations we should consider partial agenesis involving one cerebellar hemisphere (Fig. 5.19) and anomalies of the vermis. Truwit et al. describe four anomalies involving the vermis: (1) the Dandy-Walker malformation, described in text following; (2) Joubert syndrome, consisting of hypoplasia or aplasia of the vermis but without a posterior fossa cyst; (3) tectocerebellar dysraphia, which in addition to vermian hypoplasia presents an occipital encephalocele with rotation of the brainstem and cerebellum around a vertical axis; and (4) rhombencephalosynapsis (24). This rare anomaly (only 19 cases reported up to 1991) consists of the absence of the vermis, fusion of the dentate nuclei which form a half-moon or horseshoe shape around the fourth ventricle, fusion of the superior cerebellar peduncles, and an abnormal cerebellum. The cerebellar sulci and gyri cross the midline transversely because of the absence of the vermis. In addition Truwit et al. describe fusion of the fornix in the midline (24). Sagittal MRI may demonstrate the fornix in continuity with the corpus callosum. Temporal lobe hypoplasia, as manifested by enlargement of the temporal horns, may be present. The septum pellucidum may be defective or absent. Other anomalies may coexist in some cases such as corpus callosum agenesis and gray matter heterotopias.

Table 5.2.
Chiari Malformations

Chiari I

Cerebellar tonsillar ectopia (>5 mm)
Associated findings
  Hydrocephalus
  Syringohydromyelia
  Craniocervical dysgenesis

Chiari II

Lumbosacral myelomeningocele
Small posterior fossa and large foramen magnum
Downward displacement of cerebellum, pons, medulla
Cervicomedullary "kink"
Anterolateral displacement of cerebellum around brainstem
Tectal "beaking"
Common associated findings
  Agenesis of the corpus callosum
  Hydrocephalus

Chiari III
Same findings as in Chiari II but with associated occipital/high cervical encephalocoele

Anomalies Occurring Between 5 and 10 Weeks of Gestation

HOLOPROSENCEPHALY

This anomaly is included in disorders of ventral induction by van der Knapp and Valk because it involves a failure in organ development induced on the ventral side and in the rostral end of the embryo from which the face and the brain develop (4). The malformation is also termed a *disorder of diverticulation* because the initial single ventricle failed to expand into both hemispheres. Holoprosencephaly implies an incomplete separation of the two cerebral hemispheres (Fig. 5.20). Because the degree of separation of the two hemispheres varies, the three terms *alobar*, *semilobar*, and *lobar* have been created.

The most severe form is the alobar type, in which separation of the two hemispheres is completely absent and a single ventricular cavity is somewhat shapeless. There are no sylvian fissures, lissencephaly is usually present, and the falx cerebri is totally absent.

In semilobar holoprosencephaly, the ventricles have some degree of separation, the temporal horns may be partly developed, and the thalami are usually nearly fused. A rudimentary third ventricle may be incorporated into the lateral ventricles, and the septum pellucidum is absent, as in all forms of holoprosencephaly.

Lobar holoprosencephaly is easier to identify on MRI, with axial as well as coronal views demonstrating the absent septum pellucidum and incorporation of the third ventricle into the lateral ventricles. There is usually some partial direct fusion of the white matter across the midline, and the falx cerebri is only partially present. The sylvian fissures may be partially formed, and some sulcation is present. The lateral angle of the lateral ventricle is usually squared (Table 5.3).

All forms of holoprosencephaly present hypotelorism, which tends to be more pronounced in the more severe forms, in which there may only be a single eye. In some children hypertelorism may be present. The olfactory bulbs and tracts are absent. There may also be defects in the face affecting the midline structures.

SEPTO-OPTIC DYSPLASIA (DE MORSIER SYNDROME)

This relatively recently recognized entity was originally described by de Morsier in 1956 (25). The defect is probably related embryologically to holoprosencephaly and consists of absence of the septum pellucidum and hypoplasia of the

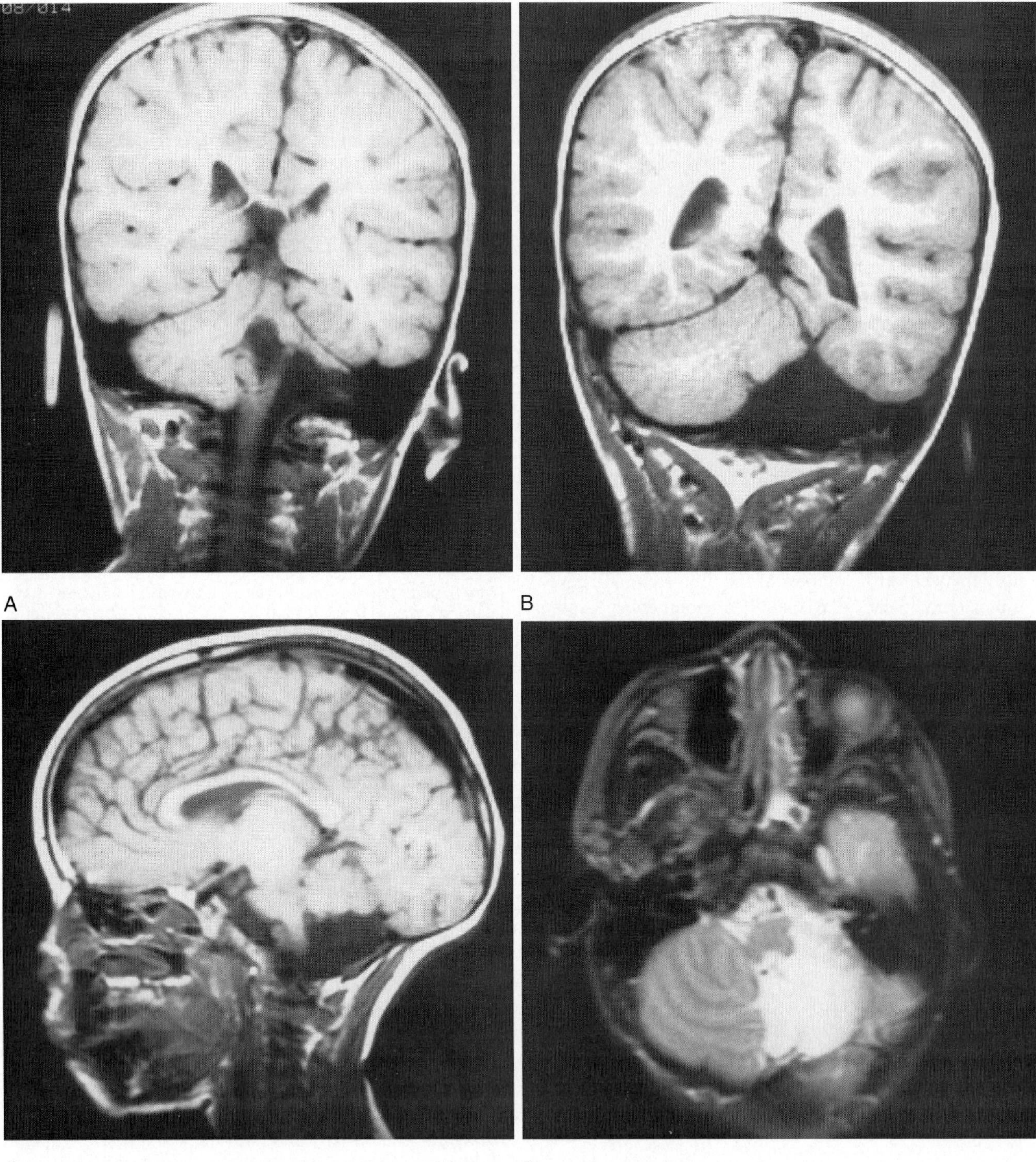

Figure 5.19. Partial cerebellar "agenesis" in 2-year-old girl. **A.** Coronal T1. The left side of the cerebellum is absent; the tentorium is lower on that side. **B.** A more dorsal T1-weighted section. The central portion of the cerebellum is present. **C.** A sagittal T1-weighted image just off the midline shows a segment of cerebellum in its upper segment (compare with B). **D.** T2-weighted axial. The left side shows only CSF intensity.

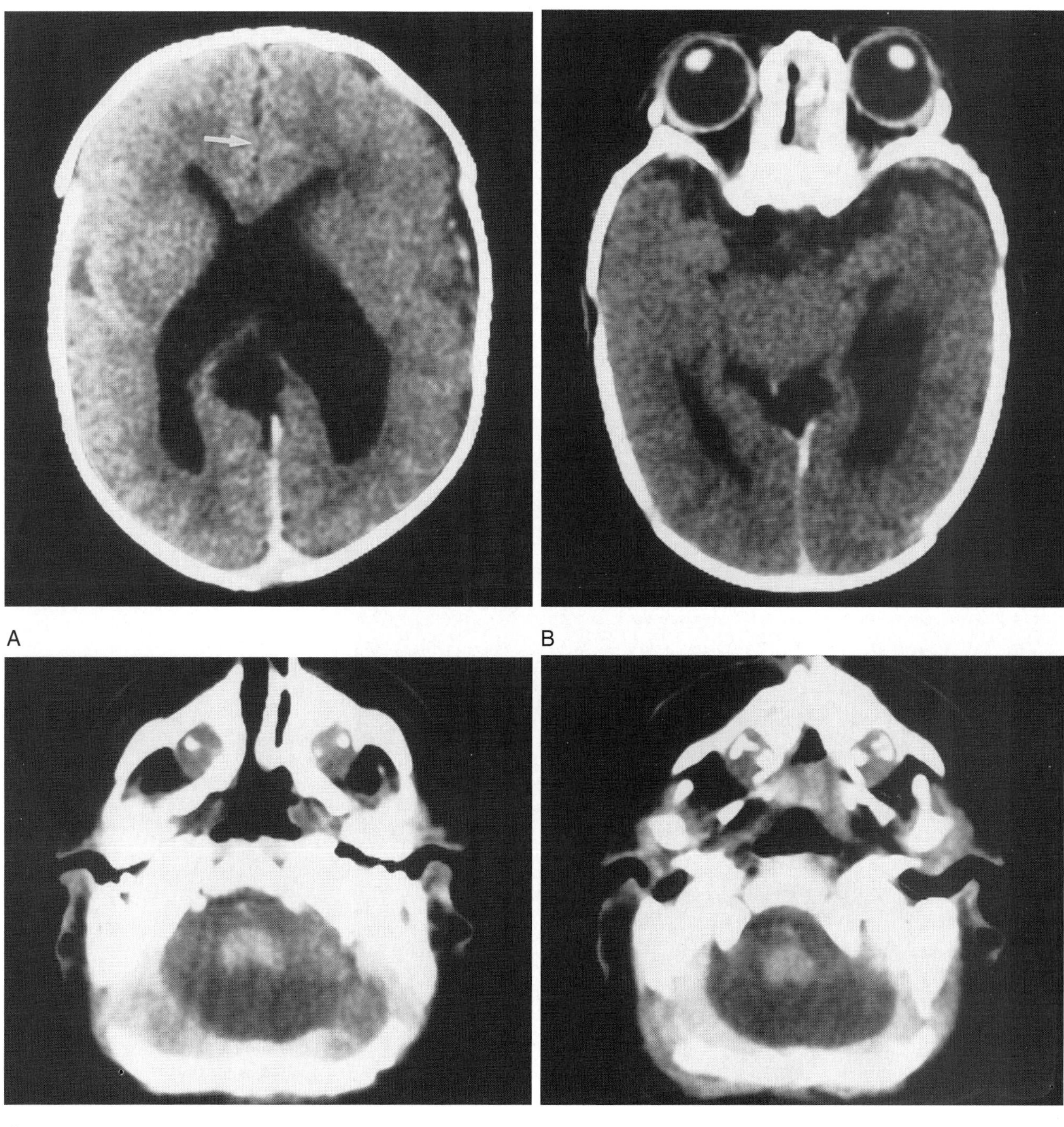

Figure 5.20. Lobar holoprosencephaly. **A.** Newborn with hypotelorism. The axial CT through the ventricles shows absent septum pellucidum, asymmetrically enlarged ventricles, and absent splenium of corpus callosum (note that the ventricular margin posteriorly abuts the CSF in cisterns). **B.** There is fusion between the thalami and the third ventricle. Rudimentary temporal horns are present. **C** and **D.** Sections through the posterior fossa failed to reveal a fourth ventricle or cerebellum, suggesting cerebellar agenesis. The interhemispheric fissure is incomplete (arrow), and the falx cerebri was only partially formed.

Table 5.3.
Holoprosencephaly

Definition	Types
Disorder of ventral induction with absent or incomplete separation of cerebral hemispheres	Alobar: absence of separation of cerebral hemispheres, single ventricular cavity Semilobar: partial separation of hemispheres and ventricles, fusion of thalamus Lobar: partial direct fusion of white matter across midline, absent septum pellucidum, partial absence of falx cerebri

optic chiasm and nerves (Fig. 5.21). Affected individuals are usually blind. According to Barkovich et al., the optic nerve and chiasm were not considered hypoplastic in about a third of their 77 patients (26). In addition, about half of their patients presented with schizencephaly. These cases were possibly not homogeneous and may represent variants of more than one congenital problem. Classification is often difficult. The ventricles may be normal or dilated. Barkovich et al. reported that white matter hypoplasia and ventricular enlargement are often seen on MRI in these patients (26). The falx cerebri is usually intact. The optic nerve atrophy may be difficult to demonstrate in the orbits because of the chemical shift artifact usually present due to the orbital fat. This appearance can be improved by use of a fat-suppression technique.

ABSENCE OF SEPTUM PELLUCIDUM

Agenesis of the septum pellucidum occurs in holoprosencephaly and in septo-optic dysplasia, but the septum pellucidum may be absent in association with schizencephaly and agenesis of the corpus callosum. Barkovich and Norman found an absent septum pellucidum in basal encephaloceles and in porencephaly/hydranencephaly (27). In addition, the septum pellucidum may be partially or completely absent in severe hydrocephalus. This is usually regarded as a rupture due to necrosis of the septum pellucidum with reabsorption. The septum pellucidum turns out to be an important structure, and when congenital absence takes place, it is usually associated with fairly severe anomalies. Its absence in the Chiari II malformation is due mostly to necrosis associated with chronic, severe hydrocephalus and not to congenital absence.

DIENCEPHALIC CYSTS

In this anomaly the considerably enlarged third ventricle bulges upward to reach the inner table of the skull in the

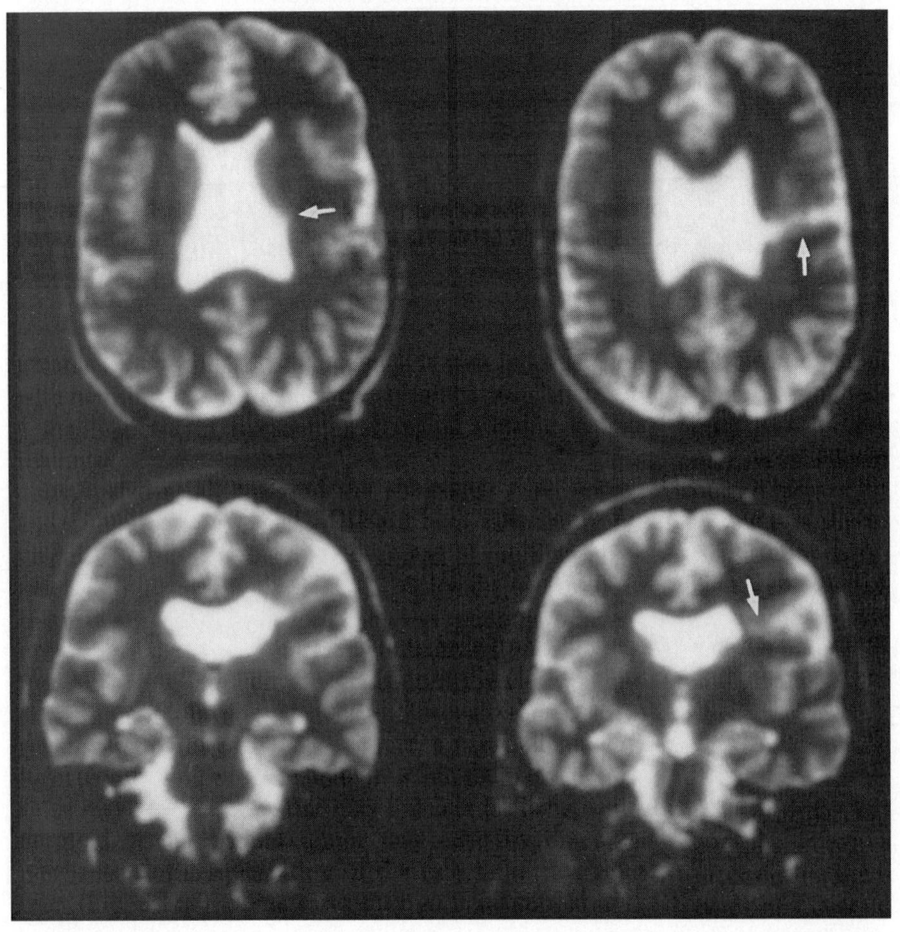

Figure 5.21. Septo-optic dysplasia (de Morsier syndrome). There is also a closed-lip schizencephaly. There is complete absence of the septum pellucidum in both axial and coronal planes. In addition, there is a bright tract going from the surface above the sylvian fissure to the ventricular wall typical of schizencephaly (closed-lip variety). In the axial image on the left, a slight bulge of the ventricular contour is seen (arrow). When this is visualized, particularly on axial CT images, a search for a closed-lip schizencephaly should be made (see also Fig. 5.28). (Courtesy of Dr. Tina Young-Poussaint, Boston, Massachusetts.)

parietal region. These cysts can be very large. They are invariably associated with agenesis of the corpus callosum, and while some believe that is a different entity (28), the association with agenesis of the corpus callosum would make this most likely a variant of the same entity (see Figs. 5.31 and 5.32). Two of the cases reported by Brocklehurst and Chir presented a scalp cyst that seemed to connect with the diencephalic cyst and was lined by fibrous tissue and not by ependyma.

OTHER ANOMALIES

Such disorders as cerebral hemihypoplasia/aplasia, lobar hypoplasia/aplasia, cerebellar hypoplasia/aplasia, and cerebellar vermis hypoplasia/aplasia are rare, and their causes are not known. One might consider an early insult involving the arteries or some inflammatory process.

DANDY-WALKER SYNDROME

Dandy-Walker syndrome is a congenital cystic dilatation of the fourth ventricle, which is presumably due to congenital atresia of the foramen of Magendie and foramina of Luschka. Cases have been reported in which some air entered the fourth ventricle during pneumoencephalography. Assuming that these were cases of Dandy-Walker syndrome, we must suspect patency of the foramina of Luschka on one or both sides. There is some degree of cerebellar hypoplasia, particularly when the lower vermis is absent. This entity is listed here because the developmental aberration which produces it may occur somewhere between the seventh and tenth weeks of gestation. However, others think it occurs between the third and fourth month or between the ninth and fourteenth weeks (29). In the first 3 months after birth, hydrocephalus is not significant, but after 3 months progressive dilatation of the ventricles leads to enlargement of the head and ultimately to the diagnosis. Associated brain malformations are frequently found, particularly agenesis of the corpus callosum and occipital encephaloceles. An interesting malformation associated with Dandy-Walker syndrome is facial angioma. Other systemic anomalies often coexist in the cardiovascular system, the most frequent of which are the cardiac septal defects. Familial cases of Dandy-Walker syndrome have been reported but are not common.

On plain lateral views of the skull, children with Dandy-Walker malformation present evidence of a high position of the groove of the lateral sinuses, which is higher than the lambda. As is well known, the torcular Herophili is well below the lambda, and the lateral sinuses start from the torcular and extend to the sigmoid sinuses and jugular fossa. The grooves of the lateral sinuses may not be formed well enough to be visible on plain films in a young child. However, the appearance of a large posterior fossa may be quite evident (Table 5.4).

CT or MRI shows the presence of a large cyst posterior to the brainstem and no evidence of a fourth ventricle.

Table 5.4.
Posterior Fossa Cystic Abnormalities

Dandy-Walker malformation
- Cystic dilatation of the fourth ventricle
- High position of tentorium
- Cerebellar vermian hypoplasia or aplasia
- Hydrocephalus
- Associated findings
  - Agenesis of the corpus callosum
  - Occipital encephalocele
  - Facial angioma

Dandy-Walker variant
- Cystic dilatation of the fourth ventricle
- Cerebellar vermian hypoplasia
- Normal size of posterior fossa
- Lesser degree of hydrocephalus than in Dandy-Walker malformation

Enlarged cisterna magna
- Large cisterna magna with normal fourth ventricle
- No associated cerebellar abnormalities of hydrocephalus

There is usually hypoplasia of the cerebellar hemispheres and an absence of the lower vermis. The cyst may grow very large posteriorly, and the remnant of the cerebellum can then be displaced forward. Hydrocephalus is usually present after 3 months of age, and the aqueduct is usually open. Contrast medium injected into the lateral ventricles will fill the cyst. The imperforate foramen of Magendie will allow a caudal bulging of the membrane of the cyst, which then projects into the spinal canal (Fig. 5.22). MRI is preferable because sagittal views demonstrate the relationships to better advantage.

The Dandy-Walker variants are related to the Dandy-Walker malformations, but they do not produce the degree of obstructive hydrocephalus that is seen in Dandy-Walker cyst. Axial and sagittal views demonstrate a direct connection of a fairly normal size or slightly enlarged fourth ventricle, absence of the lower vermis with enlargement of the vallecula, and a fairly large cystic space filled with CSF behind the cerebellum. This area freely communicates with the ventricular system, and hydrocephalus may not occur although some ventricular dilatation may well be present (Fig. 5.23).

A condition from which this entity must be differentiated is an *enlarged cisterna magna*. When an enlarged cisterna magna is present, the fourth ventricle and the vallecula are normal; the cerebellum does not give the impression of being in any way compressed or displaced. The posterior fossa is evidently more capacious than usual in these patients, and the large cistern extends to reach the undersurface of the tentorium. Occasionally, a defect in the tentorium allows the large cisterna magna to bulge upward to a certain extent (Fig. 5.24).

PREMATURE CRANIOSYNOSTOSIS

This anomaly belongs in this group because it occurs around the sixth to eighth week of gestation. It is described under the skull.

Figure 5.22. Dandy-Walker cysts in 6-day-old infant with a large head. **A.** Ultrasound revealed a large cystic structure in posterior fossa. **B.** CT cross section through the posterior fossa cysts. **C.** Axial section through the upper portion of the cyst reveals extreme degree of hydrocephalus. The cyst has a wall surrounded by thin cerebellar tissue. **D.** Reformatted sagittal view shows the extension of the cyst through the tentorial inisura and down the spinal canal. The anatomy of the brainstem is totally distorted. **E.** Only a day after surgery, the cyst has collapsed; the brain tissue in the frontal region has regained thickness, and the frontal horns are much smaller.

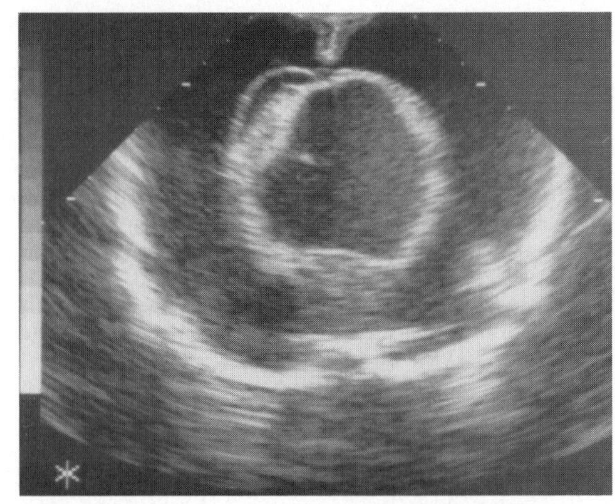

A

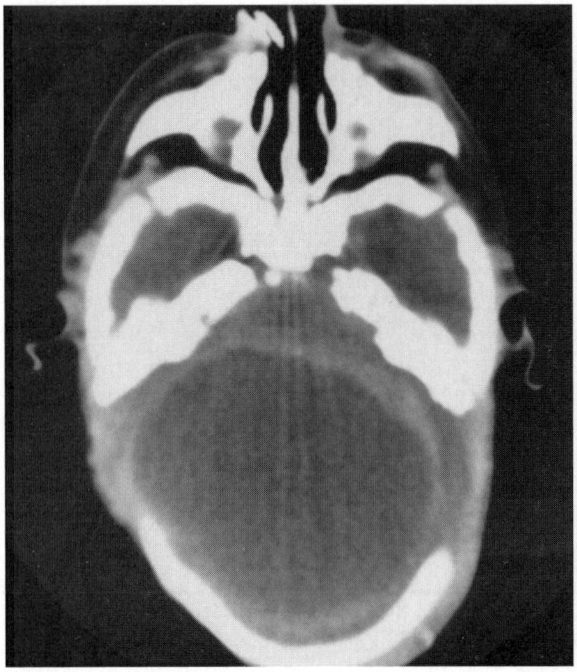

B

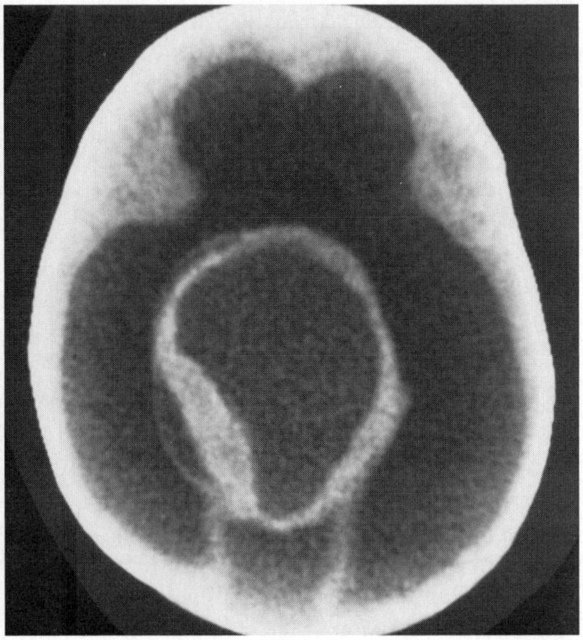

C

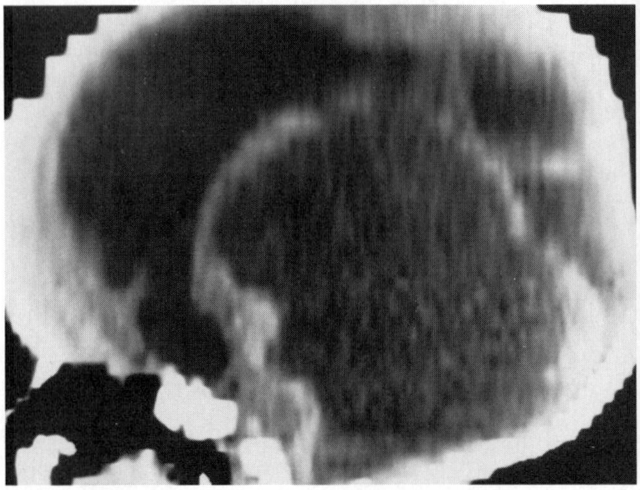

D

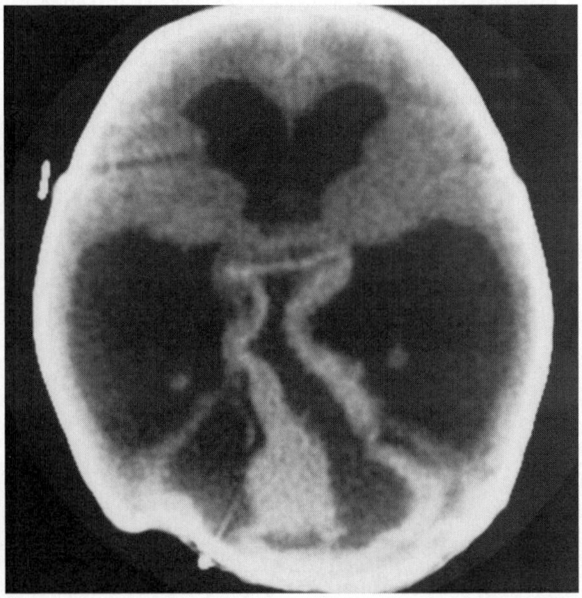

E

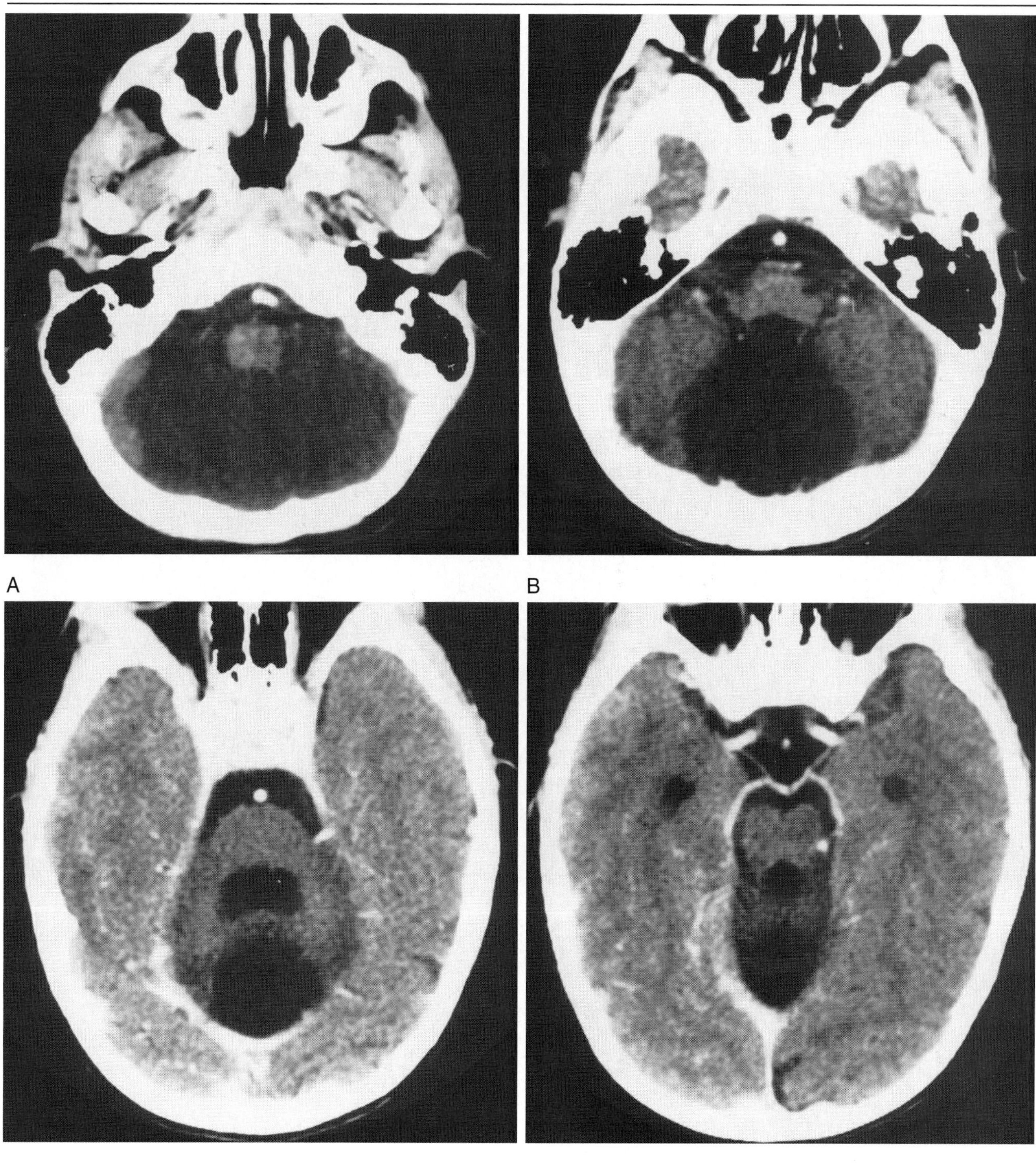

Figure 5.23. Dandy-Walker variant or posterior fossa arachnoid cyst in a 5-year-old boy. **A.** On axial CT, there is a large cystic space displacing the lower cerebellum laterally. **B.** The cyst becomes more circumscribed above A. The fourth ventricle seems to be directly continuous with the cyst. **C.** The fourth ventricle is now separated from the cysts and is enlarged. Contrast had been given and shows enhancement of the tentorium as well as of veins at the tentorial edge. **D.** The higher section shows the cysts reaching the top of the cerebellum and indenting it. Because of the apparent direct connection with the fourth ventricle, a Dandy-Walker variant is the preferred diagnosis. However, a cystogram was not performed. MRI is preferred to image these cysts and anomalies. For instance, the configuration at the foramen of Magendie cannot be shown well by CT except by reformatting, which yields less detailed sharpness (see Fig. 5.22).

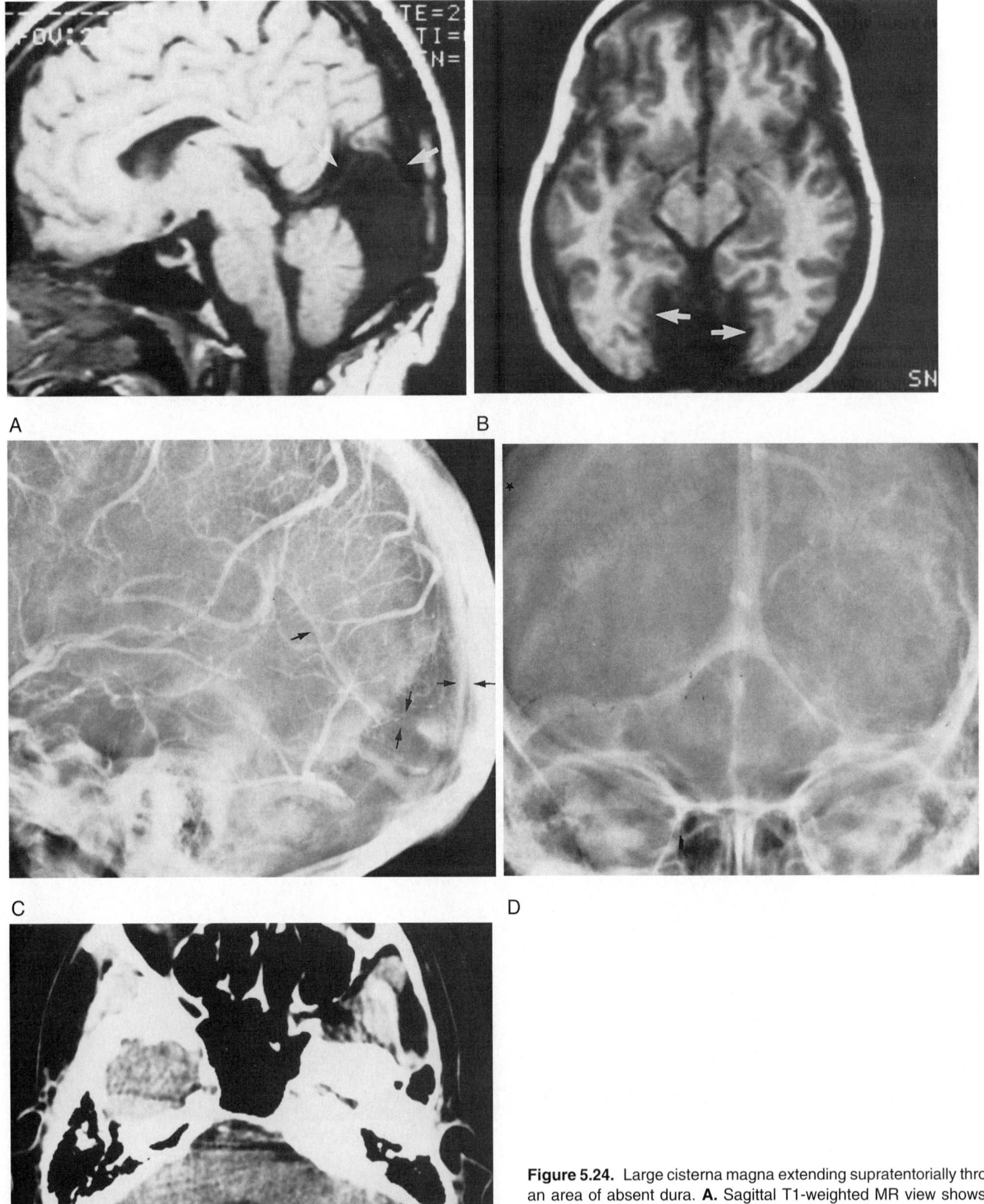

Figure 5.24. Large cisterna magna extending supratentorially through an area of absent dura. **A.** Sagittal T1-weighted MR view shows the larger cisterna magna and the upward transtentorial extension (arrows). There is no connection with any adjacent subarachnoid cisterns. The cisterna magna, on its upper aspect, is an isolated pouch behind the cerebellum and varies in size between individuals. **B.** Axial view shows lateral displacement of the occipital lobes (arrows). **C** and **D.** Venous phase (in another patient) from an angiogram demonstrates the separation of the venous flow in the posterior straight and sagittal sinuses into two channels, and absent torcular Herophili (arrows). Various degrees of cisterna magna enlargement are common. The great majority do not extend above the tentorium. **E.** Another example of simple large cisterna magna.

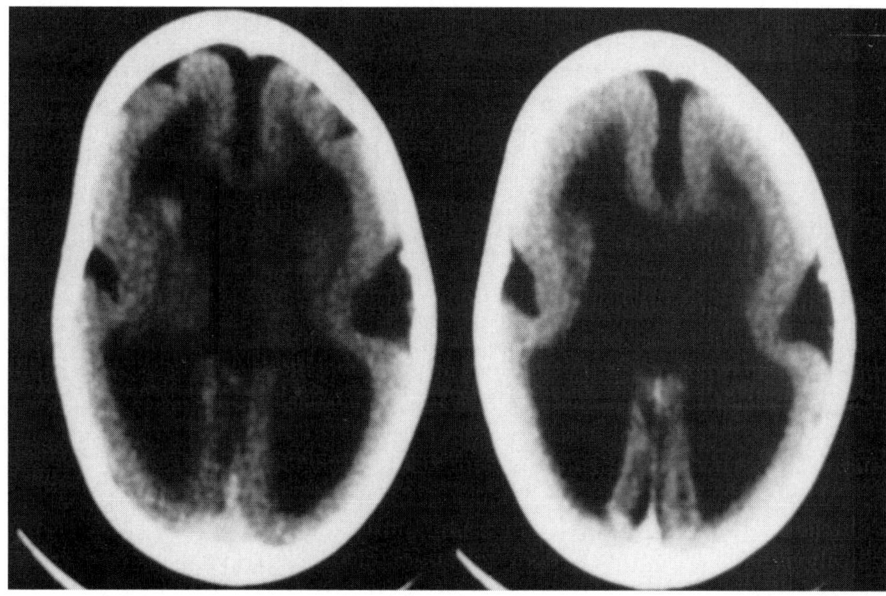

Figure 5.25. Lissencephaly. There is complete absence of cerebral sulci and gyri. There also is marked ventricular dilatation. The triangular dark shadows on each side represent a rudimentary sylvian fissure. Only in the frontal area in the image on the left can we see what look like sulci. (Courtesy of Dr. Tina Young-Poussaint, Boston, Massachusetts.)

Anomalies Occurring between 2 to 5 Months of Gestation

DISORDERS OF CELL MIGRATION

As expressed earlier, migration of cells from the germinal matrix represents a movement of neuroblasts across the white matter to form the gray matter of the brain cortex as well as the basal ganglia nuclei. Because this process is complex and is spread over a fairly long period of time, unfavorable factors may affect it.

Lissencephaly

The most severe failure of normal migration leads to essentially a smooth brain surface without gyri or with abnormally wide gyri (pachygyria) in some areas of the brain. Affected infants are severely retarded and usually do not live beyond 2 years. The anatomic configuration is really a spectrum in which various degrees of formation of abnormal gyri are present. All of the cortex is histologically abnormal, containing only four layers of cells instead of the usual six layers.

Lissencephaly may be a genetic disorder, some components of which can be found in siblings. Several syndromes have been described in lissencephaly. Byrd et al. described three types (30). In type I, the most common form is the so-called Miller-Dieker syndrome, which results from deletion of a part of chromosome 17. Type II lissencephaly is associated with a large head because of hydrocephalus, whereas an infant with type III lissencephaly has a small head. CT and MRI show either complete absence of gyri with a smooth brain surface, possibly with a rudimentary sylvian fissure, or some wide gyri, in which case the diagnosis is lissencephaly with pachygyria (Fig. 5.25, Table 5.5).

The Walker-Warburg syndrome consists of lissencephaly, congenital muscular dystrophy, and cerebellar and retinal malformations. The cerebellar malformations may be vermis hypoplasia and Dandy-Walker (present in 50 percent of patients). The disease is inherited as an autosomal recessive trait. The infant reported by Rhodes et al. died on the fifth day after birth (31). The brain presents a relatively smooth surface prior to the thirtieth week of gestation (3).

Table 5.5
Neuronal Migration Abnormalities

Lissencephaly
Most severe form of neuronal migration abnormality
Agyria or pachygyria
Pachygyria
Broad, flat gyri with shallow sulci
Polymicrogyria
Small gyri with shallow sulci
Difficult to diagnose by CT/MRI, and may be confused with pachygyria
Schizencephaly
Pia/ependyma—lined cleft extending from cortex to ventricular wall
"Open-lip" and "closed-lip" varieites exist
May be unilateral or bilateral
Cortical dysplasias
Abnormal formation, thickening, or infolding of cortical gyri
Cortical heterotopia
Abnormal gray matter foci, which may be found at any point from the subendymal lining to subcortical white matter

Pachygyria

This malformation is probably not a different entity but part of a spectrum related to failure of normal germinal matrix cell migration. By CT and particularly by MRI, broad, flat gyri are separated by shallow sulci. The entire brain may be thus configured, or the signs may be localized. Pachygyria is usually considered a somewhat less severe malformation than lissencephaly. Affected infants may live somewhat longer but always with severely retarded development.

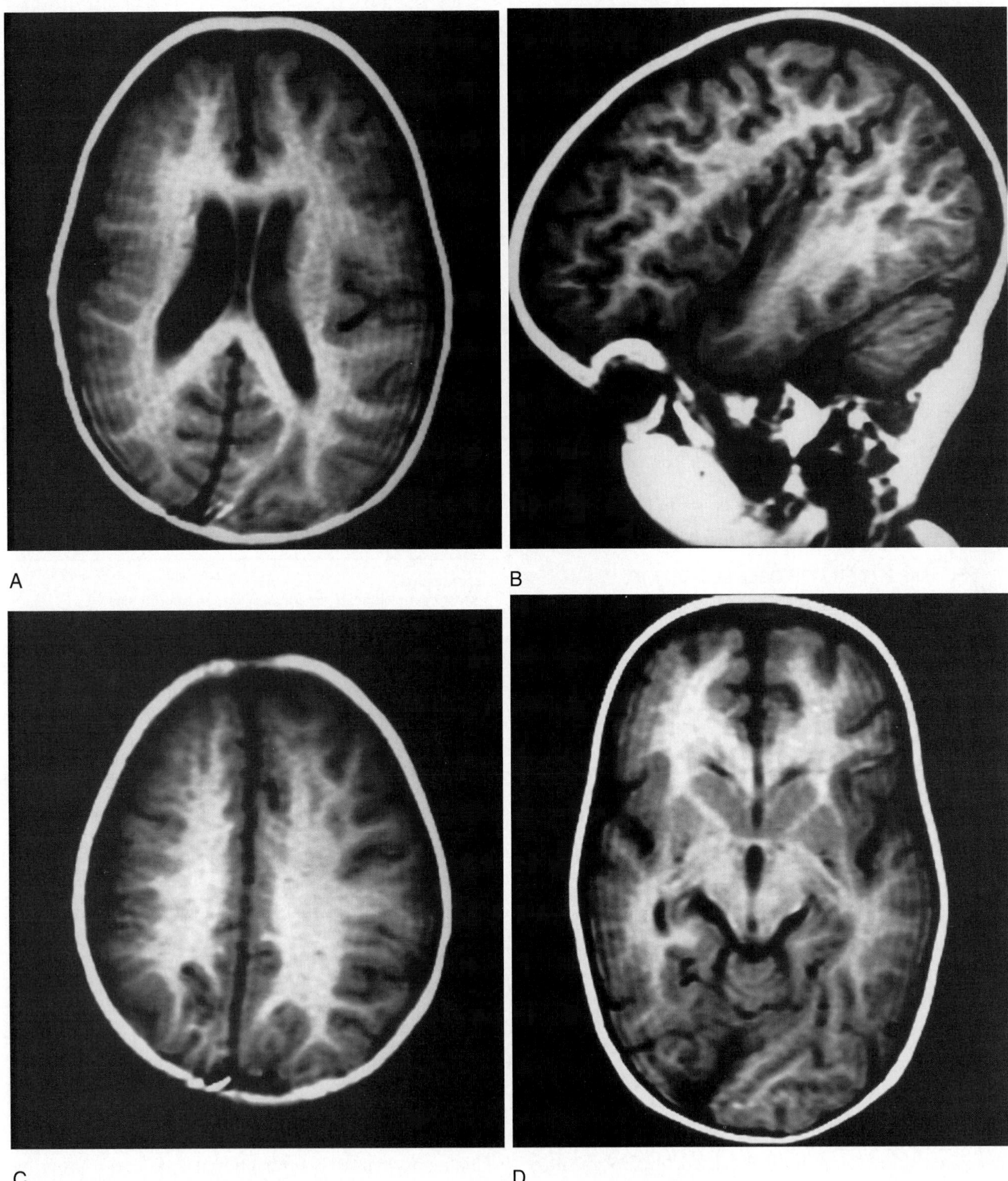

Figure 5.26. Polymicrogyria in a 2-year-old child with a seizure disorder, developmental delay, and hepatitis. **A.** The increased number of gray matter gyri on the right side as compared with the left hemisphere is evident. The sylvian fissure is not seen on the right at this level. **B.** The right-sided microgyria is also present lower down in the hemisphere, as well as higher up (**C**) compared with the left. **D.** The right anomalous sylvian fissure area shows the polymicrogyria. (Courtesy of Dr. Tina Young-Poussaint, Boston, Massachusetts.)

Infants with lissencephaly and pachygyria usually have severe seizures. Pachygyria is difficult to diagnose by CT or MRI.

Polymicrogyria

Unlike the previous two disorders, this disorder causes many small, thin, relatively shallow sulci dividing thin gyri (Fig. 5.26). On imaging studies, it may be difficult to see the separate small gyri because the sulci are so thin that there may be adhesions between the surfaces of the small gyri so that they are bunched together. They may even be confused with pachygyria on imaging studies. The areas involved by polymicrogyria are sometimes unilateral and small, and other times they may be bilateral and symmetric. When the area involved is the motor cortex, the pyramidal tracts are absent or severely stunted and spastic diplegia is present clinically (32).

Polymicrogyria may affect only one hemisphere and be associated with a hemiplegia similar to that produced by vascular occlusions occurring just before birth or at birth. The brain cortex may have a four-layered histologic configuration, or it may have other histologic abnormalities that may not be readily recognized.

CT and MRI diagnosis can be difficult for the reasons indicated earlier. The ability to do sagittal and coronal views makes MRI superior to CT examinations. Usually the cingulate gyrus, the calcarine cortex, and hippocampus are spared. Sometimes the small gyri are bunched around the sylvian fissure, which may have a more vertical position than is usually the case.

Schizencephaly

In this abnormality, a cleft in the brain extends from the cortex to the ventricular wall and is covered by pia and ependyma along its path. At one point the pia and ependyma form a seam. The term was introduced by Yakovlev and Wadsworth in 1946 (33,34). A number of theories have attempted to describe the pathogenesis of this condition. Clinically these patients may have relatively minimal to marked disability. They may be retarded and have abnormal motor function and seizures. The retardation can be relatively mild. The clefts usually occur around the central gyrus, slightly in front or in back, and the anomaly is usually bilateral. Polymicrogyria may be present around these clefts.

Two major types were originally described by Yakovlev and Wadsworth as open-lip and closed-lip schizencephaly (33,34) (Figs. 5.27 and 5.28). According to Barkovich et al., the lesion can be unilateral more often than might have been suggested by the pathology literature (35). The unilateral variety may be encephaloclastic, meaning that it may be acquired after formation of these structures but is produced by a vascular or inflammatory event. In this respect the anomaly resembles other acquired processes. Differentiation of unilateral schizencephaly with a postnatal destructive lesion such as porencephaly or large hemispheric infarcts is based on the fact that the edges of the cleft contain gray matter that can be followed along the two sides of the cleft, particularly by MRI. It is important to try to differentiate these two conditions because a disorder of cell migration may be repeated in different forms in siblings with a frequency of 5 to 20 percent.

Barkovich and Kjos have tried to correlate the severity of the clinical findings with the MRI characteristics (36). It turned out that the bilateral open-lip patients had a worse prognosis for speech and intellectual function, and those with unilateral open lip had a worse prognosis than those with unilateral closed lip.

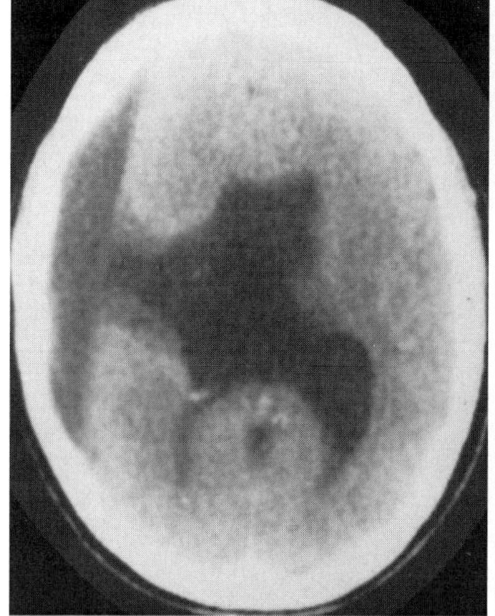

A

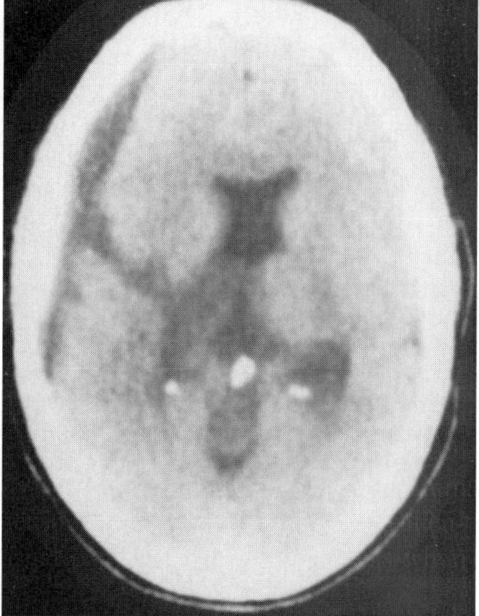

B

Figure 5.27. Open-lip schizencephaly. **A** and **B.** CT scan. There is ventricular enlargement and a broad connection between the ventricle and the subarachnoid space, which in this case is associated with an extracerebral CSF space. The right ventricle presents an outpouching extending laterally at the start of the transcerebral open track.

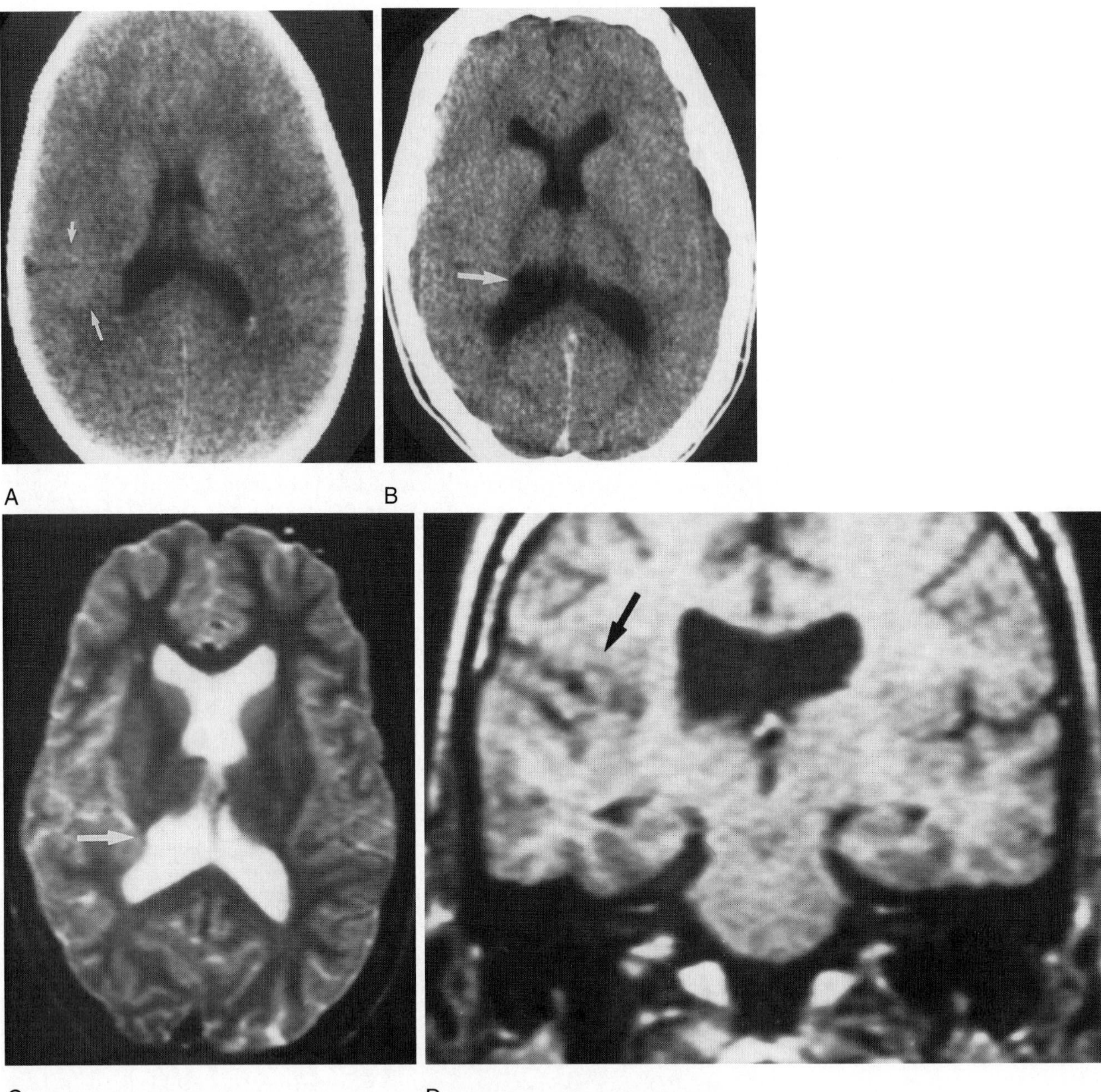

Figure 5.28. Closed-lip schizencephaly. **A.** CT axial. At the site of the junction of the transcerebral track with the ventricle there is a slight outpouching with local enlargement of the transverse diameter of ventricle. The presence of such outpouching alone in the same ventricular area should raise the question of closed-lip schizencephaly. **B** and **C.** Another patient in which a lateral outpouching of the lateral ventricular wall in the atrial region is seen on CT and MRI but without a clear-cut transcerebral track being observed. **D.** The coronal image clearly reveals a track above a somewhat caudally displaced sylvian fissure. The track is covered by gray matter on both sides; this is apparent in both the CT in A (arrows) and on the MR coronal image (black arrow).

The closed-lip schizencephaly may be difficult to see in some patients, and it may require not only axial but also coronal views (Fig. 5.28).

Porencephaly

The term *porencephaly* applies to the presence of an empty space within brain tissue that may or may not communicate with a ventricle (Fig. 5.29). Originally the term was applied to schizencephaly, but since the work of Yakovlev and Wadsworth, the latter was separated as a different entity (33, 34). Porencephaly describes a destructive process in the brain that could occur in utero as a result of some vascular or infectious injury. The injury could also occur after birth as the result of birth trauma, vascular occlusion, or infection. In fact, today the term *porencephaly* is applied to any focal dilatation of the lateral ventricles. This usage implies that the cavity in the brain is directly and broadly connected with the ventricular system.

A membrane may rarely separate the intraparenchymal cystic space from the ventricle, or a narrow communication between the cystic space and the ventricle may increase the pressure of the porencephalic cyst in relation to the ventricular pressure. This dynamic could make the cystic space grow in size with the passage of time.

Contrast material injected into the ventricles or into the subarachnoid space in the lumbar region may or may not fill the cystic space. If there is no filling, surgical establishment of a communication may be advisable, or preferably, the cystic space may be shunted. If it freely communicates with the ventricle, the chances are this static situation is related to destruction of brain tissue. In the presence of long-standing increased intraventricular pressure, true diverticula could occur in the suprapineal recess of the third ventricle, in the medial aspect of the atrium of the lateral ventricle, or, more rarely, in other locations.

Cortical Dysplasias

Cortical dysplasias may be found in children with retarded development who do not fit exactly into the classically recognized pathologic entities such as lissencephaly and schizencephaly. The lesions, presumably caused by abnormal neuronal migration, consist of relative failure of gyral formation, of focal thickening, or of abnormal infolding of the cortex. They may have overly deep sulci focally or, on the contrary, shallow sulci. While the majority of patients designated as having cortical dysplasias by Barkovich and Kjos (37) probably presented with polymicrogyria and/or pachygyria, evaluation of these pathologic conditions is rather poor by CT or MRI. As might be expected, the worse functional prognosis was in the patients who presented with bilateral diffuse cortical dysplasia. Frontal lobe involvement in the focal group was most often associated with spastic motor deficiency. The majority presented seizures, often very poorly controlled. Because the possibility of surgical intervention exists in these focal abnormalities, it is important to attempt to classify them according to Barkovich and Kjos.

Gray Matter Heterotopia

This disorder of cell migration is well known pathologically. Pneumoencephalographic diagnosis was first reported by Bergeron, who demonstrated the subependymal nodularity varying from a few millimeters to 1 to 2 cm in size (38,39). These do not grow upon later reexamination and do not calcify, such as may be seen in tuberous sclerosis. However, the abnormal gray matter masses may also be found subcortically as focal accumulations or as diffuse subcortical heterotopias (5). In the original report by Bergeron, only severely retarded children were included (38). In the recent report by Barkovich and Kjos, however, the patients with severe anatomic anomalies were excluded; thus their eight patients with subependymal heterotopia had normal speech, and six of the eight had normal intelligence (5).

MRI is preferred because gray matter isodensity in all sequences allows greater assurance that the abnormal accumulations are gray matter. On the other hand, the patients with subcortical nodular or diffuse heterotopias had a higher incidence of delayed developmental and motor impairment. A seizure disorder was present in almost all cases. The age at the time of diagnosis tended to be higher in the subependymal group than in the subcortical heterotopia group. MRI demonstrates small gray matter masses adjacent to and projecting into the ventricular lumen in the subependymal group (Fig. 5.30 and 5.33). In the subcortical group, gray matter masses are seen subcortically and sometimes a gyral pattern with subarachnoid sulci can be seen (5) (Fig. 5.30). In the diffuse heterotopias, sheets or bands of gray matter can be identified. Occasionally a large mass of heterotopic gray matter measuring several centimeters in diameter may suggest a neoplasm. The most disabling clinical manifestations may be intractable seizures, and diagnosis by imaging methods may permit a planned surgical approach. Incomplete gray matter band–heterotopia may also occur (40).

Kallman Syndrome

Kallman syndrome (KS) is clinically characterized by hypogonadotropic hypogonadism and accompanying anosmia or hyposmia. Patients present eunuchoidism, delayed puberty, gynecomastia, and microphali. KS occurs most frequently in males (1 in 10,000 births), with a male-female ratio of 4 to 1. It is a hereditary condition, and transmission can occur as an autosomal dominant, recessive, or X-linked pattern (41). It has been isolated to the Xp 22.3 portion of the X chromosome.

MRI may demonstrate absence of the olfactory bulbs, particularly well seen on coronal T1-weighted images. In addition, asymmetry of the olfactory sulci may be seen (41–45).

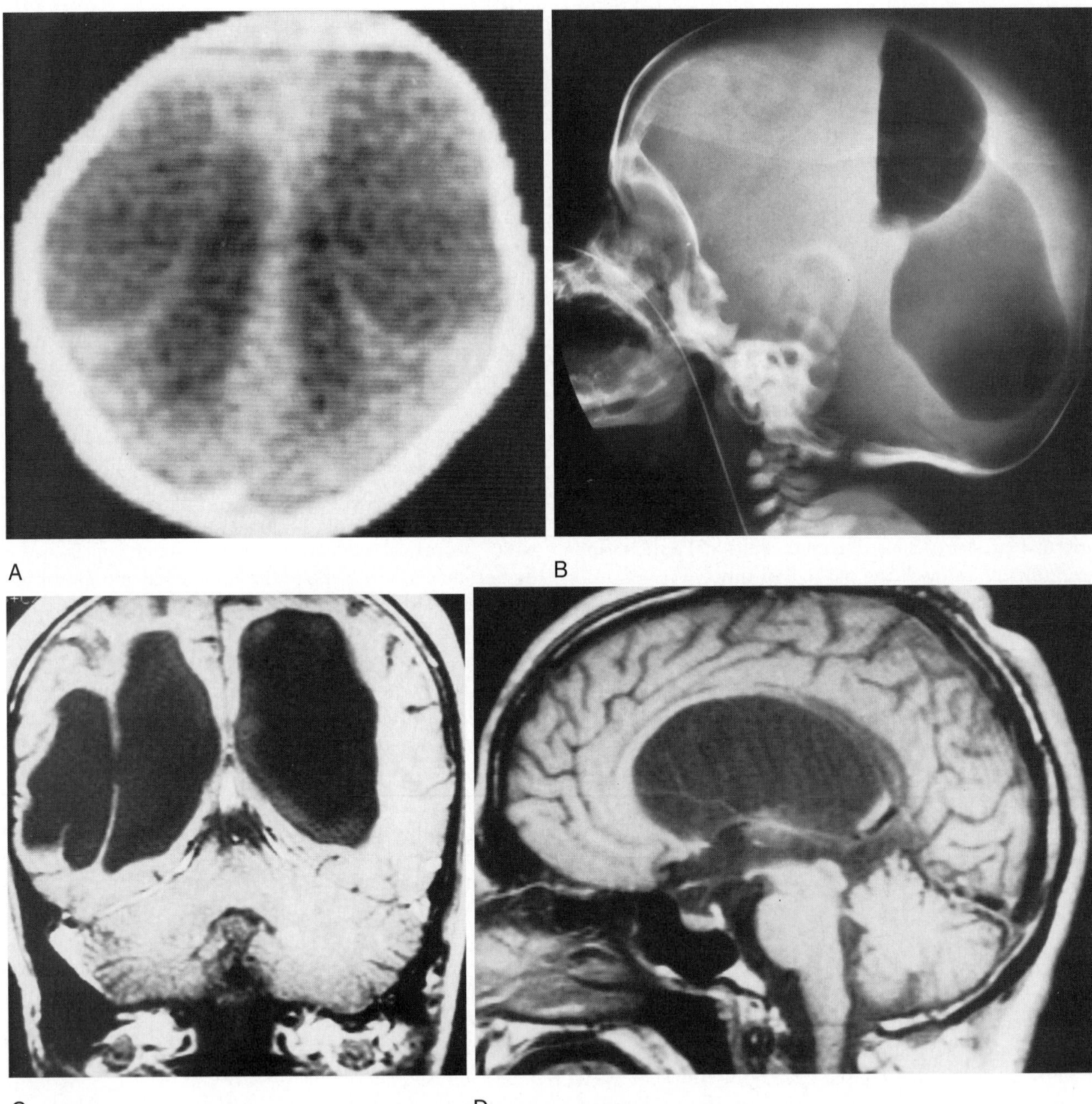

Figure 5.29. Porencephaly. **A.** Bilateral porencephalic cavities in a newborn infant. The ventricles are enlarged, and there are no calcifications in the brain tissue. **B.** Injection of air into the ventricles demonstrates communication between the ventricles and the cavities. The etiology could be some vascular or infectious intrauterine process. **C** and **D.** Porencephaly in a 28-year-old-man. **C.** The communication with the ventricle is somewhat narrow, as seen in this coronal T1-weighted MR image. **D.** Sagittal T1-weighted MR image shows narrowing of the aqueduct. The patient had aqueduct stenosis that had not been shunted. Note that there is some atrophy of the corpus callosum.

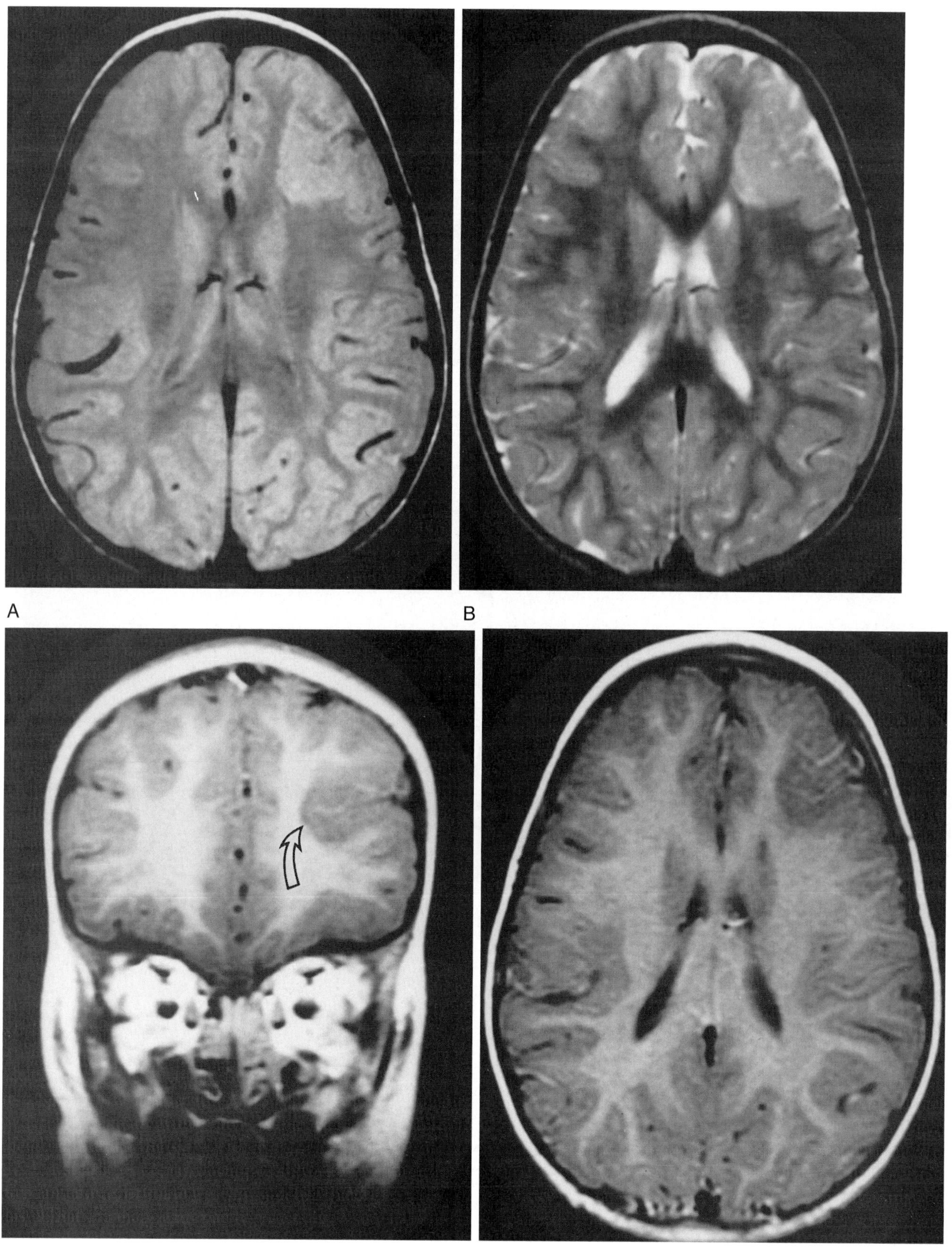

Figure 5.30. Subcortical gray matter heterotopia in a 2-year-old girl with seizures. **A** and **B.** The proton density (**A**) and T2-weighted (**B**) images show an appearance compatible with gray matter in the left frontal region. Coronal T1-weighted (**C**) and postcontrast axial (**D**) views show no evidence of uptake of contrast and, again, the appearance is like gray matter. The coronal view shows a typical gyral configuration (curved open arrow). A decision to perform surgical removal of the mass was postponed because the child was responding to anticonvulsant medication but later surgical removal was carried out.

In KS, the hypogonadism is caused by gonadotropin-releasing hormone (Gn-RH) deficiency. Embryologic studies have shown that Gn-RH originates in the olfactory placode, and in KS there is a failure of growth of the olfactory cells and nerves into the brain instead, stopping prematurely at the meninges.

CORPUS CALLOSUM ANOMALIES

Agenesis

This abnormality may be partial or complete. Development of the corpus callosum begins in the third month of fetal life and is completed during the fifth month. Because the corpus callosum develops from front to back, the entire structure is absent if the insult that causes the malformation takes place early. If the insult takes place after development of the anterior segments, the posterior aspects may be absent. This anomaly is included here because the corpus callosum, which represents a major interhemispheric commissure, is associated with cell migration events. Absence of a portion of the corpus callosum may also be secondary to destruction of an already formed structure. The falx cerebri and the inferior sagittal sinus are usually absent. The original pneumoencephalographic description was by Davidoff and Dyke (46).

Typically on MRI the corpus callosum is not present in sagittal projection, and in axial projection the lateral ventricles are separated due to the absent corpus callosum. In

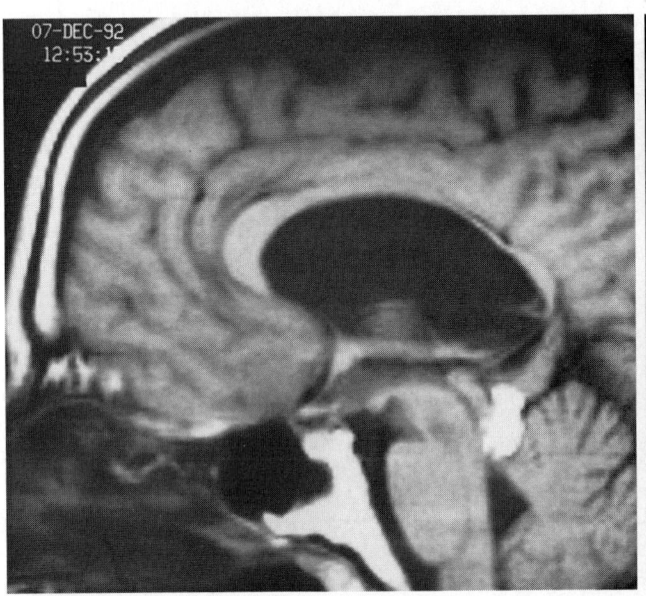

A

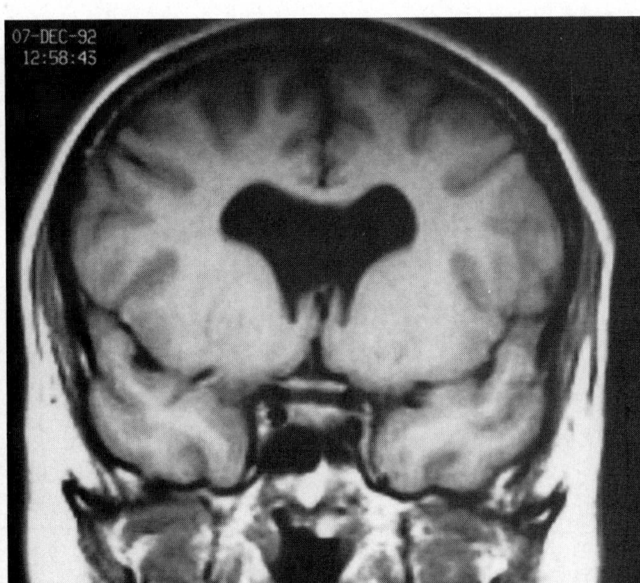

B

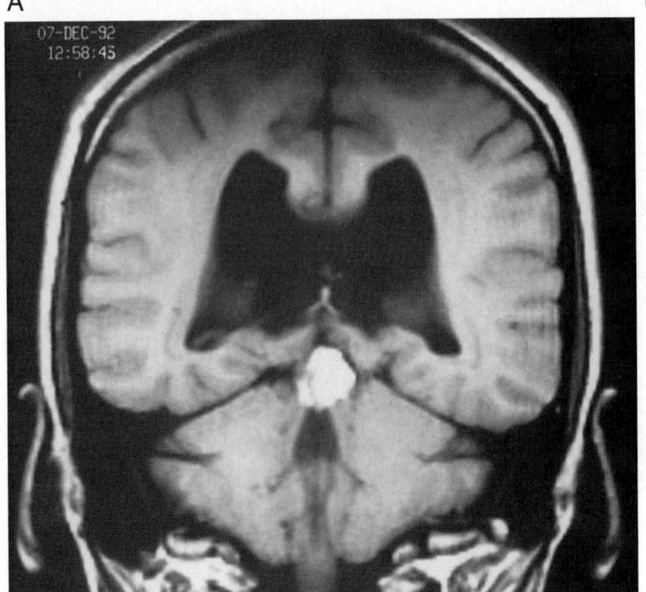

C

Figure 5.31. Partial agenesis of corpus callosum, absent septum pellucidum, and lipoma in quadrigeminal cistern. The patient, a 24-year-old man, was a college graduate and of absolutely normal intelligence. **A.** Sagittal T1-weighted image shows the very thin posterior half of corpus callosum and the absent splenium. There is a lipoma in the quadrigeminal cistern. **B.** Coronal T1-weighted image shows absent septum pellucidum with a normal optic chiasm. The ventricles are moderately enlarged. **C.** A coronal view centered more posteriorly shows the absent corpus callosum. Note that the interhemispheric fissure comes down to the ventricular level. The lipoma is well seen. (Courtesy of Dr. Eduardo Perusquia, Hospital Angeles del Pedregal, Mexico City.)

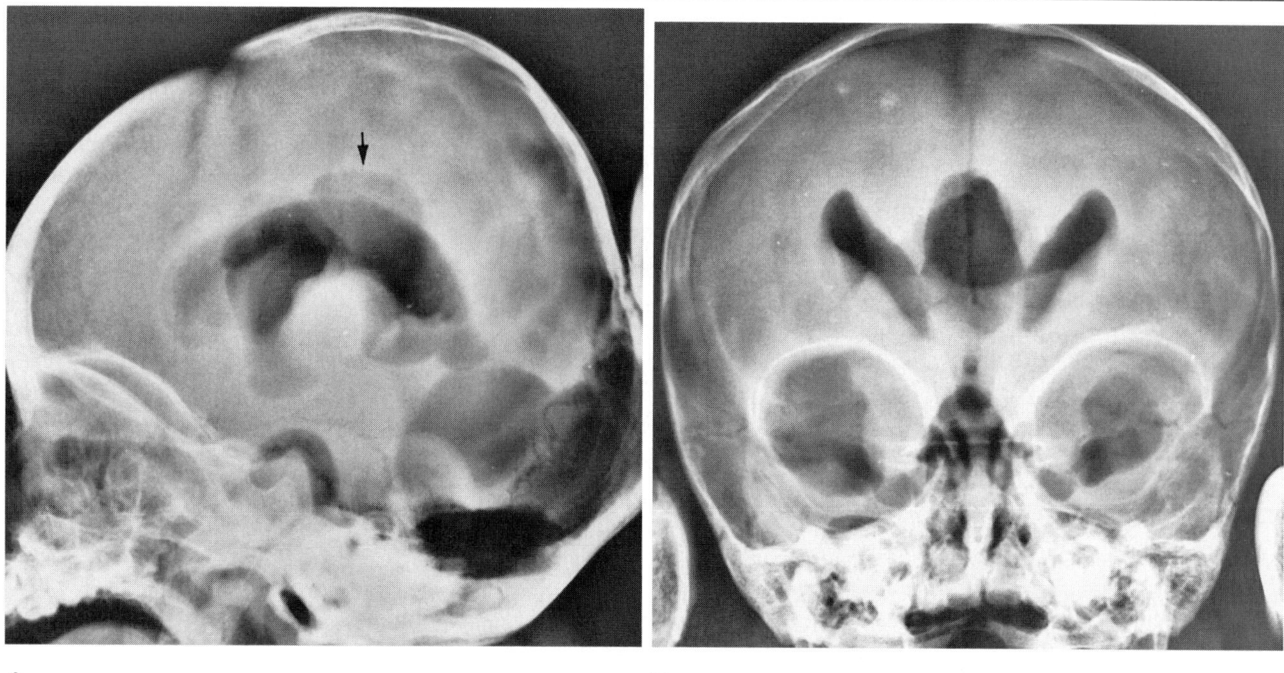

A B

Figure 5.32. Agenesis of corpus callosum with an enlarged third ventricle extending upward. **A.** Lateral view from a pneumencephalogram; **B.** Frontal view.

coronal sections, separation of the ventricles is more obvious, the lateral angles of the ventricles are directed upward, and the tips are pointed, with a hornlike configuration (Figs. 5.31 and 5.32). The medial aspect of the hemispheres in sagittal views reveals an absence of the cingulate gyrus and possibly stenogyria (narrow gyri) or true polymicrogyria. In addition, the third ventricle may be enlarged upward, sometimes forming a large midline extension that may reach as high as the inner table of the skull (see earlier text) (Fig. 5.32). Probst described, pathologically, a thickening of the inferior medial aspect of the hemisphere in these patients (47), which may represent the callosal fibers that did not cross (Probst bundle). Ventricular enlargement is often present, usually more pronounced in the atrium and occipital horns (colpocephaly).

Agenesis of the corpus callosum may be associated with other anomalies. These anomolies include cortical heterotopia (38,39) (Fig. 5.33), polymicrogyria, Chiari II malfor-

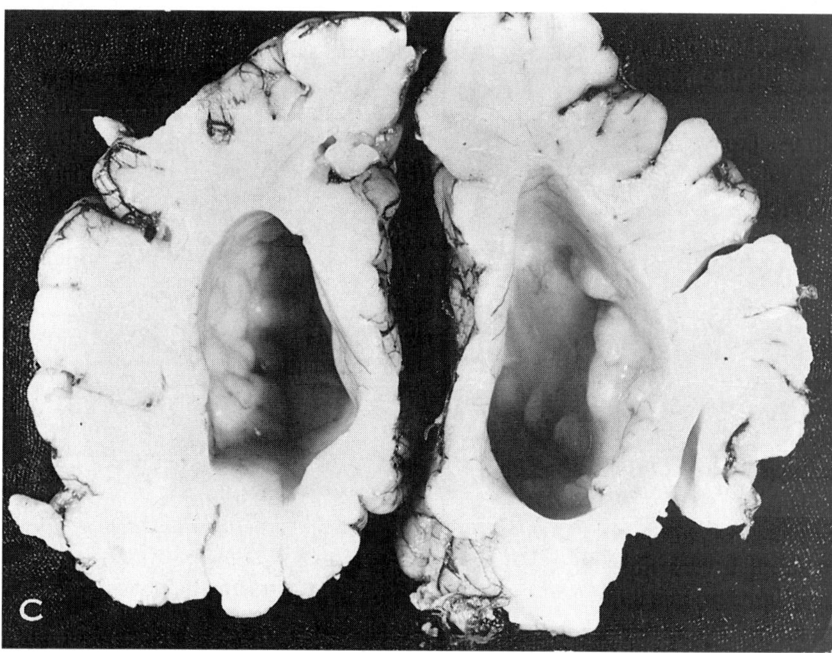

Figure 5.33. Cortical heterotopia of the lateral ventricle in a patient with agenesis of the corpus callosum (autopsy specimen).

mation, Aicardi's syndrome, holoprosencephaly, and Dandy-Walker cyst.

Aicardi's syndrome is characterized by seizures, agenesis of the corpus callosum, and ocular abnormalities (coloboma and chorioretinopathy). Other anomalies may coexist (Dandy-Walker, Chiari II) (48). Vertebral anomalies are often present. The majority of patients are female.

Agenesis of the corpus callosum is not necessarily associated with severe mental retardation. A seizure disorder is usually present, and if the malformation is partial, it may be compatible with a nearly normal intelligence (Fig. 5.31). The agenesis with associated anomalies can be expected to produce more severe forms of retardation and abnormal behavior. Corpus callosum dysgenesis is commonly associated with other anomalies of the central nervous system (49).

Corpus Callosum Lipoma

This entity is often associated with partial or complete agenesis or hypoplasia of the corpus callosum (48 percent of cases, according to Zettner and Netsky [50]) but may exist alone. It may form an irregularly oval mass, which often calcifies, or it may be flatter, extending along the sulci of the lower aspect of the hemisphere in the midline (Figs. 5.34 and 5.35). CT shows the fatty content as well as the calcification very clearly, and MRI reveals the distribution in the midline to greater advantage in the sagittal view (Fig. 5.35). Dean et al. emphasize the fact that the lipomas are more often pericallosal than callosal (51). They are often wrapped around the corpus callosum on its dorsal surface (52), or they may be somewhat more diffuse, following the sulci in the inner surface of the hemisphere (Fig. 5.35). Partial absence may be due to a vascular insult or an inflammatory process (53–55), or, like total agenesis, it could be hereditary, although in the majority of cases it is considered idiopathic.

The diagnosis can be made by CT, MRI, or ultrasound in the postnatal period. However, it is also possible to suspect the diagnosis by prenatal ultrasound (56).

Lipomas of the corpus callosum are the most common of intracranial lipomas, which may also be found in the quadrigeminal cistern, the ambient cistern, the interpedun-

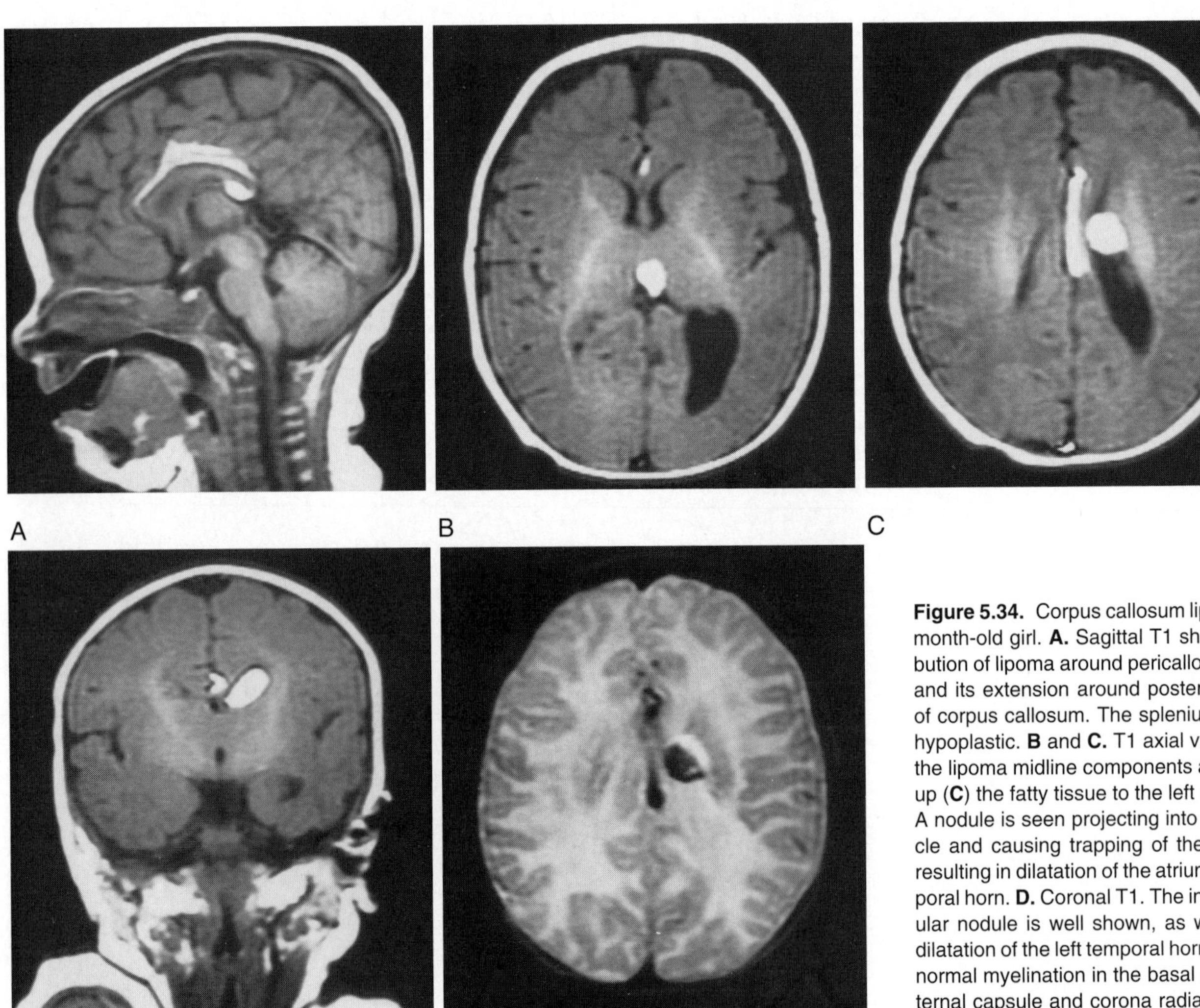

Figure 5.34. Corpus callosum lipoma in 2-month-old girl. **A.** Sagittal T1 shows distribution of lipoma around pericallosal cistern and its extension around posterior aspect of corpus callosum. The splenium may be hypoplastic. **B** and **C.** T1 axial views show the lipoma midline components and higher up (**C**) the fatty tissue to the left of the falx. A nodule is seen projecting into the ventricle and causing trapping of the ventricle, resulting in dilatation of the atrium and temporal horn. **D.** Coronal T1. The intraventricular nodule is well shown, as well as the dilatation of the left temporal horn. Note the normal myelination in the basal ganglia internal capsule and corona radiata on both sides. **E.** T2-weighted axial shows the lipoma to be very hypointense.

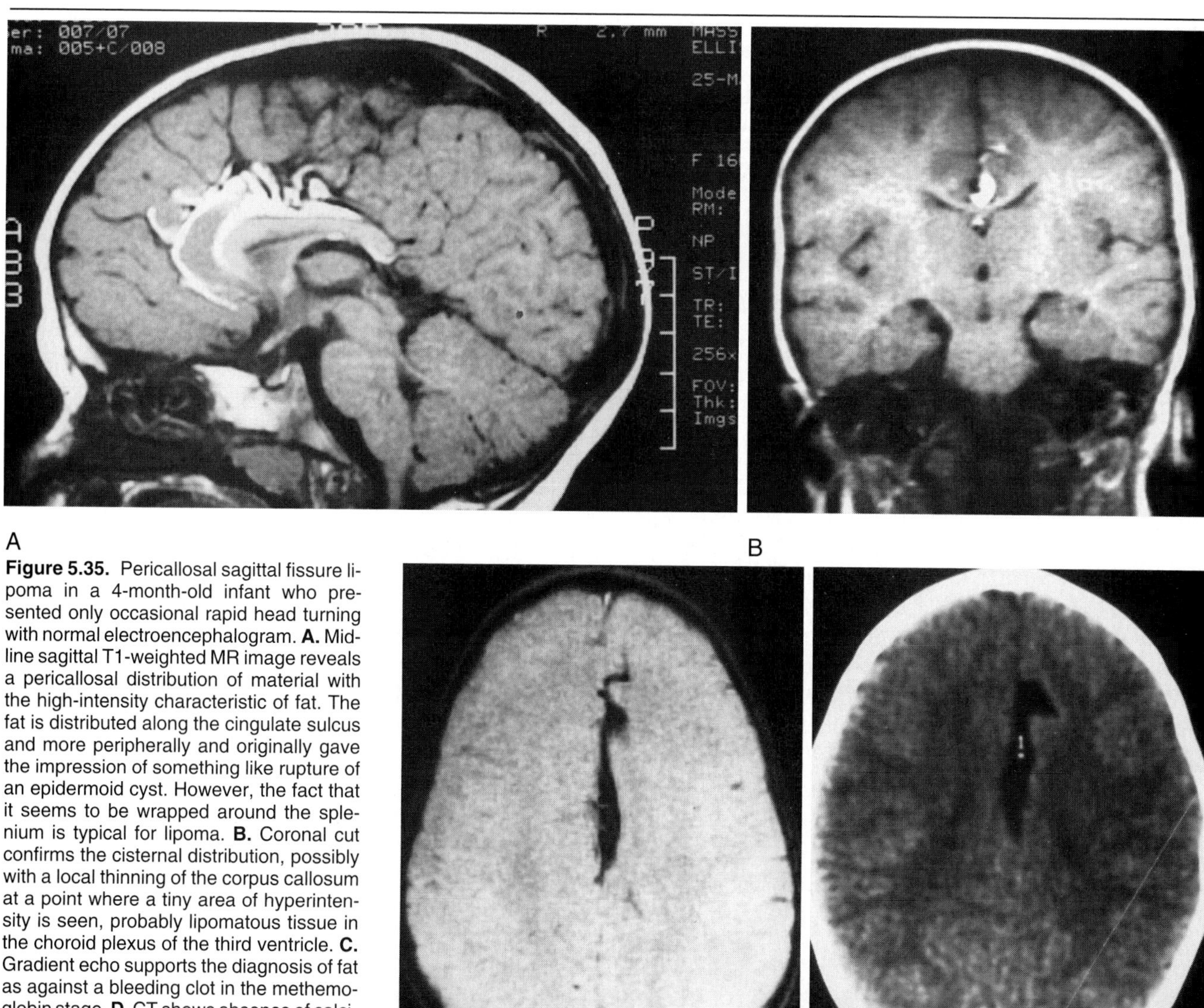

Figure 5.35. Pericallosal sagittal fissure lipoma in a 4-month-old infant who presented only occasional rapid head turning with normal electroencephalogram. **A.** Midline sagittal T1-weighted MR image reveals a pericallosal distribution of material with the high-intensity characteristic of fat. The fat is distributed along the cingulate sulcus and more peripherally and originally gave the impression of something like rupture of an epidermoid cyst. However, the fact that it seems to be wrapped around the splenium is typical for lipoma. **B.** Coronal cut confirms the cisternal distribution, possibly with a local thinning of the corpus callosum at a point where a tiny area of hyperintensity is seen, probably lipomatous tissue in the choroid plexus of the third ventricle. **C.** Gradient echo supports the diagnosis of fat as against a bleeding clot in the methemoglobin stage. **D.** CT shows absence of calcification and reduced density compatible with fat. The reading was −65 H units. Reexamination at age 15 months showed no change in configuration or size and a normal child in all respects. The occasional rapid head turning movement, occurring only once at a time, persists.

cular cistern, the perimesencephalic and sylvian cisterns, and the choroid plexus. Histologically the growths turn out to be composed of mature lipomatous tissue (Figs. 5.31 and 34).

It is probably incorrect to assume that the lipomas are in the corpus callosum. Rather, they may be associated with agenesis of the corpus callosum, but they may also occur in the midline subarachnoid space above the corpus callosum associated with minimal or no involvement of this structure. In addition, they may occur in other areas of the subarachnoid space, as indicated previously. The embryogenesis of this anomaly is probably based on the fact that the potential subarachnoid cisterns are really filled with primitive meningeal tissue, called the *meninx primitiva.* Normally, this tissue is reabsorbed completely, leaving the subarachnoid space, or if the solid material fails to be completely absorbed, it differentiates into fat, producing a mature lipoma. Lipomas are sometimes seen on CT examinations, but today, with routine MRI diagnosis, it is fairly common to see the lipomas in the various locations listed earlier because of the bright T1 appearance and the lesser brightness in the T2 images, which is characteristic of adipose tissue.

Lipomas of the choroid plexus may be associated with corpus callosum lipomas (57). Lipomas or partial agenesis is often associated with seizures, but there may be no retardation, particularly when no significant corpus callosum involvement can be demonstrated.

NEURONAL PROLIFERATION, DIFFERENTIATION, AND HISTOGENESIS (2 TO 5 MONTHS' GESTATION)

Quite a number of conditions might be included here but probably would be better described as part of a group. Among these are some congenital tumors of the nervous system, neurofibromatosis and tuberous sclerosis, von Hippel–Lindau disease, Sturge-Weber syndrome, and other less common conditions that belong with the neurocutaneous syndromes. These are described here as a group. Other conditions, such as congenital vascular malformations, are described under vascular conditions. Aqueduct stenosis is described under hydrocephalus (see Chapter 4).

Microcephaly-Micrencephaly

Micrencephaly literally means a small head. The brain usually determines the size of the skull, barring some congenital abnomalities such as premature synostosis of the bones of the skull, which, when it is generalized, could prevent normal brain growth, leading to microcephaly. This is rather unusual, however, because premature synostosis usually occurs in some of the sutures and not all at the same time, and this leads to a rather significant deformity of the skull (see under "Premature Synostosis," Chapter 19). Thus, the small head can usually be taken to mean that the brain is not growing properly. The micrencephaly could be hereditary or due to intrauterine problems such as infection or vascular disorders. The CNS is particularly vulnerable to toxoplasmosis, rubella virus, cytomegalovirus, and herpes (TORCH). All of these lead to atrophy of brain tissue, with enlargement of the ventricles and a small brain.

The size of the head can be measured in anteroposterior and transverse diameters on radiographs of the head, but the tape measure is probably more accurate and certainly easier to obtain. It can also be done by axial CT examination at the level of the lateral ventricles. Today, however, we also wish to identify any anomaly of the brain associated with micrencephaly as well as the thickness of the brain tissue left and the amount of hydrocephalus. Both CT and MR images can do this. CT is preferred because it is possible to confuse or to be unsure about hydrocephalus with stenosis of the aqueduct on MRI alone. Multiple calcifications indicate that the etiology is toxoplasmosis or cytomegalovirus infection and not aqueductal stenosis with hydrocephalus (see Fig. 4.15). MRI is not accurate when it comes to evaluating calcifications in the brain, particularly if these are small.

Familial microcephaly may be related to a number of abnormalities, some of which are described previously, or may be due to generalized hypoplasia of the brain with widened gyri and fewer convolutions. Micrencephaly without associated anomalies may well be due to an abnormal gene or to inborn errors of metabolism, but the abnormality could also be due to infectious or environmental factors. Presumably, a virus infection could destroy the immature neurons and glial cells during mitosis or during neuronal migration (58).

Megalencephaly

Enlargement of the head is usually diagnosed clinically and can be confirmed by tape measurement. In the past, a skull examination would usually be carried out in these patients. In early childhood, a widening of the sutures is evident on skull radiography. Also, calcification can be found in the presence of some chronic infections such as toxoplasmosis or cytomegalovirus; in the latter cases, however, microcephaly is more common. The other important cause of a large head is hydrocephalus.

Today, CT or MRI may be carried out, but CT is preferred because it can reveal calcifications which may be overlooked on MRI (Fig. 5.36; see Fig. 4.15). Congenital hydrocephalus is usually suspected early in infancy because enlargement of the fontanels can easily be noted clinically. Hydrocephalus is discussed elsewhere.

Megalencephaly is a term usually applied to enlargement of the brain without a significant degree of hydrocephalus. (59–61).

The normal adult brain weighs approximately 1400 g, whereas the brain of a newborn weighs about 320 g. In general, a brain size that is 2 to 2.5 standard deviations greater than normal may be considered to be large. Some notable examples of large heads in normal individuals include Lord Byron, whose brain weighed 1807 g (62). Bismarck's brain was also quite large and weighed 1790 g. In general, however, function or intelligence is somewhat disturbed in these individuals, and the majority are mentally retarded.

Achondroplastic dwarfs usually have a disproportionately large head. Megalencephaly is twice as common in males as in females. In terms of cytoarchitecture, about 25 percent show no obvious abnormality; of the remaining, about half show some neuronal abnormalities and the other half show severe malformations visible on the surface of the brain. This is the primary megalencephaly group as divided by Dekaban and Sakuragawa (63).

The secondary group is associated with metabolic processes such as mucopolysaccharidoses, gangliosidoses, sphingolipidoses, Tay-Sachs disease, various leukodystrophies, and neurocutaneous syndromes.

Unilateral megalencephaly may represent a third group. This abnormality is usually associated with mental retardation and may also be associated with hemihypertrophy of one side of the body. Cerebral gigantism (Sotos syndrome) may present an enlarged brain with enlarged ventricles and also enlargement or rapid growth of the rest of the body (60,61). Of the 12 patients reported by Barkovich and Chuang, all had seizures and some were mentally retarded (64). The white matter was usually increased and the gray matter was usually thicker (Fig. 5.37) (65). A pseudohemi-megalencephaly is produced by hemisphere brain atrophy such

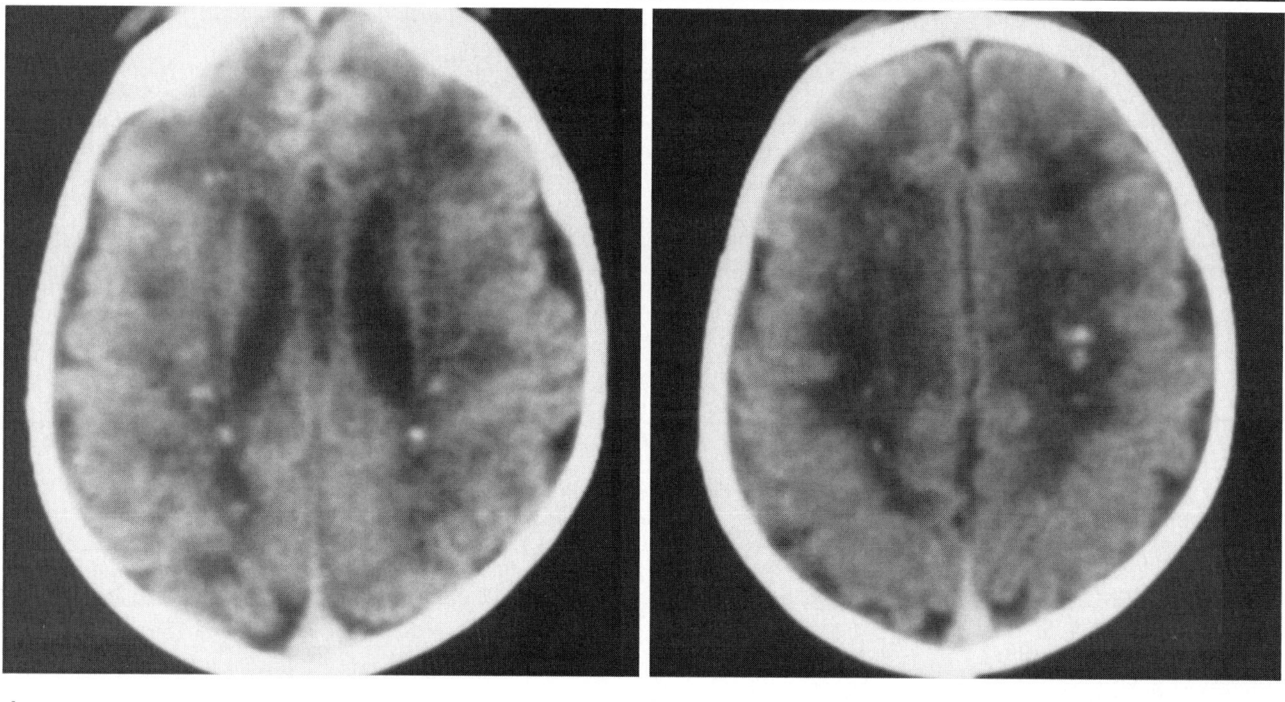

Figure 5.36. Multiple calcification in periventricular and white matter consistent with either congenital toxoplasmosis or cytomegalovirus infection in an 8-month-old infant. **A** and **B.** CT axial views showing ventricular dilatation and white matter low attenuation, as well as punctate calcifications.

as in the Dyke-Davidoff-Massom syndrome, or in incontinentia pigmenti (66).

Hydranencephaly

This term is applied to the absence of a cerebral mantle associated with fairly normal posterior fossa structures. The head is fairly normal in size, and the infant may behave normally for a number of weeks. Usually, the head begins to grow in size more rapidly than is normally expected, and this may lead to an investigation that demonstrates the complete absence of brain tissue (67). The falx may be well formed and may give the impression of a septum pellucidum.

The etiology of this condition is thought to be an obstruction of both internal carotid arteries (68). The complete absence of brain tissue may be explained by the fact that damaged parts in the fetus may be absorbed without a trace of neuronal or connective tissue repair. Reparative and inflammatory reactions do not take place before the sixth month of fetal life, according to Eicke (69). It is not surprising, therefore, that a great many congenital malformations are characterized by absence of structures or arrest of migration, union, separation, or cavitation. The developing fetal brain does not react in the same way as mature tissue.

Some remnants of the lower aspect of the frontal lobes may remain; the same applies to the temporal lobes, possibly owing to blood supply via branches of the posterior cerebral artery. The same applies to the inferoposterior aspect of the occipital lobes.

Hydranencephaly is easily diagnosed by CT or MRI. The only differential diagnosis would be with hydrocephalus due to congenital aqueductal obstruction. In the latter the carotid artery branches over the surface of the brain are normal although they may be stretched, but in hydranencephaly they are absent. Angiography usually demonstrates occlusion of the carotid arteries just above the origin of the anterior choroidal arteries.

Arachnoid Cysts

Arachnoid cysts are loculations containing CSF presumably formed within the arachnoid membrane. The cyst itself may form by splitting the arachnoid membrane, which is reinforced by a thick layer of collagen (70). The same authors have collected more than 200 cases of arachnoid cysts and reported their locations. Of these, 49 percent were in the sylvian fissure, 11 percent in the cerebellopontine angle, 19 percent in the quadrigeminal plate region and upper vermis, 5 percent in the interhemispheric fissure, 4 percent in the cerebral convexity, and 3 percent in the clival interpeduncular area.

One of the most frequent locations, as seen by CT and MRI, is the anterior aspect of the temporal fossa, which was not mentioned specifically in this group but probably is represented by the group Rengachary and Watanabe called *sylvian fissure* (70). The modern imaging diagnostic methods are superior to autopsy in detecting these cysts.

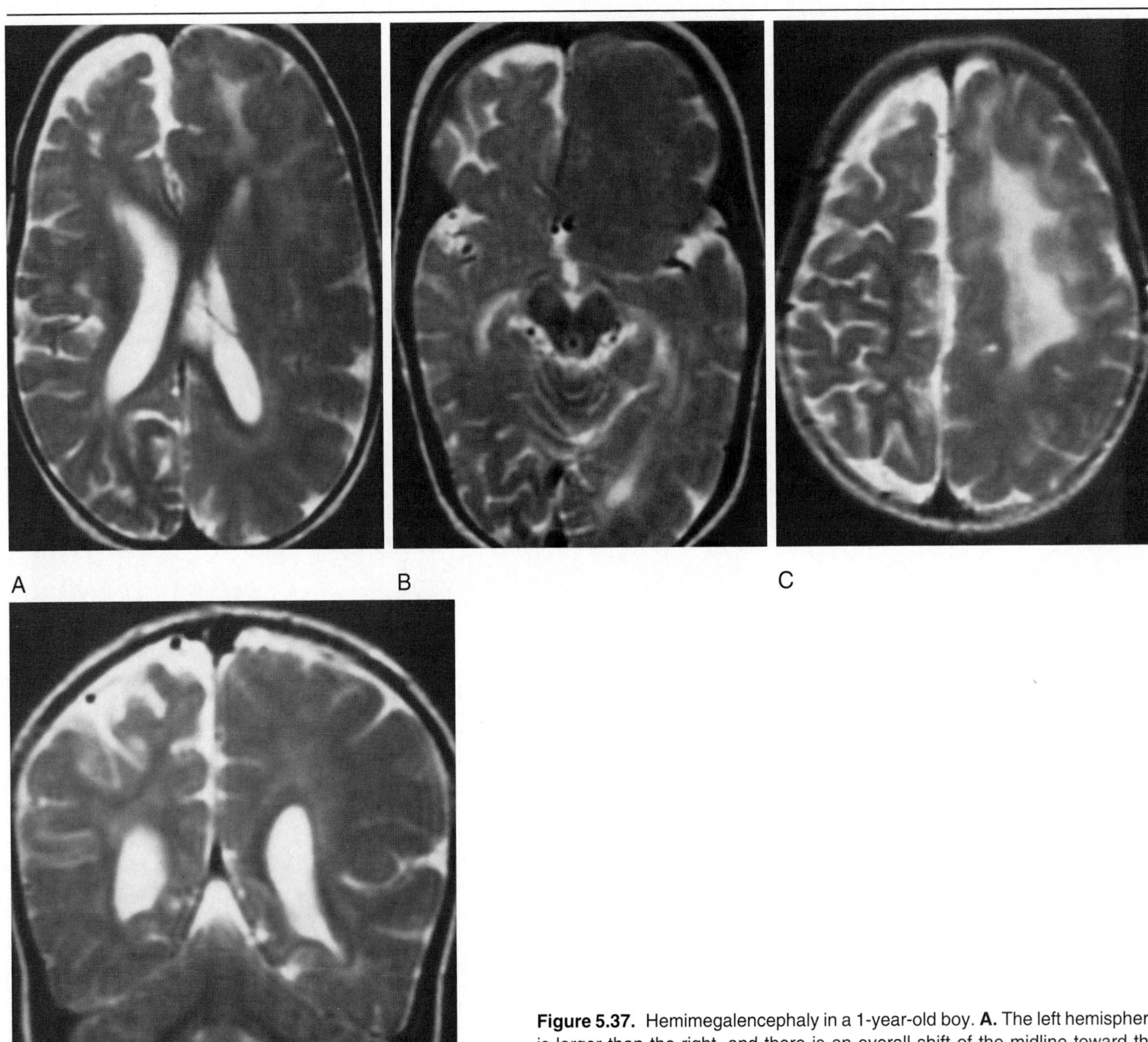

Figure 5.37. Hemimegalencephaly in a 1-year-old boy. **A.** The left hemisphere is larger than the right, and there is an overall shift of the midline toward the right. An increased space between the two ventricles anteriorly is present, possibly due to tilting of the corpus callosum or to enlargement of the fornix anteriorly. There is diminution in the number of surface sulci on the left side, also seen in a lower section (**B**). **C.** A higher section reveals signs of dysmyelination in the larger hemisphere (hyperintensity in white matter). **D.** The coronal sections confirm the presence of a smaller number of sulci on the left side. (Courtesy of Dr. Tina Young-Poussaint, Boston, Massachusetts.)

The anterior temporal cysts are often relatively small and sometimes moderate in size but produce no clinical findings. Thus they are found incidentally by CT and MRI even though some of them are quite large and displace and deform the temporal lobe. The large and moderate-size cysts were once attributed to partial agenesis of the temporal lobe. Now, however, they are believed to be associated with displacement and compression of the temporal lobe; this compression is thought to lead to hypoplasia of the temporal lobe secondary to the cyst. Hald et al. reported four children with bilateral arachnoid cysts of the temporal fossa who had glutaric aciduria type I (71). They indicate that in the presence of bilateral temporal fossa cysts, the differential diagnosis should include this disorder. Multiple cysts have also been reported in Marfan syndrome (72).

Some cysts of the temporal fossa, convexity, posterior fossa, and retrocerebellar area can grow to very large size (73) (Figs. 5.38 through 5.40).

Suprasellar arachnoid cysts may be associated with chiasmal compression. An occasional cyst will extend into the sella turcica and seem to arise directly from the sella, sug-

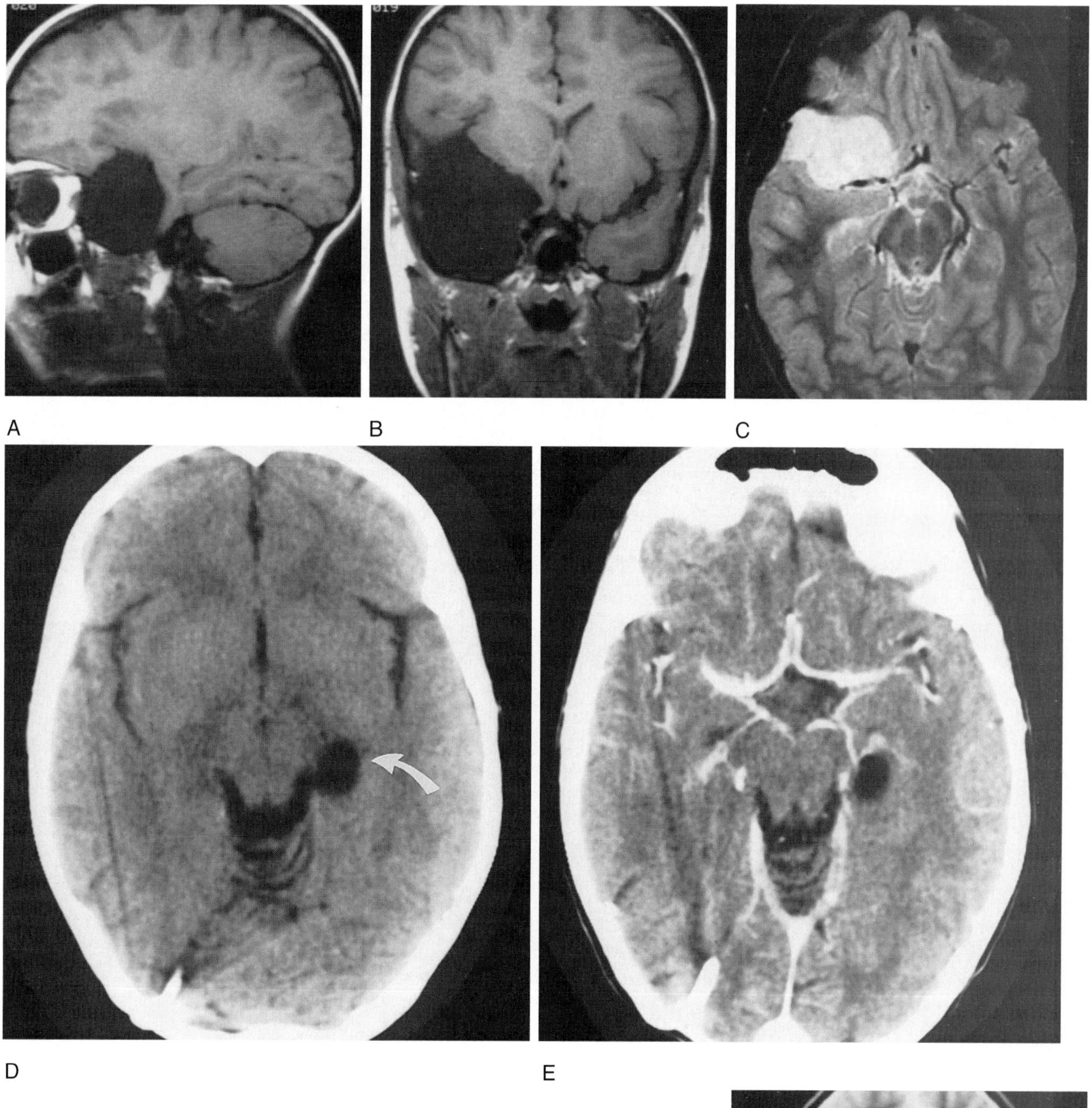

A B C

D E

Figure 5.38. Temporal fossa arachnoid cyst in an 8-year-old boy. **A.** T1 sagittal view shows enlargement of the middle fossa and posterior displacement and deformity of the anterior aspect of the temporal lobe. **B.** Coronal T1 shows elevation of the sylvian fissure, flattening and elevation of the insula. The enlargement of the middle fossa is now evident as compared with the opposite side. There is a mass effect as shown by midline shift to the left and compression of the right ventricle. **C.** Axial T2 shows the expected hyperintensity of the cyst. The middle cerebral artery is displaced dorsally. A follow-up performed 2 years later showed no increase in size, indicating equilibrium between CSF production (if CSF is in fact being produced within the cyst) and CSF absorption or extravasation through the cyst wall. **D.** Another patient in which a small choroidal fissure cyst was seen (arrow). **E.** Contrast enhancement revealed no abnormal vascularity; the choroid plexus of the temporal horn is lateral to it. It was thought that this could represent a small epidermoid tumor or an arachnoid cyst. The patient was being followed for a medulloblastoma, and reexaminations for a period of over 5 years showed no change. The diagnosis of arachnoid cyst remains the most likely. **F.** A T2-weighted axial image indicates that it behaves like CSF (arrow).

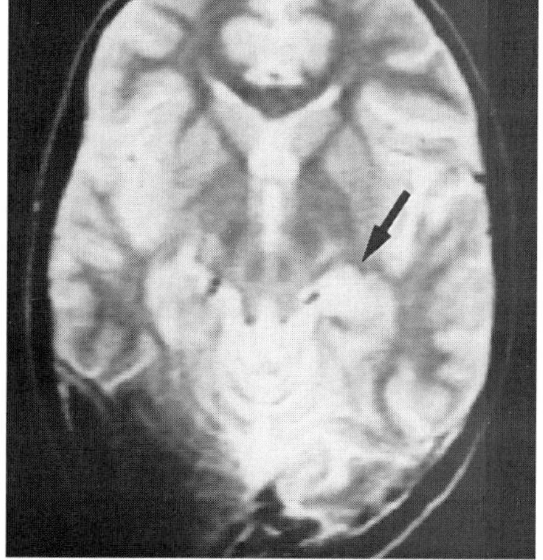

F

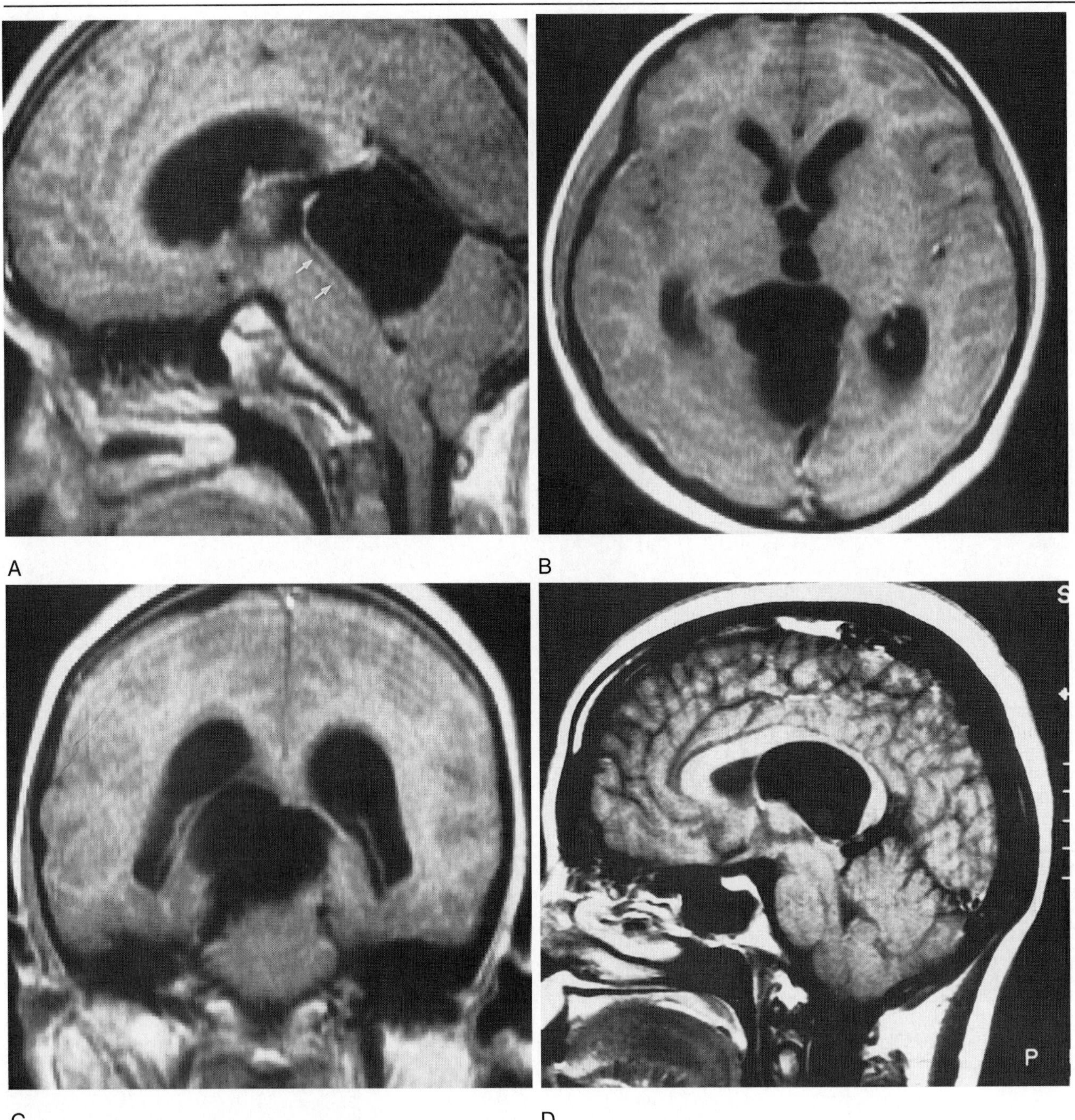

Figure 5.39. Congenital arachnoid cysts. Three cases are illustrated in different locations. The most common location is the temporal fossa–sylvian area, illustration in Fig. 5.38A–C. Another location is the superior cerebellar-quadrigeminal cistern. **A.** Sagittal midline section shows flattening and elongation of the quadrigeminal plate and narrowing of the aqueduct (arrows). Moderate hydrocephalus is present. The cerebellum is flattened and displaced caudally. **B.** Axial. **C.** Coronal section. The cyst projects more to the right of the midline and elevates the atrium of the right ventricle. **D.** Arachnoid cyst in cistern of velum interposition. The sagittal view shows the location at the roof of the third ventricle and below the corpus callosum (*continues*).

gesting a craniopharyngioma or a cystic pituitary adenoma (see Fig. 11.66).

Sometimes it is necessary to differentiate a porencephaly from an arachnoid cyst. If contrast medium is injected into the lumbar subarachnoid space and carried to the head, CT will demonstrate filling of a porencephalic cyst. On the other hand, an arachnoid cyst will not fill. Sometimes the cyst may obstruct the ventricle, particularly a retrocerebellar cyst in the posterior fossa or a cyst in the region of the quadrigeminal plate or upper vermis. In these cases the

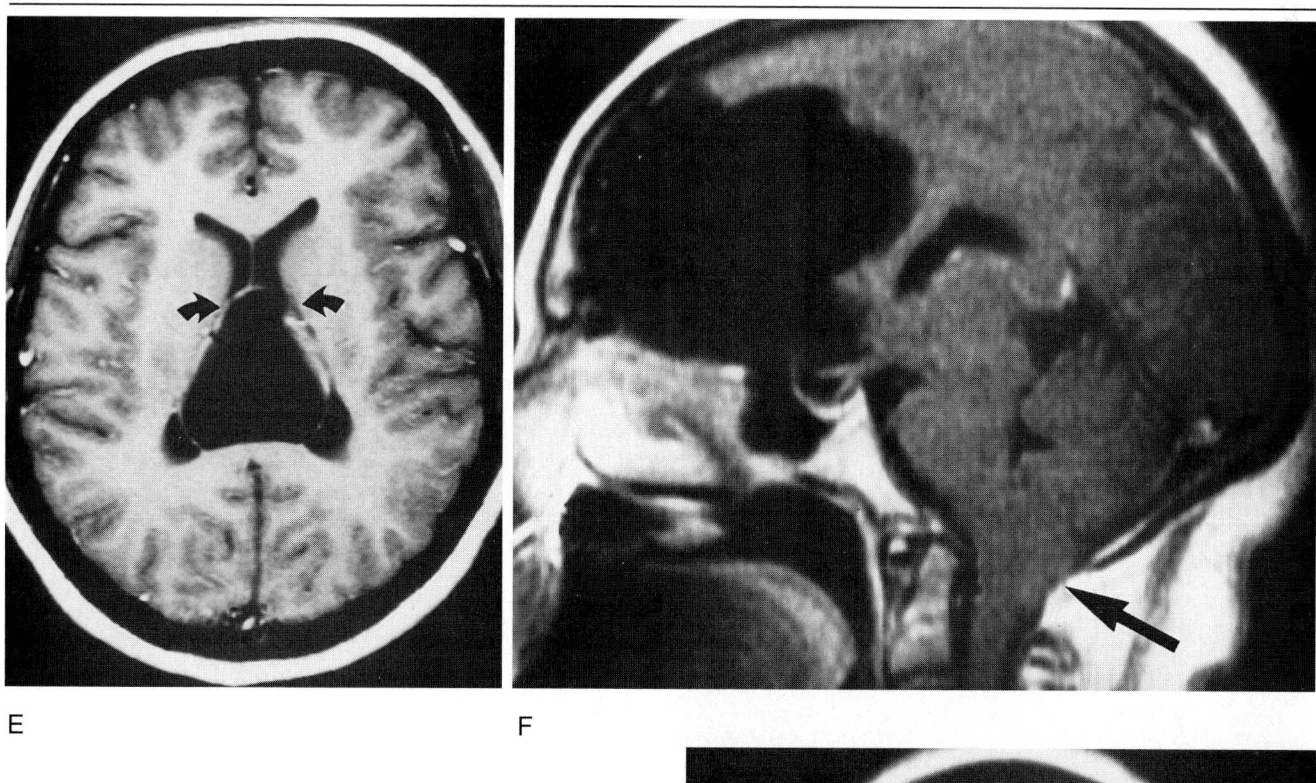

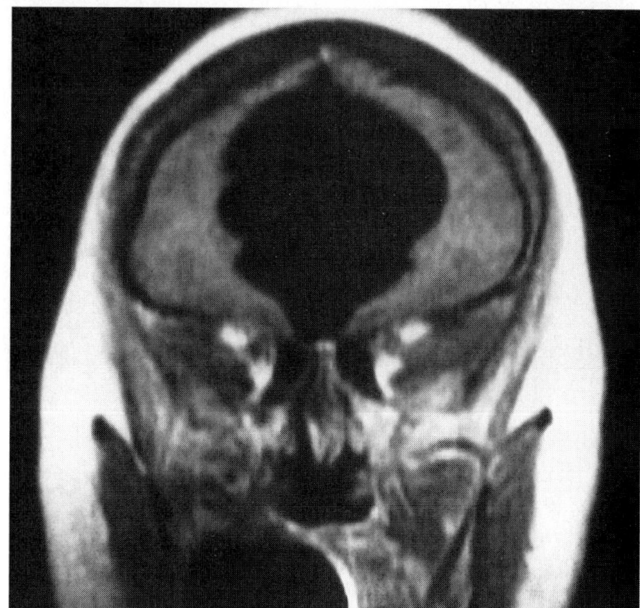

Figure 5.39. *(continued)* **E.** The axial view demonstrates the typical shape of the cistern—wider posteriorly, narrower anteriorly (arrows). **F.** Frontal interhemispheric arachnoid cyst. The sagittal view reveals the rather extensive size of the lesion, producing significant mass effect. The frontal horns are markedly displaced backward. The whole brain is rotated, and the brainstem is displaced caudally toward the posterior fossa. The cerebellar tonsils are displaced down through the foramen magnum (arrow). **G.** Coronal slice shows the interhemispheric position of the cyst. (Courtesy of Dr. José Arredondo-Estrada, Monterrey, Mexico.)

contrast medium (or air) may have to be injected into the ventricles directly in order to rule out any connection between the dilated ventricles and the cyst.

The fluid within these cysts is usually CSF. If it contains some protein, one might suggest that the origin of the cyst was postinflammatory, possibly following meningitis. (For discussion of subdural collections, see sections in Chapters 6 and 7 on inflammatory diseases and trauma.)

Arachnoid cysts can be infectious or traumatic in origin, but the majority are congenital. The embryogenesis of these cysts can be explained by the theory that the subarachnoid space is formed by expansion of the intercellular space of the meninx primitiva, which surrounds the neural tube. The clearing out of the cells of the meninx primitiva leaves space limited by the dura-arachnoid on the outer aspect and by the pia-arachnoid on the inner layer. A derangement in this embryologic process may cause formation of these arachnoid cysts, which, clinically, are found in the temporal fossa (50 to 66 percent); in the suprasellar and quadrigeminal regions (10 percent); and in the pos-

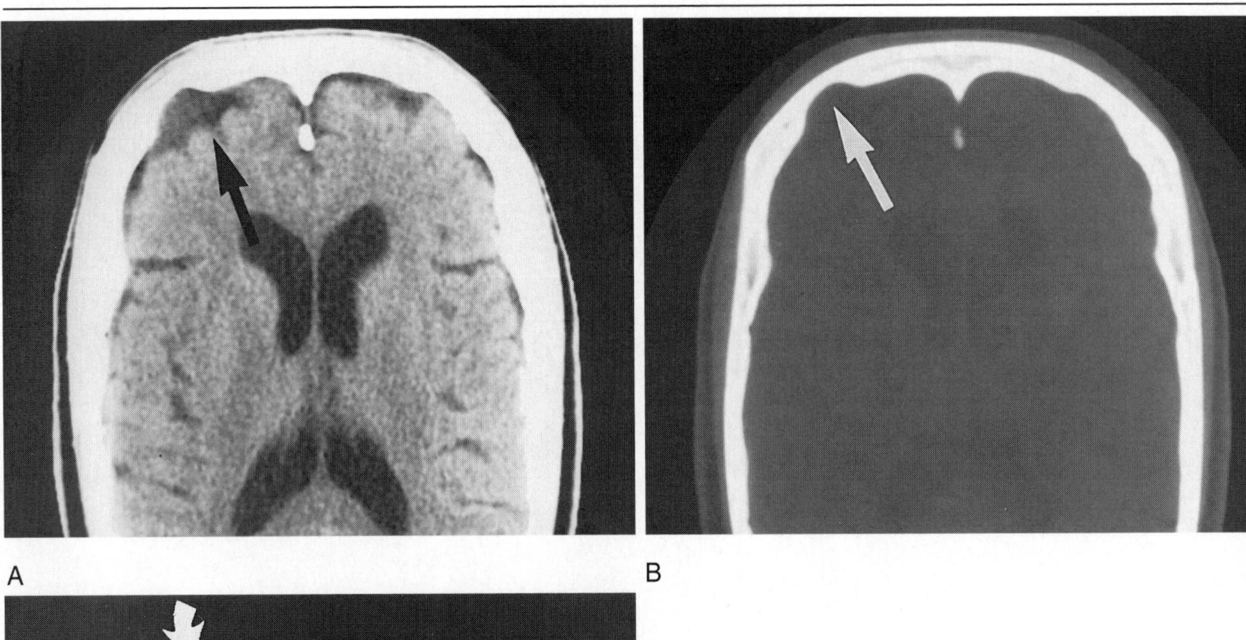

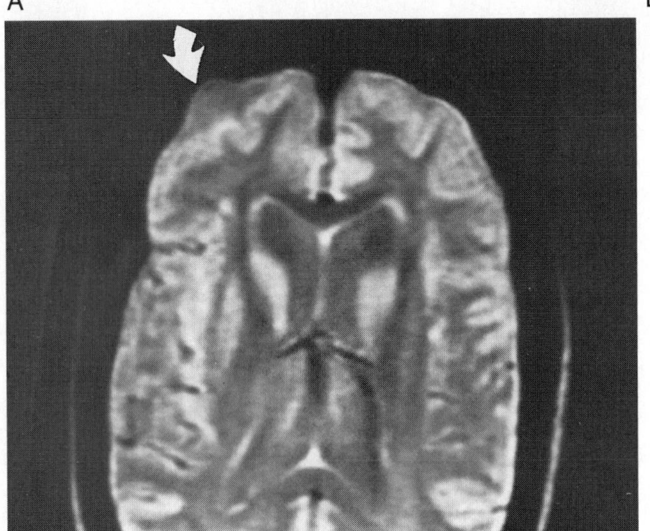

Figure 5.40. Small congenital arachnoid cyst. The collection of fluid in the right frontal region is rather small but is producing bone erosion and flattening of the adjacent brain surface. **A.** CT. **B.** CT bone window. **C.** MRI proton density image (arrow).

terior fossa and over the frontal convexities (5 percent each) (74). Of the eight middle fossa arachnoid cysts reported by Robertson et al., five were associated with hypoplasia of the temporal lobes without significant compression of the temporal lobe; three had compression of the temporal lobe and also some hypoplasia (74). A frequently associated anomaly is absence of the superficial middle cerebral vein, which dates the embryological abnormality at the sixth to eighth week of gestation (75).

Filling of these arachnoid cysts has always been controversial. Three possibilities exist: they may secrete their own fluid, they may communicate with the ventricles freely, or they may have a ball valve or flap valve effect that produces a slow egress, allowing the cyst to grow. Wolpert and Scott demonstrated by cisternography with water-soluble contrast media that some of the cysts communicate freely whereas others do not communicate, for all practical purposes, with the subarachnoid space (76). In these instances, the only way that the cyst could be seen would be via direct injection of contrast medium. These are important observations from the surgical point of view, for if a cyst does not communicate with the subarachnoid space, the cyst itself needs to be shunted. Evidently a certain percentage of the cysts can produce their own fluid, because the capacity of cells to secrete fluid can be demonstrated by electron microscopy (70), whereas other cysts do not possess electron microscopy evidence of cells capable of secreting CSF.

The majority of arachnoid cysts do not require treatment. Those that require treatment are usually associated with hydrocephalus, causing compression of the aqueduct near the quadrigeminal cistern or in the perimesencephalic cisternal space or cysts that are large enough to significantly deform and distort adjacent structures possibly with shift of the midline structures (Figs. 5.38 and 5.39). Many of these cysts are symptomatic and may be associated with a seizure disorder. The suprasellar cysts are usually associated with visual disturbances due to compression of the optic pathways.

Nowadays, with use of CT and MRI in patients with all types of symptoms, it is surprising to see how frequently the small and medium-size temporal fossa arachnoid cysts are found. In general, these cysts are considered to be unrelated to the presenting complaints and produce no significant displacement of the adjacent brain structures. Occasionally the temporal lobe may be flattened in the area but is not hypoplastic; it does, however, contain a normal-thickness gray matter and is simply adapted to the shape of the adjacent cyst.

Neuroectodermal Syndromes

The neuroectodermal syndromes, sometimes referred to as *phakomatoses* (from the Greek word *phakos*, meaning "mole" or "freckle"), are congenital disorders that involve the CNS, skin, and other organs of ectodermal origin, such as the retina. In this group are usually included the following:

- Neurofibromatosis
- Sturge-Weber syndrome
- Tuberous sclerosis
- Von Hippel-Lindau disease
- Basal cell nevus syndrome
- Osler-Weber-Rendu disease
- Ataxia-telangiectasia
- Klippel-Trenaunay syndrome
- Blue-rubber-bleb-nevus syndrome

These and other less well known disorders are included in this section. The neuroectodermal disorders are often first diagnosed by dermatologists because they see the patient first and because in many instances the skin manifestations are more florid. Further, even small skin lesions attract early attention.

Neurofibromatosis Neurofibromatosis, the most common of the neuroectodermal syndromes, is transmitted as an autosomal dominant trait, but spontaneous mutations are presumably responsible for about half of the patients. The condition is encountered in about 1 in 3000 births (77). The myriad manifestations of neurofibromatosis particularly involve the central and peripheral nervous systems. Recently, it has been possible to separate the disease into two definite groups: neurofibromatosis 1 (NF1, von Recklinghausen disease) and neurofibromatosis 2 (NF2, bilateral acoustic neurofibromatosis). They appear to be genetically distinct. NF1 has an abnormal chromosome 17, and NF2 has an abnormal long arm of chromosome 22.

The lesions found in NF1 are numerous and include optic pathways gliomas, other varieties of astrocytomas, CNS dysplasia, increased incidence of meningocele, aqueductal stenosis, arachnoid cysts, hydrocephalus, gliomas of the spinal cord, syringomyelia, osseous lesions such as sphenoid dysplasia, thinning of long bone cortex, pseudoarthrosis and neurofibromas of peripheral nerves or plexiform neurofibromas, café au lait macules, and freckling in the axillary or inguinal regions. In general a diagnosis of NF1 is made if one finds six or more café au lait macules with a diameter greater than 5 mm in prepubertal patients and greater than 15 mm in postpubertal patients; or two or more neurofibromas of any type; or freckling in the axillary or inguinal regions. A first-degree relative (parent, sibling, or child) with NF1 is also an important criterion. Pigmented hamartomas of the iris (Lisch nodules) are also found in patients with NF1 (Table 5.6).

The changes in NF2 are bilateral acoustic neuromas, multiple intracranial meningiomas, schwannomas of other cranial nerves; spinal meningiomas and schwannomas; and occasional peripheral nerve tumors. No parenchymal gliomas are found in NF2 (77–81).

The majority of these lesions are described under various specific locations such as optic gliomas (described with suprasellar lesions), the eighth nerve (acoustic) neuromas (described with posterior fossa), cerebellopontine angle lesions and meningiomas (described under "Neoplasms"). Congenital absence of the greater wing of the sphenoid has been described under "Skull." Lesions involving the spinal cord and meninges are described with the spine and spinal cord. Other abnormalities that are peculiar to neurofibromatosis are described here.

High-Intensity Lesions of Neurofibromatosis on T1- and T2-Weighted Images These patches of increased intensity, mainly on T2 images, involve certain aspects of the brain, particularly the basal ganglia region bilaterally, the optic pathways and geniculate bodies, the cerebellar peduncles, other areas in the cerebellar white matter, and the brainstem. These hyperintense patches are particularly well seen on T2 images, and they do not enhance with gadolinium.

Table 5.6.
Neurofibromatoses

Neurofibromatosis1
Related to abnormality on chromosome 17
Astrocytomas
Optic pathway gliomas
Spinal cord gliomas
Osseous dysplasia
Plexiform or peripheral nerve neurofibromas
Café au lait spots
Axillary/inguinal freckling
Pigmented hamartomas of the iris ("Lisch nodules")
Neurofibromatosis 2
Bilateral acoustic neuromas
Meningiomas of brain or spine
Cranial nerve or spinal schwannomas

They produce no mass effect, and they can be fairly well circumscribed, although some fade into surrounding tissues. They are not shown on CT (82,83). Hurst et al. considered them hamartomas or low-grade gliomas (82), whereas Bognanno et al. considered them heterotopias, or islands of dysplastic tissue (83).

While the majority of these hyperintense patches are seen on T2-weighted images, Mirowitz et al. reported a number of cases of hyperintensity in the same areas but occupying a somewhat larger territory on T1-weighted images (80). In general, the usual hyperintense patches associated with neurofibromatosis are not visible on T1 images, so we must consider that at least two types of abnormalities are responsible for these changes. Moreover, both types tend to decrease in size and may disappear completely by the age of 21, which suggests that such findings are delayed myelination (Figs. 5.41 to 5.43) (84). If this were the case in all instances, however, one would expect to have some findings on the T1 images. Some of the patches eventually develop into gliomas.

The term *hamartoma* has frequently been used, and it may well be a good expression. I prefer the term *hyperintense patches on T2 images*. Mirowitz et al. have tried to explain the hyperintense T1 patches and conclude that such lesions may represent ectopic Schwann cells in the basal ganglia, or heterotopias or hamartomas that contain Schwann cells or melanocytes, or both (80). They argue that all pigment cells throughout the body, except for those

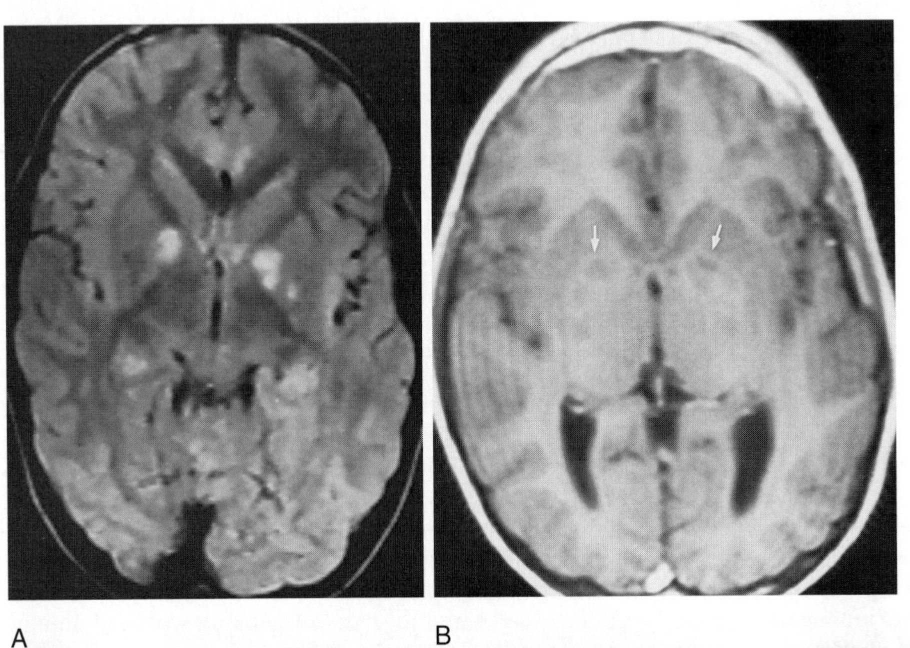

Figure 5.41. Neurofibromatosis type I in an 8-year-old boy. **A.** Proton density image. There are bright patches in the globus pallidus bilaterally and in the putamen on the left. **B.** The T1-weighted image shows low-intensity areas in the globus pallidus bilaterally (small arrows), which seem to correspond to the bright areas on T2-weighted images. **C.** CT examination also shows some hypodensity in the globus pallidus (arrow on left). **D.** Proton density image. There are other patches in the posterior hippocampal area (arrows). Another patch was seen in the upper medulla.

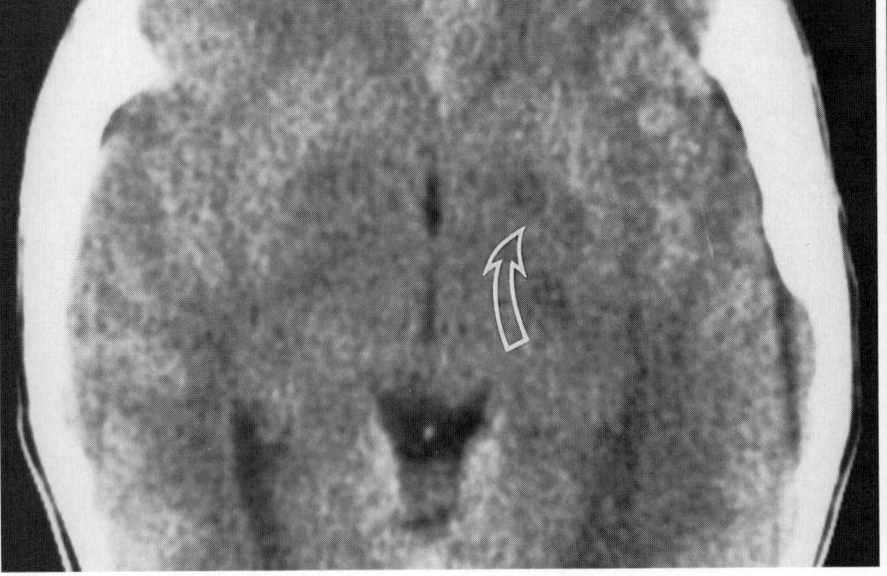

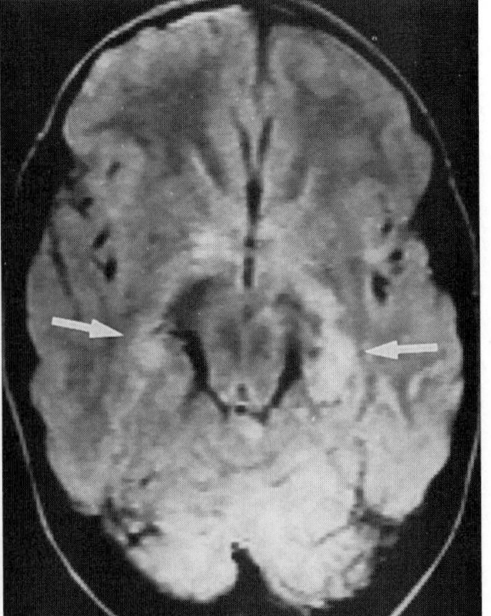

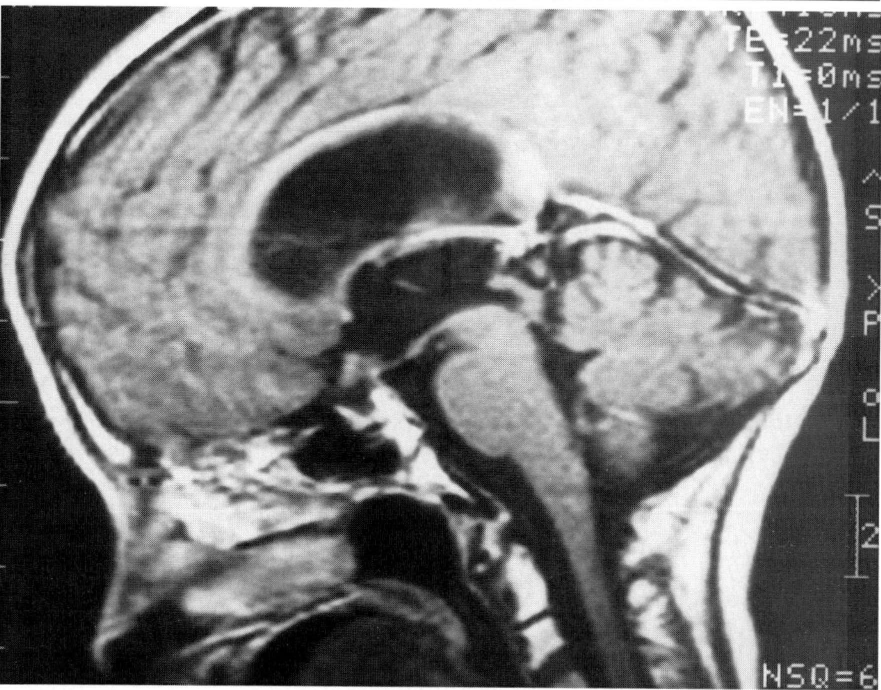

Figure 5.42. Neurofibromatosis type I. Sagittal T1-weighted image shows focal aqueduct stenosis and hydrocephalus in a 10-year-old boy with neurofibromatosis type I.

in the retina, originate as stem cells in the neural crest. These cells migrate to the leptomeninges, particularly the pia and the entire CNS. Disruption of normal migration of these cells occurs in patients with neurofibromatosis, resulting in some characteristic features such as the café au lait spots, axillary and inguinal freckling, cutaneous hyperpigmentation, and Lisch nodules in the iris. Hamartomatous collections of melanocytes have also been described in the brains of patients with neurofibromatosis, particularly in the basal ganglia. The frequency of silent lesions, particularly tumor, in patients with neurofibromatosis types I and II has been emphasized by Egelhoff et al. (85) and Elster (86).

Sturge-Weber Syndrome (Encephalotrigeminal Angiomatosis) The clinical features of this syndrome vary but include convulsions, a dermal nevus, mental retardation, glaucoma, and sometimes hemiplegia. The angioma is unilateral and is distributed along the first branch of the trigeminal nerve. The exact location may vary between patients and may be somewhat more forward, occupying the area of supply of the ophthalmic division of the trigeminal nerve. The angioma is usually present at birth (over two-thirds of the cases), and sometimes the angiomas may exist without the intracranial components or vice versa.

The fundamental cerebral lesion is a venous angioma of the leptomeninges, which is thought to result in faulty cerebral circulation. The engorged venous rather than arterial or capillary channels comprise the angiomatous malformations of the pia. The abnormal veins do not extend into the cerebral substance, but numerous intracerebral capillaries appear to be a part of the pathologic process. Vascular changes of fibrosis, hyalin degeneration, and calcification occur. Concomitantly there is loss of underlying brain cells, gliosis, and deposition of calcium in the cerebral cortex (87).

Dystrophic calcification occurs in a pericapillary distribution within the fourth layer of the cortex under the venous angioma. The calcification is probably secondary to relative anoxia of the brain cortex and, interestingly enough, may occur within a relatively short period of time. That is, calcification may be absent for several years in a child and then reexamination 3 to 6 months later will show extensive typical calcifications (88). Poser and Taveras reported on the findings by cerebral angiography in 23 of 50 patients (88). In addition to the classical capillary-venous angioma usually described pathologically in this syndrome, arteriovenous malformations, arterial thrombosis, anomalies of veins and dural sinuses, and anomalies in the territory of the external carotid circulation were demonstrated in these patients. Subdural hematoma and cerebral atrophy or hypoplasia were shown arteriographically in some cases.

Today the diagnosis is usually made by clinical observation of the skin nevus and by CT scanning. The latter demonstrates the calcifications earlier than can be seen on plain skull films and also demonstrates the presence of cerebral atrophy. If IV contrast is used, CT may demonstrate some abnormal venous channels and/or enhancement of the involved areas of the brain.

MRI is not as satisfactory as CT examinations because the calcifications cannot be evaluated. Early myelination of the white matter in the affected hemisphere has been reported on MRI (89). In addition, MRI with gadolinium enhancement may demonstrate typical leptomeningeal enhancement in the usual parietal and occipital areas when

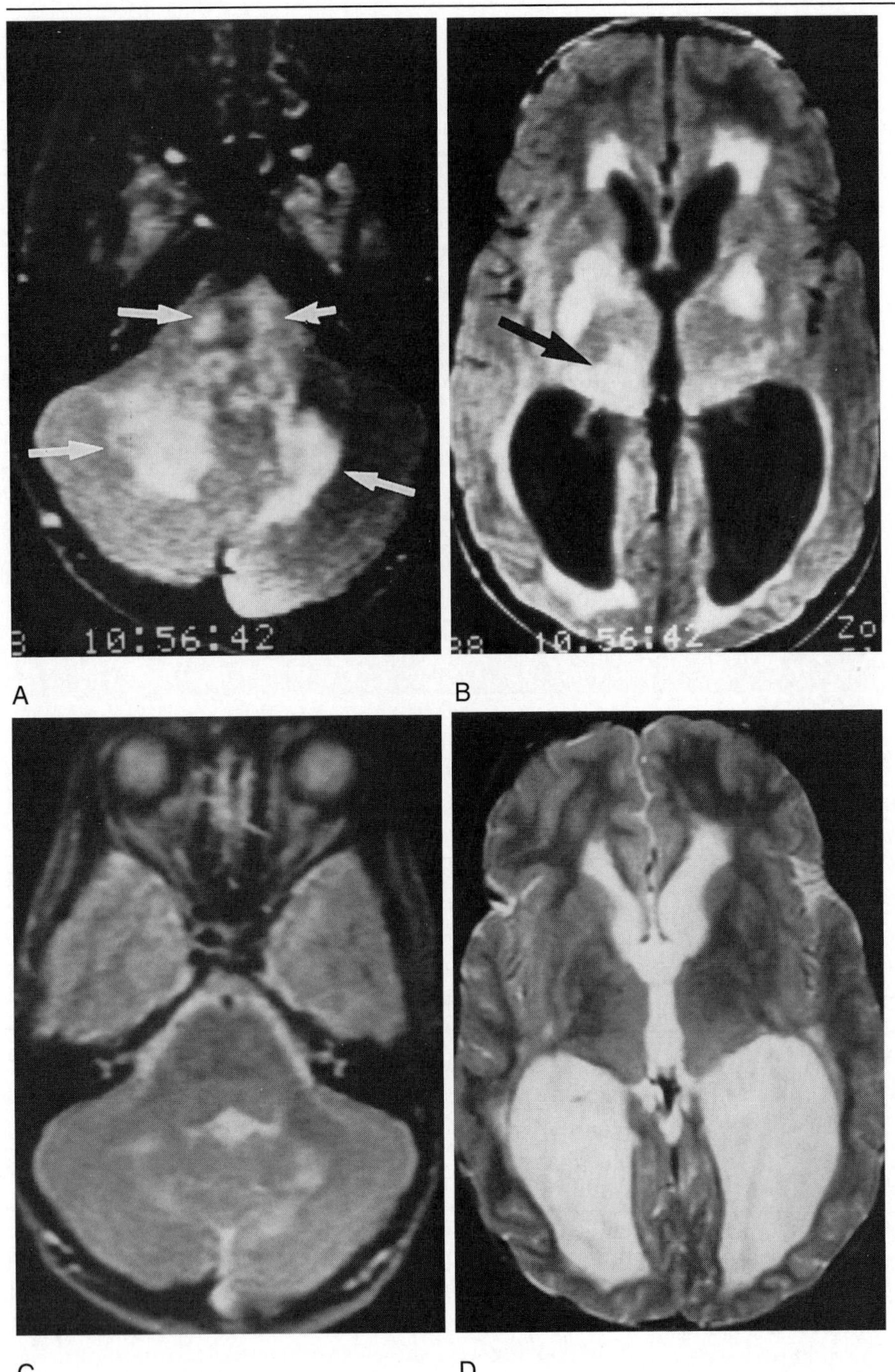

Figure 5.43. Neurofibromatosis type I in an 8 1/2-year-old boy showing disappearance of bright patches with time. **A** and **B.** T2-weighted image posterior fossa axial. There are large bright patches in the cerebellum, and there are also several patches in the pons (arrows). **C.** Reexamination 15 months later shows complete disappearance of the bright patches from the pons and incomplete clearance of the large cerebellar patches. The child was now 10. **D.** The higher T2-weighted section taken at the same time also shows disappearance of the basal ganglia and thalamic lesions. It would be inappropriate to apply the term *hamartoma* to these disappearing hyperintense patches. Are they areas of delayed myelination?

the plain MRI examination may be normal or show only minor, poorly defined changes (90) (Fig. 5.44) (Table 5.7).

The plain films of the skull show calcification in involved areas, usually the parietal and occipital lobes. Distribution of the calcifications follows a linear, often parallel, convoluted contour, evidently produced by calcification in the convolutions of the brain. Calcification is not usually observed before the age of 2. As explained previously, it may not be seen for some years and then appears within a relatively short period of time (several months) when the ap-

Table 5.7.
Sturge-Weber Syndrome

Also referred to as "encephalotrigeminal angiomatosis."

Clinical features may include mental retardation, dermal nevus, glaucoma, and hemiplegia.

Due to a pial venous angiomatous malformation.

Facial nevus (angioma) is typically unilateral and over V1 distribution.

Associated with dystrophic calcification of adjacent brain cortex.

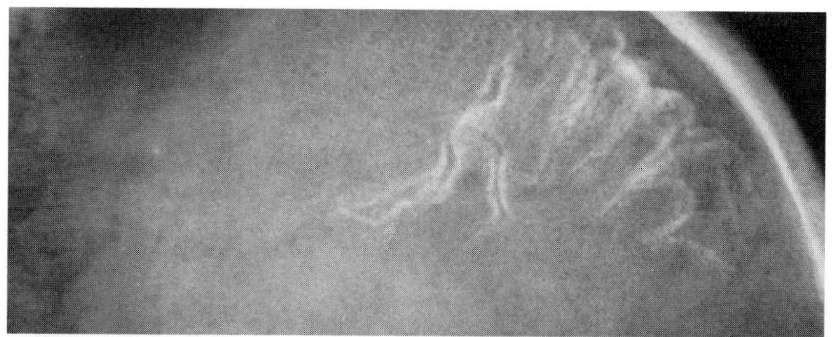

A

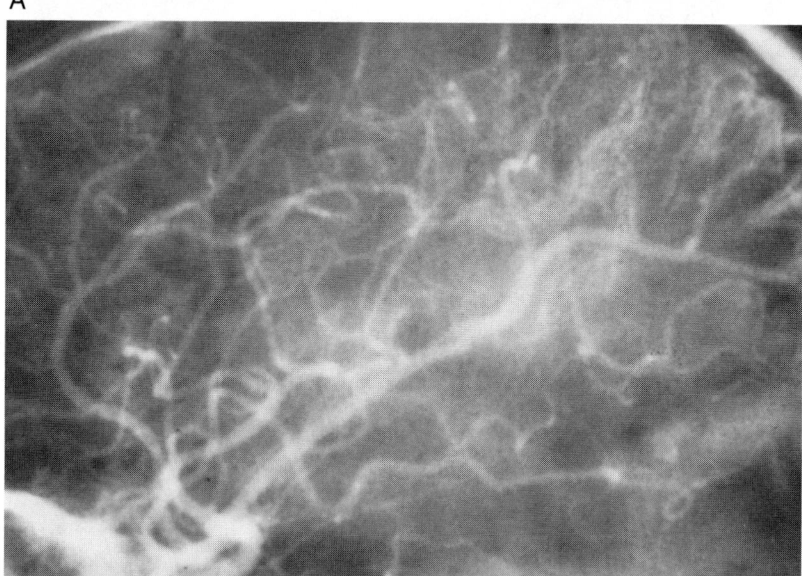

B

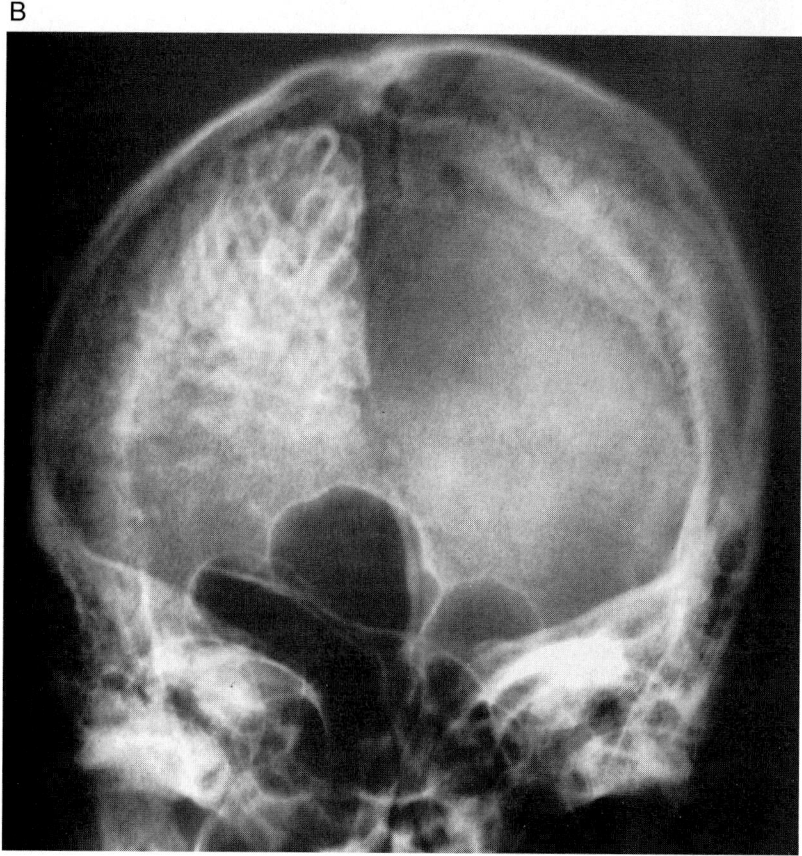

C

Figure 5.44. Sturge-Weber disease. **A.** Typical cortical calcification. **B.** Lateral view angiogram reveals only slightly increased vascularity in the abnormal area. **C.** In another patient, extensive calcification and decrease in size of the hemisphere with changes in the skull are seen. The sagittal sinus crest and groove are to the right of the midline, the frontal sinuses are overdeveloped, and the parietal bone is thicker on the right with diminished curvature as compared with the other side, all due to long-standing decrease in size of the hemisphere going back to childhood (Dyke-Davidoff-Masson syndrome) (*continues*).

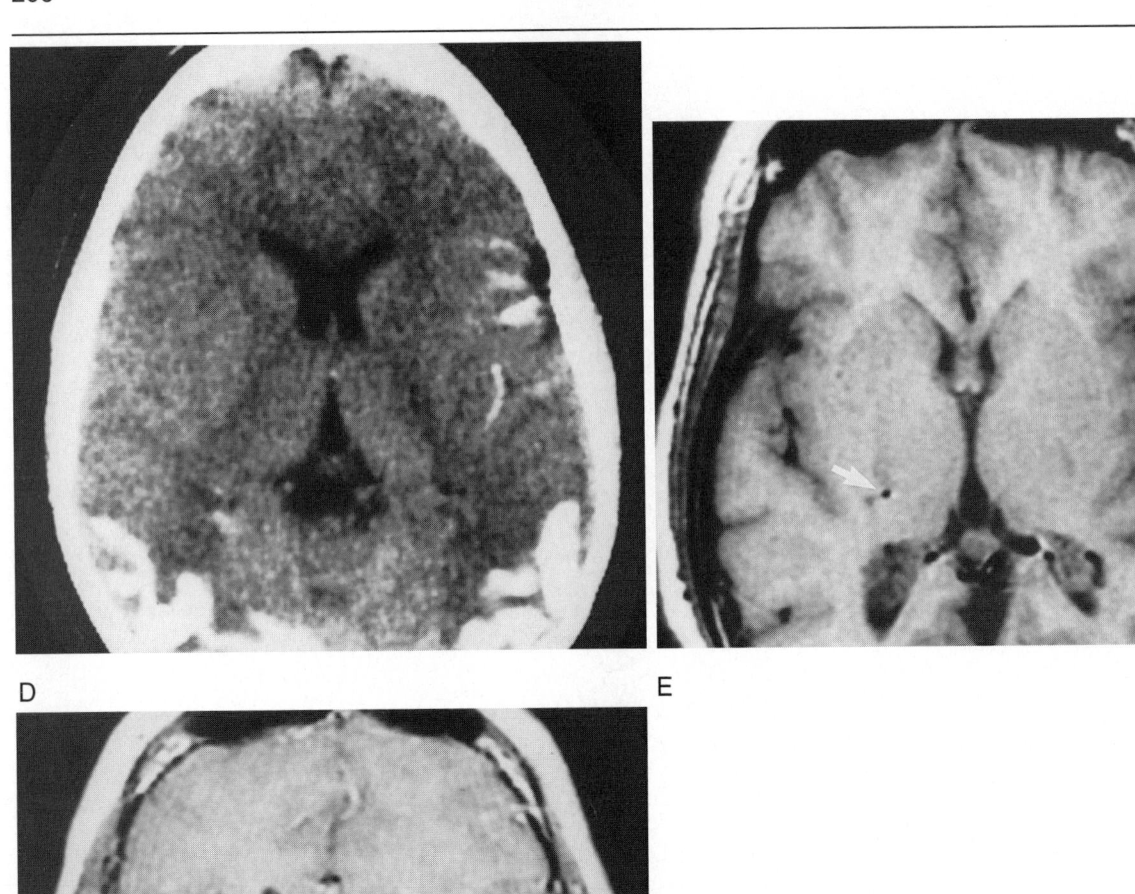

D E

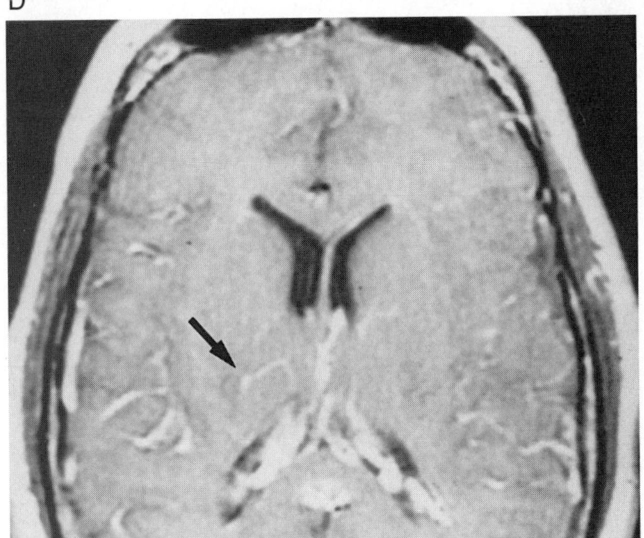

F

Figure 5.44. *(continued)* **D** to **F.** Sturge-Weber syndrome (encephalo-trigeminal angiomatosis) in a 23-year-old man. **D.** CT shows extensive bilateral cortical calcifications in the parieto-occipital region as well as less extensive cortical calcifications in the left frontal and insular region. **E.** T1-weighted MRI axial view reveals essentially no abnormalities. There may be an enlarged vein in the right lateral thalamic region to account for the flow void seen (arrow). **F.** Postcontrast axial through the same region as B shows enhancement of veins in the parieto-occipital region bilaterally. The flow void in the right thalamus is now seen to be hyperintense. There is also evidence of some enhancement in the leptomeninges over the parieto-occipital region.

propriate conditions involving certain levels of oxygen concentration in the brain tissues develop. Hemiatrophy of the brain may result in changes in the skull, secondary to the smaller brain, consisting of increased thickness of the skull, a smaller middle fossa, a slight deviation of the crista galli toward the smaller side, and enlargement of the sinuses and mastoids on the atrophic side.

Tuberous Sclerosis (Bourneville's Disease) Although Bourneville in 1880 coined the name *tuberous sclerosis*, von Recklinghausen in 1862 described cardiac rhabdomyoma in a newborn and also described the lesions found in the brain. Cardiac rhabdomyomas occur typically in patients affected with tuberous sclerosis and may be found in a fairly high percentage of the cases (about 50 percent). While tuberous sclerosis is particularly well known for its important neurologic manifestations, such as a convulsive disorder, mental retardation of a varying degree (which is occasionally absent), and tumors with obstructive hydrocephalus,

Table 5.8.
Tuberous Sclerosis

Variable degrees of mental retardation and seizures.
Extra-CNS findings include cardiac rhabdomyomas, renal or adrenal angiomyolipomas, and hepatic cysts.
Subependymal, subcortical, and cortical hamartomas.
Occasional development of giant cell tumors at foramen of Monro, causing obstructive hydrocephalus.

other organs frequently show manifestations, which sometimes become important. These include angiomyolipomas of the kidneys, which can grow to a large size; angiomyolipomas of the adrenal gland; rhabdomyomas of the heart; and changes in the liver (multiple cysts), the skin, the bones, the lungs, and the heart. Tuberous sclerosis is inherited with an autosomal dominant pattern, but many cases are thought to be a spontaneous mutation (91,92) (Table 5.8).

The radiologic findings are varied. In the brain the most characteristic lesion is the subependymal nodule, which may vary in size (Fig. 5.45). In earlier times, by pneumoencephalography, we referred to these nodules as *candle drip-*

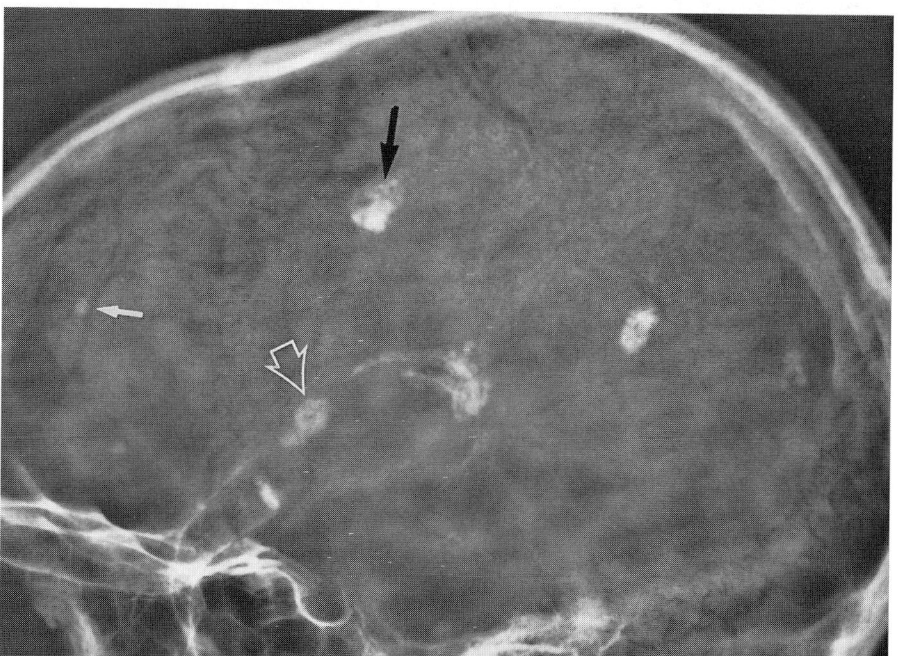

A

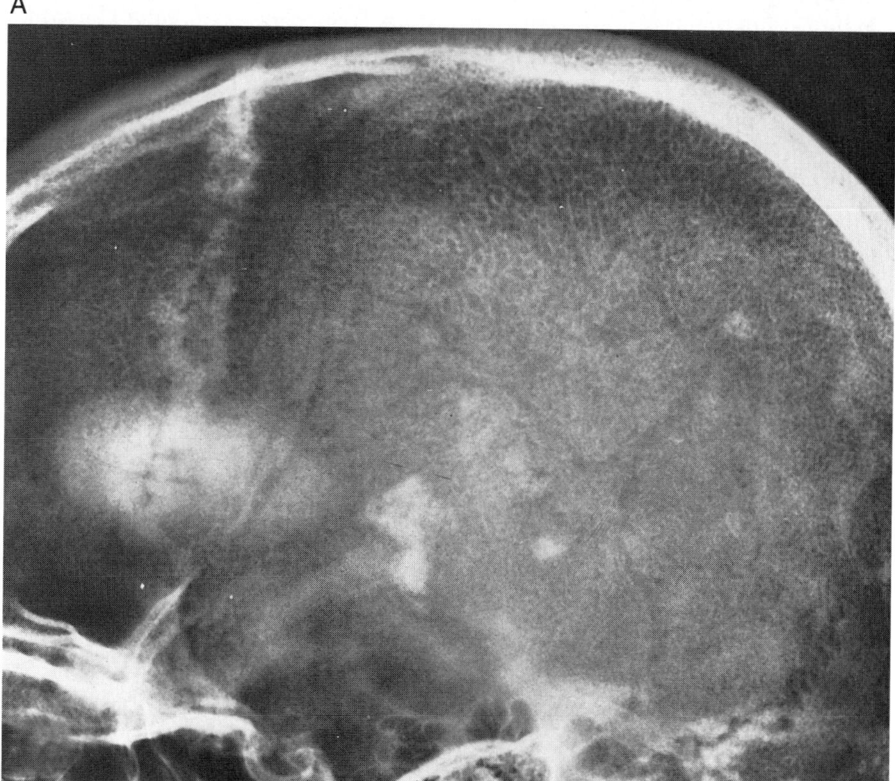

B

Figure 5.45. Tuberous sclerosis. **A.** There is extensive calcification in the cortical tubers (upper arrow), in the subependymal nodules (anterior white arrow; the lateral ventricles are enlarged), in the foramen of Monro (open arrow) and adjacent floor of the lateral ventricles. **B.** There is a large patch of sclerosis in the fronto-parietal suture region in another case.

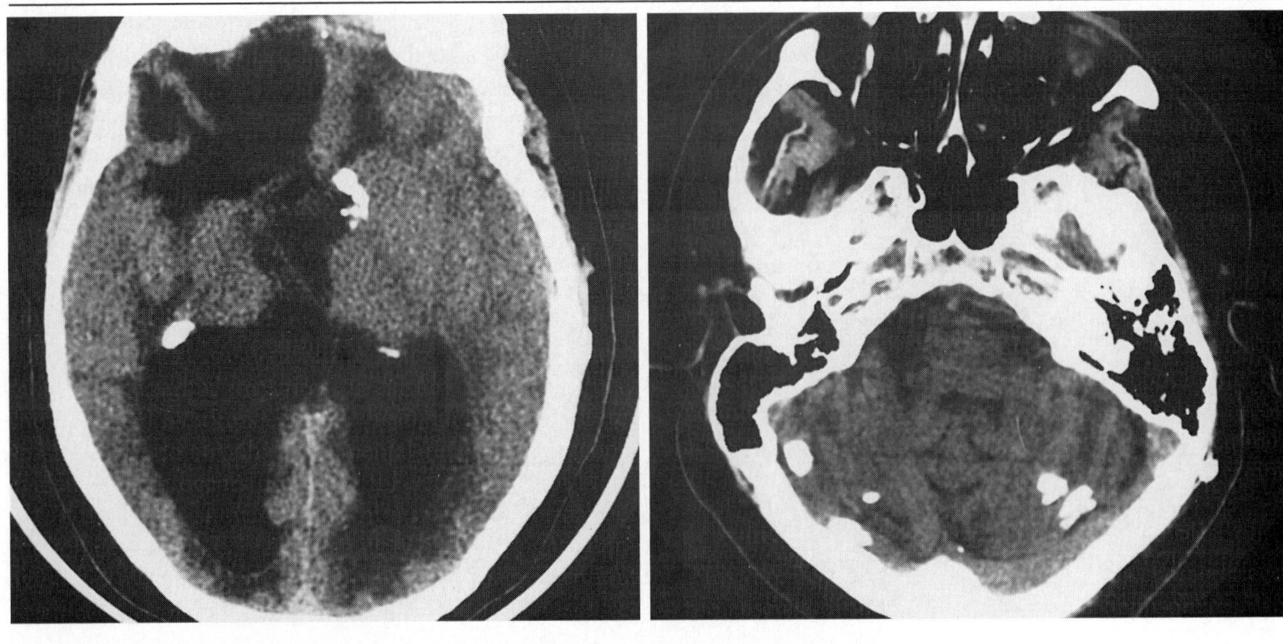

Figure 5.46. Tuberous sclerosis. **A.** Axial CT images reveal intraventricular calcifications, particularly in the region of the foramen of Monro. There is ventricular dilatation with scalloping of the ventricular margins, suggesting obstructive hydrocephalus and transependymal CSF passage. The obstruction was in the aqueduct (not shown). **B.** The posterior fossa revealed calcified tubers in the cerebellar cortex, but calcified surface tubers were not seen in the brain.

pings. They frequently contain sufficient calcium to be seen on CT of the brain, but they can also be seen on plain-film examinations of the skull when the calcification is extensive (Figs. 5.45 and 5.46). The next most typical findings are the so-called potato tumors on the surface of the brain. These tubers are hamartomas, which produce enlargement of the gyri on the surface of the brain. These changes are easily observed on autopsy specimens but are more difficult to see on CT examinations. MRI is considerably more informative about these cortical tubers. The growths are usually bright on T2 examinations, and the actual enlargement of the involved gyri can be seen (Fig. 5.47). If there is calcium, the deposits may appear as a darker area surrounded by a bright area on T2 images.

Some of the subependymal nodules are frequently located in the region of the foramen of Monro, and sometimes they degenerate into a true neoplasm.

Histologically, the surface potato tumors contain large, elongated or oval cells that resemble astrocytes. The subependymal nodules are made up of large cells that contain abundant cytoplasm. The cells are sometimes multinucleated. The tumors that may occur, most commonly near the foramen of Monro, are classified usually as giant cell astrocytomas.

Aneurysms may occur in patients with tuberous sclerosis, but these are rare.

The lesions in other organs are cysts in the metacarpals and phalanges of the hands and feet, local periosteal thickening on the shaft of some tubular bones, and patches of sclerosis in the skull (Fig. 5.45), vertebrae, pelvis, and long bones. The skin typically presents the adenoma sebaceum in the cheeks and sometimes café au lait spots. The frequency of skeletal findings is said to be fairly high, almost 50 percent of the cases, but in my experience they have been less common. Perhaps the cases I have seen did not undergo a complete skeletal examination because of the primary symptom complex being associated with the nervous system.

Von Hippel–Lindau Disease (Cerebelloretinal Hemangioblastomatosis) This disease process may be inherited as an autosomal dominant condition or may present in some patients for whom no inheritance factor can be demonstrated. The disease was originally described by von Hippel in 1904 (93); Lindau, in 1926, recognized the association of retinal angiomas with cerebellar hemangioblastoma, cysts of the kidney, lung, liver and pancreas, and tumors in the adrenal gland and kidney (94). In general, the symptoms that may bring a patient to the hospital may vary: retinal angiomas produce visual symptoms (about 16 percent of cases); cerebellar hemangioblastomas may present with symptoms of increased intracranial pressure and cerebellar signs; pheochromocytoma of the adrenal may present with paroxysmal hypertension; and renal cell carcinoma presents as a renal tumor. The retinal angiomas may be bilateral and may be multiple, but close to half of the patients have no retinal angioma (Table 5.9).

Figure 5.47. Tuberous sclerosis in a 4-year-old boy. **A.** CT shows several calcified nodules in the right ventricular wall. In addition there is an abnormal semicircular area of increased density in the right frontal region suggestive of a cortical tuber (arrows). **B.** Postcontrast T1-weighted image reveals bilateral subependymal nodules (all bright in spite of the calcification) in the ventricular wall. **C.** A T2-weighted (first echo) image passing through the ventricles slightly higher than B shows that the subependymal nodules are bright (arrows). A number of subcortical tubers are seen, and many more are seen higher up (**D**).

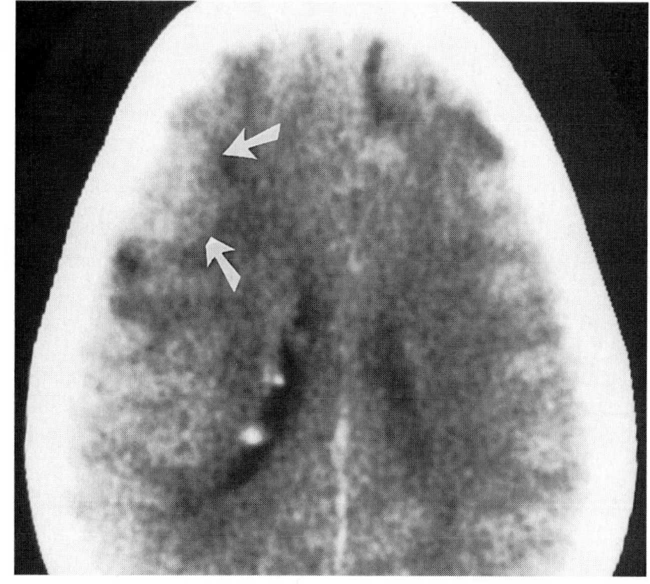

A

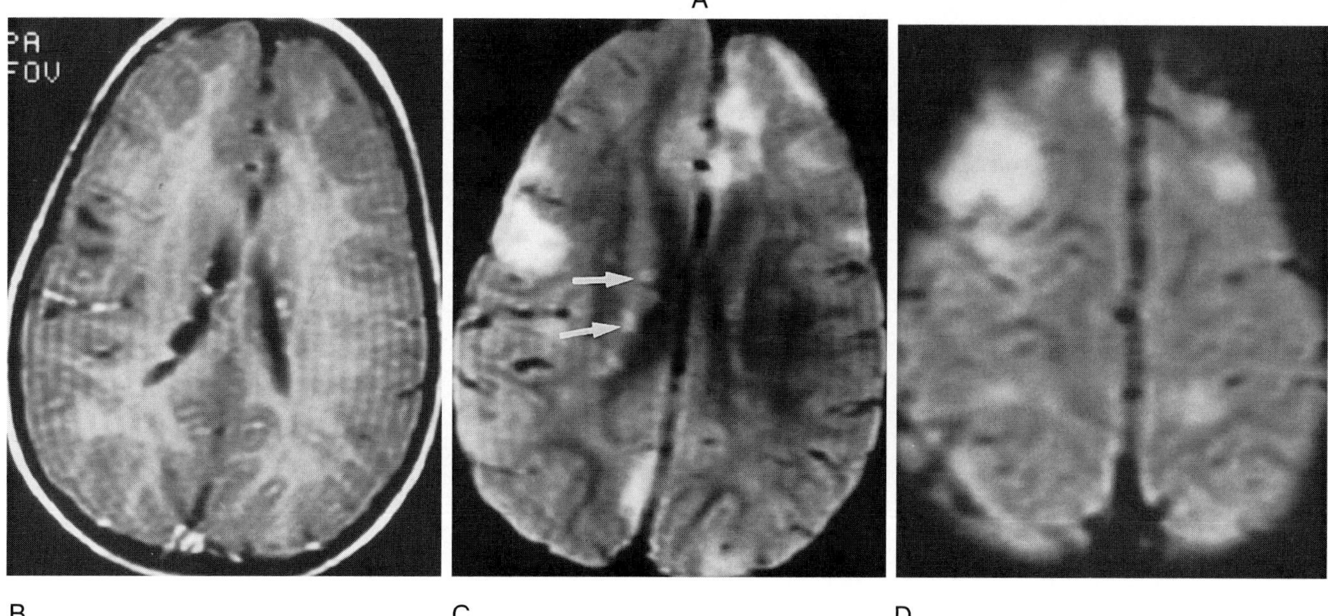

B C D

Table 5.9.
Von Hippel–Lindau Disease

Retinal angiomas
Cerebellar or spinal hemangioblastomas
Renal lesions (e.g., carcinoma, cysts)
Adrenal pheochromocytomas
Cysts in multiple organs (e.g., pancreas, liver, epididymis)

One of the most frequent lesions is hemangioblastoma of the cerebellum (close to half of all cases) or spinal cord. A cyst is usually the major part of the cerebellar or the spinal cord mass. The tumor nodules may be relatively small and may be multiple. In fact, one must look for other nodules once a nodule with an accompanying cyst is found. Multiple nodules can also exist without any associated cysts (Fig. 5.48). The hemangioblastoma nodules in the spinal cord may also be multiple (Fig. 5.49).

CT will usually show an enhancing nodule and any cyst with a nodule in its wall. The nodule enhances rather brightly, and as mentioned earlier, it may be found elsewhere in the cerebellum without an accompanying cyst. A mass effect is obvious, and the degree of hydrocephalus will depend on the size of the lesion as well as on its location in relation to the aqueduct and fourth ventricle. In a smaller percentage of the patients, only an enhancing large tumor can be found without any cystic component.

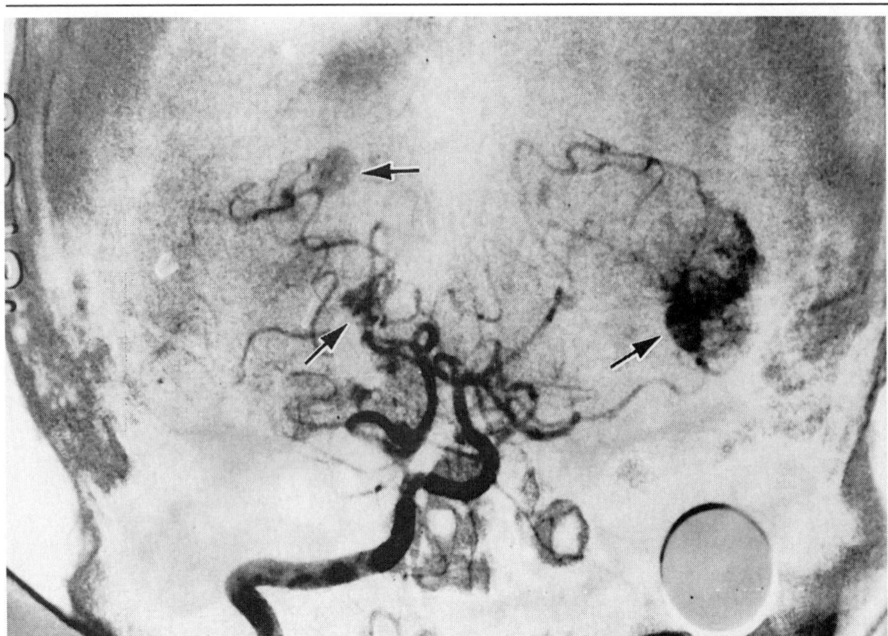

Figure 5.48. Multiple cerebellar nodules in a patient with cerebellar hemangioblastoma. The vertebral angiogram reveals at least three nodules (arrows). The patient, who had von Hippel–Lindau syndrome, also had a hemangioblastoma nodule in the spinal cord (not shown).

MRI is also quite sensitive when gadolinium enhancement is utilized. The spinal cord lesions are much better demonstrated with MRI, and syringomyelia, which most often accompanies the tumor, is easily visible. A cyst not communicating with the central canal may also be found.

Angiography usually demonstrates the tumor nodules, which, histologically, are composed of angioblasts with

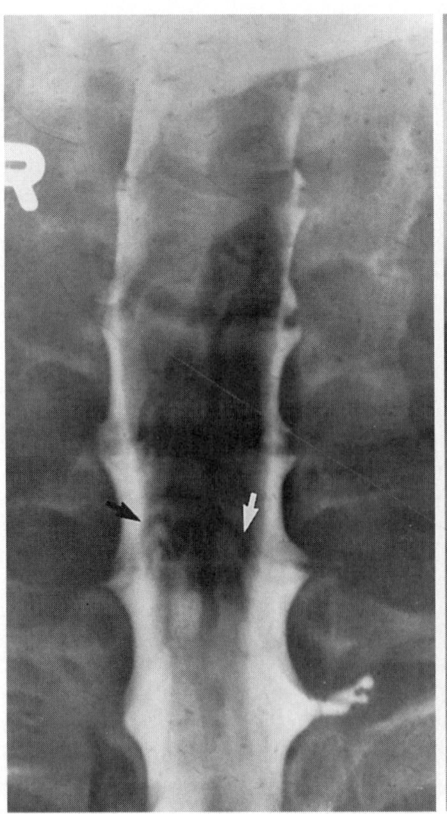

A

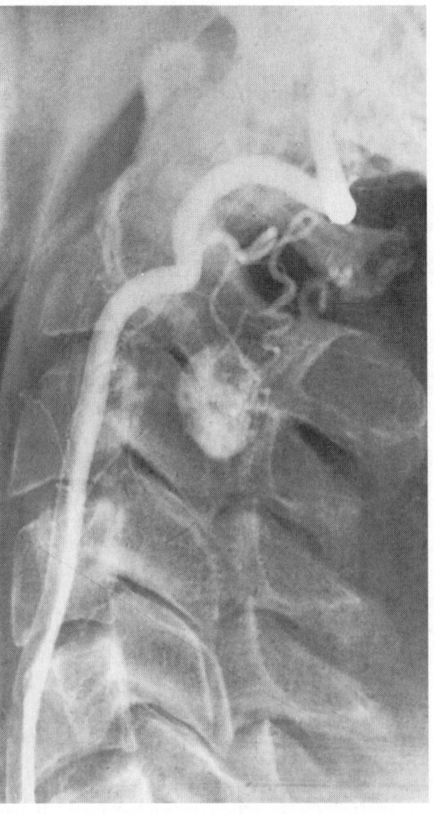

B

Figure 5.49. Hemangioblastoma nodule associated with focal syringomyelia in the cervical region. **A.** The myelogram reveals a widened spinal cord. There are enlarged vascular channels seen as radiolucent serpentine lines (arrow). **B.** Lateral vertebral angiogram reveals feeding of a nodule by branches of the vertebral artery. The association of a cyst with hemangioblastoma is common both in the cerebellum and in the spinal cord.

primitive cells that normally form the fetal blood vessels without any intervening nerve and glial tissue. In addition, there is rapid drainage of the blood out of these nodules with early filling veins.

Radiation therapy is often given to these patients, with the idea that some tiny tumor nodules may not be shown by either MRI, CT, or angiography following removal of a cystic hemangioblastoma.

Hemangioblastomas of the cerebellum are often seen without other manifestations of von Hippel–Lindau syndrome. Approximately half of patients who have developed von Hippel–Lindau syndrome will present with a renal cell carcinoma. The tumor may be bilateral and also multiple. Pheochromocytomas occur in about one-sixth of the patients and may also be bilateral.

Although supratentorial hemangioblastomas have been described, there is always considerable controversy about whether they really occur there (95). (Further details are given under "Posterior Fossa Tumors," Chapter 11.)

Ataxia-Telangiectasia (Louis-Bar Syndrome) This disease is characterized by progressive cerebellar ataxia associated with telangiectasia of the conjunctiva of the skin of the eyes. Although Louis-Bar first described the condition in 1941 (96), Sedgwick, in 1958, termed the syndrome *ataxia-telangiectasia*. In 1972 he reported over 400 cases of which some 40 had autopsy studies (97). The disease is progressive in that the infant may show no signs, the child learns to walk, and the ataxia develops slowly so that by the second decade the affected person is not able to walk and the speech is quite dysarthric. The ataxia appears before the telangiectasias in the conjunctiva and elsewhere in the skin. The disease is transmitted as an autosomal recessive condition. An interesting component of this disease is that of absent thymus and reduction of the lymphoid tissue with loss of lymphoid follicles in tonsils, adenoids, lymph nodes, and spleen. There is a strong tendency to develop malignant lymphoma. Many develop frequent pulmonary infections, which is the most frequent cause of death in these patients.

Radiologically, the only finding is that of atrophy of the cerebellum, particularly in the cortex, where there is extensive loss of Purkinje and granule cells. Patients with ataxia-telangiectasia possess a deficiency of IgA in the serum and other body fluids as well as the deficiency listed earlier in the lymphoid tissue and the thymus. Other radiologic manifestations include the signs of frequent pulmonary infections.

Osler-Weber-Rendu Disease (Hereditary Hemorrhagic Telangiectasia) This autosomal dominant vascular disorder causes multiple telangiectasias affecting the mucous membranes, intestines, stomach, liver, kidneys, skin, and nervous system. The telangiectatic vessels present marked thinning of the walls with widening of the lumen, and from there the tendency to break and to produce hemorrhage. Indeed, the most common clinical problem in this condition is multiple hemorrhages in the mucosa of the intestines, the liver, the kidneys, and the brain. The lesions in the brain may be multiple cavernous angiomas. The latter group is being diagnosed with increasing frequency as MRI is carried out more frequently, showing not only the angioma but also evidence of prior bleeding. However, the great majority of the cases where multiple angiomas of the brain are encountered have no apparent association with the Osler-Weber-Rendu disease. The disease, as well as ataxia-telangiectasia, belongs in the group of phakomatoses and is much better known by the angiographers because the vascular lesions are more common in other organs than they are in the brain (98).

Basal Cell Nevus Syndrome (Gorlin's Syndrome) This syndrome, characterized by Gorlin et al. (99), presents in childhood and has an autosomal dominant inheritance pattern with a variable degree of penetrance. The affected children have multiple basal cell carcinomas, jaw cysts, and some skeletal anomalies. The skeletal anomalies consist of bifid ribs, shortened metacarpals, usually the fourth and the fifth, kyphoscoliosis, and vertebral segmentation anomalies. The children may develop medulloblastomas. The only neuroradiologic finding is that of early calcifications in the falx and tentorium, which can be quite pronounced. (See Fig. 4.2.)

Blue-Rubber-Bleb-Nevus Syndrome The name of this syndrome comes from the combination of multiple discrete, bluish, rubbery cutaneous nevi associated with vascular malformations in other organs (including the gastrointestinal tract, lung, pleura, liver, skeletal muscle peritoneum, and CNS). Waybright et al. described a case with angioma of the CNS and thrombosis of a vein of Galen aneurysm (100). The radiologic findings are those of angioma or vascular malformation in the brain. Very few cases have been described, particularly in the neuroradiologic literature.

Klippel-Trenaunay Syndrome (Angio-osteohypertrophy) This syndrome consists of a vascular malformation of the spinal cord and meninges associated with a vascular nevus on the skin innervated by nerves originating in the corresponding area in the spinal cord. Hypertrophy of the corresponding lower extremity usually combines with enlargement of the bones and angioma. Angiography may demonstrate a normal arterial system, but venography may show varicose and enlarged veins. The angioma of the spinal meninges may bleed. Lower-extremity venography usually shows thrombosis of the deep veins; this appearance should always alert one to the possibility of Klippel-Trenaunay syndrome. Surgical stripping ligation of the superficial veins in these patients would make their condition considerably worse (101). The presence of port wine hemangiomas of the skin on the thighs, usually present in early childhood, associated with the venous anomalies described earlier makes the diagnosis almost certain.

There may be a relationship between the Klippel-Trenaunay and Sturge-Weber syndromes in that the children may present manifestations of both (102). The term *Klippel-Trenaunay-Weber syndrome* is frequently used for these patients. In the Parkes-Weber variant, arteriovenous fistulas are present in addition to varicose veins and hypertrophy of the affected parts or limbs (103).

Williams and Elster described two unusual patients with early development of brain atrophy (102); contrast enhancement with CT and MRI showed large and heavily affected leptomeningeal areas in the brain, similar to Sturge-Weber, and cortical calcifications bilaterally. One patient was a newborn, and the other was 18 months of age. The newborn exhibited marked cerebral atrophy 4 months later.

Cowden's Disease This disease is also called *multiple hamartoma syndrome*, a rare hereditary condition that causes neoplasms of ectodermal, mesodermal, and endodermal origin. Characteristically, patients also present multiple cutaneous lesions such as fibroepithelial polyps, capillary hemangiomas, and papular trichilemmomas in the face, neck, and axilla. These are surely the most typical lesions that permit the diagnosis of Cowden's disease. The association of this disease with Lhermitte-Duclos disease has been pointed out by Lloyd and Dennis (104) and demonstrated in a patient reported by Williams et al. (105). The association of manifestations of Cowden's syndrome tends to make the Lhermitte-Duclos disease a phakomatosis.

Lhermitte-Duclos disease consists of a special type of cerebellar tumor containing hypertrophic ganglion cells in the granular and molecular layers with excessive axonal myelination. This lesion is described under tumors of the cerebellum. Lhermitte-Duclos disease can be a hamartoma, or it can be a true neoplasm that may recur.

Hypomelanosis of Ito (Incontinentia Pigmenti Achromians) This neurocutaneous syndrome presents bizarre hypopigmented skin lesions and neurologic abnormalities. The diagnosis is usually made first by the dermatologist. Patients may present with multiple congenital abnormalities in the eyes, the musculoskeletal system, hair, or CNS abnormalities (in about half the cases). There may be mental retardation, psychomotor delays and seizures, language retardation, gait ataxia, and hearing defects. Williams and Elster reported a 13-year-old girl whose MRI scans revealed enlargment of a hemisphere with unilateral ventricular enlargement and extensive periventricular white matter hyperdensity on T2 images (106). Also many hyperintense small areas in centrum semiovale were visible on T1 images as low-intensity areas.

The incontinentia pigmenti (Bloch-Sulzberger syndrome) may be accompanied by microcephaly, hydrocephaly, corticospinal tract dysfunction, seizures, and ocular abnormalities (optic atrophy, cataracts, abnormal retinal pigmentation). Each of these syndromes is probably transmitted as an X-linked dominant trait, affecting girls more frequently than boys.

Wyburn-Mason Syndrome (Retinocephalic Angiomatosis) This syndrome is usually first seen by ophthalmologists because of the retinal angiomas. Patients may also present with arteriovenous malformations involving the visual pathways; arteriovenous malformations have also been found in the midbrain and basal ganglia (98).

Neurocutaneous Melanosis This rare neuroectodermal disorder is characterized by multiple congenital pigmented cutaneous nevi and melanotic thickening of the leptomeninges. The pigmented areas in the skin may reach 20 cm in diameter and may be hairy. They do not undergo malignant degeneration. The brain meningeal lesions may become neoplastic.

Gadolinium markedly enhances the involved areas, which in the patient reported by Rhodes et al. was the entire brain (107). The enhancement extended into the sulci. The case reported by Sebag et al. also had a temporal lobe mass that was typical for melanoma (bright on T1 and dark on T2) (108).

As pointed out earlier, pigmented cells arise from the neural crest, the progenitor of melanoblasts that embryologically migrate to the skin and pia mater. Most cases occur sporadically, but a familial pattern may also occur.

Maffucci's Syndrome This congenital disease is characterized by multiple enchondromas and secondary hemangiomas, phlebolithiasis, and bone malformations. The changes may affect the nervous system by virtue of compression of brain structures produced by cranial osteochondromas. Also, primary brain tumors and pituitary tumors have been reported (109). The intracranial lesions are more frequent in Ollier's disease, another form of enchondromatosis (110).

Muscular Dystrophy and Myotonic Dystrophy The Fukuyama type of congenital muscular dystrophy presents mental retardation, progressive muscle weakness, and joint contractures as typical features. It is more common in Japan (111). MRI demonstrates delayed myelination in the brain white matter, which seems to involve more extensively the frontal lobes but also involves the periventricular area in the occipital lobes (111,112). Also cerebellar abnormalities have been reported (204). Somewhat different white matter changes (patchy areas in periventricular region and farther away from the ventricular wall) have been described in *myotonic dystrophy* (113,114). Extensive calcification in the falx cerebri has also been described.

CONGENITAL METABOLIC ANOMALIES

Contrary to the anatomic malformations and neurocutaneous syndromes causing gross anomalies visible by inspection, palpation, or diagnostic imaging, congenital metabolic anomalies may or may not produce changes visible by CT, MRI, angiography, or plain films. The list of these diseases or syndromes is long and getting longer. For our purpose, however, only those conditions that present demonstrable abnormalities are described here. Since the advent of CT and MRI, the number of those conditions in which changes can be observed has grown; new observations undoubtedly will continue to appear in the literature. MR spectroscopy offers additional diagnostic possibilities, but as yet the reports are relatively few and not impressive for clinical applications (115,116).

The coverage here is not intended to be encyclopedic, but an effort has been made to cover the more frequently encountered entities. The imaging changes may not be specific, and often the neurologist will make the final diagnosis with the help of biochemical data and clinical history coupled with the physical examination. Diseases that do not appear to cause visible changes on CT or MRI are not described.

The radiologist is confronted with an examination (CT, MRI, angiography, etc.) in which a number of observations can be made. The radiologist goes from the findings on the images to the differential diagnosis. That is, for the radiologist, these findings are like the symptoms or clinical findings are to the clinician. Because of this, this rather complex and numerous group of conditions are discussed utilizing what I might call a *semiological* approach. The diseases that affect the brain white matter are described together even though their pathogenetic backgrounds are totally different. For instance, metachromatic leukodystrophy and Krabbe's disease are lysosomal storage disorders, whereas X-linked adrenal leukodystrophy is due to an enzyme defect and failure to oxidize very long chain fatty acids; Pelizaeus-Merzbacher disease is a sudanophilic leukodystrophy, and sudanophilia is a staining characteristic. Whenever possible (or desirable), a semiological approach is used in other metabolic conditions and, indeed, in other disease groups throughout this book.

Metabolic Conditions Affecting the White Matter

The normal process of myelination is a most important milestone in the developing brain. It begins in utero, as discussed earlier (see under "The Developing Brain in Infants and Children"). The white matter contains the immense majority of the myelinated fibers; for this reason, myelin disorders are usually called *white matter diseases*. The term *leukodystrophy* is usually generically applied to this group of pathologic conditions. The term *dysmyelination* applies to a condition in which the myelin sheaths of the axons in the developing nervous system fail to form or are defective. This defect is caused by some biochemical fault that blocks the synthesis or interferes with the formation of one or more components of myelin.

On the contrary, *demyelination* applies to destruction of myelin after it is formed (as in multiple sclerosis).

Looking at the entire group of congenital metabolic anomalies, the majority of these conditions presenting in childhood are clearly accompanied by changes in white matter, whether or not they are classified primarily as white matter diseases.

The following group is usually included among the white matter diseases: Alexander's disease, Canavan's disease, Krabbe's disease, adrenal leukodystrophy, metachromatic leukodystrophy, and Pelizaeus-Merzbacher disease.

As a group, these diseases are characterized by progressive mental deterioration. Patients may present with signs of slow motor development or visual and auditory symptoms, but the most prominent sign is progressive mental retardation. The degree and speed with which progression takes place varies. The metabolic abnormality is also different for each disease, and the time of onset of observable signs and symptoms varies with the type of disease. In general, the group presents an autosomal recessive pattern of inheritance.

ALEXANDER'S DISEASE

Alexander's disease (or fibrinoid leukodystrophy), the *infantile variety*, starts in the first few months after birth. The infants present with a large head and retardation. The diagnosis is made by brain biopsy, which demonstrates accumulation of Rosenthal fibers in the subependymal, subpial, and perivascular areas (117). As with Canavan's disease, enzymatic analyses and histochemical stains of muscle biopsies do not provide a diagnosis. This is contrary to the other leukodystrophies. CT and MRI do not usually demonstrate many changes. In the case reported by Shah and Ross, only a slightly hyperintense area adjacent to the frontal horn was seen on one side also involving the adjacent caudate nucleus (118). MRI demonstrated hypointensity in the same area on T1 and no enhancement after gadolinium. T2 images showed only minimal hypointensity (119).

In the case reported by Trommer et al., CT showed marked ventriculomegaly at birth with much larger occipital than frontal horns (120). At 9 months, typical lucent white matter, particularly in the frontal lobes, spared the internal capsules. Autopsy at 13 months revealed extensive demyelination and the typical widespread Rosenthal fibers in the cerebellar white matter, brainstem, and deep gray nuclei. Apparently the typical white matter changes on CT and MRI may make their appearance later. These may be located bifrontally and may spare the internal capsules. The presence of Rosenthal fibers bears no apparent relationship to the degree and location of demyelination.

Farrell et al. reported periventricular contrast enhancement in the frontal region on CT examination (121), and Valk and van der Knapp reported the same enhancement on MRI examination (122).

Grodd et al. reported variable findings with respect to the proton spectra of *N*-acetylaspartate, choline, and lactate in the two cases examined, indicating that proton MR spectroscopy (H1-MRS) may not be of value in differentiating Alexander's disease from other conditions (123).

Two other varieties have been described. The *juvenile variety* manifests itself between 7 and 14 years of age with progressive bulbar symptoms and spasticity; seizures are less prominent. The average duration to death is 8 years (from onset of symptoms). The *adult variety* begins at 15 to 70 years of age. The disorder may simulate multiple sclerosis or may be asymptomatic.

CANAVAN'S DISEASE

Canavan's disease (spongiform degeneration) (Fig. 5.50 and 5.51) is similar to Alexander's disease in that it requires a brain biopsy for diagnosis. However, evidence has suggested a deficiency in the enzyme aspartoacylase, resulting in an increase in *N*-acetylaspartic acid in urine and plasma (124,125).

Canavan's disease typically presents between 3 and 6 months of age but may present earlier. The infant may show marked hypotonia, a large head, and seizures. Later spasticity, optic atrophy, and mental retardation become evident. Death occurs usually in the second year of life.

CT and MRI show diffuse white matter abnormalities (radiolucencies on CT, hypointensity on T1-weighted images, and hyperintensity on T2-weighted images) without predilection for any particular area. The nine cases reported by Brismar et al. presented symmetric white matter changes both frontal and occipital with some sparing of the internal and external capsules (125). Later the brain cortex becomes thinner than normal, and signs of atrophy appear (including the cerebellum), which may become marked. In one case, enhanced CT showed a slight increase in density of the gray matter, which did seem to be related to the white matter changes such as seen in adrenoleukodystrophy. All cases reported by Brismar et al. demonstrated aspartoacyclase deficiency and were from Saudi Arabia (125).

A recent study by Grodd et al. reported the feasibility of assessing *N*-acetylaspartate in brain by proton MRI spectroscopy (H1-MRS) (123). H1-MRS revealed increased *N*-acetylaspartate and lack of choline-containing compounds in comparison to age-matched controls in involved areas of the brain, usually the frontal and the occipital regions, with some sparing of the internal capsule regions.

PELIZAEUS-MERZBACHER DISEASE

This rare X-linked recessive condition is characterized by the absence of myelin in the cerebral hemispheres, which

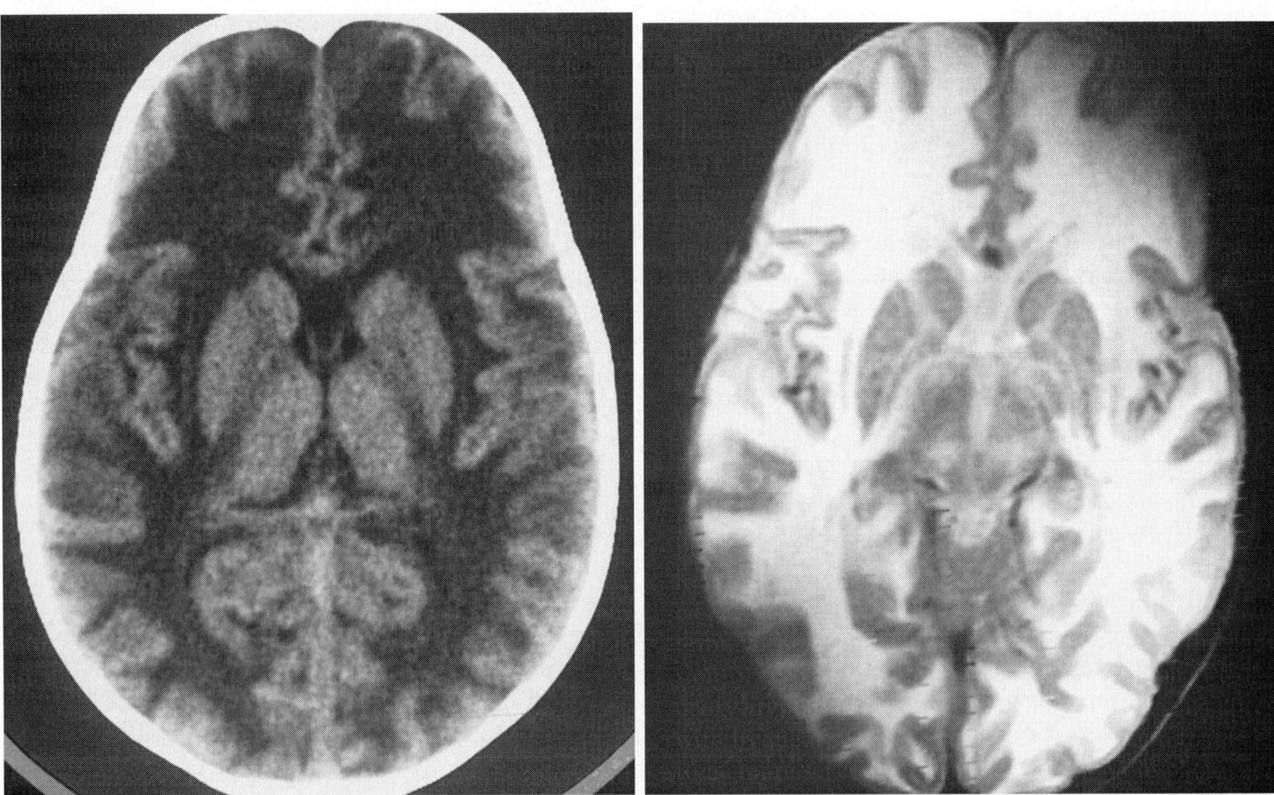

Figure 5.50. Canavan's disease in a 10-month-old macrocephalic boy who was referred for suspected hydrocephalus. **A.** CT shows normal-sized ventricles, no atrophy, but severe white matter disease. The white matter is markedly hypodense. **B.** T2-weighted MRI axial image shows severe white matter hyperintensity with some hyperintensity also in the internal capsule. The posterior fossa was also involved. There is marked reduction in gray matter thickness. (Courtesy of Dr. Jan Brismar, King Faisal Specialist Hospital and Research Center, Riyadh, Saudi Arabia [*AJNR* 1990; 11:805–810].)

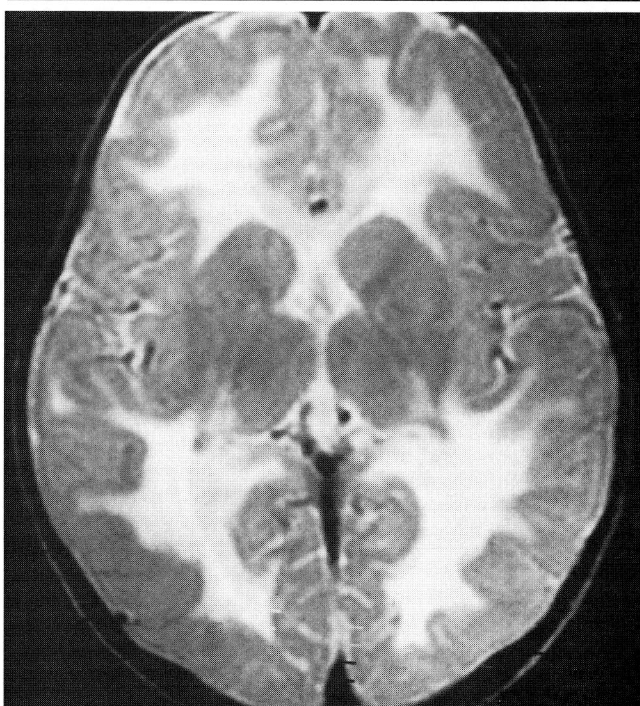

Figure 5.51. Canavan's disease in a 2-year-old mentally retarded girl with hypotonia and brisk limb reflexes. There is severe white matter disease of subcortical white matter but with normal-appearing myelination of the internal and external capsules. There was myelination, which appeared normal, in posterior fossa. This case, as well as the case in Figure 5.50, had aspartoacyclase deficiency, which, at present, is considered the best indicator of Canavan's disease. (Courtesy of Dr. Jan Brismar, King Faisal Specialist Hospital and Research Center, Riyadh, Saudi Arabia.)

suggests a failure of formation rather than destruction of myelin. Thus CT may not show any specific findings whereas MRI will show a white matter that is not bright on T1 and does not have the grayness on T2 images that normally occurs after the first year of life (126,127). The disease is more common in boys, starts in the neonatal period, and may cause death before the age of 10 years. The patients present with abnormal eye movements, shaking head, cerebellar ataxia, and retarded development.

The disease belongs in the group of sudanophilic leukodystrophies, with several forms varying according to age of onset, rate of progression of symptoms and signs, and possibly inheritance. The classic form has just been discussed, but there is an adult form with later onset, slower progression, and absence of nystagmus, a prominent sign in the earlier-onset forms. Epilepsy and moderate intellectual deterioration may occur (128). Variant forms have been mentioned by Fishman in patients who may present patchy demyelination of the CNS at autopsy and who present clinical features similar to the other forms (128).

Myelination of the brainstem and internal capsule is usually normal at birth, so that the diagnosis by MRI is not obvious early. In the succeeding weeks and months, however, the failure of myelin formation becomes obvious. Cerebral atrophy with widened sulci may be observed (Fig. 5.52).

X-LINKED ADRENAL LEUKODYSTROPHY

X-linked adrenal leukodystrophy (Fig. 5.53) is a peroxysomal disorder that affects only males and manifests itself between 4 and 8 years of age with decreasing school performance, changes in memory, and irritability. Seizures may occur. Adrenal signs (abnormal skin pigmentation, signs of adrenal insufficiency) may accompany or even precede these symptoms, or they may never appear, or they could occur without neurologic manifestations. A later onset, in adolescence or early adulthood, is also possible.

CT usually reveals decreased density of the white matter in the occipital region involving also the splenium of the corpus callosum. MRI shows signs of demyelination (high signal on proton density and T2 and low intensity on T1-weighted images) usually involving or starting in the occipital lobes, but frontal lobe involvement also occurs, sometimes prominently. Unilateral involvement in other areas, such as the internal capsule and the globus pallidus, and bilateral involvement in the caudate nucleus may present initially. Reversal of early lesions may be demonstrated following therapy such as bone marrow transplant (129).

Contrast enhancement may demonstrate a dense, enhanced margin surrounding the area of demyelination on CT and MRI (130). MRI also demonstrates lesions in the posterior fossa more clearly than CT, particularly those involving the auditory fibers and brainstem. On T2, the high-intensity margins seen on T1 gadolinium-enhanced images appear as a darker border surrounding high-intensity areas of demyelination.

Another form of adrenoleukodystrophy, *adrenomyeloneuropathy*, has a later onset (35 years of age) and symptoms of spinal cord and peripheral nerve involvement. A scoring method to classify degree of involvement has been proposed (131). Also the effects of bone marrow transplantation have been observed (132).

REFSUM DISEASE

This rare peroxysomal disorder is transmitted as an autosomal recessive condition and is caused by a deficiency of phytanic acid 2-hydroxylase, which causes phytanic acid to be accumulated in the myelin. The myelin thus affected has less viability. The peripheral myelin may be more affected than the CNS (133). The infantile form is more severe. The affected children present severe sensorineural deafness, retinitis pigmentosa, facial dysmorphism, hepatomegaly, growth retardation, and mental retardation (134).

MRI may show diffuse white matter hyperintensity in the brain and in the cerebellum on T2-weighted images, indistinguishable from other diffuse white matter diseases. Perhaps the involvement of the cerebellar white matter is more intense than in other conditions. In the cases reported by Dubois et al., there was involvement of the dentate nuclei of the cerebellum, which were hypointense on T1 and

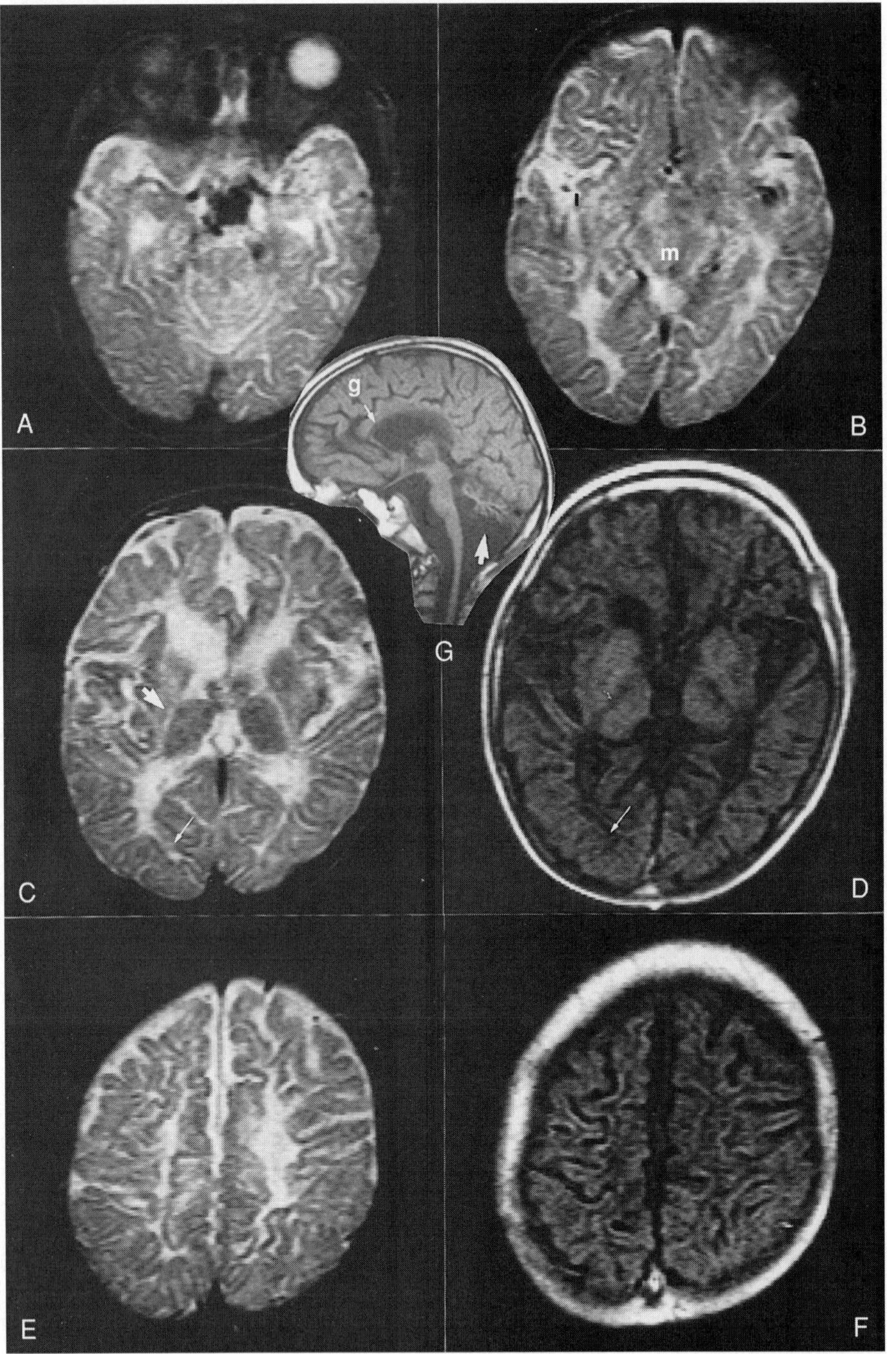

Figure 5.52. Pelizaeus-Merzbecher disease. T2-weighted (**A** to **E**), T1-weighted (**D** and **F**), and T1-weighted sagittal image (**G**) of a 10-year-old boy in vegetative condition with Pelizaeus-Merzbecher disease. No myelin present in the U fibers, the lobar and periventricular white matter, the posterior limb of the internal capsule (arrow in C), the mesencephalon (m in B), with severe atrophy of the cerebellum (large arrow in G), and very thin corpus callosum (small arrow in G). (Courtesy of J. Valk and M. S. van der Knaap, Amsterdam, Holland [AJNR 1989;10:99].)

hyperintense on T2-weighted images on one of the two children reported (134). The other had a normal MRI study in spite of a rather typical clinical picture of infantile Refsum disease. The MRI findings in these two typical and well-documented cases of infantile Refsum disease were therefore completely different from those in the two cases illustrated by Kendall (133), which tends to indicate that there is a variation in the imaging as well as in the clinical manifestations. The group of peroxysomal disorders to which Refsum disease belongs is a rather complex one, and further research continues to elucidate some of the biochemical mechanisms involved (135).

NEONATAL ADRENAL LEUKODYSTROPHY

Like the other adrenal leukodystrophies, infantile adrenal leukodystrophy (Fig. 5.54) is among the newly recognized peroxysomal disorders involving multiple enzyme deficiencies. At birth, the white matter is severely, diffusely degenerated, and cerebral atrophy occurs early. The corpus callosum is atrophic. CT shows radiolucencies in the affected white matter, and MRI shows hypointensity on T2 images of the same areas.

The basic metabolic defect in the adrenal leukodystrophies is an accumulation of very long chain fatty acids due to an impaired ability to degrade these owing to the pres-

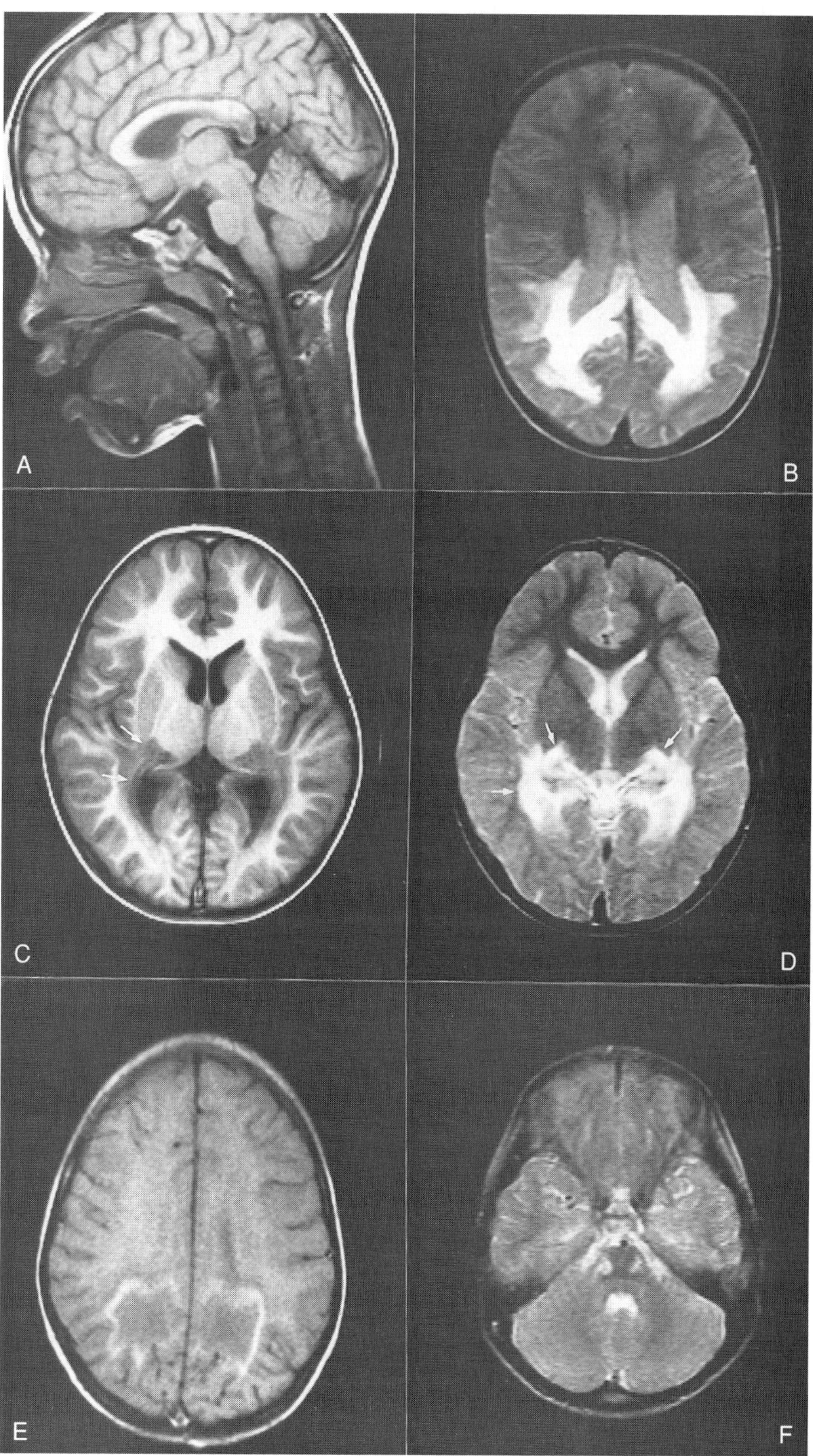

Figure 5.53. MR images almost pathognomonic for X-linked adrenal leukodystrophy in a 5-year-old boy. The images (**A** and **B**) show the involvement of the white matter in the occipital region with the involvement of the splenium of the corpus callosum. The T2-weighted image at this level (B) shows two layers of the disorder. The T1- and T2-weighted images through the ventricles (**C** and **D**) show the symmetric involvement of the lateral geniculate bodies (arrow) and the optic radiation (posterior arrow). The involvement of the descending corticospinal tracts is seen in the image through the pons (**F**). **E.** After contrast injection, the layer of active inflammation enhances and separates the regions of complete demyelination, and gliosis and partial demyelination as seen in B. (Courtesy of J. Valk and M. S. van der Knaap, Amsterdam, Holland [AJNR 1989;10:512].)

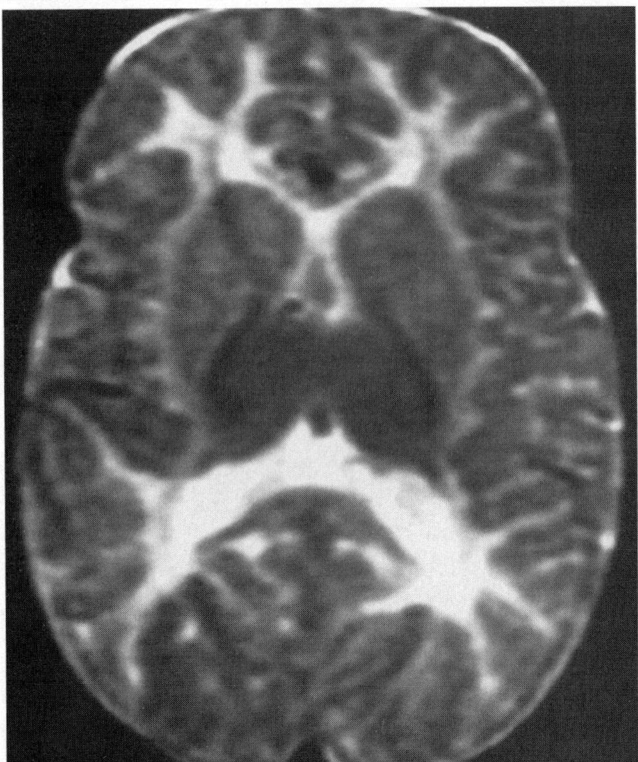

Figure 5.54. Neonatal adrenal leukodystrophy. T2-weighted axial shows very bright white matter in this 6-month-old infant. Clinically the child had a panperoxisomal disorder (class I: decreased number of peroxisomes with multienzyme involvement), considered to fall under the clinical category of neonatal adrenoleukodystrophy. He had jaundice at age 2 months. The liver was large. Zellweger's syndrome was considered, but there were no other lesions such as renal cysts, patellar ligament calcification, or gray matter migration defects.

ence of a peroxysomal defect in beta-oxidation. This leads to extensive demyelination. Calcium deposits may be observed in the oldest lesions, which usually occur in the occipital white matter (136). The subcortical U fibers are spared early. The geniculate bodies are usually involved as well as the brainstem, particularly in the corticospinal and corticobulbar tracts (Fig 5.53) (131,132).

ZELLWEGER SYNDROME

The Zellweger syndrome (cerebrohepatorenal syndrome) is a peroxysomal disorder presenting multiple organ involvement. Demyelination may occur, and a neuronal migration disorder (heterotopic gray matter, polymicrogyria) may show on MRI. The white matter volume may be decreased. This is the prototypical peroxysomal abnormality: complete absence of peroxysomes.

RHIZOMELIC CHONDRODYSPLASIA CALCIFICANS PUNCTATA

This rare autosomal recessive disorder (Fig. 5.55) causes short limbs, dwarfism, abnormal facies, psychomotor retardation, congenital cataracts, and joint contractures. These patients usually die within the first year of life. The radiographs show finely stippled epiphyses. T2 MRI may show bright periventricular white matter and subcortical changes, particularly in the occipital region (137).

METACHROMATIC LEUKODYSTROPHY

This autosomal recessive disorder usually presents in childhood (80 percent of patients), but less common juvenile and adult forms exist. Because of the deficiency of an enzyme, arylsulfatase-A, a metachromatic-staining lipid material, accumulates chiefly in the white matter but also in peripheral nervous structures. It belongs in the lysosomal diseases group along with a growing number of storage diseases (138). Patients present with gait disorders, spasticity, speech impairment, and intellectual deterioration. Death usually ensues within 1 to 4 years, but this may vary. Other organs are also involved (kidneys, pancreas, adrenal glands, liver, gallbladder).

CT shows hypointensity of the white matter, particularly in the frontal regions but also extending posteriorly. MRI shows prolonged T1 and T2 relaxation times in the white matter symmetrically. The demyelinated areas are less uniformly distributed than in other leukodystrophies, and areas of normal myelination are found as well. Ventricular dilatation and general cerebral atrophy develop (Fig. 5.56). Perhaps the one differential point to remember in comparison with other leukodystrophies is the somewhat more blotchy distribution of the demyelinating lesions found in metachromatic leukodystrophy. The patchy distribution may also be seen in adult forms of Pelizaeus-Merzbacher disease.

KRABBE'S DISEASE

Krabbe's disease (globoid cell leukodystrophy), a lipid storage disorder, is transmitted like the others as an autosomal recessive condition. Beginning early, at 3 to 6 months, the disease is manifested by irritability, rigidity followed by tonic seizures, quadriplegia, blindness, deafness, dysphagia, and progressive mental deterioration.

The disease is a lysosomal disorder due to a sphyngolipid (galactosylceramide), which accumulates in the tissues due to deficiency of the enzyme galactosylceramide-β-galactosidase. CT may show white matter lucency, and MRI will show diffuse white matter hyperintensity mostly due to demyelination although some may be due to edema (139). High-density lesions on CT may also occur in the thalamus, caudate nucleus, and corona radiata. In one of the four cases reported by Kwan et al., such lesions were visible in the cerebellum, brainstem, and subcortical white matter (140). The pathogenesis of the increased density on CT is not known but may be due to accumulation of the galactocerebrosides in the cluster of globoid cells, modified astrocytes, or histiocytes (141). The densities may disappear later when the atrophic phase supervenes. On MRI these areas may show increased or decreased

Figure 5.55. Rhizomelic chondrodysplasia punctata in a 2 1/2-month-old boy with short limbs and a relatively small head. Biochemically there was a mild hypoglycemia and severe hypocalcemia as well as decreased plasmalogen levels. **A.** The pelvis and femurs show stippled epiphyses and shortening of femurs. **B** and **C.** T2-weighted axials show hyperintensity in the white matter, particularly in periatrial region. **D** and **E.** Reexamination at 8 1/2 months again shows some hyperintensity in the periatrial region in the white matter. The ventricles are enlarged as they were previously; a large cavum septum pellucidum and vavum vergae are present, which is normal at this age. Some enlargement of the surface sulci indicative of cortical atrophy may also be present. (Courtesy of Dr. Daniel W. Williams, Bowman Gray School of Medicine, Winston-Salem, North Carolina [AJNR 1991;12:363–365].)

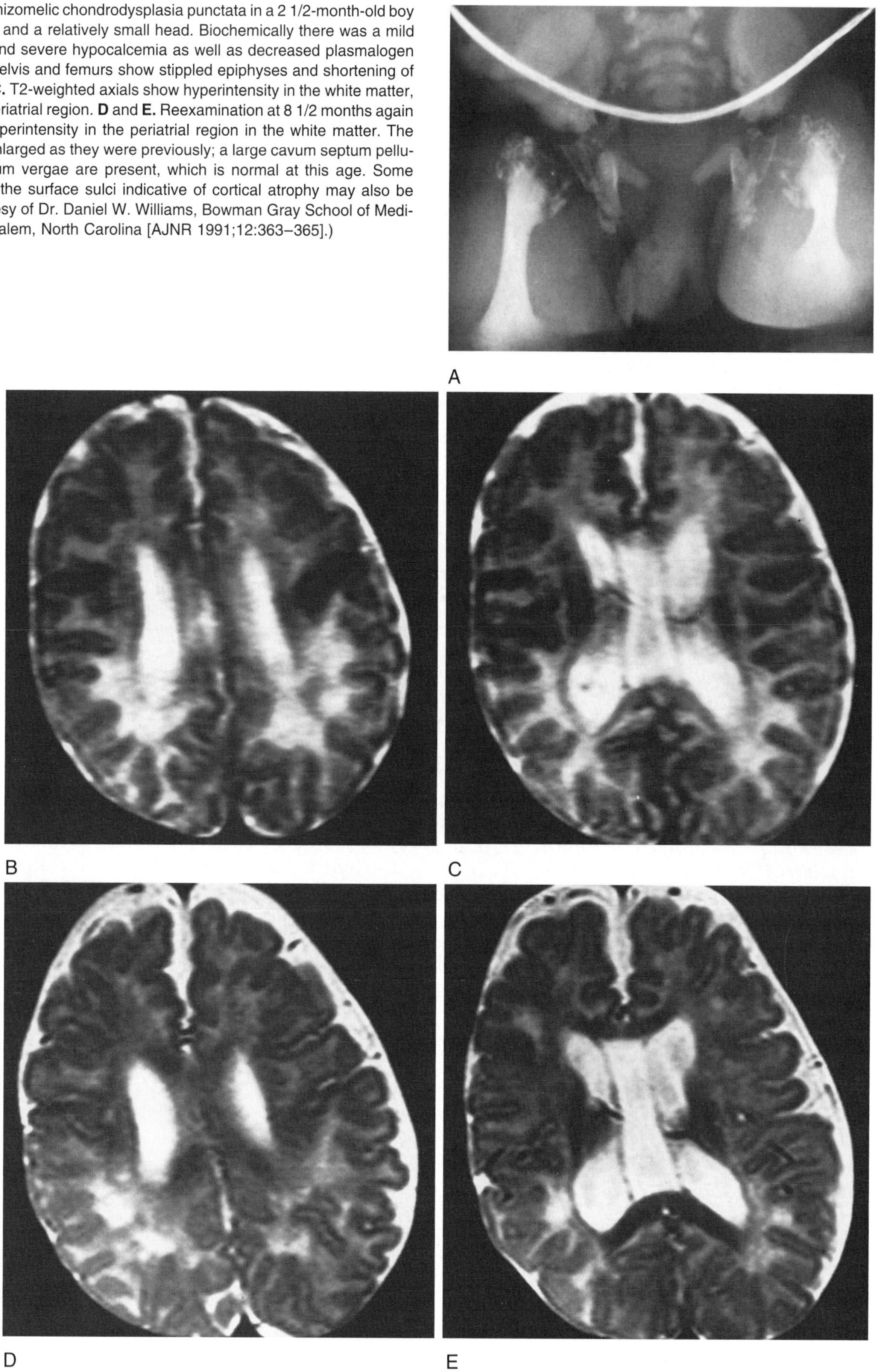

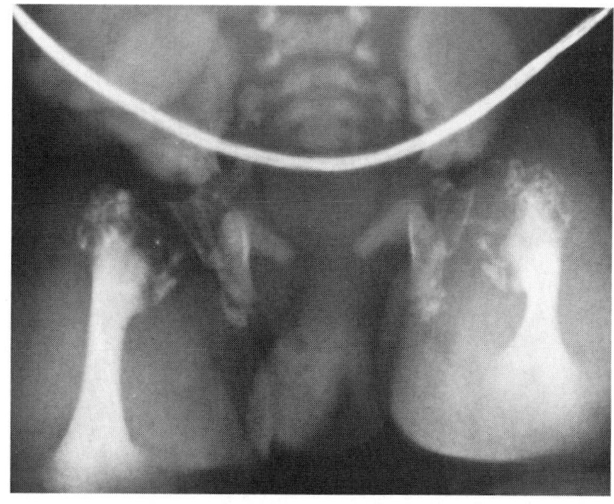

A

B

C

D

E

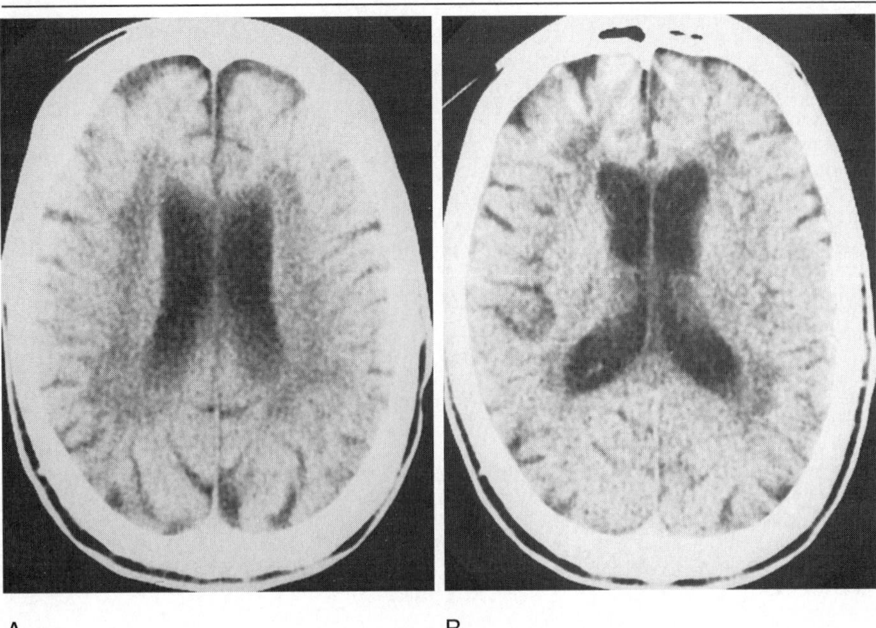

Figure 5.56. Metachromatic leukodystrophy in a 34-year-old man. **A.** A CT passing through the ventricles reveals a diffuse low attenuation in the centrum semiovale extending from frontal to occipital regions consistent with a leukodystrophy but nonspecific. **B.** A lower section shows moderate ventricular enlargement. The decreased density is not predominantly in the frontal region as is usually described in this condition. No MRI was available in the patient who was well until age 18, at which time he started showing changes in social behavior that led to the diagnosis of metachromatic leukodystrophy several years later. Since diagnosed (about 3 years previously) he has deteriorated and continues to do so in spite of adequate intake. The life expectancy is about 3 years after diagnosis of metachromatic leukodystrophy.

intensity on T1 or T2. Early examination in the infant may be normal (142).

MAPLE SYRUP URINE DISEASE

This is inherited as an autosomal recessive trait. About 75 percent of the affected children have the so-called classical form. The infant is normal for about the first week. In the second week, the infant starts to eat poorly, vomits, fails to thrive, and develops hypotonia, seizures, stupor, and finally coma. The urine has a maple syrup odor. Untreated, the condition leads to death within a few weeks. It is due to a block in the catabolic pathway of the branched-chain amino acids leucine, valine, and isoleucine.

CT or MRI will show a normal brain the first week but on the second week will show marked evidence of edema of the cerebellar white matter, posterior half of the brainstem, supratentorial white matter, and posterior limb of the internal capsule. Brismar et al. believe this is characteristic enough to allow an imaging diagnosis (143). During the second month, the edema recedes, leaving a slightly atrophic brain with some lucent lesions (on CT) or bright lesions on T2 MRI in the dorsal brainstem due to local atrophy, and also in the lenticular nucleus and thalamus. The surviving treated children show evidence of myelination in some areas, but in the centrum semiovale, myelination is usually retarded (Fig. 5.57).

PHENYLKETONURIA

This is the most common of the amino acid disorders and is detectable by examination of the blood for increased phenylalanine. Later, urine examination will show excretion of phenylpyruvic acid. The disease is due to deficiency of the hepatic enzyme phenylalanine hydroxylase, which interferes with the transformation of phenylalanine to tyrosine. The gene has been mapped on chromosome 12. Retardation (intellectual and motor) is a prominent feature observable during the first months after birth. Seizures, hyperactive behavior, and lack of coordination are frequent symptoms. Myelin is severely affected by the high phenylalanine blood concentration. If the disorder is diagnosed early after birth, treatment can prevent many of the problems. The white matter abnormalities affecting myelin seem to indicate failure of myelin formation rather than destruction. In the 15 patients reported by Pearsen et al. (144) and the 9 reported by Shaw et al. (145), the symmetric hypomyelination shown on T2-weighted images was mostly posteriorly located in the cerebral hemispheres with anterior involvement rather mild and seen only in cases where there were florid MRI-demonstrated changes. The brainstem and cerebellum showed no changes. The degree or prominence of white matter changes did not correlate with the level of mental retardation. Mild cortical atrophy was seen in half of the cases (Fig. 5.58).

MALIGNANT HYPERPHENYLALANINEMIA

A variant of phenylketonuria, in which there is an increased blood concentration of phenylalanine, worth considering here is malignant hyperphenylalaninemia due to a deficiency of dihydropteridine reductase and to a cofactor, tetrahydrobiopterin (BH_4), also a requisite for the conversion of tyrosine to dopamine and of tryptophan to 5-hydroxy-tryptamine (146,147). The patients may present with frequent seizures and mental retardation that is likely to be more severe and appear earlier than in phenylketonuria. For this reason, the term *malignant hyperphenylalaninemia* is useful. The white matter changes may be relatively mild, and only cerebral atrophy may be found early. The early changes may be reversible by appropriate therapy. The older children are likely to show more white matter abnormalities on the MRI scans. Calcification in basal gan-

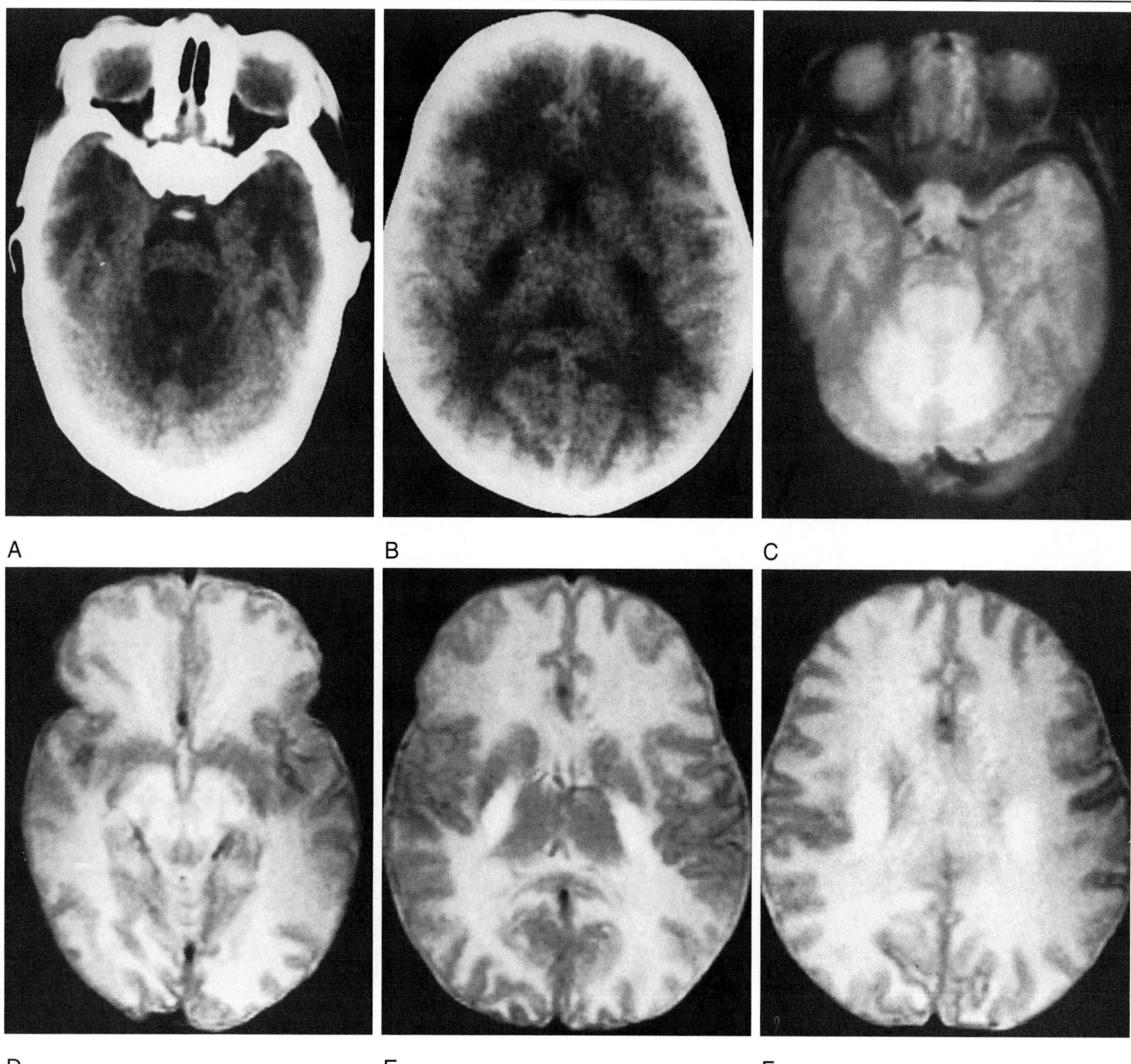

Figure 5.57. Maple syrup urine disease (MSUD) in a 27-day-old boy. The infant was already severely neurologically damaged (opisthotonus). **A** and **B.** CT images reveal low attenuation in white matter, in deep cerebellar white matter, and in dorsal brainstem. **C** to **F.** T2-weighted images 6 days later show severe edema involving the centrum semiovale (in D, E, and F), the posterior limb of the internal capsule (in E), the peduncles and the dorsal aspect of the brainstem (in C and D), and the cerebellar white matter, an appearance that is almost diagnostic of MSUD. (Courtesy of Dr. Jan Brismar, King Faisal Specialist Hospital and Research Center, Riyadh, Saudi Arabia.)

glia and in cerebral white matter has been described (147) (Fig. 5.58*C* and *D*).

NONKETOTIC HYPERGLYCINEMIA

Nonketotic hyperglycinemia (sulfatide lipidosis) is an inherited disorder of amino acid metabolism characterized by the accumulation of glycine in plasma, CSF, and urine. There is failure of normal myelination with brain atrophy and some evidence of destruction of white matter with spongy degeneration. In the cases reported by Press et al., the brainstem and cerebellum showed relatively normal myelination at birth (148). The age of onset is early (birth to 2 years); the infant may present with seizures, abnormal muscle tone, and developmental delay. MRI will show delayed myelination, a thin corpus callosum, and ventricular enlargement secondary to atrophy (Fig. 5.59).

In a recent report, Heindel et al. reported the feasibility of demonstrating a large glycine signal by proton MRI spectroscopy (H1-MRS) in brain volumes of 8 to 75 cm^3 (149). While elevated glycine levels can be demonstrated

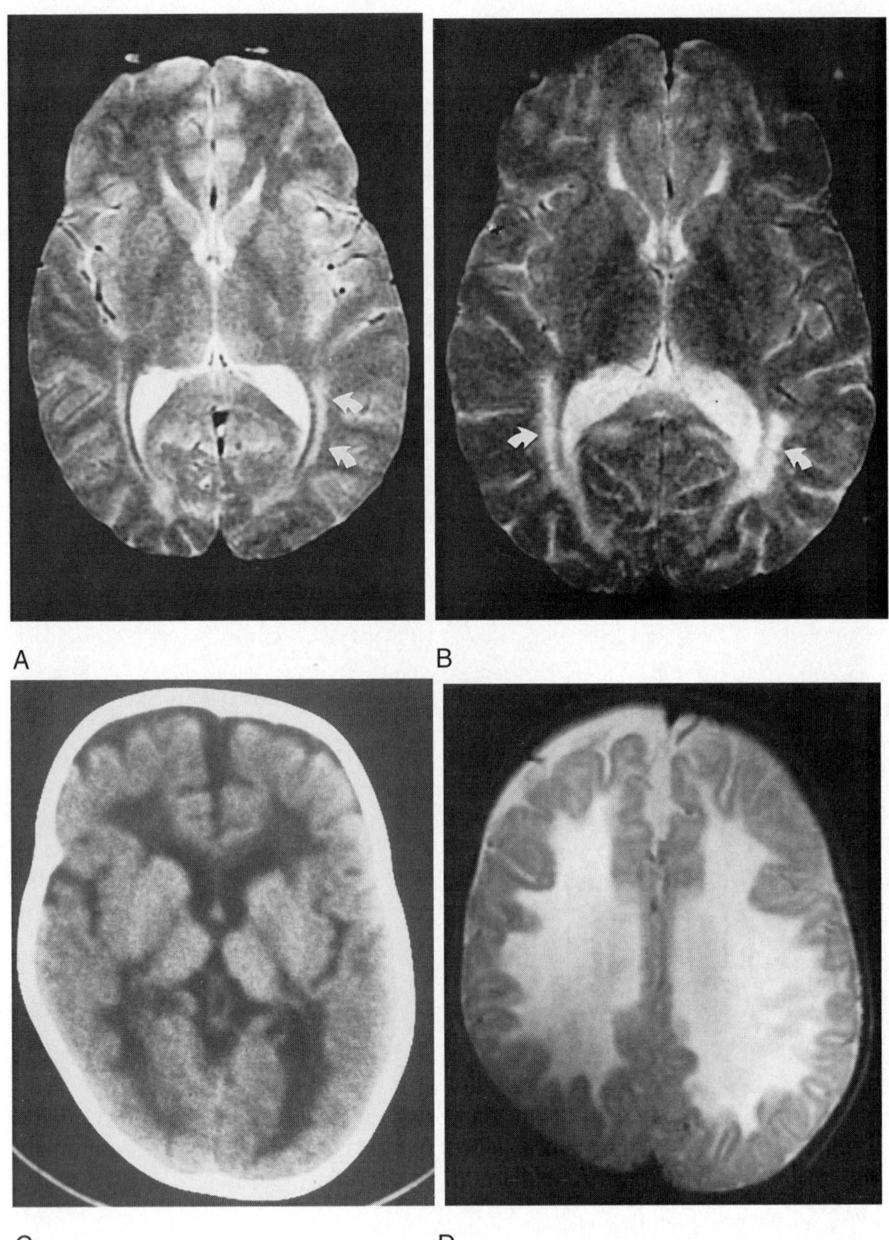

Figure 5.58. Phenylketonuria. **A.** A 17-year-old boy. T2-weighted image passing through basal ganglia shows moderate signal increase in posterior periventricular white matter about the optic radiations (arrows) bilaterally. Less severe changes are seen anteriorly. **B.** A 21-year-old man. T2-weighted axial at level of basal ganglia shows more marked high signal intensity about the optic radiations (arrows). Less severe changes are seen anteriorly, but there is questionable high intensity in the region of the corpus callosum posteriorly as well as anteriorly. These patients were not mentally retarded and were considered normal neurologically and intellectually. (Courtesy of Dr. Kenneth R. Maravilla, University of Washington School of Medicine, Seattle, Washington [AJNR 1991;12:403].) **C** and **D.** "Malignant" hyperphenylalaninemia in a 22-month-old boy with cofactor-dependent phenylketonuria and severe clinical manifestations. CT (C) and T2-weighted MR image (D) show severe white matter disease, significant widening of the brain sulci, and slight ventricular dilatation. (Courtesy of Dr. Jan Brismar, King Faisal Specialist Hospital, Riyadh, Saudi Arabia [AJNR 1990;11:135–138].)

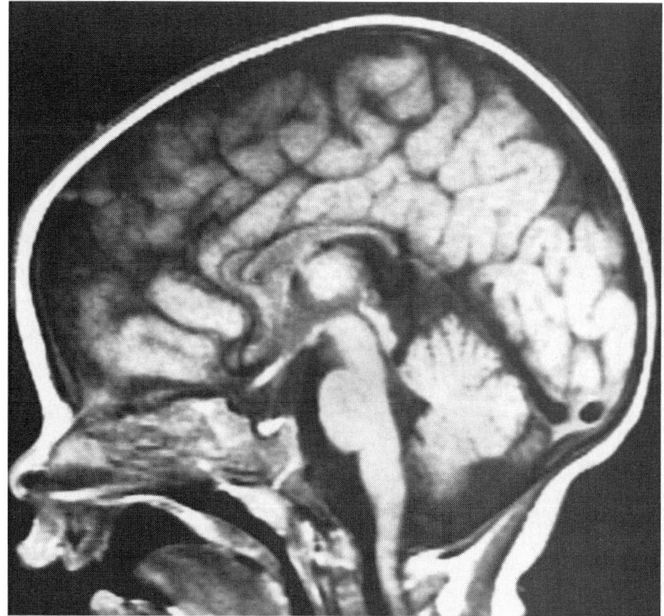

A

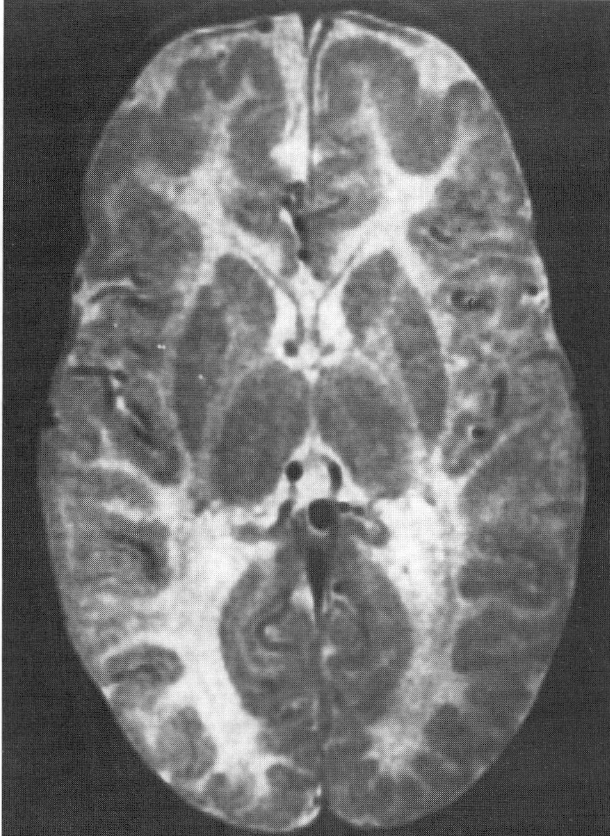

B

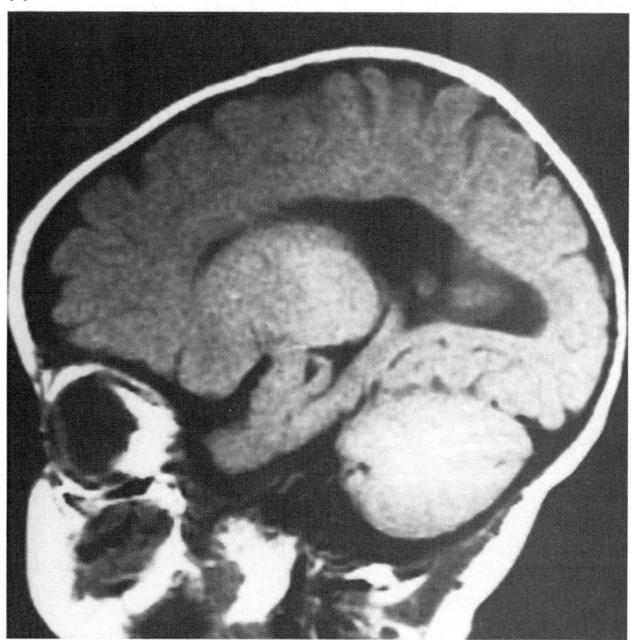

C

Figure 5.59. Nonketotic hyperglycinemia in a 4-month-old infant who presented neonatal apnea at birth. There was elevated plasma and CSF glycine. **A.** Sagittal T1-weighted image shows a thin corpus callosum and widened medial cerebral sulci consistent with volume loss. The brainstem is normal in size and reveals normal myelination. **B.** There is only minimal evidence of myelination in the internal capsule in this T2-weighted axial image. **C.** The ventricles are enlarged, particularly in the atrial region. The imaging findings are quite nonspecific; perhaps the thin corpus callosum and parenchymal atrophy, a constant finding in the seven cases reported by Press et al. (148), are the most important imaging changes. (Courtesy of Dr. John Hesselink, University of California, San Diego Medical Center, San Diego, California [AJNR 1989;10:315–321].)

by laboratory methods in the blood and CSF, H1-MRS can be used to follow the effects of treatment (such as sodium benzoate) on the glycine concentration in brain tissue, which may not parallel that of plasma and CSF.

HOMOCYSTINURIA

This congenital disease is caused by obstruction of methionine metabolism. The underlying error in the majority of cases is a cystathionine-β-synthase deficiency. There are variants. The clinical manifestations are in the skeleton (osteoporosis, so-called fish-shaped vertebrae), eye (ectopic lens, cataracts, retinal degeneration), and vascular system (leading to thromboembolism in brain, pulmonary and renal infarcts). Mild or gross intellectual retardation may be present (rarely normal). Strokes due to arterial or dural sinus thrombosis occur in about 25 percent of patients (150) (Fig. 5.60).

OCULOCEREBRORENAL SYNDROME (LOWE'S SYNDROME)

In 1952 Lowe et al. described an X-linked recessive disorder affecting boys almost exclusively and manifested by

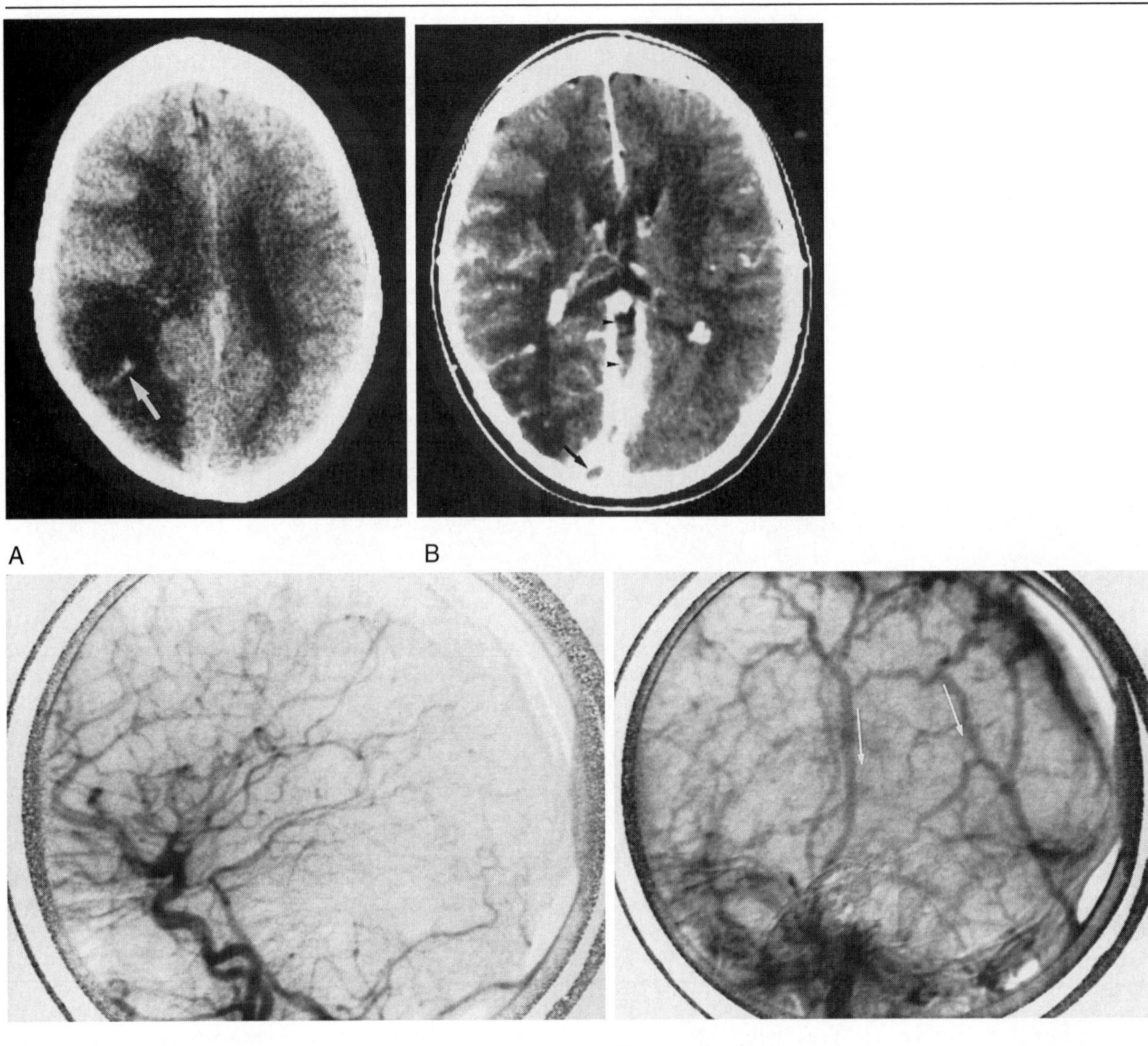

Figure 5.60. Homocystinuria in a 10-year-old girl who presented with bilateral ocular lens subluxations, learning and behavioral abnormalities, more recently left-sided focal seizures, left hemiparesis, headache, vomiting, and lethargy. The urine was positive for cystinuria. **A.** CT examination without contrast shows marked hypointensity of the white matter consistent with demyelination, and a large hypodense area in the right parieto-occipital region with a small area of hyperintensity (arrow) consistent with a venous cerebral infarction with hemorrhagic components. **B.** Postenhanced axial CT shows a delta sign in the torcular (arrow) and a filling defect in the straight sinus consistent with clotting (arrowheads). **C.** Angiography demonstrates a normal arterial phase. **D.** The venous phase shows complete reversal of normal venous flow which instead of flowing up toward the superior sagittal sinus is flowing down toward the base of the skull (arrows). Only portions of the superior sagittal sinus are filled with contrast, and the straight sinus and the internal cerebral veins and vein of Galen are not filled due to sinus thrombosis. The child was found to have homocystinuria. (Courtesy of Robert Peyster, Hahneman Medical Center, Philadelphia [Pediatr Radiol 1987;17:244–245].)

congenital cataracts, renal tubular acidosis, aminoaciduria and proteinuria, mental retardation, and hypotonia (151). The affected children have moderate ventricular enlargement. In a case reported by O'Tuama and Laster, CT showed radiolucent white matter in periventricular areas bilaterally, and MRI demonstrated bright white matter patches on T2 images (152).

GLUTARIC ACIDEMIA, TYPE 1

This autosomal recessive error in the metabolism of lysine, hydroxylysine, and tryptophan becomes manifest during the first year of life. White matter changes in frontal and occipital areas and in the putamen symmetrically are seen particularly well on MRI (high intensity on T2) but also on CT (radiolucent) (139,153) (see Fig. 5.62*G* to *J*). A typical feature is frontotemporal atrophy in both symptomatic and asymptomatic patients (154).

Peroxysomal Disorders

In the normal, peroxisomes are present in all cells and are abundant in the CNS and oligodendrocytes. Peroxisomes may be related to myelinogenesis. In the somewhat milder forms of peroxysomal defects, such as X-linked adrenal leukodystrophy, possibly only one enzyme is defective, whereas in other forms several enzymes are nonexistent or defective.

SINGLE ENZYME DEFICIENCY

X-Linked Adrenal Leukodystrophy

This condition is discussed in the section on metabolic conditions affecting the white matter.

Refsum Disease

This condition is discussed in the section on metabolic conditions affecting the white matter.

Abetalipoproteinemia

This entity is discussed in the section on metabolic conditions affecting the white matter.

MULTIPLE ENZYME DEFICIENCY

Infantile Refsum Disease

This condition is discussed under metabolic conditions affecting the white matter.

Neonatal Adrenal Leukodystrophy

This entity is discussed in the section on metabolic conditions affecting the white matter.

Hyperpipecolic Acidemia

This entity is discussed in the section on metabolic conditions affecting the white matter.

Rhizomelic Chondrodysplasia Calcificans Punctata

This entity is discussed in the section on metabolic conditions affecting the white matter.

Lysosomal Diseases

Lysosomes are minute cell bodies containing hydrolytic enzymes involved in the process of localized intracellular digestion or catabolism. Two types of lysosomal abnormalities lead to accumulation of products within the cells: the mucopolysaccharidoses and the lipid storage disorders (Table 5.10).

MUCOPOLYSACCHARIDOSES

There are a number of these, and the number identified will probably keep growing. The mucopolysaccharides (MPS) accumulate in a number of organs and tissues in the body. Mental retardation is common. The best-known types are the following:

MPS-I-H	Hurler syndrome
MPS-I-S	Scheie syndrome
MPS-I-H/S	Hurler-Scheie syndrome
MPS-II	Hunter syndrome
MPS-III-A,B,C,D	Sanfilippo syndrome
MPS-IV	Morquio's disease
MPS-VI-A,B	Maroteaux-Lamy syndrome
MPS-VII	Betaglucoronidase deficiency (Sly)

The imaging findings are briefly listed in Table 5.1. Characteristically, the head may be large and there may be ventricular enlargement, which may be related to the presence of meningeal thickening in the skull base and craniocervical junction. Meningeal thickening may be more prominent in some of the syndromes, such as Maroteaux-Lamy, than in others. The white matter changes, low-density areas in the white matter on CT and high signal on T2 MRI, are common in the various types.

LIPID STORAGE DISEASES (SPHYNGOLIPIDOSES)

In addition to the conditions listed in the following, there are two well-known and relatively frequent diseases (Gaucher disease and Niemann-Pick disease) that are not described here because they involve mostly the reticuloendothelial system and because their CNS manifestations and imaging characteristics are nonspecific, such as cerebral atrophy in Niemann-Pick disease or infections following splenectomy in Gaucher disease (155).

Metachromatic Leukodystrophy

This anomaly is described previously with the white matter diseases.

Krabbe's Disease

Also termed *globoid cell leukodystrophy*, this disease is described previously among the leukodystrophies (see under "Metabolic Conditions Affecting the White Matter").

Anderson-Fabry Disease

This alpha-galactosidase enzyme deficiency leads to accumulation of trihexoside ceramide in the walls of blood vessels as well as in various organs. In the brain this substance accumulates in the hypothalamus, amigdaloid nuclei, substantia nigra, reticular nuclei, anterior horns of the spinal cord, and sympathetic and dorsal root ganglia (156). On CT the typical appearance is that of multiple lacunar infarcts in various locations in the brain; the same is true on MRI. Clinically, the disease may manifest itself in childhood, adolescence, or early adult life; lancinating pains and dysesthesias in the extremities are typical. Chronic renal disease and cardiac ischemia, angiokeratoma of the skin,

Table 5.10.
Metabolic Anomalies (Inborn Metabolic Errors)

Type of Anomaly	Biochemical Derangement	Age of Onset	Death	Neurologic Involvement	Imaging
Lysosomal diseases (storage)					
Mucopolysaccharidoses	Deficiency of lysosomal enzymes that degrade heparan, dermatan, and keratan sulfate			Large head	All cases: large, thick skull; thick meninges, particularly in cervical area
MPS IH—Hurler syndrome	Absence of alpha-L-iduronidase activity	2–12 mo	10+ y	Mentally retarded; unique facies (ugly); low stature	Large head; possible hydrocephalus; deficient myelination; C2 sublux; gibbus
MPS IS—Scheie syndrome	Large urine excretion of heparan and dermatan sulfate; deficiency of alpha-L-iduronidase	1–10 y	30–40 y	Normal intelligence; carpal tunnel syndrome; corneal clouding; deafness + –; normal stature	Some T2 bright white matter lesions
MPS IH/S—Hurler-Scheie	Same		20–30 y	Retarded; short stature	Large sella + –, basilar impression; white matter T2 deficient myelination; basal ganglia changes
MPS II—Hunter syndrome	Same			Milder than Hurler syndrome; less severe mental retardation; deafness + –; short stature	Thick meninges in cervical hydrocephalus
MPS III ABCD—Sanfilippo syndrome	Deficient 4 enzymes involved in degradation of heparan sulfate	1–3 y	20–55 y	Short stature; keel breast; variable dementia	Hydrocephalus; cerebral atrophy
MPS IV AB—Morquio	2 enzyme deficiency; A-*N*-acetylgalactosamine 6-sulfatase. B-*P*-galactosidase keratan sulfate in urine	1–7 y		Short stature; some decreased muscle tone; paraparesis or quadraparesis	Flat vertebrae; osteoporosis; CT low-density white matter lesions; hydrocephalus; bone compression of spinal cord; hypoplastic odontoid atlantoaxial subluxation; thickened cervical meninges
MPS VI A < B—Maroteaux-Lamy	*N*-acetylgalactosamine 4-sulfatese; excrete dermatan sulfate in urine	2–3 y	25–40 y	Normal intelligence but some retarded; myelopathy due to thick cervical dura	Thick cervical meninges; C2 subluxation; hydrocephalus; some bright T2 white matter foci
MPS VII beta-glucuronidase deficiency	Beta-glucuronidase deficiency	0–12 mo		Retardation at 2–3 y	No reports
Metachromatic leukodystrophy	Accumulation of sulfatides; decreased arysulfatase A	0–2 y			Leukodystrophy
Juvenile		5–10 y	10–15 y	Progressive spasticity; loss of intellect	
Adult		30–40 y	40–60 y	Less severe	
Farber–lipogranulomatosis (rare)	Accumulation of lipoglycoprotein mucopolysaccharide ceramide acid	0–10 mo	<2 y	Minor	No neurologic findings
Cerebrotendinous xanthomatosis	Accumulation of bile acid precursor; elevated cholesterol; mitochondrial deficiency	9–10 y	+ –50 y	Progressive ataxia; dementia; cataracts	CT bilateral symmetric cerebellar hypodensities

and peripheral neuropathy are usually also present. The disease is inherited as an X-linked recessive trait.

GM1 Gangliosidosis

The CNS lesions in this condition are very nonspecific, such as atrophy, and some low-density areas in the white matter on CT, which are bright on T2 images (155). The spine shows thoracolumbar kyphosis and beaking of the vertebral bodies. Neurologic symptoms (retardation, incoordination, and spasticity) appear early. There is also a late onset type. Diagnosis is made by estimating the beta-galactosidase. Like the early onset type, this is an autosomal recessive condition.

GM2 Gangliosidosis (Tay-Sachs Disease; Sandhoff Disease)

This is a disorder of sphyngolipid metabolism in which a metabolic block due to a defect in hexoseaminidase leads to accumulation of GM2 ganglioside in brain tissue (157). Tay-Sachs disease is seen mainly in Ashkenazi Jews, and Sandhoff disease has no racial predilection. Both diseases belong in the group of amaurotic idiocy because the patients develop a cherry red spot in the macula, leading to blindness. It starts some months after birth, and the children develop mental developmental arrest and myoclonic movements as a response to sound or noise. The most important imaging characteristic is a symmetric increase in density of the thalamus, on CT, of unknown pathogenesis (158) (Fig. 5.61). The present opinion is that this appearance may be produced by calcium deposition because it is T2 dark. All 13 cases reported by Brismar et al. presented the hyperdensity, and of these 12 were diagnosed as Sandhoff disease and one as Tay-Sachs disease (157). In addition, some cases presented cerebral atrophy with ventricular enlargement, and others presented white matter disease. Both diseases are inherited with an autosomal recessive pattern. A juvenile form in which there is a "salt and pepper" pigmentation of the retina goes by the name of *Batten-Mayou* disease or *Spielmeyer-Vogt* disease.

Fucosidosis

This anomaly is due to diminished or absent alpha-L-fucosidase, an enzyme that cleaves fucose from various glycopeptides and oligosaccharides, resulting in retention and accumulation of fucose-containing substances. Fucose is also excreted in the urine. The abnormal findings relate usually to the skeleton, mild dysostosis multiplex involving the spine, pelvis, and femoral capital epiphysis (159). Kessler et al. described the CT findings in two cases in which there was CNS involvement progressing to severe spasticity (160). The patients are usually dismorphic, presenting coarse facial features that may suggest Hurler syndrome. CT may show only severe cerebral and cerebellar atrophy. One of the two cases showed scattered hypodense areas in the white matter and cerebral convolutions. The case shown in Figure 5.61*E* to *G* shows severe lack of myelination.

Mitochondrial Cytopathies

The mitochondrial cytopathies or encephalomyopathies are a heterogeneous group of disorders associated with mitochondrial dysfunction involving the central and peripheral nervous system as well as other organs (skeletal muscle, heart, endocrine glands, hematopoietic system, kidneys, and gastrointestinal tract).

Two groups may be considered: a more severe form that is usually manifested at birth or shortly afterward and that may lead to early death; this includes Leigh, Menke, Zellwager, and Alper syndromes. The second group is composed of more slowly developing abnormalities and comprises Kearns-Sayre syndrome, the MELAS syndrome, MERRF (myoclonic epilepsy with ragged red fibers), mitochondrial encephalomyopathy, and lactic acidosis (161). In the second group, diagnosis can be established by muscle biopsy, which reveals ragged red fibers with appropriate staining (Gomori trichrome) due to the accumulation of mitochondria in the muscle fiber. These conditions are mostly transmitted by non-Mendelian maternal inheritance.

LEIGH'S DISEASE (SUBACUTE NECROTIZING ENCEPHALOMYELOPATHY)

This disease (Fig. 5.62) is an autosomal recessive disorder resulting from a broad defect in mitochondrial function. The onset is insidious, and the course may be intermittently progressive for several years. It affects males more frequently than females, and onset is usually in early childhood, although adult onset cases also exist (162). There is usually psychomotor regression and cerebellar and brainstem dysfunction (ataxia, dystonia, and nystagmus). Limb weakness is often seen. Specific mitochondrial enzyme deficiencies such as pyruvate carboxylase deficiency, pyruvate dehydrogenase complex defects, and cytochrome C oxidase deficiencies have been described in Leigh's disease. Focal necrotic lesions may be found in the basal ganglia, thalamus, midbrain, medulla, and posterior column of the spinal cord, as well as in the subcortical white matter. The mammillary bodies are usually spared, which differentiates Leigh's disease from Wernicke's encephalopathy.

In the seven cases reported by Medina et al. the necrotic lesions were demonstrated in a variety of locations, most commonly the putamen, the globus pallidus, substantia nigra, periaqueductal region, inferior medulla, and periventricular white matter (163) (Fig. 5.62). Lesions were also seen in the caudate nucleus, olivary nucleus, decussation of superior cerebellar peduncles, and medial geniculate body.

MENKES' DISEASE (KINKY HAIR DISEASE)

This disease is seen in male infants and is characterized by steely hair, retardation, spastic quadriparesis, seizures, and hypothermia with an underlying defect of copper metabolism. The copper level and the ceruloplasmin in the serum

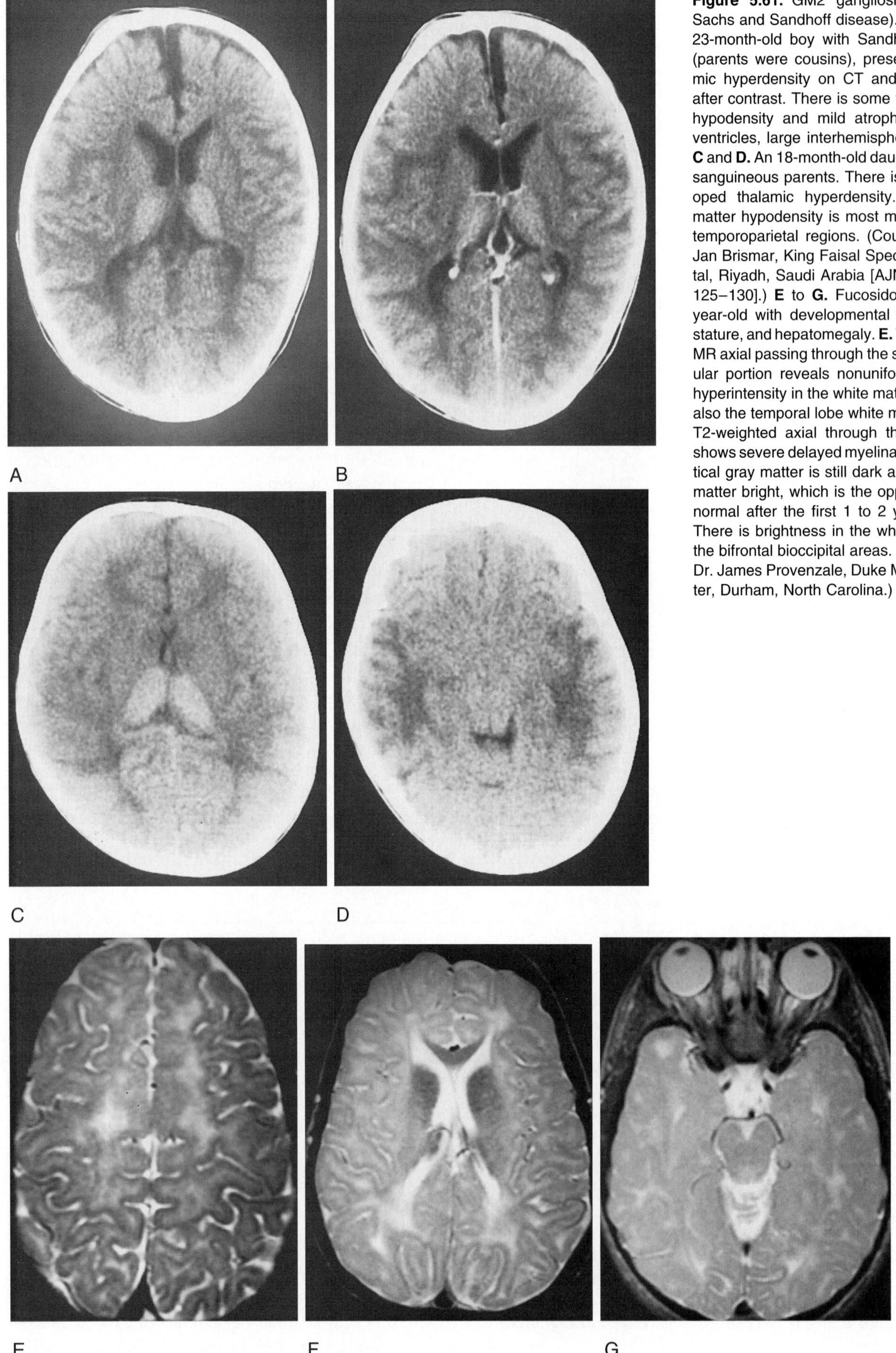

Figure 5.61. GM2 gangliosidosis (Tay-Sachs and Sandhoff disease). **A** and **B.** A 23-month-old boy with Sandhoff disease (parents were cousins), presenting thalamic hyperdensity on CT and no change after contrast. There is some white matter hypodensity and mild atrophy (enlarged ventricles, large interhemispheric fissure). **C** and **D.** An 18-month-old daughter of consanguineous parents. There is well-developed thalamic hyperdensity. The white matter hypodensity is most marked in the temporoparietal regions. (Courtesy of Dr. Jan Brismar, King Faisal Specialist Hospital, Riyadh, Saudi Arabia [AJNR 1990;11: 125–130].) **E** to **G.** Fucosidosis in a 10-year-old with developmental delay, short stature, and hepatomegaly. **E.** T2-weighted MR axial passing through the supraventricular portion reveals nonuniform areas of hyperintensity in the white matter involving also the temporal lobe white matter (**G**). **F.** T2-weighted axial through the ventricles shows severe delayed myelination; the cortical gray matter is still dark and the white matter bright, which is the opposite of the normal after the first 1 to 2 years of life. There is brightness in the white matter of the bifrontal bioccipital areas. (Courtesy of Dr. James Provenzale, Duke Medical Center, Durham, North Carolina.)

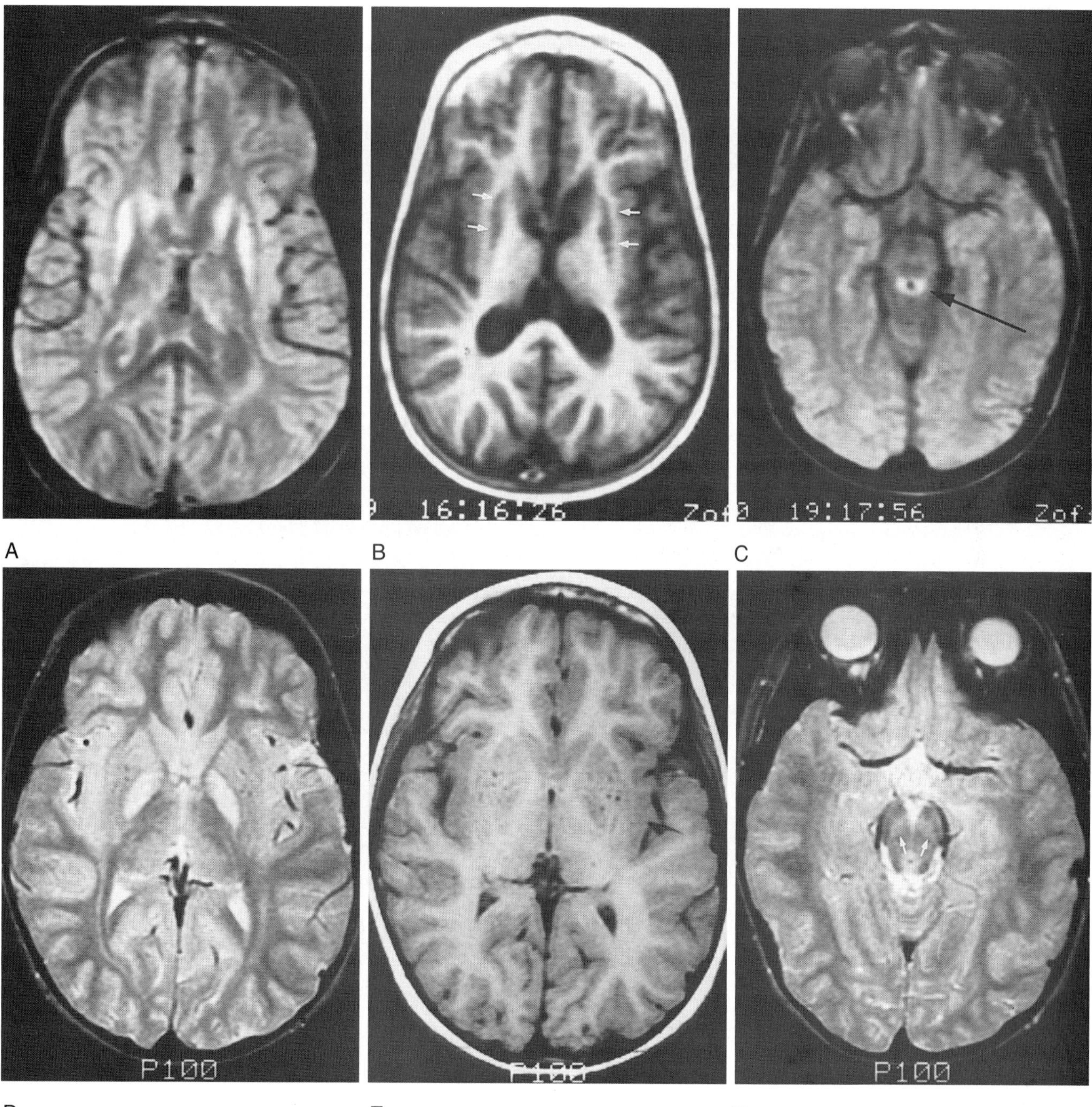

Figure 5.62. Leigh's disease. Mitochondrial encephalopathy diagnosed as Leigh's disease in 3 1/2-year-old girl with developmental arrest, then regression, seizures, optic atrophy, and hypotomia. **A.** There is signal hyperintensity in putamen bilaterally as well as in the head of the caudate nucleus on proton density images which on T1 is hypointense (arrow in B). **B.** A T_1-weighted image reveals hypointensity in the putamen. A lower section (**C**) shows periaqueductal hyperintensity on T2 (long arrow). There was no involvement of the globus pallidus. There is some hyperintensity in periventricular white matter in the frontal region. **D.** Leigh's disease in a 5-year-old girl. The diagnosis here is less clear: normal development up to the present, intractable seizure-like states, elevated CSF lactate, but normal pyruvate and no clinical signs of Wilson's disease. There is bilateral globus pallidus hyperintensity on T2. On T1 (**E**) the appearance is normal; there are prominent Virchow-Robin perivascular spaces of unknown significance. **F.** There is some periaqueductal hyperintensity on T2 (first echo) and some relative hyperintensity of the pars compacta of the substantia nigra (small arrows) (*continued*).

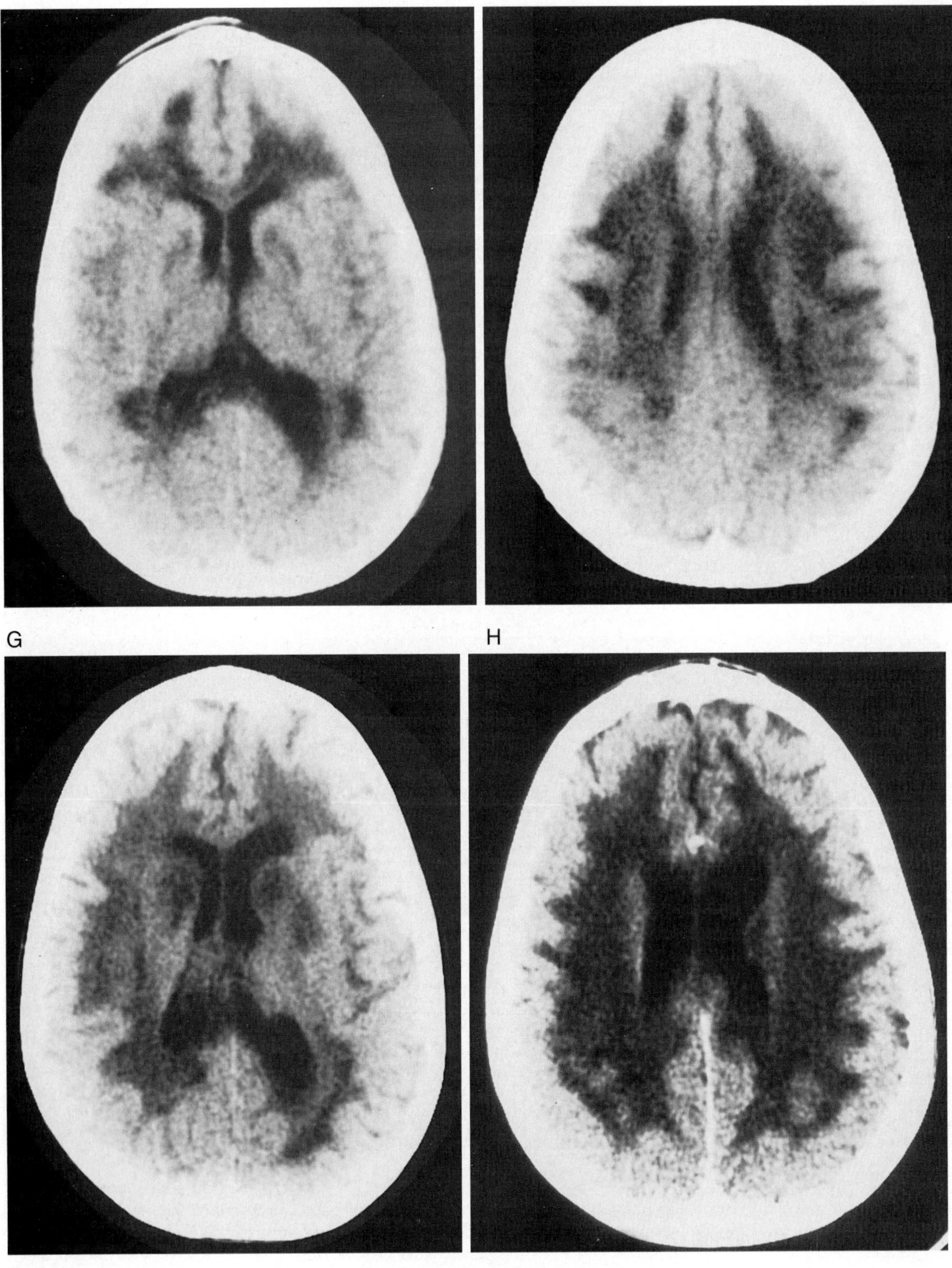

Figure 5.62. *(continued)* **G** to **J.** Glutaric acidemia and Leigh's disease in a 6-year-old boy with seizure and psychomotor retardation. **G** and **H.** CT examination at age 2 reveals white matter hypointensity in frontal and occipital area, hypointensity in globus pallidus and putamen bilaterally, and some ventricular enlargement. **I** and **J.** Reexamination at age 6 reveals considerably more hypointensity in the white matter, more involvement of the caudate nucleus and basal ganglia, and further ventricular dilatation. In addition, the child had glutaric acidemia type II, which is an unusual combination. At autopsy the distribution of the lesions in the gray matter (periaqueductal, substantia nigra, thalamus, striatum) was considered consist with Leigh's disease. However, the white matter changes where intensive demyelination was found are more consistent with glutaric acidemia. Abnormal mitochondria were found in the cardiac muscle but not in skeletal muscle.

are low. Cerebral angiography demonstrates tortuous arteries; CT and MRI demonstrate cortical atrophy, and some elongation of the arteries may be associated with the early cortical atrophy. Subdural hematomas may be found (164). The tortuous arteries may be demonstrated today with MRI angiography. Periosteal reaction in the long bones may be seen early but disappears after 1 year of age (165).

ZELLWEGER SYNDROME

See under "Conditions Affecting White Matter."

KEARNS-SAYRE SYNDROME

First described in 1958 by Kearns and Sayre (166), this mitochondrial disorder occurs more frequently in females and may be inherited as an autosomal dominant trait. Clinically it presents a triad of ophthalmoplegia, retinal pigmentary degeneration, and complete heart block. There is short stature and frequently mental deterioration. Cerebellar ataxia, facial weakness, and neurosensory hearing loss were seen in the patient reported by Demange et al. (167). Muscle biopsy reveals ragged red fibers. CT shows basal ganglia hypodensities, but MRI is likely to demonstrate more abnormalities. Hyperintense lesions on T2 images may be demonstrated in the thalamus, the globus pallidus, the dentate nucleus of the cerebellum, the superior cerebellar peduncles, and the white matter of the brain (Fig. 5.63). The location is similar to that found in Leigh's disease although probably less extensive. In the nine patients reported by Seigel et al., calcification was present in basal ganglia, thalamus, and/or cerebral hemisphere in four (168). The location of these calcifications was similar to that seen in hypoparathyroidism. Indeed, one patient, an 18-year-old woman, had clinical hypoparathyroidism, and in another, a 20-year-old woman, a diagnosis of pseudohypoparathyroidism was made in association with Kearns-Sayre syndrome. Eight of the nine cases reported by Seigel et al. had a positive muscle biopsy for ragged red fibers.

While the onset of the disease is likely to be in children up to 12 years, some cases of adult onset are seen (two of nine in Seigel et al. [168]).

MELAS SYNDROME (MITOCHONDRIAL MYOPATHY, ENCEPHALOPATHY, LACTIC ACIDOSIS, AND STROKE)

Affected patients have short stature, dementia, weakness, and sensorineural hearing loss (similar to Kearns-Sayre and

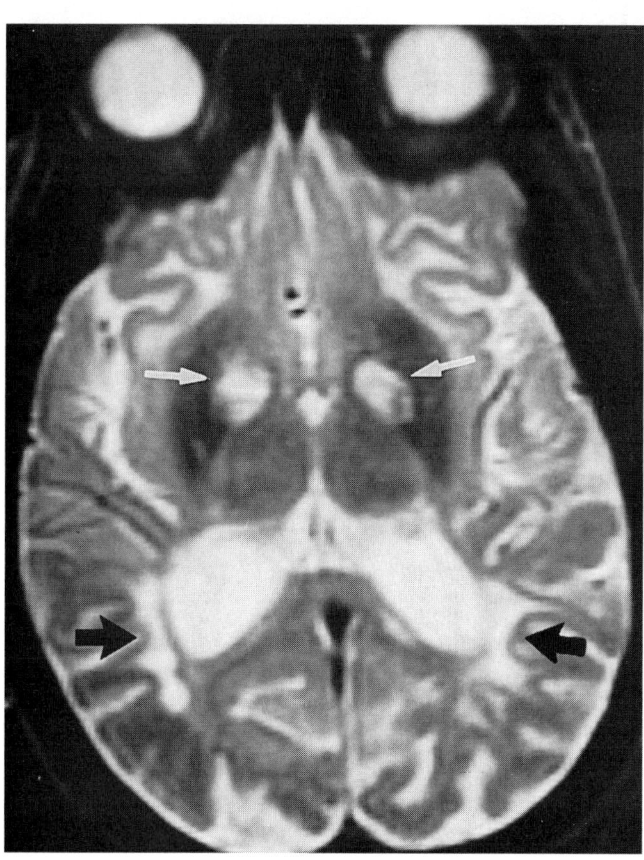

A

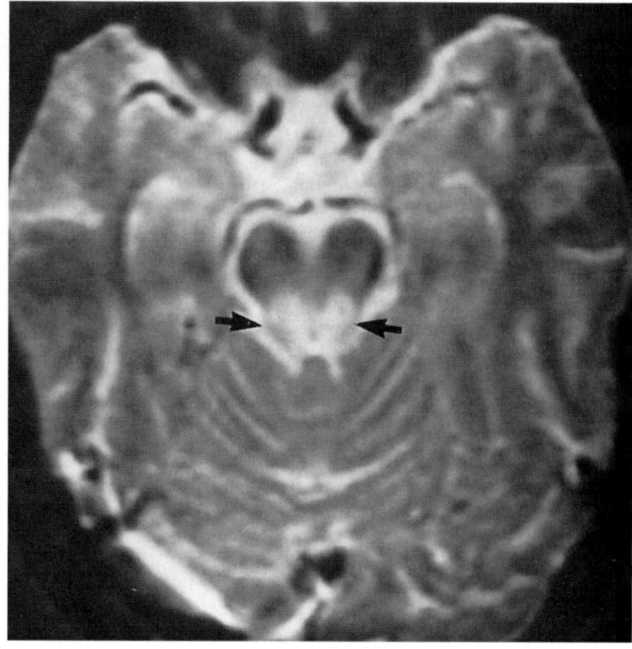

B

Figure 5.63. Kearns-Sayre syndrome in two women aged 38 and 23 who presented bilateral ptosis and limitation in eye movements. **A.** Axial T2-weighted MR image shows bilateral hyperintensity of the globus pallidus (arrows). There is also hyperintensity in the white matter around the atrium of the lateral ventricles bilaterally (arrows). **B.** Another case reveals hyperintensity in the dorsal half of the midbrain on T2-weighted image involving the periaqueductal and adjacent portion of the tegmentum of the midbrain (arrows). The latter appearance is not unlike that seen in Leigh's disease (Fig. 5.62) and Wilson's disease (Fig. 5.66). (Courtesy of Dr. James Provenzale, Duke Medical Center, Durham, North Carolina.)

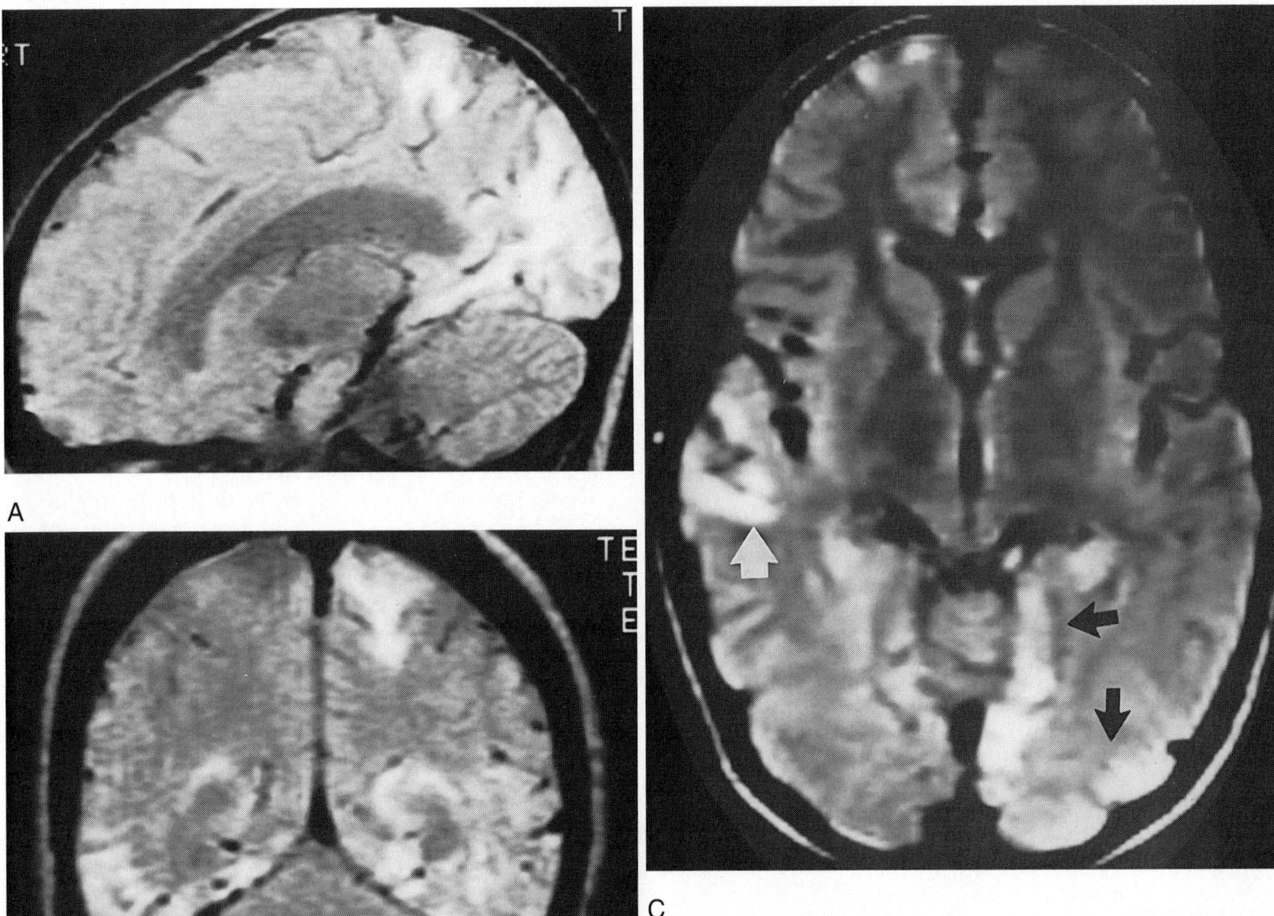

A

B

C

Figure 5.64. MELAS syndrome in a 16-year-old girl. At age 12 she developed cortical blindness, which later improved to 20/50 acuity, sensorineural hearing loss, and focal motor seizures; diagnosed as childhood multiple sclerosis. Later a mitochondrial enzymopathy was found, along with elevated lactic acid in CSF and elevated serum lactate. **A.** Proton density sagittal shows hyperintense areas in occipital and parietal regions. **B.** Coronal proton density image shows bioccipital predominantly cortical hyperintense areas, as well as cortical-subcortical lesion in left parasagittal region consistent with cerebral infarction. **C.** An MRI examination, proton density axial, done 4 years previously, was located; it showed clear cortical involvement only in the left occipital lobe and another area in the right temporal opercular region and the cortical region (arrows).

MERRF) as well as recurrent strokes and cortical blindness (Fig. 5.64). No ophthalmoplegia or heart block occurs. The CT and MRI findings are consistent with cerebral infarction (radiolucent areas with cortical involvement on CT and hyperintensity on T2-weighted MR images). One of the Allard et al. cases showed extensive calcification of the caudate nucleus head, putamen, and globus pallidus; the same authors located three other cases from the literature in which calcification was observed (169). Cerebellar involvement may also occur, but this is not usually a prominent feature. Contrast enhancement of infarcted areas was noted in one case by Allard et al., and in this case the neurologic examination could not clarify whether the patient had a subacute infarct in the hyperemic stage (169).

MELAS syndrome usually begins in childhood or early adulthood. The presence of serum lactic acidosis is an important component of this syndrome. The differential diagnosis by imaging methods alone is rather extensive. The presence of multiple infarcts tends to narrow the differential, however, because in addition to white matter abnormalities, there are focal gray matter areas of involvement, and this finding in a young individual should raise the possibility of MELAS syndrome (Fig. 5.64).

MERRF (MYOCLONIC EPILEPSY WITH RAGGED RED FIBERS)

The presence of myoclonic jerks and the absence of ophthalmoplegia and retinal degeneration make this a distinct entity, to be distinguished from Kearns-Sayre syndrome. Unlike MELAS syndrome, MERRF causes no strokes leading to cerebral infarcts. The patients have muscle weakness as well as short stature and cardiac conductive defects. CT or MRI may show cerebral and cerebellar atrophy, with the white matter yielding a low density on CT and high signal on MRI. About half of the proven cases show no significant abnormality (133,169,170).

De Volder et al. reported a case in which a positron emission tomography study that used fluorodeoxyglucose demonstrated marked decrease in glucose uptake in all gray matter structures and thalamus with relative sparing of anterior cortical regions and basal ganglia (171).

CEREBROTENDINOUS XANTHOMATOSIS

In this condition patients are deficient in a liver mitochondrial enzyme required for side-chain oxidation of cholesterol to bile salts. This causes accumulation of bile alcohols and their precursors. The serum cholesterol is normal, but the cholesterol level is high and there are increased bile alcohols in the urine. The patients may show pyramidal and cerebellar signs, may have mental retardation, and usually present xanthomas in the Achilles tendons, the knees, and the elbows; the Achilles location is the most common. CT may show decreased density in the cerebellum involving the region of the dentate nuclei bilaterally (172). Hypointensity in the same areas is shown on MRI (173). Treatment with compounds that decrease production of cholesterol is indicated. This therapy may not reverse the pathologic findings but may prevent further damage.

CYTOPLASMICALLY INHERITED STRIATAL DEGENERATION

This is a form of striatal degeneration reported by Seidenwurm et al. in which five patients, members of a family, presented Leber's type optic atrophy and various manifestations of striatal degeneration (rigidity, dystonia, gait disturbance), some with mental deterioration (174). The age of the patients varied from 3 to 18 years. The condition was inherited through the mother and was regarded as a mitochondrial disease.

The constant finding on cross-sectional imaging (CT and MRI) was the presence of putaminal low density on CT and high signal intensity on MRI T2. In two of the five patients the caudate nucleus was partially involved. Other heredodegenerative conditions may present the same findings on CT or MRI, but the distinguishing feature in this case is Leber's optic atrophy.

Disorders of Amino Acid Metabolism See Table 5.11.

MAPLE SYRUP URINE DISEASE

See "Metabolic Conditions Affecting the White Matter."

PHENYLKETONURIA

See under "Metabolic Conditions Affecting the White Matter."

MALIGNANT HYPERPHENYLALANINEMIA

See under "Metabolic Conditions Affecting the White Matter."

NONKETOTIC HYPERGLYCINEMIA

See under "Metabolic Conditions Affecting the White Matter."

HOMOCYSTINURIA

See under "Metabolic Conditions Affecting the White Matter."

METHYLMALONIC ACIDEMIA

See under "Diseases Affecting the Basal Ganglia."

GLUTARIC ACIDEMIA

See under "Metabolic Conditions Affecting the White Matter."

OCULOCEREBRORENAL SYNDROME

See under "Metabolic Conditions Affecting the White Matter."

LEUCINE METABOLISM

A deficiency of 3-hydroxy-3 methylglucaryl-coenzyme. A lyase causes an inborn error of leucine catabolism. It produces a leukoencephalopathy that on MRI involves preferentially the deep arcuate fibers (U fibers) (175). The U fiber involvement could be a specific finding for this condition.

Gray Matter Diseases

These conditions are clinically characterized by signs of neuronal dysfunction (such as seizures, intellectual deterioration, visual changes), in contrast to white matter diseases, which may present tract involvement such as loss of motor skills, spasticity, or ataxia. The understanding of all neurodegenerative diseases continues at an accelerating pace from the chemical-metabolic point of view, and the diagnosis depends on recognition of these changes rather than clinical or imaging observations alone.

NEURONAL CEROID LIPOFUSCINOSIS

Originally described as *amaurotic familial idiocy* by Batten in 1903 (176), this condition was later designated *neuronal ceroid lipofuscinosis* (Rett's syndrome) to emphasize the nature of the storage material found in this group of disorders. There is an infantile, a later infantile, a juvenile, and an adult form. Blindness and dementia as well as seizures are usually present. CT findings show only cerebral atrophy,

Table 5.11.
Amino Acid Disorders

Type of Anomaly	Biochemical Derangement	Age of Onset	Death	Neurologic Involvement	Imaging
Amino Acid Disorders					
Phenylketonuria (PKU)	Deficient hepatic enzyme phenylalanine hydroxylase; actually there are 3 components: urinary, phenylpyruvic acid, excretion	0–6 mo	—	Myelin heavily affected; increases with age; retardation; intellectual; motor	White matter changes on T2 in posterior part of brain; some atrophy
Malignant hyperphenylalaninemia	Deficiency of CO-factor tetrahydrobiopterin, BH4	0–6 mo	—	Myotonic seizures; retardation	White matter T2 lesions may be severe; mostly mild, brain atrophy
Maple syrup urine disease	Branched-chain amino acid metabolism; block in decarboxylation of amino acids leucine, isoleucine, valine	<1 wk	1 y	Vomiting; increased muscular tone; urine smells like maple syrup; convulsions; hypotonia; stupor and coma	Diffuse edema in cerebellum; brainstem and supratentorial in second week; later edema subsides; brain atrophy; slow myelination, if survival
Nonketotic hyperglycinemia	Accumulation of glycine in plasma, CSF, and urine	0–2 y		Seizures; poor muscle tone; developmental delay	Delayed myelination; thin corpus callosum; cerebral atrophy
Homocystinuria	Obstruction of methionine metabolism due to cystathionine beta-synthase deficiency	0–2 y		Eye, skeletal, vascular with thromboembolism; infarcts in brain	Infarcts in brain may be multiple; venous sinus thrombosis
Lowe's syndrome (oculocerebrorenal syndrome)	Aminoaciduria; no actual amino acid transport defect demonstrable by cultured fibroblasts	0–1 y		Mental retardation; cataracts; renal failure; like Fanconi's	White matter changes; greater in frontal seen on CT and MRI
Glutaric aciduria	Deficient metabolism of lysine, hydroxylysine, and tryptophan	0–1 y		Mental retardation	White matter brightness on T2 in frontal and occipital areas; also in putamen bilaterally
Methylmalonic and propionic acidemias	Defective conversion, in both, of propionic to succinate; ketoacidosis; elevated methylmalonic acid in blood and urine	0–2 (y ?)	Varies	Mental retardation; ketoacidosis	Some diffuse white matter lesions; tissue loss in posterior limb of internal capsule

cerebellar atrophy, and ventricular dilatation without evidence of white matter disease (177,178).

OTHER DISEASES AFFECTING GRAY MATTER

Progressive myoclonic epilepsies include the following:

1. Familial myoclonus (Unverricht-Lunborg disease). Usual onset in childhood with mild dementia.
2. Lafora's disease. Onset in adolescence, rapid severe dementia, visual loss.
3. Sialidosis. Onset in childhood, variable dementia, cherry-red spot in fundus of the eye.
4. Fukuhara's disease. Onset in childhood, variable dementia, myopathy, lactic acidosis, ragged red fibers in muscle biopsy. It belongs with the mitochondrial myopathies. All patients have myoclonus to a greater or lesser degree. CT or MRI examinations are likely to show only cerebral atrophy.
5. Rett's syndrome. Affects only girls, with onset in first year. Dementia, autistic behavior, tonic-clonic convulsions associated with hyperammonemia. "Hand-wringing" or "hand-washing" movements are typical. CT is likely to be negative or show only cortical atrophy (179).
6. Menkes' disease (see earlier).

Miscellaneous Conditions

NAVAJO NEUROPATHY

This is a disorder occurring, as a recessively inherited condition, in members of the Navajo tribe. It is classically described as presenting involvement of the extremities with weakness, corneal ulceration, failure to thrive, short stature, and scoliosis. The severity may vary. Sural nerve biopsy shows marked demyelination without evidence of regeneration. The unmyelinated axons, on the other hand, show both degeneration and regeneration.

While the main manifestations are peripheral and corneal, Williams et al. have described imaging findings on

MRI examinations involving the white matter of the cerebellum (comma-shaped lesions dark on T1, bright on T2) and also various lesions in the cerebral white matter (large patches of T2 bright lesions) (180). Because of the prohibition of postmortem studies by the Navajo tribe, autopsy data are not available. Peripheral neuropathy is seen in some of the leukodystrophies described previously (metachromatic leukodystrophy, adrenoleukodystrophy, Krabbe's disease).

PARTIAL ALBINISM

Partial albinism with immunodeficiency is a newly recognized syndrome in which, in addition to the two features implied in the name, findings involving the CNS are visible on CT and MRI. The findings in the CNS involve the white matter, in the cerebellum particularly, but also supratentorially. It is possible that the CNS manifestations represent an inflammatory process, for they tend to appear as episodes, which may recede and recur. Brismar et al. indicate that the changes in the posterior fossa tend to be more pronounced, more so than in other neurometabolic disorders (181). The patients reported have been of Arab origin. Conceivably, the albinism in northern European stock might not be recognized. The Chédiak-Higashi syndrome is similar to partial albinism with immunodeficiency and is differentiated because of the presence of giant lyposomal granules in all leukocytes (182). The white matter changes are due to demyelination, and in this respect the diagnosis would depend on the other associated conditions (partial albinism and repeated infections) (Fig. 5.65).

CONGENITAL X-LINKED AGAMMAGLOBULINEMIA

This is a congenital defect in B-cell development resulting in a severe paucity of mature B cells and decreased immunoglobulin levels. It is usually diagnosed early (2 to 4 years) because of recurrent infections, but diagnosis is not usually made unless it is suspected. In the CNS, meningoencephalitis, which may be produced by enterovirus, *Haemophilus influenzae*, and *Streptococcus pneumoniae*, to which the patients are more sensitive, may be found. In one of the cases reported by Lerner and Bilaniuk, there was extensive meningitis in brain and spinal meninges (183). In addition to antibiotics, periodic injections of gammaglobulin are necessary for treatment.

MOBIUS SYNDROME

See under "Cerebral Calcifications," Chapter 4.

CONGENITAL BILATERAL PERISYLVIAN SYNDROME

Kuzniecky et al. (184) have coined this name to be applied to an entity consisting of faciopharyngomasticatory diplegia, epilepsy, and cognitive deficits. All 31 patients collected by the authors had primarily pseudobulbar paresis. Dysarthria and restriction of tongue movements, slow motor and language development, and mild intellectual deficit were present in all. MRI revealed bilateral perisylvian and perirolandic malformations with exposure of the insula, usually symmetric (in 80 percent of cases). Pathologic correlation revealed four-layered polymicrogyria in the affected areas.

Diseases Affecting the Basal Ganglia

This is a heterogeneous group of diseases that have as a common manifestation involvement of one or more of the components of the structures usually referred to as basal ganglia, which includes the putamen, globus pallidus, caudate nucleus, amygdaloid nucleus, and claustrum. The lesions may involve not only the basal ganglia but also adjacent structures such as the thalamus, adjacent subthalamic areas, and often also the dentate nucleus of the cerebellum.

These structures react to or are involved in much metabolic activity. For instance, they are affected earliest by hypoxia, such as in carbon monoxide poisoning or circulatory failure; they undergo calcium deposition in hypoparathyroidism or pseudohypoparathyroidism; they are affected by copper accumulation as in Wilson's disease, bilirubin accumulation as in hepatic failure and kernicterus, iron accumulation in Hallervorden-Spatz and in Gerstmann-Straussler-Scheinker diseases, and calcium accumulation in Fahr's disease and in Cockayne syndrome. In addition, calcification is common in the globus pallidus as a normal variant, and cases have been described of osteopetrosis with extensive calcifications. Liver failure produces hyperintensity in the basal ganglia on T1-weighted images. See under "Systemic Diseases" affecting the nervous system (Chapter 14). Hyperintensity in the basal ganglia on T1-weighted images has also been reported in patients after several weeks or months of parenteral feeding.

In this group the following diseases are discussed:

Wilson's disease
Huntington's disease
Fahr's disease
Hallervorden-Spatz disease
Striatonigral degeneration
Striatal degeneration
Methylmalonic acidemia
Cockayne's syndrome
Membranous lipodystrophy
Gerstmann-Straussler-Scheinker disease
Kernicterus
Striatonigral degeneration
Hyperparathyroidism (described in Chapter 4)

WILSON'S DISEASE (HEPATOLENTICULAR DEGENERATION)

This disease is transmitted as an autosomal recessive trait. An inborn error of copper metabolism is responsible for the accumulation of copper in the liver and other tissues.

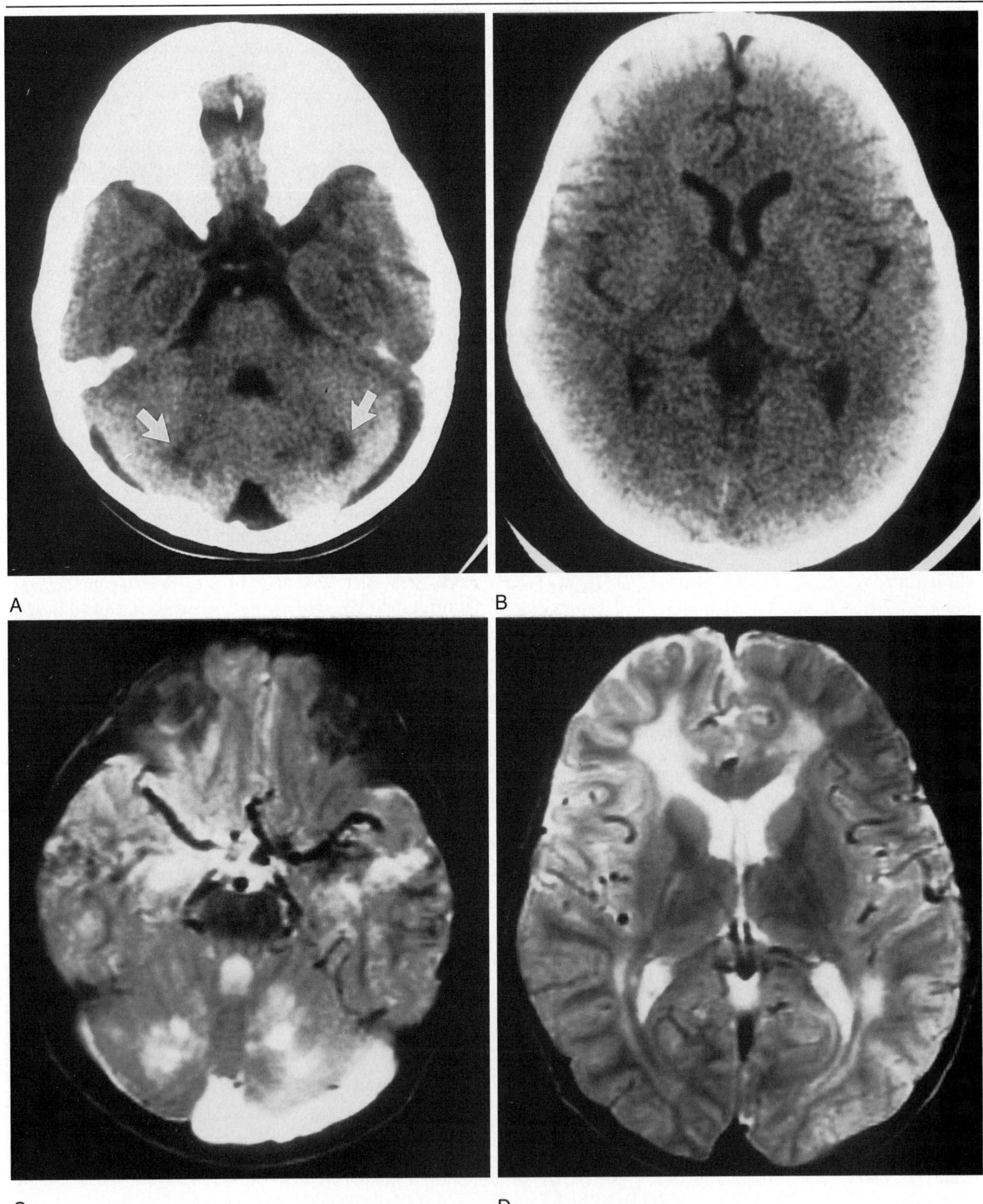

A B C D

Figure 5.65. Partial albinism and immunodeficiency in a 17-month-old boy. **A** and **B.** CT examination initially revealed low-density lesions in the cerebellum (arrows) and was otherwise normal. **C** and **D.** T2-weighted MRI 1 month later shows generalized white matter changes, sparing the peripheral subcortical white matter. (Courtesy of Dr. Jan Brismar, King Faisal Specialist Hospital and Research Center, Riyadh, Saudi Arabia [AJNR 1992;13:387–393].)

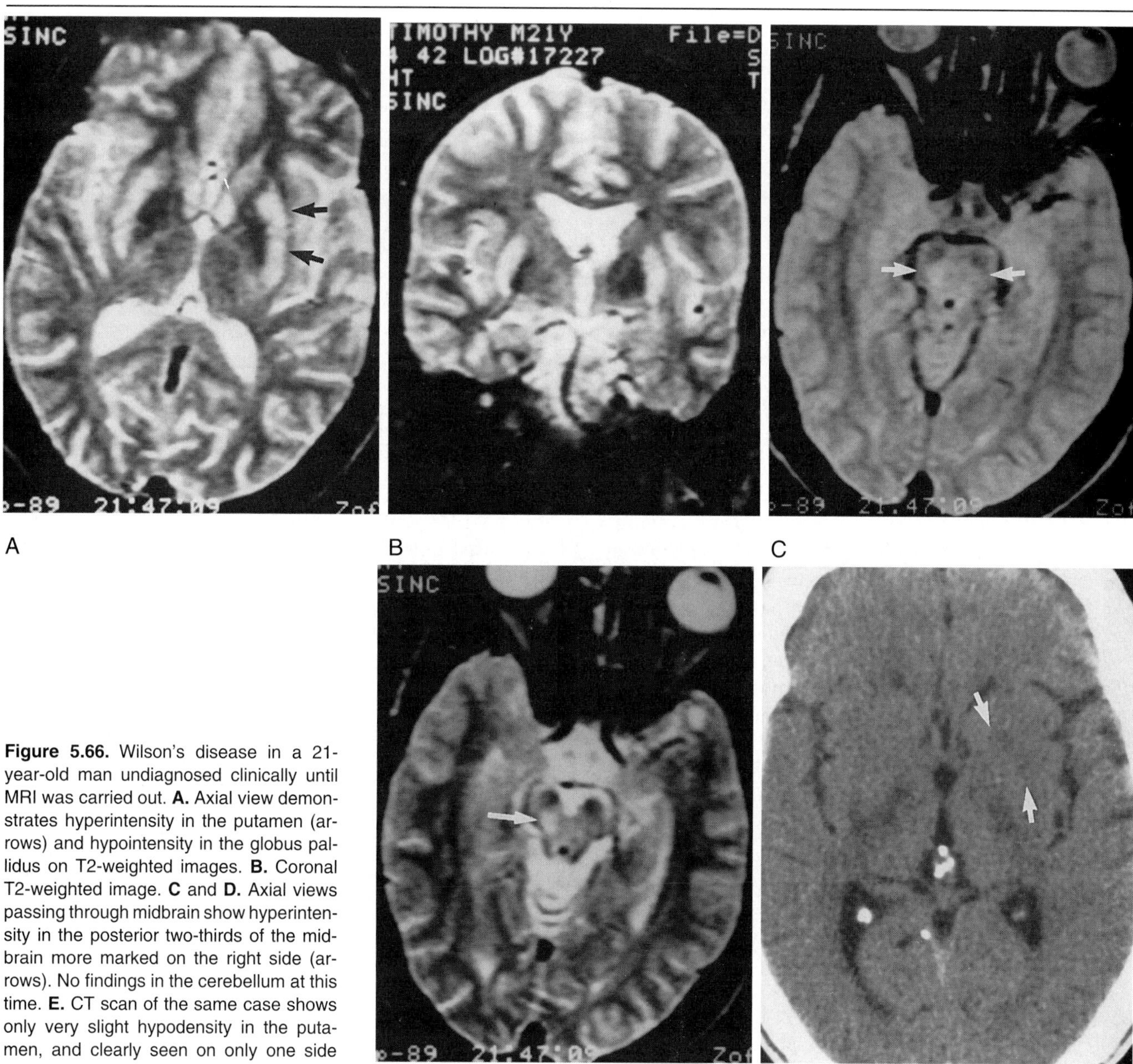

Figure 5.66. Wilson's disease in a 21-year-old man undiagnosed clinically until MRI was carried out. **A.** Axial view demonstrates hyperintensity in the putamen (arrows) and hypointensity in the globus pallidus on T2-weighted images. **B.** Coronal T2-weighted image. **C** and **D.** Axial views passing through midbrain show hyperintensity in the posterior two-thirds of the midbrain more marked on the right side (arrows). No findings in the cerebellum at this time. **E.** CT scan of the same case shows only very slight hypodensity in the putamen, and clearly seen on only one side (arrow). In general, CT may show minor changes, particularly in the early stages.

About 2 to 5 mg of copper are ingested daily. It enters the plasma, where it is linked to albumin and taken to the liver to be incorporated into a protein, mostly ceruloplasmin. Copper is excreted through the bile. Patients with Wilson's disease have a low ceruloplasmin concentration in the blood. The normal concentration of ceruloplasmin in the serum is 20 to 40 mg/100 ml. A low concentration of serum ceruloplasmin is also found in Menkes' disease.

The accumulation of copper in the liver leads to cirrhosis. In the brain, in the advanced stage of the disease, there is atrophy of the corpus striatum; there are also white matter abnormalities, which may be severe at times with cavitation as seen microscopically. Clinically the picture varies. It may start with liver failure during the first decade, but the child may first present with dystonia. The more typical signs of Wilson's disease are intention tremor, dysarthria, unusual behavior or mild dementia, drooling, and Kayser-Fleischer rings in the cornea. The last is diagnostic. The disease is often recognized during the second or third decade (Fig. 5.66).

Early diagnosis is helpful because the disease is treatable, particularly if recognized early. In addition to laboratory findings, such as low serum ceruloplasmin, which occasionally can be normal, liver biopsy may be necessary. MRI may show hyperintensity on T2 images in the putamen and globus pallidus, the caudate nucleus, and the thalamus. Some patients show hyperintensity in the brainstem, which includes the periaqueductal gray matter and red nucleus and substantia nigra. Involvement of the dentate nucleus of the cerebellum and high signal on T2 images are also found (185). The CT findings would be similar in location. Decreased attenuation may be seen in the same areas, particularly in the lenticular nuclei and thalami, but the changes in the brainstem and cerebellum may be difficult to appreciate. The accumulation of copper does not seem to produce increased density on CT. Some ventricular enlargement and widening of the sulci of the brain and cerebellum indicative of cerebral and cerebellar atrophy is observed in varying degrees on CT or MRI. In addition, on MRI, hyperintense white matter lesions are seen in some cases.

Although the final diagnosis is made by clinical and laboratory methods, the imaging findings are important because the initial clinical presentations can vary considerably. A differential diagnosis of the imaging findings includes Leigh's disease, which can present essentially the same findings on MRI, although some differences do exist; for example, thalamic involvement is fairly common in Wilson's disease but not in Leigh's disease. The presence and severity of the imaging findings vary with the age at which imaging is carried out. Wilson's disease can develop very gradually, and the patient is often not examined until late in the second or third decade of life, whereas in Leigh's disease the symptoms are usually noted early in the first decade (Figs. 5.66 and 5.67). Other conditions presenting basal ganglia abnormalities include striatal degeneration (174) and GM2 gangliosidosis (Tay-Sachs disease and Sandhoff disease), but in these only the thalamus is clearly involved. Imiya et al. reported bright lesions on T2-weighted images at the base of the pons in three cases of Wilson's disease (186), but this is somewhat unusual.

CT or MRI may be used to follow the results of therapy (usually penicillamine or triethylene tetramine). Improvement in the imaging changes, particularly in the basal ganglia but also in the ventricles, which may decrease in size, and in the cerebral hemisphere and cerebellum can be seen. Although younger patients usually respond more dramatically and demonstrate improvement on CT, older patients may also respond. There is no correlation between the severity of the imaging findings (basal ganglia hypodensity, ventricular enlargement, and cortical atrophy) and the response to treatment (187).

HUNTINGTON'S DISEASE

This is a disease affecting primarily the corpus striatum (caudate nucleus, putamen, globus pallidus). There is severe neuronal loss in these structures, less so in the globus pallidus with shrinkage of these structures. This leads to enlargement of the frontal horns of the lateral ventricles particularly involving the lateral, inferior aspect, which is typical for this condition (Figs. 5.68 and 5.69). In time, there is also some generalized atrophy of the brain. Kuhl et al. first reported decreased glucose uptake in the basal ganglia before any atrophic changes can be demonstrated by CT or MRI (188).

After onset, usually in the fourth or fifth decade of life, progression of the choreic movements, mental deterioration, and other findings is relentless until death in 10 to 15 years. Earlier onset occurs, occasionally, in childhood. The disease is inherited as an autosomal dominant trait, and the possibility of acquiring the disease from an affected, but not yet symptomatic, parent is about 50 percent. Progress has recently been announced concerning the isolation of the genetic flaw that causes Huntington's disease, located in a newly discovered gene (IT15) in chromosome 4 and consisting, apparently, in extra repeats of a three-nucleotide stretch (CA6) that inserts extra copies of the

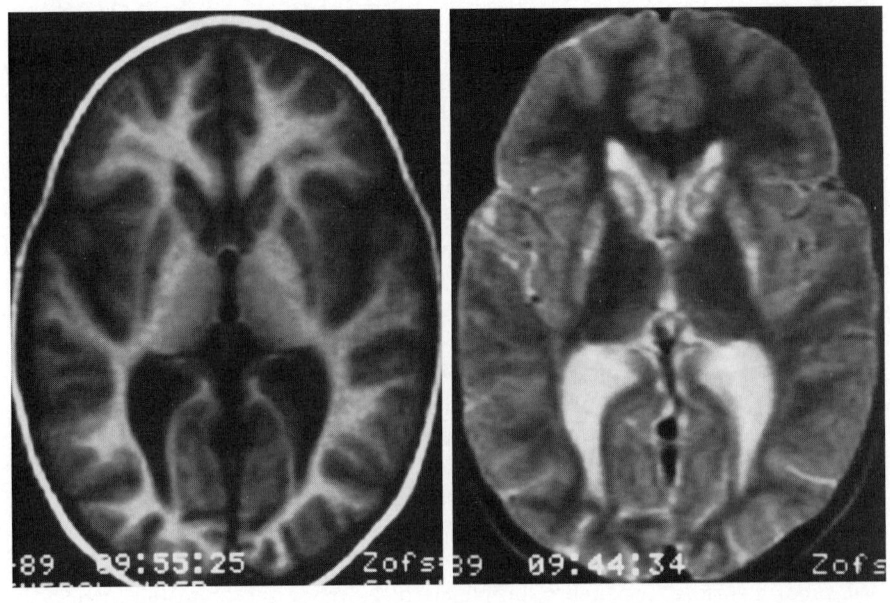

Figure 5.67. Wilson's disease in a 6-year-old girl. **A** and **B**. Only the putamen and caudate nuclei bilaterally reveal hypointensity on T1- (A) and hyperintensity on T2-weighted images (B). No other findings in this case, but the child had a history of mental retardation, liver disease, and optic atrophy.

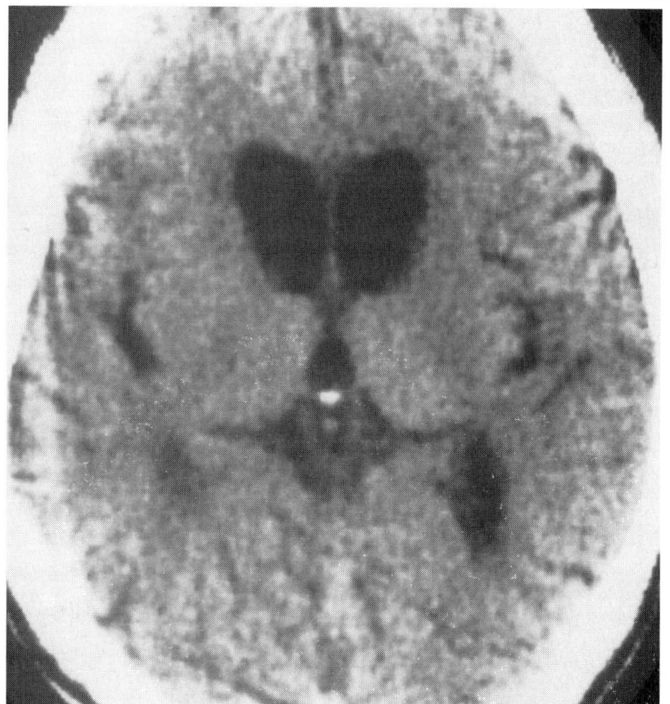

Figure 5.68. Huntington's disease in a 40-year-old man. The axial CT shows typical squaring of the frontal portion of the lateral ventricles owing to atrophy of the head of the caudate nucleus, which eliminates the normal rounded impression on the lateral inferior aspect of the frontal horns. As yet there is no significant enlargement of the sylvian fissure or of the surface sulci.

aminoacid glutamine into the gene's protein product. The gene contains 11 to 34 copies of this sequence, but in Huntington's patients the number is between 42 and 80 or higher (189).

FAHR'S DISEASE

This disorder is characterized by rather extensive calcification in the basal ganglia, a feature that is shared with other conditions. There is no abnormality of serum calcium levels and no associated endocrine disorder. Plain films of the skull may demonstrate the calcifications if they are heavy, but CT is particularly sensitive and demonstrates even small quantities of calcium, allowing for an earlier diagnosis. In most cases of Fahr's disease the calcifications are already well developed when the patients are first seen (Fig. 5.70). They are found in the globus pallidus, putamen, and caudate nucleus, and are heaviest in the globus pallidus. Calcifications are also found in the brain white matter, the dentate nucleus, and surrounding area in the cerebellum. Identical distribution of calcifications, except for the cerebellar portion, has been reported by Demirci and Sze in a case of osteopetrosis (190), and there are other reports of the same condition (191).

Histologically, the calcifications occur along capillary vessels and in the medial walls of larger arteries and veins. Although calcium is the predominant element, other elements are also present (zinc, phosphorus, iron, magnesium, aluminum, and potassium). The calcium is incorporated into proteins or bound to polysaccharides during the development

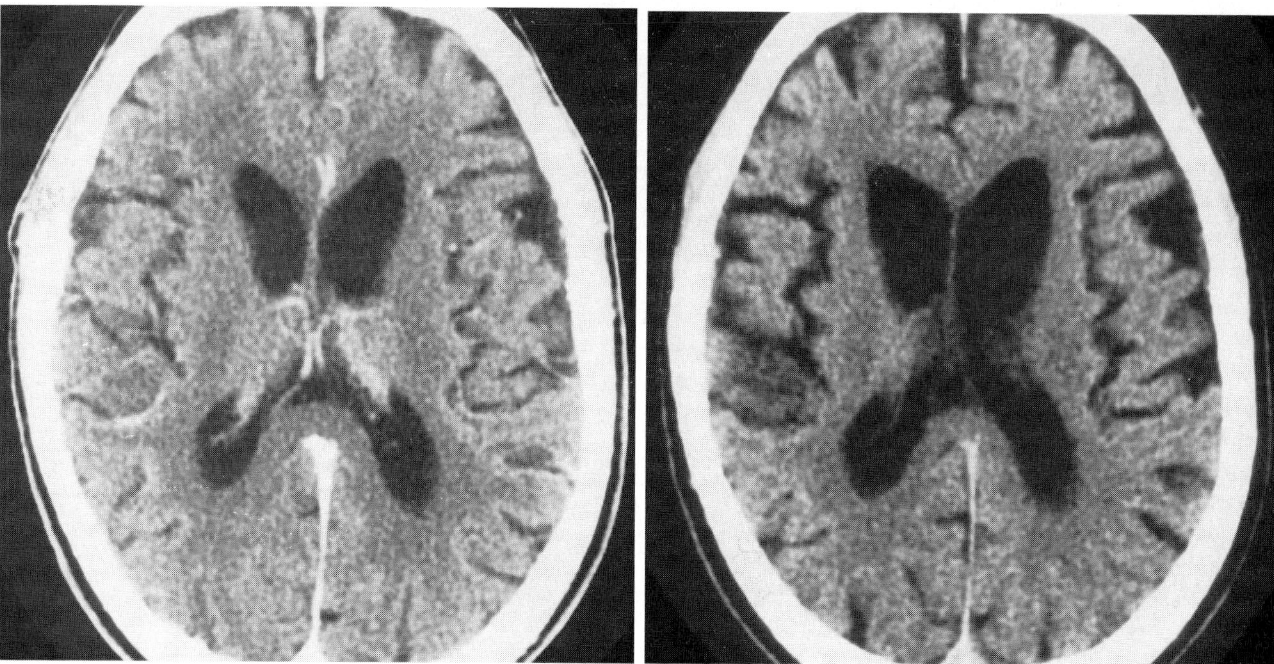

A B

Figure 5.69. Huntington's disease in a 33-year-old man. **A.** Initial study shows rounding of lateral contour of frontal horns and moderate ventricular enlargement. **B.** Reexamination 2 years later reveals progression of ventricular enlargement, and sulcal and sylvian fissure widening.

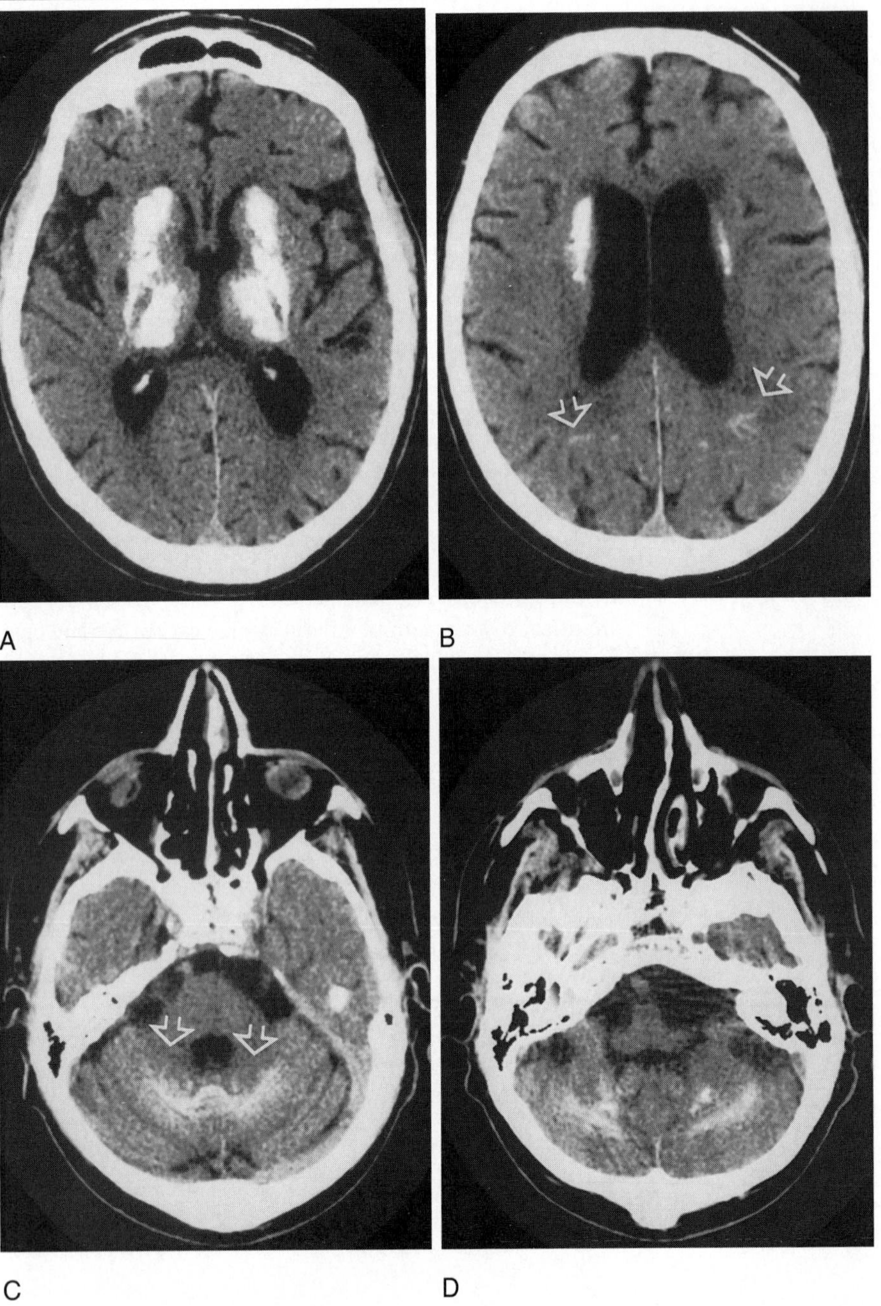

Figure 5.70. Fahr's disease. **A.** Axial CT in a 57-year-old man revealing heavy calcification in the caudate nucleus, the putamen, and globus pallidus and the thalamus bilaterally. **B.** A higher section reveals the bilateral calcification in the body of the caudate nucleus. There is also some slight calcification in the corticomedullary junction in the parietal region bilaterally (open arrows). **C.** A section through the posterior fossa reveals bilateral calcification in the dentate nuclei (arrows) and in the cerebellar substance (**D**).

and maturation of the pathologic process; these factors may well influence the MRI appearance of Fahr's disease.

On CT the findings are clear, as described previously, but on MRI the picture may vary between T1- and T2-weighted images. Low signals may be seen in some areas, and in other areas it may be T1 bright and T2 dark, whereas in other areas the T2 high signal predominates. This was particularly well shown in a case reported by Scotti et al. (192). In that case the extensive white matter, periventricular calcifications, were T2 bright, and the extensive cerebellar calcifications seen on CT were totally absent on MRI. Clinically the patients present extrapyramidal symptoms, mental deterioration, speech disturbances, and other neurologic manifestations. The patient is likely to be an adult, and the neurologic disability is progressive. Treatment attempts to arrest or to decrease the process of calcification. The disease may be transmitted as an autosomal recessive, but autosomal dominant transmission can occur in some cases (193).

HALLERVORDEN-SPATZ DISEASE

This is a disorder that most often manifests itself between 7 and 15 years of age but may also present earlier or later, characterized by the storage of iron in the globus pallidus, the substantia nigra, and to a lesser extent the red nucleus. The symptoms are gait disturbance, leg rigidity, movement slowing, and progressive mental deterioration. It is inherited as an autosomal recessive trait. CT may show decreased density in the affected areas, but MRI is much preferred because it demonstrates magnetic susceptibility in the globus pallidus and substantia nigra. The T2-weighted images demonstrate very low signals in the pallidum and substantia nigra, which is even more prominent in the special susceptibility sequence. There are no specific biochemical laboratory tests, and the clinical manifestations are not too dissimilar to other neurologic conditions involving the basal ganglia; thus, the imaging appearance is very helpful in arriving at a diagnosis. Some reported cases show low signal on T2-weighted images in the globus pallidus (194), and other reports show low intensity in the globus pallidus and in the substantia nigra (195). Ambrosetto et al. reported a bright center surrounded by low signal on T2 images in two sisters with onset in their midfifties (196).

METHYLMALONIC ACIDEMIA

This is a disorder of amino acid metabolism involving defective conversion of methylmalonyl coenzyme A to succinyl coenzyme A, which leads to accumulation of methylmalonate in the blood and urine and to ketoacidosis. The clinical presentation can occur early (weeks to months after birth) and is commonly associated with ketoacidosis without other apparent cause. Elevated methylmalonic or propionic acid levels can be demonstrated in urine and serum. Of the four cases reported by Gebarski et al., one presented at 1 month with ketoacidosis; another at 4 months with spastic quadriplegia; a third also presented with spastic quadriplegia and ketoacidosis at 2 months of age; and the fourth presented at age 17 with mild mental retardation and headache (197). Two had elevated methylmalonic acid levels, and two elevated propionic acid levels. CT showed relatively diffuse white matter change in the brain in one case. The other showed only moderate ventriculomegaly, and two did show some atrophic process in the posterior limb of the internal capsule. While these cases represent a genetically transmitted disorder of B_{12} (cobalamin) and biotin metabolism, none of the four cases mentioned here had any benefit following the administration of vitamin B_{12}. The case reported by Andreula et al., however, presented CT and MRI findings primarily in the basal ganglia, particularly the globus pallidus, with little change elsewhere and no ventricular dilatation (198). Seven of nine cases reported have had bilateral hypodensity of the pallidum on CT; for this reason it is listed among the group of disorders affecting the basal ganglia (Fig. 5.71).

COCKAYNE'S SYNDROME

Transmitted as an autosomal recessive trait, this syndrome consists of growth retardation, mental retardation, microcephaly, retinopathy, cutaneous photosensitivity, and ataxia. The cerebral pathologic changes are similar to the leukodystrophies. However, a significant difference is that the small vessels become involved by mural and extramural colloid deposits, which frequently contain iron and exhibit striking calcification. The brain is gritty on cutting, and calcification is visible on gross inspection. The deposits occur chiefly in the basal ganglia, the cerebral white matter, and the dentate nuclei of the cerebellum. Radiographs of the skull reveal a small head and may demonstrate calcifications, particularly in the basal ganglia and dentate nuclei but also in the cerebral white matter. In general, CT demonstrates these calcifications much before they become visible on plain skull films. There is also evidence of white matter lucency on CT and hyperintensity on T2-weighted images on MRI (199–201). Cortical calcifications also occur, particularly in the cerebellum; they are likely to be heavier in the older patients (Fig. 5.72).

MEMBRANOUS LIPODYSTROPHY (LIPOMEMBRANOUS POLYCYSTIC OSTEODYSPLASIA WITH PROGRESSIVE DEMENTIA)

Of the five patients reported by Araki et al., there was evidence of consanguinity in two, and a sister of another patient had a history of similar symptoms (202). The age at diagnosis may be in the third or fourth decade of life. Some mental deterioration is usually present, and fractures due to the cystic bone lesions may occur. The imaging findings on CT are calcification in basal ganglia and thalamus in some of the cases; decreased intensity of the basal ganglia and thalamus on T2-weighted images may be due to calcium and iron accumulation. Decreased signal intensity in the brain cortex on T2-weighted images could be due to calcium and iron accumulation as mentioned by Araki et al. but not well documented (202). Some increased signal intensity of the white matter on T2-weighted images may be seen. Ventricular dilatation attributed to cerebral atrophy was seen in all cases.

GERSTMANN-STRAUSSLER-SCHEINKER DISEASE

This is a rare autosomal dominant disease in which iron accumulates in the basal ganglia. In some patients, the thalamus may also be involved. T2-weighted images may show low intensity due to magnetic susceptibility effects of the iron (203).

KERNICTERUS

See below under "Perinatal Brain Damage" (Fig. 5.73).

STRIATONIGRAL DEGENERATION

Striatonigral degeneration may be described among the multiple system atrophy. It usually occurs in adults and older individuals but can be seen in children (Fig. 5.74). See under "Multiple System Atrophy" (Chapter 8).

CYTOPLASMICALLY INHERITED STRIATED DEGENERATION

See under "Mitochondrial Cytopathies."

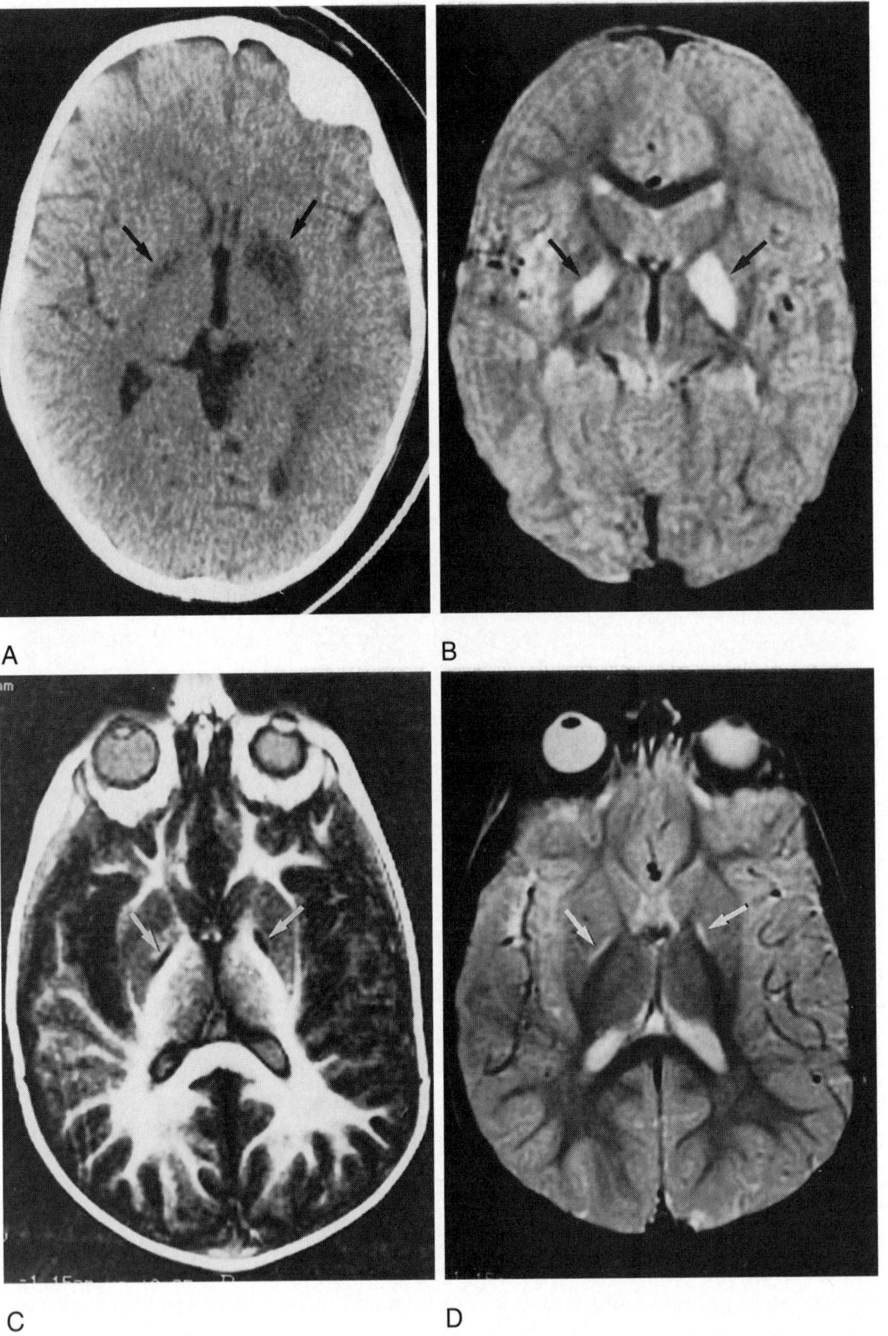

Figure 5.71. Methylmalonic acidemia in a 2-year-old girl. **A.** CT scan without contrast reveals hypodensity in the globus pallidus, more evident on the left (arrows). **B.** T2-weighted axial shows involvement of the same area in the basal ganglia. **C.** Reexamination almost 2 years later confirmed the bilateral pallidal necrosis (arrows), appearing dark on this T1-weighted inversion recovery image and bright on the T2-weighted image (**D**) (arrows). The ventricles and subarachnoid spaces are normal. The parents were cousins; at birth the girl suffered generalized seizures without hypoxia but developed normally until 24 months, at which time she presented with fever, lethargy, seizures, hypotonia, and right hemiparesis. Therapy was instituted with a low-protein diet and vitamin B_{12}. Possibly the final changes in the globus pallidus (C and D) were smaller than in the original examination (A and B). (Courtesy of Cosma F. Andreula, University of Bari, Italy [AJNR 1991;12:410].)

PERINATAL BRAIN DAMAGE

Ischemic Brain Injury

This could occur in a premature infant or in a term infant. In the premature infant there are complicating factors. Before the thirty-fourth week of gestation, the lungs are less able to provide oxygenated blood; asphyxia and ischemic brain damage are more common. The asphyxia may be classified as partial or profound. Partial asphyxia results from prolonged mild or moderate hypoxia or hypotension, which could be related to heart or lung disease, degenerated placenta, or shock. Profound asphyxia results from conditions such as abruptio placentae or cardiopulmonary arrest.

Asphyxia leads to low blood oxygen tension, acidosis, and a drop in blood pressure. In the brain, anaerobic glycolysis occurs, and acidosis and loss of autoregulation result. The lower blood pressure causes diminished brain perfusion. For further details on cerebral circulation pathophysiology see Chapter 10.

The blood vessels in the periventricular region, in the *germinal matrix*, are rich and liable to rupture as vasodilatation occurs following correction of the asphyxia. The germinal matrix has a particular area, the *ganglionic eminence*,

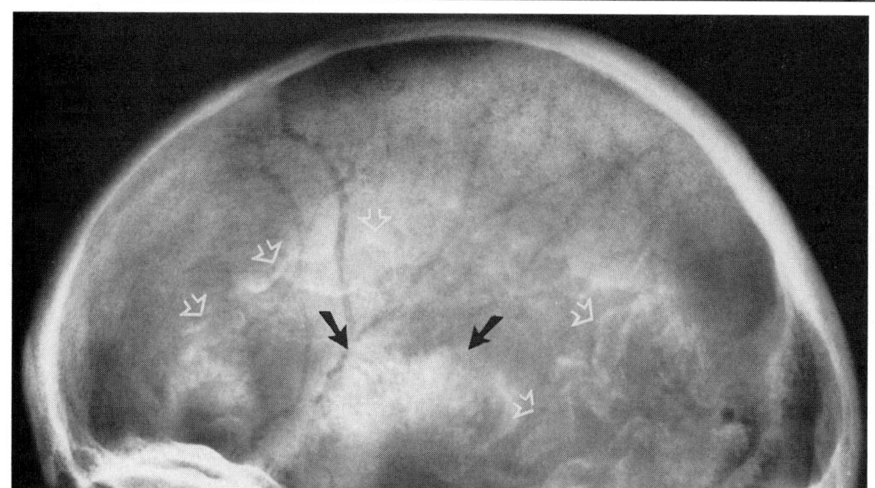

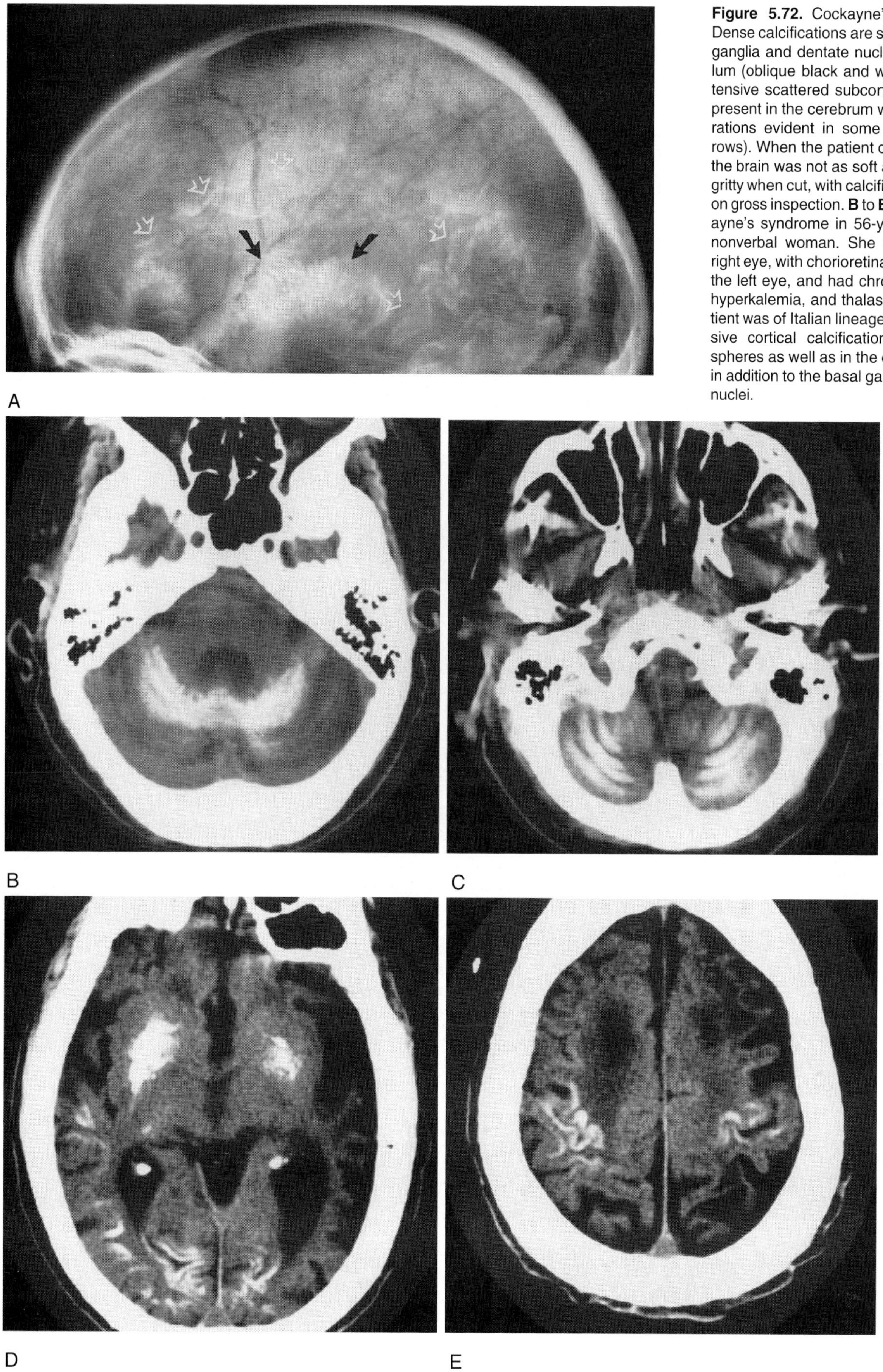

Figure 5.72. Cockayne's syndrome. **A.** Dense calcifications are shown in the basal ganglia and dentate nuclei of the cerebellum (oblique black and white arrows). Extensive scattered subcortical deposits are present in the cerebrum with gyral configurations evident in some areas (open arrows). When the patient died 2 years later, the brain was not as soft as usual and was gritty when cut, with calcific granules visible on gross inspection. **B** to **E.** Probable Cockayne's syndrome in 56-year-old retarded, nonverbal woman. She was blind in the right eye, with chorioretinal degeneration in the left eye, and had chronic renal failure, hyperkalemia, and thalassemia minor (patient was of Italian lineage). There is extensive cortical calcification in both hemispheres as well as in the cerebellar cortex, in addition to the basal ganglia and dentate nuclei.

A

B

C

D

E

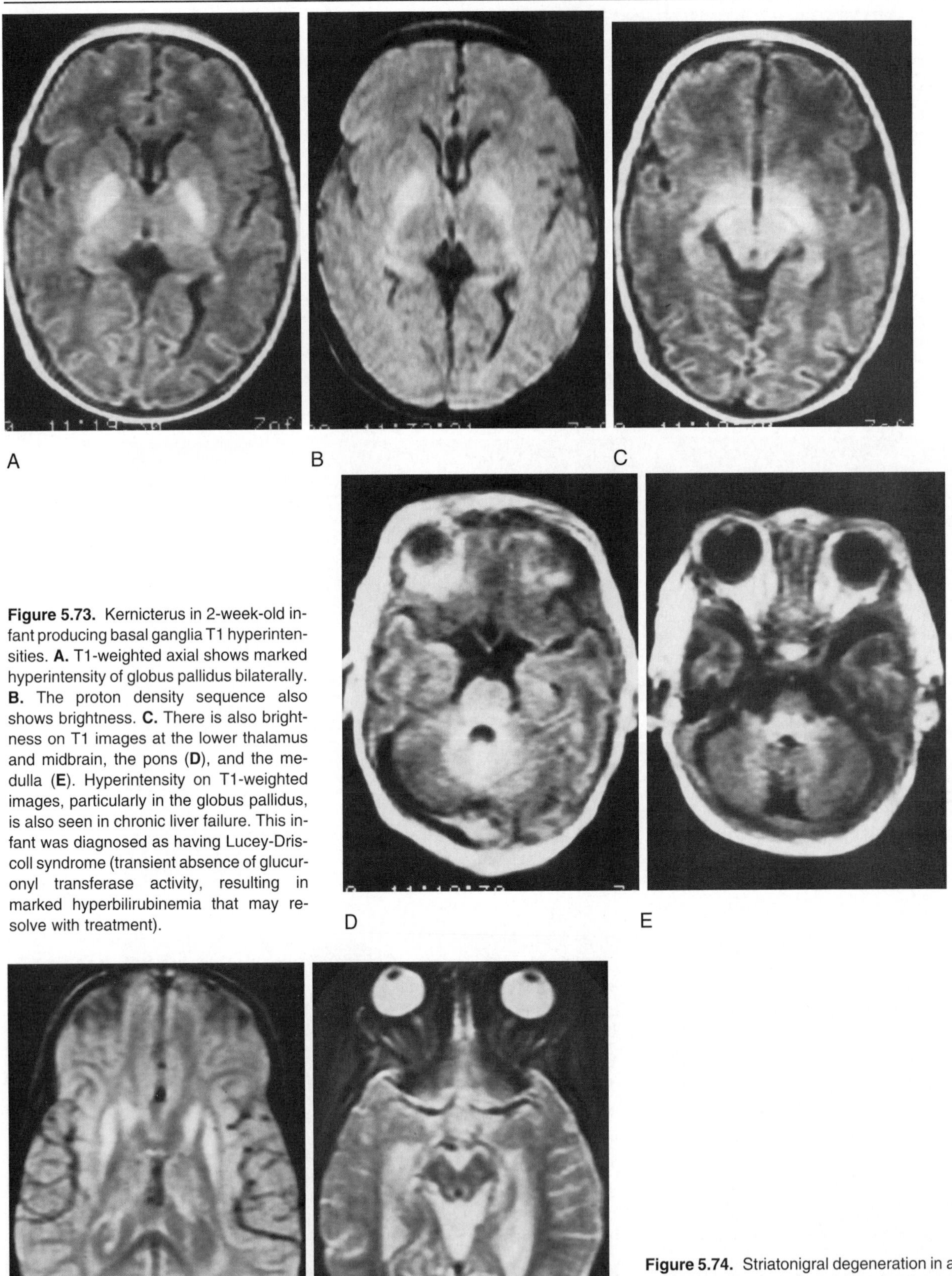

Figure 5.73. Kernicterus in 2-week-old infant producing basal ganglia T1 hyperintensities. **A.** T1-weighted axial shows marked hyperintensity of globus pallidus bilaterally. **B.** The proton density sequence also shows brightness. **C.** There is also brightness on T1 images at the lower thalamus and midbrain, the pons (**D**), and the medulla (**E**). Hyperintensity on T1-weighted images, particularly in the globus pallidus, is also seen in chronic liver failure. This infant was diagnosed as having Lucey-Driscoll syndrome (transient absence of glucuronyl transferase activity, resulting in marked hyperbilirubinemia that may resolve with treatment).

Figure 5.74. Striatonigral degeneration in a 5-year-old child. **A.** Proton density axial image shows hyperintensity in the putamen and globus pallidus as well as in the caudate nucleus. **B.** There is hyperintensity in the region of the substantia nigra in this T2-weighted axial image. A brother was diagnosed as having Leigh's disease, but at autopsy this child was considered to present striatonigral degeneration.

which is the latest to involute and thus remains vascular through most of the last trimester. The ganglionic eminence is situated over the head of the caudate nucleus on each side and is where hemorrhage most frequently occurs (204). The striothalamic sulcus area is also a frequent site of hemorrhage. The diagnosis can be made by ultrasound, which also provides for noninvasive follow-up.

The periventricular hemorrhages in premature infants are usually divided into four grades, depending on severity: grade 1: striothalamic–ganglionic eminence; grade 2: intraventricular; grade 3: intraventricular with enlargement of ventricles; and grade 4: extension of hemorrhage into cerebral hemispheres.

Ultrasound reveals the periventricular hemorrhage or regions of increased echogenicity, most frequently around the heads of the caudate nuclei (Fig. 5.75). Intraventricular hemorrhage also shows up as areas of increased echogenicity early on but later becoming somewhat less echogenic. It becomes less echogenic than the choroid plexus and usually is located in the atrium of the lateral ventricle. Parenchymal hemorrhage is seen as areas of hyperechogenicity in the brain matter, which later may become cystic. Parenchymal hemorrhage is easily diagnosed by CT (Fig. 5.76). Death is common in this group.

The white matter of the developing brain is particularly sensitive to injury, which may produce necrosis, gliosis, and disturbances in myelination. In periventricular leukomalacia (PVL) the lesions are, by definition, located in the region of the ventricles, but the term is applied more broadly to damage of the white matter away from the ventricles. The white matter of the cerebrum is most commonly affected and may involve the centrum semiovale and the subcortical areas. This leads to gliosis and diminution in the width of the white matter between the ventricular wall and the cortical gray matter. The gyri are very close to the ventricular wall; the atrium of the ventricle enlarges due to the brain atrophy.

PVL is most commonly seen in the periatrial and occipital regions; it results from ischemic lesions in the brain, as well as from periventricular hematomas. More often it involves the posterior half of the ventricular region, but it may extend to involve the body and frontal horns of the lateral ventricles. Initially, there is periventricular edema, followed by cystic changes. Again, ultrasound may show diffuse increased periventricular echogenicity, but the appearance is not diagnostic of PVL. Also, ultrasound may be negative in the presence of PVL.

CT and MRI may have to be performed to arrive at a more certain evaluation of the presence or absence of PVL. CT may show the following: (a) ventricular enlargement with irregular ventricular contour (Fig. 5.77); (b) reduced amount of white matter around the body and atrium of the lateral ventricles; and (c) prominent sulci, with the gray matter abutting or nearly abutting the ventricular wall (205) (Fig. 5.78). The ventricular wall is usually irregular, at least in the early stages. MRI may show signs of subacute hemorrhage in the periventricular region. In the chronic phase MRI will show approximately the same findings as CT. Magnetic susceptibility may be seen in the sites of hemorrhage, but the susceptibility probably will disappear after 1 year (204,206). PVL without hemorrhage will show up as periventricular hyperintensity, seen well particularly on proton density images.

In the term infant, hypoxic-ischemic lesions may result from various causes, including, in the intrapartum period, prolapse of the umbilical cord, placenta previa, placental abruption, uterine tetany, or attempts to delay progress of delivery. The lesions are usually ischemic, but may become hemorrhagic later (207).

Cerebral infarcts in the territory of the middle, anterior, or posterior cerebral arteries may occur (Fig. 5.79). Ischemic lesions in the thalamus and basal ganglia, as well as in the basis pontis, are seen particularly in the neonatal period.

CT may show hypodensity in the infarcted area; it is particularly important to look at the brain cortex, where a disappearance of the local gray-white matter differentiation may occur. The MRI appearance may be very inconspicuous because of the usual normal T2 hyperintensity of the white matter in the newborn period due to the normal greater percentage of water and no myelination. Thus the hyperintensity usually seen more easily in the white matter in ischemic lesions on T2-weighted images may not be appreciated. The expected cortical focal hyperintensity due to edema related to the ischemic lesion may be seen as an area in which it is isointense with white matter on proton density and T2-weighted images—what Barkovich calls focal "disappearance" of the gray matter.

Watershed infarctions can occur but are rare in infants. Basal ganglia and thalamic ischemia may produce uniformly hyperintense structures on proton density images, which has been termed *status marmoratus* because of the marblelike appearance. The same term may be used in the presence of preserved myelinated area (bright on T1-weighted images) surrounded by infarcted hypointense zones. Diffuse hyperintensity in the same areas on CT may also be seen due to severe metabolic changes, possibly involving calcium metabolism, as well as hemorrhage (Figs. 5.80 and 5.81).

Intrapartum Injury

In the term infant, hemorrhage is usually the result of some birth injury. The most frequent are the subdural hematomas, but subarachnoid hemorrhage also occurs, and intracerebral petechial hemorrhages are probably common but usually not clinically significant.

Subdural hematomas may occur around the tentorium due to tearing of venous sinuses near its junction with the falx cerebri or along the falx (Fig. 5.82). They may also be seen on the convexities, owing to the rupture of bridging

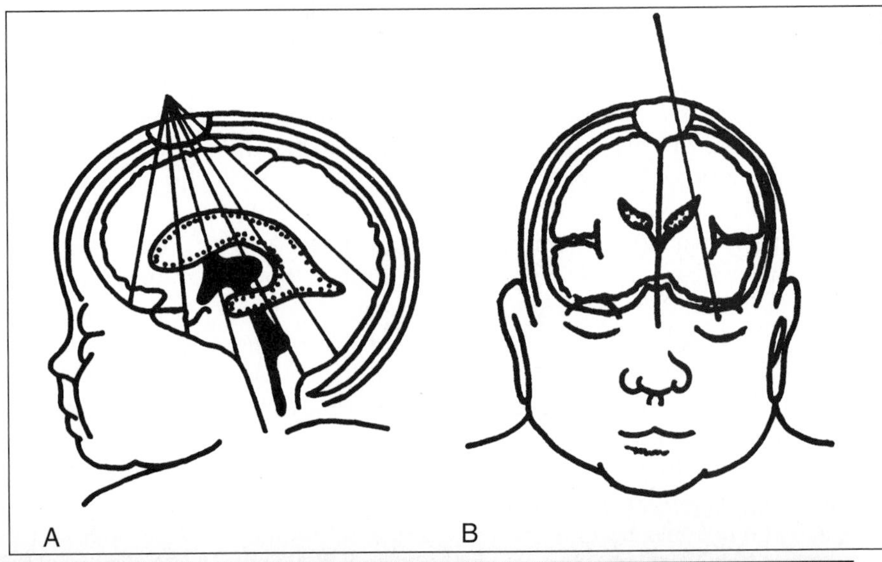

C

D

E

F

Figure 5.75. Direction of ultrasound beam through the anterior fontanel in infants **A.** Sagittal. **B.** Coronal. (Courtesy of Dr. Hans Blickman, Boston, Mass.) **C** to **F.** A hemorrhage in a premature infant demonstrated with ultrasound. **C** and **D.** Hemorrhage in the region of the choroid plexus (arrows). In D, the choroid glomus is too large, suggesting hemorrhage (grade 2) (arrow). **E** and **F.** Grade 3 intraventricular hemorrhage (arrow) (E) frontal; (F) lateral. The ventricles are hyperechoic and moderately enlarged.

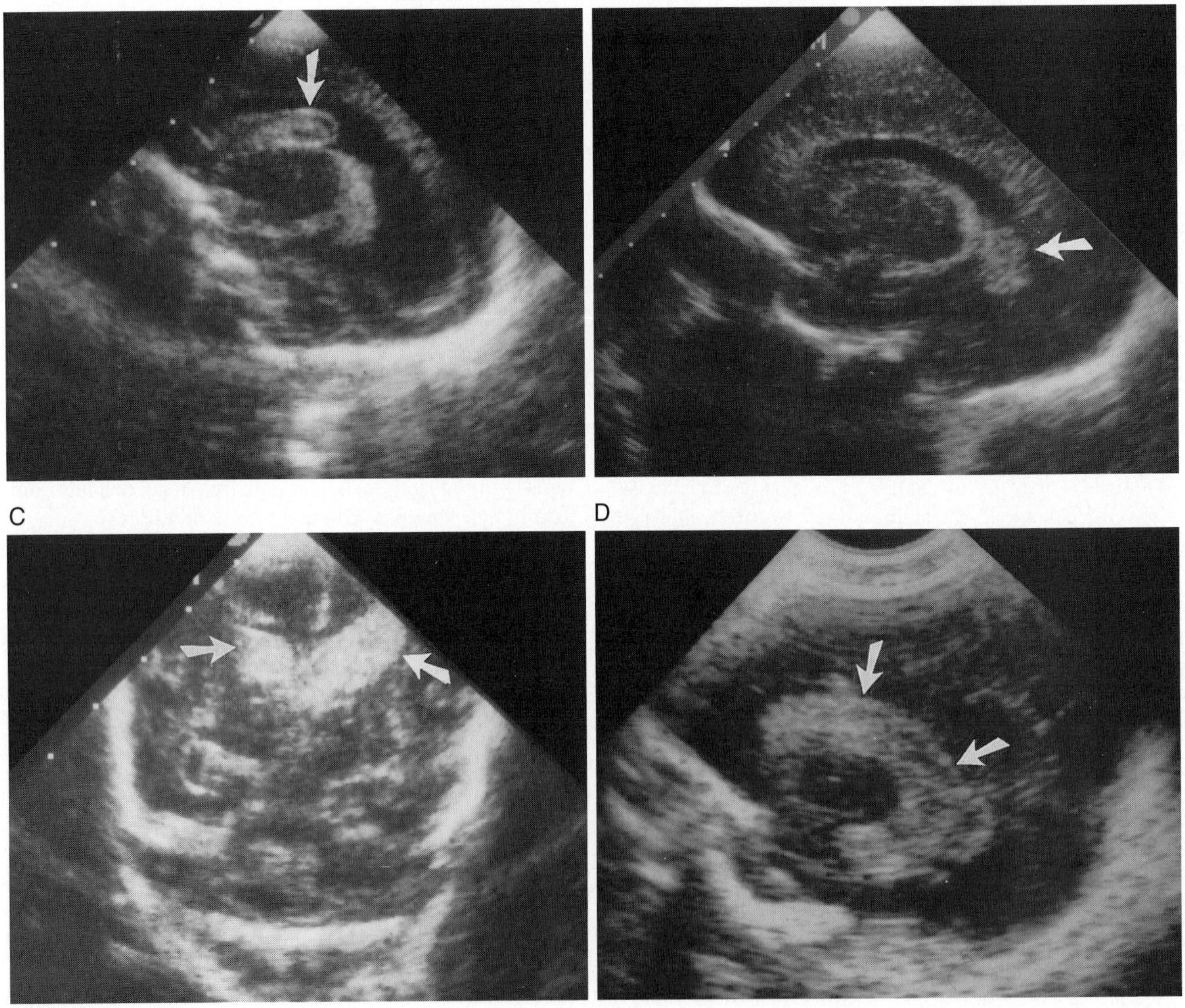

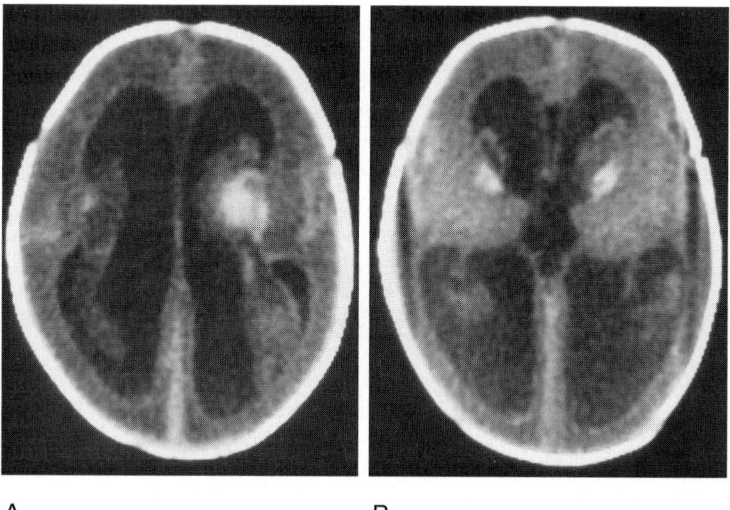

A B

C D E

Figure 5.76. Grade 4 germinal matrix hemorrhage in a 28-week premature infant. **A.** There is marked ventricular dilatation, and the hemorrhage extends into the adjacent brain parenchyma. Note that there is no development of surface sulci. **B.** A lower section reveals bilateral hemorrhage in the heads of the caudate nuclei. **C** and **D.** A Rickham reservoir was installed in the quadrigeminal cistern, causing reduction of ventricular size. The ventricular wall is hyperdense in (D), probably related to hyperemia. **E.** CT performed 4 months after birth shows considerable improvement in the hydrocephalus. Some surface sulci are now visible. The shunt tube is seen in the quadrigeminal cistern.

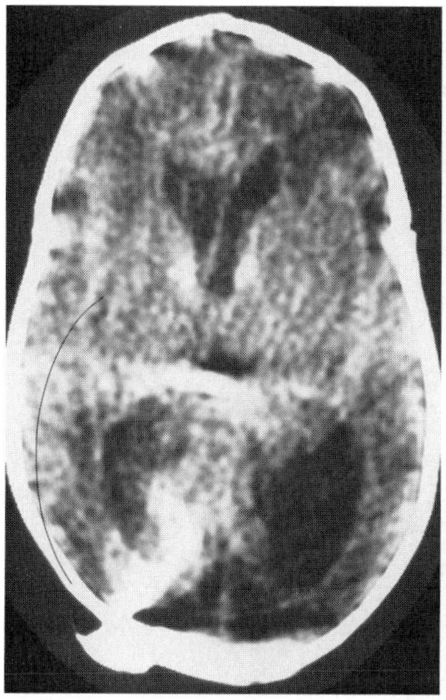

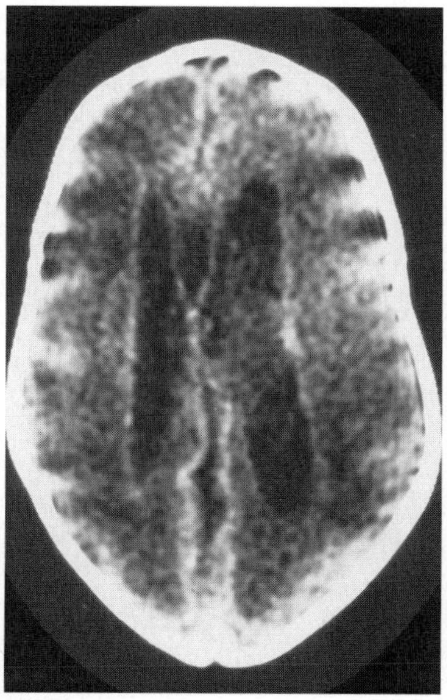

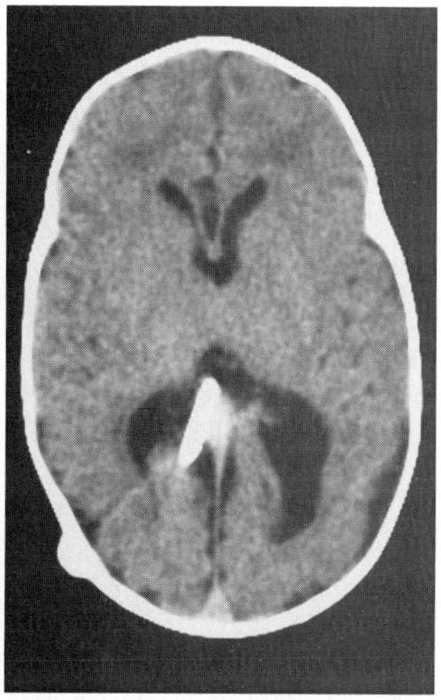

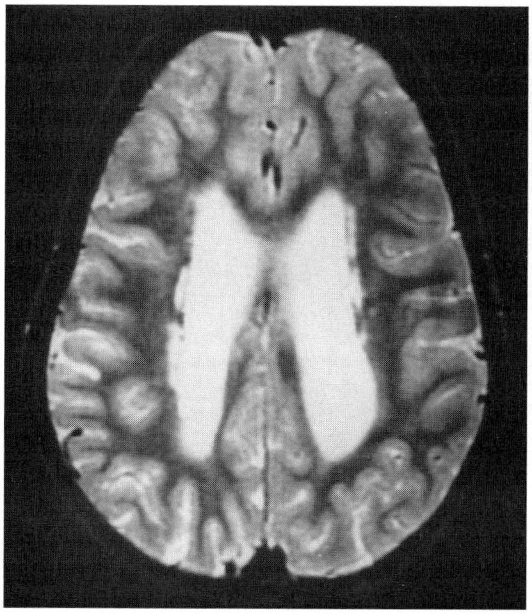

A 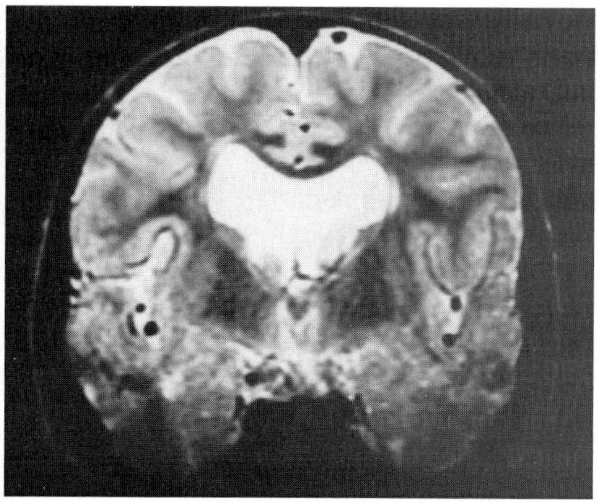 B

Figure 5.77. Periventricular leukomalacia in an 8-year-old boy, who now presents intractable seizures and spasticity. **A.** There is ventricular dilataion and marked irregularity of ventricular margin. There is a decrease in periventricular white matter. **B.** Coronal T2-weighted image showing periventricular irregularity and decrease in white matter; the cortical gyri are too close to the ventricular wall.

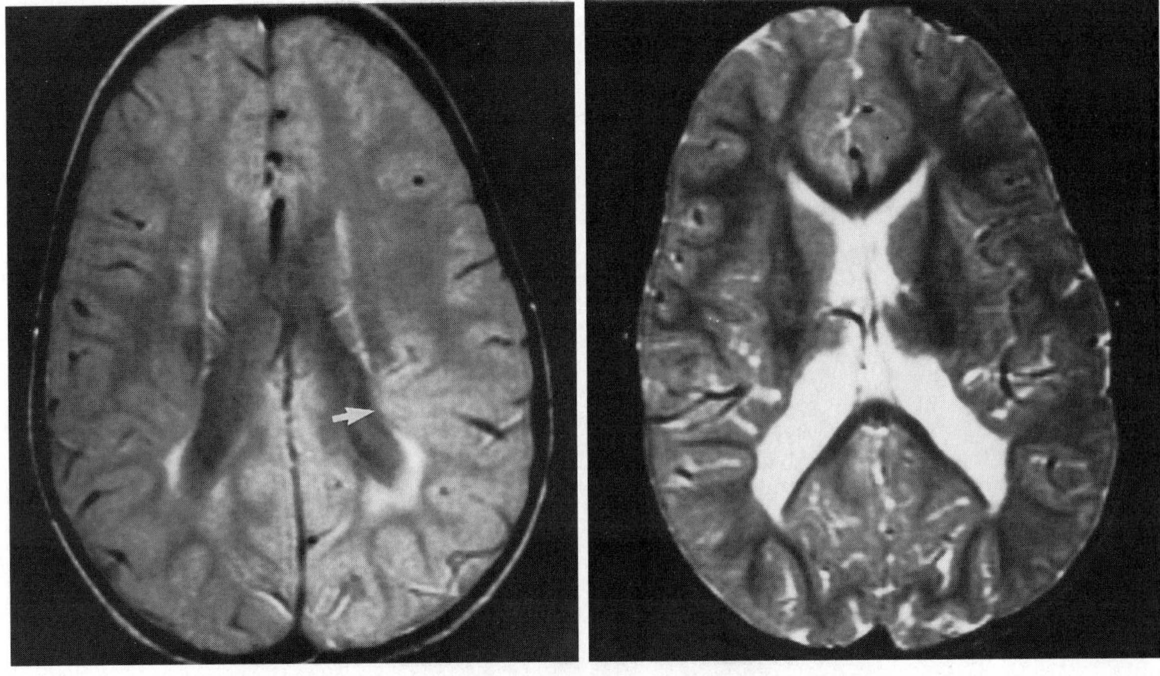

A B

Figure 5.78. Periventricular leukomalacia in an 18-month-old child with a convulsive disorder. The child was premature. **A.** A proton density axial image reveals that the gray matter indents the ventricular wall, particularly in the periatrial region, and more pronounced on the left side (arrow). **B.** T2-weighted axial view shows the bilateral scalloped irregularity of the ventricular outline due to absent white matter, allowing the gray matter to abut the ventricular wall. This appearance should not be confused with gray matter heterotopia.

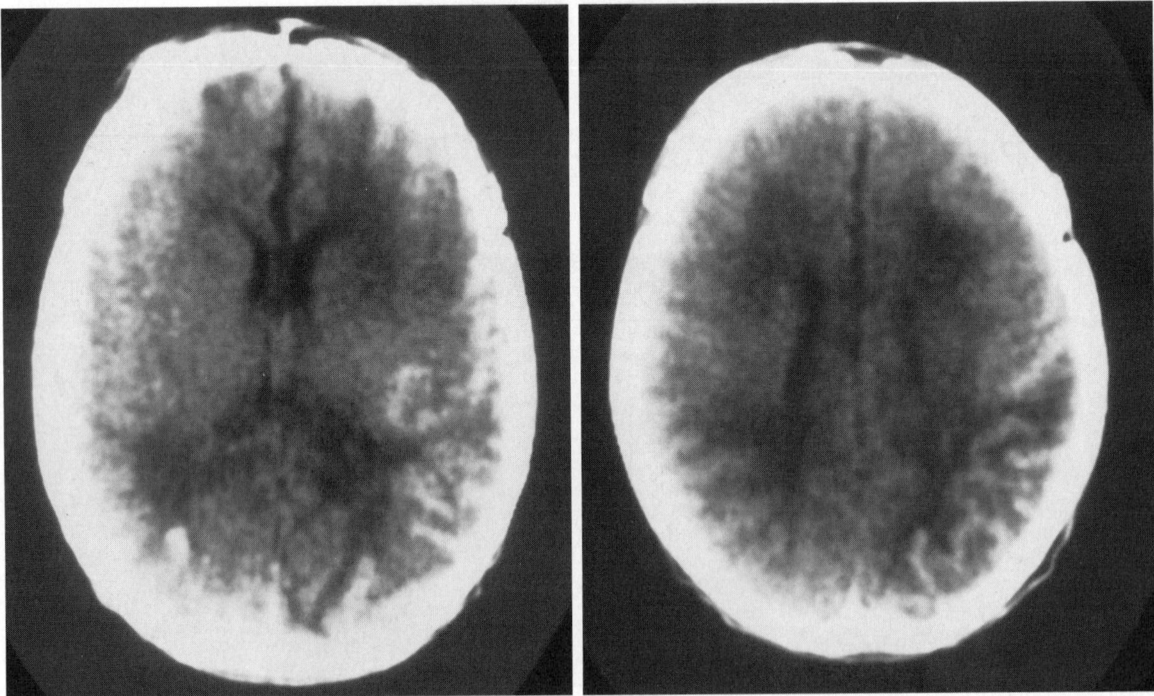

A B

Figure 5.79. Hemorrhagic infarction in full-term, 2-day-old infant born by cesarean section. **A** and **B.** CT section shows gyral hyperintensity involving the left parieto-occipital area as well as some hyperintensity on the right side. The postnatal diagnosis was meconium aspiration syndrome. Subarachnoid hemorrhage was considered, but no hyperintensity was seen elsewhere, suggestive of subarachnoid bleeding. There appears to be cortical hyperintensity in the frontal poles bilaterally as well as on the frontoparietal gyri on the right in A and B. The findings suggest asphyxia.

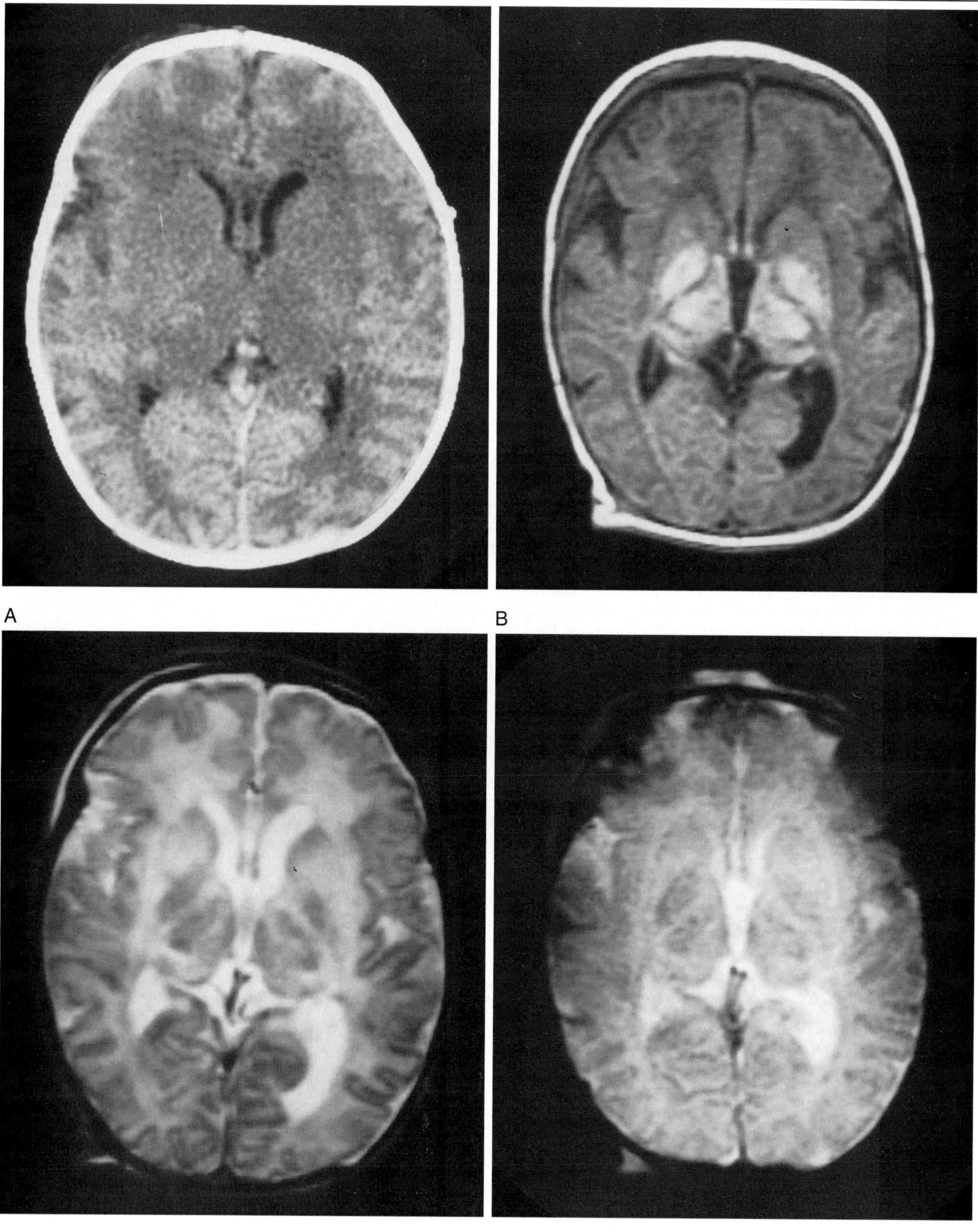

Figure 5.80. Status marmoratus in a newborn infant born by vacuum extraction. The infant had seizures, hypoxia, and pneumonia. **A.** CT done at 1 week showed low density in thalamic and basal ganglia region bilaterally. **B.** MRI examination a week later, T1-weighted axial, showed marked hyperintensity bilaterally in thalamus and globus pallidus. **C.** T2-weighted axial (4000/100) shows isointensity with gray matter in same areas. **D.** A susceptibility image (gradient echo 750/50) showed no signs of hemorrhage.

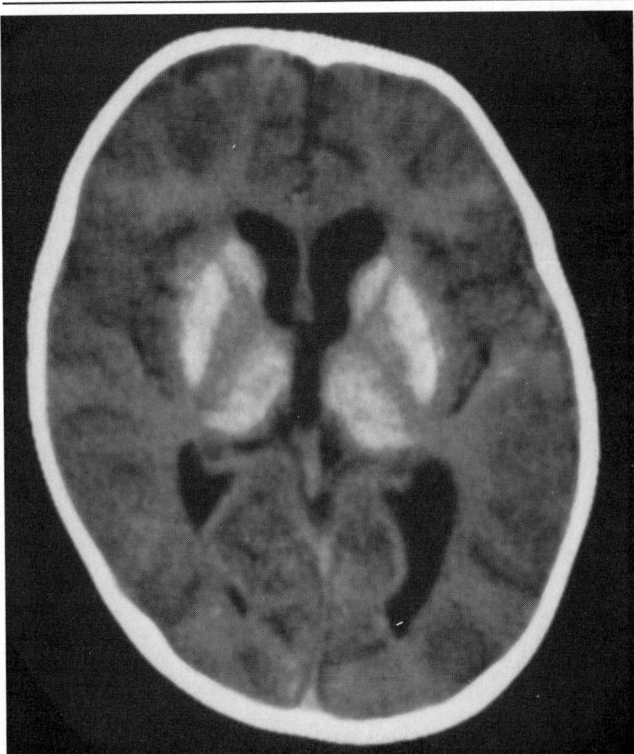

Figure 5.81. Status marmoratus on CT in a 6-month-old infant who was now comatose. CT axial demonstrates marked uniform hyperdensity in the caudate nuclei, lenticular nuclei, and thalami bilaterally, giving a marblelike appearance. The hyperintense sites may be due to diffuse calcium deposition or hemorrhage.

veins. Epidural hematomas are rare. Cephalohematomas occur on the outer surface of the bone and probably should be evacuated by drainage, when they are large, to prevent excessive local bone thickening later.

In partial asphyxia there is a tendency to preserve the circulation in the basal ganglia, the thalamus, and the brainstem during episodes of hypotension, but the hemispheric regions are hypoperfused and develop tissue damage. Occlusion of the internal carotid or the middle cererbral artery may occur at birth or in the perinatal period (Fig. 5.83). On the other hand, in severe asphyxia the complete circulatory arrest results in absent blood flow and oxygen in the entire brain. This leads to damage in the areas with highest metabolic requirements (e.g., the brainstem, thalami, basal ganglia, and corticospinal tracts, which are actively myelinating in the perinatal period). Frequently, however, the cerebral mantle shows the most severe changes, and the posterior fossa structures are the last to be affected (Fig. 5.84).

Cerebral Palsy

The hypoxic-ischemic encephalopathy of the newborn infant often results in the chronic handicapping conditions of cerebral palsy, mental retardation, learning disability, and epilepsy. Dietrich et al. described increased iron deposition, demonstrated on MRI T2-weighted and susceptibility-weighted images after ischemic-anoxic episodes in the basal ganglia, thalamus, and white matter (208).

The imaging findings in cerebral palsy can be particularly well seen on MRI (209,210). The findings vary with the pathologic etiologic factors, and include gyral anomalies, polymicrogyria suggestive of mid–second-trimester injury; isolated periventricular leukomalacia reflecting late second- or early third-trimester injury; and watershed cortical or deep gray nuclear damage consistent with late third-trimester, perinatal, or postnatal injury. Truwit et al. suggest that cerebral palsy in term infants is frequently the result of prenatal factors and less commonly related to the perinatal period (209).

Kernicterus

Kernicterus is a term applied to severe forms of icterus neomatorum. Elevation of serum unconjugated bilirubin is not usually harmful except in early infancy. At this stage of the postnatal period, bilirubin levels above 340 M mol/L(20mg/dl) may lead to kernicterus due to deposition of bilirubin in the putamen, pallidum, caudate nucleus, and substantia nigra. Survival is often followed by extrapyramidal movement disorders or by more severe cerebral palsy manifestations, sometimes with deafness and mental retardation. CT examination may be normal, but MRI may show hyperintensity in the basal ganglia, particularly the globus pallidus (see Fig. 5.73).

Cerebral Changes in Extracorporeal Membrane Oxygenation

Brunberg et al. reported on the changes in the brain in neonates with severe respiratory failure requiring extracorporeal membrane oxygenation, which they attribute to the required occlusion of the right jugular vein (212). The occlusion leads to increased venous pressure and results in subarachnoid space enlargement (21 of 31 neonates), particularly on the right side, hemorrhage (in 7 of 31), and regions of low brain attenuation in 11 of 31 infants.

There is a need to establish prognostic criteria to predict the future development and probable handicaps of the newborn child who has suffered a hypoxic-ischemic episode in the perinatal period. Clinical criteria are difficult to apply except for such severe indicators as an Apgar score of 3 prolonged. Westmark et al. in a preliminary report, have suggested that enhancement on MRI may be a possible indicator with prognostic significance (211). They found enhancement in the putamen or in the tegmentum of the midbrain in two infants followed by severe neurologic sequelae. Enhancement in the corticospinal tracts may also carry a relatively bad prognosis, whereas the absence of enhancement of any structure may carry a better prognosis. More experience is needed.

Spinal cord injury may occur secondary to excessive traction of the after-coming head during breech deliveries.

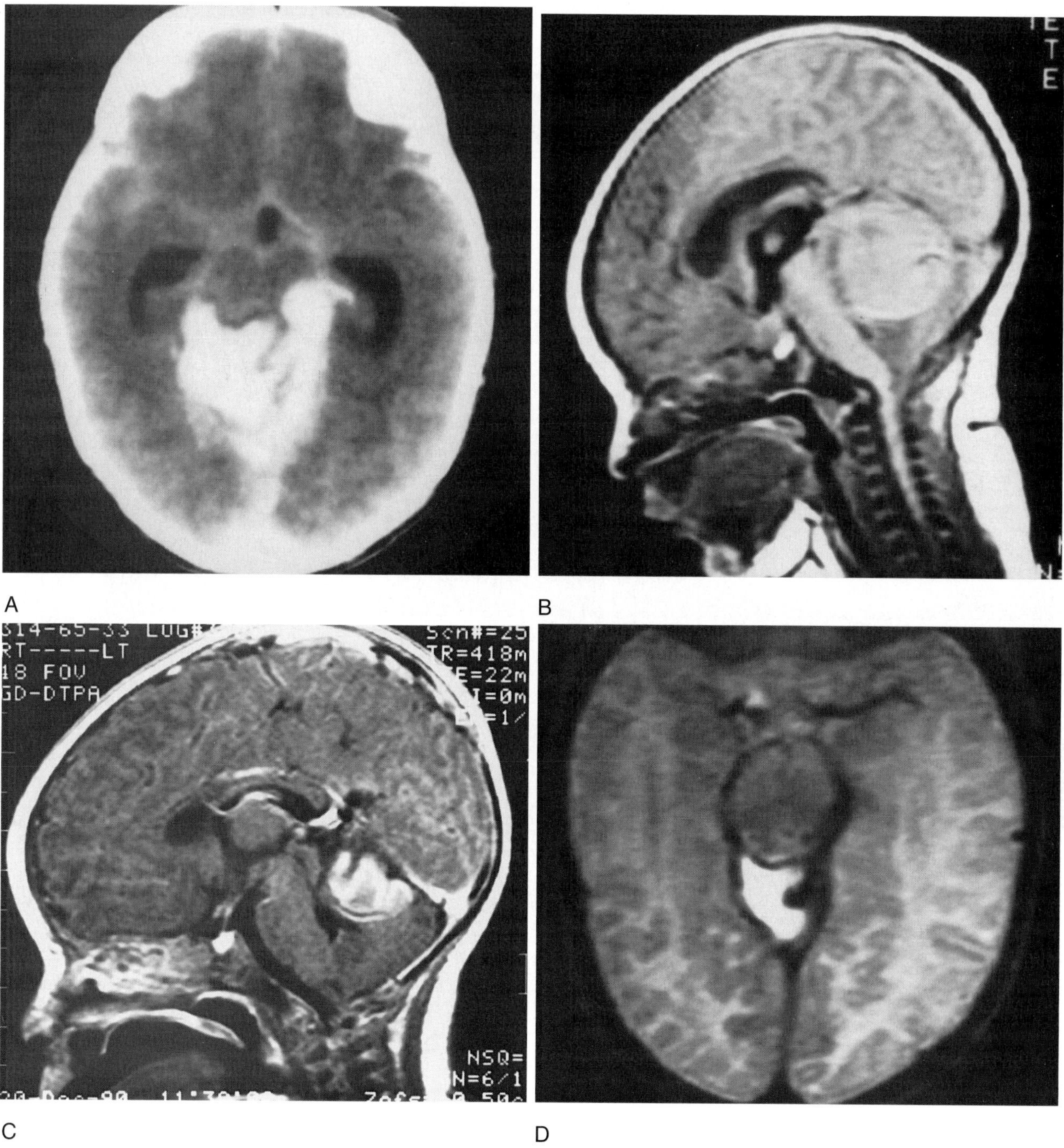

Figure 5.82. Subtentorial subdural collection in a 1-day-old term infant. **A.** CT axial shows a large peritentorial subdural hyperdensity. The infant rapidly developed hydrocephalus, which required a shunting procedure. Note large temporal horns. **B.** Sagittal T1-weighted image shows large subtentorial hyperintense area consistent with a hematoma in the methemoglobin stage. **C.** Sagittal T1-weighted image 6 weeks later shows considerable diminution in the size of the subtentorial hematoma. It is still hyperintense and shows surrounding susceptibility zone due to old blood products (**D**).

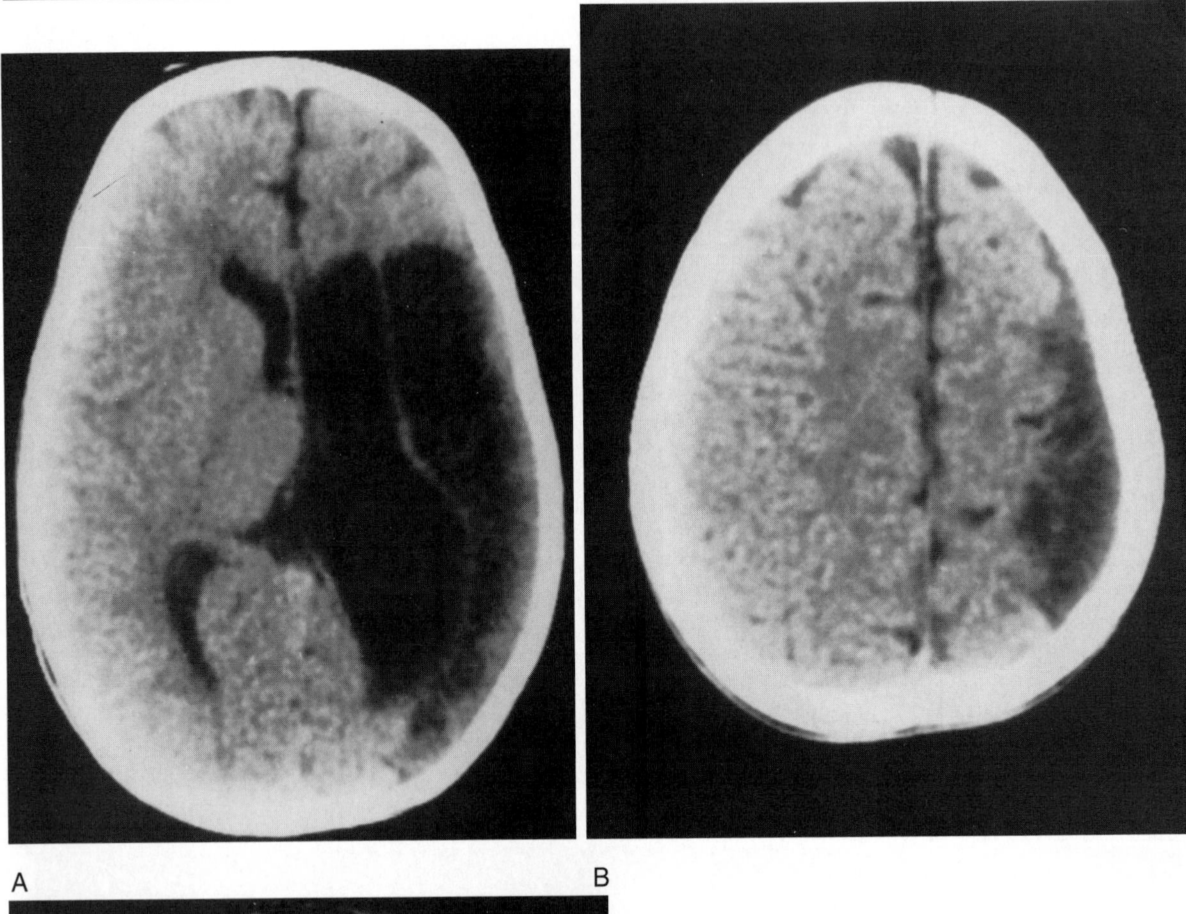

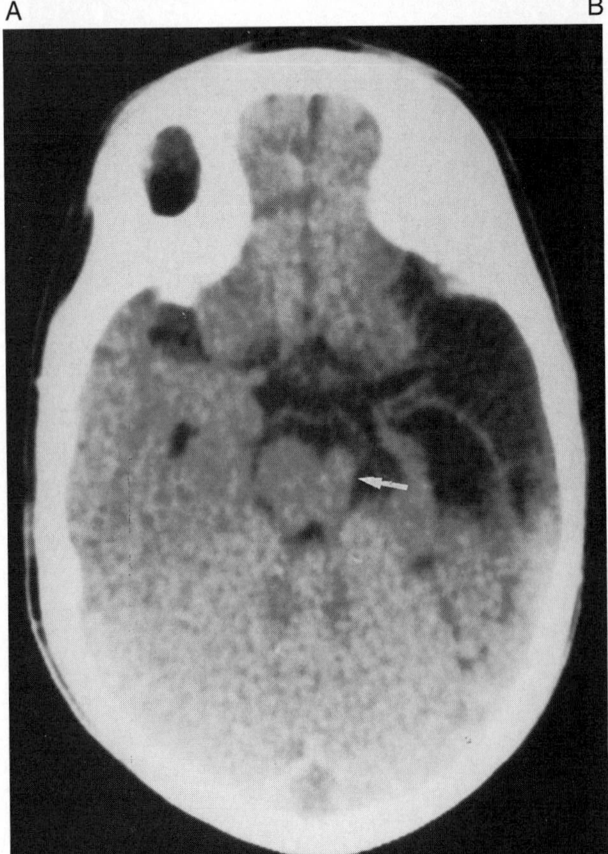

Figure 5.83. Vascular occlusion, probably occurring in utero, at birth, or in the perinatal period, producing large cerebral infarction in the middle cerebral artery territory. The hemiplegia was recognized at 3 months of age. This examination was done at 8 months. **A.** Large area of cerebral tissue loss and ventricular enlargement on left. **B.** A higher section shows the left cerebral hemiatrophy and the falx situated off center to the left. The left skull convexity is flatter than the right. **C.** A section passing through the brainstem reveals considerable decrease in size of the left side of the midbrain (arrow) due to wallerian degeneration. Because of the advanced degree of cerebral atrophy at 8 months of age with marked hemispheric hypoplasia, the child will develop what is usually called Dyke-Davidoff-Masson (DDM) syndrome (cerebral hemiatrophy with cranial hemihypertrophy).

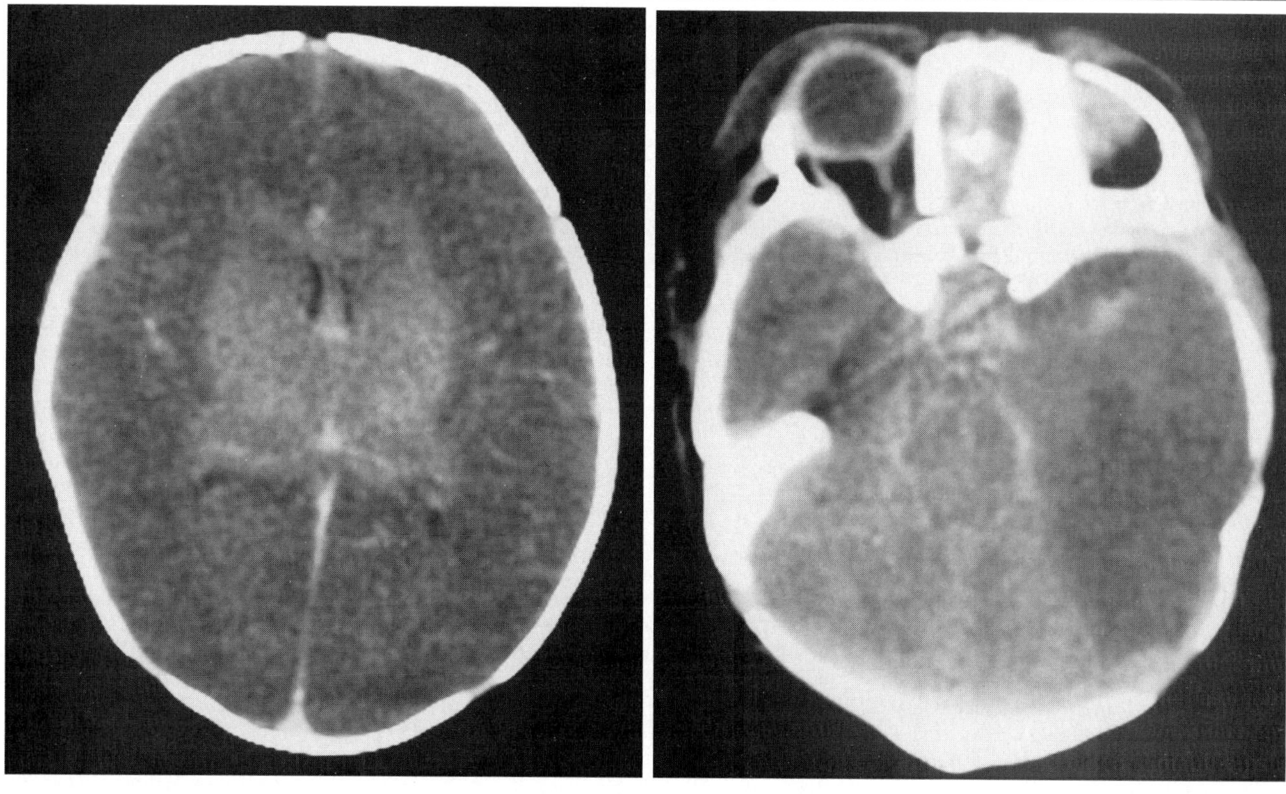

Figure 5.84. Profound asphyxia in a newborn infant. **A.** CT reveals diffuse hypointensity of the entire supratentorial structures except for the basal ganglia. This is indicative of almost total brain infarction. The ventricles are compressed due to edema. **B.** The brainstem and cerebellum have preserved normal density. The apparent difference between the two sides is caused by the tilting of the head.

REFERENCES

1. Fitz CR: Developmental abnormalities of the brain. In RN Rosenberg (ed), The Clinical Neurosciences: Neuroradiology, vol 4. New York: Churchill Livingstone, 1984, pp 215–246.
2. Laroche JC: The development of the central nervous system during intrauterine life. In F Falkner (ed), Human Development. Philadelphia: Saunders, 1966, pp 257–276.
3. Naidich TP, Grant JL, Altman N, et al: The developing cerebral surface: Preliminary report on the patterns of sulcal and gyral maturation—anatomy, ultrasound, and magnetic resonance imaging. Neuroimaging Clin North Am 1994;4:201–240.
4. Van der Knaap MS, Valk J: Classification of congenital abnormalities of the CNS. AJNR 1988;9:315–326.
5. Barkovich AJ, Kjos BO: Gray matter heterotopias: MR characteristics and correlation with developmental and neurologic manifestations. Radiology 1992;182:493–499.
6. Drayer B, Burger P, Darwin R, et al: Magnetic resonance imaging of brain iron. AJNR 1986;7:373–380.
7. Diezel PB: Iron in the brain: A chemical and histochemical examination. In Waelsch, H (ed), Biochemistry of the Developing Nervous System. New York: Academic Press, 1955, pp 145–152.
8. Volpe JJ: Neurology of the Newborn: Major Problems in Clinical Pediatrics, vol 22, ed 2. Philadelphia: Saunders, 1987.
9. Matson DD: Neurosurgery of Infancy and Childhood. Springfield, Ill: CC Thomas, 1969, pp 61–75.
10. Barkovich AJ, Vandermark P, Edwards MSB, et al: Congenital nasal masses: CT and MR imaging features in 16 cases. AJNR 1991; 12:105–116.
11. Braun M, Boman F, Hascoet JM, et al: Brain tissue heterotopia in the nasopharynx. J Neuroradiol 1992;19:68–74.
12. Weber FT, Donnelly WH, Bejar RL: Hypopituitarism following extirpation of a pharyngeal pituitary. Am J Dis Child 1977;131: 525–528.
13. Koehler PJ: Chiari's description of cerebellar ectopy (1891) with summary of Cleland's and Arnold's contributions and some early observations on neural-tube defects. J Neurosurg 1991;75: 823–826.
14. Barkovich AJ, Wippold FJ, Sherman JL, et al: Significance of cerebellar tonsilar position on MR. AJNR 1986;7:1009–1017.
15. Mikulis DJ, Diaz O, Egglin TK, Sanchez R, et al: Variance of the position of the cerebellar tonsils with age: Preliminary report. Radiology 1992;183:725–728.
16. Saez RJ, Onofrio BM, Yanagihara T: Experience with Arnold-Chiari malformation, 1960 to 1970. J Neurosurg 1976;45:416–422.
17. Naidich TP, Pudlowski RM, Naidich JB, et al: Computed tomographic signs of the Chiari II malformation: Part I. Skull and dural partitions. Radiology 1980;134:65–71.
18. Naidich TP, Pudlowski RM, Naidich JB, et al: Computed tomographic signs of the Chiari II malformation: Part II. Midbrain and cerebellum. Radiology 1980;134:391–398.
19. Naidich TP, Pudlowski RM, Naidich JB, et al: Computed tomographic signs of the Chiari II malformation: Part III. Ventricles and cisternum. Radiology 1980;134:657–663.
20. Naidich TP, Pudlowski RM, Naidich JB, et al: Computed tomographic signs of the Chiari II malformation: Part IV. The hindbrain deformity. Neuroradiology 1983;25:179–197.

21. Wolpert SM, Anderson M, Scott RM, et al: Chiari II malformation: MR imaging evaluation. AJNR 1987;8:783–792.
22. Kudryk BT, Coleman JM, Nurtagh FR, et al: MR imaging of an extreme case of cerebellar ectopia in a patient with Chiari II malformation. AJNR 1991;12:705–706.
23. Yamada H, Nakamura S, Tanaka Y, et al: Ventriculography and cisternography with water-soluble contrast media in infants with myelomeningoceles. Radiology 1982;143:75–83.
24. Truwit CL, Barkovich AJ, Shanahan R, Maroldo TV: MR imaging of rhombencephalosynapsis: Report of three cases and review of the literature. AJNR 1991;12:957–965.
25. De Morsier G: Etudes sur les dysraphies cranioencéphaliques: III. Agenesie du septum lucidum avec malformation due tractus optique: La dysplasie septo-optique. Schweiz Arch Neurol Psychiatr 1956;77:267–292.
26. Barkovich AJ, Fram EK, Norman D: Septo-optic dysplasia: MR imaging. Radiology 1989;171:189–192.
27. Barkovich AJ, Norman D: Absence of septum pellucidum: A useful sign in the diagnosis of congenital brain malformations. AJNR 1988;9:1107–1114.
28. Brocklehurst G, Chir M: Diencephalic cysts. J Neurosurg 1973; 38:47–51.
29. Hirsch JF, Pierre-Kahn A, Renier D, et al: The Dandy-Walker malformation: A review of 40 cases. J Neurosurg 1984;61:515–522.
30. Byrd SE, Bohan TP, Osborn RE, et al: The CT and MR evaluation of lissencephaly. AJNR 1988;9:923–927.
31. Rhodes RE, Hatten HP, Ellington KA: Walker-Warburg syndrome. AJNR 1992;13:123–126.
32. Norman RM: Malformations of the nervous system, birth injury and diseases of early life. In W Blackwood, WH McMenemy, DS Russell (eds), Greenfield's Neuropathology, ed 2. London: Edward Arnold Publishing, 1963, p 324.
33. Yakovlev PI, Wadsworth RC: Schizencephaly: A study of the congenital clefts in the cerebral mantle: I. Clefts with fused lips. J Neuropathol Exp Neurol 1946;5:116–130.
34. Yakovlev PI, Wadsworth RC: Schizencephaly: A study of the congenital clefts in the cerebral mantle: II. Clefts with hydrocephalus and lips separated. J Neuropathol Exp Neurol 1946;5:169–206.
35. Barkovich AJ, Chuang SH, Norman D: MR of neuronal migration anomalies. AJNR 1987;8:1009–1017.
36. Barkovich AJ, Kjos BO: Schizencephaly: Correlation of clinical findings with MR characteristics. AJNR 1992;13:85–94.
37. Barkovich AJ, Kjos BO: Nonlissencephalic cortical dysplasias: Correlation of imaging findings with clinical deficits. AJNR 1992;13: 95–103.
38. Bergeron RT: Pneumographic demonstration of subependymal heterotopic cortical gray matter in children. AJR 1967;101: 168–177.
39. Bergeron T: Radiographic demonstration of cortical heterotopia. Acta Radiol (Diagn) 1969;9:135–139.
40. Gallucci M, Bozzao A, Buratolo P, et al: MR imaging of incomplete band heterotopia. AJNR 1991;12:701–702.
41. Truwit CL, Barkovich AJ, Grumbach MM, et al: MR imaging of Kallmann syndrome, a genetic disorder of neuronal migration affecting the olfactory and genital systems. AJNR 1993;14: 827–838.
42. Yousem DM, Turner WJD, Li C, et al: Kallmann syndrome: MR evaluation of olfactory system. AJNR 1993;14:839–843.
43. Knorr JR, Ragland RL, Brown RS, et al: Kallmann syndrome: MR findings. AJNR 1993;14:845–851.
44. Bick DP, Ballabio A: Bringing Kallmann syndrome into focus. AJNR 1993;14:852–854.
45. Vogl TJ, Stemmler J, Heye B, et al: Kallman syndrome versus idiopathic hypogonadotropic hypogonadism at MR imaging. Radiology 1994;191:53–57.
46. Davidoff L, Dyke C: Agenesis of the corpus callosum, its diagnosis by encephalography: Report of three cases. AJR 1934;32:1–10.
47. Probst FR: Congenital defects of the corpus callosum: Morphology and encephalographic appearances. Acta Radiol (Diagn) Suppl 1973;331:1.
48. Igidbashian V, Mahboubi S, Zimmerman RA: CT and MR findings in Aicardi syndrome. J Comput Assist Tomogr 1987;11:357–358.
49. Barkovich AJ: Anomalies of the corpus callosum: Correlation with further anomalies of the brain. AJNR 1988;9:493–501.
50. Zettner A, Netsky M: Lipoma of the corpus callosum. J Neuropathol Exp Neurol 1960;10:305–319.
51. Dean B, Drayer BP, Beresini DC, et al: MR imaging of pericallosal lipoma. AJNR 1988;9:929–931.
52. Jinkins JR, Whittermore AR, Bradley WG: MR imaging of callosal and corticocallosal dysgenesis. AJNR 1989;10:339–344.
53. Friedman M, Cohen P: Agenesis of corpus callosum as a possible sequel to rubella during pregnancy. Am J Dis Child 1947;73:178.
54. Friedman RB, Segal R, Latchaw RE: Computerized tomographic and magnetic resonance imaging of intracranial lipoma. J Neurosurg 1986;65:407–410.
55. Loeser JD, Alvord EC: Clinicopathological correlations in agenesis of the corpus callosum. Neurology 1968;18:745.
56. Bertino RE, Nyberg DA, Cyr DR, et al: Prenatal diagnosis of agenesis of the corpus callosum. J Ultrasound Med 1988;7:251.
57. Truwit CL, Williams RG, Armstrong EA, et al: MR imaging of choroid plexus lipoma. AJNR 1990;11:202–204.
58. Larroche JC: Malformations of the nervous system. In JH Adams, JAN Corsellis, LA Duehen (eds), Greenfield's Neuropathology, ed 4. New York: Wiley, 1984.
59. Fletcher HM: A case of megalencephaly. Trans Pathol Soc London 1900;51:230.
60. Sotos J, Cutler E, Dodge P: Cerebral gigantism. Am J Dis Child 1977;131:625–627.
61. Sotos J, Dodge PR, Muirhead D, et al: Cerebral gigantism in childhood. N Engl J Med 1964;271:109–116.
62. DeMyer W: Classification of cerebral malformations. Birth Defects 1971;7:78–93.
63. Dekaban AS, Sakuragawa N: Megalencephaly. In PJ Vinken & GW Bruyn (eds), Handbook of Clinical Neurology, vol 30. Amsterdam: North-Holland, 1977, pp. 647–660.
64. Barkovich AJ, Chuang SH: Unilateral megalencephaly: Correlation of MR imaging and pathologic characteristics. AJNR 1990;11: 523–531.
65. Wolpert SM, Cohen A, Libenson MH: Hemimegalencephaly: a longitudinal MR study. AJNR 1994;15:1479–1482.
66. Castroviejo IP, Roche MC, Fernández VM, et al: Incontinentia pigmenti: MR demonstration of brain changes. AJNR 1994;15: 1521–1527.
67. Poser CM, Walsh IC, Scheinberg L: Hydranencephaly. Neurology 1955;5:284.
68. Harwood-Nash DC, Fitz CR: Neuroradiology in infants and children. St Louis: Mosby, 1976, vol 1, pp 71–169; vol 3, pp 998–1053.
69. Eicke WJ: Les Maladies inflammatoirs de l'encephale chez le foetus. In MM Heuyer, M Feld, & J Gruner (eds), Malformations congenitales du cerveau. Paris: Masson, 1959, p 81.
70. Rengachary SS, Watanabe I: Ultrastructure of pathogenesis of intracranial arachnoid cysts. J Neuropathol Exp Neurol 1982;40: 61–83.
71. Hald JK, Nakstad PH, Skjeldal OH, et al: Bilateral arachnoid cysts of the temporal fossa in four children with glutaric aciduria type I. AJNR 1991;12:407–409.
72. Robinson L, Dominguez R, Cabrera J, et al: Multiple meningeal cysts in Marfan syndrome. AJNR 1989;10:1275–1277.
73. Choi SK, Starshak RJ, Meyer GA, et al: Arachnoid cyst of the quadrigeminal plate cistem: Report of two cases. AJNR 1986;7: 725–728.
74. Robertson SJ, Wolpert SM, Runge VM: MR imaging of middle cranial fossa arachnoid cysts: Temporal lobe agenesis syndrome revisited. AJNR 1989;10:1007–1010.

75. Guidicelli G, Hassoun G, Choux M, et al: Supratentorial "arachnoid" cysts. J Neuroradiol 1982;9:179–201.
76. Wolpert SM, Scott RM: The value of metrizamide CT cisternography in the management of cerebral arachnoid cysts. AJNR 1981; 2:29–35.
77. Riccardi VM: Von Recklinghausen neurofibromatosis. N Engl J Med 1981;305:1617–1627.
78. Aoki S, Barkovich AJ, Nishimura K, et al: Neurofibromatosis types 1 and 2: Cranial MR findings. Radiology 1989;172:527–534.
79. National Institutes of Health Consensus Development: Neurofibromatosis. Arch Neurol 1988;45:575–578.
80. Mirowitz S, Sartor K, Gado M: High-intensity basal ganglia lesions on T1-weighted MR images in neurofibromatosis. AJNR 1989;10: 1159–1163.
81. Martuza RL, Eldridge R: Neurofibromatosis 2 (bilateral acoustic neurofibromatosis). N Engl J Med 1988;318:684–688.
82. Hurst RW, Newman SA, Cail WS: Multifocal intracranial MR abnormalities in neurofibromatosis. AJNR 1988;9:293–296.
83. Bognanno JR, Edwards MK, Lee TA, et al: Cranial MR imaging in neurofibromatosis. AJNR 1988;9:461–468.
84. Itoh T, Magnaldi S, White RM, et al: Neurofibromatosis Type 1: the evolution of deep gray and white matter MR abnormalities. AJNR 1994;15:1513–1519.
85. Egelhoff JC, Bates DJ, Ross JS: Spinal MR findings in neurofibromatosis type 1 and 2. AJNR 1992;13:1071–1077.
86. Elster AD: Radiologic screening in the neurocutaneous syndromes: Strategies and controversies. AJNR 1992;13:1078–1082.
87. Yakovlev PI, Guthrie RH: Congenital ectodermoses (neurocutaneous syndromes) in epileptic patients. Arch Neurol Psychiatry 1931;26:1145.
88. Poser CM, Taveras JM: Cerebral angiography in encephalotrigeminal angiomatosis. Radiology 1957;68:327–336.
89. Chamberlain MC, Press GA, Hesselink JR: MR imaging and CT in three cases of Sturge-Weber syndrome: Prospective comparison. AJNR 1989;10:491–496.
90. Elster AD, Chen MYM: MR imaging of Sturge-Weber syndrome: Role of gadopentetate dimeglumine and gradient-echo techniques. AJNR 1990;11:685–689.
91. Fitz C, Harwood-Nash D, Thompson SR: Neuroradiology of tuberous sclerosis in children. Radiology 1974;110:635–642.
92. Braffman B, Naidich TP: The phakomatoses: II. Von Hippel–Lindau disease, Sturge-Weber syndrome, and less common conditions. Neuroimaging Clin North Am 1994;4:325–348.
93. von Hippel EV: Uber eine sehr seltene Erkrankungen der Netzhaut. Graefes Arch Ophthalmol 1904;50:83.
94. Lindau A: Studien uber Kleinhirncysten: Bau, Pathogenese und Beziehungen zur Angiomatosis Retinae. Acta Pathol Microbiol Scand (Suppl 1), 93, 1926.
95. Bachmann K, Markwalder R, Seiler R: Supratentorial hemangioblastomas. Acta Neurochir 1978;44:173.
96. Louis-Bar D: Sur un syndrome progressif compremant des telangiectasies capillaires cutanies et conjonctivales symmitriques, a disposition naeroide, et des troubles cerebelleux. Confinia Neurologica 1941;4:32.
97. Sedgwick R, Boder E: Ataxia-telangiectasis. In P Vinken & G Bruyn (eds), Handbook of Clinical Neurology, vol 14. Amsterdam: North-Holland, 1972, 267.
98. Pont MS, Elster AD: Lesions of skin and brain: Modern imaging of the neurocutaneous syndromes. AJR 1992;158:1193–1203.
99. Gorlin RJ, Vickers RA, Kellen F, et al: The multiple basal-cell nevi syndrome: An analysis of a syndrome consisting of multiple nevoid basal-cell anomalies, medulloblastoma, hyporesponsiveness to parathormone. Cancer 1965:18:89.
100. Waybright EA, Sellhorst JB, Rosenbum VI, et al: Blue-rubber, bleb-nevus syndrome with CNS involvement and thrombosis of a vein of Galen aneurysm. Ann Neurol 1978;3:464.
101. Phillips GN, Gordon DH, Martin EC, et al: The Klippel-Trenaunay syndrome: Clinical and radiological aspects. Radiology 1978; 128:429–434.
102. Williams DW III, Elster AD: Cranial CT and MR in the Klippel-Trenauny-Weber syndrome. AJNR 1992;13:291–294.
103. Parkes-Weber F: Angioma formation in connection with hypertrophy of limas and hemihypertrophy. Br J Dermatol Syph 1907;19: 231.
104. Lloyd KM, Dennis M: Cowden's disease: A possible new symptom complex with multiple system involvement. Ann Intern Med 1963; 58:136–142.
105. Williams DW III, Elster AD, Ginsberg LE, et al: Recurrent Lhermitte-Duclos disease: Report of two cases and association with Cowden's disease. AJNR 1992;13:287–290.
106. Williams DW III, Elster AD: Cranial MR imaging in hypomelanosis of Ito. J Comp Assist Tomogr 1990;14:981–983.
107. Rhodes RE, Friedman HS, Hatten HP, et al: Contrast enhanced MR imaging of neurocutaneous melanosis. AJNR 1991;12:380.
108. Sebag G, Dubois J, Pfister P, et al: Neurocutaneous melanosis and temporal lobe tumor in a child: MR study. AJNR 1991;12:699–700.
109. Meyers SP, Hirsch WL Jr, Curtin HD, et al: Chondrosarcoma of the skull base: MR imaging features. Radiology 1992;184:103–108.
110. Clifton AG, Kendall BE: Intracranial chondrosarcoma in a patient with Ollier's disease. Br J Radial 1991;64:633.
111. Yoshioka M, Saiwai S, Kuroki S, Nigami H: MR imaging of the brain in Fukuyama-type congenital muscular dystrophy. AJNR 1991;12:63–65.
112. Johnson MA, Pennock JM, Bydder GM, et al: Clinical NMR imaging of the brain in children: Normal and neurologic disease. AJNR 1983;4:1013–1026.
113. Uggetti C, Sibilla L, Zappoli F, Martelli A: La risonanza magnetica dell'encefalo nella distrofia miotonica. Riv Neuroradiol 1991;4: 53–60.
114. Huber SJ, Kissel JT, et al: Magnetic resonance imaging and clinical correlates of intellectual impairment in myotonic dystrophy. Arch Neurol 1989;46:536–540.
115. Tzika AA, Ball WS, Vigneron DB, et al: Clinical proton MR spectroscopy of neurodegenerative disease in childhood. AJNR 1993; 14:1267–1281.
116. Tzika AA, Ball WS, Vigneron DB, et al: Childhood adrenal leukodystrophy: Assessment with proton MR spectroscopy. Radiology 1993;189:467–480.
117. Barrett D, Becker LE: Alexander's disease: A disease of astrocytes. Brain 1985;108:367–385.
118. Shah M, Ross JS: Infantile Alexander disease: MR appearance of a biopsy-proved case. AJNR 1990;11:1105–1106.
119. Schuster V, Horwitz AE, Kretz HW: Alexander disease: Cranial MRI and ultrasound findings. Pediatr Radil 1991;21:133.
120. Trommer BL, Naidich TD, Mauro CDC, et al: Noninvasive CT diagnosis of infantile Alexander's disease: Pathologic correlation. J Comput Assist Tomogr 1983;7:509–516.
121. Farrell K, Chuang S, Becker L: Computed tomography in Alexander's disease. Ann Neurol 1984;15:605–607.
122. Valk J, van der Knapp MS: Magnetic Resonance of Myelin, Myelination, and Myelin Disorders. Berlin: Springer-Verlag, 1989.
123. Grodd N, Krägeloh-Mann I, Klose U, et al: Metabolic and destructive brain disorders in children: Findings with localized proton MR spectroscopy. Radiology 1991;181:173–181.
124. Matalon R, Michals K, Sebesta D, et al: Aspartoacyclase deficiency and N-acetylaspartic aciduria in patients with Canavan disease. Am J Med Genet 1988;29:463–471.
125. Brismar J, Brismar G, Gascon G, et al: Canavan disease: CT and MR imaging of the brain. AJNR 1990;11:805–810.
126. André M, Monin P, Moret C, et al: Pelizaeus-Merzbacher disease: Contribution of magnetic resonance imaging to an early diagnosis. J Neuroradiol 1990;17:216–221.

127. Van der Knaap MS, Valk J: The reflection of histology in MR imaging of Pelizaeus-Merzbacher disease. AJNR 1989;10:99–103.
128. Fishman MA: Disorders primarily of white matter. In KF Swaiman (ed), Pediatric Neurology, ed 2. St Louis: Mosby, 1989, p 669.
129. Aubourg P, Blanche S, Jambaqué I, et al: Reversal of early neurologic and neuroradiologic manifestations of X-linked adrenoleukodystrophy by bone marrow transplantation. N Engl J Med 1990; 322:1860–1866.
130. Romero C, Dietemann JL, Kurtz D, et al: Adrenoleukodystrophy: Value of contrast-enhanced MR imaging. J Neuroradiol 1990;17: 267–276.
131. Loes DJ, Hite S, Moser H, et al: Adrenoleukodystrophy: a scoring method for brain MR observations. AJNR 1994;15:1761–1766.
132. Loes DJ, Stillman AE, Hite S, et al: Childhood cerebral form of adrenoleukodystrophy: short-term effect of bone marrow transplantation on brain MR observations. AJNR 1994;15:1767–1771.
133. Kendall BE: Disorder of lysosomes, peroxysomes, and mitochondria. AJNR 1992;13:621–653.
134. Dubois J, Sebag G, Agyroboulow M, et al: MR findings in infantile Refsum disease: Case report of two family members. AJNR 1991; 12:1159–1160.
135. Naidu SB, Moser H: Infantile Refsum disease. AJNR 1991;12: 1161–1163.
136. Van der Knaap MS, Valk J: MR of adrenoleukodystrophy: Histopathologic correlations. AJNR 1989;10:S12–S14.
137. Williams DW III, Elster AD, Cox TD: Cranial MR imaging in rhizomelic chondrodysplasia punctata. AJNR 1991;12:363–365.
138. Swaiman KF: Lysosomal diseases. In KF Swaiman (ed),Pediatric Neurology, ed 2. St Louis: Mosby, 1989, p 1017.
139. Wolpert SM, Barnes PD: MRI in Pediatric Neuroradiology. St Louis: Mosby–Year Book, 1992.
140. Kwan E, Drace J, Enzman D: Specific CT findings in Krabbe disease. AJNR 1984;5:453–458.
141. Banam TZ, Goldman AM, Percy HK: Krabbe's disease: Specific MRI and CT findings. Neurology 1986;36:111.
142. Finelli DA, Tarr RW, Sawyer RN, et al: Deceptively normal MR in early infantile Krabbe disease. AJNR 1994;15:167–171.
143. Brismar J, Aqeel A, Brismar G, et al: Maple syrup urine disease: Findings on CT and MR scans of the brain in 10 infants. AJNR 1990;11:1219–1228.
144. Pearsen KD, Gean-Marton AD, Levy HL, et al: Phenylketonuria: MR imaging of the brain with clinical correlation. Radiology 1990; 177:437–440.
145. Shaw DWW, Maravilla KR, Weinberger E, et al: MR imaging of phenylketonuria. AJNR 1991;12:403–406.
146. Brismar J, Aqeel A, Gascon G, et al: Malignant hyperphenylalaninemia: CT and MR of the brain. AJNR 1990;11:135–138.
147. Sugita R, Takahashi S, Ishii K, et al: Brain CT and MR findings in hyperphenylalaninemia due to dihydropteridine reductase deficiency (variant of phenylketonuria). J Comp Assist Tomogr 1990; 14:699–703.
148. Press GA, Barshop BA, Haas RH, et al: Abnormalities of the brain in nonketotic hyperglycinemia: MR manifestations. AJNR 1989; 10:315–321.
149. Heindel W, Kugel H, Roth B: Non-invasive detection of increased glycine content by proton MR spectroscopy in the brains of two infants with nonketotic hyperglycinemia. AJNR 1993;14:629–635.
150. Schwab FJ, Peyster RG, Brill CB: CT of cerebral venous thrombosis in a child with homocystinuria. Pediatr Radiol 1987;17:244.
151. Lowe CW, Terry M, MacLachlan EA: Organoaciduria, decreased renal ammonia production, hydrophthalmos, and mental retardation: A clinical entity. Am J Dis Child 1952;83:164.
152. O'Tuama LA, Laster DW: Oculocerebrorenal syndrome: Case report with CT and MR correlates. AJNR 1987;8:555–557.
153. Bergman I, Finegold D, Gartner JC Jr, et al: Acute profound dystonia in infants with glutaric acidemia. Pediatrics 1989;83:228–234.
154. Naidu SB, Moser HW: Value of neuroimaging in metabolic diseases affecting the CNS. AJNR 1991;12:413–416.
155. Blaser SI, Clarke JT, Becker LE: Neuroradiology of lysosomal disorders. Neuroimaging Clin North Am 1994;4:283–298.
156. Moumdjian R, Tampieri D, Melanson D, et al: Anderson-Fabri disease: A case report with MR, CT and cerebral angiography. AJNR 1989;10:569–570.
157. Brismar J, Brismar G, Coates R, et al: Increased density of the thalamus on CT scans in patients with GM2 gangliosidosis. AJNR 1990;11:125–130.
158. Stalker HP, Han BK: Thalamic hyperdensity: A previously unreported sign of Sandhoff disease. AJNR 1989;10:S82.
159. Brill PW, Beratis NG, Kousseff BG, et al: Roentgenographic findings in fucosidosis type 2. AJR 1975;124:75–82.
160. Kessler RM, Altman DH, Martin-Jimenez R: Cranial CT in fucosidosis. AJNR 1981;2:591–592.
161. Sandu FS, Dillon WP: MR demonstration of leukoencephalopathy: Case report. AJNR 1991;12:375.
162. DiMauro S, Servidei S, Zeriami M, et al: Cytochrome C oxidase deficiency in Leigh syndrome. Ann Neurol 1987;22:498–506.
163. Medina L, Chi TL, De Vivo DC, et al: MR findings in patients with subacute necrotizing encephalomyelopathy (Leigh syndrome). AJNR 1990;11:379–384.
164. Faerber EN, Grover EN, De Filipp GJ, et al: Cerebral MR of Menkes kinky-hair disease. AJNR 1989;10:190–192.
165. Wesenberg RL, Gwinn JL, Barnes GR Jr: Radiological findings in the kinky hair syndrome. Radiology 1969;92:500–506.
166. Kearns TP, Sayre GP: Retinitis pigmentosa, external ophthalmoplegia, and complete heart block: Unusual syndrome with histologic study in one of two cases. Arch Ophthalmol 1958;60:280–289.
167. Demange P, Pham Gia H, Kalifa G, et al: MR of Kearns-Sayre syndrome. AJNR 1989;10:591.
168. Seigel RS, Seeger JF, Gabrielsen TP, et al: Computed tomography in oculocraniosomatic disease (Kearns-Sayre syndrome). Radiology 1979;130:159–164.
169. Allard JC, Tilak S, Carter AP: CT and MR of MELAS syndrome. AJNR 1988;9:1234–1238.
170. Bertorini T, Engel WK, DiChiro G, et al: Leukoencephalopathy in oculocraniosomatic neuromuscular disease with ragged red fibers. Arch Neurol 1978;35:643–647.
171. De Volder A, Ghilain S, de Barsy TH, et al: Brain metabolism in mitochondrial encephalomyopathy: A PET study. J Comput Assist Tomogr 1988;12:854–857.
172. Peynet J, Laurent A, De Liege P, et al: Cerebrotendinous xanthomatosis: Treatment with simvastatin, lovastatin, and chenodeoxycholic acid in 3 siblings. Neurology 1991;41:434–436.
173. Dotti MT, Federico A, Signorini E, et al: Cerebrotentinaus xanthomatosis (von Bogaert-Scherer-Epstein disease): CT and MR findings. AJNR 1994;15:1721–1726.
174. Seidenwurm D, Novotny E Jr, Marshall W, et al: MR and CT in cytoplasmically inherited striatal degeneration. AJNR 1986;7: 629–632.
175. Gordon K, Riding M, Camfield P, et al: CT and MR of 3-hydroxy-3-methylglutaryl-coenzyme A lyase deficiency. AJNR 1994;15: 1474–1476.
176. Swick HM: Diseases of gray matter. In KF Swaiman (ed), Pediatric Neurology, ed 2. St Louis: Mosby, 1989, p 777.
177. Valavanis A, Friede RL, Schubiger O, et al: Computed tomography in neuronal ceroid lipofuscinosis. Neuroradiology 1980;19:35–38.
178. Vanhanen S-L, Raininko R, Santavuori P: Early differential diagnosis of infantile neuronal ceroid lipofuscinosis, Rett syndrome, and Krabbe disease by CT and MR. AJNR 1994;15:1443–1453.
179. Hagberg B, Aicardi J, Dias K, et al: A progressive syndrome of autism, dementia, ataxia, and loss of purpose hand use in girls: Rett's syndrome—report of 35 cases. Ann Neurol 1983;14:471.
180. Williams KD, Drayer BP, Johnsen SD, et al: MR imaging of leukoencephalopathy associated with Navajo neuropathy. AJNR 1990; 11:400–402.

181. Brismar J, Harfi HA, Partial albinism with immunodeficiency: A rare syndrome with prominent posterior fossa white matter changes. AJNR 1992;13:387–393.

182. Blume RS, Wolff SM: The Chédiak-Higashi syndrome: Studies in four patients and a review of the literature. Medicine 1972;51: 247–280.

183. Lerner EJ, Bilaniuk LT: Brutton-type (congenital X-limbed) agammaglobulinemia: MR imaging of unusual intracranial complications. AJNR 1992;13:976–980.

184. Kuzniecky R, Andermann F, and the CBPS group: The congenital bilateral perisylvian syndrome: Imaging findings in a multicenter study. AJNR 1994;15:139–144.

185. Aisen AM, Martel W, Gabrielsen TO, et al: Wilson disease of the brain: MR imaging. Radiology 1985;157:137–141.

186. Imiya M, Ichikawa K, Matsushima H, et al: MR of the base of the pons in Wilson disease. AJNR 1992;13:1009–1012.

187. Williams JB, Walshe JM: Wilson's disease: An analysis of the cranial computerized tomographic appearances found in 60 patients and the changes in response to treatment with chelating agents. Brain 1981;104:735–752.

188. Kuhl DE, Phelps ME, Markham CH, et al: Cerebral metabolism and atrophy in Huntington's disease determined by 18FDG and computed tomographic scan. Ann Neurol 1982;12:425.

189. MacDonald M: Novel cell containing trineucleotide repeat that is expanded and unstable on Huntington's disease chromosomes. Cell 1993;72:971–983.

190. Demirci A, Sze Y: Cranial osteopetrosis: MR findings. AJNR 1991; 12:781–782.

191. Sly WS, Whyte MP, Sundaram V, et al: Carbonic anhydrase II deficiency in 12 families with the autosomal recessive syndrome of osteopetrosis with renal tubular acidosis and cerebral calcification. N Engl J Med 1985;313:139–145.

192. Scotti G, Scialfa G, Tampieri D, et al: MR imaging in Fahr disease. J Comput Assist Tomogr 1985;9:790–792.

193. Menkes JH (ed): Textbook of Child Neurology. Philadelphia: Lea and Febiger, 1985.

194. Littrup PJ, Gebarski SS: MR imaging of Hallervorden-Spatz disease. J Comput Assist Tomogr 1985;9:491–493.

195. Mutoh K, Okuno T, Masatoshi I, et al: MR imaging of a group I case of Hallervorden-Spatz disease. J Comput Assist Tomogr 1988; 12:851–853.

196. Ambrosetto P, Nonni R, Bacei A, et al: Late onset familial Hallesvordem-Spartz disease: MR findings in two sisters. AJNR 1992; 13:394–396.

197. Gebarski SS, Gabrielsen TO, Knake J, et al: Cerebral CT findings in methylmalonic and propionic acidemias. AJNR 1983;4:955–957.

198. Andreula CF, De Blasi R, Carella A: CT and MR studies in methylmalonic acidemia. AJNR 1991;12:410–412.

199. Colabucci F, Rossodivita A, Parigi A, Colavita N: A clinical and radiological study of two brothers affected by Cockayne's syndrome type II. Diagn Radiol 1987;12:57–63.

200. Boltshauser E, Yaleinkaya C, Wichman W, et al: MRI of Cockayne's syndrome type I. Neuroradiology 1989;31:276.

201. Demaerel P, Wilms G, Verdru P, et al: MRI in the diagnosis of Cockayne's syndrome. J Neuroradiol 1990;17:157–160.

202. Araki T, Ohba H, Monzawa S, et al: Membranous lipodystrophy: MR imaging appearance of the brain. Radiology 1991;180: 793–797.

203. Kuharik MA, Farlow MR, Edwards MK, et al: MR imaging of Gerstmann-Straussler-Scheinker disease: Another cause of increased brain iron. AJNR 1988;9:1042.

204. Barkovich AJ, Truwit CL: Brain damage from perinatal asphyxia: Correlation of MR findings with gestational age. AJNR 1990;11: 1087–1096.

205. Flodmark O, Lupton B, Li D, et al: MR imaging of periventricular leukomalacia in childhood. AJNR 1989;10:111–118.

206. Kenney S, Adcock E, McArdle C: Prospective observations of 100 high-risk neonates by high field (1.5 Tesla) magnetic resonance imaging of the central nervous system: II. Lesions associated with hypoxic-ischemic encephalopathy. Pediatrics 1991;87:431–438.

207. Rorke LB, Zimmerman RA: Prematurity, postmaturity, and destructive lesions in utero. AJNR 1992;13:517–536.

208. Dietrich RB, Bradley WG Jr: Iron accumulation in the basal ganglia following severe ischemic-anoxia insults in children. Radiology 1988;168:203–206.

209. Truwit CL, Barkovich AJ, Koch TK, et al: Cerebral palsy: MR findings in 40 patients. AJNR 1992;13:67–78.

210. Volpe JJ: Value of MR in definition of the neuropathology of cerebral palsy in vivo. AJNR 1992;13:79–83.

211. Westmark KD, Barkovich AJ, Roberts TPL, et al: Patterns of MR imaging contrast enhancement in the brains of asphyxiated neonates. Paper presented at the meeting of the American Society of Neuroradiology, Nashville, Tennessee, 1994.

212. Brunberg JA, Kewitz G, Schumacher RE: Venovenous extracorporeal membrane oxygenation: Early CT alterations following use in management of severe respiratory failure in neonates. AJNR 1993; 14:595–603.

SELECTED READINGS

Adair L, Ropper A, Davis K: Cerebellar hemangioblastoma: CT, angiographic and clinical findings in seven patients. J Comput Assist Tomogr 1978;2:281–294.

Aida N, Yagishita A, Takada K, et al: Cerebellar MR in Fukuyama congenital muscular dystrophy: polymicrogyria with cystic lesions. AJNR 1994; 15:1755–1759.

Alsen AM, Martel W, Gabrielsen TO, et al: Wilson disease of the brain: MR imaging. Radiology 1985;157:137–141.

Baker LL, Stevenson DK, Enzmann DR: End-stage periventricular leukomalacia: MR evaluation. Radiology 1988;168:809–815.

Barkovich AJ, Westmark K, Partridge C, et al: Perinatal asphyxia: MR findings in the first 10 days. AJNR 1995;16:427–438.

Braun M, Boman F, Hascoet JM, et al: Brain tissue heterotopia in the nasopharynx. J Neuroradiol 1992;19:68–74.

Brown EW, Riccardi VM, Mawad M, et al: MR imaging of optic pathways in patients with neurofibromatosis. AJNR 1986;8:1031–1036.

Brunberg JA, Kanal E, Hirsch W, et al: Chronic acquired hepatic failure: MR imaging of the brain at 1.5 T. AJNR 1991;12:909–914.

Cockayne EA: Dwarfism with retinal atrophy and deafness. Arch Dis Child 1940;8:771.

Cohen MD, Edwards MK: Magnetic Resonance Imaging of Children. Toronto: Decker, 1990, p 312.

DeMyer W: Megalencephaly in children: Clinical syndromes, genetic patterns, and differential diagnosis from other causes of megalencephaly. Neurology 1972;22:634.

Donovan-Post J, et al: Asymptomatic and neurologically symptomatic HIV-seropositive individuals. Prospective evaluation with cranial MR imaging. Radiology 1991;178:131–139.

Harrington MG, MacPherson P, McIntosh WB, et al: The significance of the incidental finding of basal ganglia calcification on computed tomography. J Neurol Neurosurg Psychiatry 1981;44:1168.

Hashimoto T, et al: Abulsion of birth palsy. Radiology 1991;178:841–845.

Herskowitz J, Rasman ND, Wheeler CB: Colpocephaly: Clinical, radiologic and pathologic aspects. Neurology 1985;35:1594–1598.

Hilbert PL, Kurtz AB: Prenatal diagnosis of agenesis of the corpus callosum using endovaginal ultrasound. J Ultrasound Med 1990;9:363.

Jeffrey PJ, Monsein LH, et al: Mapping the distribution of amobarbital sodium in the intracarotid Wada test by use of Tc-99m HMPAO with SPECT. Radiology 1991;178:847–850.

Johnson MA, Desai S, Hugh-Jones K, et al: Magnetic resonance imaging of the brain in Hurler syndrome. AJNR 1984;5:816–819.

Kahn MI, et al: Volume of CSF. Radiology 1991;128:115–122.

Kingsley DPE, Kendall BE: Demyelinating and neuro-degenerative disease in childhood. J Neuroradiol 1981;8:243–255.

Kostelic JK, et al: Lumbar spinal nerves. Radiology 1991;178:837–839.

Kvicala V, Vymazol J, Nevsimalov A: Computed tomography of Wilson disease. AJNR 1983;4:429–430.

McArdle CB, Richardson CJ, Nicholas DA, et al: Developmental features on MR imaging: I. Gray-white matter differentiation and myelination. Radiology 1987;162:223–229.

McMurdo S, Moore S, Brandt-Zawadzki M, et al: MR imaging of intracranial tuberous sclerosis. AJNR 1987;8:77–82.

Moossy J: The neuropathology of Cockayne's syndrome. J Neuropathol Exp Neurol 1967;26:654.

Murata R, Nakajima S, Tanaka A, et al: MR imaging of the brain in patients with mucopolysaccharidosis. AJNR 1989;10:1165–1170.

Osborn RE, Byrd SE, Naidich TP, et al: MR imaging of neuronal migration disorders. AJNR 1988;9:1101–1106.

Pavlakis SG, Phillips PC, Di Mauro S, et al: Mitochondrial myopathy, encephalopathy, lactic acidosis, and strokelike episodes: A distinctive clinical syndrome. Ann Neurol 1984;16:481–488.

Peterson PL, Manteus ME, Lee CP: Mitochondrial encephalomyopathies. Neurol Clin 1988;6:529–544.

Pomerang SJ, Shelton JJ, Tobias J, et al: MR of visual pathways in patients with neurofibromatosis. AJNR 1987;8:831–836.

Rauch RA, Friloux LA III, Lott IT: MR imaging of cavitary lesions in the brain with Hurler/Scheie. AJNR 1989;10:51–53.

Rusenek H, et al: Alzheimer's disease. Radiology 1991;178:123–130.

Quinn N: Multiple system atrophy: The nature of the beast. J Neurol Neurosurg Psychiatry 1990;53:93–95.

Seeger JF, Burke DP, Knake JE, et al: CT and angiographic evaluation of hemangioblastoma. Radiology 1981;138:65–73.

Selekler K, Kansu T, Zileli T: Computed tomography in Wilson's disease. Arch Neurol 1981;38:727–728.

Sutton D: Radiological diagnosis of lipoma of corpus callosum. Br J Radiol 1949;22:534.

Swick HM: Disease of gray matter. In KF Swaiman (ed), Pediatric Neurology. St Louis: Mosby, 1989.

Taccone A, Di Rocco M, Fondelli P, Cottafava F: Leigh disease: Value of CT in presymptomatic patients and variability of the lesions with time. J Comput Assist Tomogr 1989;13:207–210.

Wasenko JJ, Rosenbloom SA, Duchesneau CF, et al: The Sturge-Weber syndrome: Comparison of MR and CT characteristics. AJNR 1990;11:131–134.

Wokwill F, Yakovlev P: Histopathology of meningofascial angiomatosis (Sturge-Weber disease): Report of four cases. J Neuropathol Exp Neurol 1957;16:341.

Wolpert SM, Anderson ML, Kaye EM: Metabolic and degenerative disorders. In SM Wolpert & PD Barnes (eds), MRI in Pediatric Neuroradiology. St Louis: Mosby–Year Book, 1992, pp 121 et seq.

Yakovlev PL: Pathoarchitectonic studies of cerebral malformations: III. Arrhinencephalies (holotelencephalies). J Neuropathol Exp Neurol 1959;18:22.

6

Inflammatory Diseases

Two to three decades ago it was felt that with the advent of antibiotics and the discovery of new, more effective antibiotics, infections of the central nervous system were going to decrease in incidence. Instead, there has been an impressive increase in the number of patients with infections that affect the nervous system, including the brain, spinal cord, and meninges. This increase is the result of two factors, the most important of which is the spread of acquired immunodeficiency syndrome (AIDS). As is well known, infections of various types affecting particularly the brain and its coverings are common in patients affected by the human immunodeficiency virus (HIV). In addition, as time goes on, bacteria and viruses constantly develop mutations that are usually or often more resistant to antibiotic therapy than the original strains. The chapter discusses viral, bacterial, fungal, and parasitic infections that affect the nervous system.

VIRAL INFECTIONS

Viruses represent an increasingly important chapter in the infectious diseases of humans. Their peculiar properties are different from those of other organisms that produce infectious diseases: they are very small (20 to 300 nm) and contain only one type of nucleic acid, DNA or RNA. Also, most importantly, they present no metabolic activity of their own unless they are inside a host cell.

With the exception of herpes simplex encephalitis, viral infections of all types tend to produce few pathological changes in the appearance of the brain on gross inspec-

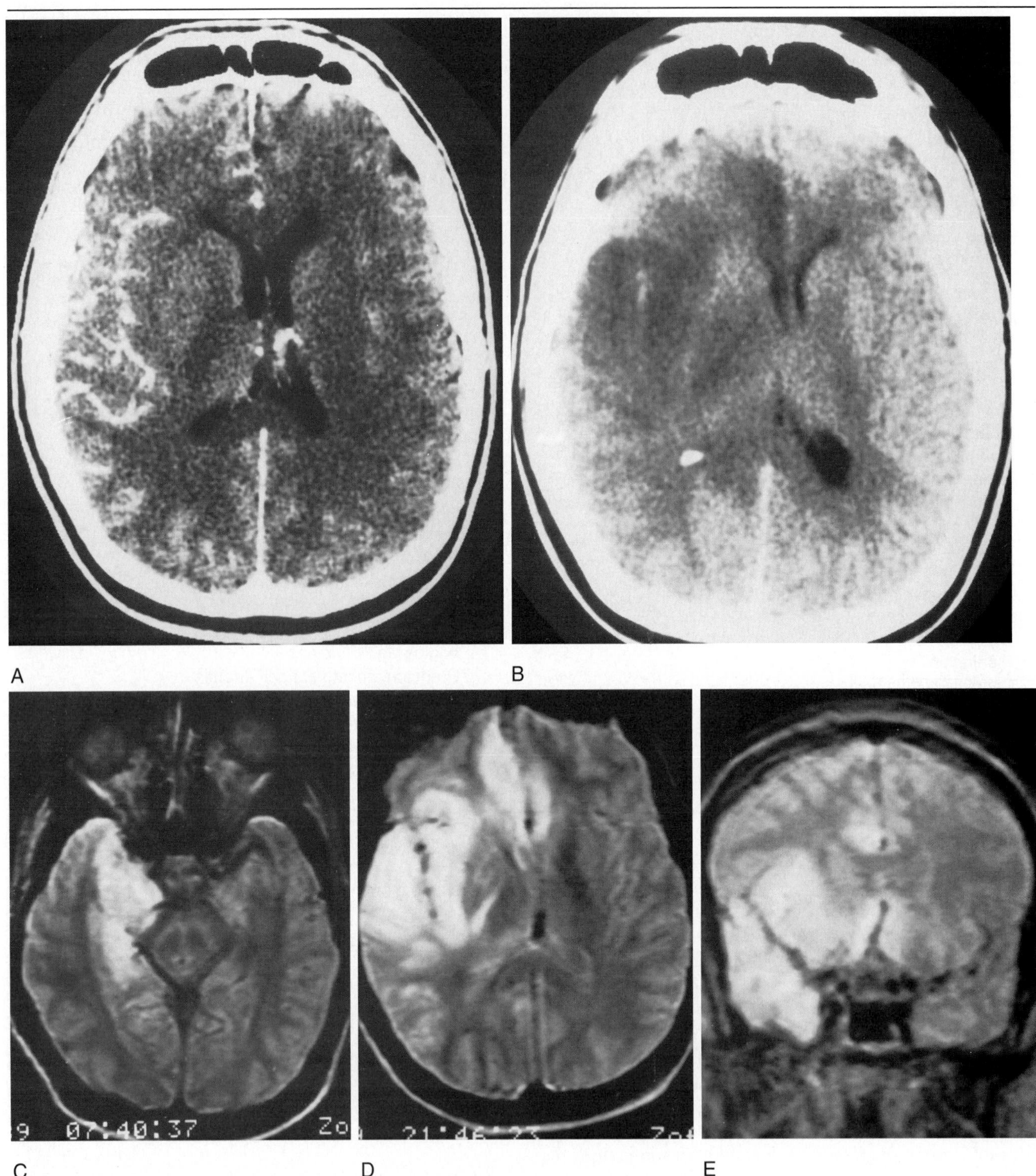

Figure 6.1. Herpes simplex encephalitis. **A.** Axial CT image after contrast shows irregular enhancement on the surface of the insula and sylvian fissure area on the right side. **B.** Examination without contrast 4 days later shows much extension of the changes; adjacent portions of the temporal and frontal lobes are now involved. **C.** Initial MRI examination reveals marked hyperintensity in the medial right temporal lobe on proton density image. **D.** Reexamination 6 days later discloses a marked increase in the edema, which now involves the temporal lobe, the frontal lobe and insula, and the medial aspect of the anterior frontal lobes on the right, but with evident involvement of the medial left frontal lobe as well. **E.** A coronal section confirms the areas of involvement.

tion, particularly in the acute stage. Microscopically, there is always an inflammatory cell infiltration that sometimes can be polymorphonuclear leukocytes, but much more commonly, and particularly in the later states, the inflammatory exudate consists almost entirely of lymphocytes, plasma cells, and large mononuclear cells (1). Inflammation in the meninges is usually mild, but perivascular infiltration with mononuclear cells in the Virchow-Robin spaces is more common and more pronounced. Sometimes significant demyelination occurs without necrosis (that is, with preservation of the axons). Necrosis is a prominent feature in some viral encephalitides and ranges from selective neuronal necrosis to infarction in large areas of the brain. Herpes encephalitis is the most common viral infection that produces infarctlike necrosis of brain tissue. St. Louis encephalitis may also produce tissue necrosis.

Inclusion bodies in the nuclei of the cells and sometimes in the cytoplasm are typical of viral infections and are found more prominently in some than in others.

Herpes Simplex Virus Encephalitis

There are two types of herpes viruses: type 1, usually found in the perioral fever blister infections, and type 2, the agent in genital herpes. Herpesvirus encephalitis is usually due to type 1 infection, and the mechanism by which the virus reaches the brain is controversial. The herpesvirus appears to live in the trigeminal ganglion in a latent state, having reached the ganglion by an initial infection in the face (2,3). Under certain conditions, which sometimes may be related to immunoincompetence, the virus may reach the inferior frontal and temporal areas of the brain, where viral encephalitis is found pathologically in most cases. In the newborn infant, the encephalitis is probably related to infection by type 2 virus due to passage through the vagina.

Herpes simplex encephalitis can be a fulminant infection with a high mortality rate and, for those who recover, with residual disabilities. Thus diagnosis and therapy as early as possible are important. Unfortunately, it was thought that magnetic resonance imaging (MRI) would show changes in the brain early enough so that the findings and somewhat typical location of the changes would provide a diagnosis quite early, earlier than on computed tomography (CT). Unfortunately, this has not turned out to be the case. Although findings may well appear on MRI earlier than on CT, they still may not provide the earliest possible start of therapy. For this reason, biopsy is still necessary in many cases, and sometimes the treatment is initiated on clinical grounds without imaging confirmation. A rise in antibody titre in the cerebrospinal fluid (CSF) is diagnostic, but it may take as long as 10 to 20 days to develop. The findings on CT or MRI may be present within 2 to 3 days after the initiation of symptoms in some patients; in others, they do not appear as early.

The diagnosis of herpes simplex encephalitis is not proven by CT or MRI examination, but involvement of the unilateral or bilateral temporal lobe and/or frontal lobe is sufficiently typical of herpes simplex encephalitis that active treatment with antiviral agents is recommended.

On CT the appearance is that of a low-absorption, diffuse area in the appropriate location, most frequently in the temporal area but also in the lower frontal area and sometimes in the superior posterior frontal areas, either unilaterally or bilaterally. On T2-weighted images, first and second echoes reveal hyperintensity in the same locations. The findings may be more dramatic on MRI than on CT, and for that reason MRI may show the findings earlier. Typically, the cortical as well as the white matter areas are involved (Figs. 6.1 and 6.2).

Pathologically, widespread necrosis of brain tissue is often accompanied by hemorrhage. Hemorrhagic components usually are not seen in the acute stage, but later the T2-weighted images are likely to show hypointense areas due to magnetic susceptibility that are typical of hemosiderin deposits. Laster et al. published the first MRI follow-up examinations following treatment for herpes simplex encephalitis (4). The scans showed a fair amount of residual change but marked improvement in relation to changes seen during the acute stage of the infection.

The degree of residual neurologic disability depends on where the maximum area of involvement is located. For instance, if the maximum lesion is in the right temporal region, the patient is likely to have fewer residual difficulties than if the lesions are in a more eloquent functional area of the brain. A large area of brain tissue destruction consistent with brain necrosis and infarction is the rule following recovery (Fig. 6.3).

Neonatal herpes simplex encephalitis is an extremely severe disease that is often followed by death. If the individual survives, he or she is likely to have severe neurologic sequelae, such as seizures, microencephaly, intracranial calcifications, and ventriculomegaly. In the neonate, changes in the brain are likely to be generalized rather than localized to the temporal and frontal regions as in the adult form (5). CT as well as MRI will show diffuse changes (radiolucent lesions on CT and hyperintense areas on T2-weighted images). In surviving infants or in newborns who may have had the intrauterine herpes simplex encephalitis, calcifications may develop that are quite different from those usually seen in patients with cytomegalovirus or congenital toxoplasmosis (Table 6.1).

Herpes simplex virus may also produce inflammation of some cranial nerves, particularly the trigeminal nerve, and in the area of the pons where the fifth cranial nerve arises (rhombencephalitis). MRI examination may demonstrate a hyperintense signal in the pons on T2-weighted images, and gadolinium enhancement may show hyperintensity in the preganglionic segment of the nerve (6). The peripheral nerves have a blood-peripheral cranial nerve barrier, and enhancement indicates loss of this barrier. In the case reported by Tien and Dillon, the patient presented numbness

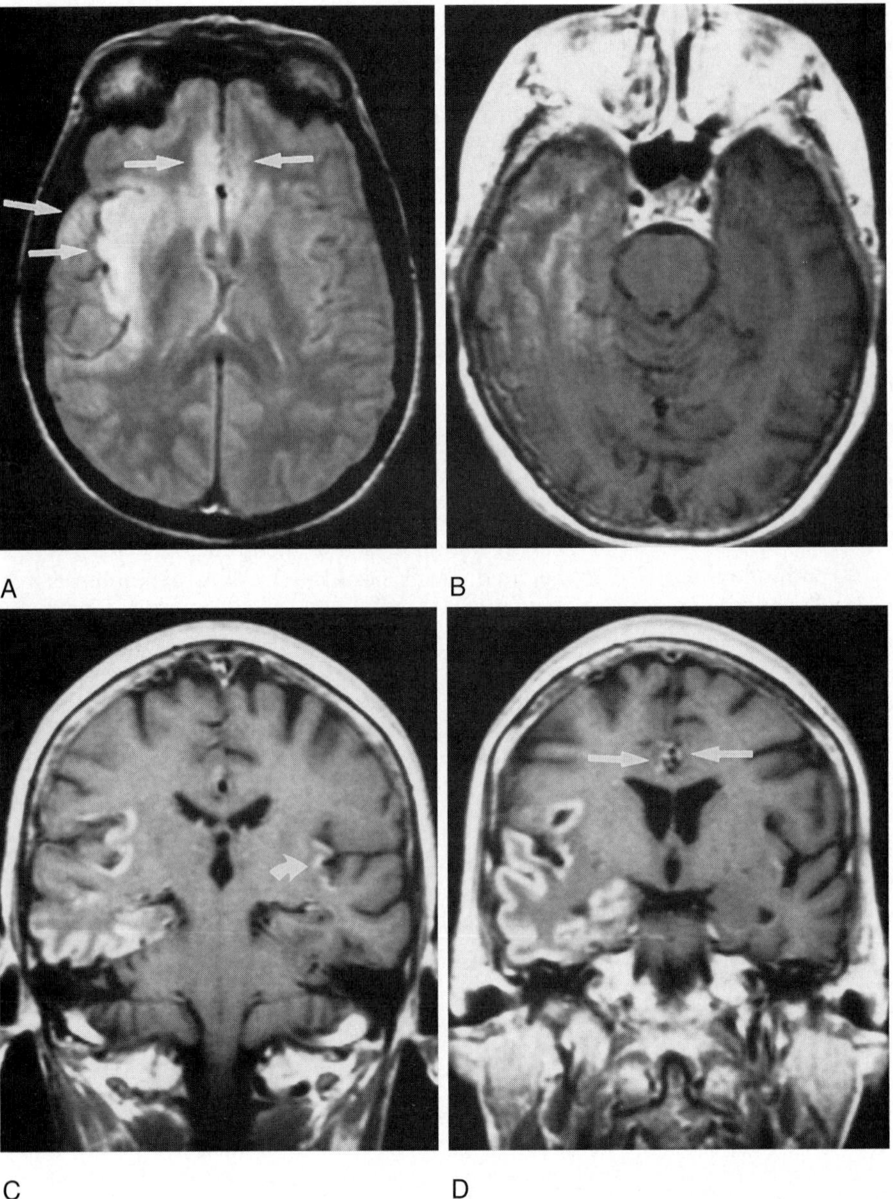

Figure 6.2. Herpes simplex encephalitis in a 61-year-old woman. **A.** Proton density axial image shows hyperintensity in the right temporal lobe and insula as well as in the frontal lobes bilaterally (arrows). **B.** Contrast-enhanced T1-weighted axial image shows gyral enhancement. **C.** Coronal postcontrast image shows the gyral enhancement, which indicates gray matter disease. There is also involvement of the insular cortex on the left side (curved arrow). **D.** Coronal section more anteriorly also shows enhancement in the frontal midline cortex bilaterally (arrows).

of the face on the corresponding side and typical herpes simplex ulcer in the oral cavity and circumoral region. MRI demonstrated hyperintensity in the pons and middle cerebellar peduncle. After gadolinium there was marked enhancement of the preganglionic segment of the trigeminal nerve and no enhancement of the pons or middle cerebellar peduncle. No treatment was applied, and the MRI findings regressed spontaneously in 6 to 8 weeks.

Ramsay Hunt syndrome (herpes zoster oticus), a viral infection of the geniculate ganglion leading to the typical clinical findings of facial paralysis, resides in the skin in and around the ears. The MRI findings are those of gadolinium enhancement of the geniculate ganglion, the adjacent portions of the facial nerve, the cochlea, the vestibule, and the semicircular canals (7). Daniels et al. reported enlargement of nerves VII and VIII on noncontrast MRI (8).

Table 6.1.
Herpes Simplex Virus (HSV) Encephalitis

HSV-1
Usually affects adults.
Confusion, lethargy, and occasionally seizures.
Temporal lobe is preferential site of involvement.
Often difficult to detect by CT during early stages of infection.
Initially subtle, nonenhancing, hypodense region on CT, progressing to more pronounced hypodensity with mass effect.
MRI is more sensitive than CT in establishing the diagnosis.
MRI findings: T1 hypointense, T2 hyperintense signal and mass effect in one or both temporal lobes and inferior frontal lobe.
HSV-2
Typically occurs in neonates; transmission is frequently during birth.
Overwelming systemic disease with CNS involvement.
Generalized findings throughout entire brain.
CT appearance: widespread hypodense abnormality.
Intracranial calcifications frequently result.
MRI appearance: diffuse T1 hypointense, T2 hyperintense signal abnormality.

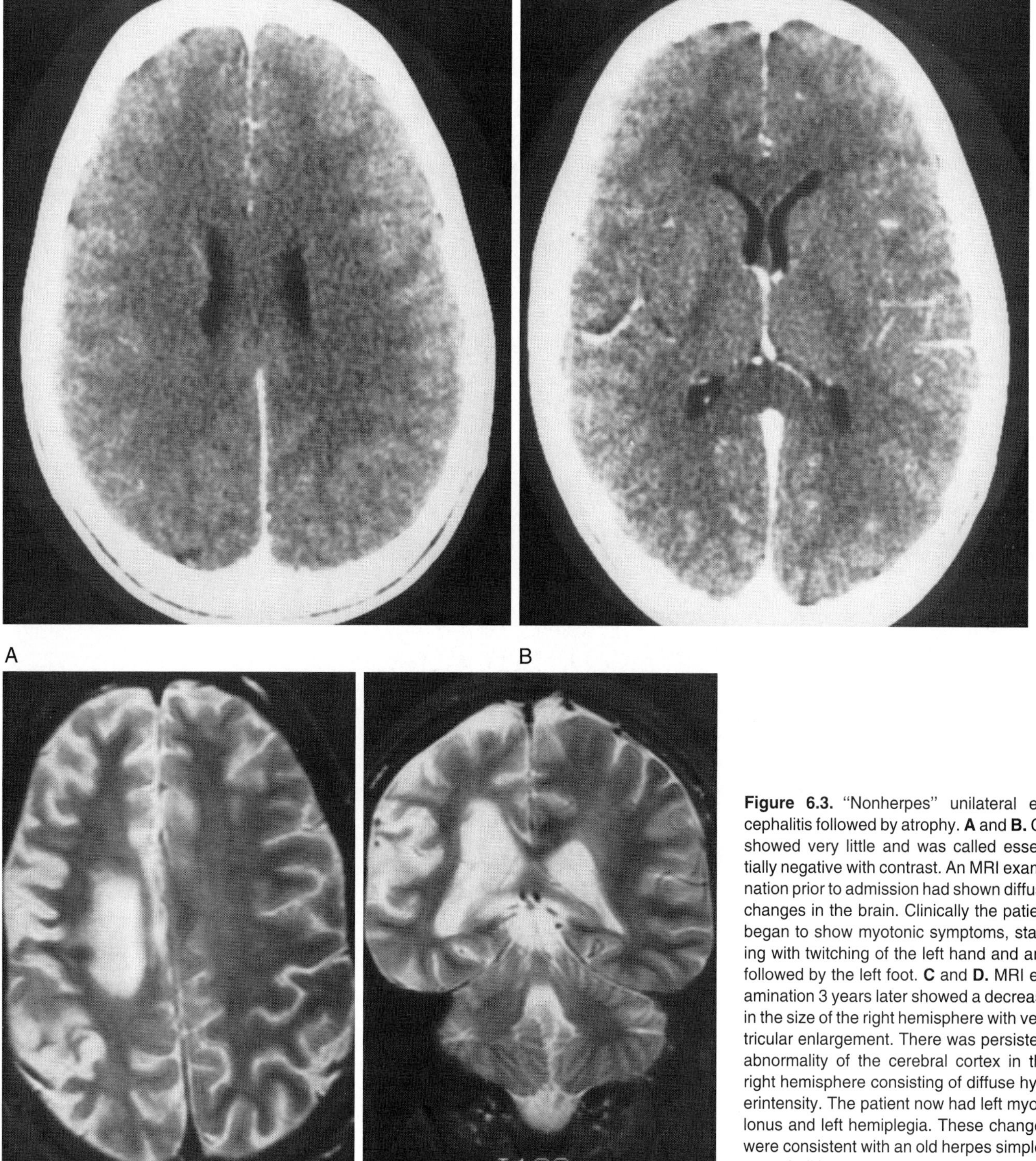

Figure 6.3. "Nonherpes" unilateral encephalitis followed by atrophy. **A** and **B.** CT showed very little and was called essentially negative with contrast. An MRI examination prior to admission had shown diffuse changes in the brain. Clinically the patient began to show myotonic symptoms, starting with twitching of the left hand and arm followed by the left foot. **C** and **D.** MRI examination 3 years later showed a decrease in the size of the right hemisphere with ventricular enlargement. There was persistent abnormality of the cerebral cortex in the right hemisphere consisting of diffuse hyperintensity. The patient now had left myoclonus and left hemiplegia. These changes were consistent with an old herpes simplex encephalitis, but this diagnosis was not made initially and it remained as an unclassified viral encephalitis.

Herpes zoster ophthalmicus may be accompanied by hemiplegia on the opposite side of involvement. This is felt to be due to an arteritic process possibly secondary to direct involvement from the adjacent inflammatory process in the region of the gasserian ganglion (9,10).

Cytomegalovirus Infection

Cytomegalovirus (CMV) is a ubiquitous DNA virus of the herpesvirus family that is the most frequent agent in fetal and neonatal viral infection. It is acquired in utero, probably through transplacental transmission from a new or re-

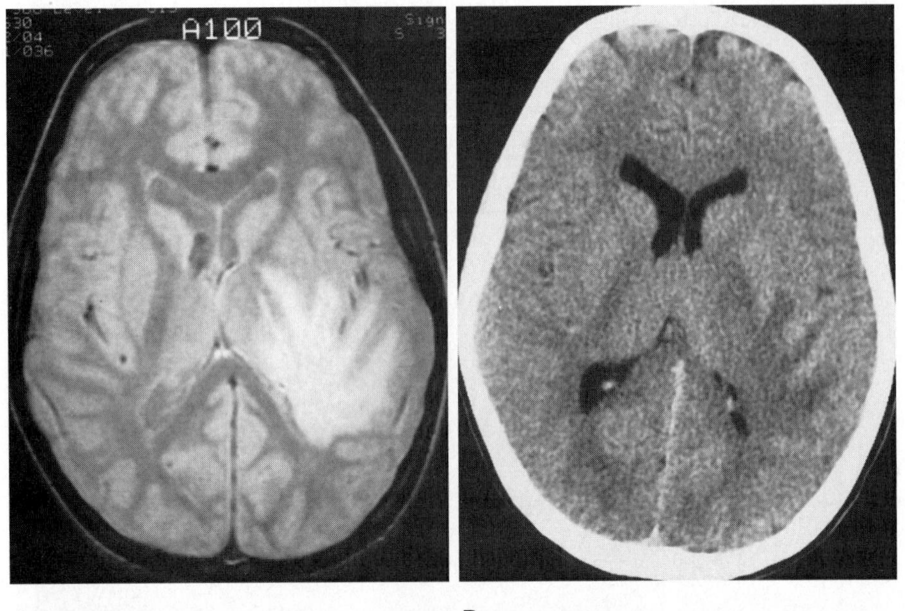

Figure 6.4. Acute disseminated encephalomyelitis (ADEM) in a 10-year-old boy who presented with flulike symptoms, right hemiparesis, and paraparesis. **A.** MRI proton density image revealed an area of diffuse edema in the left parietal region. The edema, which was primarily in the white matter, extended to follow certain fiber tracts. **B.** CT examination the following day revealed the same localization and size of the edema. **C.** Sagittal MR proton density images of the spine revealed increased intensity in the lower spinal cord and conus (arrow). **D.** T2-weighted sagittal image confirmed the spinal cord involvement (arrow). **E.** Repeat MRI examination 11 days later showed marked reduction in the edema (arrows). Interestingly enough, the perivascular CSF spaces in the lenticular nucleus were now more numerous and prominent, especially on the right side. The patient was considerably improved clinically. A rapid favorable evolution is the rule in this condition.

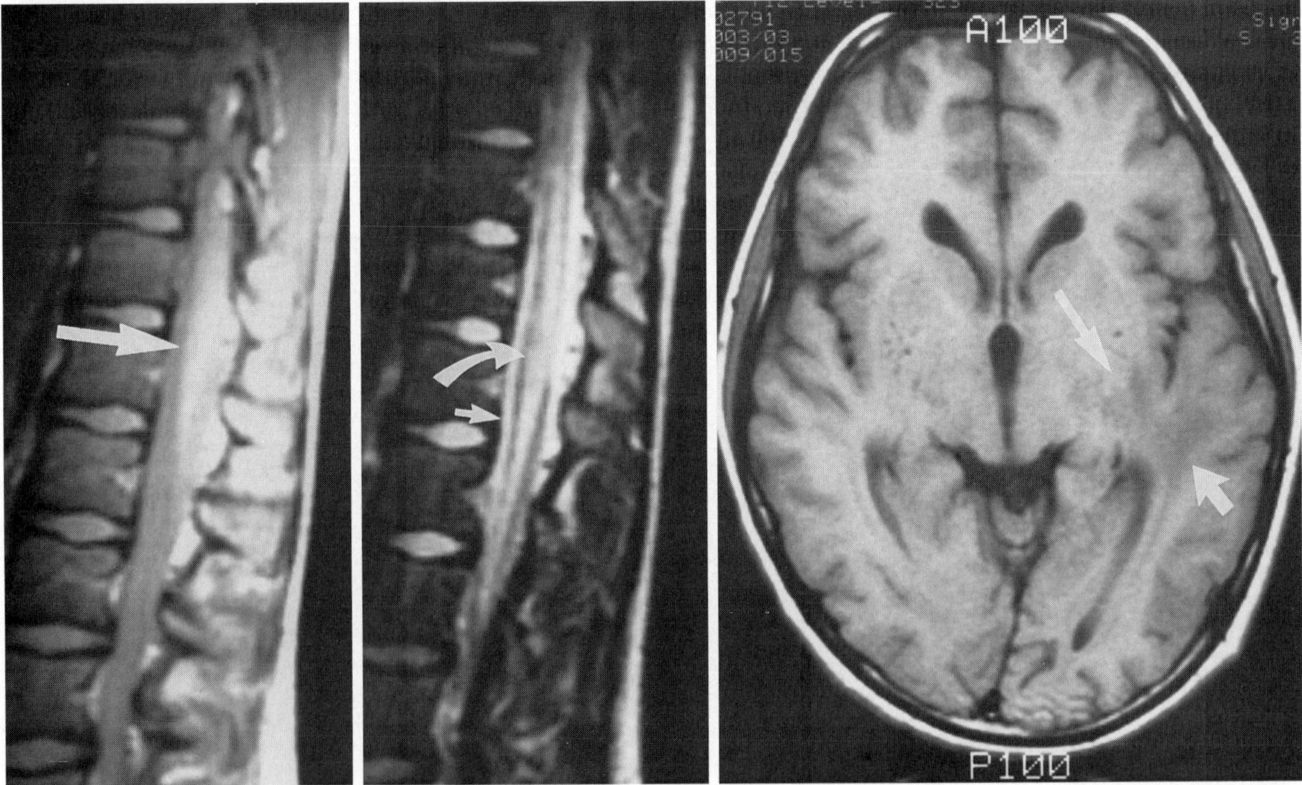

current maternal infection. The reactivated infection in the mother has a much lower incidence of central nervous system involvement in the fetus than does the newly acquired maternal infection (11). The systemic manifestations of the CMV infection in the fetus and newborn are hemolytic anemia, hyperbilirubinemia, and jaundice; thrombocytopenia; hepatosplenomegaly; and pneumonia. The CNS abnormalities are microcephaly, deafness, and ocular abnormalities. The microcephaly is associated with a severe encephalitis resulting in brain tissue necrosis, calcification, and atrophy—usually with ventricular enlargement.

Tassin et al. reported on the prenatal diagnosis of brain involvement by ultrasound (12). It is possible to show ventricular dilatation, and periventricular bright spots representing calcification (earlier, ringlike zones may be seen instead), which Tassin et al. consider characteristic of cytomegalic inclusion disease.

Poliomyelitis

Poliomyelitis virus infections are diagnosed by clinical and laboratory methods. However, bulbar poliomyelitis may produce findings in the lower brainstem that are detectable by MRI as a hyperintense area without mass effect on T2-weighted images in the medulla (13). Poliomyelitis has virtually disappeared following development of an effective vaccine. The cases seen in the United States are following vaccination, and the patients ordinarily are immunocompromised to start with. In spite of its rarity, a paralytic state in an immunocompromised adult or child who presents a hyperintense lesion on T2-weighted images in the lower brainstem without a mass should raise the question of poliomyelitis.

Acute Disseminated Encephalomyelitis

In acute disseminated encephalomyelitis (ADEM), demyelination occurs mainly in a perivenous distribution 1 to 4 weeks after an inflammatory viral disease (measles, mumps, chickenpox, rubella, whooping cough) or after vaccination. Death can occur in up to 10 percent of cases, but recovery is the rule from what is usually a monophasic condition. The disease can show a remission and relapsing type of course. It may well be directly related to a virus but is more likely related to an immunologic response. CT examination may be normal or may show minimal changes (such as scattered areas of low attenuation). MRI will show hyperintense areas on T2-weighted images in the brainstem, the centrum semiovale, the basal ganglia, or the cerebellum (Figs. 6.4 to 6.7). The number and location of the lesions vary, but when located in the periventricular white matter and centrum semiovale, they may mimic multiple sclerosis (MS). If the patient is going to show a favorable response, the lesions begin to clear within a few to several weeks (14). Cases have been reported after varicella, as have basal ganglia infarction with angiographic demonstration of middle and anterior cerebral artery narrowing (15).

Acute Hemorrhagic Leukoencephalitis

This is a fatal form with widespread abnormalities of the blood vessels, necrosis of vessel walls, and fibrinous exudation, particularly involving the small veins. The many small hemorrhages may become confluent, and there is perivascular demyelination. The lesions may be bilateral or one hemisphere may be more involved than the other.

Subacute Sclerosing Panencephalitis (SSPE)

This is an inflammatory condition occurring a number of years after measles (up to 8 to 10 years or longer). It is in fact a slow infection by the measles virus, which has remained latent after the initial infection and becomes reactivated. The serum and CSF titre of measles antibody become elevated. The disease has an insidious onset, with behavioral changes, mental deterioration, and sometimes seizures, ataxia, and myoclonus that progress to death over a period of 6 months to several years. Imaging findings are those of diffuse white matter changes (low attenuation on CT, high intensity on T2-weighted images), which later are accompanied by ventricular enlargement and cortical cerebral atrophy. The cerebellum may also show diffuse hyperintensity on T2-weighted images, and the changes may disappear later (16). The incidence of SSPE has decreased markedly since the development of antimeasles vaccine (Table 6.2).

Other Viral Encephalitides

It is not uncommon to encounter, on a clinical basis, children and adults presenting with a clinical picture consistent with encephalitis, but no specific diagnosis can be made. Many of these patients have a negative MRI, and others may present a typical picture of a diffuse inflammatory process involving chiefly the white matter in the cerebral hemispheres or the brainstem. Others may present involvement of the gray matter, usually focal, and in these cases a biopsy may be necessary to establish a final diagnosis, for it may not be possible to differentiate it from an ischemic vascular

Table 6.2.
Inflammatory Diseases of White Matter

Acute disseminated encephalomyelitis (ADEM)
- May be postinfectious or postvaccinial in origin.
- Presumed to be an autoimmune phenomenon.
- Typically monophasic but may be multiphasic.
- Subtle hypodense white matter lesions on CT.
- Optimally demonstrated on MRI, with multiple T2 hyperintense white matter foci.

Acute hemorrhagic leukoencephalitis
- Frequently fatal.
- Marked by perivascular fibrinous exudates and necrosis.
- End result is white matter hemorrhage and demyelination.

Subacute sclerosing panencephalitis (SSPE)
- Reactivation of latent measles infection, occurring years after initial exposure.
- Diffuse white matter hyperintense lesions on T2-weighted MRI.
- Subsequent cortical atrophy and ventricular enlargement.

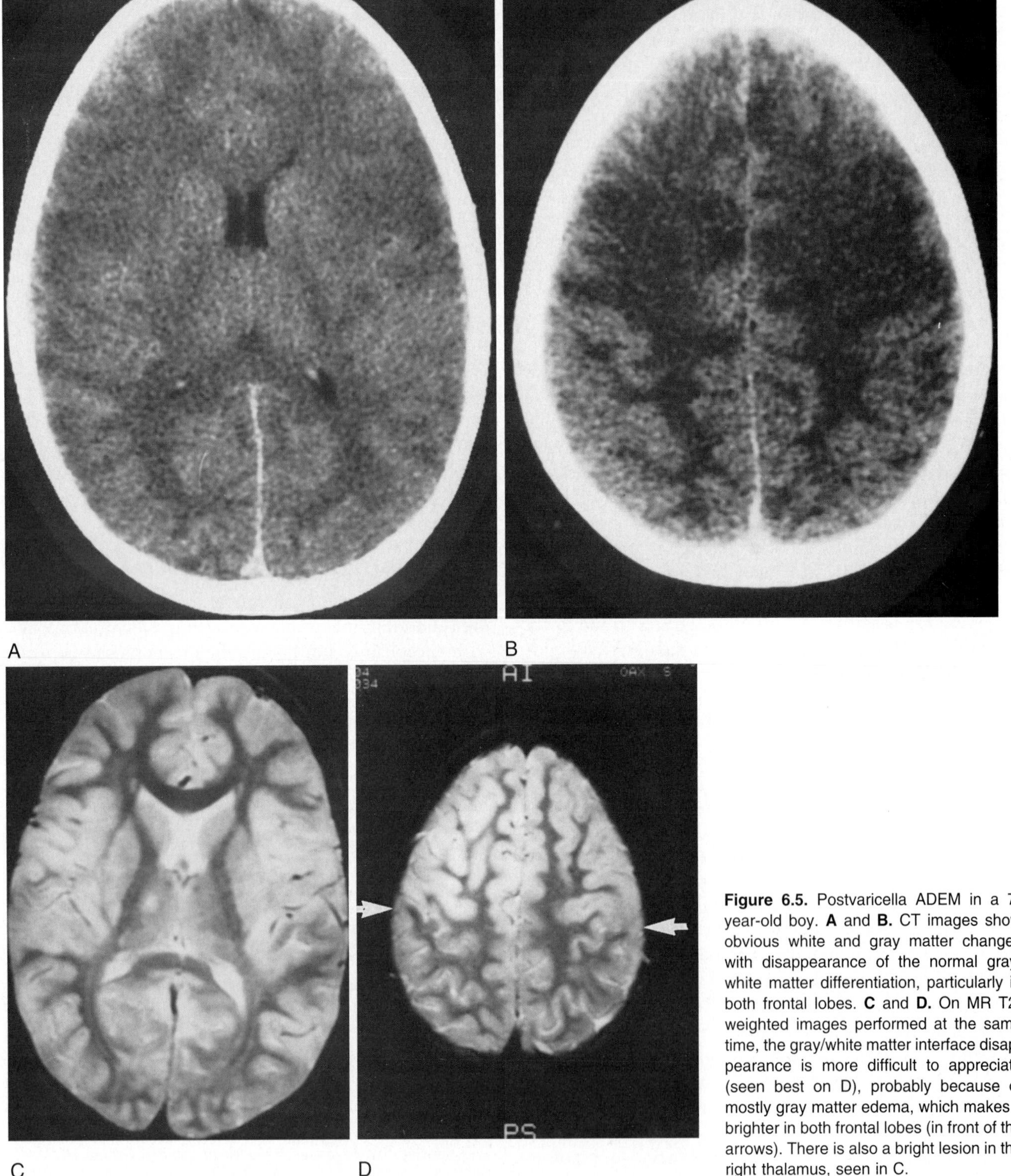

Figure 6.5. Postvaricella ADEM in a 7-year-old boy. **A** and **B.** CT images show obvious white and gray matter changes with disappearance of the normal gray/white matter differentiation, particularly in both frontal lobes. **C** and **D.** On MR T2-weighted images performed at the same time, the gray/white matter interface disappearance is more difficult to appreciate (seen best on D), probably because of mostly gray matter edema, which makes it brighter in both frontal lobes (in front of the arrows). There is also a bright lesion in the right thalamus, seen in C.

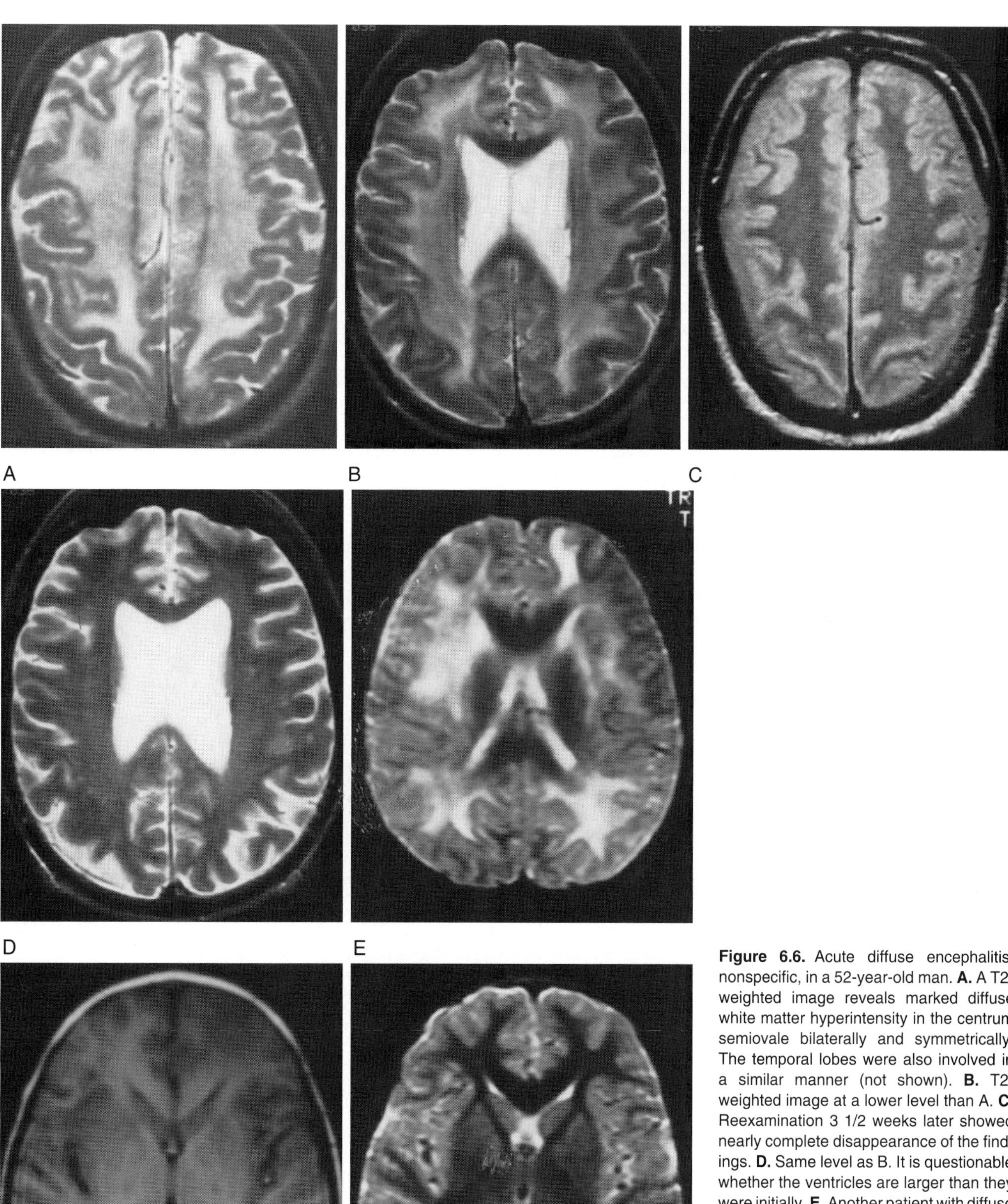

Figure 6.6. Acute diffuse encephalitis, nonspecific, in a 52-year-old man. **A.** A T2-weighted image reveals marked diffuse white matter hyperintensity in the centrum semiovale bilaterally and symmetrically. The temporal lobes were also involved in a similar manner (not shown). **B.** T2-weighted image at a lower level than A. **C.** Reexamination 3 1/2 weeks later showed nearly complete disappearance of the findings. **D.** Same level as B. It is questionable whether the ventricles are larger than they were initially. **E.** Another patient with diffuse encephalitic changes shown on a T2-weighted image. **F.** T1-weighted image after gadolinium reveals no enhancement of the involved areas. This is typical of these nonspecific encephalitides and differentiates them from herpes simplex encephalitis, in which enhancement is the rule. **G.** Repeat examination 6 months later revealed a normal T2-weighted appearance without ventricular dilatation. The patient had returned to normal.

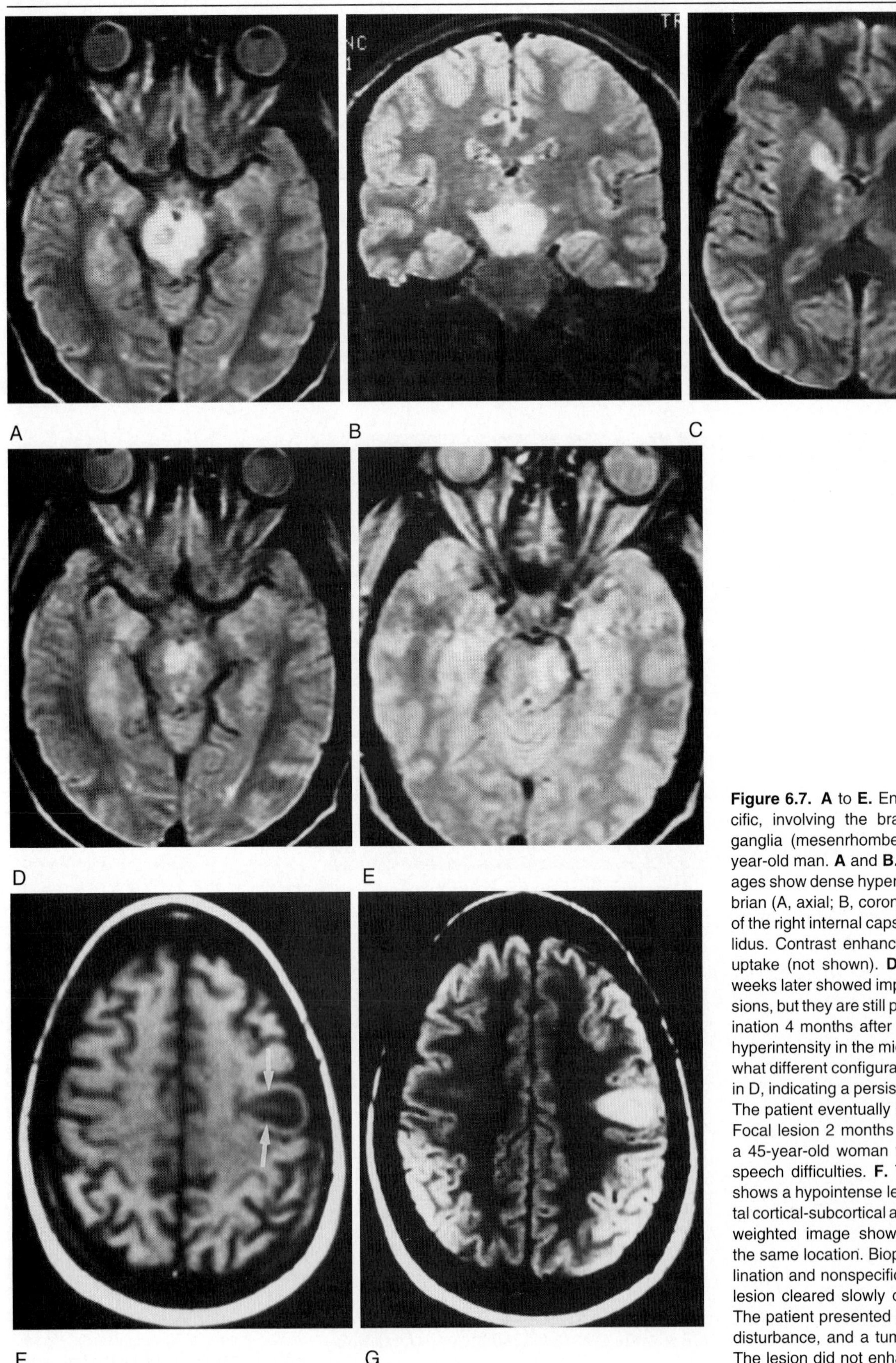

Figure 6.7. **A** to **E.** Encephalitis, nonspecific, involving the brainstem and basal ganglia (mesenrhombencephalitis) in 31-year-old man. **A** and **B.** Proton density images show dense hyperintensity in the midbrian (A, axial; B, coronal). **C.** Involvement of the right internal capsule and globus pallidus. Contrast enhancement revealed no uptake (not shown). **D.** Reexamination 2 weeks later showed improvement of the lesions, but they are still present. **E.** Reexamination 4 months after D showed residual hyperintensity in the midbrain with a somewhat different configuration from that noted in D, indicating a persistent active process. The patient eventually improved. **F** and **G.** Focal lesion 2 months after flu vaccine in a 45-year-old woman who complained of speech difficulties. **F.** T1-weighted image shows a hypointense lesion in the left frontal cortical-subcortical area (arrows). **G.** T2-weighted image shows hyperintensity in the same location. Biopsy showed demyelination and nonspecific inflammation. The lesion cleared slowly over a few months. The patient presented initially with speech disturbance, and a tumor was suspected. The lesion did not enhance with contrast.

lesion or an unusual slowly growing infiltrative neoplasm (Figs. 6.7 and 6.8*A* to *D*).

Perhaps the most important imaging characteristics in these cases are (a) that they do not enhance with gadolinium and (b) that they improve in 2 weeks to 6 months. CT may be negative or may show some decreased attenuation in the involved areas that may be difficult to evaluate.

An apparently new type of acute encephalopathy, occurring in young children (12 to 29 months), has been reported from Japan, in which no etiologic agent has been identified. In the five cases reported by Yagishita et al., the involvement was primarily in the thalami, brainstem, and cerebral and cerebellar white matter. One child died, and autopsy showed cell necrosis with little or no inflammation; three children were left with severe sequelae; only one child recovered (17).

Creutzfeldt-Jakob Disease

This is a disease produced by a slow viruslike protein called *prion* with a very long incubation period (several years). It produces brain involvement primarily in the gray matter but also in the white matter, and it results in death of the patient. Histologically, there are spongiform changes, loss of neurons and astrocytic hyperplasia, and hypertrophy of the gray matter. White matter involvement may occur in the later stages of the disease.

CT images mostly demonstrate brain atrophy (ventricular enlargement and sulcal widening), and no specific lesions are usually seen. Falcone et al. have reported increased intensity on T2-weighted images as well as thickening of the cortical gray matter in both occipital regions (18). Kovanen et al. suggest that white matter lesions would probably be demonstrated on MRI later in the disease because they are found at autopsy (19). The case illustrated in Figure 6.8*E* to *G* demonstrates hyperintensity of basal ganglia on T2-weighted images as well as some white matter diffuse hyperintensity.

Barboriak et al. reported four cases and stated that bilateral symmetric hyperintensity in the basal ganglia on T2-weighted images may be a specific sign for Creutzfeldt-Jakob disease in a patient with progressive dementia, particularly if the T1-weighted image and CT scans are normal (20). The viruslike particle (prion) that produces Creutzfeldt-Jakob disease is similar to that which produces scrapie, Gerstmann-Straussler syndrome, and kuru, a disease found in the natives of New Guinea that is uniformly fatal. Ogawa et al. suggest that fluorodeoxyglucose and positron emission tomography (PET) scanning may be useful in the early diagnosis of Creutzfeldt-Jakob disease (21).

AIDS

The virus that produces AIDS belongs to a group of more recently recognized viruses called *retroviruses.* HIV is the one that leads to production of the AIDS complex. There are two types, the HIV-1 and the HIV-2. The latter is mostly found in Africa. Another related virus, the human T-cell lymphotropic virus type 1 (HTLV-1), is found in the Caribbean area and in Japan, where it may lead to chronic myelitis and paraplegia.

Neurologic complications of HIV infection are common. The incidence was reported at 39 percent of 352 patients by Levy et al. (22) and even higher by others: 60 percent by Berger et al. (23).

AIDS ENCEPHALOPATHY

The frequency and the degree of disability resulting from what is often called *HIV encephalitis* are still under discussion. Undoubtedly, in some individuals, a direct infection by the virus in the brain may lead to impairment of cognition and memory with some behavioral abnormalities progressing to dementia (AIDS dementia complex, or ADC). In some cases, diffuse changes in the white matter or generalized atrophy can be demonstrated in the brain, but in the great majority of instances, the infections that we see in the brain are secondary. Olsen et al. indicated that ADC is more frequently associated with diffuse white matter involvement (24). They also described patchy, focal, and punctate lesions that may be produced by the virus but are more likely produced by another agent (toxoplasmosis, progressive multifocal leukoencephalopathy, lymphoma).

The HIV encephalitic manifestations have been attributed to an increase in intracellular calcium owing to the toxic effect of a protein (gp 120), a coat protein on the surface of the HIV virus. The toxic effect may be prevented by calcium channel antagonists such as nimodipine (25).

The study of Koralink et al. is revealing in that it demonstrated electrophysiological abnormalities in two-thirds of asymptomatic HIV-seropositive patients and in only 10 percent of the controls (26). MRI examinations did not show significant differences between the two groups; the same results were obtained by Cohen et al. (27). Post et al., in a study of 95 asymptomatic and 24 symptomatic HIV-positive patients, showed that MRI is likely to be negative or show only some atrophic changes and slight white matter abnormalities (28). In a subsequent study, Post et al. found no progression of detected minor changes in asymptomatic HIV-seropositive patients on repeat MRI 1 to 2 years later (29). A few neurologically symptomatic patients revealed increased abnormalities correlating with clinical deterioration. The microglial nodules with multinucleated giant cells are considered the hallmark of HIV encephalitis, but these lesions are not demonstrable by CT or MRI (30,31). Flowers et al., in 47 AIDS patients, reported a higher proportion of focal (49 percent) than of diffuse (13 percent) white matter abnormalities (32). The correlation of these findings with the clinical diagnosis of AIDS encephalopathy was not made, but the presence of cerebral or cerebellar atrophy was their most common finding (26 of 47).

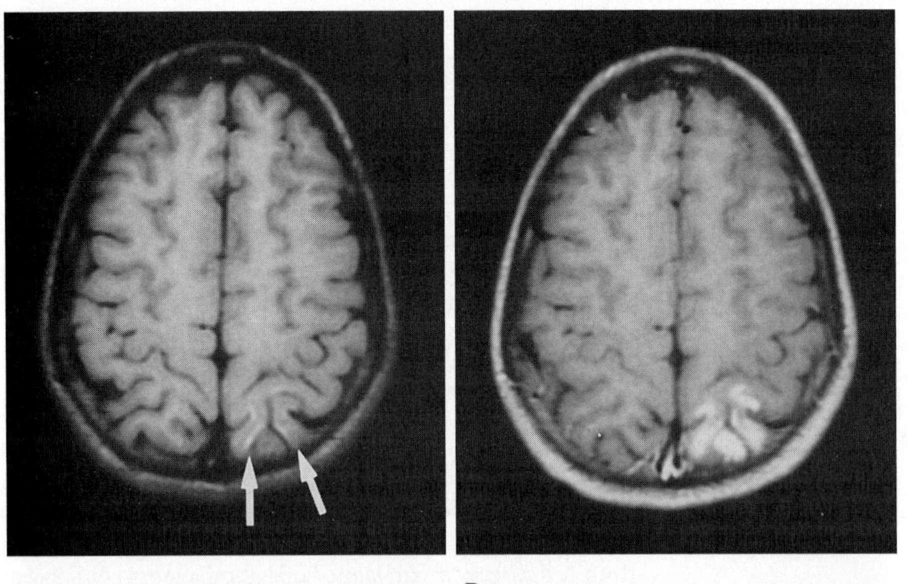

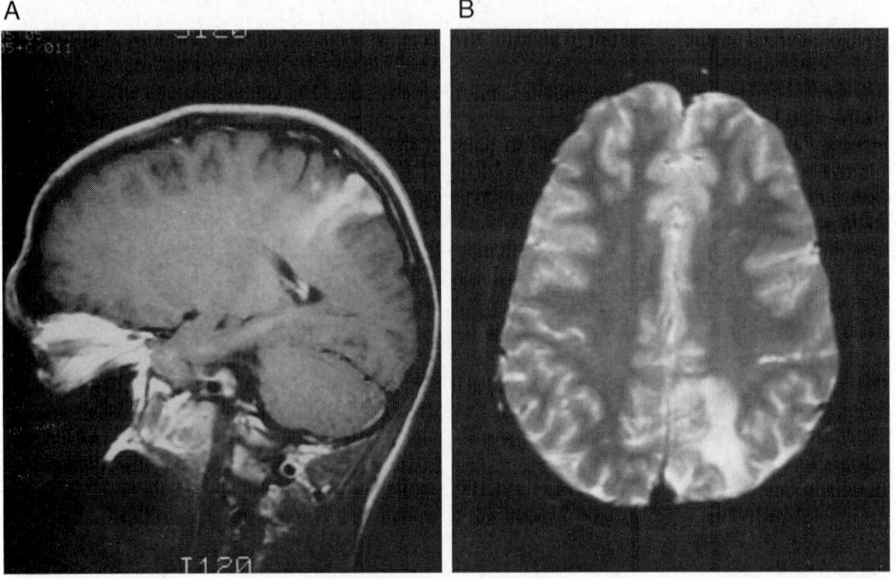

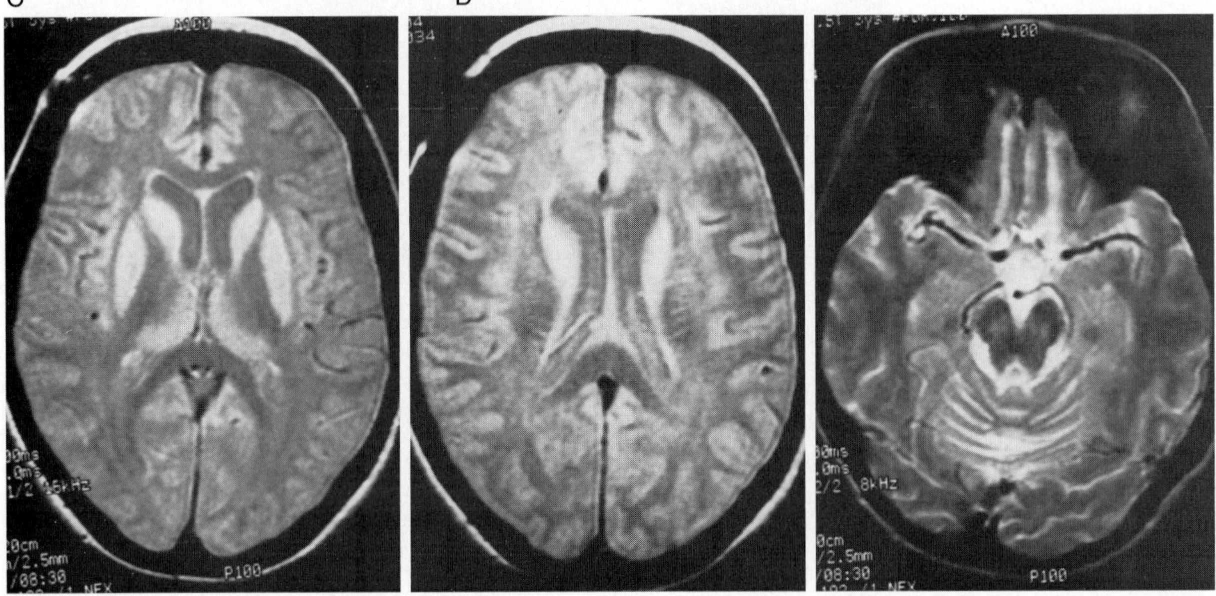

Figure 6.8. Focal encephalitis nonspecific viral, involving the white and gray matter in a 16-year-old boy. **A.** T1-weighted axial image shows slight gyriform hyperintensity in the left parietal region (arrows). **B** and **C.** Postcontrast T1-weighted image shows marked enhancement of the entire area, including the gray and white matter. **D.** T2-weighted image shows the hyperintense area extending into the adjacent white matter. **E.** to **G.** Creutzfeldt-Jakob disease in a 56-year-old woman who presented progressive gait disturbance, spasticity, speech difficulty, and paranoid ideations. The diagnosis was established by biopsy. The patient had had a meningioma removed 9 months previously. The proton density image shows hyperintensity of the putamen and caudate nucleus bilaterally. The white matter reveals irregular hyperintensity. The medial temporal lobe in G is probably normal, and the midbrain also appears to be normal in this T2-weighted image, but it presents a slight hyperintensity more on the right side.

Thus the imaging signs of HIV encephalopathy are most frequently cerebral atrophy, as manifested by ventricular enlargement and sulcal widening in the brain and/or cerebellar atrophy in a relatively young individual; diffuse hyperintensity in the periventricular white matter and centrum semiovale on T2-weighted images; and sometimes patchy focal areas of hyperintensity on T2-weighted images on MRI examinations. CT will demonstrate these as diminished attenuation, diffuse or focal, but the changes may be more subtle than on MRI. Contrast enhancement does not usually occur (Figs. 6.9 and 6.10). When there are patchy or multiple punctate areas, the diagnosis is likely to be a secondary infection or a related disease process such as lymphoma.

Kauffman et al. reported imaging findings in perinatal HIV-affected children (33). Cerebral atrophy, basal ganglia calcifications (10 of 28), and focal white matter lesions on T2-weighted images were the most common findings, and secondary infections were less common than in the adult. Neoplasms were not found.

SECONDARY INFECTIONS IN AIDS

As has become well known, a host of infections occur in patients with AIDS because of the accompanying immunodeficiency. These are *Toxoplasma gondii*, cytomegalic inclusion virus, herpes simplex virus, *Candida albicans*, *Cryptococcus neoformans*, *Aspergillus fumigatus*, *Mycobacterium tuberculosis*, atypical mycobacterium, *Nocardia asteroides* (Fig. 6.13*E* to *H*), papovavirus, and others. In addition, primary lymphoma of the brain and Kaposi sarcoma (a malignancy usually starting and spreading in the skin but which may involve viscera and the central nervous system) can afflict AIDS patients.

An etiologic diagnosis is important so that one can apply the most appropriate therapy, and for this reason biopsy is often performed. In the presence of diffuse imaging changes in the brain, antiviral therapy may be performed, particularly if the clinical symptoms suggest an early ADC. Some patients improve under this regimen (34).

Of the focal lesions, the most common etiology is *toxoplasmosis* (35). *Toxoplasma gondii* is an intracellular protozoan capable of causing a necrotizing encephalitis in immunocompromised patients, be it AIDS, organ transplantation, underlying malignancy, particularly under chemotherapy, or other states. It usually produces rounded, ill-defined areas of varying size on nonenhanced CT or MRI. Intravenous contrast usually shows ring enhancement, as for an abscess, in most of the lesions (Figs. 6.11–6.13). There is usually some surrounding edema, although some of the lesions may not show any. To avoid carrying out a brain biopsy, treatment is often applied, and if the patient improves, one can assume that toxoplasmosis is the correct diagnosis. In addition to clinical improvement, repeat CT or MRI with enhancement is necessary to verify the pathologic improvement or disappearance of the lesions. The repeat study will show partial disappearance of the lesion in 10 to 15 days or earlier. If the lesions do not show ring enhancement, differentiation from lymphoma or some other etiology is more difficult. Moreover, it should be kept in mind that more than one etiology may coexist when one is confronted with multiple lesions. In

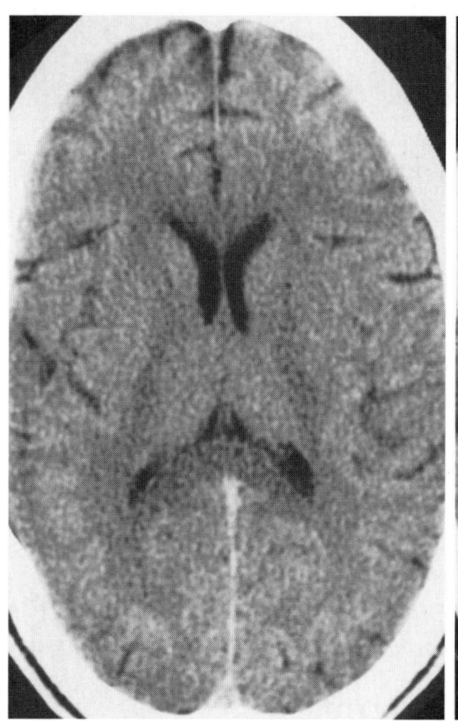
A

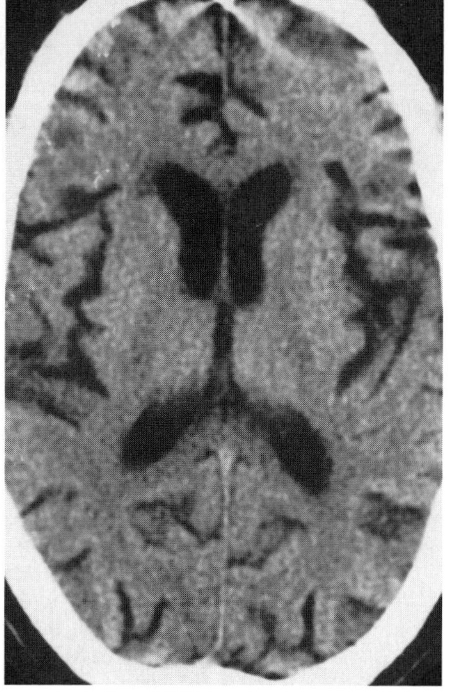
B

Figure 6.9. AIDS encephalopathy in a 32-year-old man. **A.** The examination at this time showed a normal appearance. **B.** Reexamination 15 months later showed marked atrophy. The sylvian fissures were large, the surface sulci were prominent, and the ventricles were enlarged. No other findings were evident, and the patient had not developed cerebral infections. Originally the patient presented with headaches and weakness and was found to be HIV-positive. Fifteen months later he returned complaining of headaches and stiffness of the neck, at which time only brain atrophy was detected.

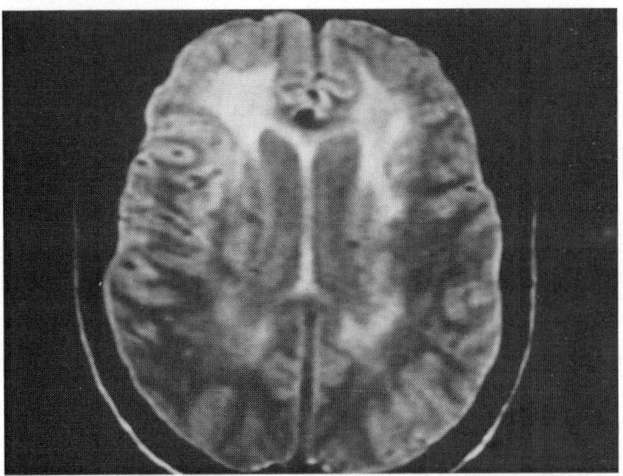

A

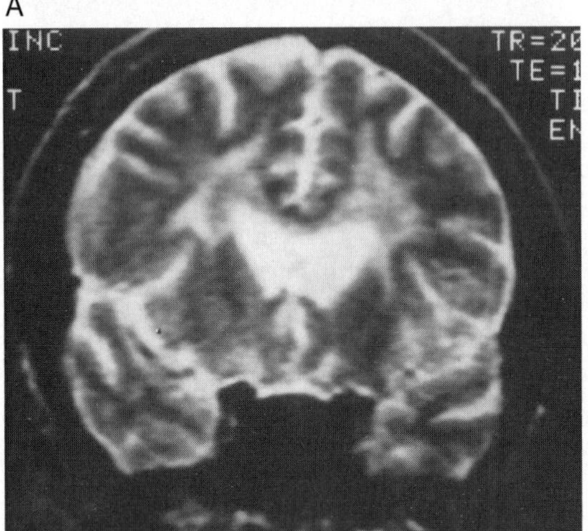

B

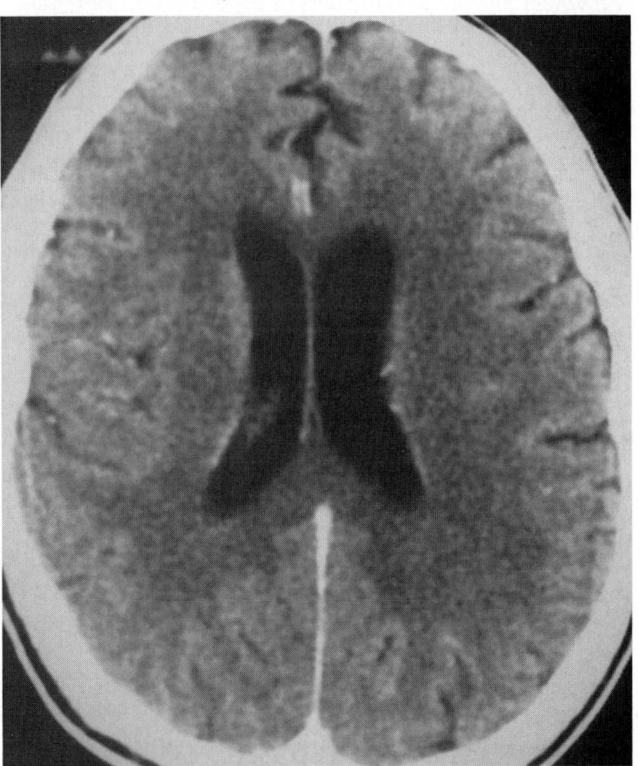

C

Figure 6.10. AIDS encephalitis in a 36-year-old-man. **A.** There is diffuse white matter hyperintensity in both frontal and parietal areas in the proton density image. **B.** The coronal T2-weighted section shows the white matter hyperintensity. The ventricles are enlarged. **C.** The CT scan is essentially normal aside from mild ventricular enlargement.

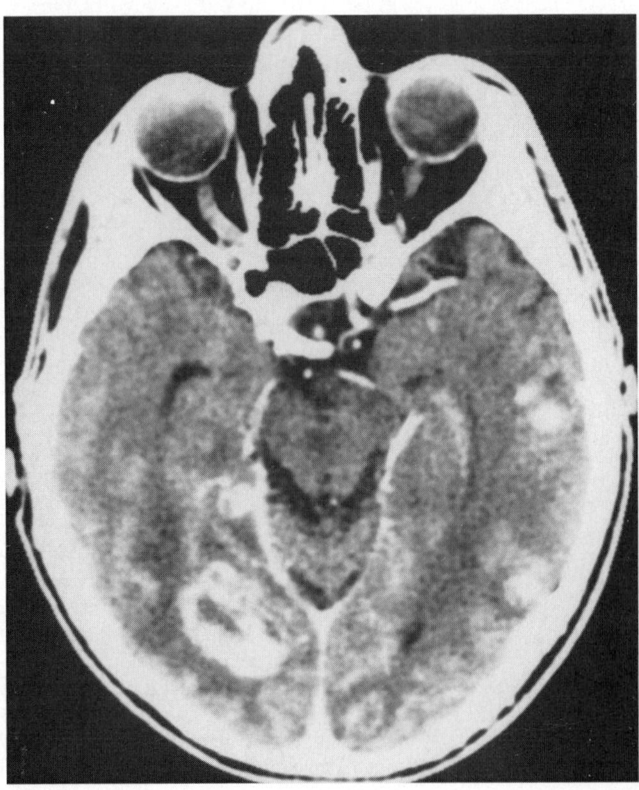

A

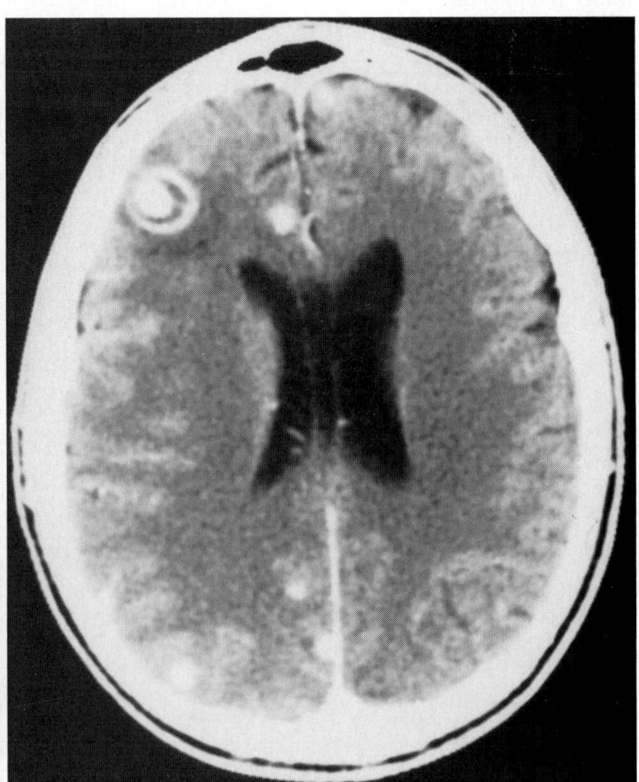

B

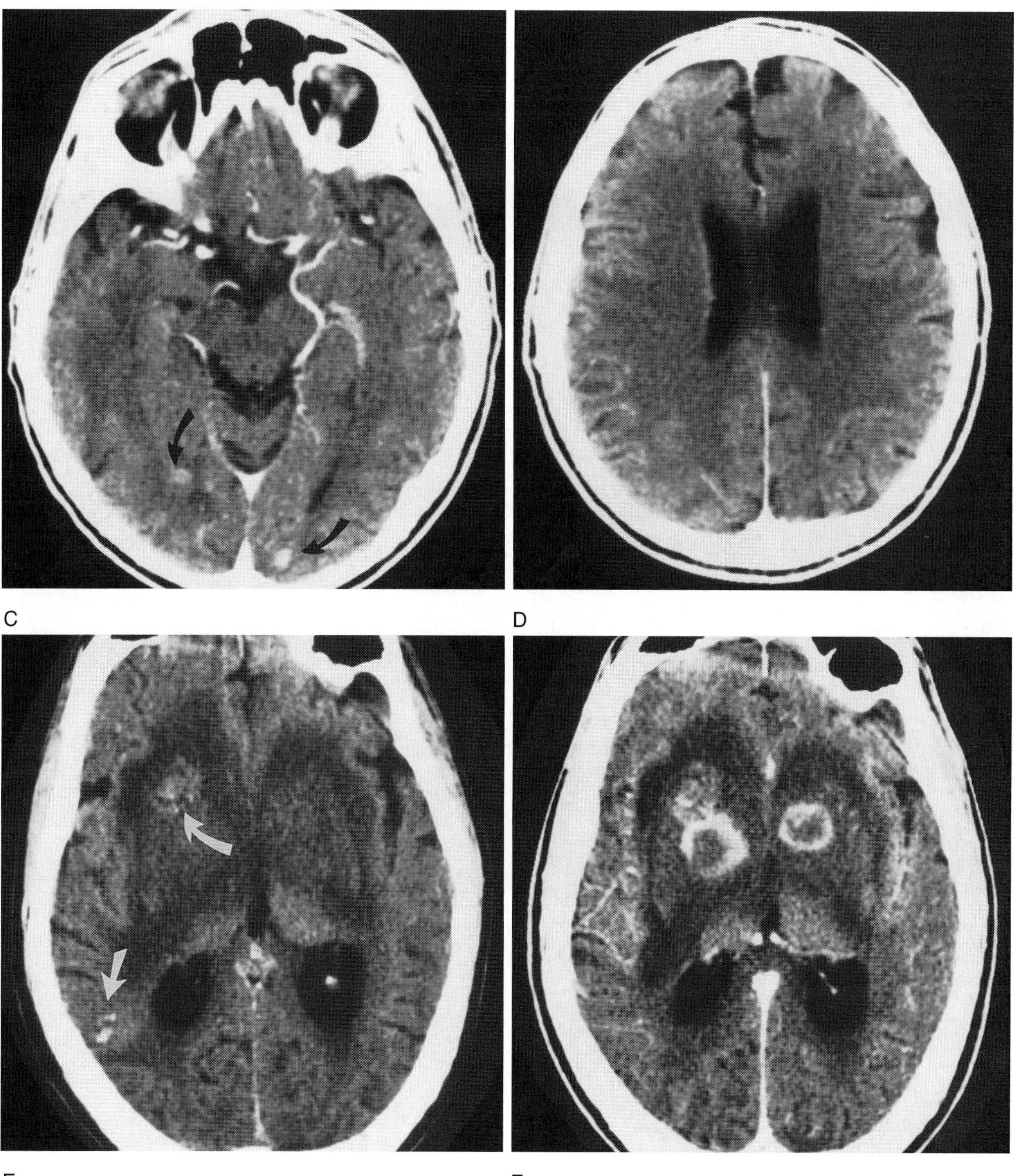

C D E F

Figure 6.11. Toxoplasmosis in an AIDS-affected man. **A.** Enhanced CT axial view reveals numerous small hyperdense areas; some are excavated and others are not. **B.** A higher section reveals other lesions. **C** and **D.** Repeat examination through the same area 3 months later following specific treatment for toxoplasmosis reveals a considerable decrease in the size and number of lesions. A few lesions still remain (curved arrows). **E** and **F.** Toxoplasmosis in a patient with AIDS showing calcifications. **E.** A noncontrast CT scan reveals calcifications: one ringlike with a calcific center (upper arrow), and the other near the cortical frontocortical area (arrow). There is edema, as shown by the surrounding low attenuation in the deep anterior lesion. **F.** After contrast two other lesions in the basal ganglia on each side are seen with ring enhancement. The calcified lesion on the right side does not enhance and most likely represents an old toxoplasmosis lesion. The basal ganglia are frequent locations for *Toxoplasma* abscesses.

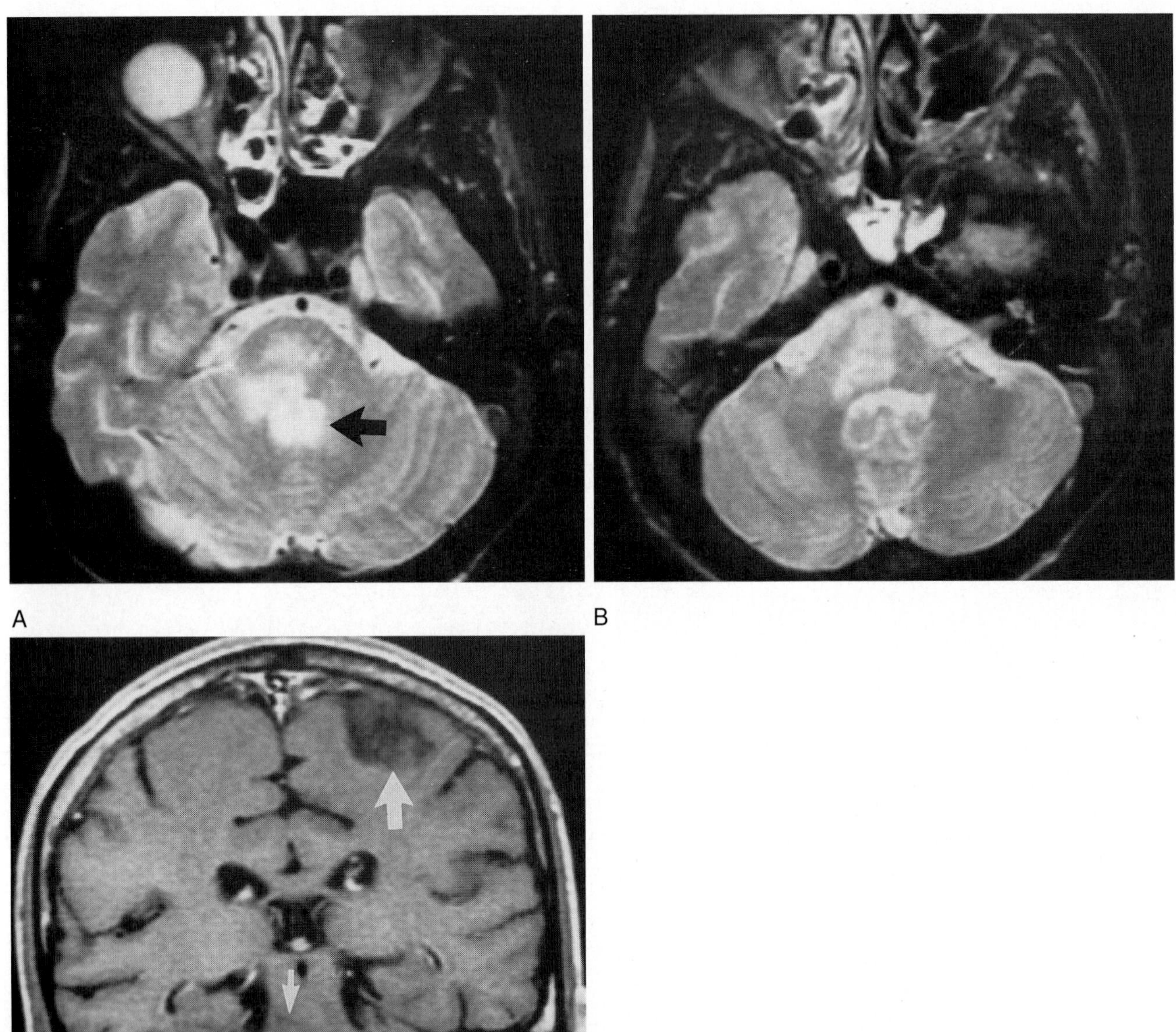

Figure 6.12. Toxoplasmosis in a 33-year-old man with AIDS. **A.** T2-weighted image shows a hyperintense area in the pons adjacent to the fourth ventricle. The fourth ventricle is shown by the black arrow. **B.** A lower section reveals that the hyperintensity extends further caudad. **C.** A postcontrast T1-weighted coronal image reveals a ringlike lesion in the pons surrounded by an ill-defined hypointense area (arrows), indicating that most of the findings on A and B are due to edema. Another lesion is present in the left parasagittal region (upper arrow).

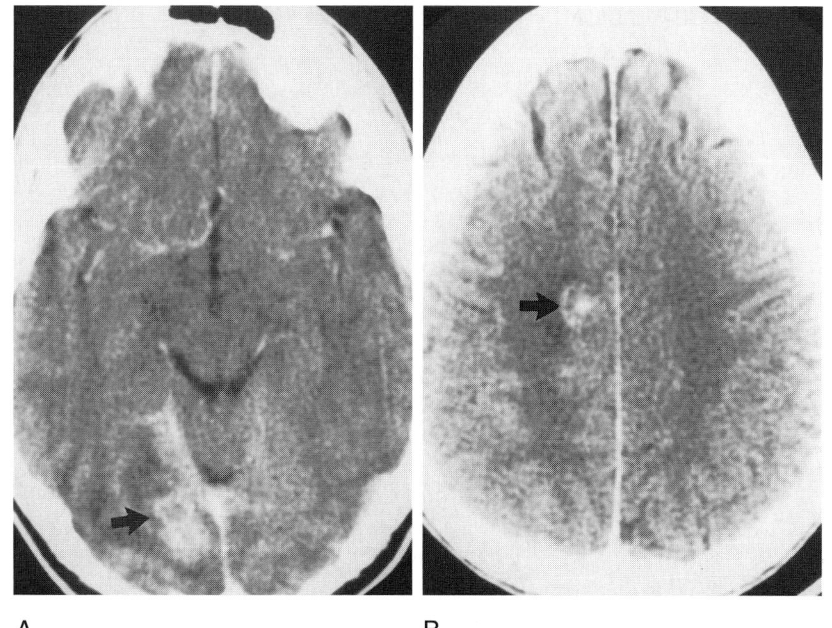

Figure 6.13. Toxoplasmosis in a patient with AIDS. **A** and **B.** Typical ring lesions seen on postcontrast CT. **C** and **D.** Reexamination 2 weeks later showed no evidence of a lesion following appropriate therapy. **E** to **H.** *Nocardia* infection in a patient with AIDS. **E.** A swelling at the top of the head was noted that on MRI examination was found to be a lesion arising in the bone and producing a subperiosteal abscess, well shown on the contrast-enhanced T1-weighted sagittal view. **F.** The T1-weighted postcontrast coronal section revealed enhancement of meninges on each side of the midline (arrows). **G.** A flow sequence was carried out that revealed absence of flow in the superior sagittal sinus (white arrow). All of the flowing vessels are bright on the image. Surface veins are well seen, and the lateral sinuses are bright bilaterally. **H.** An axial proton density image shows other lesions in the basal ganglia bilaterally. This location is common in toxoplasmosis, and a mixed infection (nocardiosis and toxoplasmosis) may well exist. This is a common problem when treating patients with AIDS. The same is often true when lymphoma in an AIDS patient is suspected. Biopsy may be required for diagnosis.

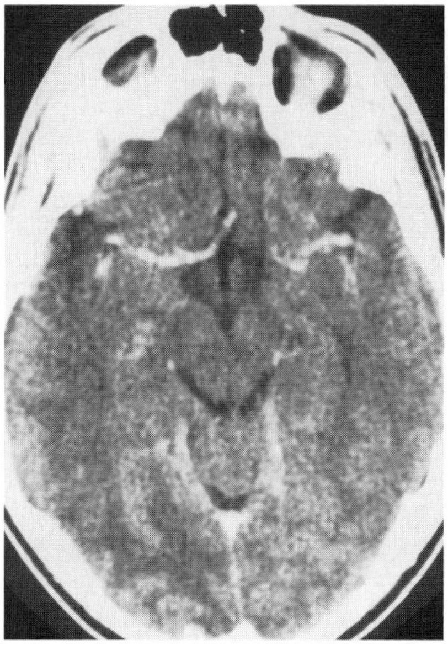

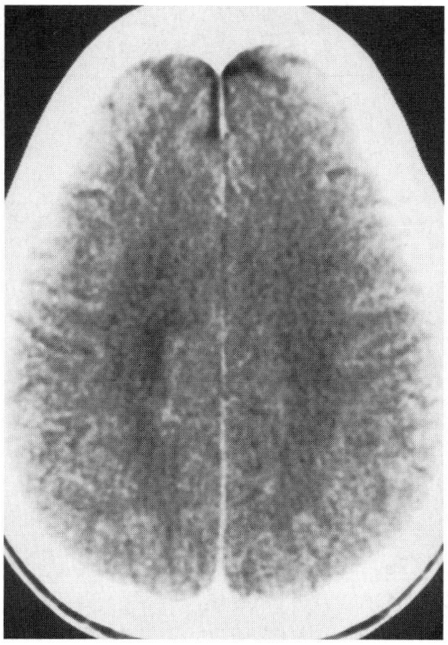

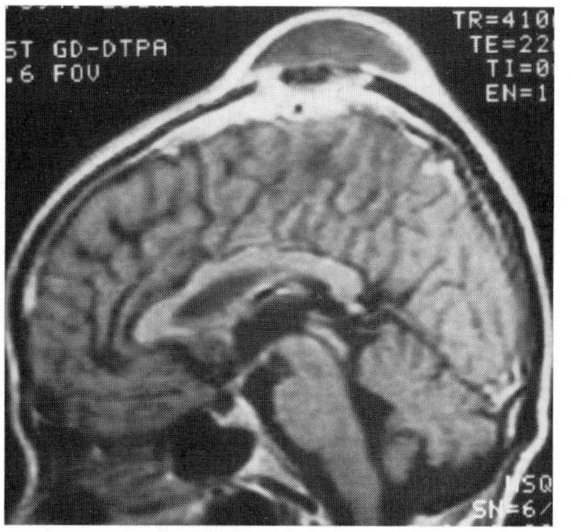

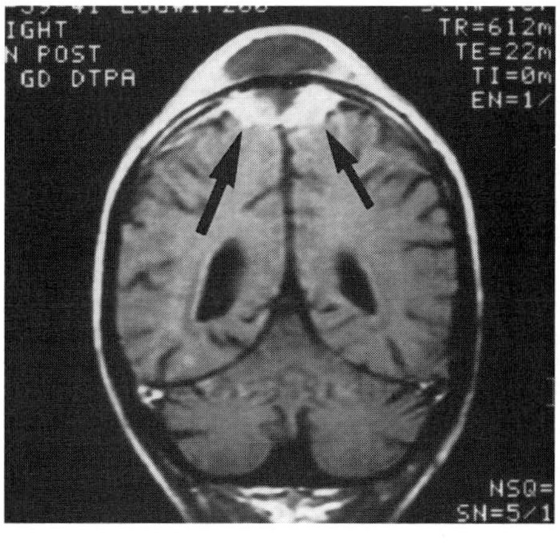

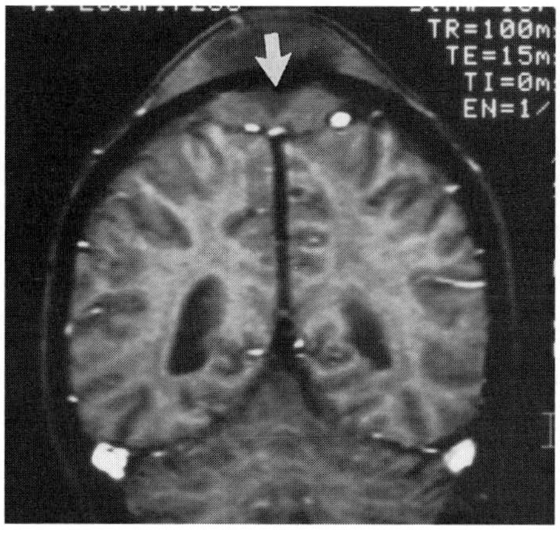

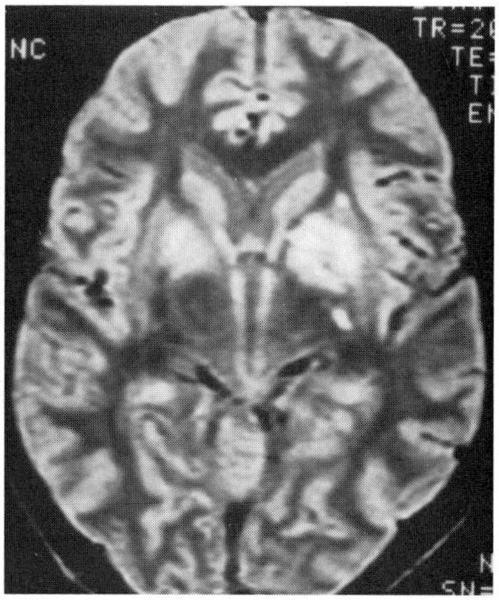

these cases, if treatment appropriate for toxoplasmosis is applied, some lesions may improve while others do not.

Bacterial infections, in addition to tuberculosis, include nocardial abscess, which produces a ring-enhancing lesion indistinguishable from other opportunistic infections in AIDS patients. Bacterial infections in AIDS patients are more common outside the nervous system. *Escherichia coli* meningitis is uncommon.

Viral infections are more common than bacterial infections in HIV patients. These include cytomegalovirus (CMV), which may also produce a diffuse encephalitis superimposed on the HIV infection.

Herpes simplex 1 and 2 viruses may also infect AIDS patients. *Aseptic meningitis* has been attributed to viral infection (herpes simplex, cytomegalovirus, Epstein-Barr virus). The HIV virus can also produce meningitis.

PROGRESSIVE MULTIFOCAL LEUKOENCEPHALOPATHY (PML)

Perhaps the most important viral complication involves the papovavirus, which produces *progressive multifocal leukoencephalopathy* (PML).

Originally described by Aström et al. (36) and Richardson (37), PML is a demyelinating condition occurring in immunocompromised individuals either secondary to some debilitating disease (such as AIDS) or because of long-term immunosuppressive therapy. Today the most frequent association is with the HIV virus. It is produced by one of the papovaviruses, the polyomavirus, JC type (named after the first patient in whom it was identified). This is a latent infection by a *slow virus* that becomes reactivated. It is estimated that 50 percent of all people are carriers of the slow virus by age 6 and 80 percent or more by middle adulthood (38). The pathogenesis of central nervous system infection in PML is not well understood. The most plausible is via the bloodstream, possibly through infected B lymphocytes (39). About 4 percent of patients with AIDS develop PML.

The lesions in PML usually involve the white matter of the hemispheres, and this distribution is ordinarily used to suggest the diagnosis when seen on CT or MRI. The changes (low attenuation on CT, low intensity on T1-weighted images, and high intensity on first- and second-echo T2-weighted images) usually start in one area of the brain and extend into the white matter of the convolutions

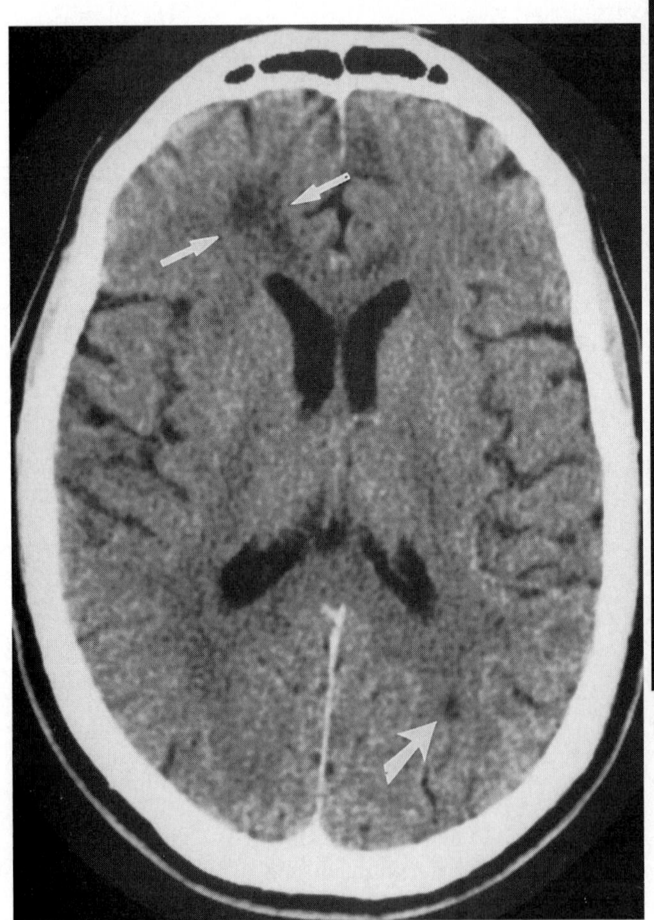

A

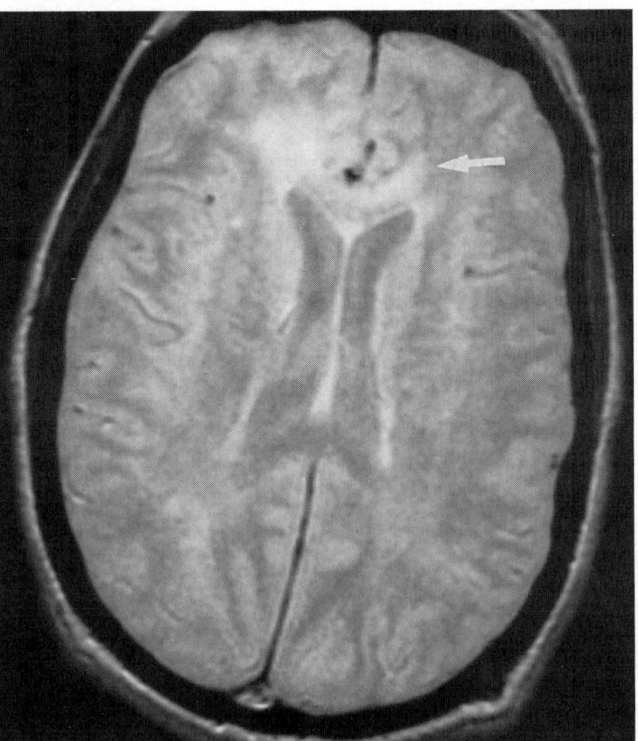

B

Figure 6.14. Progressive multifocal leukoencephalopathy (PML) in a patient with AIDS. **A.** CT image shows an area of decreased density in the right frontal white matter (arrows) that did not enhance after contrast. A tiny area of decreased density is seen in the left occipital region (single arrow). **B.** Proton density MR image shows the frontal lesion, which also extends to involve the corpus callosum and involves the opposite side (arrow). The section is above the level shown in A and does not show the occipital lesion. The two lesions did not enhance after contrast.

(Fig. 6.14). They may involve the corpus callosum, the internal capsule, the basal ganglia, and the brainstem. When they are seen in more than one area (in the right clinical setting), the diagnosis becomes almost certain (Fig. 6.14). No additional edema is associated with the changes, and thus there is usually no suggestion of a mass effect. In addition, there is no contrast enhancement MRI, although irregular ring-like enhancement has been reported (40, 41). Although ordinarily there is no mass effect, a small mass may be found at times. The same is true with gray matter involvement, which is sometimes seen on T2-weighted images. In atypical cases, brain biopsy is necessary for diagnosis. Contrast media enhancement should be used in any patient undergoing CT or MRI examination who is known to be HIV positive (42).

Cryptococcosis is found in about 5 percent of AIDS patients. *Cryptococcus neoformans* is the most common fungal disease affecting the nervous system. In a report of 35 cases, Popovich et al. reported that 43 percent had a negative CT finding (43). Of the rest, diffuse atrophy was seen in 34 percent, mass lesions (cryptococcoma) in 11 percent, hydrocephalus in 9 percent, and diffuse cerebral edema in 3 percent. All findings were nonspecific. MRI may add further information. In the basal ganglia, cryptococcus infection may show multiple small areas that are bright on T2-weighted images; these are considered characteristic (see discussion following of fungal infections) (Table 6.3).

BACTERIAL INFECTIONS

Brain Abscess

Brain abscesses may be produced by pyogenic bacteria, which were once the most common etiology. Fungal infection and toxoplasmosis may also produce abscesses or ring-enhancing lesions similar to abscesses.

A brain abscess is preceded by a local inflammatory process or cerebritis, which is later followed by necrosis and the formation of a typical abscess cavity. The abscess location may relate to the sinuses or mastoids (frontal, temporal, cerebellar), or it may be located anywhere in the brain if the abscess resulted from a hematogenous spread. Necrosis may occur relatively rapidly after the beginning of cerebritis (2 weeks) or may take a few to several months.

The pathogenic organism may be a staphylococcus, streptococcus, or pneumococcus. In abscesses complicating head trauma and in postoperative abscesses, *Staphylococcus aureus* is the most frequent pathogen. Anaerobic bacteria (or a mixture of anaerobic and aerobic) seem to be more common in abscesses arising from hematogenous spread (44). Recently, the most common underlying etiology of brain abscess is the AIDS infection, usually produced by toxoplasmosis and occasionally fungus infection or bacterial abscesses. *Listeria monocytogenes* infection should be kept in mind, particularly in patients who present no fever. This agent can produce long-term infections—8 years in a case reported in the *New England Journal of Medicine* (45).

The diagnosis of brain abscess is usually made by cross-sectional imaging, CT or MRI. Clinically the diagnosis may be suspected on the basis of the history and clinical findings, but there is such variability in the presentation and course that it is not possible to go beyond a suggestion of the possibility as part of a differential diagnosis. Commonly the patient presents only relatively mild temperature elevation, may or may not have headaches, and may or may not have any neurologic symptoms or signs that can be elicited. Thus the CT or MRI examination becomes crucial.

On CT, the appearance is that of an area of decreased attenuation produced by the cerebritis or the abscess and the accompanying edema. There is usually a mass effect, and ventricular compression or displacement of the midline structures to the opposite side may be present. Intravenous contrast usually demonstrates ring enhancement due to the loss of a blood-brain barrier in the area of the capsule of the abscess (Figs. 6.15 and 6.16). The area of necrosis and the surrounding edema do not enhance (Fig. 6.17). Abscesses can be multiple and frequently are located in the same area. The presence of scattered abscesses suggests a hematogenous infection that may be associated with endocarditis or with congenital cyanotic heart disease and intravenous drug abuse. However, the septic emboli from the heart may lodge in small arteries, which undergo changes leading to mycotic aneurysm formation. In that case, it is more common to have rupture of the aneurysm and intracerebral hemorrhage than brain abscess (Figs 6.18 and 6.44). In patients with AIDS, multiple abscesses are far more commonly due to toxoplasmosis than to pyogenic bacteria. MRI usually demonstrates hyperintensity on T2-weighted images due to the abscess itself and to the surrounding edema. Gadolinium contrast enhancement shows ring enhancement in the necrotic stage similar to CT. The T2-weighted image may show the outline of the abscess wall, which appears darker than the edema or the necrotic area. This dark appearance of the ring is attributed to the presence of paramagnetic free radicals within macrophages

Table 6.3.
AIDS-Related CNS Infections

Toxoplasmosis: Multiple ring-enhancing lesions with surrounding edema.

HIV encephalitis: Direct infection by HIV virus, resulting in diffuse white matter hypodensity on CT and hyperintense signal on T2-weighted MRI.

Cytomegalovirus: Meningoencephalitis. MRI findings of periventricular white matter hyperintensity on T2-weighted images.

Cryptococcosis: Usually produces a meninigitis, but focal cryptococcomas can be seen. Masslike collections at site of perivascular spaces at base of brain are characteristic.

Progressive multifocal leukoencephalopathy: Papovavirus related. Demyelinating process commonly involving posterior centrum semiovale. Typically nonenhancing and no mass effect.

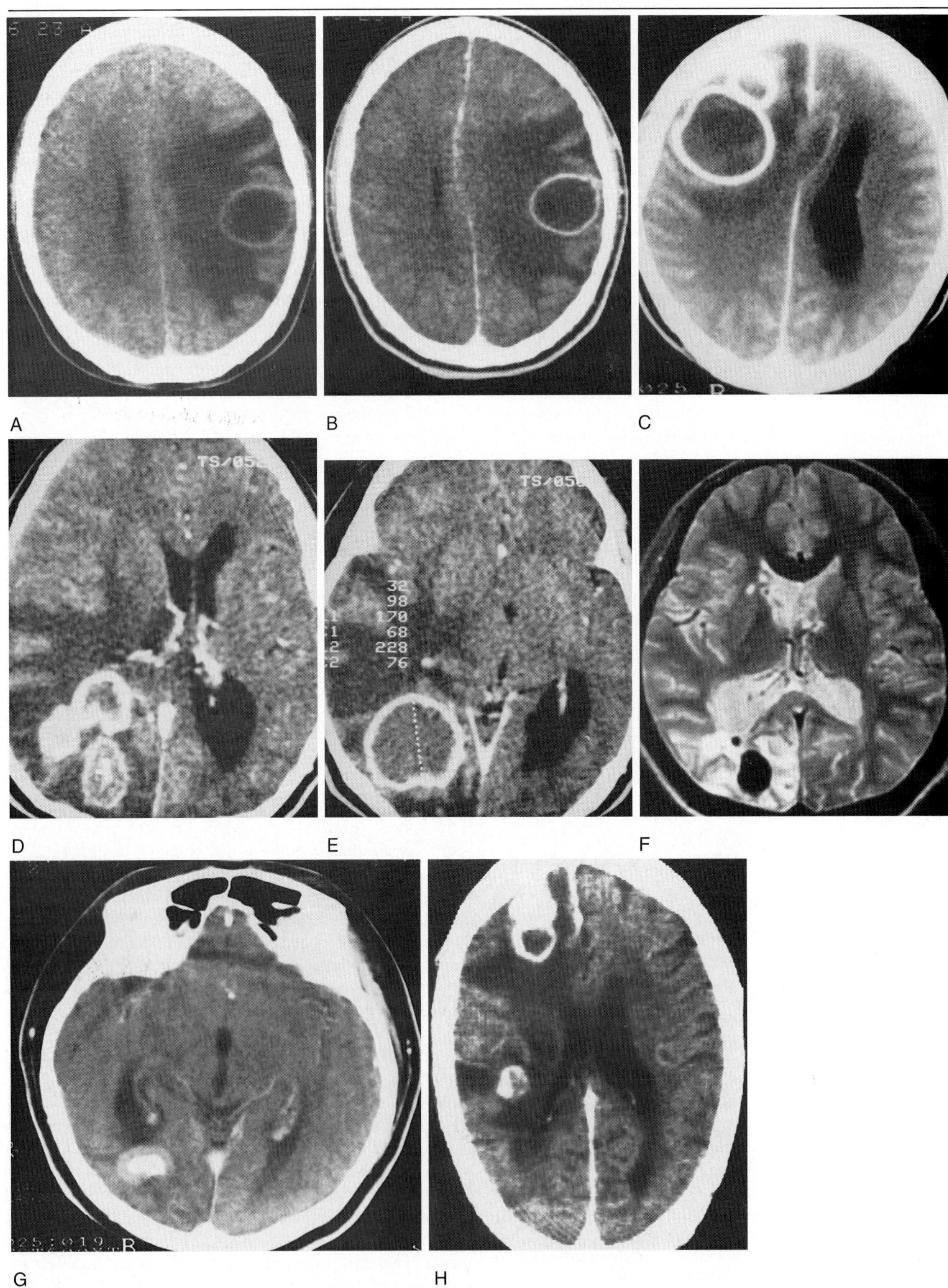
A
B
C
TS/052
D
TS/058
32
98
170
68
228
76
E
F
G
H

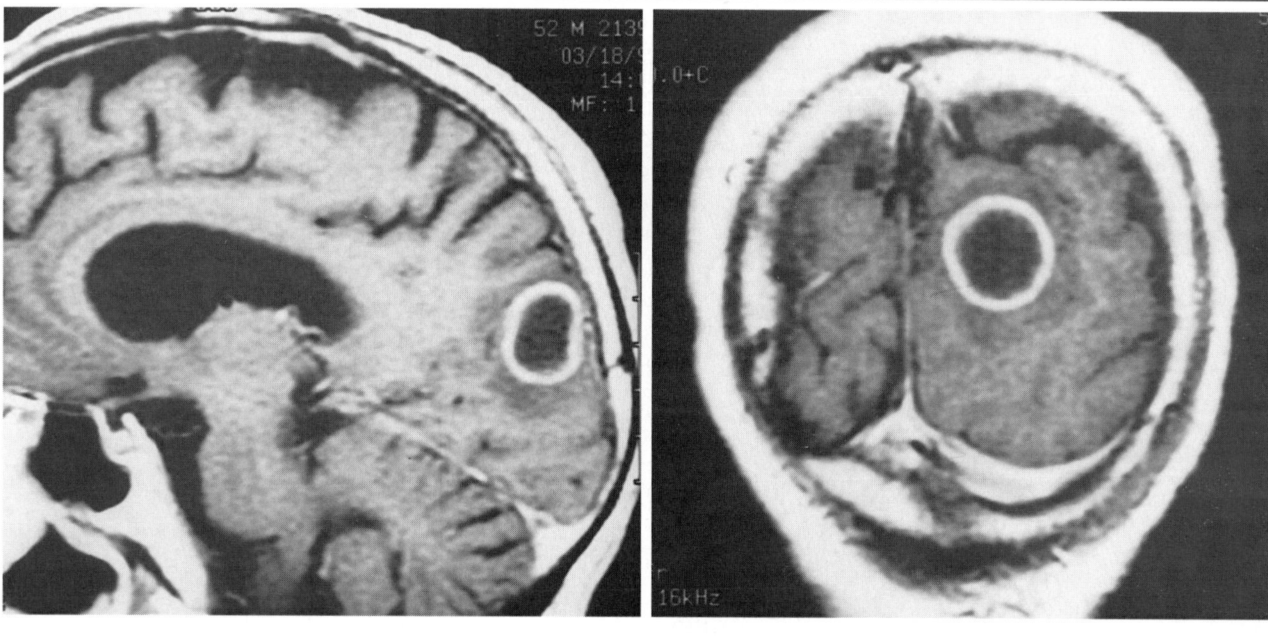

A B

Figure 6.16. Brain abscess. **A** and **B.** Postcontrast T1-weighted images in sagittal (**A**) and coronal views (**B**) show a ring-enhancing lesion surrounded by a halo of hypointensity consistent with surrounding edema. The ring itself has no sugggestion of a mass on the inner aspect of the ring, which might suggest a necrotic tumor. The appearance is consistent with a pyogenic abscess.

in the wall of the cyst (Fig. 6.17). On T1-weighted images the rim may be hyperintense; this suggests some hemorrhage but may also be related to the same phenomenon of free paramagnetic radicals within macrophages (46).

The abscess wall may be thicker on the lateral than on the medial aspect. In general, brain abscesses tend to occur at the gray/white matter junction and most commonly in the frontal and parietal lobes. The cerebellum is less commonly invoked (up to 10 percent of all brain abscesses). Toxoplasmosis abscesses in AIDS patients occur frequently in the thalamic region (Fig. 6.11) (Table 6.4).

The mycotic aneurysms usually occur in distal arteries and may be detected or, rather, suspected on contrast-enhanced CT or MRI, but they require a cerebral angiogram for final diagnosis. However, the presence of an intracerebral hemorrhage or a combination of subarachnoid and intracerebral hemorrhage in a patient at risk is strongly suggestive of a possible mycotic aneurysm (Figs. 6.18 and 6.44).

Figure 6.15. Images of brain abscesses, five cases. **A** and **B.** Pyogenic abscess of fairly recent development. **A.** Before contrast. **B.** After contrast injection. The capsule is fairly thin. Compare with a postcontrast CT of an older abscess (**C**). Note a smaller abscess cavity above. **D.** Multilocular abscess cavity. **E.** A lower-level section image reveals a single abscess cavity. **F.** MR axial proton density image taken 1 year after D and E shows a very hypointense oval area surrounded by edema. The hypointensity is seen in tuberculomas (see text). **G.** Reexamination 3 years later showed that one of the abscesses is now calcified. **H.** Multiple abscesses due to nocardia infection. (Courtesy of Drs. Jesus Taboada and Alvaro Zuluaga, Mexico City.)

Meningitis

Inflammation of the meninges may be the result of viral pyogenic organisms, tuberculosis, or fungal or protozoan infection. Viral meningitis is difficult to diagnose unless it is possible to culture the virus; the cellular response in the CSF is apt to be mild, and CT or MRI examination is usually normal. The infection tends to disappear spontaneously. The mumps virus is a common cause. Enteroviruses may also be found, particularly in epidemics (1). As to bacteria, in the infant *E. coli* infection is more frequent; in

Table 6.4.
Pyogenic Abscess

Most common responsible organisms are staphylococcus, streptococcus, and pneumococcus.
Initial infection is ill-defined cerebritis.
Progressive organization of abscess capsule by ingress of fibroblasts at periphery of infection.
End result is well-defined focus that typically has ring enhancement after CT or MRI contrast administration.
Similarities with metastases:
- Both preferentially occur at corticomedullary junction.
- Both are ring enhancing.

Features distinguishing abscess from metastases:
- Satellite ("daughter") lesions.
- Smooth inner margin of enhancing rim.
- Occasionally hypointense rim on T2-weighted MRI.
- Often slightly thicker lateral aspect of enhancing rim.

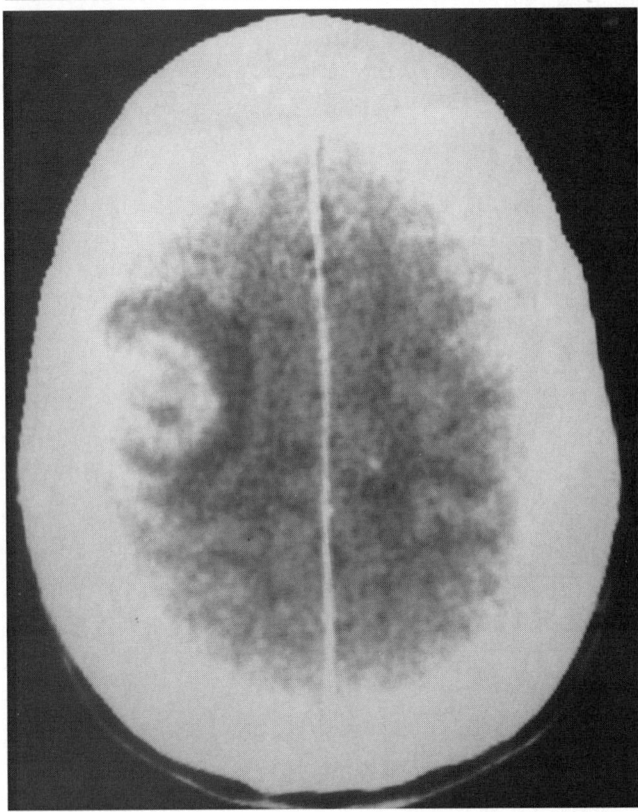

A

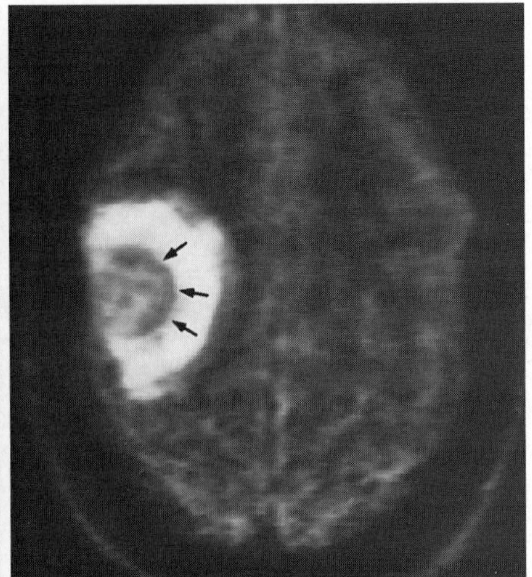

B

Figure 6.17. Cerebral abscess showing a dark rim on a T2-weighted image. **A.** Postcontrast CT scan shows the abscess surrounded by a halo of diminished density due to edema. **B.** The T2-weighted image shows a dark rim at the abscess wall (small arrows), surrounded by a hyperintense margin representing edema. The "T2-dark" border is felt to be due to the presence of paramagnetic free radicals within macrophages.

children, *Haemophilus influenzae* is most frequent; and in the adult, meningococcus and pneumococcus infections are most frequent.

Pathologic organisms reach the leptomeninges more frequently via the bloodstream, but the infection may enter via the adjacent paranasal sinuses and mastoids or by way of a penetrating injury. CSF rhinorrhea, caused by an opening of the dura matter connecting with the sinuses or mastoid, is an important route of infection. Meningitis complicating surgical procedures is another important route. Neurosurgeons fear the occurrence of infection with *Pseudomonas aeruginosa.*

Infection in the meninges can progress and spread rapidly partly because the arachnoid membrane has few capillaries. The pia allows for passage of abundant leukocytes, but the arachnoid does not, and the subarachnoid space is avascular. In the acute stage, there is marked congestion of the cortical layer; soon thereafter pus is produced in the subarachnoid space, tiny cortical abscesses develop, and some surface blood vessels may undergo fibrinoid necrosis and thrombosis. The vascular thrombosis leads to small cortical infarcts (Fig. 6.25). The infection, when severe, spreads to the ependymal surface of the ventricles. This progression is particularly frequent in neonatal meningitis, but it is not common in the less severe meningeal infections. The ventriculitis leads to ventricular enlargement (hydrocephalus) as it involves the outlets of the third and fourth ventricles. Adhesions develop in the ventricular wall leading to isolation of portions of the ventricular system. Adhesions in the subarachnoid space develop but are not very effective in limiting the spread of infection. Obliteration of the subarachnoid space occurs in the chronic stage, but in spite of them, CSF generally circulates in the supratentorial space. However, when the adhesive process involves certain crucial areas, such as the basal meninges (chronic basal adhesive arachnoiditis), the region of the incisura, or the suprasellar area, the CSF cannot pass to the supratentorial space and severe hydrocephalus results (see the discussion of hydrocephalus in Chapter 4).

Larger cortical abscesses and necrotic areas may develop. The infection may spread into the subdural space, although this is rare. Much more common is the development of subdural collections or effusions that are not pyogenic. The subdural effusions are particularly common in *H. influenzae* meningitis occurring in children. The pathogenesis of these effusions is interesting in that, at least in some cases, the fluid comes from the bloodstream, as has been demonstrated by tagging the blood with a radionuclide and recovering the radioactivity in the subdural fluid (47) (Table 6.5).

IMAGING IN MENINGITIS

CT may not demonstrate any abnormality except perhaps in more severe cases or where there is involvement of the

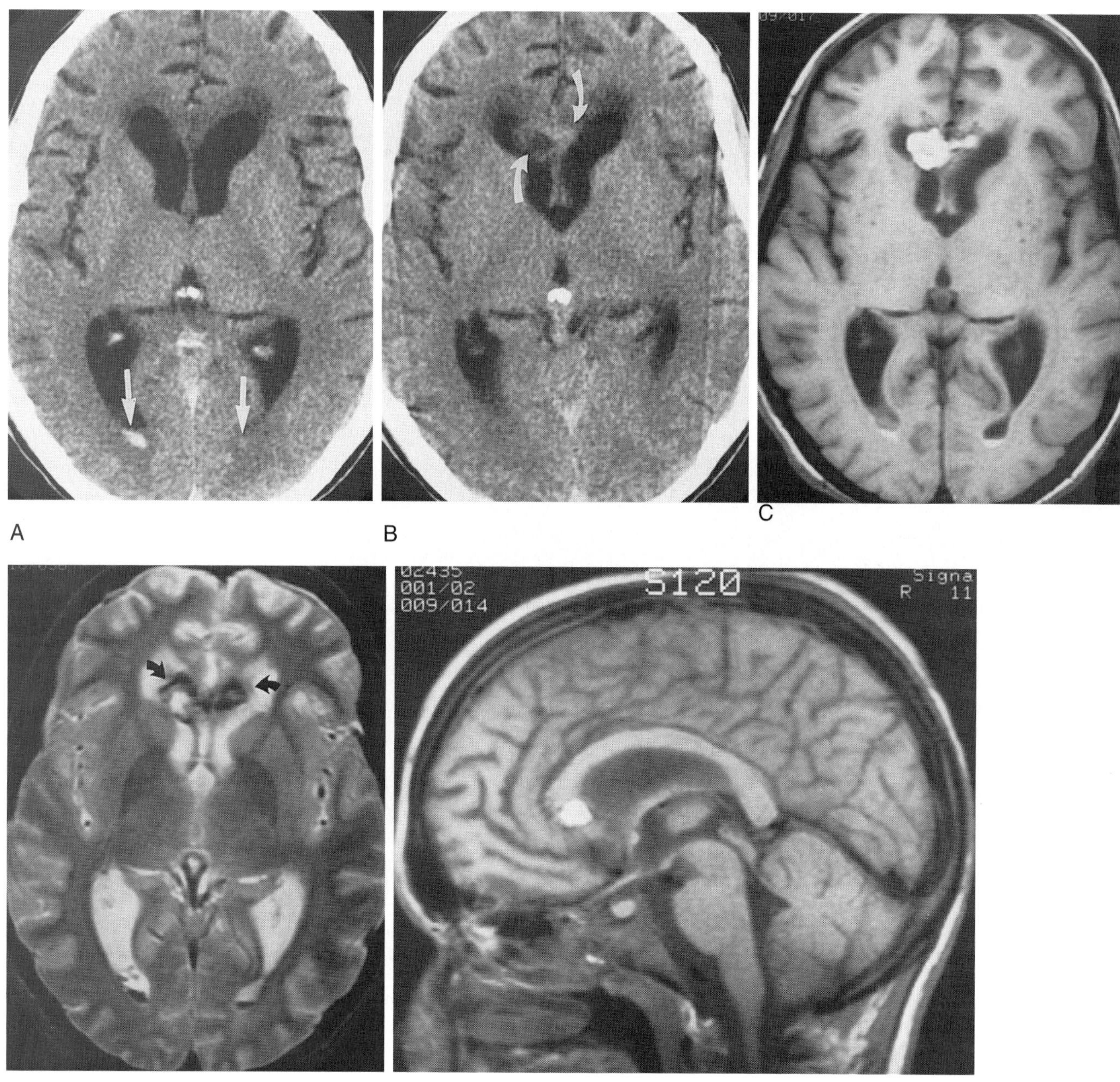

Figure 6.18. Bleeding aneurysm in a 15-year-old boy with fulminating meningococcemia. **A.** CT image shows a blood-CSF fluid level in the lateral ventricles (arrows). **B.** A slightly higher section reveals an area of decreased density surrounded by an irregular area of increased density in the frontal region (curved arrows), probably representing subacute blood. **C.** T1-weighted axial image shows a bright area in the same location as in B with extension to the left of the midline felt to represent methemoglobin. **D.** T2-weighted axial image reveals hyperintensity in a small area to the right that may represent methemoglobin (arrow). The area is surrounded by a dark halo on both sides of the midline representing older blood products (arrows) and indicating that bleeding had occurred, probably on more than one occasion. **E.** The sagittal T1-weighted image reveals the location of the hemorrhage, which was caused by rupture of an anterior cerebral artery aneurysm.

Meningitis in a 57-year-old man who presented with a defect in the posterior wall of the frontal sinuses and also had evidence of mastoid disease. (*continues*)

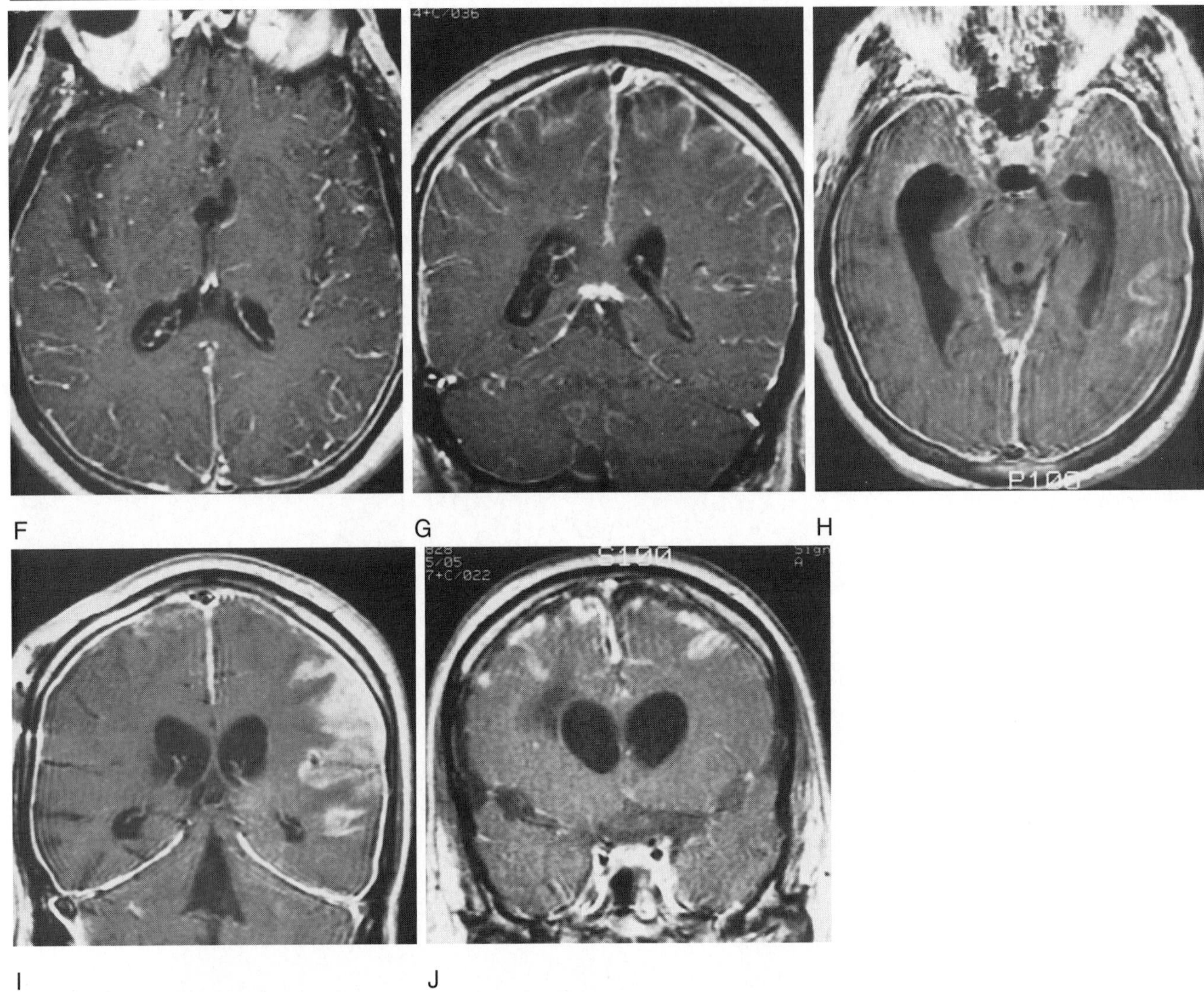

Figure 6.18. *(continued)* **F** and **G.** T1-weighted postcontrast axial (**F**) and coronal (**G**) views demonstrate diffuse enhancement of the leptomeninges; the enhancement penetrates into the intergyral sulci and the sylvian fissure. **H** and **I.** Four months later, reexamination shows uniform dural enhancement around the brain and in the falx and tentorium; the leptomeninges are not now enhancing. There is also extensive cortical enhancement in the left frontotemporal area, as well as in parasagittal areas bilaterally (**J**), which may represent cortical infarcts due to venous thrombosis and fibrinoid necrosis of cortical blood vessels. There is also moderate hydrocephalus.

suprasellar region or of the meninges around the tentorium. In more severe cases without enhancement, there may be widening of the interhemispheric fissure. With enhancement no abnormality may be observed on the brain surface because the increased density in the conical areas may be obscured by the bone. Only if the suprasellar area shows abnormalities or there is enhancement following intravenous contrast of the tentorial surface or sometimes around the belli of the pons on axial views can meningitis be suspected on CT studies. On the other hand, gadolinium-enhanced MRI may show enhancement of the meningeal surface much more clearly and in any location (Figs. 6.18 to 6.20) (48).

Ventriculitis or *ependymitis* may be seen if there is ventricular wall enhancement on CT or MRI (Fig. 6.21). Without intravenous contrast, no abnormalities are usually seen except for ventricular dilatation, but MRI may show a T2 dark outline of the ventricle and a T1 slightly hyperintense ventricular margin without gadolinium (Fig. 6.21).

In addition to the ependyma, the entire CSF within the ventricle may enhance, probably because of intraventricular cellular and inflammatory debris and extravasation of contrast through the inflamed ependyma (49). Ultrasound in infants demonstrates ventricular dilatation and increased periventricular echogenicity (50). Multiloculated hydrocephalus may result from the formation of bands and septae; this condition requires surgical management (51).

Subdural collections present a typical picture on CT or MRI. The fluid is proteinacious and may be relatively

Table 6.5
Infectious and Inflammatory Meningeal Processes

Meningitis
- Viral: Most common cause of meningitis.
- Bacterial: Pneumococcus and meningococcus are common causes in adults; *Escherichia coli* in infants.
- Fungal infections
  - Coccidioidomycosis: Predominantly basilar meningitis, extending to upper cervical region.
  - Aspergillosis: Meningitis, abscess, and granuloma formation.
  - Cryptococcosis: Meningitis may be accompaned by extension into Virchow-Robin spaces and development of parenchymal cryptococcomas.
  - Mucormycosis: Most common in diabetes, beginning as paranasal sinus infection, and osteomyelitis, often progressing to vascular thrombosis.
- Tuberculous: Thick exudates in basal cisterns are characteristic, which may progress to vascular thrombosis and infarction.
- Sequelae may include nondestructive hydrocephalus, ependymitis/ventriculitis, and (in bacterial meningitis) subdural empyema.

Neurosarcoidosis
- Granulomatous, involvement of leptomeninges.
- Predilection for surprasellar cistern, infundibulum, optic chiasm, and hypothalamic region.
- Parenchymal involvement may be seen, most commonly in the hypothalamus, adjacent to the Virchow-Robin spaces, and within white matter.

bright on T1-weighted images and irregularly darker on T2-weighted images if the protein content is very high. Follow-up of these effusions may show a difference in the intensity of the fluid, particularly if there has been some bleeding into the subdural space (Fig. 6.22).

More severe brain involvement, such as small cortical abscesses or infarcts, probably would be shown well by both imaging methods—as diminished attenuation on CT and as hyperintense sites on T2-weighted images (Fig. 6.22). Enhancement should be demonstrable with either method. Some of the cortical infarcts may be larger because of occlusion of some of the surface arteries. Infarcts secondary to venous thrombosis also occur and might be differentiated from arterial thromboses because the involved areas may not correspond to an arterial territory (Fig. 6.25).

SUBDURAL EMPYEMA

Subdural empyema should be considered a true neurosurgical emergency because the infection can progress with surprising speed, leading to thromboses and occlusion of surface veins, arteries, and dural venous sinuses. The reasons for the rapid progression are the smoothness of the subdural space, which allows for rapid movement of bacteria and pus, and the lack of capillaries in the arachnoid, so that the membrane becomes inflamed but yields relatively few leukocytes and does not easily form adhesions to localize the infection. The dura provides the granulation tissue and white blood cells. Antibiotics have little chance of reaching the space in sufficient concentration because of the relative avascularity. Wide surgical drainage is important in the management of this condition, which usually results from infection in the paranasal sinuses or mastoids, cranial osteomyelitis, or compound fractures of the skull.

Imaging may demonstrate the paranasal sinus infection while at the same time demonstrating the subdural collections. On CT the appearance is that of a thin, low-density subdural collection usually involving the midline on one or both sides of the falx cerebri as well as the

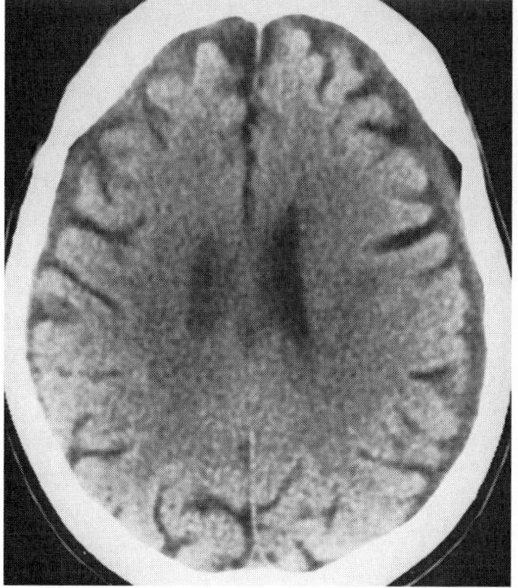
A

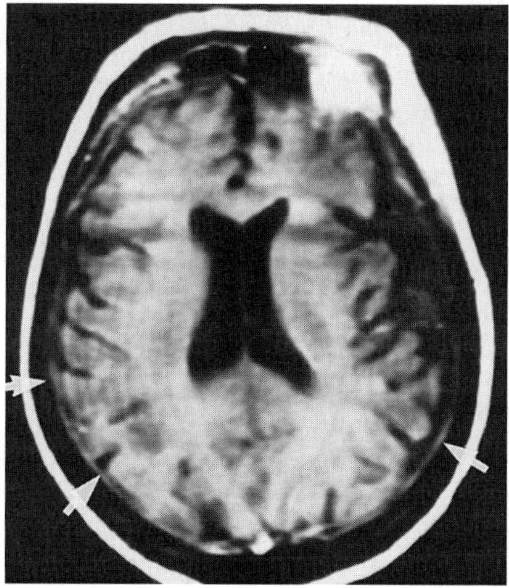
B

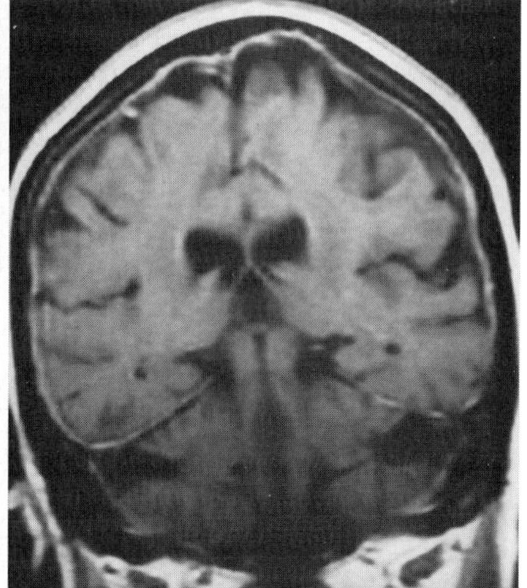
C

Figure 6.19. Meningitis in a 50-year-old man after renal transplant. **A.** CT scan shows an increase in the space between the brain cortex and the inner table of the skull. **B.** Postcontrast T1-weighted image shows meningeal enhancement around the brain (arrows). **C.** Coronal contrast-enhanced T1-weighted image reveals diffuse meningeal enhancement. The enhancement does not clearly go into any of the sulci, which may indicate that it is confined to the dura mater. There is also slight enhancement around the lateral ventricles that may be indicative of ependymitis.

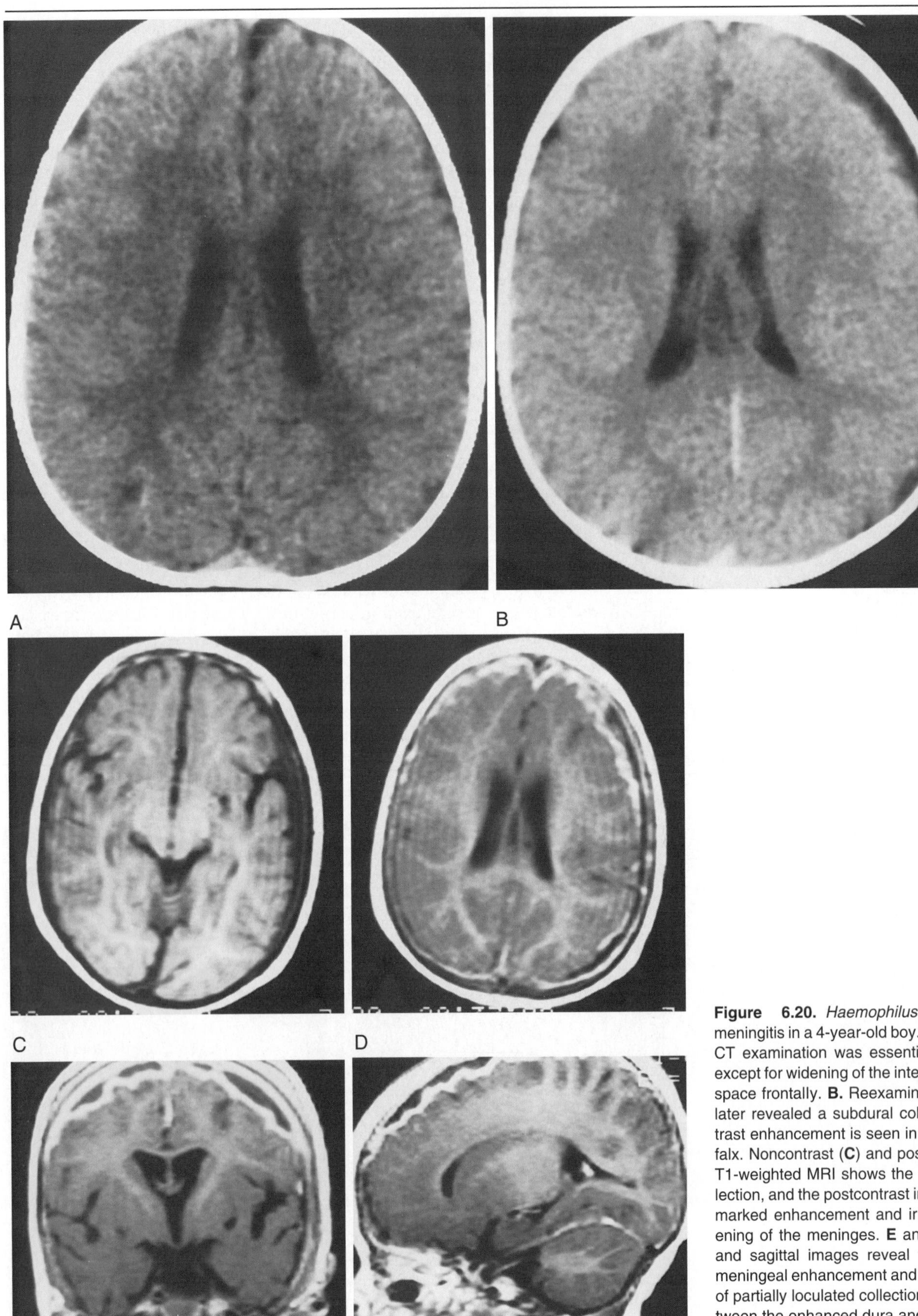

Figure 6.20. *Haemophilus influenzae* meningitis in a 4-year-old boy. **A.** The initial CT examination was essentially negative except for widening of the interhemispheric space frontally. **B.** Reexamination 1 week later revealed a subdural collection. Contrast enhancement is seen in the posterior falx. Noncontrast (**C**) and postcontrast (**D**) T1-weighted MRI shows the subdural collection, and the postcontrast image reveals marked enhancement and irregular thickening of the meninges. **E** and **F.** Coronal and sagittal images reveal the intensive meningeal enhancement and the presence of partially loculated collections of fluid between the enhanced dura and leptomeninges, which is a typical feature of *H. influenzae* meningitis.

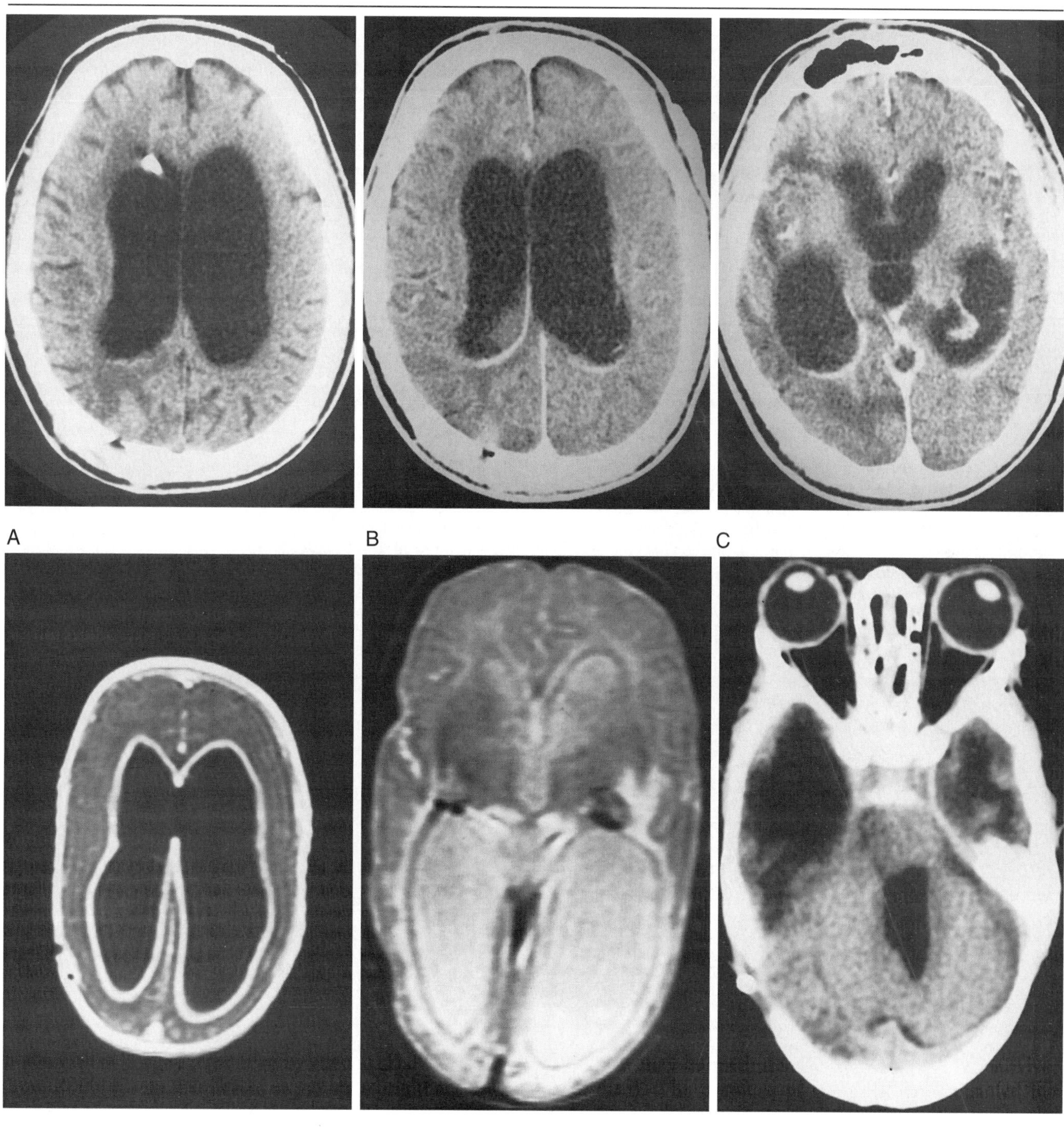

Figure 6.21. Ventriculitis (ependymitis) in a young man who had a shunting procedure and infection. **A.** Noncontrast CT scan shows dilated ventricles. A shunting tube is seen in the right ventricle. **B.** After contrast there is enhancement of the ependymal lining of the ventricles due to ependymitis. **C.** A lower section reveals that the enhancement of the ventricular lining extends to both temporal horns. Ependymitis often leads to ventricular obstruction and hydrocephalus with trapping of segments of the ventricles, which undergo considerable dilatation. This is particularly likely to occur in the temporal horns (see E and F). **D.** Ventriculitis in a young premature infant due to *Escherichia coli* infection. This postcontrast T1-weighted axial view shows marked enhancement of the ventricular wall. **E.** The axial proton density section reveals a low-intensity band corresponding to the enhanced ventricular wall on the T1-weighted image. **F.** CT scan a week later shows trapping of the right temporal horn and of the fourth ventricle. *E. coli* meningitis is usually a very severe infection leading rapidly to brain destruction.

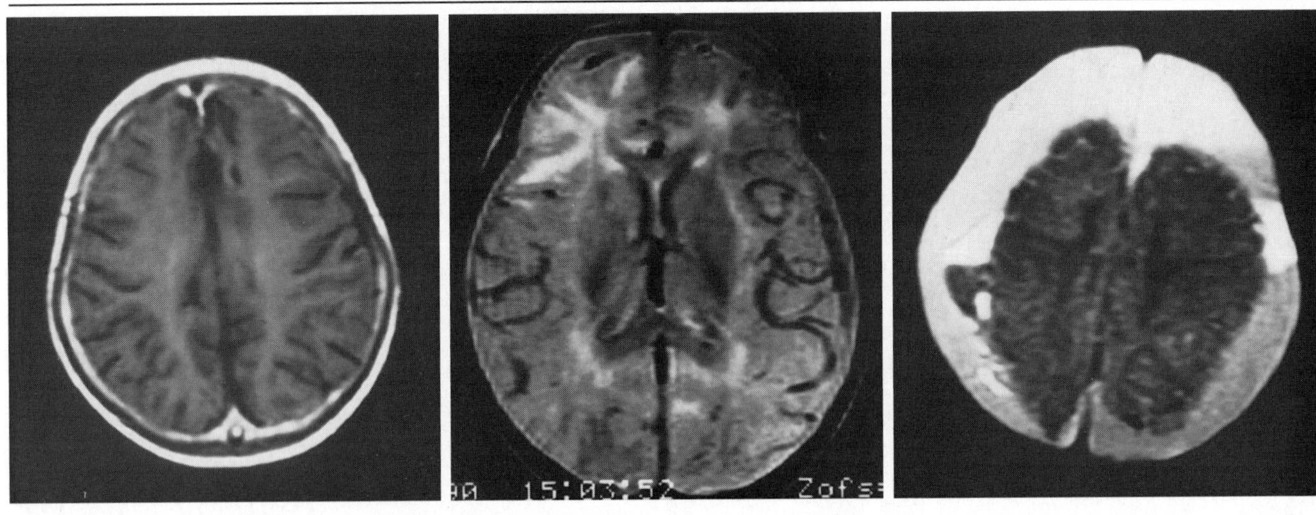

A B C

Figure 6.22. Pneumococcal meningitis in a 1-year-old girl. **A.** T1-weighted postcontrast image reveals meningeal enhancement. **B.** Axial proton density image reveals areas of subcortical edema, particularly in the frontal region. The edema is possibly due to small venous cortical thromboses, which are part of the pathology of meningitis. **C.** Large bilateral subdural collections developed. About 6 weeks after onset, the effusion was interesting in that there were different zones of brightness in this T2-weighted image, probably related to loculation and variations in the amount of protein in the fluid, and possibly to hemorrhage. By the fourth month the entire process was brought under control and the child recovered.

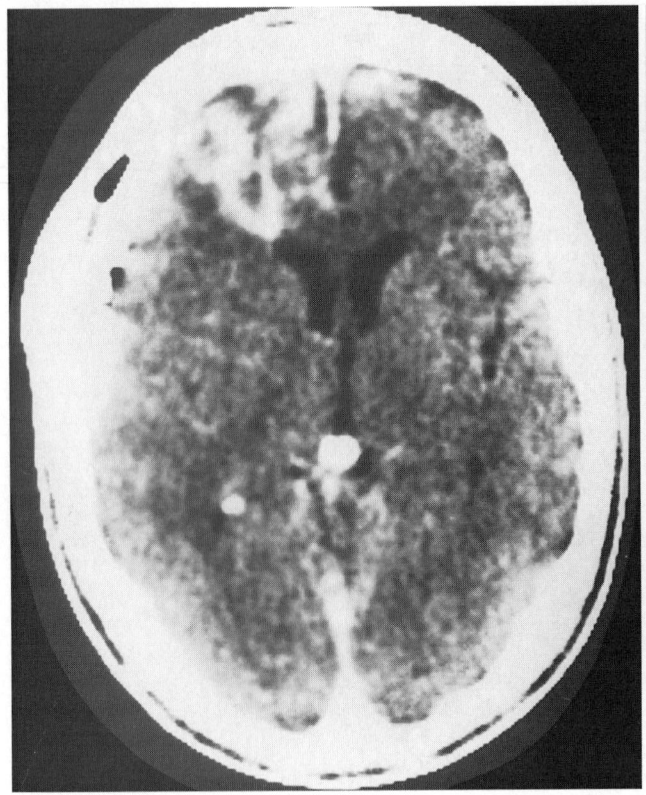

A

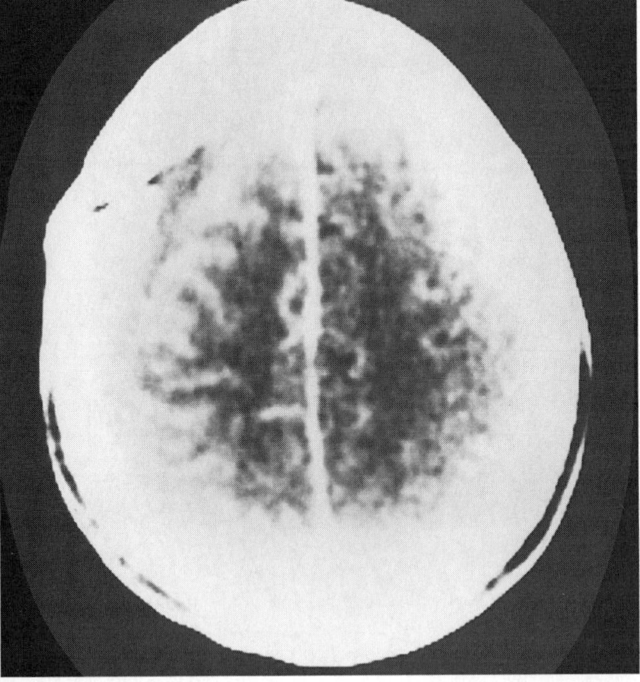

B

Figure 6.23. Subdural empyema in a patient with a frontal sinus–related infection. **A.** There is irregular contrast enhancement in the frontal region, particularly on the right side. As yet no abscess cavity is seen. **B.** An extracerebral collection is displacing the brain, and there is marked enhancement along the falx, representing extensive inflammation. The patient was rapidly becoming severely ill. In general, subdural collections associated with infection are considered emergencies because of the rapid progression of these infections, as explained in the text.

cortical surfaces and the tentorium (Fig. 6.23). Intravenous enhancement would show enhancement of the dura where it can be separated from the inner table of the skull (falx and tentorium). Edema of the cortical brain tissue is common and causes flattening of gyri and sulcal effacement on the brain surface. These changes are seen much better on MRI. Cortical infarcts due to venous and/or arterial thrombosis are easier to detect by MRI. The gradient-echo images may assist in detecting the venous occlusions. Gradient-echo flow sequences will

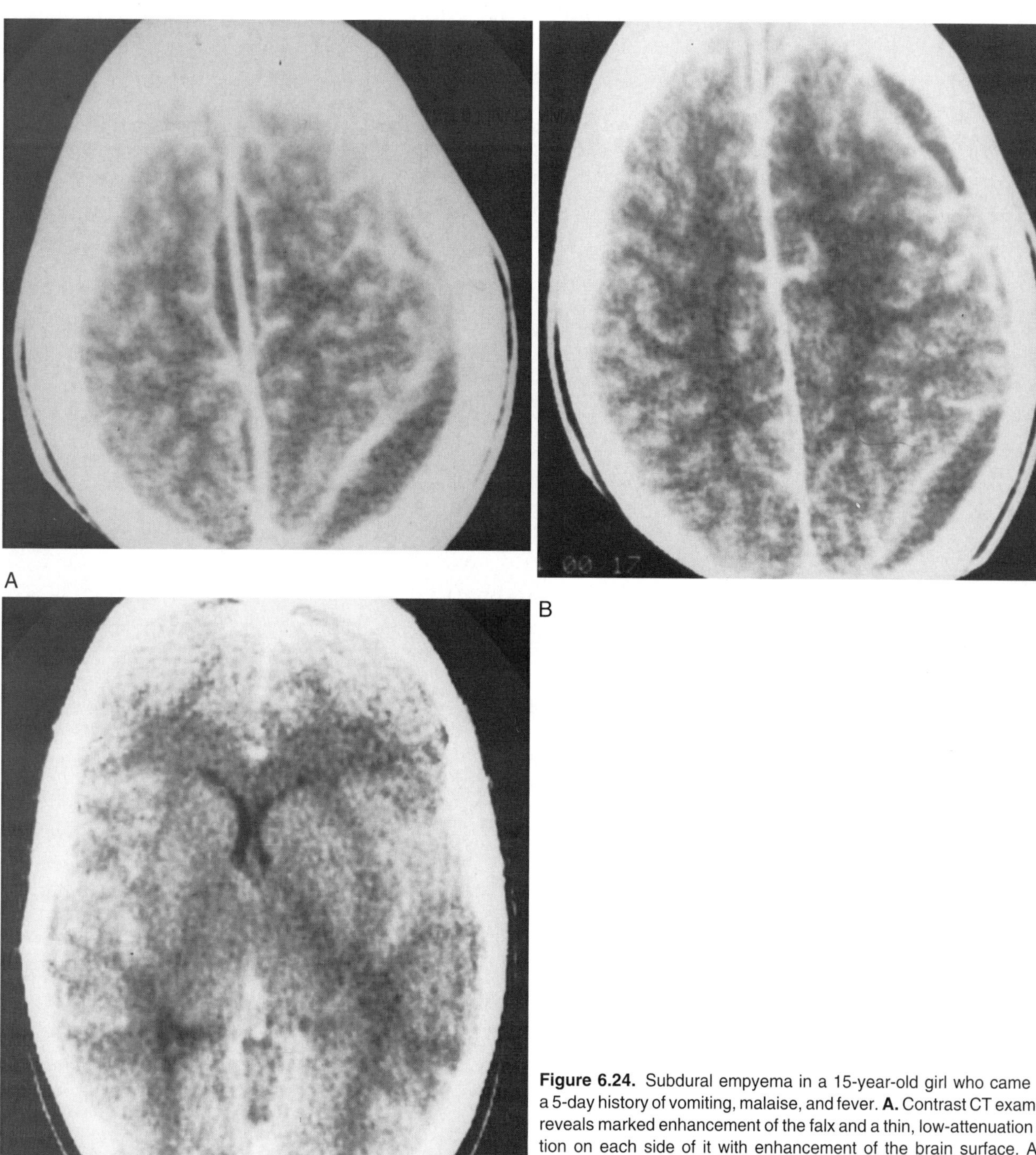

Figure 6.24. Subdural empyema in a 15-year-old girl who came in with a 5-day history of vomiting, malaise, and fever. **A.** Contrast CT examination reveals marked enhancement of the falx and a thin, low-attenuation collection on each side of it with enhancement of the brain surface. Another collection is seen in the left parieto-occipital area. **B.** Another subdural collection is seen in the left frontal region. **C.** Enhancement is also seen over the tentorium but with separate fluid collections. This appearance is almost pathognomonic for a subdural empyema and requires immediate surgical attention because of the rapidity with which the infection extends throughout the open, nonseptated subdural space.

demonstrate absent flow in the cortical veins or in the dural sinuses (52). In gradient recalled acquisition in the steady state (GRASS) sequence, possibly using a 150-ms TR and a 15-ms TE with a flip angle of 50°, the absent flow shows up dark and the flow within the vessel is bright (Fig. 6.13*E* to *H*). Zimmerman et al. (53) emphasized the intense enhancement of the dura and leptomeninges and the adjacent cortical brain as an important sign of subdural empyema (Figs. 6.23 and 6.24 [see page 287 for 6.24]).

Tuberculosis

Infection by *Mycobacterium tuberculosis* was an old common disease that decreased significantly in incidence following the development of antibiotic therapy. It has been increasing recently, partly because of incomplete therapy of existing cases, and also because of the increase in immunodeficiency states from various causes, including organ transplantation, treatment of certain malignant diseases, and AIDS.

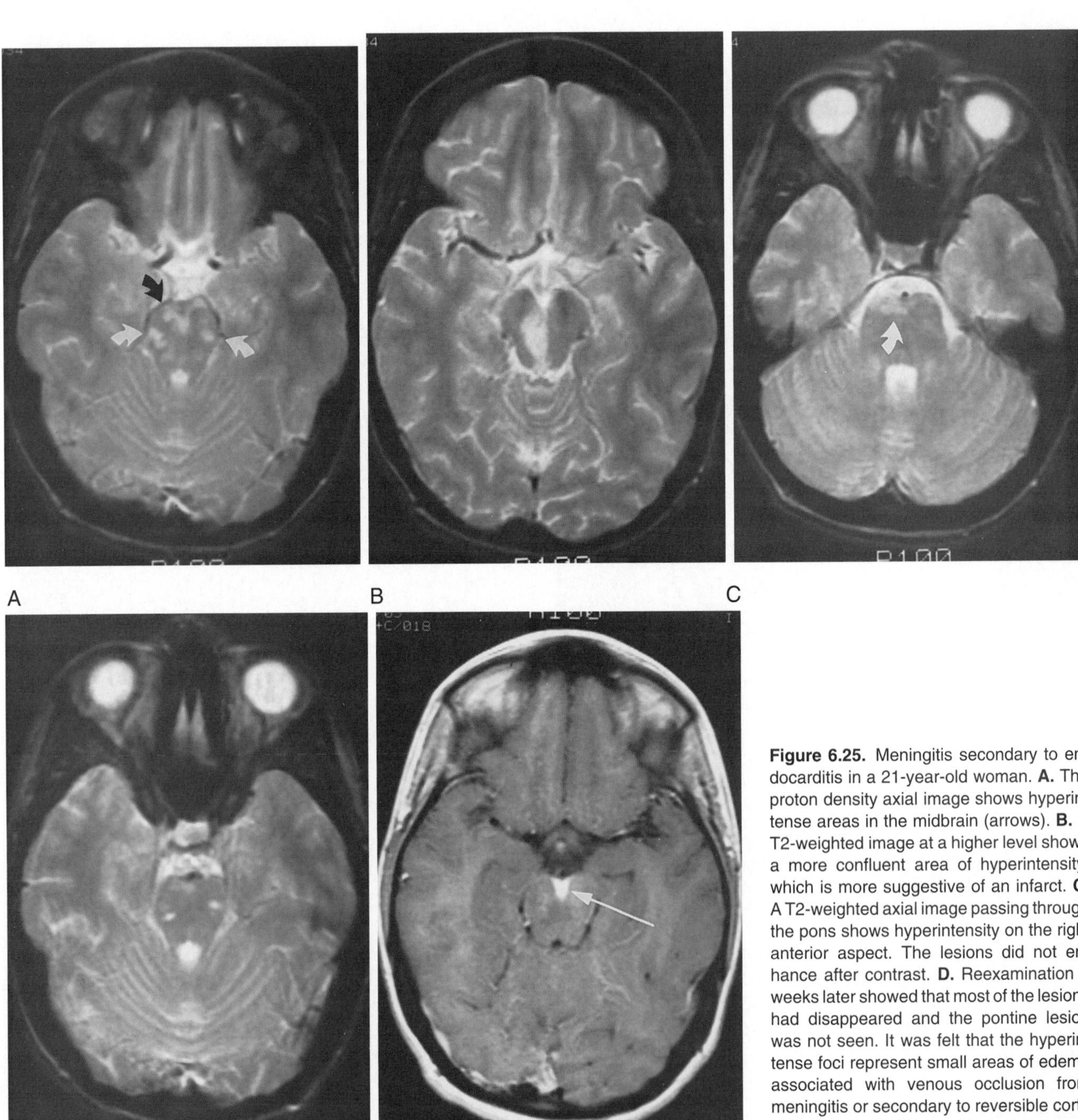

Figure 6.25. Meningitis secondary to endocarditis in a 21-year-old woman. **A.** The proton density axial image shows hyperintense areas in the midbrain (arrows). **B.** A T2-weighted image at a higher level shows a more confluent area of hyperintensity, which is more suggestive of an infarct. **C.** A T2-weighted axial image passing through the pons shows hyperintensity on the right anterior aspect. The lesions did not enhance after contrast. **D.** Reexamination 2 weeks later showed that most of the lesions had disappeared and the pontine lesion was not seen. It was felt that the hyperintense foci represent small areas of edema associated with venous occlusion from meningitis or secondary to reversible cortical ischemia. **E.** T1-weighted postcontrast axial image showed meningeal enhancement in the interpeduncular fossa (arrow).

Acute *tuberculous meningitis* is more frequent in children. It usually accompanied miliary tuberculosis, sometimes without miliary spread. In the United States it is uncommon, but in other countries it is much more common. The subacute type of tuberculous meningitis is seen more frequently in the adult and tends to occur more heavily in the basal cisterns, where it leads to the production of an exudate that is thick enough to produce narrowing of the arteries as they cross the subarachnoid space and pass through the heavy exudate to reach the surface of the brain (54). Tuberculous meningitis results either from hematogenous spread or through rupture of a cortical or subaxial granuloma into the CSF space.

Tuberculous meningitis is frequently complicated by vascular thrombosis. Arterial narrowing and occlusion, demonstrable by cerebral angiography, occurs, which leads to cortical infarcts (Figs. 6.26 and 6.47). Mycotic aneurysms also occur (55) (Fig. 6.25).

Tuberculomas are rare in the United States but frequent in many countries such as India and nations in Africa and Latin America. They occur in the subcortical region of the cerebral hemispheres, or indeed in any area of the brain or cerebellum. They may also occur in the pons. Usually they are surrounded by a large edematous area. The center usually becomes necrotic, but the lesion should not be called an abscess. True tuberculous abscesses are rare. The edema around the granuloma is indicative of an early or immature granuloma (56). The thickness of the capsule varies. Ventricular dilatation occurs frequently (Fig. 6.26).

Tuberculous meningitis in the acute stage is usually diagnosed clinically and by lumbar puncture. CT may demonstrate increased density in the suprasellar region due to the exudate, and iodide contrast may show enhancement around the tentorium and falx. In the periphery, that increased density may be difficult to detect. MRI has a much better chance of demonstrating the meningeal changes, particularly with gadolinium enhancement. The tuberculomas are interesting because they may be slightly hyperintense on T1-weighted images and hypointense on T2-weighted images (56). On T2-weighted images, the periphery may be hypointense and the center hyperintense due to necrotic material (caseous material) (Fig. 6.27). Tuberculous granulomas may be multiple. CT with contrast demonstrates a ring or a solid enhancing nodule (55). Gupta et al. consider MRI much more specific than CT because of the T2-dark (shorten T2) appearance and the hyperintense center (56).

The combination of the tuberculoma and the surrounding edema may produce a significant mass effect with ventricular compression, midline shift, and hydrocephalus in the early stages. Later the mass may decrease with diminution of the edema. Calcification may occur in the chronic stage (see Fig. 4.16 *B*).

SARCOIDOSIS

Sarcoidosis is a systemic granulomatous disease of unknown etiology. It occurs in all countries of the world, and in the United States it is more frequently seen in the southeastern part, with a predilection for blacks. Involvement of the central nervous system occurs fairly frequently, in 5 to 16 percent of cases at autopsy (57). With MRI today, the incidence may have gone up compared to that previously reported with CT scanning alone. Neurologic symptoms are present in about 3 to 9 percent of cases. The involvement of the central nervous system tends to occur frequently in the suprasellar region, the infundibulum, and the wall of the third ventricle; granulomatous leptomeningitis has a predilection for involvement in the skull base and hypothalamic region as well as the optic chiasm. The dura is often involved in this area (58). Engelken et al. reported two cases of involvement of the optic nerves only, without meningeal involvement and without systemic disease (59). In one case, the optic nerve was biopsied, and in another case the conjunctiva was biopsied, and both showed noncaseating granuloma.

Involvement of the meninges is common, and to evaluate this possibility contrast-enhanced MR T1-weighted images are needed. In fact, the diagnosis could be missed altogether without enhancement. Williams III et al. have also shown that clustered lesions in the white matter may be demonstrated in T2-weighted images; these lesions may be located near an area of meningeal involvement (60). They propose that extension into the brain parenchyma takes place by way of the Virchow-Robin spaces, and that this extension may be demonstrated in some instances with enhanced MRI. Involvement of the dura may sometimes lead to dural sinus thrombosis.

Parenchymal involvement in the brain is less common; when it occurs, it tends to be not far from the surface of the brain, and thus the mechanism may be the one just proposed (61). However, as explained earlier, the hypothalamus is frequently involved in sarcoidosis of the nervous system (Fig. 6.28). Extracerebral masses can be found, probably starting in the meninges, and it is interesting to note that the lesions enhance heavily with contrast and at the same time are "T2 dark." In other words, they present a low or very low signal on T2-weighted images (Fig. 6.29). As a matter of fact, an extra-axial mass that enhances on CT and MRI and that is T2 dark is most likely produced by sarcoidosis, although an occasional meningioma with multiple small calcifications can produce a similar image (Fig. 6.30).

Ependymitis associated with sarcoidosis may be detected by contrast enhancement because of the increased intensity on T1-weighted images.

The response to treatment with steroids and sometimes with cytotoxic drugs may be followed by CT or MRI. Two effects might be noticed for steroid therapy. One of them is an actual improvement and the other is the "steroid effect," in which the contrast enhancement decreases markedly or disappears soon after the beginning of steroid therapy, as against an actual decrease in the size of the lesion.

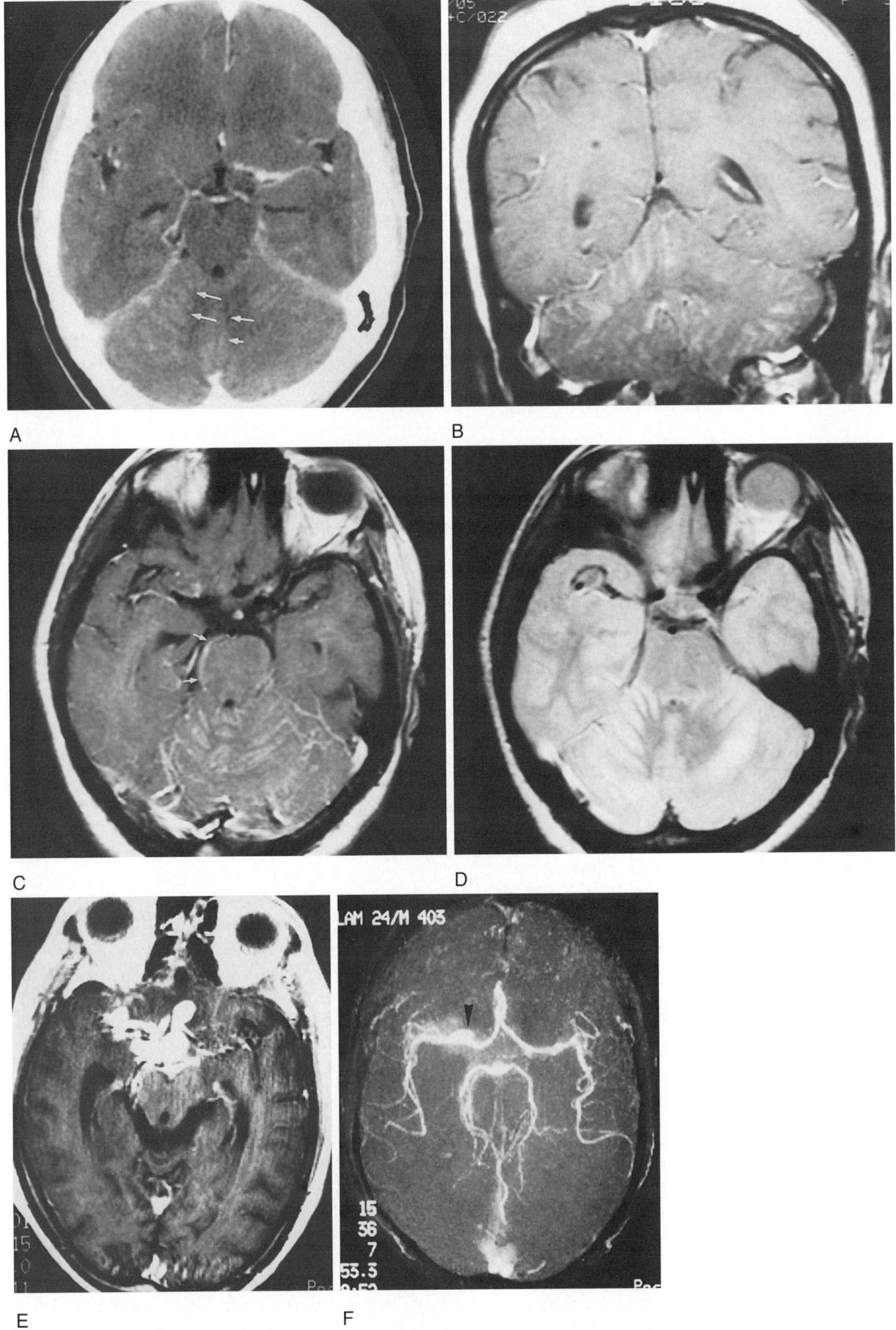
A
B
C
D
E
F
LAM 24/M 403
15
36
7
53.3

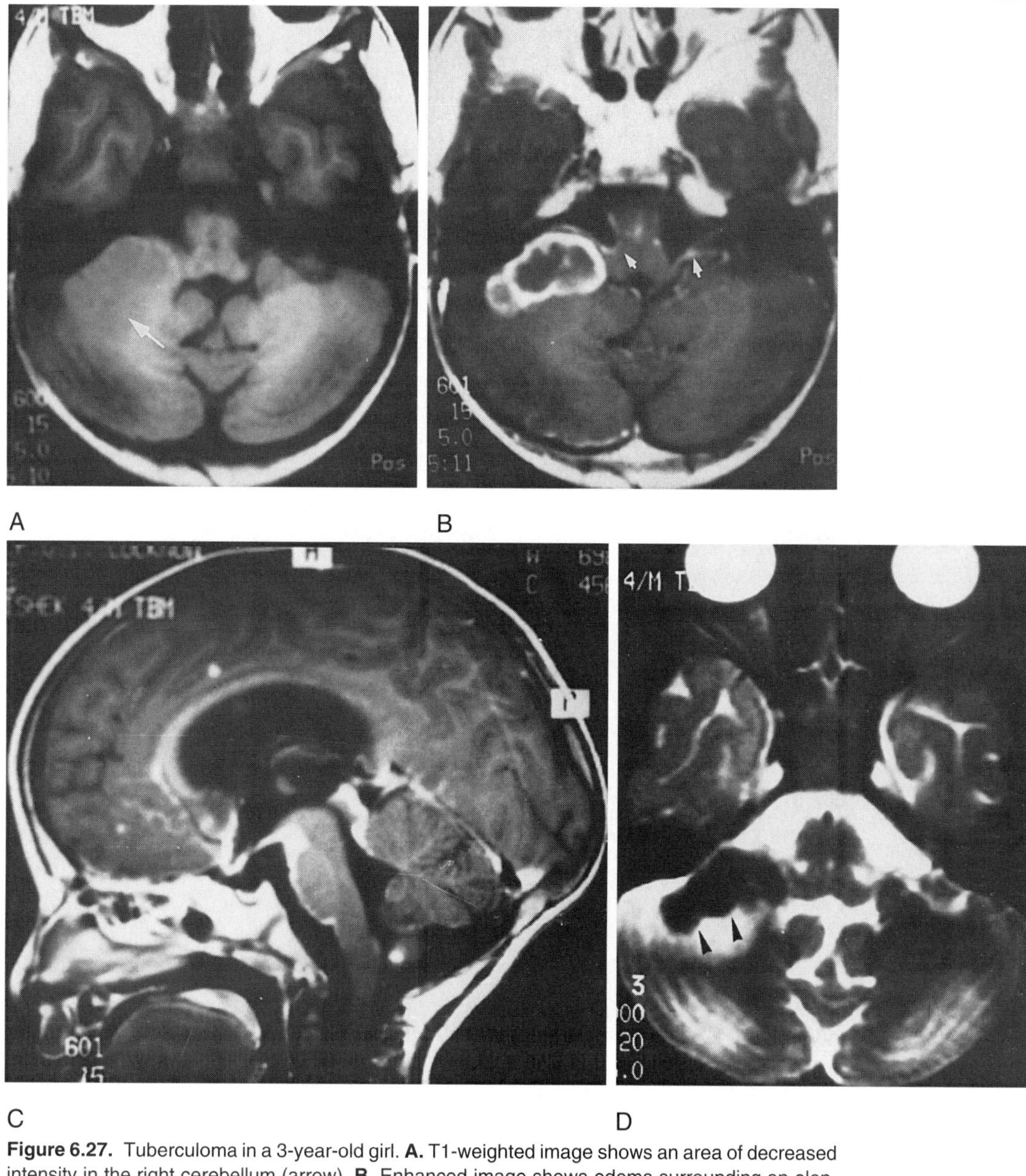

Figure 6.27. Tuberculoma in a 3-year-old girl. **A.** T1-weighted image shows an area of decreased intensity in the right cerebellum (arrow). **B.** Enhanced image shows edema surrounding an elongated area of enhancement in the cerebellum consistent with an abscess or a tuberculoma in this child, who had tuberculous meningitis. There is some enhancement of the meninges over the upper medulla and cerebellum on the other side (arrows). This is much more obvious in the sagittal enhanced image (**C**). There is marked enhancement in the suprasellar area, the lamina terminalis, and the frontal midline sulci, as well as in the interpeduncular cistern and on the anterior surface of the pons. Posteriorly, the quadrigeminal surface is markedly enhanced. **D.** A T2-weighted image of the lower cerebellum shows that the tuberculoma is hypointense (T2 dark), a feature that, according to Gupta et al. (56), is typical of tuberculomas. (Courtesy of RK Gupta, Delhi, India.)

Figure 6.26. Tuberculous meningitis in a 29-year-old woman. The patient came into the hospital complaining of headaches, nausea, and vomiting, and developed a sixth-nerve palsy and horizontal nystagmus. **A.** CT examination with contrast showed some diffuse increase in density of the cerebellar folia and vermis (arrows). **B.** Contrast MRI revealed extensive enhancement of the cerebellar folia all around the cerebellum, particularly well seen in coronal images. **C.** Axial postcontrast MRI showed the cerebellar folia pattern as well as pial enhancement around the brainstem. **D.** A proton density image demonstrated the hyperintensity of the cerebellar cortex due to edema. **E** and **F.** Another case of tuberculous meningitis. **E.** Enhanced T1-weighted image shows marked hyperintensity in the suprasellar and prepontine cisterns due to meningitis. **F.** MR angiogram reveals a pseudoaneurysm of the middle cerebral artery on the right (arrowhead). Around the area there is some hyperintensity produced by the meningitis and the thick exudate that usually accompanies tuberculous meningitis. (Images E and F are courtesy of RK Gupta, Delhi, India.)

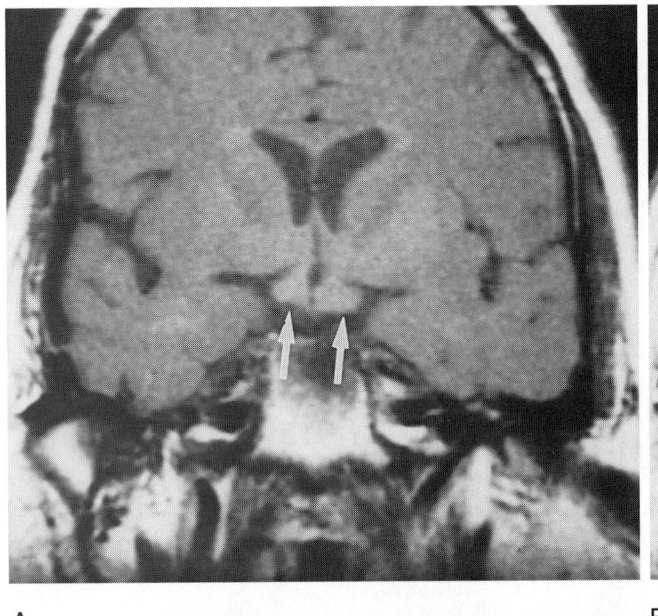

A

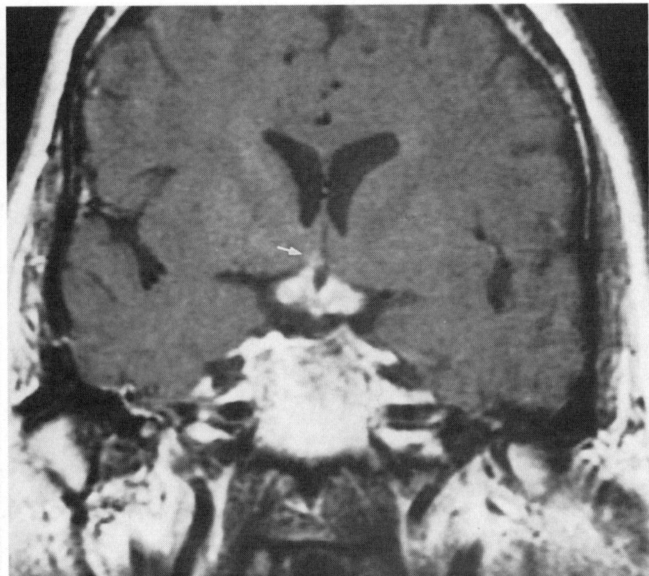

B

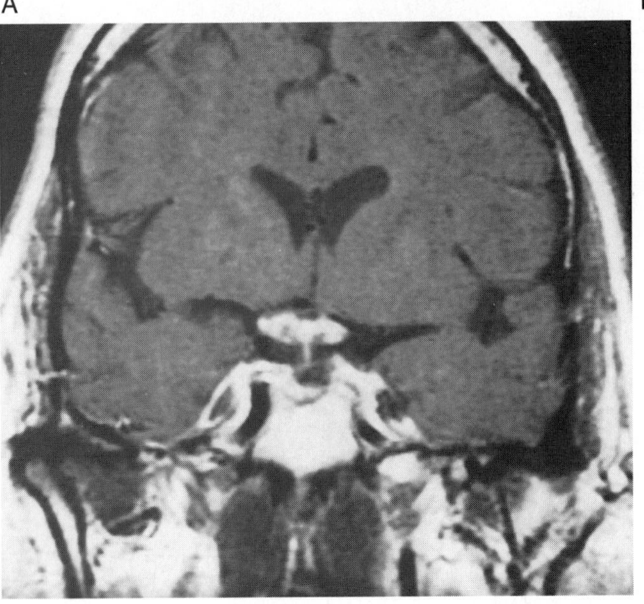

C

Figure 6.28. Sarcoidosis of hypothalamus and optic chiasm. **A.** Coronal T1-weighted image prior to contrast administration. There is thickening of the optic chiasm and adjacent hypothalamus (arrows). **B.** After contrast, there is marked enhancement and in addition some enhancement extending along the right side of the wall of the third ventricle (small arrow). **C.** A section more anteriorly shows the chiasmal enhancement. Passing below the chiasm is the pituitary stalk, which normally enhances with contrast.

When the patient is receiving steroids, it is necessary to suspend therapy several days before repeating the contrast-enhanced examination because lack of enhancement is not a reliable sign of improvement while the patient is on steroids. Involvement of the spinal cord may take place. The lesions may be detected by contrast enhancement on MRI. Involvement of the spinal nerve roots and the spinal dura may also take place (62).

Sporadic involvement of cranial nerves occurs, the most frequently involved nerve being the facial nerve. The posterior fossa may be the site of involvement, usually the cerebellum and sometimes the brainstem. Dural meningeal involvement occurs often in posterior fossa sarcoidosis, and hydrocephalus may develop as a result of basal arachnoiditis. Although the incidence of symptomatic central nervous system sarcoidosis is about 5 percent, autopsy reports indicate a higher frequency—up to 16 percent.

Intracerebral lesions in patients with sarcoidosis often tend to take on an appearance similar to that of multiple sclerosis, and from the morphological standpoint, one could not distinguish between the two on MRI. However, the sarcoid lesions are likely to enhance with gadolinium, which is usually not the case with MS lesions (although some may enhance), and the fact that they are occurring in a patient with sarcoidosis would tend to favor sarcoidosis (63). In the absence of enhancement, the differential diagnosis cannot be made unless the lesions are located near an area where there is meningeal involvement.

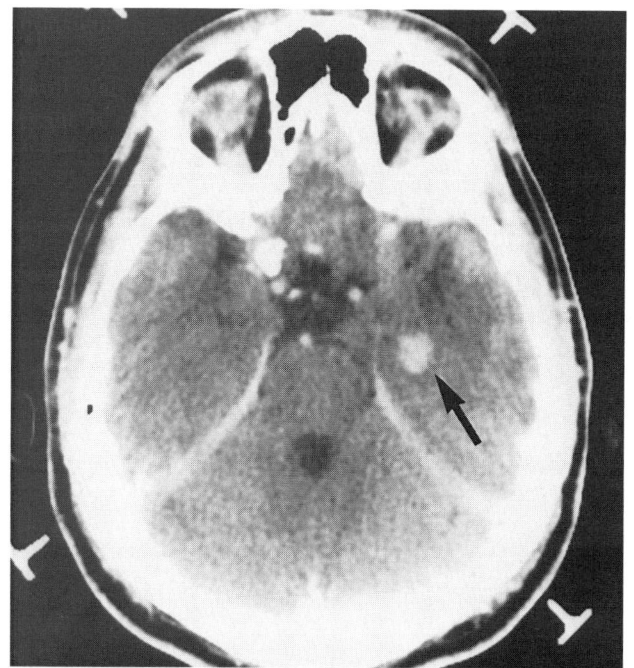

A

B

C

D

E

Figure 6.29. Atypical sarcoidosis involving the temporal lobe. **A.** Postcontrast CT scan shows a lesion in the medial left temporal lobe (arrow). There is also a low-density area anterior to the enhancing lesion. **B.** A sagittal precontrast T1-weighted view shows narrowing of the anterior aspect of the left temporal horn and enlargement of the anterior aspect of the temporal lobe as compared to the opposite normal side (**C**). **D.** Postcontrast T1-weighted axial image shows the same appearance as shown in A. **E.** A T2-weighted axial view reveals that the enhancing lesion is dark (arrow) and the rest of the pathological process is bright. One of the lesions that may be dark on T2 images is sarcoid granuloma, the diagnosis in this case. The surrounding hyperintense area is probably all edema.

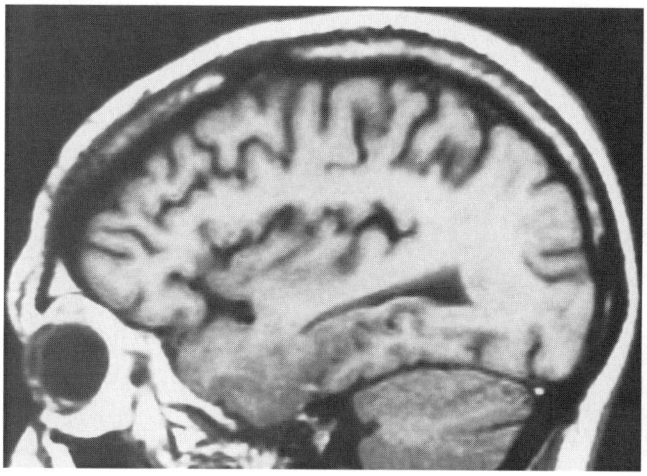

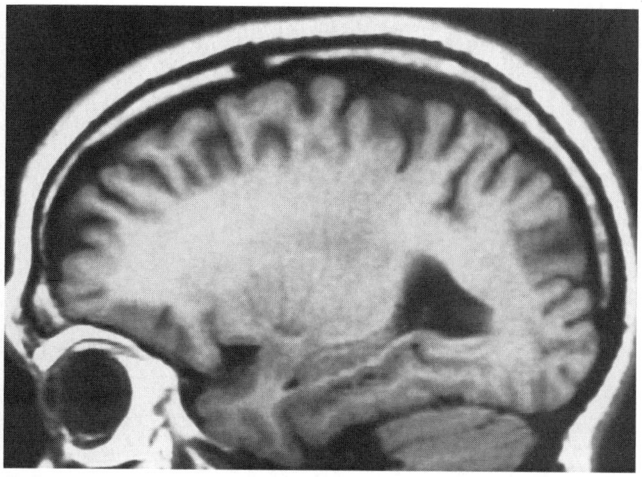

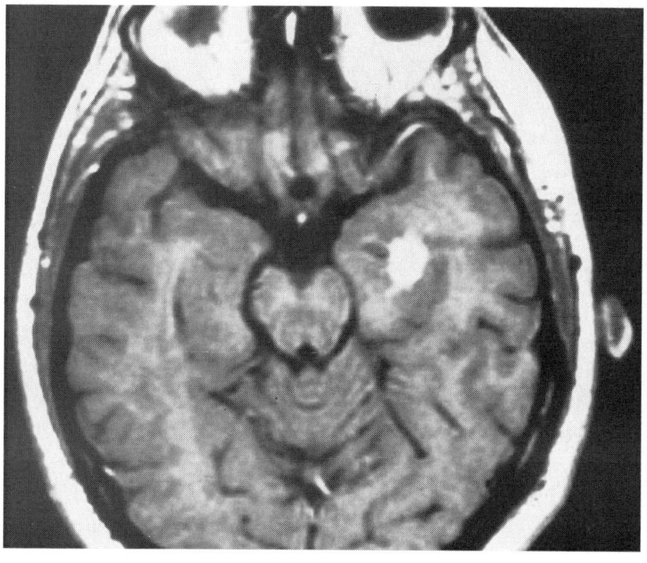

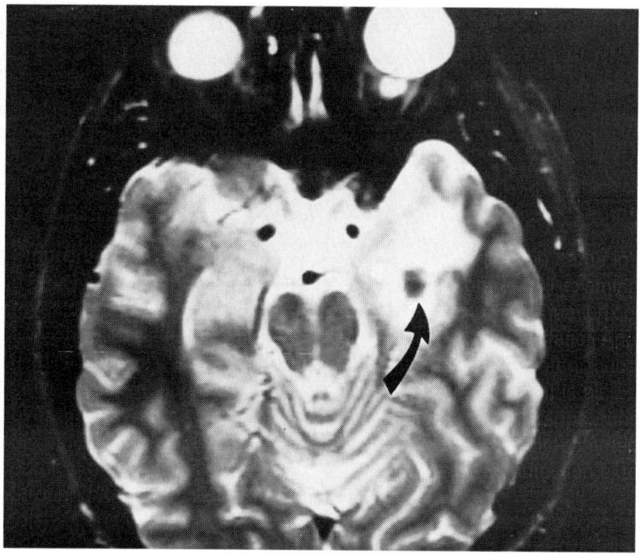

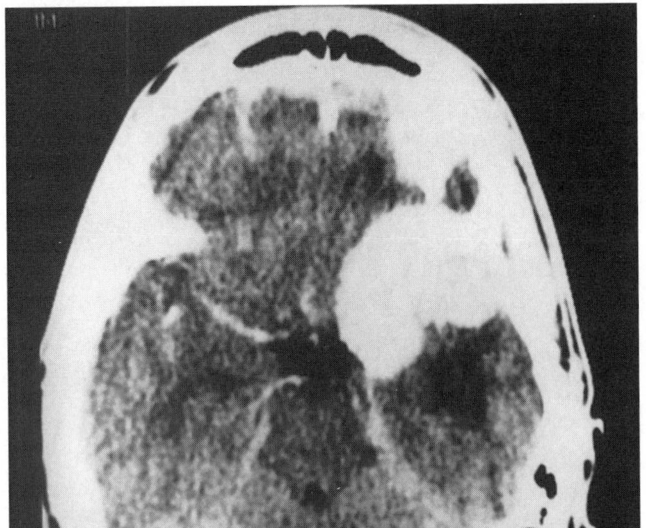

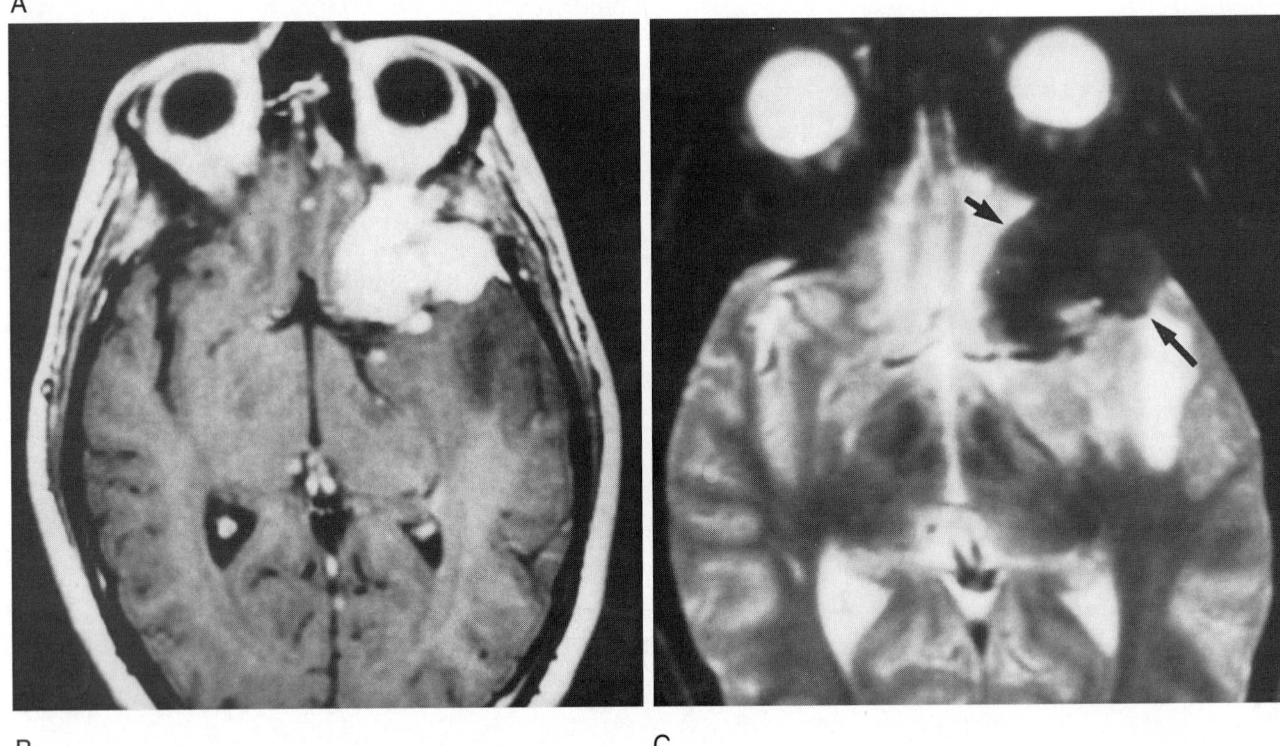

Figure 6.30. Sarcoid granuloma showing mass in temporal fossa simulating neoplasm. **A.** Contrast-enhanced CT shows hyperdense left anterior temporal mass. **B.** Enhanced T1-weighted axial MRI demonstrates the same mass shown on CT. **C.** T2-weighted axial discloses that the mass is "T2 dark," (arrows) which made the diagnosis of sarcoid granuloma a good possibility; biopsy confirmed the diagnosis.

Involvement of the calvarium also occurs in a manner similar to other bone involvement elsewhere in the skeleton (64).

SPIROCHETAL INFECTIONS

Syphilis

This has become a much less common infection since the discovery of penicillin. However, recent reports indicate an increasing number of reported cases. The secondary stage of the disease may affect the meninges. Meningovascular syphilis and acute syphilitic meningitis may be seen. The meningovascular type presents pathologically widespread meningeal thickening, lymphocytic infiltrates, and perivascular lymphocytic infiltrates around small blood vessels. The evolution from secondary to tertiary syphilis may occur with inadequate treatment, but this development almost never occurs today because patients are ordinarily treated in the first, or acute, stage. Brightbill et al. reported 35 cases, of which 32 tested HIV-seropositive. Imaging findings showed cerebral infarction (8 patients), white matter lesions (7 patients), arteritis (2 patients), gumma (2 patients), and meningeal enhancement (2 patients) (65).

In general paresis, the imaging findings are those of atrophy or diffuse tissue loss in the brain. The ventricles enlarge and the subarachnoid sulci widen. In meningovascular syphilis some cortical and deep small infarcts may be seen, and MRI can be expected to be superior to CT (66). Gummas are extremely rare but are occasionally encountered. They show contrast ring enhancement on CT with an area of central low attenuation. In the case reported by Godt et al., the ring was thick and had a small low-density central area (67). In the case reported by Agrons et al., there was a hyperintense ring image on the T1-weighted image and a hypointense image on the T2-weighted image surrounded by a large area of edema (68). CT and MR-enhanced images showed homogeneous enhancement. Gummas can be multiple (69). Pachymeningitis may occur as a tertiary manifestation. It may involve the spinal meninges, where thickening of the dura may be observed by myelography.

Lyme Disease

This is a spirochetal infection caused by *Borrelia burgdorferi*, found worldwide in various animals (deer, racoons, birds, mice). It is transmitted by ixodid ticks and can incidentally affect humans. It was originally described in Europe but is apparently more frequent in the U.S. Northeast. The deer tick (*Ixodes dammini*) is the most frequent vector.

In humans the infection usually begins with a tick bite that is likely to be quite prominent and may ulcerate. The tick may well be buried in the lesion. A few months later flulike symptoms and a characteristic rash usually develop. Weeks to months later some patients present with new neurological symptoms, frank meningitis, weakness, radiculoneuropathy, and paraparesis. The serum or CSF Lyme titre tests are likely to be positive in this stage. A third stage may occur months or even years later, when patients may develop arthritis or central nervous system dysfunction.

Six of 14 cases reported by Fernandez et al. presented MRI abnormalities, most of which consisted of bright foci on T2 images in young patients, sometimes numerous and sometimes involving the brainstem, particularly in patients with weakness or paralysis of the extremities (70). Spinal cord findings on MRI were not reported. The white matter foci are usually small and may be confused with the findings in multiple sclerosis (Fig. 6.31). In other cases the findings on MRI are those of a more diffuse encephalytic process, and some of the lesions may show ring enhancement with gadolinium (71). Meningeal enhancement may also be encountered. In a recent paper, Steere et al. discussed the frequency with which the diagnosis of Lyme disease is made when in fact the patient had other conditions, such as chronic fatigue syndrome or fibromyalgia (72). Unfortunately, a false-positive laboratory result is relatively frequent, which Steere et al. attribute to the lack of standardization of the serologic tests.

The mechanism of the neurologic symptoms is not clear. It may be immunologic or vascular, but it also includes direct involvement by the spirochete, which is found on biopsy of some lesions (71,72,73,74).

FUNGAL INFECTIONS

The fungi usually involved are either the pathogenic fungi or the saprophytes. The latter produce opportunistic infections in sensitive, immunocompromised subjects and are the most commonly encountered. The first group of infections includes coccidioidomycosis, blastomycosis, histoplasmosis, and actinomycosis. The opportunistic group includes aspergillosis, nocardiosis, candidosis, and mucormycosis.

The site of entry into the nervous system may be via the bloodstream from a lung or intestinal or skin focus, or it may be more directly from a focus in the paranasal sinus or the nose.

Coccidioidomycosis (Coccidioides immitis)

Central nervous system involvement is the most serious complication of this mycotic infection. It may produce a meningitis, more pronounced in the base leading to hydrocephalus, and vascular occlusion. The upper cervical subarachnoid space may also be involved (Fig. 6.32). Parenchymal involvement (abscess, granuloma) is found more commonly in patients with AIDS in areas where coccidioidomycosis is endemic (75).

Enhanced MRI is needed for diagnosing meningitis. When meningitis involves the sylvian and interhemispheric fissures, the intrathecal amphotericin B therapy fails to eradicate the disease because the drug does not easily reach the involved areas (75).

Blastomycosis (*Blastomyces dermatitidis*)

This infection is endemic in the southeastern United States and produces a meningitis, often more marked in the basal cisterns, that is similar to the coccidioidomycosis meningitis but occurs more frequently; it may also produce abscesses. Epidural involvement with production of a thickened dura (pachymeningitis) may also be found in the spine or intracranially, producing brain or spinal cord compression. It may also produce bone destruction at the skull base and temporal bone (76).

Candidosis

Candidosis is rarely seen in the central nervous system in vivo. However, autopsy has shown that it is among the more common fungal infections of the central nervous system (77). It usually occurs late in cases of visceral candidosis in debilitated patients. Scattered lesions may be found (small infarctlike lesions, small abscesses or granulomas, or vascular occlusions with infarcts).

Aspergillosis (*Aspergillus fumigatus*)

This infection is found more frequently in debilitated or immunocompromised patients. The types of lesions it produces are abscesses or granulomas. Sometimes the lesions

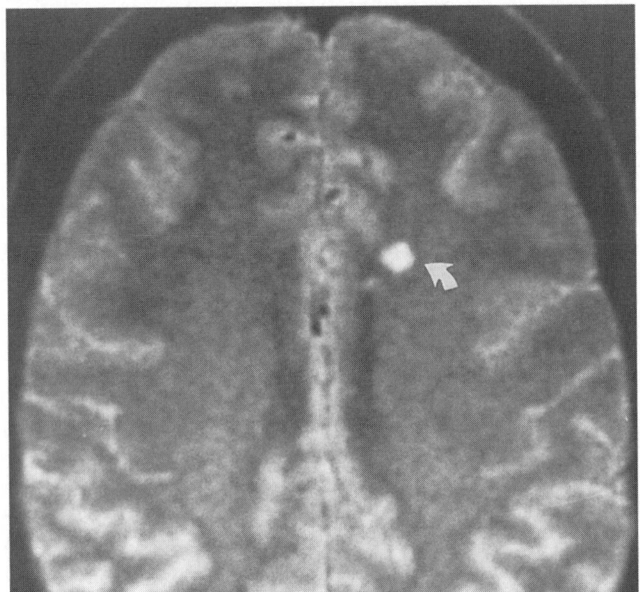

Figure 6.31. Lyme disease. **A** and **B.** There is a bright white matter lesion in the left frontal and another in the left periventricular area (arrows). The lesions are nonspecific and must be correlated with the patient's history and serologic tests. **C.** A third lesion is present in the lower midbrain (arrow). (Courtesy of Dr. Richard E. Fernandez, Toms River, NJ.)

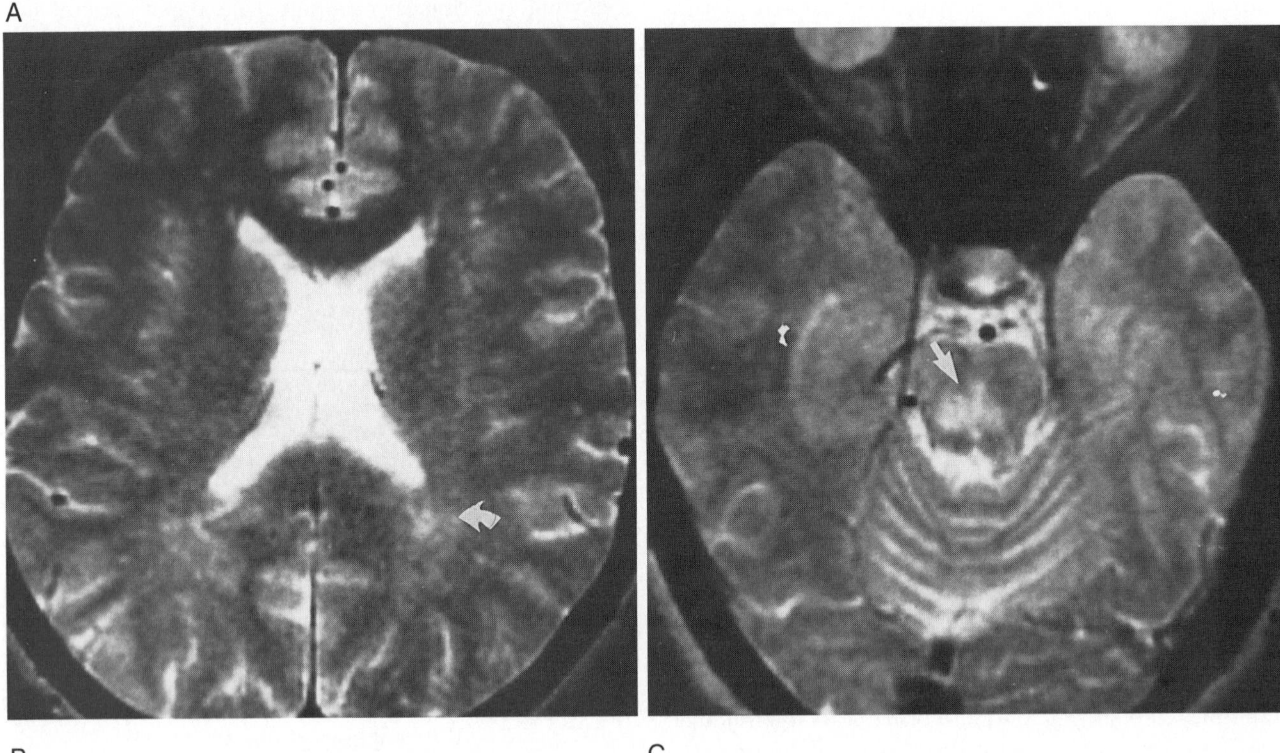

can be multiple (50 in a case reported by Meyer et al.) (78). Bone destruction of the sinus walls is common, and involvement of the orbital soft tissues is frequent (Fig. 6.46). In the author's experience this is more common with mucormycosis infections.

Histoplasmosis (*Histoplasma capsulatum*)

This is a common infection in the United States, particularly in the Midwest, and CNS involvement is rare. When it occurs the most common form is meningitis with a predilection for the basal meninges. Hydrocephalus may then result. It may also produce multiple granulomas (79,80).

Cryptococcosis (*Cryptococcus neoformans*)

This may occur spontaneously, possibly in relation to a pulmonary focus or, more frequently, as an opportunistic infection. The usual lesion is a meningitis, but frequently brain lesions are also found. Tien et al., described four imaging types observed in a group of 29 immunocompromised patients with AIDS, 1 of whom had diabetes mellitus: (a) parenchymal cryptococcomas showing as a small solid

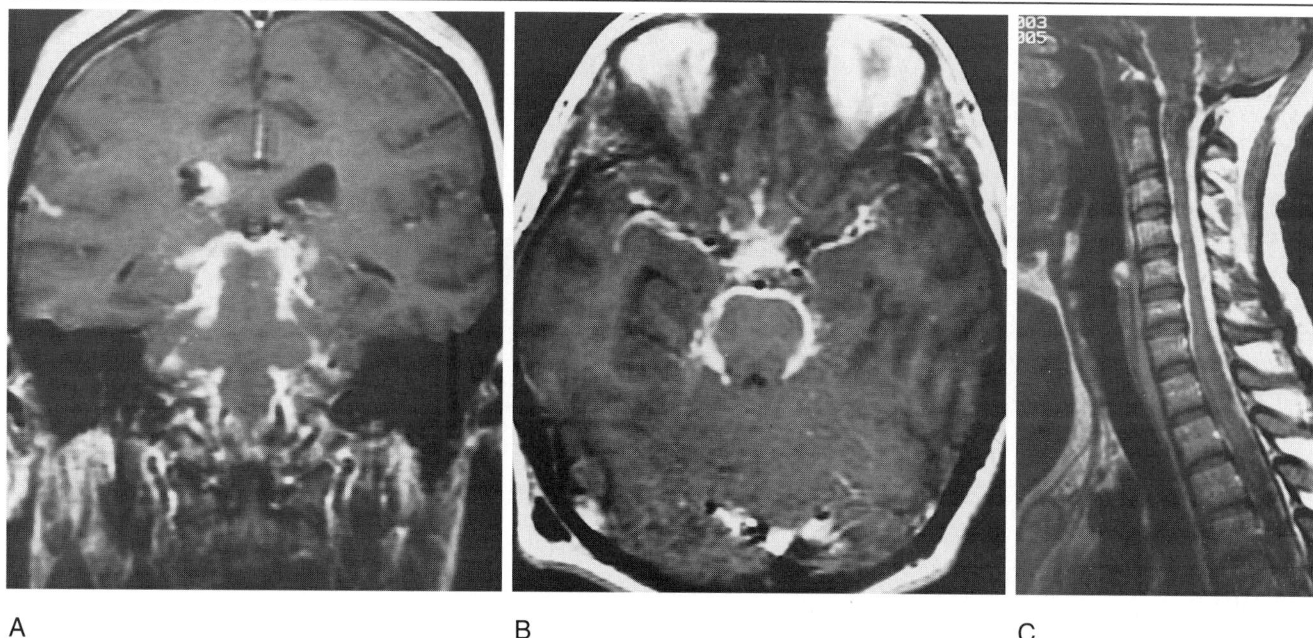

A B C

Figure 6.32. Coccidioidomycosis meningitis. **A** and **B.** Coronal and axial contrast-enhanced T1-weighted images show marked meningeal enhancement in the basal cisterns and both sylvian cisterns. There is also intraventricular enhancement on the right in A, probably due to ependymal involvement. **C.** There is considerable contrast uptake in the spinal meninges in the cervical and upper thoracic region, going up to the posterior fossa. (Courtesy of Dr. John Hesselink, University of California, San Diego Medical Center, CA; [AJNR 1992;13:1241–1245]).

or abscesslike image surrounded by edema; (2) dilated Virchow-Robin spaces manifested as punctate bright shadows in the basal ganglia on the T2-weighted image, but not enhancing on T1 postcontrast images; (3) multiple enhancing nodules in the cortex and in the meninges; and (4) a mixed pattern with two or three of the above (81). The dilated perivascular (Virchow-Robin) spaces are presumably due to cryptococcus organisms within the perivascular space (Fig. 6.33) (81).

Nocardiosis (*Nocardia asteroides*)

This produces abscesses or meningitis. Both could be recognized by MRI with contrast enhancement or on T2 images. Angiography may demonstrate arterial spasm or an arteritic pattern related to the meningitis or to true arterial involvement (Fig. 6.34).

Mucormycosis (Fungus of the Family Zygomycetes)

This is an opportunistic organism that occurs in diabetics (possibly related to the acidosis rather than to hyperglycemia), in debilitated individuals, or in patients being treated with steroids, antibiotics, or cytostatic drugs. The infection progresses rapidly, usually starting in the nose or paranasal sinuses, destroying bone at the base of the skull, and producing arterial occlusion, even of the internal carotid artery (Figs. 6.35, 6.36). It involves the dura, the basal meninges, and the brain, and is usually fatal. If it is diagnosed early, treatment may be instituted and the patient may survive (Fig. 6.35). The presence of a sinusitis accompanied by bone destruction should make one suspect a mucormycotic infection (82,83). Orbital wall and soft tissue involvement is frequent, and venous thrombosis may propagate to the cavernous sinuses. Orbital apex involvement should be carefully looked for because, if present, it indicates the need to perform an orbital exenteration as part of an aggressive treatment program.

CT is excellent in evaluating bone destruction, whereas MRI may demonstrate the soft tissue involvement somewhat better. Cavernous sinus involvement may be studied with enhanced MRI and also by using a flow study, which may demonstrate absent flow if there is sinus thrombosis (Fig. 6.13*E* to *H*).

PARASITIC INFECTIONS

Toxoplasmosis

In recent years, the most common parasitic infection in U.S. hospitals is toxoplasmosis because of the increasing frequency of AIDS. It is produced by *Toxoplasma gondii*, an obligate intracellular protozoan. Serological tests among adults in the United States and other countries show that 20 to 85 percent are seropositive (84). In newborns the infection, acquired in utero, may be quite severe. The organisms produce an ependymitis that leads to hydrocephalus. Subependymal and wider brain involvement also oc-

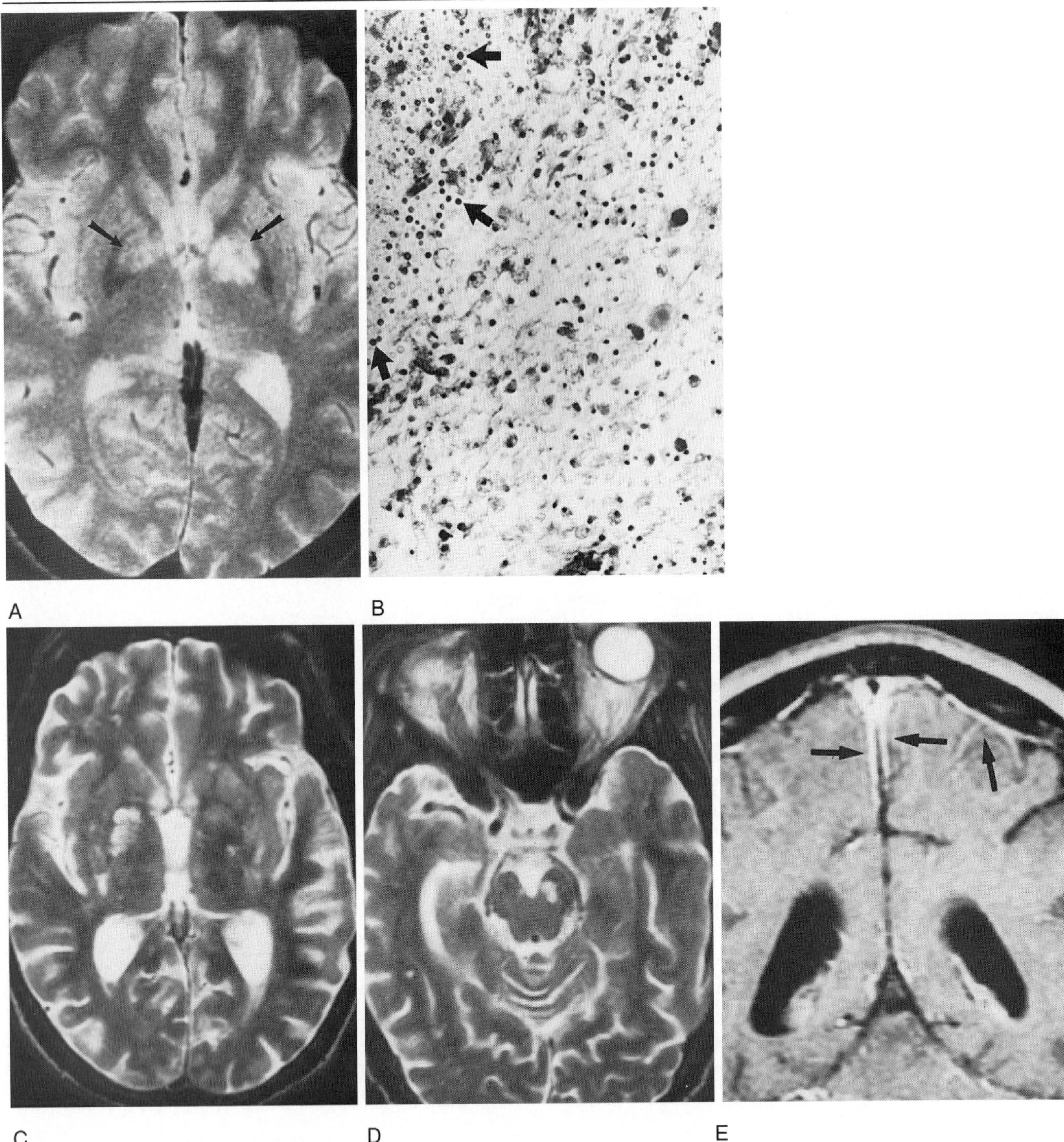

Figure 6.33. Cryptococcosis in a patient with AIDS. **A.** T2-weighted image shows numerous punctate hyperintense foci in the basal ganglia, particularly visible on the right side. On the left the appearance is similar but more pronounced, suggesting a possible cryptococcoma. These lesions do not usually enhance with contrast. The punctate appearance suggests that the changes represent lesions within the perivascular spaces (Virchow-Robin spaces). Indeed, an autopsy specimen from another patient (**B**) reveals, within this dilated perivascular space in the basal ganglia, numerous lipid-filled macrophages surrounding a pocket of darkly stained circular organisms (*Cryptococcus neoformans*) (arrows). (Courtesy of Dr. Robert D. Tien, Duke University Medical Center, Durham, NC.) **C.** Another case of cryptococcosis in a 38-year-old man who was HIV-positive. The loculated appearance in the basal ganglia region bilaterally, more on the right, is again noted in this T2-weighted axial image. **D.** Another lesion is seen in the midbrain. **E.** Evidence of meningeal enhancement on postcontrast T1-weighted images is indicative of leptomeningeal involvement (arrows). The falx (dark line between the enhanced lines) is not enhanced.

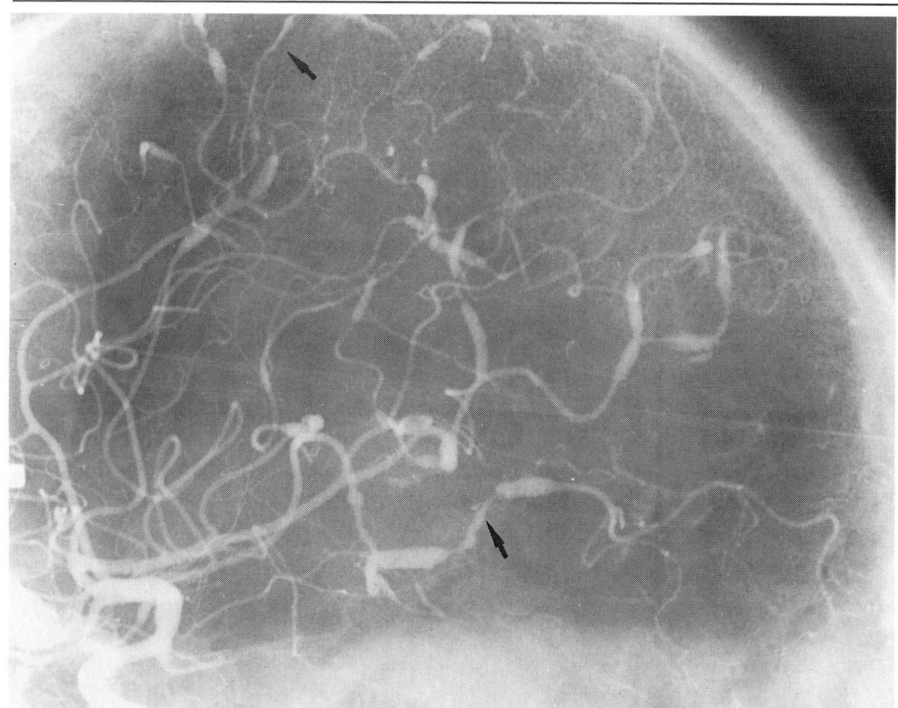

Figure 6.34. *Nocardia* meningitis associated with many areas of arterial narrowing and dilatation. Lateral view demonstrates irregularities (arrows) as well as areas of arterial dilatation. The patient had been under steroid treatment for Hodgkin disease.

curs. Infection of the fetus occurs only when the mother becomes infected during pregnancy. The cat is the parasite's definitive host and may be the source of the infestation. The frequency of seropositive adults indicates that the infection, when acquired after birth, is benign in the great majority of cases; in some cases a relatively mild illness ensues if the individual is immunologically normal. The patient may present a mild febrile illness with lymphocytosis that resolves spontaneously; in some, a more severe illness occurs (pneumonia, hepatitis, myocarditis, or encephalitis). Foci of toxoplasmosis unrelated to the cause of death are sometimes found in the brain at autopsy. In *Toxoplasma* encephalitis an inflammatory reaction occurs only if there is cell necrosis, for it is known that intracellular organisms do not elicit any inflammatory response. Persistence of *Toxoplasma* cysts after the acquisition of immunity may explain the frequent reactivation of the infection in AIDS.

As explained in the discussion of AIDS, the *Toxoplasma* abscesses may be single or multiple. They tend to occur in the basal ganglia region or elsewhere in the brain, and they usually enhance with contrast on both CT and MRI. They may be solid, but most often they produce a ring-enhancing lesion. They are usually bright on T2 images but may be iso- or hypointense (Figs. 6.11 to 6.13). Some may show signs of hemorrhage.

A therapeutic trial with antitoxoplasma medication (pyrimethamine and sulfadiazine) should show a decrease in the size of the lesions in 2 to 4 weeks. The edema may decrease or disappear and the abscess will decrease in size. If medication is maintained, complete disappearance of some lesions may occur and some may undergo calcification. The calcification is easily detected by CT, but on MRI the lesions may still be bright on T1 and T2 images, suggesting a hematoma or the result of some poorly understood paramagnetic effects; they may also be low intensity on both T1- and T2-weighted images. Absence of a favorable response with treatment indicates that the lesions are probably not toxoplasmosis, but lymphoma or some other infection.

In congenital toxoplasmosis there is usually calcification in the brain, usually more pronounced in the periventricular region; hydrocephalus due to aqueductal obstruction; brain atrophy; and often microcephaly. The ventricular enlargement was originally due to aqueductal obstruction from ependymitis, but later is mostly due to brain atrophy secondary to the encephalitis. CT is the examination of choice because the fine calcifications may go undetected with MRI (see Fig. 4.15).

Malaria

Neurologic complications of *acute malaria* occur in about 2 percent of cases (85). Hemorrhage and infarction have been reported, which are attributed to small vessel occlusion produced by the affected red blood cells. This usually occurs in patients affected by the *Plasmodium falciparum* variety. The spinal cord may also be affected.

Cysticercosis

When the embryos of *Taenia solium* lodge in the nervous system, they produce cysts containing the scolex of the par-

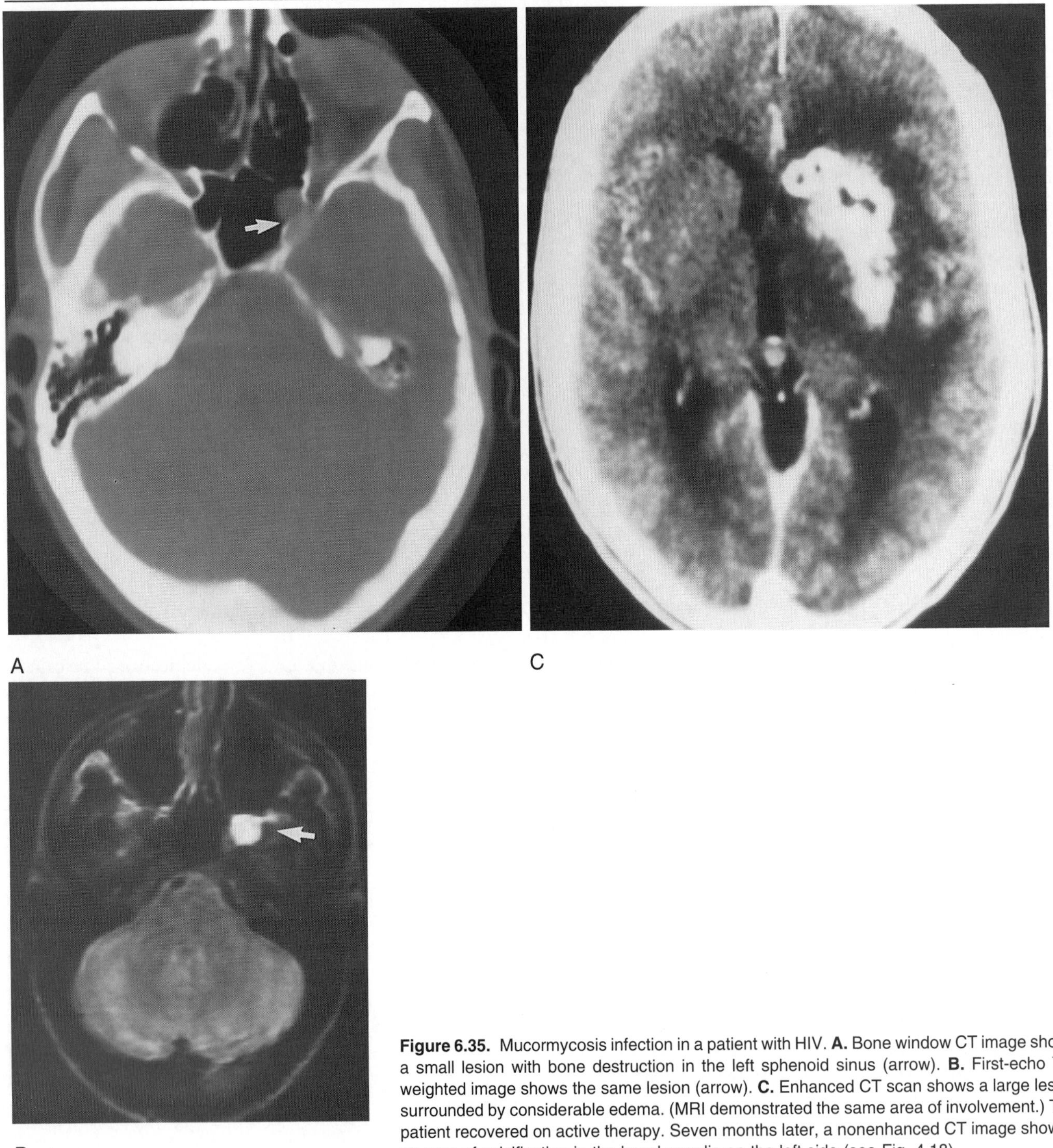

A

C

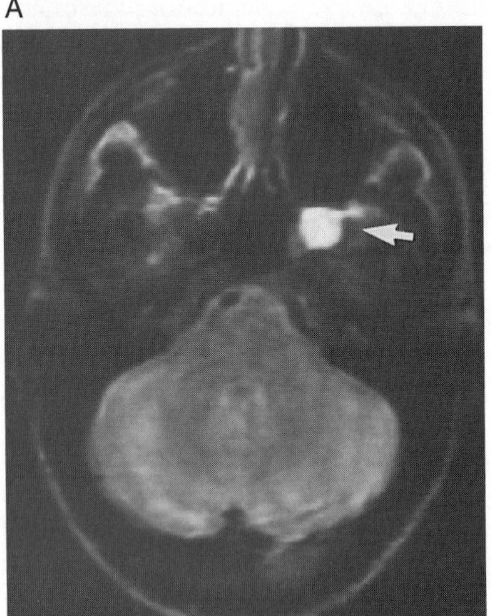

B

Figure 6.35. Mucormycosis infection in a patient with HIV. **A.** Bone window CT image shows a small lesion with bone destruction in the left sphenoid sinus (arrow). **B.** First-echo T2-weighted image shows the same lesion (arrow). **C.** Enhanced CT scan shows a large lesion surrounded by considerable edema. (MRI demonstrated the same area of involvement.) The patient recovered on active therapy. Seven months later, a nonenhanced CT image showed an area of calcification in the basal ganglia on the left side (see Fig. 4.18).

asite against one wall. The fluid in the cyst is clear as long as the larva lives, and becomes turbid and gelatinous as it dies. At this stage the vesicle, which usually is suspended in the cerebrospinal fluid spaces (subarachnoid space or ventricles) without producing an inflammatory response, provokes an inflammatory reaction that can be quite severe. The wall of the cyst becomes thicker, and the cyst becomes smaller and adherent to the surrounding meninges or ependyma. If infestation is predominantly in the basal meninges, a basal arachnoiditis results that leads to hydrocephalus. If the cysts are intraventricular, obstruction to the CSF flow will take place depending on the location of the cysts (lateral ventricles, third ventricle, fourth ventricle) (Fig. 6.37). *Cysticercus* cysts may also be found in the spinal subarachnoid space (Fig. 6.38).

Sometime after the death of the parasite, calcification takes place in typical fashion (a calcified small ring with a dot of calcification in the wall) (see Fig. 4.16). The calcifica-

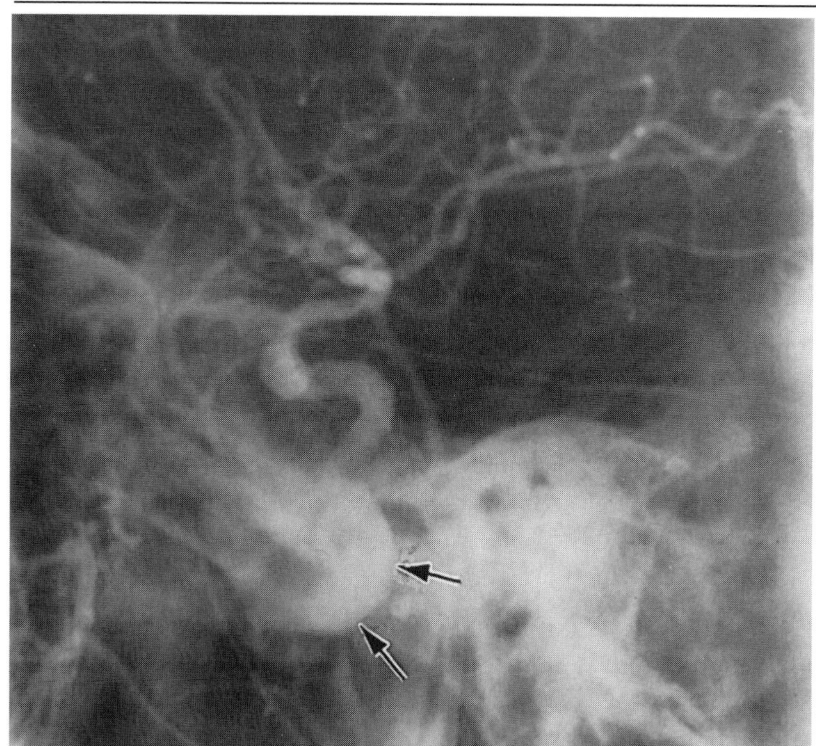

Figure 6.36. Carotid artery narrowing and aneurysm formation (arrows) in a patient with mucormycosis infection.

tions either become solid sometime later or have been solid from the start. Although the cysts are usually located in the brain cortex or in the ventricles, the brain may be directly involved. Brain tissue infestation may produce more severe clinical manifestations in the inflammatory stages, when the embryo begins to die; this is particularly so if the infestation was severe to start with. Diffuse brain edema is prominent and may lead to death from cerebral transtentorial and/or tonsillar cerebellar herniation (86).

In the case of a single lesion accompanied by edema, a tumor may be suspected and operated upon unless one thinks about cysticercosis. In both cases reported by Michael et al., the lesions were in the brain cortex, possibly a cyst in the depth of a sulcus that provoked an inflammatory reaction at the appropriate stage (87).

Contrast enhancement on CT or MRI would usually show slight to marked enhancement at the cyst wall due to the inflammatory reaction of the surrounding brain (88). In the nonenhanced MRI the fluid in the cyst is slightly hyperintense on T1 images in comparison to CSF. The presence of multiple cysts with at least one or more demonstrating a mural nodule on CT or MRI is considered almost pathognomonic for cysticercosis, and contrast study is probably not required. Edema around the cyst varies. In the early stages there is very little or no edema, but as the parasite begins to die, edema appears, and sometimes there is considerable edema around the cyst, as in the cases reported by Michael et al. (87).

The intraventricular cysts represent 17 percent of cysticercosis cases. They are usually better seen with MRI than with CT (89). Most are isointense or slightly hyperintense in relation to CSF, but some may be hyperintense on T1- and T2-weighted images. Some may enhance with intravenous contrast. An important feature of intraventricular *Cysticercus* cysts is their mobility, which is so great that they can pass from the third ventricle into the lateral ventricles through the foramen of Monro and to the fourth ventricle through the aqueduct (90,91). For this reason, neurosurgical removal must be immediately preceded by a determination of the position of the cyst by either CT or MRI. A cyst in the fourth ventricle may provoke an acute reaction with sudden ventricular dilatation and downward displacement of the cerebellar tonsils, possibly causing irreversible brain damage or death.

In the spinal canal the *Cysticercus* cysts are also mobile until they reach a stage where death of the parasite produces an inflammatory reaction in the meninges that leads to increasing neurologic disability (Fig. 6.38).

For further discussion of cysticercosis, see Chapter 4, "Cerebral Calcifications."

Paragonimiasis

The brain lesions produced by the *Paragonimus westermani* fluke are arachnoiditis, granulomas, and encapsulated abscesses. Extensive brain destruction often results, and plain films as well as CT images demonstrate calcifications that have been described as "soap bubble" in shape, which are considered characteristic (92,93,94). Ventricular dilatation and porencephalic dilatation of the ventricles from brain tissue destruction are common. The lesions are often uni-

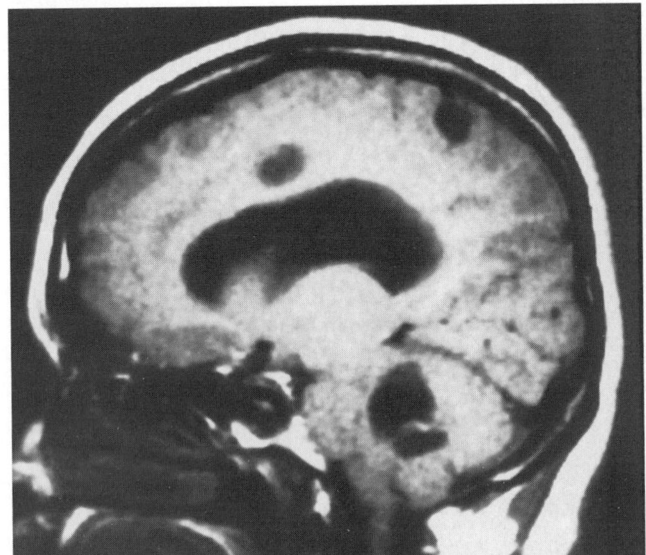

Figure 6.37. Cysticercosis. **A.** T1-weighted sagittal view. Cysts are scattered usually in or near fluid-containing spaces, such as deep in the surface sulci (giving the appearance of being intracerebral) and in the ventricles, and only sometimes in the brain tissue proper. The presence of edema seen on T2-weighted images (**B**, a proton density axial image) may indicate that the parasite is dying. **C** and **D**. The lesion in the proton density image (C) and the two lesions in the T2-weighted image (D) are all really in the depth of sulci and not in the brain tissue itself. A cyst is seen in the fourth ventricle in A; the lesion in B was originally in the wall of the temporal horn. The scolex (parasite within the cyst) is visible in some of the images (A to C). There is moderate ventricular dilatation including the fourth ventricle, which contains a *Cysticercus* cyst. Hydrocephalus (note that there is periventricular hyperintensity) could be due to fourth-ventricular obstruction or to basal arachnoiditis, a frequent complication of cysticercosis. (Courtesy of Dr. Stephen Sweriduk, Boston, MA.)

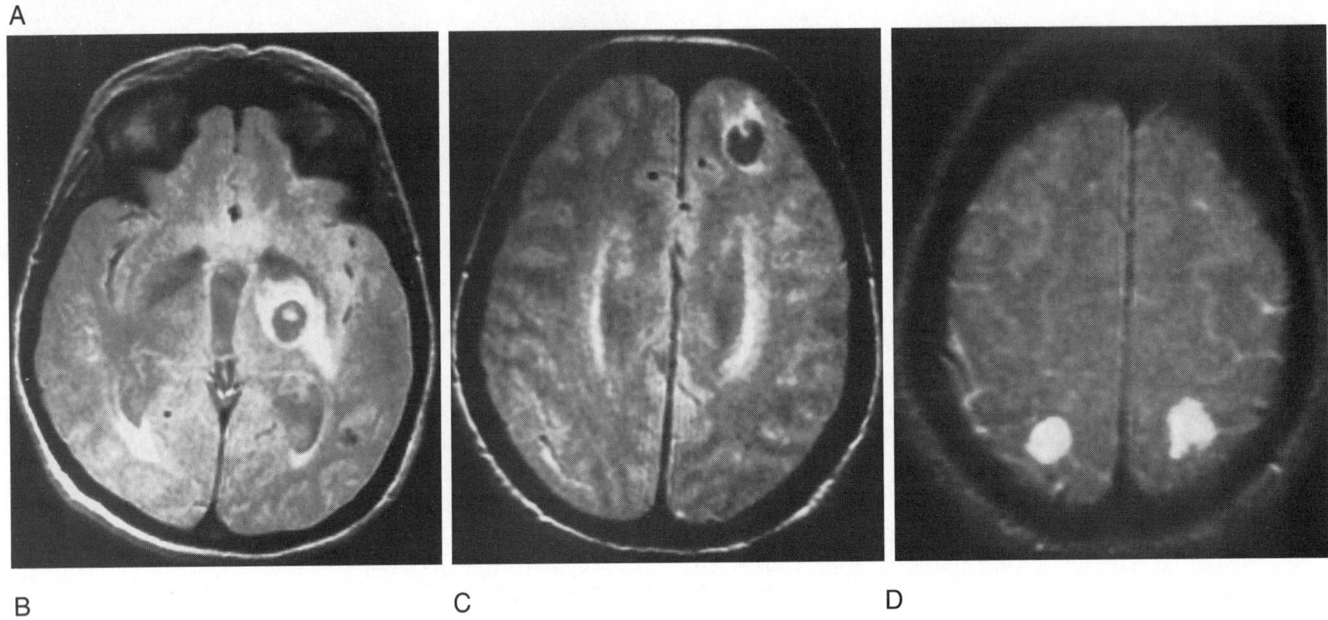

lateral. The diagnosis can be suggested from the characteristic calcifications. However, according to Oh, they are only found in 20 percent of the cases (92). The rest show punctate or small, round calcifications that can be confused with cysticercosis. The final diagnosis is made by an intradermal test that is positive for *P. westermani*, detection of ova in the sputum, or a positive complement fixation test. For further discussion of paragonimiasis, see Chapter 4.

Sparganosis

This is another parasite found in Asian countries, a pseudophyllidean tapeworm. It rarely involves the brain, but when it does, it produces white matter and subcortical lesions that may present spotty calcifications on CT. The clinical findings may be mild, but convulsions are common (95). The diagnosis is made by a serologic test.

Schistosomiasis

Schistosoma parasites are found in a number of countries in Africa, on the Mediterranean coast, and in Brazil, Puerto Rico, and Japan. All the three types encountered (*S. mansoni, S. haematobium, S. japonicum*) can involve the nervous system, perhaps more frequently the spinal cord. *S. mansoni* can affect the spinal cord more frequently but can also affect the brain. In the case reported by Schils et al. there was a mass effect with some contrast enhancement diagnosed as a malignant glioma on CT (96). Surgical intervention with partial removal revealed the true diagnosis of *S. mansoni*. The great majority of the cases involve the hepatosplenic,

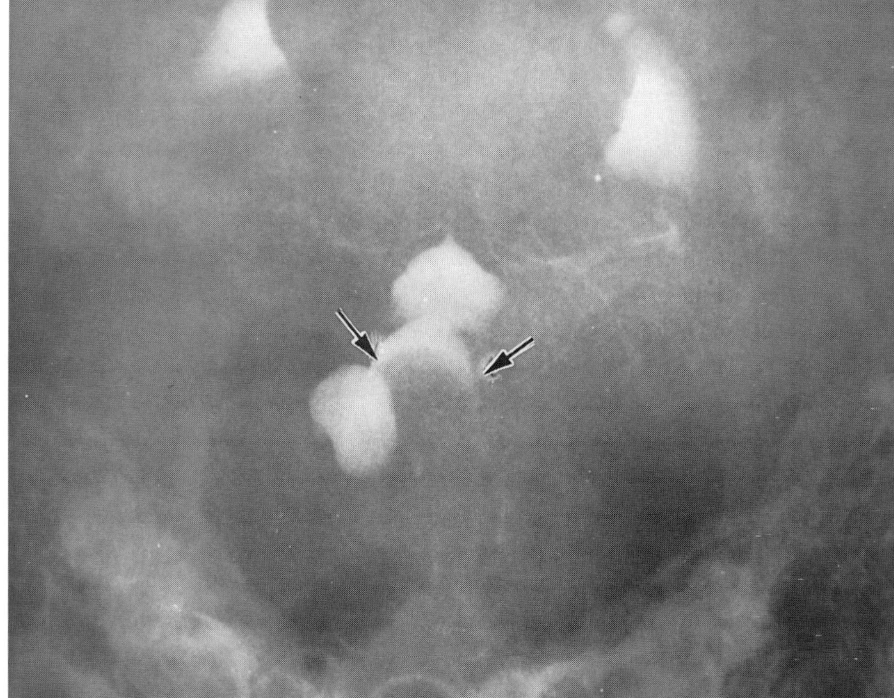

A

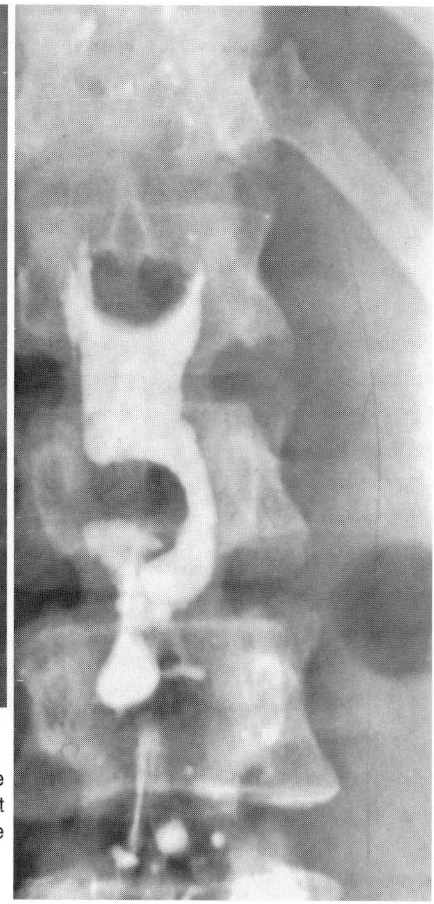

B

Figure 6.38. Cysticercosis in ventricles and in spinal subarachnoid space. **A.** The radiopaque contrast shows the parasitic cyst in the fourth ventricle (arrows). **B.** Myelography in another patient shows lesions in the upper lumbar spinal canal. Fluoroscopically the cysts moved when the table was tilted. (Courtesy of Dr. J. Rodriguez-Carbajal, Mexico City.)

pulmonary, or urinary tracts, and CNS involvement is less common. The diagnosis may be suspected in endemic regions, but it is usually not in countries where it is not seen, except in travelers. The brain lesions may be located anywhere, and the arteritic involvement may lead to cerebral hemorrhage.

Echinococcosis (Hydatid Disease)

This parasite is prevalent in Argentina, Uruguay, and Chile, the Mediterranean countries, and the Middle East and Australia. The definitive host for the adult form is usually the dog, where the tapeworm lives in large numbers in the intestines. Eggs are passed in the excreta, from which they are commonly picked up by sheep, although other mammals, including humans, may serve as the intermediate host. The usual cycle is completed by the dog's eating mutton containing the larval cysts. Shepherds are commonly affected, as are children. Only about 2 percent of patients with echinococcosis develop hydatid cysts of the brain, the majority of the larvae being filtered out in the liver and lungs.

As with cysticercosis, calcification may occur after the death of the parasite. By this time the hydatid cyst may have reached several centimeters in diameter, even in the brain. In contrast with cysticercosis, the hydatid cyst is more often solitary in the brain. Calcification, when it occurs, is chiefly about the perimeter of the cyst; however, there is often a reticular or "ground glass" type of calcium within the cyst cavity, suggesting that it may have been infected or otherwise damaged prior to death of the larva.

The cysts are easily seen by CT or MRI. They are usually unilocular, but multilocular cysts are also seen that are probably related to the presence of "daughter cysts" (Fig. 6.39). They are most frequently encountered in the supratentorial space and much less commonly in the posterior fossa or brainstem (97).

It is important to make a preoperative diagnosis of hydatid cyst because otherwise the surgeon will not be appropriately forewarned and may rupture and spread the cyst contents. This may lead to an anaphylactic reaction and/or to seeding of the "daughters" in the subarachnoid space, which would create further involvement. Fortunately, some pharmacological therapy is available (98). Although hydatid cysts are usually seen in endemic areas, they may be found in any country in travelers or in immigrants. Brain involvement in hydatidosis is seen only in about 2 to 4 percent of cases (Table 6.6).

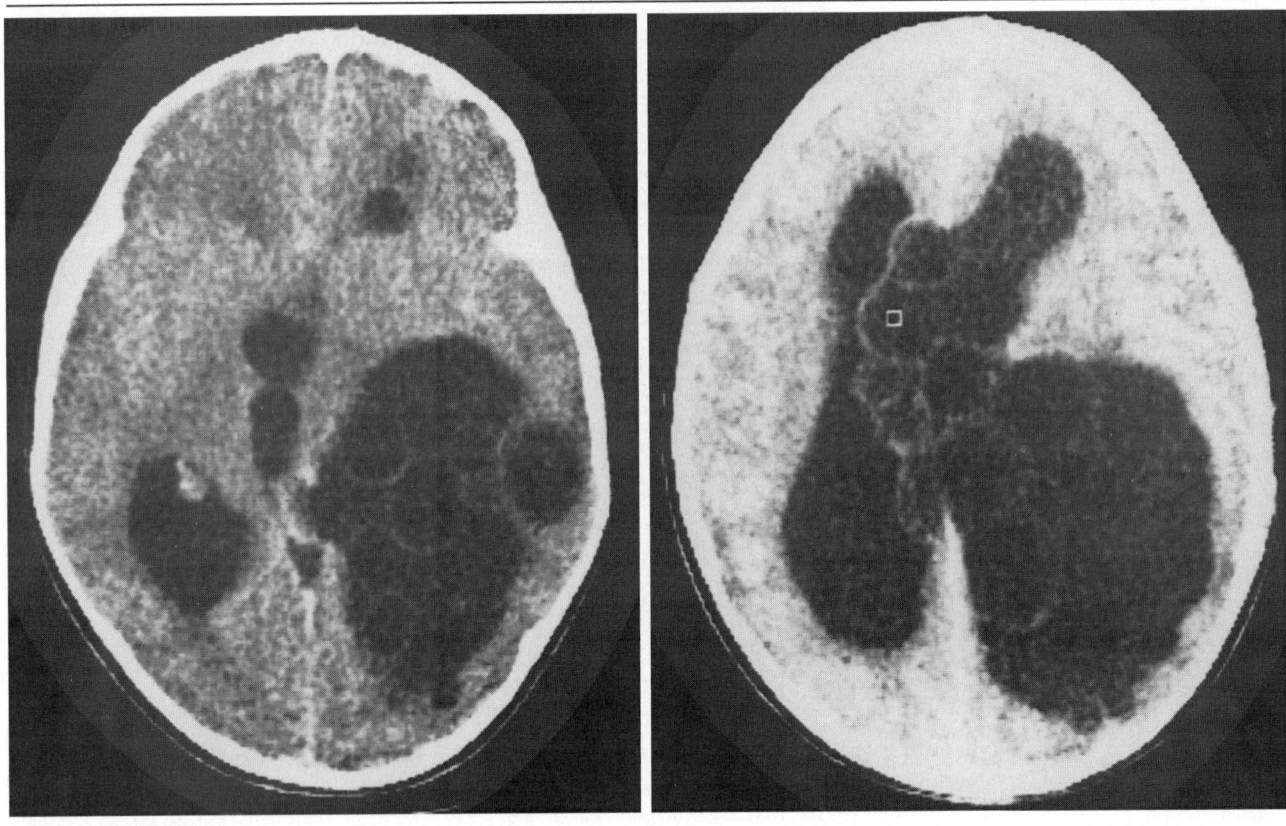

Figure 6.39. *Echinococcus* cyst. **A.** CT scan showing large multiloculated cyst within the left ventricle **B.** At a higher level, the cyst is seen to displace the septum pellucidum and project to the right of the midline. The multiloculations represent daughter cysts and further complicate the surgical procedure, for the parasites must be removed while preventing spillage, which can produce severe reactions. (Courtesy of Dr. Sergio Moguillansky, Neuquen, Argentina.)

Table 6.6.
Parasitic Infections of the CNS

- Toxoplasmosis
  - Meningitis, encephalitis, and ependymitis.
  - Multiple ring-enhancing parenchymal masses.
  - Periventricular calcification, hydrocephalus, and microcephaly commonly seen in congenital form of infection.
- Cysticercosis
  - Intracranial cyst formation with little or no inflammatory response prior to larval death.
  - Intense inflammatory changes after larval death, with decrease in cyst size, thickening of cyst wall, and eventual calcification.
  - Cysts may be located in ventricles or arachnoid spaces over brain or spinal cord, and sometimes in brain parenchyma.
- Schistosomiasis
  - Endemic regions include Africa, Brazil, and Japan.
  - Frequently coexistent pulmonary, hepatic, or genitourinary infection.
  - Involvement of brain or spinal cord.
- Echinococcosis
  - Endemic in South America, Australia, and the Middle East.
  - CNS involvement is uncommon.
  - Intraparenchymal ("hydatid") cyst formation with peripheral califications.

ADDITIONAL CONSIDERATIONS

Infection of the Choroid Plexus

In a recent paper, Mathews and Smith have pointed out that choroid plexitis is an entity, existing alone or in association with other inflammatory brain disease, that can be diagnosed by CT or MRI (99). Enlargement of the choroid plexus, in the area of the glomus and/or elsewhere, that enhances markedly on CT or MRI may be an indication of infection of the choroid plexus. In one of their cases the inflammation may have been induced by a virus; in others bacterial or fungi were proved by biopsy.

The choroid plexus may be a portal of entry for infections such as meningococcal and tuberculous meningitis. Isolated choroid plexitis is rare. The choroid plexus may also be involved in other noninfectious inflammatory processes, such as sarcoidosis, xanthogranulomas, and rheumatoid nodules (100,101). Bright, somewhat enlarged glomera of the choroid plexus are often seen bilaterally. They are bright on T2-weighted images and on CT show diminished attenuation and some peripheral calcification. They are most probably due to xanthogranuloma formation and

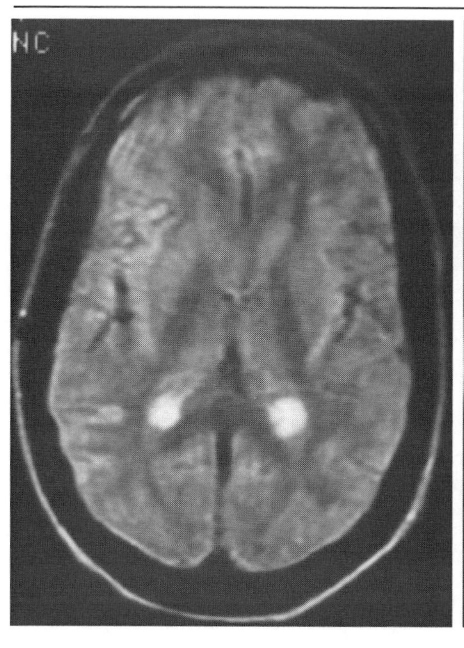

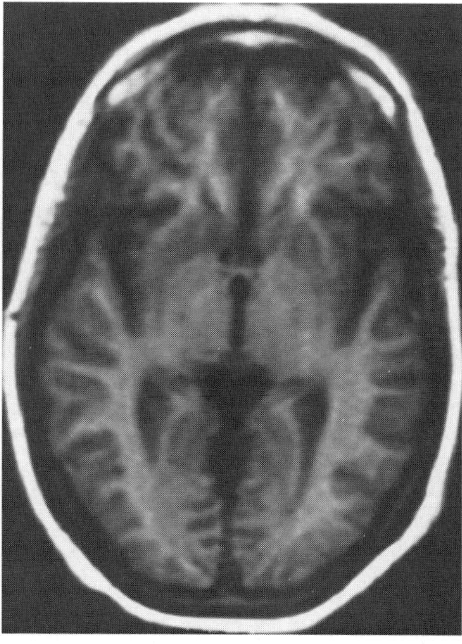

A B

Figure 6.40. Xanthogranuloma of choroid glomus. **A.** Proton density axial image showing bright choroid glomera that are larger than usual in a 20-year-old man. **B.** On a T1-weighted image the enlarged glomera are not seen. The condition is of no clinical significance.

are of no pathologic significance (Fig. 6.40)(102). The choroid plexus may be the primary site of entry into the brain for some toxins. For instance, experimentally used cyclophosphamide and heavy metals such as mercuric chloride can produce a severe hemorrhagic choroid plexitis.

Enlargement of the choroid plexus may be seen in Sturge-Weber and Klippel-Trenaunay-Weber syndromes and in patients with meningomyeloceles.

Rheumatoid nodules of the brain have been reported but are rather unusual (100). The author has not seen a case.

Cerebral Arteritis

A number of pathologic processes can affect the arteries, not only in the brain but also elsewhere in the body. There is a great variety to the types of etiologic factors that may involve the arteries (Table 6.7). The pathologic process, although involving the arterial wall, is not confined to the vessels and is commonly part of a wider process that involves the meninges and the brain tissue. This is particularly true with the infectious processes. The arterial involvement may affect mostly the intima, leading to intimal fibrosis and thickening with partial or complete obstruction, or it may affect the entire wall of the vessel, including the adventitia. It may be diffuse, involving a fairly long segment of a vessel, or it may be segmental.

ANGIOGRAPHIC FINDINGS

The angiographic findings can be divided for convenience into three types: (a) arterial narrowing, (b) arterial aneurysms, and (c) arterial occlusion.

Arterial narrowing can be produced by simple vasal spasm; which is entirely reversible, or by direct involvement of the wall, in which case the process will probably not be reversible, although this is not necessarily so. The presence of an irregular configuration in the margins of the involved vessel is probably an indication of involvement of the arterial wall rather than spasm. On the other hand, in the presence of smooth narrowing, the presence of an irritative contraction of the wall of the artery secondary to an inflammatory process involving the adjacent brain or meninges cannot be differentiated from actual inflammation of the arterial wall (Fig. 6.41). Complete reversion of the arterial narrowing to a normal appearance is not necessarily an indication of spasm as the initial cause of the arteriographic appearance. Spasm tends to be segmental, with the contracted portion of the vessel being situated

Table 6.7.
Cerebral Arteritis

Etiologies:*
1. Primary CNS arteritis
2. Due to systemic arteritis (e.g., giant cell arteritis, polyarteritis nodosa)
3. Due to systemic disease (e.g., systemic lupus erythematosus and other collagen vascular diseases)
4. Due to primary CNS causes (e.g., meninigitis)
5. Other causes (e.g., substance abuse)

Angiographic findings
- Arterial narrowing: often alternating segments of stenosis and dilatation
- Arterial occlusions (due to nonseptic or septic emboli)
- "Mycotic" aneurysms

CT findings: Often normal or small infarctions

MRI findings: Almost invariably one or more T2 hyperintense regions within gray or white matter, often within centrum semiovale or at corticomedullary junction

* Adapted from Harris et al: AJNR 1994;15:317–330 and Fauci et al: Ann Intern Med 1978;89:660–676.

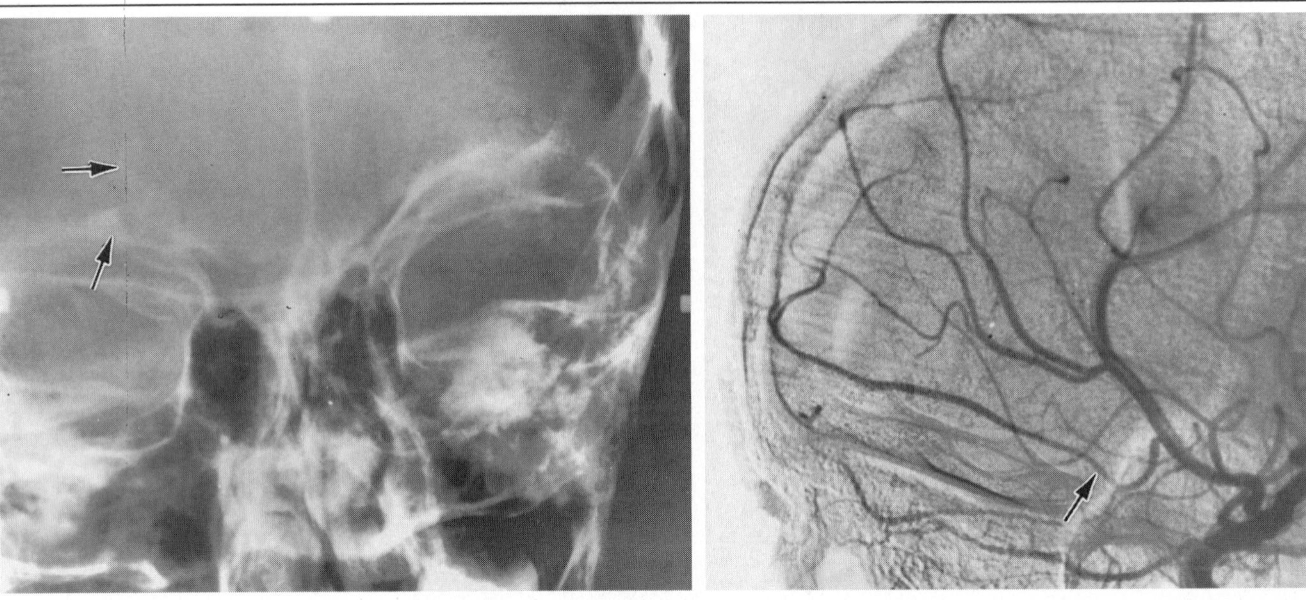

A B

Figure 6.41. Chronic abscess with calcification and localized arterial spasm. **A.** The plain film shows a faintly calcified ring (upper arrow) and some increased density in the bone as well as local loss of density in the upper margin of the orbit (lower arrow). **B.** Angiography shows local mass effect and focal narrowing of the frontopolar branch of the anterior cerebral artery (arrow). The child had fallen on a rose bush 2 years previously and a wooden spike was recovered from the chronic abscess. Focal arterial narrowing may be seen in association with infection and is felt to result from arterial spasm.

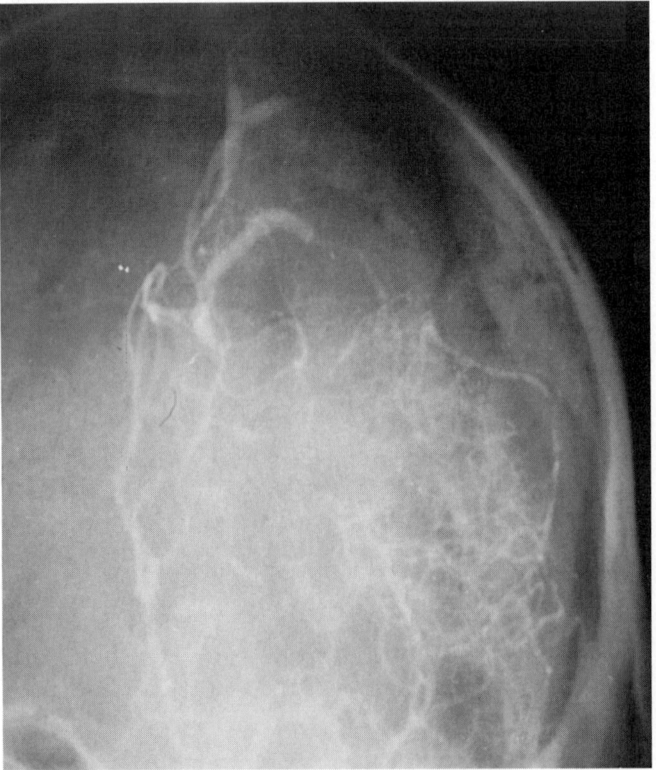

Figure 6.42. Meningitis and subdural abscess producing segmental arterial narrowing and dilatation with reversal several months later. **A.** Frontal view demonstrates midline displacement of the anterior cerebral artery and areas of dilatation on branches of the anterior cerebral artery. **B.** The dilatation and the narrowing are obvious and involve only the branches of the anterior cerebral artery. On repeat angiography after recovery, the arterial system was normal (not shown).

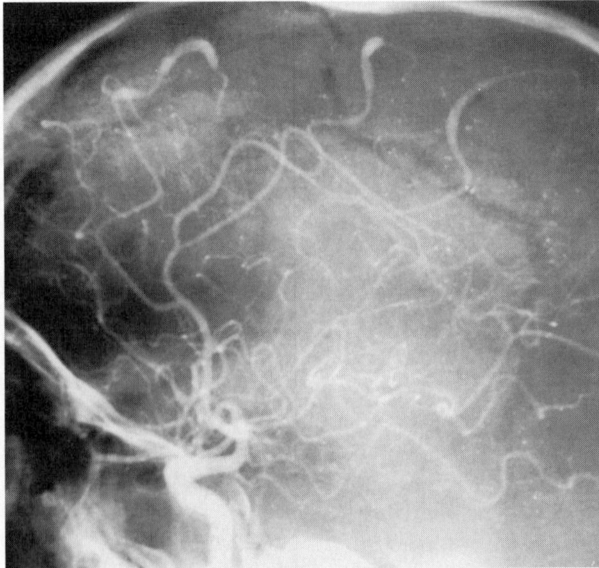

A B

between branches and a wider portion at the sites of bifurcation or at the sites of origin of branches (Fig. 6.42; see also Fig. 10.104). An almost aneurysmatic type of dilatation of the peripheral portion of branches of the anterior and middle cerebral arteries associated with areas of pronounced narrowing may take place (103–106). Inasmuch as this appearance has been described in bacterial meningitis, as well as in conditions such as *Nocardia* infection, it is likely that it represents a nonspecific appearance (Figs. 6.34 and 6.42). This arteriographic appearance is different from that seen in the cases of arterial narrowing that have been reported in addicted patients using multiple drugs, chiefly intravenous methamphetamines (see discussion following).

The "aneurysmatic dilatation" of the vessels involves the distal branches of the major arteries on the surface of the brain in meningitis. In spasm associated with subarachnoid hemorrhage, the segmental narrowing and dilatation is seen at the trunks of the major cerebral arteries. The branches may be diffusely narrow, and, more distally, the caliber of the lumen usually tends to become normal. However, on occasion, segmental narrowing and relative dilatation of the distal branches may be seen in "spasm" associated with subarachnoid hemorrhage.

Narrowing and occlusion of intracranial arteries have been described in syphilis involving the central nervous system. In a case reported by Vatz et al. there was diffuse narrowing of the supraclinoid carotid artery bilaterally and occlusion of the anterior cerebral artery on one side (107). The appearance was not dissimilar to that described in tuberculous meningitis. Irregular "beading" in the anterior

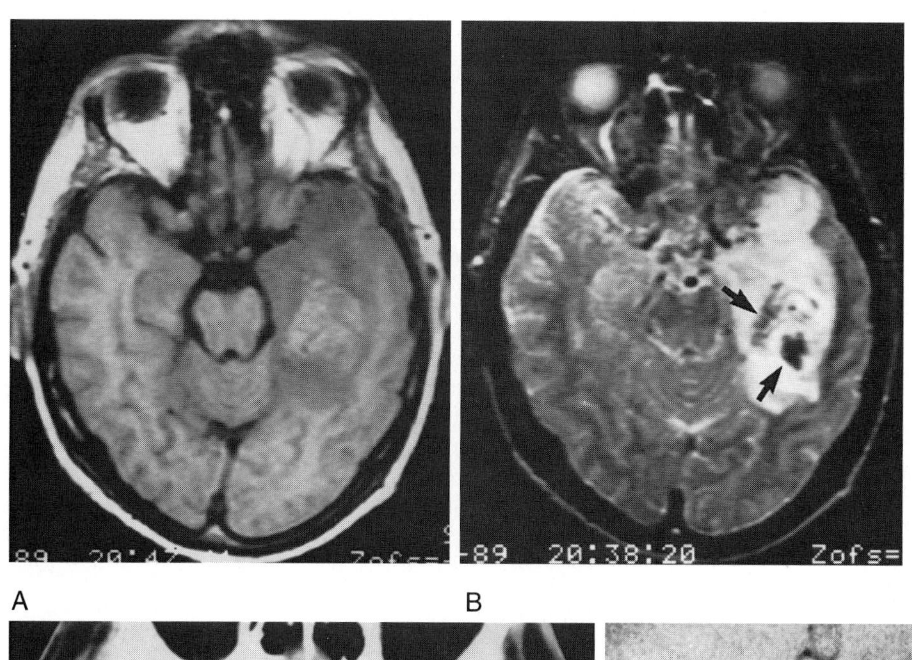

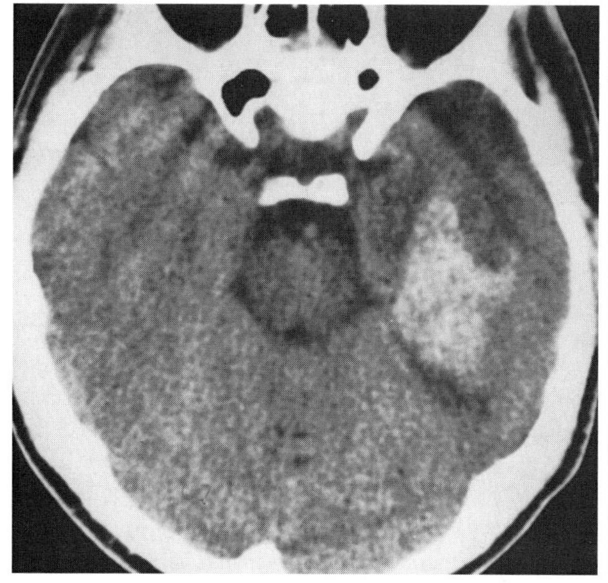

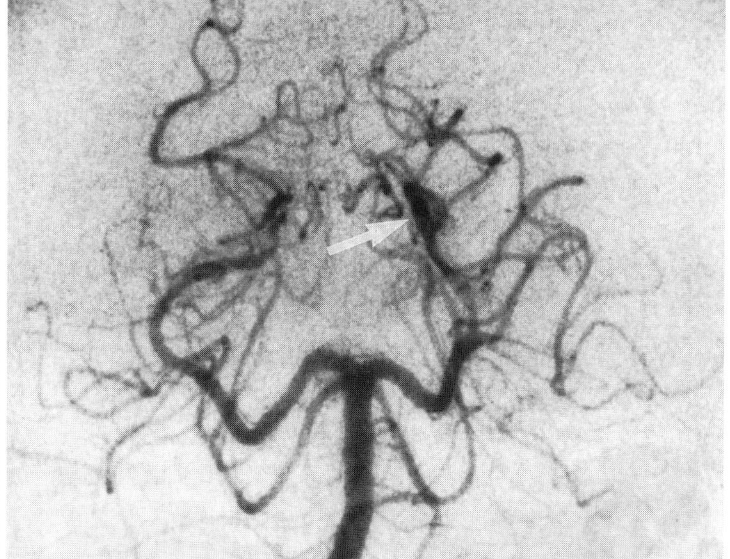

Figure 6.43. Bleeding into temporal lobe due to a mycotic aneurysm. **A.** The patient presented with headaches, difficulty speaking, and low-grade fever. MRI examination was carried out first, and the T1-weighted image revealed some decreased intensity with an irregular distribution in the left temporal lobe. The roughly square area in the dorsal side of the abnormality is actually isodense with the white matter. **B.** The T2-weighted axial image shows a large area of hyperintensity. Posteriorly, there are areas of marked hypointensity (arrows), which may be produced by calcification or by blood products. **C.** A CT examination without contrast done the following day indicated that there was a hemorrhage in the temporal lobe. **D.** Angiography demonstrated an aneurysm arising from the distal portion of a branch of the left posterior cerebral artery (arrow). This 52-year-old man was found to have a bacterial endocarditis unknown until then.

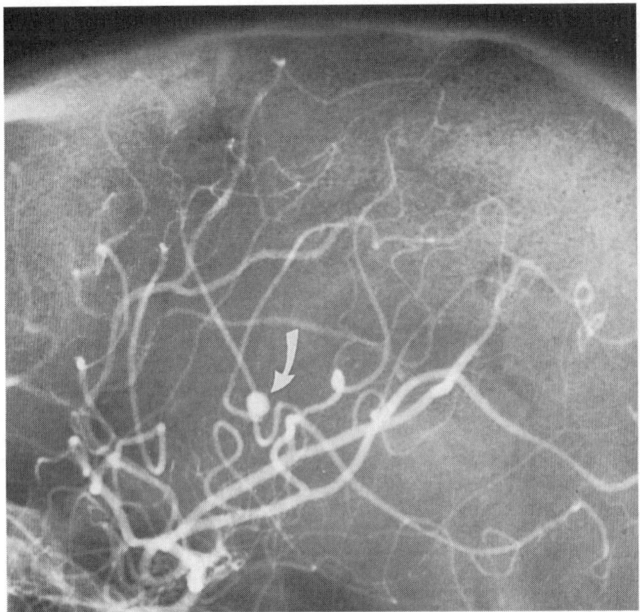

A

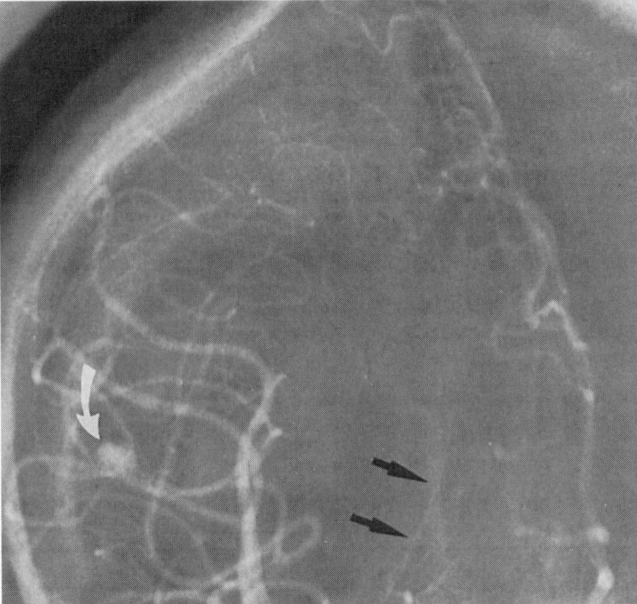

B

Figure 6.44. **A** and **B.** Angiography in a patient who presented with an acute episode of bleeding. The lateral (A) and frontal (B) views demonstrated an aneurysm in the distal portion of a middle cerebral artery branch (curved white arrows) that was associated with spreading of middle cerebral artery branches in the suprasylvian portion of the frontal lobe, and a midline shift as well as medial displacement of the lenticulostriate branches of the middle cerebral artery (black arrows). The position of the aneurysm, which originated in a distal branch of the middle cerebral artery, indicates its probably infectious origin. Spastic narrowing of segments of several arteries is noted. This may be seen in patients with intracerebral and/or subarachnoid bleeding.

and middle cerebral arteries has also been observed on angiograms in a patient with neurosyphilis (108).

Aneurysm formation is not uncommon following septic emboli and may be seen in patients with subacute bacterial endocarditis and with congenital heart disease (109). A septic embolus will lodge in one of the branches of the anterior, middle, or posterior cerebral artery and produce a local inflammatory process, causing weakening of the wall that may lead to the formation of a mycotic aneurysm. The aneurysm in turn may lead to abscess formation, or it may rupture and hemorrhage (Figs. 6.43 [see page 307] and 6.44). The formation of multiple aneurysms has been reported in patients with endocardial myxoma (110). The walls of the vessels were found to be invaded by myxoma cells. As already mentioned, pseudoaneurysmatic dilatation of arteries is not uncommon in association with inflammatory processes of the meninges and brain (Fig. 6.42). It is probably due to involvement of the wall in the inflammatory process. If recovery takes place, the involved vessel may become occluded, or it may return to normal width (111). Aneurysm formation may also be seen in the cervical portion of the internal carotid artery in conditions such as peritonsillar abscess in children (Fig. 6.45) and in mucormycosis (Fig. 6.36) (112).

Among the viral pathogens that can produce arterial involvement, herpes simplex and herpes zoster have been described (9).

Arterial occlusions of inflammatory origin involving the intracranial vessels are not uncommon. They may involve

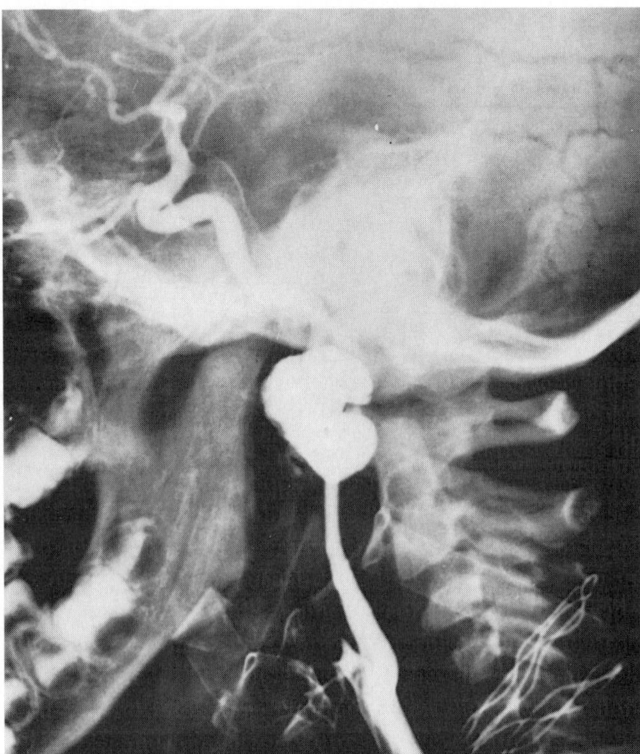

Figure 6.45. Aneurysm of internal carotid in a child with peritonsillar abscess. There is a narrowing of the internal carotid artery proximal to the aneurysm. The external carotid artery had been ligated 24 h earlier.

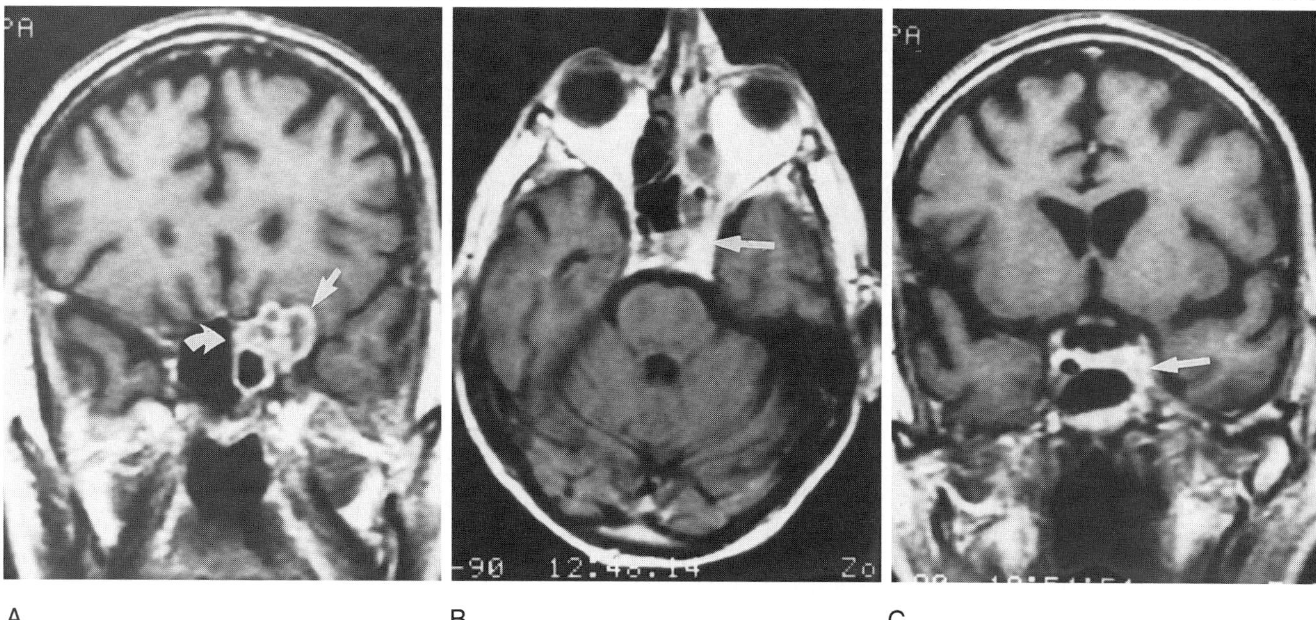

A B C

Figure 6.46. Occluded carotid in leukemic 74-year-old man with invasive aspergillosis. **A.** A postcontrast T1-weighted coronal view reveals an enhancing lesion extending to the midline and intracranially; the lesion also involves the posterior ethmoid cells (arrows). **B.** Axial postcontrast T1-weighted image shows absence of the internal carotid artery flow void (arrow) that is well seen on the right. **C.** Axial view shows that the flow void is clearly absent on the left carotid (arrow). The patient had developed a right hemiparesis.

the larger vessels, the supraclinoid portion of the internal carotid artery, and the trunks of the middle and anterior cerebral arteries, or they may involve the distal branches. The incidence of supraclinoid carotid and middle cerebral artery occlusions occurring in children owing to a nonspecific localized inflammatory process is not known (113). Complete occlusion may be produced by septic emboli, but nonseptic emboli are a much more common cause of occlusions. In a manner similar to the stenotic lesions, arterial occlusions as the result of inflammation are seen in association with meningitis and meningoencephalitis, and may be due to direct involvement of the artery with production of edema, necrosis, and granuloma formation in the arterial wall. As explained earlier, narrowing of the larger arteries at the base of the brain is common in tuberculous meningitis (Fig. 6.26), whereas occlusion of many of the finer branches of the cortex may be observed in the same patient. Carotid occlusion may be seen in invasive aspergillosis complicating other conditions (Fig. 6.46). It may be difficult by arteriography to ascertain the presence of distal occlusion, but this can be diagnosed if the peripheral branches of the middle or anterior cerebral arteries fail to empty in the correct sequence (Fig. 6.47). At the same time this may be associated with an area of hyperemia as a result of cortical infarction, as well as inflammatory granuloma. The involvement may extend to the veins and even to the venous sinuses, leading to sinus thrombosis.

The diagnosis of multiple arterial occlusions secondary to arteritis may be difficult. If the arteritis is associated with the phenomena just described, namely, the narrowing and widening of the vessel lumen in distal arteries, the diagnosis may be suggested, particularly if the wide zones are considerably wider than the usual diameter of the arterial lumen, for this phenomenon is not observed in arterial spasm associated with subarachnoid hemorrhage.

GRANULOMATOUS GIANT CELL ARTERITIS

This condition is histologically similar to temporal arteritis. However, temporal arteritis is usually localized to the temporal arteries and may involve the ophthalmic arteries, leading to blindness; it usually does not involve the arteries of the brain. On the other hand, allergic granulomatous angiitis is a generalized systemic granulomatous process that may be associated with asthma, eosinophilia, and vascular occlusions and is frequently fatal. Brain involvement may occur. The term *giant cell arteritis* has been applied to both entities because of the histological appearance. Hinck et al. reported a case of giant cell arteritis that demonstrated a beaded appearance to the anterior and middle cerebral artery branches, caused by areas of narrowing and dilatation (114). Occlusion of arteries is uncommon.

In a case of biopsy-proven temporal arteritis, the external carotid branches showed irregular narrowing (Fig. 6.48). The angiographic appearance probably is not characteristic in this condition.

Giant cell arteritis may occasionally involve the carotid artery in the neck down to its origin. The histologic appearance is different from that of Takayasu arteritis. In Takay-

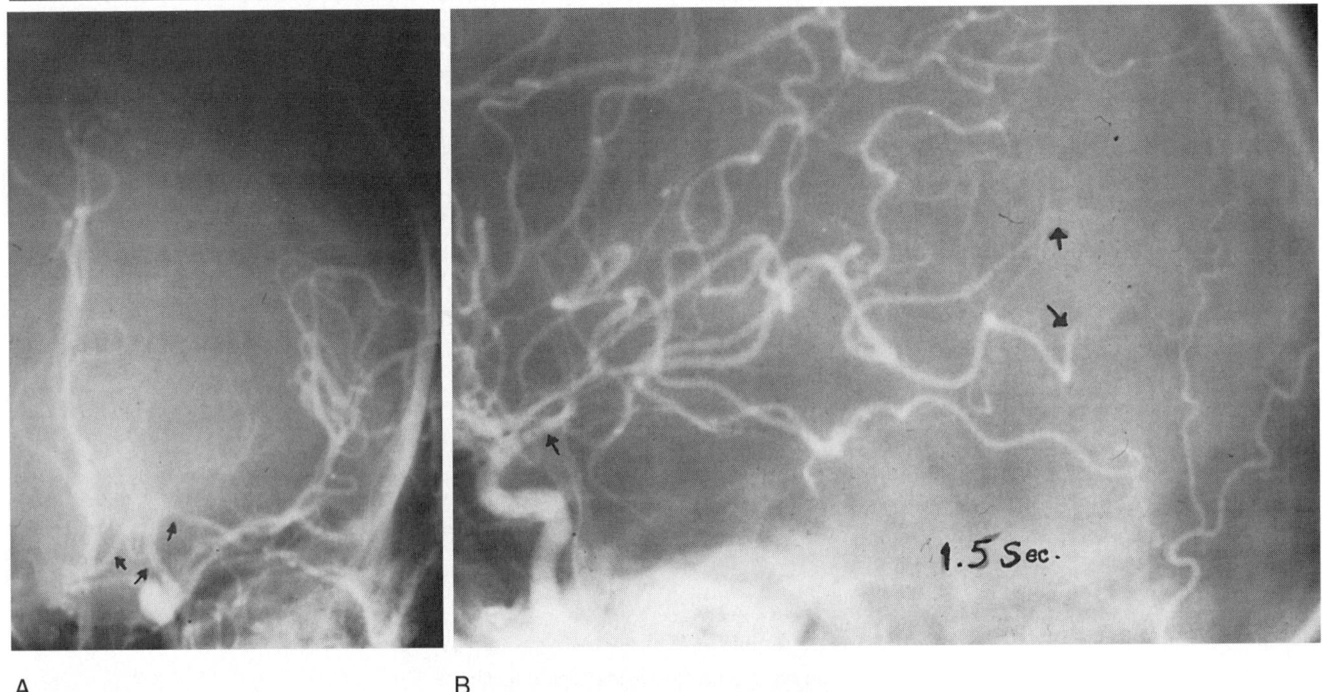

A B

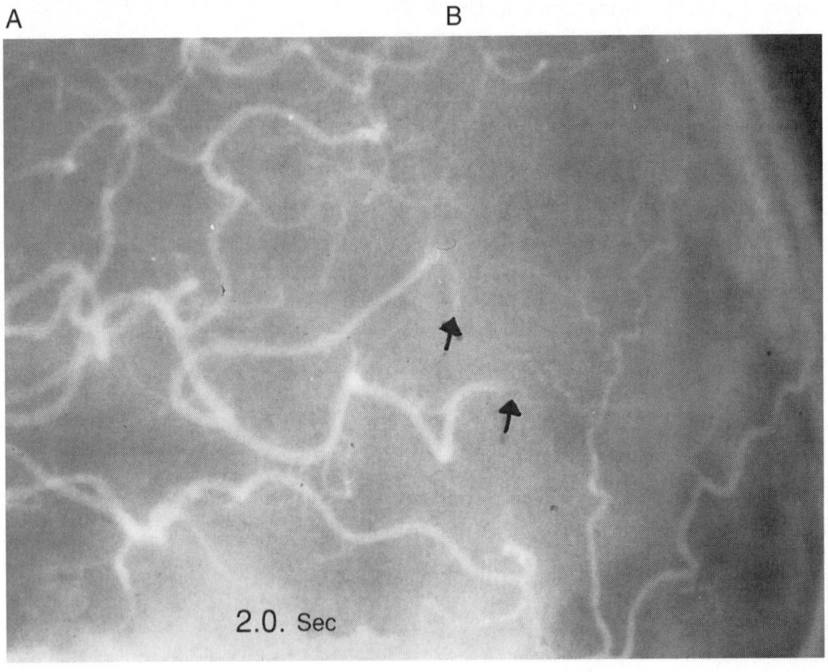

C

Figure 6.47. Arterial narrowing and occlusion in an adult patient with tuberculous meningitis. **A.** There is a uniform narrowing of the supraclinoid portion of the internal carotid artery and of the horizontal segments of the anterior and middle cerebral arteries (arrows). **B.** A film at 1.5 sec shows slow filling of branches of the middle cerebral artery in the parieto-occipital region (arrows). **C.** At 2.0 sec, slightly more filling is present. At 5.0 sec (not shown), the filling stage was still incomplete in these vessels.

asu arteritis there is a periarteritis with round cell foci that involves the media and adventitia, later involving the rest of the artery and leading to intimal sclerosis and final occlusion of the artery. The disease is seen in young female patients, and the usual site is the vessels at the base of the neck, but involvement of other arteries such as the aorta and the renal arteries is also seen occasionally.

SYSTEMIC LUPUS ERYTHEMATOSUS

In this condition involvement of the larger arteries of the brain is rare, although central nervous system manifestations are frequent. Intracranial occlusions have been described (115), and at least one case of multiple aneurysms at sites of arterial bifurcations has been seen by the author.

CT or MRI findings may demonstrate cerebral infarction of the areas supplied by the affected vessels. However, MRI may also show cortical or deep white matter lesions that disappear on reexamination at a later date. They may have been ischemic lesions, but if so infarction, which is a permanent state, did not occur. The lesions may be multiple and migratory (116). See Chapter 14.

Periarteritis nodosa likewise is only occasionally accompanied by demonstrable arteriographic findings, usually arterial narrowing or occlusion.

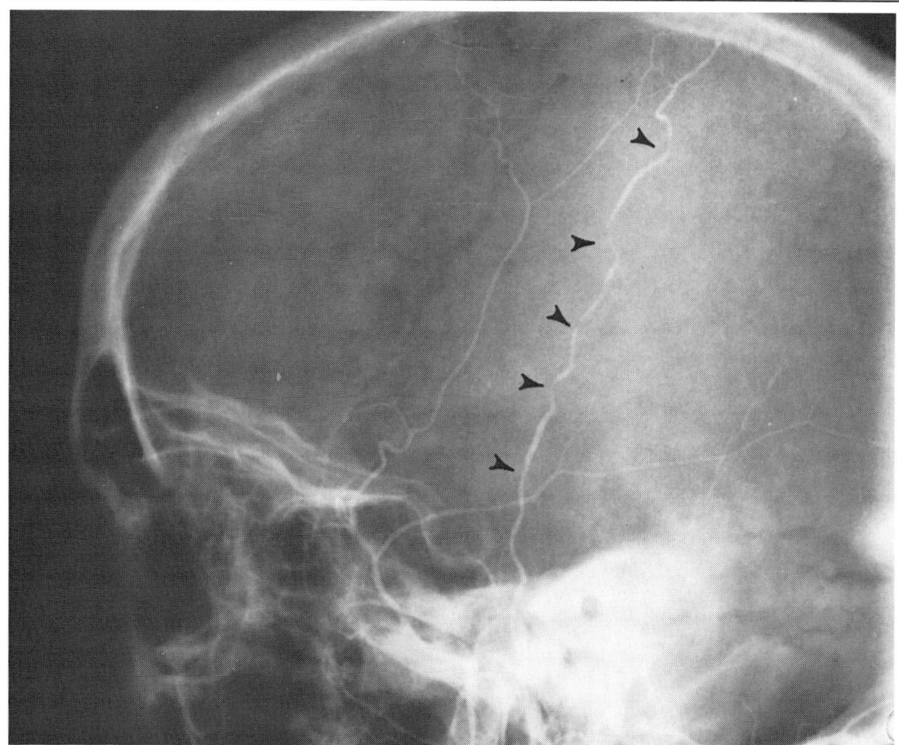

Figure 6.48. Temporal arteritis in a 65-year-old woman. There is irregular segmental narrowing of the posterior branch of the superficial temporal artery. The anterior branch is not filled. The middle meningeal artery branches are normal. The patient had blurring of vision and cordlike temporal arteries that on biopsy revealed giant cell arteritis. The internal carotid artery was occluded, but this is thought to be on the basis of arteriosclerosis.

ACUTE HEMORRHAGIC LEUKOENCEPHALITIS

In acute hemorrhagic leukoencephalitis there is acute involvement of the vessels, but in two cases in which cerebral angiography was carried out there were no demonstrable changes in the arterial contours of the visible arteries (117). This may have something to do with radiographic detail definition; no magnified serial studies were performed. In two other cases reported by Michaud and Helle, there was low attenuation and mass effect in brainstem and cerebellum, but no hemorrhage (118).

ARTERIAL CHANGES IN DRUG ABUSE PATIENTS

These changes have been reported by several authors (119,120). There is segmental arterial narrowing in arteries over the cortex of the cerebral hemispheres. The changes are probably reversible (Fig. 6.49). The drug or drugs responsible for the changes are difficult to identify because addicts often use many drugs. However, the common element in the cases that have been seen is intravenous methamphetamine. Rumbaugh et al. attempted to reproduce the findings in monkeys and were partially successful in producing arterial spasm in cortical arteries lasting 24 h (119). Histologically, some perivascular cellular infiltration was also found similar to what has been described in humans.

RADIATION ARTERITIS

Arterial narrowing may be seen following radiation therapy, particularly in children and especially if the dose levels are excessive. The arteries acquire an irregularly narrow appearance that is localized to the treated area.

MOYA-MOYA

The syndrome of multiple, progressive intracranial arterial occlusions (Moya-Moya) could be an arteritic process, but at least, in the cases that have gone to autopsy, the majority do not demonstrate any evidence of inflammation, and the cases in which any arteritic process has been seen are questionable in that the inflammation may be superimposed upon a previously diseased vessel, particularly when a child affected with this condition dies of tuberculosis with tuberculous meningitis. See Chapter 10.

ATHEROSCLEROSIS

The angiographic appearance of arteritis can in some ways be simulated by atherosclerosis. There should be no difficulty in differentiating between the two in the great majority of instances. Some cases, however, may present difficulties in differential diagnosis, particularly when the atherosclerotic lesions seem to be localized to an area involving a few vessels and do not involve the vessels at the circle of Willis, which are the most commonly involved in atherosclerosis. If, under these circumstances, the patient presents a clinical picture that is compatible with a disease causing cerebral arteritis, the differential diagnosis could be difficult.

In addition, cases of lymphoma have been described that simulate the appearance of inflammatory processes (106,108).

A diagnosis of arteritis can only be made by angiography. Cross-sectional imaging may only show the ischemic or hemorrhagic lesions, if any. Magnetic resonance angiography (MRA) cannot be used for this purpose because arterial

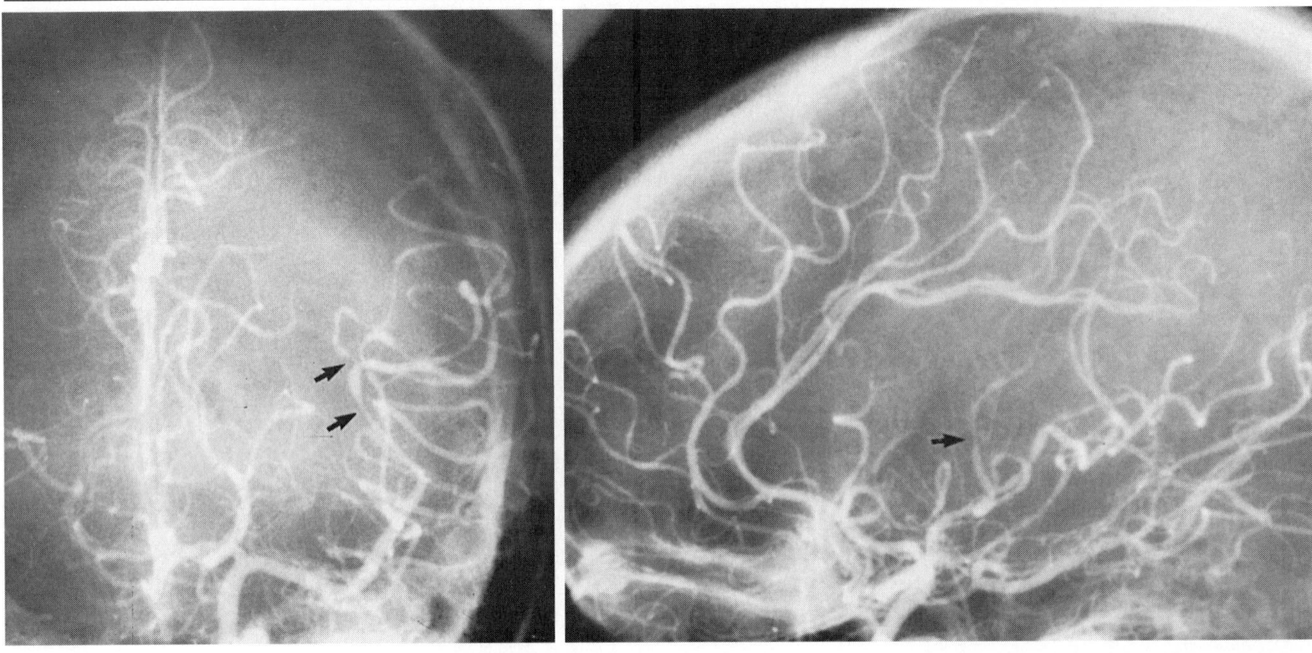

Figure 6.49. Arteritis in a drug abuse patient. The patient presented with obtundation, right hemiplegia, and aphasia, and was known to be on drugs (amphetamines, marijuana). **A** and **B** Left carotid angiogram reveals marked segmental spasm of many branches of the intracranial arteries (arrows) without narrowing of the major vessels (internal carotid artery or trunks of the anterior, middle, and posterior cerebral arteries). In the middle cerebral territory particularly, there are areas of alternating spasm and dilatation of the branches. There was rapid improvement following withdrawal of drugs.

changes are likely to be slight and often difficult to ascertain. Occlusion and severe stenotic lesions of the major arteries would be visible by MRA (Fig. 6.46).

VENOUS AND SINUS THROMBOSIS

Venous and sinus thromboses are common in association with inflammatory processes, particularly meningitis; they may occur as an isolated condition secondary to blood disorders such as polycythemia vera, or secondary to invasion of the sinuses by neoplasms such as meningioma and metastatic disease. (See Chapter 10, "Vascular Disorders," for further details.)

Sydenham Chorea

Chorea (from the Greek dance) refers to abnormal, purposeless movements thought to be due to involvement of the corpus striatum. The best known is Huntington chorea, a heredodegenerative disease described in Chapter 8. Sydenham chorea is related to rheumatic fever, a poststreptococcal infection, and the affected children usually reveal a positive throat culture for beta-hemolytic streptococcus. The disease usually resolves with minimal or no sequelae. Rheumatic heart disease may or may not accompany or follow the disease manifestations. It should be mentioned, however, that chorea may also be related to a host of other conditions, including pregnancy, lupus erythematosus, thyrotoxicosis, myeloproliferative disorders, rubella and pertussis infections, and drug reaction (phenothiazines, levodopa, phenytoin, oral contraceptives).

Kienzle et al. reported two cases of Sydenham chorea demonstrating involvement of the head of the caudate nucleus and the adjacent putamen by MRI (121). Enhancement following gadolinium administration also indicated blood-brain barrier disruption, thus proving the involvement of the corpus striatum as the cause of the choreic movements (Fig. 6.50).

The enhancement with gadolinium is attributed to the presence of a reactive vasculitis. Husby et al. have demonstrated a high incidence (about 50 percent) of positive serum for IgG antibodies, which demonstrate a high affinity for neuronal cytoplasmic antigens from the caudate and subthalamic nuclei (122).

DISEASES OF THE MENINGES

Anatomy

The meninges consist of three layers. The *dura mater*, which covers the interior of the skull, serves the twofold purpose of being an internal periosteum to the bones and a supportive membrane for the brain. It is composed of two layers, an inner or meningeal, and an outer or endos-

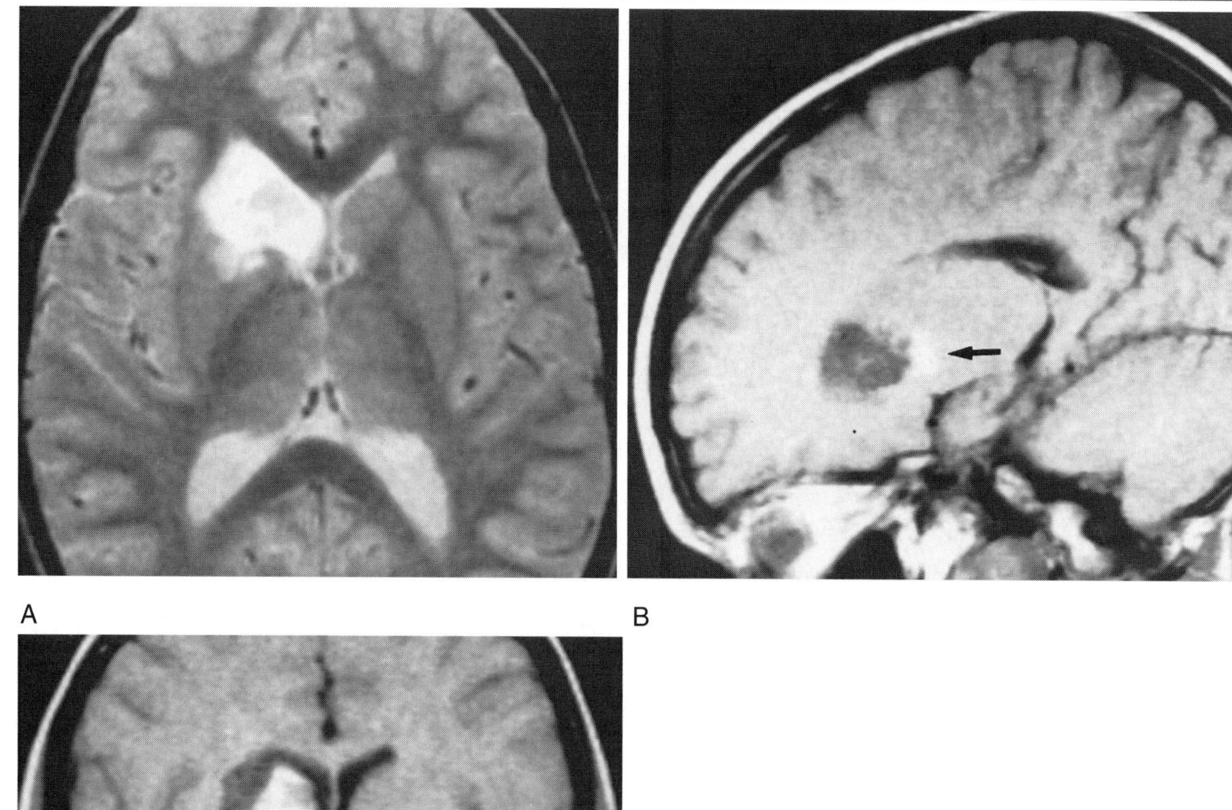

A B

C

Figure 6.50. Sydenham chorea in an 8-year-old boy with a brain lesion shown on MRI. **A.** A T2-weighted axial image shows hyperintensity in the head of the caudate nucleus and in the adjacent putamen and globus pallidus. **B.** The sagittal T1-weighted image reveals diminished intensity in the same area, except for a slightly hyperintense area behind that was felt to be produced by confluent petechial hemorrhage (arrow). **C.** A coronal post-contrast T1-weighted section shows enhancement of the lesion in the caudate nucleus surrounded by a nonenhancing edematous area. (Courtesy of Robert K. Breger, Milwaukee, WI [AJNR 1991;12:73–76].)

teal. The dura mater adheres to the inner surfaces of the cranial bones and sends blood vessels and fibrous processes into them. The dura is most adherent to the bones at the suture lines, at the base of the skull, and around the foramen magnum.

The structure of the dura mater is basically fibrous: white collagen fibers predominating with a mixture of elastic fibers.

The dura mater is well irrigated by a number of arteries: the middle meningeal artery, the accessory meningeal and meningeal branches of the internal maxillary artery, a branch from the ascending pharyngeal artery that enters the skull through the foramen lacerum, branches from the occipital artery, the posterior meningeal branches of the vertebral artery, and others. However, most of the vessels arising from these arteries go to the bone rather than to the dura mater itself.

The extradural space is virtually nonexistent in that the dura is actually partly attached to the inner table of the skull. To separate the dura from the inner table, a hemorrhage or possibly an infection or abscess would have to develop.

In the spine, the dura is separated from the surrounding bone by a space that is usually filled with the veins of the epidural plexus and by epidural fat.

The subdural space is, again, a virtual space between the dura mater and the arachnoid. However, there are no adhesions between the two membranes and they can easily become separated, as they frequently do in pathological processes such as subdural hematomas and infections.

The *arachnoid membrane* is a delicate membrane enveloping the brain and spinal cord that lies between the pia mater internally and the dura mater externally. As just explained, it is separated from the dura mater by the virtual subdural space. The arachnoid invests the brain loosely and does not dip into the cerebral sulci between the gyri or between fissures such as the sylvian fissures, but it does cover the longitudinal fissure as it follows the falx. The arachnoid membrane is thinner over the top of the brain and somewhat thicker over the basal structures; around this area there is a significant space between the arachnoid and the pia mater that forms some of the subarachnoid cisterns. As is well known, the space between the arachnoid and the pia mater is the subarachnoid space, which is filled with cerebrospinal fluid. The separation of the arachnoid and pia leaves a fairly large space in some areas, such as the cisterna magna, the cisternal spaces in front of the brainstem, the interpeduncular cistern, around the suprasellar region, where a number of cisternal spaces are usually recognized, and other spaces around the brain and in the region of the sylvian fissure.

The arachnoid granulations are relatively small projections into the venous sinuses, the superior sagittal, the transverse, and some of the other sinuses. These arachnoid granulations, the pacchionian granulations, have a function related to the absorption of cerebrospinal fluid. They can be large and tend to cause depressions on the inner table of the skull that are usually situated within a short distance from the midline on the inner table (see Fig. 19.3).

The *pia mater* invests the entire surface of the brain, dips between the cerebral gyri and between the cerebellar laminae, and invaginates into the third ventricle, where it forms the tela choroidea of the third ventricle and also the choroid plexuses of the lateral ventricles. At the fourth ventricle it forms the tela choroidea and the choroid plexus of the fourth ventricle. It is a vascular membrane containing a plexus of minute blood vessels held together by an extremely fine areolar tissue. Over the surface of the hemispheres of the brain it covers the minute perpendicular blood vessels that extend down through the substance of the brain. A small amount of cerebrospinal fluid also follows this pial covering, forming what are called the *Virchow-Robin spaces* or *perivascular spaces.* These can become larger in certain circumstances and tend to become larger in older individuals, perhaps in association with generalized tissue loss.

Both the arachnoid and the pia are composed of collagen elastin and reticulin fibers together with flattened cells usually regarded as mesothelial in type. Together they constitute the leptomeninges, as against the dura mater, which represents the pachymeninx.

The dura mater enhances normally with contrast and may be seen on both CT and MRI, particularly the latter. The enhancement is usually slight and rather smooth. The membranes appear as very thin lines without any irregularities, and the enhancement is relatively slow, so that later images are likely to show more of the dural enhancement than earlier ones.

Pathology

Enhancement and thickening of the meninges occurs in patients who have undergone intracranial surgery of almost any type. The pathogenesis of this effect is not well understood and was not really known until MRI with gadolinium enhancement was available. The meninges not only enhance but are also thicker, in some cases more than in others. The enhancement may be relatively localized to the general area where the craniotomy took place, but often both hemispheres as well as the tentorial meninges are enhanced. The enhancement is evidently more marked in the dura mater than in the leptomeninges (Fig. 6.51). One could postulate a mild inflammatory process that led to the meningeal change or the presence of a thin subdural collection of blood, but none of these actually seems to explain the findings adequately.

Meningeal enhancement can also be seen following a shunting procedure. Patients with chronic hydrocephalus who have been shunted may show considerable diffuse thickening of the cranial meninges, and the etiology of this finding is also not clearly understood (123–125). Destian et al. emphasize that the meningeal thickening can be so marked that it cannot be differentiated from a subdural collection without contrast (123). The gadolinium contrast will produce enhancement of the entire thickened membrane, which would not be the case if it were a subdural fluid collection. Meningeal thickening may be seen in chronic meningitis (Fig. 6.51 C to E).

Other causes of marked thickening of the meninges include *hypertrophic idiopathic pachymeningitis,* a rare disorder characterized by marked dural thickening. It may occur in the spine, where it has been observed since the time of Charcot and Joffroy, who were the first to describe this lesion in the cervical region (126). It can be observed intracranially, particularly in the posterior fossa. It usually enhances with contrast both on CT and MRI (Fig. 6.52) (39,127,128). With myelography it would show a separation between the pedicles and the lateral margin of the radiopaque column (see Fig. 16.81) (129). A case of Whipple disease associated with diffuse hypertrophic pachymeningitis has been seen (see Fig. 13.2). Hypertrophic thickening of the dura is also seen in some congenital lesions, such as the Maroteaux-Lamy variety of mucopolysaccharidosis (see Fig. 16.81).

Asymptomatic *rheumatoid pachymeningitis* is a rare extra-articular manifestation of rheumatoid arthritis, with nonspecific clinical symptoms and a diagnosis that could be made by exclusion in a patient who has manifestations of rheumatoid arthritis. Biopsy is usually necessary (130). As usual, the dural thickening would enhance after contrast.

In addition to postoperative enhancement and thickening of the meninges (usually the dura), cases are seen in which there is dural thickening and enhancement with gadolinium when the CSF is normal in terms of cells and protein. A number of possible etiologies have been suggested, such as viral infections, chronic intracranial hypotension (131,132), and lumbar puncture. However, the last-mentioned possibiity is questionable (133). Mittl et al. con-

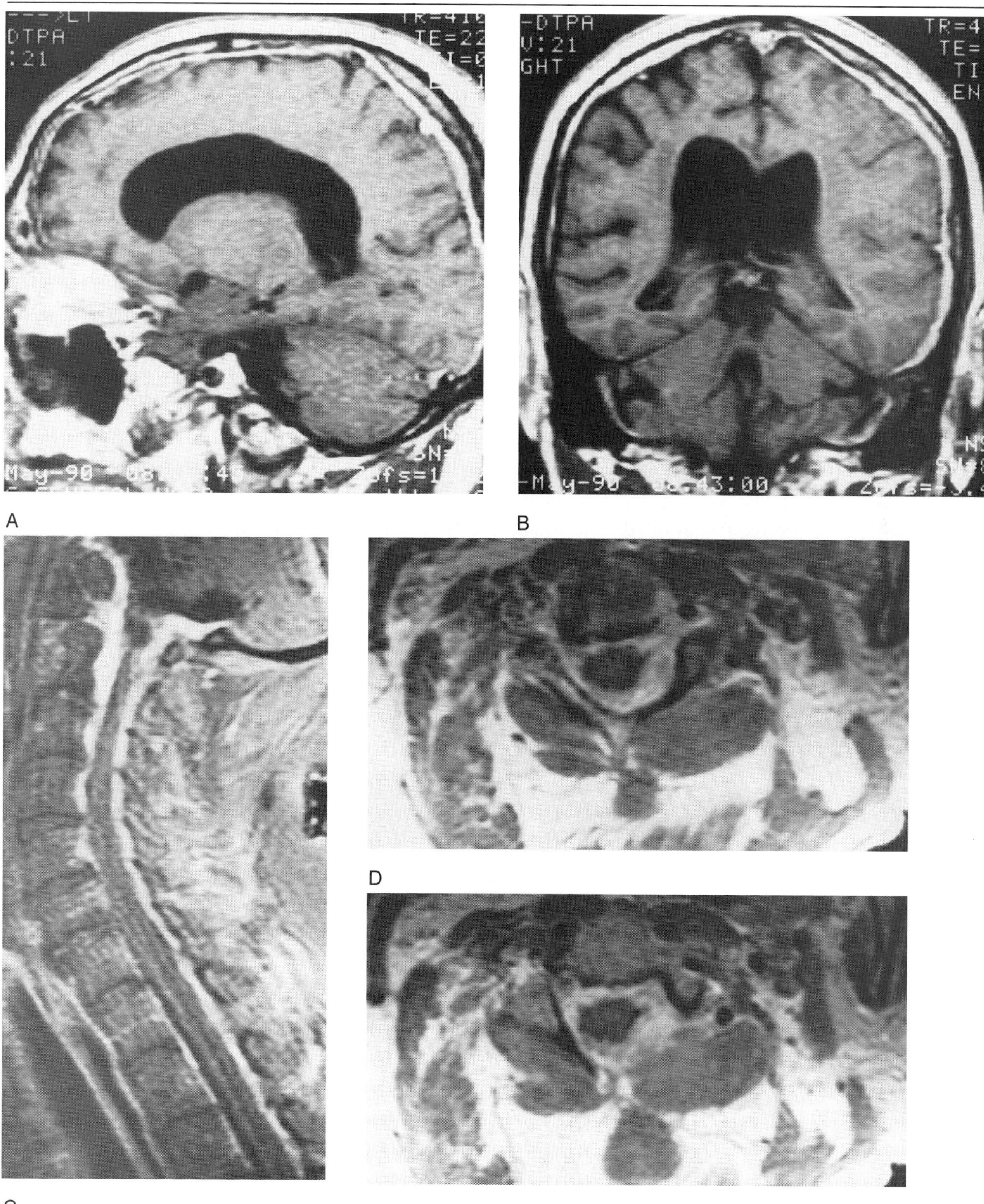

Figure 6.51. Postoperative diffuse thickening of meninges in a patient who had a posterior fossa (cerebellar) tumor removed. On sagittal (**A**) and coronal (**B**) views there is enhancement bilaterally. **C** to **E.** Meningeal thickening in a patient with chronic meningitis that is more marked in the cervical spine. The postcontrast sagittal and axial images demonstrate the marked thickening of the enhanced spinal meninges.

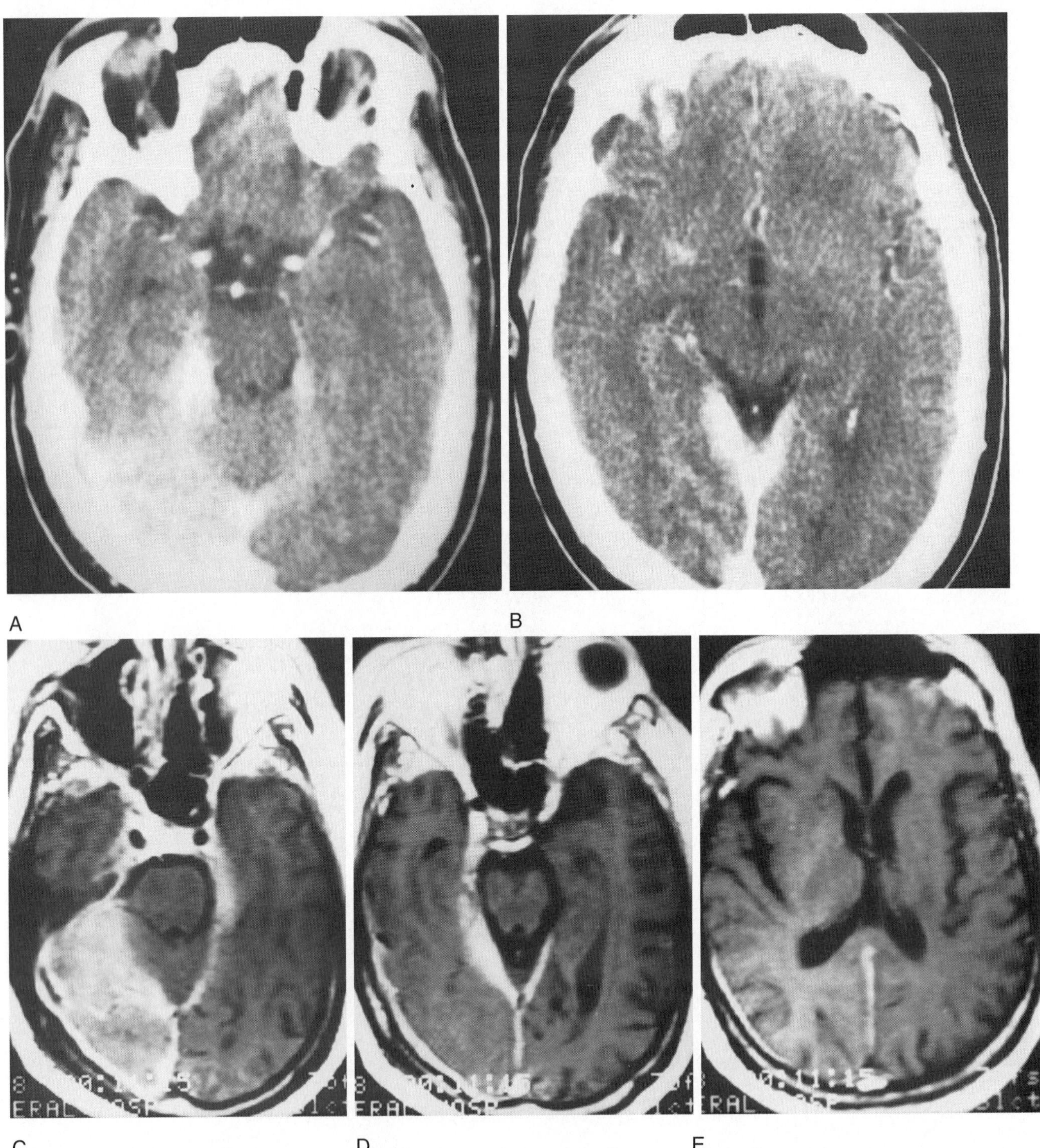

Figure 6.52. Hypertrophic pachymeningitis. **A.** There is marked thickness of the tentorium, more marked on right, as shown in this enhanced CT image. **B.** A higher section reveals the thickened enhanced tentorium. **C.** An enhanced axial T1-weighted MR image shows the enhanced thickened tentorium, particularly on the right side. **D.** A higher section. **E.** In the supratentorial space there is meningeal thickening and enhancement only over the posterior aspects of the head. The patient's symptoms were mostly headache in the back of the head, with no definite cranial nerve involvement.

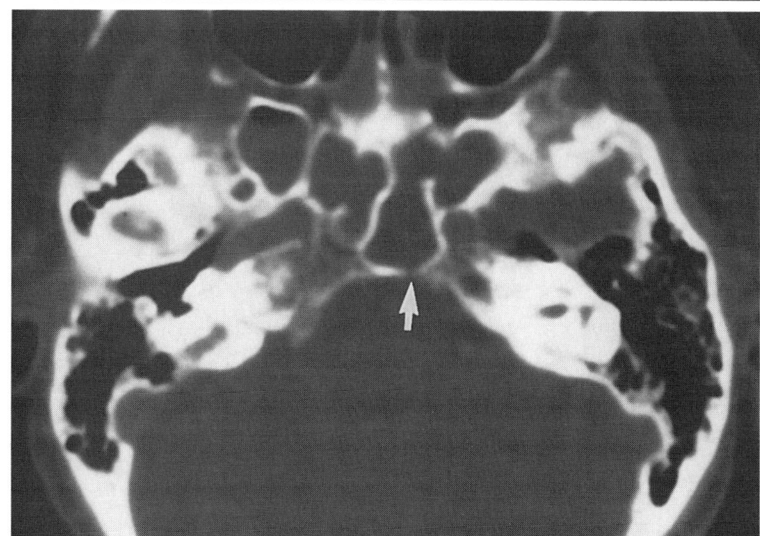

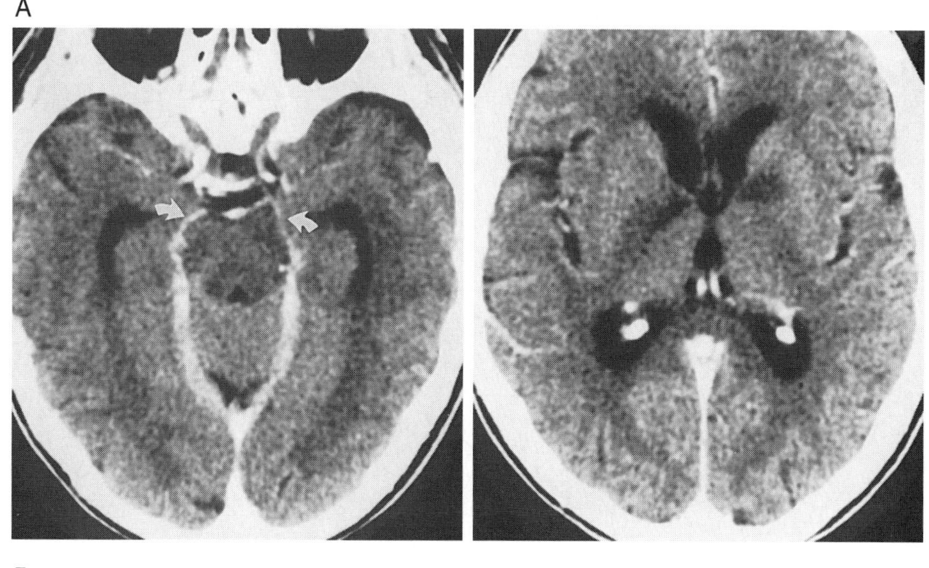

Figure 6.53. *Nocardia* meningitis in a patient with a congenital opening in the posterior sphenoid sinus. The patient died of subacute and chronic meningitis. **A.** There is a small opening in the posterior wall of the sphenoid sinus that was shown at autopsy to be a direct communication and probable path of infection to the subdural space (arrow). The sphenoid sinuses as well as some posterior ethmoid cells are almost totally fluid filled. **B.** There is a particularly heavy meningeal inflammatory reaction around the brainstem and midbrain area anteriorly (curved arrow). The lower midbrain shows diffuse diminished density (compare with the upper cerebellum more dorsally), probably due to edema and/or infarction. **C.** CT axial image shows radiolucency in the posterior limb of the internal capsule on the right and in the genu and globus pallidus on the left that was found to be due to obstruction of perforating arteries with ischemic infarction.

cluded, after examining 92 patients within a month after lumbar puncture, that meningeal enhancement must be rare or does not occur at all (133). They found 7 instances of enhancement in this group, and in each instance, except 1, there was a clear explanation of the reason for the enhancement, including sinus thrombosis, metastatic melanoma, aseptic meningitis, and neurosyphilis. However, other possible complications or sequelae, such as subdural hematomas, intracerebral hemorrhage, and prolonged CSF hypotension, do occur (134–136), and thus dural-arachnoid enhancement or thickening may well occur, though infrequently after lumbar puncture. Vascular stasis has been suggested as a possible pathogenesis. Perhaps this is a possible explanation for the apparent thickening of the dura-arachnoid in most cases where the enhancement is seen (137). Another cause, reported by Tokumaru et al. (138) and Wilms et al. (139), is that seen in nonmeningiomatous malignant lesions, as well as adjacent to meningiomas.

Meningitis

For a discussion of meningitis, see "Bacterial Infections" earlier in this chapter. The diagnosis of meningitis has been considerably assisted by the development of contrast-enhanced MRI. CT is not very helpful in a large proportion of the cases, but may be very useful to show bony defects in the wall of the paranasal sinuses and mastoids (Fig. 6.53).

Neoplasms

The primary tumor of the meninges is the meningioma, described in Chapter 11, "Intracranial Neoplasms." Meningeal carcinomatosis is usually found in the subarachnoid

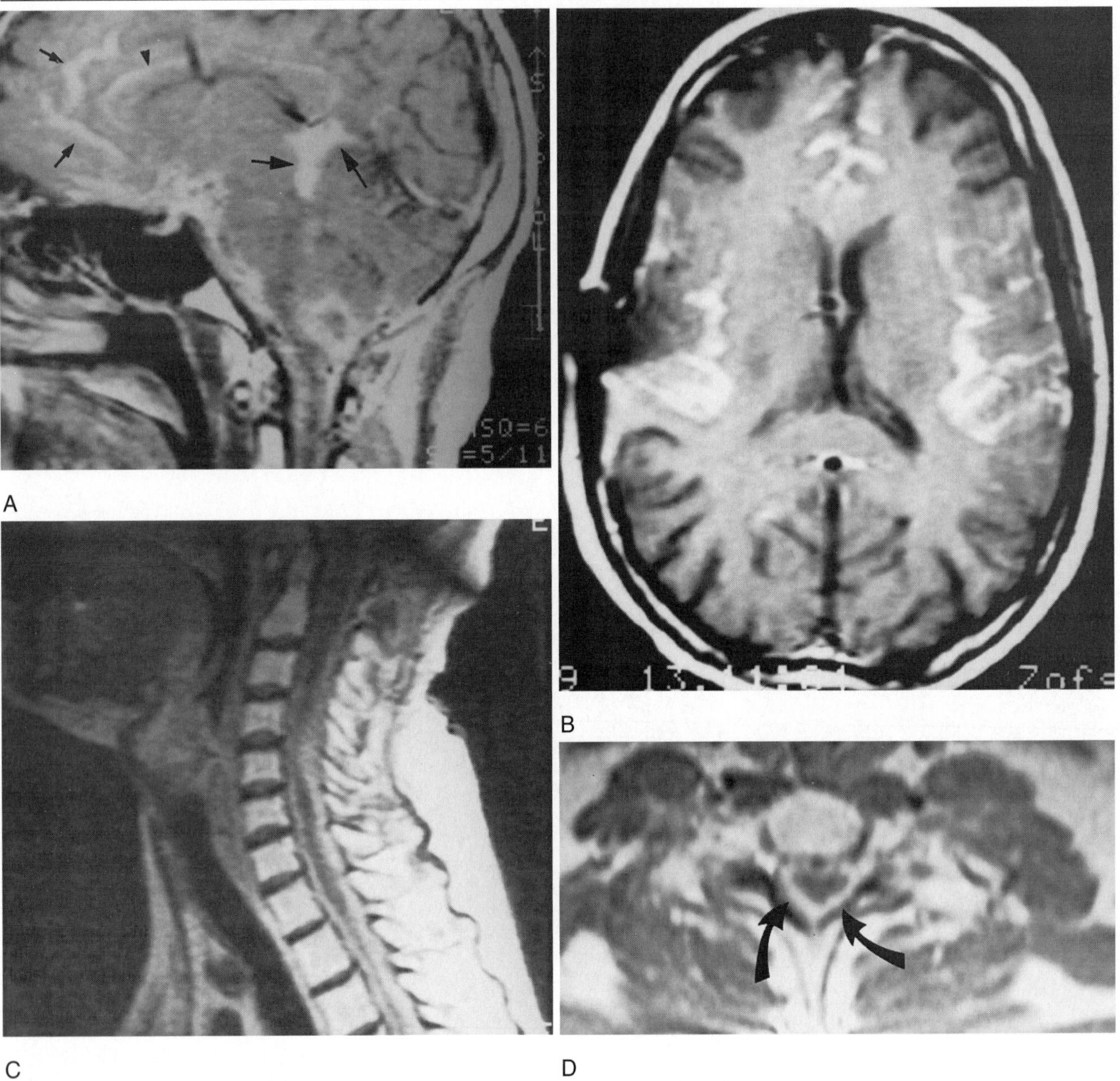

Figure 6.54. Meningeal spread of medulloblastoma in a 20-year-old man. **A.** Sagittal postcontrast image shows hyperintensity in pericallosal and callosomarginal sulci (arrow) as well as in the superior cerebellar and quadrigeminal cistern (posterior arrows) and in the cisterna magna. **B.** There is extensive enhancement in the sylvian fissure bilaterally and in the midline sulci. **C** and **D.** Extensive enhancement in the spinal leptomeninges is also present as seen in sagittal (C) and axial (D) views (curved arrows).

space and spread over the pia mater. The tumor may arise from the nervous system. Most frequently it is a medulloblastoma or pineoblastoma, and sometimes a choroid plexus carcinoma; but it may also arise outside the central nervous system, most commonly from cancer of the breast and lung (Figs. 6.54 and 6.55). The diagnosis is made easily with enhanced MRI. In these cases, involvement of the ventricular wall is also frequently found.

Meningioangiomatosis is a rare, benign, hamartomatous lesion of the leptomeninges. It has been considered to be a forme fruste of neurofibromatosis (140). The lesions can be focal over the surface but apparently extending into the brain, although they may be following the gyri. They enhance with contrast and are surrounded by an area of edema of the adjacent white matter. Calcification is usually seen on CT examination. Diagnosis is made by biopsy and is important because surgical removal results in the cure of this benign condition.

Thickening and enhancement of the dura and sometimes the leptomeninges can occur in patients with neoplasms

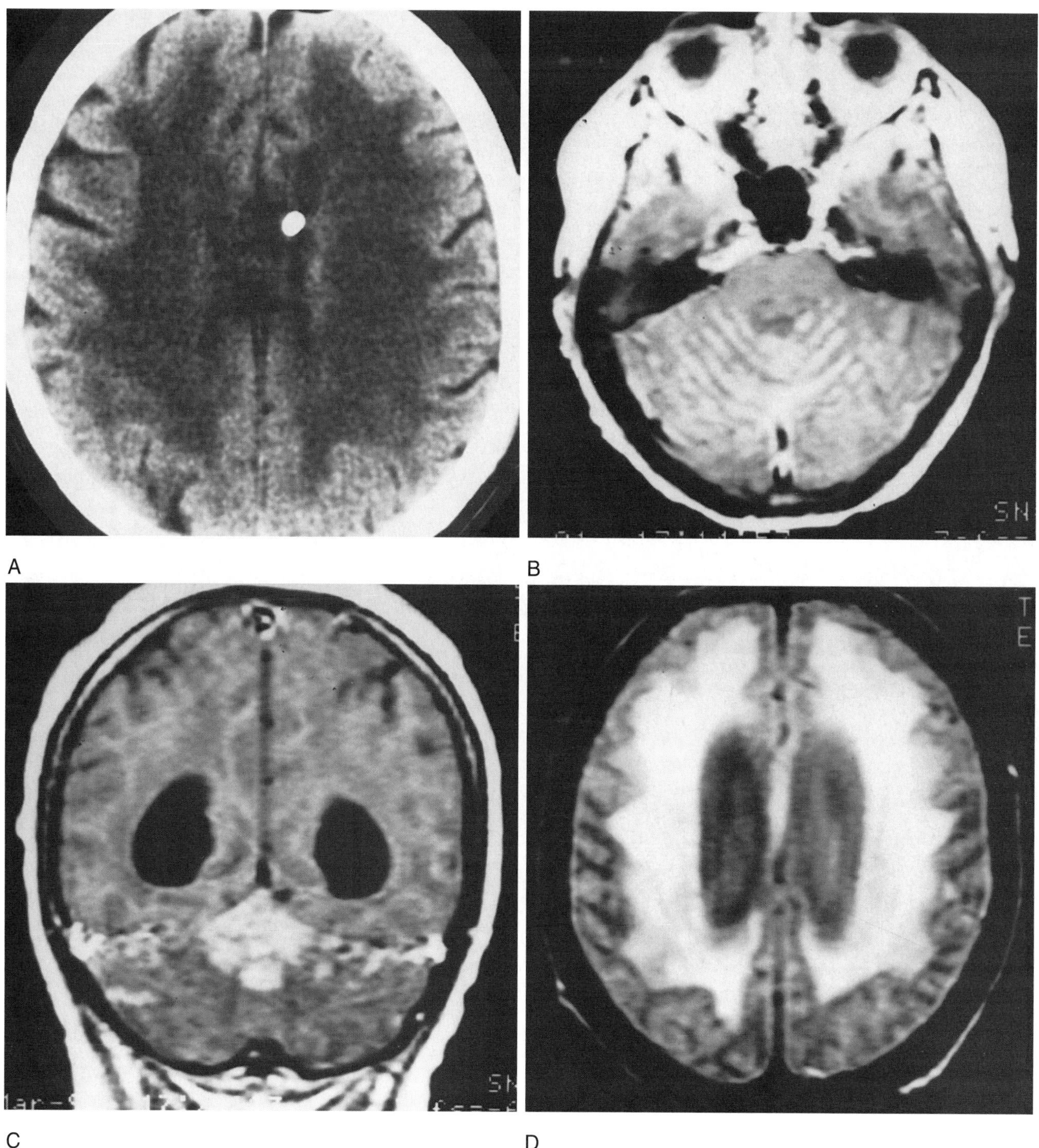

Figure 6.55. Meningeal carcinomatosis in a 70-year-old woman with breast carcinoma. **A.** Axial view shows extensive white matter attenuation, indicative of periventricular extravasation of CSF. A shunt tube was inserted recently to reduce the ventricular obstruction. **B.** Axial enhanced MRI shows the enhancement of the sulci accompanying the cerebellar folia in a V-shaped pattern. **C.** A coronal view after contrast shows the distribution of the enhanced tumor nodularity following the undersurface of the tentorium. **D.** The marked periventricular edema is shown on this proton density image. (*continues*)

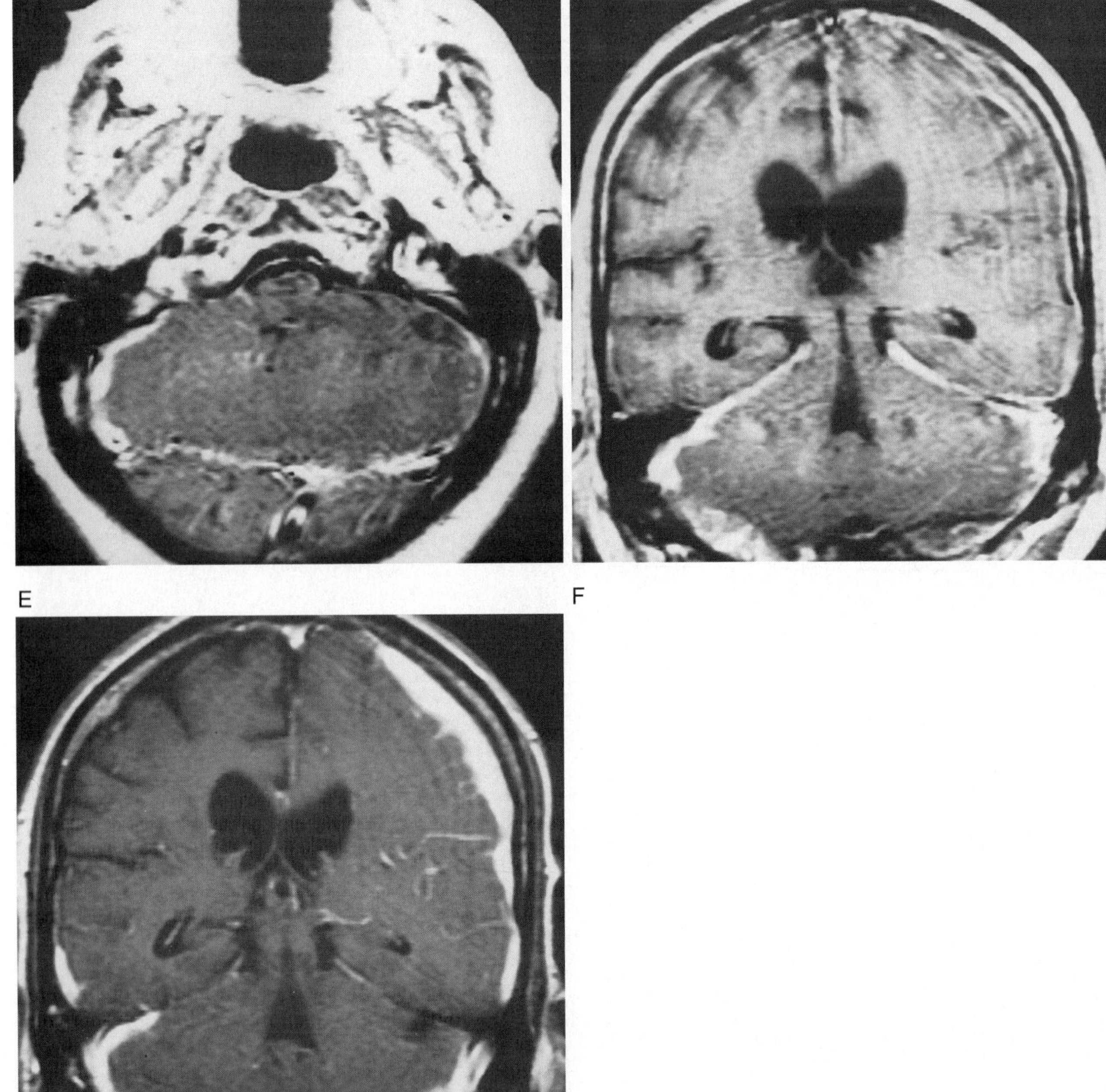

Figure 6.55. *(continued)* **E** to **G.** Another patient with meningeal carcinomatosis from cancer of the lung. **E.** Axial view. **F.** Coronal view shows enhancement and some nodularity in the thickened meninges. The patient was treated with chemotherapy, and the lesions improved. However, they became hemorrhagic in some areas, as shown in G.

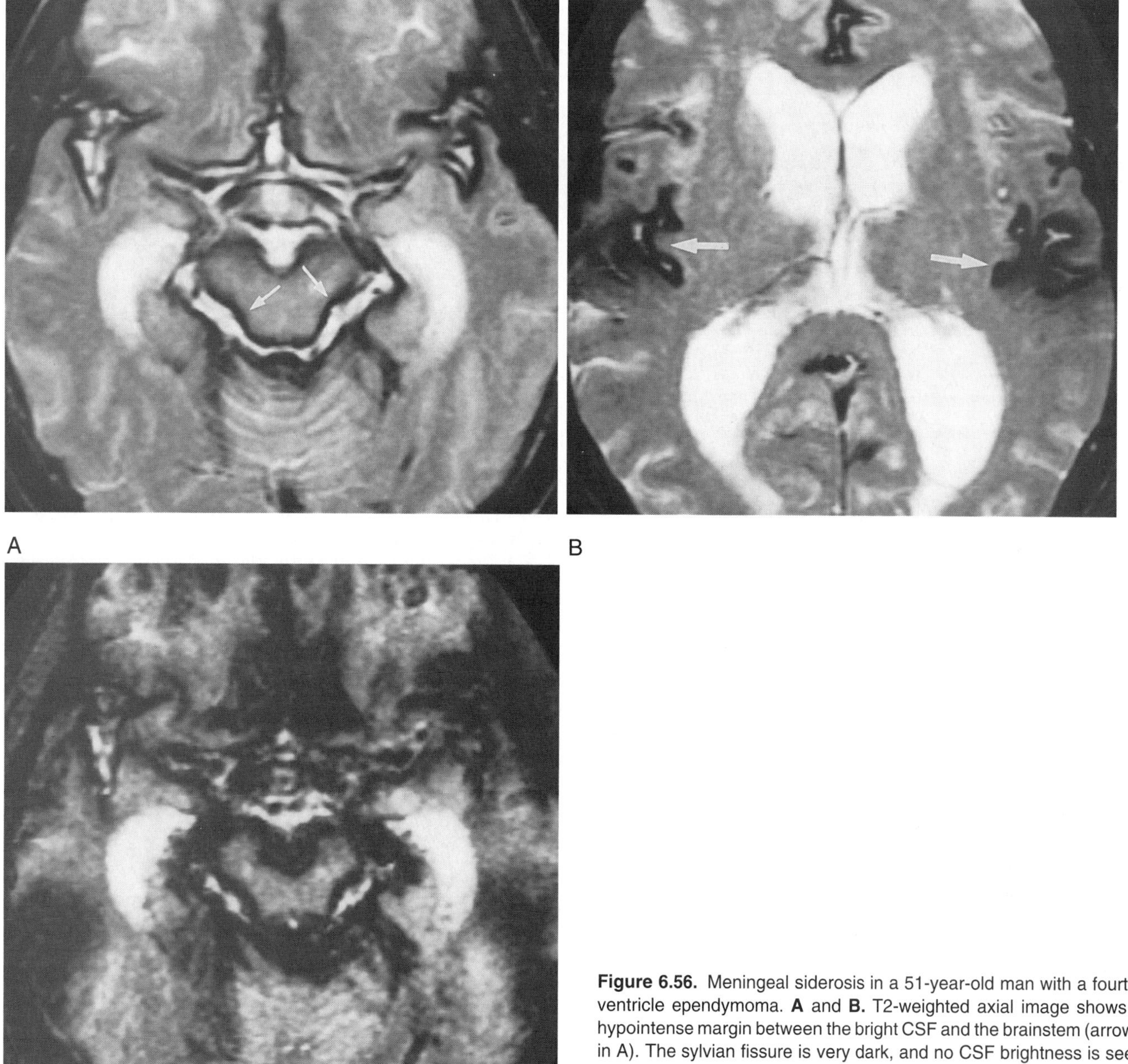

Figure 6.56. Meningeal siderosis in a 51-year-old man with a fourth-ventricle ependymoma. **A** and **B.** T2-weighted axial image shows a hypointense margin between the bright CSF and the brainstem (arrows in A). The sylvian fissure is very dark, and no CSF brightness is seen (arrows in B). **C.** A susceptibility sequence reveals marked hypointensity around the perimesencephalic cistern. The blooming effect of the hemosiderin makes the brainstem appear smaller. The hypointense halo represents hemosiderin that is deposited on the brain leptomeninges from subarachnoid bleeding. A single episode of bleeding does not usually lead to siderosis, which is likely to occur when repeated subarachnoid hemorrhage takes place.

outside the central nervous system without definite evidence of meningeal carcinomatosis. Paakko et al. reported 19 observations of patients who, all except for one, had tumors outside the central nervous system (141). As usual, there was bright enhancement that was particularly visible after contrast on MRI. Some of the patients proved to have metastatic disease in the meninges, but the majority did not have cells in the CSF. Thus the meningeal thickening and enhancement were felt to be nonspecific.

Superficial siderosis or *meningeal siderosis* of the central nervous system is a rare condition that consists in the deposition of hemosiderin on the leptomeninges, on the surface of the brain, and on the cerebeolum, brainstem, cranial nerves, and spinal cord. The deposition of hemosiderin is due to repeated chronic subarachnoid or intraventricular bleeding, and in the majority of cases the repeated bleeding was secondary to hemorrhages from tumors, especially ependymomas, vascular malformations, and subdural he-

Table 6.8.
Differential Diagnosis of Pathologic Conditions of the Meninges

Postsurgical (including post-VP shunt placement): Smooth, mild, dural thickening that enhances after contrast administration.
Meningeal thickening and enhancement seen postoperatively, focal or diffuse; also in long-standing shunts for hydrocephalus. Sometimes in cancer outside the nervous system. Hypertrophic pachymeningitis, focal or diffuse, may involve posterior supratentorial area and spine.
Infectious: Includes bacterial, viral, tuberculous, and fungal etiologies. Usually smooth enhancement but may be slightly nodular and shaggy (especially in tuberculosis).
Neoplastic
- Secondary neoplasms (carcinomatous meningitis). Usually nodular and multifocal enhancement.
- Primary neoplasms: Dural thickening and enhancement due to meningioma (common) or meningioangiomatosis (rare).

Hemorrhagic
- Superifical siderosis: Deposition of hemosiderin on leptomeninges and surface of brain and spinal cord. Most common causes are aneurysmal rupture and hemorrhage from neoplasms.

matomas. In about a quarter of the cases, no evidence of the source of bleeding was found even at autopsy (142).

The symptoms are usually hearing loss and ataxia. By MRI the diagnosis can be made because on T2-weighted images there is a dark halo surrounding the brain, particularly noticeable around the brainstem in the axial views and also in the sagittal and coronal views on T2-weighted images. The appearance may be exaggerated if susceptibility sequence images are obtained (Fig. 6.56 [see page 321]) (Table 6.8).

REFERENCES

1. Brownell B, Tomlinson AH: Virus disease of the central nervous system. In JH Adams, JAN Corsellis, LW Duchen (eds), Greenfield's Neuropathology. New York: Wiley, 1984, p 260.
2. Davis LE, Johnson RT: An explanation for the localization of herpes simplex encephalitis? Ann Neurol 1979;5:2–5.
3. Vahene A, Estrom S, Arstila P, et al: Bell's palsy and herpes simplex virus. Arch Otolaryngol Head Neck Surg 1981;107:79–81.
4. Lester JW Jr, Carter MP, Raynolds TL: Herpes encephalitis: MR monitoring of response to acyclovir therapy. J Comput Assist Tomogr 1988;12:941–943.
5. Benator RM, Magill HL, Gerald B, et al: Herpes simplex encephalitis: CT findings in the neonate and young infant. AJNR 1985;6: 539–543.
6. Tien RD, Dillon WP: Herpes trigeminal neuritis and rhombencephalitis on *Gd*-DTPA-enhanced MR imaging. AJNR 1990;11: 413–414.
7. Osumi A, Tien RD: MR findings in a patient with Ramsay Hunt syndrome. J Comput Assist Tomogr 1990;14:991–993.
8. Daniels DL, Czervioonke LF, Millen SJ: MR findings in the Ramsay Hunt syndrome. AJNR 1988;9:609.
9. Walker RJ III, El Gamal T, Allen MB Jr: Cranial arteritis associated with herpes zoster, case report with angiographic findings. Radiology 1973;107:109.
10. Rose FC, Brett EM, Burston J: Zoster encephalitis. Arch Neurol 1964;11:155–172.
11. Stagno S, Pass RF, Dworsky ME, et al: Congenital cytomegalovirus infection. The relative importance of primary and recurrent maternal infection. N Engl J Med 1982;306:945–949.
12. Tassin GB, Maklad NF, Stewart RR, Bell ME: Cytomegalic inclusion disease: Intrauterine sonographic diagnosis using findings involving the brain. AJNR 1991;12:117–122.
13. Wasserstrom R, Mamourian AC, McGary CT, Miller G: Bulbar poliomyelitis: MR findings with pathologic correlation. AJNR 1992;13:371–373.
14. Atlas SW, Grossman RI, Goldberg HI, et al: MR diagnosis of acute disseminated encephalomyelitis. J Comput Assist Tomogr 1986; 10:798–801.
15. Silverstein FS, Brunberg JA: Postvaricella basal ganglia infarctions in children. AJNR 1995;16:449–452.
16. Tsuchiya K, Yamauchi T, Furui S, et al: MR imaging vs. CT in subacute sclerosing panencephalitis. AJNR 1988;9:943–946.
17. Yagishita A, Nakano I, Ushioda T, et al: Acute encephalopathy with bilateral thalamotegmental involvement in infants and children: Imaging and pathologic findings. AJNR 1995;16:439–447.
18. Falcone S, Quencer RM, Bruce JH, Naidich TP: Creutzfeldt-Jakob disease: Focal symmetrical cortical involvement demonstrated by MR imaging. AJNR 1992;13:403–406.
19. Kovanen J, Erkinjuntti T, Livanain M, et al: Cerebral MR and CT imaging in Creutzfeldt-Jakob disease. J Comput Assist Tomogr 1985;9:125–128.
20. Barboriak DP, Provenzale JF, Boyko O: MR diagnosis of Creutzfeldt-Jakob disease: Significance of high signal intensity of the basal ganglia. AJR 1994;162:137–140.
21. Ogawa T, Inugami A, Fujita H, et al: Serial positron emission tomography with fluorodeoxyglucose F18 in Creutzfeldt-Jakob disease. AJNR 1995;16:978–981.
22. Levy RM, Bredesen DE, Rosenblum ML: Neurologic manifestations of the acquired immunodeficiency syndrome (AIDS): Experience at UCSF and review of the literature. J Neurosurg 1985;62: 475–495.
23. Berger JR, Moskowitz L, Fisch LM, Kelly R: Neurological complications in the acquired immune deficiency syndrome: Often the initial manifestation. Neurology 1984 (suppl I); 34:134–135.
24. Olsen WL, Longo FM, Mills CM, Norman D: White matter disease in AIDS: Findings at MR imaging. Radiology 1988;169: 445–448.
25. Dreyer EB, Kaiser PK, Offerman JT, Lipton SA: HIV-1 Coat protein neurotoxicity prevented by calcium channel antagonists. Channel Science April 20, 1990;248:364–366.
26. Koralink IJ, Beaumanoir A, Häusler R, et al: A controlled study of early neurologic abnormalities in men with asymptomatic human immunodeficiency virus infection. N Engl J Med 1990;323: 864–870.
27. Cohen WA, Maravilla KR, Gerlach R, et al: Prospective cerebral study of HIV seropositive and seronegative men: Correlation of MR findings with neurologic, neuropsychologic, and cerebrospinal fluid analysis. AJNR 1992;13:1231–1240.
28. Post JD, Berger JR, Quencer RM: Asymptomatic and neurologically symptomatic HIV-seropositive individuals: Prospective evaluation with cranial MR imaging. Radiology 1991;128:131–139.
29. Post JD, Levin BE, Berger JR, et al: Sequential cranial MR findings of asymptomatic and neurologically symptomatic HIV subjects. AJNR 1992;13:359–370.
30. Chrysikopoulos HS, Press GA, Grafe MR, et al: Encephalitis caused by human immunodeficiency virus: CT and MR imaging manifestations with clinical and pathologic correlation. Radiology 1990;175:185–191.
31. Grafe MR, Press GA, Berthoty DP, et al: Abnormalities of the brain in AIDS patients: Correlation of postmortem MR findings with neuropathology. AJNR 1990;11:905–911.
32. Flowers CH, Mafee MF, Crowell R, et al: Encephalopathy in AIDS patients: Evaluation with MR imaging. AJNR 1990;11:1235–1245.
33. Kauffman WM, Sivit CJ, Fitz CR, et al: CT and MR evaluation of intracranial involvement in pediatric HIV infection: A clinical-imaging correlation. AJNR 1992;13:949–957.
34. Whitley RJ: Viral encephalitis. N Engl J Med 1990;323:242–250.
35. Porter SB, Sande MA: Toxoplasmosis of the central nervous system in the acquired immunodeficiency syndrome. N Engl J Med 1992; 327:1643–1648.

36. Aström KE, Mancall EL, Richardson EP: Progressive multifocal leukoencephalopathy. Brain 1958;81:93–111.
37. Richardson EP Jr: Progressive multifocal leukoencephalopathy. N Engl J Med 1961;265:815–823.
38. Chaisson RE, Griffin DE: Progressive multifocal leukoencephalopathy in AIDS. JAMA 1990;265:79–82.
39. Mamelak AN, Kelly WM, Davis RL, et al: Idiopathic hypertrophic cranial pachymeningitis. J Neurosurg 1993;79:270–276.
40. Heinz ER, Drayer BP, Haenggeli CA, et al: Computed tomography in white-matter disease. Radiology 1979;130:371–378.
41. Wheeler AL, Truwit CL, Kleinschmidt-De Masters BK, et al: Progressive multifocal leukoencephalopathy: Contrast enhancement on CT scans and MR images. AJR 1993;161:1049–1051.
42. Tuite M, Ketonen L, Kieburtz K, et al: Efficacy of gadolinium in MR brain imaging of HIV-infected patients. AJNR 1993;14:257–263.
43. Popovich MJ, Arthur RH, Helmer G: CT of intracranial cryptococcosis. AJNR 1990;11:139–142.
44. Heineman HS, Braude AI: Anaerobic infection of the brain: Observations on 18 consecutive cases. Am J Med 1963;35:682–697.
45. Case Records of the Massachusetts General Hospital: N Engl J Med 1989;321:739–750.
46. Sze G, Zimmerman RD: The magnetic resonance imaging of infections and inflammatory diseases. Radiol Clin North Am 1988;26:839–859.
47. Rabe EF: Subdural effusions in infants. Pediatr Clin North Am 1967;50:831–850.
48. Mathews VP, Kuharik MA, Edwards MK, et al: Gd-DTPA-enhanced MR imaging of experimental bacterial meningitis: Evaluation and comparison with CT. AJNR 1988;9:1045–1050.
49. Barloon TJ, Yuh WTC, Kneppor LE, et al: Cerebral ventriculitis: MR findings. J Comput Assist Tomogr 1990;14:272–275.
50. Reeder JD, Sanders RC: Ventriculitis in the neonate: Recognition by sonography. AJNR 1983;4:37–41.
51. Nida TY, Haines SJ: Multiloculated hydrocephalus: Craniotomy and fenestration of intraventricular septations. J Neurosurg 1993;78:70–76.
52. Atlas SW, Mark AS, Fram EK, Grossman RI: Vascular intracranial lesions: Applications of gradient-echo MR imaging. Radiology 1988;169:455–461.
53. Zimmerman RD, Leeds NE, Danziger A: Subdural empyema: CT findings. Radiology 1984;150:417–422.
54. Greitz T: Angiography in tuberculous meningitis. Acta Radiol Diagn 1964;2:369.
55. Whelan MA, Stern J: Intracranial tuberculoma. Radiology 1981;138:75–81.
56. Gupta RK, Jena A, Sharma A, et al: MR imaging of intracranial tuberculomas. J Comput Assist Tomogr 1988;12:280–285.
57. Brooks BS, el Gammal TE, Hungerford GD, et al: Radiologic evaluation of neurosarcoidosis: Role of computed tomography. AJNR 1982;3:513–521.
58. Post MJD, Quencer RM, Tabei SZ: CT demonstration of sarcoidosis of the optic nerve, frontal lobes, and falx cerebri: Case report and literature review. AJNR 1982;3:523–526.
59. Engelken JD, Yuh WTC, Carter KD, Nerad JA: Optic nerve sarcoidosis: MR findings. AJNR 1992;13:228–230.
60. Williams DW III, Elster AD, Kramer SI: Neurosarcoidosis: Gadolinium-enhanced MR images. J Comput Assist Tomogr 1990;14:704–707.
61. Sherman JL, Stern BJ: Sarcoidosis of the CNS: Comparison of unenhanced and enhanced MR images. AJNR 1990;11:915–923.
62. Lexa FJ, Grossman RI: MR of sarcoidosis in the head and spine: Spectrum of manifestations and radiographic response to steroid therapy. AJNR 1994;15:973–982.
63. Smith AS, Meisler DM, Weinstein MA, et al: High-signal periventricular lesions in patients with sarcoidosis: Neurosarcoidosis or multiple sclerosis? AJNR 1989;10:485–490; AJR 1989;153:147–152.
64. NEJM case records No. 44-1988;319:1209–1219.
65. Brightbill TC, Ihmeidan IH, Post MJD, et al: Neurosyphilis in HIV-positive and HIV-negative patients: Neuroimaging findings. AJNR 1995;16:703–711.
66. Holland BA, Perrett LV, Mills CM: Meningovascular syphilis: CT and MR findings. Radiology 1986;158:439–442.
67. Godt P, Stoepler L, Wischer U, Schroeder HH: The value of computed tomography in cerebral syphilis. Neuroradiology 1979;18:197–200.
68. Agrons GA, Han SS, Husson MA, Simeone F: MR imaging of cerebral gumma. AJNR 1991;12:80–81.
69. Punt J: Multiple cerebral gummata: Case report. J Neurosurg 1983;58:959–961.
70. Fernandez RE, Rothberg M, Ferencz G, Wujack D: Lyme disease of the CNS: MR imaging findings in 14 cases. AJNR 1990;11:479–481.
71. Rafto SE, Milton WJ, Galetta SL, Grossman RI: Biopsy-confirmed CNS Lyme disease: MR appearance at 1.5T. AJNR 1990;11:482–484.
72. Steere AC, Taylor E, McHugh GL, Logigian EL: The overdiagnosis of Lyme disease. JAMA 1993;269:1812–1816.
73. Finkel MF: Lyme disease and its neurologic complication. Arch Neurol 1988;45:99–104.
74. Steere AC: Lyme disease. N Engl J Med 1989;321:586–596.
75. Wrobel CJ, Meyer S, Johnson RH, Hesselink JR: MR findings in acute and chronic coccidioidomycosis meningitis. AJNR 1992;13:1241–1245.
76. Angtuaco ECC, Angtuaco EJC, Glasier CM, et al: Nasopharyngeal and temporal bone blastomycosis: CT and MR findings. AJNR 1991;12:725–728.
77. Parker JC Jr, McClosky JJ, Lee RS: Human cerebral caudidosis. A postmortem evaluation of 19 patients. Hum Pathol 1981;12:23–28.
78. Meyer RD, Young LS, Armstrong D, Yu B: Phycomycosis complicating leukemia and lymphoma. Am J Med 1973;54:6–15.
79. Bowen BC, Post MJD: Intracranial infection. In Atlas SW, Magnetic Resonance Imaging of the Brain and Spine. New York: Raven, 1991, pp 501–538.
80. Desai SP, Bazan C III, Hummell W, Jinkins JR: Disseminated CNS histoplasmosis. AJNR 1991;12:290–292.
81. Tien RD, Chu PK, Hesselink JR, et al: Intracranial cryptococcosis in immunocompromised patients; CT and MR findings in 29 cases. AJNR 1991;12:283–289.
82. Gamba JL, Woodruff WW, Djang WT, Yeates AE: Craniofacial mucormycosis: Assessment with CT. Radiology 1986;160:207–212.
83. Centeno RS, Bentson JR, Mancuso AA: CT scanning in rhinocerebral mucormycosis and aspergillosis. Radiology 1981;140:383–389.
84. Scaravilli F: Parasitic and fungal infections of the nervous system. In JH Adams, JAN Corsellis, LW Duchen (eds); Greenfield's Neuropathology, ed 4, New York: Wiley, 1984, pp 304–337.
85. Millan JM, Millan JMS, Muñoz M, et al: CNS complications in acute malaria: MR findings. AJNR 1993;14:493–494.
86. Rodriguez-Carbajal J, Salgado P, Gutierez-Alvarado R, et al: The acute encephalitic phase of neurocystercosis: Computed tomographic manifestations. AJNR 1983;4:51–55.
87. Michael AS, Levy JM, Paige ML: Cysticercosis mimicking brain neoplasm: MR and CT appearance. J Comput Assist Tomogr 1990;14:708–711.
88. Chang KH, Lee JH, Han MH, et al: The role of contrast-enhanced MR imaging in the diagnosis of neurocysticeosis. AJNR 1991;12:509–512.
89. Ginier BL, Poirer VC: MR imaging of intraventricular cysticercosis. AJNR 1992;13:1247–1248.

90. Zee CS, Segall HD, Apuzzo M, et al: Intraventricular cysticercal cysts: Further neuroradiologic observations and neurosurgical implications. AJNR 1984;5:727–730.
91. Zee CS, Segall HD, Miller C, et al: Unusual neuroradiological features of intracranial cysticercosis. Radiology 1980;137:397–407.
92. OH SJ: Roentgen findings in cerebral paragonimiasis. Radiology 1968;90:292–299.
93. Yoshida M, Kazuhiko M, Kuga S, Anegana S: CT findings of cerebral paragonimiasis in the chronic state. J Comput Assist Tomogr 1982;6:195–196.
94. Kadoka T, Ishiichi I, Yukiko T, et al: MR imaging of chronic cerebral paragonimiasis. AJNR 1989;10:521.
95. Chang KH, Cho SY, Chi JG, et al: Cerebral sparganosis: CT characteristics. Radiology 1987;165:505–510.
96. Schils J, Hermanus N, Flament-Durant J, et al: Cerebral schistosomiasis. AJNR 1985;6:840–841.
97. Mascalchi M, Ragazzoni A, Dal Pozzo G: Pontine hydatid cyst in association with an acoustic neurinoma: MR appearance in an unusual case. AJNR 1991;12:78–79.
98. Morris DL, Dykes PW, Marriners, et al: Objective evidence of response in human hydatid disease. JAMA 1985;532:2053–2057.
99. Mathews VP, Smith RP: Choroid plexus infections: Neuroimaging appearances of four cases. AJNR 1992;13:374–378.
100. Kim RC, Collins GH, Parisi JE: Rheumatoid nodules in the choroid plexus. Arch Pathol Lab Med 1982;106:83–84.
101. Pear BL: Xanthogranuloma of the choroid plexus. AJR 1984;143: 401–402.
102. Hinshaw B Jr, Fahmy JL, Peekham N, et al: The bright choroid plexus on MR: CT and pathologic correlation. AJNR 1988;9: 483–486.
103. Lyons EL, Leeds NE: The angiographic demonstration of arterial vascular disease in purulent meningitis. Radiology 1967;88:935.
104. Ferris EJ, Rudikoff JC, Shapiro JH: Cerebral angiography of bacterial infection. Radiology 1968;90:727–734.
105. Davis DO, Dilenge D, Schlaepfer W: Arterial dilatation in purulent meningitis. Neurosurgery 1970;32:112.
106. Leeds NE, Goldberg HI: Angiographic manifestation in cerebral inflammatory disease. Radiology 1971;98:595.
107. Vatz KA, Scheibel RL, Keiffer SA, et al: Neurosyphilis and diffuse cerebral angiopathy: A case report. Neurology 1974;24:472.
108. Liebeskind A, Cohen S, Anderson R, et al: Unusual segmental cerebrovascular changes. Radiology 1973;106:119.
109. Corr P, Wright M, Handler LC: Endocarditis-related cerebral aneurysms: Radiologic changes with treatment. AJNR 1995;16: 745–748.
110. New PFJ, Price DL, Carter B: Cerebral angiography in cardiac myxomas: Correlation of angiographic and histopathologic findings. Radiology 1970;96:335.
111. Ojemann RG, New PFJ, Fleming TC: Intracranial aneurysms associated with bacterial meningitis. JAMA 1966;198:1222.
112. Price DL, Wolpow ER, Richardson EP Jr: Intracranial phycomacosis: A clinicopathological and radiological study. J Neurol Sci 1971;14:359.
113. Shillito J Jr: Carotid arteritis: A cause of hemiplegia in childhood. J Neurosurg 1964;21:540.
114. Hinck VC, Carter CC, Ripley JG: Giant cell arterisis: A case with angiographic abnormality. AJR 1964;92:769–775.
115. Trevor RP, Sondheimer FK, Fossel WJ, Wolpert SM: Angiographic demonstration of major cerebral vessel occlusion in systemic lupus erythematosus. Neuroradiology 1972;4:202–207.
116. Aisen AM, Gabrielsen TO, McCane WJ: MR imaging in systemic lupus erythematosus involving the brain. AJNR 1985;6:197–201.
117. Coxe NS, Luse SA: Acute hemorrhagic leukoencephalitis: A clinical and electron microscopic report of 2 patients treated with surgical decompression. J Neurosurg 1963;20:584.
118. Michaud J, Helle TL: Acute hemorrhagic leukoencephalitis localized to the brainstem and cerebellum: A report of two cases. J Neurol Neurosurg Psychiatry 1982;45:151–157.
119. Rumbaugh CL, Bergeron RT, Fang HC, McCormick R: Cerebral angiographic changes in the drug abuse patient. Radiology 1971; 101:335.
120. Margolis MT, Newton TH: Methamphetamine ("Speed") arteritis. Neuroradiology 1971;2:179.
121. Kienzle GD, Breger RK, Chun RWM, et al: Sydenham chorea: MR manifestations in two cases. AJNR 1991;12:73–76.
122. Husby G, van de Rijn, Zabriskie JB, et al: Antibodies reacting with the cytoplasm of subthalamic and caudate nuclei neurons in chorea and acute rheumatic fever. J Exper Med 1976;144:1094–1110.
123. Destian S, Heier LA, Zimmerman RD, et al: Differentiation between meningeal fibrosis and chronic subdural hematoma after ventricular shunting: Value of enhanced CT and MR scans. AJNR 1989;10:1021–1026.
124. Burke JW, Podrasky AE, Bradley WG Jr: Meningitis: Postoperative enhancement on MR images. Radiology 1990;174:99–102.
125. Suzuki M, Takoshima T, Kadoya M, et al: Gadolinium-DTPA enhancement of dural structures on MRI after surgery. Neurology 1992;35:112–116.
126. Charcot JM, Joffroy A: Deux cas d'atrophie musculaire progressive avec lesions de la substance grise et des faisceaux anterolateraux de la moelle epiniere. Arch Physiol Norm Pathol 1869;2:354–367, 744–769.
127. Martin N, Masson C, Henin D, et al: Hypertrophic cranial pachymeningitis: Assessment with CT and MR imaging. AJNR 1989; 10:477–484.
128. Friedman D, Flanders A, Tartaglino C: Contrast-enhanced MR imaging of idiopathic hypertrophic craniospinal pachymeningitis. AJR 1993;160:900–901.
129. Rosenfeld JV, Masson C, Henin D, et al: Pachymeningitis cervicalis hyperthrophica. J Neurosurg 1987;66:137–139.
130. Yuh WTC, Drew JM, Rizzo TJ, et al: Evaluation of pachymeningitis by contrast-enhanced MR imaging in a patient with rheumatoid disease. AJNR 1990;11:1247.
131. Pannullo SC, Reich JB, Krol G, et al: MRI changes in intracranial hypotension. Neurology 1993;43:919–926.
132. Fishman RA, Dillon WP: Dural enhancement and cerebral displacement secondary to intracranial hypotension. Neuroradiology 1993;43:609–611.
133. Mittl RL, Yousem DM. Frequency of unexplained meningeal enhancement in the brain after lumbar puncture. Am J Neuroradiol 1994;15:633–636.
134. Paulin DJ, McDonald JS, Child B, et al: Acute subdural hematoma—an unusual sequela to lumbar puncture. Anesthesiology 1979;51:338–340.
135. Mantia AM: Clinical report of the occurrence of an intracerebral hemorrhage following post-lumbar puncture headache. Anesthesiology 1981;55:684–685.
136. Grant R, Condon B, Hart I, et al: Changes in intracranial CSF volume after lumbar puncture and their relationship to post L-P headache. J Neurol Neurosurg Psychiatry 1991;54:440–442.
137. Schumacher DJ, Tien RD, Friedman H: Gadolinium enhancement of the leptomeninges caused by hydrocephalus: A potential mimic of leptomeningeal metastasis. AJNR 1994;15:639–641.
138. Tokumaru A, Toshihiro O, Tsuneyoshi E, et al: Prominent meningeal enhancement adjacent to meningioma on Gd-DTPA-enhanced MR images: Histopathologic correlation. Radiology 1990; 175:431–433.
139. Wilms G, Lammens M, Marchal G, et al: Prominent dural enhancement adjacent to nonmeningiomatous malignant lesions on contrast-enhanced MR images. AJNR 1991;12:761–764.
140. Aizpuru RN, Quencer RM, Norenberg M, et al: Meningioangiomatosis: Clinical, radiologic, and histopathologic correlation. Radiology 1991;179:819–821.
141. Paakko E, Patronas NJ, Schellinger D, et al: Meningeal Gd-DTPA enhancement in patients with malignancies. J Comput Assist Tomogr 1990;14:542–546.

142. Braachi M, Savoiardo M, Triulzi F, et al: Superficial siderosis of the CNS: MR diagnosis and clinical findings. AJNR 1993;14:227–236.

SELECTED READINGS

Angeid-Bachman E, Quint DJ: CNS non-Hodgkin lymphoma in a patient previously treated for systemic Hodgkin disease. AJNR 1990;11: 1254–1256.

Gupta RK, Gupta S, Singh D, et al: Role of MR imaging and MR angiography in the diagnosis of tuberculous meningitis. Neuroradiology. In press. 1994.

Karalnik IJ, Beaumanoir A, Häusler R, et al: A controlled study of early neurologic abnormalities in men with asymptomatic human immunodeficiency virus infection. N Engl J Med 1990;323:864–870.

King TT, Couch RSC: The diagnosis of clinical hydatid disease. Clin Radiol 1961;12:190.

Koskiniemi M, Vaheri A, Manuinen V, et al: Herpes simplex virus encephalitis, new diagnostic and clinical features and results of therapy. AJNR 1981;2:378.

Leeds NE, Rosenblatt R, Zimmerman HM: Focal angiographic changes of cerebral lymphoma with pathologic correlation. Radiology 1967;89: 10.

Seltzer S, Mark AS, Atlas SW: CNS sarcoidosis: Evaluation with contrast-enhanced MR imaging. AJNR 1991;12:1227–1233.

Soo MS, Tien RD, Gray L, et al.: Mesenrhombencephalitis: MR findings in nine patients. AJR 1993;160:1089–1093.

Spickler EM, Lufkin RB, Teresi L, et al: High-signal intraventricular cysticercosis on TI-weighted MR imaging. AJNR 1989;10:S64

7

Head Injuries and Their Complications

SKULL FRACTURES

The introduction of computed tomography (CT) and more recently magnetic resonance imaging (MRI) has revolutionized the management of head injuries. Today plain films of the skull are utilized much less frequently than was the case prior to 1973, before the discovery of CT. Today the great majority of patients are examined first with CT, and the skull examination is omitted unless there is evidence of trauma around the orbits and facial bones, where a skull examination may be desirable. Even in these areas, however, CT scanning, which can be performed in axial projections with thin slices, permitting reformatting in sagittal, coronal, or any oblique plain, are preferred. If the patient is able to cooperate, however, direct coronal views normally yield greater resolution and are preferred.

It should be pointed out, however, that CT does not show linear fractures if they are somewhat parallel to the axial direction of the plane of cut or if they are oblique to the plane but not sufficiently so to show up on the images. It is estimated that on a routine CT examination of the head in axial projection, as many as 30 to 40 percent of the fractures are not seen. However, the important aspect is the involvement of the intracranial structures, and these are usually seen in an extremely high percentage of cases by CT examination in the acute stage. Nevertheless, the presence of a fracture seen on the skull examination, or sometimes on the digital preliminary image for CT scanning, is important because it indicates the severity of the injury, which evidently was strong enough to produce a skull fracture. Nevertheless, we are most concerned with the intracranial complications because they involve the brain; we are much less concerned with fractures that do not involve the brain. An exception to this general concept is that the fractures along the base of the skull often rupture the dura mater and may lead to cerebrospinal fluid (CSF) leak and later to meningitis. This is the most important complication of a fracture that has not produced any visible intracranial complications.

Types of Fractures

Fractures may be linear, diastatic, comminuted, basal, or depressed. Table 7.1 characterizes some of these types.

Linear fractures result from a blow that first causes inbending of the skull; if the skull resists, a rebound occurs that may lead to a linear fracture (1,2). If the skull does not resist, a depressed fracture may be the result (Figs. 7.1, 7.2, and 7.3). Generally the dura bends but does not rupture, but sometimes the dura tears, and at the same time the fracture may be diastatic: that is, the margins of the bone remain somewhat separated. Under these circumstances, the arachnoid may become trapped in the diastatic fracture. If the arachnoid also tears, a subgaleal collection of CSF develops that may later disappear as the arachnoid undergoes spontaneous healing. Perhaps more often, the arachnoid does not tear and simply returns to normal position. The intact arachnoid may be trapped in the fracture, and, if so, it transmits the brain pulsations to the diastatic fracture edges and in time will produce erosion of the bones. This is the pathogenesis of the so-called growing fractures, which lead to the formation of *leptomeningeal cysts* (3). The concept is explained and illustrated in Figures 7.2 and 7.3. Unusual appearances are sometimes encountered. Bullets

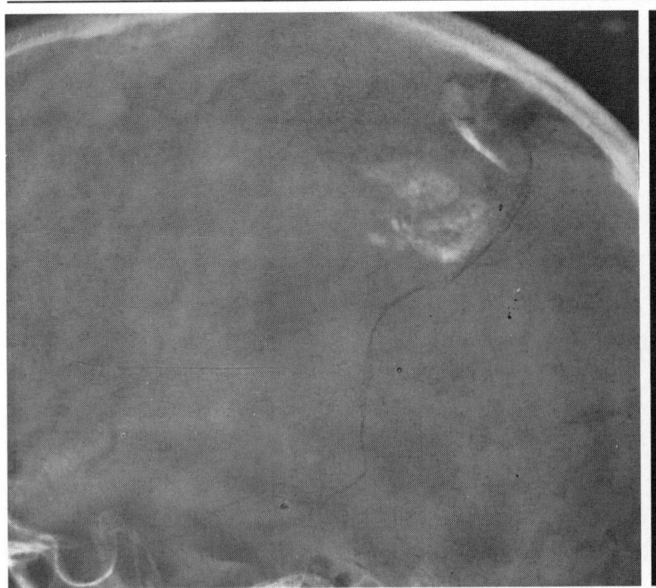

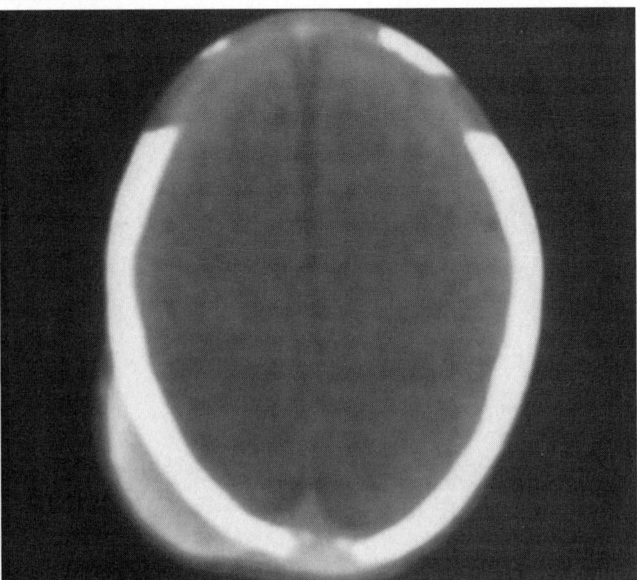

A B

Figure 7.1. Skull fractures. **A.** A long linear fracture is present, extending vertically from the midparietal region to disappear into the floor of the middle fossa. The fracture line is sharply demarcated, angular as well as curved, and exhibits a finely irregular margin at many points along its course. The sharpness of outline and density of the fracture line extending through both tables denote the recent nature of the bony injury. A 3-cm-diameter defect is present in the parasagittal portion of the parietal bone from which bone fragments have been comminuted and impacted intracranially for a distance of 4 cm. The superior longitudinal sinus may be torn by such an injury, or it may become thrombosed, as in this case. **B.** Typical cephalohematoma in a newborn. Note that the subperiosteal hemorrhage stops at the suture. No intracerebral hemorrhage was discovered. No fracture was seen, but it is assumed that a fracture occurred that is responsible for the subperiosteal hematoma.

usually produce burst fractures at the point of exit (Fig. 7.4).

Fractures through the petrous bone are best demonstrated by CT or by pluridirectional tomography (Fig. 7.5).

Infection may occur in the bone as a result of an infected open fracture (Fig. 7.6). Intracranial infection may result as a complication of a fracture that communicated with the paranasal sinuses or mastoid, causing a CSF leak, or it may be the result of a penetrating injury (Fig. 7.7).

Linear fractures of the skull heal slowly, but the time varies with the age of the patient. In infancy and early childhood, fracture lines frequently disappear in 3 to 6 months. In children 5 to 12 years of age, fractures usually heal within 1 year, whereas in adolescents healing usually takes longer. In the adult, a linear fracture usually is clearly visible for a number of months and often for a number of years; in some instances the site of a fracture may be recognized for the remainder of an individual's life. The average time, however, for healing of a linear fracture in the adult is 2 to 3 years. The fracture may be healed and still present a linear lucency with the characteristics of a fracture but be less lucent than a fresh fracture.

Depressed fractures may be diagnosed by plain films but are usually diagnosed by CT, which allows for the evaluation of intracranial complications, particularly focal brain damage.

Table 7.1.
Types of Skull Fractures

Type	Features
Linear	Least frequent skull fractures to be associated with intracranial injury. May be missed on CT. No treatment is indicated. Leptomeningeal cyst is an unusual complication.
Depressed	May be associated with dural tear or adjacent cortical contusion. Possible nidus for infection. Often surgically debrided.
Basal	May be associated with carotid dissection, CSF leak (otorrhea or rhinorrhea), meningitis, carotid cavernous fistula.

INTRACRANIAL AIR

It is interesting that the spontaneous appearance of gas within the cranial cavity following a fracture, an aerocele, a pneumatocele, or traumatic pneumocephalus, formed the basis for the first radiologic description of pneumoencephalography by Lucket in 1913 (4). The air may be located in the epidural space, in the subarachnoid space, in the brain substance, or within the ventricles. The presence of

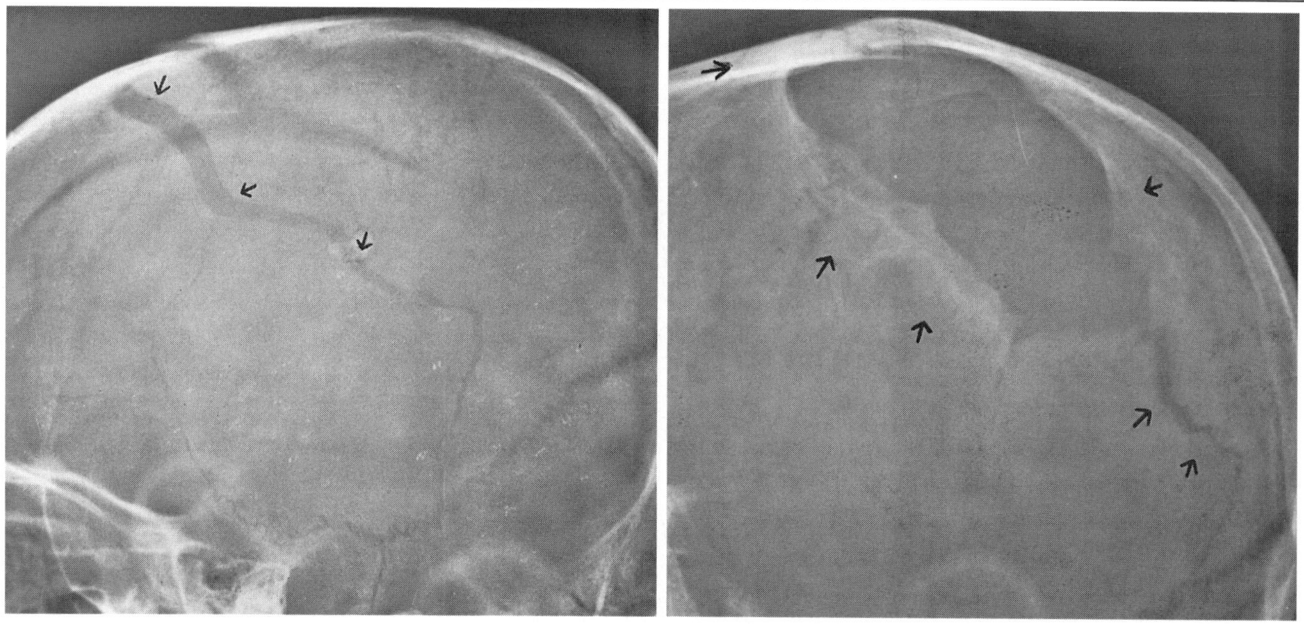

Figure 7.2. Leptomeningeal cyst. Skull fractures in children, particularly when lengthy and wide, may be associated with tearing of the dura and the development of a leptomeningeal cyst. **A.** In the case illustrated, a severe headtop injury produced a wide fracture line (arrows) that extended across the midline. The child developed bulging of the scalp in the right parietal region that became progressively larger. **B.** A skull film made 2 1/2 years after the injury reveals that, instead of healing in the normal manner, the fracture line has become much wider; the margins are scalloped in the area where marked widening has occurred (arrows). The most caudal extension of the fracture line on the same side also remains unhealed (posterior arrows). The portion of the fracture line on the opposite side of the skull appears to have healed in the usual manner.

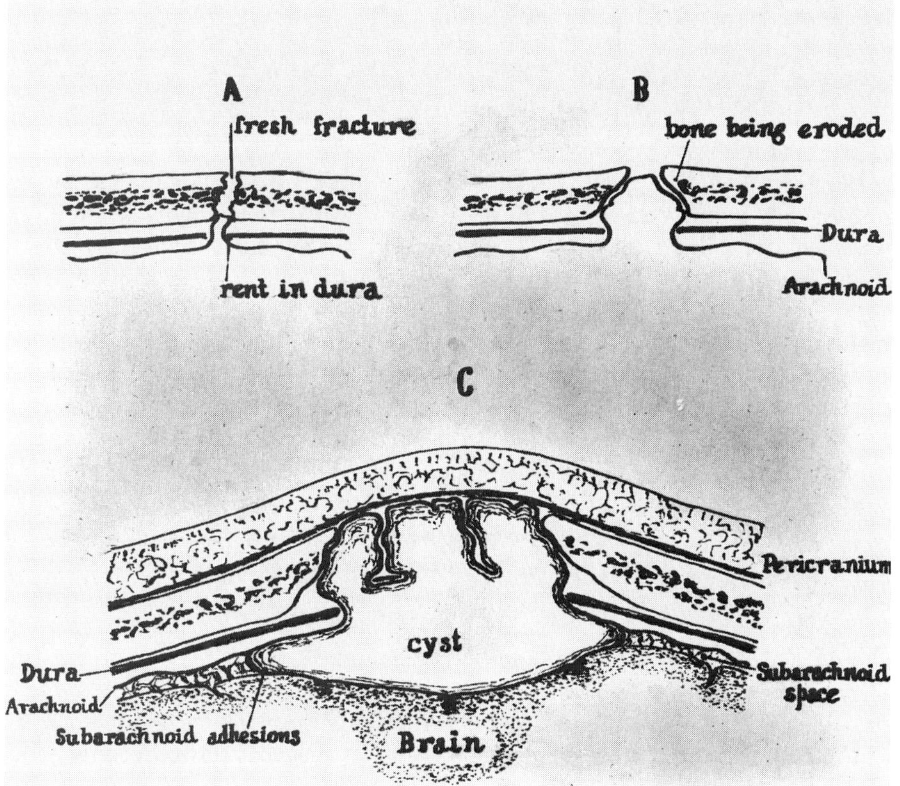

Figure 7.3. Mechanism of progressive changes with leptomeningeal cyst. The probable mechanism of production of a leptomeningeal cyst and the progressive erosion of the overlying skull are shown. **A.** The original fracture tears the dura mater, with the development of a small herniation of the arachnoid membrane through the dura. **B.** If soft tissue containing pulsating fluid is interposed, the bone does not heal in the usual manner, but the edges of the fracture line become smoother by erosion. **C.** When there is marked erosion of the bone, owing to pulsation of the cystlike collection of fluid in the partially walled-off subarachnoid space, a wide defect may be produced; an external prominence of the scalp usually is found, while internally there may be depression of the brain.

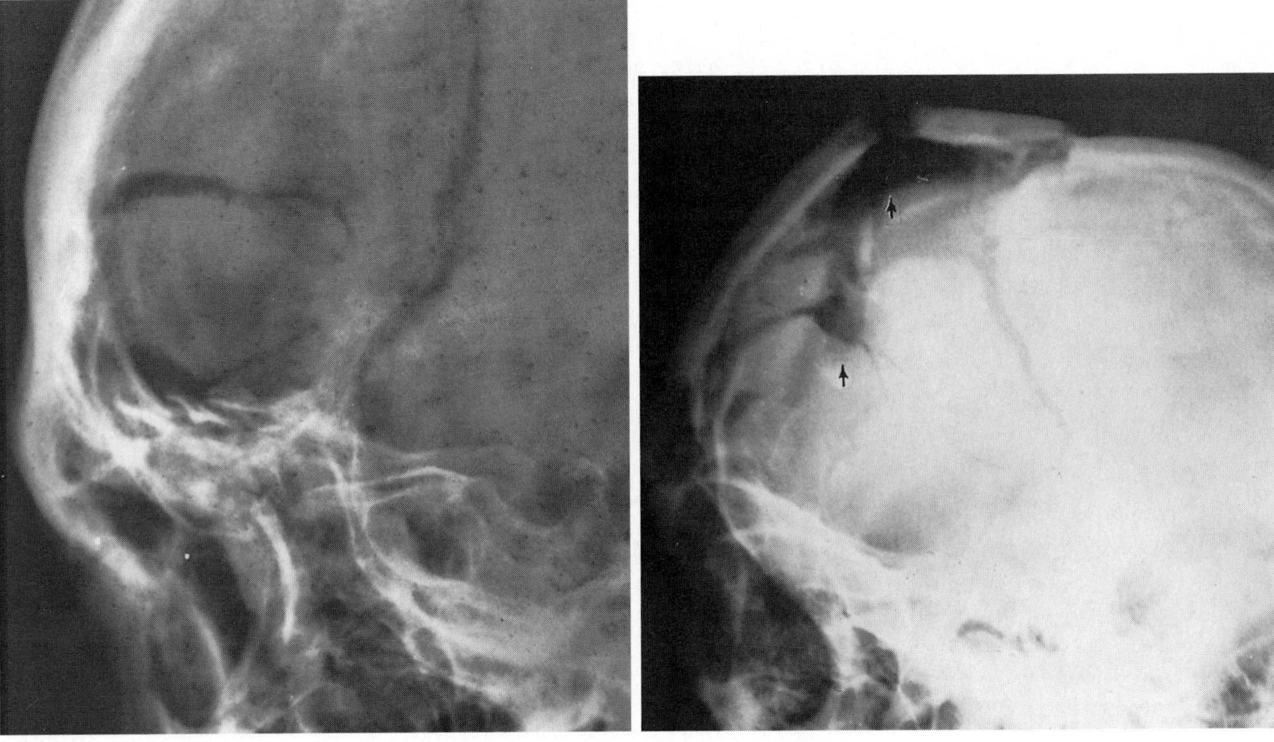

A B

Figure 7.4. Fractures in relation to paranasal sinuses. Skull fractures that involve the air sinuses of the skull, either paranasal or mastoid, are compound fractures, even though the opening to the exterior is occult. **A.** In the lateral view, a sharply demarcated fracture line is present that widens anteriorly. The inferior fracture limb is comminuted at its anterior extremity, with a few small bone fragments impacted intracranially from the sinus wall. **B.** In another case, a severely comminuted fracture of a bursting type has occurred. The fracture has resulted from perforation of the skull by a rifle bullet, and is therefore compound extracranially. The point of entrance (lower arrow), because of the greater velocity of the missile, is smaller than the point of exit (upper arrow), where a greater bursting effect is evident.

air is an indication that a fracture exists, even though not visualized by CT or plain films, and that the fracture goes through an air-containing structure: the mastoids or the paranasal sinuses. The air bubbles may be located near the fracture, but may move rapidly away from the fracture even in the epidural space (Fig. 7.8).

The presence of air bubbles in the epidural space indicates that the dura is probably intact, whereas air in the subdural or subarachnoid space, in the brain tissue, or in the ventricles would indicate that there is a rupture of the dura and the arachnoid membrane, permitting the air to pass into the subarachnoid space or beyond (Fig. 7.8 and see Fig. 7.22).

Frontal sinus fractures, which are usually well demonstrated by CT, are important. They may involve the anterior, the posterior, or both walls. Fractures involving the posterior wall are more likely to be associated with intracranial hemorrhage (5). If there is dural rupture, transient CSF leak may occur and meningitis is always a possibility. Air bubbles may be seen by CT in the epidural space or in the subdural or subarachnoid space if there is dural rupture (Fig. 7.27).

BASAL SKULL FRACTURES

Skull base fractures are difficult to demonstrate by any method. In the past, plain film tomography was utilized, but now CT is superior. It is necessary to take thin cuts (1 to 2 mm) and to reconstruct the images with bone algorithms for best results. On plain skull films taken with the patient supine and using the horizontal x-ray beam, the presence of a fluid level in the sphenoid sinus should always be taken as evidence of a possible skull fracture in the acute stage, and it is recommended that plain skull lateral views in trauma cases be made in the supine position, which is much more comfortable for the patient (Fig. 7.9). In addition to CSF leak, basal fractures may lead to the production of a carotid-cavernous fistula (Fig. 7.10; Table 7.1).

CSF RHINORRHEA

This is an important complication of skull fractures usually involving the base of the skull. In the past, basal skull fractures were not usually demonstrated by plain films, and for this reason it was (and it continues to be) recommended that one take a lateral radiograph with the patient supine

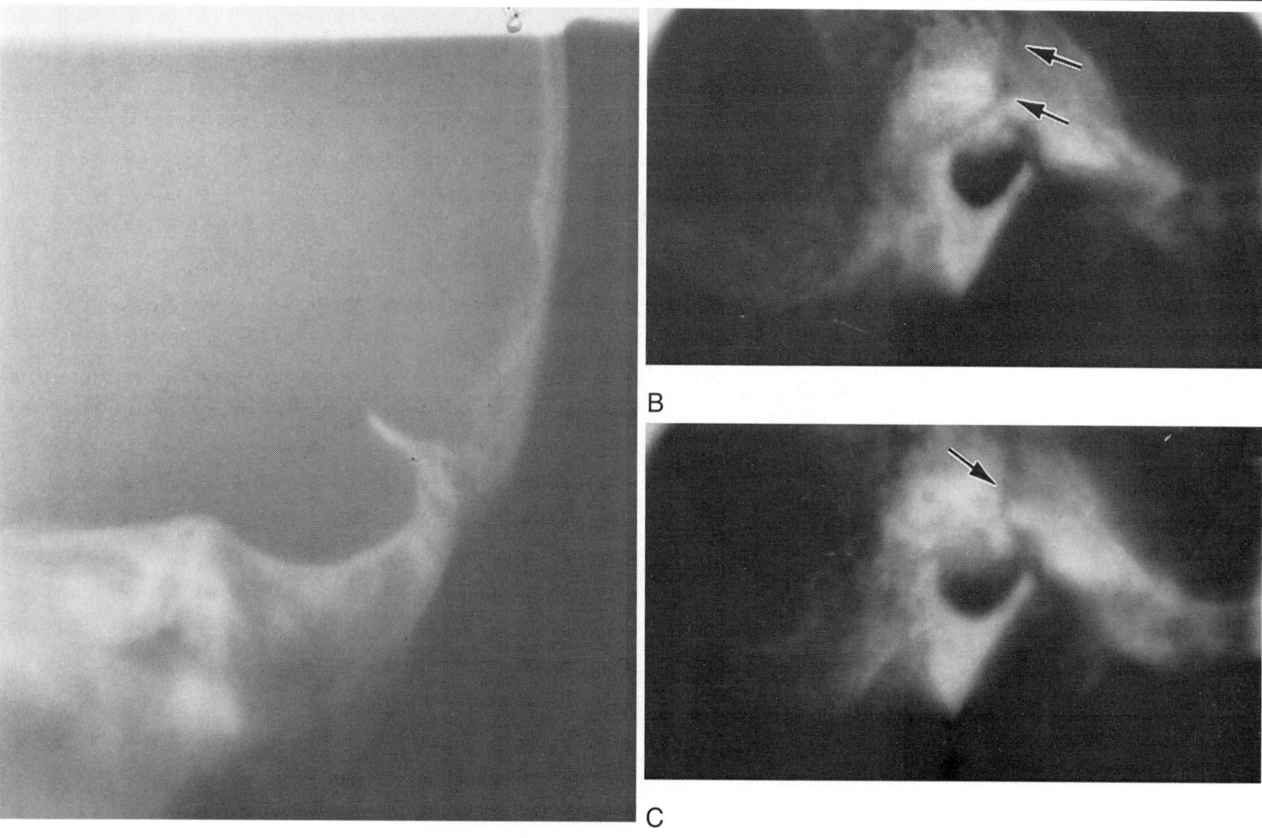

Figure 7.5. Tomographic delineation of fractures. **A.** Depressed fracture, mastoid region. There is a sharp spicule of bone projecting more than 1 cm into the cranial cavity. The plain films were less revealing than the tomograph taken in Stenvers projection. The injury was produced by direct impact over this area. **B** and **C.** Fracture of petrous portion of temporal bone not shown by ordinary radiography. There is extensive fracture of the petrous pyramid passing in front of the lateral semicircular canal and curving posteriorly through the promontory. In these cases cerebrospinal fluid can leak into the middle ear cavity and from there into the nasopharynx, as explained in the text.

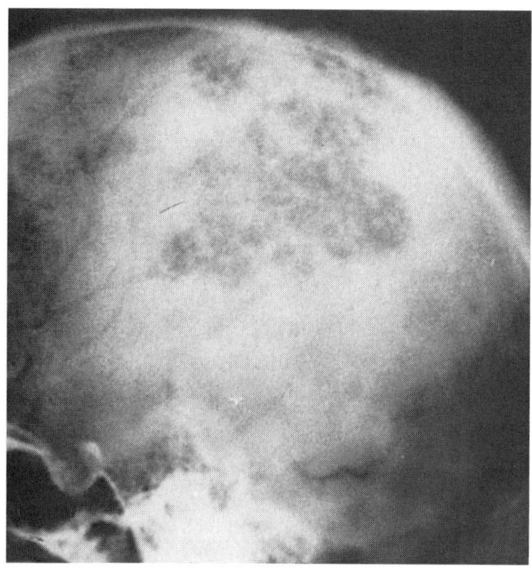

Figure 7.6. Infection following craniocerebral injury. Osteomyelitis of the skull may develop from infected scalp lacerations, even when there is no evident bony damage, and also from other causes. Irregular bone destruction with islands of sequestrated osseous tissue is found, often extending over a wide area. A latent period is seen in the radiologic manifestation of osteomyelitis of the skull, as in other areas. When chronic, there may be sclerosis about the margins of the osteolytic area. Osteomyelitis may be complicated by epidural and brain abscess.

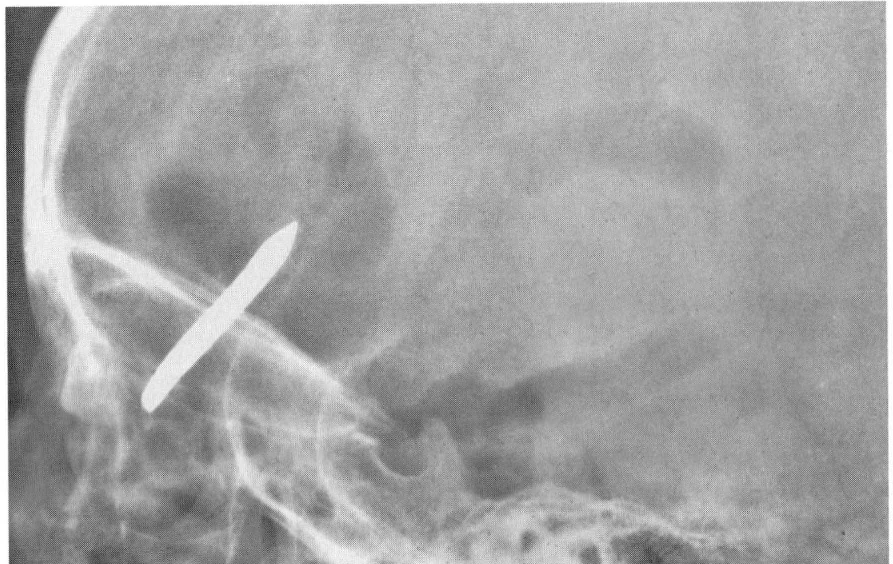

A

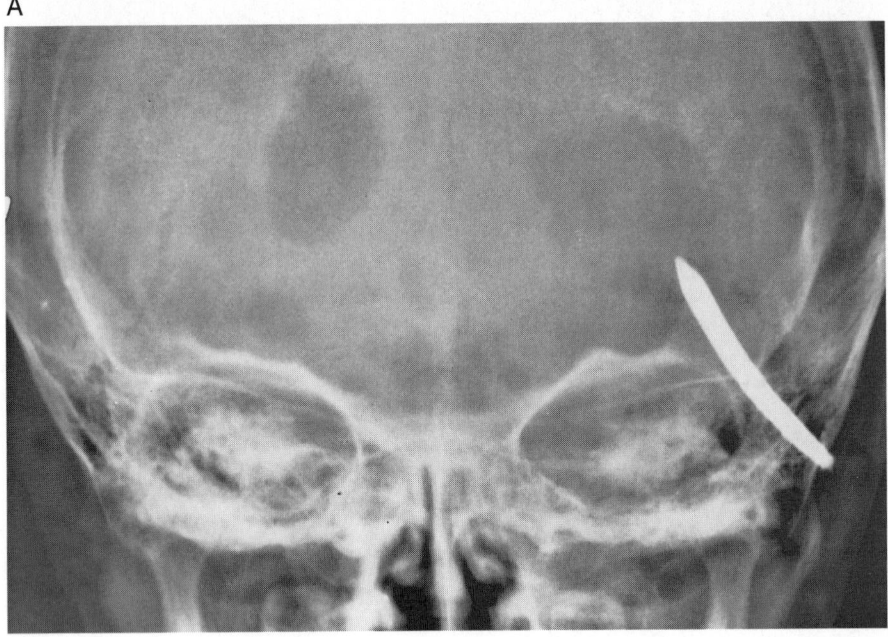

B

Figure 7.7. Ventricular infection by gas-forming organism. The child was playing in her yard while her father was cutting the lawn with a rotary power mower. The child noticed a mild stinging sensation in the region of the left temple and after a few minutes went into the house, where it was thought that she had been bitten by an insect. During the next few days the patient complained of a mild headache, developed fever, and became drowsy. The films made 10 days after the injury reveal a long fragment of a nail impacted intracranially, the tip of which is surrounded by a gas collection in the left frontal lobe.

using the horizontal beam. This would demonstrate fluid levels, if present, in the sphenoid sinuses and in other paranasal sinuses. Today CT is the procedure of choice. It is made with the patient supine and therefore will reveal fluid levels when present, but it may also reveal the fracture and any intracranial complications. However, a large proportion of basal skull fractures are not demonstrated by CT.

CSF rhinorrhea results from the rupture of the dura and arachnoid, usually at the base of the skull, where it connects with the paranasal sinuses or mastoids. The tendency is to assume that the break is in the region of the cribriform plate, but the break could be in the sphenoid bone, in which case the CSF will leak into the sphenoid sinuses and then into the nose. In the latter case, a fluid level may be seen in one sphenoid sinus (causing unilateral rhinorrhea) or in both. If the defect is anterior (posterior wall of frontal sinuses or floor of anterior fossa), the leak may be directly into the nasal cavity or into ethmoidal cells unilaterally or bilaterally. A unilateral leak indicates that the defect is only on one side. A nasal CSF leak could rarely occur following a petrous-mastoid fracture; the CSF would leak into the middle ear cavity and from there through the eustachian tube into the nasopharynx. Plain films must be made utilizing a *horizontal x-ray beam* either erect or supine. Fluid levels in the ethmoid cells indicate an anterior origin, in the frontal sinus they indicate a connection in this area,

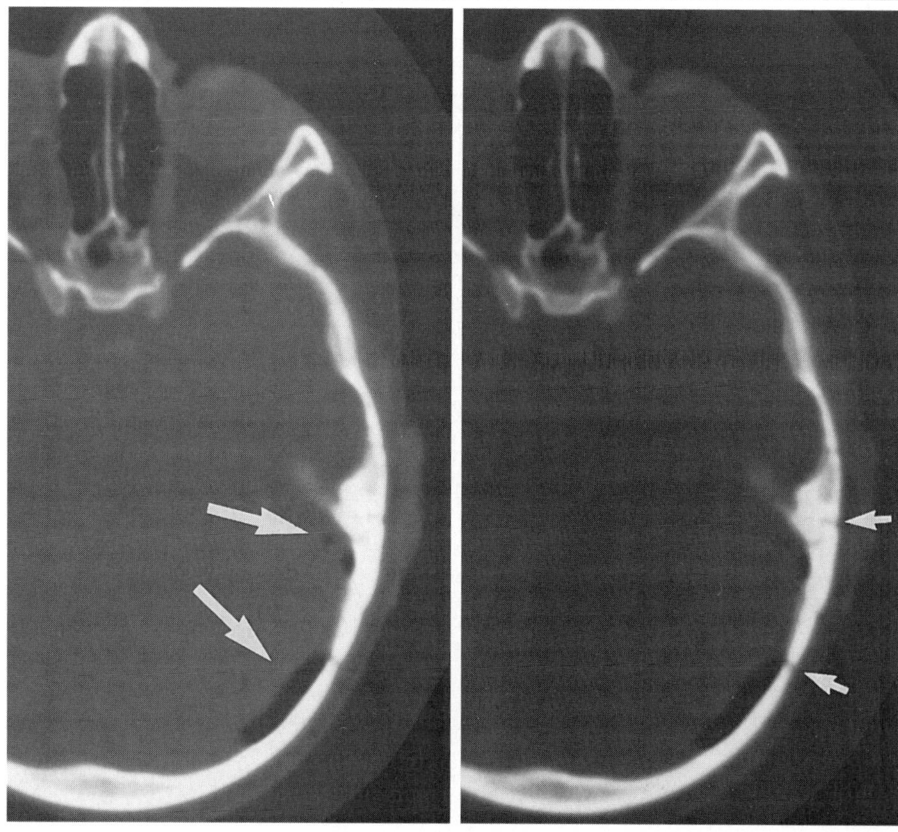

Figure 7.8. Epidural air seen in the bone window. **A.** There are two air collections following the inner table (arrows). This *always* means that there is a fracture of an air-containing sinus—in this case, the mastoid. **B.** A darker image shows the fracture line (arrows).

and in the sphenoid sinus they indicate that the break is in the sphenoid bone (Fig. 7.11). Further details may be found in Chapter 19.

Positive contrast cisternography combined with CT has been used to detect minor leaks. The patient may be positioned prone to favor the demonstration of the leak during the CT examination. Radionuclide can be injected into the lumbar spinal canal and recovered with cotton pledgets inserted on each side in the nose. This may detect a CSF leak when it is very slight and might be difficult to detect otherwise. Again, the prone position may be helpful.

More recently, El Gammal and Brooks have reported on the use of MR cisternography (6). They use a fast spin-echo technique with fat suppression, with TR 10,000, TE 200, and four repetitions. The images are videoreversed for best results (Fig. 7.12).

Extracerebral Injury

CT scanning is the method of choice to examine patients following all types of head injury in the acute stage because it can show most of the fractures and will also show the intracranial complications to best advantage. In addition, traumatized patients in the acute stage are likely to be uncooperative, and the rapid exposure on CT scanning allows for the elimination of most of the motion artifacts. CT shows the skull bones and the acute hemorrhagic complications in the epidural, subdural, and subarachnoid spaces as well as in the brain, and it will usually show focal edema and sometimes diffuse edema of the brain tissues. MRI is excellent in the subacute stage because it will reveal the posttraumatic changes in the brain much more clearly. It will also show the bleeding complications more clearly than CT, for in the subacute stage the density of the blood has diminished on CT scanning; it may be isodense with the surrounding brain tissue, or it may be hypodense. MRI will show hyperintensity on T1 and T2 images in any hemorrhagic complication in the subacute stage. It will also show brain edema, which will be hyperintense on T2-weighted images, in a much more dramatic way than CT, which reveals only relative hypodensity of the edematous area that is sometimes difficult to appreciate.

EPIDURAL HEMATOMA

A linear fracture may cross the arteries that supply the dura mater, such as the middle meningeal artery and its branches, as well as some accessory meningeal arteries. The

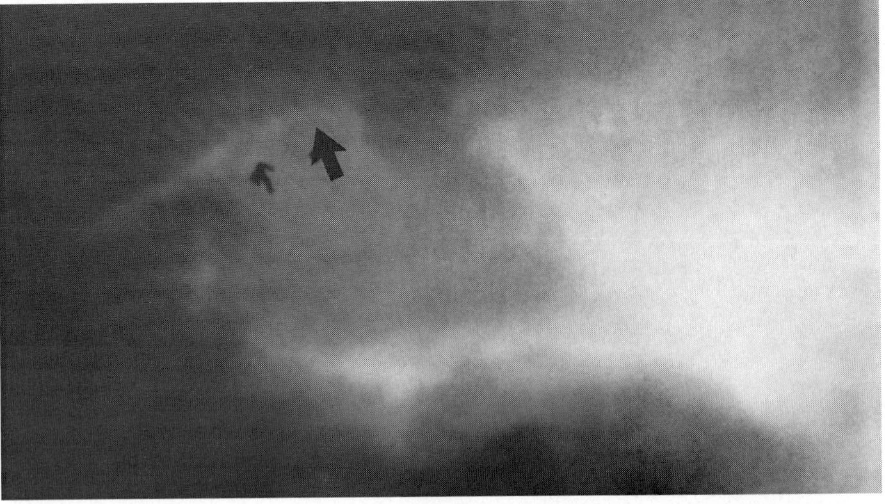

A

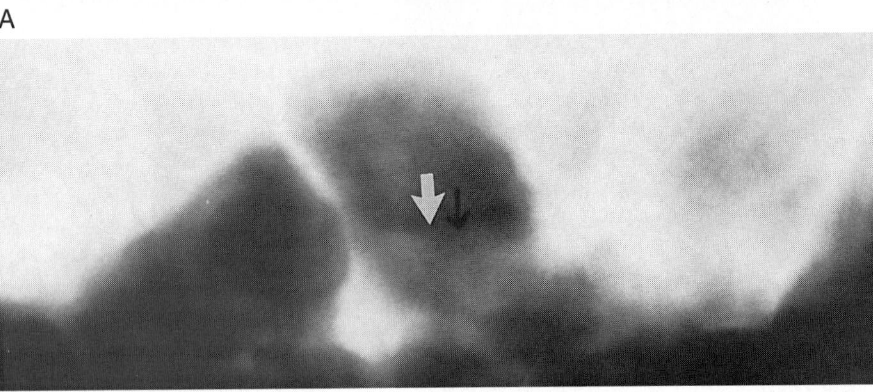

B

Figure 7.9. Basal skull fracture. **A.** Sagittal tomogram reveals fractures of the anterior fossa region just in front of the tuberculum sella and in the planum sphenoidale (arrows). The sinuses are opacified. Basal skull fractures are often difficult to demonstrate even on CT images. However, the demonstration of a basal skull fracture is not important unless there is evidence of CSF leak in the nasal area or in the ear, in which case there is the possibility of infection, particularly meningitis. **B.** Erect plain tomogram in basal plane in another case reveals a fluid level in one sphenoid sinus (arrow).

meningeal artery and its branches are contained within a groove on the inner table of the skull, for they lie on the surface of the dura mater. This anatomic arrangement allows for the rupture of the artery if a linear fracture crosses it transversely or obliquely. The rupture of the artery leads to arterial bleeding in the epidural space. Because the bleeding is occurring at the blood pressure level, it is capable of detaching the dura from the inner table of the skull, and it will usually do so until it reaches a suture line, at which point the dura is more heavily attached to the bone and usually stops the progression of the hematoma. This is typical of epidural hematomas as against subdural hematomas, as explained in text following. The configuration of an epidural hematoma, because of the dura attachments at the sutures, becomes biconvex, a characteristic configuration (Fig. 7.13). About 65 percent of epidural hematomas occur under the temporal and parietal bones, which indicates that they are related to the middle meningeal arteries and their branches (7). Venous bleeding as a result of rupture of the dural sinuses may lead to venous epidural hematomas, which are much less frequent. They ordinarily occur in the areas where the dural sinuses are found: along the superior sagittal sinus, the region of the torcular Herophili, and the lateral and sigmoid sinuses. Characteristically, these hematomas develop much more slowly—a week to 10 days or longer following the rupture—as in contrast to the arterial epidural hematomas, which develop rapidly. The classic history of an epidural hematoma is that of initial loss of consciousness, regaining of consciousness some minutes or an hour later, with a lucid period of a few hours (2 or 3), followed again by loss of consciousness. Before the second loss of consciousness occurs, it may be possible to detect dilatation of the pupil on one side because of displacement of the medial portion of the temporal lobe

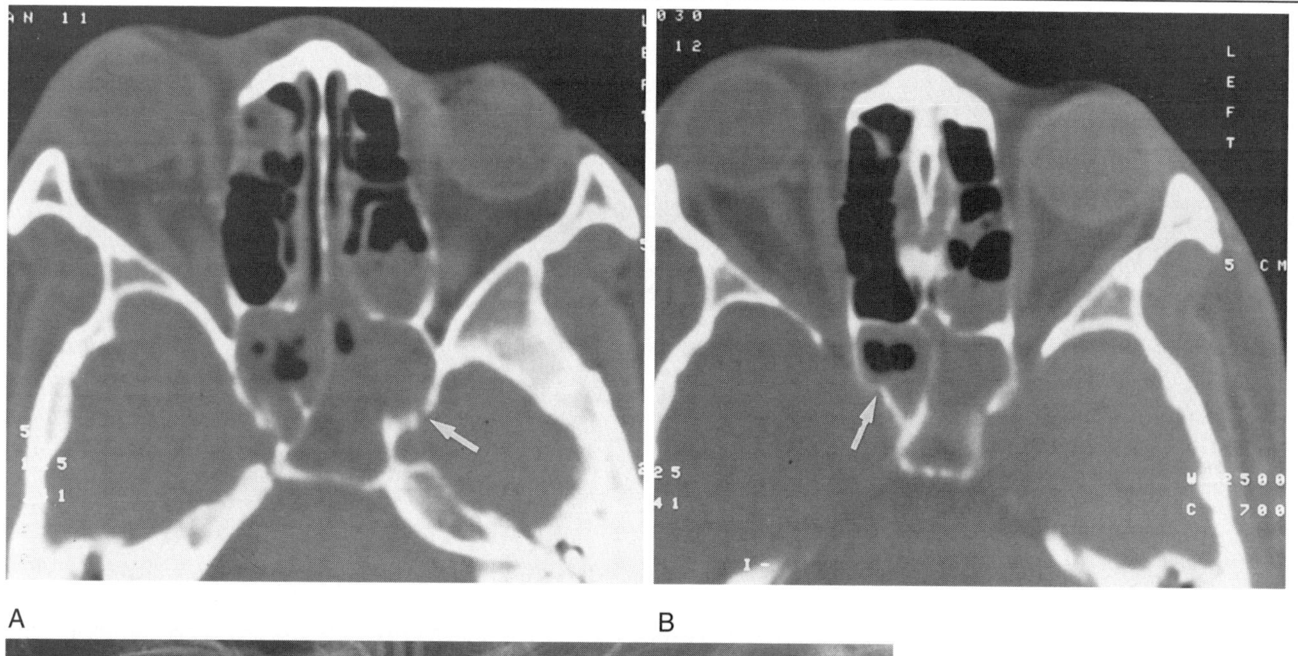

A B

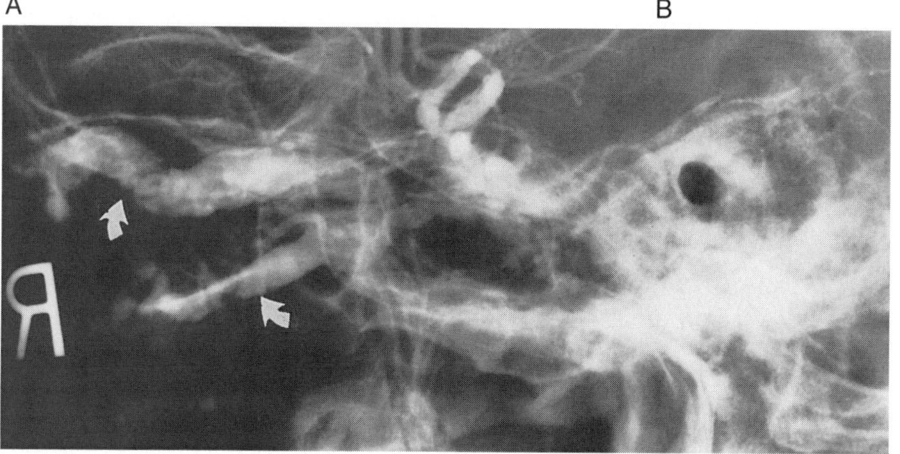

C

Figure 7.10. Basal skull fracture passing through the sphenoid bone. **A** and **B.** A fracture is seen accompanied by fluid filling the sphenoid sinuses bilaterally (arrows) and extending to the posterior ethmoid cells on the left. **C.** The patient also developed a carotid-cavernous fistula. Note the filling of the ophthalmic veins (arrows) in this late-arterial-phase carotid angiogram.

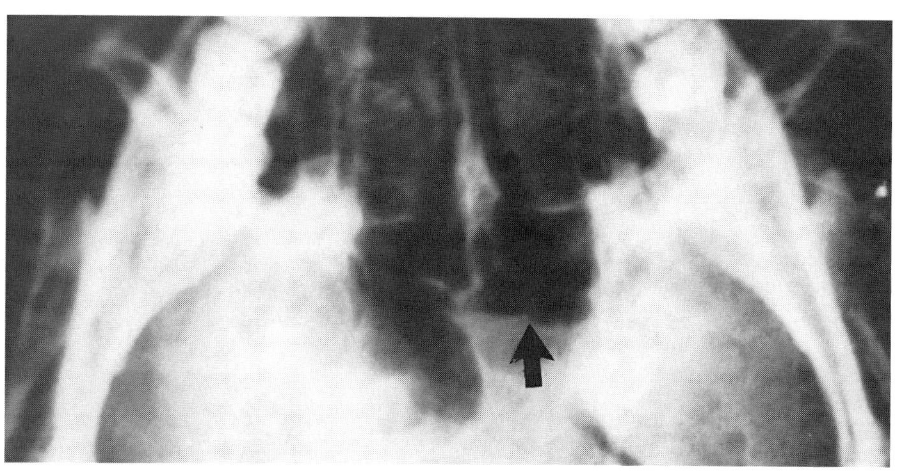

Figure 7.11. CSF rhinorrhea. The fluid level in the left sphenoid sinus (arrow) indicated that the communication was not in the ethmoid area, the more common place for CSF leak, but in the sphenoid bone. The left side had been suspected clinically because the patient indicated that the dripping was always on the left side. There had been an old head injury many years before, but on surgical intervention a small opening, probably congenital, was found in the medial aspect of the floor of the temporal fossa. The same fluid levels can be demonstrated on CT or MRI axial views, and when seen after a trauma indicate the presence of a probable basal skull fracture, which may lead to CSF rhinorrhea. The fracture is often difficult to demonstrate. The film was made with the patient sitting and the head extended against an erect Bucky stand.

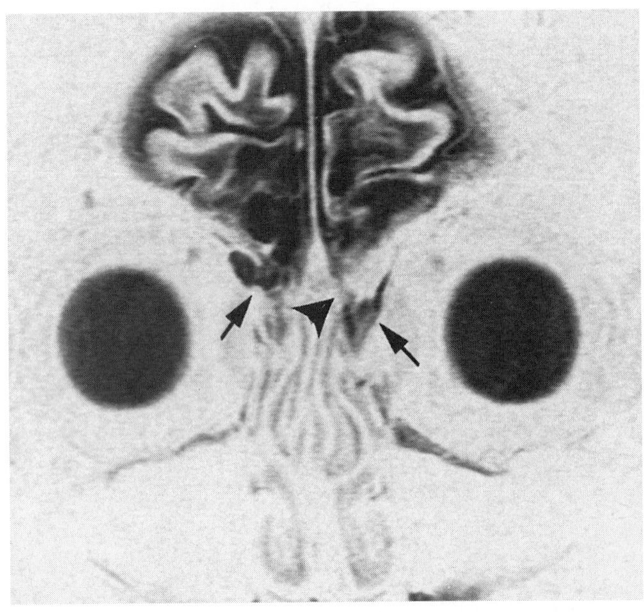

A

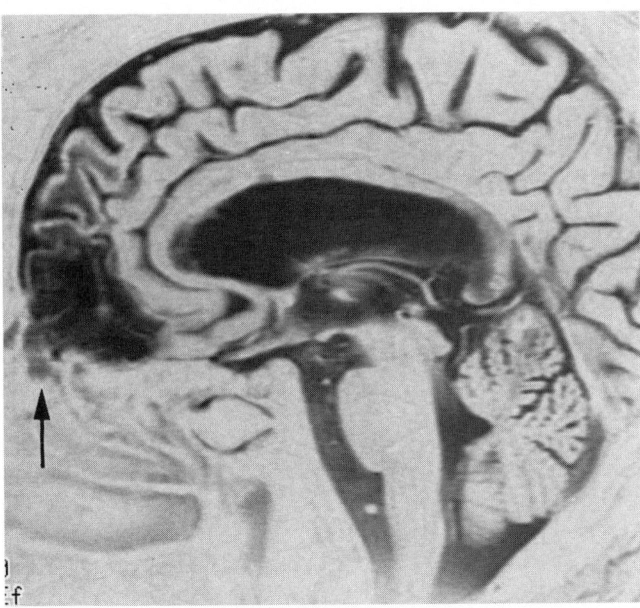

B

Figure 7.12. Posttraumatic CSF leak demonstrated by MRI cisternography. Coronal (**A**) and sagittal (**B**) views (the images are videoreversed; CSF appears black) show CSF in ethmoidal regional bilaterally (arrows). CT coronal view (**C**) shows an abnormality only on right side (arrow). The technique uses a TR of 10,000, a TE of 200, and 4 repetitions. (Courtesy of Drs El Gammal and Brooks (Birmingham): AJNR 1994;15:1647–1656, with permission.)

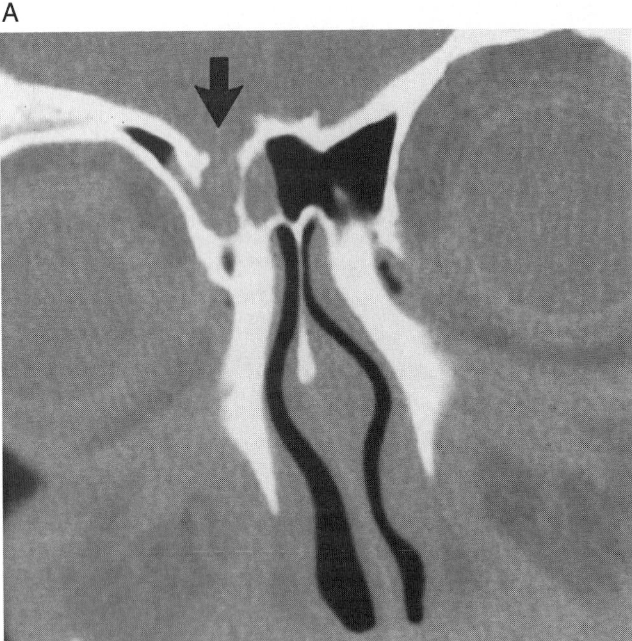

C

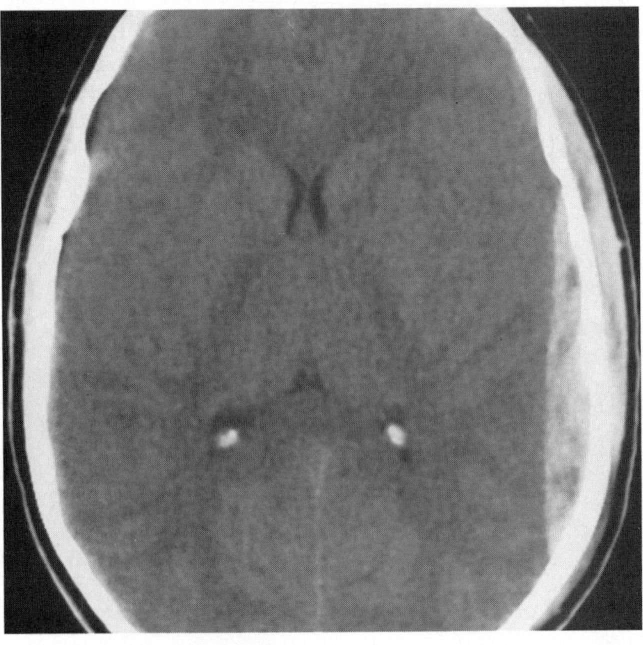

Figure 7.13. Small epidural hematoma in an infant 2 years old not necessitating immediate evacuation. The bone windows did not show a fracture of the parietal bone, but the initial digital localization image did show a transverse fracture (not shown). Because the fracture was parallel or oblique to the plane of the CT images, it was not demonstrated by CT. There is a slight degree of edema on the left hemisphere, but the epidural was followed clinically and by repeat cross-sectional images until partial resolution had occurred. Unlike with subdural hematomas, the blood collection stops at the suture lines (compare with Fig. 7.20).

and pressure on the third cranial nerve, usually attributed to hippocampal herniation. Today a CT examination would be indicated in any patient who presented loss of consciousness initially. It is a rather important consideration, for it is not possible clinically to rule out the possible presence of a rupture of the middle meningeal arteries, which may, in a few to several hours later, produce a fatal hematoma. Although a plain skull examination may show the presence of a fracture in the appropriate areas, and this may suggest a possible epidural hematoma, the absence of such visible fracture does not rule out that the patient may later develop an epidural hematoma. This is particularly true in children. In the series reported by Zimmerman and Bilaniuk in 1982, 91 percent of the patients had a demonstrated fracture, but 9 percent did not (7).

Not every fracture of the parietal bone crossing the middle meningeal artery or its branches results in the development of an epidural hematoma. Under these circumstances, the following may occur: (a) the fracture is not accompanied by injury of the dura or the vessel; (b) a false aneurysm forms in the vessel that does not lead to epidural hematoma formation; (c) the aneurysm ruptures in a few hours, or it ruptures 1 to 3 weeks later, with resultant delayed epidural hemorrhage; or (d) the vessel ruptures initially, but the blood enters the adjacent meningeal or diploic veins that ruptured at the same time, leading to an arteriovenous communication (8). In (d) the meningeal artery usually will fail to fill beyond the rupture site. Eventually, the fistula will thrombose, and the artery may become patent again (Fig. 7.14). The blood may also pass through the fracture and into the subgaleal space.

The diagnosis of epidural hematoma is easily made by CT scanning (Figs. 7.13 and 7.15). As mentioned, a venous hematoma may develop more slowly, and it may be asymptomatic and discovered only because reexamination was carried out to follow other manifestations of the head trauma (Fig. 7.16). The blood within the epidural hematoma will usually clot unless it is evacuated rapidly, and in such cases the solid portion of the hematoma will be denser than a central or more irregular area of radiolucency, which

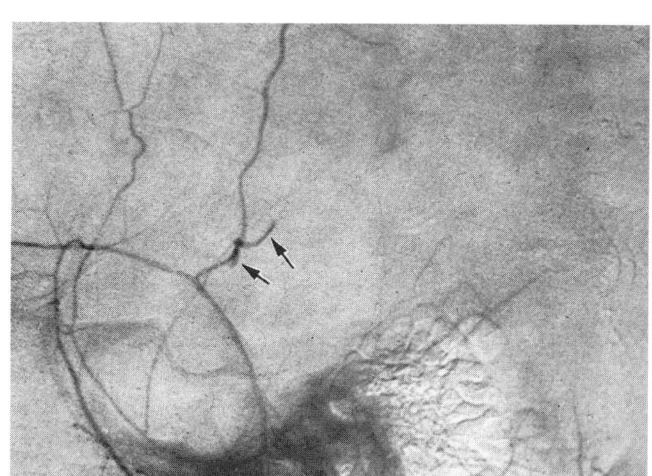

A

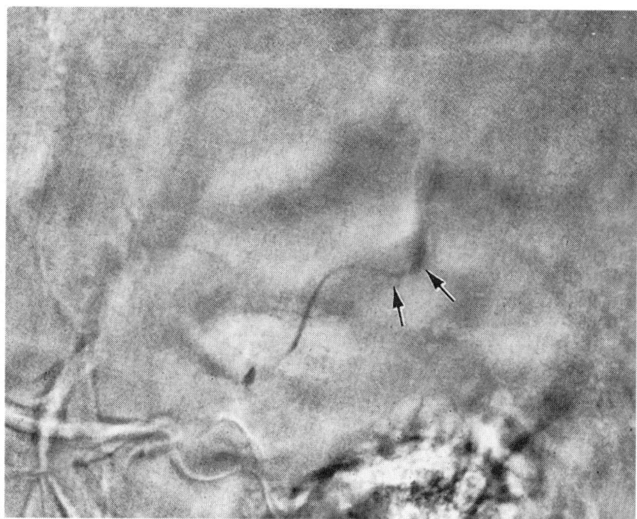

B

C

Figure 7.14. Posttraumatic aneurysm of the middle meningeal artery branch and arteriovenous communication. **A.** The lateral view shows a small aneurysm (anterior arrow) and a small vessel filling posteriorly that is probably a vein (posterior arrow). **B.** A later film reveals further filling of this vessel, which widens posteriorly. Usually the veins fill rapidly unless they are compressed by adjacent hemorrhage. **C.** The frontal film demonstrates the aneurysm more clearly (arrow).

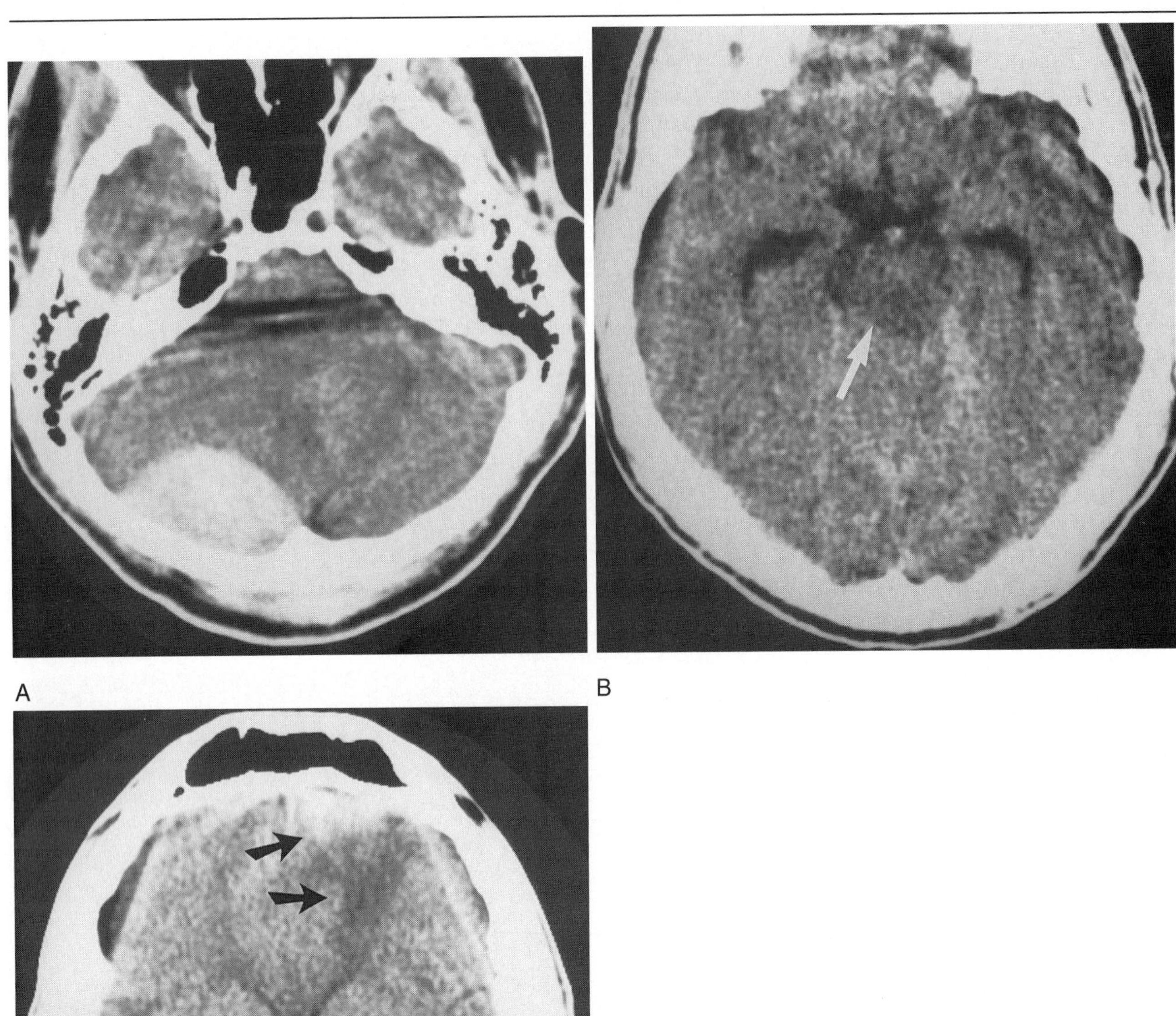

Figure 7.15. A. Epidural hematoma of the posterior fossa in an inmate who became involved in a fight. Posterior fossa epidurals are very uncommon because the area is so well protected by muscle. There is a mass effect present, and the fourth ventricle is compressed. **B.** A higher section reveals that the upper brainstem is deformed and compressed from the right and behind. The upper fourth ventricle is not seen, and the temporal horns are already moderately dilated. There is also a frontal contusion seen better in **C** (arrows). Note that in B the brainstem is hypodense in relation to the cerebellar tissue behind it, suggesting that there is diffuse edema.

may contain serum extruded from the clot. This may be more conspicuous in hematomas that develop somewhat more slowly or in venous epidural hematomas. In the latter group, contrast enhancement may reveal enhancement of the dura and adjacent areas due to granulation tissue, such as may be seen in chronic subdural hematomas. On MRI the acute epidural hematoma will be low intensity on T1 and hyperintense on T2 in the first few days. It may become hypointense on T2-weighted images before the extracellular stage of methemoglobin (Table 7.2).

CT examination is the only examination that is usually carried out in these patients in institutions where a CT scanner is available. If it is not available, cerebral angiography is required to make the diagnosis of an epidural hema-

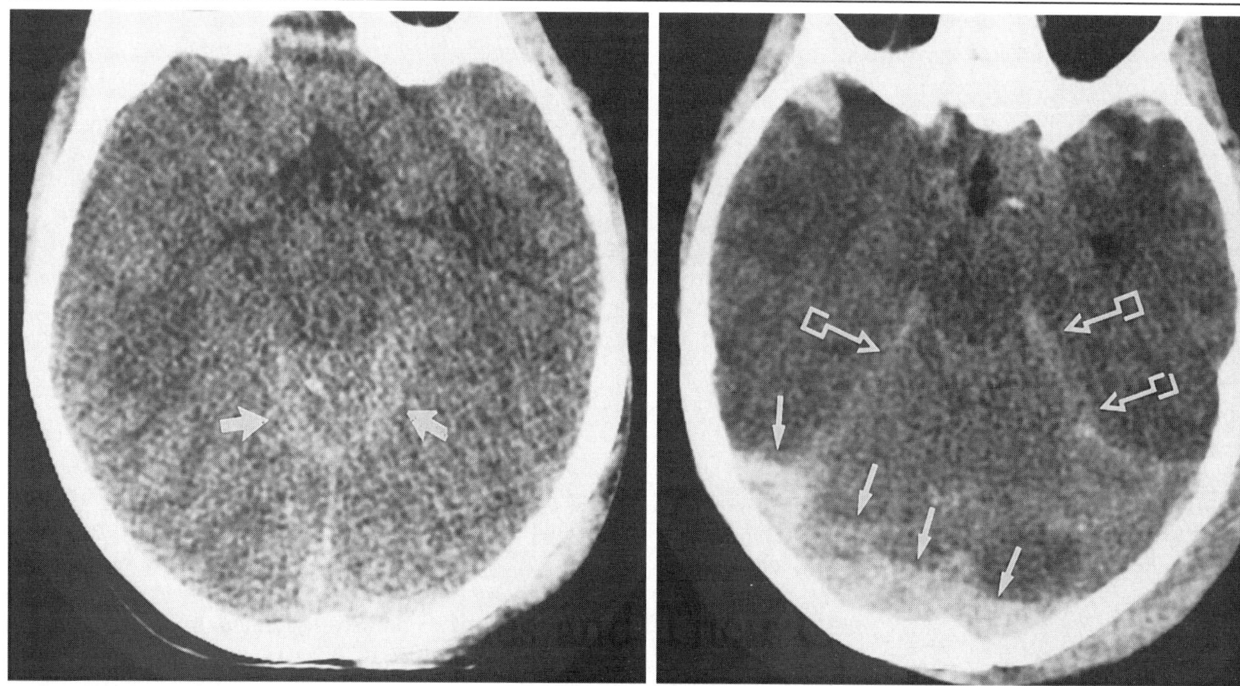

Figure 7.16. Venous epidural hematoma around torcular Herophili in a 5-year-old boy. **A.** The initial examination showed some increase in density at the edge of the tentorium consistent with subdural blood (arrows). There is no clear-cut CSF space around the brainstem. This may be due to brain edema with compression of the brainstem, or it could be produced by a small amount of subarachnoid blood that elevates the density of CSF sufficiently to make it isodense with brain structures. **B.** Repeat examination 48 hours later when the child showed clinical deterioration revealed an extracerebral dense collection behind the cerebellum and the parietal occipital lobes (arrows). There is also evidence of a subdural collection under the tentorium (open arrow). The perimesencephalic space remains poorly visible.

toma. The variations in the behavior of complete or partial rupture of the middle meningeal vessels just described can be demonstrated by cerebral angiography but not by CT scanning. Cerebral angiography is required when there are other types of complications, such as carotid-cavernous fistula or suspected posttraumatic aneurysm. Otherwise, angiography is not employed in the management of head trauma.

Some epidural hematomas are managed without surgical evacuation. Usually these are the ones that are considered small (less than 0.5 cm in thickness). The neuroradiologist should be alert for signs that might speak against a conservative management (9). Among these signs are the presence of a midline shift disproportionate to the size of the hematoma, perhaps indicating nonobvious edema; and the presence of a low-density component on CT, which may indicate active bleeding. A careful search for early hippocampal herniation should be made, and repeat CT examination to follow the progress of the hematoma should be carried out. Any increase in size, even without clinical deterioration, should be seriously considered as a possible indication for surgery.

Table 7.2.
Features of Epidural Hematoma (EDH)

85% arterial in origin.
Frequently due to posttraumatic laceration of middle meningeal artery.
Often a rapidly expanding mass lesion that requires emergency surgical decompression.
Typically biconvex, hyperdense on CT, with moderate or marked mass effect.
Usually terminates at cranial suture lines.
Hyperintense on T2-weighted MR images if less than a few days old; may also be hyperintense thereafter on T1-weighted images.

SUBDURAL HEMATOMA

Subdural hematomas are considerably more common than epidural hematomas and are considered to be secondary to rupture of the bridging veins that go from the surface of the brain and cross the subdural space to enter the superior sagittal sinus. Some subdural collections could occur in the midline due to rupture of the veins that pass from the medial brain surface to the inferior sagittal sinus at the lower edge of the falx. Because these veins are very small, usually a large hematoma does not actually occur, but a thin layer of blood around one or both sides of the falx is common. There are some exceptions, but they are uncommon.

Subdural hematomas usually occur as a result of head trauma; however, particularly in the older age group, history of trauma may not be available. In this group, brain shaking has obviously occurred, leading to shearing of the bridging veins, which are more likely to be longer because of the presence of some senile brain atrophy, but the relatively minor head trauma was overlooked or forgotten. The subdural space is normally nonexistent, and the two membranes, the arachnoid and the dura mater, are closely approximated. Nevertheless, fluid easily separates the two membranes and diffuses throughout the available subdural space. Usually it extends to the midline on both sides, but it can push apart the dura and arachnoid around the falx cerebri and then extends to the opposite side in that way. However, this does not usually happen, and when bilateral subdural hematomas are found, they almost certainly occurred independently of each other, because one cannot usually detect a significant subdural collection around the falx cerebri (Fig. 7.17).

In acute head injury, it is relatively common to find increased density of the falx, which is evidently due to the rupture of some of the small veins going from the medial brain surface to the inferior sagittal sinus. The increase in falx density is felt to be caused by an accumulation of a thin layer of blood on one or both sides of the falx. In addition, we frequently note the presence of increased density following the surface of the tentorium, which is again due to rupture of bridging veins that are probably related to the lateral sinuses (Fig. 7.18; see Fig. 7.28). The thin subdural collections over or under the tentorium and the increase in density of the falx are often seen alone, without an associated subdural hematoma on the outer surface of the brain.

In the acute stage the subdural hematoma will have the usual increased density on CT that is seen with blood, particularly clotted blood. Cases have been described in which a patient is very anemic and the subdural collection is either isodense or even slightly less dense than the brain tissue. In the absence of anemia, an isodense acute subdural hematoma may be due to the presence of disseminated intravascular coagulation (DIC) (10). The patient may reveal a normal hematocrit and red cell count but a long prothrombin time, a long partial thromboplastin time, and low fibrinogen. In the case reported by Boyko et al. there was enhancement of the hematoma with iodide contrast (10). It is important to think of DIC in patients with head trauma because it is fairly common in severe head injuries (11). The density of the subdural hematoma decreases with the passage of time, and in about 10 days to 2 weeks it may become completely isodense with the brain and thus could be overlooked on the CT scan examination. In general we pay attention to the position of the surface sulci of the brain

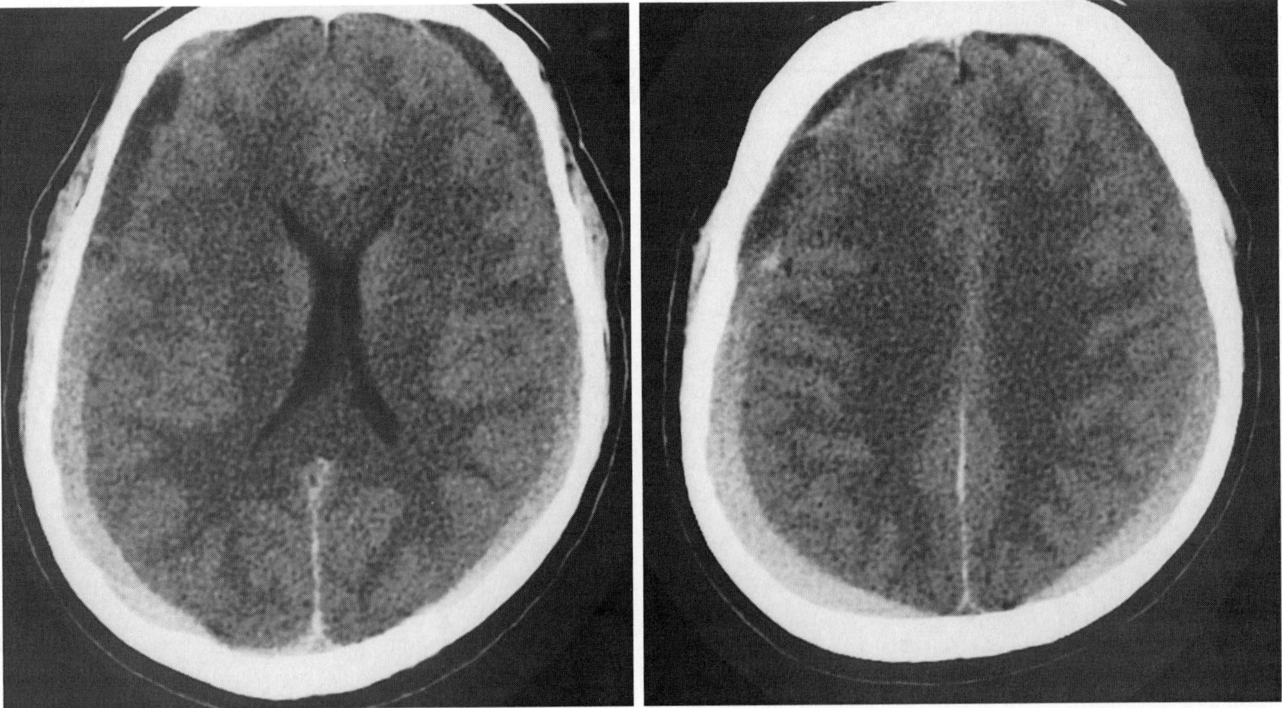

A B

Figure 7.17. Bilateral symmetrical subdural hematoma showing hyperdensity in the dependent portion (patient lying supine) and water density in the frontal regions, indicating a subacute subdural hematoma. There is only minimal midline shift to the left.

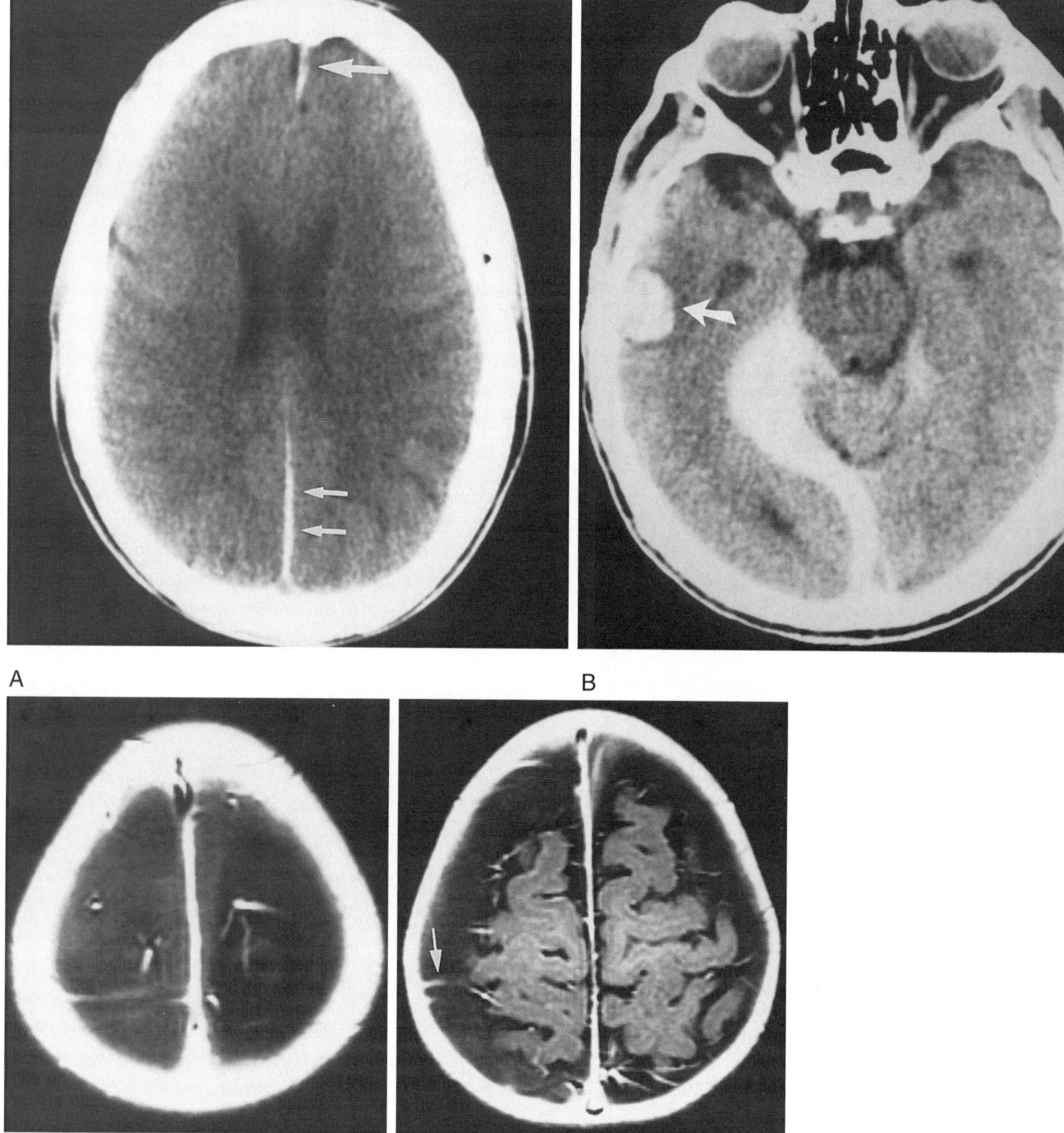

Figure 7.18. Falx and tentorial subdural collections. **A.** Increased density and thickness of the falx anteriorly and/or posteriorly in an acute head trauma patient should be carefully studied and usually means there is some subdural or subarachnoid hemorrhage around the falx (arrows). **B.** Subdural hematoma over the tentorium in another patient. The collection is usually on the upper surface, only rarely in the inferior surface. It is due to rupture of the veins draining into the lateral sinuses and is a fairly frequent finding, sometimes very subtle, after head trauma. The presence of falx or tentorial minor subdural collections is an important warning that the trauma was severe enough to require careful observation of the patient. The patient also presented hematoma in the temporal cortical-subcortical area (arrow). **C.** The bridging veins are sometimes very prominent, as shown in this case, a 4-month-old infant with an unexplained subdural hematoma who presented a bridging vein in an unusual location, much lower than usual (**D,** arrow).

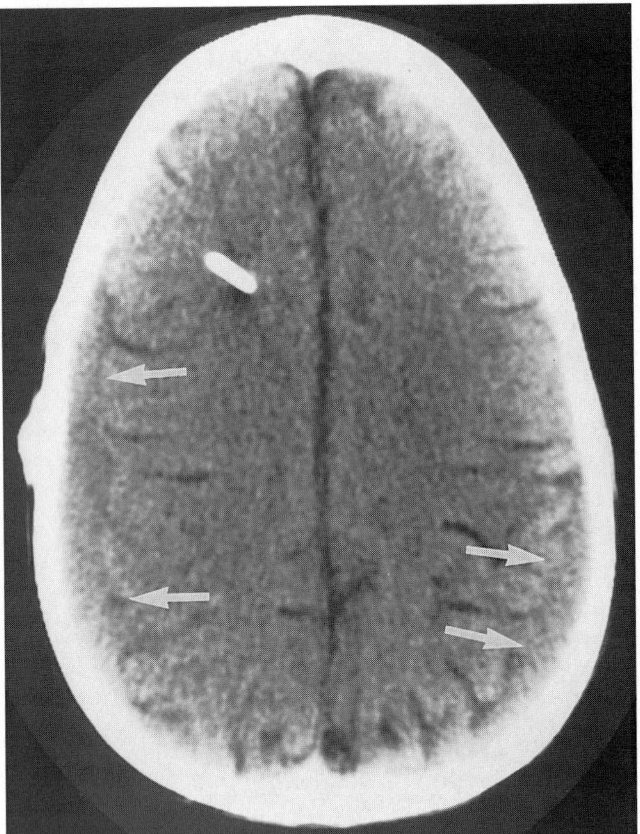

Figure 7.19. Isodense subdural hematoma on CT imaging (arrows). The hematoma does not produce a midline shift because it is bilateral, although not symmetrical. The injury had occurred about 3 weeks previously. The patient had a shunt tube because of previous hydrocephalus.

Table 7.3.
Features of Subdural Hematoma (SDH)

Approximately 90% venous in origin.
Typically less rapidly expanding than EDH.
May have considerable associated mass effect even if the thickness of the SDH is not large.
Characteristically has a lentiform shape, but may be biconvex.
Chronic SDH is common, usually due to rupture of subdural bridging veins in elderly patients.
CT appearance depends on age of SDH: may be hyperdense (acute SDH), isodense, or hypodense (chronic SDH).
Acute SDH can be hypodense in anemic patients.
Tentorial SDH or those under the temporal lobe may be difficult to diagnose on axial CT.

as these are displaced away from the inner table. If they do not clearly reach the inner table of the skull, we should suspect bilateral symmetrical isodense hematomas. Of course, if the hematoma is unilateral, the displacement of the midline structures will make the presence of a mass lesion easy to recognize (Fig. 7.19). On the other hand, MRI will always show the hematoma with extreme clarity, because if it is a subacute hemorrhage, the subdural collection will be bright on T1- and T2-weighted images (Fig. 7.20).

A chronic subdural hematoma on CT is hypodense and in time will approximate the density of the CSF. However, it is usually slightly less hypointense than CSF because it contains a certain amount of protein. On MRI, the intensity of the subdural collection may also become waterlike and be almost equal to that of the CSF in the ventricles: that is, on T1 it will be low intensity like the lateral ventricles, and on T2 it will be bright (Fig. 7.20; Table 7.3).

It is important to point out that a subdural collection of CSF density is a somewhat frequent occurrence in acute head injury. It cannot be blood because it is very hypodense; it cannot be an old subdural collection because it probably was not observed on the first CT scan on admission. I believe it probably represents a rupture of the arachnoid membrane that allows for leakage of CSF into the subdural space. The fluid collection usually disappears in a week or two, but sometimes it seems to become a regular subdural collection that increases in size. This indicates the presence of increased protein, which attracts fluid and allows the amount to increase over time (see Fig. 7.21*A* to *C*). In this case some hemorrhage must have occurred or at least can be postulated, even though it may not have been demonstrated. The rupture of the arachnoid as a cause of these acute hypodense subdural collections is suggested for lack of a better explanation and because of the CSF-like density of the fluid. It is more commonly observed after 50 years of age but is also seen in younger patients. Rapid appearance and disappearance of subdural and epidural hematomas within 24 hours has been reported by Kurowia et al. with CT follow-up (12).

SUBARACHNOID HEMORRHAGE

Subarachnoid hemorrhage is seen in moderately to markedly severe head injuries. It is less common than epidural or subdural hematomas. The presence of subarachnoid hemorrhage may be focal, in the area of a fracture, and may indicate that there has been trauma to the surface vessels or, more likely, that there has been an injury to the brain surface—a contusion or a laceration. A subarachnoid hemorrhage may also be seen in the midline following rupture of the very small veins going from the medial surface of the hemispheres to the inferior sagittal sinus. As explained earlier, this hemorrhage could be in the subdural space, but it may also be in the subarachnoid space. Subarachnoid bleeding may also be seen in the newborn as a result of severe head deformation during birth, and in this case it may be located around the tentorial surface or around the falx. In general, the bleeding in the subarachnoid space is not excessive but rather relatively mild, and CT examinations of good quality are required (see Fig. 7.25). Sometimes only isodensity of the CSF is seen, and this will obliterate the normal separation between the CSF density and the brainstem and surrounding areas of the base of the brain. It is rather rare for trauma to cause a false aneurysm

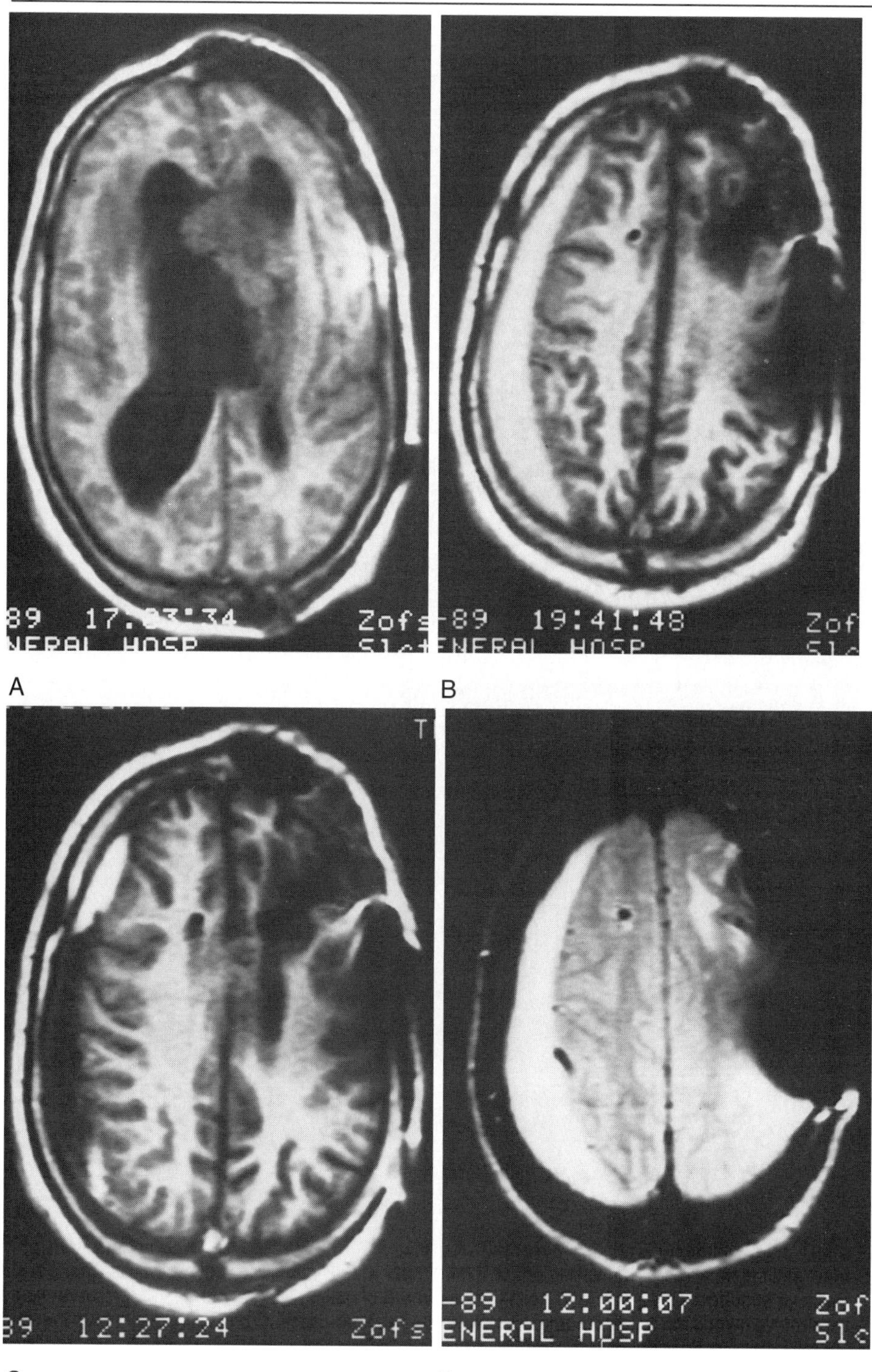

Figure 7.20. Subdural hematoma. **A.** No subdural hematoma was seen on MRI at this time. The patient had an intraventricular tumor that later required shunting to relieve the associated hydrocephalus. **B.** Possibly as a result of the shunting and a relatively minor head trauma, the patient, a 24-year-old man, developed a subdural hematoma that on T1-weighted images was hyperintense. Artifacts are seen on the left side from metal on the skin related to the shunting. **C.** Reexamination 3 months later showed that the subdural hematoma was now hypointense, although there was a bright component in the frontal region—probably a more recent hemorrhage. **D.** On proton density and T2-weighted images the hematoma was bright in both examinations because methemoglobin would be bright and a hygroma, now present in the third examination, would also be bright. If the hygroma contains enough protein, it will be bright on a proton density image, as may be the case here. If the hygroma approaches the CSF, it will follow CSF intensity.

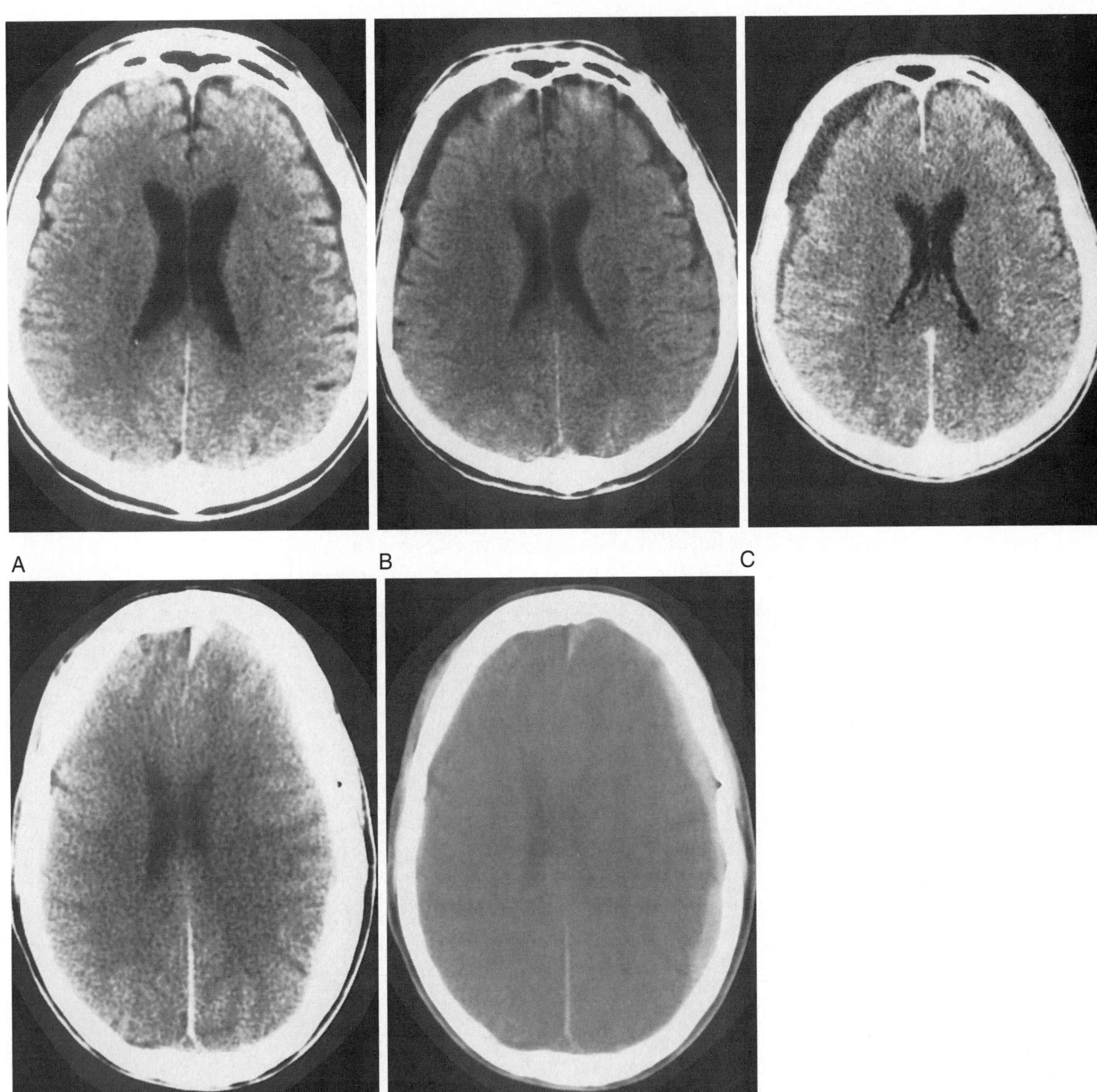

Figure 7.21. Acute subdural hygroma. **A.** This 45-year-old patient was involved in a motor vehicle accident and in the first examination revealed a bilateral subdural hygroma. The patient was not anemic and had no brain atrophy. **B.** Six days later the subdural collection had increased in size. **C.** Twenty days after B, the collection was smaller on the left but slightly larger on the right. Both collections cleared spontaneously. The pathogenesis of these "subdural hygromas" occurring in the acute stage after head trauma is of interest. There may be a rupture of the arachnoid, which allows the leakage of CSF into the subdural space. Otherwise it is difficult to explain why the collections are usually CSF-like in density. **D** to **G.** Subdural hematoma, acute, seen only on subdural windows. **D.** The standard window on CT for photography (window level 40, window width 80) does not show a subdural collection. However, there is hyperdensity in the falx anteriorly and posteriorly, suggesting that there is some subdural blood there. **E.** A subdural window (window level 40, window width 350 or 250) reveals a subdural collection on the left side. (*continues*).

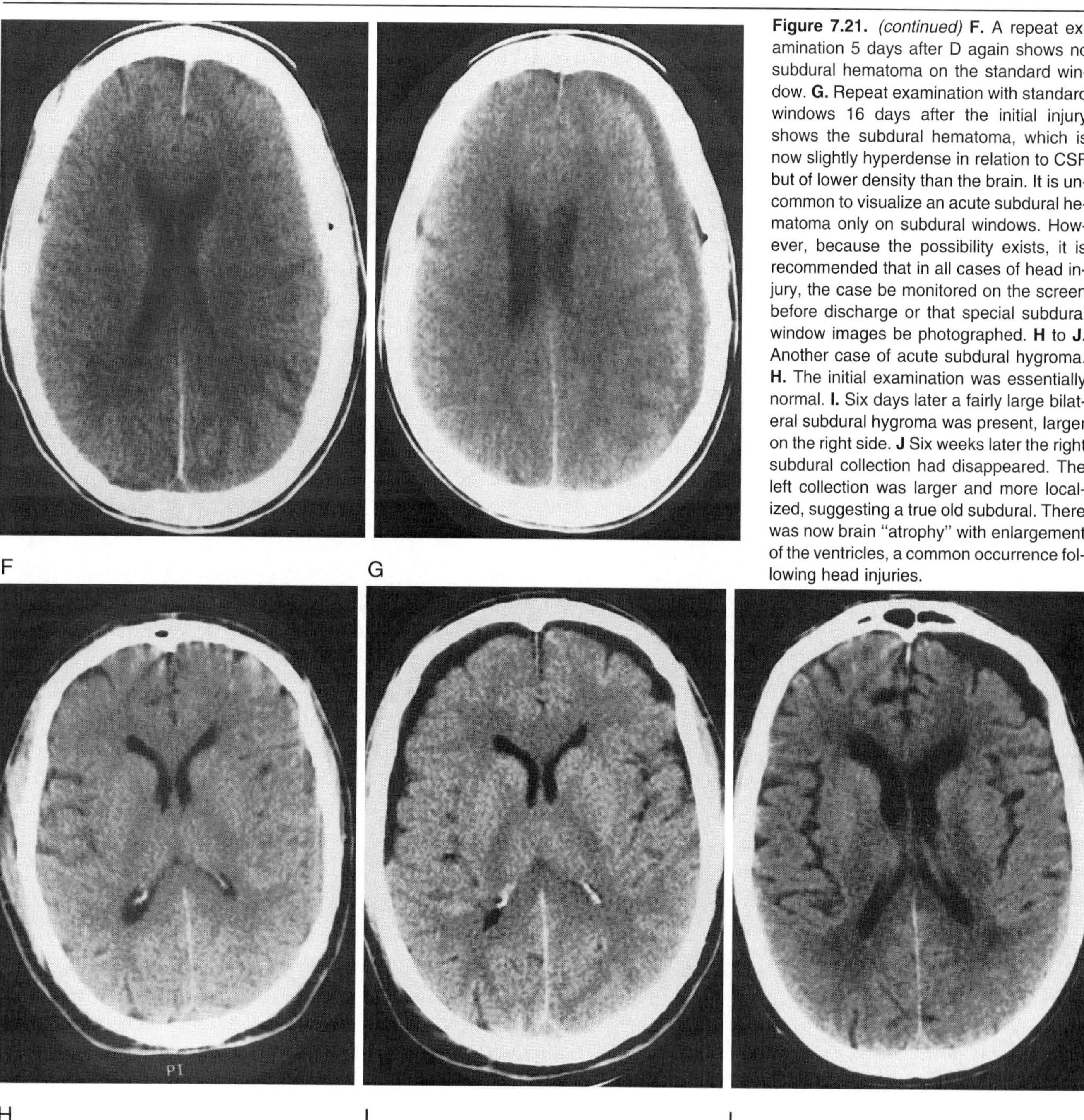

Figure 7.21. *(continued)* **F.** A repeat examination 5 days after D again shows no subdural hematoma on the standard window. **G.** Repeat examination with standard windows 16 days after the initial injury shows the subdural hematoma, which is now slightly hyperdense in relation to CSF but of lower density than the brain. It is uncommon to visualize an acute subdural hematoma only on subdural windows. However, because the possibility exists, it is recommended that in all cases of head injury, the case be monitored on the screen before discharge or that special subdural window images be photographed. **H** to **J.** Another case of acute subdural hygroma. **H.** The initial examination was essentially normal. **I.** Six days later a fairly large bilateral subdural hygroma was present, larger on the right side. **J** Six weeks later the right subdural collection had disappeared. The left collection was larger and more localized, suggesting a true old subdural. There was now brain "atrophy" with enlargement of the ventricles, a common occurrence following head injuries.

that then ruptures (see Fig. 7.38). Another source of subarachnoid blood seen on CT scanning is the presence of posttraumatic intraventricular hemorrhage with the blood escaping through the outlet foramen of the fourth ventricle and extending into the subarachnoid space (Fig. 7.22).

TRAUMATIC BRAIN INJURIES

The response of the brain to trauma is related to the type of injury. For instance, in the case of direct, blunt trauma, there is likely to be a localized lesion in the brain that could be (a) simple edema, (b) edema associated with petechial hemorrhages, (c) contusion, (d) brain laceration accompanying the contusion, (e) local hemorrhage, or (f) local or diffuse axonal injury. The same phenomenon may be repeated in several areas where the head has hit something, or has been hit, in the same accident. One area may present only edema, and another may represent contusion, hemorrhage, or axonal injury (Figs. 7.23, 7.24, and 7.26).

The term *pulping* of the brain is applied to indicate the presence of hemorrhage, edema, and necrosis of brain tissue. In severe head injuries, it is often found in the anterior poles of the brain (both frontal and both temporal lobes).

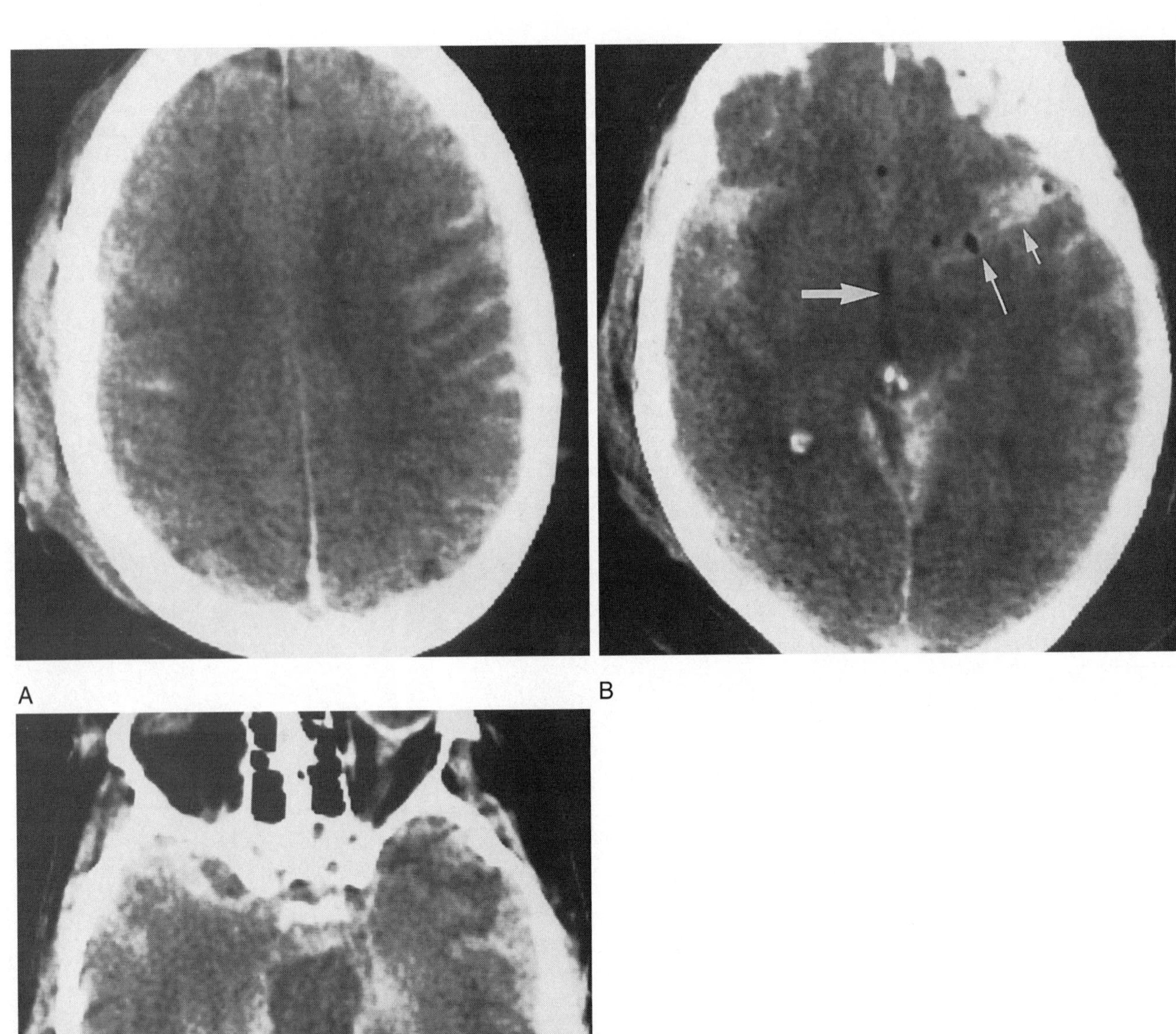

Figure 7.22. Posttraumatic subarachnoid hemorrhage. **A.** There is hyperdensity over the cortical sulci with a typical configuration for subarachnoid hemorrhage. **B.** A lower section reveals intracerebral hemorrhagic foci and gas bubbles as well as air in the third ventricle (arrows), indicating that there is a fracture through the sinuses, although these could also be produced by a penetrating injury. **C.** There is evidence of blood over the tentorium, usually indicating a subdural hematoma. The patient also had facial and orbital fractures passing through the sinuses.

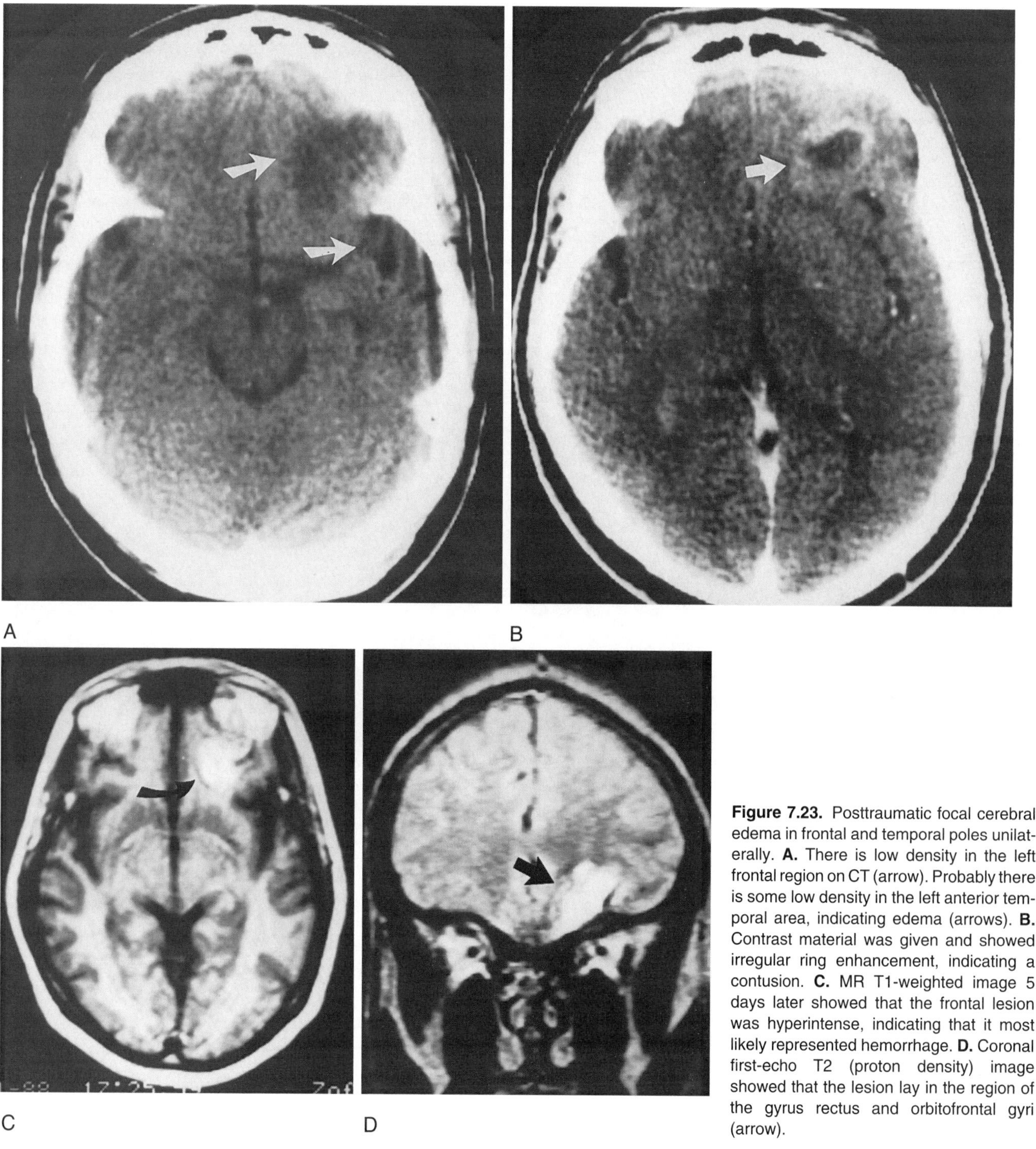

Figure 7.23. Posttraumatic focal cerebral edema in frontal and temporal poles unilaterally. **A.** There is low density in the left frontal region on CT (arrow). Probably there is some low density in the left anterior temporal area, indicating edema (arrows). **B.** Contrast material was given and showed irregular ring enhancement, indicating a contusion. **C.** MR T1-weighted image 5 days later showed that the frontal lesion was hyperintense, indicating that it most likely represented hemorrhage. **D.** Coronal first-echo T2 (proton density) image showed that the lesion lay in the region of the gyrus rectus and orbitofrontal gyri (arrow).

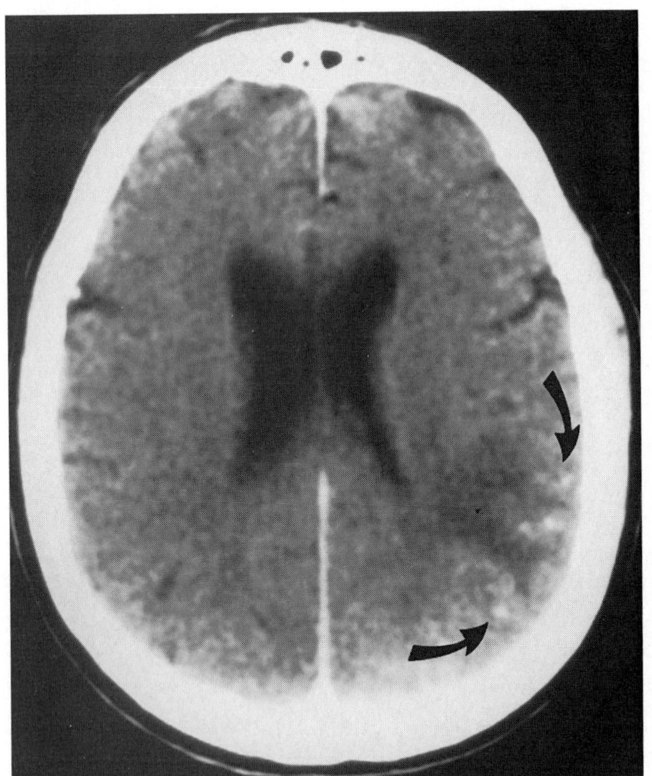

A

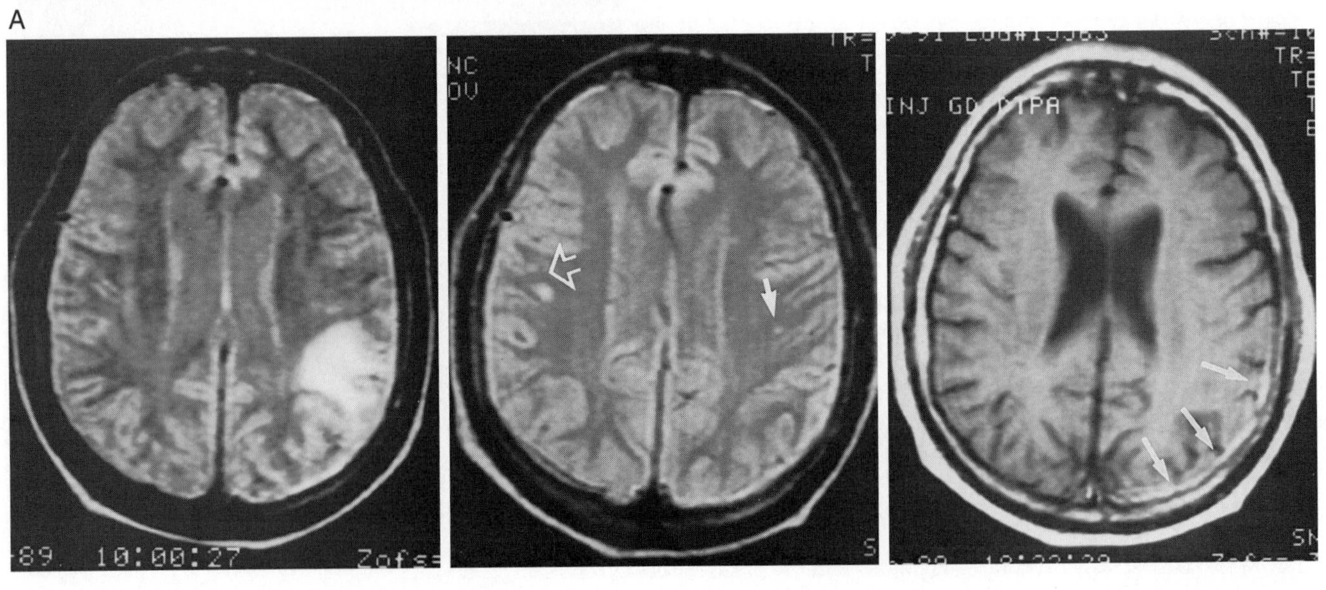

B C D

Figure 7.24. Brain contusion in a 40-year-old man. **A.** Axial CT scan shows the presence of cortical and subcortical edema in the left parietal region. The edema is associated with a number of punctate hyperintensities, representing confluent petechial hemorrhage (arrows). **B.** Several days later an MR proton density image showed hyperintensity representing edema in the left parietal region. The edema involves the cortex as well as the subcortical tissues. **C.** MR proton density image 6 weeks later showed disappearance of the left parietal edematous area with residual minor bright spots (arrow), but also showed bright spots in the opposite hemisphere not previously observed. These represent changes in the brain related to the trauma, probably a contrecoup effect (open arrow). **D.** A postcontrast T1-weighted axial image now showed uptake in the left parieto-occipital region, representing a small residual subdural collection or meningeal thickening (arrows).

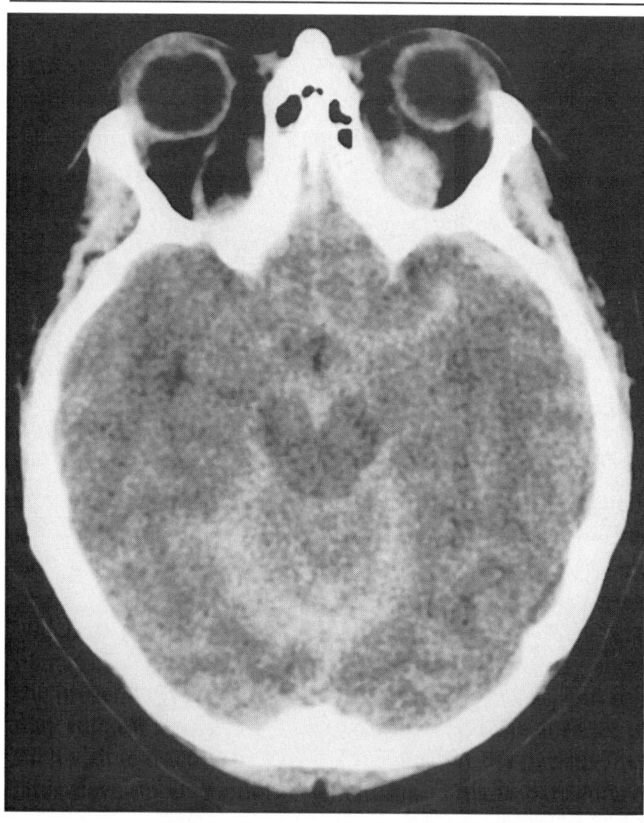

A

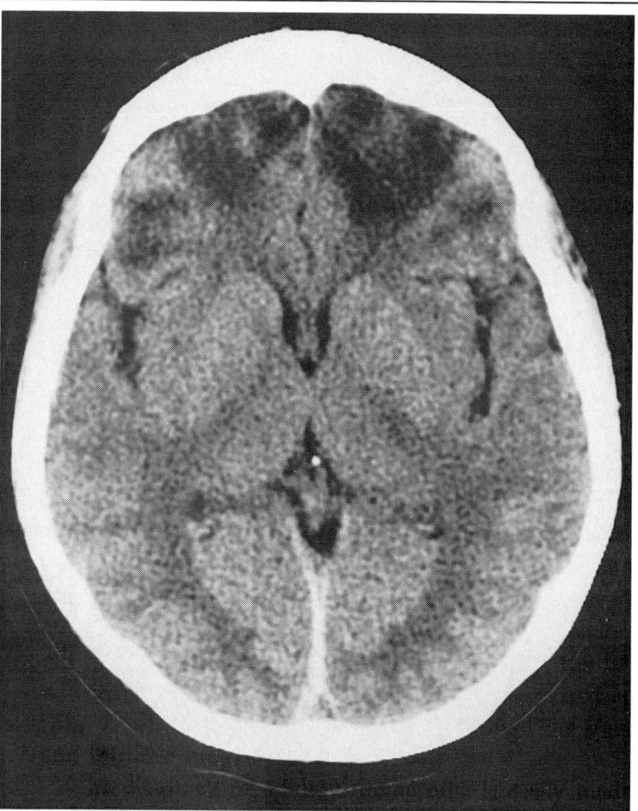

B

Figure 7.25. Posttraumatic subarachnoid hemorrhage in a 33-year-old woman hit by a car. **A.** The initial image showed a moderately severe generalized subarachnoid hemorrhage. **B.** Reexamination 7 days later revealed disappearance of the subarachnoid blood density, but now there was extensive bifrontal low density not seen on the initial examination, representing marked edema that was probably due to contusion. No hemorrhagic lesions were seen. Bifrontal involvement is common, either as a result of direct injury or as a contrecoup injury following an occipital injury. The same is true of the temporal tips.

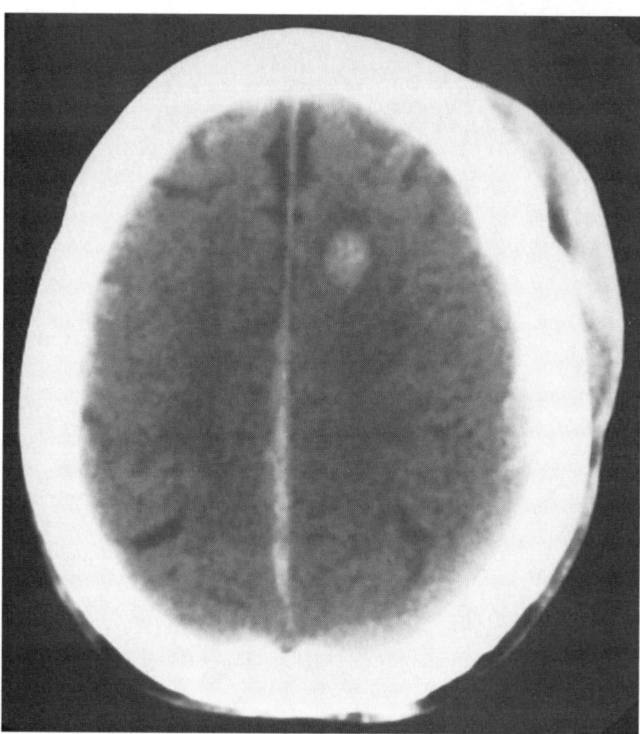

Figure 7.26. Subcortical hemorrhagic lesion. There is a subcortical hemorrhage, as well as a subdural hematoma around the falx. The patient had other hemorrhagic lesions related to a cortical contusion.

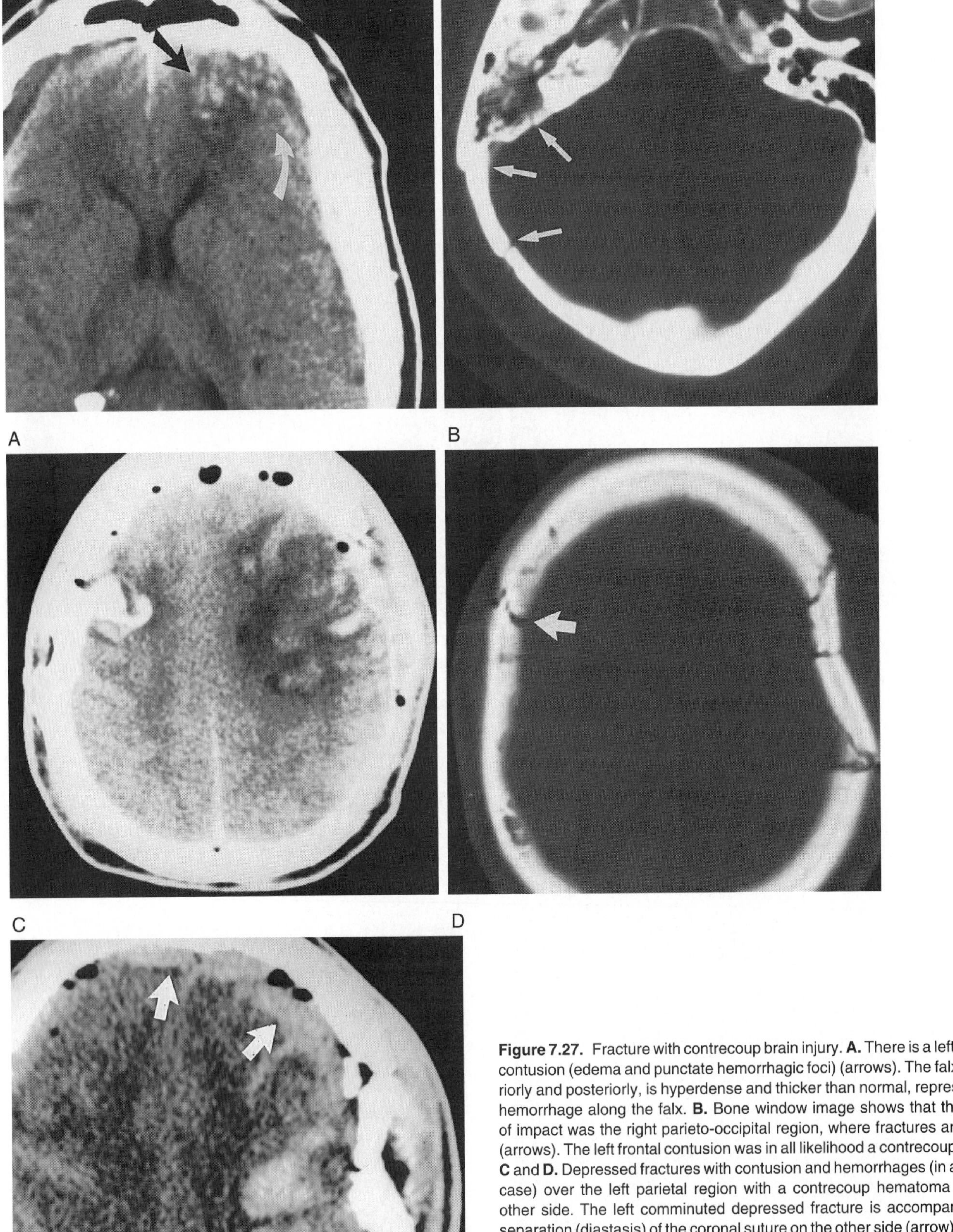

Figure 7.27. Fracture with contrecoup brain injury. **A.** There is a left frontal contusion (edema and punctate hemorrhagic foci) (arrows). The falx, anteriorly and posteriorly, is hyperdense and thicker than normal, representing hemorrhage along the falx. **B.** Bone window image shows that the point of impact was the right parieto-occipital region, where fractures are seen (arrows). The left frontal contusion was in all likelihood a contrecoup effect. **C** and **D.** Depressed fractures with contusion and hemorrhages (in another case) over the left parietal region with a contrecoup hematoma on the other side. The left comminuted depressed fracture is accompanied by separation (diastasis) of the coronal suture on the other side (arrow). There is also air in the subdural or epidural space, indicating a fracture traversing the wall of an air-containing sinus. There is diffuse bifrontal brain edema (**E**) and an epidural hematoma crossing the midline frontal region (arrows). Unlike a subdural hematoma, it does not get into the interhemispheric space.

This can occur as a result of a blow to the head against the frontal region, but it also may be seen as a *contrecoup* injury. For instance, the patient may have a fracture in the occipital region, having fallen backwards, and yet have extensive bilateral frontal edema and/or contusion (Fig. 7.25). Both temporal lobes may also be involved by contrecoup injury. Contrecoup effect may be found anywhere in the brain, however (Fig. 7.27).

Edema and Contusion

In the great majority of cases posttraumatic brain edema is focal, and in a much lower percentage of cases it is generalized. If generalized, it probably is related to a more severe injury. Focal edema manifests itself as uniform decreased density on CT scanning and as uniform decreased density on T1-weighted MRI or as high intensity on T2-weighted images. A contusion is diagnosed when there is hyperdensity mixed with hypodensity on CT scanning. A contusion is difficult to diagnose on MRI in the acute stage because the streaks of hemorrhage would be obscured by the surrounding edema. In focal injuries the contusion and the edema may produce a mass effect. This will produce displacement of the midline structures toward the opposite side, or it may produce deformity of certain structures such as the lateral ventricles, with or without a midline shift. Diffuse cerebral edema may be difficult to recognize on a CT examination in the acute stage, but both CT and MRI give certain signs that should be looked for. One of them

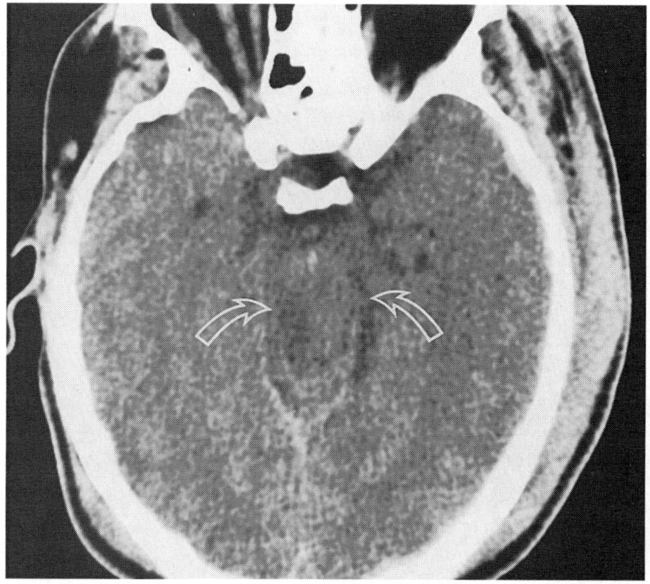

A

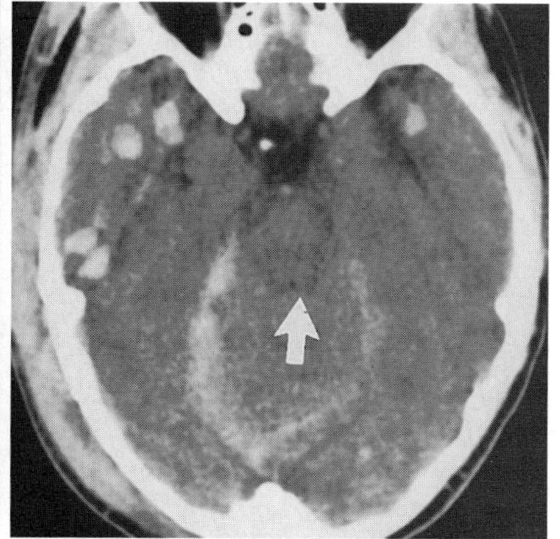

B

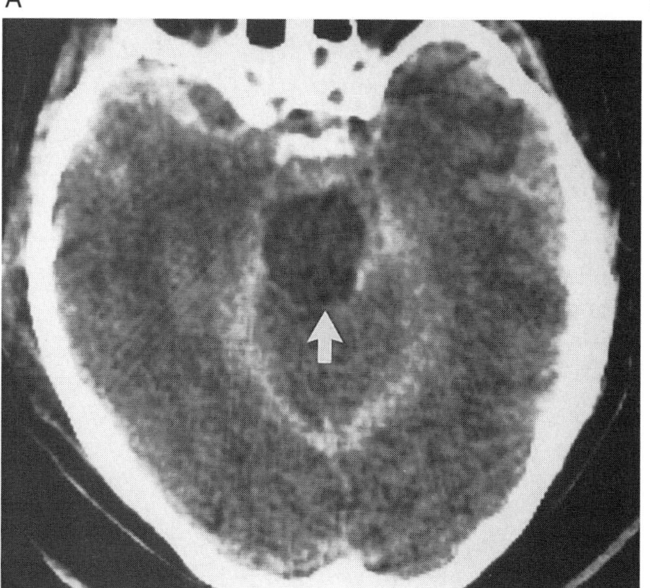

C

Figure 7.28. Posttraumatic tightening of the brainstem, three cases. **A.** Generalized edema producing bilateral compression and deformity of the midbrain due to hippocampal swelling bilaterally. The perimesencephalic CSF space is almost nonexistent (arrows). **B** and **C.** Again, the perimesencephalic CSF space is not seen or is extremely thin, also in the posterior aspect (arrow) over the quadrigeminal plate. In B and C there is evidence of a subdural hematoma over the tentorium. B shows a number of hemorrhagic foci in the corticomedullary area of the brain, which represent shear-strain injury.

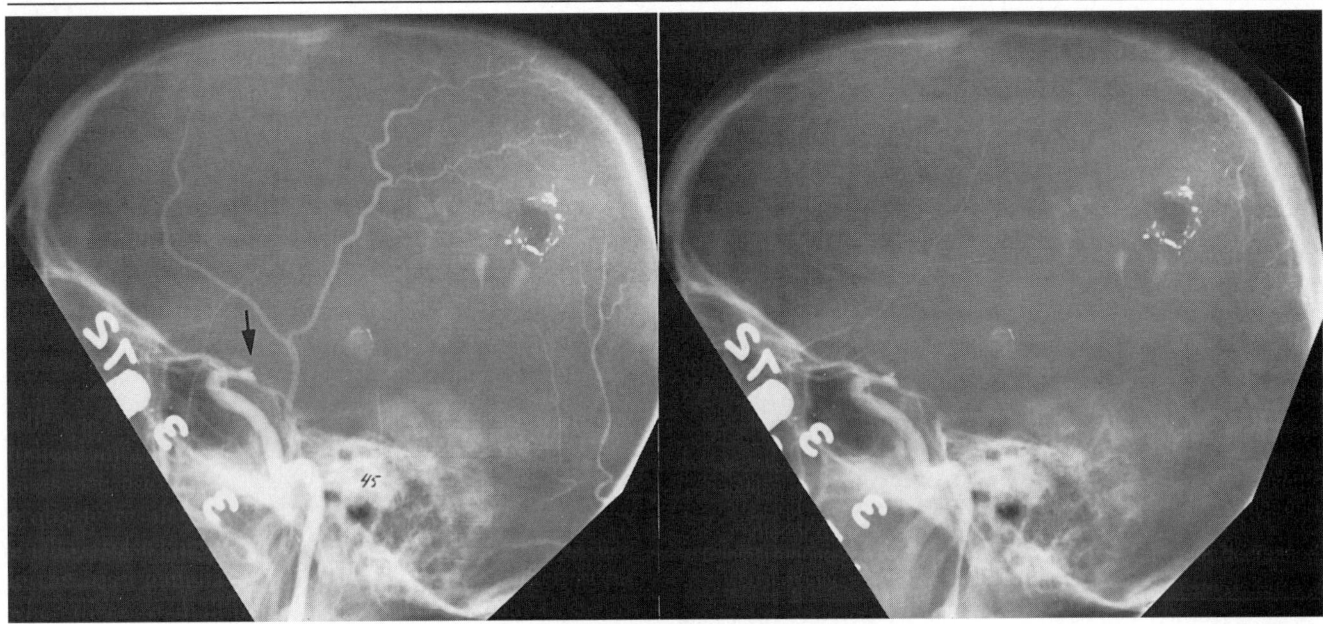

A B

Figure 7.29. Arrest of circulation due to brain edema following a bullet wound. **A.** The early film, 3.0 sec after contrast injection, reveals the internal carotid artery filling up until it enters the subarachnoid space (arrow). The external carotid branches are filled. **B.** At 9.0 sec the circulatory arrest of the internal carotid artery continues. It is caused by extremely high increased intracranial pressure, higher than the systolic blood pressure, and is indicative of brain death. The patient died several hours later. The opposite carotid artery was similarly obstructed.

is a decrease in the size of the lateral ventricles, another is a decrease in the radiolucency of the white matter of the cerebral hemispheres in relation to the gray matter (gray/white matter relationship), and another is a decrease in the size of the perimesencephalic cistern and of the cistern behind the quadrigeminal plate. It is also possible to detect a decrease in the size of the prepontine cistern, because when there is generalized edema, there is a downward displacement of the brainstem that results in a forward displacement of the belli of the pons. We should also carefully note the presence of displacement of the medial aspect of the temporal lobes toward the midline. As explained in Chapter 4, the medial displacement of the temporal lobes on one or both sides may result in downward transtentorial herniation. This causes compression of the midbrain and may lead to further deterioration of the patient's condition (Fig. 7.28; see Figs. 4.32 and 4.33). One should be careful in diagnosing generalized edema in a posttraumatic situation in young individuals because they often have a relatively small perimesencephalic cisternal space. Displacement and compression of the brainstem against the edge of the tentorium of the opposite side may cause an ipsilateral hemiparesis due to a Kernohan notch (13).

Cerebral edema can become an extremely important clinical problem and requires immediate treatment, for it can generate a vicious cycle that will continue to raise the intracranial pressure until it reaches a level above the systolic pressure, which produces arrest of circulation and brain death. This can be proved beyond doubt by cerebral angiography (Fig. 7.29) or by electroencephalography, which demonstrates absence of electrical activity in the brain. If MRI is available, MR angiography may also be used, but at present it is not considered conclusive because slow flow may simulate absent flow on MR angiography. The excessive rise in intracranial pressure first produces a marked rise in systolic blood pressure. The intracranial pressure increases in waves, and a vasomotor paralysis may take place while the arterioles and capillaries remain dilated. This tends to increase the edema because there is loss of autoregulation of the brain circulation. The generalized edema may be treated by hyperosmolar solutions intravenously. Sometimes a large craniectomy may have to be performed to reduce the intracranial pressure acutely. However, this is often followed by brain herniation through the large defect and by itself is not necessarily effective. Venous thrombosis and occlusions often occur as a result of marked generalized edema. (Further details on cerebral edema may be found in Chapter 4.)

Intracerebral Hematoma

These hematomas may occur in shear-strain injuries (see text following) and in the acute stage are not usually large, although some may be. They can cause delayed worsening of the patient's clinical condition. Two groups of such patients must be considered here:

1. Head injury patients who talk and then deteriorate into coma within a relatively short period of time (14). Of a group of 211 patients reported by Lobato et al., 42 percent had an intracerebral problem (contusion/hemorrhage), 38 percent had an extracerebral hematoma, and about 20 percent showed no focal lesions (presumably shear-strain injuries or diffuse axonal injury).
2. Delayed traumatic intracerebral hematomas (Spat-Apoplexie). This is an entirely different group from that described above. These patients deteriorate and frequently die within 7 to 12 days after the original trauma (Fig. 7.34). The delayed hemorrhage may be due to brain softening that involves the wall of an artery, with eventual rupture of the artery (15). Other mechanisms have been suggested.

McPherson et al. reported on the relation of brain contusion and hematoma to the type and site of fracture as well as the presence of a skull fracture demonstrable by plain films and/or CT (16). Of the 850 patients with a demonstrated fracture, contusion and/or hematoma was found in 71 percent, compared with 46 percent in the 533 patients in whom no fracture was demonstrated. Hematomas were more common in association with lateral and occipital fractures. Occipital fractures were often associated with frontal contusion and less frequently with occipital brain contusion, but frontal fractures were rarely associated with posterior brain damage.

The hematomas resulting from contusion or from shear-strain injuries are hyperdense on CT in the acute stage and slowly decrease in density, essentially becoming invisible in about 10 to 20 days. On the other hand, MRI shows isointensity on T1-weighted images and hyperintensity on T2-weighted images in the acute stage. In the subacute stage the hemorrhage becomes T1 hyperintense and at first T2 dark, only to become T2 bright a few days later. It remains T1 and T2 bright for a few to several weeks. Eventually it becomes T1 iso- or hypointense and T2 dark because of the magnetic susceptibility effect produced by iron in the residual hemosiderin.

Shear-Strain or Axonal Injury

The shear-strain deformation of the brain is felt to be responsible for most of the serious injuries of the brain that occur as a result of head trauma: the diffuse axonal injuries (DAI). In today's society, deceleration injuries as a result of automobile or motorcycle accidents are extremely common. The brain, suspended, so to speak, in CSF inside a rigid cavity, is subject to considerable linear and rotational shaking during deceleration head injuries. The shaking of the brain may occur in the anteroposterior direction, in a coronal direction, in an axial direction, or in a combination of these. Because of partial adhesions and fixations of various parts of the brain, the deep and superficial portions may not move at the same rate and may even move in opposite directions. This causes shear strains, which lead to actual axonal injury and rupture. These may manifest themselves on cross-sectional images as areas of focal edema or hemorrhage occurring most frequently at the junction of the gray and white matter but they may also occur in deep structures, the brainstem, and the corpus callosum. The hemorrhagic areas or the areas showing focal edema are frequently bilateral and widespread (Figs. 7.30 and 7.31)

The hemorrhagic lesions are usually well demonstrated on CT examinations in the acute stage. MRI may not show them clearly in the acute stage, but they may be suspected because of the brightness on T2-weighted images. Interestingly enough, in the presence of a rather well-developed indication of extensive shear-strain injuries to the brain, soft-tissue swelling is often not demonstrated on the initial CT examination. This emphasizes the importance of the rotational mechanisms of injury already mentioned as against a strike against a local area of the brain, which is likely to produce a focal area of contusion and edema. In fact, the head may not have struck directly, and yet the axonal injuries may be severe, all of which has been demonstrated experimentally in animals (17).

It should be emphasized that axonal injuries may not be seen in an initial CT examination but may be shown on MRI examination several days later. Gentry et al. indicated a rather high incidence (48 percent) of all primary head trauma cases in their series (18). Of special interest is that shear-strain injuries are much more common in younger individuals. Children and adolescents under 20 years of age in the group of head injuries reported by Lobato et al. had a 39 percent incidence of nonfocal mass effect (diffuse brain damage), whereas in patients over 40 years of age, only 30 percent had a nonfocal traumatic injury (14).

The majority of diffuse axonal injury lesions occur in the white matter of the hemispheres, but they may occur in any area of the brain, and in fact may also involve the cerebellum and the brainstem.

Corpus Callosum Injury

The corpus callosum is probably the second most common site of shear-strain injuries (19). The mechanism is most likely a shear strain secondary to rotation. A rigid falx is probably an important component of the mechanism of corpus callosum injury. It seems to occur more frequently posteriorly than anteriorly, and this is attributed to the fact that the brain can move laterally under the falx more freely anteriorly than posteriorly. There may be hemorrhage in the corpus callosum, although it may only be edema. The fornix, which is attached to the corpus callosum on its undersurface, may become separated from it as a result of the injury. Injuries of the corpus callosum are much more easily seen by MRI than by CT, particularly in the subacute stage some days or a week after the injury.

Intraventricular hemorrhage is common in injuries of the corpus callosum, and indeed in shear-strain injuries in general. It should be looked for carefully, for often it is quite inconspicuous and can be easily overlooked. The intraventricular hemorrhage is attributed to a shearing rupture of the subependymal veins (Fig. 7.31).

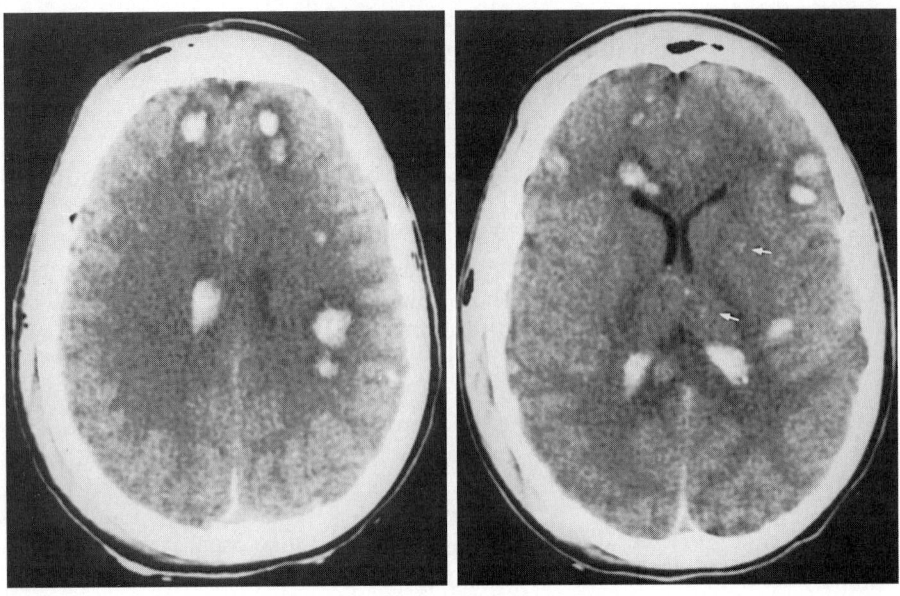

Figure 7.30. Shear-strain injury in a 17-year-old boy who was involved in an auto accident. There was no fracture. **A.** Section showing a number of hemorrhagic foci located mostly at the gray/white matter junction. **B.** A lower section passing through the ventricles reveals more hemorrhagic foci, including small foci in the thalamus and putamen on the left (small arrows). The focal hemorrhages are surrounded by a low-density halo, representing edema. Shear-strain injuries are seen more frequently in younger trauma patients.

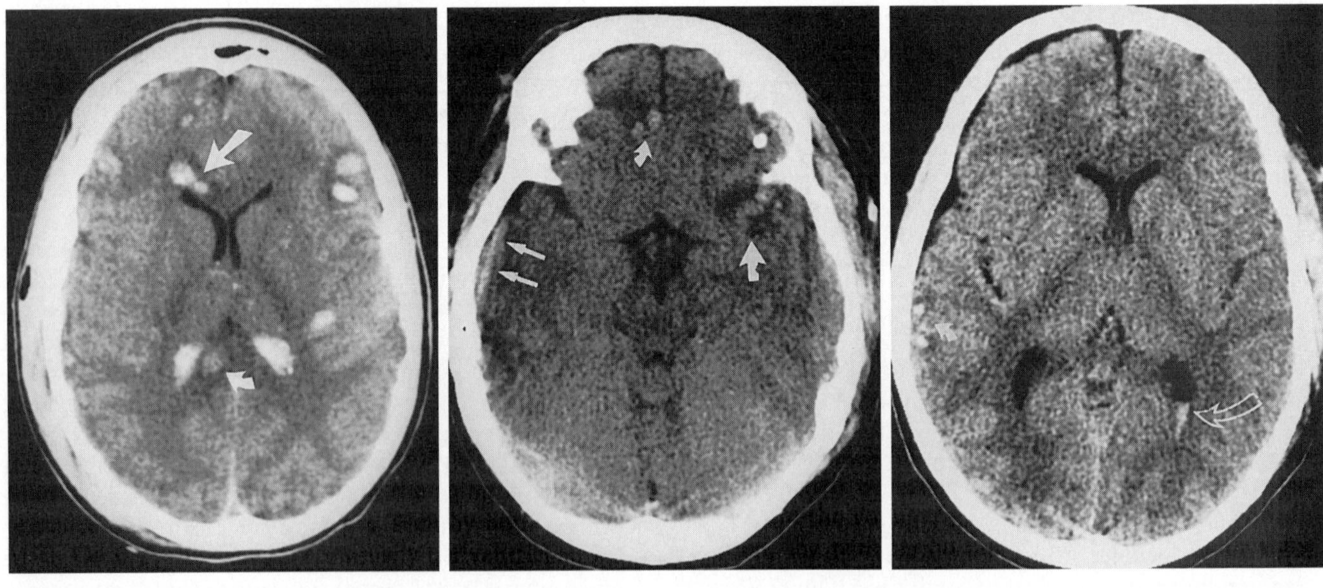

Figure 7.31. Shear-strain injury. **A.** Same case as Figure 7.30. Corpus callosum hemorrhagic foci are well seen on CT in the genu and in the splenium (arrows). Corpus callosum lesions are generally shown much better with MRI. **B** and **C.** Another case, this one of a 16-year-old boy presenting a left temporal contusion (arrow). **B.** A small right subdural hematoma is visible (2 arrows). **C.** There are multiple hemorrhagic foci due to shear-strain injury (curved arrows) and intraventricular bleeding (open arrow). There is also a small acute subdural hygroma on the right.

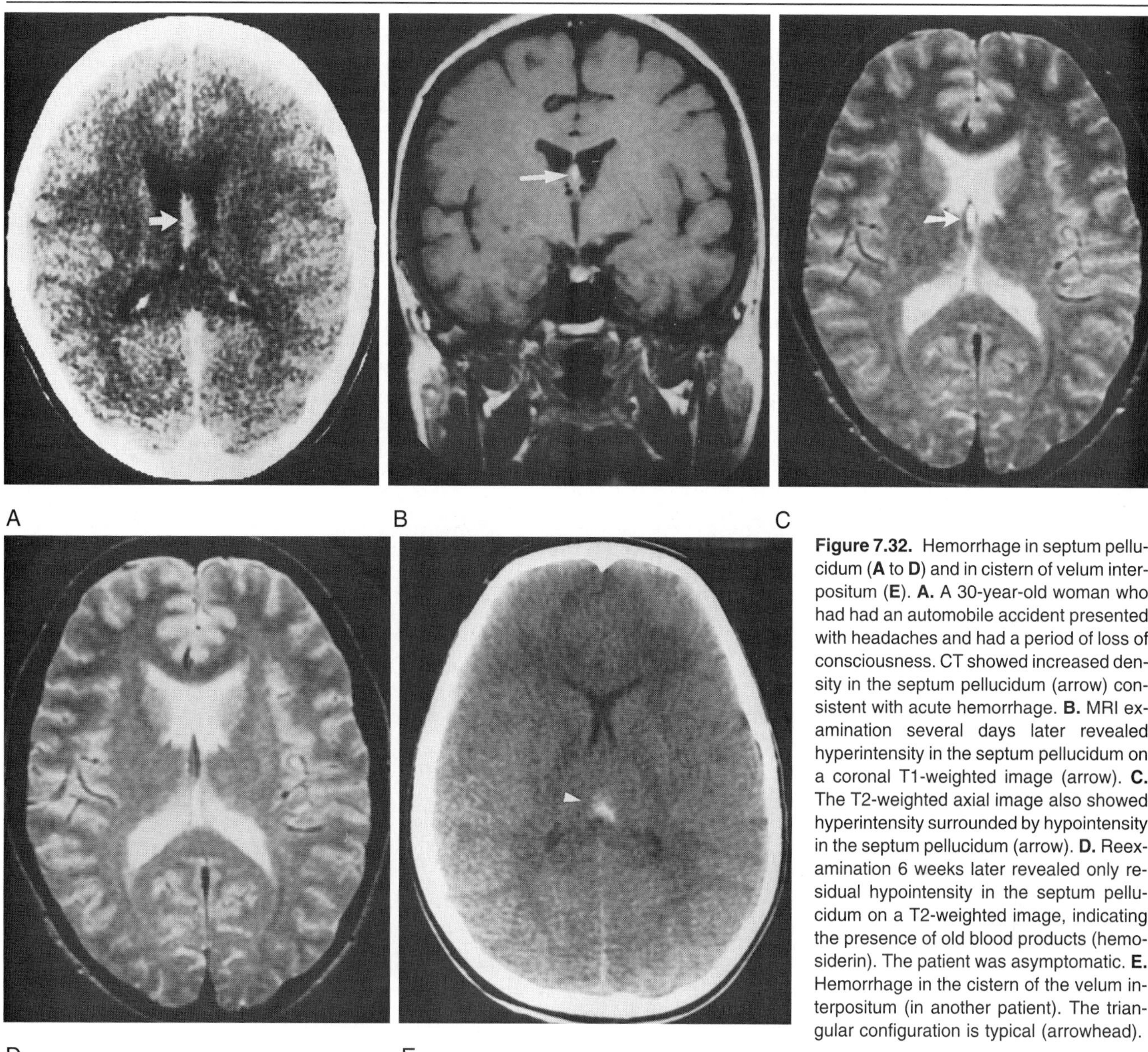

Figure 7.32. Hemorrhage in septum pellucidum (**A** to **D**) and in cistern of velum interpositum (**E**). **A.** A 30-year-old woman who had had an automobile accident presented with headaches and had a period of loss of consciousness. CT showed increased density in the septum pellucidum (arrow) consistent with acute hemorrhage. **B.** MRI examination several days later revealed hyperintensity in the septum pellucidum on a coronal T1-weighted image (arrow). **C.** The T2-weighted axial image also showed hyperintensity surrounded by hypointensity in the septum pellucidum (arrow). **D.** Reexamination 6 weeks later revealed only residual hypointensity in the septum pellucidum on a T2-weighted image, indicating the presence of old blood products (hemosiderin). The patient was asymptomatic. **E.** Hemorrhage in the cistern of the velum interpositum (in another patient). The triangular configuration is typical (arrowhead).

The septum pellucidum and the fornix may be involved in shearing injuries, usually together with corpus callosum injury. The septum pellucidum may be involved alone (Fig. 7.32). In this case there was no clinical or imaging evidence of involvement of either the corpus callosum or the fornix, and the patient was and remained well after the acute traumatic episode. Hemorrhage may also occur in the cistern of the velum interpositum as a manifestation of shear-strain injury of the deep structures, usually in young subjects (Fig. 7.32*E*).

Brainstem Injury

For over 100 years brainstem injuries were described pathologically at autopsy in the majority of cases. In spite of the advent of CT scanning in 1973, imaging of the brainstem was often covered by artifacts that prevented a clear evaluation of brainstem injury. As the technology of CT scanning continued to improve, we began to see the presence of hemorrhage and contusion in the brainstem (20). However, MRI is much more likely to demonstrate these injuries, particularly in the subacute stage or several days after the initial trauma.

Since the patient is likely to be moving and very uncooperative in the initial acute stage, CT scanning is the examination of choice at this time. When there is brainstem injury, corpus callosum injury is also likely because brainstem injury is usually associated with DAI. Thus when DAI is suspected, one should also look for lesions indicating involvement of the corpus callosum and the deep cerebral white matter, and vice versa. *Primary involvement* of the

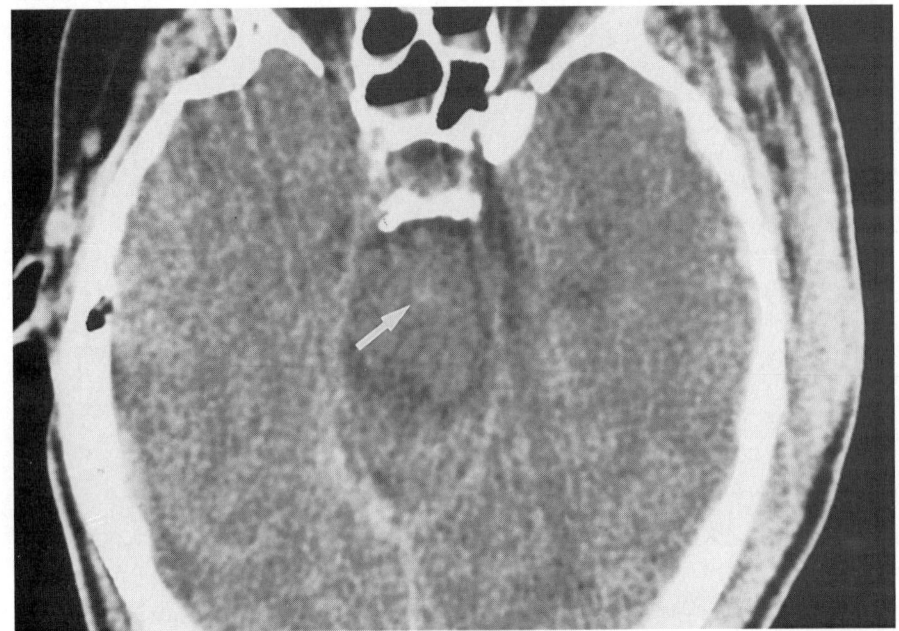

A

Figure 7.33. Severe head injury with multiple effects on the brain (edema, hemorrhage, extracerebral blood) in a 56-year-old woman. **A.** Axial CT view showing tightening of the CSF space around the brainstem, which is flattened and deformed from the generalized increase in the size of the intracranial tissues. This increase is usually caused by brain edema, but may also be due to extracerebral collections (subdural, epidural). The brainstem is more radiolucent than the surrounding tissue, possibly because of edema, and its center presents a small hyperdense area, probably a small hemorrhage (arrow). **B.** Coronal T2-weighted MR image made 8 days after A shows diffuse increased brightness of the white matter due to edema (or hemorrhage) in the right side of the midbrain and pons (arrows). A shear-strain injury is seen in the right parasagittal region (upper arrow) and in the left thalamus. A left subdural hematoma is also visible. **C.** Axial proton density image reveals edema (or hemorrhage) in the right side of the brainstem. The temporal lobe white matter is not as edematous as the frontoparietal white matter. Focal edema cannot be differentiated from hemorrhage (in the methemoglobin stage) unless a T1-weighted image is available. If it is bright on T1, the lesion is a hemorrhage. The patient was in a coma.

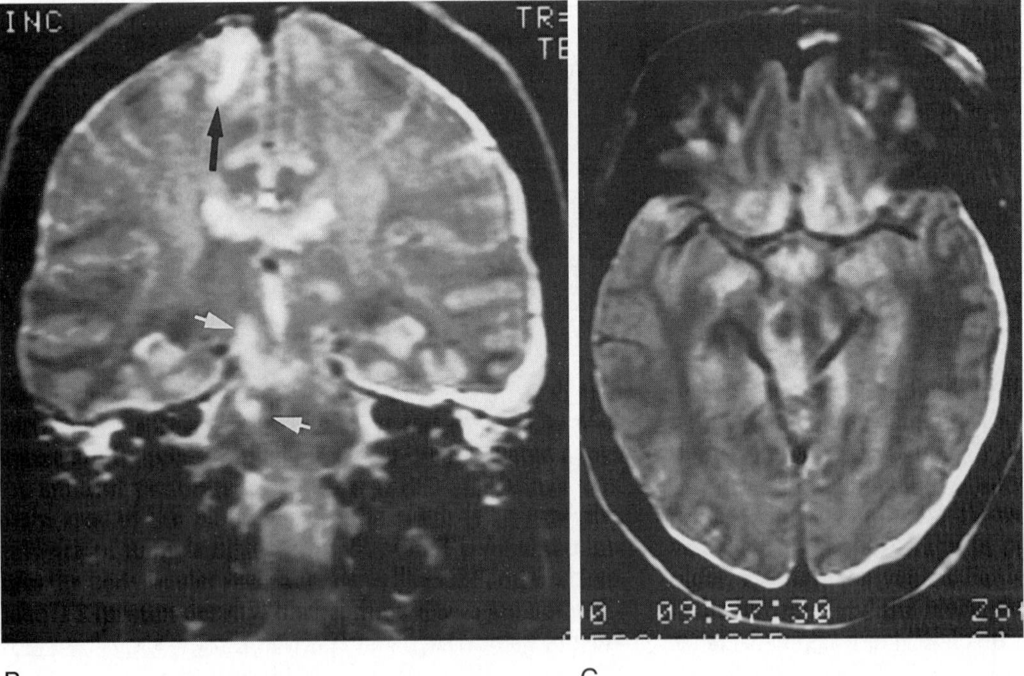

B C

brainstem is the result of the primary traumatic episode. However, *secondary involvement* of the brainstem also occurs, more frequently because of brain swelling and extra- or intracerebral hemorrhage, which displace the brain and cause hippocampal herniation and brainstem compression (see discussion of cerebral edema in Chapter 4).

Brainstem injury lesions tend to occur in the dorsolateral aspect of the upper brainstem and tend to spare the ventral aspect, according to Gentry et al. (21). The lesions are usually edematous without hemorrhage, and for this reason may not be seen well on CT, particularly if there happens to be an artifact in the area (Figs. 7.33, 7.34). Multiple petechial hemorrhages may also involve the brainstem in the periaqueductal region as well as the cerebral central white matter and the thalamus and hypothalamus. These hemorrhages may be caused by the rupture of numerous

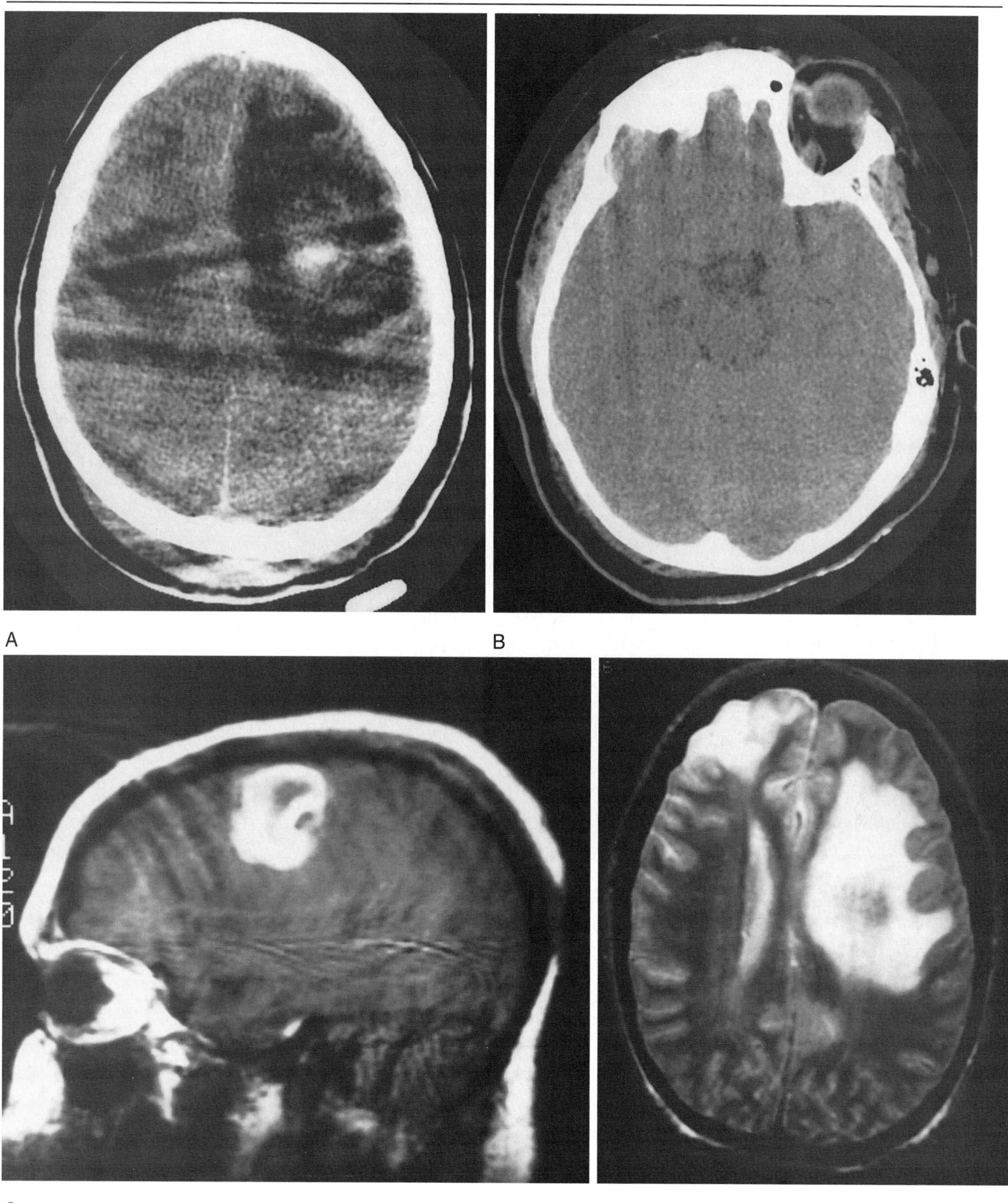

Figure 7.34. Delayed posttraumatic intracerebral hematoma after severe head injury. **A.** The initial examination showed a large left frontal contusion with a small irregular hemorrhagic area. **B.** There was some diffuse brain edema with loss of gray/white matter differentiation and loss of perimesencephalic CSF space. **C.** Thirty days later there was a large hemorrhagic lesion in the left frontal lobe, shown on this T1-weighted image. The hemorrhage is in the methemoglobin stage, and there is irregular central low intensity suggestive of deoxyhemoglobin, also seen in the axial T2-weighted view (**D**).

penetrating blood vessels. This may yield an increased density of the posterior midbrain but few direct signs on CT. In the subacute stage MRI may demonstrate hyperintensity on T1- and T2-weighted images, but edema may accompany the changes, thus making it difficult to recognize the exact pathology present. The presence of diffuse petechial hemorrhages carries a bad prognosis.

Edematous or hemorrhagic changes in the anterior lateral aspect of the midbrain are typical for secondary brainstem compression associated with hippocampal herniation. Infarct or hemorrhage may occur in the central tegmental region of the brainstem as a result of transtentorial herniation.

Subcortical Gray Matter Injury

These are less common, usually hemorrhagic, lesions due to head injuries (18). They tend to be hemorrhagic in most cases because of the high vascularity of this region and probably result from shearing rupture of some of these small vessels. They are more common in the thalamus than in the basal ganglia (see Fig. 7.30) and most often occur when there are multiple hemorrhagic lesions due to shear-strain injuries in the rest of the brain. (Table 7.4).

TRAUMATIC VASCULAR INJURIES

Until the development of CT, cerebral angiography was a nearly routine procedure in any case of head injury where there was a clinical suspicion of intracranial injury. Today only patients suspected of having a vascular complication are subjected to cerebral angiography, but it is most important to be alert to possible vascular damage that can be diagnosed only by angiography. A more complete discussion focused on the therapeutic approach is given in Chapter 18.

The vascular injuries that may occur are traumatic dissection of the internal carotid or vertebral arteries, arterial aneurysms, arterial spasm, thrombosis, carotid-cavernous fistula, and dural sinus laceration. Table 7.5 outlines the characteristics of carotid dissection, vertebral dissection, and carotid-cavernous fistula.

Table 7.4.
Intra-axial Traumatic Injuries

Cortical contusion
- May occur at site of impact (coup) or 180° from impact (contrecoup). Approximately 50% are hemorrhagic.
- Initially nonhemorrhagic contusions may convert to hemorrhagic type, usually over the course of days.
- May have considerable mass effect and edema.
- Inferior frontal and temporal lobes are preferential sites of injury.
- Hemorrhagic contusions are hyperdense on CT and usually initially hyperintense on T2-weighted images.

Diffuse axonal injury (DAI) (shear-strain injury)
- Preferential distribution is at corticomedullary junction.
- May occur even in absence of impact injury.
- More easily detected by MRI than by CT.
- Typical appearance is hypointense and/or hyperintense round or oval lesions on T2-weighted images in white matter, corticomedullary junction, or corpus callosum.

Deep gray matter injury
- Hemorrhagic or nonhemorrhagic lesions in basal ganglia or thalamus.
- Associated with worse prognosis than cortical contusion.

Brainstem injury
- Dorsolateral aspect of pons is preferred site of involvement.
- Primary brainstem injury occurs at time of initial trauma.
- Secondary brainstem injury occurs subsequent to initial trauma and may result from hypoxic/ischemic compromise or transtentorial herniation.
- Frequently associated with corpus callosum DAI.

Table 7.5.
Traumatic Arterial Injury

Carotid dissection
- Usually occurs in cervical portion of internal carotid artery often extending distally into petrous segment.
- May occur following direct trauma or "trivial" trauma.
- Petrous or supraclinoid segment dissections are often associated with adjacent fractures.
- Multiplicity of appearances: narrowing of arterial lumen, luminal irregularity, pseudoaneurysm formation, intimal flap.
- May produce ischemia or infarction due to embolization.
- Typical appearance on MRI is hyperintense mural signal on T1- and T2-weighted images with narrowing of arterial flow void.

Vertebral dissection
- Posttraumatic vertebral dissections most commonly occur at C1-C2 vertebral body level.
- Extension into intracranial vertebral artery segment may be accompanied by subarachnoid hemorrhage.

Carotid-cavernous fistula
- Direct (high-flow) and indirect (low-flow) types.
- Direct type is often due to penetrating trauma or to rupture of intracavernous aneurysm.
- Results in arterialization of the venous system draining the cavernous sinus and enlargement of the superior ophthalmic vein, and of inferior or superior petrosal sinus.
- Clinical manifestations are chemosis, proptosis, and often decreased visual acuity.

Dissection

Injuries to the branches of the external carotid arteries were described in text preceding on epidural hematomas. The most important arterial lesions, both because they are relatively frequent and because they need treatment, are arterial dissections. Posttraumatic dissections of the carotid or vertebral arteries usually occur in the neck from a direct blow to the neck or from hyperextension of the neck, which causes extreme elongation of the carotid or vertebral arteries and rupture of the inner wall. In the vertebral artery the dissection may be associated with a fracture of the cervical vertebrae. The last several cases of vertebral dissection that have come to the author's attention resulted from a basketball striking the turned neck. Dissections sometimes occur following relatively trivial injuries such as rapid head turning.

An arterial dissection may cause diffuse narrowing of the arterial lumen and the formation of emboli, which could produce intracranial arterial occlusions (Fig. 7.35). The typical dissection leads to the formation of a false lumen that can be shown by angiography or by MRI (Figs. 7.36 and 7.37). MRI is particularly useful for diagnosing carotid

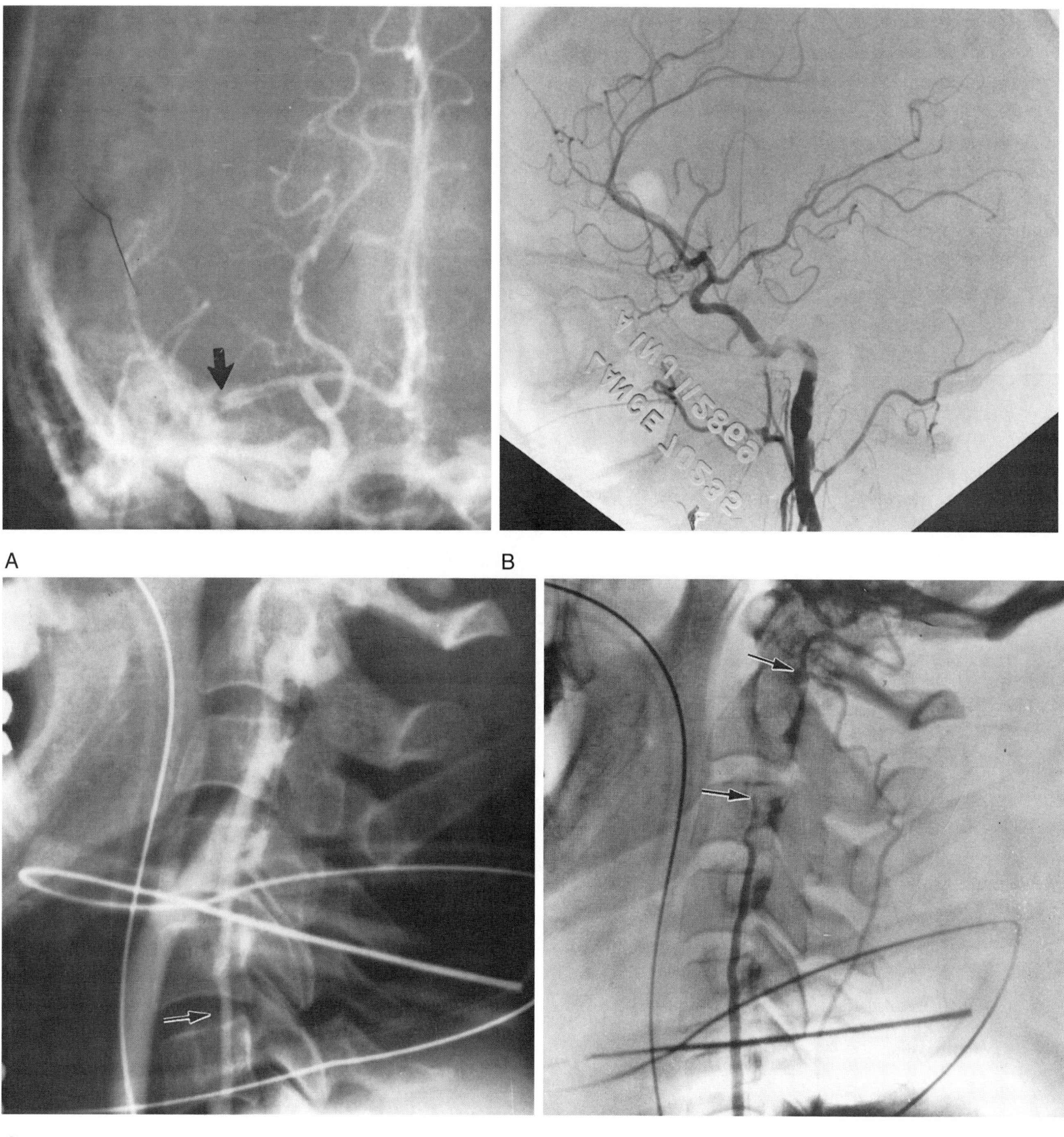

Figure 7.35. Dissection of carotid and vertebral arteries and arterial emboli due to hyperextension injury. **A.** The frontal carotid angiogram demonstrates an embolus in the trunk of the middle cerebral artery and partial occlusion more distally (arrow). **B.** The lateral view demonstrates the partial occlusion of the middle cerebral vessels and in addition reveals irregularity of the lumen of the cervical internal carotid artery owing to damage to the arterial wall, most probably due to hyperextension. **C** and **D.** Bilateral vertebral injections demonstrate bilateral narrowing and compression of the artery on the right (C, arrow). On the left side there is intravascular coagulation (D, arrows). The basilar artery filled much later. The patient recovered with some residual deficit after a stormy course of several weeks.

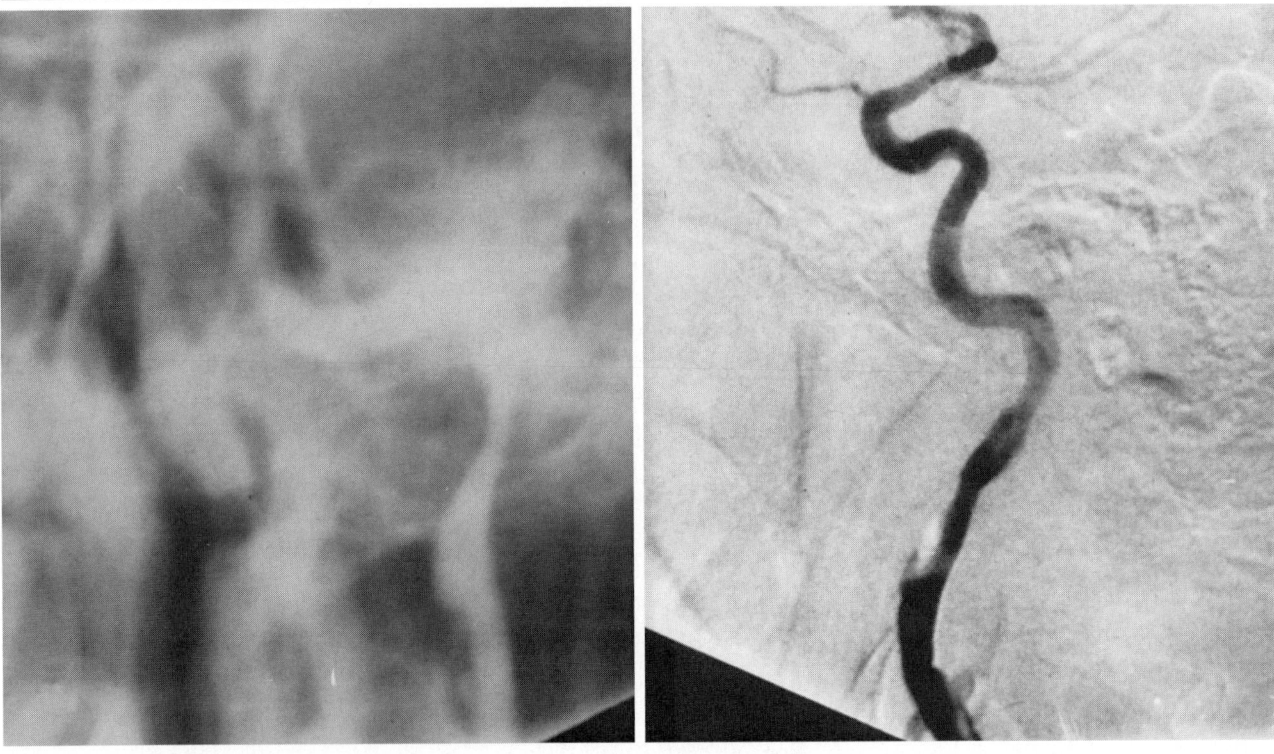

Figure 7.36. Hyperextension injury of the internal carotid artery in the neck. Frontal (**A**) and lateral (**B**) projections reveal irregular narrowing of the lumen of the carotid artery in a patient who had been in an automobile accident. The injury consists of intimal tear and intramural dissection. Sometimes a pseudoaneurysm may form. If the intramural clot becomes organized, the arterial lumen will remain narrow or the artery may become occluded. If the blood remains liquid, angiography will show false lumens with irregular widening of the artery, as outlined by contrast, as in the case shown in Figure 7.35B. MRI will show the false lumen well (see Chapter 10).

or vertebral artery dissections, for it usually demonstrates a T1 and T2 hyperintense collection partially surrounding a narrowed lumen presenting a flow void (22, 23). In successive slices the bright half-moon–shaped hyperintense area may change its relationship to the flow void because the dissection is often spiral shaped.

Fat around the carotid arteries may be a source of confusion, but this can easily be eliminated using a fat-suppression technique, which would eliminate the fat signal. The dissection may extend to involve the vessels at the base of the skull, and again MRI will show the bright intramural hematoma well on T1-weighted images (Fig. 7.37). Intracranial dissections may also involve the internal carotid artery or components of the circle of Willis (24–26).

Aneurysm

Posttraumatic intracranial aneurysms of the cerebral arteries are infrequently observed. They may be directly associated with a fracture or may occur at a site unrelated to the fracture (27). The pseudoaneurysms directly related to the fracture may have been produced by an outbursting or outbending of the skull, which then fractures and momentarily permits the brain to herniate through the separated bone. The bone then recoils, trapping some brain tissue and surface vessels, veins, or arteries. This implies that the dura ruptured at the same time (Fig. 7.38). The vessel may remain trapped in the fracture or it may simply return, but the result is injury to the vessel wall with formation of a false aneurysm. Formation of an arteriovenous communication is described by Rumbaugh et al. as very rare (27). As is well known, venous injury or rupture is considerably more frequent and is in fact the mechanism that explains the frequent occurrence of subdural hematomas.

Laceration and Occlusion

Arterial lacerations and occlusions also occur and may be expected to occur more frequently in open head injuries and missile-type injuries. They lead to either immediate or delayed intracranial hemorrhage or to cerebral infarction if thrombosis occurred. Local brain edema alone without hemorrhage may clear completely and leave few or no sequelae. If associated with hemorrhage, it will leave an area of atrophy demonstrable by CT or MRI. An infarct leaves a better-defined permanent area of abnormality on CT or MRI.

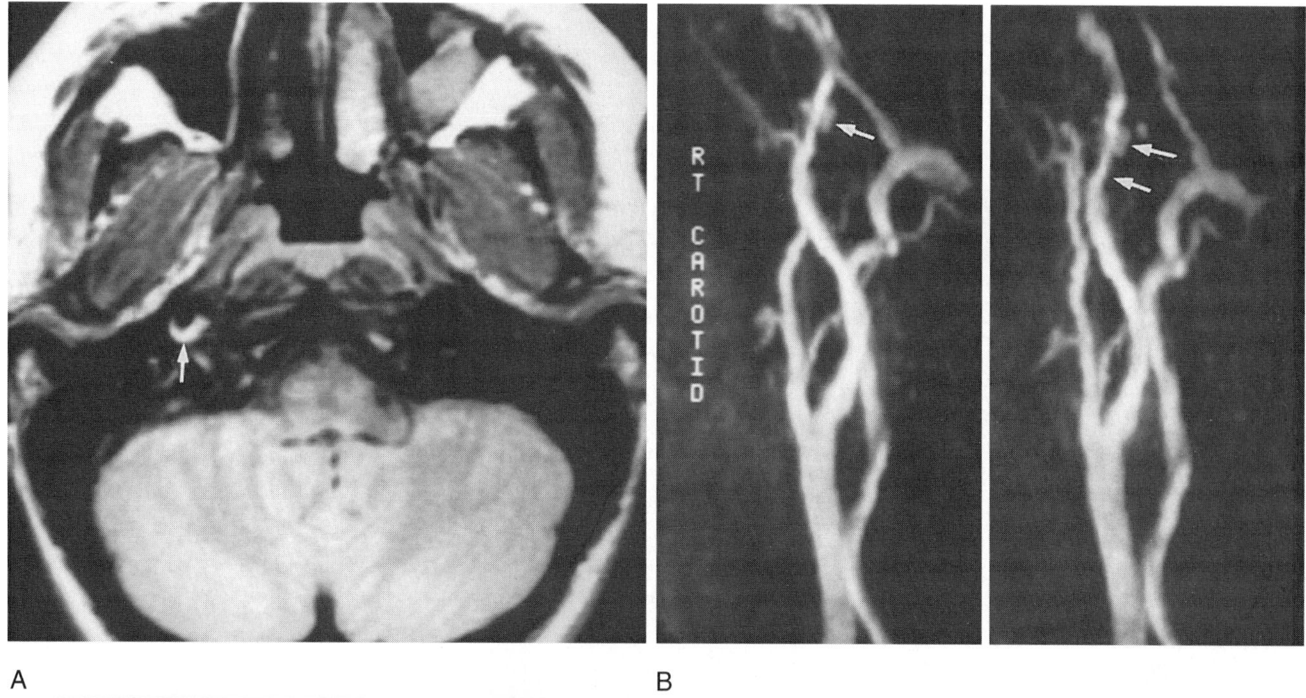

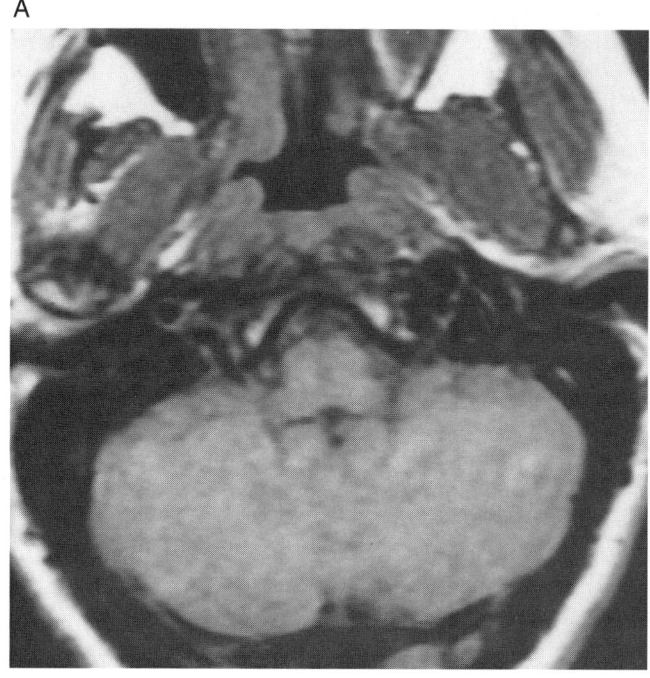

Figure 7.37. Traumatic dissection of cervical internal carotid artery. **A.** Axial T1-weighted view demonstrates a hyperintense half-moon configuration around the reduced lumen of the right internal carotid artery (arrow), representing a small hematoma in the wall of the artery. **B.** MR angiography of the right side demonstrates narrowing and irregularity of a portion of the right internal carotid artery with a suggestive double lumen in a short segment (arrows). **C.** Reexamination 8 months later shows almost complete disappearance of the hyperintensity around the right internal carotid artery. The residual hyperintensity could be produced by a slight amount of fat surrounding the vessel. The image was not fat suppressed.

Carotid-Cavernous Fistula

The carotid-cavernous fistula may be posttraumatic in onset and may be due to rupture of the intracavernous carotid in an artery that was normal prior to the injury, but it may also occur somewhat spontaneously following rupture of a preexisting intracavernous aneurysm. The rupture may be provoked by a head injury not necessarily associated with a basal skull fracture. A carotid-cavernous fistula may also be due to a dural arteriovenous malformation involving the wall of the cavernous sinus. CT and MRI can be utilized to make a diagnosis of a carotid-cavernous fistula, but angiography is needed to separate the two major types and to apply appropriate therapy, which in the last several years has been via an endovascular approach (see Chapter 18).

CT and MRI diagnosis can be made because there is enlargement of the cavernous sinus, enlargement of the superior ophthalmic vein on one or both sides, and moderate proptosis usually evident clinically where pulsations may be evident. Swelling of the preseptal orbital soft tissues

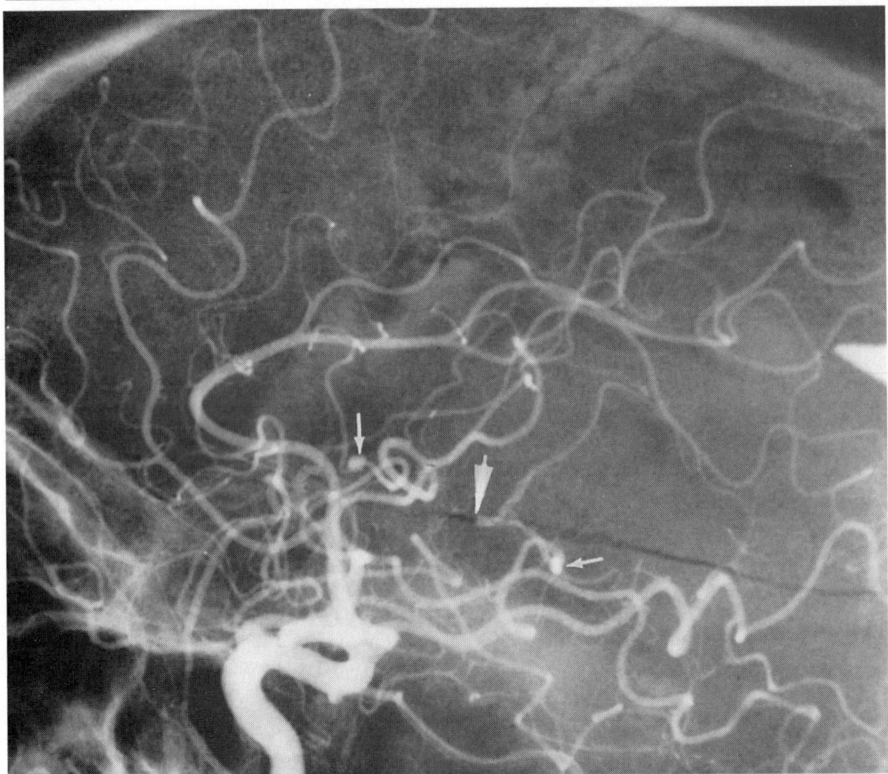

Figure 7.38. False posttraumatic aneurysms of branches of the middle cerebral artery. The small aneurysms (arrows) are seen along the fracture line. The mechanism is not clear, but probably the pial vessels, following dural rupture, were pushed out at the time of injury, became temporarily trapped in the diastatic fracture, which would be more diastatic at the instant of trauma, and so were injured as the fracture borders came closer together.

and enlargement of extraocular muscles may also be observed. The "low-flow" carotid-cavernous fistulas may follow a smaller rent in the artery such as may occur when a small intracavernous branch is severed. This type must be differentiated from the arteriovenous dural malformation (Table 7.5).

Dural Sinus Laceration

Dural sinus laceration may occur and may lead to the formation of an epidural venous hematoma, which usually develops more slowly than an arterial epidural hemorrhage and is consequently less dangerous. The epidural venous hematoma tends to occur when the laceration is situated in or around the torcular. It can be differentiated from a subdural hematoma because it displaces the sinus away from the inner table of the skull, whereas a subdural collection would not. The dural sinus laceration may also lead to occlusion of the sinus.

Brain Death

For a discussion of brain death, see Chapter 10.

DELAYED EFFECTS OF HEAD INJURY

Mild head injuries may not reveal any initial findings on cross-sectional images but may show some slight ventricular enlargement 6 to 8 weeks later. This is particularly true if unconsciousness occurred at the time of injury. Possibly the best example of mild posttraumatic brain atrophy is that seen in boxers. Both cortical atrophy and ventricular enlargement are seen (28). Rupture of the septum pellucidum may be observed in some boxers.

The ventricular enlargement may be unilateral or bilateral. More severe head injuries almost always show ventricular enlargement later. In the presence of brain contusion or hemorrhage, focal atrophic changes may be expected as a permanent sequela. Any persistent disability would depend on the location of the initial focal injury. More severe head injuries may leave a host of clinical deficits, up to total disability and a permanent comatose state. Brainstem injuries may leave the patient unable to ambulate properly as well as dysarthric, with disturbed eye movements and deafness. Psychiatric symptoms may well accompany or persist following head injuries. Some 50,000 deaths yearly in the United States alone are related to head injuries, and the amount of persistent disability is significant (29).

Gentry has attempted to evaluate MRI findings and compare them with the results of the clinical Glasgow Coma Scale in order to develop a method of predicting final outcome (18). The presence of lesions due to diffuse axonal injury is the most important criterion, and although the number of these lesions per se is insufficient to predict final outcome, the association with a mass effect causing transtentorial herniation, midbrain deformity, and intrinsic secondary brainstem injury tends to correlate with final outcome (2). Brainstem injury caused by severe midline shift and transtentorial herniation also correlates with poor prognosis, and the speed with which appropriate therapy is applied is significant in this respect.

REFERENCES

1. Numerow LM, Kreek JP, Wallace CJ, et al: Growing skull fracture simulating a rounded lytic calvarial lesion. AJNR 1991;12:783–784.
2. Mirvis SE, Wolf AL, Numaguchi Y, et al: Post traumatic cerebral infarction diagnosed by CT: Prevalence, origin, and outcome. AJNR 1990;11:355–360.
3. Taveras JM, Ransohoff J: Leptomeningeal cysts of the brain following trauma with erosion of the skull: A study of seven cases treated by surgery. J Neurosurg 1953;10:233.
4. Lucket WH: Air in the ventricles of the brain following a fracture of the skull: Report of a case. Surg Gynecol Obstet 1913;17:237.
5. Olson MO, Wright DL, Hoffman HT, et al: Frontal sinus fractures: Evaluation of CT scans in 132 patients. AJNR 1992;13:897–902.
6. El Gammal T, Brooks BS: MR cisternography: Initial experience in 41 cases. AJNR 1994;15:1647–1656.
7. Zimmerman RA, Bilaniuk LT: Computed tomographic staging of traumatic epidural bleeding. Radiology 1982;144:809–812.
8. Schechter MM, Zingesser LH, Rayport M.: Torn meningeal vessels: An evaluation of a clinical spectrum through the use of angiography. Radiology 1966;86:686.
9. Hamilton M, Wallace C: Nonoperative management of acute epidural hematoma diagnosed by CT: The neuroradiologist's role. AJNR 1992;13:853–859.
10. Boyko OB, Cooper DF, Grossman CB: Contrast-enhanced CT of acute isodense subdural hematoma. AJNR 1991;12:341–343.
11. Grabowski EF, Zimmerman RD: Disseminated intravascular coagulation and the neuroradiologist. AJNR 1991;12:344.
12. Kurowia T, Harushi T, Hiroyuki T, et al: Rapid spontaneous resolution of acute extradural and subdural hematomas. J Neurosurg 1993; 78:126–128.
13. Jones KM, Seeger JF, Yoshino MT: Ipsilateral motor deficit resulting from subdural hematoma and a Kernohan notch. AJNR 1991; 12:1238–1239.
14. Lobato RD, Rivas JJ, Gomez PA, et al: Head-injured patients who talk and deteriorate into coma. J Neurosurg 1991;75:256–261.
15. Elsner H, Rigamonti D, Corradino B, et al: Delayed traumatic intracerebral hematoma; "Spat-Apoplexie." J Neurosurg 1990;72: 813–815.
16. McPherson BCM, Macpherson P, Jennett B: CT evidence of intracranial contusion and haematoma in relation to the presence, site and type of skull fracture. Clin Radiol 1990;42:321–326.
17. Gennarelli TA, Thibault LE, Adams JH, et al: Diffuse axonal injury and traumatic coma in the primate. Ann Neurol 1982;12:564–574.
18. Gentry LR, Godersky JC, Thompson BH: MR imaging of head trauma: Review of the distribution and radiopathologic features of traumatic lesions. AJNR 1988;9:101–110.
19. Gentry LR, Thompson B, Godersky JC: Trauma to the corpus callosum: MR features. AJNR 1988;9:1129–1138.
20. Tsai FY, Teal JS, Quinn MF, et al: CT of brainstem injury. AJNR 1980;1:23–29.
21. Gentry LR, Godersky JC, Thompson BH: Traumatic brain stem injury: MR imaging. Radiology 1989;171:177–187.
22. Goldberg HI, Grossman RI, Gomori JM, et al: Cervical internal carotid artery dissecting hemorrhage: Diagnosis using MRI. Radiology 1986;158:157–161.
23. Brugieres P, Castrec-Carpo A, Héran F, et al: Magnetic resonance imaging in the exploration of dissection of the internal carotid artery. J Neuroradiol 1989;16:1–10.
24. O'Sullivan RM, Robertson WD, Nugent RA, et al: Supraclinoid carotid artery dissection following unusual trauma. AJNR 1990;11: 1150–1152.
25. Kitani R, Itouji T, Noda Y, et al: Dissecting aneurysms of the anterior circle of Willis. J Neurosurg 1980;52:11–20.
26. Parkinson D, West M: Traumatic intracranial aneurysms. J Neurosurg 1980;52:11–20.
27. Rumbaugh CL, Bergeron RT, Kurze T: Intracranial vascular damage associated with skull fractures. Radiology 1972;104:81–87.
28. Jordan BD, Jahre C, Hauser A, et al: CT of 338 active professional boxers. Radiology 1992;185:509–512.
29. Sosin DM, Sacks JJ, Smith SM: Head injury–associated deaths in the United States from 1979 to 1986. JAMA 1989;262:2251–2255.

SELECTED READINGS

Holbourn AHS: Mechanics of head injuries. Lancet 1943;2:438–441.

Holbourn AHS: The mechanics of brain injuries. Br Med Bull 1945;3: 147–149.

8

Degenerative Conditions

THE AGING BRAIN

Over many years there has been considerable discussion of whether the brain does in fact decrease in size or whether there is a decrease in cerebral blood flow with advancing age. Following the introduction of cross-sectional imaging, it began to appear that in fact there is a decrease in brain mass with aging. Both computed tomography and magnetic resonance imaging (MRI) show a widening of the surface sulci and an enlargement of the ventricles that is most likely associated with shrinkage or loss of brain tissue. Considerable variability exists among individuals, and it is not possible to predict whether an individual of an appropriate age (e.g., 70 years) will have loss of brain mass or how great this loss will be (1). Whether there is tissue loss or diminution is generally a subjective judgment.

Cerebral Atrophy

The term *cerebral atrophy* is used loosely in reports of imaging examinations, and it is recommended that it be used with more caution, since it is strictly a subjective impression on the part of the observer. Measurements exist for the lateral ventricles and the third ventricle, but they are rarely taken. There are no clear criteria for the sulci, and the radiologist is left to form his or her own criteria as to what looks too wide for the patient's age. At the present time it is best to base one's judgments on personal experience.

It is generally stated that the ventricular size is more or less stable or increases very slowly up to age 60 and then gradually increases with age. Ventricular volume is about twice that normally encountered at age 35 as the individual reaches the age of 65 (2–4). It is possible to measure or to quantitate sulcal size by MRI, which was not possible with CT because of beam-hardening artifacts. T1 inversion recovery axial images have shown that sulcal size (extraventricular cerebrospinal fluid [CSF]) increases by about 25 percent between ages 30 and 65. Individual variations are common; some individuals show a remarkable preservation of normal ventricular size, but they represent the exception rather than the rule.

Kohn et al. described a method for estimating ventricular CSF and total CSF volume as well as brain volume by MRI (5). The accuracy was high for ventricular and brain volume and less so for total CSF volume. The method could be used clinically to evaluate progression or regression of pathologic processes affecting the CSF.

The corpus callosum is smaller in women than in men, but this difference probably has to do with the brain being larger in males. The corpus callosum becomes smaller in generalized cerebral atrophy, and the decrease in the area of the corpus callosum is not due to advancing age but to the atrophic process (6).

Cerebral blood flow decreases with advancing age. This has been a rather controversial subject over a number of years; however, it is now generally agreed that there is diminution of local cerebral blood flow. It may be that the flow diminution is related to the decrease in brain mass, just discussed (7). On the other hand, de Leon et al. reported that there is no decreased glucose consumption in normal aging as measured with positron emission tomography (PET) scanning and 11C-2 deoxyglucose (DG) (8).

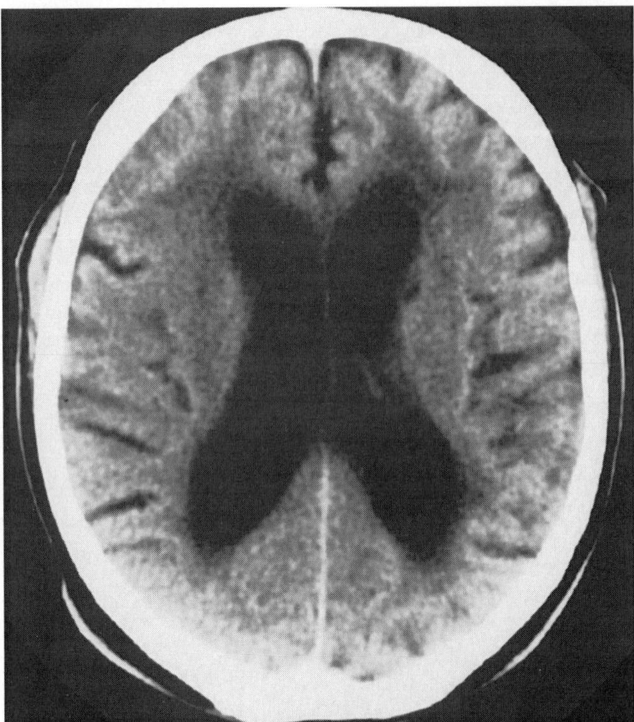

Figure 8.1. Periventricular low density more pronounced in the frontal region bilaterally and less so in the bioccipital region in a 75-year-old patient who had known moderate ventricular dilatation for at least 10 years and no evidence of normotensive hydrocephalus.

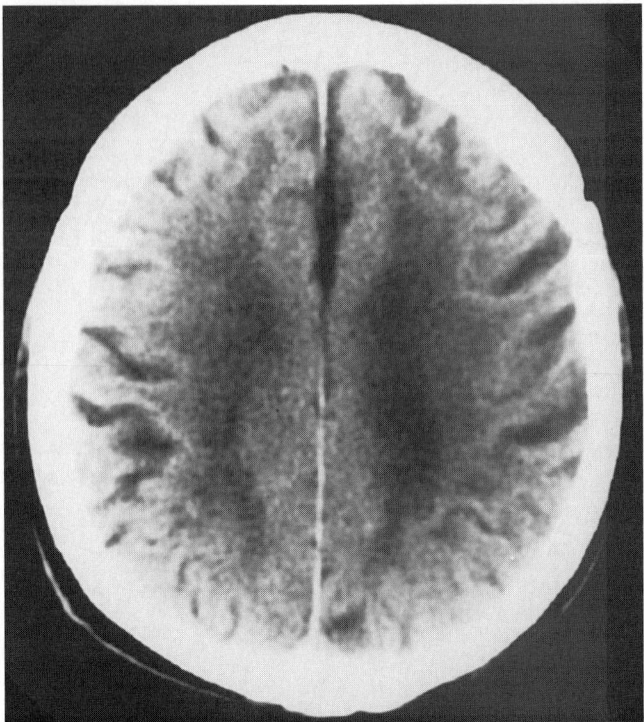

Figure 8.2. White matter hypodensity on CT involving the centrum semiovale bilaterally. The hypodensity is fairly uniform. This appearance was known to have existed for more than 5 years in this patient. There is marked sulcal enlargement indicative of a decrease in the size of the gyri throughout.

Diffuse White Matter Changes

Another frequent phenomenon in the aging brain is the presence of white matter changes, seen by both CT and MRI. On CT, the changes are usually periventricular and low density; they are fairly uniform in density, but they may be more pronounced in the frontal and occipital periventricular areas. In some patients the changes are very pronounced and may spread uniformly around the ventricles, extending farther into the centrum semiovale (Figs. 8.1 and 8.2). This type of change is usually reported as secondary to microvascular leukoencephalopathy, but actual pathological correlation is scant. On MRI the changes are more dramatic on T2-weighted images because they are bright and very conspicuous. They can be uniform or patchy, presenting the same distribution as shown on CT.

Bright White Matter Foci on T2-Weighted Images (Leukoaraiosis)

These hyperintense lesions are common in patients after 60 years of age. They are less frequently encountered between 50 and 60 and are usually not encountered under 50 years of age. They are so frequently observed in patients over 60 that a careful description is usually not carried out in the usual reports of MRI examinations. They are subcortical, periventricular, fairly well circumscribed, rounded or oval, and measure up to 2 cm in diameter (Fig. 8.3). The lesions could be confused with multiple sclerosis (MS) lesions, but their occurrence in the aged separates the patients from the younger group usually affected by MS. In addition, the patients do not present symptoms or signs compatible with MS. If they do, MS must be part of the differential diagnosis (9–11).

The lesions should be evaluated in the first-echo (proton density) T2 image to differentiate the bright spots from perivascular (Virchow-Robin; V-R) spaces. In the proton density image (long repetition time, short echo time), the CSF is essentially isointense or hypointense in relation to brain tissue: the V-R spaces, which are CSF spaces around the blood vessels, are isointense and not visible, whereas on T1-weighted images, the V-R spaces are clearly hypointense (Fig. 8.4). This is an important differential point. If a lesion is seen on T1-weighted images, it is considered to be a V-R space, a lacunar infarct, an area of gliosis, a small cyst, or some other lesion.

What are these hyperintense white matter foci? A number of studies have been carried out to try to determine their nature (12–15). In the studies of Awad et al. an effort was made to correlate the small lesions observed in vivo on the T2-weighted image with autopsy material of the same patients (12,13). Only patients of appropriate age (60 to 84) were studied. They found that the lesions were associated with arteriosclerosis, dilated perivascular spaces, and

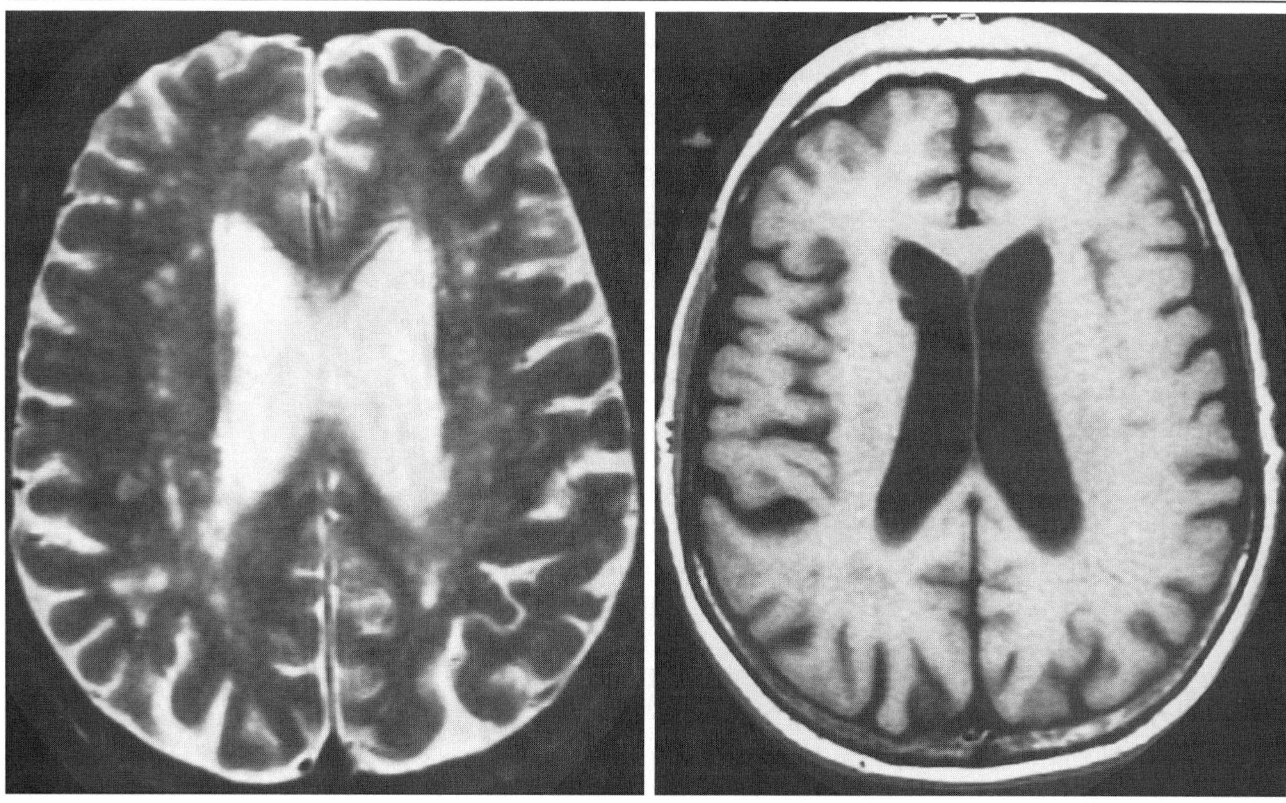

Figure 8.3. Bright white matter foci in a 75-year-old man. **A.** There are many small and medium-size bright patches in the white matter seen in this T2-weighted axial image. **B.** The findings are not demonstrated in the T1-weighted image. This fact differentiates the bright foci from dilated perivascular spaces, which are seen well on T1-weighted images. In the right frontal region there is a small outpouching, which represents a lacunar infarct in the caudate nucleus, a frequent location for lacunae.

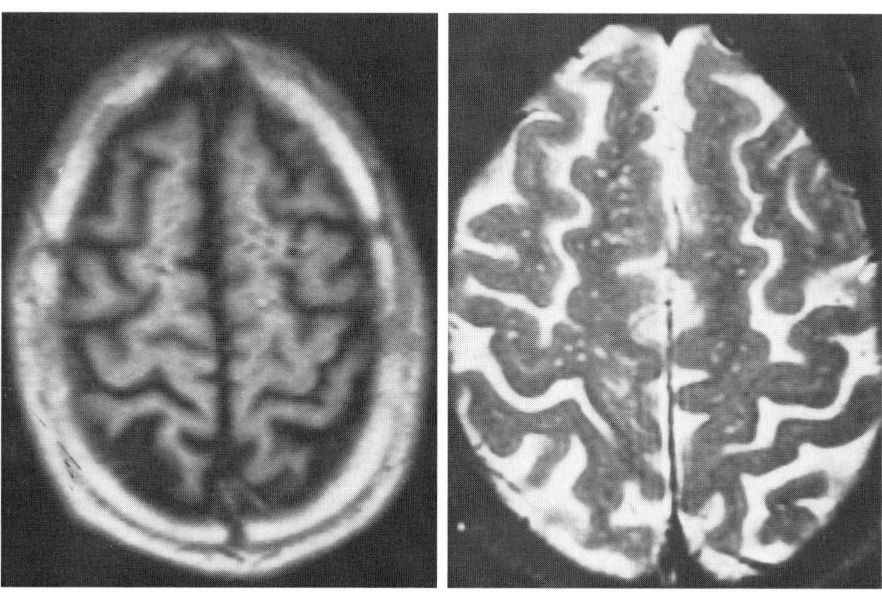

Figure 8.4. Perivascular (Virchow-Robin) spaces in upper-hemisphere white matter. **A.** T1-weighted axial image reveals numerous hypointense, small, round dots in the upper white matter. On proton density images they were not visualized (not shown). **B.** T2-weighted image shows the same spots as hyperintense, indicating that they are behaving like CSF. Prominent Virchow-Robin spaces are much more frequently encountered after the sixth decade and probably represent some degree of atrophy with enlargement of the CSF space around the blood vessels. This appearance probably does not warrant application of the term *état criblé*. It is seen usually in the upper white matter and is fairly frequent (see Fig. 8.5).

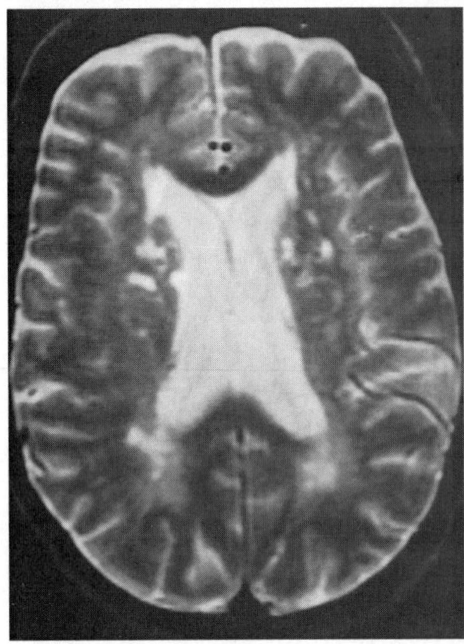

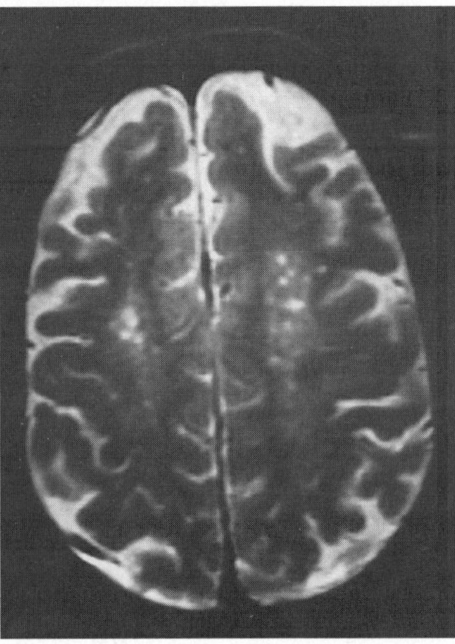

A B

Figure 8.5. A, B. Large numbers of enlarged Virchow-Robin spaces (état criblé), T2-weighted images at two different levels. The case shown in Figure 8.4 probably would not qualify for the diagnosis of état criblé because they are uniform in size and located high in the hemisphere.

vascular ectasia. An exaggeration of the number of dilated perivascular spaces carries the term *état criblé.* The V-R spaces are frequent in the area of the brain situated above the anterior perforated substance. If there is shrinkage of brain around the blood vessels, the result is an extensive network of tunnels filled with CSF. On T1-weighted images the perivascular spaces are dark, like CSF; on the first-echo T2 (proton density) image, these spaces are not ordinarily visible, whereas on the T2-weighted images (second echo) they appear as bright spots, usually round and relatively small, but sometimes surprisingly large (Fig. 8.5). Occasionally very large V-R spaces are encountered (Fig. 8.6). In general, enlarged V-R spaces are more numerous in the upper portion of the centrum semiovale (Fig. 8.4) in the aged. It might be mentioned here that enlarged V-R spaces may be found in the brainstem, most frequently in the region of the substantia nigra. They may be unilateral (50 percent) or bilateral and symmetrical (50 percent) (16).

Thus the bright foci on T2-weighted images may be produced by foci of demyelination, foci of incomplete demyelination, ischemic lesions (lacunes), gliotic foci, some inflammatory or vascular lesion, or trauma, or dilated perivascular spaces. Which of these possible etiologies might be favored depends on the number and location of the lesions. The great majority of the time, if they are fairly numerous, they are idiopathic and may represent areas of incomplete demyelination, which are not seen on CT or on T1-weighted images.

The white matter patches are more numerous in demented patients and also more frequently found on MRI than in nondemented patients of the same age group (17). However, in the study of Bowen et al. subcortical white matter patches were found in 98 to 100 percent of patients with vascular-type dementia, but only in 50 percent of patients cataloged as Alzheimer dementia (18).

There is a tendency to observe white matter brightness on first- and second-echo T2-weighted images in the periventricular area bilaterally in patients in their sixties and older. Of these periventricular locations the most frequent is the bifrontal and the bioccipital regions (Fig. 8.7). However, a brightness on T2 images in the bifrontal region is also commonly found in younger individuals and may be considered a normal finding. Sze et al. have found a histologic change called *ependymitis granularis* that represents patchy loss of the ependyma in the frontal horns with astrocytic gliosis (19). They postulate that flow of interstitial fluid within this region of the brain tends to converge at the dorsolateral angle of the frontal horns, which contributes to increased water locally.

The periventricular brightness on T2-weighted images represents an increase in water in the surrounding tissues. The accumulation of water may represent transependymal extravasation of CSF, such as occurs in the presence of hydrocephalus or any process that causes intraventricular increased pressure, focal or generalized (Fig. 8.8; also see Fig. 4.47). It may also be caused by edema or other unknown factors.

There is an extensive differential diagnosis to be considered with respect to the interpretation of these bright white matter foci. In younger individuals, particularly under age 50, we must conclude that the presence of bright white matter foci on T2-weighted images is due to some pathological process, either past or present.

Multiple small foci are found in cases of migraine in individuals in their third and fourth decades. Similarly, foci may be found in children and young adults as a result of head trauma. In the absence of these two etiological factors, one must consider other conditions, of which prior inflammation is the most common. Prior vascular insults would be unusual in the young. However, certain conditions occur in this age group. MS represents the most important condition that must be differentiated; for the many other conditions that must be considered, see discussions on inflammatory conditions, parasitic, vascular, and congenital diseases; autoimmune diseases; metastatic neoplasms; and postoperative and postirradiation therapy, elsewhere in this book (Table 8.1). Hazardous occupations such as professional boxing and compressed-air tunnel work may increase the number of T2-bright white matter foci (20).

Symmetric (sometimes unilateral) small hyperintense areas on T2-weighted images are seen in a fairly high proportion of normal adults in the posterior limb of the internal capsule. These are isointense on proton density and hypointense on T1-weighted images. A lesion would be hyperintense in the proton density image (21).

In summary, it may be stated that the hyperintense white matter foci seen frequently in the elderly have a varied histopathological representation. Some are frankly small infarcts, some represent areas of gliosis, some are foci of complete or incomplete demyelination, and some represent small cystic areas. It is likely that they are related to microvascular changes in the white matter of the brain (22). More diffuse periventricular changes in the white matter are frequently seen, and some may represent a more severe form of the same condition. Although we are currently attributing the diffuse white matter to microvascular changes, good histopathologic proof is lacking. It must be pointed out, however, that the periventricular diffuse white matter changes are seen well on CT images as diffuse periventricular low attenuation whereas the hyperintense foci are not. Does this mean that they are histologically different, or only different in size?

It is known that increased water is well seen on CT, whereas partial or complete demyelination is poorly shown. Most of the areas of demyelination associated with MS are not seen on CT images even though they may be well developed. Because the diffuse changes being discussed here are so well seen on CT as a diffuse decreased density in the periventricular white matter, one would have to conclude that increased water is the major pathologic change present. Another aspect that has not been elucidated is whether the white matter hyperintense foci are fixed lesions or whether they may change or disappear and be replaced by other foci. The author tends to look upon them as areas of partial demyelination, which would mean that they most likely represent fixed lesions.

Moody et al. have recently described the strong association of periventricular venous collagenosis, a frequently observed degenerative disease in the elderly, with the periventricular bright white matter patches seen on MRI T2-weighted images that are frequently referred to as *leukoardiosis* (23). The possibility that partial obstruction of venous flow is involved in the accumulation of water in the white matter is an attractive hypothesis, for, as discussed previously, the images favor a simple increase of water in the tissues, particularly in the diffuse white matter changes that are seen on CT as well as on MRI.

The V-R spaces represent CSF surrounding the small vessels that penetrate the brain cortex. They are known to be more numerous in the region of the anterior perforated substance, but are also found in the white matter of the centrum semiovale, more frequently in older individuals. On axial views they are seen mostly behind the anterior commissure. Sometimes they may be extremely numerous in the white matter of the centrum semiovale and dilated, in which case we may use the term *état criblé* (Fig. 8.4 and 8.5). As previously mentioned, large, single V-R spaces are sometimes found, usually in the region of the anterior commissure and lower basal ganglia. As discussed earlier, they are CSF-filled spaces and therefore would be seen as dark, round spots on T1-weighted images, as isodense with CSF on first-echo T2 (proton density) images, and as bright, round spots on second-echo T2 images. If there is any pathology associated with dilated V-R spaces in the white matter, they may be partially bright on first-echo images, becoming brighter on second echo.

Table 8.1.
Differential Diagnosis of Incidental White Matter Hyperintensities on T2-Weighted Images

Virchow-Robin spaces: Isointense with CSF on long TR/short TE images; adjacent to anterior commissure and in subcortical regions.

Ependymitis granularis: Located adjacent to frontal horns of lateral ventricles in young individuals.

Leukoaraiosis: One of many names given to essentially benign hyperintense white matter lesions in elderly individuals. May be due to small regions of demyelination or gliosis or, in some cases, small infarcts. In young people may be associated with old trauma, migraine, or prior encephalopathies.

Lacunar infarcts: May be found in periventricular white matter but also commonly found in deep gray matter structures and brainstem.

DEMENTIA

Dementia can be simply defined as an organic loss of intellectual function. The prevalence of dementia is increasing as the proportion of older individuals in our population increases. Dementia afflicts about 2 percent of the population between 65 and 70 but affects 20 percent of people above 80. Thus we may expect an increasing number of demented people as the longevity of the population continues to increase. In a recent study, dementia was present in nearly one-third of unselected 85-year-olds in Sweden (24). About half of these appeared to have vascular dementia, which is considered more amenable to prevention or treatment than Alzheimer disease.

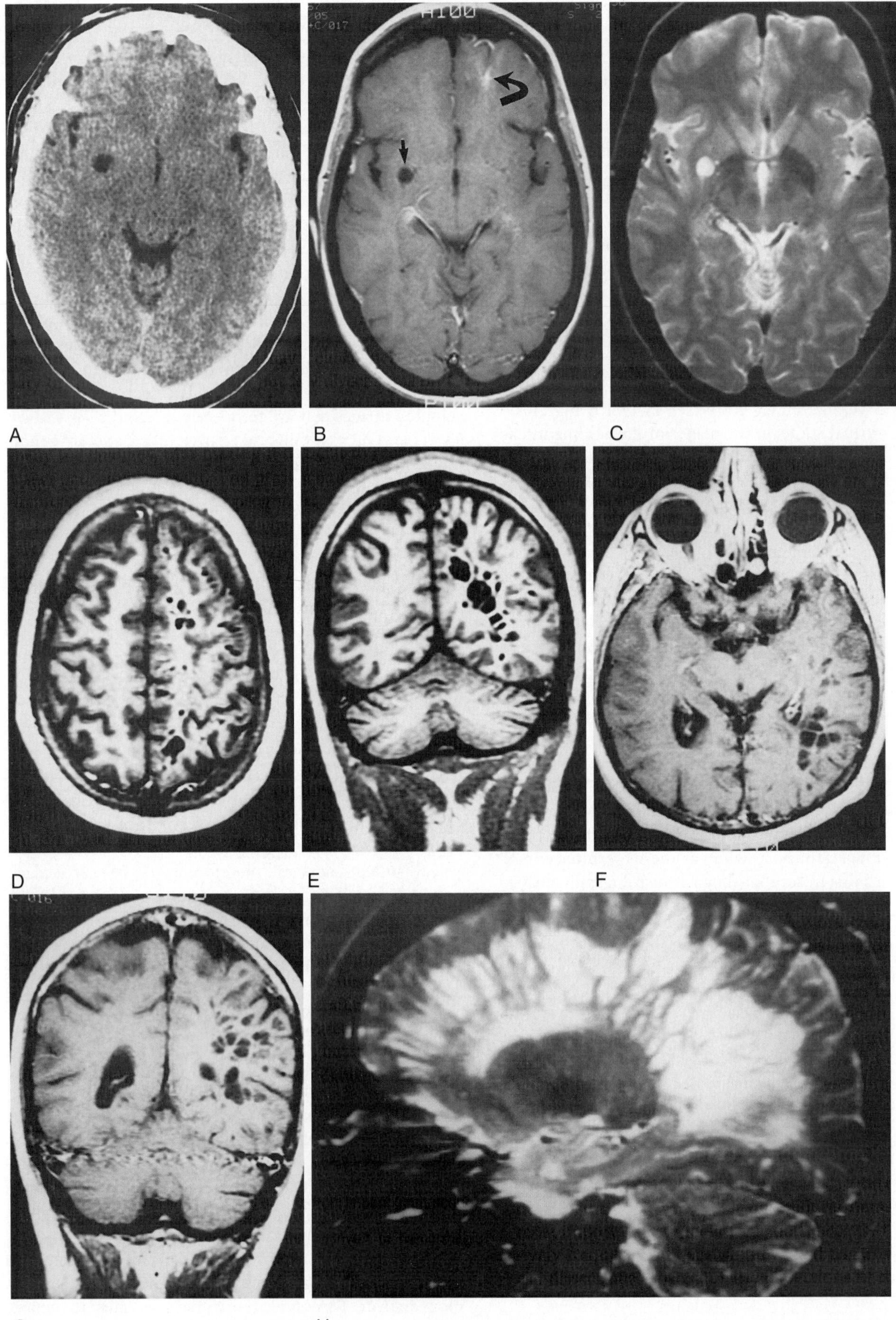
A
B
C
D
E
F
G
H

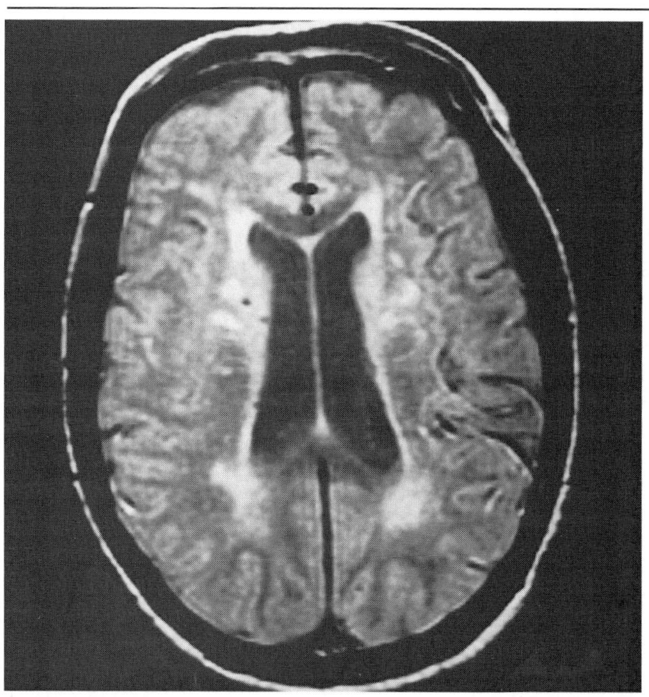

Figure 8.7. Periventricular brightness, more pronounced in mainly the frontal and bioccipital areas in a 68-year-old man. Axial proton density image. There are also a number of nonspecific, bright white matter foci.

Dementia is a clinical diagnosis and has a number of etiologic factors.

Alzheimer Disease

Alzheimer disease is the most common of the dementias. We used to speak of senile dementia of the Alzheimer type to separate the later-onset from the earlier-onset cases, which were referred to as Alzheimer disease or (AD). However, the tendency today is to refer to all patients as AD. The first manifestation is the gradual onset of forgetfulness or loss of anterograde memory, which refers to the inability to recall recent events. This is followed by language disturbances, visuospatial disorientation, and ideomotor apraxia. The course of the illness progresses until death, which occurs in 5 to 7 years (25).

The classic histologic appearance in AD is neuritic plaques in the cerebral cortex. They may be very numerous and may increase to occupy one-third to one-half of the cortex (26). "The plaques consist of grossly enlarged neuritic processes mingled with astroyctes and microglia and, in the majority, a demonstrable central deposit of amyloid" (26). The other classic manifestation is neurofibrillary degeneration. The changes are more extensive in the temporal lobe hippocampal formation, as previously expressed. Atypical features are common, and the occurrence of amyloid angiopathy should be mentioned in particular. Amyloid angiopathy may occur alone (see Chapter 10, "Brain Vascular Diseases"), but the histologic findings may also be associated with AD. As indicated previously, the earliest and usually most extensive changes occur in the hippocampus and the amygdala. Also, neurofibrillary degeneration (tangles) and loss of neurons are found within these areas and within subcortical regions such as the nucleus basalis of Meynert, the locus ceruleus, and the dorsal raphe (27). The earliest neuronal loss occurs in the entorhinal cortex in the parahippocampal gyrus (28). Another point of interest is the frequency with which these pathological changes are found in persons with Down syndrome in their fifth and sixth decades. Persons affected with Down syndrome

◄

Figure 8.6. Large perivascular space in basal ganglia region, four examples. **A.** CT examination shows a 1.0-cm round hypodense image in the right basal ganglia region, felt to represent a large perivascular space (Virchow-Robin space). **B.** In another patient, this T1-weighted, gadolinium-enhanced image shows a 1.0-cm hypointense image (arrow) in the same location as in A, with an enhanced central dot consistent with a blood vessel (probably too faint to be seen on the reproduction). This patient also had a small vascular malformation in the left frontal region (curved arrow). **C.** T2-weighted image reveals a hyperintense area consistent with CSF in the region of the right basal ganglia and anterior perforated substance. Other small, round dots are seen in the same area, which is situated in the region of the anterior commissure, where Virchow-Robin spaces are most frequently seen. **D** and **E.** Another patient with greatly dilated Virchow-Robin spaces only in one hemisphere. The patient (age 21) was neurologically normal and remained so on follow-up of several years. T1-weighted axial (**D**) and coronal (**E**) images show the multiple low-intensity, cystlike areas in the white matter. This and a few other patients from the same area in Brazil may well harbor an unusual infectious or parasitic agent. **F** and **G.** Images of a 57-year-old man, also neurologically intact, who was diagnosed with migraine. The images show dilated perivascular spaces unilaterally. **H.** Lateral T2-weighted image of another patient reveals the markedly dilated Virchow-Robin spaces. The fanlike distribution (perpendicular to the ventricular wall) is characteristic of the small perforating vessels in the white matter. (Courtesy of Dr. Luiz Bacheschi and Alvaro Magalhaes, University of São Paulo Medical School, Brazil.)

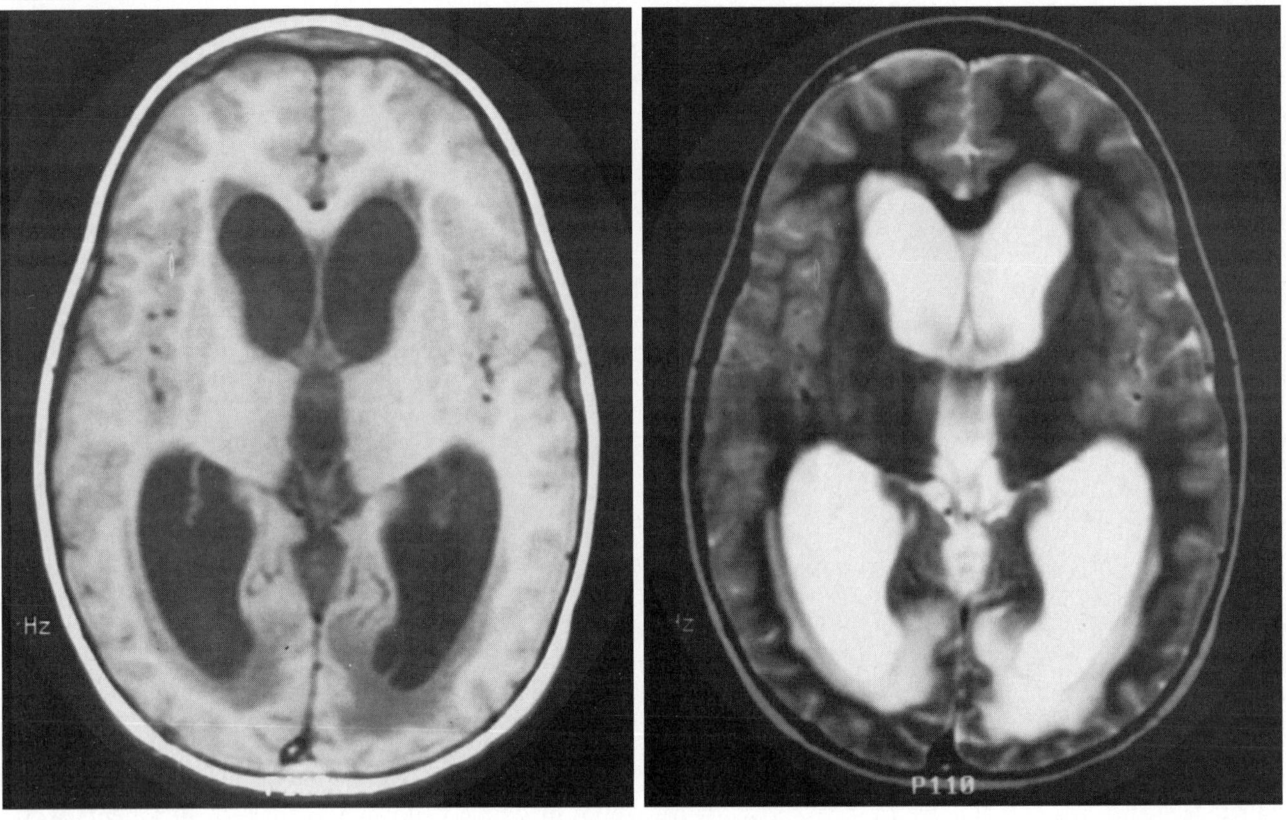

Figure 8.8. Periventricular changes associated with communicating hydrocephalus in a young patient. **A.** The transependymal passage of fluid is low intensity in this T1-weighted image. **B.** On a T2-weighted image the periventricular fluid is bright. The communicating hydrocephalus was secondary to poor CSF absorption related to meningeal disease.

develop Alzheimer disease with great frequency in their fifties.

Efforts are ongoing to locate the gene in the specific chromosome that controls the disease inheritance (presumably an autosomal dominant mode), but at present there is no universal agreement that this has been accomplished (29). The earlier-onset cases are more likely to present a family history. They also progress more rapidly and present more language disturbance (30).

From the imaging point of view it is often difficult to find anything more on CT or MRI examinations than a generalized decrease in brain mass, which in an early case of AD is essentially similar to that of a normal patient of the same age: that is, there is some ventricular dilatation and some widening of the surface sulci. The difference between the normal aged individual and a patient affected with AD becomes manifest on follow-up examinations because the patient with AD continues to lose tissue at a much more rapid rate (3,4). In AD there is greater involvement of the hippocampus than in the normal aged individual. Atrophy is noticeable on CT or MRI and is manifested as temporal horn enlargement and as an increase in the prominence of the hippocampal fissure. The changes in the temporal horn and hippocampal area are caused by a particularly noticeable involvement of the hippocampus, the amygdala, and adjacent white matter. Kido et al. carried out measurements of the temporal horns and also evaluated the size of the sylvian fissure in a series of AD and normal age-matched controls (31). If the anteroposterior diameter of the tip of the temporal horn measured more than 3 mm, it was considered enlarged, and was found to be so in the majority of the AD patients as against the controls. It was also found, however, that subjective evaluation by simple observation was as accurate as measurement. The same was true of enlargement of the sylvian fissure, which was found more commonly in the AD patients. The combination of the two findings (unilateral or bilateral temporal horn enlargement and sylvian fissure enlargement) is suggestive of a diagnosis of AD (Figs. 8.9 and 8.10). A diagnosis cannot be made on the basis of diagnostic imaging; rather, it is made on clinical grounds, and the imaging studies are used to support the diagnosis. Imaging is used particularly to exclude other possible diagnoses, such as multi-infarct dementia or diffuse vascular disease in the white matter.

Rusinek et al., with a special program for MRI that estimated volume of white matter, gray matter, and CSF,

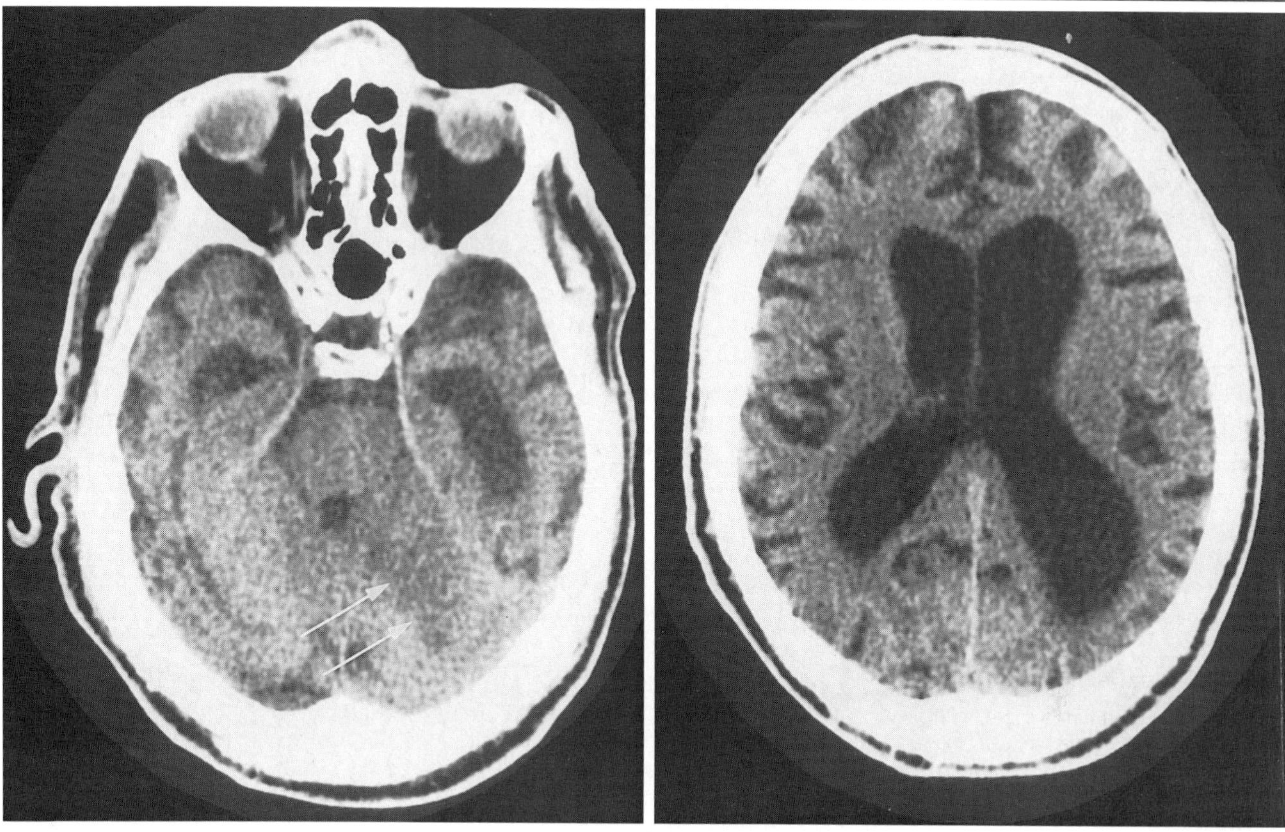

Figure 8.9. CT of a 68-year-old man with a clinical diagnosis of Alzheimer disease. **A.** Section through the temporal fossa shows marked enlargement of the temporal horns. **B.** A higher section reveals moderate to marked ventricular enlargement and widening of the surface sulci. The appearance is consistent with general brain tissue loss. The enlargement of the temporal horns is seen more frequently in patients with Alzheimer-type dementia but is not diagnostic. There is no significant periventricular decrease in density in the white matter. An incidental finding is the presence of hypodensity in the upper right cerebellum in A, felt to represent a cerebellar ischemic infarction (arrows).

found that the percentage of gray matter in AD patients as against normal individuals was reduced (44.9 percent ± 4.4), whereas in normal individuals the figure was 50.2 percent (32). The most significant reduction occurred in the temporal lobes (13.8 percent), which was found to be statistically significant ($P < .001$).

Perhaps more promising than CT or MRI is the use of techniques capable of demonstrating brain metabolism, such as PET. Using ^{18}Fl deoxyglucose, it is possible to demonstrate decreased metabolism of glucose, which, in early AD is found only in the biparietal cortical association areas and in more advanced cases is also found in the frontal and temporal cortical areas (Fig. 8.11). This has also been shown by a method utilizing single photon emission tomography (SPECT) to demonstrate cerebral blood flow with 123 I-N-isopropyl-p-iodoamphetamine (123 I-IMP) (33–35). The same decrease may also be shown with MRI functional imaging (36).

Concerning the possibility of changes in energy metabolism occurring in AD, the work of Bottomley et al. with P-31 NMR spectroscopy yielded negative results with respect to the concentration and relative ratios of phosphocreatine, nucleoside triphosphate, inorganic phosphate, phosphomonoester, and phosphodiester in whole axial sections of the cerebral hemispheres (37). These negative results could not be explained by the cerebral atrophy, and there was no correlation with the severity of dementia. McClure et al. reported elevated levels of phosphodiesters (PDE) and glutamate, and elevated phosphomonoesters (PME) early in the disease (38). Gonzalez et al. also reported somewhat different findings, such as an increase in the PME-PDE ratio (39). Gonzalez et al. have speculated that these findings reflect changes in the biophysical state of membrane phospholipids in AD.

In summary, the atrophic changes found in Alzheimer disease cannot be differentiated from those of an elderly normal patient, particularly in the early stages. If there are changes suggestive of greater temporal lobe atrophy (enlargement of the temporal horn, unilaterally or bilaterally) and atrophy of the hippocampal gyri (40,41) (enlargement

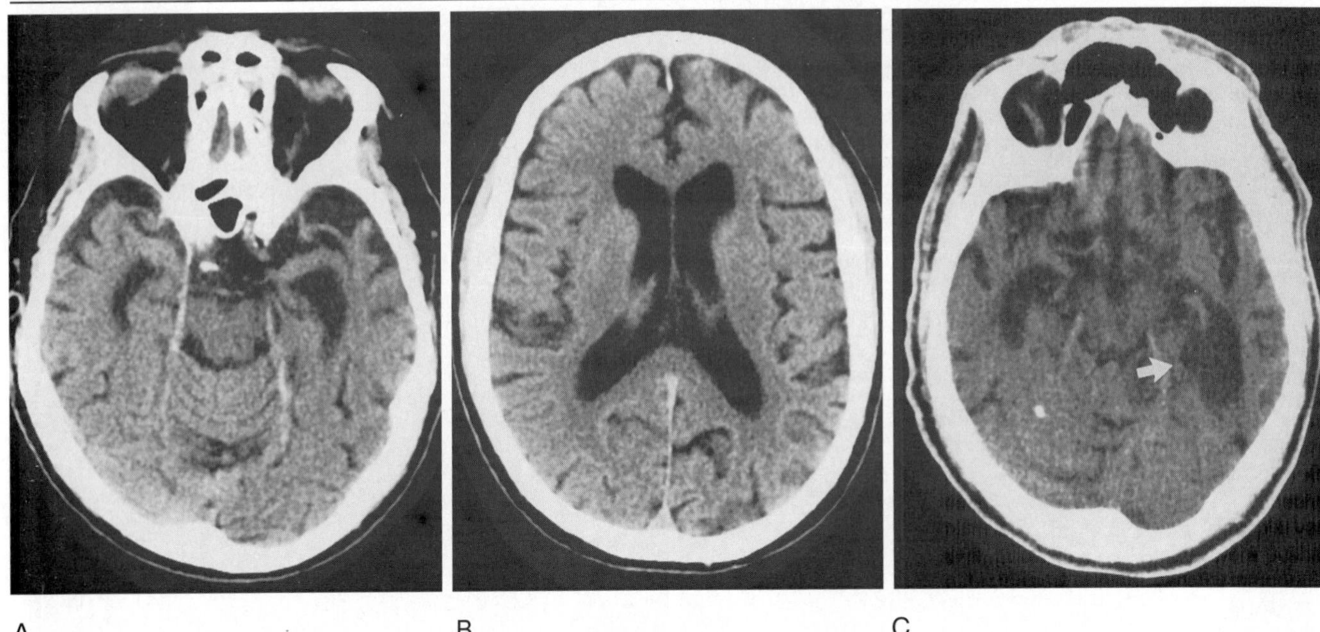

Figure 8.10. CT of an 82-year-old man with a clinical diagnosis of Alzheimer-type dementia. **A.** There is bilateral asymmetrical enlargement of the temporal horns. Some low attenuation is seen in the region of the choroidal fissure (medial temporal) on the left side. **B.** A higher section shows moderate ventricular enlargement, but the sylvian fissures and the surface sulci are not particularly enlarged for an 82-year-old man. There is no significant periventricular low density, which is ordinarily associated with microangiopathic changes in the white matter. **C.** Alzheimer disease in another patient demonstrates the enlarged temporal horns and the widened medial hippocampal-choroidal fissure on the left side (arrow).

of the temporal choroidal fissure) (42), and these are associated with some enlargement of the sylvian fissure and some degree of ventricular dilatation, the diagnosis may be suggested. If a follow-up examination is obtained, the AD patient is likely to show demonstrable progression, whereas the normal patient will probably remain nearly unchanged. As discussed, studies of blood flow or glucose metabolism utilizing PET or SPECT may be somewhat more reliable (43) (Table 8.2).

A promising imaging approach in the early diagnosis of AD is MR proton spectroscopy, in which the height of the peak representing *N*-acetylaspartate (NAA) is compared with the normal. NAA is directly related to the number of neurons, and, as there is a decrease in the number of viable neurons in AD, a decrease in NAA is to be expected (44).

In general, the diagnosis is made clinically and by clinical follow-up to show progression, but the clinician is always faced with the need to exclude other disease processes, and

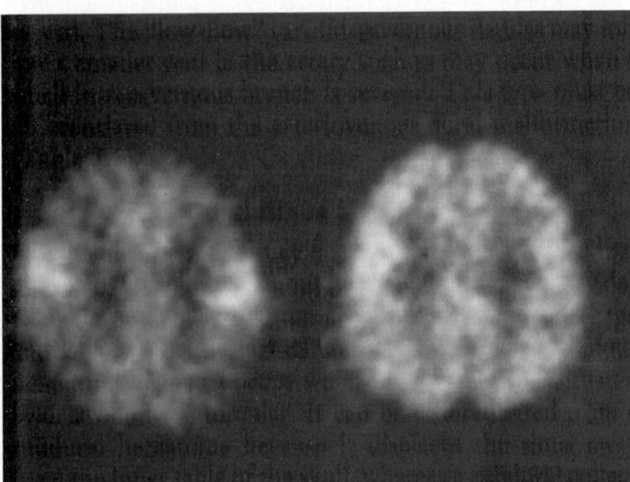

Figure 8.11. Alzheimer disease, PET scan. The image on the left is an affected patient. There is decreased fluorodeoxyglucose consumption in the bifrontal and biparietal areas consistent with the diagnosis of advanced Alzheimer-like dementia. On the right is a normal patient for comparison. In A, the bright area bilaterally in the hemispheres is the normal uptake of fluorodeoxyglucose; compare with normal image in B.

Table 8.2.
Differential Diagnosis of Dementias

Alzheimer disease: Usually nonspecific findings of diffuse atrophy. Often with more prominent atrophy of hippocampus and amygdala resulting in enlargement of temporal horns, and hippocampal fissure. Sylvian fissures usually enlarged. PET and SPECT show hypometabolism or hypoperfusion in biparietal areas primarily; also bifrontal.

Multi-infarct dementia: Multiple infarctions in brain cortex and subcortical/periventricular white matter.

Binswanger disease: Microangiopathic encephalopathy with diffuse, often confluent white matter regions of hyperintense signal on T2-weighted images. Definitive diagnosis is made only by histopathologic analysis.

Pick disease: Preferential involvement of frontal lobes compared with temporal lobe involvement. Hypometabolism or hypoperfusion is frontal rather than biparietal.

for this reason imaging examination is usually necessary. Several of these disease processes are discussed in text following.

Multi-Infarct Dementia

Multi-infarct dementia is a condition that can be diagnosed by CT or MRI because of the presence of multiple focal areas of involvement, some of which clearly involve the brain cortex (Fig. 8.12). The white matter also will show signs of periventricular hyperintensity on MRI or diminished attenuation on CT. There will also be bright white matter patches on T2-weighted images and generalized signs of loss of brain mass (ventricular dilatation and widening of the surface sulci), but the multifocality of the changes that are similar to infarcts and that involve the cortical gray matter would suggest a specific diagnosis of multi-infarct dementia in the presence of the appropriate clinical syndrome.

Lacunar Infarcts

Lacunar infarcts are common and are caused by occlusion of perforating small arterial branches. On cross-sectional imaging they are particularly visible in the basal ganglia, in the immediate periventricular wall, and in the external capsule region and in the centrum semiovale. Loeb et al. concluded that patients with lacunar infarcts suffer from dementia 4 to 12 times more frequently than the normal population (45). Thus the frequency with which lacunae are observed in the elderly should not lead us to underestimate their clinical importance (see Chapter 10, "Brain Vascular Disorders," "Ischemic Infarction").

Binswanger Disease

Like AD, Binswanger encephalopathy cannot be diagnosed by imaging changes alone. The presence of a marked degree of periventricular hyperintensity is usually attributed to microvascular changes in the white matter (microangiopathic encephalopathy), but with insufficient pathologic proof, for the changes could be produced by increased water in the tissues, of unknown etiology (as discussed earlier). The author has recently had an opportunity to follow a patient who, 8 years previously, presented extensive periventricular and centrum semiovale hyperintensity on MRI and corresponding changes on CT, but who was mentally normal and remained so for all that time; he then developed signs of forgetfulness that clinically were considered consistent with Binswanger encephalopathy (Fig. 8.13). Subsequently, he presented signs of remission, similar to that previously described (46). The pathologic findings in Binswanger encephalopathy include athero- and arteriosclerosis of the cerebral vessels, sharply delimited areas of necrosis, and diffuse demyelination of the deep white matter, as well as small infarcts in the basal ganglia and thalami. Interestingly enough, the corpus callosum is not involved. Moody et al. attribute this fact to the peculiar blood supply to the corpus callosum, which consists mainly of short arteries with the absence of long, penetrating arterioles or arteries (47). The cerebral cortex is preserved, in spite of the fact that Binswanger encephalopathy is thought to be a variety of multi-infarct dementia. Pure cases of Binswanger chronic progressive subcortical encephalopathy are difficult to find. On the other hand, extensive periventricular white matter changes broadly involving the periventricular area and extending laterally to involve the external capsule are relatively common in individuals over 70 years of age who show no significant signs of a dementing disorder (Fig. 8.7) (48,49,23).

Cerebral Autosomal Dominant Arteriopathy with Subcortical Infarcts and Leukoencephalopathy

Among the vascular conditions, a relatively recently recognized disease, deserving special mention, that can be associated with dementia is cerebral autosomal dominant arteriopathy with subcortical infarcts and leukoencephalopathy (CADASIL). It affects adults in their fourth to sixth decades of life (mean age about 43 years) and is characterized by recurrent subcortical ischemic strokes, in nonhypertensive individuals, leading some patients to dementia. It is different from multi-infarct dementia in that it affects younger subjects and is familial. CT and MRI show white matter disease and subcortical areas consistent with ischemic lesions. Tournier-Lasserve et al. have indicated that the disease locus has been assigned to chromosome 19 q 12 (50). Of 57 living members analyzed in one family, 11 had suffered recurrent strokes. Three developed pseudobulbar palsy and subcortical dementia (50,51).

Pick Disease

Pick disease is a rare type of dementia that can only be diagnosed pathologically. By CT or MRI, there may be greater involvement of the frontal lobes, represented as enlargement of the frontal horns to a greater extent than the rest of the lateral ventricles. The temporal lobes are often involved, usually together with the frontal lobes

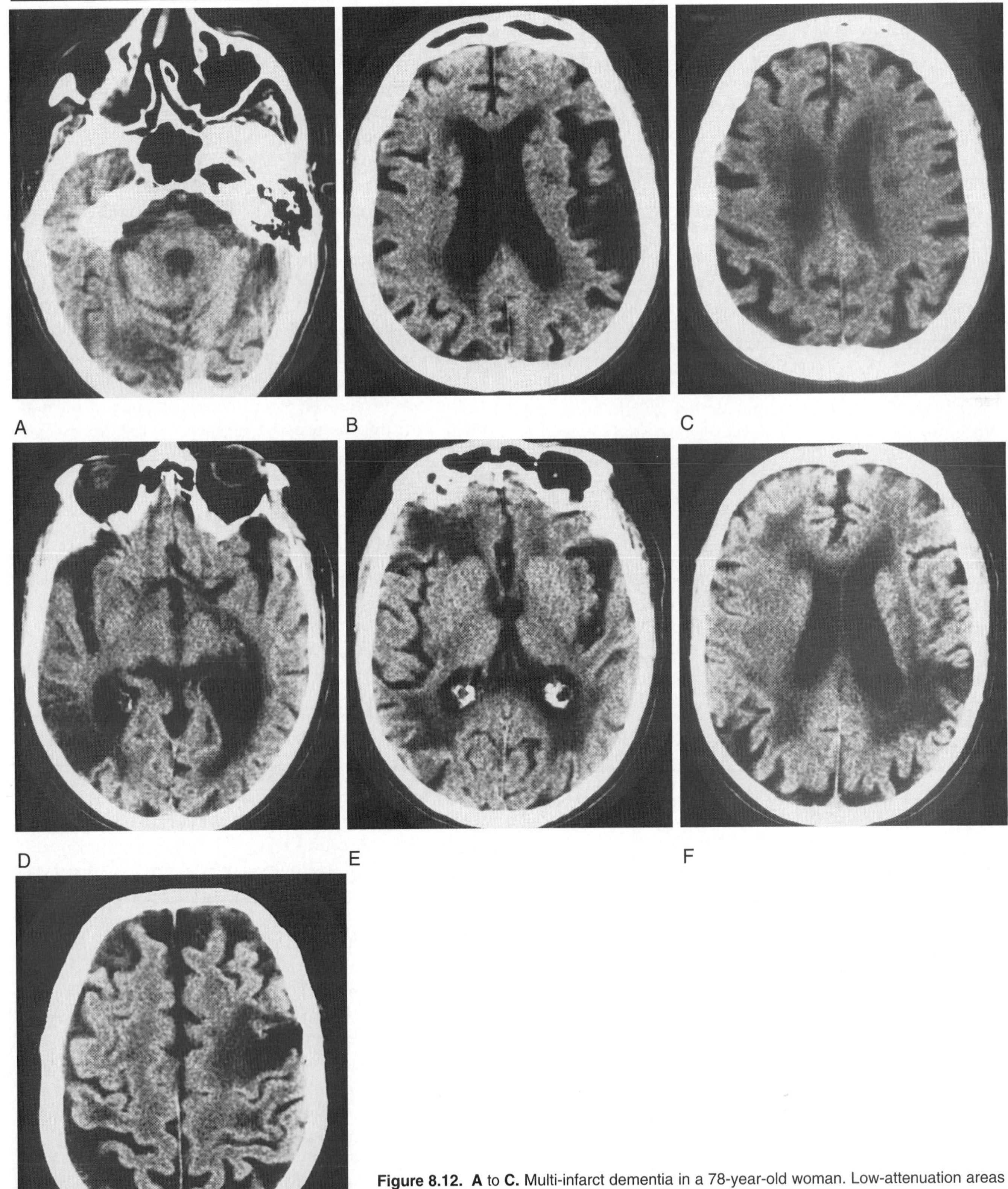

Figure 8.12. **A** to **C.** Multi-infarct dementia in a 78-year-old woman. Low-attenuation areas due to ischemic infarcts are seen in the right occipital, right corona radiata, and frontal area and in the left sylvian fissure area and deep white matter. There is also considerable generalized tissue loss. **D** to **G.** Multi-infarct dementia in a 65-year-old man. Four large areas of infarction are seen in the right parieto-occipital area, right anterior and deep frontal area, and left parietal and left frontal area, as well as diffuse white matter hypodensity consistent with small-vessel disease in the white matter. Marked generalized atrophy is also present.

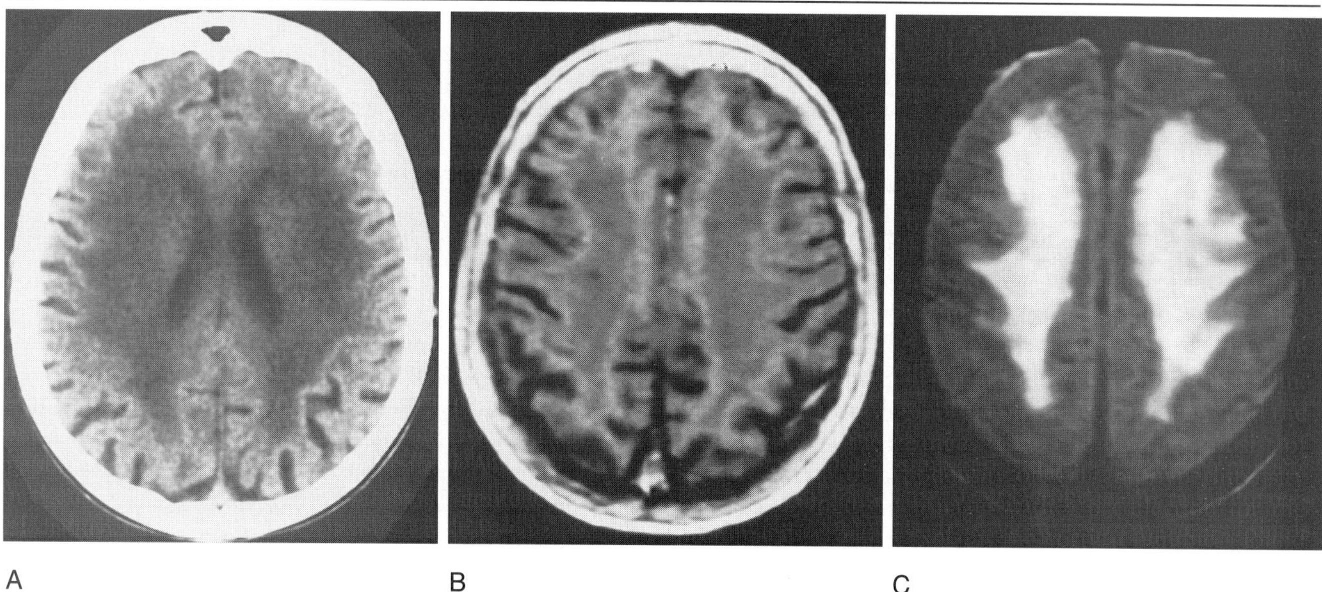

Figure 8.13. Binswanger disease in an 80-year-old woman. **A.** CT shows a marked degree of hypodensity in the periventricular region and centrum semiovale. **B.** T1-weighted axial image shows essentially the same appearance as the CT image. **C.** A T2-weighted image shows the marked hyperintensity in the white matter consistent with diffuse microvascular disease.

(frontotemporal atrophy) (52). Heredity is more commonly involved in this condition than in AD. PET studies show decreased metabolic activity much as in AD, but the decreased activity is localized to the frontal and temporal lobe cortex.

Other Conditions Associated with Dementia

A number of other conditions may be accompanied by a dementing syndrome, such as various poisons, liver or renal failure, severe inflammatory and posttraumatic states, and in fact any severe state that can affect the nervous system. However, these dementias are acute or subacute and usually improve if appropriate treatment is applied. Brown et al. reported a case of Whipple disease in which the patient presented only with a 2-year history of progressive dementia and weakness and no symptoms outside the CNS (53). They stress the importance of considering such disease processes in the differential diagnosis. The diagnosis in this particular case was made by brain biopsy.

Mixed cases of dementia are probably more common than is generally recognized, especially in the elderly. The brain is probably especially susceptible to factors that impair cognition. These include vascular disease, alcoholism, chronic pulmonary disease, some degenerative brain disorders, Parkinson disease, and others (54). Loeb et al. reported a much higher incidence of dementia in patients presenting with lacunar infarcts as compared with the general population on an average follow-up of 4 years (45). This would emphasize the fact that the presence of multiple lacunar infarcts should be considered a predisposing factor for the development of vascular-type dementia.

MISCELLANEOUS DEGENERATIVE CONDITIONS

This heterogeneous group of conditions includes Parkinson disease; Shy-Drager syndrome; progressive supranuclear palsy; cerebellar and brainstem degeneration, including olivopontocerebellar degeneration; Friedreich ataxia; cerebellar cortical degeneration; and others. Wallerian degeneration and amyotrophic lateral sclerosis also warrant discussion.

Parkinson Disease

This is a common condition seen in middle or late life that progresses rather slowly. It may occur in families but is usually sporadic. Clinically the diagnosis is relatively easy to make because of the relative stiffness, the stooped posture, the fixed facial expression, and the rhythmic tremor. Pathologically, the most regularly observed changes involve the melanin-containing nerve cells in the brainstem (substantia nigra, locus ceruleus). Nerve cell loss with reactive gliosis of varying degrees can be demonstrated. Other histological changes may be observed, such as Lewy bodies (eosinophilic intracytoplasmic inclusions). Parkinson disease can be considered a neuronal system disease involving mainly the nigrostriatal dopaminergic system. There is a decrease of dopamine in the caudate nucleus and putamen (55).

On MRI, changes can be found in the substantia nigra, particularly in the pars compacta, which becomes thinner or disappears altogether (22). Although these findings may be found in some typical examples of Parkinson disease patients, the majority do not present a clear enough picture of these findings demonstrable on T2-weighted images.

There is also hypointensity of the putamen, presumably associated with iron accumulation seen on T2-weighted images (22). In Parkinson disease there is increased hypointensity also extending to involve a larger area of the putamen. However, this again turns out to be a soft finding in practice.

Hyperintense foci may be found sometimes in the putamen and globus pallidus in some Parkinson patients. However, these are also found in normal age-matched controls.

Shy-Drager Syndrome

This syndrome is characterized by autonomic nervous system failure. The prominent features are postural (orthostatic) hypotension, urinary incontinence, inability to sweat, muscular rigidity and tremor, and sexual impotence in the male. The syndrome affects both sexes about equally and occurs sporadically in the sixth and seventh decades. Pathologically, there is rather widespread symmetrical neuronal degeneration affecting the caudate nucleus, the substantia nigra, and the locus ceruleus pontis; there are also findings involving the spinal cord (loss of cells from the ventral and lateral horns) (56). In some cases imaging findings in the involved structures may be expected, particularly in the more advanced cases, since the disease is progressive. Although no specific imaging findings have been described, Savoiardo et al. have found some increased hypointensity in the globus pallidus and putamen and in the substantia nigra similar to that found in Parkinson disease (57). (See text following under "Multiple System Atrophy.")

Progressive Supranuclear Palsy

Originally described by Steele et al. (58), this syndrome consists of progressive paralysis of vertical eye movements, dysarthria, and muscular rigidity, particularly involving the muscles of the neck. It occurs in the fifth to seventh decades and leads to death in 5 to 7 years. Pathologically there is evidence of neuronal loss in the globus pallidus, the red nucleus, the substantia nigra, the tectum and periaqueductal gray matter, and the dentate nucleus of the cerebellum. The cerebral cortex is not affected. Males are affected twice as often as females.

Imaging findings are usually well developed: there is periaqueductal atrophy; the quadrigeminal plate is thinner, particularly the upper portion; the aqueduct is larger than usual; and the pars compacta, the brighter band separating the pars reticulata of the substantia nigra from the red nucleus, becomes narrower in a manner similar to what has been described in Parkinson disease (59). The narrowing of the brighter pars compacta may be due to the accumulation of iron, for gliosis, when replacing neuronal loss, should also be bright on T2-weighted images.

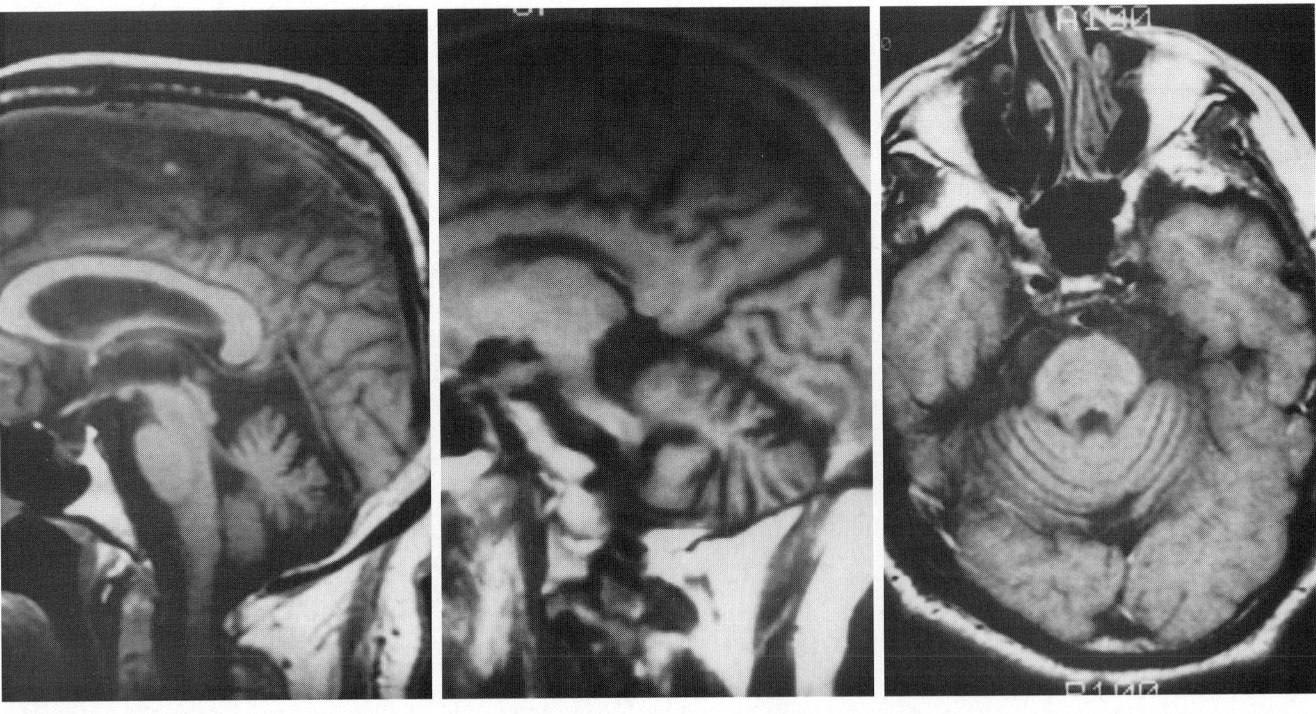

Figure 8.14. Cerebellar atrophy in a 65-year-old patient with progressive cerebellar symptoms. **A.** Midline sagittal section reveals vermian atrophy. The sulci are widened. **B.** A section lateral to the midline reveals widened sulci and a relatively small cerebellar hemisphere. **C.** Axial T1-weighted image reveals the widened sulci, usually indicative of thinning of the cerebellar folia.

Degenerative Conditions Affecting the Cerebellum

Cerebellar atrophy is frequently encountered in the elderly. It may be related to vascular disease, to toxic effects such as alcohol or drugs, or (most commonly) to unexplained causes. Cerebellar atrophy is usually manifested on CT or MRI as a slight or moderate increase in the size of the fourth ventricle, an increase in the size or prominence of the vermis folia, and an increase in the size of the transverse cerebellar fissure, which on axial CT images is usually shown as an area of decreased density symmetrically arranged on each side of the midline (Fig. 8.14). Minor degrees of cerebellar atrophy are more difficult to evaluate. On axial CT images, a slight degree of cerebellar vermis atrophy is suspected when more than four sulci can be counted over the top of the vermis. More marked degrees of cerebellar atrophy show an increase in the CSF space all around the cerebellum. MRI is particularly good in diagnosing cerebellar atrophy because the sagittal images demonstrate vermian atrophy particularly well and show the enlargement of the fourth ventricle (Fig. 8.14).

Olivopontocerebellar atrophy (OPCA) probably occurs as two main varieties: one that presents an autosomal dominant inheritance, and a recessive or sporadic variety that has not been as extensively studied pathologically. However, since there are a number of different clinical manifestations and pathologic distributions of the lesions, imaging examination is important. Some patients present pure cerebellar ataxia similar to that seen in atrophy of the cerebellar

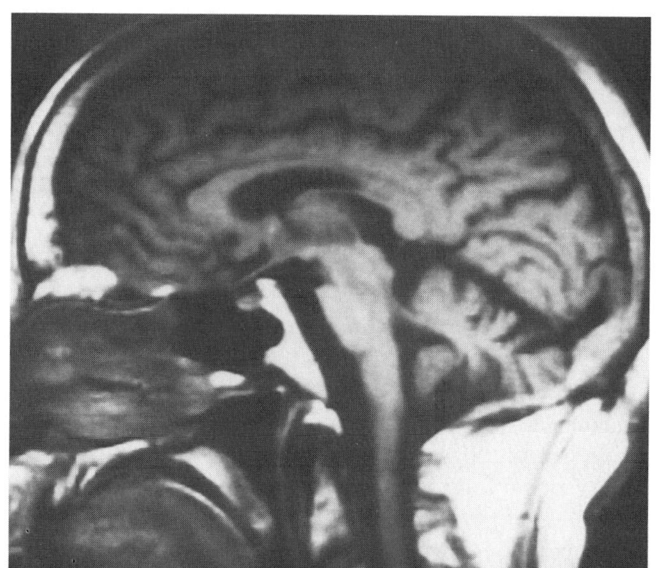

A

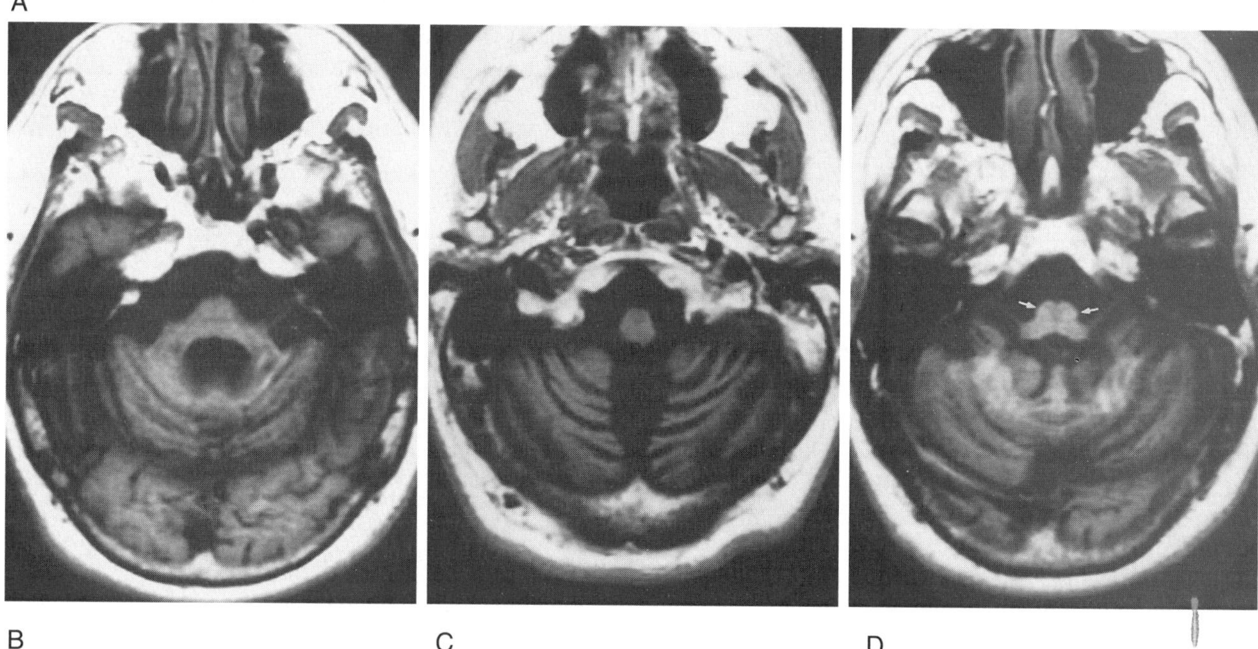

B C D

Figure 8.15. Pontocerebellar atrophy in a 56-year-old man. **A.** Midline sagittal T1-weighted view shows flattening of the belli of the pons and atrophy of the cerebellar vermis. **B.** Axial T1-weighted view reveals enlargement of the fourth ventricle, atrophy of the middle cerebellar peduncles and of the pons, and prominent cerebellar sulci. The prepontine cistern is very large. **C.** There is considerable enlargement of the cerebellar sulci and of the vermis sulci, as shown in this axial T1-weighted view. **D.** A section slightly higher than C shows that the medullary olives are not decreased in size, indicating that secondary atrophy of the olivary nuclei has not occurred (arrows). Compare with Fig. 3.30*B* under normal anatomy.

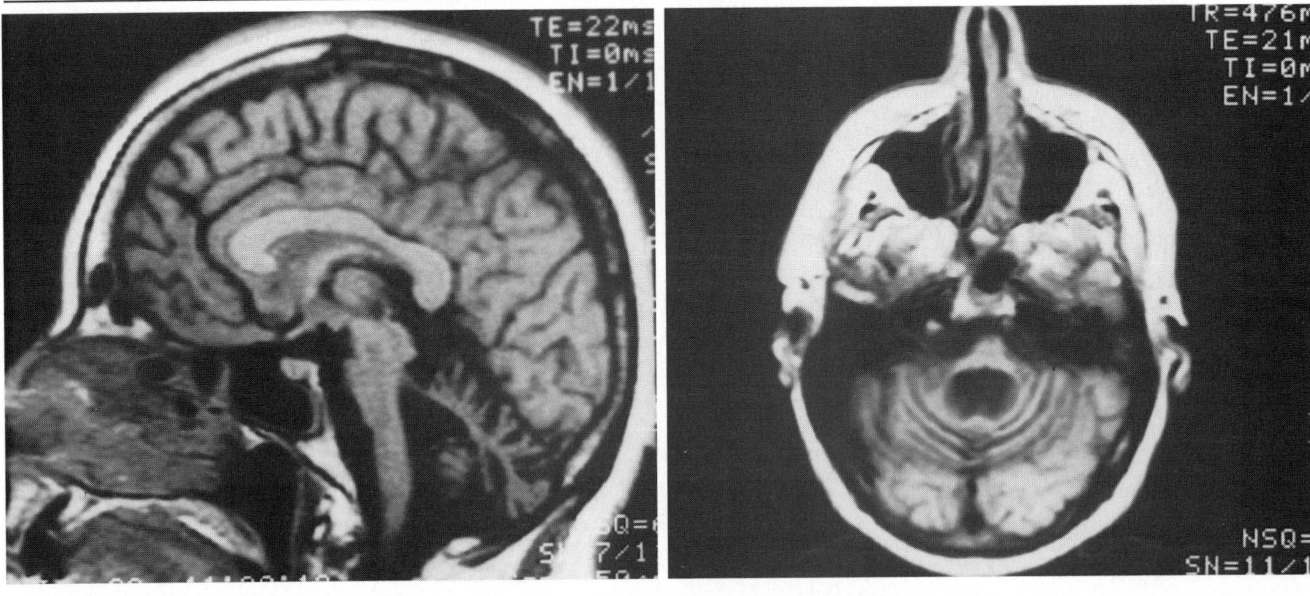

Figure 8.16. Sagittal (**A**) and axial (**B**) projections showing pontocerebellar atrophy. There is an even greater degree of atrophy of the pons and cerebellum and greater enlargement of the fourth ventricle than that shown in Figure 8.15.

cortex (which usually leads to secondary atrophy of the olivary nuclei). Other patients may present features resembling Parkinson disease. Pathologically, there is a decrease in the size of the belli of the pons as well as of the middle cerebellar peduncles. Cerebellar cortical atrophy is usually present. In the medulla there is atrophy and loss of neurons in the inferior olive. This change is secondary, and for this reason the name of the syndrome could be shortened to *pontocerebellar atrophy.*

Imaging usually shows flattening of the belli of the pons in lateral MR images, as well as diminution in the size of the pons; a decrease in the size of the medulla is usually observed. Transverse axial images on CT or MRI show pontine atrophy, enlargement of the fourth ventricle, and cerebellar atrophy (Figs. 8.15 and 8.16). OPCA can occur from the first to the fifth decade, and patients usually live for 8 to 15 years after onset. Along with Shy-Drager syndrome and striatonigral degeneration, OPCA may be considered part of multiple system atrophy, discussed in text following.

As noted, there are a number of nonspecific and somewhat more specific conditions causing cerebellar decrease in mass or true degeneration. Among these might be listed *cerebello-olivary degeneration,* which is difficult to differentiate from OPCA. However, CT or MRI, particularly on sagittal images, may demonstrate a predominance of atrophy in the anterior vermis. The age of onset is similar to that of OPCA, but evolution may be slower (Table 8.3).

Friedreich ataxia (spinocerebellar degeneration) is an autosomal recessive (also dominant) ataxic condition with an age of onset usually between 10 and 20 years. It is progressive, and affected children cannot walk within 5 years of onset. Kiphoscoliosis and pes cavus are typical manifestations. MRI may demonstrate spinal cord atrophy, particularly well shown in the cervical portion, but cerebellar atrophy may be only mild or cannot be ascertained because the primary pathology is cell loss in the dorsal root ganglia and secondary degeneration in the posterior columns and spinocerebellar tracts.

Other causes of cerebellar degeneration or atrophy as shown by cross-sectional imaging include alcohol abuse; toxicity from certain drugs, such as phenytoin (Dilantin) when used for a long time for the treatment of epilepsy, or cytosine arabinoside (60); and paraneoplastic disorders. However, by far the most frequently observed cerebellar atrophy is seen in the elderly and is not necessarily associ-

Table 8.3.
Differential Diagnosis of Nondementing Degenerative Diseases

Parkinson disease: Extrapyramidal dysfunction marked by tremor, rigidity, and "masklike" facies. MR findings of decrease in size of substantia nigra (pars compacta) and hypointensity of putamen on T2-weighted images.

Shy-Drager syndrome: Autonomic dysfunction manifested by postural hypotension, urinary incontinence, and nonspecific MR features.

Progressive supranuclear palsy (Steele-Richardson-Olszewski syndrome): Characterized by paresis of vertical gaze, dysarthria, and rigidity. MR findings include atrophy of the periaqueductal region and pars compacta of the substantia nigra.

Olivopontocerebellar degeneration: Clinical manifestations include ataxia and extrapyramidal dysfunction. MR findings include atrophy of the pons, medulla, and cerebellum, and enlargement of the fourth ventricle.

Table 8.4.
Considerations in Diagnosis of Cerebellar Atrophy

Age related
Related to toxins, including alcohol, phenytoin, some forms of chemotherapy
Paraneoplastic syndromes
Degenerative disorders (e.g., olivopontocerebellar degeneration)
Disorders of energy metabolism (e.g., mitochondrial encephalomyopathies)

ated with cerebellar manifestations. It may well be simply an aging phenomenon similar to cerebral atrophy and showing extreme variability between subjects (Table 8.4).

Marchiafava-Bignami Disease

Marchiafava-Bignami disease is a progressive degeneration involving the corpus callosum. It is seen in alcoholics, chiefly in Italy in consumers of crude red wine, but may be seen occasionally in other countries. The patients may present progressive intellectual deterioration, confusion, tremor and rigidity, hallucinations, and convulsions. Thinning of the corpus callosum may be seen on MRI, particularly in coronal and sagittal projections. See Chapter 9.

Multiple System Atrophy

This is a degenerative condition occurring sporadically in adults in which a variable combination of extrapyramidal, cerebellar, and autonomic nervous system changes occur. There are no biochemical markers, and the diagnosis is strictly based on clinical findings. Cloft et al. have presented evidence of some findings on MRI that may help in diagnosing this condition (61). They reported tapering of the anterior aspect of the pons on sagittal T1-weighted images, narrowing of the middle cerebellar peduncles, enlargement of the fourth ventricle, and reduced dimensions of the brainstem and cerebellum. The findings are not unlike those found early in patients with pontocerebellar degeneration, but these patients nevertheless may present a somewhat different clinical picture neurologically.

The concept of multiple system atrophy is now broadly applied to a group of four entities that heretofore have been described separately: (a) striatonigral degeneration; (b) Shy-Drager syndrome; (c) olivopontocerebellar atrophy; and (d) parkinsonism-amyotrophy syndrome (62). Lesions involve the neostriatum, the substantia nigra, the cerebellum, the inferior olives, the basal pontine nuclei, and the intermediolateral horn cells and anterior horn cells of the spinal cord. In striatonigral degeneration there is a Parkinsonlike syndrome that does not respond to levodopa because of cell loss. The presence of cerebellar symptoms would lean the diagnosis toward olivopontocerebellar atrophy. The latter presents degeneration of the olives, pons, and cerebellum and neuronal loss in the neostriatum and substantia nigra. When there is involvement of the intermediolateral horn cells, the case may fit the Shy-Drager syndrome (63). However, the separation between these syndromes may be difficult. Response to levodopa makes the diagnosis less clear; some cases may be difficult to differentiate from progressive supranuclear palsy.

Imaging findings may be helpful in arriving at a clinical diagnosis. Perhaps olivopontocerebellar atrophy is the variant that presents the best-developed imaging findings (64) (see text preceding and Figs. 8.15 and 8.16). The other variants do not reveal specific findings.

Motor Neuron Diseases

Local involvement of the motor cortex of the brain as well as the motor fibers and the pyramidal tract is a very common result of vascular, inflammatory, traumatic, and neoplastic conditions, but primary diseases of the motor system are uncommon. Among the few that are worth describing is *amyotrophic lateral sclerosis* (ALS), a disease that occurs in all parts of the world, and almost twice as frequently in males in middle age. It rarely starts before the age of 35 and starts with weakness, commonly accompanied by pain in one or more extremities. The disease is progressive, leading within a few to several years to complete disability and death. The cerebellum is not involved. The muscles become profoundly atrophic. The pathological findings consist in loss of the motor neurons, particularly in the anterior horn cells of the spinal cord, more noticeable in the cervical and lumbar enlargements, and in the hypoglossal nuclei. Changes in the white matter of the spinal cord are variable; usually there is degeneration of the pyramidal tracts that can be traced upwards to the white matter of the cerebral hemispheres, as well as in the lateral corticospinal tracts (65). MR T2-weighted images may demonstrate some diffuse hyperintensity in the brainstem following the pyramidal tract through the internal capsule and into the centrum semiovale.

Among the other diseases affecting the motor system may be listed *primary lateral sclerosis*, a disease that resembles amyotrophic lateral sclerosis but in which the primary pathology is in the large pyramidal cells of the precentral gyrus. This is accompanied by degeneration of the corticospinal and corticobulbar projections. It occurs sporadically, affecting the same age group as ALS, and leads to death within a similar period of time. The author has not seen an example of this disease, but findings on MRI may be expected to show changes involving the motor pathways on T2-weighted images. Another disease is *spinal muscular atrophy* (SMA), of which there are two main forms: the infantile form (Werdnig-Hoffmann disease), a severe, rapidly fatal condition (infants die within the first year), and the juvenile form, which runs a slow course. There are also other varieties of SMA. *Hereditary spastic paraplegia*, a rare disorder, is inherited as an autosomal dominant trait. It is clinically characterized by spastic paraparesis that progresses very slowly, sometimes permitting an essentially normal life span.

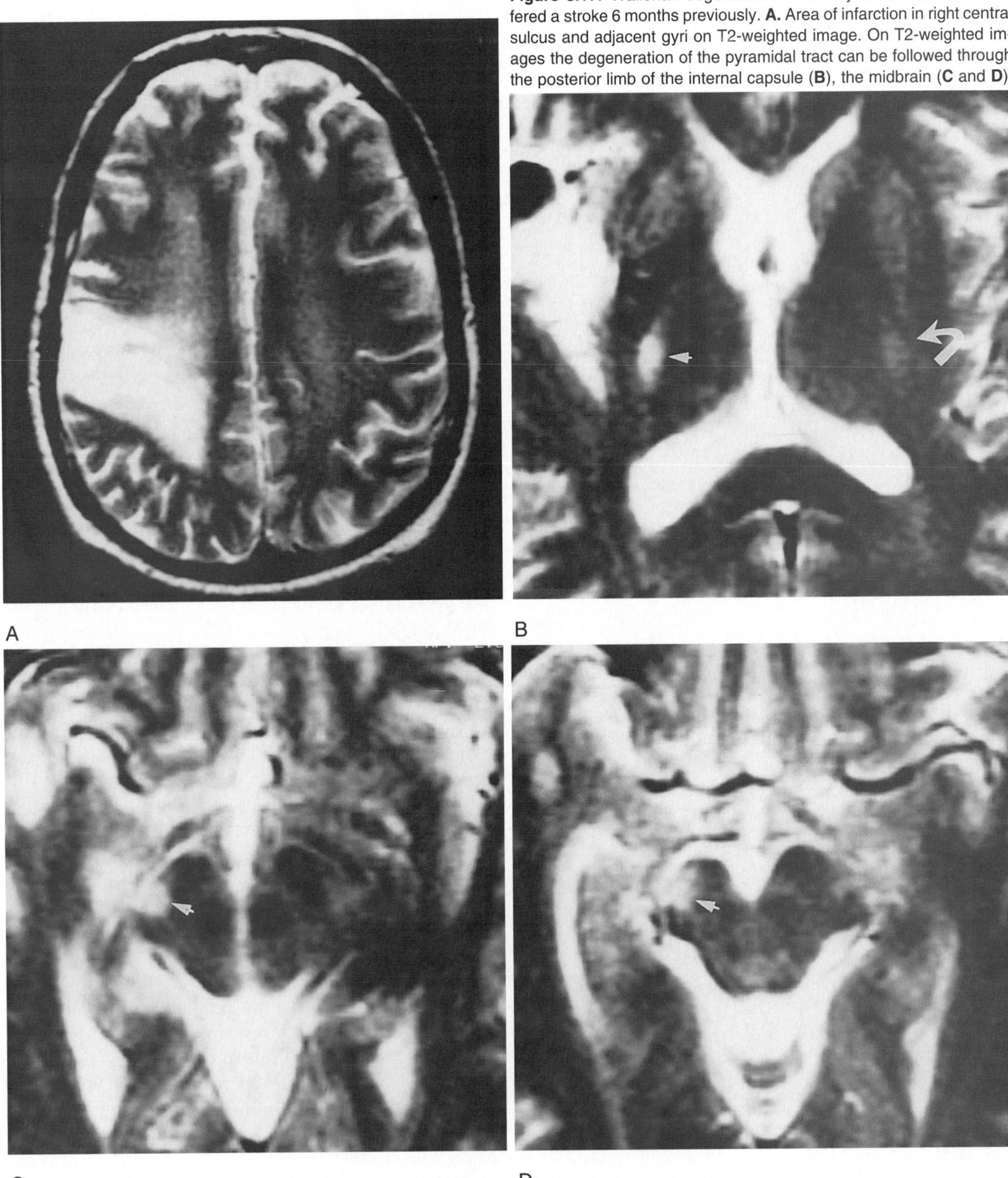

A B C D

Figure 8.17. Wallerian degeneration in a 42-year-old man who suffered a stroke 6 months previously. **A.** Area of infarction in right central sulcus and adjacent gyri on T2-weighted image. On T2-weighted images the degeneration of the pyramidal tract can be followed through the posterior limb of the internal capsule (**B**), the midbrain (**C** and **D**),

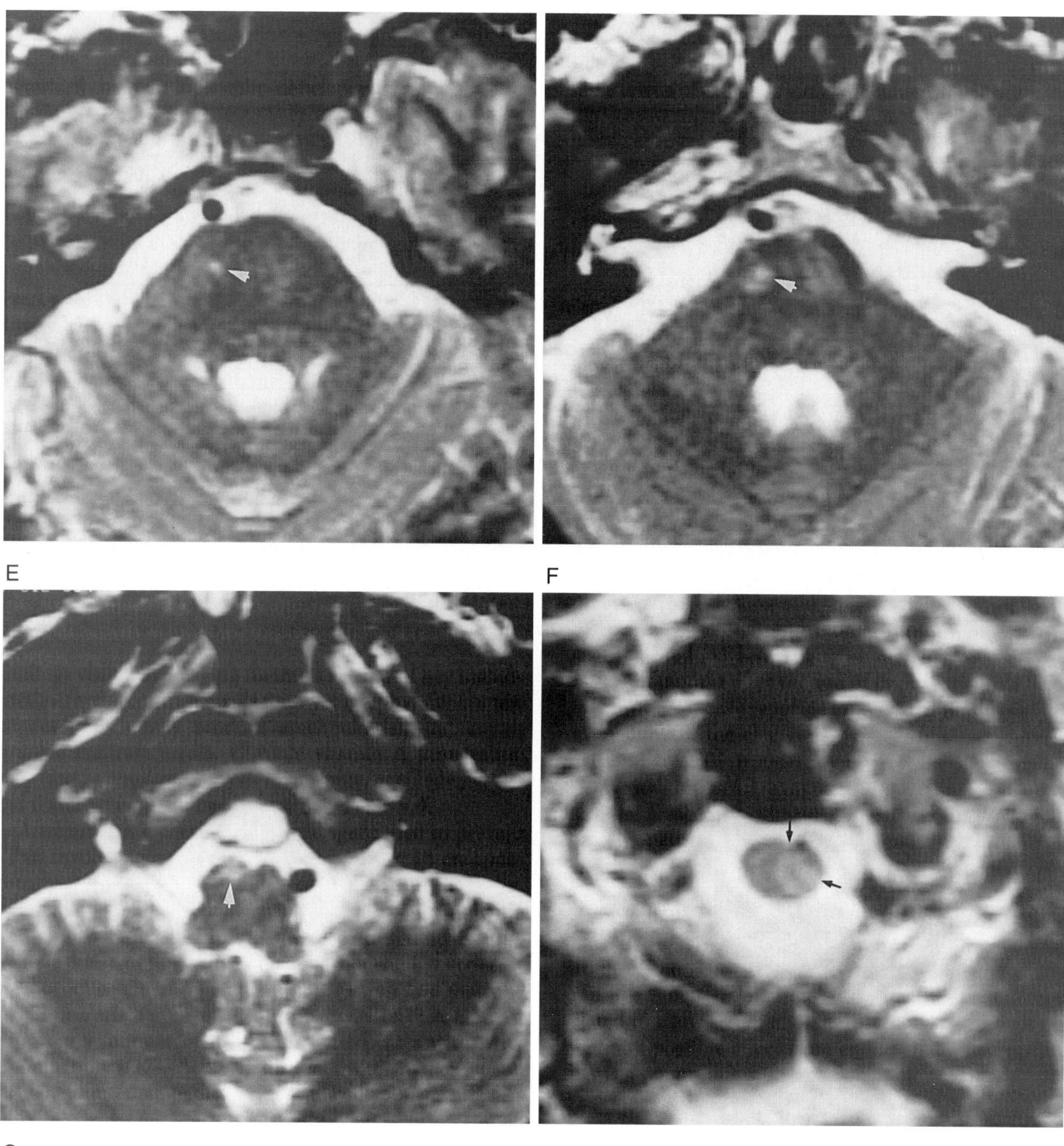

Figure 8.17. *(continued)* the upper pons (**E**), the lower pons (**F**), the upper medulla (**G**), and the lower medulla after decussation on the left side (**H**) (arrows). Note that on the left side there is a slightly hyperintense area in the internal capsule (curved arrow), in the same relationship with the adjacent structures presented by the focus of wallerian degeneration on the right internal capsule. The degenerated area marks the position of the corticospinal tract in the posterior limb of the internal capsule. The slightly hyperintense area on the left side is a frequent finding in normal individuals, and at present there is no clear explanation as to its histogenesis.

Juvenile amyotrophy of the distal upper extremity typically causes unilateral atrophy of the muscles of the distal forearm and hand. The condition occurs sporadically, almost always in boys. All seven of the cases reported by Biondi et al. were males ranging in age between 15 and 31 (66). All were or had been extremely active in sports, but no particular relation to an injury can be traced.

MRI reveals evidence of local cord atrophy on T1-weighted images in both the sagittal plane and the axial plane. The unilateral cord atrophy is subtle but can be well demonstrated. The atrophic process progresses up to a point and then arrests. There is no clinical evidence of pyramidal tract involvement. Five of the cases studied by Biondi et al. showed focal spinal cord findings on MRI in the cervical cord at the level of the fifth and sixth cervical vertebrae.

Wallerian Degeneration

Following the death of a neuronal cell body, there is degeneration of the entire arborization of the neuron, axon, and axonal branches and dendrites. Cell death occurs most frequently in the brain as a result of cerebral infarction, but may also be seen following hemorrhage, in cerebral neoplasms, and in demyelination. Kuhn et al. reported demonstrating wallerian degeneration on MRI also in a patient with movement disorder (67). The axons degenerate prior to the myelin sheath, a process that occurs rather rapidly, in a matter of 4 or 5 days. The entire degenerative phenomenon is completed in a year or in several years, depending on the location of the initial injury. In peripheral nerves, the process is completed more rapidly than in the central nervous system. Kuhn et al. describe four stages in the process of wallerian degeneration (68). In stage 1 there is degradation of the axon with little biochemical change; this lasts about 4 weeks and generates no imaging changes. In stage 2 (4 to 14 weeks) there is myelin protein breakdown. "Myelin lipids remain intact, and the tissues become more hydrophobic. The high lipid-protein ratio results in hypointense signal on T2W images." In stage 3 the tissues become more hydrophilic, and there is myelin lipid breakdown and gliosis. The chronic stage ensues, and the MR images become dark on T1-weighted images and bright on T2-weighted images. Stage 4 occurs 1 to several years later, and in this stage the appearance may be simply atrophy better seen in the brainstem, although in some instances some T2 brightness may remain (Figs. 8.17 [see pages 382–383] and 8.18).

On CT the only abnormality visible, with very few exceptions, is a decrease in the size of the corresponding aspect of the brainstem. This is because the degeneration follows the fiber tracts through the internal capsule, the midbrain, the pons, and the medulla along the pyramidal tract. By MRI, however, it is possible to follow the degenerative process through all these areas (Figs. 8.17 and 8.18). The lesion is low intensity on T1-weighted images and high intensity on T2-weighted images in the chronic stage. However, there is a stage when these appearances may be reversed; that is, the track of degeneration is bright on T1-weighted images and dark on T2-weighted images (stage 2), as discussed in the preceding paragraph (Fig. 8.18).

NEUROIMAGING IN PSYCHIATRIC CONDITIONS

Neuroimaging examinations have become an important component of the work-up of psychiatric patients. This has been increasingly recognized since the introduction of MRI, MR spectroscopy, and MR functional neuroimaging. Usually the imaging examinations are needed to exclude organic brain disease, and this can be done quickly and noninvasively by CT, and/or MRI.

The abnormalities represented by a histopathologic condition are likely to be visible with the imaging methods. The abnormalities related to a metabolic derangement are much more difficult to elucidate. Some may well be diagnosed by functional imaging methods in the future. PET offers the possibility of carrying out metabolic studies, and MR functional imaging offers a new approach to studying anatomy and physiology combined.

Abnormalities of glucose metabolism, as shown by PET and fluorodeoxyglucose, have been described in affective disorders and in schizophrenia (69–72).

Cerebral atrophy is a frequent finding in a high proportion of cases, particularly in the elderly, but it is nonspecific. There are ways of estimating, by MRI or CT, the relative percentage of the gray matter, the white matter, and the CSF (1). Focal asymmetries, such as may be produced by atrophy (or hypertrophy?) of a section of a cerebral hemisphere, can be seen. Shenton et al. have described such an asymmetry in patients with schizophrenia demonstrated by MRI (73). Others have used CT and MRI techniques to measure the temporal lobe as well as other structures (74–76).

Lesions such as hypoplasia of cerebellar vermis lobule have been reported in autism (77); the changes were evaluated in the sagittal MR images, and there were no corresponding signal changes.

Study of therapeutic drugs can be assisted by tagging the drugs with carbon 11 and using PET scanning to determine their localization and concentration in the brain. MR spectroscopy can be used for a similar purpose if the drug contains a paramagnetic compound such as fluor or lithium. For instance, the amount of lithium concentration in patients on long-term lithium therapy varies among subjects and cannot be predicted by the concentration in the serum (78). As mentioned earlier, proton MR spectroscopy can be used to study neuronal loss in AD because *N*-acetylaspartate is found only in the neuronal cells (38). Many organic diseases have psychiatric manifestation, and these have been discussed when appropriate.

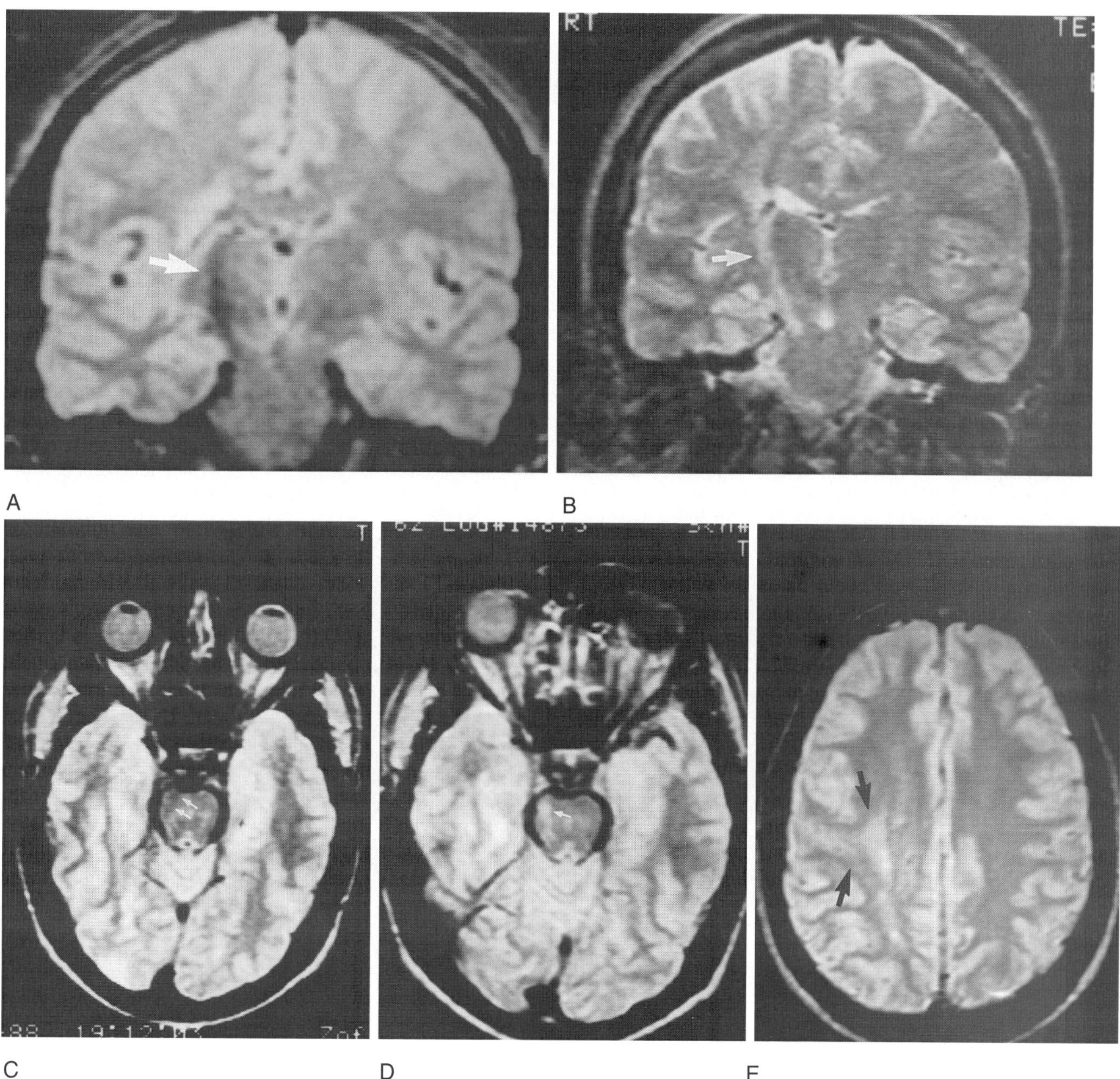

Figure 8.18. Wallerian degeneration as seen by MRI. **A.** This 31-year-old man developed a fronto-parietal infarction and within 2 months showed hypointensity on T2-weighted images along the pyramidal tract (arrow). **B.** Reexamination 4 months later shows that the same area is now hyperintense (arrow). In the brainstem the region of the peduncle of the midbrain was hypointense on T2-weighted images early on (**C**) (arrows) and hyperintense a few months later (**D,** arrow). **E.** Location of the original infarct in the right posterior frontal region (arrows).

We can expect that efforts that will tend to clarify the significance of anatomic, metabolic, and chemical deviations from the normal will continue as the availability of in vivo imaging technology increases.

Further details may be found in Chapter 14, "Selection of CT versus MR and Functional Neuroimaging."

REFERENCES

1. Malko JA, Hoffman JC, Green RC: MR measurement of intracranial CSF volume in 41 elderly normal volunteers. AJNR 1991;12: 371–374.
2. de Leon MJ, George AE, Reisberg B, et al: Alzheimer's disease: Longitudinal CT study of ventricular change. AJNR 1989;10: 371–376.
3. Gado M, Hughes CP, Danziger W, Chi D: Aging, dementia, and brain atrophy: A longitudinal computed tomography study. AJNR 1983;4:699–702.
4. George AE, de Leon MJ, Rosenbloom S, et al: Ventricular volume and cognitive deficit: A computer tomographic study. Radiology 1983;149:493–498.
5. Kohn MI, Tanna NK, Herman CT, et al: Analysis of brain and cerebrospinal fluid volumes with MR imaging. Radiology 1991;178: 115–122.
6. Rauch R, Jinkins JR: Change in corpus callosum size with advancing age in the presence and absence of cerebral atrophy in neurologically intact adults. Paper presented at the annual meeting of the American Society of Neuroradiology, Vancouver, 1993.
7. Imai A, Meyer JS, Kobari M, et al: LCBF values decline while LR values increase during normal human aging measured by stable xenon enhanced computed tomography. Neuroradiology 1988;30: 463–472.
8. de Leon MJ, George AE, Ferris SH, et al: Positron emission tomography and computed tomography assessment of the aging human brain. J Comput Assist Tomogr 1984;8:88–94.
9. Kobari M, Meyer JS, Ichijo M, et al: Leukoaraiosis: Correlation of MR and CT findings with blood flow, atrophy, and cognition. AJNR 1990;11:273–281.
10. Hendrie HC, Farlow MR, Austrom AG, et al: Foci of increased T2 signal intensity on brain MR scans of healthy elderly subjects. AJNR 1989;10:703–707.
11. Fazekas F, Kleinert R, Offenbacher H, et al: The morphologic correlate of incidental punctate white matter hyperintensities on MR images. AJNR 1991;12:915–921.
12. Awad IA, Spetzler RF, Hodak JA, et al: Incidental subcortical lesions identified on magnetic resonance imaging in the elderly: I. Correlation with age and cerebrovascular risk factors. Stroke 1986;17: 1084–1089.
13. Awad IA, Johnson PC, Spetzler RF, Hodak JA: Incidental subcortical lesions identified on magnetic resonance imaging in the elderly: II. Postmortem pathologic correlations. Stroke 1986;17:1090–1097.
14. Braffman BH, Zimmerman RA, Trojanowski JQ, et al: Brain MR: Pathologic correlation with gross and histopathology: 1. Lacunar infarction and Virchow-Robin spaces. AJNR 1988;9:621–628.
15. Braffman BH, Zimmerman RA, Trojanowski JQ, et al: Brain MR: Pathologic correlation with gross and histopathology: 2. Hyperintense white matter foci in the elderly. AJNR 1988;9:629–636.
16. Elster AD, Richardson DN: Focal high signal on MR scans of the midbrain caused by enlarged perivascular spaces: MR-pathologic correlation. AJNR 1990;11:1119–1122.
17. Brandt-Zawadzki M, Fein G, Dyke CV, et al: MR imaging of the aging brain: Patchy white-matter lesions and dementia. AJNR 1985; 6:675–682.
18. Bowen BC, Barber WW, Loewenstein DA, et al: MR signal abnormalities in memory disorder and dementia. AJNR 1990;11:283–290.
19. Sze G, DeArmond SJ, Brandt-Zawadzki M: Foci of MRI signal (pseudo lesions) anterior to the frontal horns: Histologic correlation of a normal finding. AJNR 1986;7:381–387.
20. Fueredi GA, Czarnecki DJ, Kindwall EP: MR findings in the brains of compressed-air tunnel workers: Relationship to psychometric results. AJNR 1991;12:67–70.
21. Mirowitz S, Sartor K, Gado MG, et al: Focal signal-intensity variations in the posterior internal capsule: Normal MR findings and distinction from pathologic findings. Radiology 1989;172:535–539.
22. Braffman BH, Grossman RI, Goldberg HI, et al: MR imaging of Parkinson disease with spin echo and gradient echo sequences. AJNR 1988;9:1093–1099.
23. Moody DM, Brown WR, Challa VR, et al: Periventricular venous collagenosis: Association with leukoaraiosis. Radiology 1995;194: 469–476.
24. Skoog I, Nilson L, Palmertz B, et al: A population-based study of dementia in 85-yr-olds. N Engl Med 1993;328:153–158.
25. Adams RD, Victor M: Principles of Neurology, ed 4. New York: McGraw-Hill, 1989.
26. Tomlinson BE, Corsellis JAN: Aging and the dementias. In JH Adams, JAN Corsellis, LW Duchen (eds), Greenfield's Neuropathology, ed 4. New York: Wiley, 1984, p. 973.
27. Mann DMA: The neuropathology of Alzheimer's disease: A review with pathogenetic, aetiological and therapeutic considerations. Mech Ageing Dev 1985;31:213–255.
28. Van Hoesen GW, Human BT, Damasio AR: Entorhinal cortex pathology in Alzheimer's disease. Hippocampus 1991;1:1–8.
29. Henderson VW, Finch CE: The neurobiology of Alzheimer's disease. J Neurosurg 1989;70:335–353.
30. Seltzer B, Sherwin I: A comparison of clinical features of early and late onset primary degenerative dementia. Arch Neurol 1983;40: 143–146.
31. Kido DK, Caine ED, Le May M, et al: Temporal lobe atrophy in patients with Alzheimer's disease. AJNR 1989;10:551–555.
32. Rusinek H, de Leon MJ, George AE, et al: Alzheimer disease: Measuring loss of cerebral gray matter with MR imaging. Radiology 1991;178:109–114.
33. Cutler NR, Haxby JV, Daura R, et al: Clinical history, brain metabolism, and neuropsychological function in Alzheimer's disease. Ann Neurol 1985;18:298–309.
34. Ohnishi T, Hoski H, Nagamachi S, et al: Regional cerebral blood flow study with 123I-IMP in patients with degenerative dementia. AJNR 1991;12:513–520.
35. Hellman RS, Tikofsby RS, Collier D, et al: Alzheimer's disease: Quantitative analysis of I-123-iodoamphetamine SPECT brain imaging. Radiology 1989;172:183–188.
36. Gonzalez RG, Fischman AJ, Guimaraes AR, et al: fMRI in evaluation of dementia: Correlation of abnormal dynamic cerebral blood volume measurements with changes in cerebral metabolism measured by 18FDG PET. AJNR, in press.
37. Bottomley PA, Cousius JP, Pendrey DC, et al: Alzheimer dementia: Quantification of energy metabolism and mobile phosphoesters with P-31 NMR spectroscopy. Radiology 1992;183:695–699.
38. McClure RJ, Kanfer JN, Panchalingam K, et al: Magnetic resonance spectroscopy and its application to aging and Alzheimer's disease. Neuroimaging Clin N Am 1995;5:69–86.
39. Gonzalez RG, Guimaraes AR, Moore GJ, et al: Quantitative in vivo ^{31}P magnetic resonance spectroscopy of Alzheimer's disease. Alzheimer Dis Assoc Disord, in press.
40. Doraiswamy PM, McDonald WM, Patterson L, et al: Interuncal distance as a measure of hippocampal atrophy: Normative data on axial MR imaging. AJNR 1993;14:141–143.
41. Early B, Escalona PR, Bouko OB, et al: Interuncal distance measurements in healthy volunteers and in patients with Alzheimer's disease. AJNR 1993;14:907–910.
42. de Leon MJ, Golomb J, George AC, et al: The radiologic prediction of Alzheimer disease: The atrophic hippocampal formation. AJNR 1993;14:897–906.
43. Newberg AB, Alvari A, Payer F: Single photon emission tomography in Alzheimer's disease and related disorders. Neuroimaging Clin N Am 1995;5:103–123.

44. Guimaraes AR, Schwartz P, Prakash MR, et al: Quantitative in vivo ^{1}H nuclear magnetic resonance spectroscopy imaging of neuronal loss in rat brain. Neuroscience, in press.
45. Loeb C, Gandolfo C, Croce R, et al: Dementia associated with lacunar infarction. Stroke 1992;23:1225–1229.
46. DeReuck J, Crevits L, DeCoster W, et al: Pathogenesis of Binswanger chronic progressive subcortical encephalopathy. Neurology 1980;30:920–928.
47. Moody DM, Bell MA, Challa VR: The corpus callosum, a unique white matter tract: Anatomic features that may explain sparing in Binswanger disease and resistance to flow of fluid masses. AJNR 1988;9:1051–1059.
48. Lotz PR, Ballinger WE, Quisling RG: Subcortical arteriosclerotic encephalopathy: CT spectrum and pathologic correlation. AJNR 1986;7:817–822.
49. Jack CR, Mokri B, Laws ER, et al: MR findings in normal pressure hydrocephalus: Significance and comparison with other forms of dementia. J Comput Assist Tomogr 1987;11:923–931.
50. Tournier-Lasserve E, Joutel A, Melki J, et al: Cerebral autosomal dominant arteriopathy with subcortical infarcts and leukoencephalopathy maps to chromosome 19 q 12. Nature Genetics 1993;3: 256–259.
51. Mas JL, Dilouya A, de Recondo JA: Familial disorder with subcortical ischemic strokes, dementia and leukoencephalopathy. Neurology 1992;42:1015–1019.
52. Groen JJ, Heckster REM: Computed tomography in Pick's disease: Findings in a family affected in three consecutive generations. J Comput Assist Tomogr 1982;6:907–911.
53. Brown AP, Lane JC, Marayama S, Vollmer DG: Whipple's disease presenting with isolated neurological symptoms: Case report. J Neurosurg 1990;73:623–627.
54. Larson EB: Illnesses causing dementia in the very elderly. N Engl J Med 1993;328:203–205.
55. Beal MR, Richardson EP Jr, Martin JB: Degenerative diseases of the nervous system. In Harrison's Principles of Internal Medicine, ed 12. New York: McGraw-Hill, 1991.
56. Oppenheimer DR: Diseases of the basal ganglia, cerebellum and motor neurons. In JH Adams, JAN Corsellis, LW Duchen (eds), Greenfield's Neuropathology, ed 4. New York: Wiley, 1984.
57. Savoiardo M, Strada L, Girotti F, et al: MR imaging in progressive supranuclear palsy and Shy-Drager syndrome. J Comput Assist Tomogr 1989;13:555–560.
58. Steele JC, Richardson JC, Olszewski J: Progressive supranuclear palsy. Arch Neurol 1964;10:333–359.
59. Brown R, Polinsky RJ, Di Chiro G, et al: MRI in autonomic failure. J Neurol Neurosurg Psychiatry 1987;50:913–914.
60. Miller L, Link MP, Bologna S, et al: Cerebellar atrophy caused by high-dose cytosine arabinoside: CT and MR findings. AJR 1989; 152:343–344.
61. Cloft HJ, Brunberg JA, Yobbagy J, Gilman S: Multiple system atrophy: Structural alterations demonstrated with MR imaging. Paper presented at the annual meeting of the American Society of Neuroradiology, Vancouver, 1993.
62. Quinn N: Multiple system atrophy: The nature of the beast. J Neurol Neurosurg Psychiatry 1989 (special suppl):78–89.
63. Fahn S: Parkinson's disease and other basal ganglion disorders. In AK Asbury, GM McKhann, WI McDonald (eds), Diseases of the Nervous System—Clinical Neurobiology. Philadelphia: Saunders, 1992.
64. Savoiardo M, Strada L, Girotti F, et al: Olivopontocerebellar atrophy: MR diagnosis and relationship to multisystem atrophy. Radiology 1990;174:693–696.
65. Friedman DP, Tartaglino LM: Amyotrophic lateral sclerosis: Hyperintensity of the corticospinal tracts on MR images of the spinal cord. AJR 1993;160:604–606.
66. Biondi A, Dormont D, Woitzner JI Jr, et al: MR imaging of the cervical cord in juvenile amyotrophy of distal upper extremity. AJNR 1989;10:263–268.
67. Kuhn MJ, Johnson KA, Davis KR: Wallerian degeneration: Evaluation with MR imaging. Radiology 1988;168:199–202.
68. Kuhn MJ, Mikulis DJ, Ayoub DM, et al: Wallerian degeneration after cerebral infarction: Evaluation with sequential MR imaging. Radiology 1989;172:179–182.
69. Phelps ME, Mazziotta JC, Gerner R, et al: Human cerebral glucose metabolism in affective disorders: Drug-free states and pharmacologic effects. J Cereb Blood Flow Metab 1983;3(suppl):S7–S8.
70. DeLisi LE, Buchsbaum MS, Holcomb HH, et al: Increased temporal lobe glucose use in chronic schizophrenic patients. Biol Psychiatry 1989;25:835–851.
71. Wiesel FA, Wik G, Sjögren I, et al: Regional brain glucose metabolism in drug free schizophrenic patients and clinical correlates. Acta Psychiatr Scand 1987;76:628–641.
72. Widen L, Blomqvist G, Greitz T, et al: PET studies of glucose metabolism in patients with schizophrenia. AJNR 1983;4:550–552.
73. Shenton ME, Kikinis R, Jolesz FA, et al: Abnormalities of the left temporal lobe and thought disorder in schizophrenia. New Engl J Med 1992;327:604–612.
74. Brown R, Colter N, Corsellis JAN, et al: Postmortem evidence of structural brain changes in schizophrenia: Differences in brain weight, temporal horn area, and parahippocampal gyrus compared with affective disorder. Arch Gen Psychiatry 1986;43:36–42.
75. Falkai P, Bogerts B, Rosumek M: Limbic pathology in schizophrenia: The entorhinal region—a morphometric study. Biol Psychiatry 1988;24:515–521.
76. Colter N, Battal S, Crow TJ, et al: White matter reduction in the parahippocampal gyrus of patients with schizophrenia. Arch Gen Psychiatry 1987;44:1023.
77. Courchesne E, Yeung-Courchesne R, Press BA, et al: Hypoplasia of cerebellar vermal lobules VI and VII in autism. New Engl J Med 1988;318:1349–1354.
78. Gonzales RG, Guimaraes AR, Sachs GS, et al: Measurement of human brain lithium in vivo by MR spectroscopy. AJNR 1993;14: 1027–1037.

SELECTED READINGS

Baloh RW, Yee RD, Honrubia V: Late cortical cerebellar atrophy: Clinical and occulographic features. Brain 1986;109:159–180.

Burger PC, Burch JG, Kunze V: Subcortical arteriosclerotic encephalopathy (Binswanger's disease): A vascular etiology of dementia. Stroke 1976;7:626–631.

Hachinski VC, Potter P, Messby H: Leukoaraiosis. Arch Neurol 1987; 44:21–23.

Heier LA, Bauer CJ, Schwartz L, et al: Large Virchow-Robin spaces: MR-clinical correlation. AJNR 1989;10:929–936.

Johnson KA, Davis KR, Buonanno FS, et al: Comparison of magnetic resonance and roentgen ray computed tomography in dementia. Arch Neurol 1987;44:1075–1080.

Kuhn MJ, Taveras JM: Small bright foci on T2-weighted magnetic resonance images and associated disorders. In JM Taveras, J Ferrucci (eds), Radiology: Diagnosis/Imaging/Intervention. Philadelphia: Lippincott, 1985, chap 40, vol 3.

Loes DJ, Biller J, Yuh WTC, et al: Leukoencephalopathy in cerebral amyloid angiopathy: MR imaging in four cases. AJNR 1990;11: 485–488.

Osborn RE, Alder DC, Mitchell CS: MR imaging of the brain in patients with migraine headaches. AJNR 1991;12:521–524.

Soges LJ, Cacayorin ED, Petro GR, Ramachandran TS: Migraine evaluation by MR. AJNR 1988;9:425–429.

Tracey I, Phil D, Carr CA, et al: Brain choline-containing compounds are elevated in HIV+ patients prior to onset of AIDS dementia complex: [1]H magnetic resonance spectroscopic study. Neurology, in press.

9

Toxic and Iatrogenic Conditions

TOXIC ENCEPHALOPATHY

In the complex world in which we live, many factors can affect the brain—not only the adult brain, but particularly the developing brain in utero and in early infancy, when it is much more vulnerable. With Valk et al. we will divide the origin of the agents that may produce a toxic encephalopathy into two main categories: endogenous and exogenous (1).

Endogenous Agents

Endogenous agents are included in the inborn errors of metabolism. Typical examples are maple syrup urine disease, phenylketonuria, and globoid cell leukodystrophy (Krabbe disease). These have been described in Chapter 5, "Congenital Metabolic Anomalies."

Exogenous Agents

The exogenous toxic agents include (a) *external toxic* substances, the largest group, and (b) those processes within the body, but outside the central nervous system, that produce toxins that can cross the blood-brain barrier, which Valk et al. classify as *exogenous-internal.* (See Table 9.1.)

EXOGENOUS-INTERNAL AGENTS

The exogenous-internal group includes some of the known toxins such as the diphtheria bacteria and *Escherichia coli,* which are capable of producing an encephalopathy. It also includes such conditions as Wilson disease, which is characterized by ceruloplasmin deficiency. The deficiency causes encephalopathy secondary to copper accumulation in the globus pallidus and other related areas (see Chapter 5). Hepatic encephalopathy is seen in hepatic failure and produces findings in the basal ganglia (T1 hyperintensity) believed to be a toxic effect from hyperammonemia (see under Chapter 13, "Systemic Diseases Affecting the Central Nervous System"). Central pontine myelinolysis results from hyponatremia and is usually related to chronic alcoholism. The precipitating factor may be rapid correction of the hyponatremia by aggressive intravenous fluids (see Chapter 4, "Myelin and Demyelination").

EXOGENOUS-EXTERNAL AGENTS

Among the exogenous-external agents, which are the most numerous, there are a number of well-known toxic agents and others that are less well known.

Carbon Monoxide

Carbon monoxide produces a hypoxic state in the brain (Table 9.2). The most common areas to show early changes by CT or MRI are the white matter of the centrum semiovale (23 of 60 cases in the series of Miura et al. (2) examined by CT only) and of the globus pallidus (18 of 60 cases). More severe cases will show loss of the normal gray/white matter differentiation due to diffuse brain edema and patchy areas of cortical gray matter involvement on MRI. The ventricles are usually compressed. The changes may be seen within 8 h and are more clearly developed at 24 h. The causes in the series of Miura et al. (2) and of Kim et al. (3) were natural gas inhalation for suicide or accidental smoke inhalation, inhalation of automobile exhaust, and inhalation of domestic coal gas. In the Kim et al. series, globus pallidus hypodensity was the most common finding. Death is frequent, and moderate to severe disability may persist; some remain in a permanent vegetative state. Severe white matter changes carry a poor prognosis, and the same is true of extensive globus pallidus low density extending to the adjacent internal capsule. Delayed encephalopathic changes may be observed (4).

Methyl Alcohol (Methanol)

Methyl alcohol intoxication may produce changes in the putamen bilaterally that may be hemorrhagic because of necrosis. The localization in the putamen is typical (5).

Table 9.1.
Exogenous Toxic Substances Affecting the CNS

External toxins
- Alcohol
- Substances of abuse
- Carbon monoxide
- Methyl alcohol
- Lead
- Arsenic
- Organic mercury

Internal toxins
- Microorganisms (e.g., diphtheria, *E. coli*)
- Elements (e.g., Wilson disease)
- Disorders of sodium balance

Source: Adapted from Valk et al: AJNR 1992;13:747–760.

Lead

Lead encephalopathy occurs in children, and in adults a neuropathy develops. The lead encephalopathy may present edema that might be seen on CT or MRI, but the most important contribution of imaging is in detecting hyperdensity of the epiphyseal area of the long bones in growing children. Organic lead compounds, mostly tetraethyl lead, may be toxic at lower levels. It is the agent that produces encephalopathy (lesions in the hippocampus) in gasoline sniffers and in workers around storage tanks that formerly contained leaded gasoline.

Arsenic

Arsenic produces a peripheral neuropathy and does not involve the brain.

Organic Mercury and Other Toxins

Organic mercury intoxication may occur by eating contaminated fish (Minamata disease) or by eating seed that has been treated with a methyl mercury fungicide. Neuropathology shows degeneration of the granular layer of the cerebellum and patchy loss of cells in the cerebral cortex, particularly in the region of the calcarine fissure. Magnetic resonance imaging (MRI) made with a magnetic susceptibility technique will show changes in these areas (1,6). This is an excellent example of what Valk et al. refer to as *selective vulnerability*, for the most prominent clinical symptoms are cerebellar ataxia and constriction of the visual fields (Fig. 9.1).

A number of metals and compounds to which workers may be exposed are toxic and may affect the central or peripheral nervous system (manganese, tellurium, platinum [used in chemotherapy as cisplatin], thallium, triethyltin, trimethyltin, aluminum, gold, and cadmium). However, there are no specific imaging findings.

A number of industrial agents may also cause neurologic involvement, mostly neuropathy. They may be polymerizers (acrylamide, allyl chloride, etc.) or various chemicals and solvents: barium in soluble salts, toluene diisocyanate, hydrogen cyanide (accidental inhalation), toluene (inhalation in solvent mixtures [7]), and others.

Table 9.2.
Carbon Monoxide Poisoning

CT and MR findings seen within first 24 h.

Combination of focal findings (globus pallidus and centrum semiovale) against backdrop of diffuse brain edema.

Globus pallidus hypodensity on CT or hyperintensity on T2-weighted MRI is most specific finding.

Involvement of white matter pathways is associated with poor prognosis.

Alcohol

Chronic alcoholism may produce important changes in the brain (Table 9.3). These changes may be partly due to malnutrition. Some alcoholics obtain as much as 50 percent of their calories from ethanol, and some develop serious nutritional deficiencies, particularly for protein, thiamine, folate, and pyridoxine (8). Some alcoholics develop neurologic manifestations and signs of malnutrition whereas others do not; this difference may be due to some poorly understood genetic factors.

Alcoholic cerebellar degeneration is a relatively common occurrence in chronic alcoholics. It may occur in well-nourished alcoholics (9) without other neurologic manifestations, but may be associated with a polyneuropathy. The vermis seems to be more involved than other parts of the cerebellum.

Wernicke encephalopathy is seen most commonly in chronic alcoholics but also occurs in other conditions: starvation, hepatic failure, malignancies, disseminated tuberculosis, chronic hemodialysis, inadequate parenteral nutrition, persistent vomiting, hyperemesis gravidarum, and anorexia nervosa, or refusal to eat (10). The symptoms vary but include confusion, apathy, encephalopathy, gait ataxia, and conjugate gaze defects. The onset may be abrupt, with double vision and truncal ataxia. MRI may assist in the diagnosis. Atrophy of the mammillary bodies is fairly specific. Enhancement of the mammillary body may be the only sign in the acute stage (11). In the acute stage, low density in the periaqueductal area and around the third ventricle may be seen on computed tomography (CT). T2-weighted images show hyperintensity in these areas that

Table 9.3.
Alcohol Intoxication

Cerebellar degeneration
- Preferential involvement of cerebellar vermis.

Wernicke encephalopathy
- Due to thiamine deficiency of any cause.
- Characterized clinically by confusion, gait ataxia, and conjugate gaze deficits.
- Sites of involvement include periaqueductal gray matter, mammillary bodies, thalamus, and hypothalamus.
- Periaqueductal region appears hypodense on CT, hyperintense on T2-weighted MR images.
- Bithalamic hyperintensities on T2-weighted MRI may be seen.

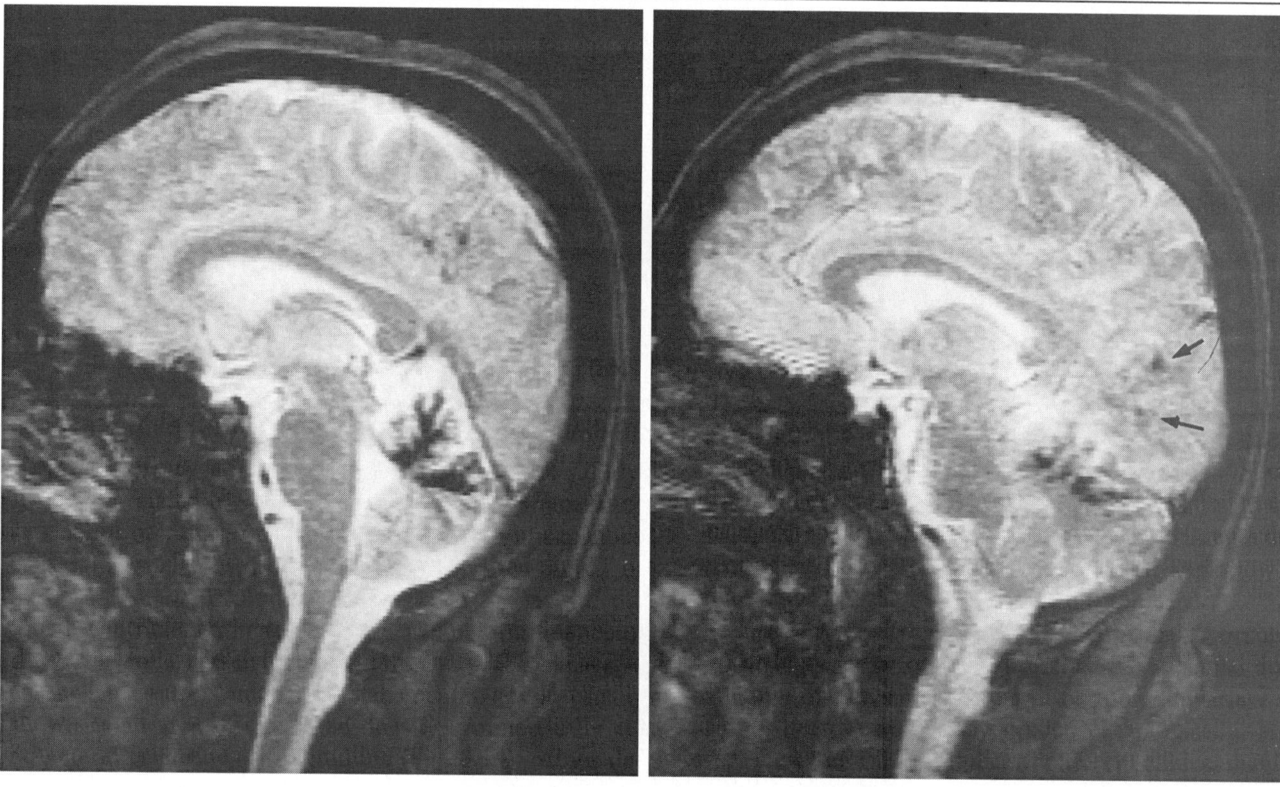

Figure 9.1. Mercury poisoning. **A** and **B.** Sagittal proton density weighted images show marked hypointensity in the cerebellar white matter and patchy areas of hypointensity in the medial parieto-occipital region involving also the area of the calcarine fissure (arrow in B). The location of the magnetic susceptibility changes is typical of mercury poisoning. (Courtesy of Jacob Valk and M. S. van der Knaap, Free University Hospital Amsterdam, Holland; AJNR 1992;13:747–760, with permission.)

tends to improve in the chronic stage or after treatment with thiamine (12). The lesions seen on MRI are sometimes bithalamic, and may sometimes disappear altogether (13). Following treatment, some of the changes tend to persist. Gallucci et al. indicate that the aqueduct may remain dilated because of atrophy of the periaqueductal area, and the third ventricle is enlarged (12) (Fig. 9.2).

Korsakoff psychosis is often associated with Wernicke encephalopathy. It affects learning ability and memory more than other qualities, so the individual may appear otherwise normal. When a Wernicke-affected patient (usually a man) recovers, he or she may remain amnesic, in which case the term *Wernicke-Korsakoff syndrome* is appropriate (14). Patients may die in the acute stage of the disease, and autopsy usually shows lesions in the thalamus and hypothalamus, symmetrically, as well as in the periaqueductal region and in the floor of fourth ventricle. Various degrees of necrosis are found, and hemorrhagic lesions are encountered in 20 percent of cases, but these might be agonal (14).

It should be remembered that minor degrees of Wernicke encephalopathy in the absence of alcoholism are probably far more common than we are used to thinking because of the frequency of prolonged courses of dialysis, intravenous hyperalimentation, gastric plications in the treatment of marked obesity, and prolonged use of dextrose and water without vitamin supplementation for long-term illnesses (11).

As indicated earlier, other forms of alcohol, such as methanol, are severe poisons and produce cerebral changes rapidly (15). Putamenal necrosis and hemorrhage, and diffuse white matter changes are encountered. Death or total disability may ensue.

Marchiafava-Bignami disease is also a syndrome that is associated with alcohol. It was first described in heavy drinkers of Italian red wine, but was later described as occurring outside Italy (France, Americas). Corpus callosum demyelination is the most characteristic feature and can be seen on MRI (16). See also Chapter 4, "Myelin and Demyelination."

Drug Abuse

This is a large chapter in medicine and neurology, but most of the hallucinogens, stimulants, opiates, and sedatives do not produce findings that can be observed on CT or MRI. The sympathomimetic drugs, cocaine and amphetamine,

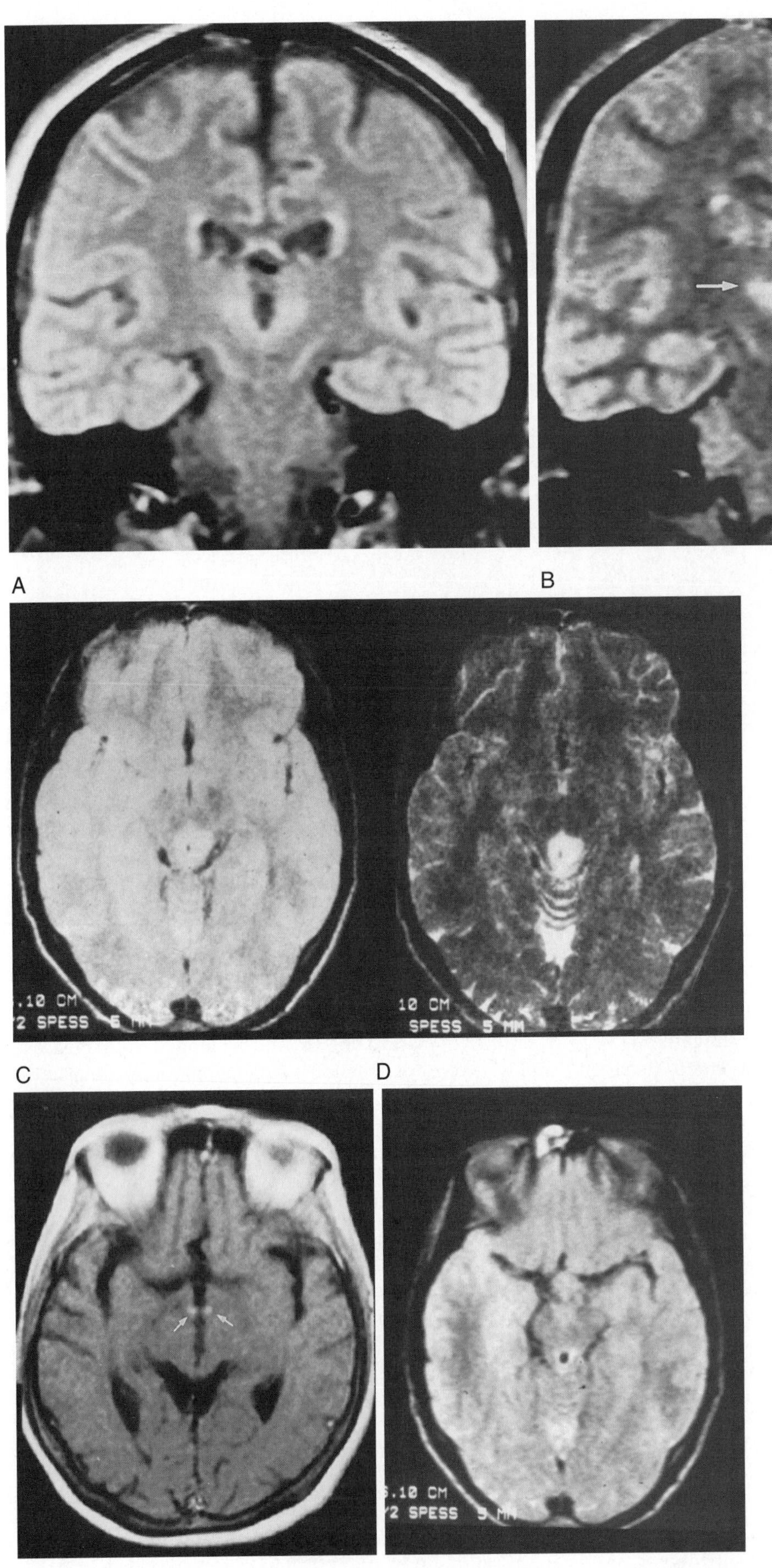

Figure 9.2. Wernicke encephalopathy. **A** and **B.** Coronal proton density images in a 39-year-old alcoholic woman, who developed abrupt bilateral third-nerve palsy, stupor, and ataxia, show hyperintensity around the third ventricle in A and in the hypothalamus (wing-shaped) around the lower half of the third ventricle in B (arrows). **C** and **D.** Proton density and T2-weighted axial images show marked hyperintensity in periaqueductal region of the midbrain. **E.** There is hyperintensity of the mammillary tubercles (arrows). On CT examination (not shown) the changes consist of hypodensity in the hypothalamus and in the periaqueductal region, a picture similar to what is seen on T1-weighted MR images. The changes tend to disappear with vitamin B therapy and elimination of alcohol, but atrophy in the involved areas usually occurs. The aqueduct becomes larger (**F**), the third ventricle also becomes larger, and the mammillary tubercles become much smaller. (Courtesy of Dr. Massimo Gallucci, Universita dell Aquila, Italy; AJNR 1990;11: 887–892, with permission.)

may be associated with strokes (17), and these are usually attributed to arterial spasm and/or vasculitis. In the experimental work of Wang et al., arterial spasm in animals was observed when the two drugs were used in combination and was not demonstrated when either one was used alone (18). Cerebral hemorrhage and subarachnoid hemorrhage have been reported in cocaine addicts (19–22). Cocaine in the pregnant mother leads to severe congenital anomalies in the fetus (23).

Vascular changes (arterial spasm) have been reported in amphetamine abusers both angiographically and pathologically (Fig. 9.3) (24,25). Heroin inhalation may cause leukoencephalopathy (26).

SELECTIVE VULNERABILITY

In dealing with toxic and iatrogenic disease, the concept of *selective vulnerability* is important in that many toxic substances and food or vitamin deficiencies affect specific areas of the brain or the peripheral nervous system. The thiamine deficiency related to *Wernicke encephalopathy* affects specifically the hypothalamus, the mammillary bodies, the dorsal medial thalamus, and the periaqueductal matter (Fig. 9.2). Chronic mercury poisoning affects the cerebellum and the cortical brain matter in the visual cortex (Fig. 9.1). The globus pallidus is affected early in carbon monoxide poisoning. The basal ganglia are particularly vulnerable to ischemia, as well as to many other toxic or metabolic agents. Thus pathologic changes are frequently observed in these areas by CT or MRI, particularly the latter, in a number of disease states (Wilson disease, hypoparathyroidism, Leigh disease, Fahr disease, liver failure, kernicterus).

Myelin is a frequent example of selective vulnerability. It has a high lipid content and a slow turnover and is particularly sensitive to the accumulation of lipophilic substances and to lipid peroxidation. *Hexachlorophene encephalopathy*, found in infants with skin problems who are washed with hexachlorophene solution, is an example (due to greater permeability of infants' skin). The vacuolating myelinopathy associated with hexachlorophene has also been reported in women using vaginal tampons, and in burned patients in which these antiseptic solutions were used (1).

Central pontine myelinolysis is another interesting example of selective vulnerability; the low serum sodium and the rapid correction of this state lead to an osmotic myelinolysis that may also involve, less frequently, the thalami, putamina, caudate nuclei, and subcortical white matter (see Chapter 4, "Myelin and Demyelination," and Fig. 4.65).

CENTRAL NERVOUS SYSTEM (CNS) REACTIONS TO MEDICAL AND SURGICAL TREATMENT

These include reactions to pharmaceutical agents, radiation injury to the nervous system, and postoperative changes.

Pharmaceutical Agents

Pharmaceutical agents are known to produce neurotoxic effects in inappropriate dosages or in sensitive individuals. The list is fairly long, but the agents that would produce

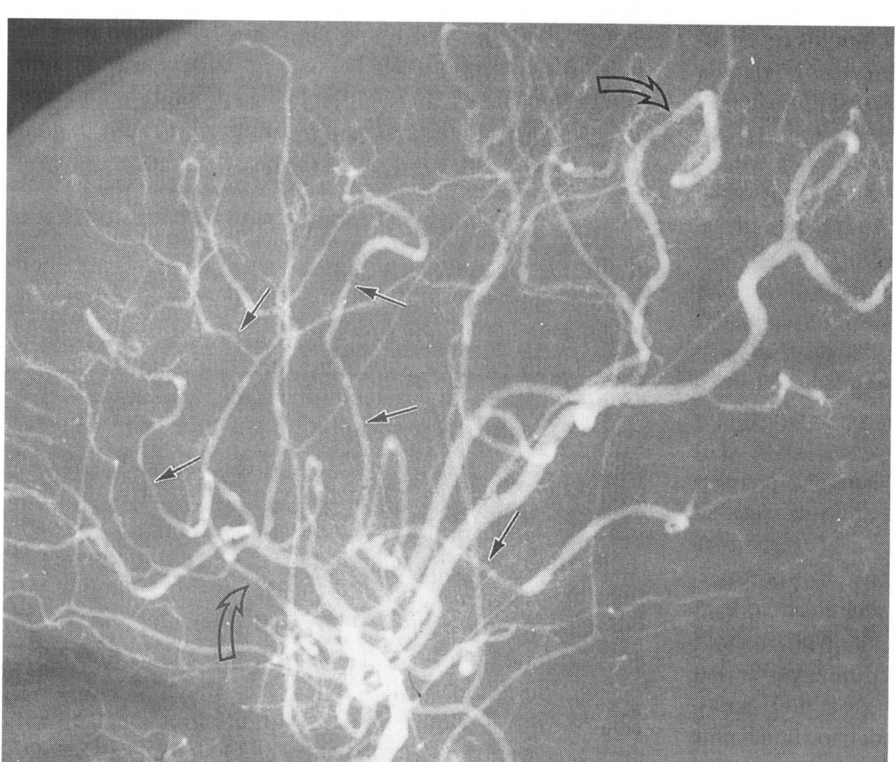

Figure 9.3. Extensive segmental spasm in a patient addicted to drugs (amphetamine, marijuana). There are a number of narrowed areas in the distal arteries (arrows). Such areas usually indicate arterial spasm. The patient was brought in with obtundation, right hemiplegia, and aphasia. There was rapid improvement following the withdrawal of drugs.

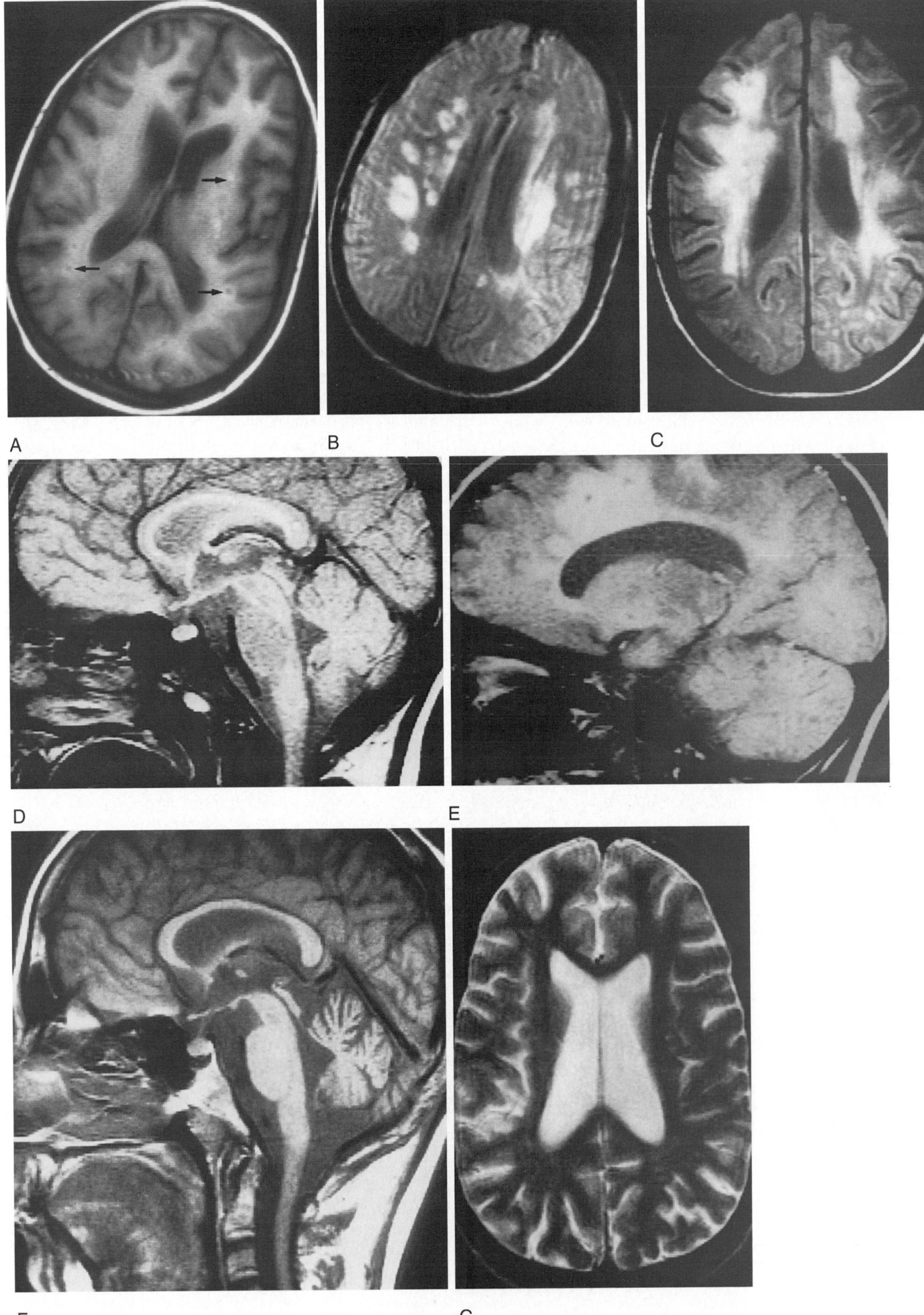

A
B
C
D
E
F
G

Table 9.4.
Therapeutic Agents that May Produce CNS Reactions

Methotrexate
Chemical arachnoiditis
Disseminated necrotizing leukoencephalopathy
Cyclosporin A
Encephalopathy, seizures, cortical blindness
Reversible white matter hyperintensities on T2-weighted imaging
Phenytoin
Cerebellar atrophy
Vitamin A intoxication
Pseudotumor cerebri syndrome (papilledema, visual disturbance, headache)

findings visible by imaging methods are few. They include methotrexate, contrast media for myelography, spinal anesthetics (which may produce arachnoiditis), and angiographic contrast media. Chronic vitamin A intoxication may cause a *pseudotumor cerebri* syndrome, papilledema, visual disturbances, and headaches. See Table 9.4.

Methotrexate, a chemotherapeutic agent used to prevent CNS involvement in leukemia, can produce an encephalopathy whether injected intravenously or intrathecally. Methotrexate inhibits the enzyme dihydrofolate reductase and prevents folic acid from converting to tetrahydrofolic acid. It does not normally cross the blood-brain barrier. It may produce chemical arachnoiditis as well as a disseminated necrotizing leukoencephalopathy. Ebner et al. have reported a number of well-documented cases with MRI examinations (27). Acutely, diffuse white matter edema may be found that, pathologically, may demonstrate spongiosis of white matter and chronic edema. Interestingly enough, the edema seems to spare the basal ganglia. Later, cerebral atrophy as well as persistence of white matter lesions indicative of tissue loss are found (Fig. 9.4). In milder cases the brain may return to a nearly normal state (28). Calcification in the cortex and subcortical areas may be seen later (29). Chemical arachnoiditis (or arachnoidal adhesions) may be produced by intrathecal methotrexate and also by myelographic agents and spinal anesthesia (see Chapter 16).

Figure 9.4. Methotrexate-induced encephalopathy in a 15-year-old girl with osteogenic sarcoma of distal tibia. Neurologic dysfunction started about 2 weeks after the seventh high-dose methotrexate treatment, with convulsions, intermittent loss of consciousness, generalized seizures, and status epilepticus. **A.** T1-weighted axial images show a number of hypointense foci (arrows) in white matter bilaterally surrounded by slightly hyperintense halo (arrows). **B.** Proton density weighted images showed numerous hyperintense patches in the white matter, which 4 weeks later became confluent (**C**). **D** and **E.** Sagittal proton density equivalent images (1600/60), showed hyperintense changes in the medulla, midbrain, corpus callosum, and cingulate gyrus, as well as the cerebellum. **F** and **G.** Sagittal T1-weighted and axial T2-weighted images 4 years later showed disappearance of lesions. The ventricles are moderately enlarged, as previously, but the cerebellum now shows moderate atrophy. (Courtesy of Professor F. Ebner, Karl-Franzens-University, Graz, Austria; AJNR 1989;10: 959–964, with permission.)

Phenytoin (Dilantin), a classic anticonvulsant, may produce cerebellar involvement resulting in cerebellar atrophy that is demonstrable by CT or MRI. The ataxia may improve following discontinuation of the medication, but the atrophy remains (30).

Cyclosporin A is known to present neurotoxic effects. It is an important immunosuppression agent that is used in organ transplantation, usually in liver transplants but also in renal, cardiac, and bone marrow transplants. The symptoms consist of seizures and altered mental status; cortical blindness and speech and motor disturbances have also been reported (31,32). The symptoms may occur 1 week to several months after the use of cyclosporin A is begun.

Truwit et al. have reported on the MRI findings and the reversibility of the changes (33). The findings consist of scattered areas of hypodensity on CT and hyperintensity on T2-weighted MR images with a predilection for the occipital area, which explains the cortical blindness found in some patients. The lesions are mostly reversible and may be due to focal cerebral edema induced by paroxysmal hypertension in a patient who may have some disruption of the blood-brain barrier (Fig. 9.5). The occipital predilection tends to favor this theory in view of the occipital localization of the acute hypertensive encephalopathy changes seen in eclampsia. The other theory is that the effects are related to a low serum cholesterol level (32). Truwit et al. suggest a possible effect from endothelin, a neuropeptide that is a potent diffusible vasoconstrictor (33).

Radiation Effects in the Brain and Spinal Cord

It is well known that with full therapeutic dosages of radiation, the brain tissue around the treated neoplasm may present irradiation changes (Table 9.5). The brain, because of its low rate of cell division, which involves only the glia, is considered to be among the more radioresistant tissues. However, radiation effects are frequently encountered following treatment for brain neoplasms, and sometimes for cancer of the nasopharynx, the orbits, the olfactory area, or the frontal sinuses (34). The mechanism is direct injury to macromolecules and, particularly in the presence of oxygen, the formation of peroxide and superoxide free radicals.

Table 9.5.
CNS Radiation Effects

Spectrum of changes ranging from edema and demyelination to coagulative necrosis.
White matter involved more than gray matter.
Predominantly white matter hyperintensities on T2-weighted MR images.
Severe cases enhance after contrast administration.
PET scanning most reliable method for distinguishing residual or recurrent tumor from radiation necrosis.

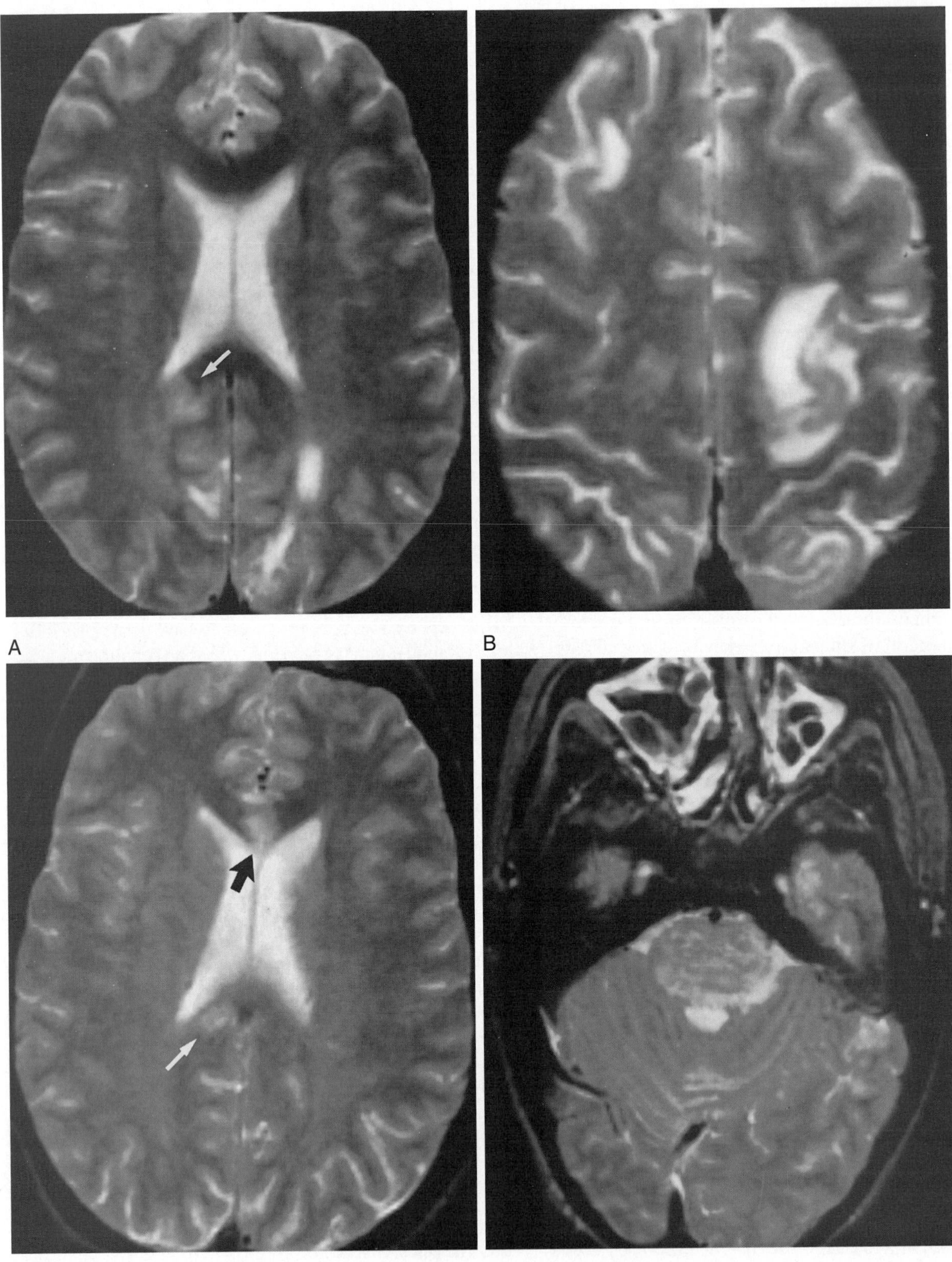

Figure 9.5. Cyclosporin neurotoxicity. **A** and **B.** The patient is a 33-year-old woman following cardiac transplant and treatment with cyclosporin A; the neurotoxicity was manifested by generalized seizures with right arm involvment preceded by severe headache. There is involvement of the splenium of the corpus callosum (arrow), and there are hyperintense subcortical white matter patches in both hemispheres. The patient was placed on phenytoin therapy and improved. The white matter changes disappeared. Subsequently, the cyclosporin dosage was increased, and about 2 weeks later the patient had another episode of seizures and headache; examination again demonstrated involvement of the splenium and now also the rostrum of the corpus callosum (**C**). In addition, there is hyperintensity in the pons on T2-weighted images (**C** and **D**). The phenytoin therapy was reinstituted, and the patient improved. All lesions disappeared in 2 weeks. (Courtesy of Charles L. Truwit, University of Minnesota, Minneapolis; AJNR 1991; 12:651–659, with permission.)

Some areas, such as the brainstem and the spinal cord, are more sensitive to radiation than others.

Early changes may occur in the first 2 to 4 weeks but are usually not seen in clinical practice because the treatment is started with low dosages that are slowly raised in subsequent visits. Thus we are concerned with later effects. The delayed effects may present as an acutely developing space-occupying lesion affecting the white matter more than the gray matter. Histologically edema, demyelination, and necrosis are found. In severe cases there is a coagulative necrosis of all elements. The vessels may show endothelial proliferation and perivascular fibrosis. The majority of cases show hyperintensity of the white matter on T2-weighted MR images. In many cases the T1-weighted image shows no hypointensity and the CT images may be normal or nearly normal (Fig. 9.6) (35). The white matter edema may be localized to the treated area, or the entire hemisphere may show changes if it was exposed to a high dose of radiation. If the whole brain was treated, the edema may involve both hemispheres. This is a chronic edema that does not enhance after contrast and is not associated with an increase in the size of the involved area. There is usually no midline shift or displacement of structures (Fig. 9.6). On the contrary, cases in which there is a coagulative necrosis show a mass effect and marked enhancement with contrast, making it difficult to differentiate between tumor recurrence (or tumor extension from an adjacent tumor) and radionecrosis.

In cases of coagulative necrosis, CT and MRI are not helpful, and it is necessary to use a different approach to diagnosis and therapeutic decision making. At the author's institution, we use positron emission tomography (PET) scanning with fluorodeoxyglucose. A malignant tumor is hypermetabolic and would show increased uptake, whereas radionecrosis would show no metabolic activity (Fig. 9.7) (36). An effort has been made to develop other means of differentiating between tumor and radionecrosis, and single photon emission tomography (SPECT) has been proposed. SPECT shows increased blood flow through a recurrent tumor, whereas radionecrosis would not show an increase. Also, if a dual isotope is used, the tumor may show increased thallium uptake (37). More recently, MRI measurement of blood volume may lead to other methods, all of which would tend to decrease the need for PET scanning.

Postoperative Changes

Acute postoperative changes are extremely variable and depend on the type of surgery performed. In the immediate postoperative period, there is swelling of the brain in the local area, and a subdural collection of fluid may be present.

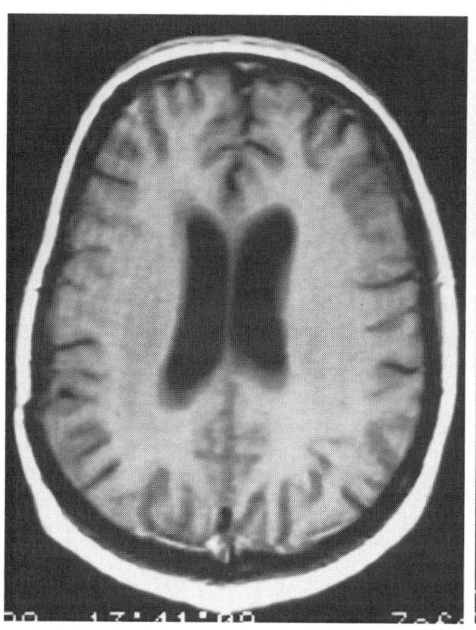
A

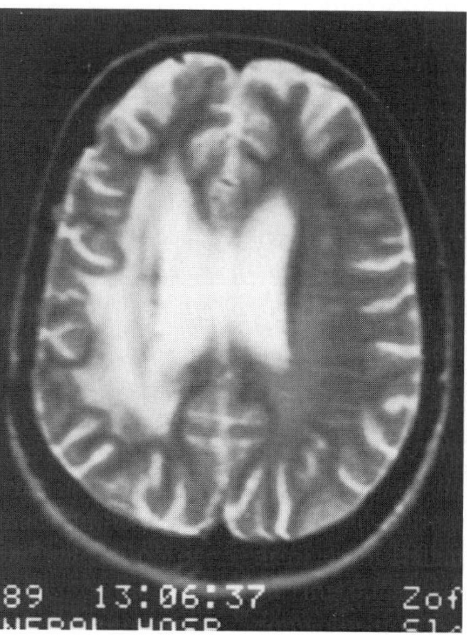
B

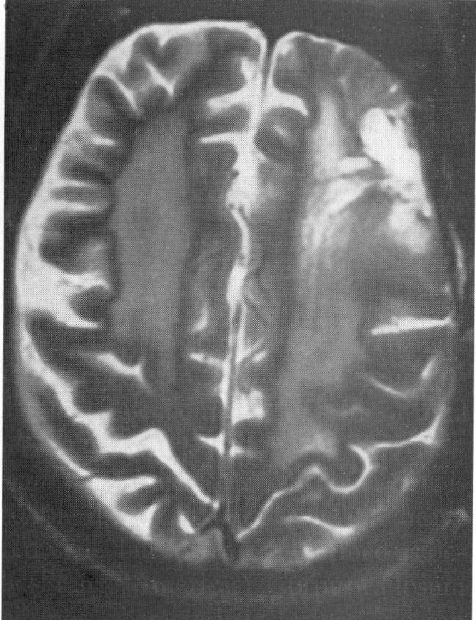
C

Figure 9.6. Radiation effects on the brain. The patient had been treated with radiation following partial surgical removal of an astrocytoma 3 years previously. He was clinically stable. **A.** The T1-weighted image was essentially normal, and postcontrast images showed no change (not shown). **B.** The T2-weighted image showed extensive white matter hyperintensity in the treated hemisphere only. CT was negative, except for the moderate ventricular enlargement (not shown). The T2 hyperintensity evidently represents a chronic state in which there is either mild diffuse demyelination or a mild increase in water, primarily in the white matter but insufficient to cause changes on T1 MRI or on CT. The white matter of the opposite hemisphere shows a slight diffuse increase in intensity indicative of some radiation effect. **C.** Another patient with a glioblastoma who had received whole-brain radiation therapy 18 months previously. There is uniform bilateral white matter hyperintensity. The old tumor site is seen in the left frontal region.

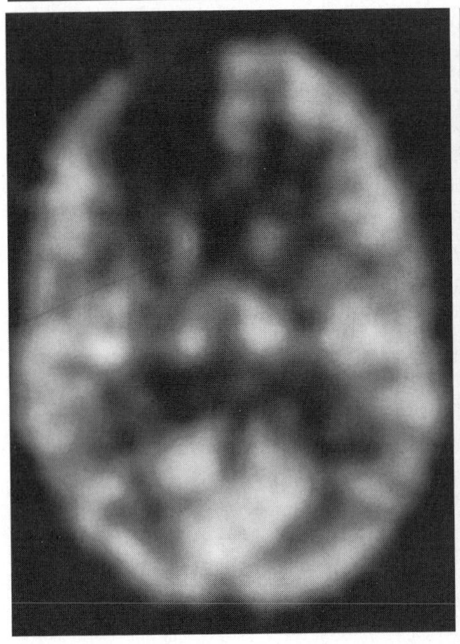

A B

Figure 9.7. Radionecrosis versus tumor recurrence studied by PET scanning. **A.** Right frontal glioblastoma was treated with radiation therapy, and about 16 months later, CT as well as MR scanning (not shown) showed considerable uptake suggestive of recurrent glioblastoma. PET scanning with ^{18}Fl deoxyglucose showed no evidence of metabolism in the lesion, which was all due to radionecrosis. **B.** A similar clinical situation in the left frontal area in another patient. This time there is marked hypermetabolism, indicative of active tumor regrowth.

Usually some air is also present in the subdural space. Blood is commonly present in the surgical bed but is usually slight. CT is preferred in this period because the patients may be uncooperative and would show motion on MRI examinations.

In patients operated on for tumor removal, intra- or extracerebral, the question may be asked about residual tumor. In the intracerebral tumor, this question is always difficult to answer because normal tissues enhance in the early postoperative period and the enhancement may last for 2 to 3 weeks or longer. After that time brain tissue enhancement is probably due to residual tumor. In extracerebral tumors (usually meningiomas), residual tissue enhancement is usually neoplasm.

In aneurysm surgery, the most important complication is occlusion of a vessel, which may lead to ischemic infarction. This is more common in anterior communicating aneurysms. However, in many instances, the changes are related to arterial spasm and subsequent ischemia. The usual imaging finding is hypodensity on CT and hypo- and hyperintensity on T1- and T2-weighted images, respectively. This is commonly found in the territory of the anterior cerebral artery because of the frequent problems in anterior communicating aneurysm surgery often associated with arterial spasm.

In the posterior fossa, edema is important, and postoperative examinations are performed to determine the presence of ventricular dilatation, which may necessitate a shunting procedure.

Postoperative hemorrhage, in both the supratentorial and infratentorial spaces, is easily diagnosed by CT.

Edema is sometimes pronounced and may be related to vascular compromise and to tissue retraction during the surgical procedure. A mass effect is usually present, and usually the edema and the mass effect subside within the next week or so after the surgical procedure.

REFERENCES

1. Valk J, Van der Knaap MS: Toxic encephalopathy. AJNR 1992;13: 747–760.
2. Miura T, Mitomo M, Kawai R, et al: CT of the brain in acute carbon monoxide intoxication: Characteristic features and prognosis. AJNR 1985;6:739–742.
3. Kim KS, Weinberg PE, Suh JH, et al: Acute carbon monoxide poisoning: Computed tomography of the brain. AJNR 1980;1:399–405.
4. Chang KH, Han MH, Kim HS, et al: Delayed encephalopathy after acute carbon monoxide intoxication: MR imaging features and distribution of cerebral white matter lesions. Radiology 1992;184:117.
5. Aquilonius SM, Bergstrom K, Erickson P, et al: Cerebral computed tomography in methanol intoxication. J Comput Assist Tomogr 1980;4:425–428.
6. Kirogi Y, Takahashi M, Shinzato J, et al: MR findings in seven patients with organic mercury poisoning (Minamata disease). AJNR 1991;15:1575–1578.
7. Caldemeyer KS, Pascuzzi RM, Moran CC, Smith RR: Toluene abuse causing reduced MR signal intensity in the brain. AJR 1993; 161:1259–1261.
8. Diamond I: Alcohol neurotoxicity. In AK Asbury, GM McKhann, MI McDonald (eds), Diseases of the Nervous System—Clinical Neurobiology. Philadelphia: Saunders, 1992.
9. Estrin WJ: Alcoholic cerebellar degeneration is not a dose-dependent phenomenon. Alcohol Clin Exp Res 1987;11:372–375.
10. Doraiswamy PM, Massey EW, Enright K, et al: Wernicke-Korsakoff syndrome caused by psychogenic food refusal: MR findings. AJNR 1994;15:594–596.
11. Shogry ME, Curnes JT: Mamillary body enhancement on MR as the only sign of acute Wernicke encephalopathy. AJNR 1994;15: 172–174.
12. Gallucci M, Bozzao A, Splendiani A, et al: Wernicke encephalopathy: MR findings in five patients. AJNR 1990;11:887–892.
13. Donnal JF, Heinz ER, Burger PC: MR of reversible thalamic lesions in Wernicke syndrome. AJNR 1990;11:893–894.

14. Victor M: MR in the diagnosis of Wernicke-Korsakoff syndrome. AJNR 1990;11:895–896.
15. Glazer M, Dross P: Necrosis of the putamen caused by methanol intoxication: MR findings. AJR 1993;160:1105–1106.
16. Chang KH, Cha SH, Han MH, et al: Marchiafava-Bignami disease: Serial changes in corpus callosum in MRI. Neuroradiology 1992; 34:480–482.
17. Golbe LI, Merkin MD: Cerebral infarction in a user of free-base cocaine ("crack"). Neurology 1986;36:1602–1603.
18. Wang AM, Suojanen JN, Colucci VM, et al: Cocaine and methamphetamine induced acute cerebral vasospasm: An angiographic study in rabbits. AJNR 1990;11:1141–1146.
19. Wojack JC, Flamm ES: Intracranial hemorrhage and cocaine use. Stroke 1987;18:712–715.
20. Lichtenfeld PJ, Rubin DB, Feldman RS: Subarachnoid hemorrhage precipitated by cocaine snorting. Arch Neurol 1984;41:223–224.
21. Massachusetts General Hospital—Case Records. Case 27-1993. N Engl J Med 1993;329:117–124.
22. Jacobs IG, Roszler MH, Kelly JK, et al: Cocaine abuse: Neurovascular complications. Radiology 1989;170:223–227.
23. Heier LA, Carpanzano CR, Mast J, et al: Maternal cocaine abuse: The spectrum of radiologic abnormalities in the neonatal CNS. AJNR 1991;12:951–956.
24. Rumbaugh CL, Bergeron RT, Scanlan RL, et al: Cerebral vascular changes secondary to amphetamine abuse in experimental animals. Radiology 1971;101:345–351.
25. Bostwick D: Amphetamine induced cerebral vasculitis. Hum Pathol 1981;12:1031–1033.
26. Tan TP, Algra PR, Valk J, et al: Toxic leukoencephalopathy after inhalation of poisoned heroin: MR findings. AJNR 1994;14: 175–178.
27. Ebner F, Ranner G, Slavc I, et al: MR findings in methotrexate induced CNS abnormalities. AJNR 1989;10:959–964.
28. Wending LR, Bleyer WA, DiChiro G, et al: Transient severe periventricular hypodensity after leukemia prophylaxis with cranial irradiation and intrathecal methotrexate. J Comput Assist Tomogr 1978;2:502–505.
29. Peylan-Ramu N, Poplack DG, Blei CL, et al: Computer assisted tomography in methotrexate encephalopathy. J Comput Assist Tomogr 1977;1:216–221.
30. Schaumberg HH: Chemical neurotoxicity. In AK Asbury, GM McKhann, WI McDonald (eds), Diseases of the Nervous System—Clinical Neurobiology. Philadelphia: Saunders, 1992.
31. Rubin AM, Kang H: Cerebral blindness and encephalopathy with cyclosporin A toxicity. Neurology 1987;37:1072–1076.
32. De Groen PC, Aksamit AJ, Rakela J, et al: Central nervous system toxicity after liver transplantation: The role of cyclosporine and cholesterol. N Engl J Med 1987;317:861–866.
33. Truwit CC, Denaro CP, Lake JR, et al: MR imaging of reversible cyclosporin A-induced neurotoxicity. AJNR 1991;12:651–659.
34. Chieng PU, Huang TS, Chang CC, et al: Reduced hypothalamic blood flow after radiation treatment of nasopharyngeal cancer: SPECT studies in 34 patients. AJNR 1991;12:661–665.
35. Dooms GC, Hecht S, Brant-Zawadzki M, et al: Brain radiation lesions: MR imaging. Radiology 1986;158:149–155.
36. Di Chiro G, Oldfield E, Wright DC, et al: Cerebral necrosis after radiotherapy and/or intraarterial chemotherapy for brain tumors: PET and neuropathologic studies. AJNR 1987;8:1083–1091.
37. Schwartz RB, Carvalho PA, Alexander E III, et al: Radiation necrosis vs high-grade recurrent glioma: Differentiation by using dual-isotope SPECT with 201 T1 and 99m TC-HMPAO. AJNR 1991;12: 1187–1192.

SELECTED READINGS

LeQuesne PM: Metal neurotoxicity. In AK Asbury, GM McKhann, WI McDonald (eds), Diseases of the Nervous System—Clinical Neurobiology. Philadelphia: Saunders, 1992.

O'Brien CP, Urschel HC III: Neurologic consequences of drug abuse. In AK Asbury, GM McKhann, WI McDonald (eds), Diseases of the Nervous System—Clinical Neurobiology. Philadelphia: Saunders, 1992.

Zeiss J, Velasco ME, McCann KM, et al: Cerebral CT of lethal ethylene glycol intoxication with pathologic correlation. AJNR 1989;10: 440–442.

10

Brain Vascular Disorders

The brain uses 20 percent of the circulating oxygenated blood because of its avid need for oxygen to perform its functions, even though the mass of the brain in relation to the rest of the body represents only about 2 percent of the body mass. It is therefore not remarkable that vascular diseases of the brain compose a very high percentage of the symptom-producing neurologic conditions. Strokes are one of the most important sources of disability in the old age group, but they are also frequently encountered in younger individuals. Strokes may be due to arterial occlusions, venous occlusions, hemorrhage, rupture of saccular aneurysms, inflammatory conditions involving the arteries, and arterial dissections. In addition, vascular changes involving the small vessels of the brain are a source of mental disability ranging from memory defects to dementia. Anomalous conditions such as arteriovenous malformations as well as cavernous angiomas may produce cerebral hemorrhage or may lead to epileptic seizures. The neurologist must always keep vascular disorders at the top of the list of etiologic processes that lead to neurologic symptoms.

Circulatory problems that could not be recognized or cataloged previously can now be diagnosed because of the increasing number of new approaches. One of the earliest approaches was ultrasound examination of the carotid artery and of the periorbital circulation for indirect signs of pathology. Then, after the development of computed tomography (CT), it was possible to study the effects of ischemia in the brain that lead to cerebral infarction, as well as the changes in white matter that we now attribute to small-vessel disease, particularly that involving the periventricular region. The advent of magnetic resonance imaging (MRI) was another milestone. Not only have we increased our ability to see the brain changes produced by cerebral ischemia, but we are now able to perform magnetic resonance angiography (MRA). This technology is progressing rapidly, and we can anticipate further developments in this area. Cerebral angiography still remains the gold standard for demonstrating direct arterial involvement, in both the cervical portion of the internal carotid or vertebral arteries and the intracranial portion of the carotid artery and all of its branches or the basilar artery and its branches. Physiologic studies using radionuclide indicators with both single photon and positron emitters can be carried out to study cerebral blood flow, and studies with MRI also allow us to evaluate local cerebral blood volume and circulation time. All of these methods are discussed in text following, and their relative contribution to our knowledge of physiology and pathophysiology is evaluated.

EXAMINATION METHODS

Computed Tomography

At the time of this writing CT scanning remains the most valuable examination method in the acute stage. As a patient arrives, it is most important to determine whether there is a hemorrhage in the brain or in the subarachnoid space. Since many of these patients are uncooperative upon arrival at the hospital facility, CT scanning is the method of choice because it will not only show the hemorrhage but will also yield a satisfactory examination in a patient who may be moving and is uncooperative. The patient may arrive presenting symptoms or signs suggestive of a focal ischemic lesion that may well turn out to be hemorrhagic. In general, it is not possible to determine by neurologic examination alone whether the patient has a cerebral parenchymal hemorrhage or an ischemic lesion. CT scanning clarifies this issue with an accuracy that is extremely high: parenchymal hemorrhage is revealed with almost 100 percent accuracy, and the absence of hemorrhage indicates that the lesion is probably an ischemic event. Thus the first examination that should be performed is a CT scan. The examination is carried out without contrast enhancement, and a routine axial set is sufficient. The use of contrast media is not indicated if the clinical impression is that of an acute cerebral vascular problem.

Contrast media injections are not utilized except in the subacute stage to determine whether there is a break in the blood-brain barrier, as is seen in cerebral infarction after 10 days. It has been said that the injection of contrast media can be harmful to a patient who has a cerebral infarction, particularly if it is in the hyperemic stage (1). The approach at the Massachusetts General Hospital has been to not use contrast, but we do not hesitate to use it when it is considered necessary. The author has never encountered a case in which there was a very strong indication that the patient was made worse simply by the injection of intravenous contrast media. Whisson et al. have shown blood-brain barrier effects in animals with induced acute hypertension injected with nontoxic contrast media (2).

SPIRAL CT ANGIOGRAPHY

Following the development of spiral CT, a number of publications have appeared demonstrating the clinical use of spiral (helical) CT angiography (CTA) (3–7). This modality provides images of the true lumen of the arteries, as opposed to MRA, in which flow is being imaged. It is slightly invasive in that it requires continuous injection of contrast material at the rate of 2 to 4 ml/sec during the exposure time, which would normally last about 30 to 40 sec, for a total of 100 to 120 ml. At the common carotid artery bifurcation, where heavy calcification is often present, the true lumen of the stenosed internal carotid artery may be difficult to discern, but special computer programs are available to separate the lumen from the calcium (Fig. 10.8). The axial images may be helpful in this respect. CTA may also be useful for visualizing intracranial arteries and saccular aneurysms (7,8). CTA requires careful manipulation of the data for best results. Usually 3-mm collimation is used with 1-mm reconstruction and a 3-mm table speed. The filming is started 15 to 20 sec after beginning the intravenous injection. Maximum intensity projection (MIP) reformations, as well as shaded surface display

(SSD), are used. The latter yields images with a three-dimensional effect that is useful. Infinite variation in the degrees of rotation is possible through adequate manipulation of the data (Fig. 10.112*C* to *H*).

Magnetic Resonance Imaging

CROSS-SECTIONAL IMAGING

MRI is capable of demonstrating the ischemic changes associated with cerebral infarction earlier than CT scanning, partly because of the more dramatic changes seen on T2-weighted images, which consist of hyperintensity involving the ischemic areas in both the white and gray matter. On T1-weighted images, the changes may show up, but the hypointensity in the involved area is less conspicuous. On CT the appearance is that of decreased attenuation due to the presence of edema; in general, this shows up very clearly, but the ability of MRI to demonstrate increased interstitial water in the tissues appears to be greater. Special MRI techniques might be used to diagnose the ischemic lesions earlier. With the present ordinary techniques, the difference in the MRI and CT detection time following the appearance of symptoms is not very great. If such techniques as diffusion-weighted imaging were applied, brain tissue changes might be demonstrated considerably earlier, within a few hours (9,10). For further details, see the discussion of diffusion imaging in Chapter 2 and functional neuroimaging in Chapter 14. The early diagnosis of an ischemic lesion is important as we strive to develop treatment approaches to reduce tissue damage in ischemic brain disease.

In general, MRI examination is carried out only if it is considered necessary, particularly in the presence of a negative CT examination in a patient who has definite symptoms and signs of neurologic deficit consistent with ischemic disease. MRI may clarify a diagnosis by demonstrating the usual flow voids of open arteries on routine examination. In an open artery there is a well-developed flow void in the neck. At the base of the skull, it is important to look for the flow void of the carotid siphon, (intracavernous and supraclinoid portions) in all available sequences.

Contrast enhancement sometimes may be used in the same way as with CT but in general is not considered necessary except in some atypical cases when the breakdown of the blood-brain barrier may be considered of diagnostic significance.

MAGNETIC RESONANCE ANGIOGRAPHY

All MRA flow-imaging techniques fall into two categories: phase-contrast and time-of-flight (TOF) angiography (Table 10.1). Both techniques are satisfactory and may be considered complementary, leaving the choice of one or the other to individual considerations in a given case. The type of equipment available may also influence the choice of technique.

When the carotid and vertebral circulation in the neck is being studied, TOF imaging is preferred. TOF imaging is based on the fact that when a specific slice is imaged, the flowing blood will have moved past the slice when the echo is received, and thus the unsaturated blood moving into the slice being imaged provides the signal. The thinner the slice, the more likely it is that the flowing blood has completely moved out of the slice. In general, the slices are very thin, around 1.5 mm.

Table 10.1.
Relative Advantages of MRA Techniques

Time-of-flight (TOF) technique
Duration of study is usually shorter than that of phase contrast (PC)
Foreknowledge of proper velocity encoding setting (as in PC MRA) is not necessary
Phase-contrast technique
Allows determination of directional flow
Sensitivity to flow in all directions
Absolute determination between flow and substances with short T1 (e.g., thrombus)
Velocity encoding can be tailored for slow or fast flow

A number of variations of these techniques have been published, and the reader is referred to these for further details not considered appropriate in this text, for the techniques will continue to evolve and rapidly become obsolete, being replaced by other variants (11–20).

Artifacts are common because of patient breathing and swallowing or any movement. In spite of the frequent artifacts, however, the images can usually be interpreted (Fig. 10.1). The data can be collected two-dimensionally or three-dimensionally. The images are presented starting with one lateral view followed by a series of images rotated approximately 10° passing through the frontal projection and ending with the opposite lateral view (Fig. 10.1). In addition, the axial images (raw data) are available for comparison to make the interpretation more accurate. T1-weighted images are also made that show the flow voids of the flowing arteries. These are used to check on any questionable changes seen on the TOF images. The 180° presentation of the images is indispensable for a more complete visualization of the anatomy because of overlapping of the arteries.

What we are imaging in the carotid and vertebral arteries is the flow and not necessarily the lumen of the arteries. Thus flow artifacts are frequent and may lead to misinterpretation unless we are familiar with them. Turbulence may result in absence of the flow image in a specific location. For this reason, when there is arterial narrowing resulting in increased flow speed and turbulence, there may be disappearance of the flow image for a short segment. The absent flow image in a short segment usually indicates significant narrowing of the lumen (21) (Figs. 10.2 and 10.3).

In the cervical region, phase-contrast images are used as scout images prior to TOF images, but usually not as the diagnostic study because they show the veins as well as the arteries, and the arterial images then tend to be confused.

The technique of MRA has been progressing quite rapidly. A number of variations have been described, and we

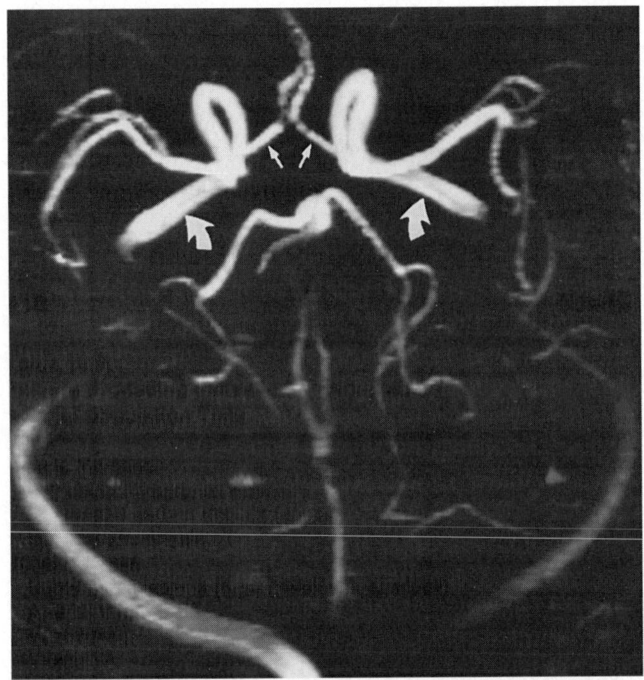

A

Figure 10.1. Normal intracranial magnetic resonance angiogram (MRA), phase contrast. The presentation in rotation of each image at 10° starting with the left sagittal image is helpful and allows one to visualize the proximal vessels with a fair amount of detail. **A.** Collapsed view looking at the vessels as a base view. Intracavernous carotid artery (curved arrows). The small arrows point at part 1, the anterior cerebral arteries. The anterior communicating artery is not directly visible, and the posterior communicating arteries are not seen. The middle cerebral arteries are seen up to a point around the bend into the sylvian fissure and only for a short distance beyond. The posterior cerebral arteries are well seen as they pass around the brainstem. Posteriorly, the two lateral sinuses are well seen, the right better than the left. **B.** Left lateral view showing the superimposed internal carotid arteries; the basilar artery is well seen, and so are their respective branches. The internal cerebral vein and the vein of Galen, the straight sinus, and the superior sagittal and lateral sinuses are well seen. **C.** Rotating the image to the left at 20°. The internal carotid arteries are now separated; the basilar artery is partly superimposed on the left carotid artery. **D.** A 90° view shows the two internal carotid arteries and the basilar artery bifurcations. The superior longitudinal sinus is superimposed on the right carotid system, as is expected in phase-contrast MRA images. **E.** View 10° past D showing the anterior cerebral artery on the right above the bifurcation of the basilar arteries. The superior sagittal sinus is now to the left. **F.** Image is rotated to the right lateral view, and the two internal carotid arteries are again perfectly superimposed.

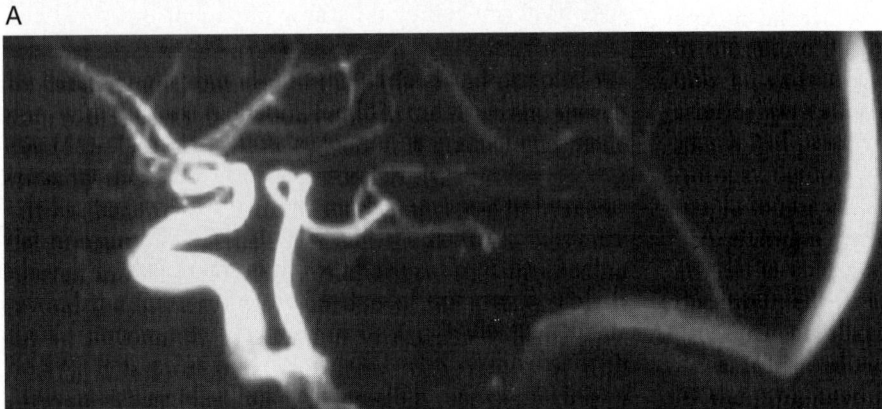

B

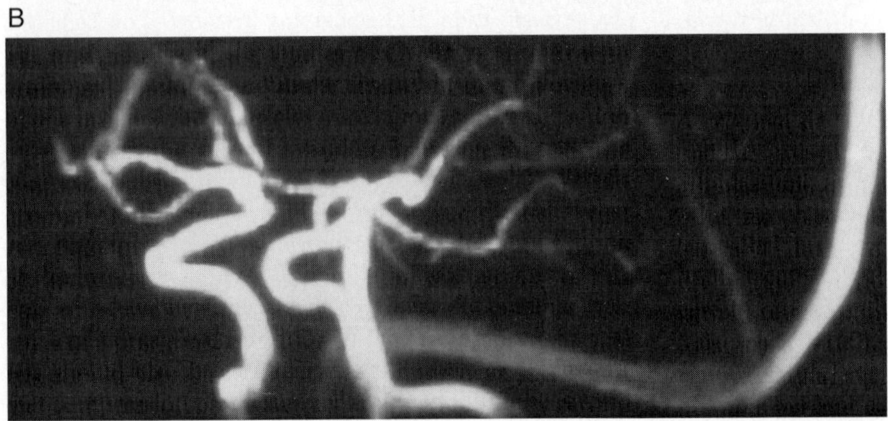

C

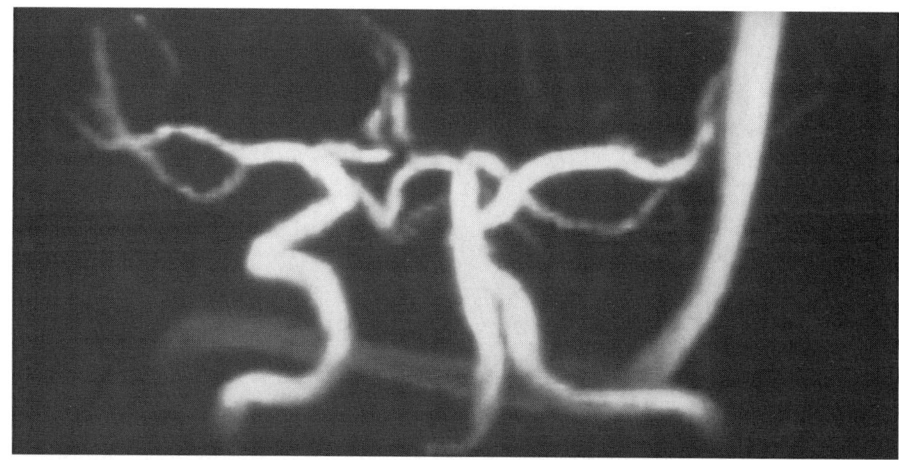

D

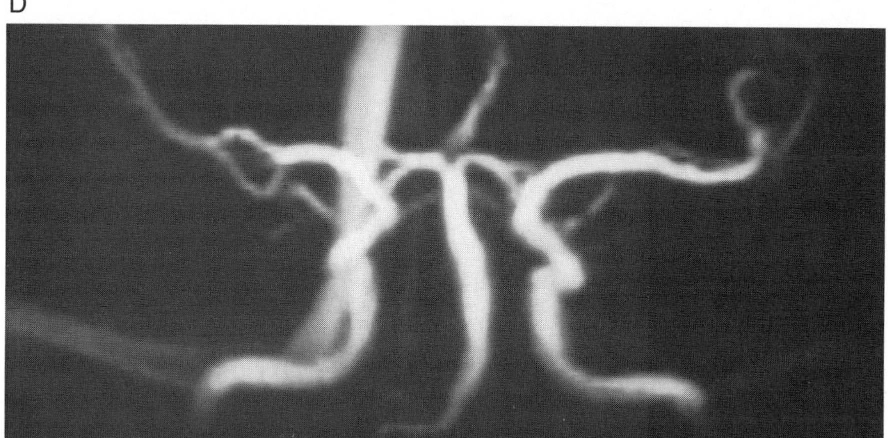

E

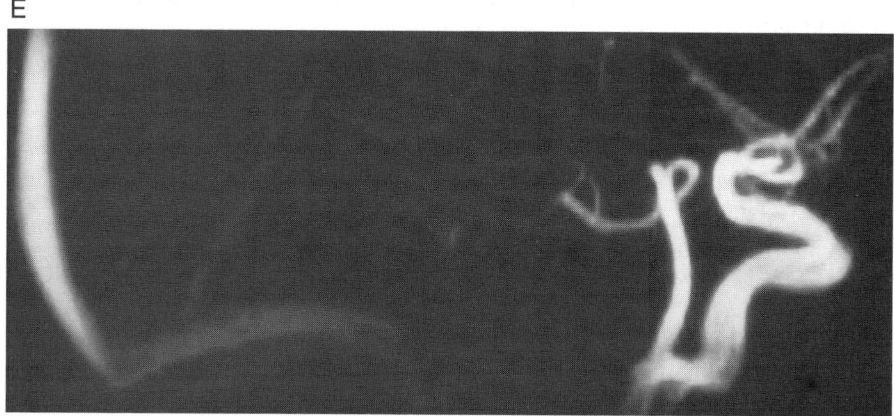

F

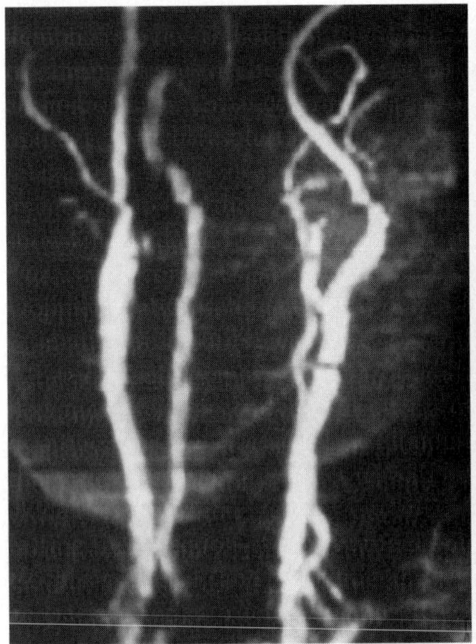

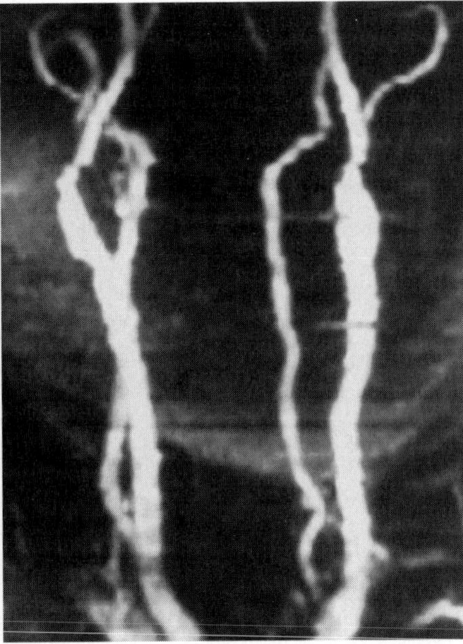

A B

Figure 10.2. Artifacts in time-of-flight (TOF) imaging of cervical arteries. Because of swallowing and breathing, there are often irregularities passing straight across the lumen of the artery. Movement will cause a complete lack of registration. These artifacts are seen in both the carotid and vertebral arteries.

can expect continued improvements in the results (22–25). These techniques are all based on flow and are handicapped by slow flow. Wright et al. have described a flow-independent technique, but this will require a great deal of clinical trial to determine its potential usefulness (26).

The use of MRA is increasing in the investigation of possible stenotic lesions in the neck; along with other noninvasive studies of carotid disease (Doppler ultrasound, sonic color flow imaging, velocity measurements, periorbital Doppler, oculoplethysmography), it may obviate the need for cerebral angiography if the findings in the two groups of studies are in accord (27). Some surgeons are now operating on the basis of these noninvasive findings alone without angiography.

The degree of stenosis present is overestimated by MRA, but sonographic tests may be used to correct the error. This is important because endarterectomy should not be performed simply to correct a narrowed artery, but only when there is demonstrated a symptomatic, hemodynamically significant stenosis or one in which the residual lumen of the artery is of the order of 1.0 mm or less. The size of the residual lumen can be estimated by sonographic approaches with a fairly high degree of accuracy. At the Massachusetts General Hospital (MGH) surgery is performed only in the presence of symptomatic or hemodynamically significant stenosis. Otherwise, the patient is placed on a platelet adhesiveness control agent or on anticoagulants, if deemed necessary, and followed. If the residual lumen is estimated at 2.0 to 2.5 mm, follow-up is recommended at 18 to 24 months; if the residual arterial lumen is estimated at 1.5 mm or less, the follow-up examination should be at 6 to 9 months; and if at 1.0 to 1.25 mm, at 4 months. Under these circumstances surgery is usually recommended.

In a long-term clinical evaluation of the noninvasive battery of tests used in the MGH laboratory, the accuracy of the residual lumen estimate as compared to that of cerebral angiography is above 90 percent (28). Sometimes the residual lumen cannot be estimated and the artery is declared occluded if the lumen falls below 1.0 mm. In these cases angiography may demonstrate total occlusion or a very small residual lumen, which indicates that endarterectomy should be considered.

Whereas in conventional angiography we advocate measuring the arterial lumen in millimeters across the narrowest portion, this is not possible with MRA. The method recommended by Barnett et al. (29) and Fox (30) is preferable (Fig. 10.4). In this case a percentage of arterial lumen narrowing is calculated. When the arterial lumen is down to 1.0 mm or below, it usually causes narrowing of the artery beyond the stenosis, in which case the percentage of narrowing is declared as 90 to 99 percent.

In MRA, narrowing of the lumen of the carotid artery beyond the stenosis may be observed when the lesion may not actually be hemodynamically significant. This is because only flow is being imaged and the flow in the peripheral portion of the artery may fall below a level that can be imaged by the usual TOF technique. The laminar flow in the carotid artery is faster in the center of the artery and slower in the periphery.

Turbulent flow in a wider-lumen artery occurs at a much higher flow speed than in a smaller-lumen artery. For this reason, when there is stenosis in the proximal carotid artery, there may be turbulence, which would tend to decrease the intensity of the image or eliminate it altogether (Figs. 10.3 and 10.5).

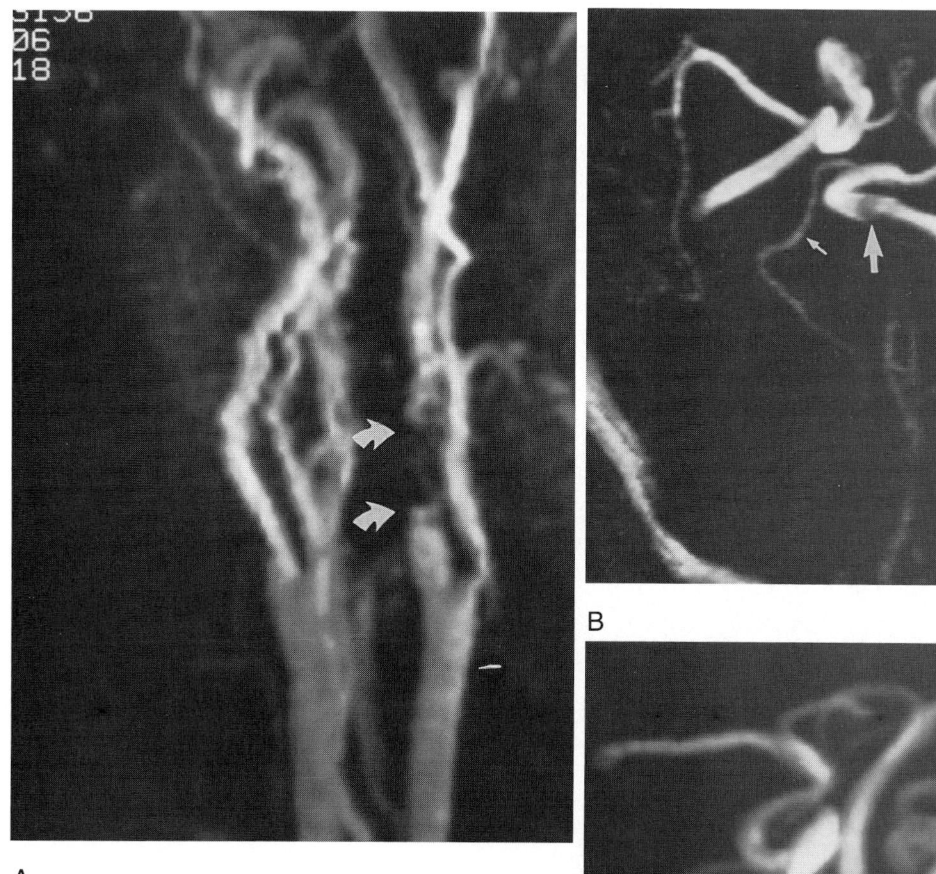

A

B

C

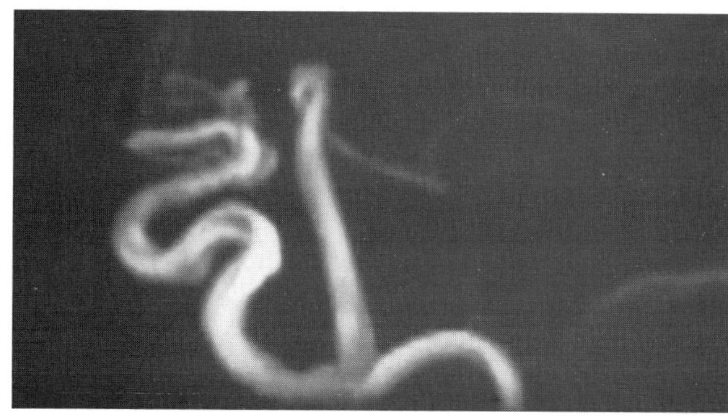

D

Figure 10.3. MRA in a 65-year-old man. **A.** There is an area of signal loss measuring about 1.5 cm in length near the origin of the left internal carotid artery (arrows). The lumen of the artery is again seen above, indicating that the absent signal is secondary to arterial narrowing and turbulence. The narrowing is probably around 70 percent of the lumen because there is no diminution in the diameter of the lumen above the signal loss when compared to the other side. **B.** The collapsed axial view of the head shows the fairly symmetrical configuration of the carotid siphons and proximal middle cerebral arteries. There is asymmetry in the size of the posterior cerebral arteries as shown by the flow (small arrows). There is a dominant left vertebral artery, and where the right vertebral artery joins the left, there is a short area of absent flow, believed to be due to focal turbulence rather than focal disease. **C.** Frontal view showing the basilar artery between the two carotid arteries. No narrowing of the basilar artery is seen. **D.** Direct lateral view shows that the two internal carotid arteries are superimposed; the basilar artery is well seen and in normal position.

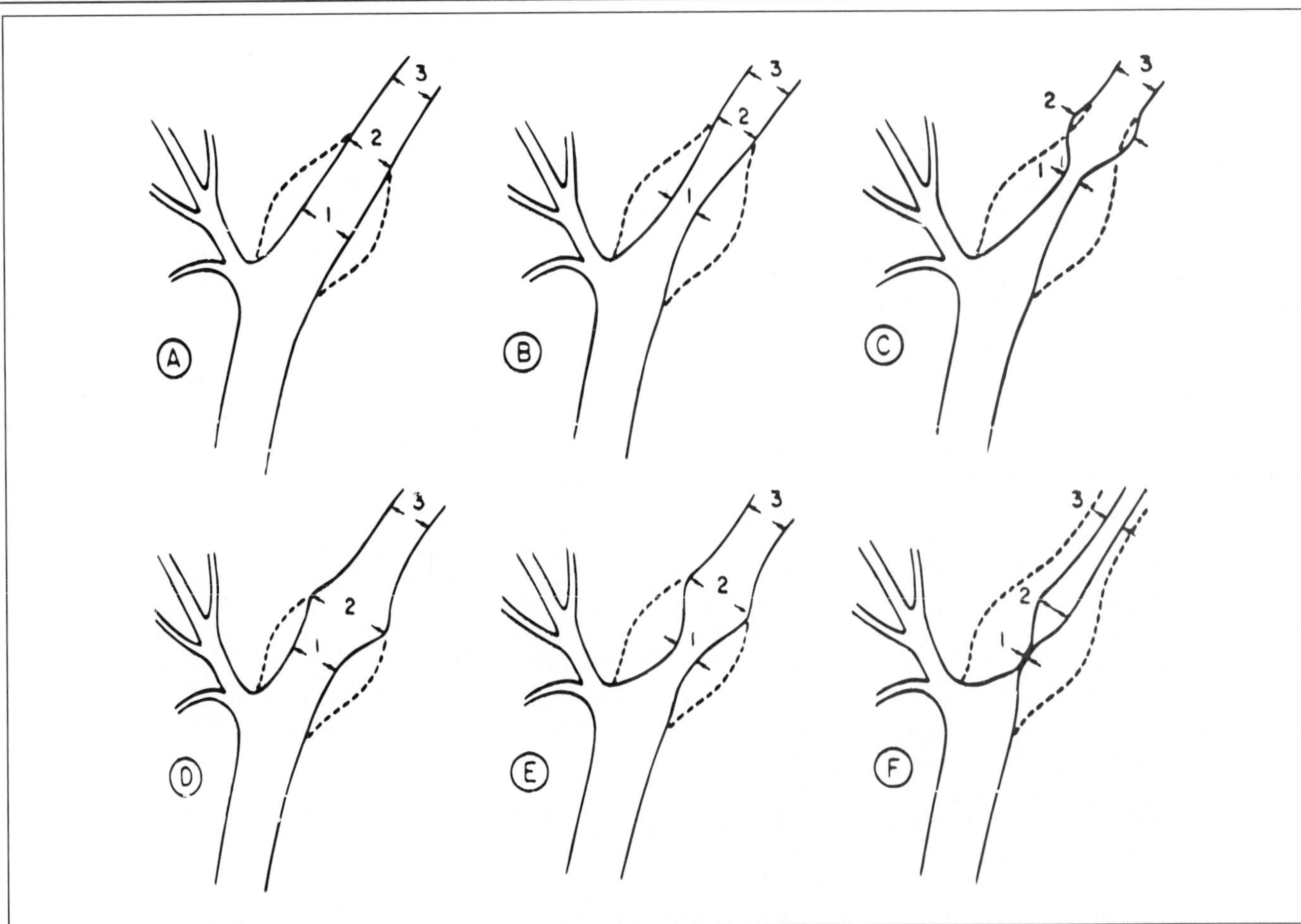

Figure 10.4. The view showing the most severe narrowing of the internal cartoid artery (ICA) was used to calculate the stenosis, with the measurement of the site of greatest narrowing (measurement 1) used as the numerator and that of the proximal normal ICA (measurement 3) used as the denominator. Site 2 represents the value for the distal carotid bulb. The formula for data analysis was (1 − [measurement 1/measurement 3]) × 100 percent. **A** to **F** depict the more common combinations of plaque location, bulb changes, and altered diameter of the distal artery. Calculated percentages of stenosis for panels A to E, by using measurement 1 as numerator and measurement 3 as denominator, are 0 percent for panel A, 40 percent for panel B, 70 percent for panel C, −10 percent for panel D, and 50 percent for panel E. In panel F, the distal narrowing from reduced flow flaws the calculation, and 99 percent is the assigned value. (Courtesy of Barnett et al., Stroke 1991;22:711–720, with permission.)

Since the overestimation of lumen narrowing by MRA as compared to conventional angiography is not the same in all cases, one cannot establish an applicable percentage to correct the error, and, as already mentioned, it would be necessary to depend on ultrasound correlations to arrive at a more accurate value for the stenosed lumen (31,32). The total disappearance of the lumen (signal loss) on MRA does not mean occlusion; it usually correlates with a high degree of stenosis, but the lumen may actually be totally occluded. Absent signal in a segment of the artery followed by reappearance higher up is taken to mean that there is at least a 70 percent stenosis (21) (Fig. 10.3). This statement is based on the use of the MIP algorithm.

The vertebral arteries are seen routinely on MRA. In general, no particular effort is made to visualize the origin of the vertebral arteries because if the subclavian arteries are included in the image, it is usually not possible to show the upper portions of the vertebral arteries as they join to form the basilar artery, owing to limitations imposed by surface coil design and other factors. In addition, the edge of the field shows little detail because of signal drop-off. Furthermore, narrowing of the vertebral arteries at their origin, although common, appears to have little clinical significance in most cases. Also, if the field of view is moved down, the upper portion of the internal carotid arteries is cut off. Further details are discussed in text following.

MRA of the intracranial circulation is being used with increasing frequency. Again, a TOF or a phase-contrast technique can be used. In the head, the visualization of the

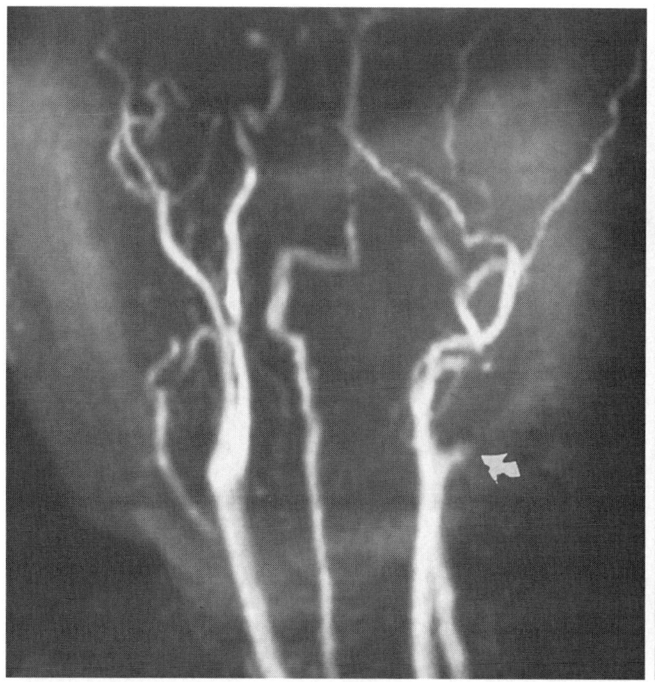

A

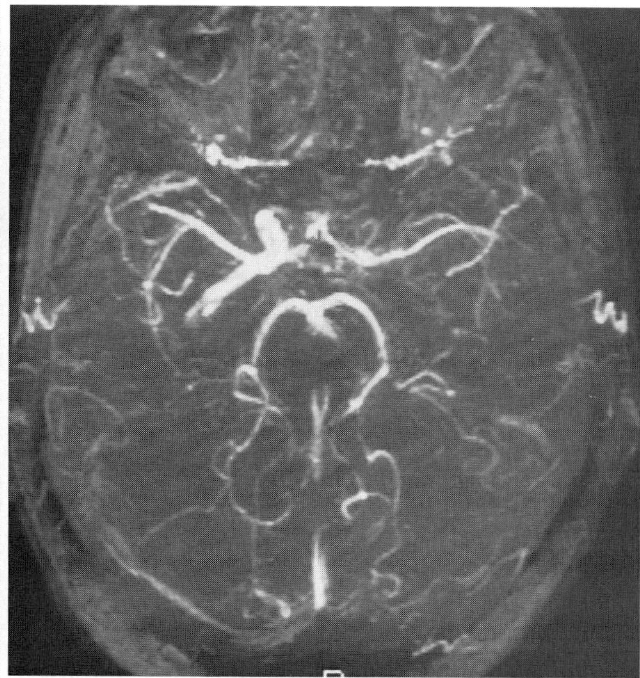

B

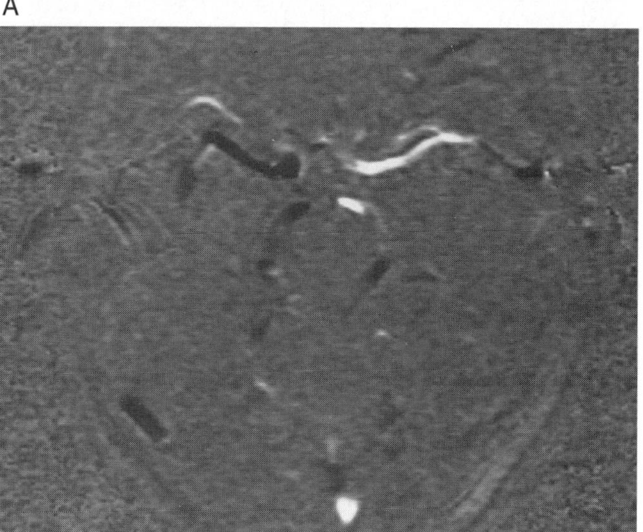

C

Figure 10.5. Total occlusion of left internal carotid artery in the neck of a 44-year-old woman who came in complaining of aphasia for 24 h but had no weakness of extremities. **A.** MRA revealed absent flow in the left internal carotid artery except for a short segment at its origin (arrow) in this TOF image. **B.** The collapsed view of the circle of Willis (three-dimensional TOF) shows absence of the carotid siphon on the left; the anterior and middle cerebral artery trunks on the left show good flow. **C.** Directional flow image (right-to-left bright; left-to-right dark) shows that the flow in the middle cerebral artery trunks is normal; that is, the blood is flowing from left to right on the right side, the normal side, and from right to left on the left side. This means that there is adequate collateral circulation through the anterior communicating artery. If the anterior communicating and posterior communicating arteries were defective, the flow would probably take place by way of leptomeningeal anastomoses and the flow in the middle cerebral trunk would be reversed (both middle cerebral arteries would be dark or both would be bright).

veins by phase contrast is not as troublesome as in the neck; only the superior sagittal sinus and the straight and lateral sinuses are usually seen if the minimum imaging speed is set at 40 cm/sec. If the speed is set lower, other venous channels may be imaged.

Only the arteries near the base of the brain are imaged by intracranial MRA: the supraclinoid carotid arteries, the carotid bifurcation, and the middle and anterior cerebral arteries. The detail is quite satisfactory in these arteries (Fig. 10.6). Sometimes one or both posterior communicating arteries may be seen, but that would depend on whether flow is actually taking place during imaging. The intracranial portion of the vertebral arteries and their junction to form the basilar artery are usually well seen, and the posterior inferior cerebellar arteries are often seen but not in all cases. The anterior inferior cerebellar arteries are often seen, and the posterior cerebral arteries are seen in all cases. When the posterior cerebral artery originates from the carotid artery (fetal anatomic variant), the initial segment of the posterior cerebral artery may not be seen on that side. The superior cerebellar arteries are usually seen. One can see more vessels by cutting down the minimum speed, but this tends to add artifacts and overlapping veins. The lower speed may be used when one wants to see the middle cerebral arteries more peripherally, such as when looking for an aneurysm, or when there is vascular occlusion. However,

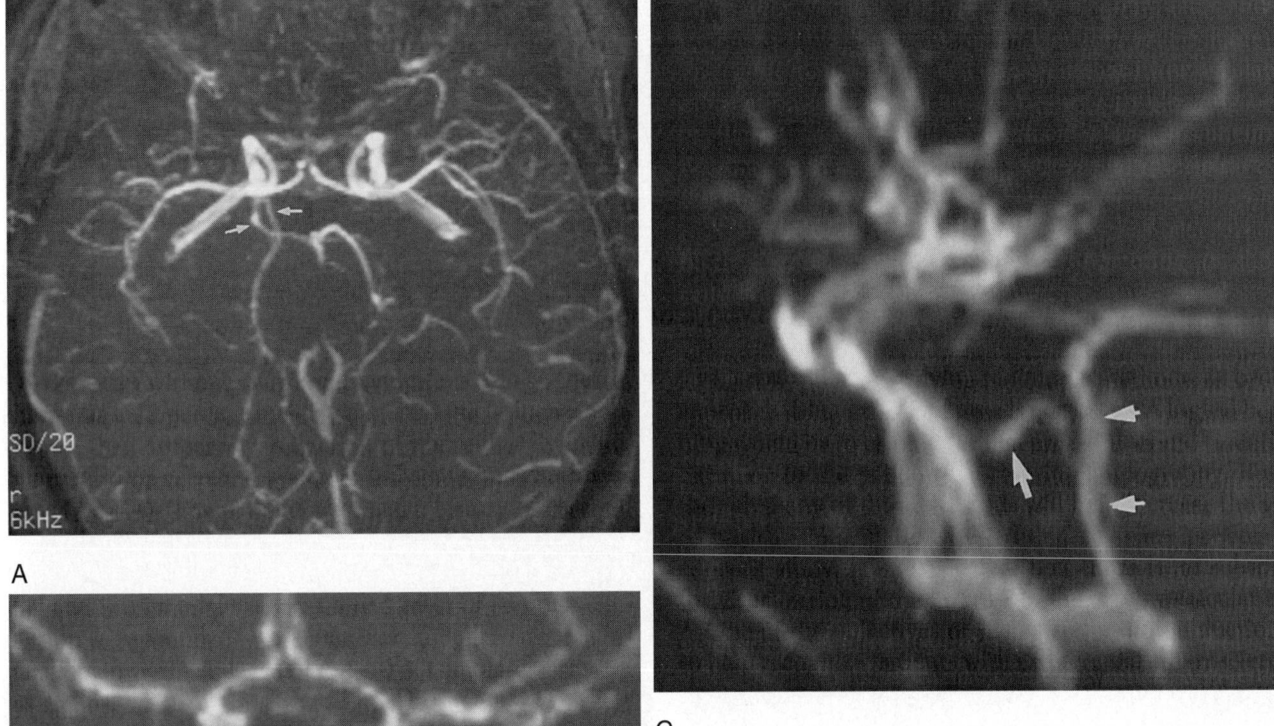

Figure 10.6. MRA demonstrating a persistent trigeminal artery. **A.** Collapsed axial view shows a posterior communicating artery joining the distal segment of the posterior cerebral artery (medial arrow) and another artery, which originates more proximally, joining the basilar artery (lateral arrow). **B.** A frontal-oblique view shows the connection between the precavernous right internal carotid and the basilar artery (arrows). **C.** A sagittal slightly oblique view shows the connection (arrow) between the internal carotid and the basilar artery (posterior arrows).

the detail in the branches of the middle or anterior cerebral arteries is always suboptimal, and no conclusions can usually be reached. One wonders if future technical refinements will eliminate this limitation or whether this is technically unsolvable.

The TOF technique is also used to visualize the major intracranial arteries, and at present we are using it in preference; the resolution is slightly better and the veins are not usually seen. The accuracy of MRA in demonstrating stenoses and occlusions of major intracranial arteries is quite good, according to Heiserman et al. (33). The diagnosis of occlusion is fairly accurate when compared to conventional angiography.

The introduction of a technique that allows separation of the right from the left or of the anterior from the posterior circulation is very useful. It is used whenever the superimposition of all the vessels makes interpretation difficult. In the General Electric Systems this is referred to as interactive vascular imaging (IVI) (Fig. 10.7).

The direction of flow can be recorded by using a special phase-imaging technique. This may be useful, for instance, when there is an intracranial vascular occlusion and the elucidation of collateral circulation becomes important. In visualizing arteriovenous malformations it is possible to separate arterial feeders from draining veins, although we rely on conventional angiography to obtain this information.

Normally the flow direction in the posterior communicating arteries is from the carotid to the posterior cerebral arteries, as shown by Ross et al., who demonstrated it in 36 out of 50 normal patients (34). In only 3 of the total of 39 in which flow in these arteries was demonstrated by MRA was it posterior to anterior. However, in the 15 cases with occlusive disease, reversal of flow (posterior to anterior) was the rule on the same side when the internal carotid was occluded.

Flow imaging with a gradient-echo technique can be used to image flowing vessels. This will produce a conventional anatomic image with the flowing vessels. The technique is used to demonstrate thrombosis of venous sinuses

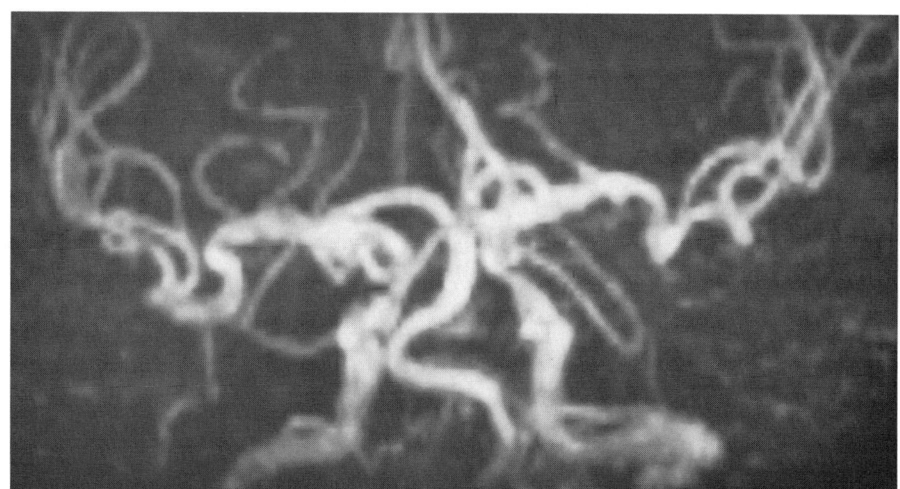

A

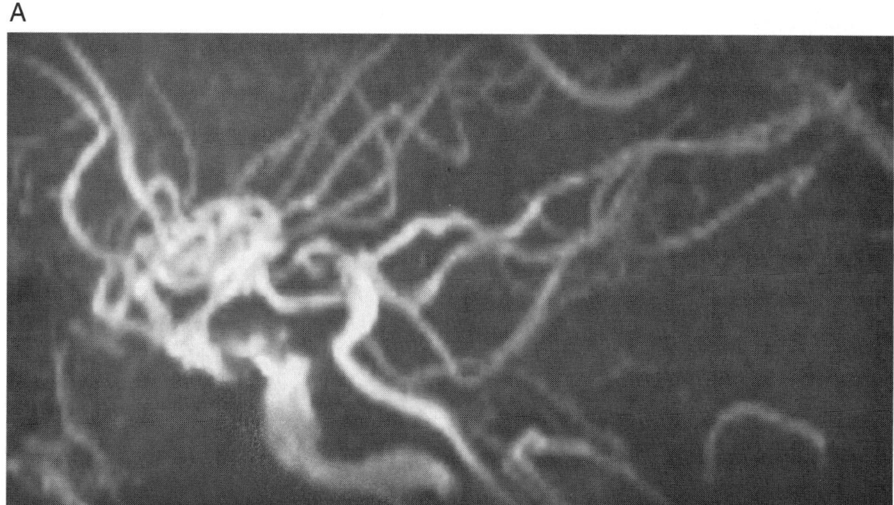

B

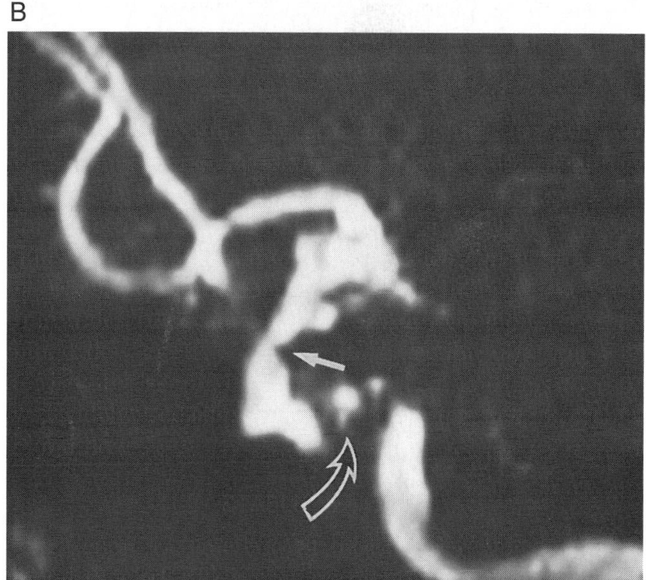

C

Figure 10.7. Interactive vascular imaging (IVI) to avoid superimposition of tortuous vessels. **A.** Frontal MRA image shows tortuous vessels and difficulties in ascertaining disease in the carotid siphon, particularly difficult in sagittal view (**B**). **C.** IVI of the left carotid artery shows that there is irregular flow in the left siphon in its proximal portion (open arrow) and a narrowed area in the supraclinoid segment (solid arrow). The anterior cerebral artery can be followed in its entirety, which is not possible in the sagittal view (B).

or of larger arteries such as the carotid, middle cerebral, or basilar and vertebral arteries. It cannot be used to demonstrate thrombosis of branches of the middle cerebral or anterior or posterior cerebral arteries.

MRA can be used to measure flow velocities of intracranial vessels, such as the middle cerebral artery, as described by Mattle et al. (35). This can be done by applying a modification of dynamic bolus tracking. It may give information that is useful in determining flow velocities in vasospasm, arteriovenous malformations, and occlusive disease.

The veins of the brain can be studied separately from the arteries through the use of a special MRA technique that requires gadolinium contrast, as shown by Chakeres et al. (36). This is sometimes useful clinically, for instance, to demonstrate more thoroughly the venous component of the arteriovenous malformation in the study of dural sinus thrombosis, and to visualize surgically relevant venous structures in tumors. Mattle et al. use a different technique from that described by Chakeres et al., and employ no intravenous contrast (35).

Ultrasonic Techniques

The first technique developed to examine the carotid circulation was probably the periorbital Doppler approach to demonstrate reversal of flow in the supraorbital and supratrochlear arteries in the presence of severe stenosis or occlusion of the internal carotid artery. Following the development of high-resolution transducers, it was possible to image the carotid artery directly. Today it is possible to image the flow in the carotid artery and simultaneously to show antegrade and retrograde flow with color Doppler as well as to record peak systolic velocities. Continuous-wave Doppler is also useful and turns out to be very reliable in estimating residual lumen size.

B-mode sonography of the carotid bifurcation, Doppler flow measurements and measurements of peak systolic and diastolic flow velocities, and continuous-wave Doppler of the carotid arteries are direct tests. The indirect tests include the periorbital Doppler examinations, which include testing the direction of flow in the supraorbital and supratrochlear arteries and palpating the superficial temporal and facial arteries to determine the effects of their compression on the palpated pulse of the supratrochlear and supraorbital arteries for a more complete evaluation of flow direction. They also include occuloplethysmography, which is carried out in a few laboratories, such as the neurovascular laboratory at the MGH (28,31,37). This technique adds confirmatory data that tend to increase certainty in some pathologic states. Further details about correlation with MRA are given in text preceding.

Transcranial Doppler examination is being used with increasing frequency, and as we learn to perform and to interpret the findings, its accuracy is increasing. It is truly a noninvasive method that, combined with other tests, has significant usefulness. It also represents, along with the battery of tests just mentioned, a practical way to follow patients who harbor atherosclerotic lesions but who are for the most part asymptomatic. With transcranial Doppler it is possible to obtain information regarding flow velocities in the ophthalmic arteries, the supraclinoid portions of the internal carotid arteries, the basilar arteries, and the intracranial portions of the vertebral arteries as well as in the middle cerebral arteries and in the anterior cerebral arteries. Obtaining flow velocities is extremely valuable in the diagnosis and follow-up of arterial spasm after subarachnoid hemorrhage. The posterior cerebral arteries can also be probed regarding flow velocities, although these vessels are more difficult to examine.

Other tests exist that have been used in the past or may still be used by some institutions. *Thermography* of the face was extensively used at the MGH but was abandoned because of the variability of the appearance of the thermal images. *Ophthalmodynamometry* was carried out for a number of years but has been largely discontinued. It was a difficult test to perform and interpret accurately. *Bruit analysis* consists of producing a frequency spectrum of the sound to isolate the highest frequency sound components of the bruit. The narrower the lumen, the greater the high-frequency component is likely to be. This is a sophisticated method but requires special equipment. Because fairly accurate estimates of residual flow can be obtained with the methods listed in text preceding, this approach never gained popularity. *Ocular plethysmography* is considerably easier to perform and probably much more accurate than ophthalmodynamometry because it eliminates the subjective factors.

CEREBRAL CIRCULATION, PHYSIOLOGIC CONSIDERATIONS

In order to understand MRA better, it may be useful to review in detail the physiology of cerebral circulation as demonstrated by cerebral angiography. In general, pathologic changes in circulation are not readily observed in MRA because we are imaging a steady state rather than an induced change provoked by the injection of contrast. Nevertheless, changes *are* present that could be interpreted if we understood cerebral circulation physiology more thoroughly.

It has been an accepted fact for many years that the current of blood through a vessel is faster in the center of the vessel than it is in the periphery near the walls. However, this concept has been challenged; it is now postulated that the flow of blood resembles more a square wave than a parabolic curve. The only slower or relatively stationary area is that layer of plasma adjacent to the arterial wall. The flow through blood vessels cannot be subjected to the usual mathematical analyses because blood is a non-Newtonian fluid: it circulates with a pulsatile and turbulent flow through elastic tapering tubes and is subjected to varying degrees of peripheral resistance (38). Where two arteries come together carrying blood, such as the two vertebral arteries forming the basilar artery, the current of blood opacified with contrast substance can usually be followed along the same side of the vessel, whereas nonopacified blood will continue on the other side for variable distances. Sometimes one can see the opacified flow changing from one wall to the other, but it still remains separated from the current of nonopacified blood coming from the other vertebral artery. This is a very important phenomenon, because there is a tendency to call a basilar artery that appears narrow abnormal. This narrowing may be simply a manifestation of incomplete filling with opacified blood. A basilar artery cannot be considered completely filled unless sufficient regurgitation into the opposite vertebral artery takes place so that mixing of opacified and nonopacified blood occurs in the contralateral vertebral artery. In this case, contrast substance is washed up toward the basilar artery from both sides, and opacification should be complete.

It is commonly observed that when the internal carotid artery is injected, the contrast substance is rapidly washed out of the lumen by the bloodstream except along the most dependent wall. The contrast substance, being heavier than the blood, tends to remain for a longer period of time along the dependent side of the artery. The slower the flow of blood, the greater the chance of having the heavier contrast substance lag along one wall of the vessel. A similar phenomenon is also frequently observed in the veins. It is not uncommon to find that the posterior sides of the veins are denser than the rostral sides when the patient lies in the supine position. *It is surprising how rapidly the contrast material can settle from the blood.* For this reason, attempts at studying the changes in the viscosity of blood induced by the contrast substances at low shear rates have been frustrating. The contrast layers out very rapidly, and it has been difficult or impossible with present instrumentation to maintain the state of turbulence necessary to keep the contrast mixed with the blood. Nevertheless, these studies need to be carried out because it is likely that a change in viscosity is one of the important effects of contrast substances on the blood. This is a particularly important consideration when examining patients suffering from conditions associated with increased blood viscosity, such as polycythemia vera.

It is possible for one of two branches to opacify less well than the other following bifurcation of an artery. Observations in the frog mesentery reported by Knisely and coauthors indicate that at the point of bifurcation of a vessel, the blood cells may continue together in one branch, and only plasma may continue in the other (39). It is also possible that with the help of gravity, a contrast substance may better fill the more dependent of two branches of a cerebral artery. With increases in the speed of flow, increased turbulence is produced at the point of bifurcation, and this condition tends to mix the radiopaque substance with the nonopacified blood. However, if the flow is relatively slow, the chances of the previously described phenomenon's occurring are enhanced. Schechter and Elkin demonstrated better filling of an aneurysm arising from the posterior wall of a vessel when the patient was placed in the supine versus the prone position, and vice versa if the aneurysm arose from the anterior wall of the artery (40).

The actual caliber of the arteries as seen in angiographic films often appears greater when the injection is made into the internal carotid artery than when it is made into the common carotid artery. This is probably a manifestation of more complete filling. Since the flow tends to be in the center of the vessel, if the lumen is not completely and rapidly filled with contrast substance, the periphery of the vessel may never become completely opacified. It therefore appears narrower in the angiogram. In making physiologic observations on arteriograms, it is therefore of the utmost importance to consider the factors of laminar flow, injection time, position of the needle, and amount of contrast substance injected (Table 10.2). Factors that cannot be controlled are arteriosclerosis, speed of blood flow in a given patient, presence of anomalies in the circle of Willis, status of intracranial pressure, systemic blood pressure, and arterial spasm.

Table 10.2.
Contrast Angiography Artifacts Related to Injection Technique

Incomplete opacification (inflow of nonopacified blood)
Dependent settling of contrast material
Differential opacification of arterial branches beyond the point of a bifurcation
Apparent slight differences in arterial caliber depending on whether the common carotid artery (CCA) or the internal carotid artery (ICA) is injected
"Standing waves"

The local stimulation of an arterial or venous wall by the contrast material is said to affect the size of the lumen. Greitz found dilatation of surface cerebral veins occurring during the passage of contrast (either Urokon or Renografin) in the course of carotid angiography (41). He concluded that the widening is real and not due to laminar flow and that it is observed in the veins but not in the arteries. Greitz does not speculate as to the significance of these findings. Huber and Handa, on the other hand, found significant increases in the diameter of the smaller arteries of the brain (1.5 mm or less) occurring during the arterial phase of the angiogram observed in a single serial following the injection of 6.0 ml of Urografin (Renografin) (42). The same authors observed enlargement of arteries of the external carotid system in routine cerebral angiograms; they attribute this to laminar flow and state that the periphery of the artery fills better in the late arterial phase, thus making the artery appear wider. However, in view of the earlier considerations, this may be true vasodilatation. It is known that the somatic vessels respond more readily to the vasodilating effect of contrast material than do cerebral vessels.

Vascular Phases

As the contrast substance is observed passing through the brain, it is customary to refer to three phases in the angiogram, as originally suggested by Moniz (43). These are the *arterial* phase, the *intermediate*, capillary, or mixed phase, and the *venous* phase.

ARTERIAL PHASE

The arterial phase lasts approximately 1.5 sec (it varies between 1.0 and 2.5 sec). A time greater than 2.5 sec should be considered abnormal if one can eliminate a technical artifact, such as poor positioning of the needle or a prolonged injection time. The arterial phase, of course, *cannot be shorter than the injection time.* Therefore, one cannot speak of a prolonged arterial phase unless the injection time is controlled. Actually, as the arterial phase is observed on the serialogram, one can see the proximal arteries filling first. As the serial proceeds, the distal arteries become well filled, while the carotid siphon and proximal anterior and middle cerebral arteries begin to empty. The emptying process then gradually takes place in the periphery. Thus one can speak of *arterial filling* and *arterial emptying* phases.

It is important to observe the arterial filling phase in the serialogram because this very often gives a clue to the presence of a neoplasm as well as of an arterial occlusion. The arterial emptying phase is important in cases of multiple small emboli and of damage to the perforating vessels arising from the larger arterial branches and extending centrally (see text following).

The arterial transit time is much faster in the internal carotid system than in the external system. In fact, the arterial circulation time is nearly twice as fast in the internal as in the external carotid artery in the average case. For this reason it is possible to inject the common carotid artery, and, in a normal case, there usually is no interference with visualization of the intracranial vessels. This relationship may change under certain conditions, such as the presence of increased intracranial pressure and vascular occlusions (see text following).

INTERMEDIATE PHASE

The intermediate or mixed phase (so-called capillary phase) is not very well defined. It corresponds to the period of time when the terminal branches of the arteries are seen and perhaps nothing else is apparent aside from very faint delineation of the origins of some of the frontal veins. Occasionally, a true capillary phase exists in that no arteries and no veins are visible. This phase lasts between 0.5 and 1.0 sec, but is quite variable. In many normal cases, it is so poorly defined that the terminal branches of the arteries are seen, followed immediately by the filling of the veins without any intermediate stage.

VENOUS PHASE

The venous phase begins when the first branches of the superficial cerebral veins are visualized and lasts possibly 4 or 5 sec. Of course, the venous phase actually continues until all of the contrast material is out of the veins, which takes a variable length of time. It is somewhat dependent on the speed of the injection and on the amount of contrast material used. In fact, it may be difficult to determine when all of the veins are completely empty. For these reasons the so-called venous circulation time is of little importance clinically.

The frontal veins usually fill just before the parietal veins. This is probably related to the distance that the contrast agent has to travel in the arteries. The arteries supplying the frontal lobe are a little shorter, and therefore the contrast substance reaches the capillary stage and the veins a little sooner than in the parietal and occipital regions. The same is true of the arterial filling phase, in which the frontal arteries may be completely filled but the parietal arteries are not. *If the parietal veins fill before the frontal veins, an abnormal condition should be suspected;* this could indicate that there is either a slowing of circulation in the frontal region or an increased speed of circulation in the parietal region. The former may be seen with neoplasms or with thromboses. The latter may be seen with vascular neoplasms, with arteriovenous malformations, and sometimes with arterial occlusions where collateral flow becomes established or where there is an increase in the speed of circulation associated with local vasodilatation ("luxury perfusion").

The deep cerebral veins usually fill later than the superficial cerebral veins. Approximately 4 to 8 percent of the time, the deep cerebral veins fill earlier than the superficial ones, but whenever this is noted, the possibility of an abnormal increase in the speed of circulation through the deep veins must be considered. In approximately 20 percent of normal individuals, the deep veins can be seen simultaneously with the superficial ones in the early venous phase of the angiogram (44). The deep cerebral veins remain filled for a longer time than the superficial veins in the later stages of the venous phase. The late films of a serialogram are usually the best for study of the deep veins without the obstacle of overlying surface veins. Leeds and Taveras observed that the sylvian veins filled at the same time as the frontal veins in 46 percent of cases and were the first veins to fill in 17 of 100 normal angiograms reviewed (44).

Circulation Time

ARTERIAL CIRCULATION TIME

The time from the maximal concentration of contrast agent in the carotid siphon to the time when only terminal branches of the arteries remain filled is called the *arterial circulation time*. It is slightly more rapid in the frontal region. The medians reported by Leeds and Taveras are as follows: frontal 1.0 sec, insular area 1.25 sec, parietal 1.5 sec, parieto-occipital 1.25 sec (44). The regional variation is related to the length of the arteries supplying these areas from the carotid siphon. It is common, in normal cases, for the arteries in the posterior parietal and parieto-occipital areas to remain filled for an even longer period of time, sometimes for several seconds more, than the frontal arteries. The significance of this observation is not clear. It could conceivably be a gravitational effect, with the heavier contrast material staying in the posterior vessels because the patient is lying supine. It could be speculated that a lower circulation rate exists in this area because the patients are under sedation and there is reduced cortical sensory activity. Certainly no such regional differences in flow as studied by diffusible indicators have been detected in human patients. It must be said, however, that the degree of definition attainable with the cerebral angiogram cannot be equaled by the external counting methods when considerable overlap between adjacent areas exists. The probes "see" a core of brain tissue that is also partly "seen" by the adjacent probes, and the Compton effect is exaggerated when relatively low-energy isotopes such as xenon 133 are used. It could be imagined that keeping the eyes closed during the examination could reduce occipital cortical activity. Ingvar and Risberg demonstrated increased blood volume (using a radioactive blood pool indicator) in the occipital region in cats during photostimulation, as compared to the resting state (45). More recently, increased blood flow in regional areas after various forms of stimuli have been demonstrated with diffusable indicator techniques (46, 47) Thus photostimulation and arm movements have caused increased regional flow in the occipital and in the posterior frontal areas, respectively. This is also demonstrable with functional MRI techniques (see Chapter 14).

ARTERIOVENOUS CIRCULATION TIME

The *angiographic circulation time* is different from the carotid-jugular circulation time that is used clinically and which is measured either by sampling jugular blood following carotid injection of a nondiffusible indicator (5 to 8 sec) or by carotid artery and jugular vein counting after the intravenous injection of a radioactive isotope (7 to 10 sec). Thus, references to arteriovenous circulation times found in the literature must be evaluated in terms of the method employed. The arteriovenous circulation time described below has a mean value of 4.25 sec; the carotid-jugular circulation time has a mean value twice that long (48).

Greitz proposed a different method of measuring the circulation time angiographically (49). The progress of the contrast material in the serialogram is studied and the film showing the greatest *beginning* concentration in the carotid siphon is selected. The error in picking the right film is probably no more than ¼ sec. The maximal concentration of the contrast material in the parietal veins is then determined. This, again, is not too difficult to detect in a serialogram. The first film showing a *decrease* in the contrast density in the parietal veins as compared with the previous one indicates that the maximal concentration has been passed. The time from the *maximal concentration of the contrast substance in the carotid siphon to maximal concentration in the parietal veins is called the circulation time.* We would prefer the name *arteriovenous circulation time* when this method is used to differentiate it from the circulation time measured in the arteries, as described in text preceding, and also the contrast transit times of the capillary and venous phases.

The mean arteriovenous circulation time is 4.13 sec according to Greitz, with a standard deviation of plus or minus 0.74 sec (49). If it is greater than 6 sec, the arteriovenous circulation time is considered to be definitely prolonged. Using their technique, Leeds and Taveras (44) found that the arteriovenous circulation time had a mean value of 4.37 sec and a standard deviation of 0.83 sec, essentially equal to the values recorded by Greitz. In a group of normal children, the average arteriovenous circulation time was 3.3 sec, that is, slightly shorter than in adults (50).

The cerebral arteriovenous circulation time measured by Greitz's method represents an average and applies specifically to the parietal area. It is advantageous, however, to study serial cerebral angiograms with a view toward estimating the *regional* circulation time (i.e., frontal, sylvian, parietal, occipital, deep). Thus, shortening or lengthening of one regional arteriovenous circulation time can become an important clue to the presence of disease in the absence of other abnormalities on the angiogram.

Similarly, the filling sequence of the subependymal veins may be important. As shown by White and Greitz, the sequence of filling of the subependymal veins is related to whether they drain only white matter, gray substance, or a mixture of the white and gray matter (51). The slowest-filling veins, such as the septal vein, drain pure white matter. In contrast, the earliest-filling veins drain pure gray matter. The appearance times of those draining both gray and white substance fall in between. Deviations from the normal may have pathologic significance.

Factors Influencing Circulation Time

INCREASED CIRCULATION TIME

The arterial circulation time is frequently increased (prolonged) in the presence of increased intracranial pressure. Lengthening of the arterial and arteriovenous circulation times is found in approximately one-half of patients with intracranial hypertension.

One of the common causes of prolonged circulation time in cerebral angiography is a low arterial carbon dioxide tension (P_{CO_2}), ordinarily due to hyperventilation. This is often associated with apprehension during the procedure. For this reason, the arterial P_{CO_2} should be measured whenever prolonged circulation time is encountered; otherwise, a false impression of a pathologic process might be gained. Correlations between P_{CO_2} values and circulation times have been excellent (52). If P_{CO_2} values are normal and the circulation time is prolonged, it can be reasonably concluded that disease is present. Circulation time changes have been found also with procedures performed under general anesthesia (53).

The presence of a neoplasm or other type of space-occupying mass, such as an abscess, may produce a *local slowing of the circulation.* The arteries in the region of a mass may fill more slowly than elsewhere, and the veins would then also fill more slowly. Such local prolongation of circulation is most commonly observed angiographically with tumors situated in the frontal and parietal regions. This is true regardless of whether the tumor mass is intracerebral or extracerebral in location (44).

Arterial thrombosis is a frequent cause of localized slow circulation. Slowing also occurs in the prethrombotic stage of severe atherosclerosis. There is no significant difference in cerebral blood flow (CBF) in older patients up to the sixth decade as compared with young adults, in the absence of atherosclerosis (48). Later, there is a reduction in cerebral blood flow, but this was felt to be due to atherosclerosis and not to aging per se by Sokoloff (54) (Table 10.3).

However, the question of blood flow reduction with advancing age has been somewhat controversial. Tachibana et al., utilizing a stable xenon inhalation and CT imaging technique, conclude that there is a reduction in CBF in the aged in all areas, particularly in the frontal area including

Table 10.3.
Factors Producing Increased (Prolonged) Arterial Circulation Time

Diffuse increase
- Increased intracranial pressure
- Decreased carbon dioxide tension
- General anesthesia

Focal increase
- Some mass lesions (e.g., neoplasm, abscess)
- Arterial thrombosis
- Vasospasm
- Vasculitis

the basal ganglia, but also in the parietal and occipital region, with the least reduction found in the visual and speech area (55). The blood flow reduction is gradual and made worse by the presence of atherosclerosis.

It has been reported that a marked increase in intracranial pressure may actually prevent the contrast substance injected into the internal carotid artery from proceeding beyond the intracavernous portion of the artery. This is not an uncommon observation in extremely ill patients (56,57). It is most often associated with trauma or with intraventricular bleeding. It is possible that the taking of very late serial films routinely would show that the contrast substance eventually gets into the cerebral vessels; but this was not the case in the studies of Greitz et al. (58) with prolonged filming (see "Brain Death" in text following). In one instance the ventricles were tapped and the injection repeated; on the second injection following the tap, the contrast substance entered the intracranial vessels promptly (56). This would tend to confirm the belief that very high intracranial pressure influences the lack of filling of the intracranial vessels. Since all of the patients of this type who have been observed have died, the possible existence of a preagonal condition leading to spasm of the vessels should also be considered. Amundsen et al. suggest that compression of the supraclinoid portion of the carotid siphon could occur; in one case, they were able to fill the intracranial carotid by increasing the amount of contrast and the force of the injection (53). It is hard to conceive of the intracranial pressure being higher than the blood pressure for a period of time. Presumably, infarction and irreversible chemical changes that eventually lead to death could produce a degree of generalized cerebral edema resulting in an intracranial pressure actually higher than the systolic blood pressure.

Occasionally, when angiography is performed while the patient is moribund, the serialogram shows stasis within the arteries throughout a program covering a period of approximately 6 to 7 sec; no filling of the veins takes place, since the arteries are filled even on the last film. It is obvious that there is a great slowing of circulation in the brain, possibly as a result of sludging of the blood in the capillaries. In one case, an extreme slowing of the circulation was noted in a patient who had an acute episode suggesting subarachnoid hemorrhage. The injection was repeated, and the serial study was continued for 15 additional sec; the last films still showed distal arteries filled. There were also a few superficial veins, poorly outlined; the deep veins were never seen. This patient died several hours later and was found to have intraventricular bleeding and a large clot under the temporal lobe. It was felt that intravascular agglutination in this patient contributed to blocking of the capillaries. In some of the patients in whom this phenomenon has been observed, autopsy revealed multiple venous thromboses.

A block at the level of the capillaries has been observed by the author in a patient in whom the arteriogram showed only an extremely prolonged arterial phase; in 7 sec the arteries were still fully filled, although some contrast substance had passed beyond the arteries into the capillaries. Autopsy demonstrated the presence of numerous microscopic tumor emboli from a carcinoma of the lung.

A *prolonged injection time* may cause an increase in the arterial circulation time but will not cause an increase in the intermediate and arteriovenous circulation time. Because of generalized filling of arteries and veins on the same films, it is possible to tell that this is an artifact produced by the prolonged injection. It is always necessary to consider the possibility that the changes in circulation observed at cerebral angiography are due to technical problems.

DECREASED CIRCULATION TIME

A regional decrease in the circulation time (acceleration) may be caused by tumors that shunt the blood, such as glioblastoma multiforme, metastatic carcinoma, and a few other neoplasms. It may also be seen in cerebral infarction (so-called luxury perfusion syndrome [59]), in localized brain trauma (brain contusion), in brain abscess, and in certain other conditions such as in status epilepticus with focal seizures (60). It is commonly produced by an arteriovenous fistula, such as in the cavernous sinus. Inhalation of 5 to 8 percent carbon dioxide decreases circulation time (61). As mentioned above, routine determination of the arterial P_{CO_2} during cerebral angiography is helpful in achieving greater accuracy in the interpretation of the alterations of physiology as observed in the angiogram. Huber and Handa reported accelerated circulation when papaverine was injected into the carotid circulation (42) (Table 10.4).

Table 10.4.
Factors Producing Decreased Arterial Circulation Time

Diffuse decrease
- Metabolic causes (e.g., increased carbon dioxide tension)

Focal increase
- Arteriovenous malformations and carotid-cavernous fistulas
- Some mass lesions with "shunt vascularity"
- Cerebral infarction
- Cerebral contusion

Caliber of Intracranial Arteries

The diameter of the intracranial arteries is dependent on blood flow through the brain. The diameter increases under conditions that increase cerebral blood flow, such as a high arterial P_{CO_2}, and decreases when the arterial CO_2 tension lowers, such as in hyperventilation or when breathing 100 percent oxygen. The latter response has been recommended for use to obtain better visualization of the arteries during angiography (62,63). The studies reported by Du Boulay and coauthors were carried out under general anesthesia using intermittent positive pressure ventilation (IPPV) with hyperventilation (62). With this technique, the slowing effect on the circulation time is probably more profound than that produced by hyperventilation alone because of the induced increase in intrathoracic pressure and the resultant increase in venous pressure. The slowing of the circulation allows for greater concentration of the contrast material in the blood, and the expanded time (two to three times longer) allows a longer period of observation. Du Boulay and coauthors recommend taking films at 1-sec intervals for 15 sec. The present author does not use general anesthesia for cerebral angiography. Breathing 100 percent oxygen has a similar (though less pronounced) effect on the circulation time.

Papaverine increases vessel diameter, according to Huber and Handa, who made direct measurements on cerebral angiograms (42). The same authors observed that the diameter of the smaller intracranial arteries, even without papaverine, is larger in the late arterial phase as compared with the early arterial phase of the same serialogram. They attribute this change to a vasodilating effect of the contrast material (Urografin 60 percent). As mentioned earlier, Greitz did not observe this increase in the diameter of the arteries (41).

Measurement of Cerebral Blood Flow

The study of regional cerebral blood flow to be correlated with the cerebral angiographic findings in patients suffering from various brain abnormalities has been receiving increasing attention, particularly with regard to vascular lesions. In the original description by Kety and Schmidt, total brain blood flow in terms of milliliters per 100 g of brain per minute was determined by the use of nitrous oxide, which the subject breathed until saturation was thought to have been achieved (approximately 10 min) (64). This method was an important advance, but it proved to be of limited value for clinical applications. Lassen and Ingvar described a method for measuring regional cerebral blood flow after the intracarotid injection of krypton 85 (65). Later xenon 133 was introduced, and this method was widely used among investigators interested in cerebral blood flow.

STABLE XENON CT

The xenon 133 method of measuring regional cerebral blood flow (rCBF) is now obsolete. It has been replaced by stable xenon inhalation and CT scanning, which not only eliminates the radioactive component but also permits separation of cortical from deep structures with high resolution. Tachibana et al. and Meyer et al. use a 35 percent concentration of xenon and 65 percent oxygen to avoid the anesthetic effects of xenon (55,66).

POSITRON EMISSION TOMOGRAPHY

If one knows the volume of blood flow per 100 g of tissue per minute and the oxygen difference between the arterial blood and the blood sampled from the jugular vein, it is possible to determine the oxygen consumption of the brain by positron emission tomography (PET). Until recently, it was not possible to determine regional oxygen consumption. The use of water tagged with oxygen 15 and oxyhemoglobin tagged with oxygen 15 has permitted not only the determination of regional blood flow by the use of an ideal tracer (water), but also calculation of the regional oxygen consumption (67–70).

PET scanning has the advantage of yielding information on brain metabolism that is not possible by any other method. This includes cerebral oxygen consumption and the cerebral oxygen extraction fraction, both extremely important in determining brain tissue viability. For instance, local circulation could be reduced, but if the reduction is not too great (see text following), viable tissue is capable of increasing the oxygen extraction fraction to maintain energy metabolism. Vice versa, there may be increased perfusion through the local area, but if the brain tissue is not viable, the oxygen extraction fraction would decrease to almost zero. The same would be true of glucose metabolism measured with 18F fluorodeoxyglucose or with 11C deoxyglucose. pH measurements can also be obtained that would help estimate lactacidosis such as results from anaerobic glucose metabolism (71,72).

Oxygen 15 has the disadvantage of being a cyclotron-produced positron emitter, which is expensive. It has a 511-kev value, which causes shielding problems for the probes. Additionally, oxygen 15 has a half-life of only 2 min and must therefore be immediately utilized. However, oxygen 15 is still the only agent that permits calculation of regional oxygen utilization.

SINGLE PHOTON EMISSION TOMOGRAPHY

A less expensive and potentially much more widespread technique is that of single photon emission tomography (SPECT). It is possible to measure CBF and cerebral blood volume with this technique, but tissue oxygen consumption cannot be measured. As we strive to develop effective treatment of ischemic stroke as early as possible, the information related to tissue oxygen consumption, an indicator of tissue viability, is crucial.

MAGNETIC RESONANCE FUNCTIONAL IMAGING

Yet another method that is now receiving attention is *functional imaging by magnetic resonance* (MRFI). This allows for the determination of cerebral blood volume and the speed of cerebral circulation, which would allow us to calculate CBF (but not tissue perfusion) following the intravenous injection of a bolus of gadolinium (or another paramagnetic indicator) (73). MR rapid imaging techniques such as echoplanar techniques are required for this purpose. Although it may be theoretically possible to calculate oxygen consumption by MRI, to date this has not been accomplished.

CEREBRAL VASCULAR REACTIVITY

The ability of the cerebral circulation to adjust itself to changes in the arterial carbon dioxide tension is reflected as its reactivity. Normally, an increase in CBF takes place when the patient breathes 5 to 8 percent CO_2 in oxygen. If no increase occurs under these circumstances, it can be concluded that the cerebral circulation is incapable of responding to this strong stimulus; that is, the vessels are probably maximally dilated (usually to compensate for ischemia). This lack of reaction can be called *loss of cerebral vascular reactivity* (74–76).

Carbon dioxide inhalation turns out to be a very uncomfortable method for the patient. A better method of provoking increased CBF is through the use of acetazolamide (Diamox). The combination of high-resolution rCBF (utilizing xenon/CT) and the acetazolamide challenge has been proposed by Rogg et al. (77).

LOSS OF AUTOREGULATION

Autoregulation is the usual ability of the normal brain to adjust CBF to the blood pressure. If the blood pressure rises, blood flow in the brain does not increase in a normal subject because of inherent mechanisms that produce arterial and arteriolar contraction, and thus impede high pressure flow in the various areas of the brain (78). When there is brain damage such as occurs with infarcts and certain other lesions, the affected area of the brain usually loses its ability to adjust blood flow when there is an elevation of the blood pressure (79).

Lassen introduced the term *luxury perfusion* to denote increased circulation through an area of infarcted brain that he could detect by external measurements of regional CBF (59). Lassen attributes this to a lowered tissue pH, a posthypoxic acidosis with vasoparalysis. The same phenomenon had been noted earlier in angiograms by the authors (80). It was observed angiographically that there was an increased circulatory rate, with early filling of the basal vein, in infarcts in the territory of the middle cerebral artery. Vasodilatation of the cerebral cortical vessels following occlusions was also demonstrated. Later, Cronqvist et al. and others reported on this phenomenon as observed angiographically (81). In the series of cases reported by Taveras et al., an increased circulatory rate with early-filling veins was found in 35 percent of the cases (82). In no case was an accelerated rate observed angiographically beyond 15 days following the onset of hemiparesis. Thus the luxury perfusion syndrome is something that occurs often and disappears approximately 2 weeks after the initial insult (see text following for further details).

The term *luxury perfusion* has been challenged because it is really not true perfusion of brain tissue but rather *nonnutritional flow.* The brain tissue is probably being bypassed either by true arteriovenous connections or by a very dilated capillary bed. Indeed, the same phenomenon can be observed with radioactive indicators when the probe is placed over the internal carotid artery bifurcation; that is, a high peak is recorded that in calculation yields, erroneously, a higher blood flow value for that area. Moreover, when an occluded vessel is shown to be producing the infarct, increased speed of circulation with early-filling veins is not observed unless the contrast material somehow reaches the area of infarction. In other words, if the afferent vessels are occluded, the veins do not fill early (or do not fill at all) in the area. It may be that the increased circulatory rate is observed only after an occluded artery reopens (by lysis) and that in the area of tissue damage a local loss of autoregulation then takes place.

It is worth noting that in the acute stage of infarction, there is depression of the CBF in the entire hemisphere, even though the lesion is well localized. The opposite hemisphere may show a diffuse decrease in CBF as well. The reason is not clearly understood, but it is certainly an important phenomenon of cerebral infarction.

Consideration has to be given also to the possible influence of cerebrospinal fluid (CSF) pressure on capillary blood flow. If there is loss of autoregulation in the brain, a relatively minor increase in CSF pressure may produce profound changes in blood flow. The capillaries become unable to function if CSF pressure approaches capillary pressure (83).

BRAIN DEATH

With the widespread availability of equipment to sustain vital functions, it has become important to determine whether an individual may be technically dead, that is, whether the brain has ceased to function even though the heart continues to beat and the lungs ventilate. The question poses a number of ethical problems that are difficult to resolve. Although the clinical signs usually suggest total brain infarction, a dilemma often exists. If it is possible, however, to be sure that the brain is functionless, the ethical questions are largely dispelled. Brain death is associated with complete or almost complete cessation of circulation, which leads to generalized cerebral infarction. An isoelectric electroencephalogram (EEG) tracing is usually found in such cases; however, the EEG can be isoelectric when there is not complete cessation of circulation, and vice versa.

Neuroradiologists are familiar with the fact that when carotid angiography demonstrates failure of a contrast agent to enter the intracranial portion of the circulation in significant quantity, this indicates that the patient will surely die. This method of visualizing the cerebral circulation is not used as frequently as it might be, possibly because it has not yet been incorporated as an intensive care routine. Heiskanen collected 100 cases in which failure of the contrast material to enter the cranial circulation was followed by death in all but two instances, and these two patients did not show the usual clinical signs of brain death (84).

Because there is a possibility that technical difficulties during direct puncture could result in nonfilling because of intramural injections, Greitz et al. have convincingly demonstrated that if an aortocranial angiogram is performed by injecting the contrast into the aortic arch via a femoral catheter, one can be sure that the contrast will reach any vessel that may still be open (58). Moreover, both external carotid arteries will be opacified, and this fact means that the contrast agent entered the common carotid arteries. Greitz et al. recommended that serial films be made for a long period (30 sec) and that a second injection and serial filming be performed 30 min later in order to eliminate the possibility of temporary or intermittent nonfilling. If under these circumstances there is no significant intracranial filling, it is a sure indication of total brain infarction (58).

Although radioactive nuclides and angiography with contrast agents are the most reliable methods of determining brain death, there are practical difficulties in using standard techniques in an unresponsive, apneic patient.

Braunstein et al. have shown that technetium pertechnetate injected intravenously can be used to determine the existence of absent brain circulation with a high degree of accuracy (85). In the normal case, a high peak, lasting about 10 sec, is recorded, and this peak is absent in cases of total brain infarction.

Occlusive and Stenotic Lesions

CLINICAL AND PATHOLOGIC CONSIDERATIONS

The "stroke syndrome" may be produced by a variety of conditions involving the vessels of the brain. Among these may be listed (a) stenotic and occlusive lesions of the extracranial and intracranial arteries (thrombosis and embolism); (b) intracranial hemorrhage due to rupture of an artery, an aneurysm, or an arteriovenous malformation; (c) systemic hypotension; (d) venous and dural sinus thrombosis; and (e) conditions of undetermined origin.

The stenotic and occlusive lesions of the extracranial and intracranial vessels may be due to localized atheromatous changes. They are usually found at arterial bifurcations and may be part of a generalized degenerative process with more pronounced changes in certain focal areas. The lesions may also develop as the result of an inflammatory process of the vessel. In some cases, arteritis is associated with a known inflammatory disease, such as syphilis, or develops from embolism of pyogenic or tuberculous origin. At other times, cerebral arteritis may be part of a disease of undetermined origin, such as lupus erythematosus (rarely) and polyarteritis nodosa. It may also occur as a solitary arteritic process of unknown etiology (see "Inflammatory Disease," Chapter 6).

STROKES IN YOUNG PEOPLE

A recently recognized relationship between strokes in the young and the presence of antiphospholipid antibodies (APLAs) deserves consideration here. APLAs are immunoglobulins of the immunoglobulins G, M, and A (IgG, IgM, and IgA) with activity against axionic and neutral phospholipids. The two most widely recognized are the lupus anticoagulant and the anticardiolipin antibodies. The patients usually present a false-positive VDRL test. APLAs have been reported with an increasing frequency in patients with systemic lupus erythematosus and other clinical disorders, including infection, neoplasms, AIDS, and primary immunodeficiency, and after treatment with certain drugs. The term *lupus anticoagulant* is probably a misnomer, for it is associated with increased coagulability and not with bleeding (86,87). Patients with either secondary or primary APLA syndromes have an increased frequency of thromboembolism. Brey et al. found a high incidence of APLA syndrome in young patients with stroke (as high as 45 percent) (88). Although patients with APLAs may have other neurologic manifestations (migraine, seizures, chorea, Guillain-Barré syndrome, multiple sclerosis, Degos disease), a positive anticardiolipin test is found much more frequently in patients with ischemic brain conditions than in patients with other neurologic disorders (89).

Thus it behooves us to include in our reports the possibility of APLA syndrome in any young patient who presents with a stroke (90). This is particularly true because recurrent ischemic episodes may be preventable by appropriate anticoagulant medication such as warfarin (Coumadin).

Another condition needing consideration when encountering a stroke in a young patient is cerebral autosomal dominant arteriopathy with subcortical infarcts and leukoencephalopathy (CADASIL). It affects adults in the fourth to sixth decade of life (mean age about 43 years) and is characterized by recurrent subcortical ischemic strokes in nonhypertensive individuals and leads some patients to dementia. CT and MRI show white matter disease and subcortical areas consistent with ischemic lesions. Tournier-Lasserve et al. indicate that the disease locus has been assigned to chromosome 19 q 12 (91). Of 57 living members analyzed in one family, 11 had suffered recurrent strokes. Three developed pseudobulbar palsy and subcortical dementia (91,92). The affected individuals do not show atherosclerosis or amyloid angiopathy. The transmission of this disease is consistent with an autosomal dominant pattern of inheritance.

PATHOPHYSIOLOGIC CONSIDERATIONS

Local circulatory arrest due to occlusion of a brain arterial channel leads to local brain ischemia. The occlusion may be due to embolus or to focal atherosclerosis, dissection, spasm, or trauma. The occlusion may be temporary or permanent, but most larger artery occlusions are temporary and last a few minutes to several hours. The collateral cerebral circulation ordinarily takes over the blood supply to the involved area, and this takes place very rapidly. However, if the occluded artery is terminal, as are some of the perforating brain arteries (lenticulostriate and others), or if the collateral circulation cannot be established because of propagation of thrombus beyond the site of occlusion, brain ischemia develops; in addition, the availability of collaterals varies among individuals or may be affected by disease. The blood supply in the affected area would then drop. It has been stated, based on the experimental situation, that if local blood flow in the affected tissues falls below a certain level, a cascade of changes begins to occur. The normal blood flow is about 50 ml/100 g brain tissue/min. If it falls below 18 ml, first the spontaneous and evoked electrical activity ceases, causing weakness, paralysis, aphasia, and so forth. If the low blood flow remains for more than 30 min, *cytotoxic edema* begins, first in the gray matter at a blood flow of 20 to 22 ml/100 g/min and in the white matter at a lower level of flow (93,94). In cytotoxic edema there is accumulation of water in the cell body. This is attributed to ion pump dysfunction, which allows increased intracellular sodium and potassium. The decreased blood flow causes a decreased oxygen supply, which leads to depletion of adenosine triphosphate (ATP). To preserve energy metabolism, the cells initiate anaerobic glycolysis, but this is a very ineffecient pathway for energy production, yielding only about 5 percent of the ATP normally yielded by the aerobic oxidative pathway. The anaerobic glycolysis leads to lactic acidosis. The membrane-bound ion pump failure resulting from the low ATP levels allows for an accumulation of sodium, potassium, hydrogen, and calcium ions in the cells, which leads to an increase in the osmotic gradient for water and increased intracytoplasmic water.

Vasogenic edema is the passage of water from the capillaries into the extracellular space. In order for vasogenic edema to occur, there must be damage to the capillary endothelium. This takes some time to develop, 3 to 6 h or longer, depending on the percentage reduction in blood flow. In addition, there must be some residual or reestablished blood flow. The greater the hydrostatic pressure, the greater the potential for vasogenic edema once there is capillary wall damage. For that reason, an embolic occlusion in which the occluding embolus becomes lysed after a number of hours may lead to more vasogenic edema than an atherosclerotic occlusion. In spite of the capillary wall damage, the blood-brain barrier is not necessarily broken until much later, 8 to 10 days. (At least one cannot demonstrate passage of iodide- or gadolinium-based contrast media into the extravascular space until after 1 week in the majority of cases, as discussed in text following.)

Table 10.5.
Major Forms of Cerebral Edema

- Cytotoxic edema
  - Accumulation of intracellular water
  - Due to ischemia-related dysfunction of cell membrane
  - Characteristically seen in cerebral infarction
- Vasogenic edema
  - Accumulation of water in extracellular space
  - Related to damage of capillary endothelium
  - Can be due to a wide variety of causes other than infarction (e.g., mass lesions)

Thus it may be concluded that there is already some cytotoxic edema present when the patient arrives in the hospital, because cytotoxic edema begins to develop within 30 min to 1 h after the onset of symptoms. If the involved area is large enough, 3 to 5 cm in diameter or larger, it should be possible to detect the edema by cross-sectional imaging methods, particularly MRI, and less efficiently by CT. However, the accumulation of cytotoxic edema occurs gradually and may take a few to several hours to become detectable. It is now possible to demonstrate cytotoxic edema by diffusion imaging techniques. At Massachusetts General Hospital it is being carried out routinely and found to be highly accurate and extremely useful clinically. (See text following under "Therapeutic Considerations," page 458. See also Chapter 4 for further discussion on cerebral edema. Table 10.5 summarizes the two major forms of cerebral edema.)

Irreversible cell damage and neuronal death begin in 30 to 60 min if the blood flow reduction is 40 percent or greater (95). The cell bodies first swell up, as explained in text just preceding, because of cell membrane damage that allows the passage of sodium and calcium ions into the cytoplasm. The passage of calcium ions into the cell is tightly regulated, and once this excessive intake occurs, cell death is sure to occur. The cell membrane ruptures and allows passage of intracellular water and proteins into the extracellular compartment. Membrane rupture of glial cells also occurs.

Once dead tissue is present, macrophages invade the area, and regenerating capillaries devoid of tight junctions, and thus permeable to water and larger molecules, begin to form. Capillary proliferation begins in the periphery of the infarct about the third day and reaches a maximum in 7 to 10 days (96,97), at which time contrast enhancement, usually of the infarct, can be observed on CT or MRI.

CLINICAL STROKE STAGES

Clinically the stroke syndrome can be divided into several stages or types. First, there are *transient ischemic attacks*, (TIAs), which may be produced by stenotic or ulcerative lesions of the extracranial vessels and also by disease of the intracranial vessels. The attacks may also be associated with other conditions, such as cardiac arrhythmia. A TIA is diagnosed when the symptoms last from a minute to perhaps

5 to 30 minutes. Beyond that it may last an hour to several hours, in which case the term *reversible ischemic neurologic deficit* (RIND) may be used, instead. The TIA may consist of weakness, numbness, transient monocular blindness (TMB), dysarthria, transient dizziness, confusion, and other transient manifestations difficult to define (98).

This is the stage at which the diagnosis should ideally be made because the obstruction, if extracerebral, may lend itself to removal of the cause, in many instances leading to complete recovery. Between the attacks of circulatory insufficiency the patients may be entirely normal. The symptoms may evolve from the carotid or the vertebral-basilar circulation. There may be no evidence of permanent damage to the brain resulting from such attacks.

The second stage, or *intermittent progressive type*, indicates that the patient did not quite recover from an ischemic attack, and days or sometimes weeks later another attack occurs from which the patient recovers even less. At any time the patient may have a third, fourth, or more attacks, which eventually will leave him or her hemiplegic. *Advancing stroke* (or *stroke in evolution*) constitutes the third type. The term may be applied to a clinical evolution in which the patient's condition, following the first partial involvement of his or her functions, continues to deteriorate over a period of hours or within a day or two. The condition is similar to the intermittent progressive type but differs from it in that the increase in functional deficit takes place more steadily and usually more rapidly.

The final type is the *completed stroke*. Siekert defined the completed stroke as a state in which the neurologic deficit is stable and persistent over a period of hours or days. If the patient is completely disabled, it is easy to determine that a completed stroke exists (99). On the other hand, the stroke process may reach termination when only a partial, or even a minimal, deficit has occurred. Undoubtedly, some of these patients belong in the intermittent progressive stroke category, since a patient who has partial neurologic involvement may later have another attack with advancement toward greater disability.

On examination of the brain, the pathologist usually finds evidence of a cerebral infarct, sometimes multiple infarcts. Whether an infarct develops after an arterial obstruction depends on the sufficiency or insufficiency of the anastomoses to supply the needs of the part. If they are insufficient, then the tissue becomes ischemic and may be permanently damaged.

The word *infarct* means "to stuff," that is, with interstitial fluid and with blood. Edema is usually maximal within 24 to 48 h. A distinction is often drawn between pale and red infarcts; however, as long ago as 1846, Rokitansky contended that there is no fundamental difference between the two. He believed that each was an area stuffed with blood and red from dilatation of anastomotic vessels in the beginning; depending on the efficiency of the collateral circulation, the infarct might remain red or might become pale. In the cerebral cortex anastomoses are abundant; the central or ganglionic vessels are more of the nature of "endarteries" in their reaction to acute occlusions.

In a permanently damaged area, necrosis ensues. In the central nervous system, necrosis is colliquative rather than coagulative. Therefore, an infarcted area may soon become liquefied and absorbed so that a brain cyst (pseudocyst) forms. This may be a large area of porencephaly or a small lacuna, depending on the size of the original lesion.

True hemorrhage into an infarcted area may occur either from overdistention of vessels in the early stages or, later, from vasal necrosis in the softened tissue undergoing liquefaction. Cerebral hemorrhage may also be associated with a disturbance of the blood-clotting mechanisms, and is not uncommon in patients receiving anticoagulant treatment. Hypertension contributes. Occasionally, arterial occlusion, with or without intracerebral hemorrhage, is due to medial necrosis of the arterial wall, the lesion being similar to that found in the aorta (100).

Some neoplasms, particularly metastatic tumors and some glioblastomas, may cause a sudden occurrence of neurologic findings very suggestive of a vascular accident. Intracerebral hematomas occurring spontaneously, or from an aneurysm or arteriovenous malformation, often produce clinical findings similar to those resulting from vascular occlusions. These are usually well demonstrated by CT or MRI. On the other hand, angiography can show the presence of an extracranial stenotic lesion of the carotid artery for which surgical treatment may be indicated. At the same time, some caution must be exercised in attributing neurologic disorders to extracranial atheromatous lesions found angiographically. Some stenotic lesions of the internal carotid and vertebral arteries, and even of the common carotid and subclavian arteries, occur without producing symptoms; that is, the patient's old or recent history does not reveal any cerebrovascular accident. Martin et al., after a study of 100 embalmed cadavers over 55 years of age, reported an 11 percent incidence of complete occlusion of at least one major artery, either the internal carotid, the common carotid, or the vertebral artery (101). In 3 patients there was occlusion of two major extracranial arteries. A few of these patients had a history of neurologic disease in the past, but the material was an unselected, consecutive series. Fisher, in 1954, found a 9.5 percent incidence of occlusion or severe stenosis of the cervical carotid arteries in a large necropsy series (102). In the series of Martin and coauthors, an additional 29 percent of their cases had partial occlusions in which one or more of the four major vessels were at least 50 percent reduced in caliber (103).

Because the incidence reported by these authors was so high, angiographic studies were performed on cadavers under conditions that more closely simulated those existing in vivo (104). A contrast substance of moderate viscosity was used that did not pass readily through the capillaries. It was possible, therefore, to distend the major vessels to a degree similar to that encountered in the living subject. A pressure ranging between 120 and 200 mmHg was used during the injection. A total of 130 cadavers were studied.

Of 121 cases without neurologic symptoms prior to death, there was a 22 percent incidence of stenotic lesions with a greater than 50 percent reduction of the caliber involving the carotid or vertebral systems, and sometimes both systems (7 cases). The patients who had a history of cerebral ischemia (9 cases) prior (but not necessarily related) to death all had stenotic lesions involving both the extracranial and intracranial vessels. Only 6 cases of complete occlusion were found, of which one was thought to be preagonal. The lower incidence (4 percent) of complete occlusion (as against 11 percent as found by Martin and coworkers [103]) is more in keeping with the author's daily experience in cerebral angiography. The author has only infrequently encountered carotid occlusions when performing cerebral angiograms in older patients without related clinical manifestations.

From the preceding discussion, it is evident that the general incidence of partial or complete extracranial arterial obstruction is lower than that described in the pathologic specimens but is still surprisingly high. This increases the difficulty of establishing a cause-and-effect relationship between carotid atherosclerosis and cerebral ischemia. Ultimately, all symptoms are provoked by circulatory failure at the local, or intracranial, level, and *it is more than likely that the majority are due to embolic phenomena.* Some strokes are undoubtedly caused by hypotension, such as those associated with myocardial infarction. The development of an obstructing lesion in the neck also may promote an occlusion in an intracranial vessel. If both an extracranial carotid artery and an intracranial branch are involved by arteriosclerosis, the lowering of pressure resulting from progression of the cervical lesion might provoke completion of occlusion in the intracranial artery. The same result can follow application of a clamp to the internal carotid artery in the neck for the treatment of an aneurysm. If the clamp is released promptly, the neurologic deficit usually disappears, but sometimes it persists. In addition to lowering of pressure, another mechanism is clot formation above the clamp, with embolism, which would explain continuation of the deficit. Also among the many causes of stroke are emboli from cardiac lesions. Fragments of valvular or mural thrombi may embolize from the left cardiac chambers. Bacterial endocarditis is a less common cause since the advent of antibiotics. Neoplastic emboli may be derived from a left atrial myxoma. Emboli from other parts of the body may occur when there is a pulmonary or cardiac shunt.

Multiple arteriosclerotic lesions of the intracranial and extracranial vessels probably are the rule rather than the exception. Because of the problem of multiplicity of lesions, all of the extracranial vessels, as well as the intracranial vessels, must be studied to ensure a complete diagnosis prior to surgical intervention.

SEQUENCE OF EXAMINATION

Since there are a variety of procedures available for the examination of patients suspected of having cerebrovascular disease, not all involving radiologic methods, an orderly approach using groups of tests is necessary. A logical beginning would be to use studies that are painless and essentially harmless to the patient before using angiography. But although many of these methods will help increase the yield of positive information by helping to select patients for contrast study, it often evolves that there is no substitute for visualization of the interior of the cerebrovascular tree.

One of the objectives of such a series of examinations is to help recognize patients with extracranial atherosclerosis, since surgical reconstruction of one or both carotid arteries in the neck is now being performed with greater skill and safety in the treatment of major vessel atherosclerosis causing ischemia. It goes without saying that careful neurologic and neuro-ophthalmologic evaluations are essential. The finding of retinal artery emboli is often helpful in detecting extracranial cerebrovascular lesions.

The concept of using noninvasive techniques early in the evaluation of cerebral ischemia entails the early use of CT. It has long been recognized that calcification in the cavernous and supraclinoid portions of the internal carotid artery is an indication of arteriosclerosis. Angiographic and pathologic correlation has shown, however, that, in many of these cases, the lime deposits are in the tunica media (Mönckeberg type) and that there is not significant narrowing of the arterial lumen by intimal disease. More important is calcification in the region of the carotid bifurcation as seen on soft-tissue films of the neck. More than one-half of the patients who have calcification 1 cm or more in length along both the medial and lateral walls of the cervical carotid bifurcation have significant narrowing of the internal carotid artery at its origin. In addition, calcification and ulceration are degenerative changes often occurring together, and many patients with less than the heavy calcification just described can be shown to have ulcerative atheromatous changes at angiography. Calcification may at times be so extensive that there is an angulation of the internal carotid artery with a sharp reduction in caliber at the site of a kink between the flexible and calcified portions of the vessel. It might be advocated that a soft-tissue radiograph of the neck be made a part of the routine procedure in evaluating patients with suspected extracranial atherosclerosis. This examination is usually omitted partly because the presence of calcification does not correlate often enough with the presence of atherosclerotic narrowing of the carotid lumen. The presence of bruit on auscultation of the carotid bifurcation region is usually considered an adequate substitute and possibly more informative in terms of suggesting a significant stenosis. More recently, the presence of heavy calcification has been found to interfere with the examination of this carotid bifurcation when the spiral or helicoid CT technique with contrast enhacement is used. It may be possible, technically, to separate the Hounsfield number of the calcium from that of the iodide contrast material so as to arrive at a more accurate estimate of the narrowed lumen of the internal carotid artery (Fig. 10.8).

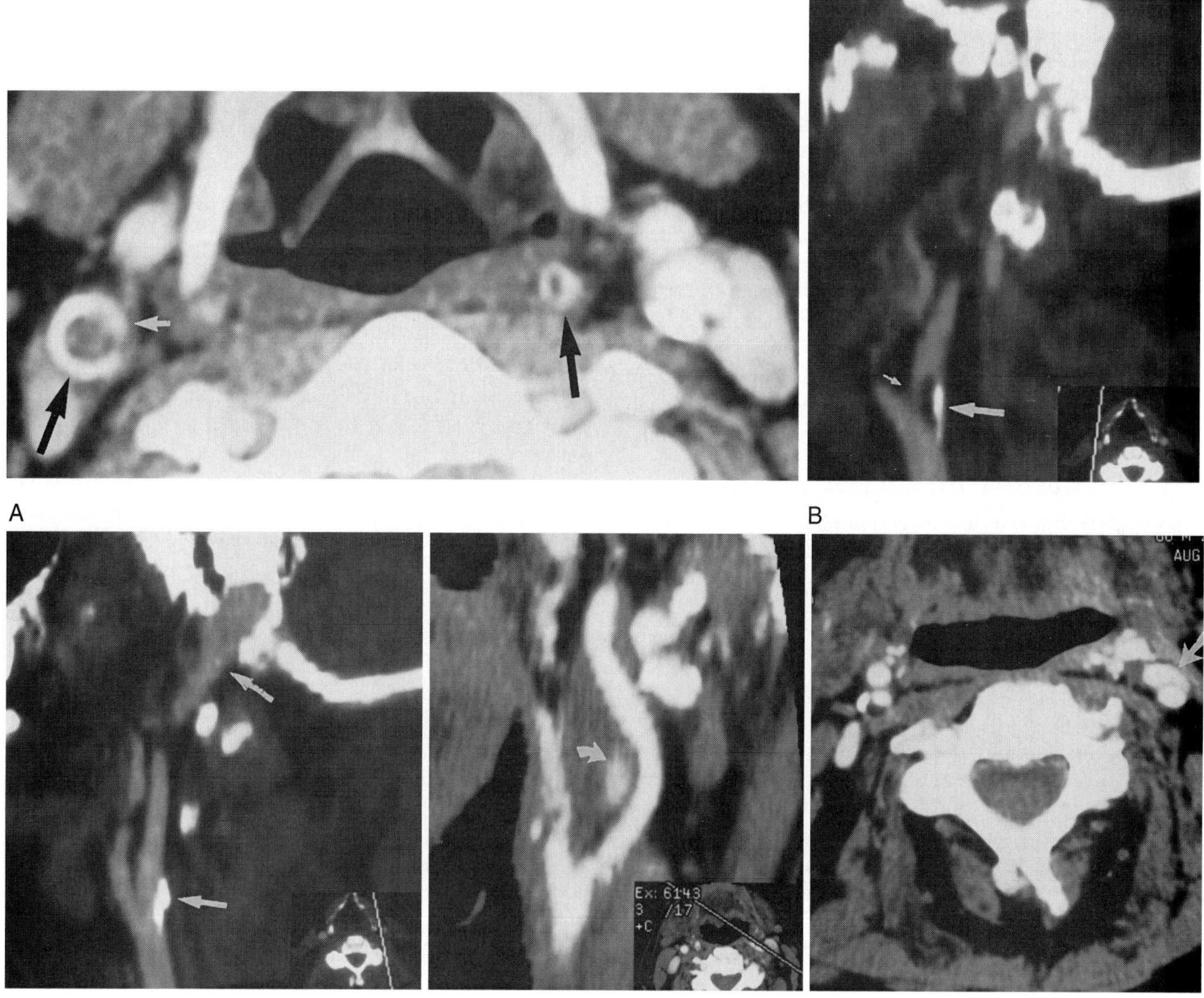

C D E

Figure 10.8. Spiral CT angiography of carotid artery bifurcation. **A.** Axial view after contrast shows a calcified plaque on both sides, larger on the right (arrows). The center of the circumferential calcified arterial wall is filled with a noncalcified plaque. The lumen is represented by a small area of contrast shown by the white smaller arrow. **B.** Sagittal view of right carotid artery shows the top of the common carotid artery, its bifurcation, the presence of a calcified arterial wall (large arrow), and a noncalcified plaque. The lumen is narrow and measures 2.0 mm in residual diameter (small arrow). **C.** On the left side there is a calcified plaque, but it is not producing narrowing of the arterial lumen (lower arrow). The upper arrow points at the jugular bulb and the upper jugular vein. **D** and **E.** Spiral CT angiography in another case demonstrating calcification in wall of internal carotid artery. **D.** Oblique reconstruction reveals narrowing of internal carotid artery above the common carotid bifurcation and the presence of a large calcified plaque (arrow), which was not seen by MRA. **E.** Axial view shows that the calcified plaque (arrow) is larger than the arterial lumen.

Imaging Findings

TRANSIENT ISCHEMIC ATTACKS

In TIAs, it is presumed that the period of ischemia leading to the production of symptoms did not last long enough to produce permanent damage to the brain tissue. The pathogenesis of the TIA is not really known. It may be a circulatory insufficiency lasting for several minutes, or it may be a small platelet-fibrin aggregate coming possibly from an atherosclerotic plaque, from an ulceration in the plaque, or from an unknown source. Because these white emboli usually fragment and do not obstruct the vessels for a long enough period of time, the symptoms are transient. They could also be produced by a red embolus, which is small enough to proceed directly to a relatively small vessel and to fragment rapidly. The theory of white emboli is somewhat important and has been seen in one case in which the retina was followed ophthalmoscopically for 20 to 30 min until disappearance was recorded (105). If such is seen to produce a receding scotoma in the eye, presumably the same could occur in the brain; nevertheless, there is no agreement as to the actual cause of TIAs. In the RIND, the symptoms last longer, possibly several hours or half a day, and are followed by complete recovery. In these cases one would suspect that a true red embolus may well have gone into the cerebral circulation but fragmented early and so did not produce a permanent deficit. In these cases, again, an ischemic lesion may not be detected by CT or MRI, but in some cases a lesion is found. It is in these two types of cases, TIA and RIND, that a thorough study of the cerebral circulation is worth pursuing. Normally one would start with a CT scan, followed by noninvasive examinations: Doppler ultrasound of the carotid arteries, periorbital Doppler, measurements of the peak velocities of the carotid artery systems, and possibly other noninvasive examinations. Transcranil Doppler may also be useful, as well as oculoplethysmography. Following this, particularly if an abnormality is found in the extracranial vessels or around the base of the skull, MRI examination with MRA may be useful. MRA may confirm or reinforce the findings found with the ultrasound noninvasive tests, and if a lesion is demonstrated that might require surgical intervention, a cerebral angiogram may then be performed. Today angiography is usually carried out, but in some cases, now that ultrasound noninvasive tests and MRI may complement each other, we may omit cerebral angiography if there is no discrepancy between the two.

ISCHEMIC INFARCTION

A CT examination is usually carried out on the patient's arrival at the hospital, which allows us to rule out the presence of a cerebral hemorrhage. In the first 24 to 48 h following an ischemic episode, the CT scan may be negative (Figs. 10.9 and 10.49). Sometimes, if one looks very carefully at the examination, it may be possible to detect very minor changes, such as minimal differences in the density of the white matter or of the adjacent gray matter, minimal disappearance of the outline of the structures of the basal ganglia–internal capsule region when one compares one side to the other, and sometimes loss of the outline of the sulci in the cerebral surface, loss of the insular ribbon, again comparing one side with the other (106). An early sign may be hyperintensity of one or more of the major arteries due to thrombus (Fig. 10.9*C* to *E*). Findings consistent with cerebral ischemic infarction when the patient arrives or up to 12 h after the beginning of symptoms are an indication of an extensive infarction that will be considerably more manifest within the next day or two. In other words, large infarcts are seen earlier than smaller ones on CT or MRI (Fig. 10.10).

In a comparison study of CT and MRI in patients examined within the first 24 h after onset of symptoms, Bryan et al. found a positive CT reading in 58 percent and a positive MRI reading in 82 percent of cases (107). An ischemic infarction on CT is seen as an area of decreased attenuation involving the white matter and the adjacent gray matter in the cerebral cortex or in the region of the internal capsule and basal ganglia. The decreased attenuation is likely to become better defined in 3 or 4 days or longer and usually ends up fairly well demarcated in about a week or 10 days (Table 10.6). Sometimes it may be possible to see the "fogging effect," which will decrease the lower attenuation and bring the diseased area to a level approaching the surrounding normal brain. This phenomenon is attributable to reopening of capillary blood vessels in the region and to hyperemia, and is not an indication that the patient is improving. Later a regular permanent scar will be formed in the infarcted region where there is disappearance of normal structure, gliosis, and many small cystic spaces, which is why the density of an old infarct approaches that of CSF. We are concerned by the lack of ability to detect reliably an ischemic lesion in the brain by CT scan in the first 24 to 48 h. The same is true of MRI; although the changes on the proton density and T2-weighted images can be seen somewhat earlier than on CT, they cannot be seen early enough to make a difference. At the present time there is no real treatment for strokes in the very early stage, but we are all looking for it and hoping

Table 10.6.
CT and MR Imaging of Infarctions

CT imaging findings in early nonhemorrhagic infarction
- Blurring of outlines of basal ganglia and internal capsule
- Loss of outline of cortical sulci
- Indistinctness of gray/white junction
- Loss of insular ribbon

Early (first 24 h) MRI findings of infarction*
- Absence of arterial flow void
- Arterial enhancement
- Brain swelling on T1-weighted images
- Hyperintense signal (due to cytotoxic edema) on T2-weighted images
- Diffusion imaging shows slow diffusion

* Adapted from WTC Yuh, MR Crain: Neuroimag Clin North Am 1992;421–439.

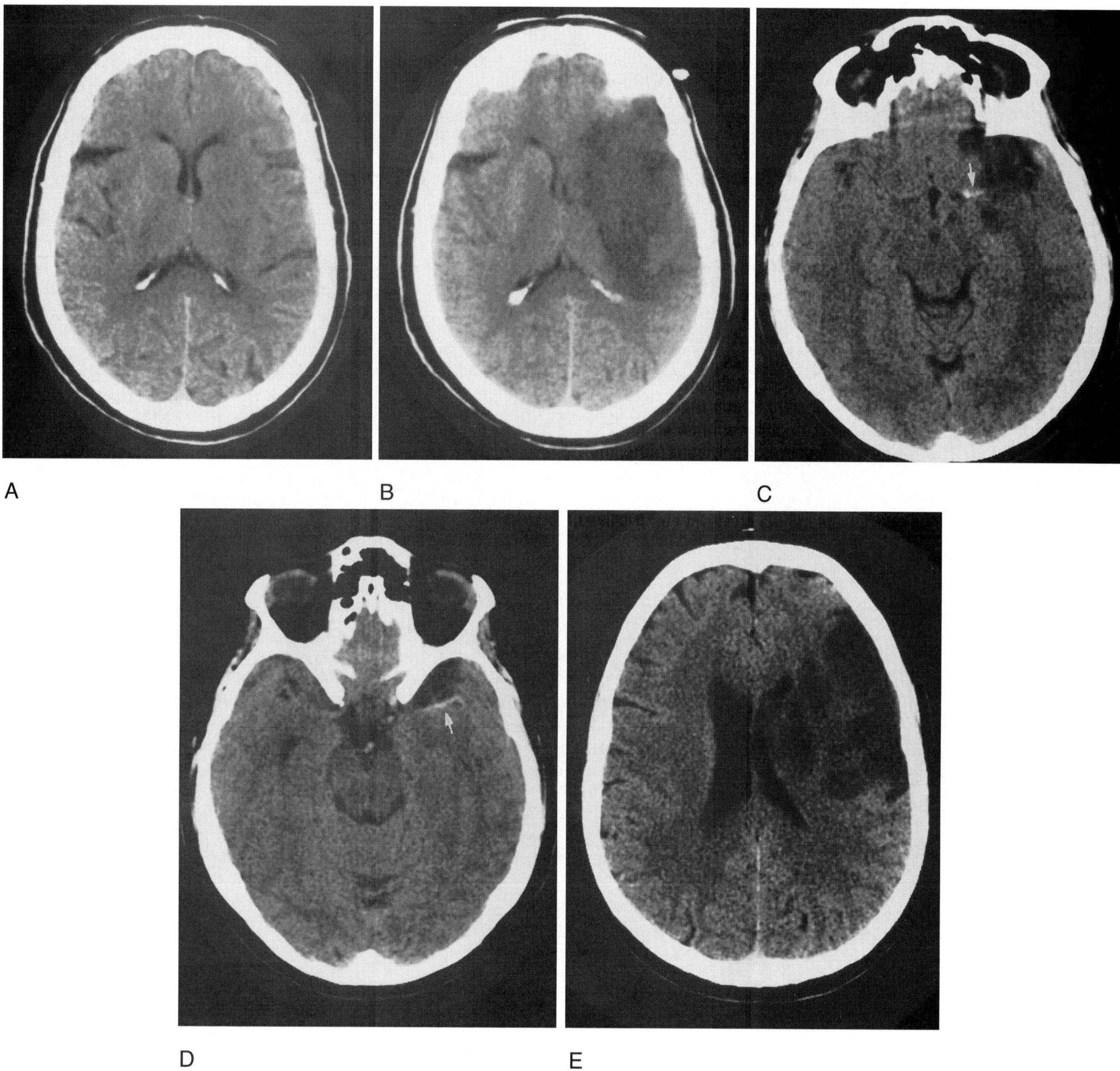

Figure 10.9. Cerebral infarction. **A.** Less than 24 h after onset of symptoms there is only a slight reduction in the density of the basal ganglia and a loss of the normal contrast between the lenticular nucleus and the internal capsule. There is also some decreased attenuation at the anterior aspect of the head of the caudate nucleus. The sylvian fissure and insular surface are not as well seen on the left as on the right, possibly because of mild edema. **B.** Two days later there is an extensive hypodense area primarily involving the frontal lobe but also involving the basal ganglia and internal capsule, but sparing the thalamus. The appearance suggests that an obstruction of the trunk of the middle cerebral artery is affecting the perforating branches as well as the superior division of this vessel. **C** to **E.** Middle cerebral artery thrombosis seen on plain CT. **C** and **D.** There is marked hyperdensity in the trunk of the middle cerebral artery (arrow), indicative of a thrombus. Moderate hyperintensity is often seen in normal individuals because the artery is surrounded by the cerebrospinal fluid in the sylvian cistern, particularly in older subjects. Thus it is necessary to compare the relative density between the sides. **E.** Four days later a large infarct with mass effect compressing the lateral ventricle is seen. The mass effect is due to edema; there is no evidence of hemorrhage.

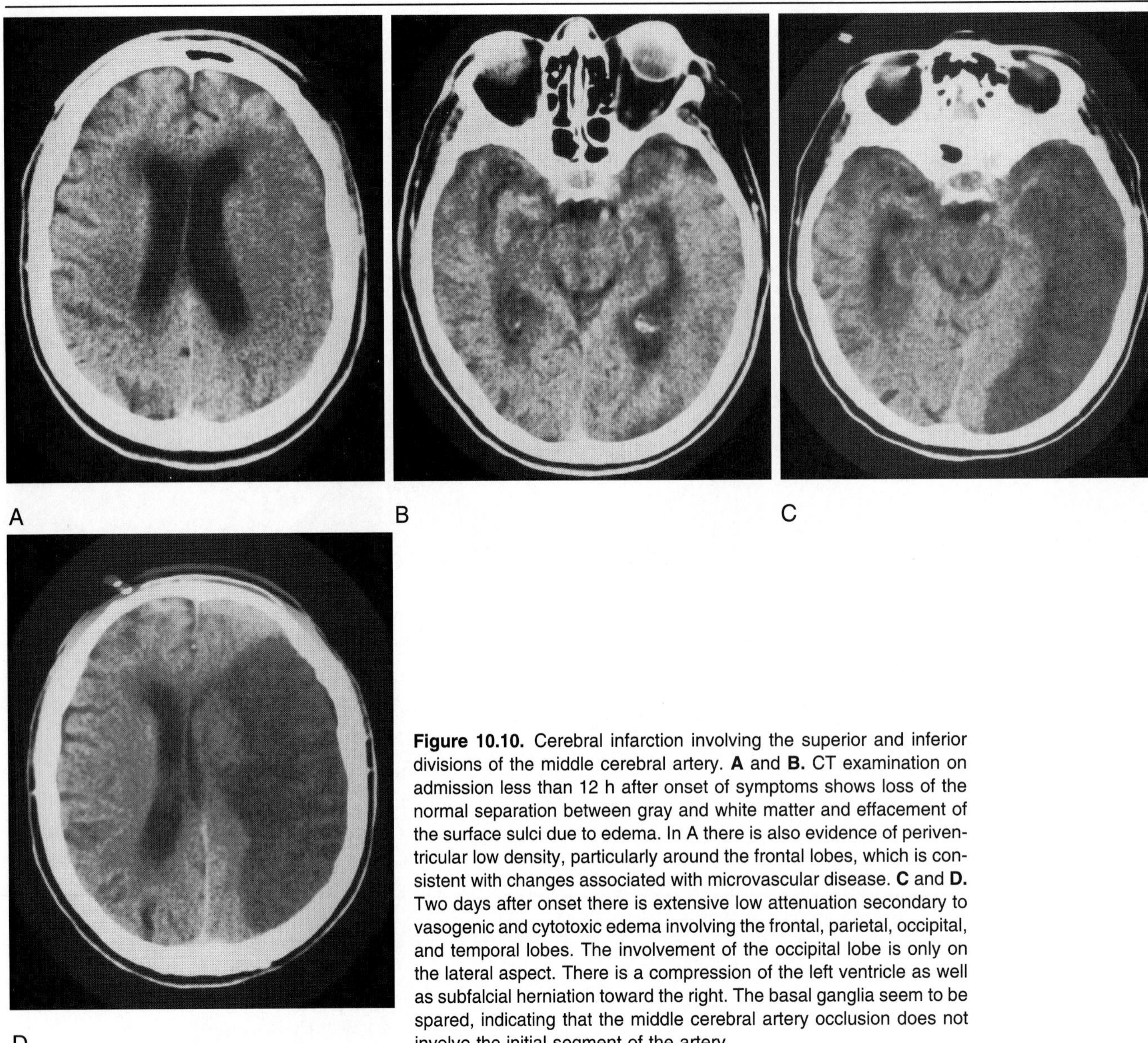

Figure 10.10. Cerebral infarction involving the superior and inferior divisions of the middle cerebral artery. **A** and **B.** CT examination on admission less than 12 h after onset of symptoms shows loss of the normal separation between gray and white matter and effacement of the surface sulci due to edema. In A there is also evidence of periventricular low density, particularly around the frontal lobes, which is consistent with changes associated with microvascular disease. **C** and **D.** Two days after onset there is extensive low attenuation secondary to vasogenic and cytotoxic edema involving the frontal, parietal, occipital, and temporal lobes. The involvement of the occipital lobe is only on the lateral aspect. There is a compression of the left ventricle as well as subfalcial herniation toward the right. The basal ganglia seem to be spared, indicating that the middle cerebral artery occlusion does not involve the initial segment of the artery.

that a well-accepted method can be developed to treat these patients at this stage. Among these is controlled hypertension. Early diagnosis is a requirement, and diffusion-weighted imaging offers this possibility. It requires some special instrumentation, such as echoplanar imaging or other rapid imaging techniques because these patients are often uncooperative and may move during the examination. Also needed is cerebral perfusion measurement.

In the acute stage, the first week to 10 days, the blood-brain barrier is intact, and if contrast medium were administered intravenously, there would be no extravasation outside the blood vessels into the brain tissue. Starting about a week to 10 days later, there is disruption of the vessel walls. This permits the contrast to pass outside the vessel walls, and CT can now demonstrate increased density in the tissues (Fig. 10.11). Actually, the blood-brain barrier breakdown is attributed to the formation of new capillaries devoid of tight junctions in the infarcted area (see text preceding under "Pathophysiologic Considerations"). This happens much more markedly in the gray matter than in the white matter because there are three to four times more blood vessels in the gray matter. Contrast enhancement of the infarcted areas can be seen usually between 10 and 20 days and occasionally longer than that. When it is seen longer than 20 days following the initial symptoms, there may have been other secondary areas of infarction that occurred at a later date. This is probably common in the embolic infarction in which the initial embolus lodges in larger vessels; later it breaks into small fragments, which pass into smaller arteries, and still later further fragmentation takes place along with passage into other smaller branches. The speed of lysis of the embolus varies with the

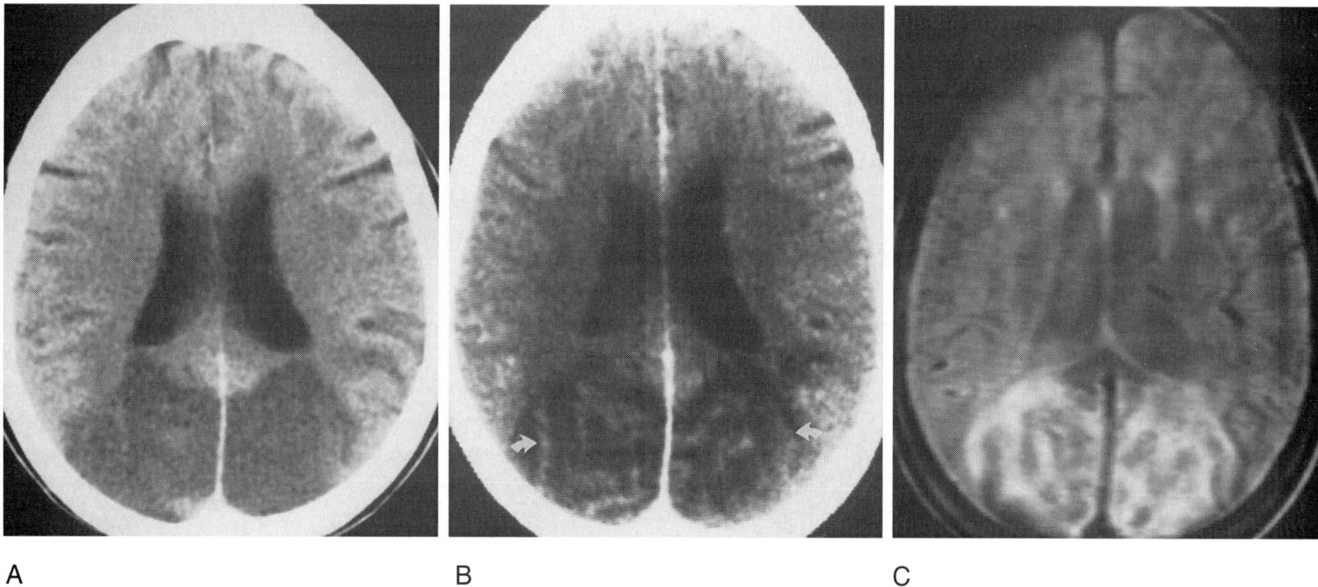

A B C

Figure 10.11. Bioccipital infarct in the territory of the posterior cerebral arteries in a 79-year-old woman. **A.** CT scan performed less than 2 days after onset of difficulty walking, right gaze preferred, and incontinence. **B.** CT with contrast done 4 days later shows contrast uptake with a gyral pattern (arrows). **C.** First-echo T2-weighted image shows hyperintensity with a gyral pattern in both occipital areas involving the medial side of the lobes.

type of embolus and the patient. Because the localization is always in the gray matter, the contrast enhancement has a characteristic gyral configuration similar to that of the convolutions of the brain surface. Enhancement in the deep basal ganglia would also be seen if contrast enhancement were to be used in the deep infarction.

MRI is also used in the acute and subacute stages. Ordinarily it is done after the CT scanning, particularly when the initial CT examination is negative. In some cases MRI may show early changes when CT is negative (Fig. 10.12). Perhaps the earliest change seen by MRI involves the disappearance of the signal void of the involved artery, more frequently the middle cerebral artery and its branches (108) but also sometimes the supraclinoid portion of the internal carotid artery.

The administration of an MRI contrast may enhance our ability to visualize the slowly flowing arteries, for they may enhance on postcontrast T1-weighted images (109). However, contrast enhancement is rarely used in these cases, since CT is usually performed first to exclude hemorrhage. MRI is not carried out in the acute period unless there is some doubt about the diagnosis on clinical grounds.

Because both CT and MRI, particularly the latter, show the anatomic distribution of the ischemic lesion, which may be supplied by a number of different arteries, it is felt to be useful to show arterial territories supplied by the different arteries (Figs. 10.13 to 10.17). This is important because the clinical correlation is much better if one tries to identify the involved vessels. A careful search can be made of the area where the clinical symptoms and neurologic signs suggest.

The findings on MRI are hypointensity on T1-weighted images and hyperintensity on the first- and second-echo T2-weighted images. T2-weighted images are considerably more sensitive than T1-weighted images and for this reason are favored. The hyperintensity is due to the presence of increased water from vasogenic and cytotoxic edema in the tissues and is seen in the white matter as well as in the adjacent gray matter. Ischemic changes in the brain leading to cerebral infarction characteristically involve the gray matter, usually the cerebral convolutions. They may also involve the gray matter in the basal ganglia and thalamus. However, these changes are almost always more pronounced, or at least easier to appreciate, in the white matter and in the region of the basal ganglia and the internal capsule (Figs. 10.18 and 10.19).

MRI is more sensitive than CT in the first 24 h after onset, when it may show some change in 82 percent of cases as against only in 58 percent by CT, as reported by Bryan et al. (107). However, the examination times after onset of symptoms were not as well defined in this study as one might desire. MRI is known to be more sensitive than CT in detecting changes in the early period. In general, the detectability is partly related to the size and location of the infarct. Large infarcts are almost always seen early on both CT and MRI; small infarcts involving the cortical and subcortical areas in the region of the sylvian fissure may not be seen by either method early but will become apparent later. The proton density weighted image is best for demonstrating early changes. The very early changes, less than 6 h after onset, are not usually shown, and the author advocates the use of diffusion-weighted

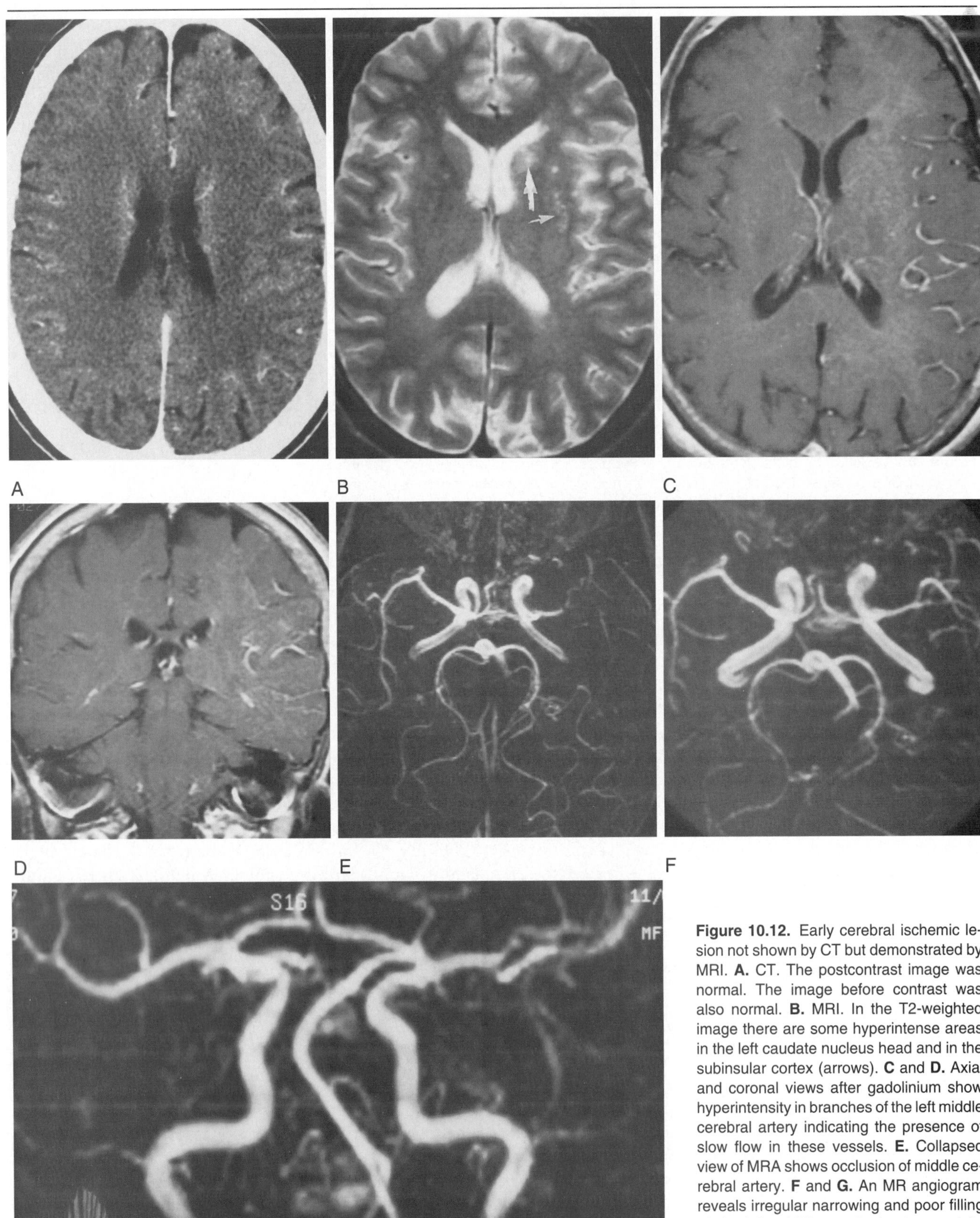

Figure 10.12. Early cerebral ischemic lesion not shown by CT but demonstrated by MRI. **A.** CT. The postcontrast image was normal. The image before contrast was also normal. **B.** MRI. In the T2-weighted image there are some hyperintense areas in the left caudate nucleus head and in the subinsular cortex (arrows). **C** and **D.** Axial and coronal views after gadolinium show hyperintensity in branches of the left middle cerebral artery indicating the presence of slow flow in these vessels. **E.** Collapsed view of MRA shows occlusion of middle cerebral artery. **F** and **G.** An MR angiogram reveals irregular narrowing and poor filling of the left middle cerebral artery and its branches, indicating partial recanalization 24 h after E.

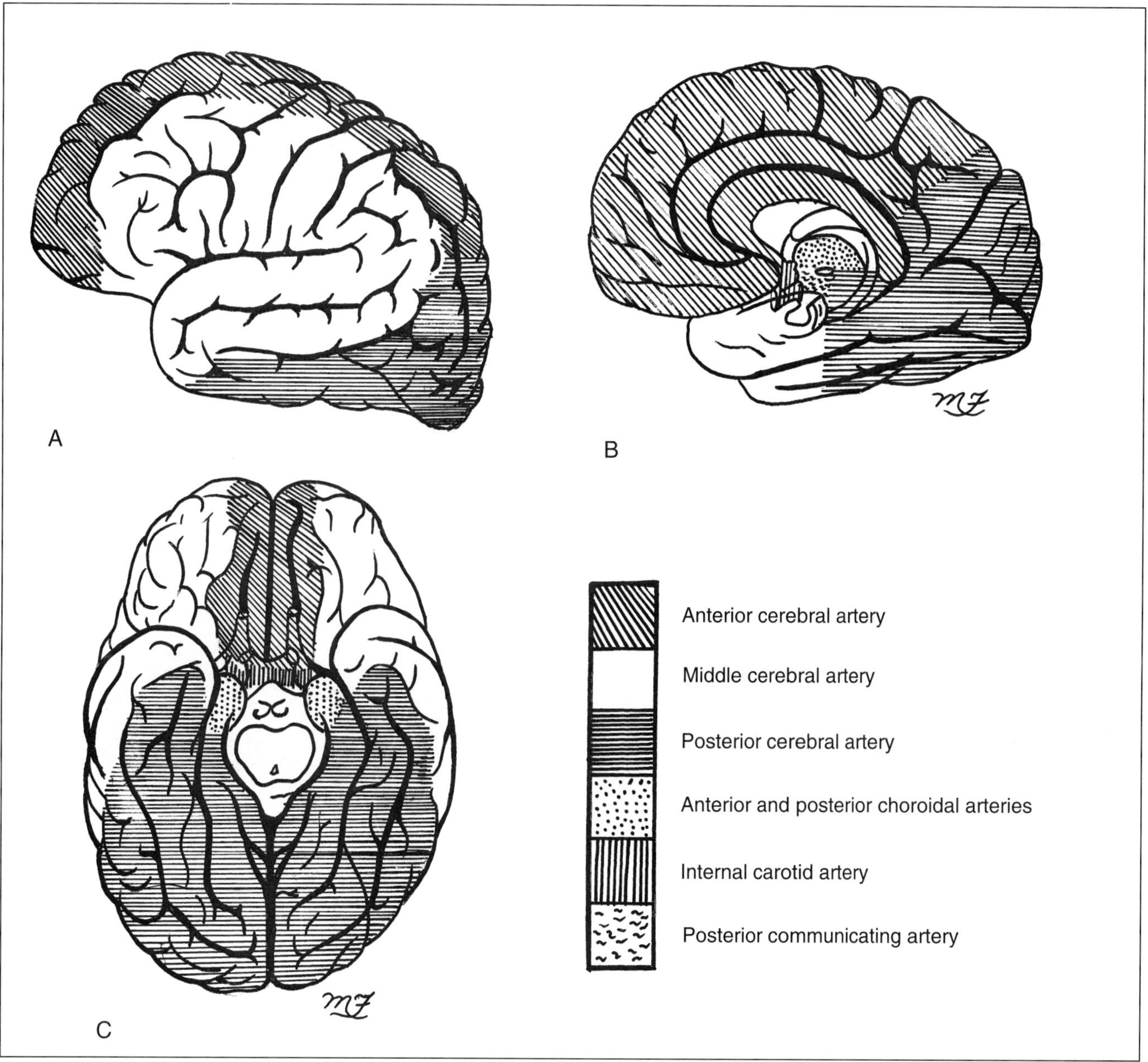

Figure 10.13. Arterial blood supply zones of arteries of the brain. **A.** Lateral surface of hemispheres. **B.** Medial surface of hemispheres. **C.** Basal surface of hemispheres. **D.** Key to vascular zones. (Modified from JM Taveras and F Morello: Normal Neuroradiology, Chicago: Year Book, 1979.)

Anterior cerebral artery
Middle cerebral artery
Posterior cerebral artery
Posterior choroidal artery
Posterior communicating artery
Anterior choroidal artery
A
B

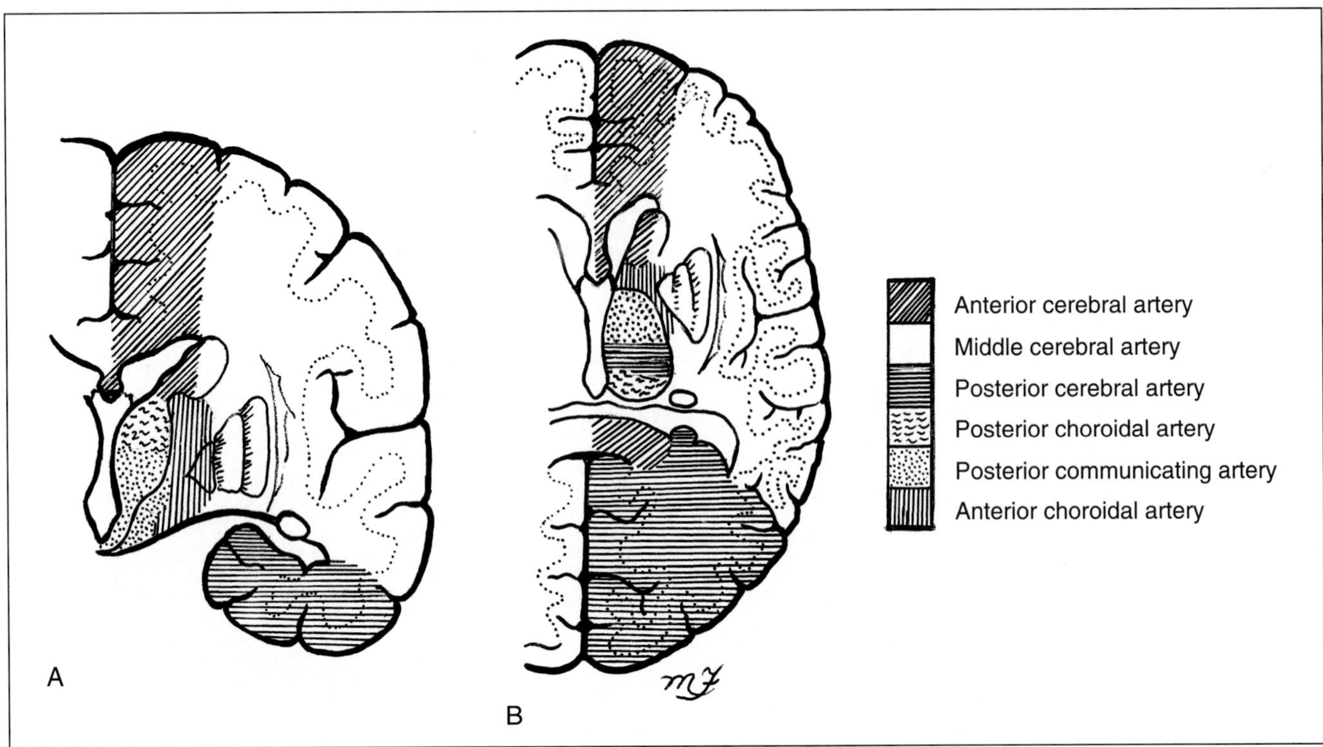

Figure 10.14. Arterial blood supply zones of cerebral hemispheres (after Lazorthes). **A.** Coronal cross section. **B.** Axial cross section. **C.** Key to vascular zones.

B
Anterior cerebral artery
Posterior cerebral artery
Anterior and posterior choroidal arteries
Posterior communicating artery
Internal carotid artery
A

Figure 10.15. Arterial blood supply zones of arteries of the brain. Hypothalamus and third ventricle regions. **A.** Sagittal view. **B.** Inferior view. **C.** Key to vascular zones.

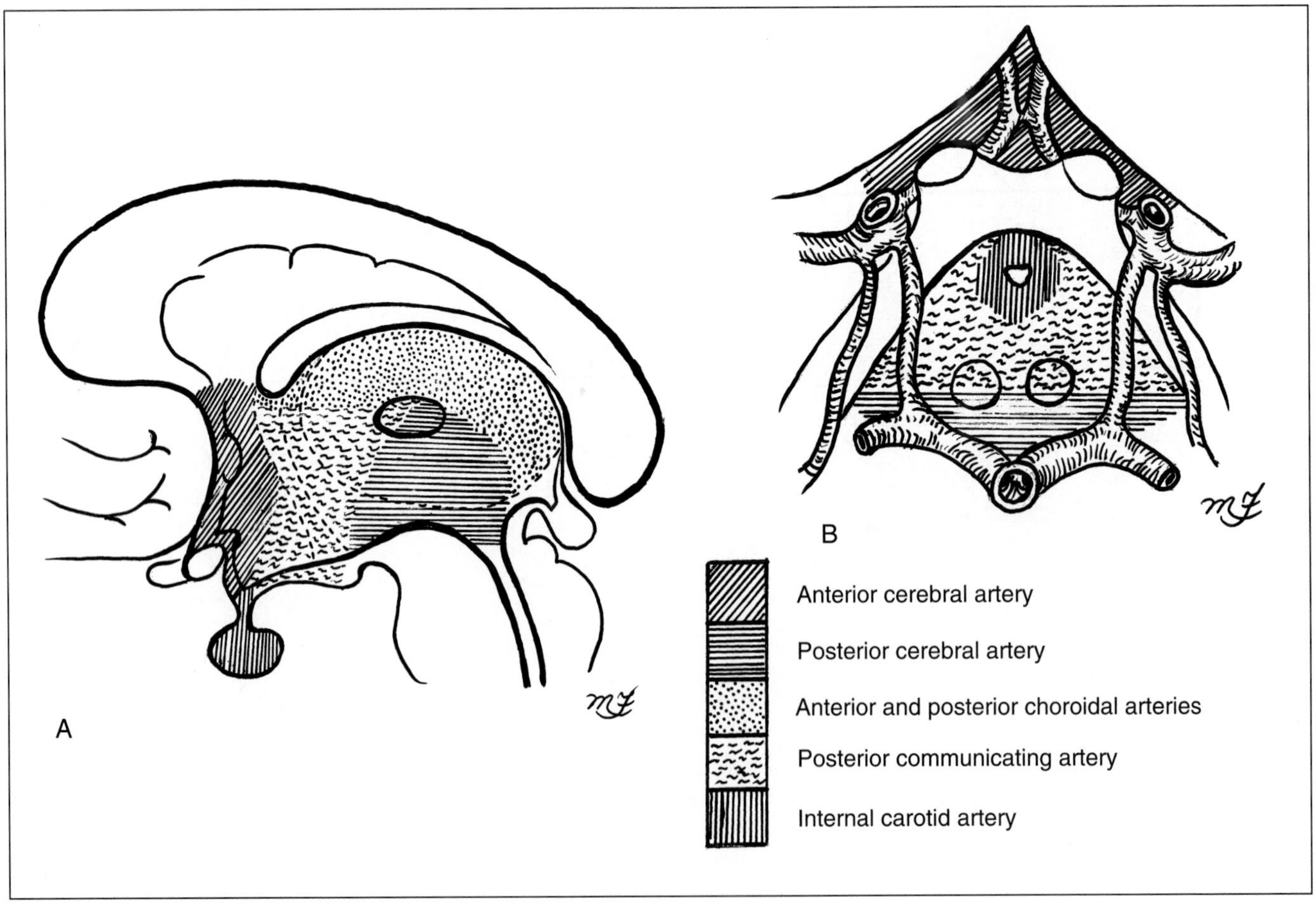

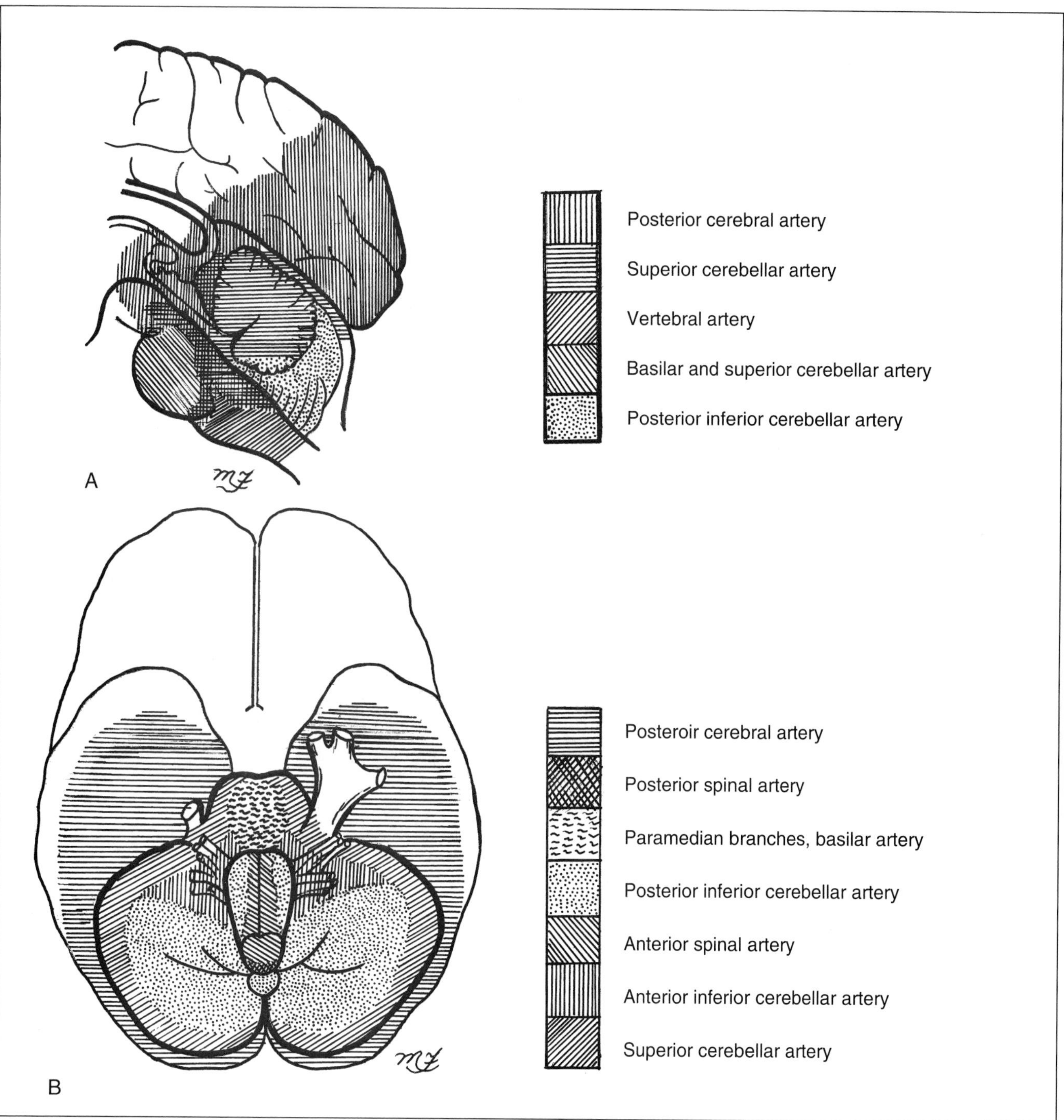

Figure 10.16. Blood supply zones, vertebral and basilar arteries. **A.** Lateral view. **B.** Basal view. (Modified from JM Taveras and F Morello: Normal Neuroradiology, Chicago: Year Book, 1979.)

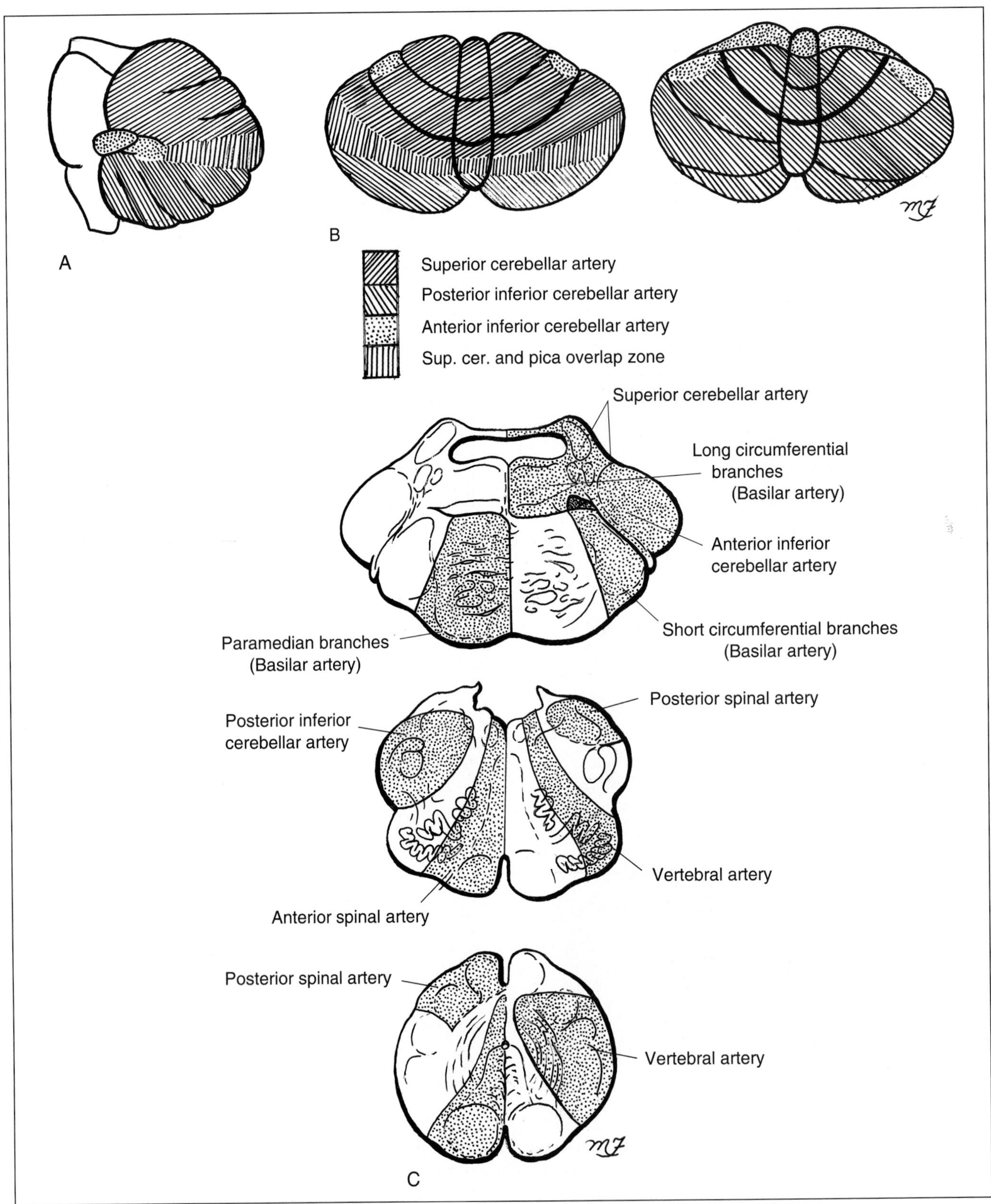

Figure 10.17. Arterial supply zones. **A.** Cerebellum, lateral view. **B.** Cerebellum, superior aspect (left) and inferior aspect (right). **C.** Blood supply zones of pons and medulla. (A and B modified from JM Taveras and F Morello: Normal Neuroradiology, Chicago: Year Book, 1979).

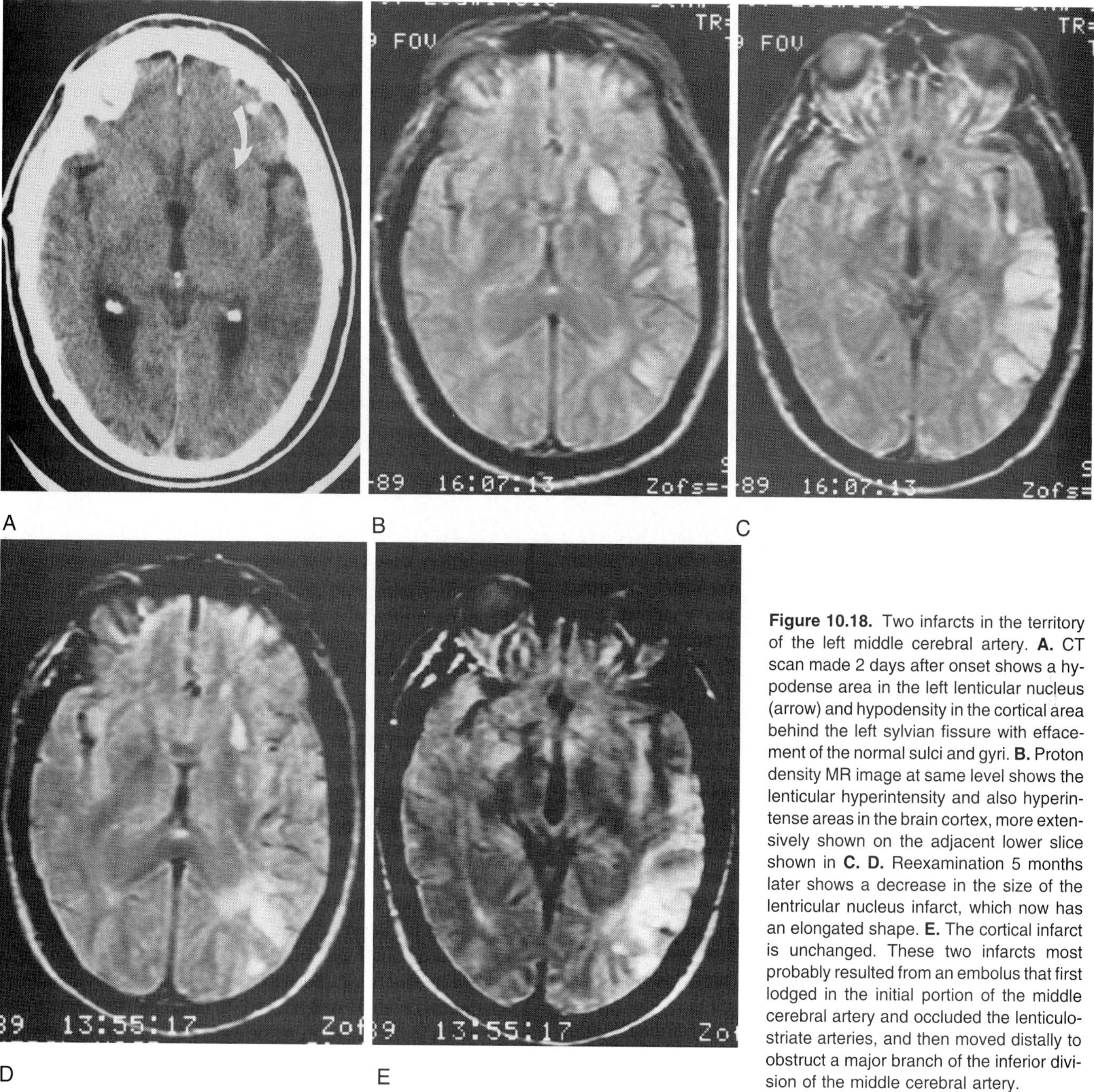

Figure 10.18. Two infarcts in the territory of the left middle cerebral artery. **A.** CT scan made 2 days after onset shows a hypodense area in the left lenticular nucleus (arrow) and hypodensity in the cortical area behind the left sylvian fissure with effacement of the normal sulci and gyri. **B.** Proton density MR image at same level shows the lenticular hyperintensity and also hyperintense areas in the brain cortex, more extensively shown on the adjacent lower slice shown in **C. D.** Reexamination 5 months later shows a decrease in the size of the lentricular nucleus infarct, which now has an elongated shape. **E.** The cortical infarct is unchanged. These two infarcts most probably resulted from an embolus that first lodged in the initial portion of the middle cerebral artery and occluded the lenticulostriate arteries, and then moved distally to obstruct a major branch of the inferior division of the middle cerebral artery.

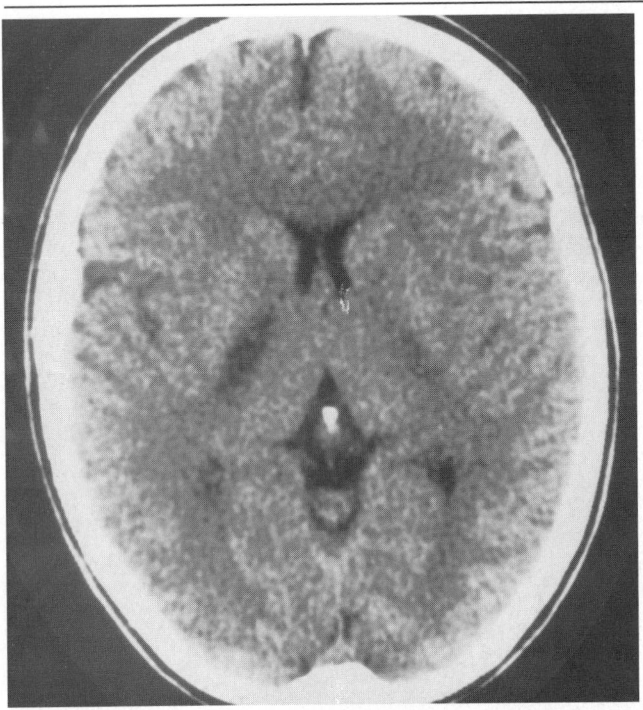

A

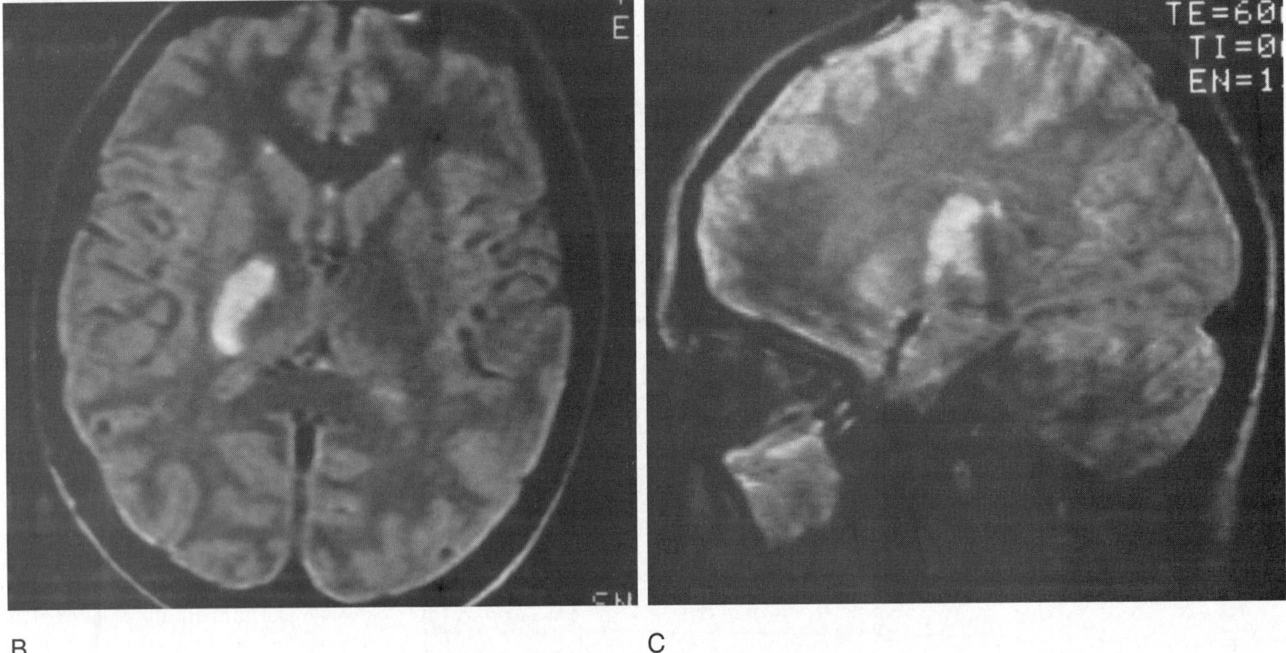

B C

Figure 10.19. Infarct in posterior limb of internal capsule in 28-year-old woman who was on contraceptives for 10 years. **A.** CT shows hypodensity in the right posterior limb of the internal capsule. **B.** Proton density MR image shows the infarct to be hyperintense, and the edema also extends into the adjacent thalamus. **C.** Sagittal proton density image shows the position of the infarct. The obstructed vessel is probably the anterior choroidal artery. The patient also smoked two packs of cigarettes per day and had an elevated cholesterol level and a high level of low-density lipoproteins.

imaging for that purpose (Figs. 10.20 and 10.21). In some reports indicating the possibility of MRI diagnosis within 3 h after sudden onset of symptoms that are felt to be due to cerebral embolism, half of the patients suffered from atrial fibrillation (110). However, these cases seem to be composed mostly of patients with large infarcts, which are known to be detected early.

The majority of infarcts occur in the cerebral hemispheres, but they may also occur in the cerebellum or in the brainstem. Cerebellar infarcts may be in the territory of the posterior inferior cerebellar artery, the superior cerebellar arteries, or the anterior inferior cerebellar arteries (Figs. 10.22 to 10.24). On CT examinations it is common to see low-attenuation areas along the horizontal fissure of the cerebellum that could be confused with infarction. One needs to remember that CT images are nearly always axial and so are partly parallel to the horizontal fissure of the cerebellum; this tends to exaggerate this appearance (Fig.

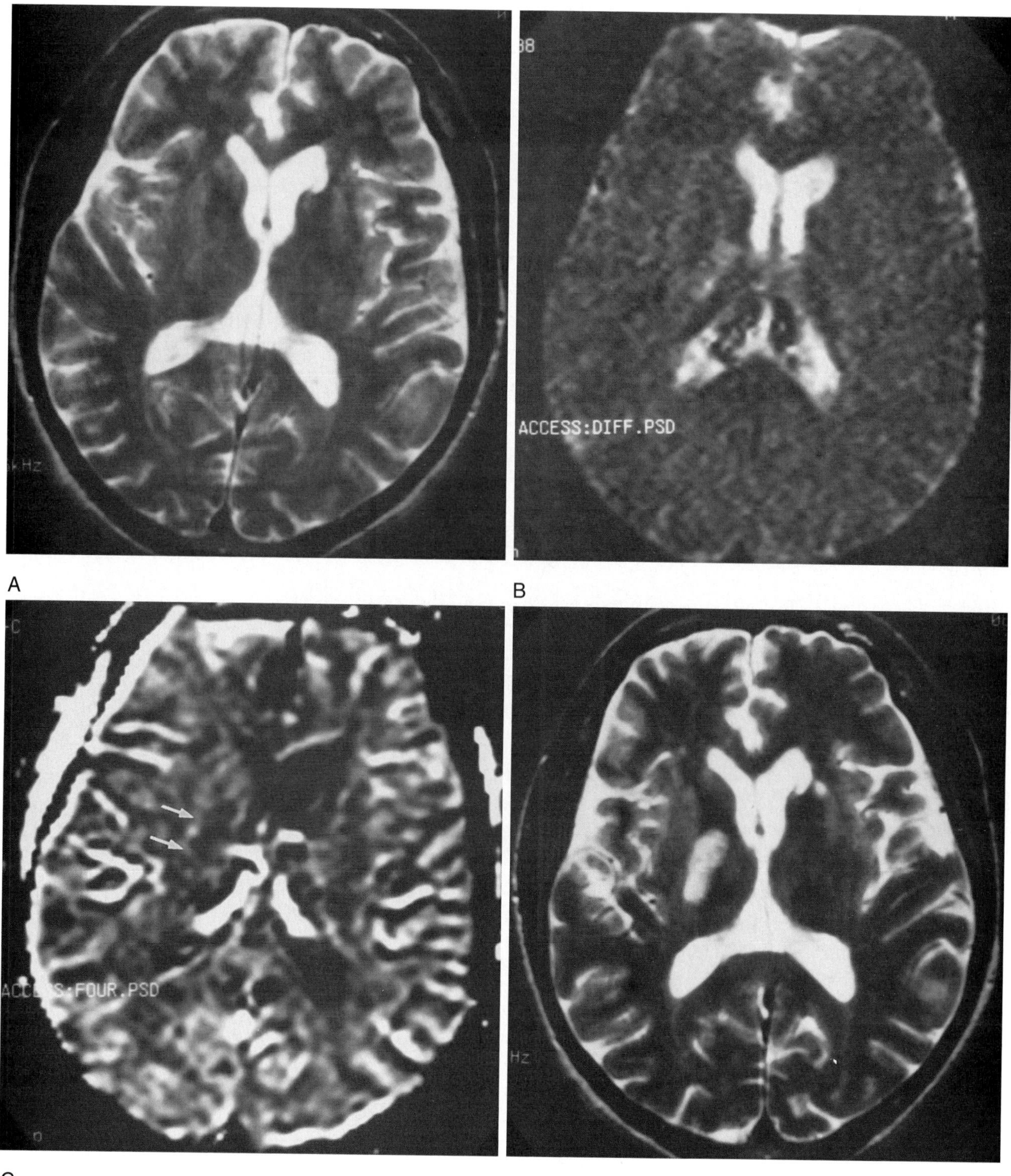

Figure 10.20. Deep infarct not shown by CT or usual MRI at about 8 h but shown by diffusion imaging. **A.** Initial T2-weighted MR image shows no abnormality. **B.** Diffusion imaging done at the same sitting reveals an abnormal diffusion area in right thalamic region. A perfusion image **(C)** was also done, which revealed hypoperfusion in the involved area (arrows). **D.** Repeat MR image several days later now shows the thalamic lesions. The lacune adjacent to the left frontal horn was present earlier.

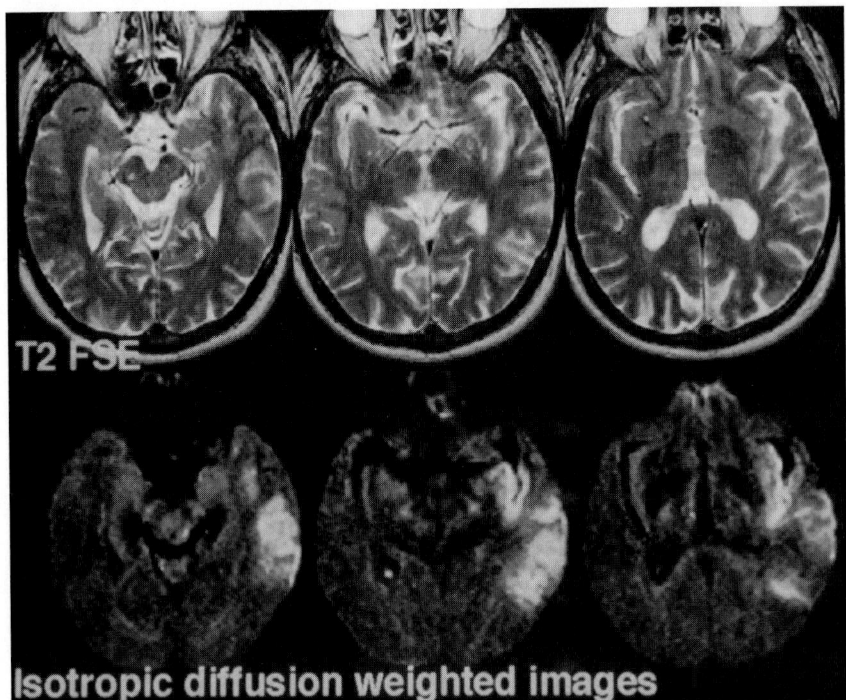

A

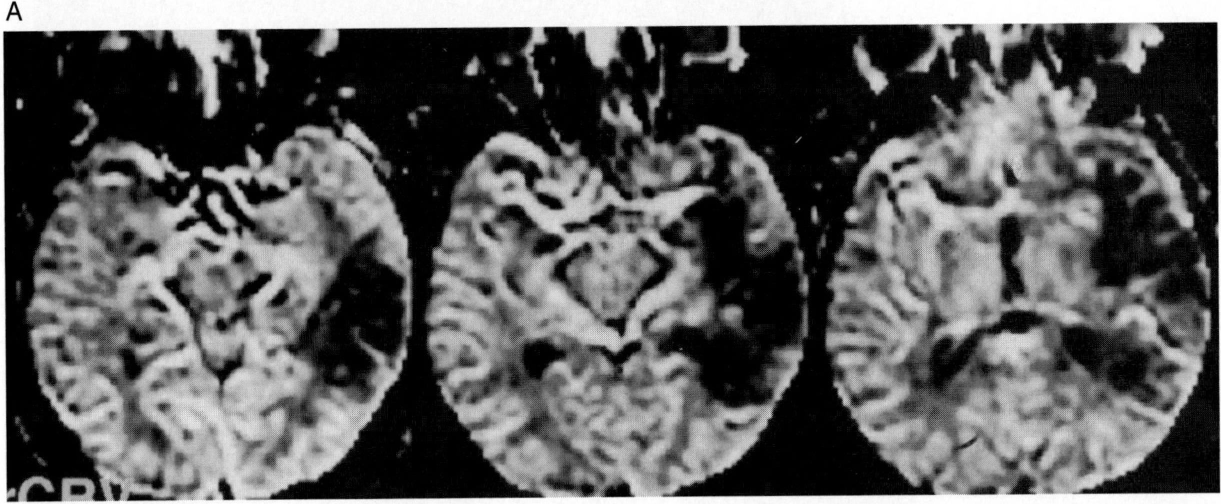

B

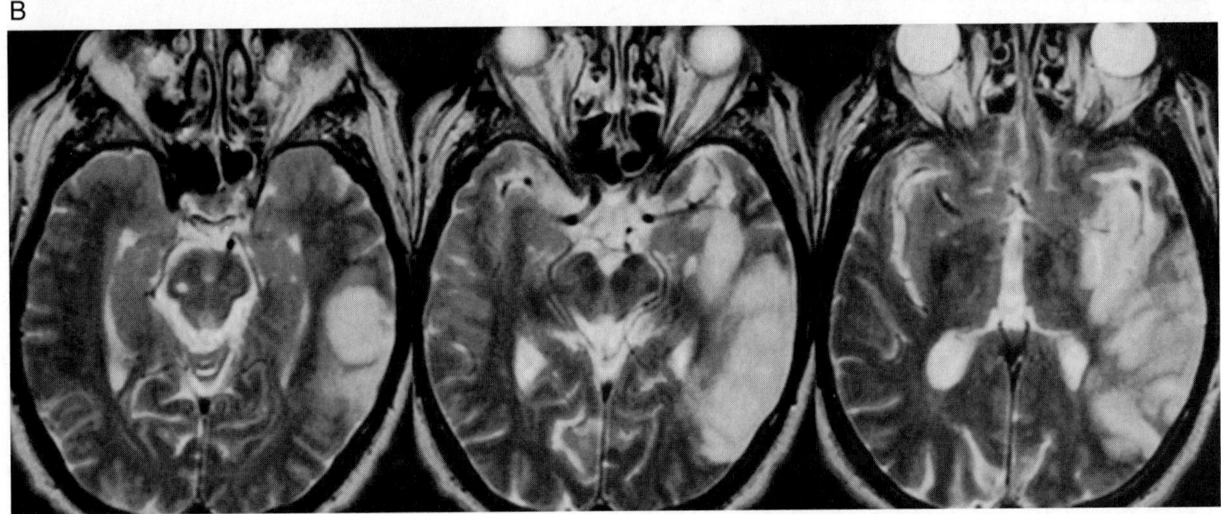

C

Figure 10.21. Early ischemic lesion not shown by CT or usual MRI and demonstrated by diffusion-weighted imaging and also by perfusion imaging. **A.** Top images T2 weighted; bottom images diffusion-weighted, showing left hyperintense area. **B.** Perfusion imaging with gadolinium demonstrates large area of hypoperfusion in same area as A (bottom row). **C.** T2-weighted axial image taken 3 days later reveals the ischemic area. (Courtesy of Dr. Greg Sorenson, Massachusetts General Hospital, Boston.)

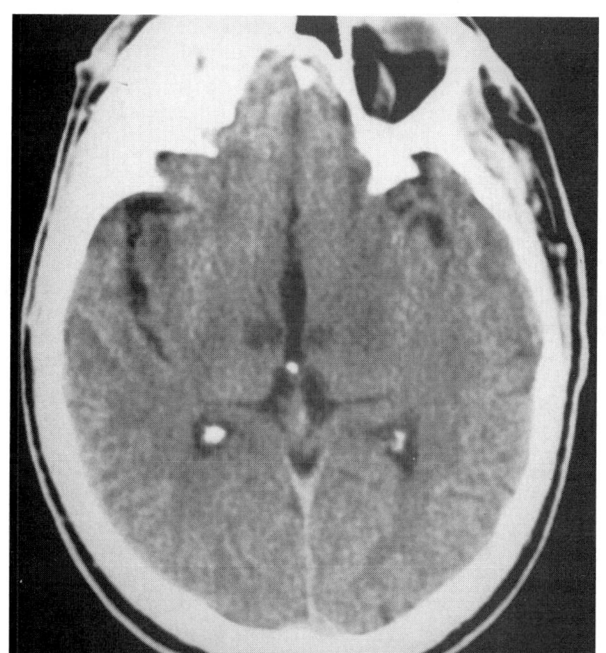

A

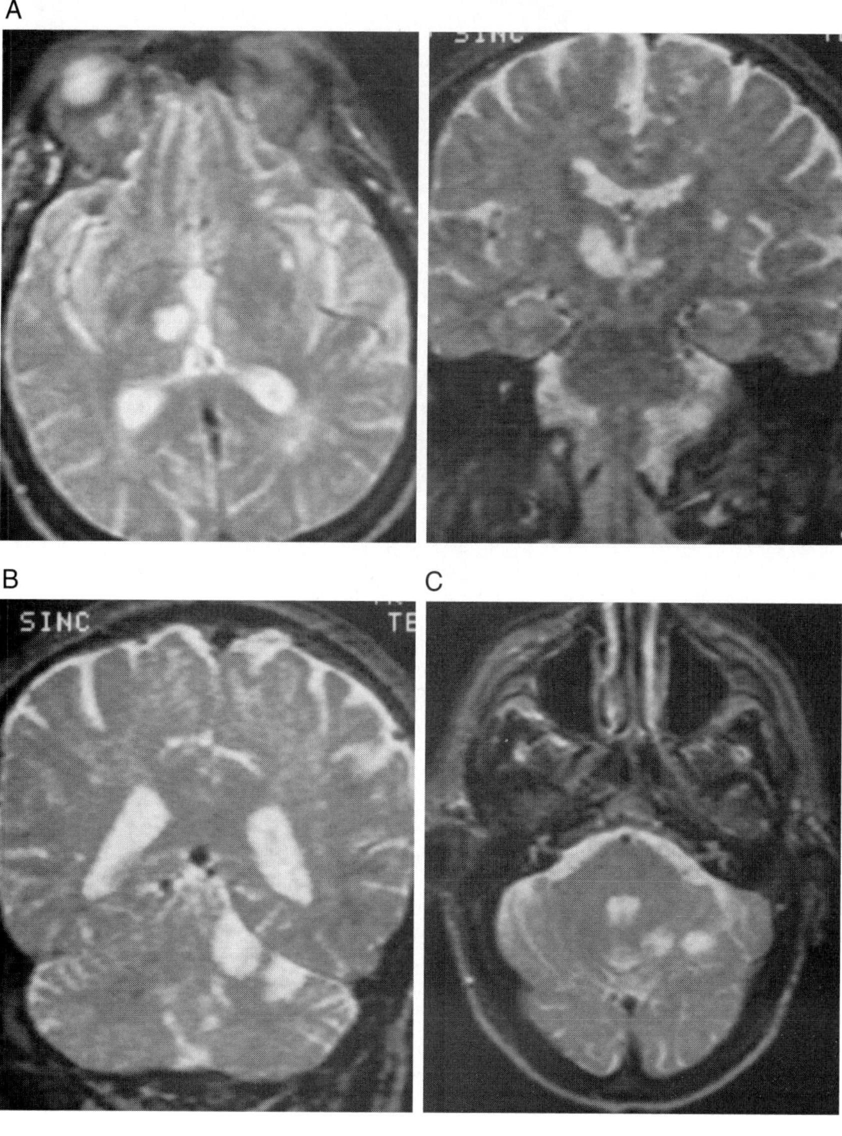

B C D E

Figure 10.22. Bilateral thalamic infarcts and cerebellar infarcts in a 71-year-old man with atrial fibrillation. **A.** Axial CT image showing two symmetrical areas of low density on each side of the midline in the thalamus. **B.** T2-weighted axial MR image confirms the lesions; the right side is larger. **C.** Coronal T2-weighted image shows the configuration of the lesions. **D.** There was also evidence of infarction in the left upper cerebellum, seen best on coronal T2-weighted images. **E.** Axial view also shows infarction. The pons is normal. The relatively symmetrical infarcts are due to thalamic branches arising from the proximal posterior cerebral arteries, sometimes as a common trunk (artery of Percheron) supplying both sides and sometimes as two separate perforating branches. The infarct in the left upper cerebellum also suggests that the occluding embolus originally lodged at the bifurcation of the basilar artery involving the left superior cerebellar artery.

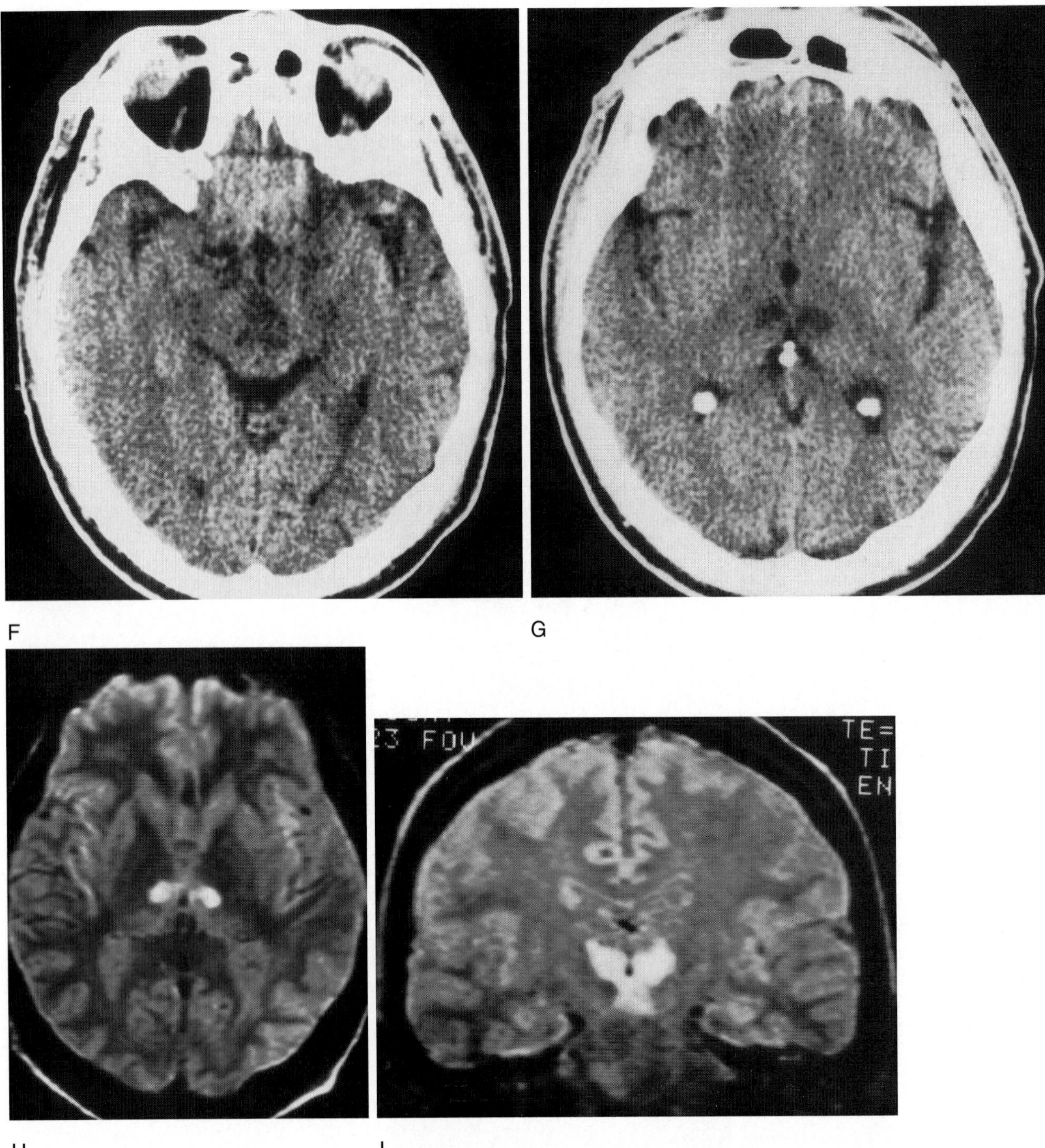

Figure 10.22. *(continued)* **F** to **I.** Another example of bilateral thalamic infarction due to occlusion of the artery of Percheron, which arises from the origin of the posterior cerebral arteries. **F** and **G.** CT showing involvement of upper midbrain. Axial (**H**) and coronal (**I**) MR proton density images.

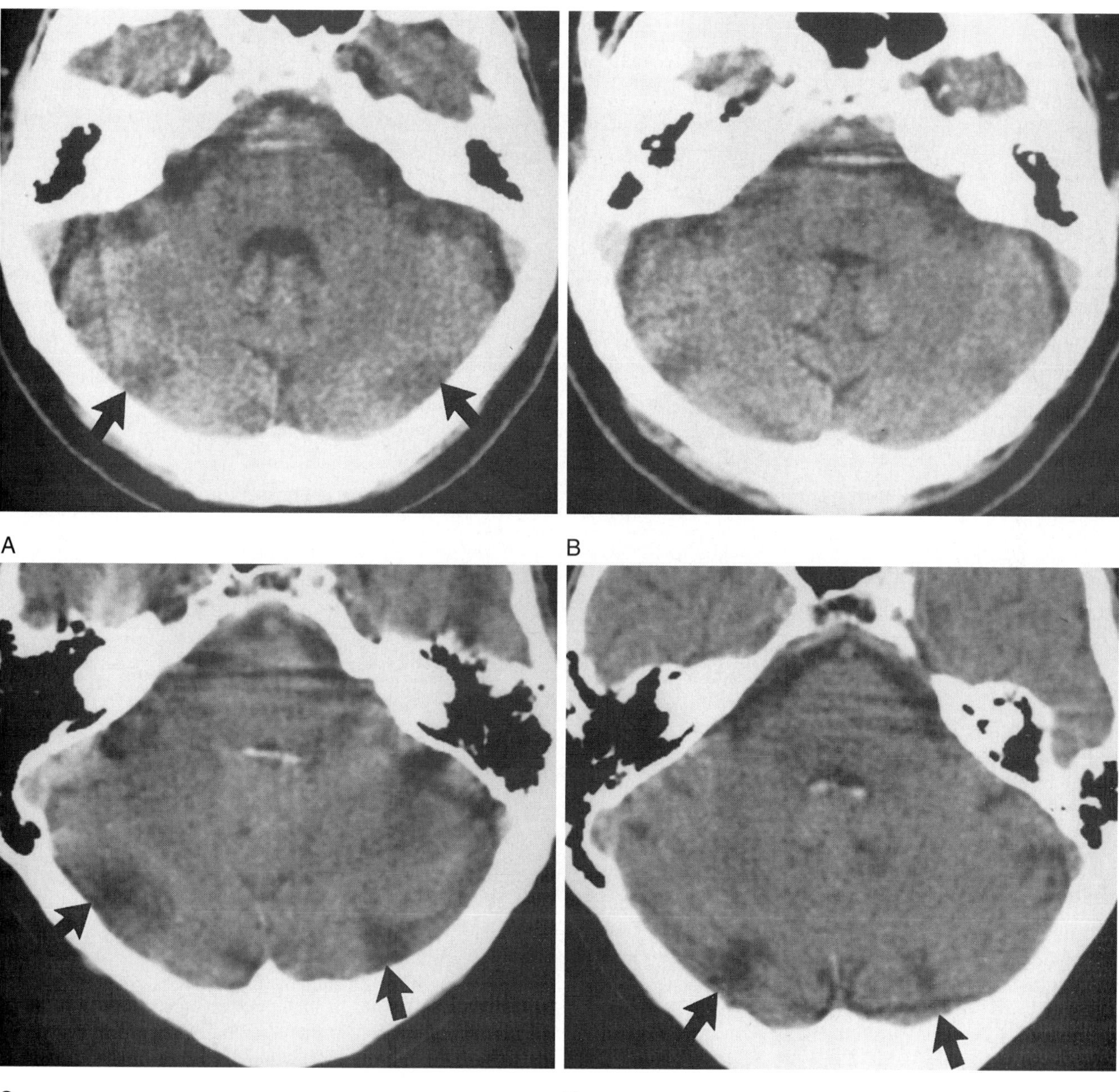

Figure 10.23. Horizontal fissure of cerebellum suggesting infarct. **A.** A hypodense area in the cerebellum is seen on both sides, representing the horizontal fissure of the cerebellum (arrows). The fissure becomes more prominent when there is some degree of cerebellar atrophy. If the head is slightly canted in the scanner, it will be seen on one side and not on the other. **B.** A lower slice showing the apparent abnormality more laterally. **C.** View of another patient with cerebellar atrophy whose head was canted in the CT unit. There is a low-density area of the horizontal fissure that is larger on the right side (the lower side). In this case it may be more difficult to rule out an infarct. **D.** However, the next higher slice shows that the two low-intensity areas approach the midline symmetrically, although the right side still remains wider because of the head canting, which brings the fissure closer to being parallel to the slice plane (arrows).

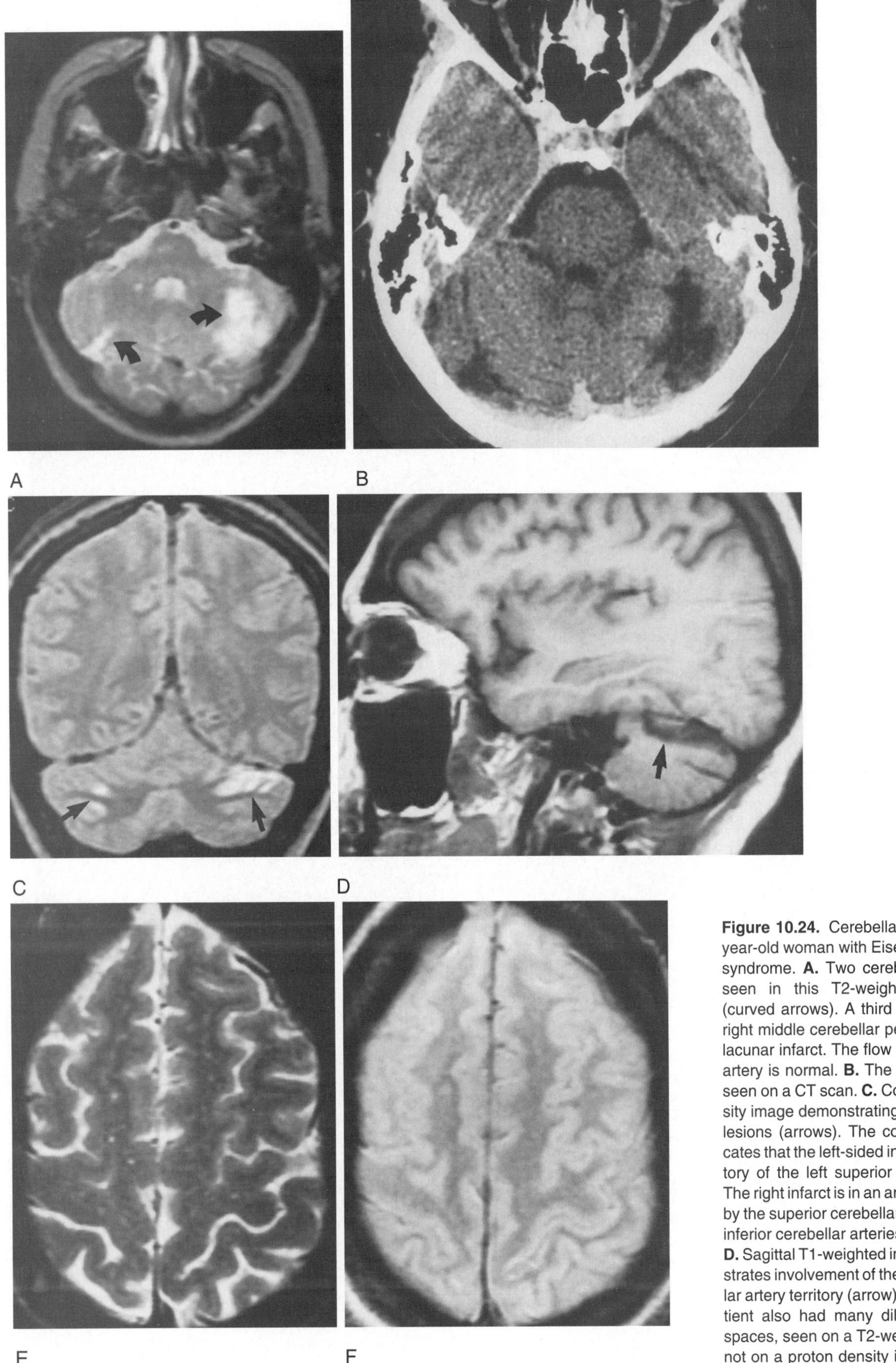

Figure 10.24. Cerebellar infarcts in a 36-year-old woman with Eisenmenger cardiac syndrome. **A.** Two cerebellar infarcts are seen in this T2-weighted axial image (curved arrows). A third bright spot in the right middle cerebellar peduncle may be a lacunar infarct. The flow void in the basilar artery is normal. **B.** The same infarcts are seen on a CT scan. **C.** Coronal proton density image demonstrating the two ischemic lesions (arrows). The coronal image indicates that the left-sided infarct is in the territory of the left superior cerebellar artery. The right infarct is in an area jointly supplied by the superior cerebellar and the posterior inferior cerebellar arteries (see Fig. 10.16). **D.** Sagittal T1-weighted image also demonstrates involvement of the superior cerebellar artery territory (arrow). **E** and **F.** The patient also had many dilated perivascular spaces, seen on a T2-weighted image and not on a proton density image (F).

10.23). The appearance is also exaggerated by the presence of some degree of cerebellar atrophy common in the older age group.

Brainstem infarcts are seen considerably better with MRI than with CT because of the known problems on CT related to beam-hardening artifacts, which usually go through the pons and lower midbrain and are nearly unavoidable in routine examinations (Fig. 10.25). Thus, whenever a suspicion exists that a brainstem infarct may be present, an MRI examination should be recommended. In general, proton density images (first-echo T2-weighted images or long TR, short TE) are the best for visualizing ischemic changes in the brain, and if the lesion is not apparent on the first echo and is only seen in the second echo, it may be only an artifact rather than edema in the brain tissue. It is not uncommon to see bright areas in the brainstem only in the second echo, in which case they may be considered artifacts or at least probably of no pathologic significance. If they are pathologic, they probably represent cystic spaces such as may occur from old lacunes, and not acute or recent lesions. A lacune may not be seen in a proton density image (isodense); the same would be true with a small cystic space of unknown etiology. The T1-weighted sagittal views would probably demonstrate the lacune or

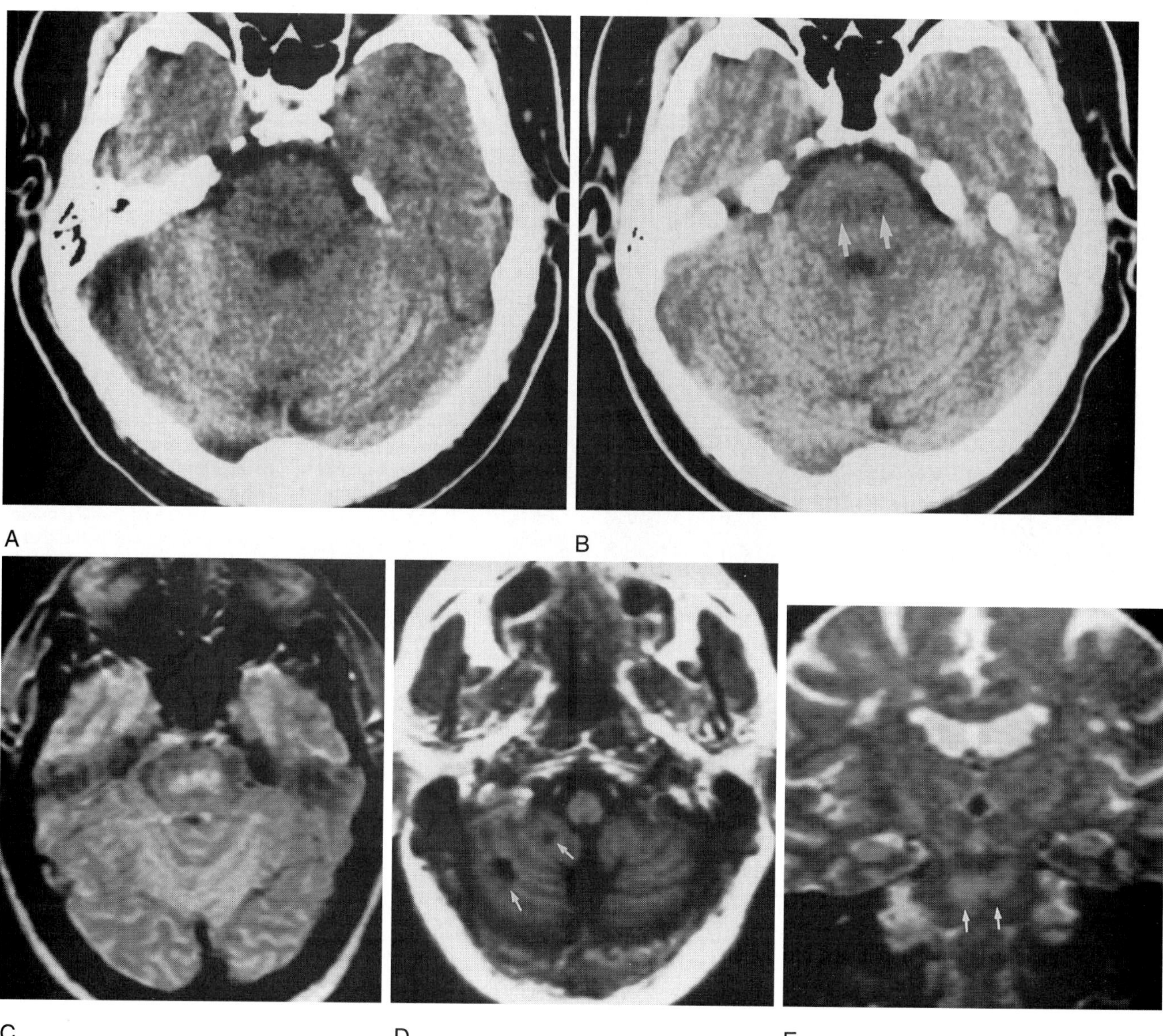

Figure 10.25. Brainstem infarcts. CT axial views through the pons were at first negative (**A**) and became positive 4 days later (**B**). **C.** Axial proton density MR image shows the same lesion in both sides of the pons due to occlusion of bilateral perforating branches. **D.** A lower T1-weighted section shows two ischemic lesions in the cerebellum (arrows). **E.** The coronal T2-weighted image shows that the pontine ischemic lesion is localized to the midpons (arrows).

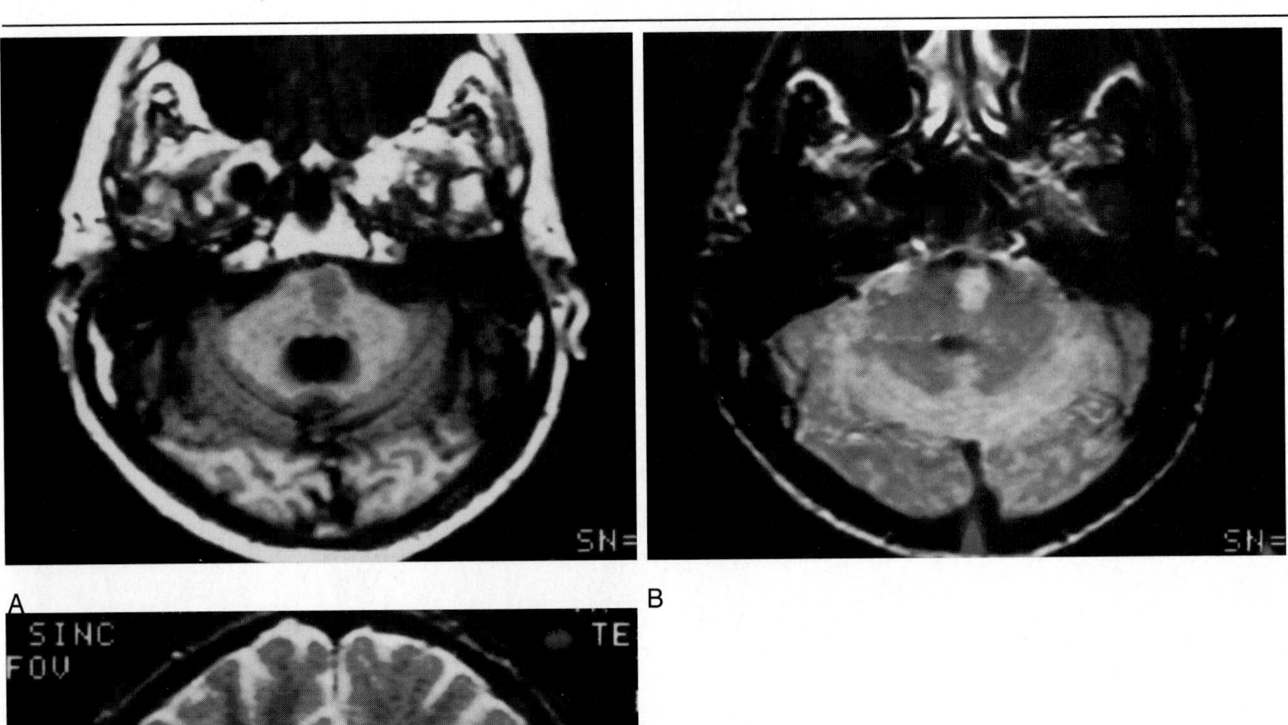

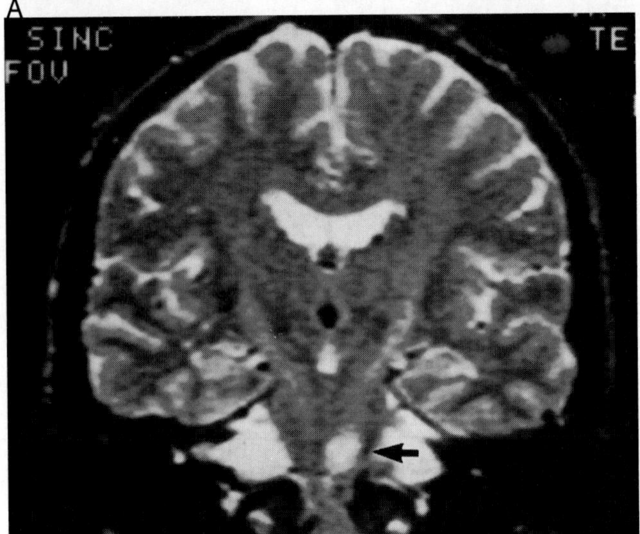

A B C

Figure 10.26. Pontine infarct in a 61-year-old woman. **A** and **B.** The T1-weighted image shows a low intensity and the T2-weighted image a high-intensity lesion in the pons just to the left of the midline. The CT examination did not show the lesion because of interpetrous artifacts in this area (not shown). **C.** Coronal T2-weighted image shows the lesion well (arrow). The obstructed vessel is presumably a perforating branch arising from the basilar artery. In general, brainstem infarcts tend to involve one side or the other and are frequently sharply demarcated in the midline, as shown in A. The appearance shown in Figure 10.25 indicates a more extensive involvement.

small cyst as a low-intensity area. This would then appear as high intensity on the second echo because it is mostly filled with fluid and has minimal residual glial tissue; its intensity follows that of CSF. Small cystic spaces may also be related to perivascular CSF (Virchow-Robin) spaces, and these should be differentiated from lacunes.

Brainstem infarcts are usually considered to be related to perforating branches from the basilar artery and are usually longer in the anteroposterior diameter than in the transverse diameter. They often start at the midline and for the most part are rather small (Fig. 10.25). In the pons they may sometimes extend to both sides and be located in the central portion, and sometimes they are longer in the transverse direction (Fig. 10.26). Infarcts in the medulla can also be seen by MRI and ordinarily cannot be seen by CT. The clinical localization and the correlations with the findings on MRI are sometimes exquisite (Fig. 10.27).

EDEMA IN ISCHEMIC INFARCTION

Vasogenic and/or cytotoxic edema occurs in all cases of ischemic infarction and is the reason that infarctions become visible on CT or MRI. Although in most cases the edema is insufficient to cause a mass effect, in many instances the infarct is associated with sufficient accumulation of intracellular and extracellular fluid that a mass effect is produced. The swelling may be very slight, such as obliteration of sulci on the brain surface or flattening of the adjacent ventricular wall in infarctions that involve the periventricular white matter. However, in some instances the edema is sufficiently pronounced to produce a midline shift (Fig. 10.10). These are usually larger infarcts and in general may indicate a poorer prognosis in terms of recovery of function. In general, infarcts accompanied by much edema are usually seen by CT or MRI upon the patient's arrival to the hospital, within several hours after onset of

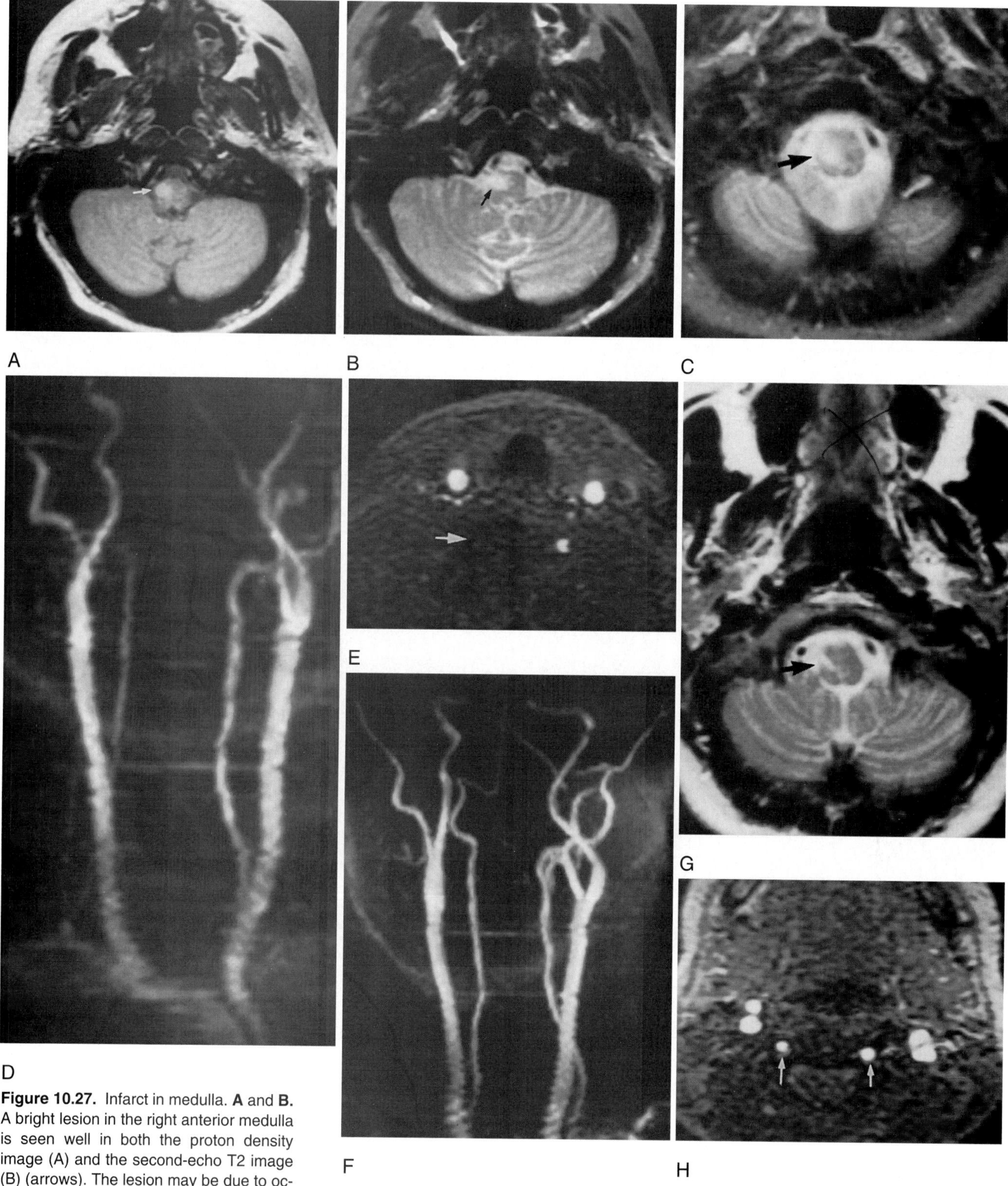

Figure 10.27. Infarct in medulla. **A** and **B.** A bright lesion in the right anterior medulla is seen well in both the proton density image (A) and the second-echo T2 image (B) (arrows). The lesion may be due to occlusion of a branch arising from the posterior inferior cerebellar artery. The patient also had an intracavernous carotid aneurysm. **C.** Another example of a lateral medullary infarct with MRA. T2-weighted axial image shows a hyperintense lesion in the right side of the medulla (arrow). **D.** MRA reveals a normal left vertebral artery, and the right vertebral artery shows only some flow in segments. **E.** The axial raw-data image shows absent flow (arrow). **F.** Repeat MRA 5 months later shows reappearance of right vertebral flow. The patient was clinically improved. **G.** Axial T2-weighted image 5 months later shows the permanent infarcted area to be smaller than it was originally (arrow). **H.** Raw-data axial image shows both vertebral arteries. Medullary infarction is more frequently related to vertebral than to posterior inferior cerebellar artery occlusion.

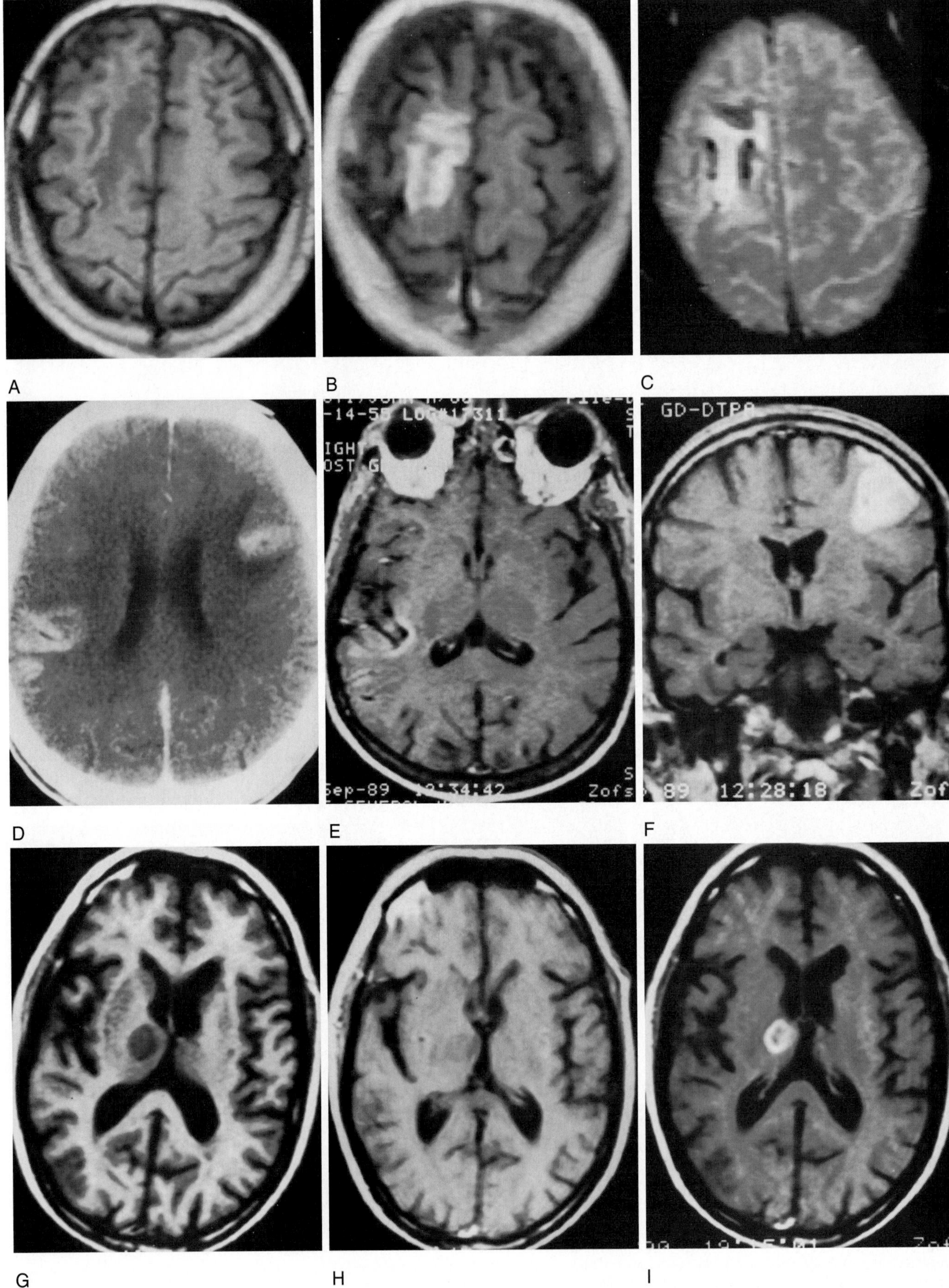
A
B
C
GD-DTPA
12:28:18
D
E
F
G
H
I

symptoms. Although the total abnormality may not be visible, other signs indicate the abnormalities (Fig. 10.9).

PROGNOSIS IN CEREBRAL INFARCTION

Kummer et al. found prognostic significance in the extent of parenchymal hypodensity, the presence of local brain swelling, and the hyperdense middle cerebral artery sign as shown by CT within the first 5 h after onset of symptoms in patients with middle cerebral artery trunk occlusions (111). They found that, at this early stage, local brain swelling and more than 50 percent hypodensity of the middle cerebral artery territory had a high predictive value for a fatal outcome. In general, it is known that any patient who presents positive CT findings of an infarct early after onset of symptoms has a poor prognosis for recovery of function, and death is common in this group, particularly if the involved area is large. The smaller the ischemic zone, the better the prognosis for functional recovery. Lacunar infarcts are usually asymptomatic; at least, no specific history can be elicited in the majority of cases.

USE OF CONTRAST MEDIA IN THE STUDY OF CEREBRAL INFARCTION

Contrast media are sometimes used to study cerebral infarction, but only when there is a specific question to be answered. The configuration of an infarct is extremely variable. By the same token the clinical presentation of an ischemic lesion in the brain may be atypical, and in some of these cases the use of contrast may be required to exclude other lesions, such as an inflammatory process or a new neoplasm. As expressed in text preceding, an infarct will not take up contrast material in the first 6 to 10 days (sometimes earlier) following the appearance of symptoms. After this date there is a breakdown of the blood-brain barrier and leakage of contrast into the brain tissue. The leakage is into the gray matter and not usually into the white matter (at least it is less visible in the white matter) because there are so many more capillaries in the gray matter of the brain. On CT the enhancement is obvious and presents a gyriform configuration similar to the cerebral convolutions (Figs. 10.11 and 10.28). Enhancement can also be seen in areas away from the cerebral cortex that involve deep structures or the cerebellum or brainstem (112). The enhancement will always be during the time when the breakdown in the blood-brain barrier exists. It should be remembered that the enhancement of a lesion that is originally ischemic might be seen at different times; that is, a lesion that usually enhances between 10 to 20 days following the initial episode may enhance at 25 to 35 days. This may occur because of additional arterial occlusions, which lead to new areas of infarction that then enhance at a later date. This phenomenon could be encountered more often if contrast media were used more frequently than they are in ischemic brain lesions. We usually do not need to use contrast media to diagnose ischemic infarctions, and it has been stated, as expressed earlier, that the intravenous injection of contrast could be harmful if there is breakdown of the blood-brain barrier (113). If enhancement in a patient with infarcion is going to be used, it might be well to recommend nonionic contrast in the presence of cerebral infarction. Contrast enhancement on MRI examination is similar to that of CT; that is, it is observed after a week following the appearance of symptoms (Table 10.7). Crain et al. reported that they observed two patterns of enhancement: (a) progressive enhancement, seen in the usual infarct; and (b) early or intense parenchymal enhancement (before 7 days) (109). The latter was observed in patients who often presented a lesser degree of ischemic insult with little or no neurologic sequelae, which is contrary to what one might expect. It is quite possible that these patients may have had a "silent stroke" several days before (114). Crain et al. also reported frequent arterial enhancement in the middle cerebral artery territory in the first several days after onset that was usually not observed after a week (109).

Elster reported on 100 cases of brainstem and deep cerebral infarctions and found that in 43 cases enhancement was present after 6 days from clinical onset, and in one case lasting to day 80 (112).

Figure 10.28. Enhancing infarct in a 77-year-old man with atrial fibrillation. **A.** T1-weighted axial image shows typical hypointensity in the right frontal region. **B.** T1-weighted image after intravenous contrast shows marked enhancement with gyral configuration in the same region. **C.** T2-weighted image shows hyperintensity in the infarct, but in addition there is marked hypointensity in the region of the gray matter, indicating that there is magnetic susceptibility consistent with prior hemorrhage, although clinically the patient did not have signs consistent with a hemorrhagic infarction. **D** to **I.** Enhancing multiple infarcts in a 60-year-old man, two cases. **D.** Postcontrast CT scan shows enhancement of two infarcts on opposite sides, evidently produced by a vascular accident, most probably embolic, occurring about 10 days previously. The event must have occurred at the same time because of the enhancing characteristics, also seen with MR postcontrast images (**E** and **F**). **G.** In another case a right thalamic lesion is seen on a T1-weighted image. **H.** Contrast was given, and the lesion became isointense. **I.** Two weeks later the contrast examination was repeated, and now the T1-weighted postcontrast image shows marked enhancement typical of an ischemic infarct in the subacute stage.

LOCATION OF INFARCTS AND MATCHING WITH VASCULAR TERRITORIES

As shown in Figures 10.13 through 10.17, the area where the lesion is seen on CT or MRI is usually indicative of

Table 10.7.
CT and MRI Contrast Enhancement of Cerebral Infarction

Due to breakdown of blood-brain barrier, attributable to proliferation of new capillaries lacking tight junctions
Usually seen between days 10 and 20 after infarction
Predominates in gray matter
Typically gyriform in configuration

Table 10.8.
Vascular Territories of the Anterior Circulation

Middle cerebral artery
Superior (anterior) division: lateral portions of anterior and middle aspects of frontal lobes and lateral aspect of temporal lobe
Inferior (posterior) division: lateral portion of posterior aspect of frontal lobe, parietal lobe, and occipital lobe
Anterior cerebral artery
Medial aspect of frontal and parietal lobes
Anterior portion of hypothalamus
Rostrum of corpus callosum, anterior portion of putamen, caudate head
Posterior cerebral artery
Medial aspect of temporal lobe
Medial aspect of occipital lobe
Thalamus
Medial lenticulostriate arteries
Lentiform nucleus, caudate nucleus, internal capsule
Lateral lenticulostriate arteries
Caudate nucleus
External capsule
Anterior choroidal artery
Cerebral peduncle
Globus pallidus
Posterior limb of internal capsule
Optic tract and optic radiation
Lateral geniculate body

the artery or arteries that have become occluded. Thus a review of these images is recommended (see Tables 10.8 and 10.9).

Because the middle cerebral artery and its branches are the most frequently affected vessels, one is likely to encounter many more examples of middle cerebral artery territory infarcts than infarcts of the other arteries. We often speak of the two major subdivisions of the middle cerebral artery: the anterior or superior division and the inferior or posterior division. By definition, the anterior division would produce the typical changes of cerebral infarction in the anterior aspect of the brain, mainly the anterior, middle, and posterior aspects of the frontal lobes, and the posterior or inferior division would involve more the posterior aspect, the parietal lobe and the posterior frontal lobe. Typically, the inferior division involves the occipital lobe on its lateral and posterior aspects but does not usually involve the medial portion of the lobe, which is normally supplied by the posterior cerebral artery. The posterior cerebral artery would produce ischemic changes on the medial aspect of the occipital lobe and may extend into the posterior temporal lobe because it yields an anterior temporal branch. In addition, the trunk of the posterior cerebral artery gives origin to thalamic branches. Sometimes a single branch may give rise to an artery (the artery of Percheron [115]), which supplies both inferior posterior thalami (Fig. 10.22). There are other perforating arterial branches arising from the posterior communicating artery that supplies the thalamus. The anterior cerebral arteries supply the anterior aspect of the frontal lobe, particularly on the medial side, and also follow the medial superior surface of the frontal lobes. Thus an anterior cerebral artery occlusion will produce an infarct that is located parallel to the midline (Fig. 10.114). The anterior cerebral artery also supplies the anterior portion of the hypothalamus, as shown in Figure 10.15. The central branches of the anterior cerebral artery arising from the first segment (A1) pass through the anterior perforated substance and supply the rostrum of the corpus callosum, the septum pellucidum, the anterior part of the putamen, and the head of the caudate nucleus. The most important of these central branches is the artery of Heubner.

Table 10.9.
Vascular Territories of the Posterior Circulation

Basilar artery
Anterior portion of brainstem
Posterior inferior cerebellar artery
Inferior and lateral aspects of cerebellum
Lateral portion of medulla
Dentate nucleus of cerebellum
Superior cerebellar artery
Pons
Superior aspect of cerebellum
Superior medullary velum
Anterior inferior cerebellar artery
Anterolateral aspects of inferior surface of cerebellum
Inferolateral aspects of pons

The perforating branches of the middle cerebral artery that arise from the first segment (M1) also rise and enter the brain through the anterior perforated substance. There are two sets. The medial striate branches ascend through the lentiform nucleus and supply it as well as the caudate nucleus and the internal capsule. The lateral striate branches ascend in the region of the external capsule and then immediately traverse the lentiform nucleus to supply the caudate nucleus. (For greater detail on the anatomy of the lenticulostriate arteries, see Chapter 17.)

The anterior choroidal branch of the internal carotid artery gives branches to the cerebral peduncle on each side and also supplies branches to the globus pallidus, the posterior limb of the internal capsule, the optic radiation, the optic tract, the hypocampus, the fimbria, and the lateral geniculate body.

In the posterior circulation, the vertebral arteries give rise to the posteroinferior cerebellar arteries (PICA), which supply the inferior and lateral aspect of the cerebellum on each side. These branches anastomose with the anterior inferior cerebellar as well as with the superior cerebellar arteries, which are branches of the basilar artery. The PICA also give branches to the medulla and to the choroid plexus of the fourth ventricle and supply the dentate nucleus of the cerebellum. The area that the PICA supplies in the medulla lies dorsal and lateral to the olivary nucleus.

The basilar artery is most important because it supplies the major portion of the brainstem. It gives numerous short branches that perforate the anterior surface of the brainstem from the midbrain down to the upper medulla (Figs. 10.25 and 10.26). These are usually considered terminal branches, and when they become obstructed, they produce small infarcts or lacunes. The basilar artery gives rise to the anterior inferior cerebellar artery, which is somewhat variable but usually is found on both sides. It supplies the anterolateral parts of the inferior surface of the cerebellum, the inferior and lateral aspects of the pons, and sometimes the upper medulla. The posterior cerebral and the superior cerebellar arteries represent the terminal branches of the basilar arteries. In addition, small thalamoperforating branches arise from the top of the basilar and proximal posterior cerebral arteries (Figs. 10.22 and 10.23). The superior cerebellar artery arises near the top of the basilar artery. It supplies the superior aspect of the cerebellum after going around the brainstem on each side. Anastomoses exist between the superior cerebellar arteries and the anterior inferior and posterior inferior cerebellar arteries. The superior cerebellar arteries also give branches to the pons, the pineal body, and the superior medullary velum.

In addition, the vertebral arteries give branches to the spinal cord via the anterior spinal and the posterior spinal arteries. The vertebral arteries also have muscular branches, and anastomoses exist between these branches and branches of the external carotid arteries. The vertebral arteries also yield the radicular arteries, which supply the spinal cord.

LACUNAR INFARCTS

In 1965, Fisher described the lacunes and the clinical syndrome that is likely to accompany them (116). The syndrome usually consists of purely motor or purely sensory symptoms, ataxia with hemiparesis, clumsy hand syndrome, and dysarthria. These symptoms usually clear completely in a relatively short period of time. CT or MRI may demonstrate these lesions, but in the early stages they may well go undetected because of their small size. A subsequent examination, possibly several days later, may show signs of a small infarction, which weeks or months later becomes a small, sharply outlined dark area well seen by CT and hyperintense on MR on T2-weighted images (Figs. 10.42 and 10.43). The most frequent location for lacunar infarcts is the region of the basal ganglia, the internal and external capsules, the immediate periventricular region around the lateral ventricles, and less frequently the centrum semiovale.

Lacunes may also be seen in the brainstem. They are presumed to be due to occlusion of perforating branches. The occlusion is probably due to atherosclerosis, but it may also be due to small emboli. CT and MRI have clarified the problem considerably, for what was thought to be lacunar syndromes in the past sometimes turns out to be something different, such as larger emboli or infarcts, hemorrhage, tumor, inflammatory disease of the arteries, and even systemic disease.

Both the lenticulostriate arteries and the perforating branches of the basilar artery that supply the brainstem are considered terminal arteries, and an occlusion of one of these arteries will lead to the production of a small infarct that may well be a lacunar infarct, or sometimes to a larger infarct. These are called *lacunar infarcts* if they are smaller than 10 mm in diameter and *small infarcts* if they are larger than that.

HEMORRHAGIC INFARCTION

A hemorrhagic infarction is usually seen some days following the initial ischemic episode, at a time during its evolution when the walls of arterioles and capillaries become disrupted and local blood pressure is restored in the area of the infarction—possibly between the fourth and tenth day or even later. Under these circumstances, it is easy to see how leakage of blood in the damaged area of the brain can occur. For this reason, it is felt that the majority of infarcts that become hemorrhagic are embolic. The embolus would be partly lysed, and the fragments would move more distally, lysing and fragmenting farther. Experimentally, most emboli lyse and fragment in a few hours, and thus there is no hemorrhagic infarct because the walls of the blood vessels are still preserved. Thus the conversion of an ischemic infarction into a hemorrhagic infarction is the exception rather than the rule and involves a number of factors, some of which may well be connected with delay in the lysis and fragmentation of the clots, and possibly with some disturbance in the coagulation mechanisms.

The use of heparin or some other anticoagulant would favor the production of hemorrhage. Sometimes the entire area of the infarct appears to becomes hemorrhagic (Figs. 10.29 and 10.30). *We used to fear the production of a hemorrhagic infarction, but now that we follow these lesions with CT and particularly MRI, we find some evidence of extravasation fairly frequently in patients who are progressing satisfactorily, and it does not usually lead to a large hemorrhage.* (Fig. 10.28). Hemorrhagic infarction can be diagnosed particularly well with MRI because the blood is usually in the methemoglobin stage, bright on both T1- and T2-weighted images. The distribution of brightness in the cortical area of the brain is typical for hemorrhagic infarction (Fig. 10.30).

On CT the hemorrhagic infarction shows up as an increased density, particularly in the brain cortex. If the hemorrhage is relatively slight, it may not be seen by CT or is seen as a slight increase in density that may be attributed to the "fogging effect" previously described (Fig. 10.30). The hyperintensity on T1-weighted images associated with hemorrhage in infarction is often seen in the periphery of the central ischemic area, where circulation may be restored earlier (117).

Boyko et al. found T1 hyperintensity in postischemic infarction not due to hemorrhagic conversion at the same time that histologic examination or autopsy confirmation revealed no blood or significant iron accumulation, such as might be expected if there had been a hemorrhage (118). Moreover, no calcification was present that might be con-

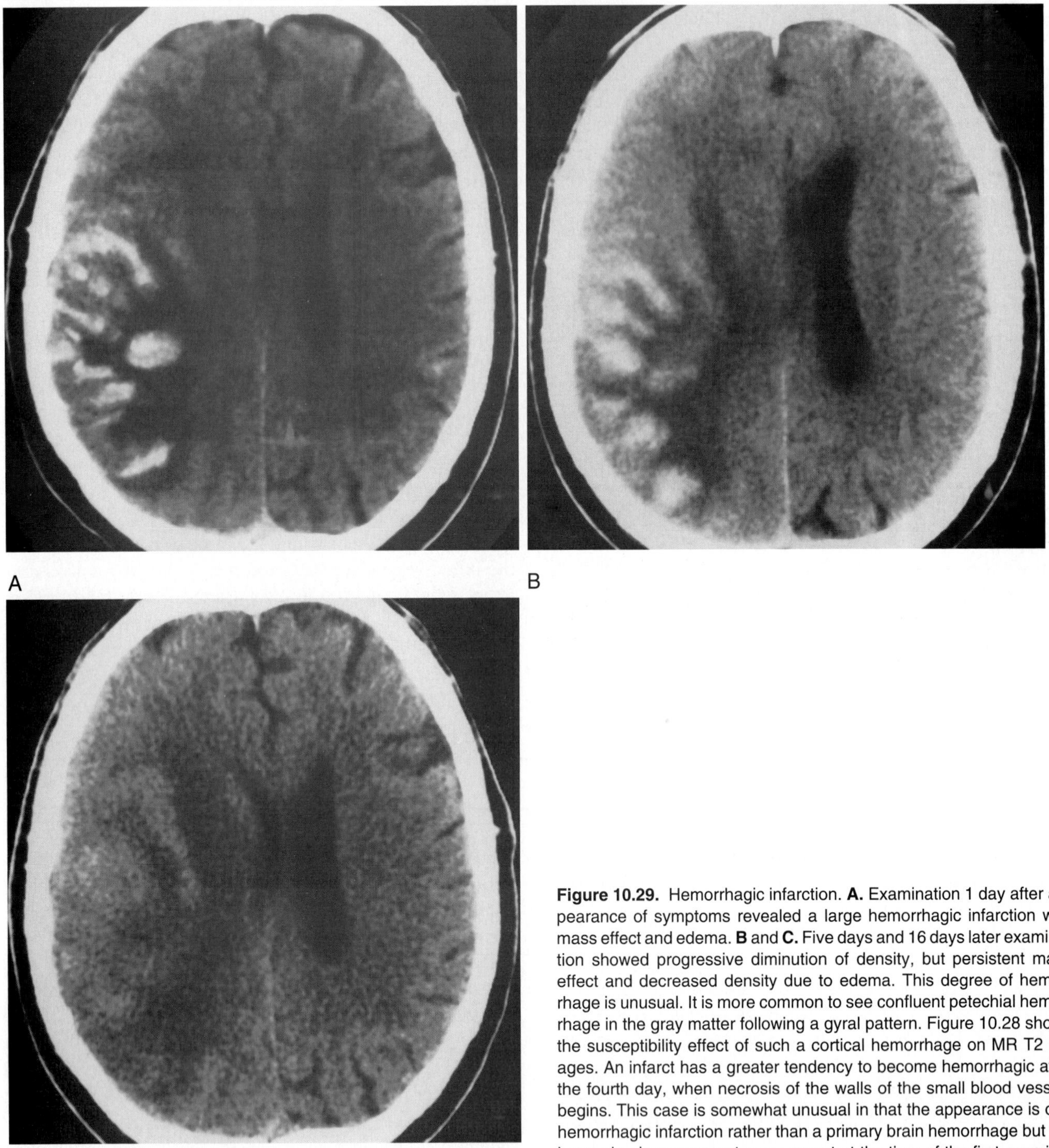

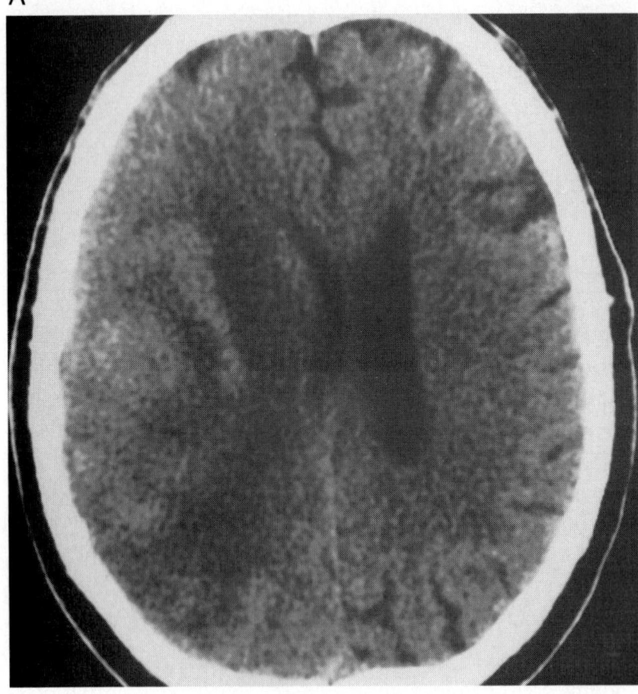

Figure 10.29. Hemorrhagic infarction. **A.** Examination 1 day after appearance of symptoms revealed a large hemorrhagic infarction with mass effect and edema. **B** and **C.** Five days and 16 days later examination showed progressive diminution of density, but persistent mass effect and decreased density due to edema. This degree of hemorrhage is unusual. It is more common to see confluent petechial hemorrhage in the gray matter following a gyral pattern. Figure 10.28 shows the susceptibility effect of such a cortical hemorrhage on MR T2 images. An infarct has a greater tendency to become hemorrhagic after the fourth day, when necrosis of the walls of the small blood vessels begins. This case is somewhat unusual in that the appearance is of a hemorrhagic infarction rather than a primary brain hemorrhage but the hemorrhagic component was present at the time of the first examination. This means that some infarcts are hemorrhagic from the start.

sidered the possible reason for the T1 shortening effects, such as has been reported by Araki et al. (119), Henkelman et al. (120), and others. The pathogenesis is not known, but Boyko et al. (118) proposed that T1 shortening is due to denatured proteins and cellular components, somewhat similar to what is produced by high protein concentration. Thus the differential diagnosis of bright T1 images includes cerebral infarction in addition to calcification, intra- and extracellular methemoglobin from cerebral hemorrhage, mucin, and high protein and lipid/cholesterol concentrations.

CEREBRAL HEMORRHAGE

This is a common problem and results from many causes. It may be seen as the initial finding on CT or MRI following the onset of neurologic symptoms. In general, it may

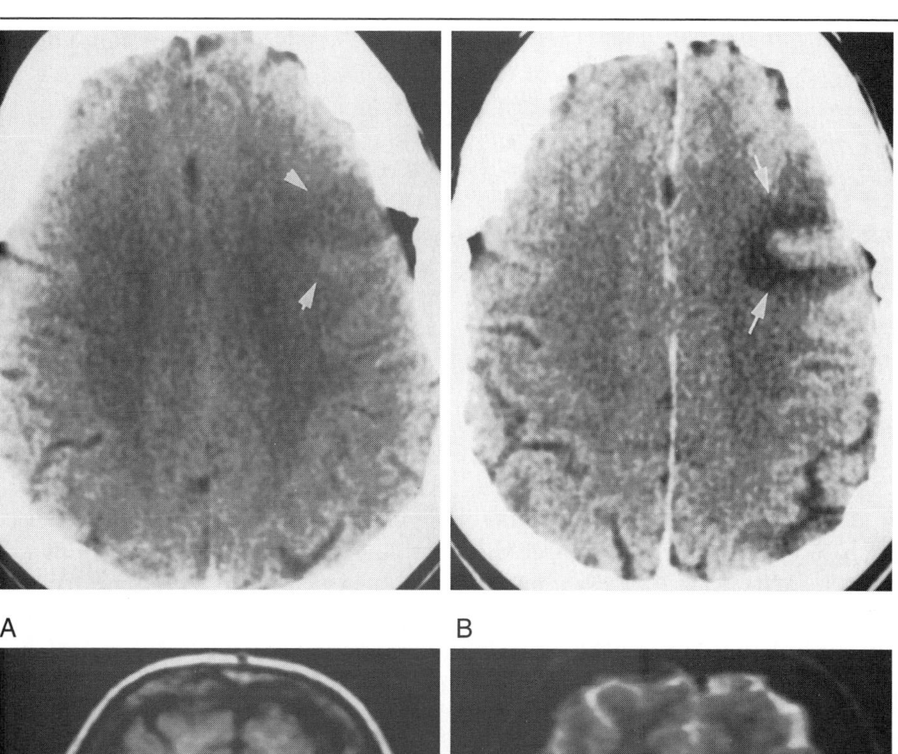

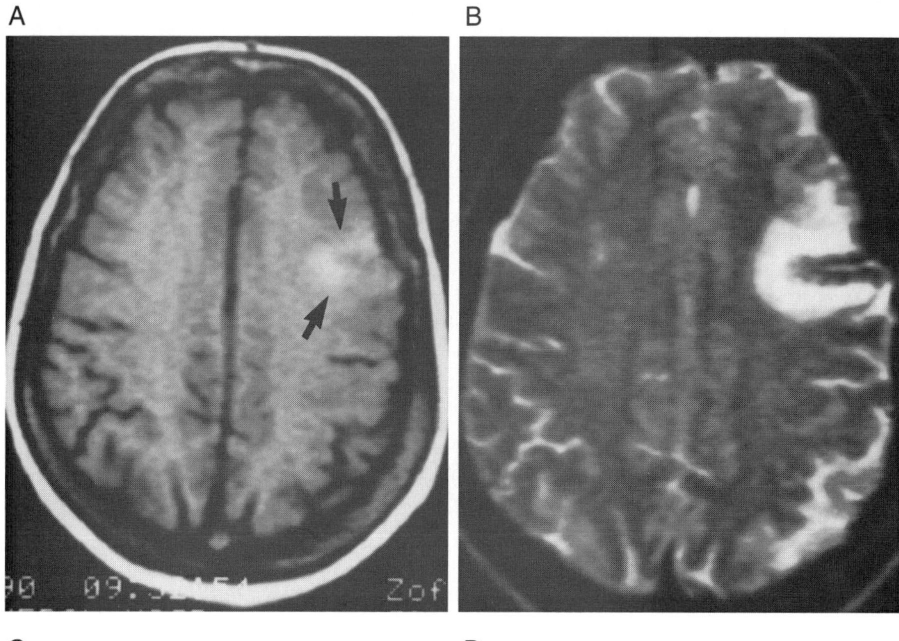

Figure 10.30. Hemorrhagic infarct. **A.** CT shows an infarct in the left frontal region. **B.** Four days later there is a hyperdense area surrounded by low density (arrows). **C.** T1-weighted MR image done on the same day as B shows hyperintensity in the area of infarction consistent with blood in the methemoglobin stage. **D.** T2-weighted image shows hyperintensity but larger than the zone shown in C because of surrounding edema. There is a low-intensity area on the cortical side that may represent blood in the deoxyhemoglobin state. More blood is shown on MRI than might be suspected on CT, where the hyperdensity is rather slight and questionable for hemorrhage.

not be possible clinically to differentiate between ischemia and hemorrhage, and an imaging examination is needed for this purpose. If the patient complains of headache at the onset and is hypertensive, this favors a hemorrhage as against ischemia. Ordinarily the patient is brought into a facility and a CT examination is carried out. One of the most important reasons for a CT is precisely to determine whether we are dealing with an ischemic lesion or with a hemorrhage. Whereas the majority of patients in their sixth or seventh decade presenting with a hemorrhage have systemic hypertension, many other hemorrhages in the brain may be seen in younger individuals. These may be related to hypertension but may also be related to arteriovenous malformations, arterial aneurysms, occult vascular malformations or angiomas, infectious processes associated with mycotic aneurysms, hemorrhagic metastasis, thrombosis of the superior sagittal sinus or of the superficial and deep cerebral veins, cerebral vasculitis, and possibly some other conditions, such as leukemia, systemic conditions such as lupus erythematosus, and general conditions that may be associated with disturbance of the clotting mechanisms of blood. A condition in the elderly that we must remember is amyloid angiopathy. This is probably more common than we suspect and should be considered whenever a hemorrhage occurs in an unusual location or whenever there are multiple hemorrhages (Table 10.10).

On CT the cerebral hemorrhage will appear as an area of increased density in various locations. In the hypertensive hemorrhage, the location is the area of the basal ganglia and thalamus (Fig. 10.31). However, hemorrhages can occur in

Table 10.10.
Major Causes of Intraparenchymal Hemorrhage

Hemorrhagic infarction (frequently embolic)
Hypertensive hemorrhage
Vascular malformations (arteriovenous malformations, cavernous angiomas)
Intratumoral hemorrhage
Vasculitis
Cortical venous infarction secondary to dural sinus thrombosis
Aneurysms (usually subarachnoid hemorrhage)
Mycotic aneurysm
Amyloid angiopathy
Bleeding dyscrasias or anticoagulation therapy

almost any location. If the location of the hemorrhage is in the basal ganglia, the classical area for hypertensive hemorrhages, we are probably dealing with just that. However, if it is in another location, other etiologic possibilities must be considered, and if the patient is on anticoagulants, the hemorrhage is likely to occur in areas other than the basal ganglia.

Whereas the blood is hyperdense in the initial stage, it soon begins to decrease in density, so that in about 48 to 72 h it is significantly less dense than initially, and in about 10 days the density will have completely disappeared or mostly disappeared and become isodense. If the surgeon explores the brain at that point, he or she will find a large hemorrhage in that area even though nothing may be seen by CT scanning. In other words, the disappearance of the density on CT does not mean that the clot has disappeared, even though there may not be much of a mass effect present. On the other hand, the hemorrhage is best seen by MRI at this time. Of course, if the hemorrhage is small, it is likely to disappear sooner on CT. Eventually the hemorrhage will be replaced by brain tissue disruption and some surrounding edema, which will turn the hemorrhage into a radiolucent or low-attenuation area. Following the initial hemorrhage, the density may be surrounded by a radiolucent area that may appear from several hours to a day later, and this dark halo will increase in size due to surrounding edema. This phenomenon is quite variable; sometimes the surrounding edema is larger than at other times, but it will usually be present. The hemorrhage will sometimes acquire a ring configuration in which there is some density in the periphery and less density in the center, and it will be surrounded by an area of edema. This appearance is uncommon. The cavity of an old hemorrhage may present a slit configuration, which is considered typical.

Roda et al. have recently described what they consider a distinct entity, that of an encapsulated intracerebral hematoma that is characterized by a gradual clinical onset and which presents a well-defined capsule at operation (121).

MRI AND CEREBRAL HEMORRHAGE

At this point it would be worthwhile to describe in detail the diagnosis and evolution of hemorrhage as seen by MRI. We may divide the MRI appearance of intraparenchymal

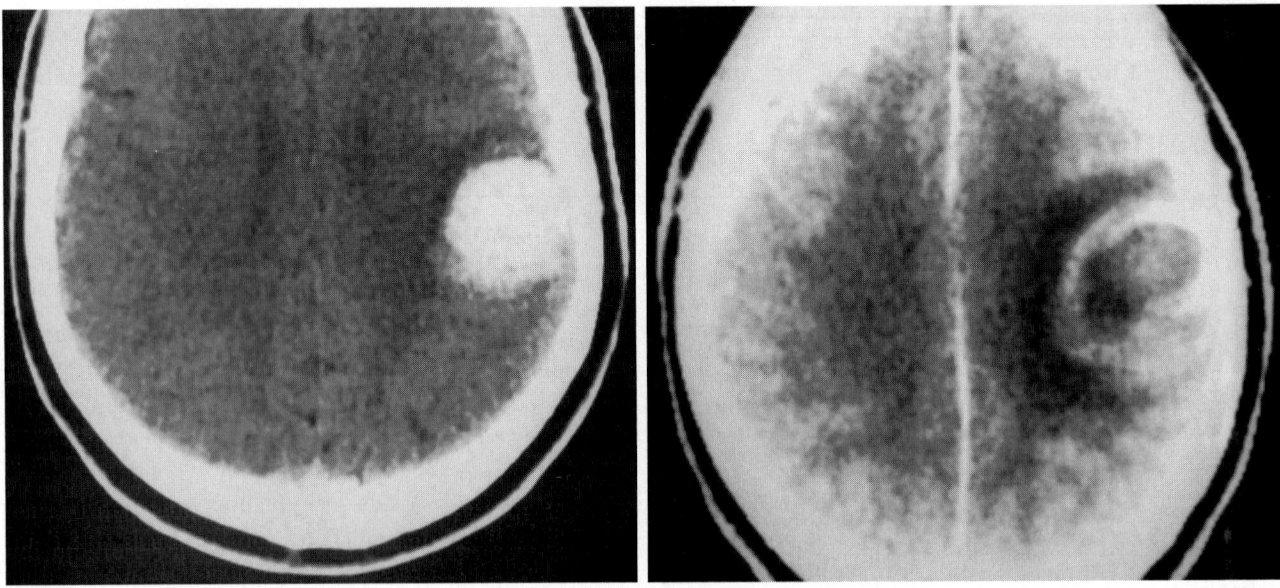

A B

Figure 10.31. Cerebral hemorrhage on CT. **A.** There is a hematoma in the left posterior frontal cortex surrounded by a thin halo of hypodensity consistent with edema. **B.** Twenty-four days later, the hematoma is low density and is surrounded by a hyperdense rim in this enhanced CT scan. There is also a wide hypodense band from edema. The evolution is according to the majority of hematomas as seen by CT; the enhanced rim with contrast is the usual appearance (see Fig. 10.101; also see Fig. 10.33, an MR image of the same case).

brain hemorrhage into various stages following the initial bleeding episode (122–124). These stages are related to the fact that in the brain we are usually dealing with arterial hemorrhage.

In the stage of fresh hemorrhage, presumably arterial, the *oxyhemoglobin* behaves essentially like water; that is, it is low intensity on T1-weighted images, isointense on proton density images, and hyperintense on T2-weighted images.

The next stage is the conversion of the oxyhemoglobin into *deoxyhemoglobin* (four unpaired electrons), which indicates that the oxygen will be disappearing from the extravasated blood. However, in the brain this does not occur as rapidly as it might occur in other tissues, and it may also occur more rapidly in some hemorrhages than in others. In this stage, the hemorrhage will be low intensity on T1-weighted images, isointense on proton density images, and *hypointense on T2-weighted images.* It might be said that if there is partial conversion only, the portion that is deoxyhemoglobin will be low intensity but the portion that remains as oxyhemoglobin will be hyperintense on T2-weighted images.

Stage 3 involves *methemoglobin* (with five unpaired electrons). In this early stage the methemoglobin may be all intracellular, and some of the blood may still be in the deoxyhemoglobin stage. On T1-weighted images the hematoma may be bright or a combination of isodense and bright; on proton density images the hematoma may be isodense or bright, and on T2-weighted images it will be dark.

The next stage (stage 4) is that of *extracellular methemoglobin,* now associated with lysis of the blood cells and dilution of the methemoglobin. The hematoma will now be bright on T1-weighted images, bright on proton density images, and bright on T2-weighted images. This stage can last for a relatively long time in the brain because the exchange of the surrounding brain tissue with the hematoma is quite limited, in contrast to what happens in other tissues. It is possible for the hematoma to remain bright for one or several months. In general, however, the next stage is probably taking place partially or slowly (Table 10.11).

The next stage (stage 5) is caused by *further degradation of hemoglobin* to hemosiderin and ferritin. These molecules have high numbers of unpaired electrons, as many as 10,000 in their molecules. The result is a rather marked degree of magnetic susceptibility that will yield a very low intensity on T2-weighted images and maybe also on proton density and even on T1-weighted images. The conversion of the hemoglobin to hemosiderin usually starts in the periphery, and that is the area where one might expect to see the hypointensity first (Fig. 10.36). From there it will progress toward the center.

In general, the changes tend to occur first on the periphery of the blood clot and from there progress toward the center. Thus, in the methemoglobin stage, it may be possible to see a hyperintense outer portion and a hypointense inner portion that can be quite irregular; the opposite will occur when the blood is continuing to degenerate to hemosiderin. It must be pointed out that clotted blood may have a very high hematocrit, as much as 90 percent, and that the high concentration of protein will cause a decrease in the number of protons and therefore a decrease in signal on both T1- and T2-weighted images. The higher the protein content, the lower the T2 image intensity is likely to be because of the mobility of the protons, which is decreased in the presence of higher protein. More diluted blood with a lower hematocrit will have a higher signal in these hemorrhagic lesions, and as the blood becomes clotted, the changes will not be as neatly differentiated as they are in the stages previously described. The stages in brain hemorrhage occurring with time are illustrated in Figures 10.30 to 10.36.

It is true that in the ordinary clinical situation CT scanning presents the simplest way to diagnose brain hemorrhage. However, if the patient presents sometime after the onset of neurologic symptoms, the CT examination may only show an area of decreased density in the brain, and it will not be possible to tell whether it represents an older hemorrhage or an ischemic infarct that is older than 2 weeks. On the other hand, MRI examination will definitely establish that this is a hemorrhagic lesion because it is most likely to be still in the stage of methemoglobin, with T1-bright and T2-bright images. In addition, it may present a halo of hypointensity consistent with hemosiderin. The same will be true if the lesion is several weeks old. At that stage it is possible that all of the methemoglobin may have disappeared, but the hemosiderin, which produces a rather

Table 10.11.
MR Images of Hemorrhage

	Signal		
Fresh Blood	*T1*	*PD*	*T2*
1. Fresh hemorrhage	Low	Iso	High
2. Deoxyhemoglobin	Low	Iso	Low
3. Methemoglobin (early intrcellular)	High	?High	Low
3a. Combined methemoglobin and deoxyhemoglobin	High, Iso	High, Iso	High, Low
4. Methemoglobin (extracellular)	High	High	High
4a. Combined methemoglobin and hemosiderin	High	High	High, Low
5. Hemosiderin	Iso or Low	Iso or Low	Low

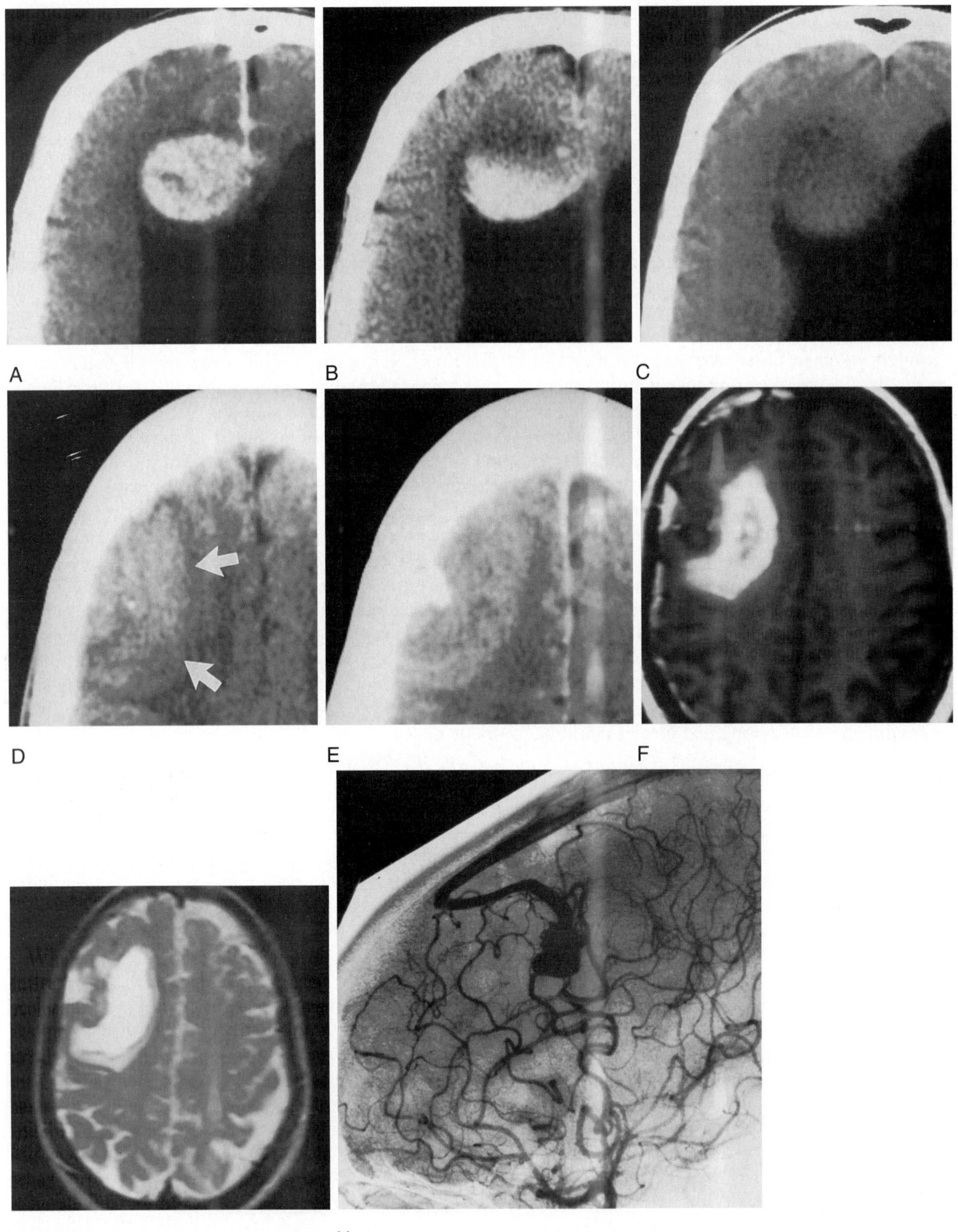

Figure 10.32. Juxtaventricular cerebral hemorrhage seen on CT. **A.** The first examination demonstrates a hematoma in the right frontal region compressing the frontal horn of the lateral ventricle. **B.** Reexamination 5 days later reveals a fluid level due to erythrosedimentation in a hematoma that is at least partly liquid (patient lying supine). **C.** Reexamination 10 days after B shows that the hematoma is nearly isodense with the surrounding brain, although there is slight hypodensity in the anterior aspect and a slight hyperdensity posteriorly, again due to sedimentation of some red blood cells. **D** to **H.** Encapsulated intracerebral hematoma in a 60-year-old woman complaining of headaches and left extremity weakness. **D** and **E.** CT without and with contrast shows a mildly hyperintense area in the right frontal region (arrows), which after contrast (E) shows slight enhancement and presents an area of greater enhancement against the inner table of the skull. This was thought to represent a meningioma. **F.** T1-weighted image shows marked hyperintensity consistent with subacute hemorrhage. There are also hyperintense areas around the brain, suggesting subdural blood in the methemoglobin stage. **G.** T2-weighted image shows hyperintensity. **H.** Lateral cerebral angiogram discloses an unsuspected arteriovenous malformation.

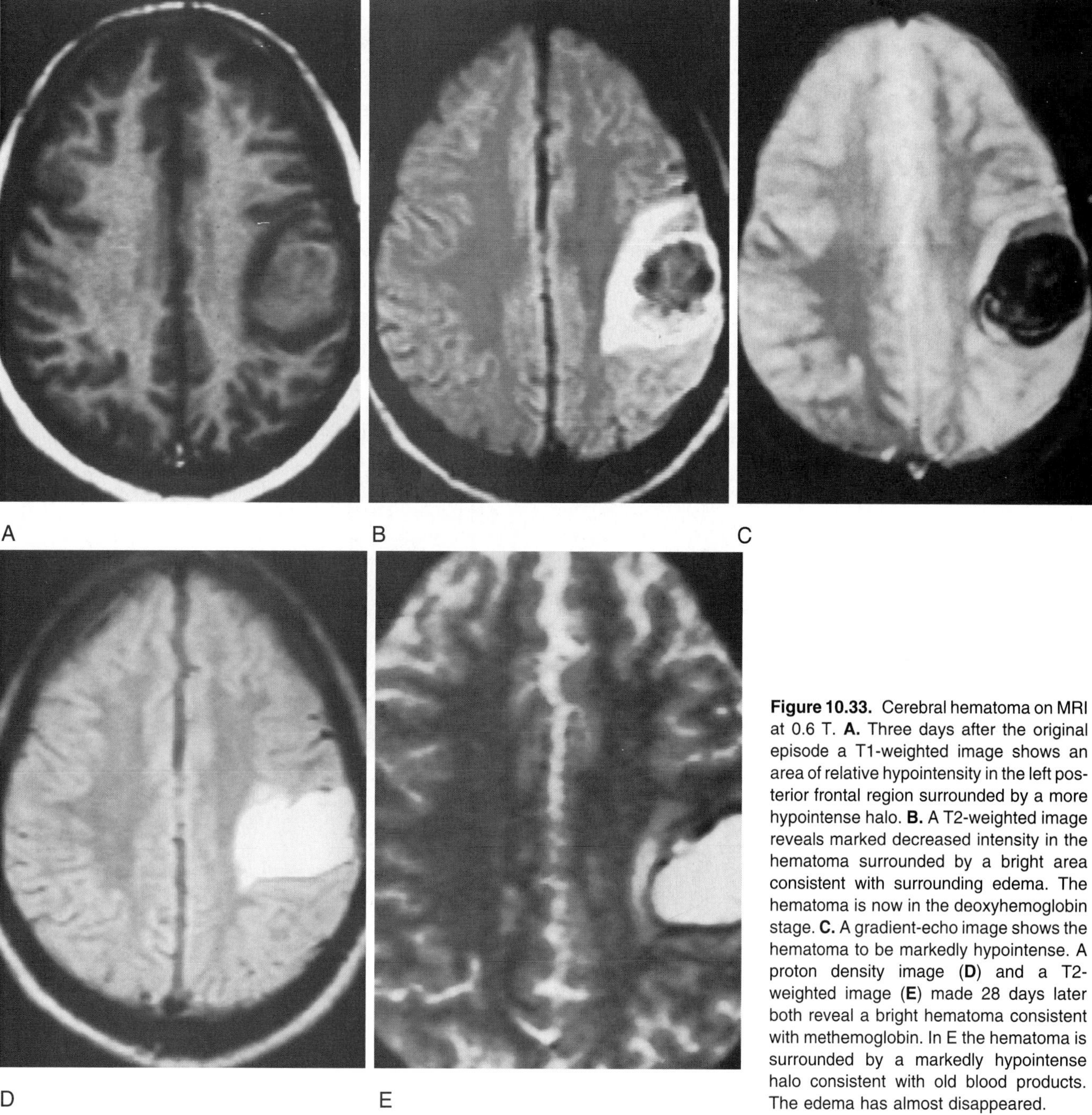

Figure 10.33. Cerebral hematoma on MRI at 0.6 T. **A.** Three days after the original episode a T1-weighted image shows an area of relative hypointensity in the left posterior frontal region surrounded by a more hypointense halo. **B.** A T2-weighted image reveals marked decreased intensity in the hematoma surrounded by a bright area consistent with surrounding edema. The hematoma is now in the deoxyhemoglobin stage. **C.** A gradient-echo image shows the hematoma to be markedly hypointense. A proton density image (**D**) and a T2-weighted image (**E**) made 28 days later both reveal a bright hematoma consistent with methemoglobin. In E the hematoma is surrounded by a markedly hypointense halo consistent with old blood products. The edema has almost disappeared.

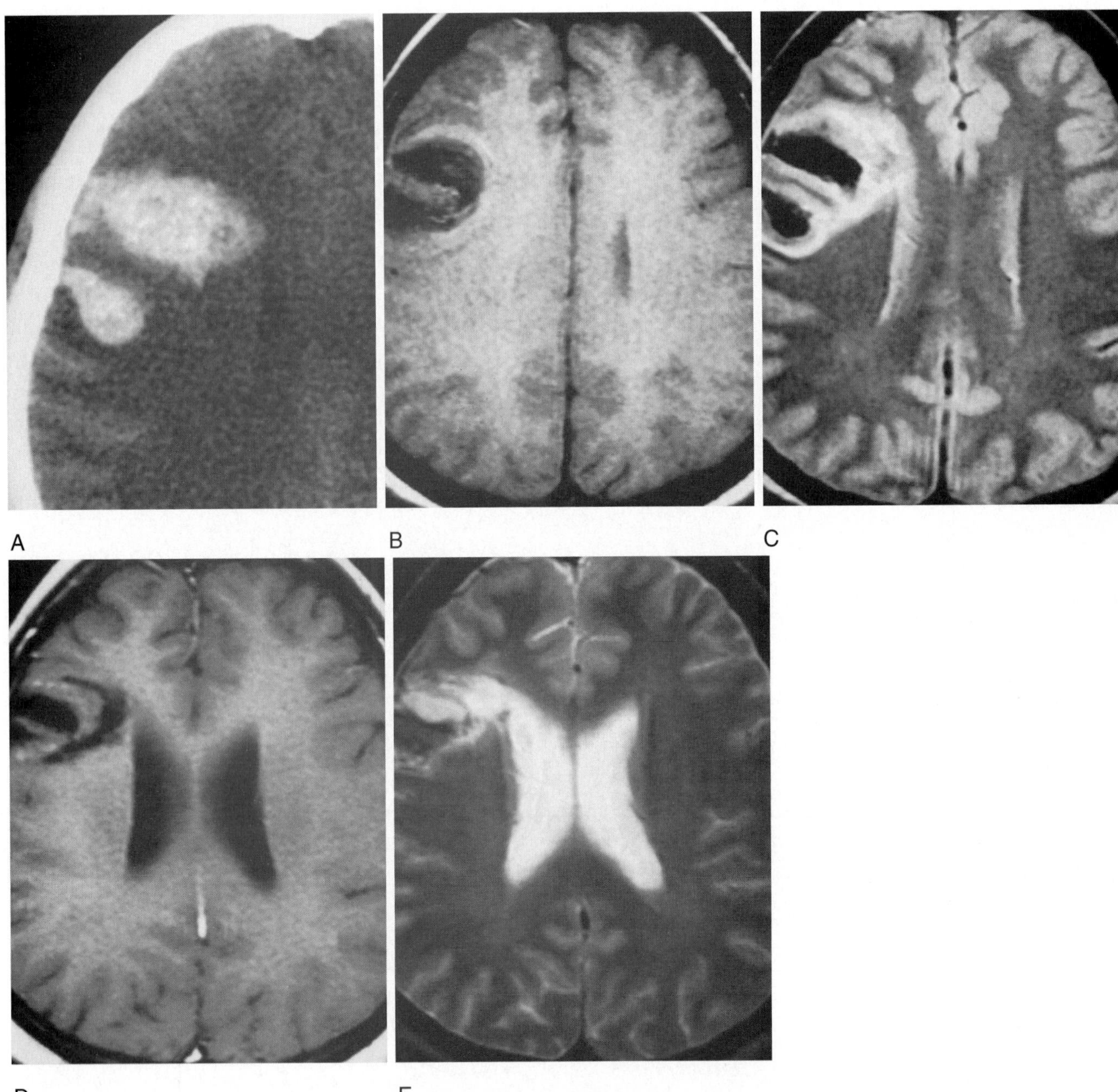

Figure 10.34. Cerebral hematoma in a 26-year-old woman. **A.** In the acute stage CT reveals fresh hematoma. Three days later MRI shows the hematoma to be hypointense on a T1-weighted image (**B**) and markedly hypointense on a T2-weighted image (**C**), which is consistent with deoxy-hemoglobin. The hematoma is surrounded by an edematous area. **D.** Reexamination with contrast 3 months later shows a few areas of enhancement consistent with small vessels, and low intensity in the center and in the periphery of the hematoma consistent with cyst formation in the center and gliosis and chronic edema in the periphery. **E.** T2-weighted image shows brightness in the rostral portion of the old hematoma consistent with cyst formation, and a low-intensity area dorsally consistent with old blood products. The presumed diagnosis was a vascular malformation, but none could be clearly demonstrated, even though the slight vascular enhancement is suggestive. Cavernous angiomas sometimes self-destruct when they hemorrhage.

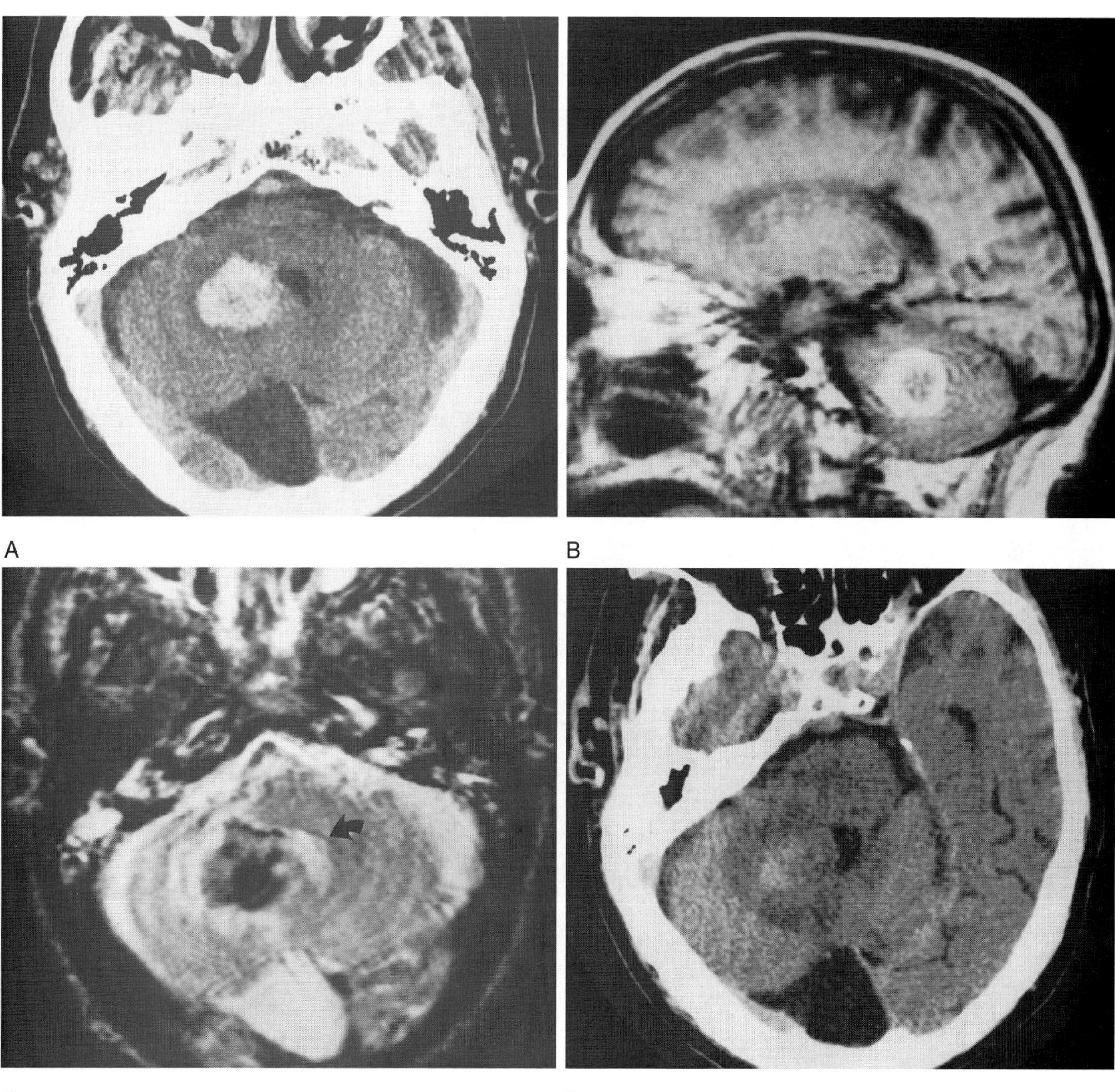

Figure 10.35. Cerebellar hemorrhage in an 82-year-old man. **A.** CT demonstrates a hyperdense area adjacent to the fourth ventricle, which is compressed but not completely obliterated. **B.** T1-weighted sagittal image 7 days later shows the hematoma to be bright peripherally and isointense centrally. The brightness suggests some conversion to methemoglobin, probably in the intracellular methemoglobin state. **C.** MR T2-weighted axial image 7 days later shows a very low intensity in the hemorrhage indicative of deoxyhemoglobin. The hematoma is surrounded by some edema (surrounding bright area). The fourth ventricle (arrow) is compressed to about the same extent as in the initial examination in A. The bright area posteriorly in C represents the cisterna magna. **D.** CT performed 14 days after A shows that the hematoma is almost isodense and is surrounded by some edema.

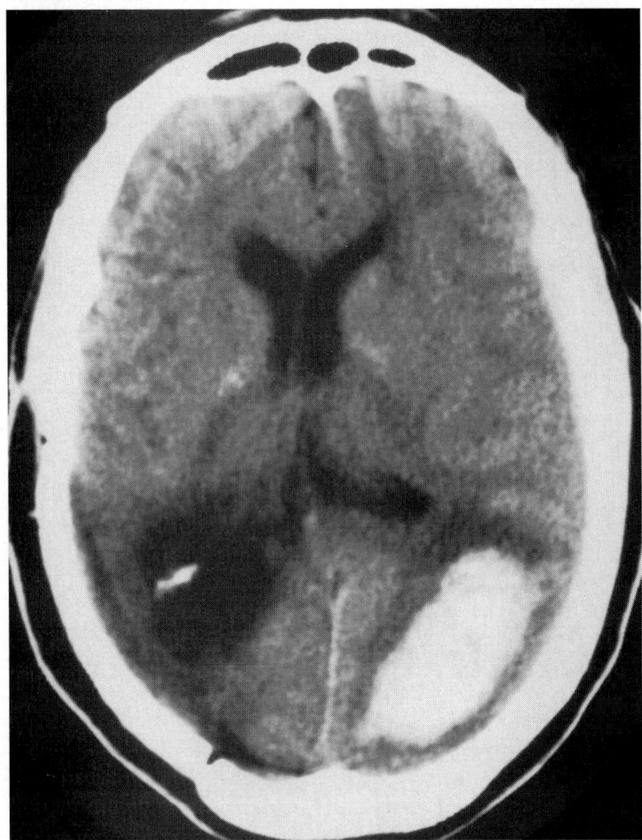

A

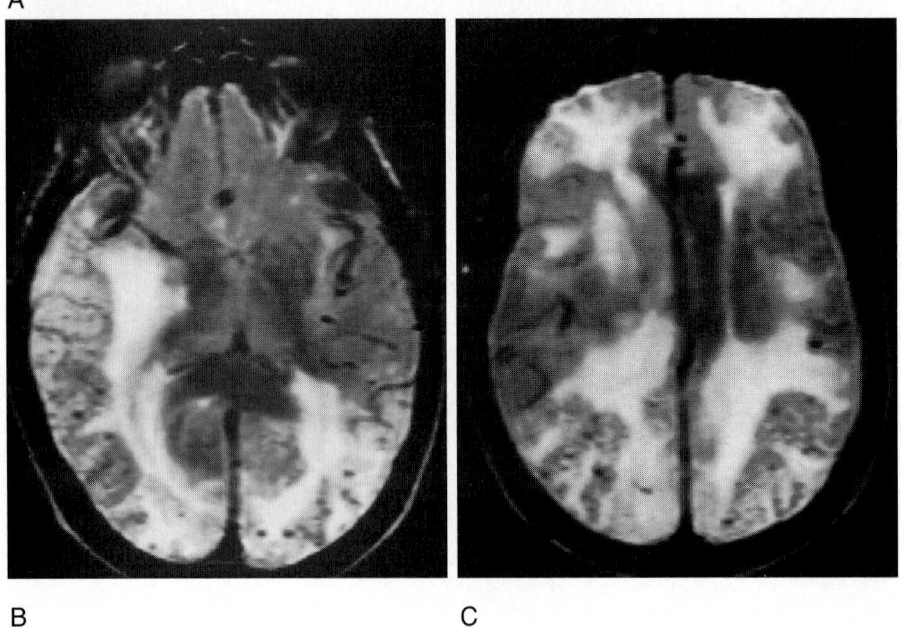

B C

Figure 10.36. A. Recurrent hematoma on opposite side in a 75-year-old man with amyloid angiopathy. There is a new hematoma in the left parieto-occipital region surrounded by a halo of edema. There is also evidence of an old markedly hypodense lesion on the opposite side with displacement of the midline to the right side due to cerebral atrophy. **B** and **C.** Another case of amyloid angiopathy proven at autopsy. T2-weighted MR images reveal numerous small T2-dark areas consistent with magnetic susceptibility related to hemosiderin or old blood products from multiple hemorrhages in a 75-year-old patient. There was also evidence of leukoencephalopathy, which is a recently recognized feature of cerebral amyloid angiopathy. (Case records of the Massachusetts General Hospital, N Engl J Med Case 27-1991;325:42–54.)

marked magnetic susceptibility effect with shortening of the T2, is characteristic of hemorrhage.

In this connection, certain disease processes, such as amyloid angiopathy, may present more than one and sometimes numerous areas of magnetic susceptibility representing repeated old hemorrhages (Fig. 10.36). The same is true of traumatic lesions of the brain, in which hemorrhages are common and sometimes multiple. Again, the magnetic susceptibility will remain and thus can be detected, for hemosiderin tends to be picked up by the surrounding cells and to remain in the area for a very long period of time, possibly for the rest of the patient's life.

Old hemorrhage, particularly in the subarachnoid space and particularly if repeated, may generate hemosiderosis

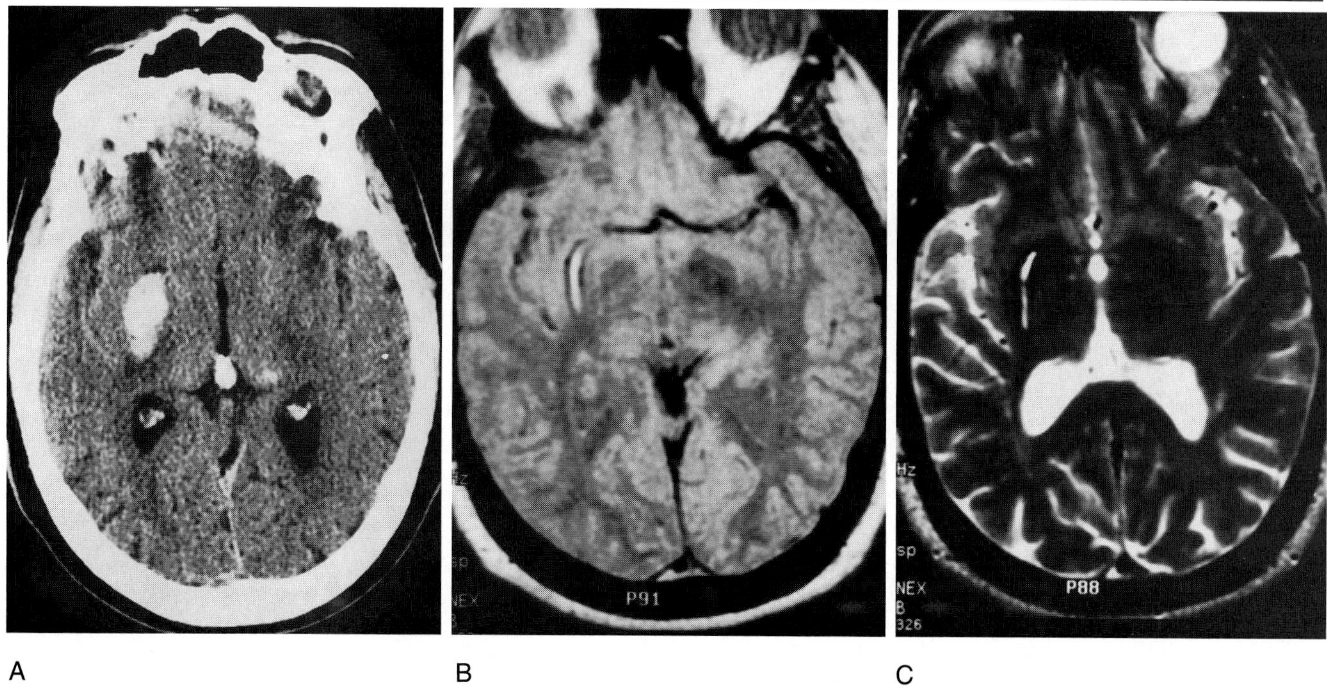

A B C

Figure 10.37. Cerebral hemorrhage showing a slit-shaped area of tissue loss. **A.** Typical hypertensive-type hemorrhage in right thalamic basal ganglia region. **B** and **C.** Six months later MRI shows a slit-shaped scar, bright on T2-weighted images, surrounded by an area of hypointensity due to old blood products.

in the meninges. Meningeal siderosis will show up on T2-weighted images as a dark halo surrounding the surface of the cerebral structures, between the structure surfaces and the bright CSF surrounding them. It is more apparent in the area of the midbrain and brainstem because there is more CSF surrounding these structures (see Fig. 6.56).

Sequelae of Cerebral Infarction and Hemorrhage

An infarct will produce a permanently damaged area in the brain that can easily be shown on CT or MRI. In general, it is possible to state whether an ischemic lesion is old or recent because old infarcts are more sharply outlined at the periphery of the lesions and their density on CT and their low intensity on MRI approach that of CSF. On the other hand, an acute or subacute infarction is less well circumscribed, and its density and signal characteristics are less like CSF. There may be different areas of intensity within the abnormality in recent infarctions. The diagnostic problem arises when there is no typical clinical history, for in the presence of a good history of cerebral ischemia, the clinical correlation makes the interpretation obvious. However, sometimes there may be a lesion that looks like a very old infarct in a patient with new symptoms. In some of these cases there is a history of an old ischemic lesion, and the new symptoms may be due to a recent ischemic insult in the same area. If old images are available for comparison, an added abnormality may become visible and represents the recent ischemic area producing new symptoms. An old hemorrhage may leave an area of permanent tissue loss; the area often has an elongated configuration, which is usually referred to as a *slit-shaped scar*. On CT the slit scar is low density; MRI may show, in addition to low intensity on T1-weighted images, an area or halo of susceptibility (T2 dark) surrounding the slit scar, which is usually T2 bright (Fig. 10.37). Wallerian degeneration also takes place, becoming visible after a number of weeks (Fig. 10.38).

A bilateral anterior cerebral occlusion will leave a well-defined area of tissue loss bifrontally (Fig. 10.39).

A middle cerebral artery occlusion involves most of the hemisphere and affects the frontal, parietal, and temporal lobes (Fig. 10.49). An infarct involving the basal ganglia and internal capsule area may be produced by an occlusion of the initial segment of the middle cerebral artery or by occlusion of the internal carotid artery secondarily involving the middle cerebral artery (Figs. 10.40 and 10.41).

Lacunar infarcts are usually considered to be related to obstruction of perforating branches of the middle, posterior, posterior communicating, and anterior cerebral arteries; they usually are seen best as scars rather than in the acute stage (Figs. 10.42 and 10.43).

Basilar artery occlusions may involve the supratentorial or the infratentorial branches or both, depending on the location of the obstruction (Fig. 10.50).

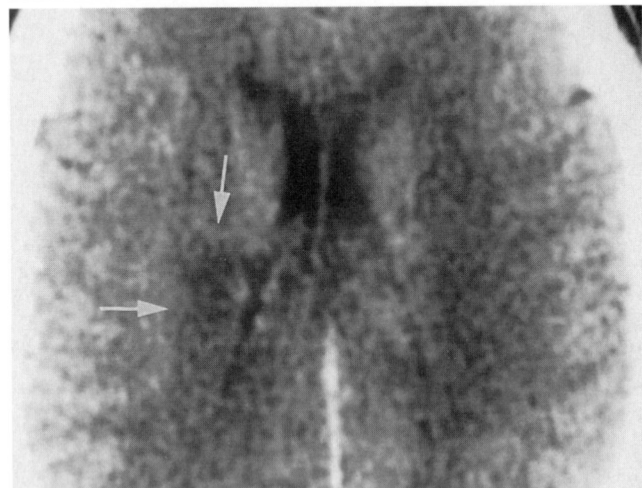

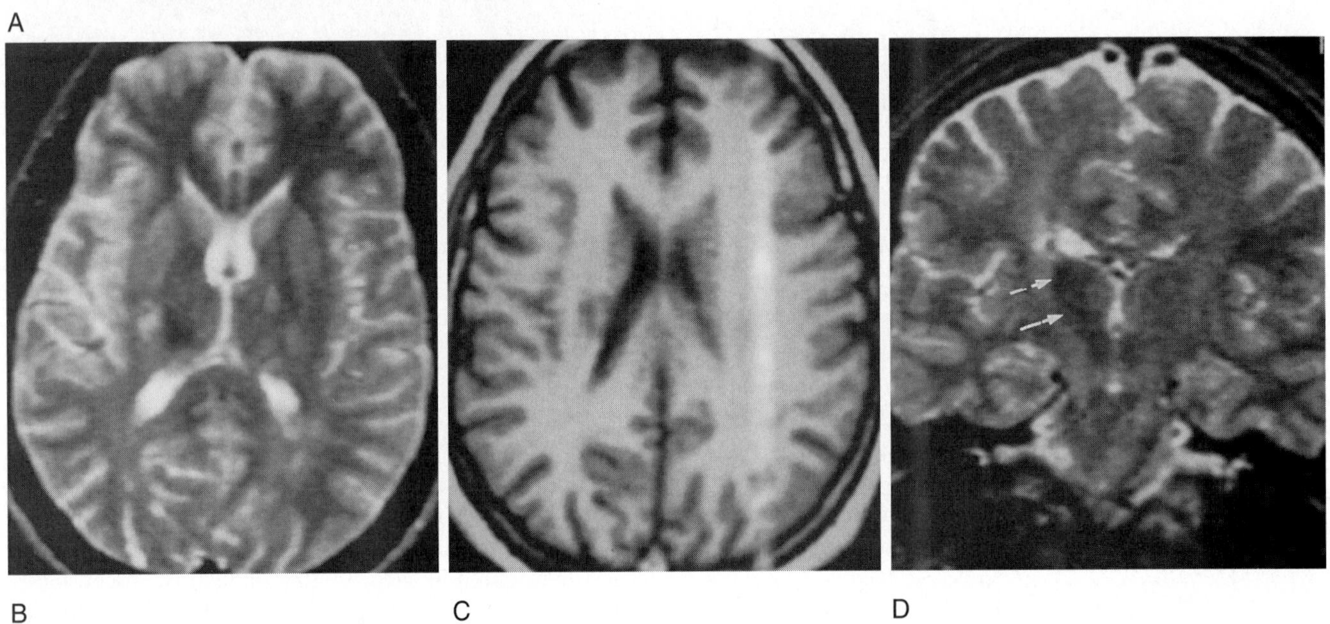

Figure 10.38. Cerebral infarct followed by fixed scar and wallerian degeneration. **A.** CT showing a low-density area on the right side adjacent to ventricles (arrows). **B.** MRI shows that the lesion extends to involve the posterior limb of the internal capsule. **C.** Reexamination 11 weeks later shows a low intensity on T1-weighted axial image in the previous area of infarction. **D.** Coronal T2-weighted image shows a low intensity in the pyramidal tract region extending to the upper brainstem (arrows). The low intensity on T2-weighted image represents the early period of wallerian degeneration (see Figs. 8.17 and 8.18).

Therapeutic Considerations

In the acute stage, the permanent brain scar may be smaller than the initial area of involvement seen on CT or MRI because of the disappearance of some peripheral edema around the central core. An ischemic brain lesion always contains a core in which cell death will surely occur and a peripheral area or penumbra where the ischemia is less severe and where there is cell viability. If it is possible for some blood supply to reach this area, function will be restored. The treatment of cerebral ischemia is directed toward saving as much viable tissue around the central core as possible by various means, such as by lowering blood viscosity, raising blood pressure, and using anticoagulants (usually heparin) and possibly other pharmaceutical products now being evaluated. Among these are calcium channel blockers, which limit the access of extracellular calcium to the nerve cells' interior and, in addition, may have a beneficial effect by improving circulation in the "penumbra" area surrounding the core of the infarct (125). Thus nimodipine, nicardipine, and levemopamil will be receiving special attention, and controlled clinical trials are on the way. Unfortunately, in experimental animals these agents are effective if they are administered within 1 to 4 h after the stroke, and most patients are brought in too late after the onset, which may have occurred during sleep. Moreover, the trials should be limited to those patients who are likely to benefit, and this excludes the massive infarctions.

Again, by CT or MRI, it is often not possible to ascertain early enough the amount of brain damage present. The advent of diffusion imaging by MRI may well allow us to see an infarct much earlier than is possible with conventional MRI. This will require the use of new techniques such as echoplanar imaging, which is emerging from industrial and clinical research. Thrombolytic agents, such as

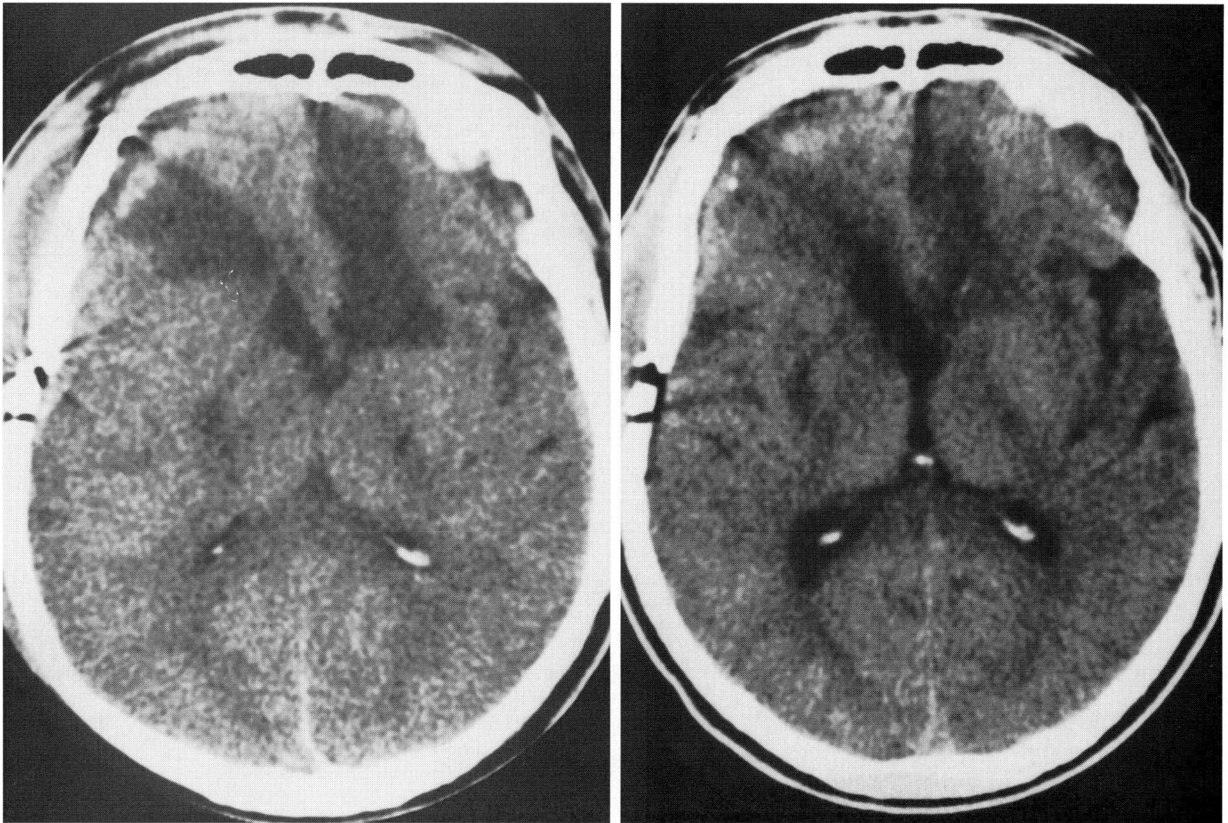

Figure 10.39. Anterior cerebral artery infarction. The patient had an anterior communicating aneurysm. It was surgically clipped, but arterial spasm developed in both anterior cerebral arteries. **A.** There is bilateral involvement in the frontal lobes in a fairly typical location for anterior cerebral artery occlusion or severe, prolonged spasm. **B.** Repeat examination 2 weeks later shows some improvement in that the total area of involvement is somewhat smaller, but the patient will undoubtedly have a permanently damaged area bifrontally.

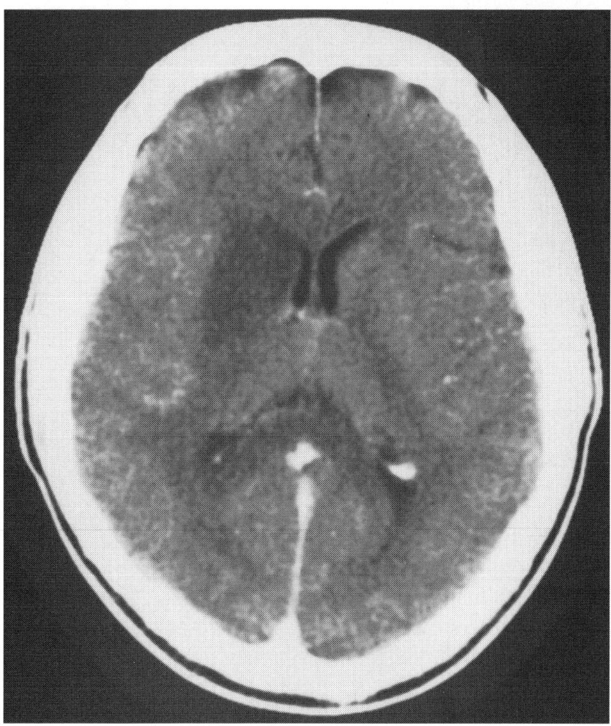

Figure 10.40. Infarct involving head of caudate nucleus, putamen, globus pallidus, anterior limb of internal capsule, and external capsule in a 19-year-old patient. There is a hypodense area adjacent to the frontal horn of the right lateral ventricle. The ventricle is being compressed as a result of edema.

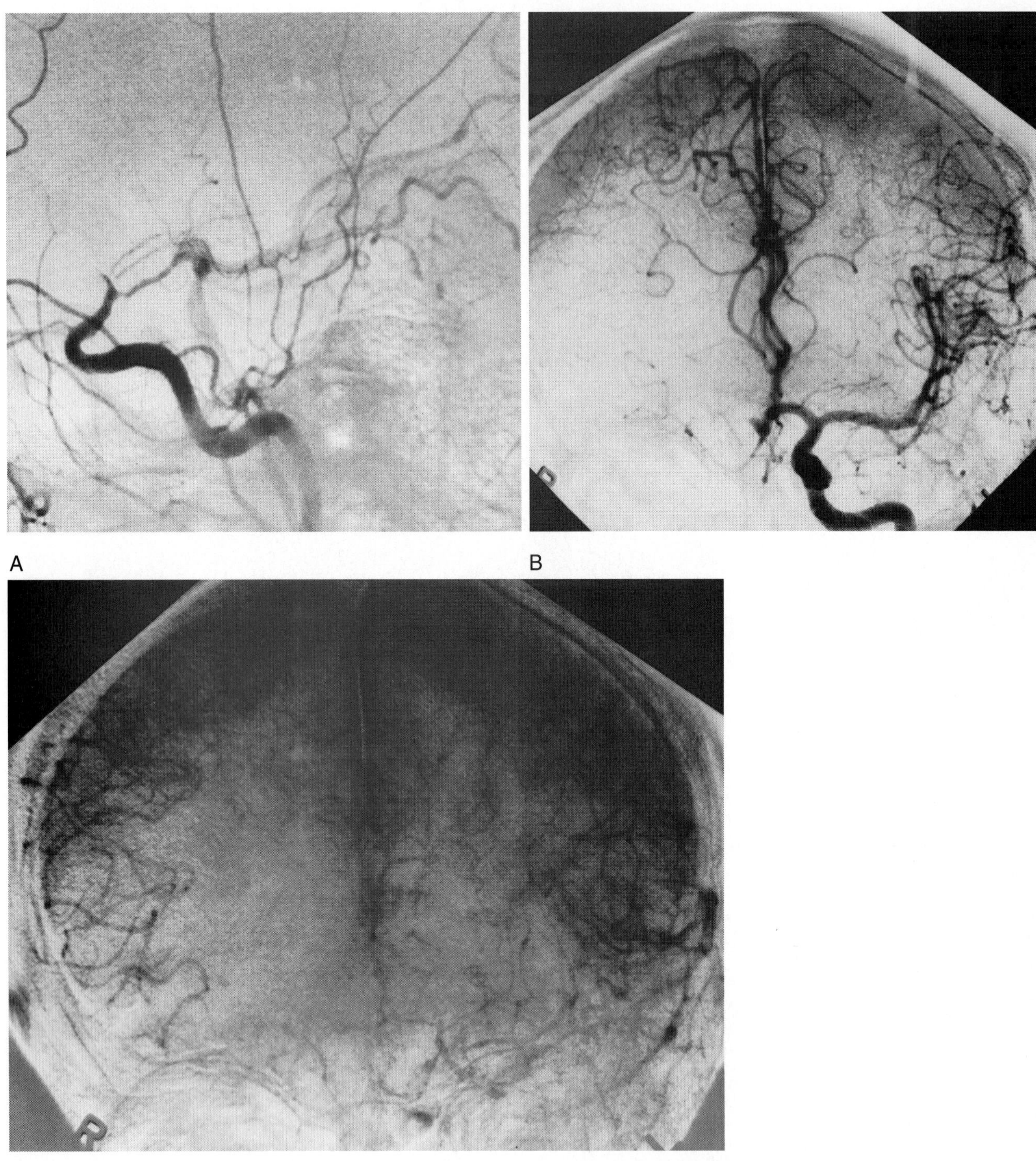

Figure 10.41. Angiography in patient shown in Figure 10.40 demonstrating occlusion of the internal carotid artery. **A.** Right carotid angiography demonstrates an occlusion of the internal carotid artery above the level of the origin of the anterior choroidal artery. **B.** Frontal view after injection of left carotid shows bilateral filling of anterior cerebral arteries with filling of middle cerebral artery branches on the surface due to the leptomeningeal anastomoses. **C.** The only portion of the middle cerebral artery that did not fill was the first, horizontal segment in this 3-sec delayed arterial phase. The infarcted area involved the territory irrigated by the perforating (lenticulostriate) branches of the middle cerebral trunk.

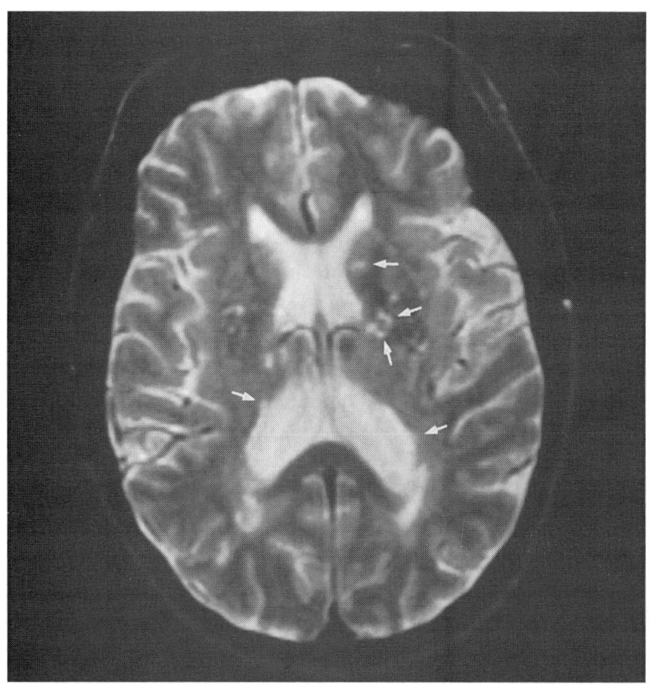

Figure 10.42. Lacunar infarcts. T2-weighted image shows a number of bright, small spots, most of them not corresponding to dilated Virchow-Robin spaces. There are periventricular small, bright areas (arrows), a frequent location for lacunes (arrows); they are also in the thalamus and in the head of the caudate nucleus. Most lacunar infarcts occur in the basal ganglia region and in the immediate periventricular margin, as well as in the thalamus and are seen best as old lacunes rather than in the acute stage.

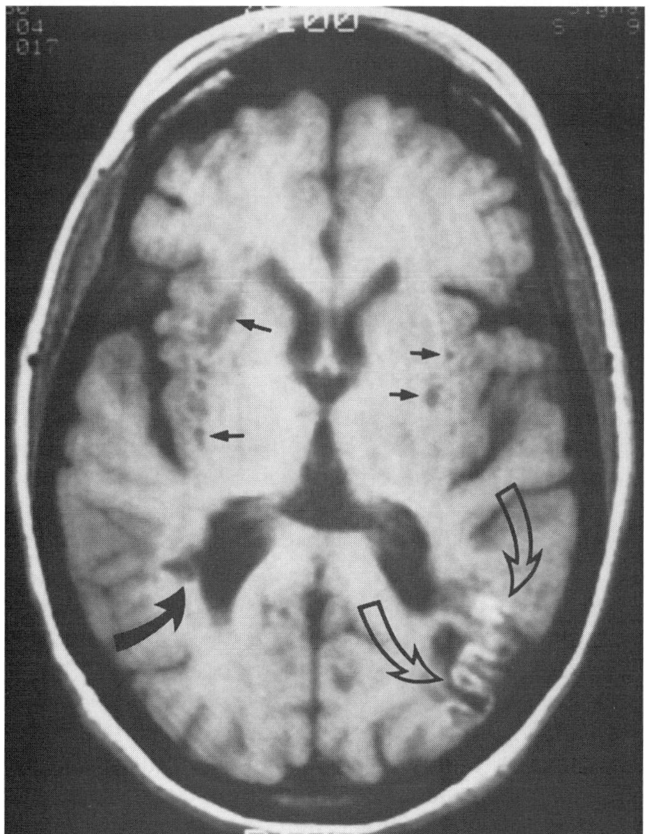

Figure 10.43. Multiple lacunar infarcts in a 52-year-old woman. There are a number of low-intensity small and medium-sized spots in the basal ganglia and external capsule region (arrows), as well as in the periventricular area (curved arrow). In addition, there is a small, slightly hemorrhagic infarct in the left parieto-occipital region (open arrows). The patient was developing signs of dementia. Multiple lacunar infarcts are associated with an increased incidence of dementia.

streptokinase and urokinase, and tissue plasminogen activator (t-PA) have received some attention, particularly after the success of these drugs in treating myocardial infarction (126). The early experience in stroke was disappointing because of cerebral hemorrhage as a complication. More recently, intra-arterial injection by superselective catheterization of the involved arteries is being tried. Only a small percentage of stroke patients are suitable for this approach, partly because it must be done early and partly because it requires angiographic confirmation and a high degree of skill in the use of these techniques, which is not always available.

In the chronic stage the most important consideration is that of carotid endarterectomy, both to treat signs of cerebral circulation insufficiency, as evidenced by repeated transient ischemic attacks, and to correct the insufficiency in a patient who already may have had a nondisabling stroke. The North American Symptomatic Carotid Endarterectomy Trial provided evidence of the usefulness of this surgical approach in patients who had a 70 percent or greater stenosis of the internal carotid artery (29, 127).

CEREBRAL ANGIOGRAPHY IN STROKE: THE COLLATERAL CIRCULATION OF THE BRAIN

There are important communications between the branches of the cerebral arteries and also between the external carotid artery and the internal carotid artery systems. The presence and the efficiency of the collateral circulation determine whether an infarct will be produced following an occlusion of an intracranial artery and will also determine at least the size of the infarct. For this reason, even though this topic is based on angiographic observations, it is worth discussing here.

There are three groups of collateral circulations that can be considered here: (a) the circle of Willis; (b) the anastomoses between the branches of the anterior, middle, and posterior cerebral arteries on the surface of the brain, called *meningeal arterial anastomoses;* and (c) anastomoses between the extracranial and intracranial arteries. Of these, the most important are the circle of Willis and the end-to-end anastomoses between the anterior, middle, and posterior cerebral arteries. The extracranial-to-intracranial anastomoses become activated more slowly and function only in chronic or slowly developing occlusions (Table 10.12).

Table 10.12.
Major Forms of Arterial Collateral Circulation

Circle of Willis
- Anterior communicating artery
- Posterior communicating artery

Anastomoses between distal branches of major arteries (pial-pial collaterals)

Extracranial-intracranial anastomoses
- Via branches of the external carotid artery (including from muscular branches of the vertebral artery) principally supplying the ophthalmic artery
- Intrapetrosal and intracavernous internal carotid artery (ICA) branches
- Transdural anastomoses, especially via the middle meningeal artery

Circle of Willis

It is well known that the arterial connections between the two anterior cerebral arteries through the anterior communicating artery, and those between the internal carotid and the posterior cerebral arteries through the posterior communicating arteries, are not always symmetrically developed. For instance, the anterior cerebral artery in its first segment proximal to the anterior communicating artery can be small on one side, sometimes quite small, and this will interfere with the cross circulation between the two sides. The same is true with the posterior communicating artery, which can be small on one or both sides. Moreover, the posterior cerebral artery may originate from the internal carotid artery, an anatomical variant called *fetal-type posterior cerebral artery*. In this case the segment between the junction of the posterior communicating to the posterior cerebral artery and the basilar artery is quite small. These asymmetries in the circle of Willis are important in cases where hypotension develops on one arterial system, which would then call for collateral flow from the opposite side. The variation in the size of the components of the circle of Willis is shown in Figure 10.44.

Anastomoses Between Intracranial Arteries

Of great physiologic and clinical significance are the direct end-to-end anastomoses between the branches of the anterior, middle, and posterior cerebral arteries. The channels are physiologically available for bidirectional flow at all times. They are naturally and readily utilized to support general circulation whenever there is a lowering of arterial pressure in one area that demands a reversal of the usual direction of flow. In a manner similar to that operating in the circle of Willis, the circulation of blood can be reversed very rapidly in these small arteries following occlusion of a major vessel by an embolus or thrombus.

Because many of the branches of the anterior and middle, as well as the posterior cerebral, arteries anastomose with one another directly, the flow of blood must stop at some point in these vessels. The anterior cerebral artery flow is upward and backward along the medial surface of the hemisphere to the parasagittal margin of the brain. Thence, it travels laterally and downward for a short distance, as the branch vessels curve outward onto the lateral hemispheric surface. In the middle cerebral branches, the flow of blood is upward to reach the superior portion of the hemisphere. Usually the middle cerebral branches can be followed at angiography only to a point 2 to 3 cm below the upper edge of the hemisphere. Beyond this point they ordinarily are not visible. This is clearly shown in cases where there is no contrast filling of one anterior cerebral artery, but in which flow is normal as a result of both anterior cerebral arteries filling from the contralateral side. At such junction

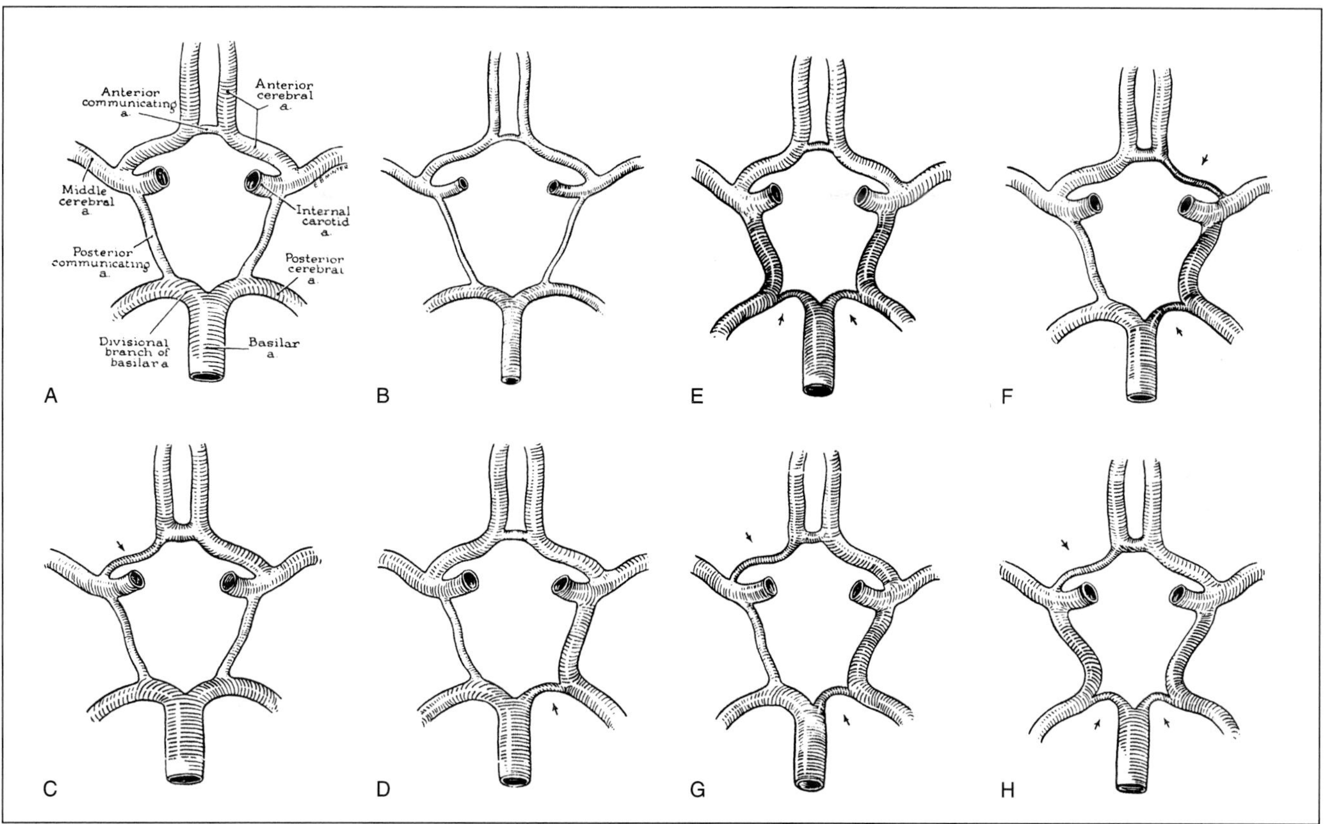

Figure 10.44. Incidence of various forms of the circle of Willis found at autopsy. **A.** Group I, 18 percent. **B.** Group II, 6 percent. **C.** Group III, 25 percent. **D.** Group IV, 16 percent. **E.** Group V, 11 percent. **F.** Group VI, 8 percent. **G.** Group VII, 8 percent. **H.** Group VIII, 8 percent. (Based on Hodes et al: Am. J Roentgenol 1953;70:61–82.)

points ("watershed areas"), the pressures in the anastomotic vessels between the anterior and middle cerebral arteries become equalized, and no flow results except toward the perforating branches that supply the brain (Fig. 10.45). If, however, the pressure is lowered in either the middle or the anterior cerebral system, retrograde flow into the territory of the hypotensive vessel will occur and can be followed on serial films. As mentioned, retrograde flow can be established only if there is no propagation of the occlusion by intravascular clotting distally from the site of obstruction, since extension will cause obliteration of the arterial branches (Figs. 10.46 and 10.66).

Undoubtedly the configuration of the circle of Willis is a very important factor in the development of symptoms following intracranial arterial occlusions. The presence of a hypoplastic segment of the circle on the critical side of an occlusion may be crucial. At other times, a major anomaly of the arteries may be present that influences the clinical picture.

Watershed Infarction

As already explained, there are end-to-end anastomoses between the branches of the anterior, middle, and posterior cerebral arteries on the surface of the brain. These anastomoses permit the bidirectional flow of blood if there is a decrease in pressure in one main artery or the other. The middle cerebral arteries supply the external surfaces of the frontal, parietal, and occipital lobes, and the anterior cerebral artery supplies the medial surface of the hemispheres extending up to the upper surface of the hemisphere and slightly on the outer surface. In one area there is an equalization of the arterial blood pressure between the branches of the anterior, middle, and posterior cerebral arteries. This is most apparent over the outer surface of the frontal and parietal lobes, where a parasagittal fringe exists that extends from the lateral aspect of the frontal pole to the posterior parieto-occipital areas. If there is an occlusion of the middle cerebral artery or of the important branches of the middle cerebral artery, the hypotension created by this occlusion will provoke flow of blood through these end-to-end anastomoses from the anterior cerebral artery and sometimes from the posterior cerebral artery to the outer surface. This can easily be demonstrated by cerebral angiography provided there has been no propagation of clot within the obstructed vessels distally, as explained earlier (Figs. 10.45 and 10.46).

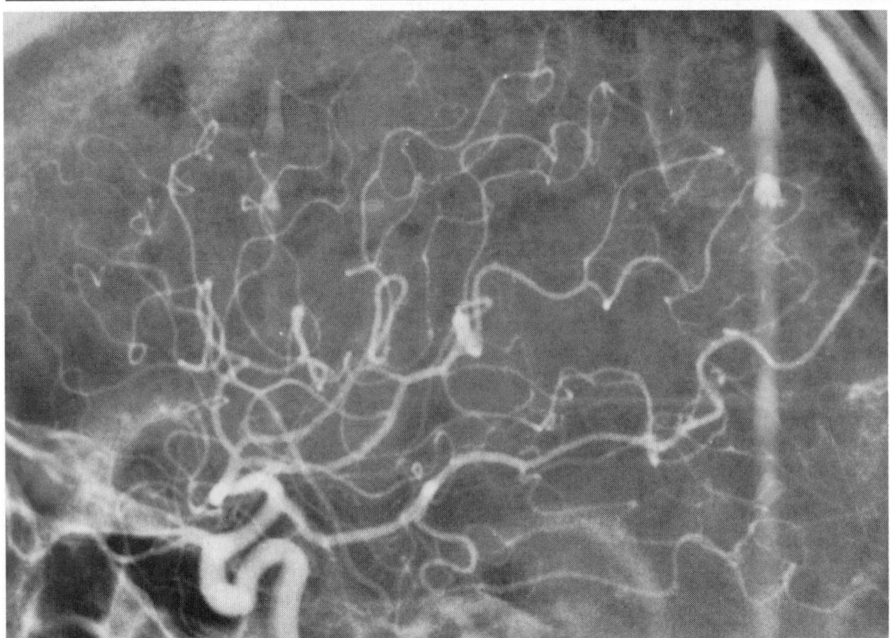

Figure 10.45. Lateral view of cerebral arteries in which there was no filling of the anterior cerebral artery, presumably because of hypoplasia of the initial segment of that artery, with both anterior cerebral arteries filling from the opposite side. At 1.25 sec, the filling of the middle cerebral artery branches has extended as far as it will go toward the top of the hemisphere. The anterior cerebral artery branches normally come down on the outer hemisphere for a short distance after reaching the upper margin. In this case they are not visible because they are not opacified.

When there is lowering of the blood pressure in the entire hemisphere, such as may occur, for instance, in an occlusion of one internal carotid artery in a patient who has insufficient collateral circulation through the circle of Willis, there will be a uniform lowering of the blood pressure in that hemisphere. Under these circumstances the parasagittal area, the area where the branches of the middle and the anterior and posterior cerebral arteries anastomose, will have a more severe lack of oxygenated blood than the other portions supplied by these arteries. Consequently, an ischemic infarction may occur that extends parasagittally, starting in the frontal pole and extending all the way back to the occipital pole (Fig. 10.47).

Several examples of infarcts produced by occlusion of the internal carotid artery (Fig. 10.48), the middle cerebral artery (Fig. 10.49), and the basilar artery (Fig. 10.50) are shown. Figure 10.51 provides an example of infarction in the basal ganglia secondary to cardiac arrest. An example of carotid artery occlusion with collateral circulation is shown in Figure 10.52.

Anastomoses between Extracranial and Intracranial Arteries

Circulation from the extracranial arteries to the intracranial vessels may take place by way of the ophthalmic artery, the most common route. Branches of the ophthalmic artery anastomose with those of the superficial temporal, external maxillary, and internal maxillary arteries and with branches of the middle meningeal artery as well. Since the ophthalmic artery is a sizable branch of the internal carotid system, reverse circulation can be established fairly easily (128). It probably requires some time, however, for full collateral circulation to be established by way of the ophthalmic artery. How long this takes cannot be stated, but it may be as much as a few weeks before there is voluminous flow. There is not good correlation between the presence of collateral circulation through the ophthalmic artery and the degree of recovery from a stroke following occlusion of the internal carotid artery in the neck (129).

The collateral circulation through the orbit cannot become established unless the obstruction is proximal to the origin of the ophthalmic artery and unless the carotid siphon remains patent (Fig. 10.52). Filling of the portion of the internal carotid artery proximal to the origin of the ophthalmic artery indicates that this segment is patent. In the majority of these cases, flow can be reestablished by endarterectomy and surgical reconstruction of the carotid artery in the neck. On the other hand, if no circulation can be demonstrated in the internal carotid artery below the ophthalmic origin, the chances of reestablishing flow by carotid reconstructive surgery are much less (130).

Another course for external-internal carotid collateral supply is through the intrapetrosal and intracavernous branches. These vessels play an important role in maintaining patency of the internal carotid artery proximal to the ophthalmic origin (Fig. 10.52). Many of the anastomoses are between meningeal branches of the internal and external carotid systems.

Transdural anastomoses constitute a third source of collateral supply from the extracranial to the intracranial arterial networks. Anastomosis between a branch of the middle meningeal artery and a division of the middle meningeal artery can occur directly through the subdural space. In one case, following intracranial ligation of the internal carotid artery, good filling of many of the branches of the middle cerebral artery took place via this route (131). Many cases

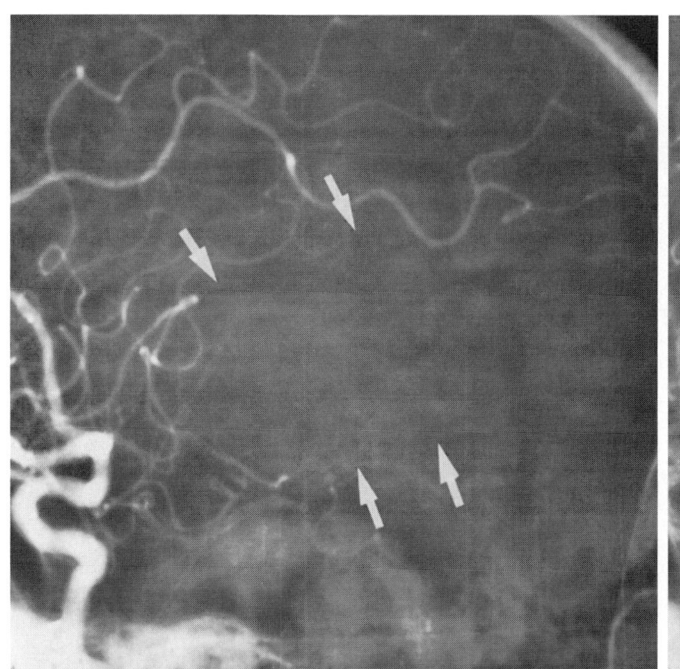
A

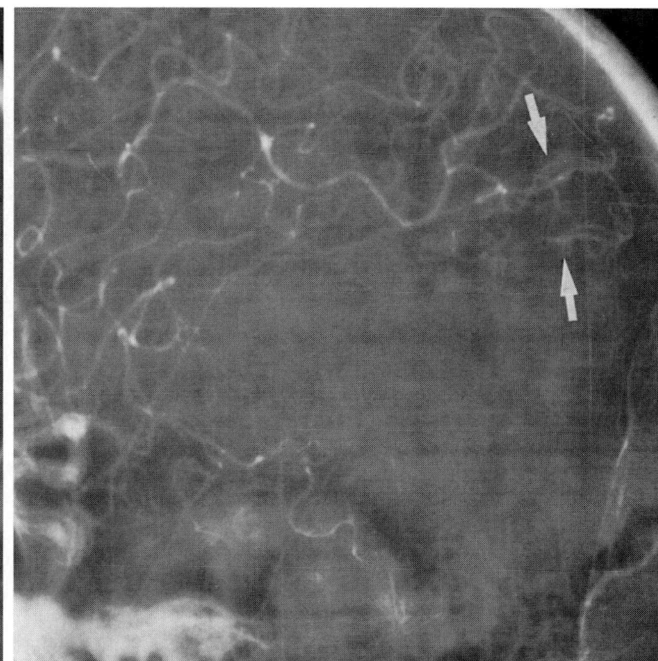
B

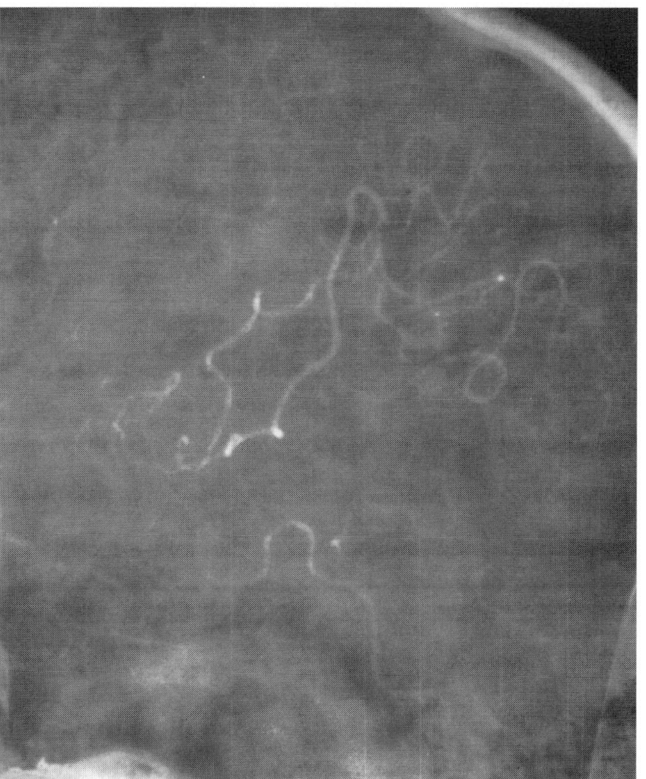
C

Figure 10.46. Thrombosis of branches of middle cerebral artery simulating tumor. **A.** A film made at 1.0 sec shows an avascular zone in the retrosylvian area (arrows). **B.** A film made at 1.5 sec discloses a persistence of the avascular area with some fine vessels in this region. **C.** A film made at 2.5 sec now discloses retrograde filling of branches of the middle cerebral artery (from the anterior cerebral artery), which fill the avascular area. In B it is already possible to see the prominent branches of the anterior cerebral artery, which have turned downward after reaching the upper margin of the hemisphere (arrows).

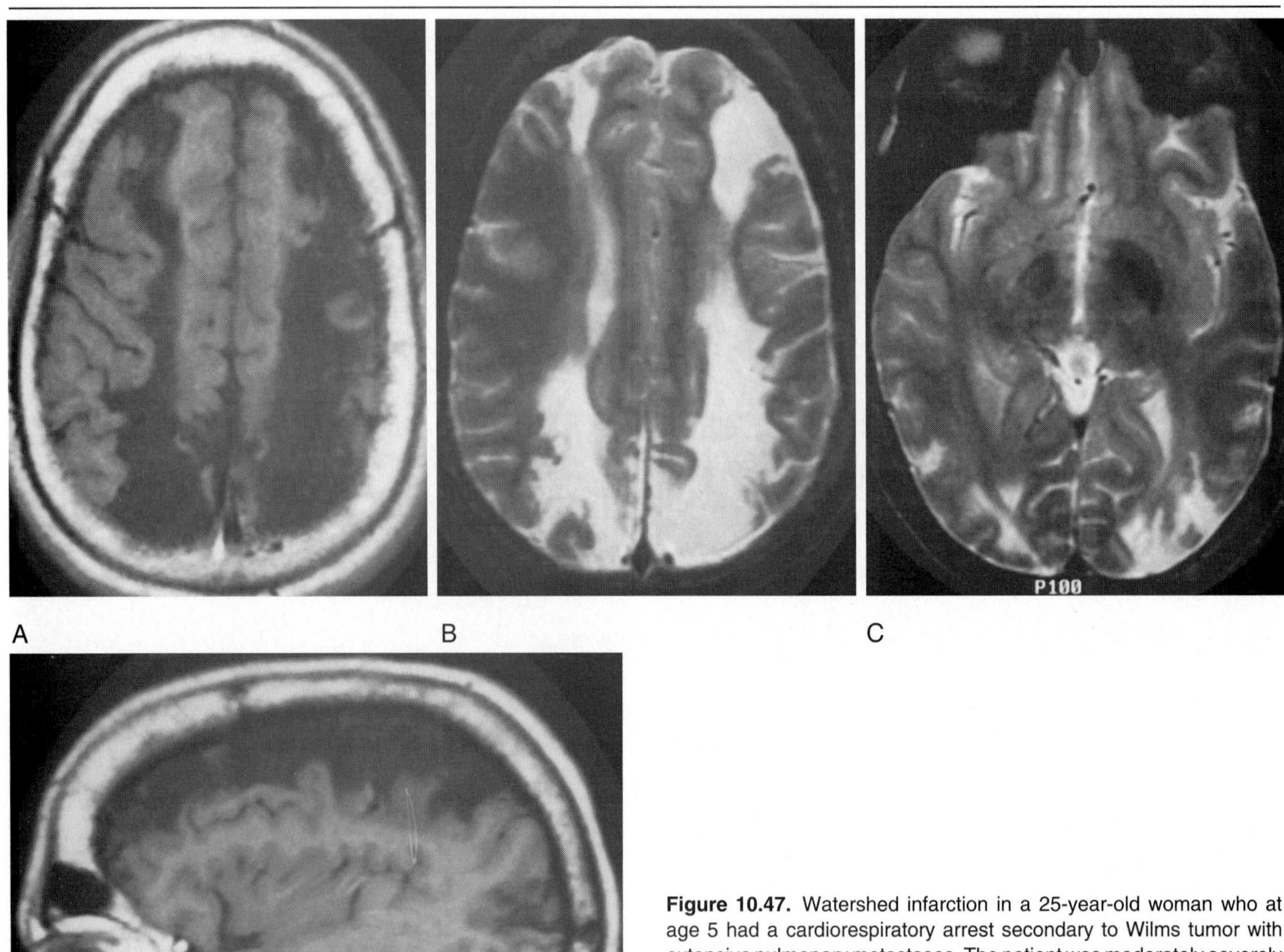

Figure 10.47. Watershed infarction in a 25-year-old woman who at age 5 had a cardiorespiratory arrest secondary to Wilms tumor with extensive pulmonary metastases. The patient was moderately severely handicapped. **A.** T1-weighted axial image shows the bilateral paracentral infarctions. **B.** T2-weighted axial image shows identical findings extending from the frontal to the occipital region. **C.** Axial T2-weighted image passing through the basal ganglia shows relative preservation of these areas. **D.** Sagittal view shows the destruction along the top of the hemisphere. Compare with Figure 10.114, which shows a bilateral anterior cerebral artery occlusion. In that figure the hypodensity extends to the midline, whereas in watershed infarction it is separated from the midline.

have been seen with more extensive communications following old thromboses (Fig. 10.53). Enlargement of the middle meningeal channels can even be visible on plain skull films (Fig. 10.54). Mount and Taveras applied the term *rete mirabile of man* to these transdural anastomotic pathways that may develop over the vault, in the posterior fossa, on the surface of the tentorium and falx cerebri, and around the base of the skull (131). Although the *retia mirabilia* are normally functional in some animals (such as the cat, the ox, and the pig), the anastomoses in humans are "potential" communicating channels that become important clinically only in the presence of long-standing occlusion of the internal carotid system. The term *transdural external-internal carotid anastomoses* is preferable to designate these compensatory pathways (132). Under certain circumstances (see text following) these channels may constitute the only open pathways for support of cerebral circulation (Fig. 10.53).

An important collateral pathway for both the carotid and vertebral-basilar circulations is through the muscular branches of the vertebral artery. The muscular branches can become greatly enlarged, and sizable intercommunications may develop with branches of the external occipital artery and other divisions of the external carotid system. If a common carotid lesion is present, blood may flow proximally to the carotid bifurcation and thence into the internal carotid artery. If a cervical internal carotid occlusion occurs, the vertebral artery may feed reverse flow in the ophthalmic artery through muscular branch communications with the external occipital and internal maxillary ar-

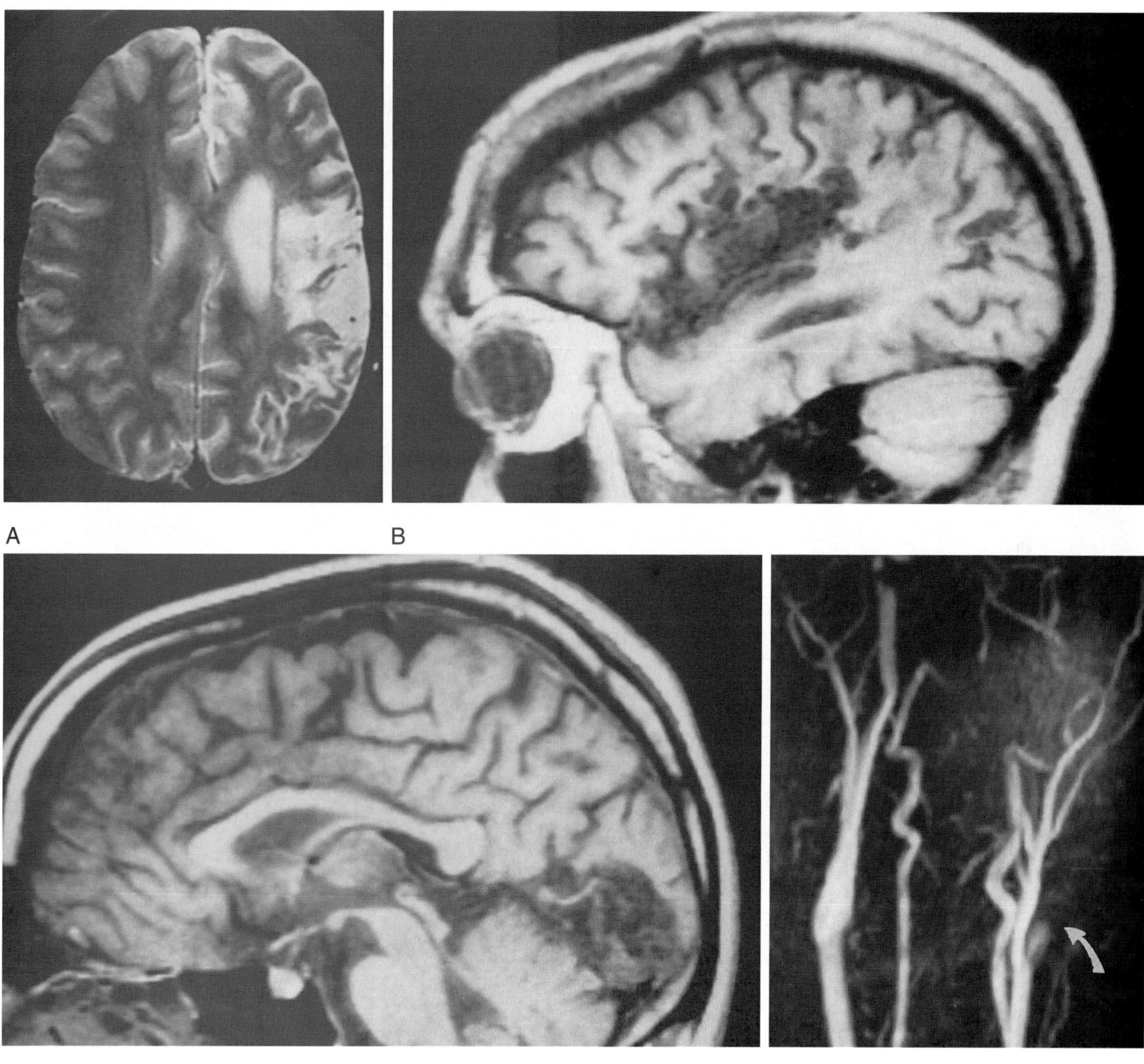

Figure 10.48. Middle cerebral artery territory infarction associated with internal carotid artery occlusion. **A.** T2-weighted axial MR image shows extensive hyperintensity in the left middle cerebral artery territory (superior and inferior division). The midline is displaced to the left, indicating an old lesion with atrophy. **B** and **C.** Sagittal T1-weighted MR image reveals the atrophic changes in the suprasylvian as well as in the occipital area. **D.** An MRA reveals occlusion of the left internal carotid artery (arrow). Whether an infarct will in fact occur after proximal internal carotid occlusion depends on whether it occurred slowly or rapidly or whether an embolus may become lodged in the middle or anterior cerebral artery. The infarct usually occurs in the middle cerebral artery territory. If there is no embolic phenomenon, the configuration of the circle of Willis (see Fig. 10.44) determines whether an ischemic lesion will occur.

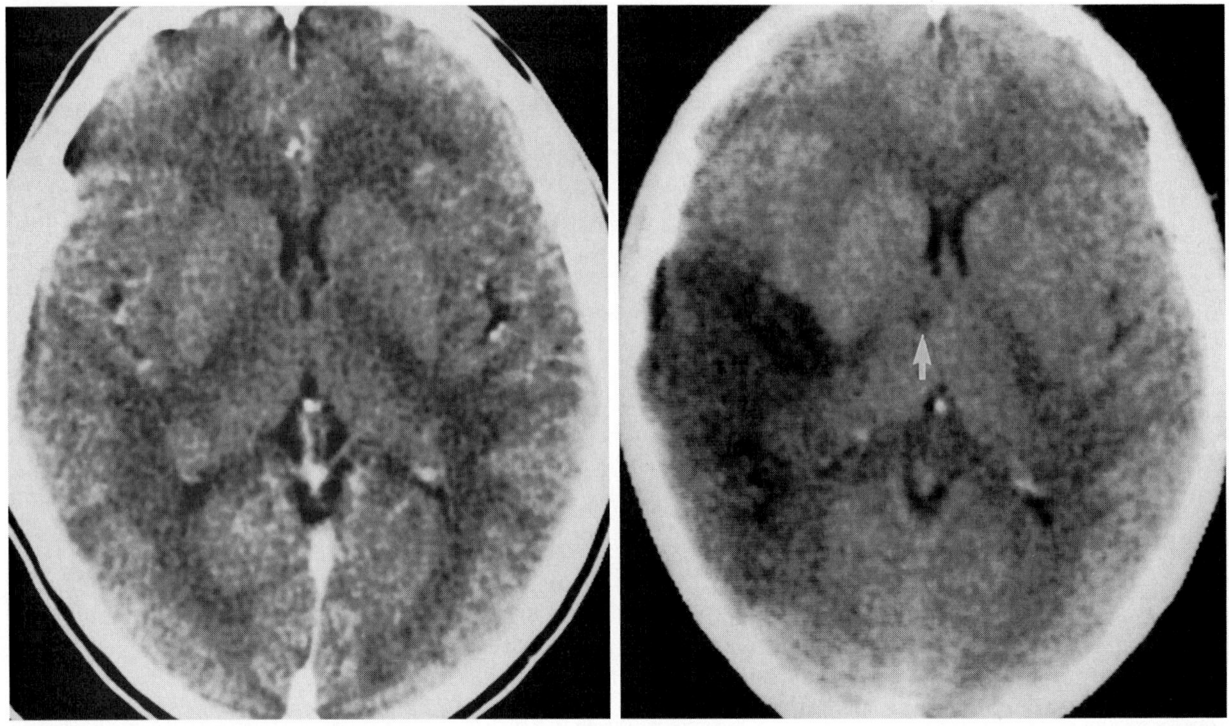

Figure 10.49. Infarct in middle cerebral artery territory. The patient was a 43-year-old man who came in complaining of left arm weakness and left facial droop. **A.** The CT scan on admission was completely normal. **B.** Reexamination 2 days later revealed a large low-density area in the inferior division territory of the right middle cerebral artery. There was also a small ischemic area in the right thalamus (arrow).

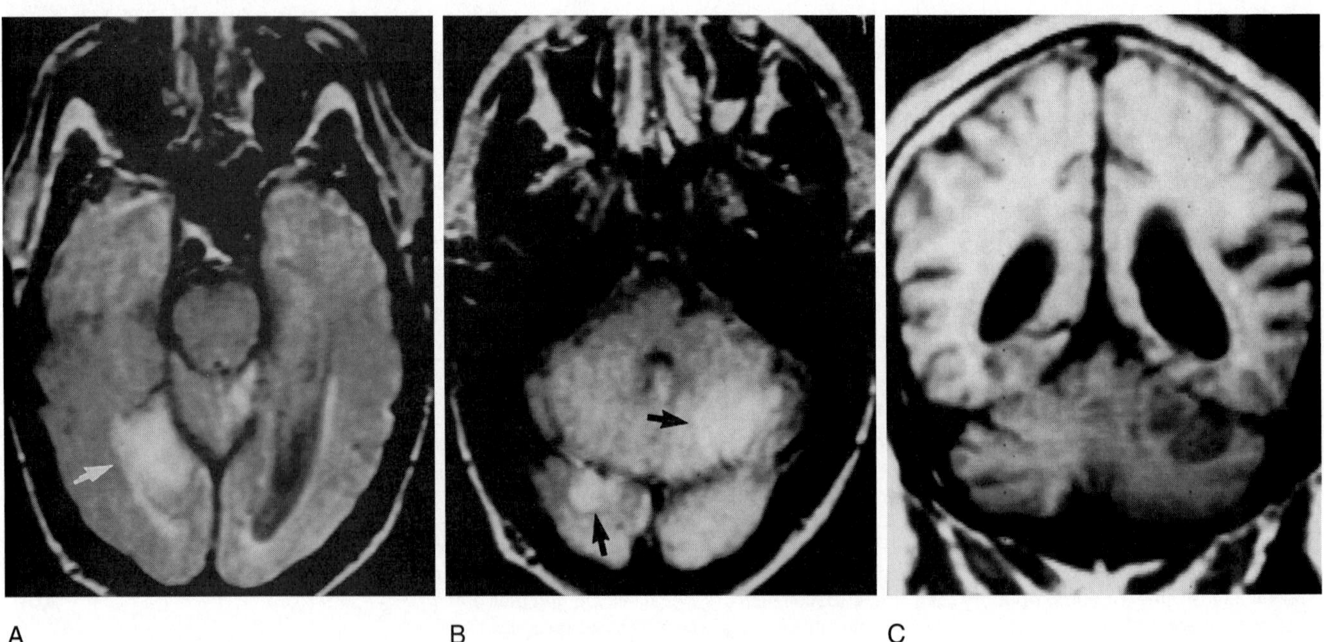

Figure 10.50. Infarcts involving the territory of the bifurcation of the basilar artery. **A.** Proton density image shows a hyperintense lesion in the right occipital lobe (arrow). **B.** A lower proton density axial image shows a left cerebellar infarction. **C.** A coronal section reveals the subtentorial position of the right cerebellar ischemic area. The lesions involve the right posterior cerebral and the left superior cerebellar artery territories; this is typical for an occlusion, probably embolic, at the top of the basilar artery.

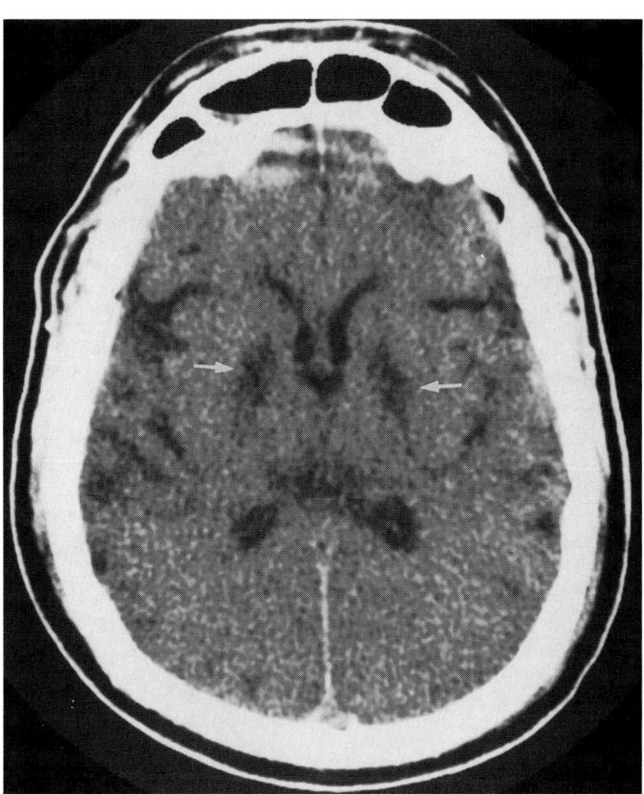

Figure 10.51. Bilateral basal ganglia ischemic lesions following cardiac arrest. There is bilateral low density in the globus pallidus, as well as loss of gray/white matter density differentiation. The basal ganglia are particularly sensitive to hypoxia and are often the earliest to demonstrate ischemic damage. The appearance is similar to what is seen in carbon monoxide poisoning.

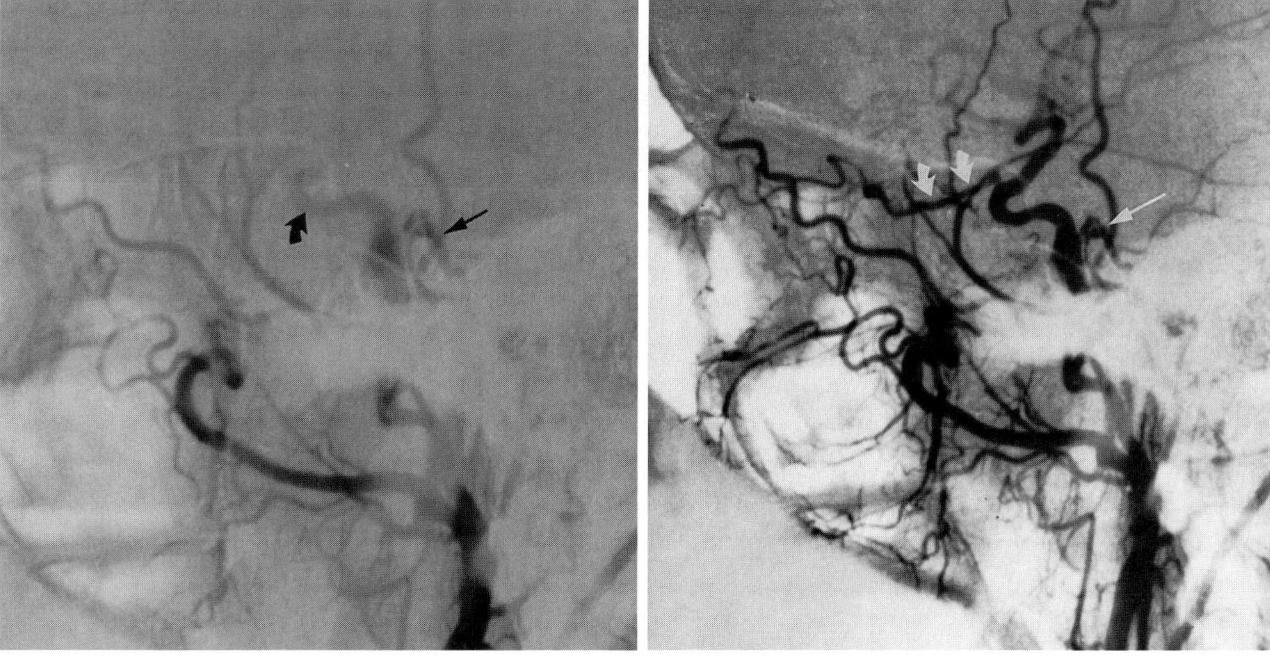

Figure 10.52. Occlusion of the internal carotid artery with collateral circulation by way of the intracavernous and ophthalmic artery branches. **A.** In the serialogram, the carotid siphon (curved arrow) filled first via the meningohypophyseal branches (arrow). **B.** Later, the ophthalmic artery also filled the siphon and the anterior and middle cerebral branches.

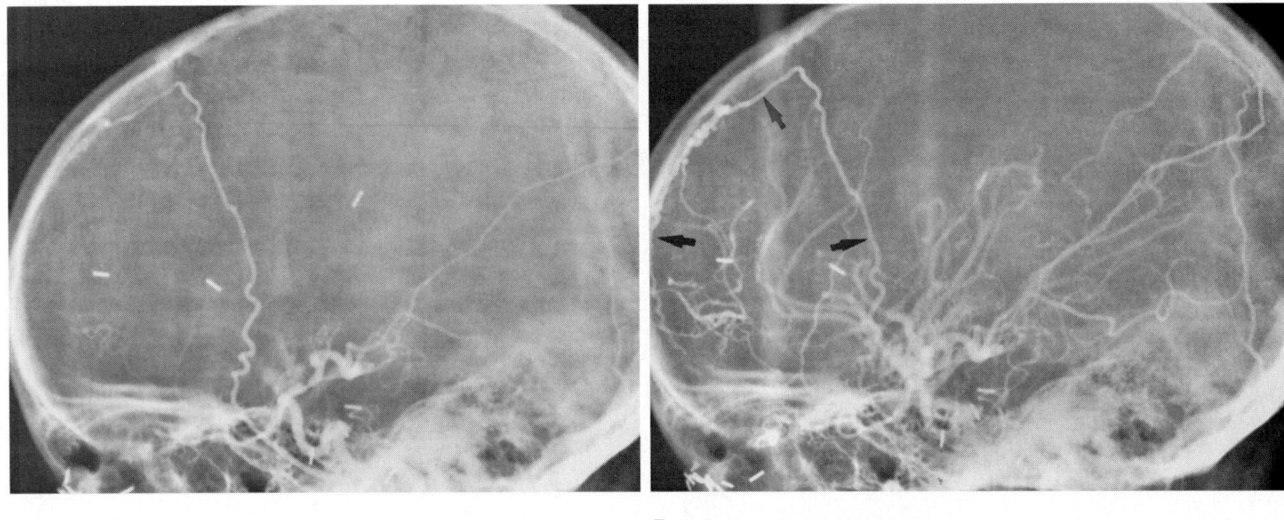

A B

Figure 10.53. Moya-moya. Multiple progressive intracranial arterial occlusions with marked development of transdural anastomoses in an 8-year-old girl with bilateral internal carotid and bilateral vertebral thrombosis. **A.** The early arterial phase shows rapid filling of external carotid branches. **B.** Later, the enlarged anterior and middle meningeal channels also anastomose with each other (arrows).

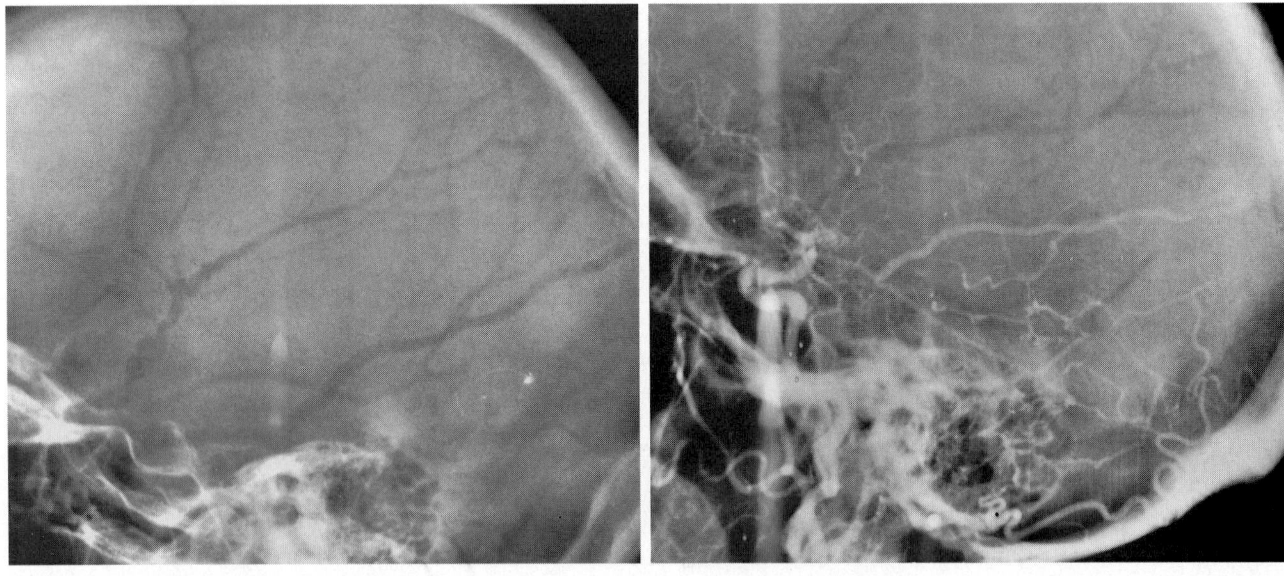

A B

Figure 10.54. Enlarged middle meningeal artery channels in the skull and transdural arterial anastomoses in a 31-year-old woman with multiple, progressive, intracranial arterial occlusions (Moya-Moya). Both internal carotid and both vertebral arteries eventually became occluded. **A.** There is extensive enlargement of the middle meningeal channels in the skull. **B.** The filling of intracranial branches from the enlarged meningeal arteries is well seen. The internal carotid arteries were occluded at the bifurcation. There is also filling via transdural collaterals in the posterior fossa.

teries. If low pressure develops in the vertebral artery from a proximal stenosis, collateral circulation takes place in the opposite direction from the carotid system and from the contralateral vertebral artery. Collateral circulation from the vertebral artery to the intracranial circulation may also develop through its meningeal branches.

EXTRACRANIAL ARTERIES

Occlusion of the internal carotid artery at its origin, that is, at the bifurcation of the common carotid artery, is a frequently encountered lesion (Figs. 10.55 and 10.56). The diagnosis is generally simple by angiography. MRA may show the total occlusion of the internal carotid artery above the bifurction of the common carotid, but one cannot be sure that total occlusion actually is present, for it may be a very severe stenosis; the same is true with ultrasound and Doppler noninvasive tests (Fig. 10.55).

Although not extracranial, another site of obstruction by thrombosis is in the distal internal carotid artery, usually in the region of its bifurcation intracranially, as seen occasionally in young adults or in children. It is uncommon to find occlusion of the internal carotid artery between these

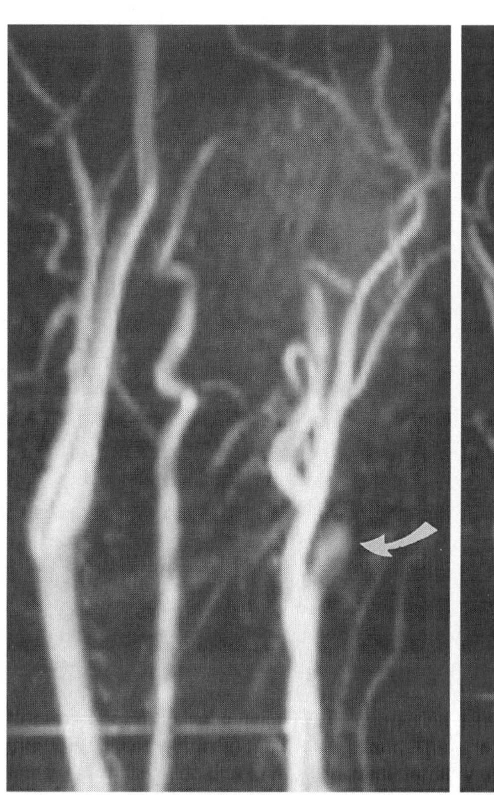

A

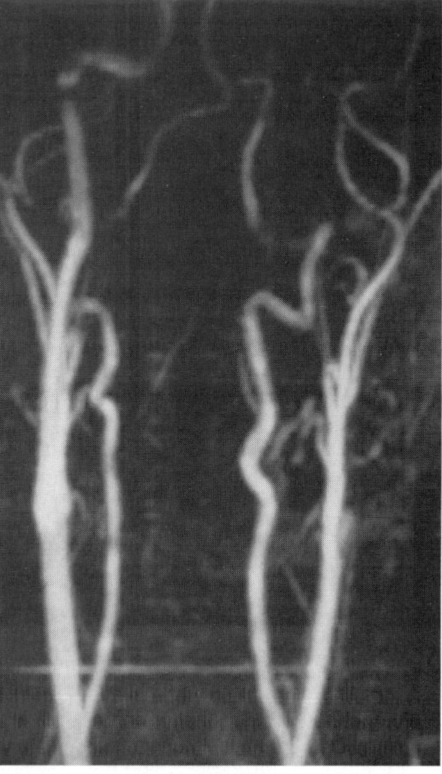

B

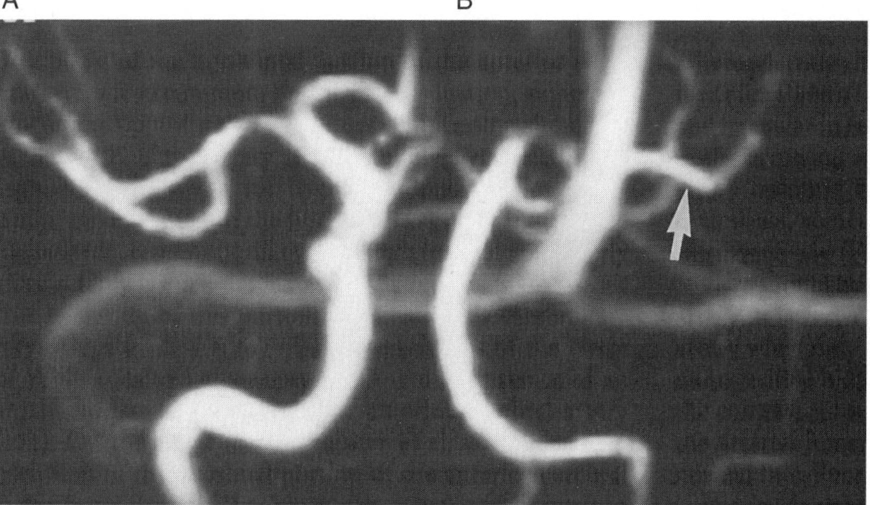

C

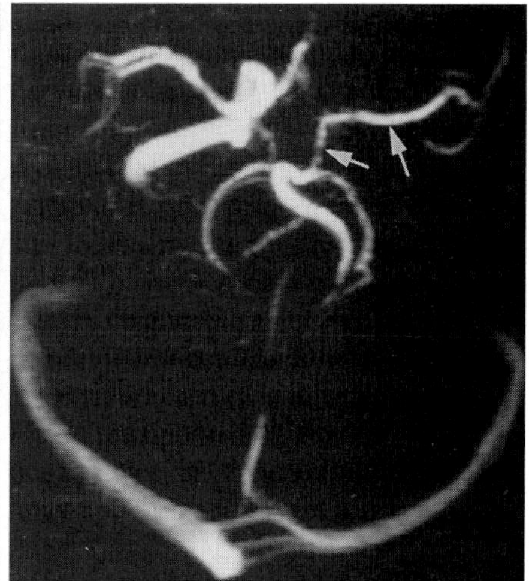

D

Figure 10.55. Occlusion of left internal carotid artery on MRA. **A.** There is only a stump of the left internal carotid artery at the bifurcation of the common carotid artery (arrow). **B.** Both vertebral arteries are well seen, as well as their junction to form the basilar artery. **C.** Intracranial vessels show no left internal carotid artery, but flow is visible in the left middle cerebral artery (arrow). In this phase-contrast flow image, the sagittal sinus is superimposed; the lateral venous sinuses are also seen. **D.** The collapsed view confirms the absent left carotid artery flow. The left posterior communicating artery fills the left middle cerebral artery (arrows). The occlusion was confirmed by conventional angiography. The absence of filling anywhere above the cervical segment would tend to indicate that there is no significant flow through the upper portion of the artery.

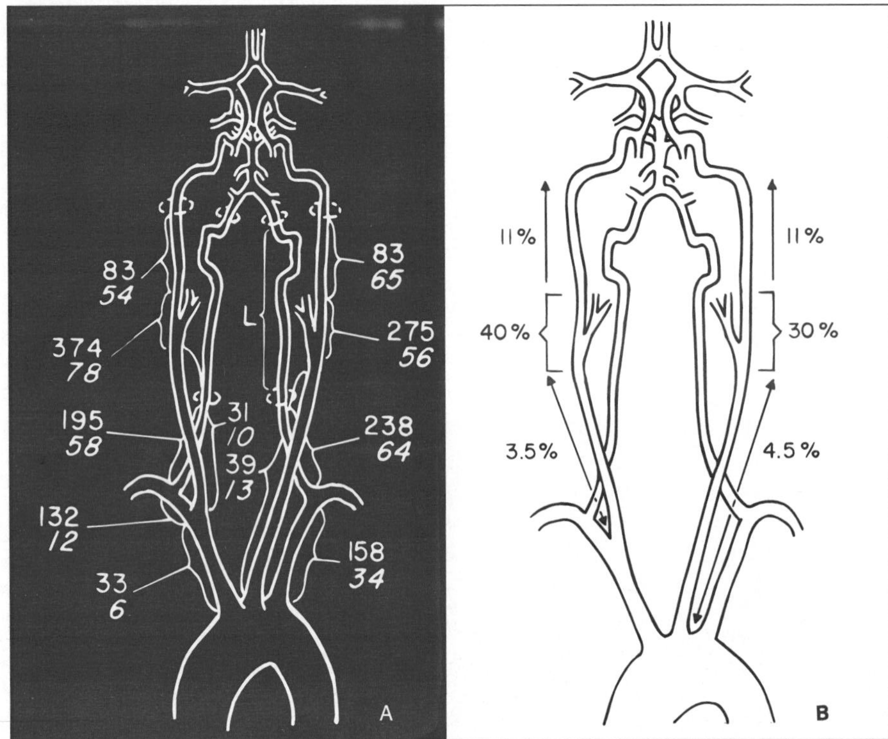

Figure 10.56. Locations of surgically accessible extracranial atherosclerotic lesions. **A.** The sites of 2090 stenotic (roman numbers) and occlusive (italic numbers) lesions are shown. Of these, 555 were in the vertebral circulation and 375 in the brachiocephalic trunks. The letter *L* emphasizes the frequent involvement of the intraosseous vertebral artery by the "ladder effect." (Reproduced by permission from C Lyons: Progress Report of the Joint Study of Extra Arterial Occlusion, p 226. In CH Millikan (ed), Cerebral Vascular Diseases, Fourth Conference, © Grune & Stratton, Inc., New York, 1965.) **B.** The numbers from A are reduced to percentages for the carotid lesions in the three principal segments of involvement.

two areas with patent proximal and distal ends of the vessel, although Lyons collected more than 100 such lesions (133). Occlusions in this region are usually secondary to direct trauma, to infection (as from a peritonsillar abscess), to a dissecting aneurysm, or to a cervical hyperextension injury to the wall of the internal carotid artery. On the other hand, it is common to find propagation of a thrombus starting at the siphon and progressing proximally or, vice versa, starting at the origin of the internal carotid artery and progressing distally. The distal portion of the internal carotid artery tends to remain open when occlusion of the proximal portion has occurred under certain circumstances. Taveras et al. have shown that by retrograde flow through the ophthalmic artery, the distal internal carotid artery remains patent in patients with surgical occlusion of the internal carotid artery in the neck (128).

Under more natural circumstances, in which spontaneous thrombosis of the proximal portion of the internal carotid artery takes place, a thrombus tends to propagate fairly rapidly, often within a few hours. The lumen of the internal carotid artery may be obliterated as far as the origin of the ophthalmic or posterior communicating branches. At other times, the distal part of the artery remains patent as far proximal as the cavernous or petrosal anastomoses between the internal and external carotid systems. The thrombus probably propagates because no flow of blood takes place in the cervical portion of the internal carotid artery. A reversal of flow occurs in the supraclinoid portion of the internal carotid artery down to the ophthalmic artery, owing to pressure from the opposite side. If the circle of Willis is not adequate, the flow is from the ophthalmic artery to the siphon. The thrombus tends to stop below the ophthalmic artery, although this is not always so. The rapid propagation of a thrombus to the nearest branch is an important reason for prompt surgical intervention in the cases where an amenable occlusion of the proximal portion of the internal carotid artery is demonstrated. Surgical intervention has not commonly been carried out because patients are usually not brought into the hospital and not studied soon enough after the beginning of symptoms.

It has been stated that if surgical correction of an occlusion is performed a day or two after initiation of symptoms there is great danger of precipitating a hemorrhagic infarction and death (134). However, experiences at the Neurological Institute of New York (135) and at MGH (136), where many of these surgical interventions have been carried out in the acute stage with excellent results, clearly contradict this opinion, provided that no infarct is visible by CT or MRI. It is unlikely that a very recent (less than 24 h) bland infarct would be converted into a hemorrhagic one simply by raising the local blood pressure and improving flow (116). In the postoperative period many of these patients have a tendency to develop transient hypertension that may well lead to hemorrhage. It is this latter tendency that must be avoided postoperatively, and careful monitoring of blood pressure is indispensable.

In the presence of cerebral infarction *that is visible on CT or on MRI*, surgery to remove an atherosclerotic plaque in the internal carotid is considered hazardous because of the possibility of hemorrhage as blood flow through the opened artery increases. If surgery is considered important, it may be postponed for 6 weeks or longer.

Thrombosis of the common carotid artery is less common. It may occur just proximal to its bifurcation so that the external carotid as well as the internal carotid artery are occluded. Obstruction also may develop at its origin from the innominate artery on the right side and from the aorta on the left side. Of the 409 cases of completed stroke reported by Gurdjian et al. and studied by angiography, there were only two instances of occlusion of the common carotid artery, indicating its relative infrequency (137). In the same series, there were 68 cases of internal carotid occlusion, 5 of which were bilateral. However, in a joint study of extracranial arterial occlusions, there were 23 common carotid thromboses among 450 complete occlusions reported by Lyons, a 5 percent incidence (Fig. 10.56) (133).

Proximal vertebral occlusions are frequently seen and formed 27 percent of Lyons's series. The obstruction is most often at the origin of the artery from the subclavian trunk. If there is no vertebral "stump," it may be difficult to differentiate absence from occlusion of the vertebral artery, although with congenital absence, the contralateral vessel may be very large, depending on posterior cerebral artery requirements. Adequate presentation of contrast material to the orifices of both vertebral arteries is essential in studying patients who show evidence of basilar artery insufficiency.

The possibility of involvement of major arteries *proximal* to the common carotid and vertebral arteries should be kept in mind. Of 149 cases of stenotic and occlusive lesions reported by Crawford et al., the internal carotid artery was involved in 93, the common carotid artery in 12, the innominate artery in 14, the subclavian artery in 21, and the vertebral artery in 9 cases (138). Moreover, in the same

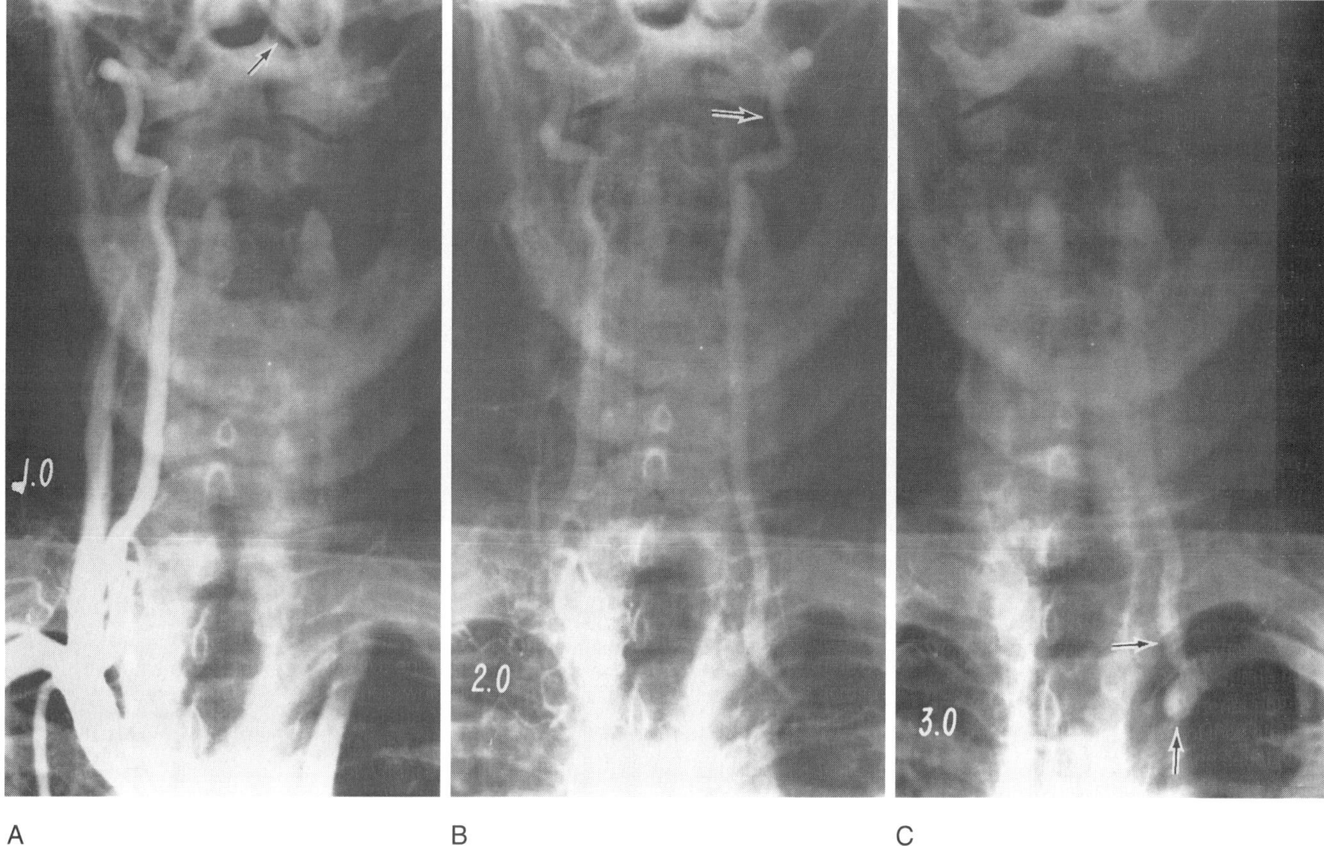

A B C

Figure 10.57. Subclavian steal syndrome. Stenosis or occlusion of the subclavian artery proximal to the origin of the vertebral artery often results in a disturbance of the flow dynamics in the ipsilateral vertebral artery and in the basilar artery. Radiologically, to establish a diagnosis of "subclavian steal," the contrast medium must be shown to flow in a retrograde manner in the vertebral artery ipsilateral to the subclavian lesion, and it must also be seen to clear out in retrograde. **A.** In the case illustrated, a film made 1.0 sec after a right retrograde brachial injection shows complete opacification of the right vertebral artery and regurgitation of contrast into the distal left vertebral artery (arrow). **B.** At 2.0 sec, antegrade clearing of the right vertebral artery is taking place while retrograde opacification of the left vertebral artery (arrow) continues proximally to its origin. **C.** After 3.0 sec, the right vertebral artery has cleared antegrade and the left vertebral artery is now clearing retrograde. Only the most proximal part of the left vertebral artery (upper arrow) remains well opacified, the contrast having largely passed into the left subclavian artery where the distal stump of the occluded vessel is well opacified (lower arrow).

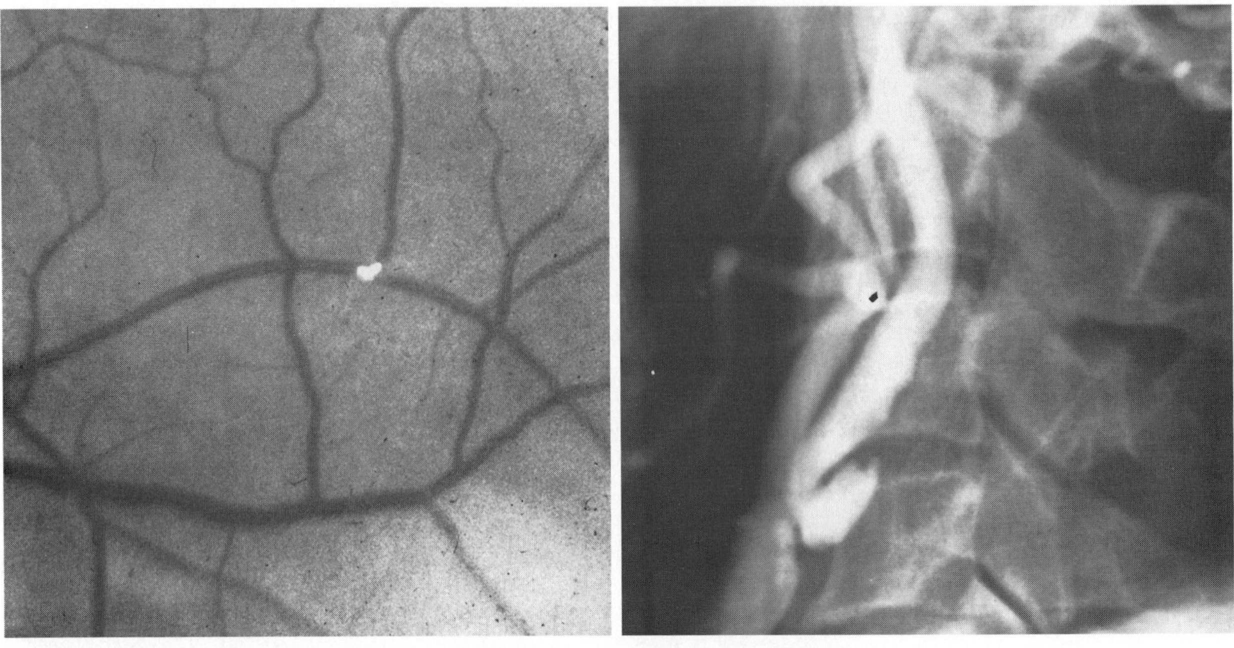
A B

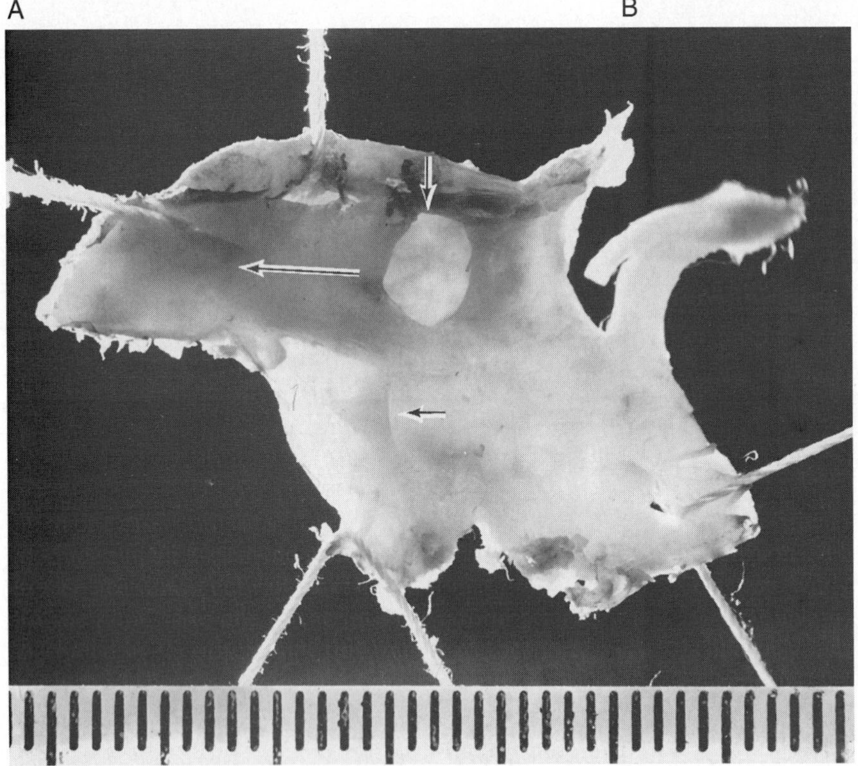
C

Figure 10.58. Atherosclerotic cervical carotid ulceration. **A.** A retinal photograph reveals an embolus lodged at a distal bifurcation of the superior temporal artery of the retina. A complete obstruction was not produced, but intravascular agglutination caused by slow flow was observed in branches distal to the lesion. **B.** A giant atheromatous ulcer is present along the posterior wall of the internal carotid artery at its origin. The crater measured 15 mm length and 7 mm depth and had a distinct neck with overhanging edges, as evident in this profile view of the lesion. The rostral and caudal margins of the ulcer cavity are irregular owing to mural thrombi. **C.** The surgical specimen removed by endarterectomy has been opened along its anterior wall; the common carotid portion of the specimen is on the reader's right. Near the origin of the channel of the internal carotid artery (transverse arrow) the almost circular mouth of the ulcer (large vertical arrow) is shown. The thin base of the large cavity beyond is seen through transillumination. In such cases, the base may be almost at the adventitia because of atrophy of the muscular and elastic tissues of the tunica media, but even such deep ulcers are almost always entirely within the very thick atheromatous lesion of the intima. The orifice leading to the external carotid artery (short horizontal arrow) has not been opened. The appearance of the specimen is to be compared with the angiographic findings in B.

cases, the lesions involving the common carotid, the innominate, and the subclavian arteries were segmental in nature and restoration of circulation in many instances was possible by surgical means. In the same series, 83 of the 93 cases involving the internal carotid artery were considered segmental. As mentioned earlier, occlusive disease of the extracranial vessels may involve more than one vessel. The subclavian steal syndrome is the result of occlusion of the subclavian artery proximal to the origin of the vertebral artery on either side, but more commonly on the left (Fig. 10.57).

Obstructive lesions of a *stenotic* type involving the extracranial vessels are common. A lesion may be visible only on the frontal or only on the lateral angiogram. For this reason frontal and lateral views are necessary to diagnose arterial narrowing with certainty. If the stenosis is due to a lesion involving the periphery of the vessel, a concentric narrowing is produced that may be shown on either the frontal or the lateral projection. On the other hand, if, as is commonly the case, the narrowing is produced by a plaque situated only on one side of the vessel, it may be obscured in one projection. The outline of the lumen in the stenotic segment is usually irregular as seen in profile by angiography, because the tunica intima is rough in this region. The beginning of a stenotic segment is generally fairly abrupt, and it can frequently be traced to its beginning and end at sharply defined points. Contrariwise, if the narrowing is due to spasm, it is usually of greater length and begins smoothly and gradually at both ends; the lumen of the vessel is seen to decrease progressively in size and then to widen again.

The ulcerated lesions are commonly found in the aorta and some of its larger branches, including the carotid arteries, in the neck (139). An atheroma is usually defined as an arteriosclerotic plaque in which fatty softening predominates. When such softening reaches the luminal surface of the plaque, grumose material is extruded into the bloodstream, leaving a cavity, or ulcer niche, in the atheroma. Subsequently, varying amounts of lipoidal material may be repeatedly released from below the surface of the atheroma through the ostium, and in this way a collar-button–shaped ulcer may be formed (Fig. 10.58). The excavations may be multiple and vary from microscopic to large size, sometimes being larger than 1 cm.

Thrombosis frequently occurs within carotid ulcers. In some cases, white thrombi develop that are composed of clumps of fibrin and platelets. At other times, red thrombi develop that contain masses of red cells as well. In addition, mural thrombi may form on a carotid atheroma apart from a site of ulceration. At times, such aggregates of fibrin and cellular material may build up to a large size and remain attached to the atheroma only by a pedicle, constituting a polypoid thrombus (Fig. 10.59).

As early as 1906, Chiari described ulceration of the extracranial carotid arteries and suggested a relationship of the lesions to encephalomalacia caused by the detachment of thrombotic fragments. One of the early neurologic correlations of extracranial carotid disease and vascular lesions of the brain was made by Hunt (140). From the above description, it is evident that the emboli may be of several types. First, the atheromatous material evacuated into the carotid lumen during the formation of an ulcer may block a cerebral artery. Such emboli are composed chiefly of cholesterol and other lipid material, so they usually fragment and become dispersed after only temporarily blocking a vessel. Fragments from white thrombi may also disappear relatively rapidly (141). Fragments of other thrombi may produce more prolonged occlusion until there is organization of the embolus and recanalization of the vessel.

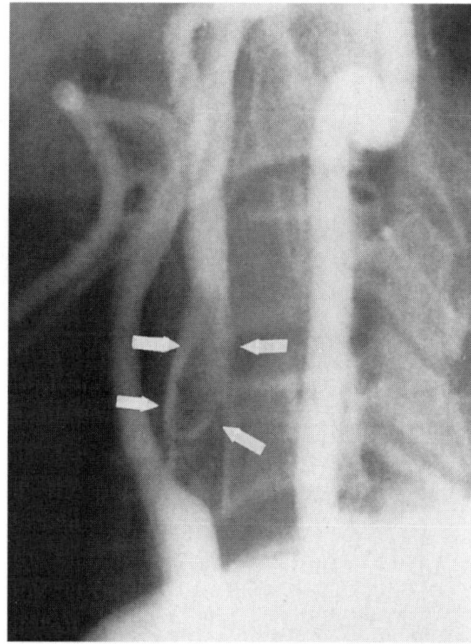

Figure 10.59. Polypoid thrombus in internal carotid artery. A tight stenosis at the origin of the internal carotid artery is shown. The vessel opacifies well distally, however, an intraluminal filling defect is shown just beyond the zone of narrowing. In this lateral angiogram, a cuff of contrast material (arrows) is present in front of, and behind, the radiolucent shadow, and similar evidence of its position free in the vasal lumen was found in other projections.

The fragmentation of thrombi and the carrying of particles distally to the eye or brain by the bloodstream can usually explain the occurrence of TIAs. Fisher reported a case of transient partial blindness (scotomas) occurring in the same eye and in a similar manner several hundred times (105). Ophthalmoscopic examination during one of these attacks revealed a white thrombus occluding a retinal artery and later fragmenting and moving distally into the retinal branches until it completely disappeared in 2 to 3 h. Similar phenomena are likely to occur in the brain. Indeed, in the study of Wood and Correll such an embolism accounted for 54 percent of patients coming to endarterectomy for TIAs, as compared with 46 percent of the patients with stenosis without ulceration (142). In patients who present with a history of *several* TIAs, it is common to find a tightly stenotic (1.5-mm diameter or less) lesion, often irregular, possibly with tiny "ulcerations" in the plaques. It is less

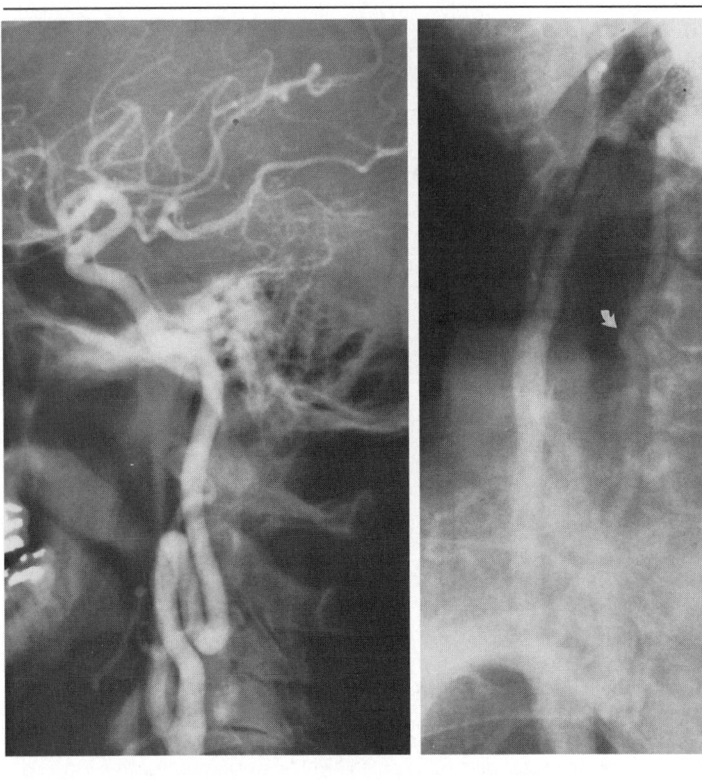

A B

Figure 10.60. Buckling of carotid and vertebral arteries. **A.** Tortuosity and coiling of the internal carotid artery are sometimes encountered, and the clinical significance is questionable. When bilateral, it has been said that circulatory changes could occur upon head turning. **B.** Cervical spondylosis can cause kinking of the vertebral arteries (arrow), and in these cases twisting of the neck may interfere with normal flow of blood.

common to demonstrate a simple ulcerated plaque producing nonhemodynamically significant obstruction (lumen of 2.0 mm or larger). The significance of this observation is difficult to analyze, but it may be either that hemodynamically significant lesions per se play an important part in the production of TIAs, or that thrombi are more likely to form in tightly stenotic lesions. Indeed, when occlusion occurs in these tight lesions, the thrombus appears to form first in the area of maximum stenosis.

The embolic theory explains the frequent absence of angiographically demonstrable occlusions in patients who are symptomatic, particularly if some time (1 to 2 weeks or longer) has elapsed between the appearance of symptoms and the performance of an angiogram. It also explains the frequent absence of obstructed vessels at autopsy. It is necessary to postulate that lysis of the obstructing agent takes place. On the other hand, a study of a group of patients with angiographically demonstrable middle cerebral branch occlusions by Kishore et al. showed double the incidence of irregular and ulcerated extracranial carotid plaques compared with those patients with normal or smoothly stenosed arteries (143).

Care should be taken to examine closely the origins of the *vertebral arteries* since there is usually a slight curve at the points of origin that may obscure stenotic lesions. Atherosclerosis of the distal vertebral artery, prior to its entering the dura, may also be seen. Narrowing of the intraosseous portion of the vertebral artery may be produced by osteophytes arising from the vertebral column (Fig. 10.60*B*); at other times, there may be multiple atherosclerotic plaques along the intraosseous portion of the vertebral artery, producing a "ladder effect." Occasionally, there is an extreme degree of osteophytosis originating in the articular facets, which causes the vertebral artery to be quite irregular in its course. Many clinicians believe that this may be a significant cause of obstruction, particularly upon turning the head, and that it may explain the occurrence of "dizzy spells" in older individuals following motion of the head and neck. The general significance of such changes, however, is hard to evaluate. When head turning is suspected of producing vertebral artery insufficiency, it is the author's custom to take films not only in neutral position but also with the head forcibly turned to the opposite side, and sometimes turned to the same side as the osteophytosis. When obstruction does occur, it is most commonly seen at the level of C5 or C6. The author has seen only a few instances of obstruction of the vertebral artery during this manueuver. Obstruction on head turning may also occur at C1-C2 (144).

How often cerebrovascular insufficiency results from an occlusive or stenotic lesion of the vessels of the neck is not known. It has been stated that over 30 percent of stroke patients have their symptoms owing to lesions of the extracranial vessels (137). Others have estimated it to be lower, approximately 20 percent (145), or higher, perhaps as much as 40 percent (135).

Extracranial carotid and vertebral tortuosity and kinking are often seen in patients with arteriosclerosis. Elongation of a vessel with mild tortuosity but without kinking may not be clinically significant unless it is associated with narrowing of the lumen by an atheroma. Occasionally, severe tortuosity of the upper cervical internal carotid artery results in markedly redundant loops (Fig. 10.60). This is sometimes found in young subjects without arteriosclerosis. Because of the frequency of the bilateral and symmetrical involvement of the two internal carotid arteries by the coiling process (especially in children), it is felt that a congenital factor could be the basis of this entity; later on in life this could be exaggerated by increased blood pressure and the vascular elongation of arteriosclerosis. Martin et al. found one thrombotic occlusion among four patients with marked kinking coming to necropsy; in others there was increased atherosclerosis on the lesser curvature sides of the tortuosities (103). Metz et al. found a 16 percent incidence of redundancy among 1000 angiograms reviewed (146). There was a strong suggestion that recurrent cerebrovascular episodes were more common in patients with kinks than in a normal control group.

The effect of carotid coiling on blood flow is variable. The carotid blood flow measured during operation using the electromagnetic flowmeter shows that only when such loops are grossly excessive is there an observable effect on the circulation; in some cases the effect is associated with rotation of the head.

Dissection of Carotid and Vertebral Arteries

Traumatic dissections of the internal carotid or vertebral arteries are well known (see Chapter 7). Spontaneous dissection can also occur and should be suspected, particularly in relatively young patients (147, 148). Up to the last several years angiography was the only method that permitted an accurate diagnosis, although CT could be used without and with contrast to attempt a noninvasive diagnosis. On CT, the postcontrast axial views of the neck can demonstrate lack of enhancement of the portion of the carotid artery lumen occupied by the hematoma; only the open lumen enhances (148). MRI is far superior, however, and the diagnosis can be made with certainty because of the bright T1 and T2 images produced by the arterial wall hematoma (Fig. 10.61). The spiral configuration of the dissection can be imaged on a series of slices, also by conventional angiography (Fig. 10.62). Vertebral artery dissections may also occur spontaneously. Fat surrounding the vessels is easily eliminated by utilizing a fat-suppression technique.

Dissection on angiography causes narrowing of the arterial lumen over a relatively long segment that may or may not stop at the carotid canal at the base of the skull. The author has seen a case of carotid dissection apparently provoked by hemorrhage into a pituitary adenoma (see Fig. 11.60). Bilateral dissections are occasionally observed. Clinically the patients may present with head and neck pain, TIAs, and hemiparesis. A Horner syndrome is commonly found on examination. Pseudoaneurysms are sometimes seen on angiography, and irregular narrowing of the lumen is common (Table 10.13). For further details, see Chapter 7.

Among the conditions to be considered along with carotid artery dissection is Raeder syndrome, which usually presents with unilateral headache and facial pain; a Horner syndrome is usually detected (149). There is involvement of the first and second divisions of the fifth nerve. The syndrome may well be related to fibromuscular dysplasia and may be associated with dissection of the internal carotid artery. Narrowing of the distal cervical and intracranial internal carotid arteries is shown by MRA or by conventional angiography. In the case reported by Castillo et al., the opposite carotid artery was affected by fibromuscular dysplasia (149). *Fibromuscular dysplasia* of the internal carotid artery may be unilateral or bilateral (65 percent of cases) (Fig. 10.63). The condition is usually discovered on angiography upon investigation of other conditions, usually in women, and represents an incidental finding. Nevertheless, it may be found in patients with spontaneous dissection of the carotid artery (150).

Displacement, narrowing, and even occlusion of the internal carotid artery may be produced by tumors at the base of the skull. Occlusion of the internal carotid artery may also be produced by severe inflammatory diseases (peritonsillar abscess, severe fungal infection such as mucormycosis [see Fig. 6.36], and invasive aspergillosis).

Major Cerebral Arteries

Occlusion of the intracranial portion of the *internal carotid artery* is not as common as that of the cervical portion. It usually occurs just above the origin of the posterior com-

Table 10.13.
Craniocervical Arterial Dissection

Angiography appearance
- Most commonly irregular arterial narrowing beginning in cervical segment of internal carotid artery or high cervical portion of vertebral artery
- Often extends into intracranial segment of the artery
- Arterial narrowing may terminate in occlusion
- May appear as subtle region of luminal narrowing or irregularity or be associated with pseudoaneurysm formation
- Other findings may include slow arterial flow and branch occlusions

MR imaging appearance
- Usually seen as an eccentric, circumferential "collar" of hyperintense signal surrounding an arterial flow void, which may increase the external diameter of the artery
- Arterial lumen diameter may be normal or narrowed

Clinical findings
- Headache is most common symptom
- Oculosympathetic paresis ("Horner syndrome") is present in about 15% of internal carotid artery dissections
- Transient or permanent neurologic deficits
- Vertebral artery dissection can be manifested by occipital headache or neckache, neurologic ischemic syndromes, or (in intradural dissections) subarachnoid hemorrhage

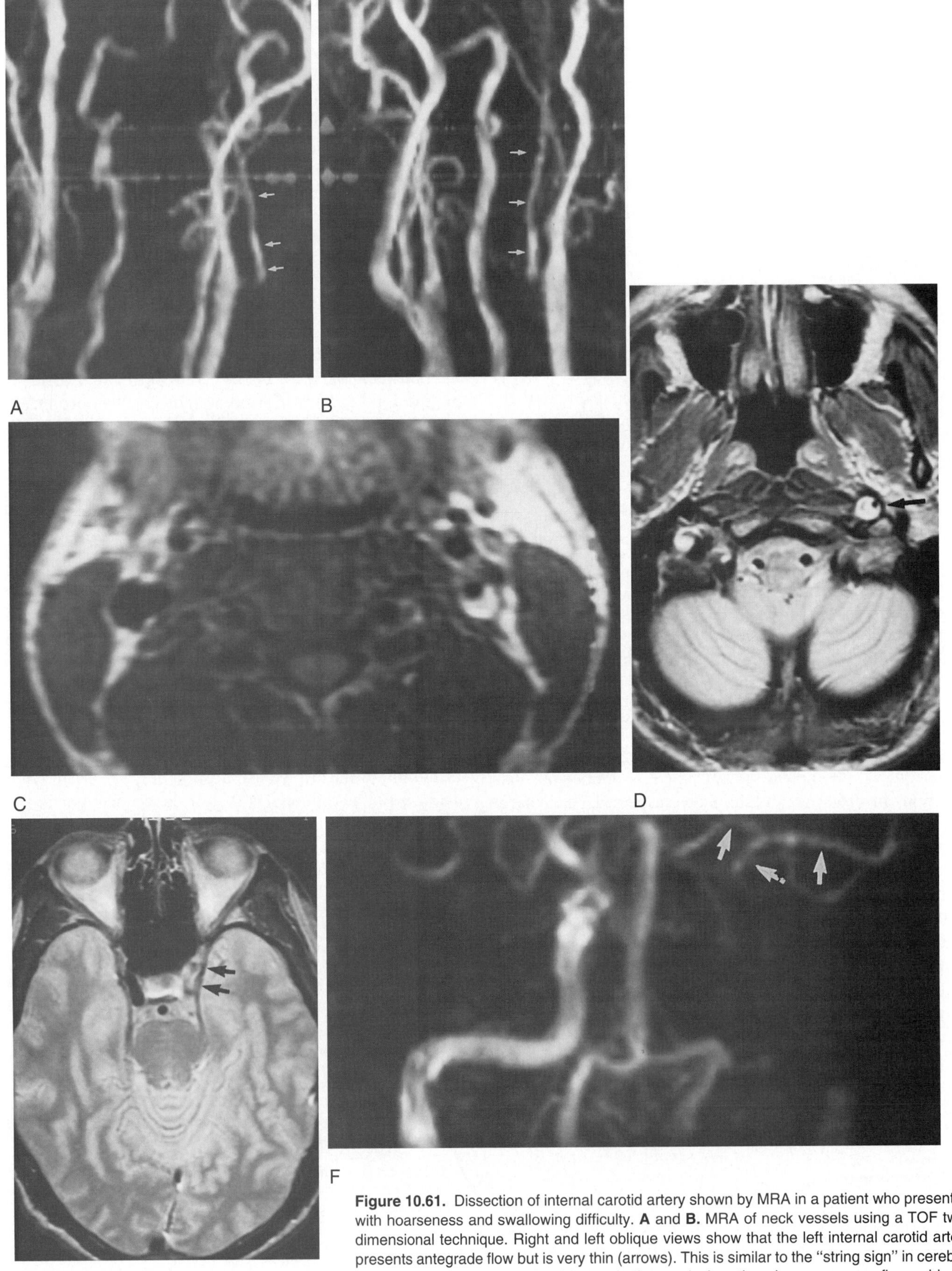

Figure 10.61. Dissection of internal carotid artery shown by MRA in a patient who presented with hoarseness and swallowing difficulty. **A** and **B.** MRA of neck vessels using a TOF two-dimensional technique. Right and left oblique views show that the left internal carotid artery presents antegrade flow but is very thin (arrows). This is similar to the "string sign" in cerebral angiography. **C.** A T1-weighted image in the cervical portion shows a narrow flow void surrounded by a bright, thick "half-moon" representing blood in the methemoglobin stage in the wall of the artery.

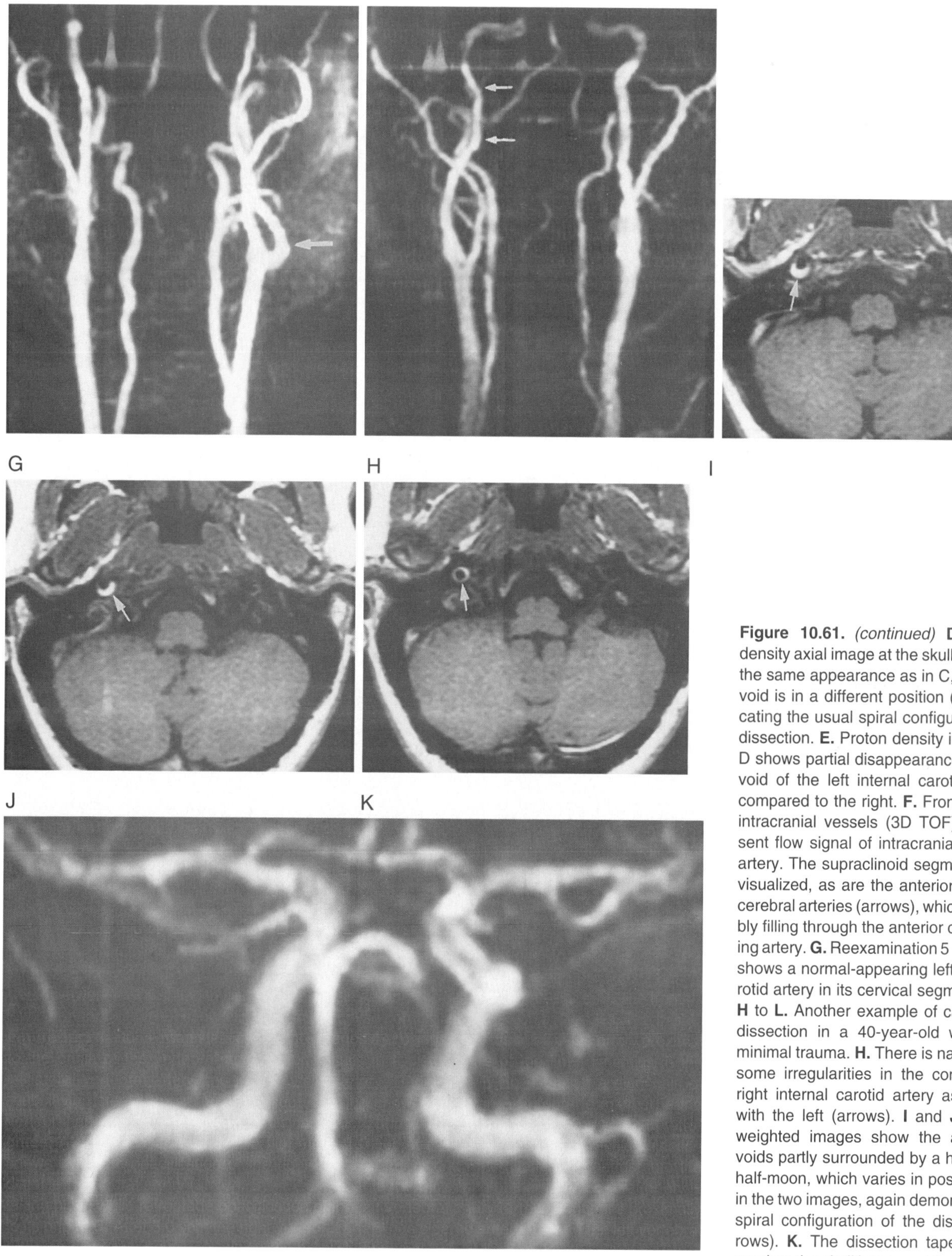

Figure 10.61. *(continued)* **D.** A proton density axial image at the skull base shows the same appearance as in C, but the flow void is in a different position (arrow), indicating the usual spiral configuration of the dissection. **E.** Proton density image above D shows partial disappearance of the flow void of the left internal carotid artery as compared to the right. **F.** Frontal image of intracranial vessels (3D TOF) shows absent flow signal of intracranial left carotid artery. The supraclinoid segment is faintly visualized, as are the anterior and middle cerebral arteries (arrows), which are probably filling through the anterior communicating artery. **G.** Reexamination 5 months later shows a normal-appearing left internal carotid artery in its cervical segment (arrow). **H** to **L.** Another example of carotid artery dissection in a 40-year-old woman with minimal trauma. **H.** There is narrowing and some irregularities in the contour of the right internal carotid artery as compared with the left (arrows). **I** and **J.** Axial T1-weighted images show the arterial flow voids partly surrounded by a hyperintense half-moon, which varies in position slightly in the two images, again demonstrating the spiral configuration of the dissection (arrows). **K.** The dissection tapers off as it reaches the skull base, and the intracranial arteries have a normal configuration (**L**).

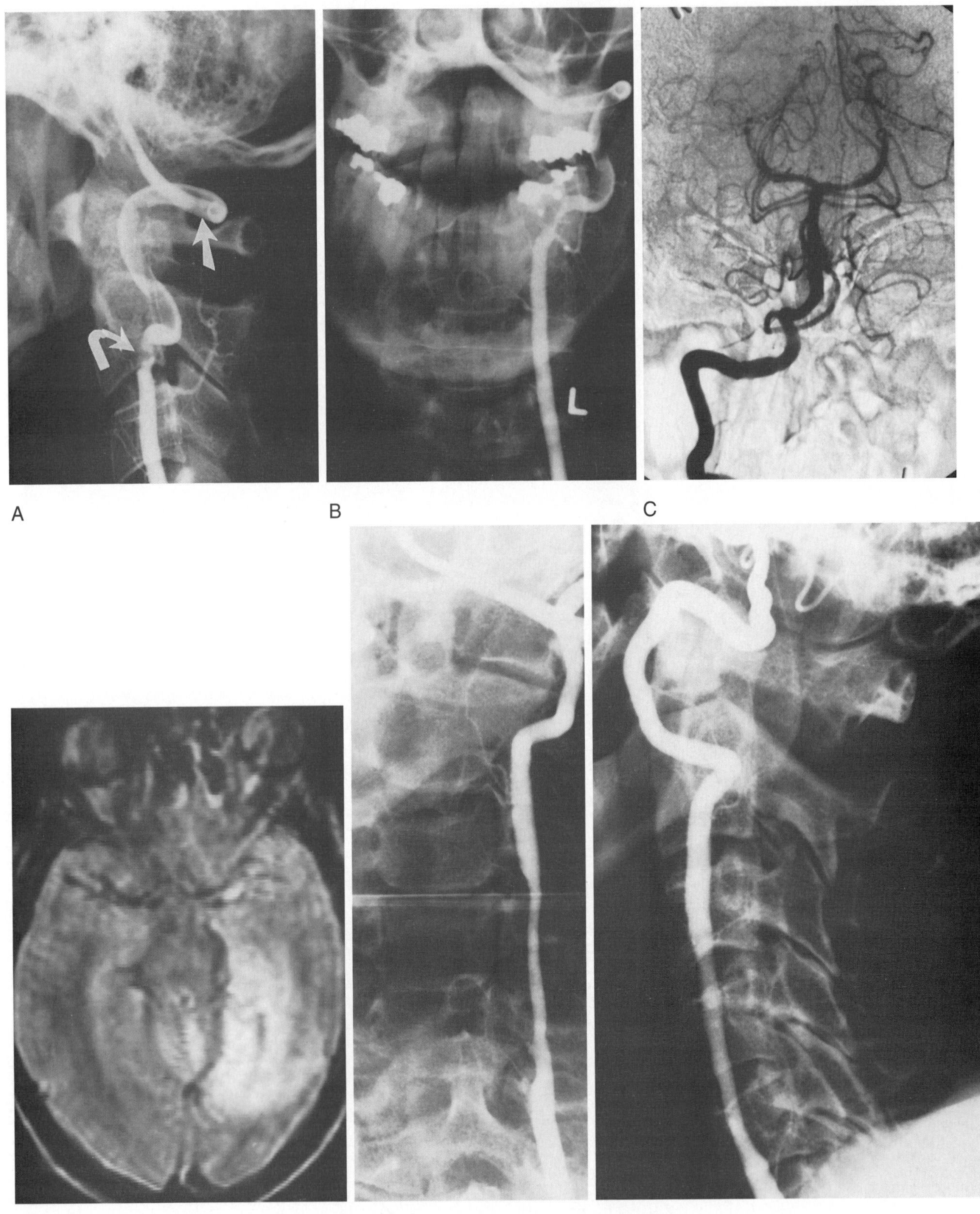

Figure 10.62. A to **D.** Dissection of vertebral artery in a 29-year-old man hit by an elbow while playing basketball. Lateral (**A**) and frontal (**B**) views reveal an area of incomplete filling from C2-C3 to atlas (arrows). **C.** Angiogram of right vertebral artery shows normal filling. **D.** MR proton density axial image shows hyperintensity in the left upper cerebellum and in the territory of the left posterior cerebral artery due to infarction. Evidently an embolus had occluded the bifurcation of the basilar artery, but the embolus had been lysed by the time the angiogram was performed. The patient's symptoms had partially improved by then. **E** and **F.** Spontaneous vertebral dissection in a 48-year-old man seen angiographically in frontal (E) and lateral (F) projections as a narrowed segment.

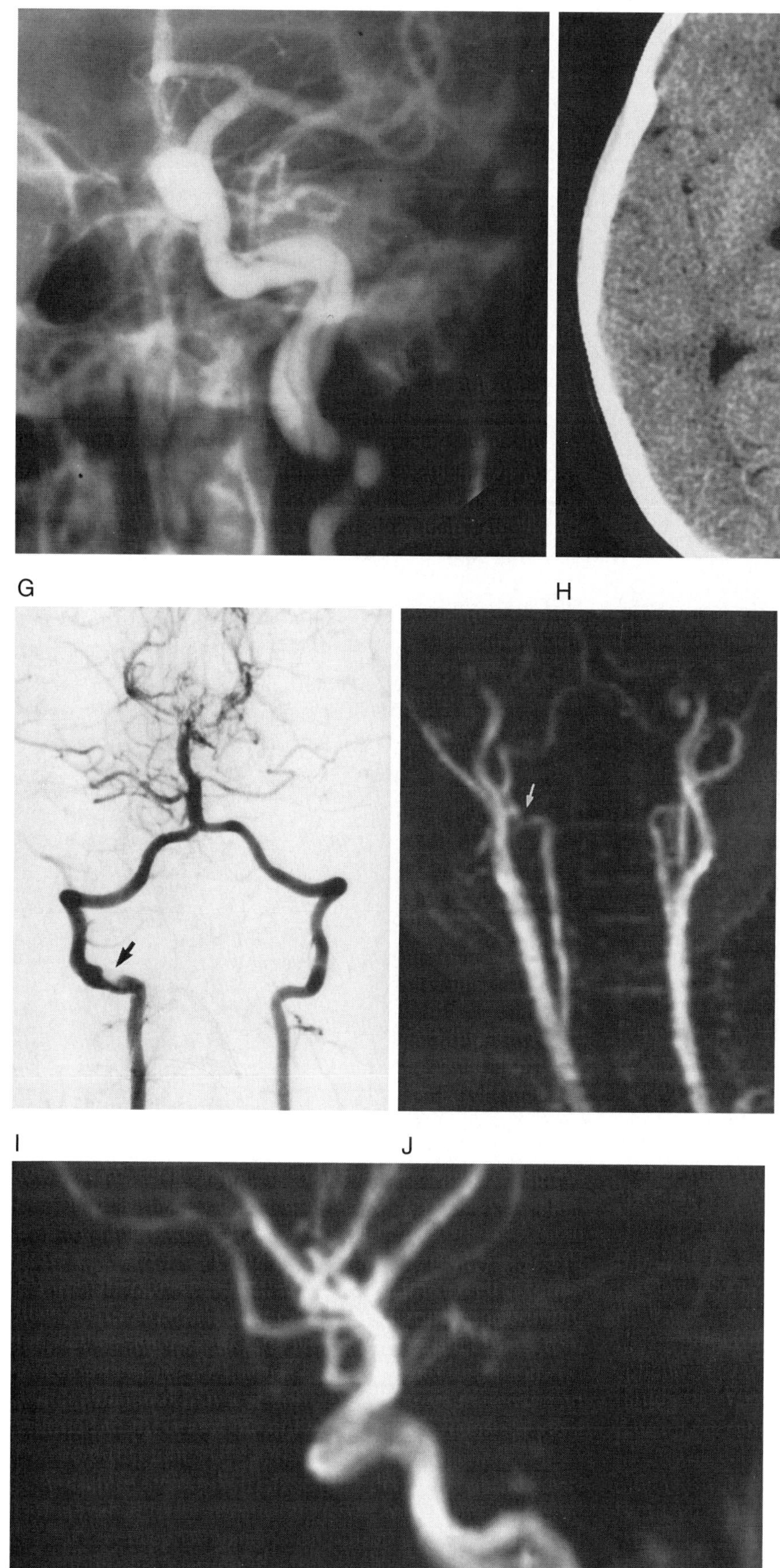

G H I J K

Figure 10.62. *(continued)* **G.** Dissection of internal carotid artery beginning in the distal one-third and extending through the carotid canal. Both the true and false lumens are visualized. When the false lumen does not fill, the appearance is that of a long narrowed segment, which has been referred to as the "string sign" (see Fig. 10.61 *A* and *B*). **H** to **K.** Dissection of vertebral artery following minor trauma episode in a 7-year-old boy. **H.** View showing a thalamic infarct produced by emboli through the basilar artery and thalamus-perforating artery. **I.** Vertebral angiography demonstrates a focal narrowing of the right vertebral artery that is associated with an area of dilatation attributed to a dissection of the vertebral artery (arrow). The basilar artery shows partial obstruction at its upper end with poor bilateral filling of the posterior cerebral and superior cerebellar arteries. **J.** MRA performed a few weeks after I shows the same local narrowing at the right vertebral artery shown in I (arrow). **K.** Sagittal MRA image shows no flow in the basilar artery. This could be due to poor flow distally or to further obstruction in the basilar artery. The minimal signs of dissection in this case points out the need to look for minor findings when searching for dissection of the carotid or vertebral arteries.

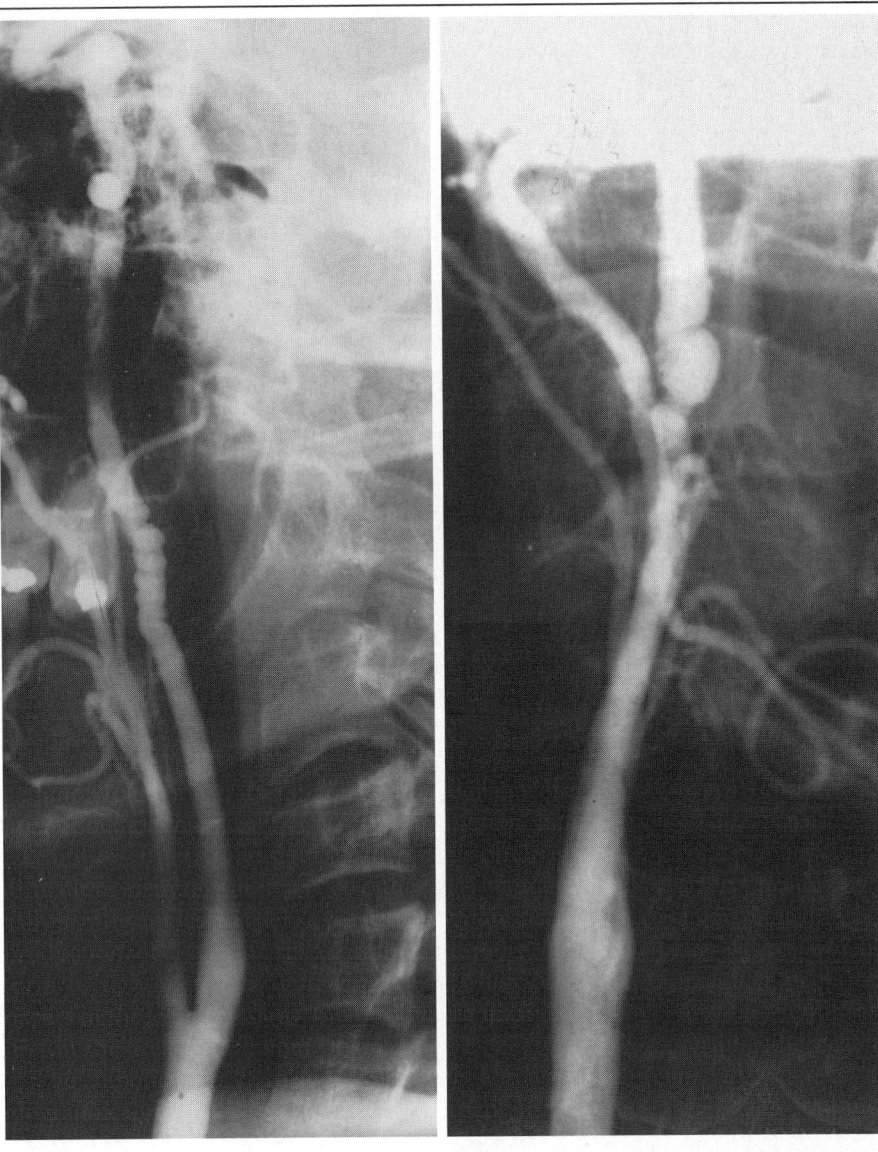

Figure 10.63. Fibromuscular dysplasia. **A.** The mid and distal cervical segments of the left internal carotid artery exhibit alternating bands of circumferential narrowing and widening of the arterial lumen. The appearance has been likened to a string of beads. **B.** On the right side (same case as A) there is a sacculation of the artery between two deeply constricting grooves. The patient was a young woman who had symptoms of ischemia of the right cerebral hemisphere but who refused surgical intervention.

municating artery. Arteriosclerotic narrowing, with irregular plaques in the walls of the artery, is common in this region. Such stenoses may be found in the intrapetrosal, intracavernous, and supraclinoid segments of the vessel. *Primary occlusion of the supraclinoid portion of the internal carotid is found almost exclusively in children and in relatively young subjects* (Fig. 10.64; see also Fig. 10.54). When found in the elderly, it is accompanied by disease of the proximal carotid artery as well. On MRA what is usually observed is an absent flow signal in the supraclinoid portion of the internal carotid (Fig. 10.65). Care should be taken to avoid possible artifacts.

Occlusion of the *middle cerebral artery* most often occurs in its horizontal portion, either immediately distal to its origin or at the site of the first branching. The first large branch of the middle cerebral artery, normally the orbitofrontal or anterior temporal branch, is usually well filled (Fig. 10.66). In the author's experience, in children, occlusion of the middle cerebral artery happens more frequently than obstruction of the internal carotid artery. When the middle cerebral artery is thrombosed, there is usually very good opacification of the anterior and posterior cerebral arteries on the same side. Collateral circulation by way of the meningeal arterial anastomoses is established through direct end-to-end intercommunications between the anterior and the middle cerebral arteries. If there is stenosis of the anterior cerebral artery coexisting with occlusion of the middle cerebral artery, the principal collateral circulation is established by way of the posterior cerebral artery.

Occlusion of the *anterior cerebral artery* may take place in its proximal or distal portions. Care should be taken not to diagnose thrombosis of the proximal horizontal segment merely on the basis of lack of filling from one side, since

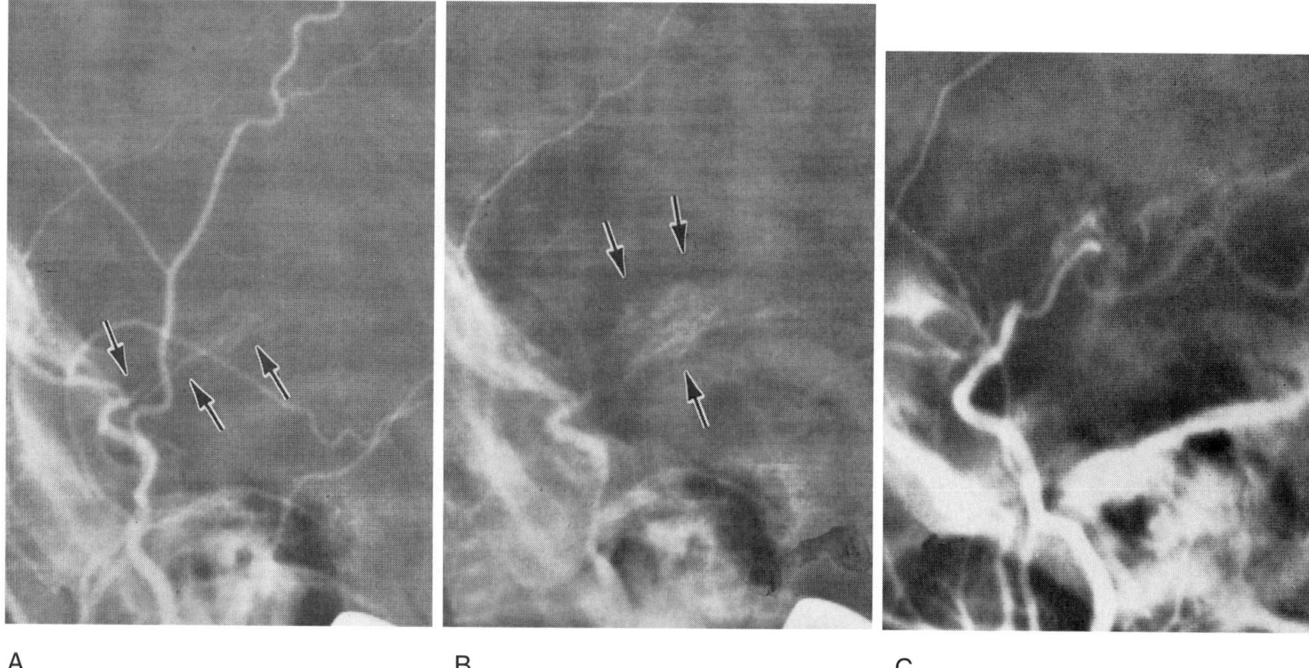

Figure 10.64. Two instances of acute supraclinoid internal carotid artery occlusion in children. **A** and **B.** Occlusion in a 20-month-old infant. There is filling of the anterior choroidal artery and marked vasodilatation due to hypoxia in the territory of the anterior choroidal artery. **C.** Occlusion in a 3-year-old child, just distal to the origin of the posterior communicating artery.

hypoplasia of the horizontal portion of the anterior cerebral artery is so common. For further evaluation, angiography on the opposite side with cross compression should be carried out. If the artery is only mildly hypoplastic, the segment will usually fill from the opposite side when compression is used. If the horizontal segment is markedly hypoplastic, it may not fill even though it is not completely atretic. Only a small percentage of patients actually have a true occlusion of this portion of the anterior cerebral artery. Riggs made a study of 1647 specimens of the circle of Willis obtained at autopsy and found no instance of an absent horizontal portion of the anterior cerebral artery (151). On the other hand, Webster et al. concluded that occlusion of the proximal portion of the anterior cerebral artery is not rare (152). This position, however, is open to question, since the opinion was drawn from angiographic material that did not have the benefit of serialographic studies and routine ipsilateral neck compression when the contralateral side was being injected.

Occlusion of an anterior cerebral artery is easier to demonstrate angiographically in the distal portion than in the proximal portion. In cases of anterior cerebral thrombosis, collateral circulation is often seen over the medial surface of the brain from branches of the posterior cerebral artery (Fig. 10.67). At other times, anastomotic channels over the superior surface of the hemisphere may be seen extending from the middle cerebral artery arborization.

Thrombosis of the *basilar artery* and of the intracranial portion of the *vertebral arteries* occurs frequently. Marked atherosclerotic changes are commonly found in both arteries (Fig. 10.68). The vessels become elongated, tortuous, and irregular in contour (Fig. 10.69). There may be areas of both narrowing and dilatation of the lumen. As the basilar artery becomes elongated, it may project upward higher than usual, sometimes indenting the inferior aspect of the third ventricle (Fig. 10.70).

Care should be taken in diagnosing stenosis of the basilar artery. It is very common to see laminar flow in the basilar artery when only one vertebral artery is injected, since the nonopacified blood from the opposite side tends to confine the contrast substance to one side of the vessel. Therefore, the arterial lumen may appear narrow when it is actually normal in caliber.

In some instances the posterior inferior cerebellar artery is unusually well visualized. This also should not be interpreted as evidence that distal occlusion of the basilar artery is present, since one vertebral artery may terminate as the PICA. A good vertebral injection usually produces some regurgitation of the contrast substance into the opposite vertebral artery. A diagnosis of thrombosis of the basilar artery probably should not be made unless some regurgitation takes place. Thrombosis of the basilar artery is often found just proximal to the bifurcation of the artery. The lesion may also develop above the junction of the two vertebral arteries but is less frequently encountered at that site. At other times, the thrombosis may start in the trunk of the artery and propagate distally. In cases of occlusion of the basilar artery, collateral flow via the anastomoses be-

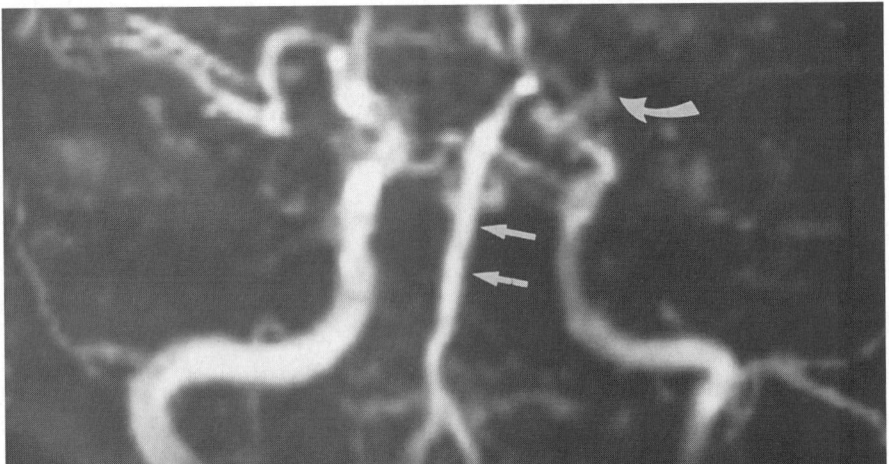

A

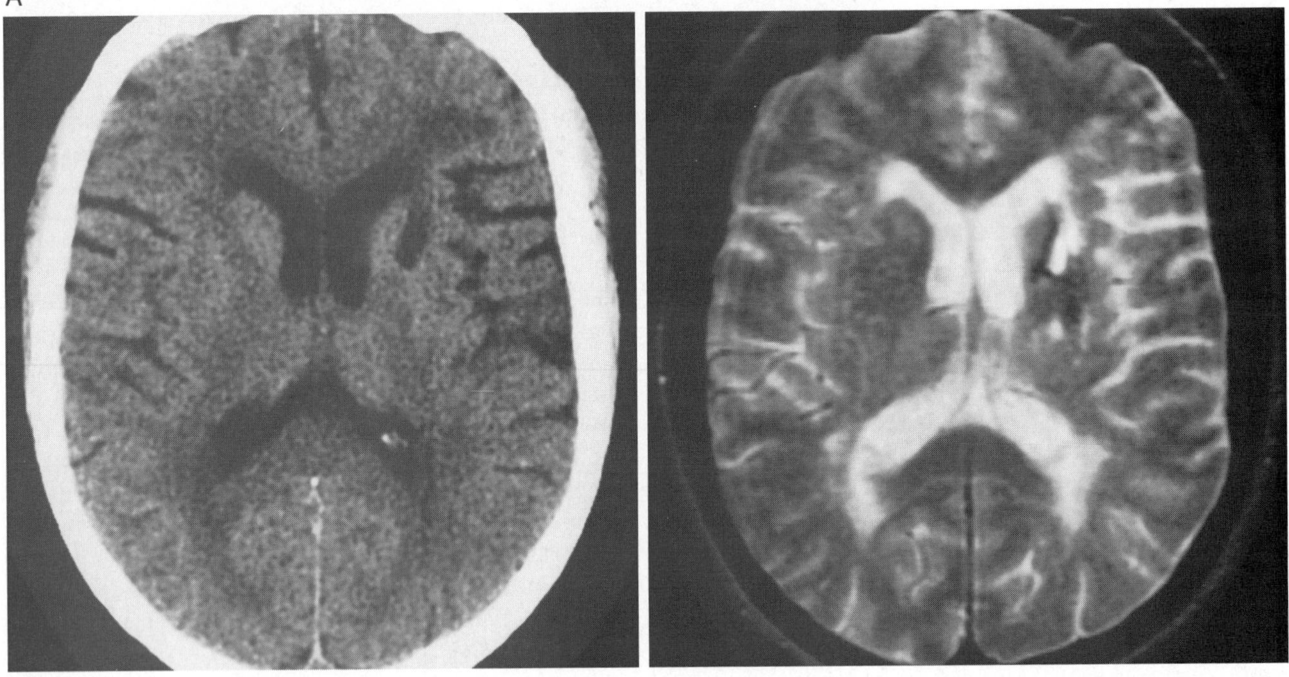

B C

Figure 10.65. Supraclinoid carotid artery occlusion shown by MRA in a 65-year-old woman. **A.** The left internal carotid artery shows attenuation of its flow pattern as compared to the right. At its supraclinoid portion a complete disappearance of flow is observed (arrow). The middle cerebral artery and the initial segment of the anterior cerebral arteries are not seen. The basilar artery flow is normal (two arrows). **B.** CT axial image shows an infarct involving the anterior limb of the internal capsule and also slightly the posterior limb. **C.** T2-weighted axial image shows the area of old infarction accompanied by low-intensity areas consistent with old blood products. Internal carotid artery occlusion often leads to ischemic infarction in the basal ganglia–internal capsule areas, involving primarily the perforating branches arising from the internal carotid artery and the middle cerebral artery trunk.

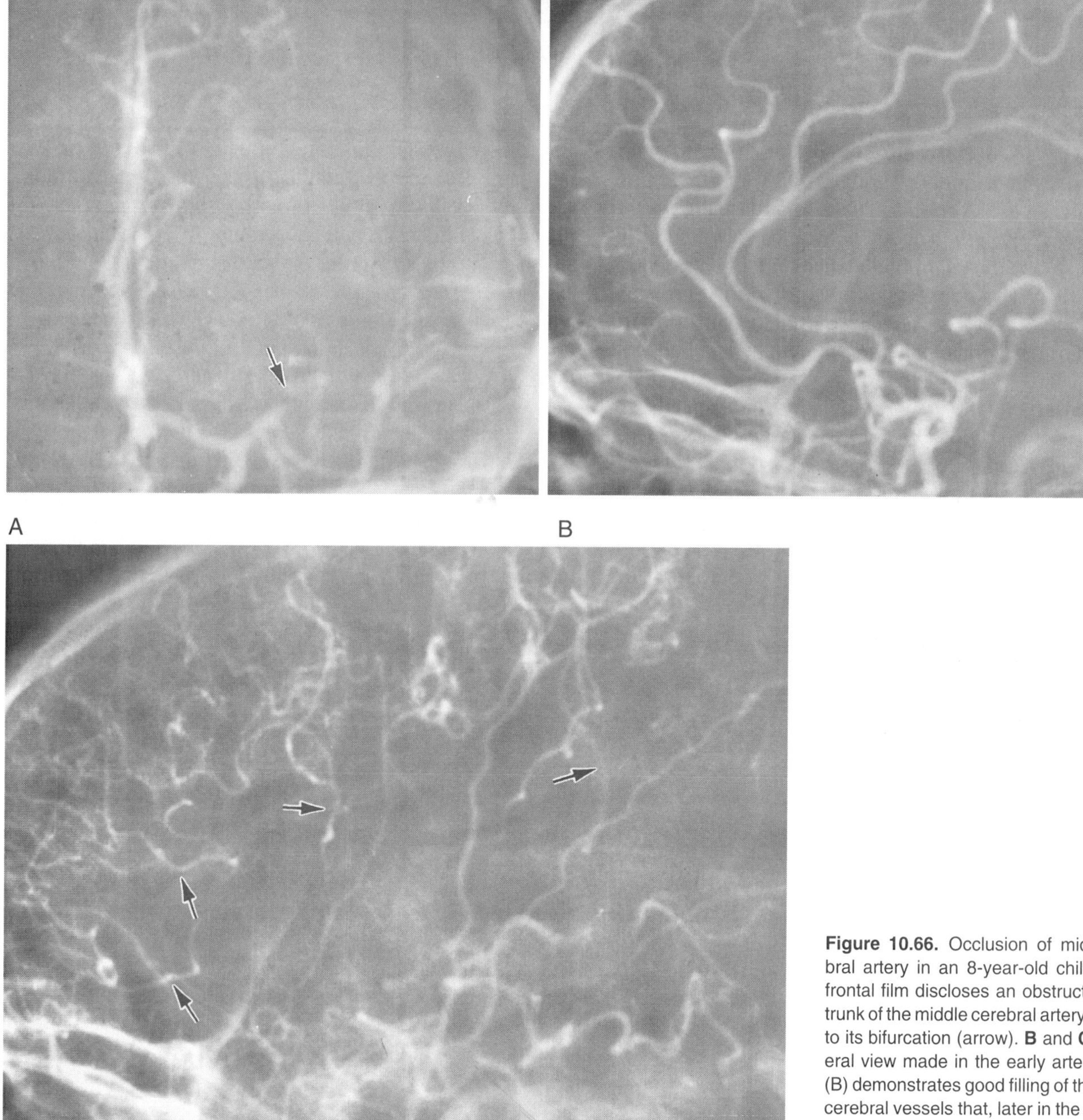

Figure 10.66. Occlusion of middle cerebral artery in an 8-year-old child. **A.** The frontal film discloses an obstruction of the trunk of the middle cerebral artery just distal to its bifurcation (arrow). **B** and **C.** The lateral view made in the early arterial phase (B) demonstrates good filling of the anterior cerebral vessels that, later in the serial (C), are shown to supply (in retrograde manner) the branches of the middle cerebral artery (arrows).

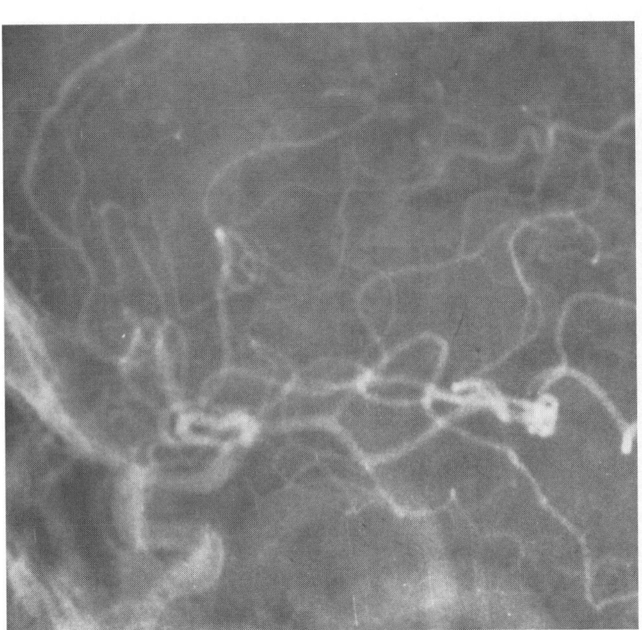

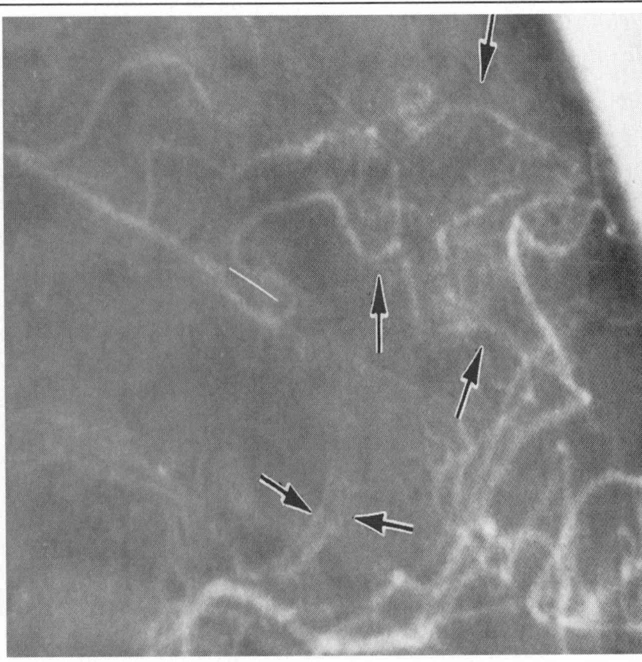

A B

Figure 10.67. Bilateral occlusion of pericallosal arteries with collateral circulation from vertebral system. **A.** The right and left angiograms reveal nonfilling of both pericallosal arteries. The callosomarginal arteries and at least the anterior and middle internal frontal branches of these arteries are filled. **B.** A vertebral angiogram reveals retrograde flow by way of anastomoses between the parieto-occipital branches of the posterior cerebral arteries and the branches of the pericallosal arteries (upper arrows). There is also filling of the arteries of the splenium (or posterior pericallosal arteries) that anastomose with the terminal branches of the pericallosal arteries (lower arrows).

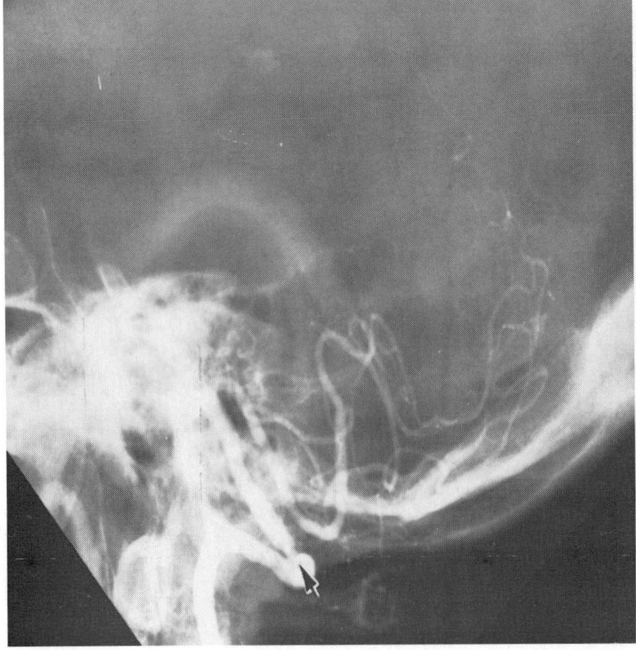

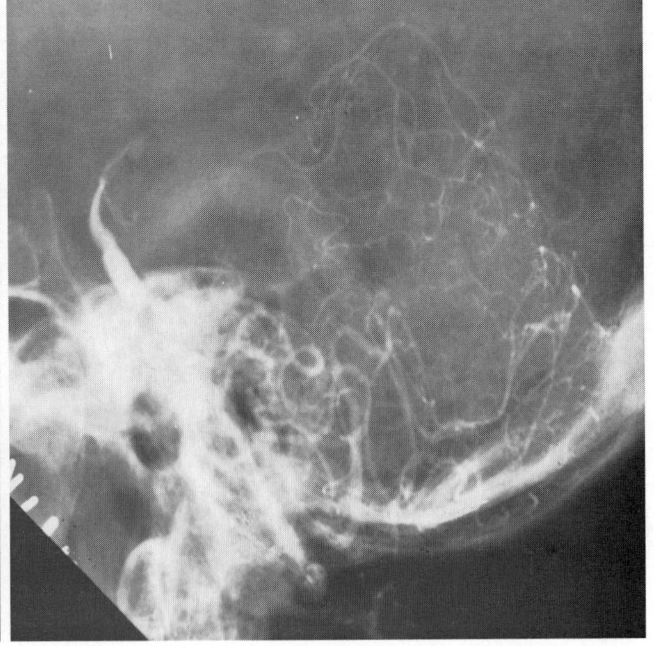

A B

Figure 10.68. Thrombosis of upper basilar artery with excellent collateral circulation from the PICA. **A.** Lateral vertebral angiogram shows that there is a narrowed segment in the vertebral artery (arrow). **B.** At 2 sec there is already almost complete filling of the superior cerebellar territory through anastomoses between the two arterial territories. The patient was admitted with signs of a posterior circulation stroke but had marked recovery.

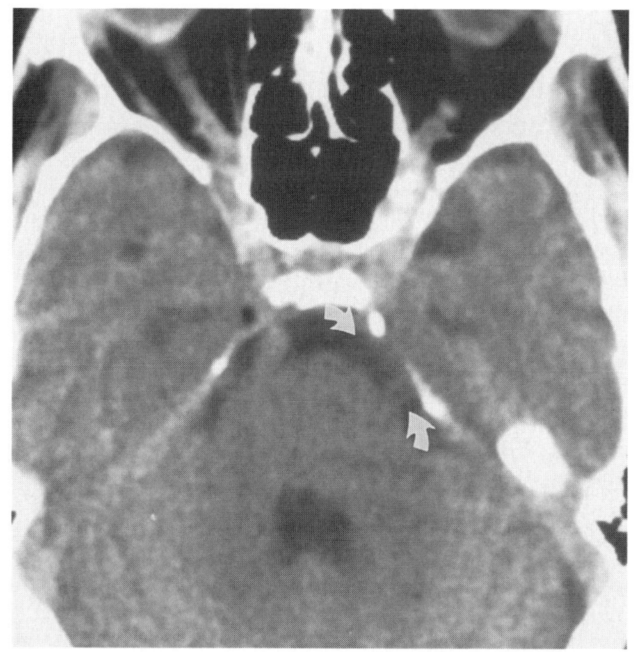

A

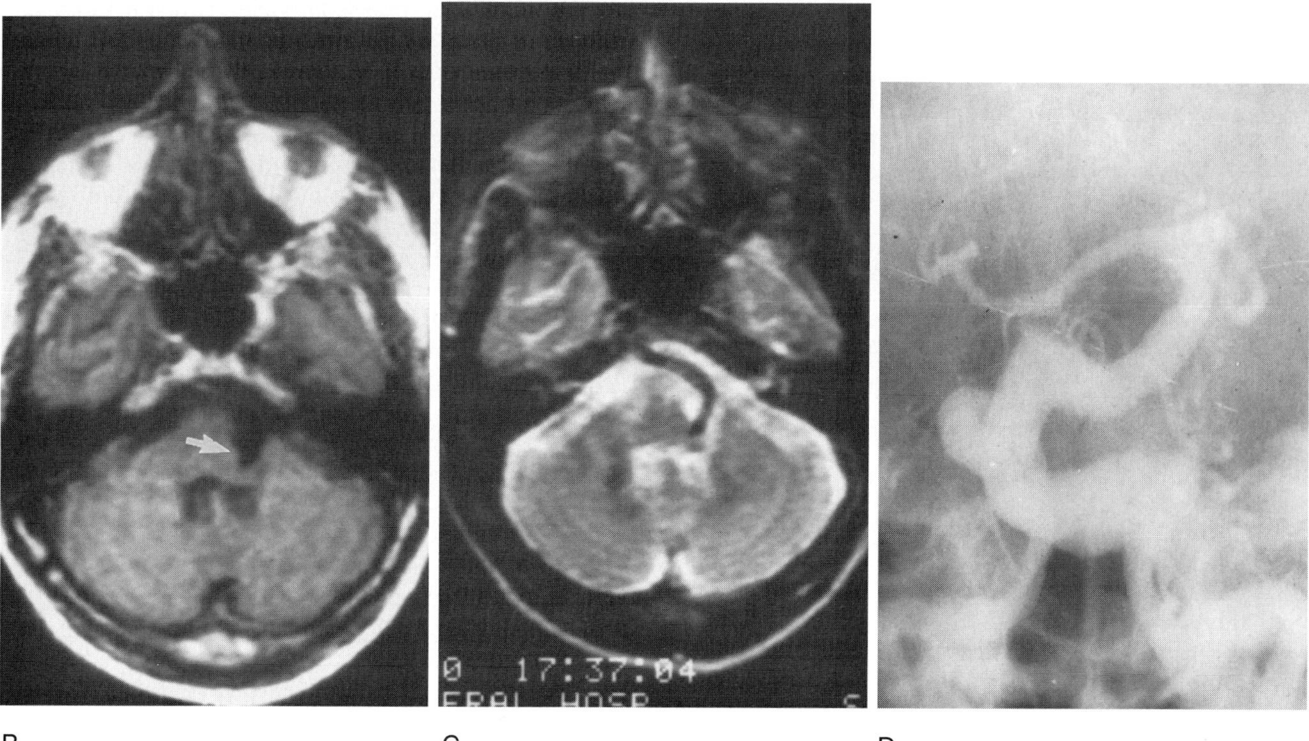

B C D

Figure 10.69. Elongated, tortuous vertebrobasilar arteries suggesting a mass on CT. **A.** Axial CT image shows suspicion of a mass in the left lateral pontine region (arrows). **B.** T1-weighted MR image shows an apparent defect in the left pontine region (arrow). **C.** T2-weighted axial image shows a large flow void due to an elongated tortuous basilar artery. Vascular flow voids are usually seen much better on T2-weighted images. **D.** Angiogram in another case showing extreme tortuosity and enlargement of the basilar artery with aneurysmal dilatation.

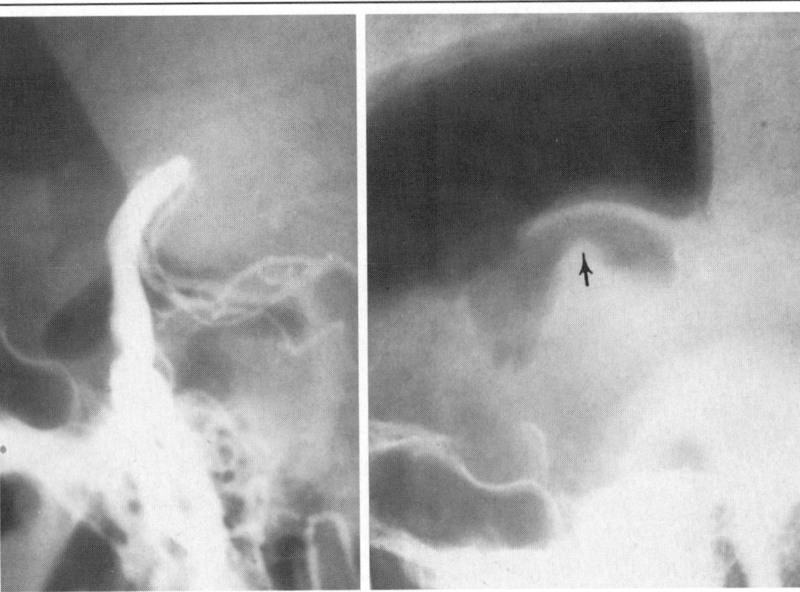

Figure 10.70. Indentation of the third ventricle produced by an elongated basilar artery. The indentation is close to the foramen of Monro (arrow) and may be responsible for the ventricular dilatation noted. (**A**, angiogram; **B**, from an air ventriculogram.)

tween the vermian and hemispheric branches of the posterior inferior cerebellar arteries and branches of the superior cerebellar arteries can be demonstrated on serialograms. The demonstration of these collateral pathways confirms the presence of partial or total occlusion of the basilar artery (Fig. 10.68). In these cases, carotid angiography usually shows filling of both posterior cerebral and superior cerebellar arteries from the anterior circulation. Such collateral flow through the circle of Willis helps confirm the presence of stenosis or occlusion of the basilar artery. MRA may demonstrate absence of flow in the basilar artery. This means that there may be occlusion or diminished flow of a significant degree in the basilar artery but is not diagnostic of basilar artery occlusion (Fig. 10.71).

MULTIPLE PROGRESSIVE INTRACRANIAL ARTERIAL OCCLUSIONS (MOYA-MOYA)

This term has been applied to a syndrome of progressive intracranial occlusions encountered in children and young adults (132). The syndrome consists of a progressive occlusion of the internal carotid artery in its intracranial portion, as well as of the trunks of the middle and anterior cerebral arteries on both sides. The occlusion occurs slowly, affecting the anterior two-thirds of the circle of Willis (153) and usually (but not always) sparing the posterior cerebral and basilar arteries. Since the circle of Willis is no longer useful to provide blood for the cerebral tissues, circulation must be reestablished by way of anastomoses on the surface of the brain and through the central arteries.

The three factors of (a) slow development, (b) occurrence in children or young adults, and (c) obstruction of the circle of Willis are believed by the author to be responsible for the surprising development of anastomoses via the deep perforating vessels at the base of the brain. These anastomoses were emphasized by many of the original writers who reported cases of this condition (153–155). Subarachnoid hemorrhage is frequent, and the enlargement of the perforating branches is so marked that the lesion has been suggested to come from some vascular malformation (Figs. 10.72 and 10.73). However, the same vasodilatation can be observed in other areas of the brain in association with more peripherally placed occlusions and in association with the transdural anastomoses.

The syndrome is not confined to the Japanese but it is evidently more frequent among them. The author has seen many cases in this country in both white and black subjects. One case was seen in an infant with Down syndrome, and several examples of occurrence in siblings have been reported. The children often become mentally retarded (about 50 percent of the cases), they may have varying degrees of neurologic involvement, alternating hemiparesis, often very mild, or they may lead normal lives until a complication—such as subarachnoid hemorrhage—causes a cerebral angiogram to be performed. The present author has stopped using the term *moya-moya* because this is believed to be an occlusive disease. The original designation of *moya-moya* (by Japanese authors), *congenital basal telangiectasia*, and other terms were based on the concept of a congenital origin of the syndrome; however, this is surely an acquired condition.

The syndrome provides the best examples of transdural internal-external carotid anastomoses, as well as of cortical arterial anastomoses, owing to the obstruction of the circle of Willis (Figs. 10.53, 10.54, and 10.72). Subarachnoid, subdural, or intracerebral hemorrhage may result from rupture of the dilated arterial channels. The subdural hemorrhages are likely to be severe because they are arterial in origin, usually caused by rupture of the transdural arterial anastomoses.

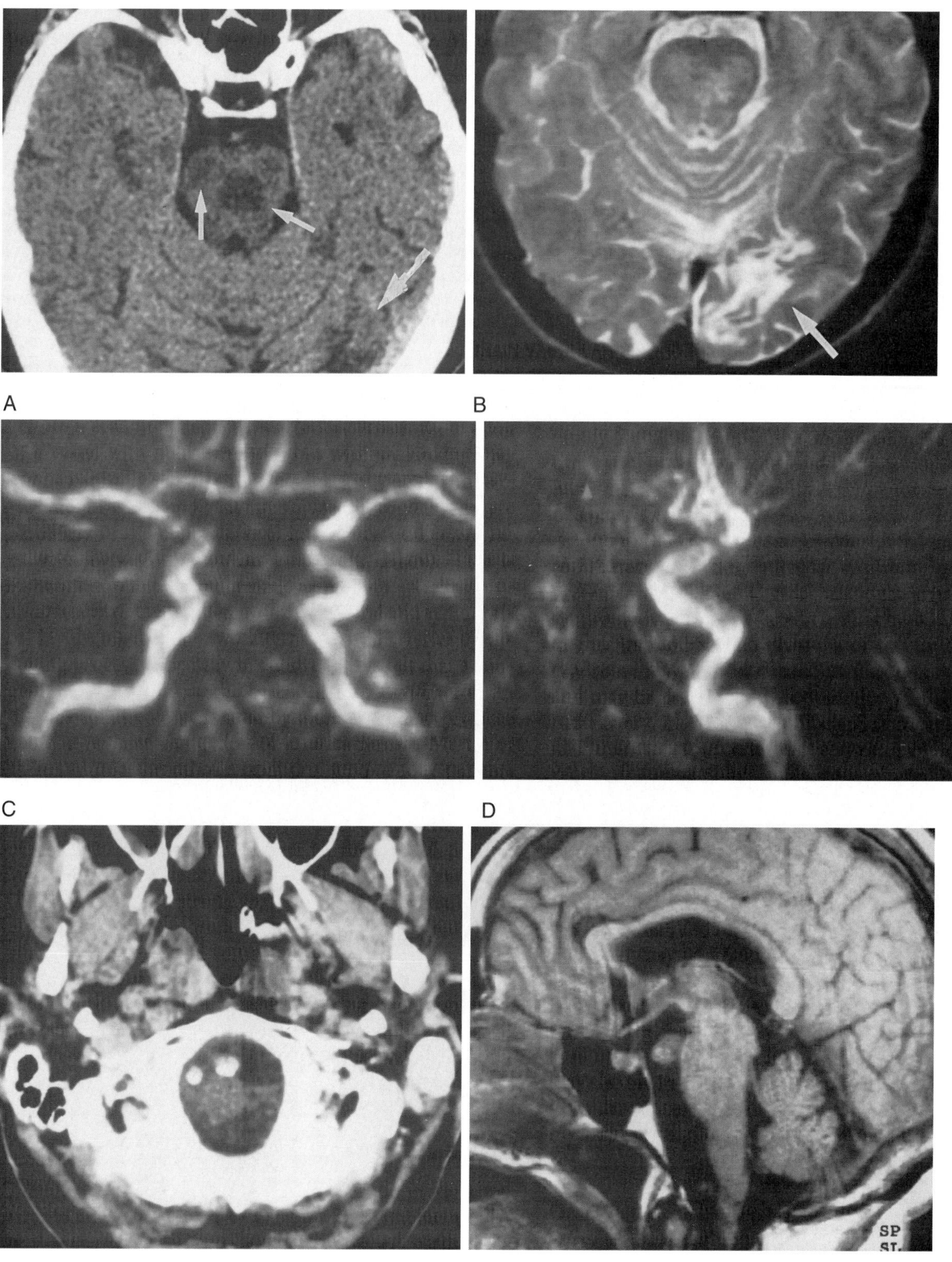

Figure 10.71. Occlusion of basilar artery in a 76-year-old woman. The patient was admitted with an acute onset of dysarthria and decreased consciousness, followed by bilateral arm and leg weakness; she later became nonverbal. **A.** CT axial image shows hypodense areas in the upper pons consistent with ischemic changes that were not present a few days previously. There is also an ischemic lesion in the left occipital lobe (arrows). **B.** T2-weighted axial MR image shows the same areas seen in A to be hyperintense (pontine as well as occipital areas). **C.** Coronal MRA view shows both carotid arteries and their branches but no basilar artery, which is indicative of absent flow. **D.** A direct sagittal view shows the two carotid arteries superimposed, but no basilar artery. The site of the occlusion cannot be determined, only the absence of flow. **E** to **H.** Images on another patient. Axial CT scan (**E**) and sagittal MR T1-weighted image (**F**) show a dilated tortuous basilar artery.

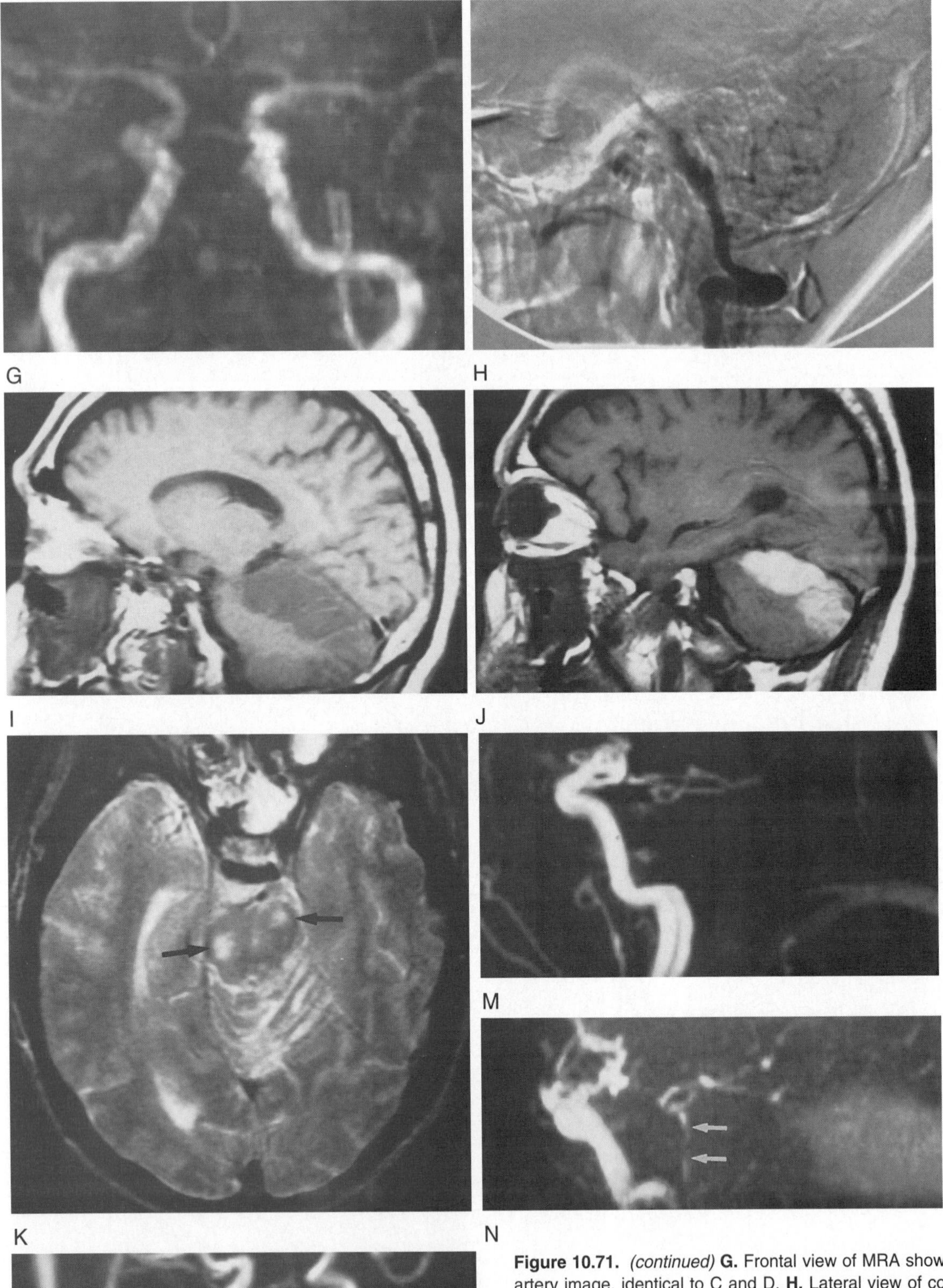

Figure 10.71. *(continued)* **G.** Frontal view of MRA shows an absent basilar artery image, identical to C and D. **H.** Lateral view of conventional cerebral angiogram shows the basilar artery up to its upper portion where the occlusion took place. There was absent flow on MRA, indicating that there was insufficient flow to generate an image, but the artery was in fact open to its uppermost portion. **I** to **N.** Another example of basilar artery thrombosis with conversion of cerebellar infarct into a hemorrhagic one. **I.** Sagittal T1-weighted view reveals a low-intensity area in the territory of the superior cerebellar artery. **J.** T1-weighted sagittal view taken 10 days later shows hyperintensity in the area, evidently due to hemorrhagic conversion of the infarct. The patient was actively treated with anticoagulation.

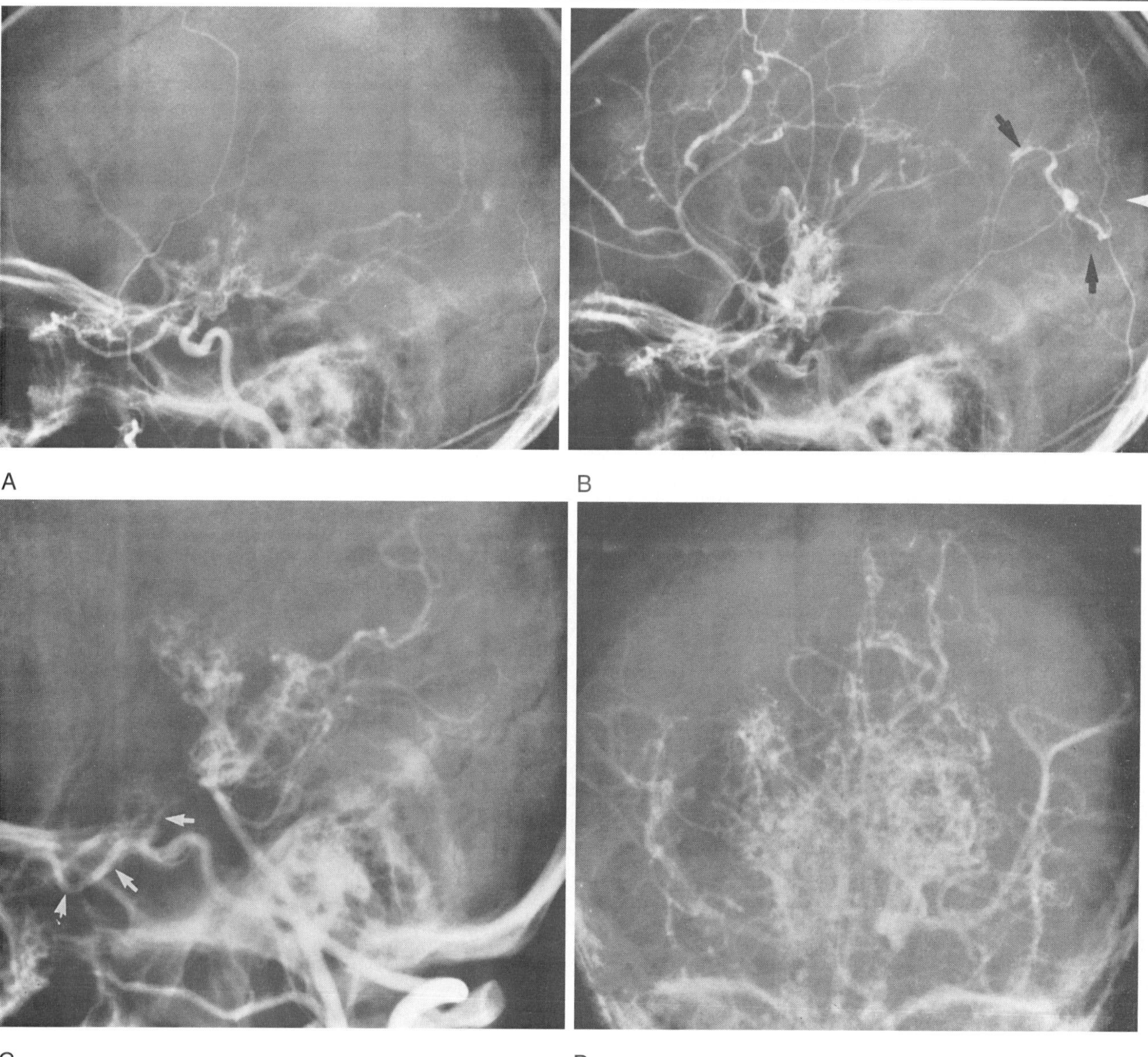

Figure 10.72. Multiple progressive arterial occlusions (Moya-Moya) in a 3-year-old child. **A** and **B.** A left carotid angiogram shows a left internal carotid arterial occlusion. There is a fine network of vessels at the base of the brain on both sides representing dilated perforating branches of the internal carotid and posterior communicating arteries, which supply most of the cerebral circulation. The ophthalmic artery is enlarged and has extensive enlargement and proliferation of its branches, some of which anastomose with meningeal branches, which in turn anastomose with cortical arteries across the subdural space. **B.** Prominent transdural anastomoses are filling (arrows). Transdural anastomoses are also supplied by the tentorial branch of the meningohyophyseal artery and by the anterior branch of the middle meningeal artery. **C.** A right brachial study shows changes in the carotid system resembling those found on the left (arrows). The basilar artery is preserved and provides a basal arterial network that resulted in filling of the middle cerebral branches on both sides. **D.** The frontal view (later phase than C) shows filling of most middle cerebral branches on both sides. The basal network appears to be more efficient in this instance than the surface (subpial) anastomoses.

Figure 10.71. *(continued)* **K.** Axial T2-weighted image shows brainstem infarcts bilaterally (arrows). **L.** MRA demonstrates absent flow in the basilar artery. **M.** Sagittal view of MRA shows the absent basilar artery flow. Some filling of the posterior cerebral arteries is seen through the posterior communicating arteries. **N.** Repeat MRA 10 days later shows that there is now some flow in the basilar artery (arrows), which may account for the hemorrhagic conversion of the infarct in the cerebellum. The hemorrhagic infarction is seen posteriorly.

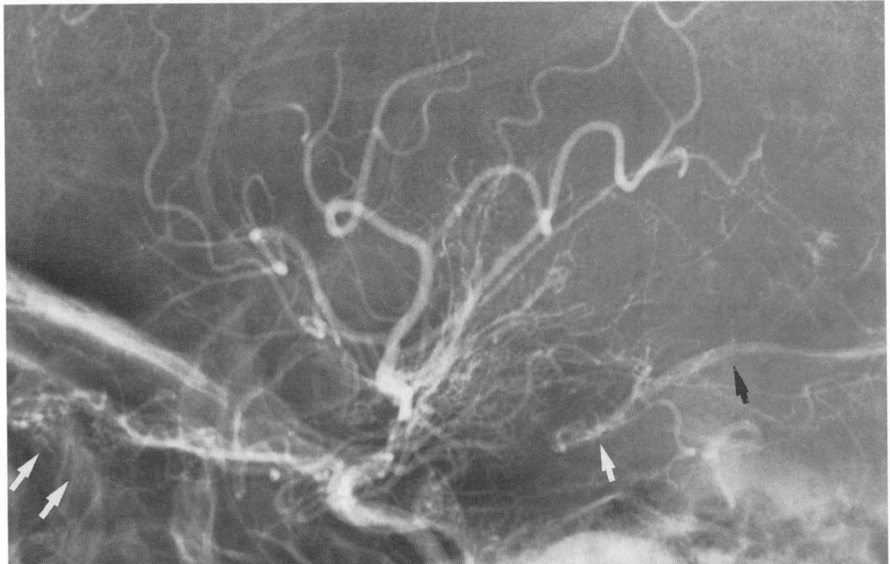

A

Figure 10.73. Multiple progressive intracranial arterial occlusions (Moya-Moya) in a 28-year-old woman. **A.** A left carotid angiogram shows a supraclinoid occlusion of the internal carotid artery with collateral bypassing via numerous enlarged perforating vessels. The posterior cerebral artery (arrows) fills by the same route. The ophthalmic artery shows extensive arborization with many new small vessels. **B.** Right brachial angiography demonstrates an internal carotid occlusion on the right side also. The basilar artery is narrow. The initial segments of the posterior cerebral arteries are becoming stenotic. **C.** The frontal film confirms the bilateral stenosis of the posterior cerebral arteries (arrows).

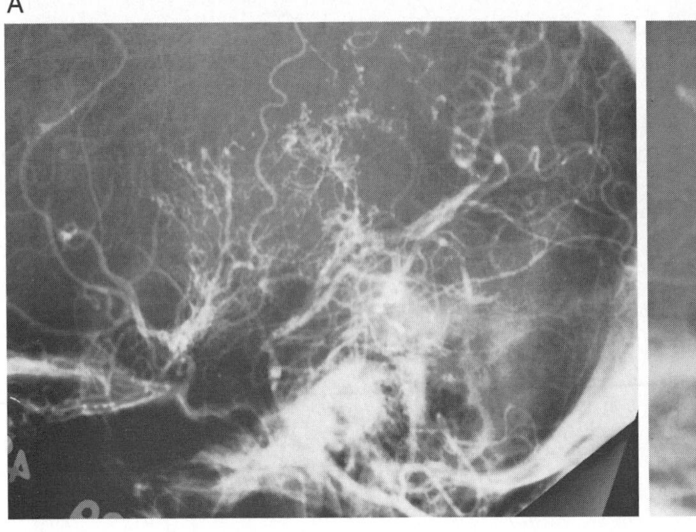

B

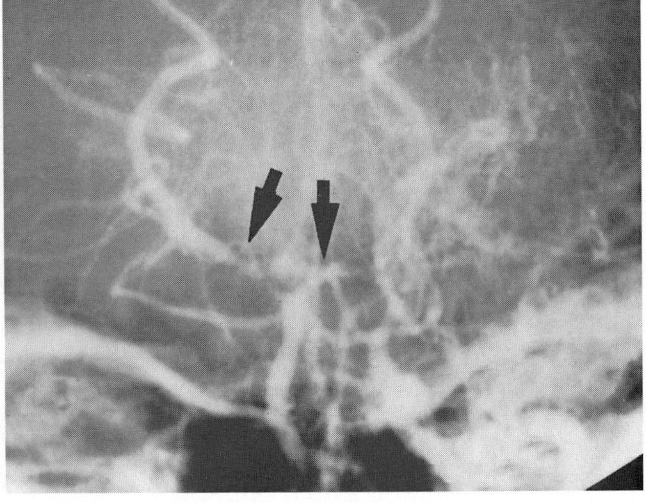

C

In one case, both carotid and both vertebral arteries were occluded in an 8-year-old girl and the cerebral circulation took place almost entirely via transdural anastomoses (156). In the same case, one of the internal carotid arteries was occluded at its origin, and this must have occurred very early in life because tomography demonstrated poor development of the osseous carotid canal in the corresponding petrous pyramid.

The etiology of this condition is unknown. It is felt that an inflammatory origin is most likely. However, pathologically, it has not been possible to demonstrate inflammation that would suggest a nonspecific arteritis. The most frequently encountered appearance has been a thickened intima with marked narrowing or actual occlusion of the lumen of an involved artery (157). Intimal thickening is nonspecific, and involvement of the other arterial layers has been atypical or sometimes totally absent. For these reasons, the entity is described here with the stenoses and occlusions. The diagnosis may be suspected on MRI if linear flow voids are seen bilaterally that do not have a configuration suggesting an arteriovenous malformation in a child or young adult. Angiography is usually required for diagnosis. Cerebral infarctions may be found. As just mentioned, the child may present with an intracerebral hemorrhage owing to rupture of some of the collateral deep channels, which is easily detectable on CT images.

HEMOGLOBIN SS, SICKLE CELL ANEMIA

Multiple intracranial arterial occlusions may be encountered in these cases, and the appearance may be somewhat similar to that seen in Moya-Moya. The history would differentiate between the two. The vascular occlusions have been attributed to red cell clumping and vasa-vasorum occlusion. However, the latest concept is that the vascular occlusions result from a progressive vasculopathy due to hyperdynamic blood flow (high-flow angiopathy) caused by the anemia and increased cardiac output (Fig. 10.74).

The occluded arteries tend to be major, such as the internal carotid bilaterally, and multiple small infarcts are not usually demonstrated on CT or MRI, which speaks against the theory of small-vessel occlusion due to sickling (158–160). Large infarcts are often encountered. White matter lesions in young patients with sickle cell disease are seen frequently.

Sneddon syndrome is a rare disease consisting of diffuse livedo reticularis and cerebral vascular lesions. It is a progressive, occlusive, noninflammatory arteriopathy involving medium-sized vessels occurring in younger adults (30 to 50 years of age) (161). Perhaps the most prominent clinical sign is that of livedo reticularis, a diffuse bluish mottling in the skin of the extremities, but which in these patients may be seen in the face and trunk; for that reason, dermatologists would frequently see the patient first. The CT or MRI examination may show multiple areas of ischemic infarction, particularly well shown on MRI. Cortical atrophy seen in young individuals with this condition may be related to prior ischemic lesions. In the case report by Blom, cerebral angiography demonstrated evidence of multiple branch arterial occlusions in the middle and posterior cerebral artery territories with collateral circulation from pial arterial anastomoses, as well as from transdural arterial external-internal carotid anastomoses that were indicative of chronicity (162).

The appearance is different from Moya-Moya in that the latter involves predominantly the major vessels (bifurcation of the internal carotid artery occluding the origins of the anterior and middle cerebral arteries), but at first glance the multiple collaterals, the progressive course, and the young age of the patients may be confusing (163). Pathologically there is evidence of arterial occlusions (shown on skin biopsy of the extremities), but no arteritic changes. In this respect it is similar to the pathology of Moya-Moya. Arteriography of the extremities usually shows arterial occlusions with collaterals. Occlusion of the central retinal artery has been frequently reported (164, 165).

BRANCHES OF MAJOR CEREBRAL ARTERIES

The diagnosis of occlusion of the principal branches of the anterior, middle, and posterior cerebral arteries can be made from serial angiographic films. If such films are not made, it is possible to confuse the lack of filling of a given branch with an anatomic variant or even a small tumor. Adequate films usually demonstrate the presence of *collateral flow* into the area normally supplied by the obstructed vessel. In the case of thrombosis of a middle cerebral branch, collateral flow most often comes from the anterior cerebral arterial branches, and retrograde filling of the obstructed territory usually can be traced on serial films (Figs. 10.46 and 10.66). In anterior cerebral branch occlusions, the middle cerebral subdivisions, which anastomose directly with those of the anterior cerebral artery, may be the source of collateral supply. In the author's experience, however, the posterior cerebral artery is a more common source of collateral supply for the anterior cerebral area (Fig. 10.67). In one instance of proximal thrombosis of branches of a posterior cerebral artery, there was retrograde filling of the posterior temporal branch by way of intercommunications between the parieto-occipital division of the posterior cerebral and the middle cerebral arteries. When the occluded branches do not fill by collateral flow, *propagation of a thrombus* into these branches may have occurred.

Propagation of a thrombus from the original site of obstruction may cause the branches of the cerebral arteries to remain occluded for a period of time. There is no way in which blood can get to the area supplied by these vessels inasmuch as the perforating branches arising from them will also be occluded. Eventually the thrombus may disappear, but the damage to the territory of this vessel will persist as a cerebral infarction. After the thrombus is dissolved, filling of the previously obstructed portions of the vessels may then take place; however, since damage to the perforating vessels has already occurred, capillary block will probably be permanent in the infarcted area. There will be a persistence of the contrast material in the vessels filled by collateral flow. This phenomenon, which we have come to call "stasis in the collaterals," is evidently the result of blockage of the perforating branches arising from those cerebral arteries that are visible by angiography.

Single-branch occlusions of the cerebral arteries, particularly branches of the middle cerebral artery, may also be diagnosed accurately by angiography. The diagnosis is based on the demonstration of local stasis in the 1 or 2 cm of the occluded vessel distal to the last branching and retrograde flow into the area of the occluded vessel. It may take several seconds for the segment beyond the occlusion to fill in a retrograde manner from an adjacent territory. This type of diagnosis requires careful scrutiny of the areas in question because the arteries that fill by retrograde flow may be confused with veins. Additionally, in the parieto-occipital region, care should be taken not to confuse the usual late emptying that takes place in this area with pathologic opacification. The late emptying may be caused by slower regional flow or by the longer length of these arteries. It is also possible that the last amount of contrast material of the injection tends to persist in the posterior arteries by gravity, the contrast material being heavier than the blood.

Alertness must be continually exercised to detect obstructed branches of the cerebral vessels. Any *delayed filling* or *delayed emptying* of these branches should always be considered abnormal, with the possible exception just mentioned of the parieto-occipital region. In normal cases, physiologic slow filling and emptying is quite uniform and involves several branches; the vessels do not taper but are of even caliber. When a vessel fills slowly because of ob-

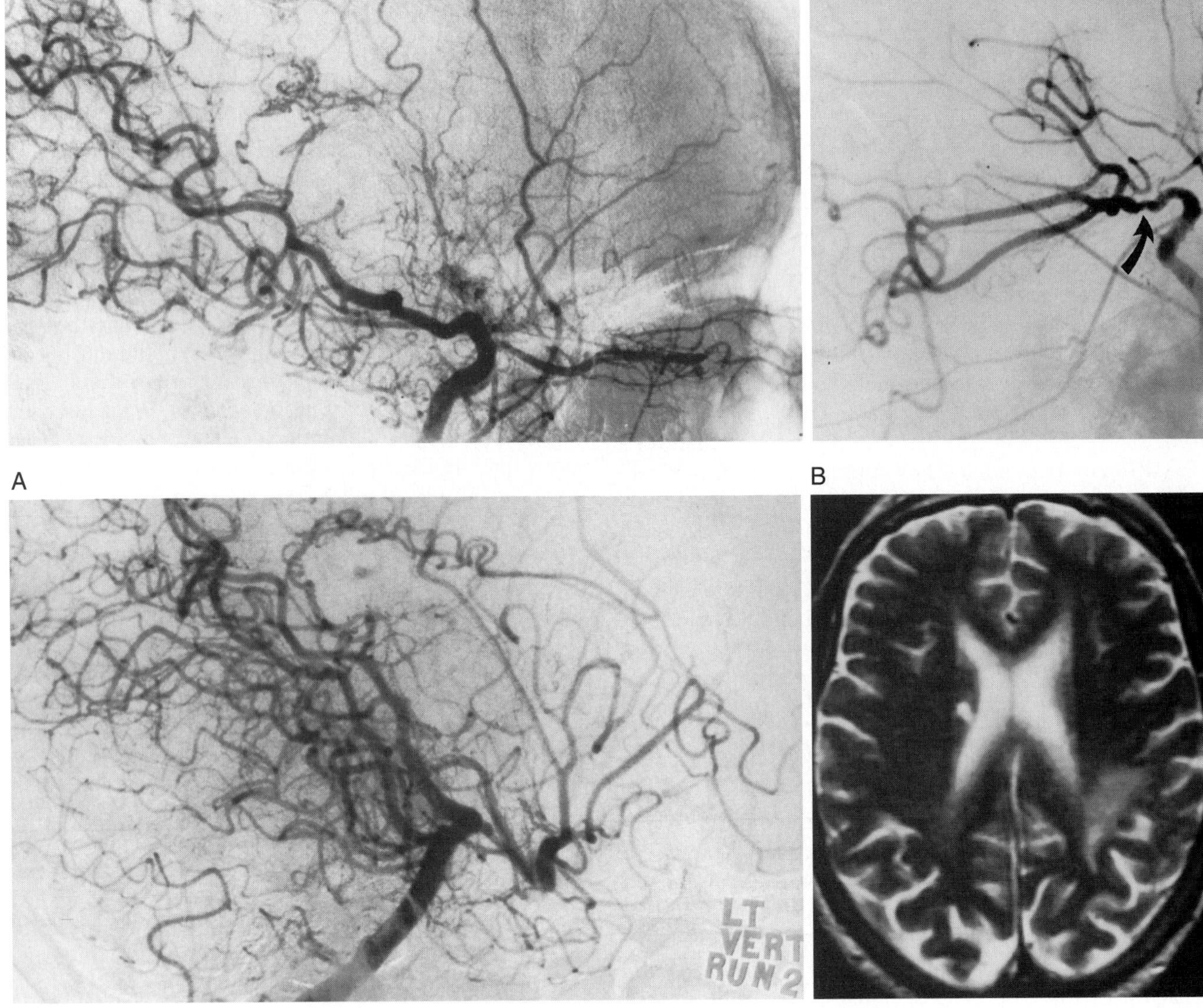

Figure 10.74. Arterial occlusions associated with hemoglobin SS, sickle cell anemia. **A.** Left carotid angiography in a 15-year-old boy presenting with right hemiparesis reveals carotid occlusion distal to the posterior communicating artery with excellent filling of the posterior cerebral artery and branches. The deep perforating branches are particularly well filled, and there is some filling of the leptomeningeal anastomoses in this early film. **B.** Right carotid angiogram in a 6-year-old boy presenting with a right-sided stroke. The supraclinoid carotid is irregular and narrow (arrow). The anterior cerebral artery does not fill and did not fill on angiography of the left carotid, indicating possible occlusion. **C.** Vertebral angiogram in a 13-year-old male presenting with a stroke. There is occlusion of the left carotid in its supraclinoid portion proximal to the origin of the posterior communicating artery. (Courtesy of Dr. Ramon E. Figueroa, Augusta, GA.) **D** to **F.** Stroke in a 72-year-old woman due to arteritis. The patient presented with aphasia. **D.** MRI demonstrated a left posterior frontal, predominantly subcortical, hyperintensity. A lacunar infarct is seen in the right caudate body.

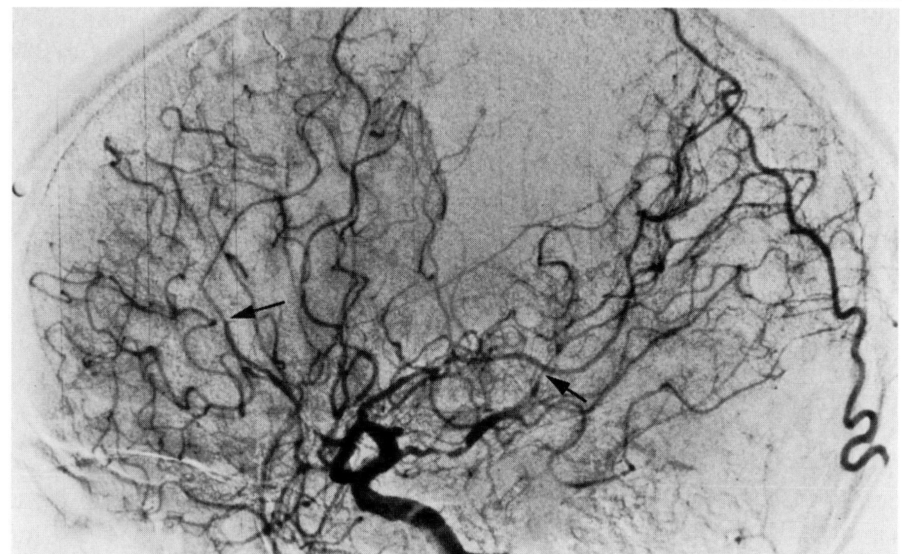

E

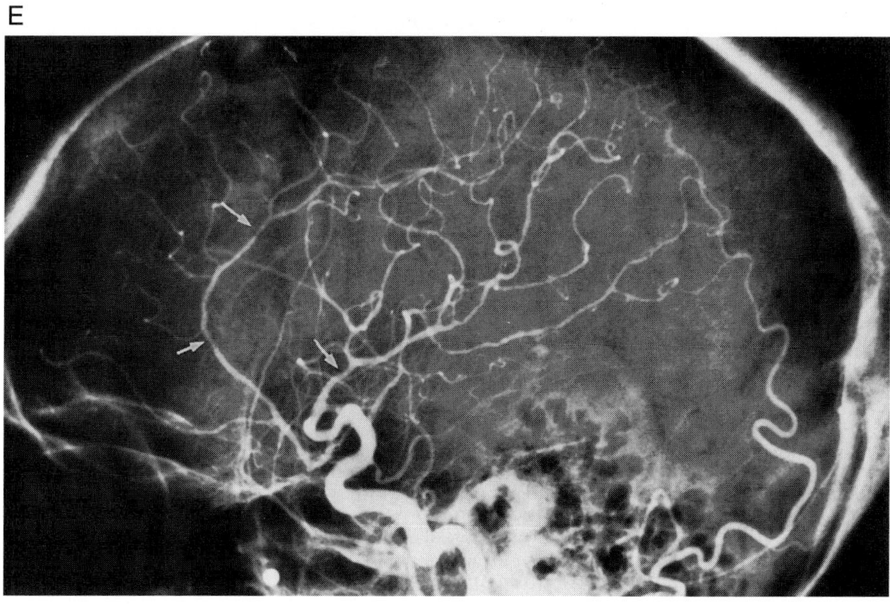

F

Figure 10.74. *(continued)* **E.** Cerebral angiography demonstrated an avascular area in the left posterior frontal region associated with irregularity in the caliber of the larger arteries (anterior and middle cerebral and their branches [arrows]). **F.** The right carotid artery system also revealed areas of stenosis combined with areas of normal or slightly widened lumen (arrows), considered typical of arteritis (see Chapter 6 for further discussion).

struction, it presents an *advancing tapered end*, unless a cupped deformity produced by a recent embolus is outlined by the head of the opaque column. The thin streak of contrast material may move peripherally during the serial.

Ring suggested a method for facilitating the recognition of occluded arterial branches (166). Although that author's method is useful in suspecting arterial obstruction from a single film, the pathophysiologic changes observed on a serialogram are far more helpful in establishing a diagnosis of arterial occlusion.

Occlusion of the *posterior inferior cerebellar* branch of the vertebral artery is a well-recognized clinical entity (Wallenberg syndrome). The diagnosis by angiography, however, is tenuous because there are so many anatomic variants, including absence of this artery. It is possible that thrombosis of the PICA or some of its branches may at times be a part of stenosis of the vertebral artery from which it arises, in which case the vertebral trunk is deformed.

MRA is not helpful in diagnosing occlusion of branches of the middle cerebral artery because nonvisualization of branches beyond a short distance past the bifurcation or trifurcation of the middle cerebral artery trunk is not reliable. Also, collateral circulation cannot usually be ascertained. However, an infarct in the appropriate territory may be seen.

CEREBRAL ARTERITIS

Arteritis of cerebral vessels is another condition that cannot be diagnosed by MRA and requires the use of angiography, but ischemic lesions may be seen on MRI or on CT images

(Fig. 10.74*D* to *F*). Arteritis has been discussed in Chapter 6. The diagnosis of arteritis of cerebral vessels is important because of the possibility of causing rapid improvement in the patient's symptoms through intra-arterial injection of vasodilators such as nimodipine and papaverine through superselective catheterization, as recently reported by Dr. Oscar Solis (personal communication).

MINOR CEREBRAL ARTERIES

It has been demonstrated by anatomic dissections that there are direct end-to-end anastomoses between branches of the anterior, middle, and posterior cerebral arteries on the surface of the brain. This fact is repeatedly confirmed angiographically. Whether anastomoses exist between such small "end" arteries as the lenticulostriate and other perforating branches of the cerebral vessels has not been shown. Intercommunication between the anterior and posterior choroidal arteries was demonstrated by Wollschlaeger and Wollschlaeger (167). It is probable that anastomoses for the perforating vessels exist by way of the capillary bed, but the pathways are insufficient to carry the circulation from one territory to another, at least in the acute stage of ischemia.

On cerebral angiograms in cases of thrombosis, it is common to see dilatation of many small, perforating branches of the cerebral arteries that are not generally apparent. The dilatation is due to high local carbon dioxide tension and tissue acidosis in the acute stage (59). Later, enlargement of the vessels is usually an indication of the development of the collateral circulation. The case shown in Figure 10.64*A* and *B*, in which a thrombosis of the internal carotid artery occurred just above the level of the origin of the anterior choroidal artery, illustrates extreme dilatation of the branches of the anterior choroidal artery, which produces a relatively wide area of staining in the angiogram. The evidence of increased vascularity remained on the serialogram for several seconds, and it is likely that there was stasis here within the arterioles. The enlargement of numerous small perforating branches is sometimes so pronounced that it suggests the presence of a tumor (see text following).

Whether small vessels will become dilated and be visible in the angiogram probably depends on the status of arteries distal to the site of obstruction. That is, if a thrombus propagates within the branches of the obstructed main vessel, the perforating branches arising proximal to the obstruction probably will become dilated and may succeed in supplying at least a part of the ischemic area. On the other hand, if arteries beyond the point of obstruction remain patent, blood supply can be affected by retrograde flow from anastomoses on the surface of the brain.

Sometimes the presence of small, dilated perforating branches of the cerebral vessels adjacent to an area of thrombosis is helpful in differentiating a neoplasm from an edematous area secondary to occlusion of vessels. These small branches remain dilated and tend to surround each one of the larger arteries or groups of arteries with a "halo" of fine vascularity. In early stages of vascular occlusion, there usually is cerebral edema, which may be localized. In some cases it may be sufficiently pronounced to suggest a tumor. A midline shift may be present, and sometimes it is very marked. It takes approximately 2 weeks for edema to disappear, provided that no subsequent vascular occlusion occurs, such as takes place in the intermittent progressive type of stroke syndrome.

DISAPPEARANCE OF ARTERIAL OCCLUSION

On the basis of numerous angiographic examinations in patients with stroke, for many years it has been felt by the author, as well as by others, that emboli are the most common direct cause of intracranial arterial occlusion. The embolic theory is particularly logical in cases where multiple branch occlusions are demonstrated. It explains the lack of evident intracranial occlusions at autopsy in the face of severe, fatal strokes. Because emboli can disappear by lysis, cerebral angiography may show vascular obstruction early in the course of the illness, and patent vessels later. The chances of demonstrating occluded vessels are thus greater in the early evaluations. Many authors have reported the disappearance of an obstruction in the intracranial arteries (168, 169). If the disintegration of occlusions is not encountered more commonly, it may be because examinations are not usually repeated for investigative purposes only.

If the emboli are composed of red thrombotic material, they first fragment and later are destroyed by lysis. In the experimental animal such lysis occurs in 6 to 24 h. If the embolic material is made up of fibrin and platelet aggregates, it will break up and disappear in minutes or perhaps in an hour or two.

At times, the actual embolus is clearly discernible. Emboli often get caught at a site of bifurcation, obstructing both branches (Fig. 10.75). When several branches are occluded, it is almost certain evidence of an embolic occlusion. The original occluding clot may have been single, but on fragmentation particles are carried more distally, so that more than one smaller branch becomes occluded. Thus it is important to look for evidence of multiple branch occlusions. A concave shape of the head of the contrast column is observed only occasionally. If the obstruction is complete, the contrast material more often progresses slowly distally in the occluded vessel and presents a tapered configuration as it advances. The concave configuration of an embolus is usually seen at a bifurcation when there is only a partial block and in the larger vessels, such as the trunks of the middle and anterior cerebral arteries. A primary thrombus within the lumen of an artery can sometimes be perceived if it is not producing complete obstruction.

The earlier an angiogram is carried out after onset of symptoms, the greater are the chances of demonstrating an obstructed intracranial artery (170).

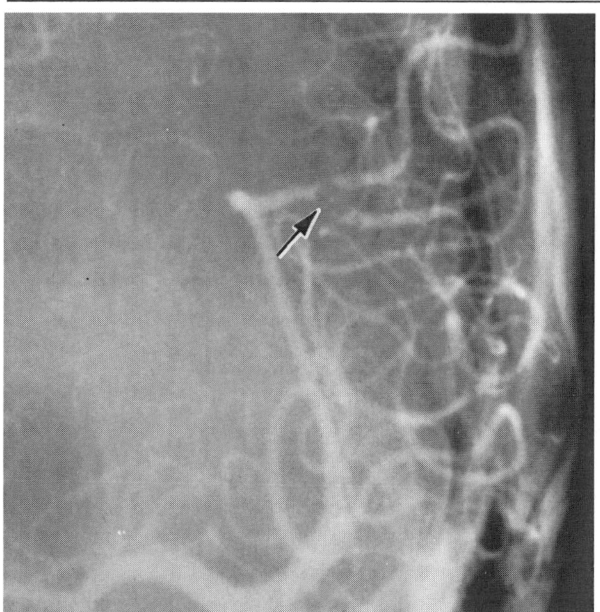

Figure 10.75. Saddle embolus in branches of the middle cerebral artery (arrow).

ANGIOGRAPHIC SIGNS OF CEREBRAL INFARCTION

The diagnosis of cerebral infarction is made by CT or MRI examination, as explained in text preceding. However, findings may be encountered on angiography, and for this reason it is considered useful to briefly describe some of the findings encountered on serial cerebral angiography.

1. *Arterial occlusions.* These were demonstrated in 19 out of the 40 cases of Taveras et al. (82).
2. *Effect of a mass secondary to swelling of the brain.* The edematous mass may be localized or may involve the entire hemisphere. It generally indicates a poorer prognosis and may be associated with a hemorrhagic infarction.
3. *Slowing of circulation.* This may be manifested as slow filling and emptying of one or more arterial branches opacified either directly or by collaterals. The slowing of the circulation may involve the entire hemisphere or, indeed, the entire brain. When the entire hemisphere is affected, it constitutes an important phenomenon that is poorly understood (171). (See Table 10.14.)

   Both the arterial and the arteriovenous circulation time are increased in patients with thrombosis. It is the author's impression that, proportionately, the arterial circulation time is increased more than the arteriovenous circulation time. The *collateral arterial circulation time,* measured as the time from appearance to disappearance of collateral channels, may last from 2 to 6 sec. A circulation time over 4 sec, however, is considered as excessively slow.

   Usually the contrast substance is still visible in collateral channels when it has disappeared from other arterial branches. In some cases, stasis and narrowing of the collateral vessels are observed. Pronounced stasis suggests thrombosis or sludging within distal branches or changes in brain tissue resulting in capillary block, either of which may impede normal flow. The phenomenon of *generalized stasis* in collateral channels is thought to indicate a bad prognosis. On the other hand, local stasis in collateral channels is not necessarily associated with a poor outlook. It is likely that local stasis is associated with damage to the perforating branches supplying the brain, with consequent diminished flow, and is one of the indications of an area of cerebral infarction.
4. *Local increase in the speed of circulation.* This is an important phenomenon that is attributed to the vasodilation occurring as a result of lowered oxygen tension with resultant decrease in tissue pH. The term *luxury perfusion syndrome* had been applied to this occurrence by Lassen (59). Angiographically it manifests itself by *early filling of local veins* and by vasodilatation, which produces dilated small arteries and various degrees of capillary blush that sometimes may simulate a tumor (Figs. 10.76 and 10.77). Whenever dilated small vessels ("anoxic vasodilation") and early venous filling are seen, they indicate *distressed cerebral circulation* locally. At times, the changes may be more generalized. Early-filling veins are seen only in the first 2 weeks following arterial occlusion. In the cases reported by Taveras et al., they were seen in 12 out of 30 cases, all in the first 2 weeks and in none of those examined after 15 days (82).

   It is surprising how quickly cerebral ischemia causes vasodilation. In one case in which an embolus was accidentally injected with the contrast material during carotid angiography, the embolus lodged in a distal branch of the middle cerebral artery. The serialogram disclosed that in 2 sec there was local early venous filling (Fig. 10.78). Thus vasodilation as a response to local lowering of tissue oxygen tension occurs extremely rapidly.
5. *Capillary blush or stain that is sometimes pronounced enough to suggest tumor.* It may be worth mentioning at this point that local hyperemia of the brain may be associated with status epilepticus. The hyperemia manifests itself on the angiogram as a blush with disruption of the local normal venous filling pattern. In the author's experience, it is seen only when the angiogram is performed while the patient is still in status and disappears soon thereafter (60). The same phenomenon has been observed by Yarnell et al. (172).
6. *An old infarct may be associated with local disruption of the arterial pattern.* The appearance may be entirely normal if there has been lysis of emboli.

Table 10.14.
Angiographic Findings in Stroke

Angiographic Findings in Stroke
Arterial occlusions
Displacement of vessels due to mass effect of the infarction
Slow arterial filling and emptying
Early venous filling
Occasionally increased capillary blush

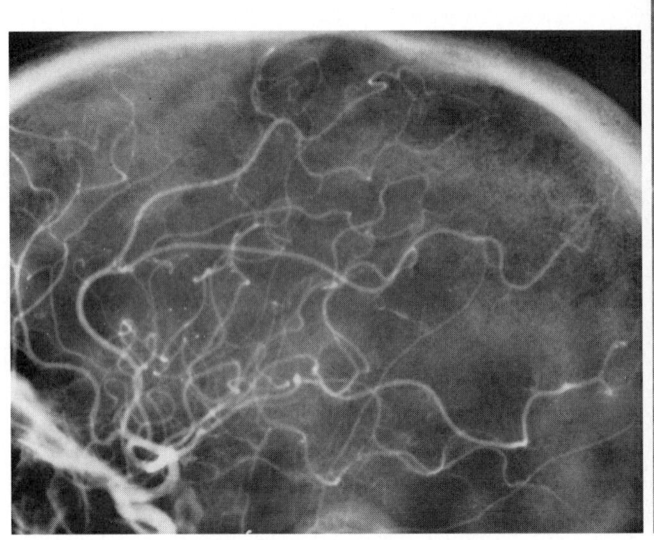

A

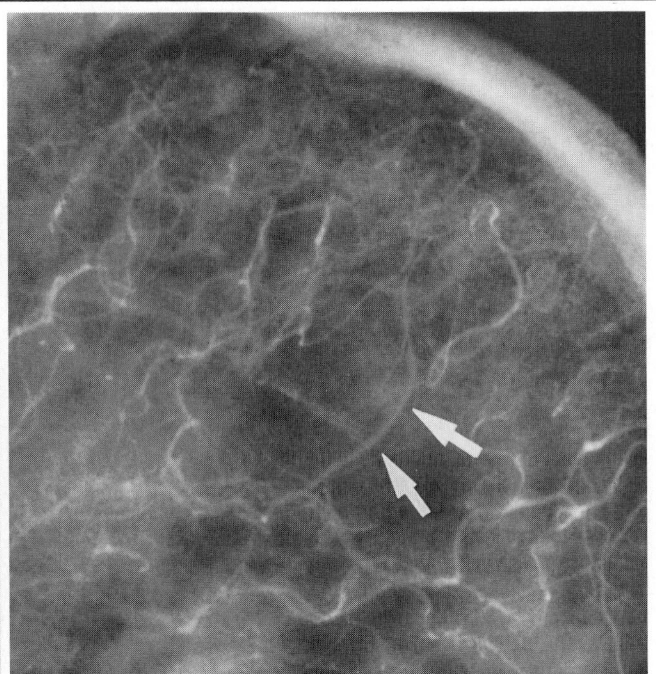

B

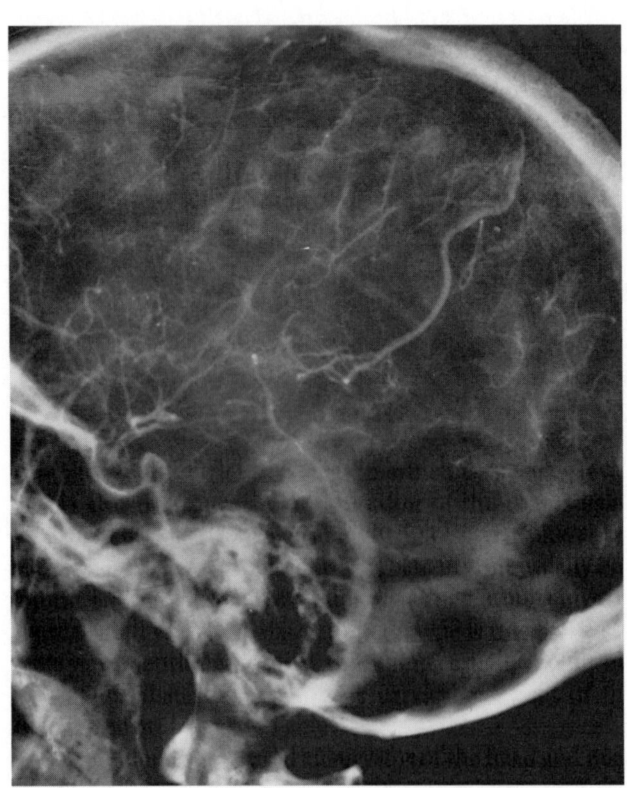

C

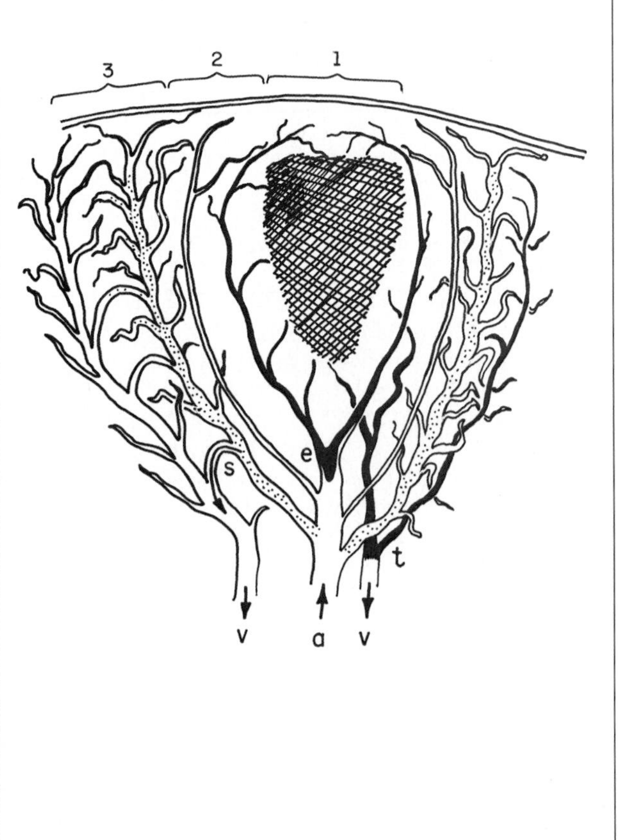

D

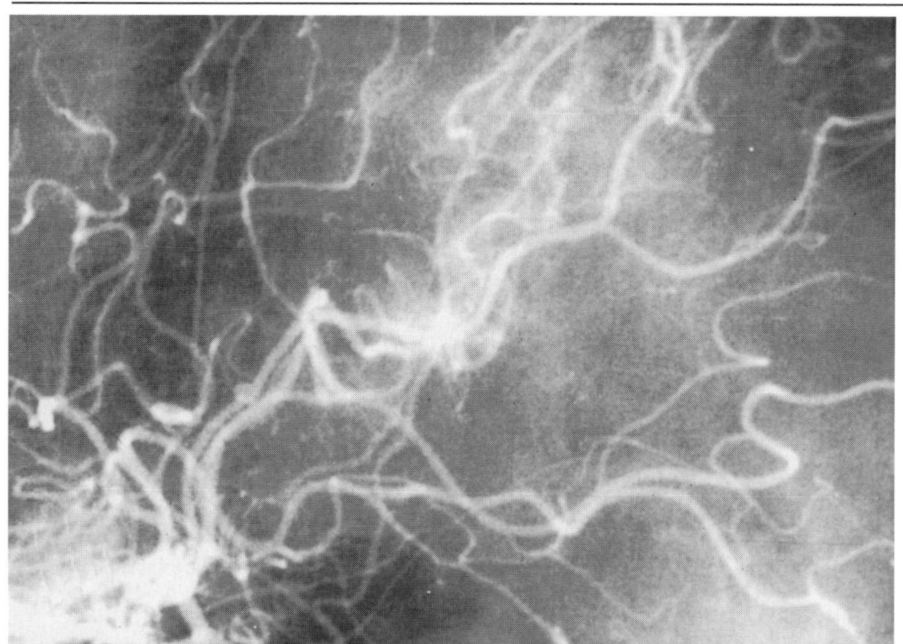

A

Figure 10.77. Luxury perfusion and early-filling vein in cerebral infarction. There is marked hyperemia as well as early filling of the vein in the posterior frontal region (arrows).

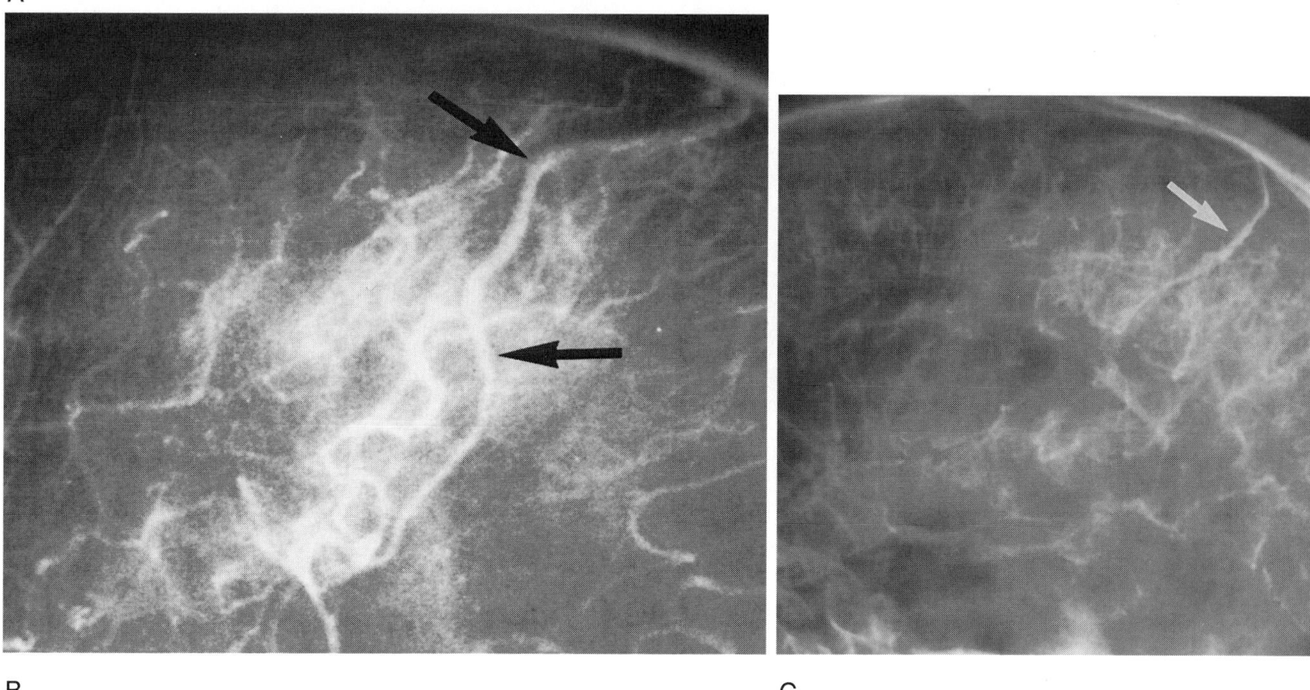

B C

Figure 10.76. Early-filling veins in cerebral infarction. **A.** There is an avascular area in the parietal region. **B.** The film made in the late arterial phase shows early filling of a superficial parietal vein (arrows) before any other vein is opacified. **C.** The early venous phase confirms the fact that the vein shown in B fills earlier than the others and now is denser than any other. An increased density of any vein, regardless of size, may be an indication of early filling and when observed requires careful scrutiny in the serialogram. **D.** The diagram shows some features of an infarct. A feeding artery (*a*) is occluded by an embolus (*e*). One draining vein (*v*) is filled with a secondary thrombus (*t*). The resulting central zone (*1*) is ischemic. Outside this is a zone of extravasation or edema (*2*) with thin, stretched, but patent vessels. If collateral circulation is adequate, a peripheral area of hyperemia develops (*3*); in this zone "shunts" (*s*) may open between the enlarged arterioles and patent venules.

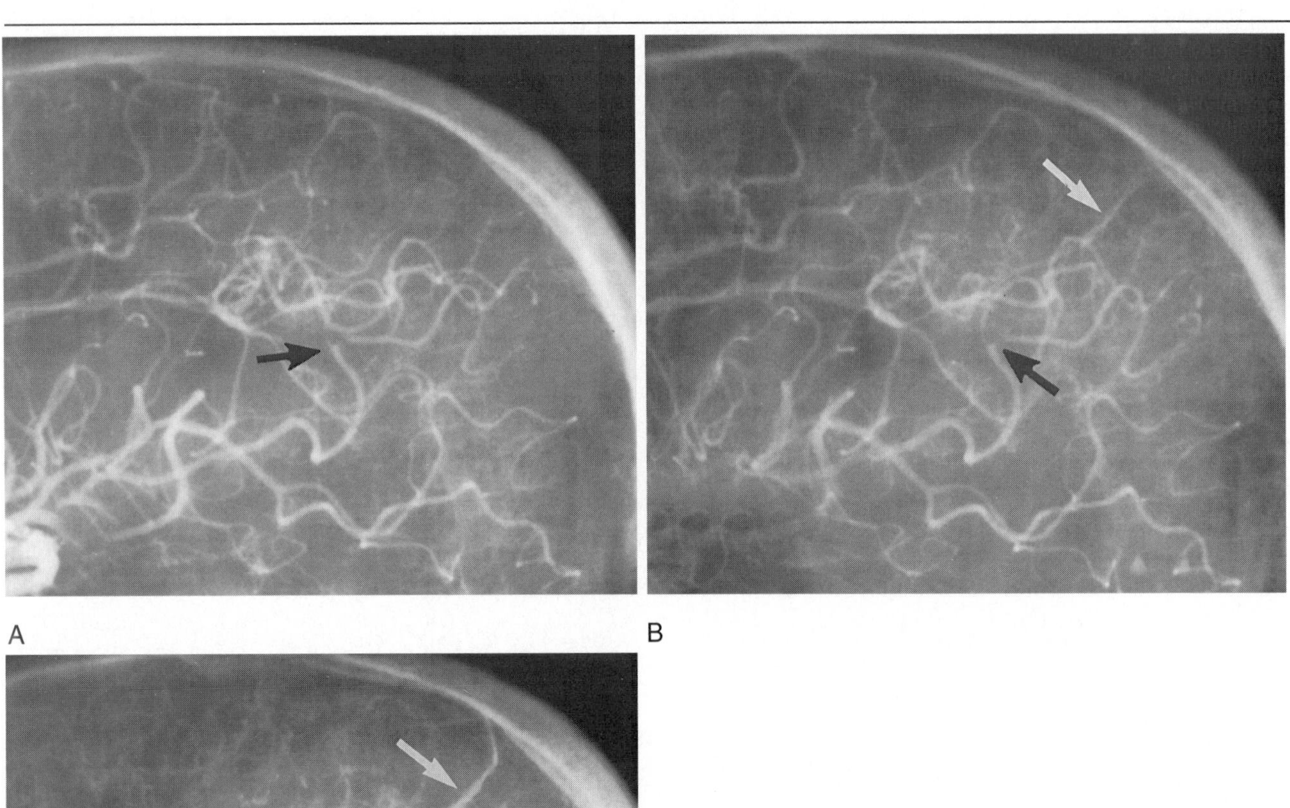

A B

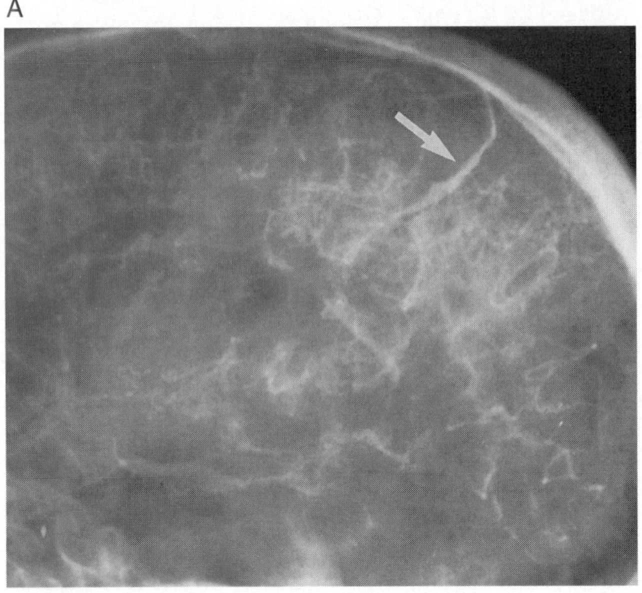

C

Figure 10.78. Early-filling vein appearing only seconds after inadvertent injection of "needle embolus" during angiography. **A.** At 0.5 sec the arterial phase is normal except for a filling defect at the bifurcation of the angular branch of the middle cerebral artery (arrow) and slower filling of the arteries beyond the "saddle embolus." **B** and **C.** At 2 sec further arterial filling beyond the embolus has occurred, indicating that the embolus (arrow in B) is only partially obstructing at this time. There is already filling of a parietal vein (white arrow in B), which becomes clearer on a film made 1 sec later (arrow in C).

CEREBRAL ARTERIOSCLEROSIS

The degree and frequency of involvement of the intracranial arteries vary in different parts of the world. In Japan, for instance, the frequency of atherosclerosis of the intracranial arteries is higher than in the United States and European countries. Elongation of the arteries is a common manifestation of arteriosclerosis. The basilar artery is one of the most frequently observed examples of this manifestation. However, branches of the vertebral-basilar system as well as of the internal carotid arteries frequently show elongation that results in increases in the curves of the arteries as they course to their destinations. Tortuosity of certain arteries may be seen in younger subjects that is not necessarily associated with arteriosclerosis. The tortuosity of some of the arteries of the posterior fossa has been associated with certain symptoms, such as hemifacial spasm and trigeminal neuralgia (173, 174). The condition may be corrected by surgical mobilization of the tortuous artery. Although angiography is the method ordinarily employed to study these cases, recent reports indicate the feasibility of utilizing MRA (175, 176). Flow voids produced by tortuous arteries may be demonstrated on coronal images of the brainstem near the root entry zone of the facial (seventh) nerve. The artery may be a tortuous vertebral or a posterior inferior (PICA) or anterior inferior cerebellar (AICA) artery. The demonstration can be improved by superimposing a coronal collapsed view of an MRA on the T1-weighted coronal image, as shown by Tien and Wilkins (176). CT examination with small quantities of air in the cerebellopontine angle has also been proposed and sometimes yields information not readily demonstrated by angiography (177).

CEREBRAL VEINS AND DURAL SINUSES

Thrombosis of the dural sinuses and of the deep veins is probably more common than is recognized. The obstruction causes increased intracranial pressure, which is the most common manifestation. Frank hemiplegia suggesting stroke is uncommon, but a variety of neurologic manifestations, including convulsions, may be encountered. As a result of obstruction of a sinus, there is back-pressure of blood in the cerebral veins, which leads to hypoxia of cerebral tissue and even to hemorrhage.

Sinus thrombosis may be the result of inflammation, such as meningitis, either tuberculous or nonspecific. It may be seen following an infection of the mastoid or paranasal sinuses, or it may be associated with dehydration and cachexia, particularly in infants and young children. Venous thrombosis also may be seen in the postpartum period and in some cases may be associated with hemic disorders, such as polycythemia and sickle cell disease. Birth control pills often cause alterations of clotting factors. A small percentage of women taking oral contraceptives have strokes that may be produced by venous thromboses or arterial occlusions (178). The stroke is often preceded by severe headaches, which should serve as warnings against the further ingestion of contraceptive pills.

Retrograde thrombosis of cerebral veins starting at the sinuses is not uncommon. In the case of thrombosis of the lateral sinuses, only intracranial hypertension may result. Extrinsic pressure on the sinus may produce the same effect. Occlusion of the superior longitudinal sinus by meningiomas may not lead to retrograde venous thromboses because it occurs slowly. Sinus occlusion may also result from direct invasion of the sinus by an adjacent malignant bone lesion, such as a neuroblastoma (see Fig. 6.13*E* to *H*). Trauma is also an important cause of obstruction of the dural sinuses.

Dural sinus thrombosis can be diagnosed by CT if typical findings can be demonstrated. The "empty delta" sign has been described as a typical appearance (179) and consists of enhancement of the periphery of the superior sagittal sinus on an enhanced CT scan and failure to enhance the central portion because of clotting (Fig. 10.79).

Care should be taken in interpreting the delta sign. Ulmer and Elster have demonstrated that, in a postcontrast examination in which a delay occurs between contrast injection and CT scanning (possibly 20 to 50 min), the dural enhancement in the wall of the sinus will simulate a delta sign almost exactly like the one seen in dural sinus thrombosis (180). The dura enhances routinely and in some patients more than in others. As the blood concentration of contrast decreases and that of the dura increases, the dura in cross section may be denser than the flowing blood.

In addition to the "empty delta" sign, venous thrombosis may be seen as hyperdense veins near the superior sagittal sinus before contrast injection. Small or larger hemorrhages may be observed in the same areas. Venous infarction manifested as edema may be seen. Deep venous thrombosis may be seen in association with straight sinus occlusion, and in that case central edema may be seen simulating a mass. Accompanying hemorrhage should help in making a diagnosis. CT with contrast or MRI without or with contrast would probably lead to the proper diagnosis.

In young infants the lateral and superior sagittal sinuses in the region of the torcular are usually fairly dense, without contrast material, in relation to brain density. This is a normal appearance and should not be confused with possible thrombosis of the dural sinuses. It is probably related to the fact that the newborn infant has a high concentration of water in the brain tissue, which would make the blood-containing sinuses relatively denser (see Fig. 5.11).

Sinus as well as venous thrombosis can be suspected and usually diagnosed by MRI (181, 182). MRI is frequently being used when searching for dural sinus thrombosis, but care must be taken because flow-related artifacts are common. Sze et al. have described a spin-echo technique using T1- and T2-weighted images in axial, sagittal, and coronal views (183). Hyperintensity on T1- and T2-weighted images raises the question of clotting within the sinuses, which should be differentiated from flow-related enhancement. A gradient-echo flow sequence is probably the easiest and most useful. Venous MR angiography has also been suggested. Flow appears as a high-intensity area, and lack of flow would be low intensity (Figs. 10.80 and 10.81; see also Fig. 6.13*E* to *H*). However, conventional angiography is still needed when doubt remains following CT or MRI examination (Table 10.15).

Sonography has been suggested in the newborn, and an echogenic pattern of the torcular has been described (184). Cerebral angiography is often needed to obtain a definitive

Table 10.15.
Dural Sinus Thrombosis

Most common causes
- Dehydration
- Intracranial infection
- Oral contraceptive use or postpartum state
- Hypercoagulable states

Clinical manifestations
- Pseudotumor cerebri syndrome (headaches, papilledema, visual disturbance)
- Infarction due to retrograde venous thrombosis

CT imaging findings
- Occasionally hyperdense cortical veins and infarction on noncontrast CT
- "Empty delta" sign on contrast-enhanced CT

MR imaging findings
- Usually hyperintense signal within dural sinus on T1- and T2-weighted images

Contrast angiography findings
- Nonopacification of dural sinus, occasionally enlargement or nonopacification of superificial or deep veins

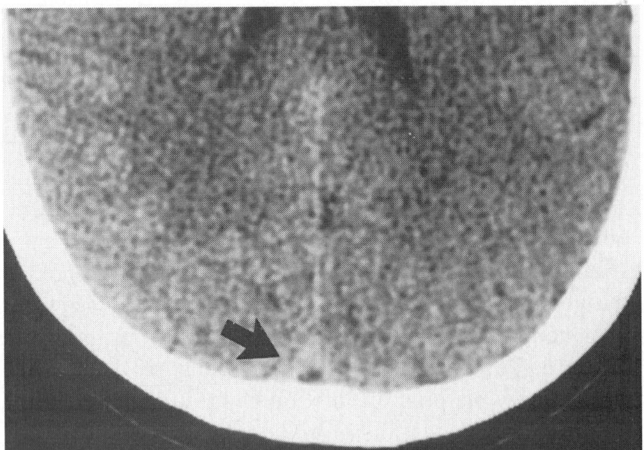

Figure 10.79. Thrombosis of superior sagittal sinus. "Empty delta" sign on enhanced CT. **A.** Prior to enhancement (arrow). **B.** After enhancement. There is evidence of thickening of the falx, and the wall of the sinus is thick. A hypodense center is seen (arrow). **C.** The hypodensity along the center of the sinus is well seen in the top image (arrows).

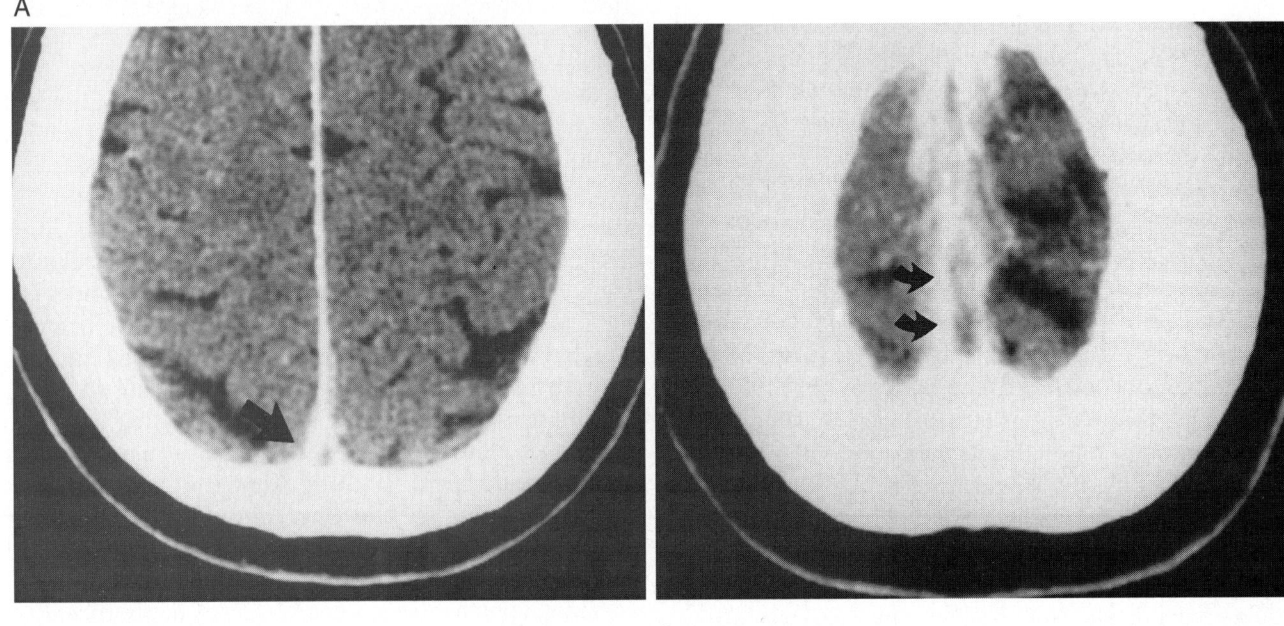

diagnosis in suspected cases because the diagnosis may be only suspected on CT or MRI. Examples of angiographic appearances are shown in Figures 10.82 and 10.83.

Cavernous sinus thrombosis is an important complication of infection in the periorbital area and in the nasal and paranasal sinuses, and is due to retrograde progression of infection through veins of the orbit and face that may drain through the cavernous sinuses (Fig. 10.84). The diagnosis can be made by CT without and with contrast. Enlargement of the sinus on the thrombosed side may be demonstrated. The thrombosed portions will not enhance. In the presence of an appropriate clinical history, the appearance is diagnostic. However, other lesions, particularly neoplasms (lymphoma, metastasis), may present a similar configuration on CT. Other more indolent inflammatory conditions, such as the Tolosa-Hunt syndrome, may also present enlargement of the sinus on one side (see Fig. 11.68).

Carotid angiography may be used to demonstrate an obstruction of the dural sinuses, particularly if an increased amount of contrast material is used and compression of the side opposite the injection is carried out. Occlusion of the sinuses may also be demonstrated by means of a sinogram. Doppler ultrasonography has been advocated by Brisman et al. to measure blood velocity in the superior longitudinal sinus (185).

The angiographic findings may be divided into two categories. First, the carotid and vertebral injections almost invariably demonstrate a normal arterial pattern, with the possible exception of some lengthening of the arterial phase. The obstruction of the sinuses may not be too clearly shown unless good bilateral filling is obtained by compressing the contralateral carotid artery and an increased amount of contrast is injected. The sinus obstruction may be partial, but the thrombosis may extend to the cortical veins (Fig. 10.83). In the deep venous thromboses there is

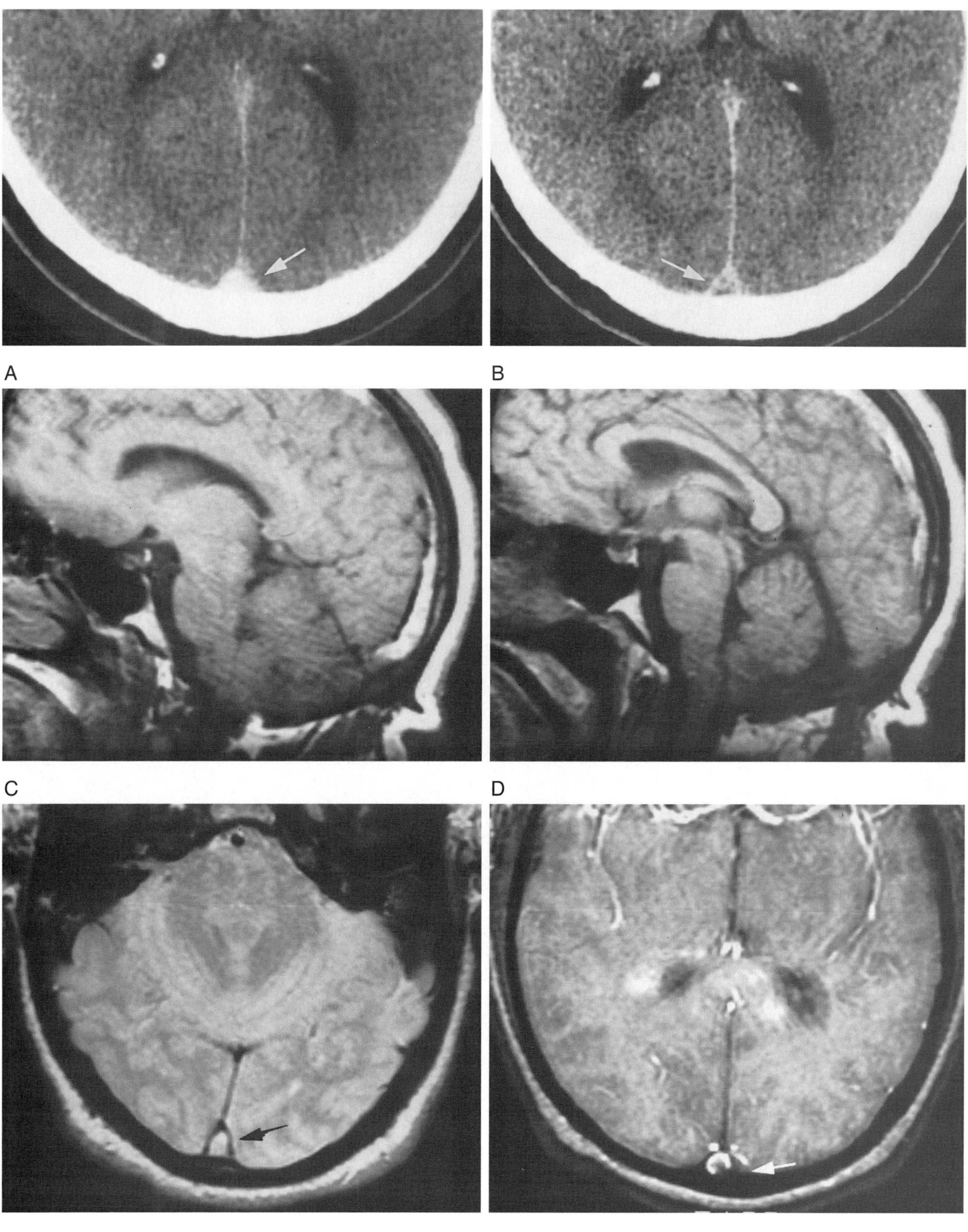

Figure 10.80. Thrombosis of superior sagittal sinus in a 42-year-old woman who also had pulmonary emboli. **A.** The first CT examination with contrast showed a normal appearance. The superior sagittal sinus was completely opacified (arrow). **B.** Repeat examination 6 days later with contrast now shows that the wall of the sinus is opacified but the lumen is not, indicating possible lack of flow ("empty delta" sign) (arrow). An MRI carried out at that time shows a bright superior sagittal sinus on T1-weighted image (**C** and **D**). A proton density axial image (**E**) revealed no evidence of a flow void in the sinus, which was hyperintense (arrow). **F.** A flow sequence axial image shows partial flow in sinus combined with absent flow (arrow).

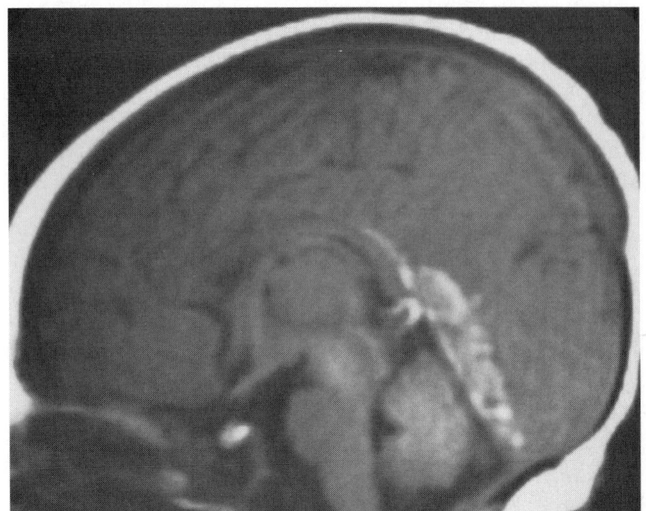

A

Figure 10.81. Thrombosis of straight sinus and draining veins in a 6-day-old infant, probably associated with dehydration. **A.** Sagittal T1-weighted image shows hyperintensity in straight sinus and in subependymal veins, consistent with clot formation. **B.** Axial T2-weighted image shows diffuse hyperintensity in the posterior half of both hemispheres and marked hypointensity in the region of the straight sinus, consistent with intracellular methemoglobin in view of the bright signal in A. **C.** A CT done the following day reveals hyperdensity in the anterior half of the straight sinus and in the internal cerebral veins, shown also in **D.** Subependymal vein thrombosis is also shown by CT in **E.** The infant was immediately placed on active anticoagulant therapy and recovered.

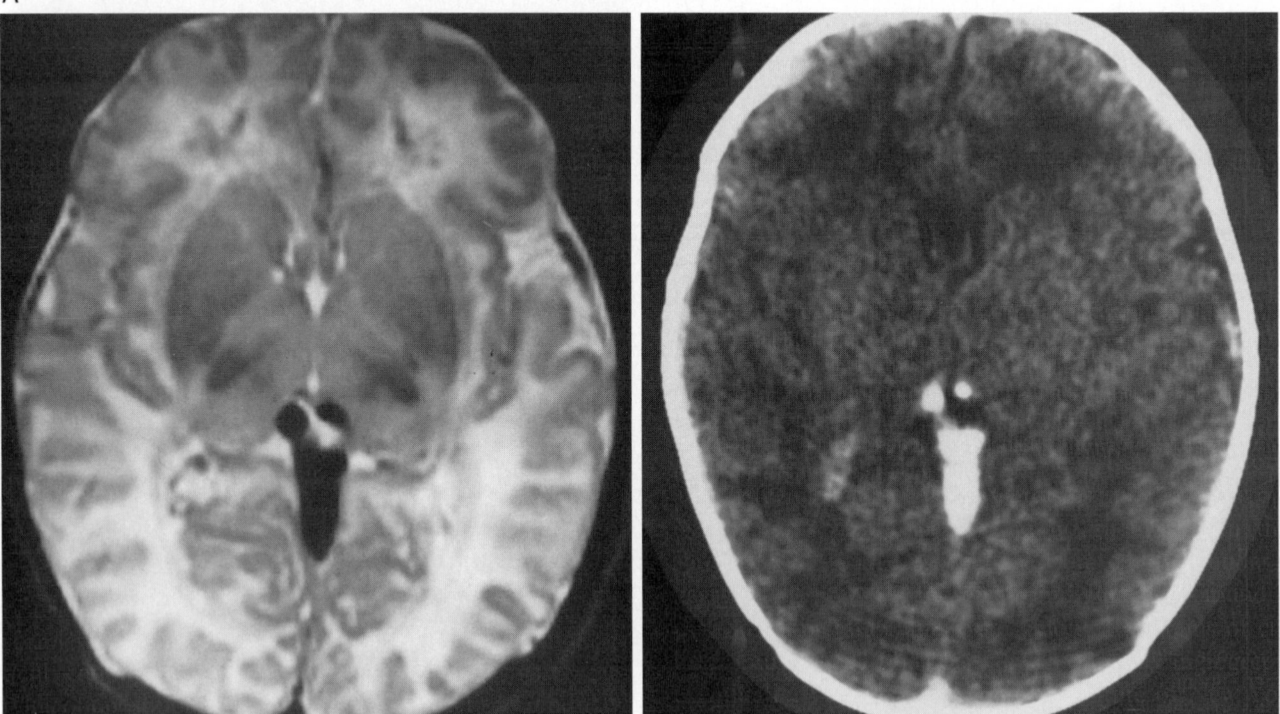

B C

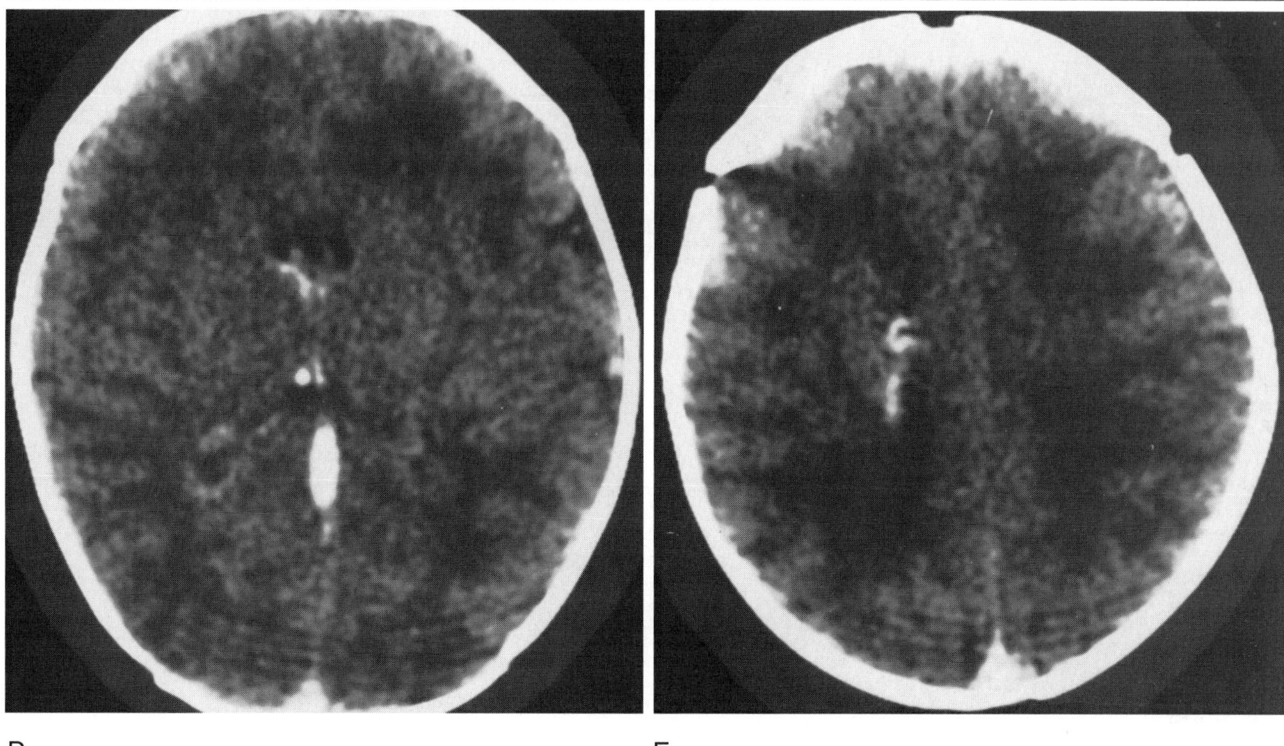

D E

Figure 10.81. *(continued)*

central edema of the brain, usually bilateral but sometimes more pronounced unilaterally, which may lead to an erroneous diagnosis of tumor (Fig. 10.82*D* and *E*). Failure of filling of the deep veins or of the straight sinus associated with delayed venous emptying and collateral venous flow is usually encountered (Fig. 10.82).

Second, jugular venography may be used to confirm the findings of sinus thrombosis (Fig. 10.83). When opacification of the jugular vein is carried out (while compressing the vein below the injection site), some intracranial filling of the lateral sinus on the same side and of the superior sagittal and straight sinuses is normally obtained, provided that a sufficient amount of contrast (about 15 to 20 ml) is employed. Sometimes a clot can even be demonstrated within the jugular vein (Fig. 10.83).

The venous phase of the angiogram may show enlargement of many of the superficial venous channels that usually are not conspicuous. This is due to enlargement of numerous small anastomotic veins (joined like a network) between the superior and the inferior major draining veins. The appearance of these veins is characteristic of sinus occlusion (Fig. 10.82*A* and *B*). If the patient survives, recanalization of the sinuses is the rule, but this may take some time to be accomplished. The margins of a recanalized sinus usually are irregular. In some cases, angiography after recanalization may show only the residual dilated network of surface veins. When this is found, a diagnosis of old sinus thrombosis is justifiable even if no clear history is obtainable, for the thrombotic episode may have occurred during infancy.

Thrombosis of the sinuses and of the jugular veins may be found in children with a diagnosis of *pseudotumor cerebri.* Thus an angiogram should be performed with a long series of exposures and a careful search made for partial or complete sinus or jugular veins occlusion. Jugular venography should be performed as well, possibly via the brachiocephalic veins, to detect lower obstructions to the jugular flow, if it appears indicated (186, 187).

ARTERIAL ANEURYSMS

General Considerations

An aneurysm is usually defined as an abnormal dilatation of an artery. In the past, luetic aneurysms of the aorta were the most commonly encountered lesions. Now that luetic aneurysms have been eliminated, in large part through the use of antibiotics, cerebral lesions are the most commonly encountered aneurysms in the human body. In most cases, the lesions are found along the course of medium-sized arteries at the base of the brain. At other times, however, small arteries are affected by the development of miliary or microaneurysms, especially in patients with hypertension. In patients with arteriovenous malformations, venous aneurysms may develop.

Arterial aneurysms may be considered in relation to their general location, which influences the symptoms they pro-

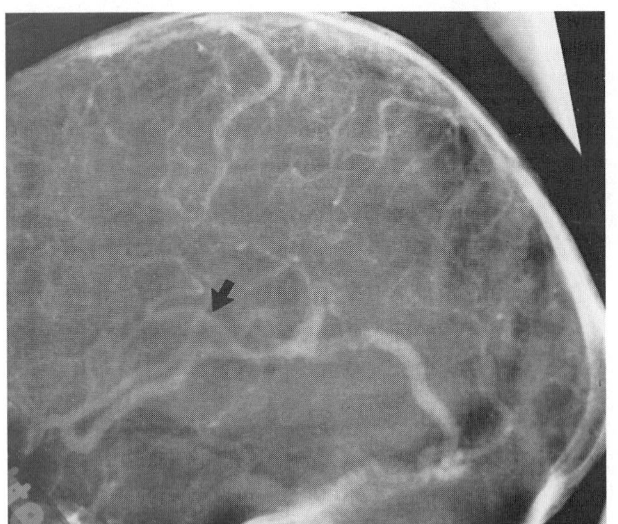

Figure 10.82. **A** to **C.** Sinus thrombosis showing extension 1 week later. **A.** There is obstruction of the superior longitudinal sinus posteriorly. The straight sinus is not seen, but the deep veins are visualized (arrow). **B.** Reexamination a week later, following a course of urokinase after which the child seemed to improve, reveals better visualization of the cortical veins, but there is now thrombosis of deep veins (arrows) that previously appeared to be normal. There are now numerous cortical veins serving as collateral channels to bypass the obstructions. **C.** The frontal venogram also shows failure of the superior longitudinal sinus to opacify (arrow). **D** and **E.** Deep venous thrombosis in a 15-month-old infant. **D.** The lateral venous phase from the carotid angiogram demonstrates complete absence of deep venous filling. Most of the deep circulation is draining by way of the large vein of Labbé. Fine subependymal veins are seen outlining part of the ventricular wall (arrows). **E.** Lateral view from a vertebral angiogram demonstrates widening of the curve of the lateral posterior choroidal arteries (arrows) indicative of a central mass effect due to edema.

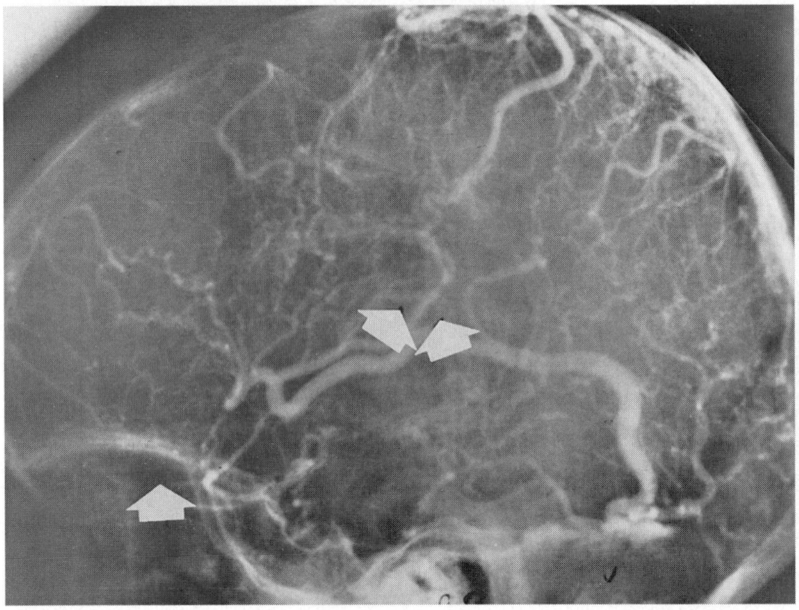

A

B

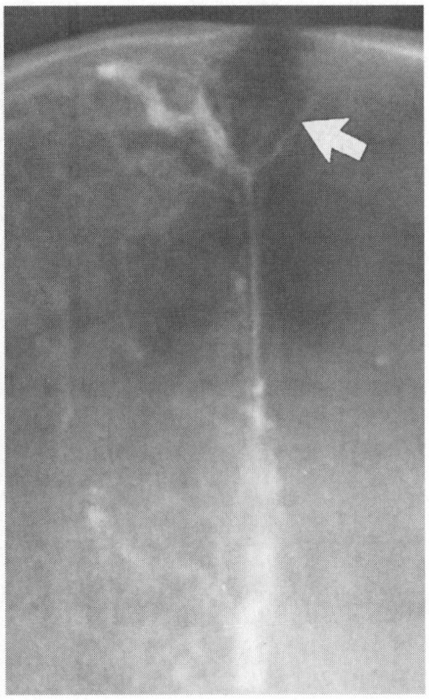

C

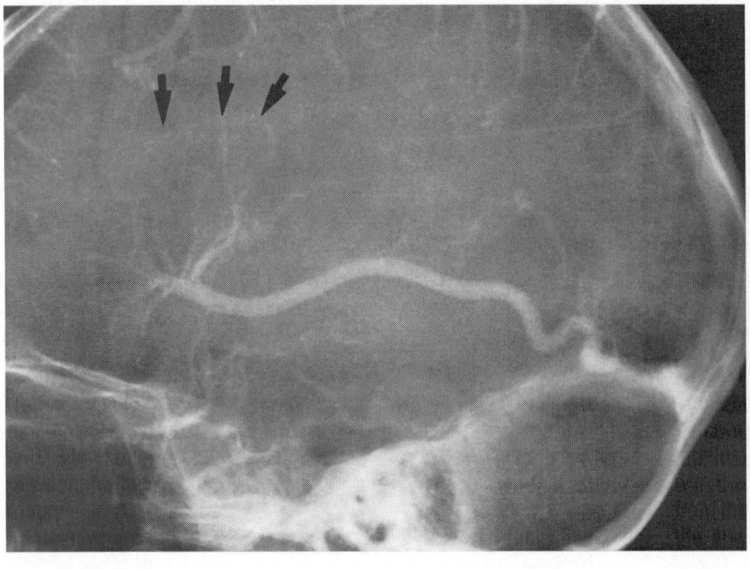

D

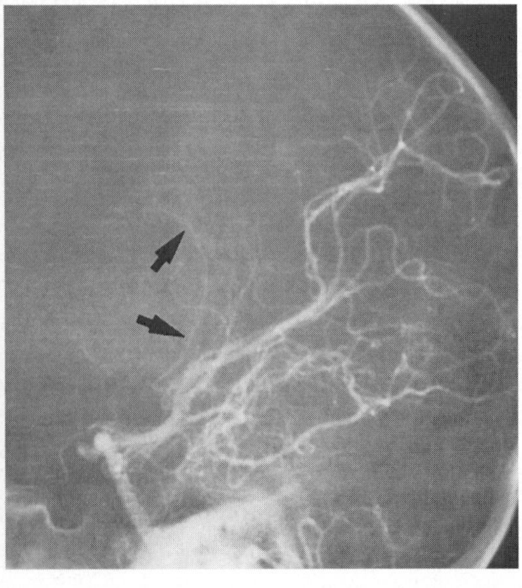

E

Figure 10.83. Almost complete thrombotic occlusion of superior longitudinal sinus extending into cortical vein in a 45-year-old man. **A.** Normal arterial phase. **B.** Occlusion of the vein of Trolard is present before it joins the superior sagittal sinus (arrow). **C.** The frontal view of the venous phase discloses a radiolucency within the sinus with contrast outlining both walls of the sinus (arrows). **D.** The oblique view confirms the appearance and demonstrates patent inferior longitudinal and straight sinuses (arrow). The deep veins are normal (small anterior arrow). The illness started with headache, paresthesias in the right arm, and a generalized convulsive seizure. **E** to **I.** Thrombosed cortical vein without evidence of superior sagittal sinus occlusion in a patient who suffered a convulsive seizure. **E** and **F.** Precontrast sagittal and postcontrast coronal T1-weighted images reveal a hyperintense oval cortical lesion, which was thought to represent a thrombosed vein (arrow).

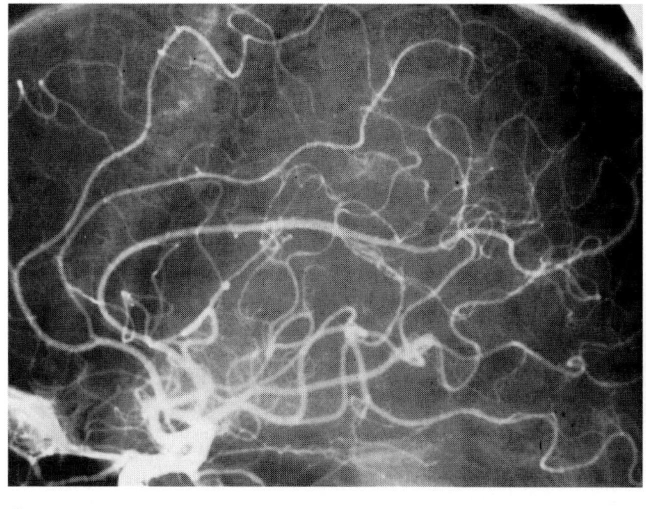

A

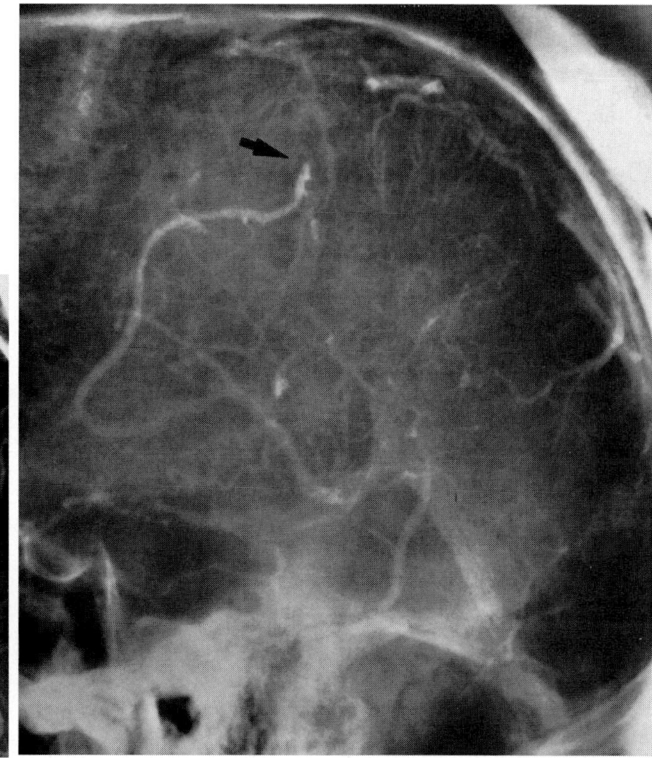

B

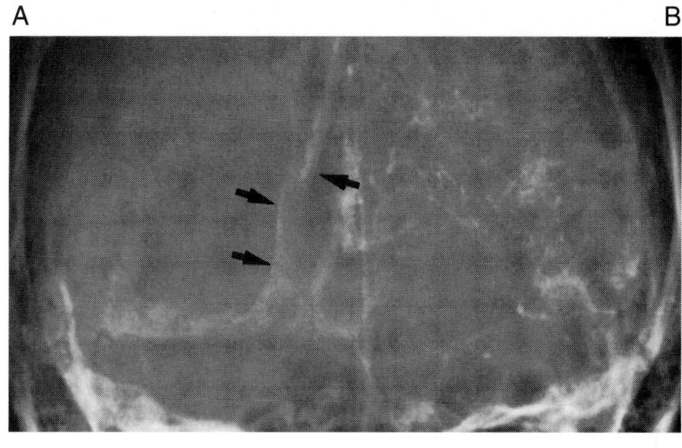

C

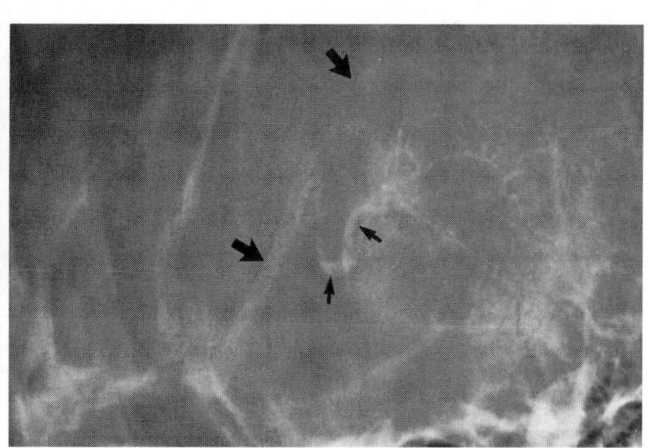

D

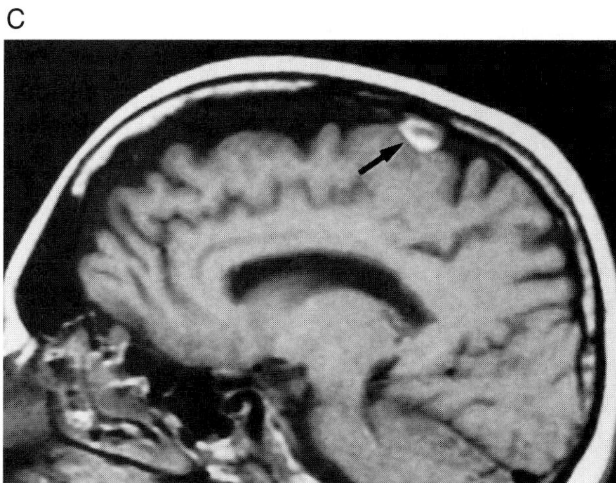

E

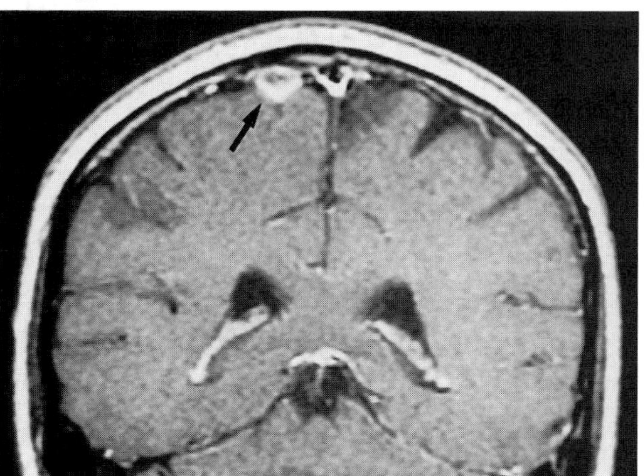

F

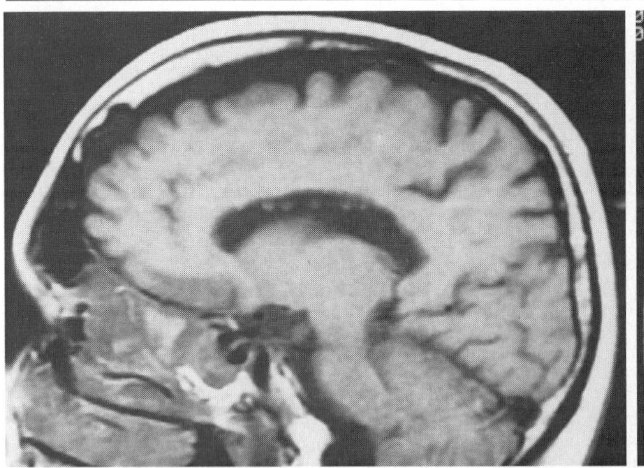

G

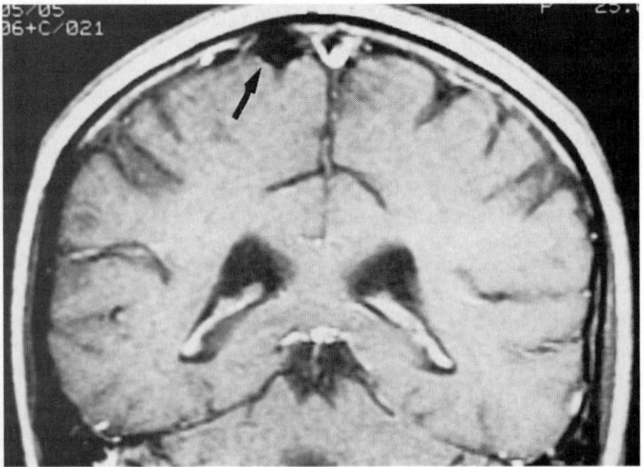

H

I

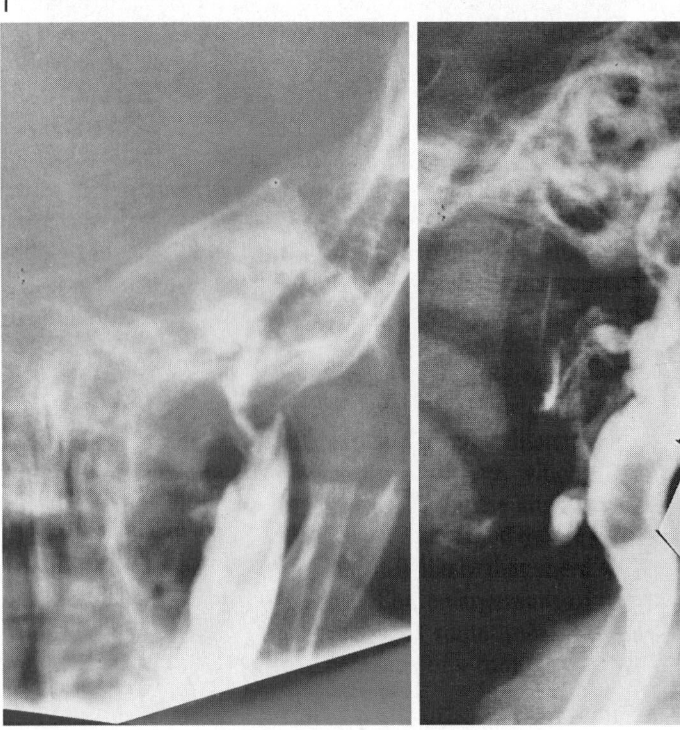

J

K

Figure 10.83. *(continued)* **G** and **H.** Repeat examination 4 months later without and with contrast showed disappearance of the hyperintense lesion. In the coronal postcontrast view there is a hypointense area in the location of the previously demonstrated abnormality (arrow). **I.** Coronal T2-weighted image shows evidence of magnetic susceptibility consistent with old blood products. **J** and **K.** Thrombus in jugular vein in a child with dural sinus thrombosis (same case as in Fig. 10.82 A to C). **J.** The jugular venogram shows failure of contrast to enter the jugular bulb. **K.** There is a clot hanging within the jugular vein (arrows).

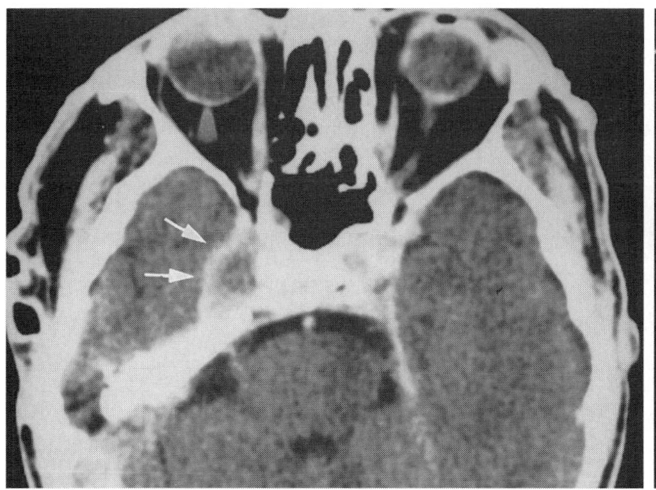

A

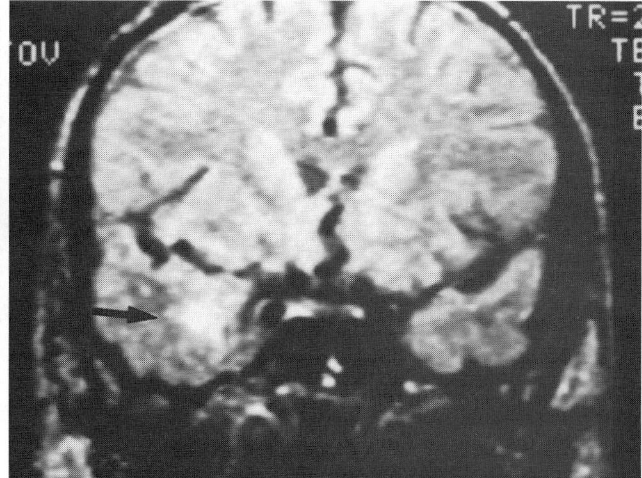

B

Figure 10.84. Thrombosis of cavernous sinus. A. Enhanced CT scan shows bulging of the right cavernous sinus as compared to the other side (arrows). There is enhancement of the periphery but not of the central portion of the sinus. B. MR proton density weighted shows hyperintensity in the medial right temporal lobe (arrow) due to edema. The normal carotid flow void is present. C. Repeat contrast CT examination several weeks later shows a decrease in the bulging right cavernous sinus, but there is still enhancement of the wall extending posteriorly toward the tentorial edge.

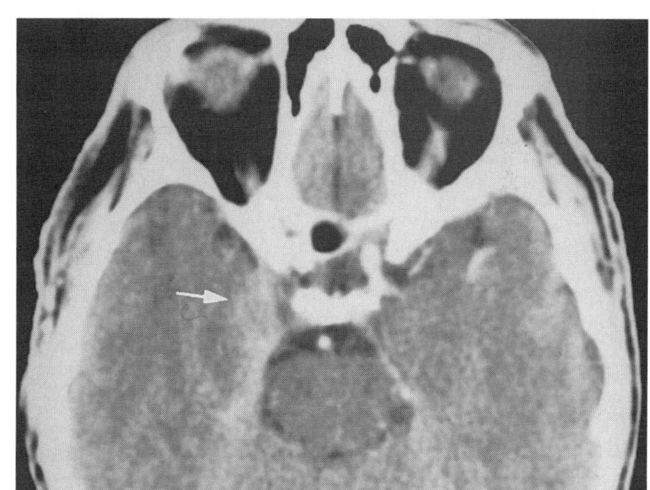

C

duce, or according to their presumed mode of origin. If the former grouping is used, they could be classified as (a) cervical, (b) intracranial extradural, or (c) intracranial intradural. Aneurysms of the major cervical arteries may present only as pulsating masses; at other times a spontaneous dissection may develop, producing severe pain and cerebral ischemia. Intracranial extradural aneurysms are principally those of the cavernous sinus, which may produce mass effects or a carotid cavernous fistula if the aneurysm ruptures. Although some intracranial intradural aneurysms may present as mass lesions, the vast majority are encountered because of subarachnoid hemorrhage. Indeed, in 72 percent of patients with subarachnoid hemorrhage, an arterial aneurysm is the cause of the bleeding. Arteriovenous malformations were found to account for 10 percent of subarachnoid hemorrhages, and primary intracerebral hemorrhages to account for 12 percent of cases of subarachnoid bleeding; in 6 percent of cases a subarachnoid hemorrhage remained unexplained in spite of thorough angiographic investigation.

From the etiologic standpoint, it is thought that the majority of aneurysms develop as a result of a congenital anomaly, presumably a congenital weakness of the vessel wall, permitting a localized berrylike evagination to occur (Fig. 10.85). A second type of aneurysm is the result of atherosclerosis, which produces a fusi-form dilatation of one of the larger arteries. Intracranially, the basilar artery is most frequently affected. The third type is caused by trauma, but such lesions are also referred to as "false" aneurysms since they are the result of dehiscence of the vascular wall. The congenital or saccular lesions and the atherosclerotic fusi-form dilatations are considered "true" aneurysms because elements of all three of the arterial layers can be identified, at least microscopically, even though with the saccular aneurysms the tunica media is developmentally defective. Fourth, an aneurysm may develop because of embolism, the smaller peripheral arteries of the brain being most frequently affected. The arterial wall may be partially destroyed by a septic embolus with the development of a "mycotic" aneurysm. Neoplastic emboli frequently occur

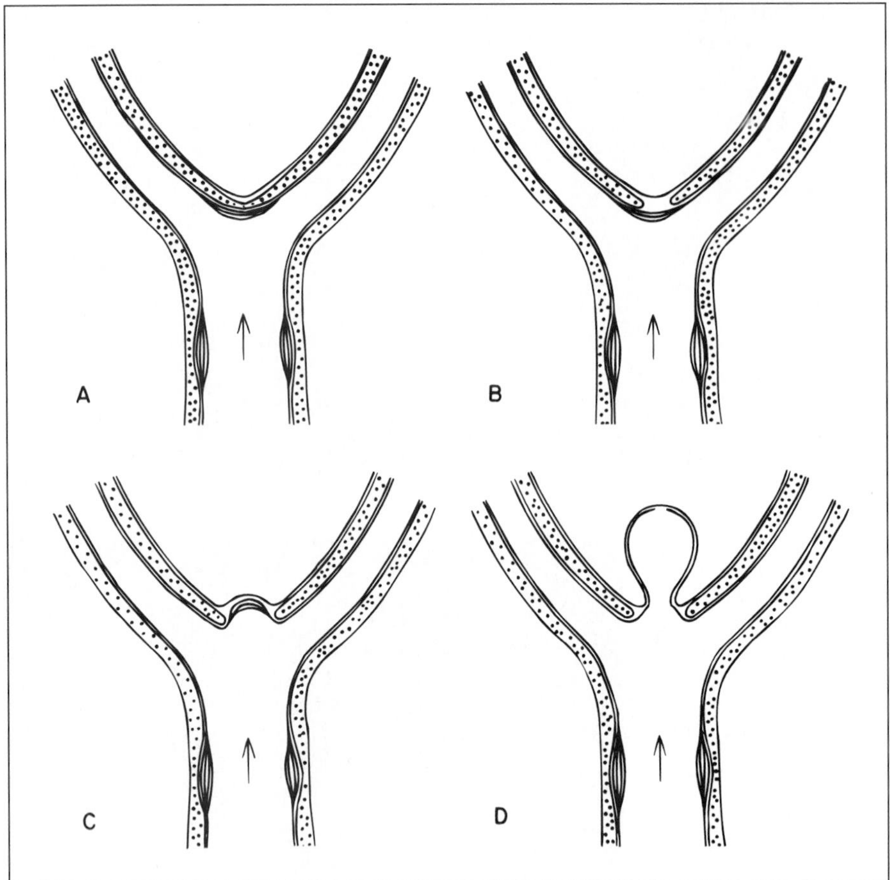

Figure 10.85. Mechanism of the development of an aneurysm. **A.** The bifurcation of a normal artery is represented. The stippled portion of the vessel wall indicates the lamellae of smooth muscle and elastic tissue of the tunica media disposed circularly around the vessel. The sites of the intimal pads are also shown. **B.** A medial defect is present in the fork of a faulty artery with discontinuity of the muscular and elastic fibers. **C.** Evagination of the tunica intima and tunica adventitia has begun at the site of the medial defect. **D.** A well-developed saccular aneurysm is now present in the fork of the artery. The tunica intima is stretched to the point of discontinuity. The lumen is contained at the fundus only by the connective tissue and external elastic lamina of the tunica adventitia.

in patients with atrial myxoma, in which case the arterial wall is also destroyed by proliferation of the tumor cells. A fifth aneurysmal lesion, also involving the peripheral cerebral vessels, is the miliary or microaneurysm, usually encountered in hypertension and in occlusive lesions involving the small vessels. A sixth etiologic type is the dissecting aneurysm mentioned in text preceding, usually found involving the distal portion of the cervical segment of the internal carotid artery (Table 10.16).

The incidence of arterial aneurysms of the head and neck may be higher than we think. Reliable statistics are available only for intracranial saccular or berry aneurysms. The first clear idea of the frequency of aneurysms was established by Crompton, who carefully searched at autopsy for aneurysms studied by angiography during life (188). Using this correlation, he found that approximately 7 percent of patients coming to necropsy have saccular aneurysms. By carrying out postmortem cerebral arterial injections routinely, radiographing the brain, and then dissecting the brain, Wollschlaeger and Wollschlaeger found that 10.6 percent of approximately 1000 patients dying of all causes in their institution had saccular aneurysms (167). Some other investigators have reported the incidence to be as high as 14 percent, and this would seem to be a reasonable figure if all types of aneurysms are included.

Of interest in Wollschlaeger's data are that (a) slightly more than 20 percent of the aneurysms found had ruptured while almost 80 percent were unruptured; (b) more unruptured aneurysms were found in men than in women, whereas the clinical incidence of bleeding stands at two to one in favor of women; and (c) there is an increased number of aneurysms with advancing age, with rupture most common between 40 and 60 years. The available statistics on the occurrence of aneurysms in children indicate a low incidence. Riggs and Rupp, who found a 9 percent incidence of aneurysms in 1437 necropsy examinations of the brain, had no aneurysms in their series among the 102 specimens from children under 10 years of age (189). Housepian and Pool also found no cases of intracranial aneurysm among the brains of children examined (190); however, among the angiographic examinations at the Neurological Institute of New York, approximately 1 percent of patients with aneurysms have been under the age of 10 years.

From comparative pathologic studies, subarachnoid hemorrage is known to be a rare occurrence in animals. Aneurysms are found most frequently in primates and in other animals with relatively large brains (see text following under "Intracranial Intradural Aneurysms").

Table 10.16.
Types of Aneurysms, by Etiology, and Associated Conditions

Type of Aneurysm	Factors	Associated Conditions	Comment
1. Berry	Media or elastic defects and or degeneration, flow stresses, arteriosclerotic vascular disease	Ehlers-Danlos, familial, adult polycystic disease, coarctation of the aorta, arteriovenous malformations, fibromuscular disease, agenesis of the carotid, arterial anomalies of the carotid	Occurs at branching points of proximal intracranial cerebral arteries
2. Atherosclerotic	Medial degeneration or absence	Atherosclerosis and hypertension, corpus callosum lipoma	Usually occurs on the vertebral basilar system
3. Trauma (dissections and penetrating)	Spontaneous dissection of cystic degeneration of media		Vertebral site most common, young age, headache, antecedent trauma
	Penetrating trauma		Usually fatal
4. Mycotic	Septic degeneration of media	Subacute bacterial endocarditis, cerebral infarctions	Treat infection, serial angiogram, if aneurysm grows → treat
5. Tumor	Tumor invasion of media	Atrial myxoma	
6. Dissecting	Trauma (?spontaneous)		Diagnosed by MRA, angiography

Cervical Aneurysms

Aneurysmal lesions affecting the major vessels of the neck may be congenital, dissecting, or traumatic. In the case of *congenital* lesions very large sacculations may develop that present as gradually enlarging pulsatile masses, usually in the upper neck. The majority encountered by neuroradiologists arise from the internal carotid artery. In some cases, similar lesions arise from the external carotid system; at other times, such an aneurysm can originate from a branch of the thyrocervical trunk or other neck vessels. Multiple aneurysms are sometimes encountered (191).

The saccular lesions usually develop near the midportion of the cervical internal carotid artery. In some cases, there is an adjacent kink or knuckle of the vessel, which some investigators believe is caused by a congenital band. This kinking, together with histologic study of the vascular structures when excised, supports the belief that such aneurysms are on the basis of a congenital mural defect. A congenital band deforming the artery from the time of embryonic development could conceivably be related to a medial defect of the vessel wall occurring at a site where no arterial branching occurs.

At angiography, a large, oval sac filling with contrast material is usually observed along the course of the internal carotid artery, most frequently at the C3 or C4 vertebral level (Fig. 10.86). In some cases, the artery curves around the aneurysmal sac and, beyond the ostium of the aneurysm, continues cephalad in an essentially normal manner. In one case, there was a double aneurysm, one along each limb of a sharply kinked vessel. At other times, the proximal portion of the internal carotid artery may be displaced and buckled by the mass of the saccular lesion.

Dissecting aneurysms have been described in text preceding. See also Chapter 7. Angiographically, the abnormality involves the mid and distal thirds of the cervical internal carotid artery. Characteristically, the common carotid bifurcation and the origin of the internal carotid artery appear normal. Narrowing of the vessel usually begins 2 to 3 cm distal to the origin of the internal carotid artery. If contrast material passes through the affected segment of the vessel, the lumen usually returns to a normal appearance before reaching the base of the skull. The dissection may extend into the intraosseous portion of the artery (see Figs. 7.35 to 7.37).

Occasionally, the false lumen of the dissection joins the normal lumen of the vessel at both ends of the lesion (Fig. 10.62). In such cases, both the true and false lumens of the vessel are opacified with the intima, and that portion of the tunica media central to the dissection appearing as bandlike filling defects between the two lumens. More often, however, the false lumen is closed distally so that a thrombus develops in this compartment. In such cases, only the residual true lumen is visualized, and this appears as a long, irregular tapering of the vessel either to a point of maximal narrowing or to complete occlusion. The resultant long, narrow column of contrast material has been described as a "stringlike" deformity. When seen to involve the distal internal carotid artery without atheromatous changes being present, it is considered characteristic of a dissecting aneurysm.

Traumatic aneurysms of the vertebral, as well as the carotid, arteries are frequently encountered. Stab wounds are the most common cause of such false aneurysms; such an injury may also produce an arteriovenous fistula (Fig. 10.87). False aneurysms resulting from penetrating injuries usually have an irregular configuration and surface contour because they are bounded by tissue planes or fibrous tissue from an adjacent organized hematoma. In wartime, shrapnel wounds of the neck that lacerate only part of an arterial wall are a common cause of large false aneurysms. Arteriovenous fistulas also frequently result from such injuries. Any of the vessels of the neck may be affected, depending on the location of an injury.

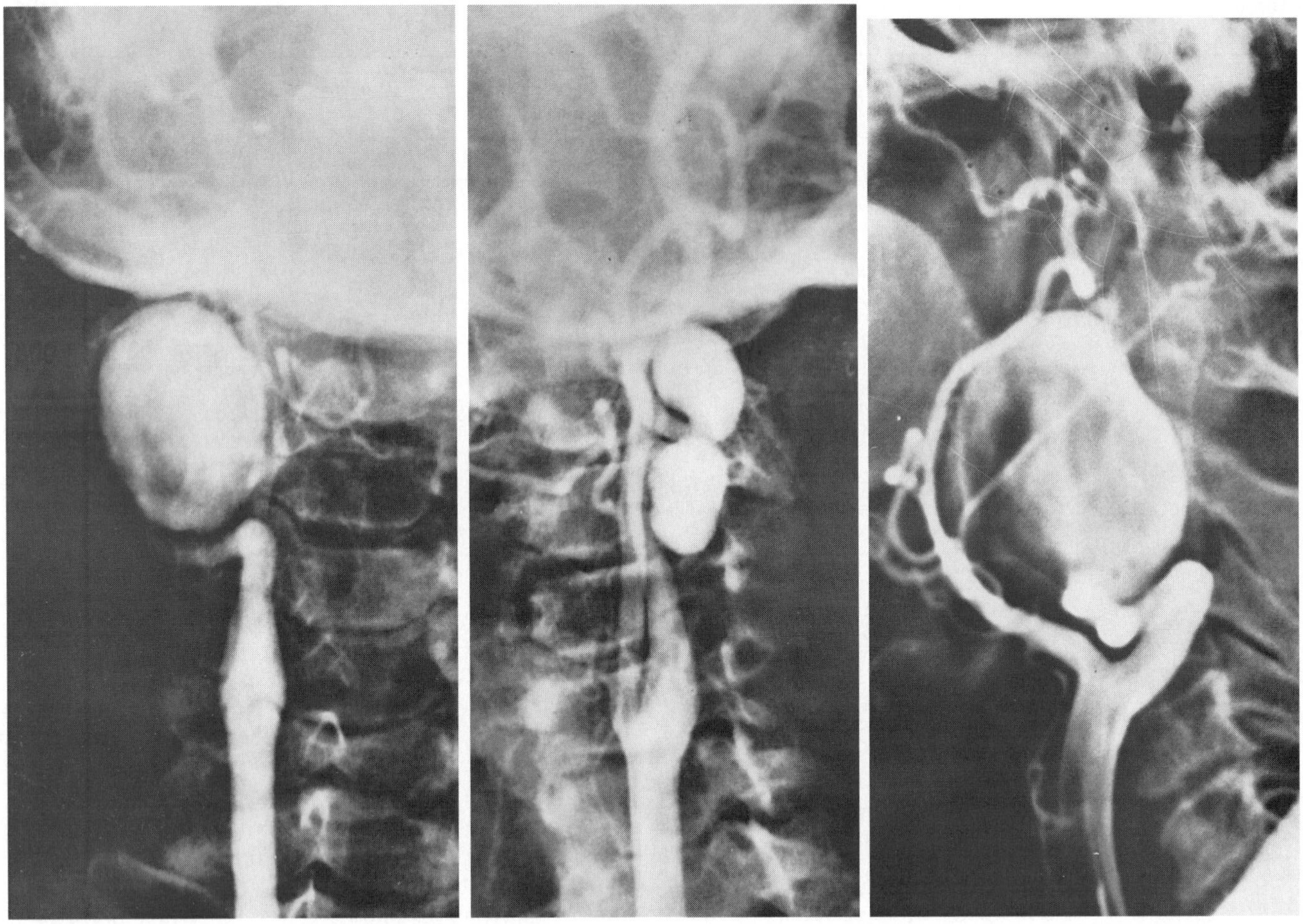

A B C

Figure 10.86. Saccular cervical aneurysms. **A.** A large, oval sac fills with contrast material from the internal carotid artery at the level of C3. The artery deviates laterally around the aneurysm as it courses cranially. The patient had been aware of a fullness in the region of the right carotid bulb for many years but only shortly before admission had she appreciated a mass in the neck. **B.** A double aneurysm, one along each limb of a sharply kinked internal carotid artery, is shown on the left side in the same case as A. The patient had been completely unaware of any abnormality in the left side of the neck. **C.** In another case, a very large saccular aneurysm is shown arising from the distal cervical internal carotid artery at the C2 and C3 vertebral levels. The patient had appreciated a slowly enlarging pulsatile mass in the neck for many years but had no other symptoms.

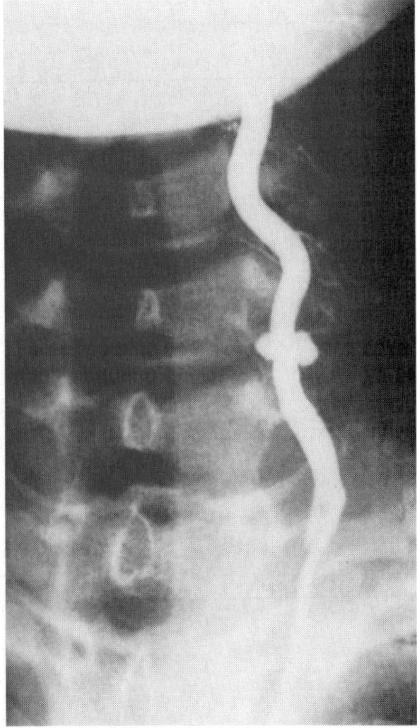

Figure 10.87. False posttraumatic aneurysm of the left carotid artery resulting from a stab wound of the neck 1 month prior to the angiogram.

As described earlier, the diagnosis of arterial dissection can be made by MRI because the intramural blood collection is hyperintense on T1- and T2-weighted images. This is seen particularly well in axial views, where the hyperintense semilunar image surrounds the flow void produced by the remaining true lumen of the artery (Fig. 10.61; see Fig. 7.37).

Intracranial Extradural Aneurysms

Almost all of the lesions in the extradural group are *cavernous carotid aneurysms.* The lesions are saccular in type and congenital in origin, presumably arising in connection with the numerous intracavernous minor branchings of the internal carotid artery. In approximately one-fourth of the cases, cavernous carotid aneurysms are bilateral; indeed, the early report of Blane concerned such bilateral lesions (Fig. 10.88) (192).

If such an aneurysm ruptures, a carotid-cavernous fistula results. In the absence of trauma, the spontaneous rupture of a saccular aneurysm is the most common cause of an arteriovenous fistula in this location. After a fistula has developed, it may be difficult or impossible to demonstrate the original sacculation by angiography because of surrounding dural sinus opacification, unless the arterial aneurysm had attained considerable size prior to rupture. The condition is given further consideration in text following under "Arteriovenous Fistulas" in the section "Arteriovenous Lesions," and also in Chapter 7.

The second principal manifestation of a cavernous carotid aneurysm is its mass effect. Occasionally symptoms may develop because of blockage of the cavernous sinuses. Some cavernous aneurysms become extremely large. This is possible because as they expand, usually upward, they are covered by the dural wall of the sinus, which helps prevent early rupture. Rarely, they may act as an extracerebral subfrontal tumor in the anterior fossa. More often, they expand into the suprasellar cistern; an aneurysm must always be included in the differential diagnosis of suprasellar tumors (Fig. 10.91). Less frequently, such a lesion may extend laterally and backward. Also, infrequently, the expansion of such aneurysms may so thin the overlying dura that the aneurysms rupture intracranially to produce a subarachnoid hemorrhage or intracerebral hematoma. In many cases, a large portion of the aneurysmal lumen may be filled by organized thrombus, and a shell of calcium about its periphery may allow diagnosis from plain skull films. In spite of the organized thrombus and calcification, many such lesions continue to enlarge slowly throughout life. Erosions of the superior orbital fissure, the lateral aspect of the sella turcica, and of the clinoid processes are sometimes found.

Cranial nerves are often compressed because of the expanding mass of a cavernous carotid aneurysm. Within the cavernous sinus, the internal carotid artery lies chiefly below and medial to the oculomotor nerve (Fig. 10.89). A rather similar relationship pertains to the trochlear nerve, whereas the abducent nerve is very close to the lateral wall of the carotid artery, along the transverse course of the vessel in the cavernous sinus. Extraocular movements and other functions may be impaired by compression of one or more of these cranial nerves by a cavernous aneurysm. A medially projecting aneurysm is occasionally seen to encroach upon the cavity of the sella turcica, producing enlargement of the sella.

The diagnosis of intracavernous carotid aneurysm can be made by MRI. The T1- and T2-weighted images may show the sac, and MRA may demonstrate the aneurysm. Partial thrombosis within the aneurysm is common in these locations (Figs. 10.88 and 10.90).

Intracranial Intradural Aneurysms

MASS LESIONS

Fusiform lesions resulting from atherosclerosis were among the earliest intracranial aneurysms described (193), and, although they are not nearly as common as congenital saccular lesions, they are occasionally encountered in the course of examination of older individuals. The major vessels at the base of the brain, particularly the basilar artery, are most commonly affected. The basilar artery is frequently found to be ectatic to a marked degree; the vessel is also usually elongated and tortuous. As noted earlier, the increased mass of the artery may produce indentation of the floor of the third ventricle and interference with the circulation of CSF (Fig. 10.70). Occasionally, the vertebral artery may undergo aneurysmal atherosclerotic dilatation. A greatly elongated and ectatic vertebral artery may press on cranial nerves and even simulate a cerebellopontine angle tumor clinically and on CT (Fig. 10.69). Basilar and vertebral fusiform aneurysms may displace the brainstem backward and upward; it may also be displaced laterally by eccentric aneurysmal dilatation of an elongated S-shaped basilar artery. Some lesions indent and compress the brainstem. They seldom rupture, but there are often symptoms of ischemia. Apparently the orifices of branch vessels become occluded by the intimal disease. At times, the carotid siphon is grossly ectatic and tortuous. The enlargement may extend into the proximal segments of the main branches of the internal carotid and basilar arteries, and elements of the circle of Willis may be involved.

When they become large without rupturing, true *saccular* aneurysms of principal arteries at the base of the brain produce mass effects, even more often than fusiform aneurysms, which may be silent. A large supraclinoid aneurysm of the carotid siphon frequently extends medially and upward to compress the optic chiasm and hypothalamus (Fig. 10.91). There may even be obstruction at the foramen of Monro. In many instances, a large portion of the aneurysm is filled by mural thrombus so that there is much more

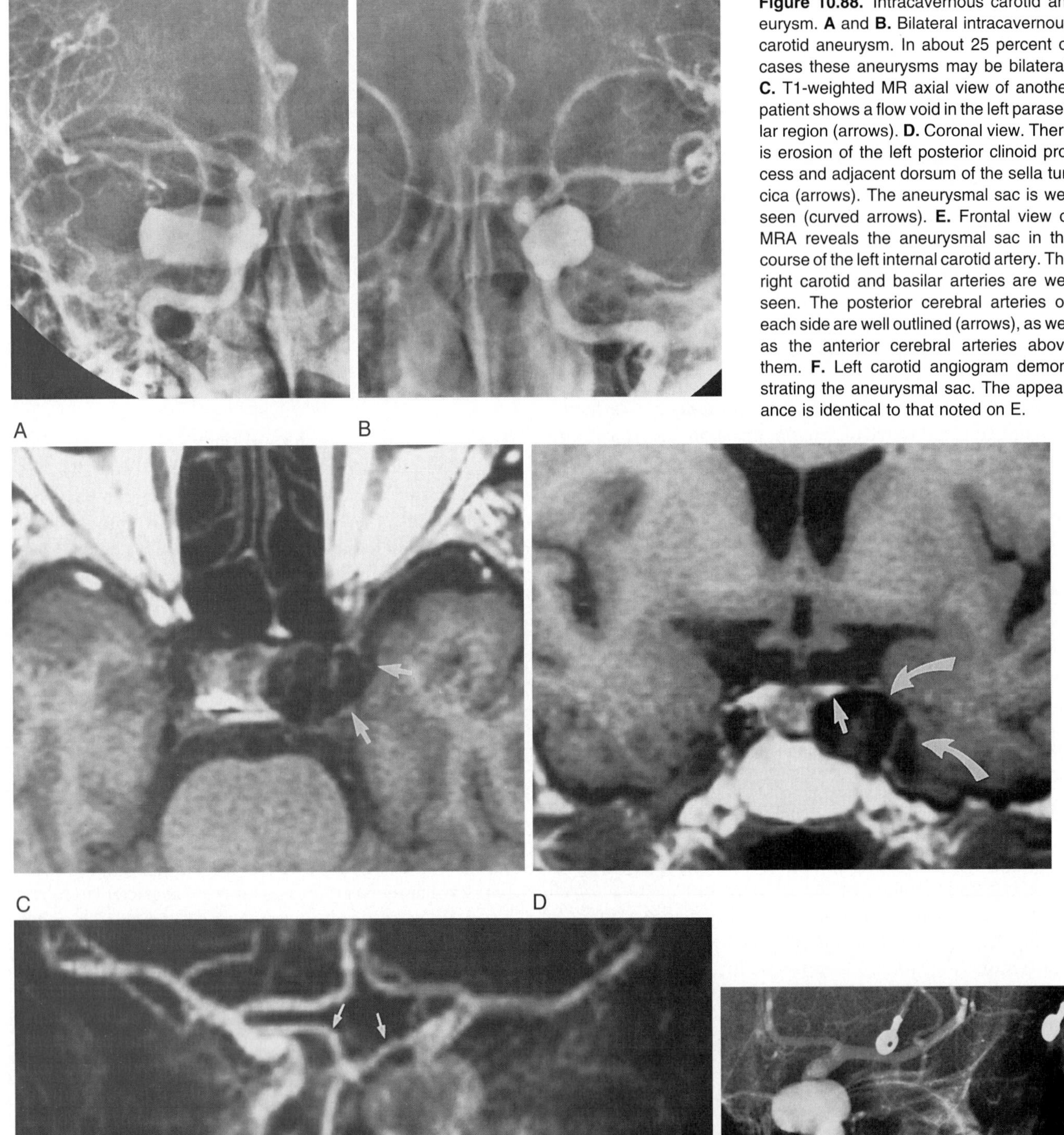

Figure 10.88. Intracavernous carotid aneurysm. **A** and **B.** Bilateral intracavernous carotid aneurysm. In about 25 percent of cases these aneurysms may be bilateral. **C.** T1-weighted MR axial view of another patient shows a flow void in the left parasellar region (arrows). **D.** Coronal view. There is erosion of the left posterior clinoid process and adjacent dorsum of the sella turcica (arrows). The aneurysmal sac is well seen (curved arrows). **E.** Frontal view of MRA reveals the aneurysmal sac in the course of the left internal carotid artery. The right carotid and basilar arteries are well seen. The posterior cerebral arteries on each side are well outlined (arrows), as well as the anterior cerebral arteries above them. **F.** Left carotid angiogram demonstrating the aneurysmal sac. The appearance is identical to that noted on E.

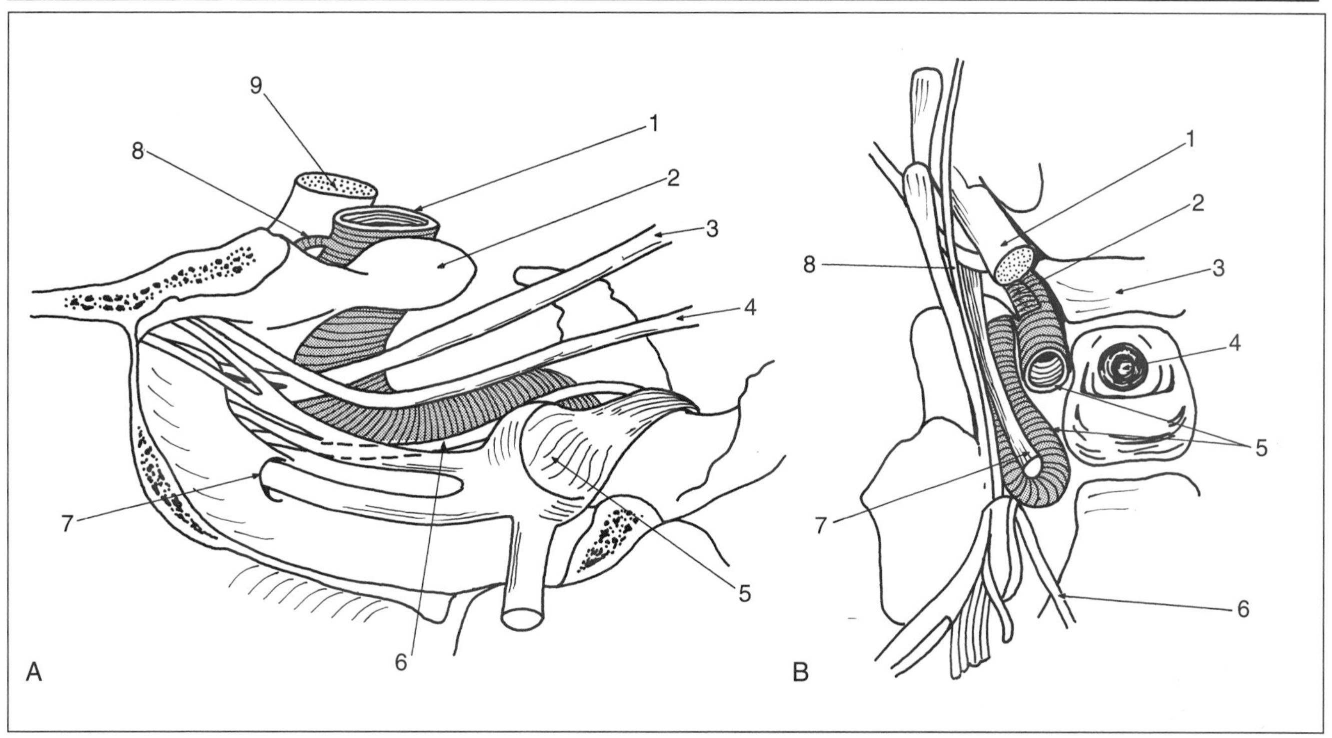

Figure 10.89. Relationship of structures in cavernous sinus. **A.** The left cavernous sinus area is viewed laterally: (1) internal carotid artery, (2) anterior clinoid process, (3) oculomotor nerve, (4) trochlear nerve, (5) trigeminal ganglion, (6) abducent nerve, (7) foramen rotundum, (8) ophthalmic artery, and (9) optic nerve (see also Fig. 17.8). **B.** The left cavernous sinus is drawn from above: (1) optic nerve, (2) ophthalmic artery, (3) tuberculum sellae, (4) pituitary stalk, (5) internal carotid artery, (6) abducent nerve, (7) oculomotor nerve, and (8) trochlear nerve.

vascular displacement than can be accounted for by the size of the opacified lumen at angiography.

Occasionally, an aneurysm arising at the origin of the ophthalmic artery may be encountered. Such a lesion may arise either intradurally or extradurally. Similarly, its expansion may occur within the subarachnoid space or extradurally along the course of the vessel toward the optic foramen. In the latter instance, erosion of the inner end of the optic canal may be visible on plain skull radiographs or on CT. Such an aneurysm can compress the optic nerve against the bony edge of its canal.

Surprisingly large aneurysms can develop along the course of the middle cerebral artery (Fig. 10.92*A*). Although many middle cerebral aneurysms bleed when they are relatively small, occasional aneurysms along the course of this vessel over the anterior perforated substance and between the temporal lobe and insula become sufficiently enlarged to act as tumors. In the case illustrated in Figure 10.92*B* and *C* a middle-aged man developed headache and temporal lobe seizures as the only manifestations of his lesion. Calcification in the wall of giant aneurysms is common and can be seen on CT, sometimes even on plain radiographics (see Fig. 4.7).

A posterior communicating aneurysm is a common cause of third-nerve palsy. The aneurysms often grow backward and downward from their origin in the fork of the internal carotid and posterior communicating vessels (Fig. 10.93). Such an extension causes compression of the oculomotor nerve as it passes from the subarachnoid space into the lateral wall of the cavernous sinus, the piercing of the dura occurring between the anterior and posterior clinoid processes. Since the oculomotor nerve is superior to the other orbital nerves, it is the neural structure most often affected by enlarging unruptured aneurysms in this area (Fig. 10.89).

Saccular aneurysms of the basilar artery may become very large. Their massive proportions are probably related to the frequent development of a large, organized thrombus about the periphery of the lumen. Circulation in the lumen of the lesion may constitute a relatively small part of its total volume (Fig. 10.94*E* and *F* and Table 10.17).

At angiography, an estimation of the true size of the mass may be gained from the displacements of adjacent vessels and the circumferential course of the basilar arterial branches around the lesion and the displaced and deformed brainstem. Basilar artery aneurysms often imbed themselves deeply in the anterior or anterolateral aspect of the brainstem. Long tract signs are frequently produced. The aqueduct of Sylvius may be displaced far backward and narrowed, and the floor of the posterior part of the third ventricle may be invaginated. Narrowing of the iter frequently produces hydrocephalus involving the lateral and third

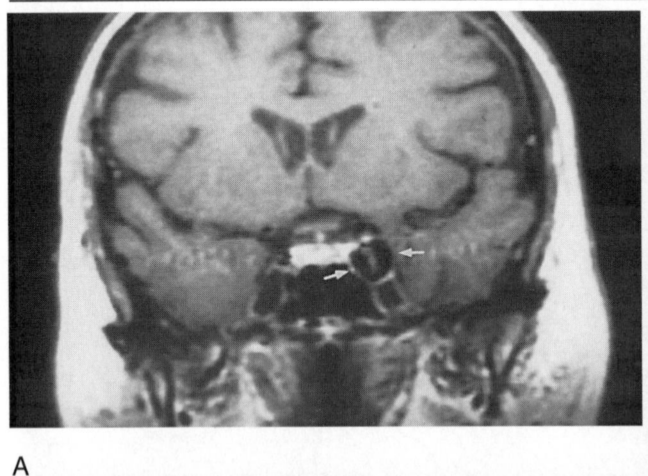

A

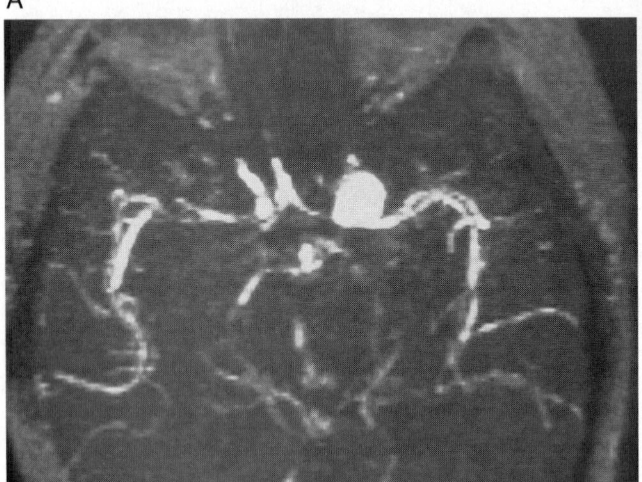

C

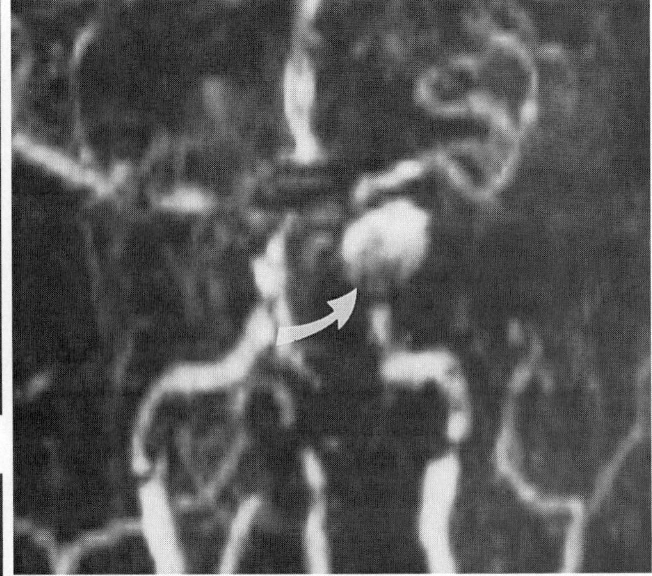

B

Figure 10.90. Intracavernous aneurysm shown by MRI and MRA. **A.** T1-weighted coronal image with contrast shows a flow void in the left cavernous sinus, much larger than the normal carotid flow void (arrows). **B.** Frontal image shows the aneurysmal sac in the left intracavernous portion of the carotid artery with an area that is not bright inferiorly, probably because of clotting (arrow). **C.** Axial view from MRA shows the aneurysmal sac.

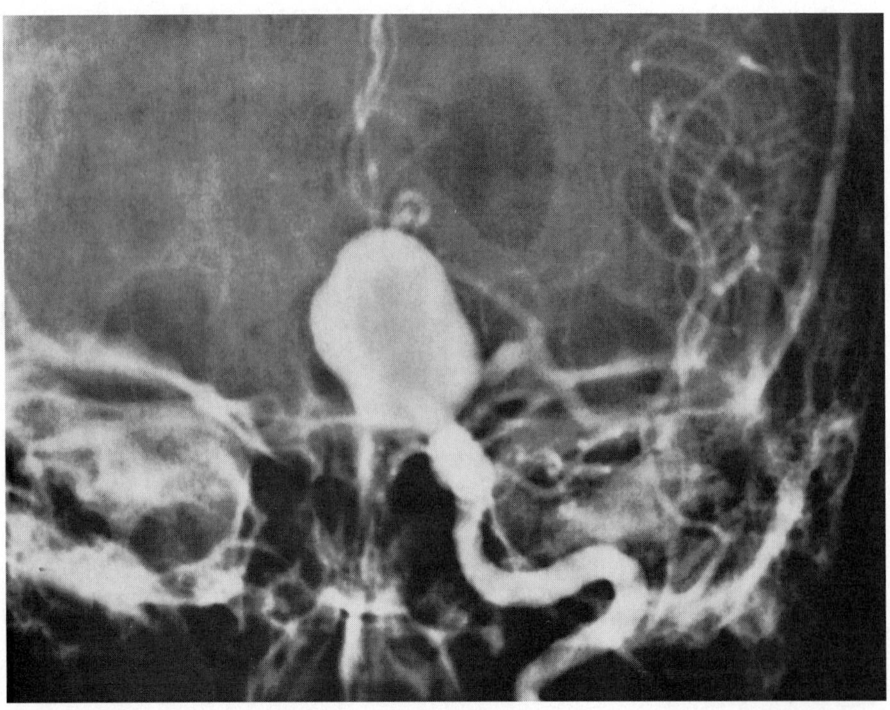

Figure 10.91. Giant carotid supraclinoid aneurysm producing bitemporal hemianopia. There is marked elevation of the proximal anterior cerebral artery and lateral displacement of the carotid siphon and of the bifurcation of the internal carotid artery. Probably there is a clotted unopacified portion as well.

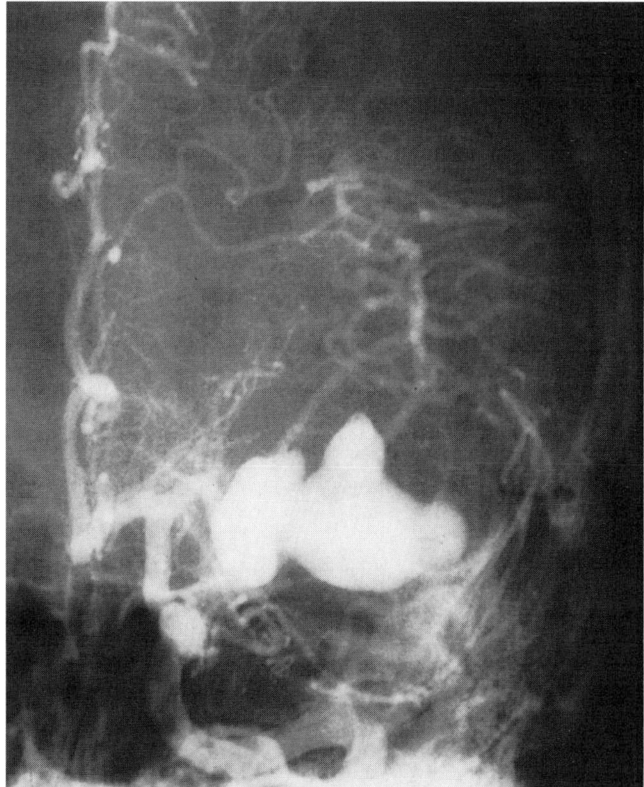

A

B

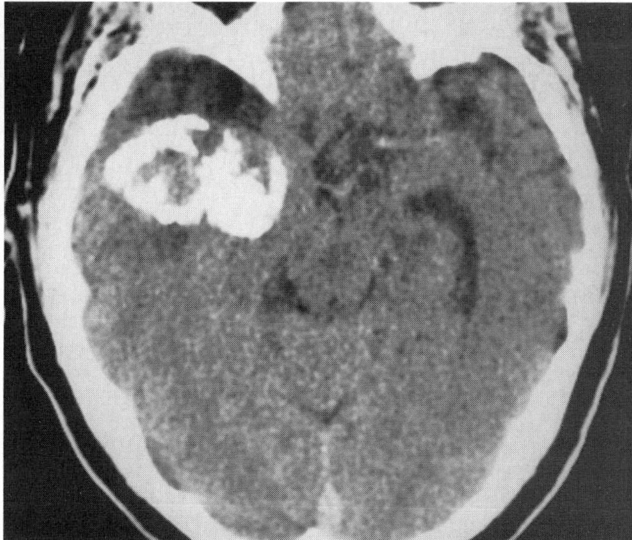

C

Figure 10.92. Large middle cerebral aneurysm. **A.** A very large multilobular aneurysm of the left middle cerebral artery is present with a sizable mass effect. There is a square shift of the anterior cerebral artery and local displacements, resulting in an avascular zone around the opacified lumen, suggesting the presence of a thick mural thrombus. The lesion had never bled; it was found in a middle-aged man who developed headache and temporal lobe seizures and who was thought to have a neoplasm. **B** and **C.** Giant middle cerebral aneurysm, with a calcified wall and partial thrombosis of the lumen. There is a large arachnoid cyst anteriorly that is probably related to arachnoidal adhesions to the wall of the aneurysm. A mass effect is present with compression of the right frontal horn and a midline shift.

Table 10.17.
Intracranial Intradural Aneurysms

Types
Saccular: usually at major branch points
Mycotic: frequently distal to branch points
Fusiform: usually found at base of brain
Most common sites
Anterior communicating artery
Middle cerebral artery bifurcation
Posterior communicating artery
Internal carotid artery bifurcation
Basilar artery tip

ventricles. There also may be interference with CSF circulation at the tentorial incisura. Such a large basilar artery aneurysm occasionally ruptures into the brainstem, even after having been present for very prolonged periods of time, during which it has acted as a slowly expanding anterior extra-axial mass.

Some of the larger aneurysms can be identified by CT. With this technique, increased radiation absorption may be caused by a calcified shell, a densely organized mural thrombus, blood, or a blood clot in the lesion; or the density of an unclotted aneurysm may be enhanced by contrast enhancement techniques.

BERRY ANEURYSMS

By far the most commonly encountered lesion of all is the *saccular* or *berry* aneurysm, arising from the circle of Willis

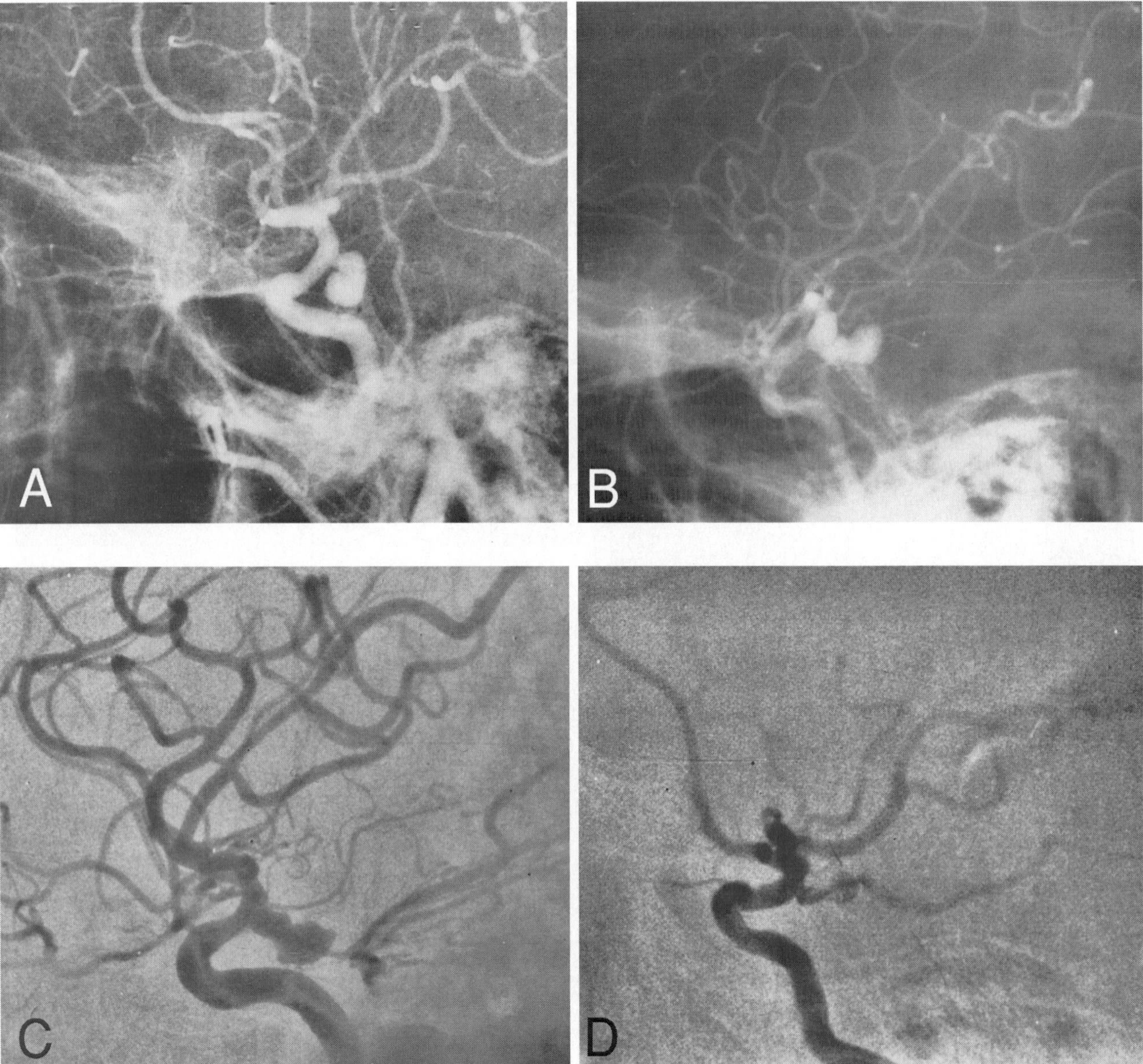

Figure 10.93. Posterior communicating aneurysms producing ophthalmoplegia. Aneurysms arising from the internal carotid artery at the usual site of origin of the posterior communicating artery, or in the fork between the two vessels, are referred to as posterior communicating aneurysms. **A.** The lateral angiogram shows an aneurysm arising at the point where the posterior communicating artery is usually seen. It extends backward and then downward onto the roof of the cavernous sinus. The remainder of the four-vessel study revealed a large posterior communicating artery on the contralateral side, but the ipsilateral artery was never visualized, suggesting that the aneurysm is "replacing" the communicating vessel. **B.** In another case, a trilobed aneurysm arises by a wide neck from the internal carotid artery. As in A, the lesion appeared to be of the "replacement" type, and an ipsilateral posterior communicating artery was never opacified. **C.** A magnification-subtraction angiogram discloses an irregular aneurysm extending backward and downward from the carotid siphon. The posterior communicating artery is stretched, and it could be traced from its junction with the posterior cerebral artery rostrally to a normal-appearing origin from the carotid siphon; the communicating vessel is visualized through the shadow of the aneurysm beside which it courses. **D.** In another case, resembling C, a normal-appearing posterior communicating artery is visualized through the shadow of an aneurysm. This establishes that the communicating artery does not fill through the aneurysm and that the lesion arises in the fork between the internal carotid and posterior communicating arteries. Such differential filling of an aneurysm and an adjacent vessel can often be demonstrated by fast filming in the early arterial phase of the angiogram.

Figure 10.94. Basilar artery aneurysm, three cases. **A.** CT scan shows subarachnoid blood in the basal cisterns. A round low-density area is seen in the interpeduncular cistern (arrows) that was later shown to represent the aneurysmal sac. There is already evidence of enlargement of the temporal horns due to ventricular dilatation. **B.** Vertebral angiography demonstrated the aneurysmal sac. **C.** MRA of another patient showing an aneurysmal sac at the top of the basilar artery. **D.** Sagittal T1-weighted image shows elevation of midline structures around the third ventricle and deformity of the anterior aspect of the midbrain structures due to displacement by a large aneurysmal sac (arrows). **E** and **F.** Basilar bifurcation aneurysm. **E.** The frontal bibrachial angiogram reveals the opacified lumen of a saccular aneurysm of the top of the basilar artery extending to the left of the midline. The segments of the posterior cerebral arteries extending around the brainstem are greatly stretched and widely separated. The proximal portions of the superior cerebellar arteries are displaced downward and stretched laterally, more marked on the left.

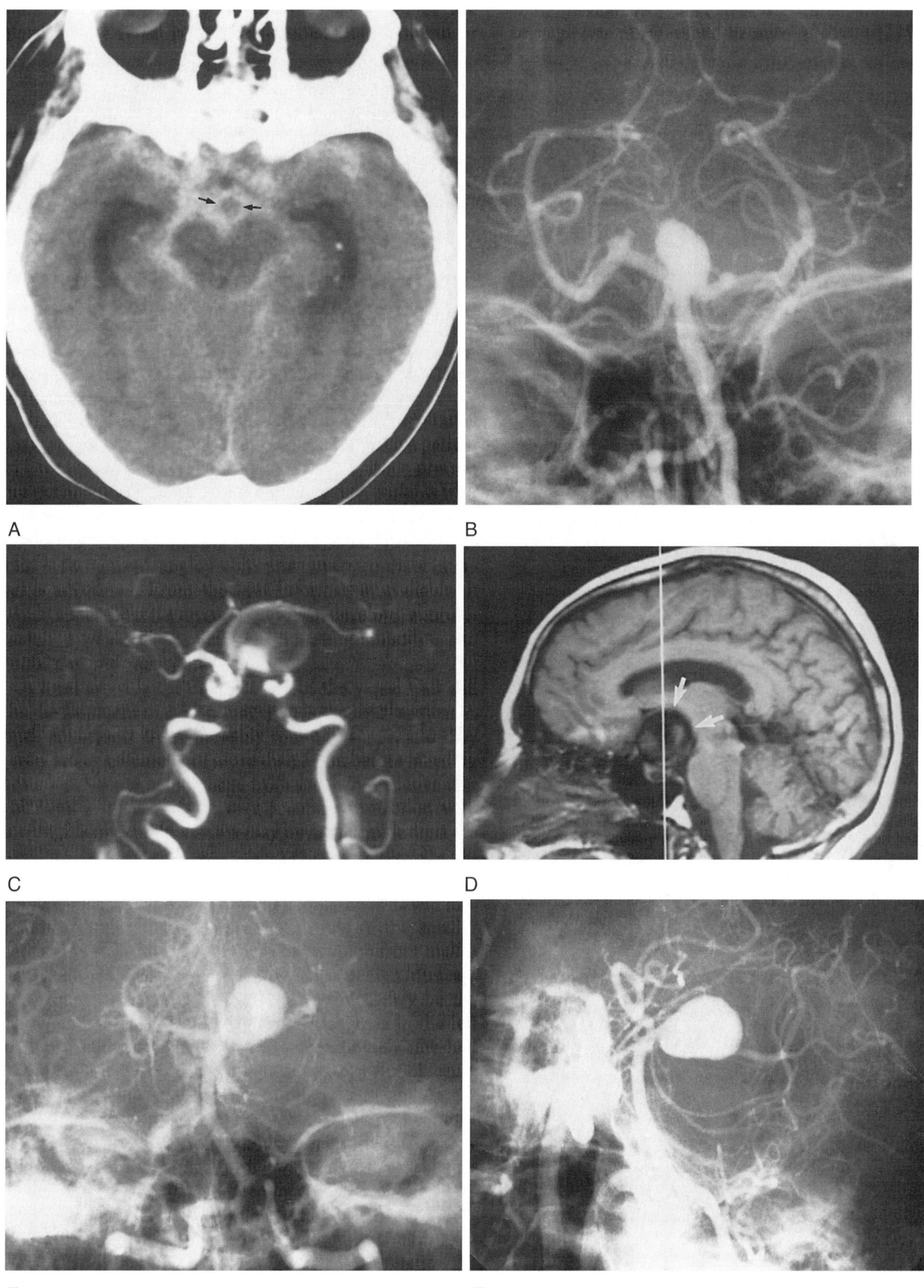

Figure 10.94. *(continued)* **F.** A 45° oblique film shows to good advantage the deformity of the left superior cerebellar vessels. The findings indicate a lesion of considerably more volume than is represented by the opacified patent lumen and denote a very large aneurysm, with a mural thrombus, that is displacing and deforming the brainstem.

and the medium-sized arteries along the base and infoldings of the brain. Credit appears to belong to Blackall (194) for first clearly describing a case of rupture of an intradural aneurysm, according to Bull (195). Pathologic studies then formed the basis for most of the investigations concerning aneurysms for more than 100 years. Good and complete angiography has now given more information about the importance of aneurysms and the complications of their rupture in living subjects.

The theory that intracranial aneurysms originate because of developmental defects in arterial walls is widely accepted. It is also generally recognized that an aneurysm is usually found in the fork between two arterial branches. At a point of normal branching, the wall between the two limbs opposite the channel of the undivided vessel usually contains the average amount of muscular and elastic tissue in the tunica media. In addition, there are extra layers of intimal cells in the fork, usually referred to as "intimal pads." A collarlike intimal pad is also present proximal to the point of bifurcation of an artery (Fig. 10.85). In the cerebral vessels of humans, the tunica media is often defective at the fork of a dividing vessel, containing less smooth muscle than in an average normal artery and also having poorly developed elastic fibers. The finding of such medial defects led Forbus to the conclusion that these were the bases for the development of aneurysms (Fig. 10.85) (196).

Another congenital theory of origin is based on the embryologic studies of Padget (197, 198). She found many arterial channels in the fetus in early stages of development that later disappeared. It was suggested that at the sites where these "experimental vessels" arise, a relative weakness of the arterial wall remains that later may become the site of development of a saccular aneurysm. Where a fetal vessel becomes smaller but does not disappear, a weakness in the parent vessel could also remain; the presence of an aneurysm through which a branch artery fills, which is the case with some intracranial saccular lesions, might well be explained in this way.

In further support of the congenital origin of most intracranial aneurysms is the fact that anomalies of the circle of Willis are commonly associated with these saccular lesions. Anomalies outside the brain also occur, such as polycystic kidneys (199) and coarctation of the aorta (200).

As noted earlier, intracranial aneurysms are not common in animals other than primates. Medial defects were found by Crompton in a great many species of animals at the same sites as in humans, but they were smaller (201). In addition, the tunica media was thicker and contained more elastic fibers, and the adventitia was denser and also contained more elastic fibers, especially over the medial defects, than in humans. The intimal pads of animals contain muscle, and elastic fiber degeneration is less frequent than in humans. There is more longitudinal stress in the human because of the larger multifolded brain, resulting in longer and poorly supported arteries. The report of Stehbens concerning a chimpanzee that died of a subarachnoid hemorrhage is of interest because the animal had 8 berry aneurysms (202).

In addition to the basic anatomic defects, the age of the patient and arterial hypertension are important factors in the initiation, growth, and rupture of cerebral berry aneurysms (138). With advancing age, elastic degeneration gradually increases. The degeneration appears first beneath the intimal pads around the arterial bifurcation, then in the more superficial elastica over the medial defects, and finally becomes diffuse along the arterial trunks. Approximately two-thirds of patients with ruptured aneurysms have hypertension. The degree of atherosclerosis is found to be exactly what should be expected in such a high fraction of hypertensive patients, according to Crompton (201). The same investigator found large medial defects to be much commoner at middle cerebral arterial forks than at other sites, apparently accounting for the greater frequency of aneurysms at the middle cerebral bifurcation than elsewhere. Aneurysms may also develop at sites of arterial fenestration, when there is forking and then rejoining of a vessel not normally divided (Fig. 10.95). Tunica media defects are frequently found in the forks of a fenestration.

Controversy exists concerning the incidence of aneurysms associated with fenestration of various intracranial arteries. Out of a total of 59 cases, Campos et al. found 21 instances of vertebrobasilar aneurysms arising in a fenestration in the basilar artery (203). On the other hand, Sanders et al. found 38 fenestrated arteries (16 basilar, 10 vertebral, 9 middle cerebral, 3 anterior cerebral) in 37 patients, out of a total of 5190 cerebral angiograms (204). A total of 13 aneurysms were found in 7 of these patients, but in only 1 was the aneurysm at the fenestration site. Thus patients with fenestrations have an increased incidence of aneurysms, but, with the exception of basilar artery fenestrations, the aneurysm may not be at the fenestration site.

SUBARACHNOID HEMORRHAGE

This is the most frequent and most common manifestation of intracranial aneurysms. The rupture of an aneurysm leads to an intracranial hemorrhage, usually in the subarachnoid space. The blood is mixed with CSF and is usually more pronounced in the immediate neighborhood of the aneurysm; the concentration of blood will decrease as it is farther away. The blood is visible on CT, and the visibility is partly dependent on the amount of bleeding that has taken place by the time the CT examination is carried out. The bleeding may have occurred through a very small puncture of the aneurysmal wall, which may well seal off promptly only after a few cubic centimeters of blood have escaped. At other times the bleeding continues for a longer period, in which case fairly large accumulations of blood can take place before tamponade of the aneurysm occurs. In the great majority of cases, the bleeding is in the subarachnoid space because all of the large blood vessels of the brain are located either in the subarachnoid space or on the surface of the brain.

Aneurysmal rupture occurs most frequently between the ages of 40 and 60, and experience shows that it is more

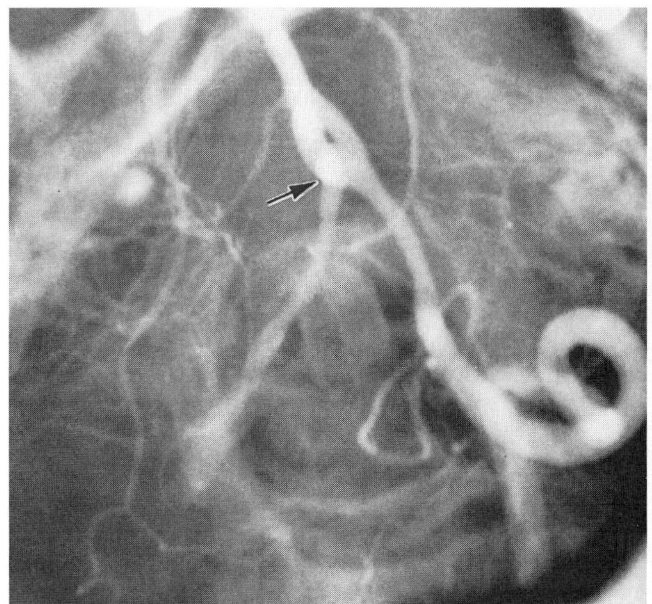

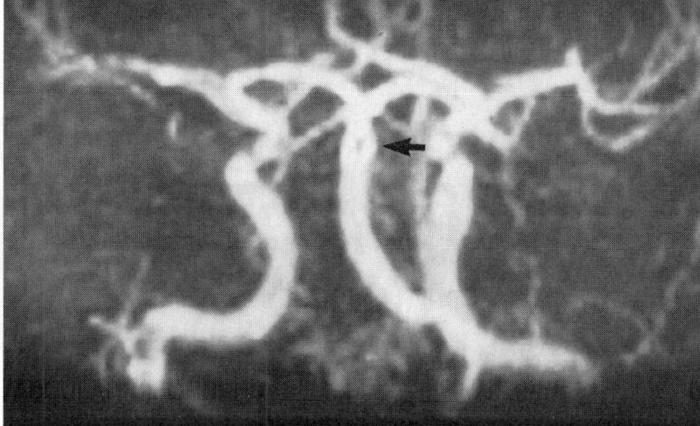

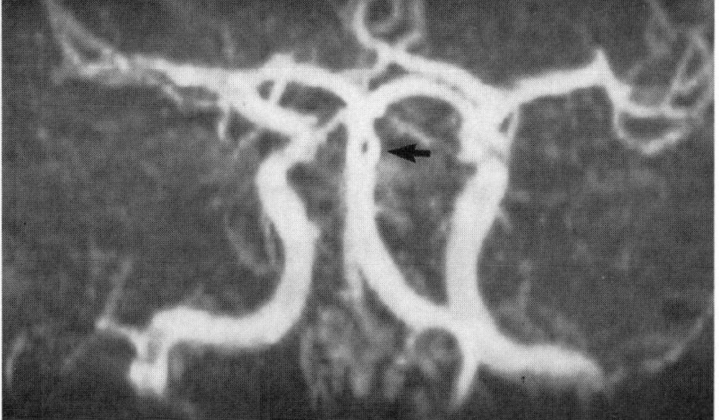

B

Figure 10.95. A. Fenestration of basilar artery and arterial aneurysm. The basilar artery immediately after its origin is divided into two branches that then join together again to form a common trunk. An aneurysm is seen arising from the site of the first junction of the two vertebral arteries (arrow). Although fenestration of the basilar artery is known to be associated with aneurysms, a recent report indicates that the incidence of saccular aneurysms is lower than had been thought; in a large series of angiograms it was only 7 percent. (See Sanders, Sorek, Mehta: AJNR 1993;14:675–680.) **B.** Fenestration of basilar artery without an aneurysm demonstrated by MRA (arrows). Two views in frontal projection are shown rotated 10° from each other.

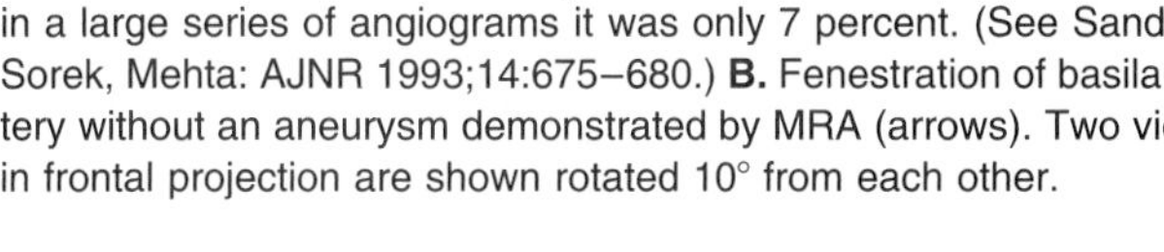

Table 10.18.
Aneurysmal Rupture Clinical Grading Scale

Grade I: asymptomatic or mild headache
Grade II: moderate or severe headache, nuchal rigidity, oculomotor paresis
Grade III: confusion, drowsiness, mild focal signs
Grade IV: stupor or hemiparesis
Grade V: coma

Source: Adapted from EW Hunt, RM Hess: J Neurosurg 1968;28:14–20.

Table 10.19.
CT Findings of Subarachnoid Hemorrhage

Positive findings present in 95% of cases
False-negative studies may be due to small amount of hemorrhage (e.g., "sentinel hemorrhage") or delay in imaging
Hemorrhage site is usually localized to site of aneurysmal rupture:
- Anterior interhemispheric fissure (anterior communicating artery aneurysms)
- Lateral perimesencephalic cistern (posterior communicating artery aneurysms)
- Sylvian fissure (middle cerebral artery aneurysms)
- Prepontine cistern (basilar tip aneurysm)

Intraparenchymal hemorrhage may be seen
Ventricular enlargement may be present even soon after aneurysmal rupture

frequently found in females. A subarachnoid hemorrhage presents itself as a sudden onset of headache that is often described by the patients as the worst headache of his or her life. The severe headache may well be accompanied by transient loss of consciousness and sometimes by vomiting. In some patients the loss of consciousness may last longer or may be deeper. We therefore need a method for classifying the severity of patients' symptoms at the time that they are first seen by a physician. One grading system exists that ranges from grade 0, no subarachnoid hemorrhage, patient intact; to grade 5, which is deep coma and decerebrate rigidity (Table 10.18).

The diagnosis of subarachnoid hemorrhage is made by CT, which should be performed as soon as possible. In the absence of available CT equipment, one should perform a spinal puncture to look for evidence of blood in the CSF (Table 10.19)

CT is about 95 percent accurate in detecting evidence of subarachnoid hemorrhage. The CT findings are as follows:

1. A definite hyperintense area in the neighborhood of the aneurysm that bled (Fig. 10.96).
2. A large subarachnoid hemorrhage with blood accumulation in the area and subarachnoid blood elsewhere (Fig. 10.97).

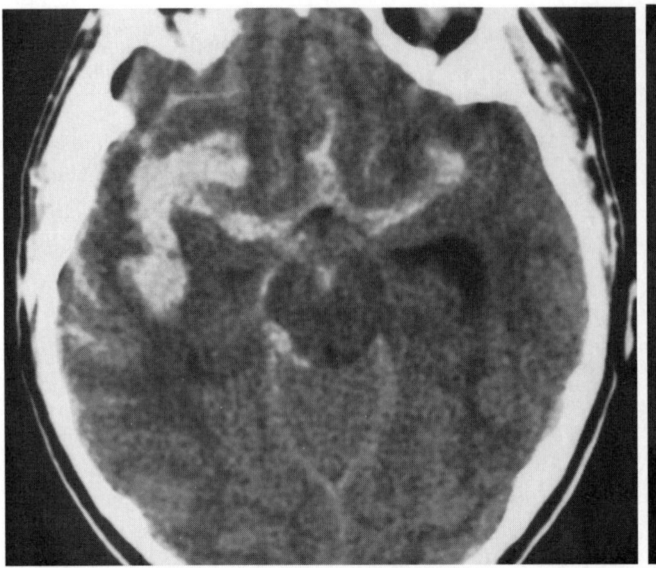

A

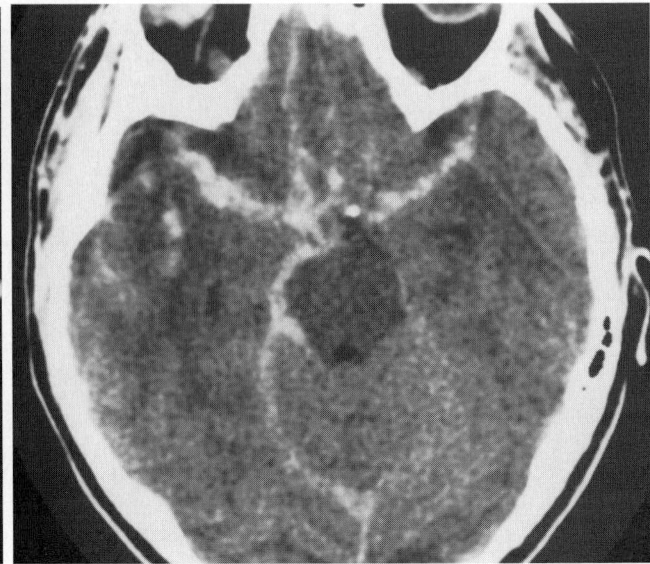

B

Figure 10.96. Subarachnoid hemorrhage in the right sylvian fissure area with extension. **A** and **B.** The blood collection is largest in the right sylvian region. There is extension to the other side, to the interhemispheric fissure, and to the lateral aspect of the perimesencephalic cistern and the tentorial edge. **C.** Cerebral angiography shows that the aneurysm arose at the site of bifurcation or trifurcation of the right middle cerebral artery.

C

3. If the amount of blood is small or if the examination is delayed some hours or a day or two, the only thing visible may be a decrease in the contrast between the brain and the CSF in the basal cisterns and in the suprasellar cisterns (Fig. 10.98).
4. No blood discernible in the subarachnoid space but a small amount of blood in the lateral ventricles (Fig. 10.99). The latter is seen in patients with an anterior communicating aneurysm where bleeding occurred

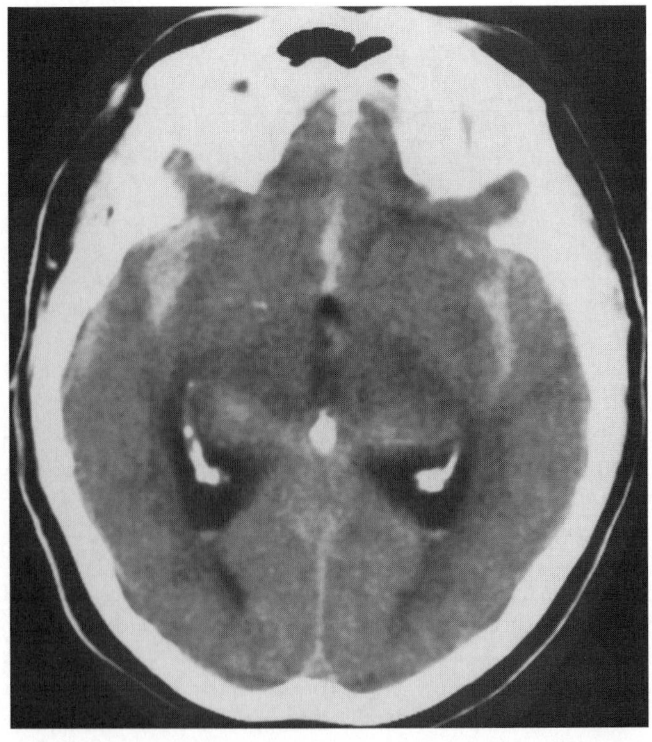

Figure 10.97. Subarachnoid hemorrhage. There is blood in both sylvian fissures, in the midline interhemispheric fissure, and in the suprasellar and perimesencephalic cisterns (seen in a lower cut, Fig. 10.94A) due to an aneurysm at the top of the basilar artery. Also, there is a small amount of blood in both lateral ventricles. With this amount of blood, the likelihood of arterial spasm developing in 5 to 10 days is high.

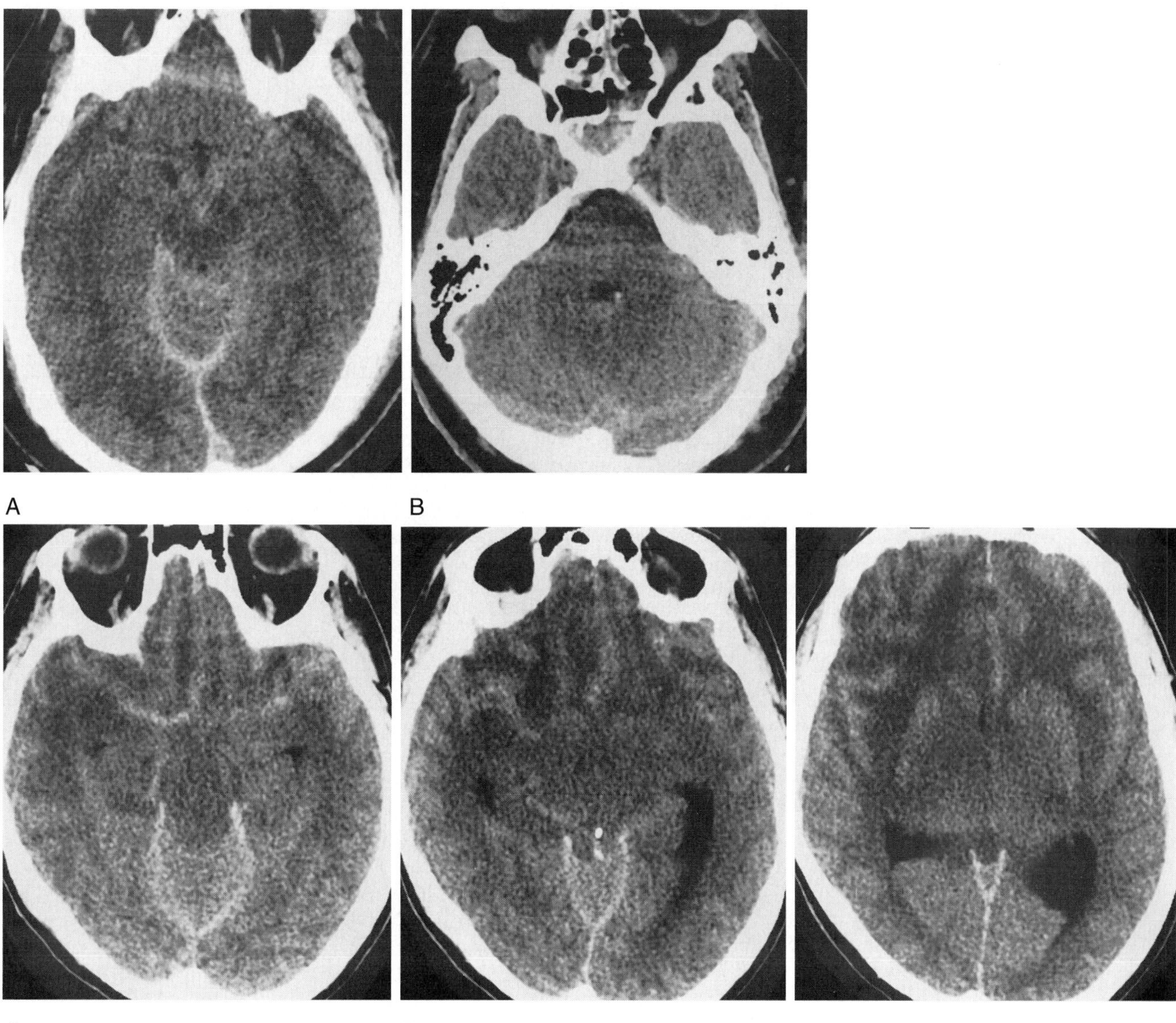

Figure 10.98. Subarachnoid hemorrhage with loss of contrast between the CSF and the brain structures. **A.** In the suprasellar space and around the midbrain the outline of the interpeduncular cistern and perimesencephalic space cannot be seen. Some brightness over the superior cerebellar cistern is suggestive of blood. **B.** The prepontine cistern cannot be seen. Care should be taken when looking for suspected subarachnoid hemorrhage to compare the relative densities of the CSF and brain structures. A decrease in contrast between the two should be carefully weighed, for it may be due to a small amount of blood, not sufficient to be hyperdense (see Fig. 10.97). **C** to **E.** Image of pseudosubarachnoid hemorrhage in a patient with diffuse encephalitis. The patient, a 40-year-old man, was stricken suddenly with a severe headache. The clinical diagnosis was possible subarachnoid hemorrhage. **C.** CT examination revealed relatively hyperdense areas in the region of the perimesencephalic and tentorial margin as well as in the suprasellar and medial sylvian fissure region. **D.** There is some enlargement of the left lateral ventricle and a relative hyperdensity, suggesting possible subarachnoid blood in the surface sulci. **E.** The same appearance as in D. A diffuse hypodensity of the brain tissue, particularly in the anterior two-thirds of the brain, was also noted. The "hyperdensity" noted in the surface sulci of the brain was felt to be due to the diffuse decrease in density of the brain tissue, but an angiogram was performed to rule out an aneurysm, and it was negative. Later the patient died, and autopsy revealed diffuse acute encephalitis.

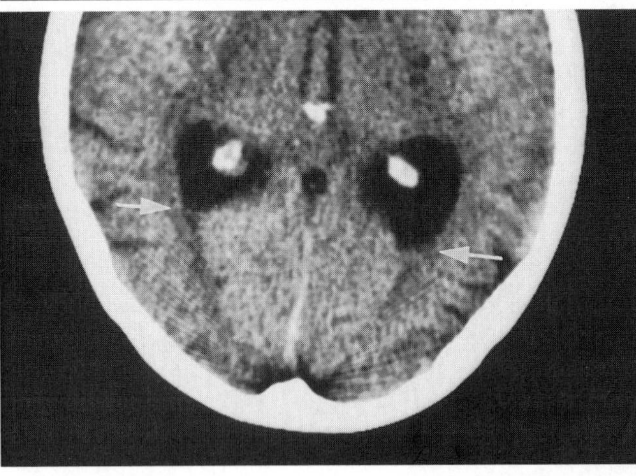
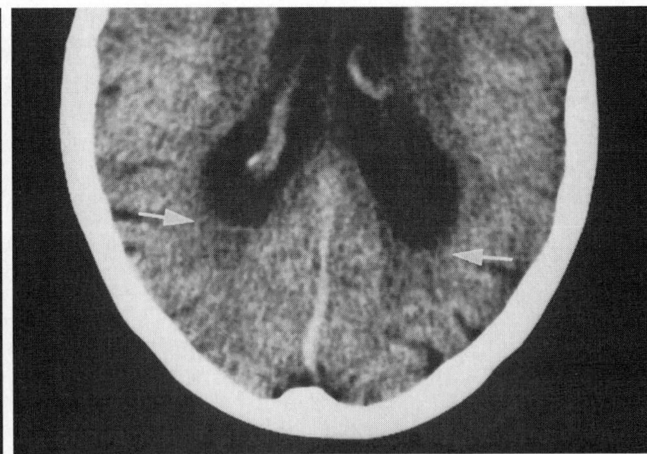

A B

Figure 10.99. Subarachnoid hemorrhage showing only a slightly hyperdense fluid level in moderately dilated vertricles. **A.** The occipital horns show hyperdensity in relation to the CSF with the suggestion of a fluid level (arrows). **B.** A higher section again shows the fluid level and the posterior portion of the ventricles, which are isodense to the surrounding cerebral tissue (arrows). In looking for subarachnoid hemorrhage, it is essential to look for occipital horn hyperdensity on CT because some early bleeding can occur in the ventricles, possibly through early rupture of the lamina terminalis in an anterior communicating aneurysm, or possibly because the subarachnoid bleeding occurred a few days previously and the extracerebral portion is no longer visible, whereas the intraventricular portion remains visible for a much longer period.

directly into the medial wall of the lateral ventricles or into the anterior wall of the third ventricle.

5. Enlargement of the ventricles might take place rather rapidly in patients with subarachnoid hemorrhage. This enlargement may be due to interference with the passage of CSF through the suprasellar cisterns, to obstruction of the aqueduct by a blood clot, or to rapid interference with absorption of CSF over the brain convexity.
6. Subdural bleeding from the aneurysm with or without subarachnoid bleeding (Fig. 10.100). Subdural bleeding in combination with subarachnoid bleeding is not rare. Subdural bleeding alone is much less common, and in either case the bleeding is due to rupture of the arachnoid leading to passage of blood into the extraarachnoidal space.
7. Intracerebral bleeding (Fig. 10.101) occurs whenever an aneurysmal sac is partly imbedded in the brain substance. It is often seen in the anterior communicating aneurysms, the sacs of which usually project away from the larger of the two anterior cerebral arteries often supplying both anterior cerebral arteries. It may also occur in basilar artery aneurysms, and in general, whenever the aneurysmal sac is partly embedded in the brain tissue.

There are other causes of subarachnoid hemorrhage in addition to intracranial saccular aneurysms. Heinz indicates that 75 percent of patients with spontaneous subarachnoid hemorrhage have an intracranial aneurysm, and 5 percent have an arteriovenous malformation (205). A number of conditions may be associated with subarachnoid hemorrhage, such as deficiency of coagulation factors, also related to the clinical use of anticoagulants; uncommon diseases such as fibromuscular dysplasia and Moya-Moya; sickle cell anemia (50 percent may have an aneurysm in addition to occlusive lesions); collagen vascular disease (lupus erythematosus, polyarteritis nodosa); and drug abuse (cocaine, amphetamine, and phencyclidine), because of the hypertension the drugs produce. The perimesencephalic subarachnoid hemorrhage is probably the one where an aneurysm is most frequently not demonstrated and where repeat angiography may be omitted (206–208).

In their description of nonaneurysmal perimesencephalic subarachnoid hemorrhage, Rinkel et al. emphasized that the blood tends to remain in the premesencephalic area and ex-

Figure 10.100. Subdural bleeding from a supraclinoid carotid aneurysm. **A.** CT scan shows hyperdensity along the left side of the tentorium extending to the midline posteriorly (arrows). No subarachnoid hemorrhage is seen. **B.** T1-weighted coronal MR image shows some subdural hyperintensity over the left convexity consistent with subdural hemorrhage (arrows). It is situated medial to the bright bone marrow fat. **C.** A T2-weighted axial image shows magnetic susceptibility or a flow void in the left parasellar region (arrow). There is also a fluid level in the occipital horns bilaterally, representing a small amount of blood due to intraventricular bleeding; the dark portion on T2 means that it is probably slightly clotted and in the deoxyhemoglobin state. Bleeding may have occurred a few days previously and the history was not clear. It was decided to do an MRA, which revealed a saccular image of intermediate intensity that displaced the supraclinoid carotid upward (**D**) in the coronal plane and displaced it forward in the sagittal view (**E**). The sac is posterior (arrow).

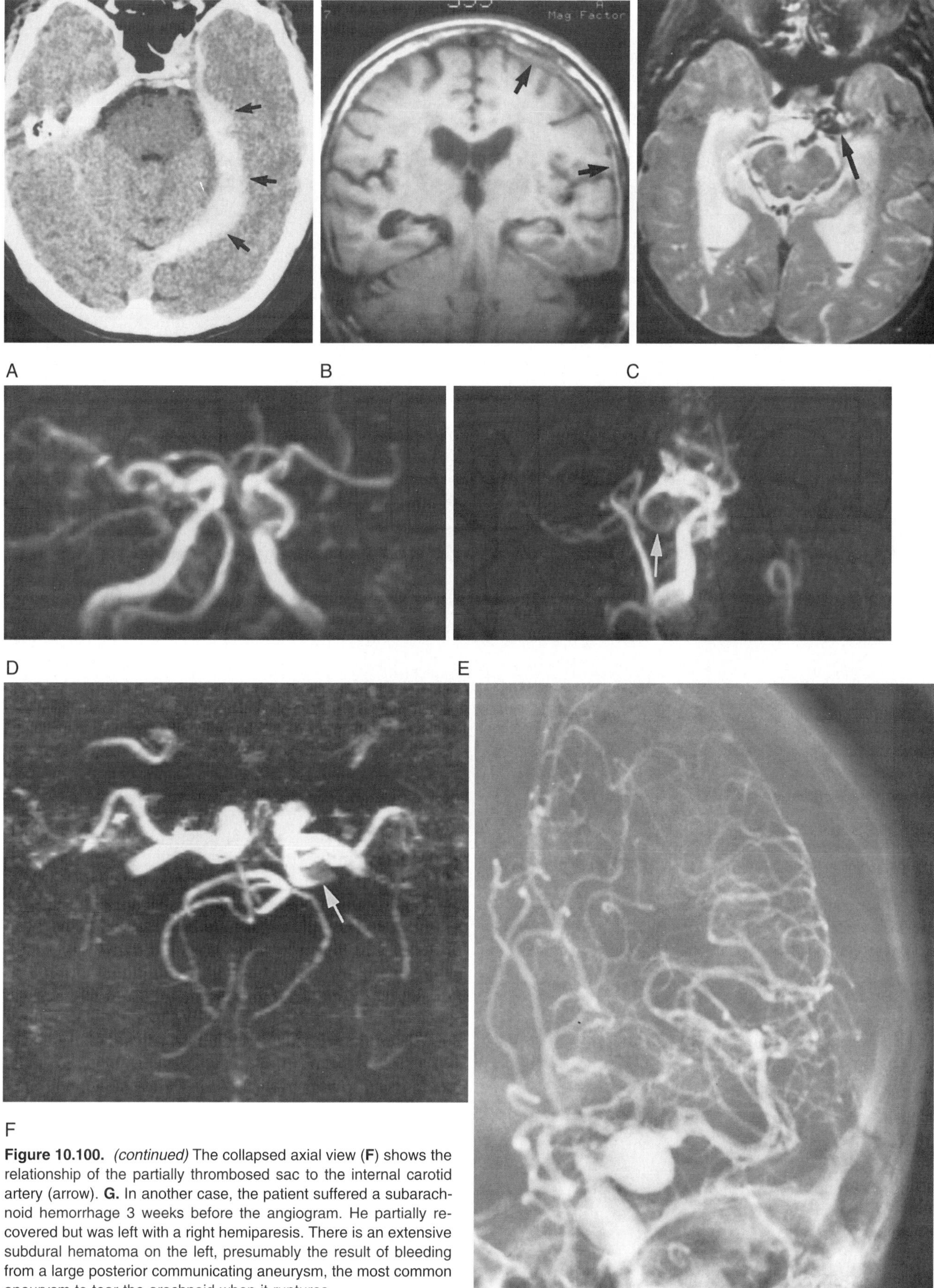

Figure 10.100. *(continued)* The collapsed axial view (**F**) shows the relationship of the partially thrombosed sac to the internal carotid artery (arrow). **G.** In another case, the patient suffered a subarachnoid hemorrhage 3 weeks before the angiogram. He partially recovered but was left with a right hemiparesis. There is an extensive subdural hematoma on the left, presumably the result of bleeding from a large posterior communicating aneurysm, the most common aneurysm to tear the arachnoid when it ruptures.

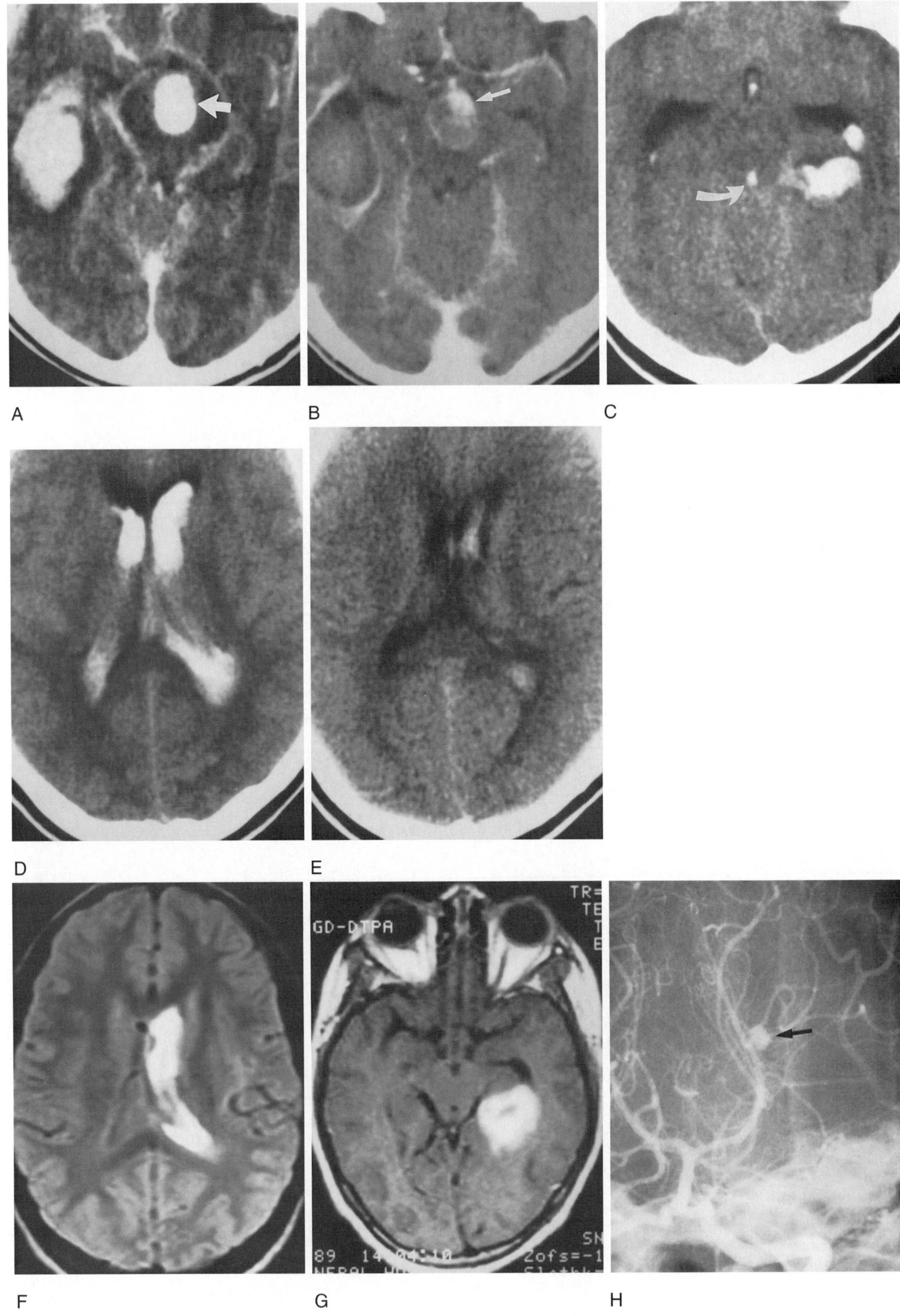
A
B
C
D
E
F
GD-DTPA
G
H

tend laterally, but only sometimes reaching the quadrigeminal cistern; it extends forward over the suprasellar cistern and medial sylvian cisterns but never to the lateral aspect of the sylvian cisterns (207). Unfortunately, a basilar tip aneurysm could produce a similar blood distribution, although it is usually more extensive and may reach the lateral aspects of the sylvian cisterns or show frank intraventricular blood. The etiology of perimesencephalic subarachnoid hemorrhage could be a rupture of some of the fine arterial branches supplying the thalamus (thalamoperforating and lenticulostriate arteries) and adjacent structures.

In cases of multiple aneurysms, CT examination is also very valuable when determining which aneurysm has bled, for there is probably more blood near and around the aneurysm that has ruptured.

It is important to remember that an aneurysm often presents a minor or premonitory leak before a larger rupture may occur 24 h to several days or 2 to 4 weeks later (209). The minor leak produces headache or hemifacial or periorbital pain on the side of the aneurysm; but in the cases reported by LeBlanc (34 out of a total of 87 patients with subarachnoid hemorrhage from an intracranial aneurysm), none were diagnosed even though half of them saw a physician prior to the major hemorrhage (209). Another important observation is that CT was frequently negative because the amount of blood was insufficient to produce visible hyperdensity. On the other hand, a spinal puncture revealed blood in the CSF in almost all cases.

There has been considerable misunderstanding about the frequency of aneurysms at various sites because some think of aneurysms as having clinical importance only when they have ruptured or caused neurologic changes, whereas others think in terms of total incidence. If all aneurysms are considered, both ruptured and unruptured, then the middle cerebral bifurcation is the most common site for aneurysms to be found (Fig. 10.102). Aneurysms arising from the internal carotid artery, at the site of origin of the posterior communicating artery, are the second most frequent. An almost equal percentage applies to the forks between the anterior communicating artery and the two anterior cerebral arteries. The fourth most common location is at the bifurcation of one of the carotid arteries into the anterior and middle cerebral arteries. Together, these four locations (middle cerebral, posterior communicating, anterior communicating, and carotid bifurcation) account for 90 percent of berry aneurysms. The distribution of the remaining 10 percent comprises the basilar bifurcation (2 percent), the vertebral artery at the posterior-inferior cerebellar arterial origin (2 percent), lesions of the basilar trunk probably arising at the site of origin of one of the pontine branches or an "experimental vessel" (1 percent), the distal anterior or middle cerebral artery (2 percent), and the proximal and distal portions of the posterior cerebral artery (3 percent).

As already noted, only a minority of aneurysms rupture. The location of an aneurysm affects the probability of its bleeding. Anterior communicating aneurysms, for example, carry the highest risk for the production of a subarachnoid hemorrhage. In a group of 525 patients, each with a single aneurysm and a subarachnoid hemorrhage, McKis-

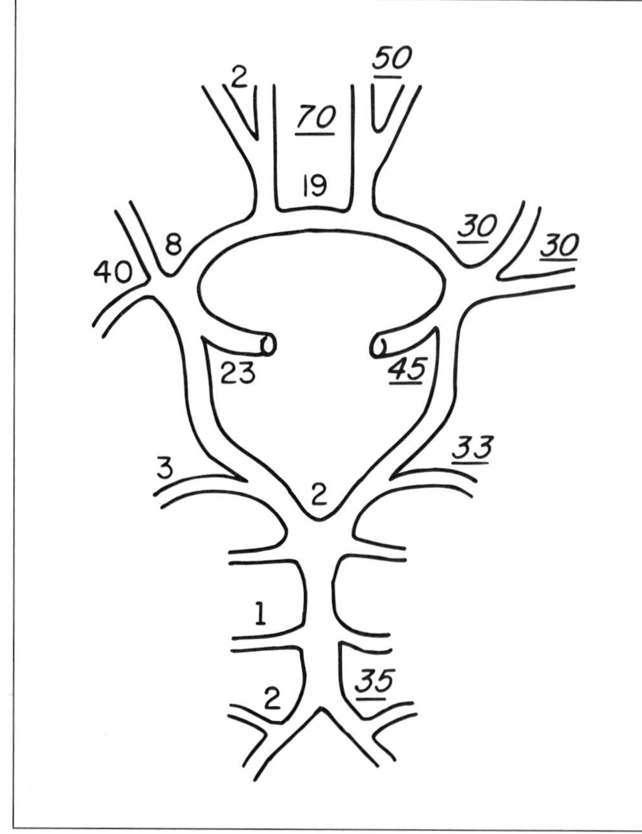

Figure 10.102. Anatomic distribution of intradural aneurysms. The ordinary numbers on the viewer's left denote the frequency of occurrence of berry aneurysms at various sites in percentage, both ruptured and unruptured. The numbers in italics (underscored) indicate the probability of an aneurysm at a certain site having ruptured if a patient with subarachnoid hemorrhage has two or more aneurysms.

Figure 10.101. Bleeding basilar artery aneurysm producing hematoma in the temporal lobe. **A.** There is extensive hemorrhage. The oval aneurysm is filled with fresh clot (arrow), and there is a large hematoma in the right temporal lobe. **B.** Reexamination 14 days later with contrast shows that the aneurysmal sac is filled with old clot and only the anterior aspect shows evidence of contrast material (arrow). The temporal hematoma is now slightly hypodense and there is enhancement of its capsule. **C** to **H.** Intracerebral bleeding from a posterior cerebral artery aneurysm. **C.** Axial CT. There is a hematoma in the region of the atrium of the left ventricle indicating that the aneurysm ruptured into the ventricle. The patient rapidly became severely ill, and ventricular drainage was necessary. There is a small blood clot in the aqueduct (arrow). The temporal horns are dilated. **D.** The lateral ventricles are filled with blood. **E.** Reexamination 10 days later shows only a small amount of residual opacity, as is usual on CT scans. **F.** MRI shows that there is considerably more residual blood in the ventricle than was suspected on CT. **G.** The intracerebral hematoma is still large. **H.** Vertebral angiography shows an aneurysm arising from the left posterior cerebral artery (arrow).

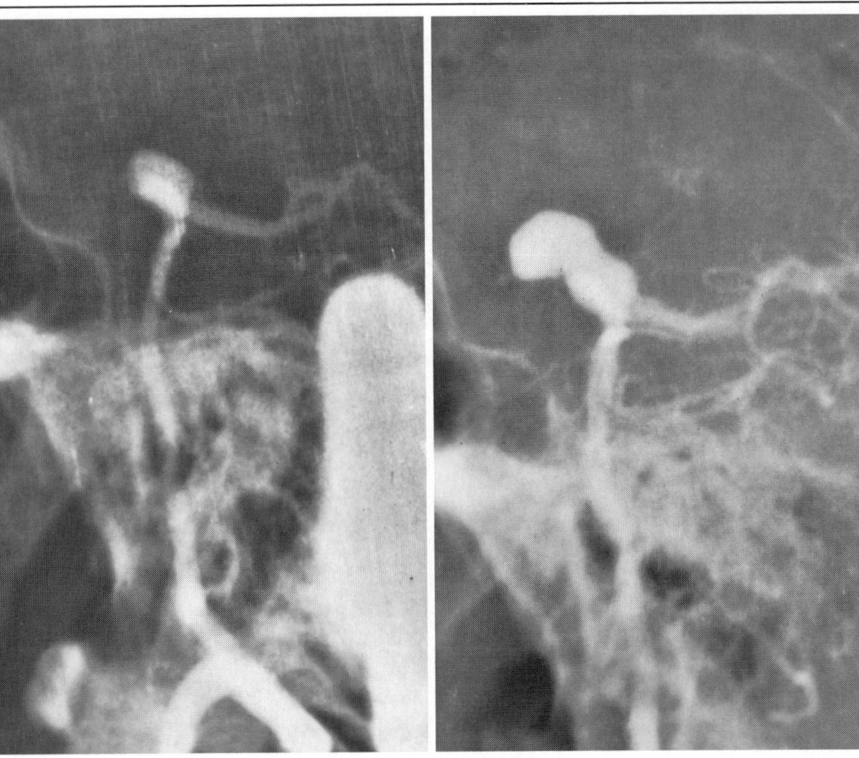

Figure 10.103. Enlargement of aneurysm between two examinations. **A.** An aneurysm is demonstrated at the bifurcation of the basilar artery. **B.** Angiography performed 3 months later because of recurrent severe headache revealed that the aneurysm had doubled in size and had become bilocular; enlargement during a brief interval through the development of a new loculus indicates deterioration of the wall of the sac that may be ominous.

sock et al. found that the offending lesion was on the anterior communicating artery more than one-third of the time (210). An aneurysm at the site of origin of the posterior communicating artery has the second highest probability of bleeding among the more frequently occurring lesions, the rare peripheral aneurysms having a slightly higher bleeding tendency.

Although aneurysms have certain features in common, they are all different with regard to their shape, size, and to a lesser extent their direction of growth. It is important to assess angiographically the orifice or mouth of the aneurysm, the neck or cervical portion formed by the proximal third of the sac, the body or middle third, and the fundus or apex of the lesion. The vast majority of aneurysms rupture through the apex. Perhaps 10 percent rupture laterally from the body of the sac, whereas a rupture through the neck is rare.

Size is also important in the assessment of rupture. The great majority of aneurysms rupture when they are between 5 and 15 mm in diameter. It is unusual for an aneurysm less than 4 mm in its smallest diameter to produce a subarachnoid hemorrhage. Larger multiloculated aneurysms are much more likely to rupture than smaller unilocular lesions; however, size is more important than multiloculation. Many unruptured aneurysms also have more than one loculus at their domes. The presence of multiple apices or secondary bubbles or pseudopods on the surface is indicative of the pattern of past growth of the aneurysm but does not predict its future prospect for rupture. In addition, some loculations are caused by external structures crossing the aneurysm rather than changes in the wall of the lesion.

An aneurysm may rupture with extravasation of blood through the intima but not beyond the wall of the vessel. At other times a local thinning and bulging of the wall may occur without intramural hemorrhage; in this way the pseudopods or multiloculations of the surface are produced. In these cases the size of the aneurysmal sac increases rapidly and the patient may complain of headache, or there may be involvement of the cranial nerves that are adjacent to the aneurysm (Fig. 10.103).

Cerebral angiograms carried out as soon as the patient is brought into the hospital usually show the aneurysm, and only rarely has the contrast material been seen to spurt out of the ruptured sac. For the most part, cerebral angiography does not appear to cause significant deterioration of the patient's condition when carried out at almost any stage of the clinical course.

The incidence of bleedings from aneurysm is greatest in the sixth decade of life, and is in the range of 12/100,000/year in North America. This brings the estimated number of patients in the United States to nearly 30,000/year. The incidence throughout the world varies from 0.5/100,000 for Hong Kong Chinese to 15.7 for Finn and 17.5 for the Japanese. Besides age, smoking, atherosclerosis, diet, and genetic predisposition no doubt play a role.

The mortality and morbidity of aneurysm rupture remain high. Close to half of the patients will be dead within the first 3 months. More than half of the patients will have

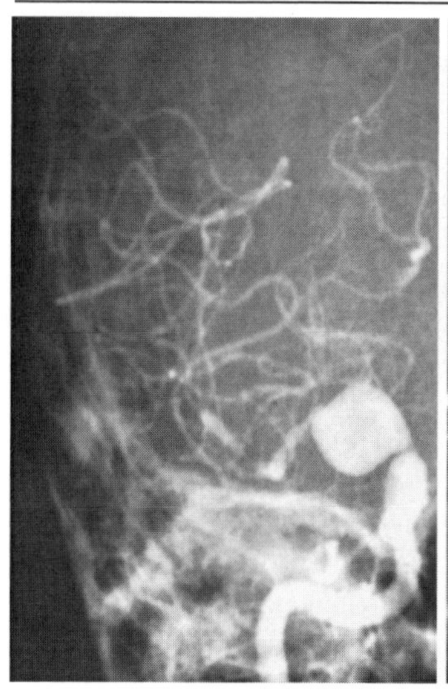
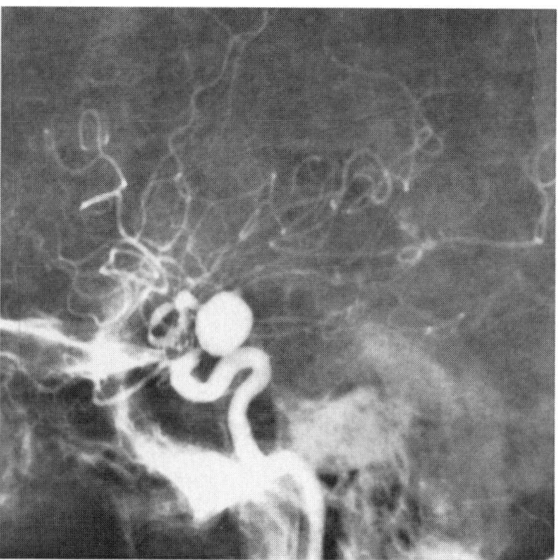

A B

Figure 10.104. Severe spasm after bleeding of aneurysm. **A.** An angiogram made 6 days after a subarachnoid hemorrhage reveals a large saccular aneurysm at the bifurcation of the internal carotid artery with marked spasm both proximal and distal to the lesion. The carotid siphon narrows markedly in the supraclinoid region. The middle cerebral trunk exhibits segmental spasm, and several of the branches have a beaded appearance. The anterior cerebral artery fills poorly. **B.** The proximal part of the anterior choroidal artery is elevated by a local subarachnoid hematoma. Slowing of the circulation and edema of the entire right hemisphere were present, and the patient died of infarction 2 days after the angiogram.

major disability, and only a third who leave the hospital will ever enjoy the quality of life they had before they bled. There does not appear to be any activity that promotes bleeding, with the exception of the second trimester of pregnancy.

In a study in Finland, Pakarinen reported a 43 percent mortality rate from the first bleeding (211). The possibility of rebleeding within the first week was 13 percent and within the first month 64 percent. Also, the mortality from a second bleed was higher (65 percent).

What to do with unruptured aneurysms represents a medical problem. The great majority will not rupture. Nevertheless, when found, the patient may become extremely worried, particularly if there is a family history, and a therapeutic decision may have to be made. According to a study by Wiebers et al., saccular aneurysms less than 10 mm in diameter have a very low probability of rupturing (212). Yet a high percentage of ruptured aneurysms are found to be less than 10 mm in diameter. The question may be raised as to whether a recently developed aneurysm may not have a higher probability of rupture. If an aneurysm is found, follow-up is recommended within a year, and if growth is demonstrated, treatment should be considered.

Arterial Spasm

It is very common to see arterial spasm in the region of a ruptured aneurysm. It is common also for all of the major vessels on the side of the lesion to be involved by spasm with poor filling of minor branches. Spasm may be seen affecting the carotid systems bilaterally, and the basilar branches as well when diffuse spasm is present; however, it often is most severe in the neighborhood of the bleeding lesion. In occasional cases spasm may be seen only contralateral to a ruptured aneurysm.

Arterial spasm after subarachnoid hemorrhage (SAH) is a major source of morbidity and mortality, and a considerable amount of effort has gone into elucidating the etiology and pathogenesis of the vascular lumen narrowing. Whether spasm will occur and how severe it will be may be related to the amount of blood, as shown by Fisher et al. (213). There is good correlation between the site of accumulation of more blood and the subsequent demonstration of arterial narrowing, and a larger hemorrhage is accompanied by a higher incidence and severity of spasm.

Arterial narrowing indicative of spasm is seen predominantly in the first 3 weeks after bleeding of ruptured intracranial aneurysms, and, according to Bergvall and Galera, it is maximal between 6 and 12 days (Fig. 10.104) (214). Thereafter, the incidence of spastic narrowing decreases (215).

The actual cause of spasm has remained controversial. It is evidently provoked by the presence of fibrinogen degradation products, which generate changes in the arterial wall (216, 217). Because normal cerebral arterial vasoconstriction is calcium dependent, calcium antagonists have been tried. These have produced minor improvement but not sufficient to warrant routine use (218). Many other efforts to elucidate the pathophysiology of cerebral arterial spasm and to prevent and treat it have been fruitless up to the present. The same is true with preventing rebleeding. The use of antifibrinolytic agents and of induced hypertension may decrease the incidence, but also may increase the incidence of thrombolitic complications. For these reasons early surgical management is the most highly recommended approach in those patients who are in a satisfactory clinical grade.

PERIPHERAL ANEURYSMS

Lesions arising from the secondary or tertiary branchings or branches of the major cerebral arteries can be considered

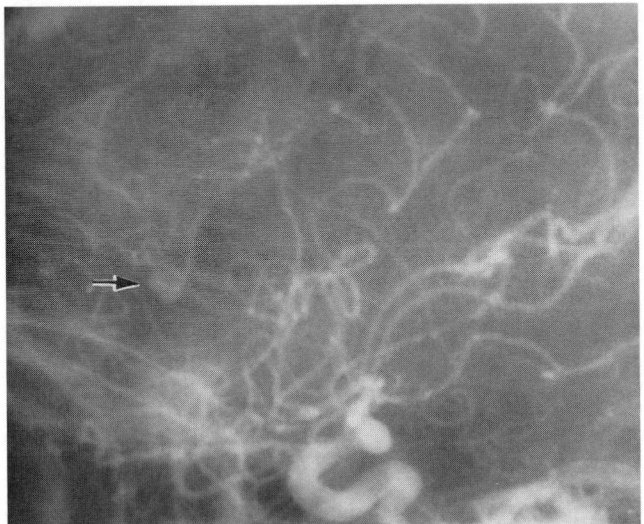

A

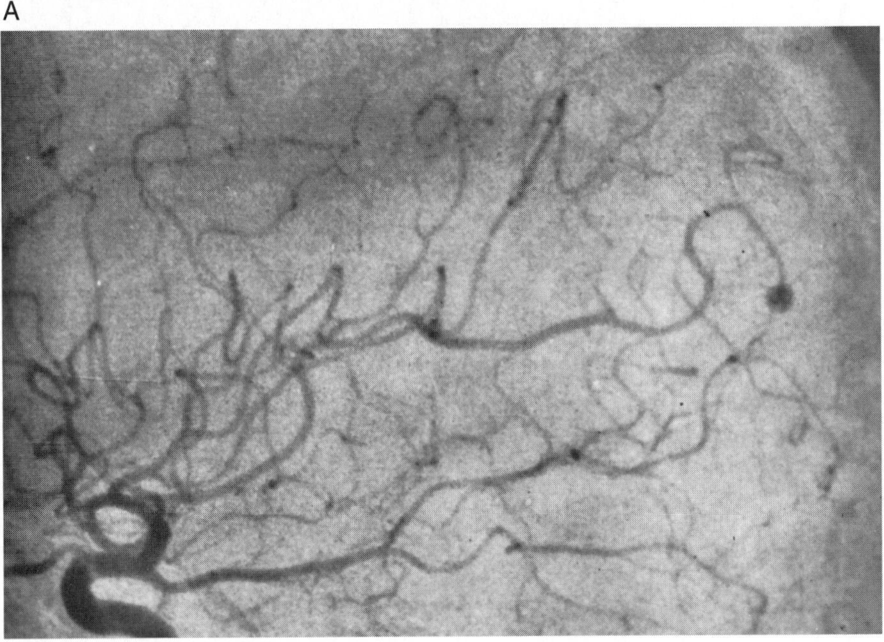

B

Figure 10.105. Peripheral aneurysms. **A.** A distal anterior cerebral "congenital" aneurysm at the genu of the artery is present (arrow). The proximal segments of the anterior cerebral artery exhibit spasm, as does the supraclinoid part of the carotid siphon. **B.** A man who had been on antibiotic therapy for 4 weeks because of subacute bacterial endocarditis suddenly developed numbness of the left arm and left side of the face. The angiogram discloses a mycotic aneurysm of the distal angular branch of the middle cerebral artery.

peripheral. These aneurysms may be congenital in origin. They may also be the result of embolism and trauma. Traumatic aneurysms are considered in Chapter 7.

The peripheral congenital aneurysms are usually found at secondary or tertiary branchings of the anterior and posterior cerebral arteries. For some reason, they are not as frequently seen along the distal segments of the middle cerebral artery. The lesions are saccular in type and have the other features frequently observed with berry aneurysms of the circle of Willis (Fig. 10.105). Large aneurysms are seldom seen peripherally. Most often such lesions attain a size of 5 to 6 mm in diameter, which are their average proportions when the patient is seen with a subarachnoid hemorrhage. There would appear to be a very strong tendency for such congenital peripheral lesions to bleed; they are seldom seen as an incidental finding in patients with brain tumors, or with aneurysms elsewhere that have bled.

Embolic aneurysms may be either infective or neoplastic. The middle cerebral arterial branches are most commonly affected. Before the advent of antibiotics, mycotic aneurysms accounted for at least 5 percent of intracranial aneurysms. Delayed or inadequate treatment of bacterial endocarditis is now associated with most cases, although such lesions can occur in drug addicts. Of the patients who have active subacute bacterial endocarditis, one-third have visceral emboli and one-half of the latter are to the brain. Congenital cardiac lesions may be complicated by infection and result in septic emboli lodging in distal cerebral arterial branches.

In many cases, hemorrhage from a mycotic intracranial aneurysm leads to death; it is not unusual for such a patient to have no clinically recognizable embolic episode preceding the hemorrhage. At other times, however, patients with bacterial endocarditis have neurologic problems of strokes or meningoencephalitis when first seen. If an embolic episode is recognized, angiography after an appropriate interval is advocated. From the best information available, it would appear that if a mycotic aneurysm develops, approximately 3 weeks elapse between the septic embolism and rupture of the aneurysm.

A local arteritis with destruction of the vessel wall and the development of a false aneurysm is the usual sequence. Such aneurysms are remarkably round in shape, and they rarely attain a diameter of more than 5 mm before bleeding ensues. Since the hemorrhage from such a destructive vascular lesion may be fatal, or a secondary infection with meningitis or a brain abscess may develop, the lesions are usually treated by surgical excision as soon as they are detected (Fig. 10.105B).

Occasionally, a sizable group of neoplastic cells will metastasize as an embolus and lodge in one of the smaller cerebral vessels. Such tumor cells often come from malignant pulmonary lesions, but occasionally a benign intracavitary tumor of the heart, a cardiac myxoma, may be the cause. The tumors, the majority of which arise in the left atrium, frequently embolize, and approximately one-half of the emboli are cerebral. The myxomatous emboli cause arterial occlusions and damage to the walls of the vessels. Cerebral infarction and hemorrhage are common complications. The embolic myxomatous cells invade and destroy the normal elements of arterial walls, and because their growth is slow and accompanied by connective tissue proliferation, false aneurysms may develop. New et al. described 3 such cases and reviewed the literature on the subject (219). They also gave a detailed correlation of angiographic and pathologic findings. The radiologic abnormalities include irregular filling defects in major and minor cerebral arterial branches, occlusions of vessels, a delay in circulation of contrast material, and the presence of fusiform and saccular aneurysms, chiefly of the middle cerebral arterial tree (Fig. 10.106). The patient may also present with recurrent episodes of hemorrhagic cerebral infarction demonstrable on CT or MRI (220).

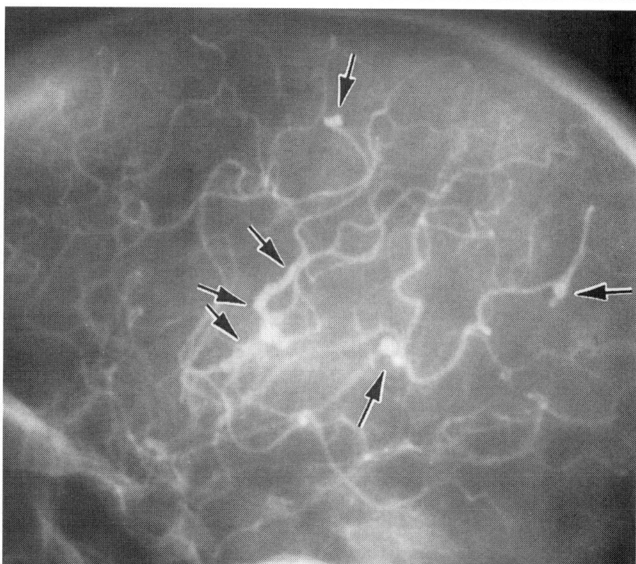

Figure 10.106. Neoplastic embolic aneurysms. Multiple peripheral cerebral aneurysms have developed in a patient with an established diagnosis of intracavitary cardiac myxoma. The rostral and inferior three arrows point to a lengthy middle cerebral segmental fusiform dilatation. The upper and posterior three arrows indicate more localized and rounded abnormal dilatations or false aneurysms. (Courtesy of Dr. P. F. J. New, Boston, Mass.)

MULTIPLE ANEURYSMS

The first clear description of multiple berry aneurysms of the brain was published by Thomson (221). Approximately one-third of patients with aneurysms have multiple lesions. The great majority of these patients have two aneurysms. In some cases, however, a large number of lesions may be present (Fig. 10.107). The author has encountered one case with 14 aneurysms and another patient with 11 lesions.

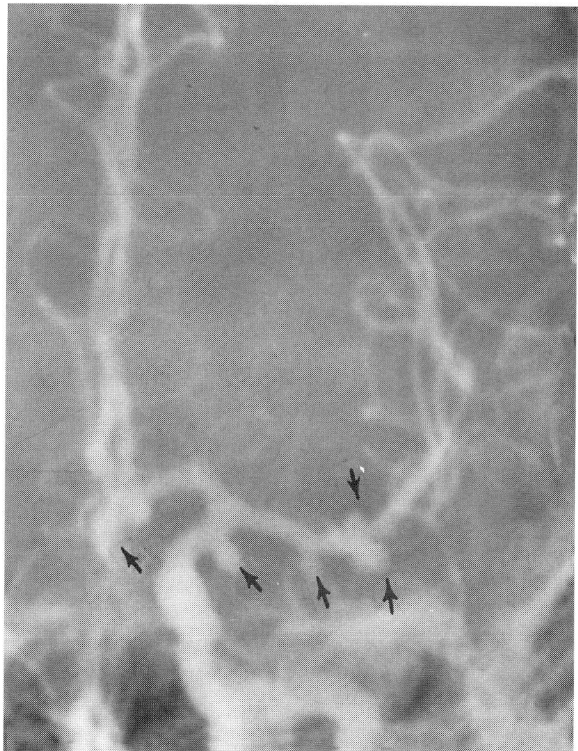

Figure 10.107. Multiple aneurysms. Five aneurysms are demonstrated by left carotid angiography alone; one is at the anterior communicating site, one at the posterior communicating location, and three in the proximal middle cerebral arterial branchings (arrows).

It is important to be able to identify a bleeding aneurysm among multiple lesions in order to avoid a delay in proper treatment or the institution of inappropriate treatment. In patients with multiple aneurysms the problem of finding angiographic clues as to which aneurysm has caused the subarachnoid hemorrhage may arise when there are no neurologic findings to localize the hemorrhage. Through a radiologic-pathologic correlative study of a large number of cases of multiple aneurysms, well documented anatomically, Wood found that it was possible to identify the ruptured aneurysm from the angiogram in 95 percent of instances (222).

Prior to CT, the decision as to which of two or three aneurysms had bled was always difficult to make from angiography alone, and surgical approaches to the wrong aneurysm were not uncommon. Since the advent of CT, the diagnosis of which aneurysm had ruptured became much more secure because there is usually a larger amount of blood near the aneurysm that has ruptured (Fig. 10.96). In the occasional doubtful cases, one might depend on the presence of other signs, such as arterial spasm or aneurysmal sac size (Table 10.20).

Greater size is the most frequent common denominator among aneurysms that have bled in patients with multiple lesions. In 87 percent of the patients studied by Wood (222), it was found that the larger of two aneurysms (or the largest of more than two aneurysms) was the lesion that had ruptured. These observations were confirmed by the pathologic studies of Crompton (201), who found that in 88 percent of patients with multiple aneurysms, the largest aneurysm had ruptured.

If one has the advantage of observing the appearance of multiple aneurysms on successive angiograms made either a few days or many months apart, changes in the size and shape of the aneurysms may be significant findings. When one aneurysm is observed to increase in size or to develop loculations between two examinations while other aneurysms remain essentially unchanged, the enlargement is reliable evidence of aneurysmal rupture.

It might be expected that the location of an aneurysm is significant with regard to its probability of rupture in that the more proximal lesions are subjected to greater pressure and flow. Jain observed that in ipsilateral multiple aneurysms in which one lies distal to the other on the same artery or a branch of the artery, the proximal aneurysm ruptures two-thirds of the time (223). For example, if middle cerebral and internal carotid aneurysms are present on the same side, the carotid aneurysm ruptures more often. (A notable exception, already mentioned, is the site of the anterior communicating artery, where an aneurysm, in association with a lesion at any other location, ruptures in 70 percent of instances.)

The categories shown in Figure 10.108 may be useful for showing more clearly some possible combinations of bleeding and nonbleeding multiple aneurysms.

Table 10.20.
Multiple Aneurysms: Neuroimaging Findings Helpful in Determining Site of Rupture

Site of hemorrhage as demonstrated by CT
Largest aneurysm demonstrated by angiography
Irregular aneurysm contour
Aneurysm closest to site of vasospasm

CEREBRAL ANGIOGRAPHY

Angiography is carried out soon after the patient undergoes CT examination. By CT, the diagnosis of subarachnoid hemorrhage has been made, and the probable location of the aneurysm has been determined. If the patient is in good clinical condition—grade 0 to 2—an angiographic diagnosis is needed to decide on the type and the timing of treatment to be applied. In grades 3, 4, and 5 it is necessary to know the location and the size of the aneurysm in order to make a decision as to management. However, if the patient is grade 3, it may be useful to wait for a day or two to determine the evolution of the patient's clinical condition.

If CT indicates the probable side of the lesion, the carotid artery on that side is injected first (approximately 90 percent of aneurysms fill from the carotid circulation). The aneurysm may be readily seen, but it is important to look for signs of arterial spasm, for, if spasm is present, it is wise to refrain from further injections to avoid adding any possible irritant to the spastic vessels. The use of nonionic contrast media is preferred. If spasm is present, it is best to postpone further angiography of the other vessels (carotid and vertebrobasilar) because in the presence of spasm, the treatment will usually be postponed for several days.

The author advocates simultaneous anteroposterior (AP) and lateral serialograms with each injection of contrast to minimize the total amount of contrast to be used.

If no aneurysm is demonstrated in the first injected carotid artery, the other side is done next, but it may be useful to perform a frontal view with compression of the opposite carotid artery in the neck before removing the catheter. In this way the collateral circulation across the anterior communicating artery is tested and, in addition, the anterior communicating artery region may be better visualized. It should be remembered that in spite of apparent excellent filling of the opposite side with compression, an aneurysmal sac may not fill (Fig. 10.109). The same applies to aneurysms arising from the vertebral artery prior to the origin of the basilar artery. If regurgitation is obtained from a vertebral injection into the opposite side and the contrast reaches the origin of the PICA, one can hope to have obtained sufficient visualization in the great majority of cases. Unfortunately, a small aneurysm may not fill sufficiently, and for that reason it is recommended that each vertebral artery be injected separately. Recent reports indicate that it is possible to demonstrate an aneurysm by MRA that was not seen by conventional angiography (205, 224).

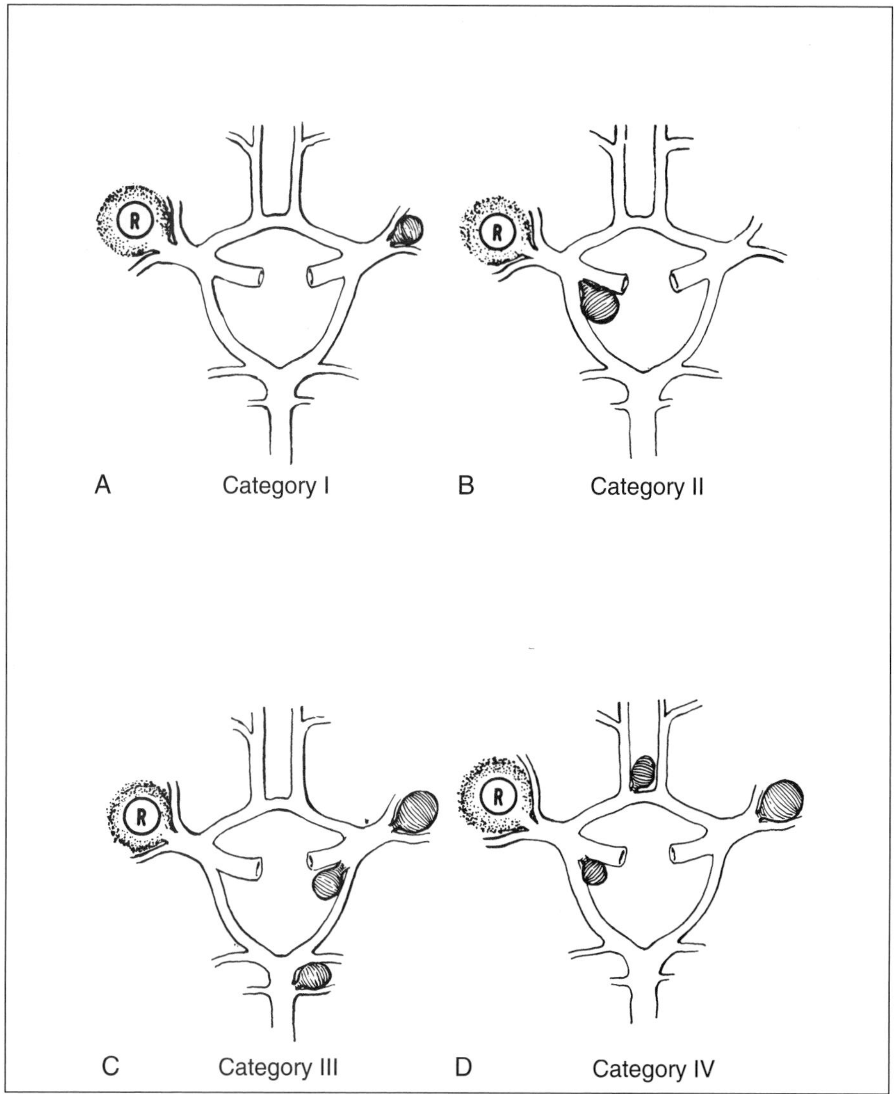

Figure 10.108. Schematic portrayal of multiple aneurysms. Cases can be placed in one of the four categories shown according to the relationship of the ruptured (R) and unruptured aneurysms. Patients with two aneurysms are in category I or II, depending on whether the lesions are in different systems or in the same major vascular system, respectively. **A.** Bilateral aneurysms of the middle cerebral arteries are shown. **B.** An unruptured aneurysm of the posterior communicating artery is on the same side as a ruptured lesion of the middle cerebral artery. Similarly, patients with more than two aneurysms can be placed in category III or IV, depending on whether the ruptured aneurysm is isolated on one major cerebral arborization (**C**), or whether one or more unruptured lesions occur with it on the same system (**D**).

In some cases, aneurysms arising in the fork between the internal carotid and posterior communicating arteries may not fill at carotid angiography but may be seen after catheter injection of the vertebral artery with carotid compression. Information is also gained about potential flow through the posterior communicating artery if carotid ligation is to be performed.

Positioning and filming are tailored to the needs of the individual case. Inasmuch as angiography is performed with an intent to apply the proper surgical treatment, a study of the exact relationship of the vessels to the aneurysmal wall, neck, and orifice is essential. An effort should be made to determine all points of diagnosis before removing the catheter. Many cases require several injections before a complete study is made. It is in this type of case that simultaneous biplane angiography is extremely useful, not only by shortening the time of the examination but also by diminishing the amount of contrast material that must be injected. At least 10 min, and preferably more, should be allowed to elapse between successive full size injections, usually of 8 ml of contrast material. Smaller amounts are used for more selective injections.

The arterial phase, recorded at about 2 exposures per second, is, of course, the most important, and in some cases it

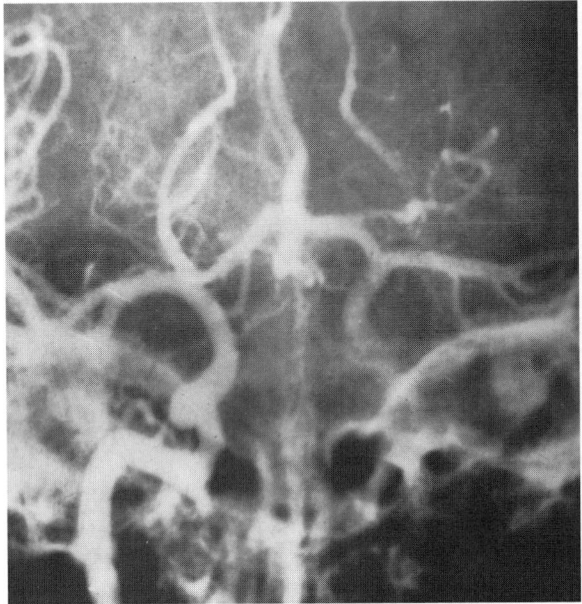

A

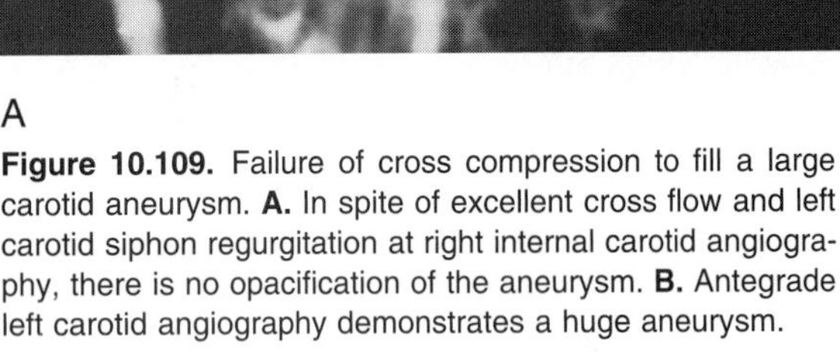

Figure 10.109. Failure of cross compression to fill a large carotid aneurysm. **A.** In spite of excellent cross flow and left carotid siphon regurgitation at right internal carotid angiography, there is no opacification of the aneurysm. **B.** Antegrade left carotid angiography demonstrates a huge aneurysm.

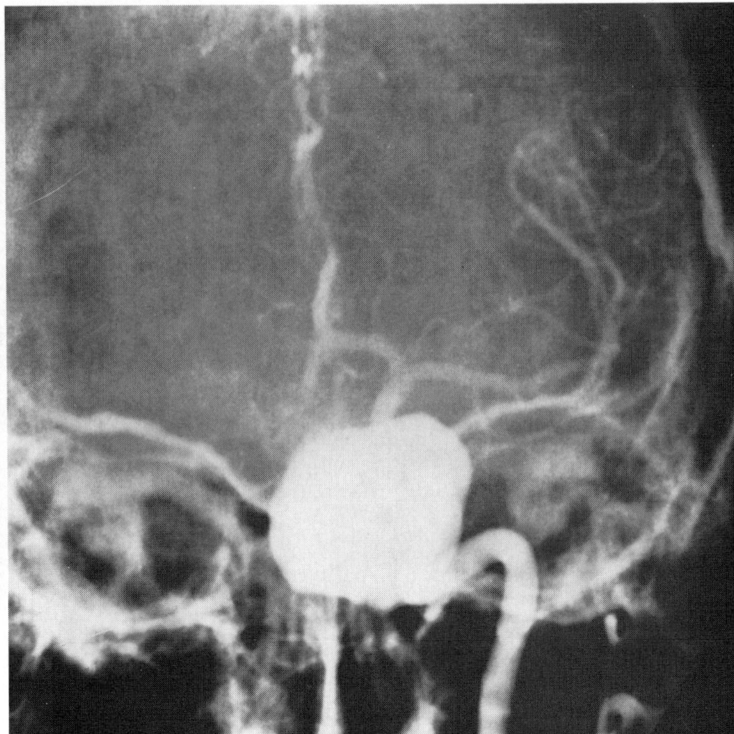

B

is desirable to obtain the first films at 4 frames per second in order to observe the filling pattern of an aneurysm and better visualize its orifice and the neck. The first series includes frontal and lateral views taken in the standard angiographic projections. (The AP view is angled 12° above the orbitomeatal line.) If these films show no evidence of spasm, then additional injections are made on the same side if necessary. An oblique view with 25° to 30° rotation of the head away from the side being injected is taken almost routinely. This oblique film serves to visualize, in another plane, aneurysms that may have been seen on the initial series as well as to "uncoil" the vessels in case another aneurysm may be hidden because of tortuosity. The contralateral oblique view is essential for visualizing the anterior communicating artery territory. This standard frontal oblique position also serves to open the U loop formed by the anterior and middle cerebral arteries. In addition to projecting the anterior cerebral arteries apart and opening the U loop, it shows the posterolateral and anteromedial walls of the supraclinoid segment of the internal carotid artery in profile. The simultaneous off-lateral projection is often suboptimal but frequently gives information when there is tortuosity from arteriosclerosis. Displacements caused by hematomas are difficult to recognize in such nonstandard projections. It should go without saying that, after the first standard frontal and lateral serialograms, the x-ray beam should be coned or collimated as narrowly as practicable.

The value of additional special views is difficult to overestimate. The reverse oblique frontal view is a widely advocated projection that is made by turning the head ipsilateral to the side of injection. This projection is particularly important for aneurysms in the region of the posterior communicating artery, which are often superimposed on the parent vessel in the standard angiographic frontal projection and may be even further obscured in the standard oblique projection, especially if such an aneurysm projects posteriorly and medially.

A transorbital view is extremely useful for studying the horizontal portion and genu of the middle cerebral artery as well as the bifurcation of the internal carotid artery. A small aneurysm in the bifurcation or trifurcation of the middle cerebral artery may be largely obscured by the trunk and branches of the vessel in the standard frontal projection but may be demonstrated well in orbital films. For such middle cerebral lesions, a transorbital study that is a straight anteroposterior view with the vertical x-ray beam projected through the center of the orbit is usually adequate (Fig. 10.110). The bifurcation or trifurcation of the middle cerebral artery and the divergence of its branches should be projected through the central portion of the orbital cavity, minimizing the number of the superimposed shadows.

Perorbital views of aneurysms more medially situated can be obtained by applying simple geometry to the first series of standard angiograms. In the lateral view, a line is drawn parallel to the orbitomeatal line through the aneurysm. Another line is drawn from the estimated pupillary point to meet the first line in the aneurysm

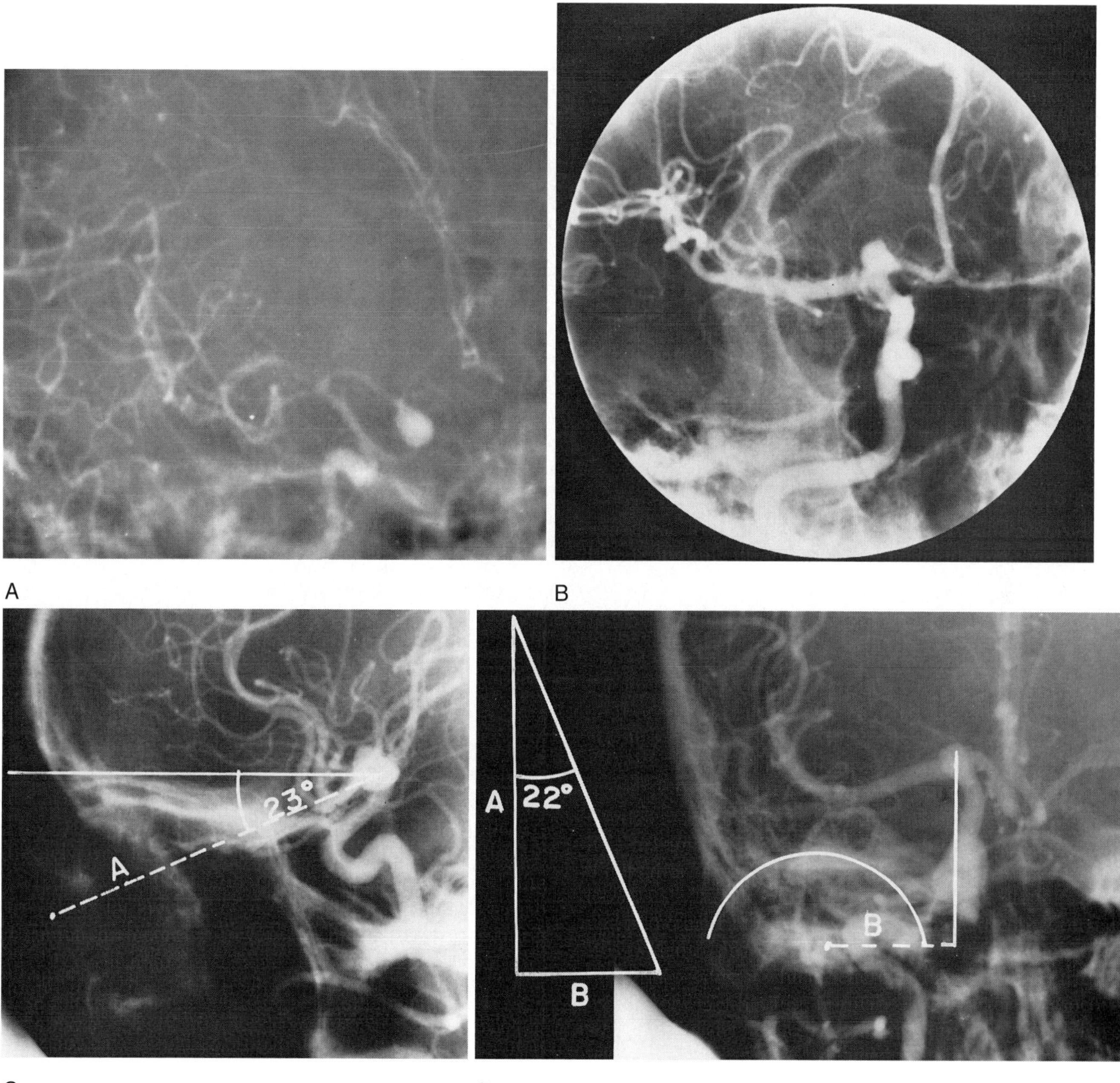

Figure 10.110. Techniques of head rotation and tube angulation in studying aneurysms. **A.** The standard frontal oblique angiogram is made with the head rotated 25° contralateral to the side of injection. The point of origin and a profile view of the neck of an anterior communicating aneurysm are often best seen in this projection. **B.** A carotid bifurcation aneurysm is projected through the center of the orbit and visualized free of overlying bone shadows. However, the orifice was wide and a well-defined neck was never seen in profile. **C.** In the same case as B, the method of determining tube angulation is shown. A line is drawn parallel to the orbitomeatal line through the aneurysm, and another line is drawn from the estimated pupillary point to meet the first in the aneurysm shadow. In this case the x-ray tube had to be angled 23° caudocranially to project the aneurysm through the orbit. **D.** In the same case as B and C, the method of determining the degree of required head rotation for the projection illustrated in B is shown. The distance from the pupillary point to the parasagittal plane of the aneurysm is measured and used as the base of a triangle. The distance from the pupillary point to the aneurysm in the lateral view (C) is plotted as the height of the triangle. The measurement of the smaller acute angle will indicate how much ipsilateral rotation of the head is required to bring the medially situated aneurysm behind the center of the orbit (the angle of rotation needed to project the aneurysm along the hypotenuse rather than the long side of the triangle).

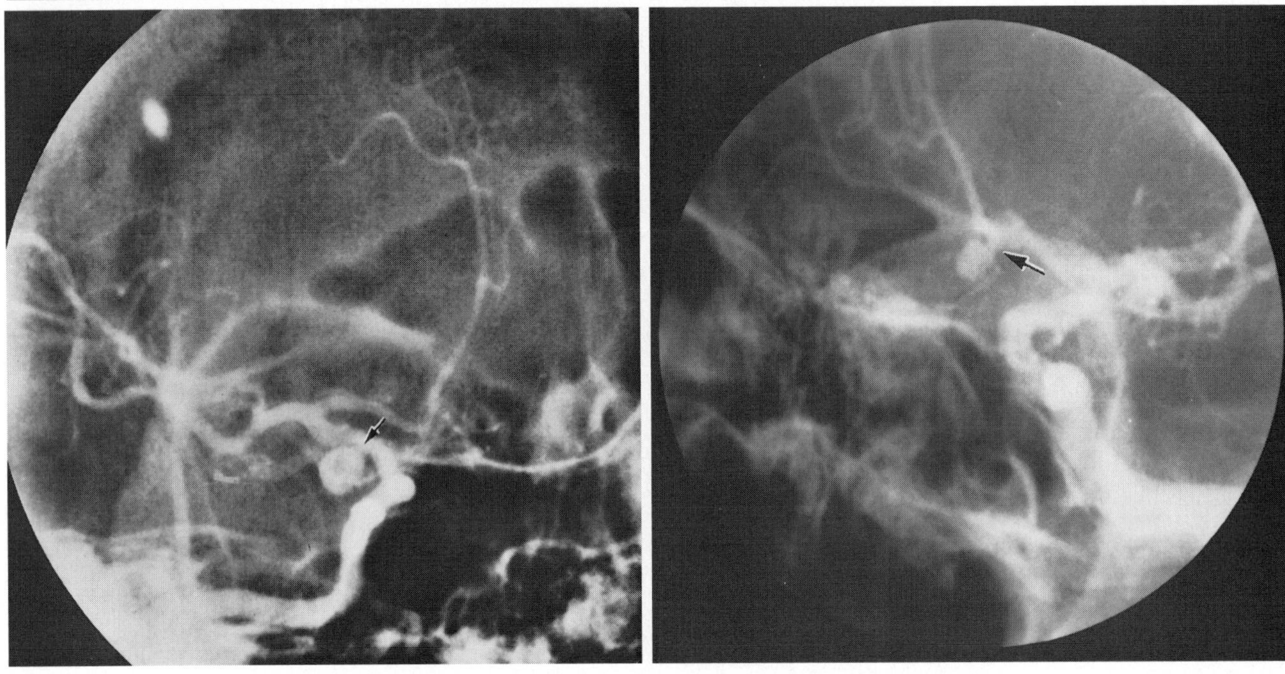

Figure 10.110. *(continued)* **E.** The perorbital technique is used to show the neck of a posterior communicating aneurysm (arrow). **F.** A more marked angulation was required to demonstrate the neck of an anterior communicating aneurysm (arrow). Nonsubtraction films are used in this illustration to show the relationship with the bony contours more clearly.

shadow. The angle formed by the lines indicates the degree of caudocranial angulation of the x-ray tube that must be used for an anteroposterior angiogram to project the aneurysm through the center of the orbit. In the frontal view, a line is drawn through the aneurysm in the sagittal plane. A second line is constructed from the parasagittal line to the center of the orbit. If the oblique line from the lateral view and the transverse line from the frontal view are drawn at right angles to each other and a hypotenuse constructed, the small acute angle produced will indicate the degree of rotation of the head that is required to bring the center of the orbit into line with the aneurysm. Using this rotation of the head and angulation of the tube, a virtually bone-free depiction of the aneurysm is obtained (Fig. 10.110).

Some middle cerebral artery aneurysms extend almost straight forward or at only slight angles from the axis of the transverse portion of the vessel. In these cases the aneurysm will overlie the bifurcation or trifurcation of the artery in the straight orbital view. In some cases, an axial or base view may show such an aneurysm in profile so that its neck can be seen. At other times, however, this projection does not throw the aneurysm completely clear. If the aneurysm could be seen without the superimposition of other vessels, particularly the anterior cerebral group, the lateral view would show the neck of such an aneurysm satisfactorily. In order to visualize the lesion satisfactorily, a 30° off-lateral view is recommended.

The 30° off-lateral projection for middle cerebral artery aneurysms can be easily obtained in one of several ways. If the patient is on a table that can be readily moved in relation to the head support, the foot of the table can be turned toward the side being injected until the axes of the head and body make an angle of 30° with their original line. The tube and film are not moved (Fig. 10.111). The same view can be accomplished by moving the tube and film changer 30° and leaving the patient in his or her original position. Another possibility is to tilt the head and neck 30° away from the side being injected, leaving the axis of the body as well as the tube and film in their original position. Any of these arrangements causes the genu of the middle cerebral artery to be projected well above the horizontal limbs of the anterior and middle cerebral arteries and above the region of the anterior communicating artery. It is often possible to then see the aneurysmal neck and its point of origin from the parent vessel in profile.

The full axial or submentovertical view is often very helpful in visualizing several types of intradural aneurysms as well as those in the cavernous sinus. The difficulty and danger of positioning the patient for this type of projection are lessened when the carotid artery is opacified via a femoral catheter. In addition to being useful in studying middle cerebral artery lesions, this approach can give valuable information concerning aneurysms of the anterior and posterior communicating sites. One can visualize the neck of the aneurysm and gain important information about the

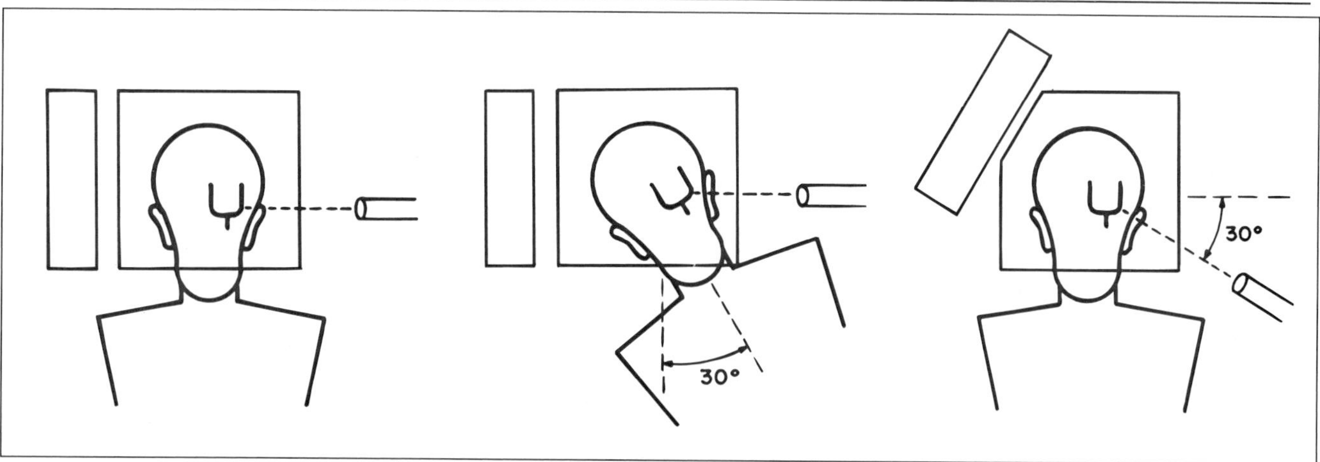

Figure 10.111. Methods of obtaining off-lateral projections of middle cerebral aneurysms. From the straight lateral view, the genu of the middle cerebral artery can be projected higher by moving the patient or by moving the tube and film as shown in the sketches (see text).

relationship of the lesion to surrounding vessels. For example, an aneurysm arising in the fork between the internal carotid artery and the posterior communicating artery may lie either medial or lateral to the latter vessel (Fig. 10.112). If the lesion is medial, the posterior communicating artery may have to be sacrificed in order to clip the aneurysm. In other cases, when the exact point of origin of a lesion in the anterior communicating region is shown, preoperative plans can be made for preserving (or altering) circulation through the circle of Willis.

The axial view is also quite valuable for demonstrating details of aneurysms arising along the vertebrobasilar system. The major vessels are visualized free of mastoid and petrosal shadows in this projection. At other times, a Caldwell or Waters projection may give the best view of a vertebral or basilar lesion face-on with minimal foreshortening of the vertebrobasilar shadows. Straight lateral views of posterior fossa aneurysms may give inadequate details about the lesions even with subtraction, which must be used liberally. A 45° oblique view often throws such lesions into good profile (Table 10.21).

Table 10.21.
Special Views Useful in Angiographic Evaluation of Aneurysms

Reverse oblique frontal view: posterior communicating artery aneurysms
Transorbital view: ICA bifurcation, MCA bifurcation
Oblique frontal projection: anterior communicating artery aneurysm
Submentovertex view: posterior communicating artery or basilar tip aneurysm

RADIOLOGIC DIAGNOSIS OF ANEURYSMS

The actual angiographic diagnosis of an aneurysm is extremely easy once it has been demonstrated on films made in proper projections. Aneurysms may be overlooked if all the vessels are not carefully scrutinized in frontal and lateral projections; an error also may result when poorly visualized arteries are not studied further by making a second injection and rotating the head in the most desirable direction to uncoil a loop of the vessel. A common error of commission is incorrect interpretation of a vessel seen end on, which may give the impression of an aneurysm. A segment of vessel seen end on, however, is always denser than the same vessel immediately proximal or distal. Since the lumen of the vessel is visualized containing a column of contrast substance possibly 0.5 to 1.0 cm in length, it obviously must be denser than the vessel itself, which only measures 0.2 cm. On the other hand, an aneurysm has no more density than the parent vessel and, in fact, the density of the aneurysmal sac on films is usually less than that of an artery of the same diameter.

In addition to the technical and interpretational pitfalls already mentioned, there are also natural causes of diagnostic error. These may be physiologic or anatomic. The most common natural phenomenon accounting for diagnostic failures is a disturbance of cerebral circulation caused by subarachnoid hemorrhage. When there is spasm, the vessels are narrowed in caliber and are poorly visualized by the reduced circulation and delay in filling of vessels. The spasm is usually most severe in the neighborhood of a ruptured aneurysm, but distant spasm may also occur (a) throughout the entire arborization of the vessel on which a ruptured aneurysm is situated, (b) throughout the entire ipsilateral cerebral hemisphere, or (c) bilaterally or generalized throughout the brain. In the majority of cases, however, the vascular narrowing is greatest in, or limited to, the neighborhood of a ruptured aneurysm, and in some cases an aneurysm will not be visualized because of the spasm. In 2.5 percent of the cases studied by Perret and Bull, the aneurysm that had caused the subarachnoid hemorrhage was not outlined because of spasm (225). When

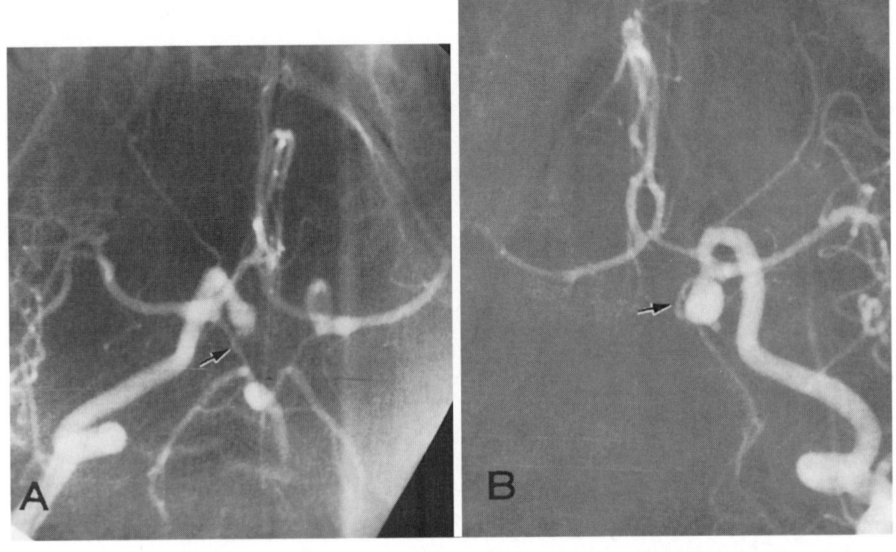

A B

Figure 10.112. Axial projection with subtraction. **A.** An aneurysm arising from the right internal carotid artery projects backward and medially and is shown to lie medial to the posterior communicating artery (arrow). **B.** In another case, an aneurysm arising in the fork between the left internal carotid and posterior communicating arteries is shown to lie lateral to the communicating vessel (arrow). **C** to **H.** Complex aneurysm and aneurysm near the base of the skull demonstrated by CT angiography (CTA). **C.** Conventional angiography demonstrates a left middle cerebral trifurcation aneurysm. The relationship of the sac to the arterial branches is difficult to visualize. **D.** MRA shows the aneurysmal sac. **E.** CTA reveals the aneurysmal sac with greater detail than MRA. A slowly filling aneurysm and branches may not show as well with MRA as with CTA. **F.** Shaded surface display provides a much better understanding of the relationship of the sac to the trifurcation branches and to other smaller branches crossing the surface of the aneurysm.

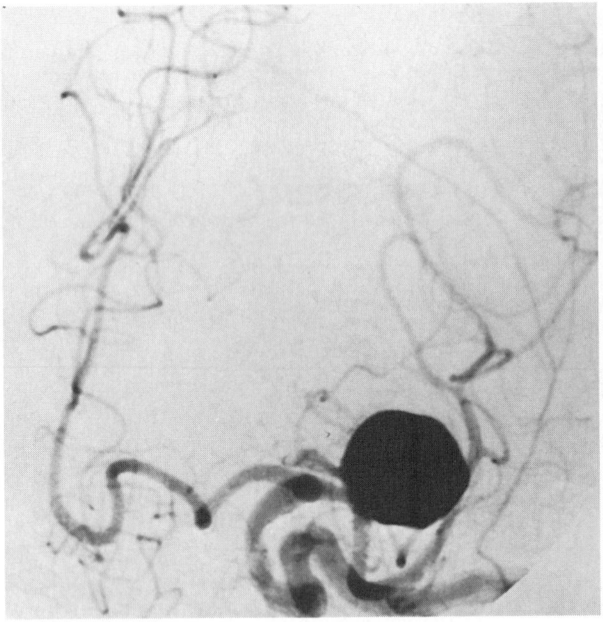

C 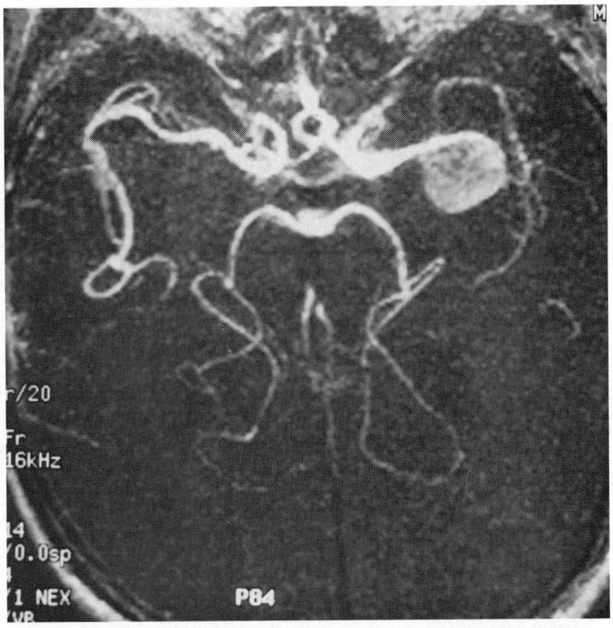 D

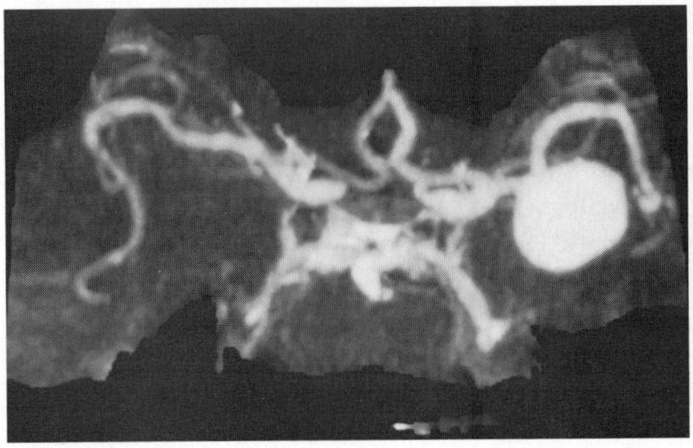

E 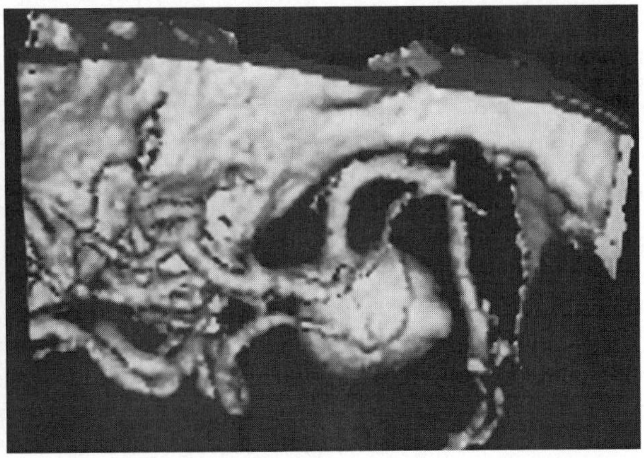 F

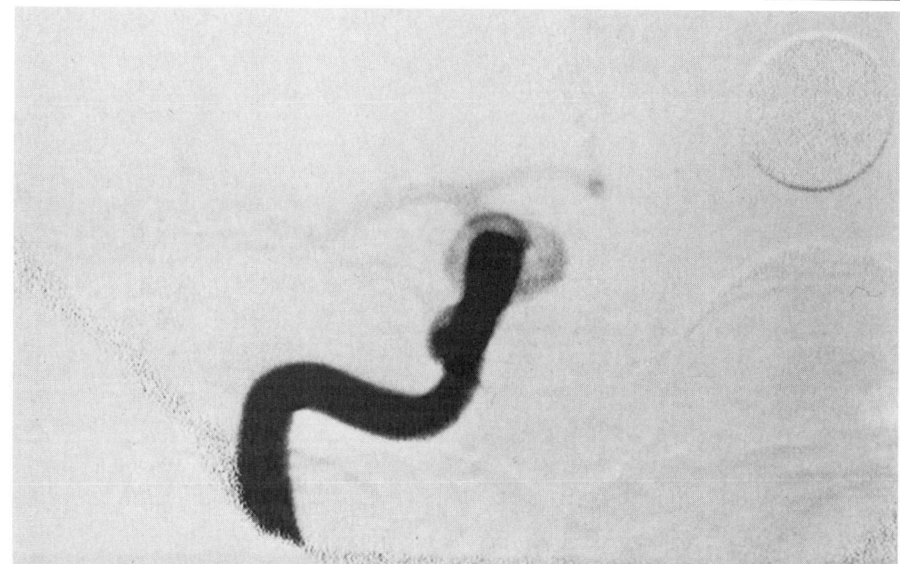

G

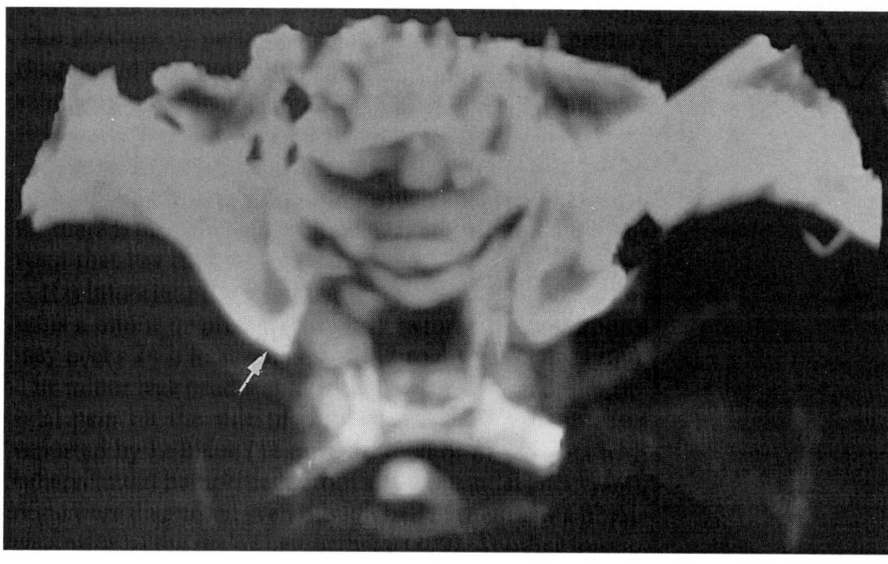

H

Figure 10.112. *(continued)* **G.** MRA of another patient presenting an aneurysm near or at the origin of the ophthalmic artery. **H.** CTA reveals the erosion of the medial aspect of the right anterior clinoid process (arrow) and the relationship of the sac with the surrounding bones at the skull base. This information was extremely useful to the neurosurgeon.

no cause for a subarachnoid hemorrhage is demonstrated at angiography, and significant spasm is observed, it is recommended that the examination be repeated after a few days (usually 5 or 6 days). The repeat examination is not only useful for diagnosis but is valuable for prognosis and is a guide to the selection of an optimal time for the institution of surgical treatment. If spasm is present in a patient with subarachnoid hemorrhage without an aneurysm being opacified, this is strong evidence that a ruptured aneurysm is indeed present even if it is not seen initially. The vessel eliciting the greatest degree of spasm should be examined first at the time of the repeat study, 5 or 6 days after the initial examination. Spasm of significant degree may persist for as long as 3 or 4 weeks after a bleeding episode. According to the studies of Bergvall and Galera, spasm is most severe between 6 and 12 days after a subarachnoid hemorrhage (214). They found that the circulation time was often prolonged for 4 to 5 weeks. As noted in text following, spasm is likely to occur and be more severe earlier in patients whose hemorrhage results in an intracerebral hematoma, that is, during the first 6 days.

In a small percentage of patients, angiography fails to demonstrate an aneurysm that is later shown to be present and no cause for the failure is evident. It appears probable that, in a majority of instances, nonfilling of an aneurysm is related to anatomic factors if faulty radiographic technique can be excluded. The most common similarity, among aneurysms found at necropsy that do not fill by angiography during life, is that the size of the orifice is small in relation to the volume of aneurysm.

Table 10.22.
Causes of False-Negative Angiography for Intracranial Aneurysms

Faulty angiographic technique
Overlap of vessels
Vasospasm
Thrombosed aneurysm

Another important reason for failure of aneurysms to fill is that they undergo thrombosis. Some aneurysms that are opacified can be seen to contain a thrombus in the lumen of the lesion. A double density may be found with the fundus being irregular in outline or a zone of reduced contrast density being present about the periphery of the lumen. A fibrinoid clot develops at the point of bleeding soon after it occurs, and this is probably the reason that bleeding points and even extravasation of contrast material are not seen more frequently. It is not known how often small aneurysms undergo self-extinction following rupture by closing the lumen to blood flow from the parent vessel through thrombosis. The number of cases may be significant. It is probable that such an event accounts for the better prognosis for patients in whom no cause is ever found for a subarachnoid hemorrhage (Table 10.22).

MRI and MRA are also very useful in the study of aneurysms, particularly those that have not bled, or if the angiographic study is postponed in a patient with known subarachnoid hemorrhage. Huston et al. reported a positive diagnosis in 87.5 percent of cases using TOF technique in aneurysms that were 5.0 mm or larger. However, the percentage drops considerably in aneurysms only 3 mm in size to the point where they were confidently identified only retrospectively from prior angiography (226). The three-dimensional TOF technique seems preferable to the phase-contrast technique (227).

The relatively recent advances in CT technology make it possible to attempt a diagnosis of aneurysm at the same time that the initial examination is carried out and a subarachnoid hemorrhage is demonstrated. A diagnosis probably cannot be made if the blood clot is too large because the clot would tend to obscure the postcontrast CT findings. Aoki et al. suggest a three-dimensional technique with appropriate reconstruction (8). A supraorbitomeatal plane can be used to minimize radiation exposure to the lens; 1.5-mm contiguous sections for a total thickness of about 3.5 to 4.0 cm are made while injecting a 60 percent concentration of one of the tri-iodinated contrast media at the rate of 1.0 ml/sec. The exposure can be made with a conventional unit, which permits a dynamic set of contiguous exposures, or, preferably, with the spiral CT technique (injecting 2.0 ml/sec), which would allow for a much more rapid examination. Aoki et al., using this technique, demonstrated 15 out of 15 aneurysms shown by conventional angiography (8).

CT angiography carried out with the spiral (helical) technique is particularly useful in the study of aneurysms, already demonstrated by angiography, located at the base of the skull. It assists the surgeon in determining the exact relationship with osseous structures at the base of the skull for surgical planning (Fig. 10.112*C* to *H*).

COMPLICATIONS OF ANEURYSMAL RUPTURE

The volume of blood that extravasates when an intracranial aneurysm ruptures is relatively small in comparison with the hemorrhages from aneurysms in other parts of the body. The acute appearance of blood in the subarachnoid space is not, in itself, a threat to life. On the other hand, death may rapidly ensue when there is trauma to important centers in the brain by a rapidly dissecting hemorrhage. Complications more often occur later because of the secondary compression and displacement effects of a hematoma, the prolonged occurrence of cerebral ischemia leading to infarction, or the development of both hematoma and infarction. Infarction, through the development of associated edema, may produce a mass effect that at times exceeds that of a hematoma. Either may cause a cerebral herniation.

Hematoma

The rupture of approximately two-thirds of cerebral aneurysms results in the formation of hematomas, which may be large or small. In fewer than one-half of patients in whom an intracerebral hematoma develops, the lesion is caused by a direct dissection of blood into the cerebral substance from the ruptured aneurysm. In the majority of the cases there is first an extravasation into the subarachnoid space, with subsequent or indirect dissection into the cerebral substance. In a small number of patients (2 percent) the rupture of an aneurysm may be accompanied by tearing of the arachnoid, with direct hemorrhage into the subdural space or dissection of subarachnoid blood between the arachnoid and dura mater (Fig. 10.100). Many patients with ruptured aneurysms have hematomas that remain confined to the subarachnoid space, where they produce the effects of a localized extracerebral mass.

Certain patterns of subarachnoid hematoma formation and of intracerebral dissection are found with aneurysms in specific locations. These patterns have been worked out pathologically and can be recognized by angiography, as described in text following. However, it is more satisfactory to diagnose and follow intracerebral hematomas by CT once the cause of bleeding has been established.

Not only are aneurysms of the anterior communicating artery responsible for subarachnoid hemorrhage more often than lesions at any other single site, but the rupture results in an intracerebral hematoma more often than with lesions at other sites. Inferior frontal or olfactory hemorrhages may dissect upward, and break into a frontal horn of the ventricular system (Fig. 10.113).

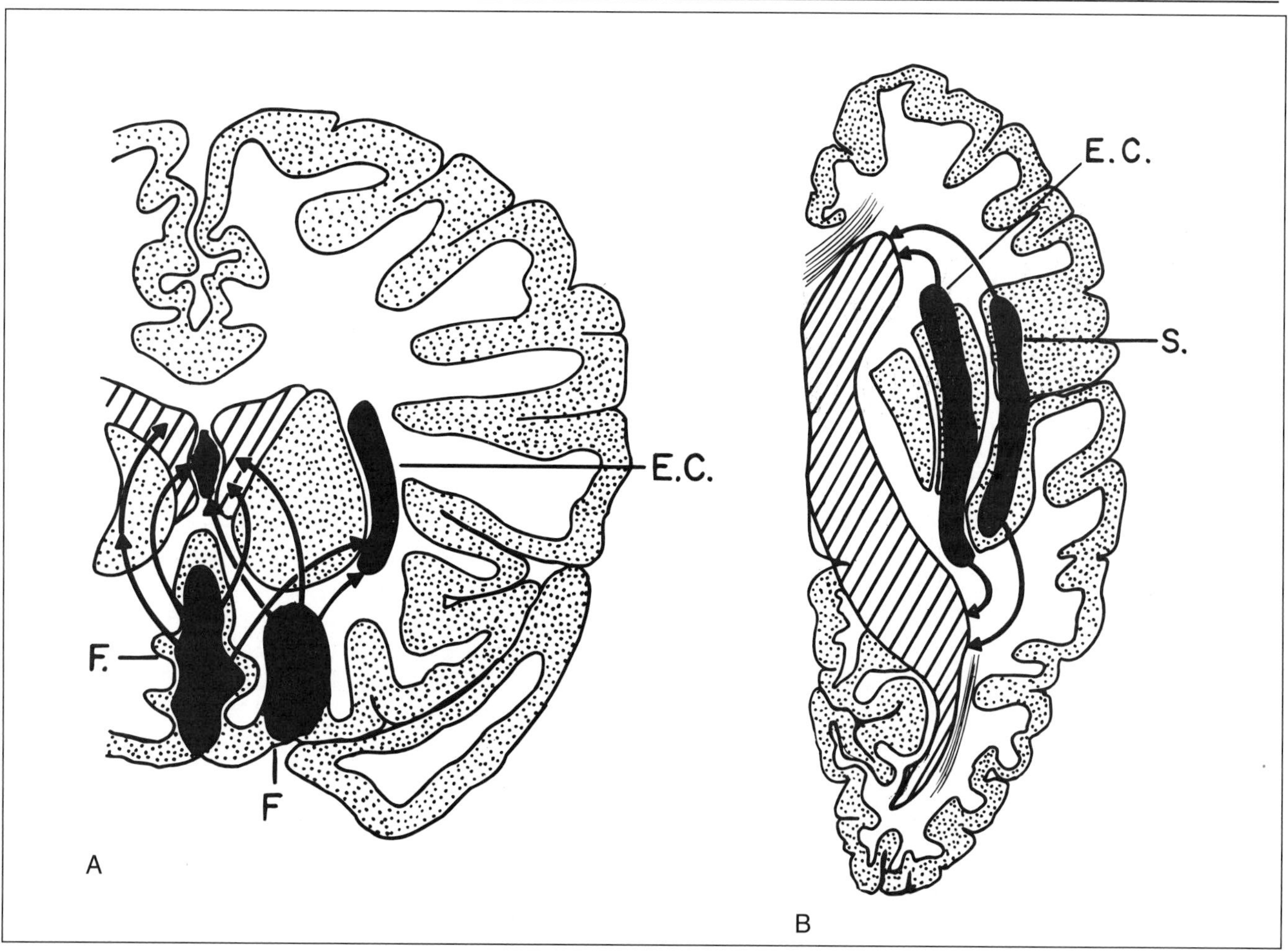

Figure 10.113. Patterns of development and dissection of hematomas. **A.** In the coronal section are shown the more common sites of hematomas developing from anteriorly and inferiorly situated carotid bifurcation, anterior communicating, and anterior cerebral aneurysms. F: Frontal lobe primary intracerebral hematoma that usually dissects in the directions of the arrows; IF: interfrontal subarachnoid hematoma that frequently ruptures secondarily into the cerebral substance; EC: external capsule, a frequent site of hematoma extension. **B.** The transverse section of the right cerebral hemisphere shows the frequent locations of intracerebral and subarachnoid hematomas from aneurysms of the middle cerebral artery. EC: External capsule, common site of occurrence of primary intracerebral hematomas; S: Sylvian subarachnoid space over the insula.

At other times an anterior communicating artery aneurysm may rupture into the subarachnoid space between the medial surfaces of the frontal lobes and form an interfrontal subarachnoid hematoma. Such hematomas may dissect upward into the septum pellucidum, often distending the potential cavum between the layers of the septum pellucidum. At any point the dissecting subarachnoid hematoma may burst into the substance of the frontal lobe or into the ventricular system. Anterior communicating artery aneurysms are also the most common lesions to produce injury of the hypothalamus.

Less frequently, extension of an interfrontal hematoma may pass around the corpus callosum to form a hematoma in the callosal sulcus or in the intercingulate region. Dissection into the corpus callosum itself may take place, and occasionally an intracerebral hematoma developing primarily in the frontal lobe, or extending into it from the subarachnoid space, may dissect laterally into the external capsule. Aneurysms of an anterior cerebral artery distal to the circle of Willis produce hematomas in the proximity of the lesion. The more proximal anterior cerebral aneurysms most often rupture into the frontal lobe substance, whereas the more peripheral aneurysms produce hematomas in the callosal sulcus or in the cingulate fissure.

Aneurysms extending upward and forward from the bifurcation of the internal carotid artery often are imbedded in the frontal lobe and rupture directly into its substance; thence the hematoma may burst into a frontal horn of a lateral ventricle. Aneurysms at the bifurcation that extend backward and upward may rupture into the hypothalamic nuclei or through the lamina terminalis into the third ventricle.

Aneurysms of the cerebral segment of the internal carotid artery, which usually arise at the site of origin of the posterior communicating artery and extend backward, most often rupture into the anterior temporal lobe substance, and thence into the temporal horn. At other times, a subarachnoid hematoma may develop above the uncus and dissect along the choroidal fissure into a temporal horn. The hemorrhage may also extend beneath the uncus. Bleeding from the fundus of a forward-pointing aneurysm may result in a subarachnoid collection beneath the frontal lobes.

Middle cerebral artery aneurysms often result in the formation of a hematoma deep in the sylvian fissure over the central lobe or island of Reil. Such sylvian hematomas then may dissect into the external capsule (Fig. 10.113). There also may be direct rupture into the external capsule or into the frontal or temporal lobe. A hematoma may dissect forward from the external capsule or from the frontal horn of a lateral ventricle. At other times there may be dissection backward from the external capsule or temporal lobe with rupture into the atrium of a lateral ventricle.

Correlating well with the pathologic changes, CT demonstrates the hematomas extremely well, particularly in the acute stage. MRI may show them even better in axial, coronal, and sagittal views, particularly in the subacute stage. Angiography will demonstrate displacement of vessels corresponding to effects of mass lesions, but these findings will not be described here because CT or MRI examination is sufficient to diagnose the presence, size, and location of the hematoma (Fig. 10.101*A* and *B*).

Aneurysms at the rostral end of the basilar artery may rupture directly into the third ventricle, the lesions often being imbedded in the structures forming the posterior portion of the ventricular floor. At other times a hematoma may form in the cisterna interpeduncularis. Such a subarachnoid hematoma may then dissect caudad into the midbrain and pons, following the course of perforating branches of the basilar and posterior cerebral arteries. A posteroinferior cerebellar aneurysm may produce a hemorrhage in the brainstem and in the subarachnoid cisterns. Some PICA aneurysms are peripheral in position and produce a cerebellar hematoma in the proximity of the lesion.

It is generally accepted that the second bleeding of an aneurysm is more likely to result in serious complications, or even a terminal event, than is the first rupture. One important reason is that a second rupture usually occurs directly into the brain substance because the first hemorrhage produces subarachnoid adhesions in the neighborhood of the aneurysm or the development of adhesions binding the sac of the aneurysm to the pia mater. In a high percentage of fatal intracerebral hemorrhages, there is bleeding into the ventricular system. Under such circumstances, the ventricles may become rapidly distended with blood, which is evident on CT.

Infarction

Cerebral infarction is a more common fatal complication of the rupture of an intracranial aneurysm than intracerebral hematoma formation. In some cases, infarction can be produced by a hematoma. At times, an intracerebral hematoma compresses vessels, producing ischemia; very frequently such a hematoma evokes spasm with the same result. Whenever early, severe spasm is found after a subarachnoid hemorrhage, CT usually shows fairly extensive subarachnoid and/or intracerebral hemorrhage.

In a group of 159 cases coming to necropsy following the rupture of an aneurysm, 75 percent had significant infarction (228). Cortical infarction was found to occur almost twice as frequently as ganglionic infarction. The infarction associated with ruptured aneurysms is pale and ischemic, not hemorrhagic in type.

Cerebral infarction occurs most often after the rupture of aneurysms (a) of the internal carotid artery where the posterior communicating vessel originates, (b) of the middle cerebral artery, and (c) of the anterior communicating artery, and in that order of frequency. The order is just the reverse of that found for intracerebral hematomas, according to Crompton (228). Aneurysms at the origin of the posterior communicating artery produce infarction over a wider area than other aneurysms, probably because they are more proximal on the carotid arterial vascular tree. The infarcted area is most often found in the distribution of the middle cerebral artery, which is the main continuation of the internal carotid. The rupture of aneurysms at the posterior communicating level also produces more ganglionic infarcts than aneurysms at other sites. Bilateral infarction occurs frequently after the rupture of aneurysms of the anterior communicating artery. Such infarction is usually in the cortical distribution of the anterior cerebral arteries and, although the survival rate is relatively high, many patients exhibit mental changes (Fig. 10.114). The hematoma combined with the accompanying edema may produce a mass large enough to provoke hippocampal transtentorial herniation in the same manner as posttraumatic edema and hemorrhage or neoplasms.

Hydrocephalus

A sizable number of patients who have a subarachnoid hemorrhage develop hydrocephalus. The onset may be acute or gradual. Acute ventricular dilatation occurs when the initial hemorrhage extends directly into the ventricular lumen. Acute enlargement may also develop when an intracerebral hematoma dissects by pressure necrosis through the ventricular wall.

Follow-up CT scanning is necessary to follow ventricular size, for when there is ventricular dilatation, the patients will do poorly. If the ventricles continue to enlarge over a period of 24 to 72 h, a temporary ventricular shunt is required to maintain intracranial pressure within normal ranges (Fig. 10.114*C* to *F*).

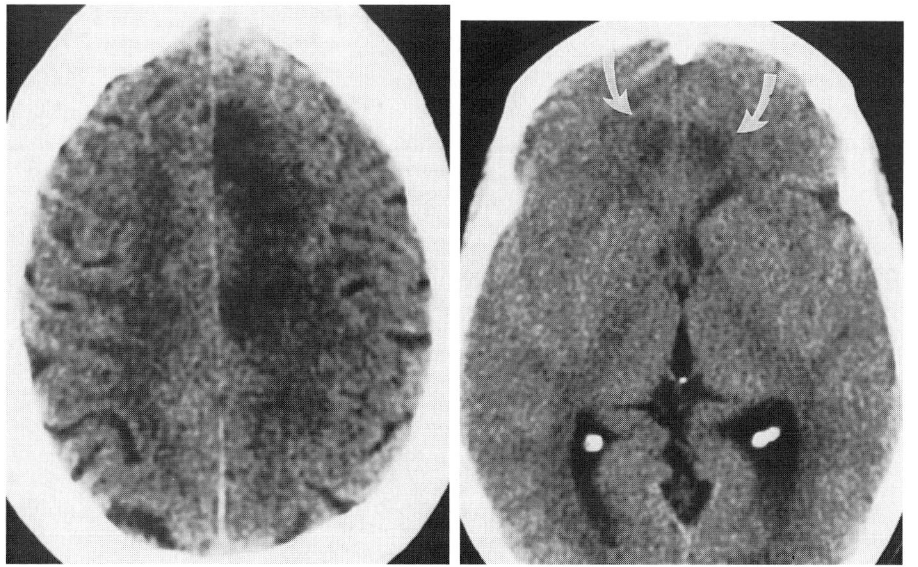

Figure 10.114. Cerebral ischemia in territories of both anterior cerebral arteries due to spasm in a patient with multiple aneurysms in the anterior cerebral arteries. **A.** There is bilateral hypodensity on each side of the midline and reaching the falx. This is typical of anterior cerebral artery involvement as against watershed ischemia, which does not reach the midline (compare with Fig. 10.47). **B.** Two weeks later the edema had improved, and only a small bilateral low density in the frontal region remained as a permanent infarction (arrows). **C** to **F.** Bleeding PICA aneurysm leading rapidly to hydrocephalus requiring shunting. Frontal (**C**) and lateral (**D**) angiography reveals a saccular aneurysm arising from the right PICA. **E.** The initial CT showed a subarachnoid hemorrhage not limited to the posterior fossa, with blood in the fourth ventricle. **F.** In less than 48 h the ventricles had become considerably larger, necessitating rapid installation of a shunt.

A

B

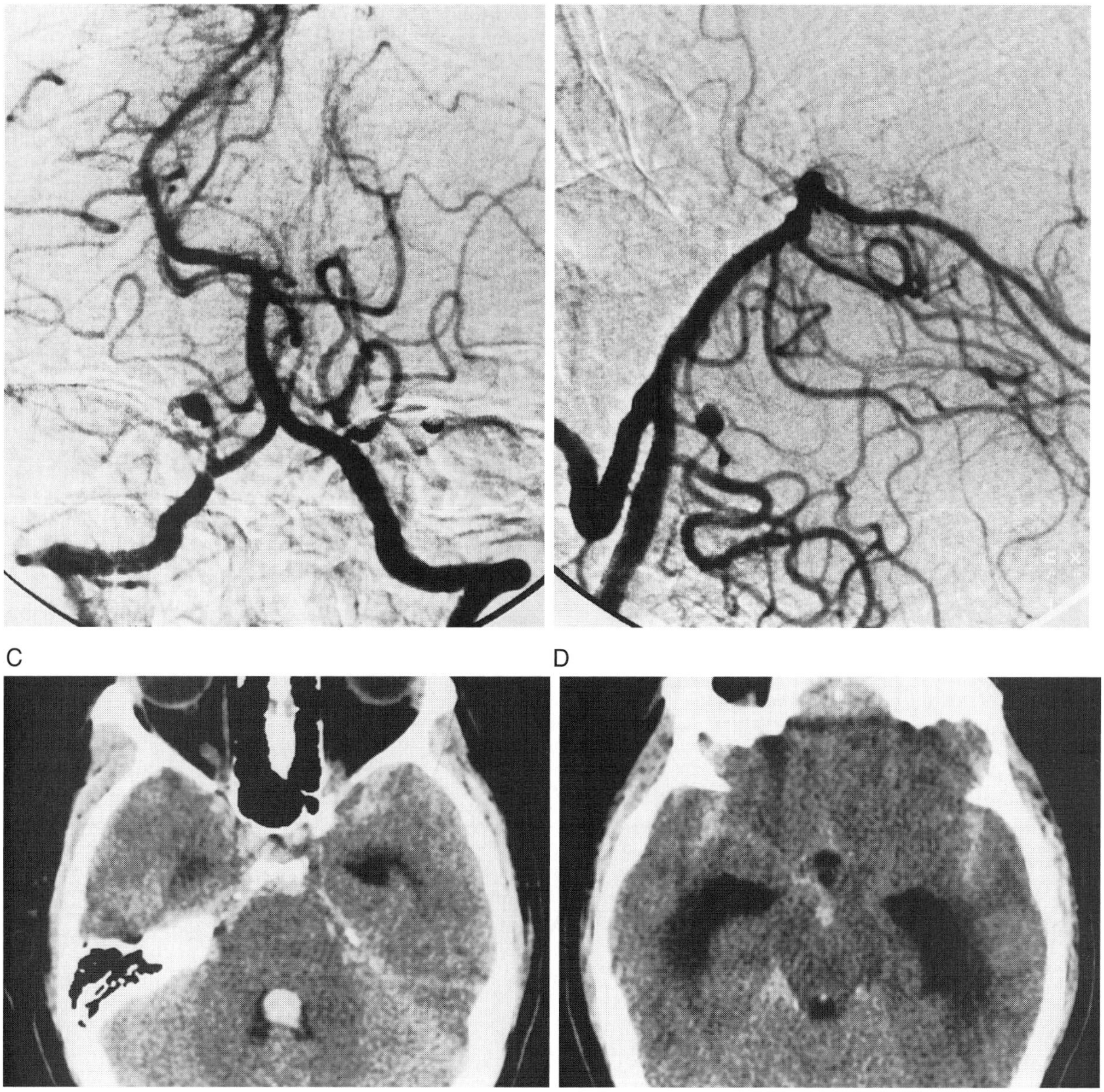

C

D

E

F

The cause of the dilatation is not always clear. Sometimes intraventricular bleeding may produce aqueductal blockage or interfere with normal passage of CSF through the fourth ventricle and ventricular outlets or through the tentorial incisura, but most often a mechanical cause cannot be seen. Probably the most important factor is the blockage of the arachnoid granulations by blood cells interfering with the absorption of fluid and of the protein in the fluid. Since this may occur acutely and may improve or disappear later, shunting is usually not required permanently.

Hyponatremia is a frequent cause of complications after subarachnoid hemorrhage and should be considered in the presence of neurologic deterioration. There is a decrease in total blood and plasma volume, which should be corrected by fluid replacement. Fluid restriction in these cases could be dangerous and might lead to cerebral infarction (229).

In most cases in succeeding days, the dilatation of the ventricular system develops gradually without dramatic symptoms. The changes often begin slowly after an interval of apparent clinical improvement. Patients who develop only mild ventricular enlargement may remain asymptomatic.

In most instances in which gradual hydrocephalus occurs, it begins within 1 month after the subarachnoid hemorrhage. In the patients who develop symptoms, the manifestations can be rather similar to normal pressure hydrocephalus. Headache, decline in level of consciousness, and general deterioration in the clinical state may occur, and CT or MRI will show ventricular enlargement with evidence of transependymal passage of CSF (periventricular hypodensity on CT or hyperintensity on T2-weighted images). Graff-Radford et al. showed that the incidence of hydrocephalus after subarachnoid hemorrhage may be increased by the use of antifibrinolytic drugs preoperatively (230). Galera and Greitz carried out serial carotid angiography on 100 consecutive patients with proved subarachnoid hemorrhage caused by the rupture of an arterial intracranial aneurysm (231). In the group, one-third of the patients developed ventricular dilatation, and more than one-half of these had symptoms. The most prominent change was dementia, sometimes accompanied by gait disturbances and a spastic paraparesis. A surprisingly large number with more advanced hydrocephalus had epileptic seizures and developed hypertension when they had been normotensive before the subarachnoid hemorrhage. It was felt that arterial spasm and the occurrence of an intracerebral hematoma as well as the number of hemorrhages contributed significantly to the development of hydrocephalus.

Therapeutic Considerations: Carotid Ligation

Carotid ligation or balloon occlusion is sometimes required in the treatment of certain aneurysms, particularly some giant aneurysms. In these cases it is important to determine whether the patient will tolerate the vascular occlusion, which is usually related to the configuration of the circle of Willis.

Cases have been reviewed to determine angiographic features that may indicate the patient's ability to tolerate occlusion of the internal carotid or common carotid artery. Several combinations of findings were encountered in the preoperative angiograms that are thought to have significance. It is known that whether a patient is able to tolerate ligation of the internal or the common carotid artery is dependent on the anatomy of the circle of Willis. Figure 10.44 indicates the configurations of the circle of Willis encountered in 1647 specimens, according to Hodes et al. (232). As is now well recognized, a perfectly symmetrical circle is encountered in only 18 percent of cases. The majority of specimens exhibited one or more components of the circle of Willis that were hypoplastic in relation to the other components. The pathways of collateral circulation will therefore depend to a significant extent on the relative caliber of the components of the circle of Willis, if the occlusion is in the cervical portion of the internal carotid artery. As indicated in a preceding section, "Occlusive and Stenotic Lesions," the collateral circulation on the surface of the brain is more important in occlusions that are distal to the circle of Willis.

Certain criteria derived from the two carotid angiograms of the overall study have been found helpful as a guide to determine whether a patient is capable of tolerating ligation of the internal carotid or of the common carotid artery (233).

1. If, on the initial carotid angiogram, there is noted smallness of the trunk of the anterior cerebral artery on the side *opposite* the one to be ligated, this is evidence of insufficient collateral circulation; none of the seven patients who had a small or a nonvisualized horizontal segment of the anterior cerebral artery contralaterally had sufficient collateral circulation for immediate ligation of the internal carotid artery. Smallness of the horizontal portion of the anterior cerebral artery on the side of the aneurysm is not necessarily an indication of insufficient collateral circulation (Fig. 10.115).
2. Bilateral demonstration of the posterior cerebral arteries is an indication of deficient collateral circulation; only one patient in five tolerated ligation of the internal carotid artery. Similarly, filling of both posterior cerebral arteries, when one internal carotid artery is injected and the other is compressed, is an indication of deficient collateral circulation (group V and sometimes group IV in Fig. 10.44).
3. Bilateral filling of the anterior and the middle cerebral arteries, when the opposite side is compressed, is an indication of sufficient collateral circulation for ligation of the common carotid artery. On the other hand, it is not sufficient grounds for ligation of the internal carotid artery; 13 of 24 patients did not tolerate internal carotid ligation.

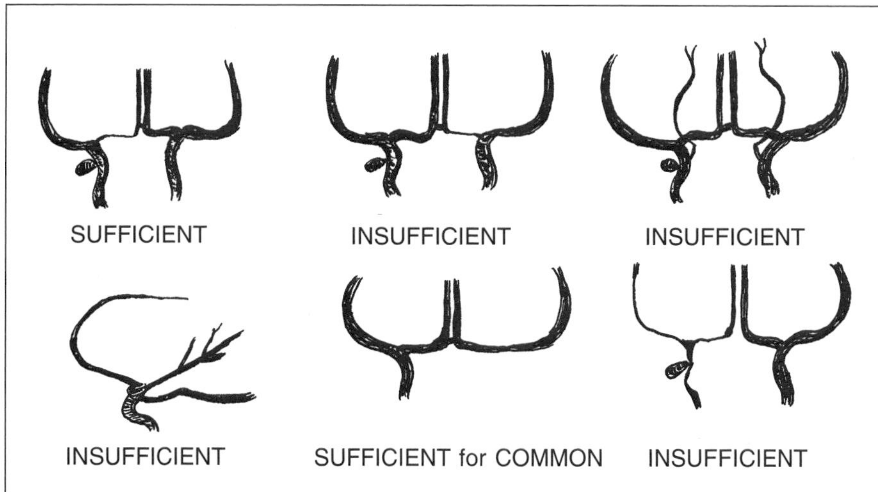

Figure 10.115. Importance of collateral circulation in patients with aneurysms. The sketches explain the angiographic findings that were found to be of statistical significance in the evaluation of the collateral circulation across the circle of Willis from preoperative angiograms in patients with intracranial aneurysms (see text). Ligation of the internal carotid artery was not tolerated in most cases with the angiographic findings as shown.

4. Diffuse spasm on the side of the lesion suggests insufficient collateral circulation for any type of ligation while the spasm lasts. It is possible that if spasm later disappears, ligation may be carried out.

Two of the 31 patients who were analyzed had insufficient collateral circulation for carotid ligation, but showed no preoperative evidence of this deficiency based on the criteria just listed. In 29, the radiologic criteria of adequacy or inadequacy of collateral circulation were substantiated by postoperative results (233).

Whether the patient will tolerate internal carotid occlusion can be determined by placing an occluding balloon during angiography with the patient awake. More sophisticated evaluations can also be made through the Wada test (see under "Endovascular Therapeutic Neuroradiology," Chapter 18). If the patient does not tolerate occlusion, a bypass procedure is carried out, usually an external carotid branch to an internal carotid branch.

ARTERIOVENOUS LESIONS

This section discusses arteriovenous fistulas and various vascular malformations. Arteriovenous fistulas and malformations deserve diagnostic consideration and are also discussed under "Endovascular Therapeutic Neuroradiology," Chapter 18.

Arteriovenous Fistulas

The best known of these is the carotid-cavernous fistula (CCF), in which there is a direct communication between the internal carotid artery and the cavernous sinus owing to a rupture of the carotid artery. The rupture could be related to a preexisting aneurysm or may be provoked entirely by trauma. It is possible that a preexisting aneurysm ruptured as a result of a traumatic episode.

The internal carotid artery passes through and is contained within the cavernous sinus for a distance of about 1.0 to 1.5 cm. Clinically, the most prominent symptoms of a carotid-cavernous fistula are pulsating exophthalmos and a bruit that is very annoying to the patient. These symptoms usually begin within 24 h after the development of the fistula, but occasionally they begin several weeks or several months later. In addition to these symptoms, the patient may present chemosis, extraoccular palsies, and loss of vision. Sometimes bilateral pulsating exophthalmos develops as the result of the presence of an anastomosis between the two cavernous sinuses. In one of the author's cases, flow through the circular sinus resulted in a pulsating exophthalmos only on the side opposite the fistula (Fig. 10.116*B*).

The initial diagnosis is suspected clinically and can be confirmed by CT with contrast or by MR and MRA (Fig. 10.118). With angiography, many presumed carotid-cavernous fistulas have been found to be indirect shunts through dural arteriovenous malformations (234). Complete selective angiography is essential for a correct diagnosis. It should be possible in most cases, however, to differentiate readily the classic carotid-cavernous fistula (Fig. 10.116) from an indirect one (Fig. 10.117) because with the former there is high flow, rapid venous filling, and often a steal from the intracranial circulation.

The angiographic demonstration of an arteriovenous fistula is relatively easy. The contrast substance can be seen to leave the internal carotid artery in the early arterial phase of the angiogram. Filling of the cavernous sinus and its venous communications ordinarily occurs while the contrast material is still being injected. Thus the internal carotid artery and internal jugular vein are visualized coursing parallel in the neck. There is reversal of flow in the ophthalmic veins, which ordinarily drain into the cavernous sinus, owing to increased intracavernous pressure resulting from the carotid artery opening into the sinus. Dilated, elongated superior and inferior ophthalmic veins usually are opacified, together with their tributaries (Fig. 10.116). In

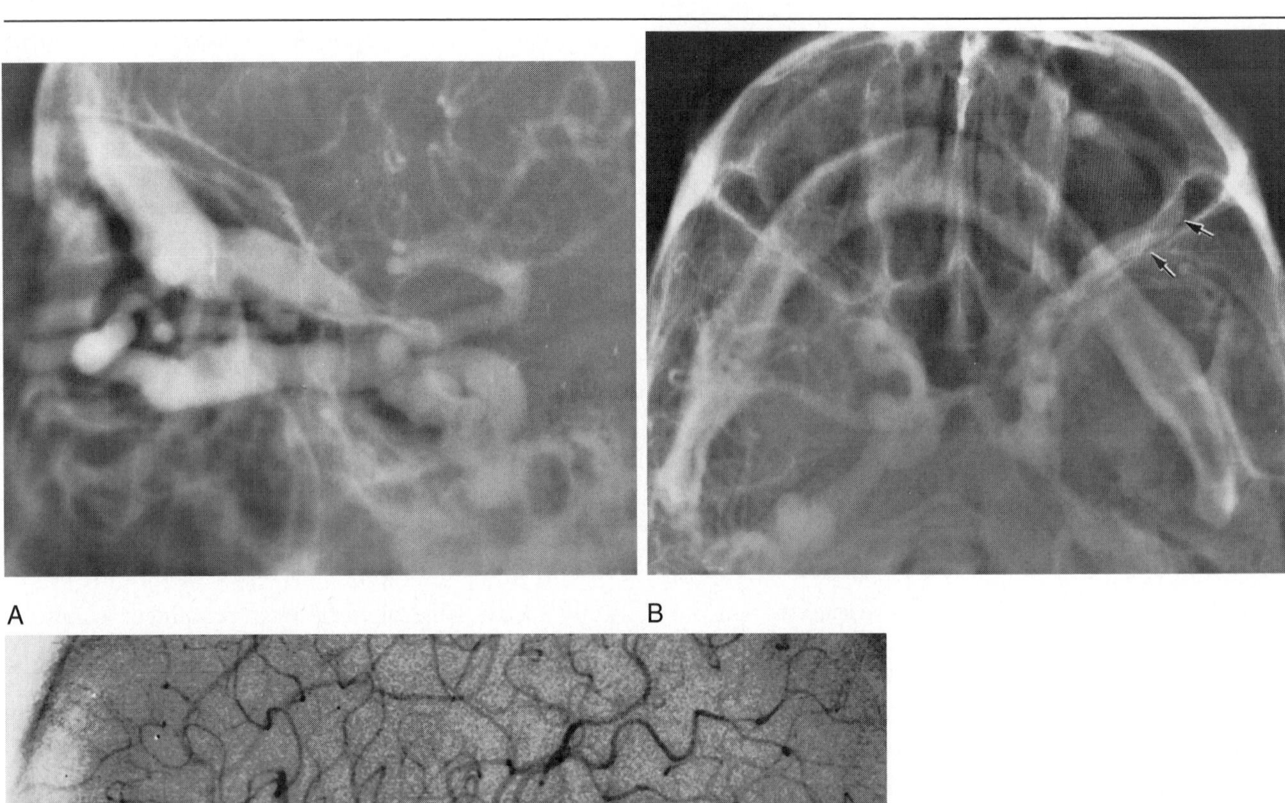

A B

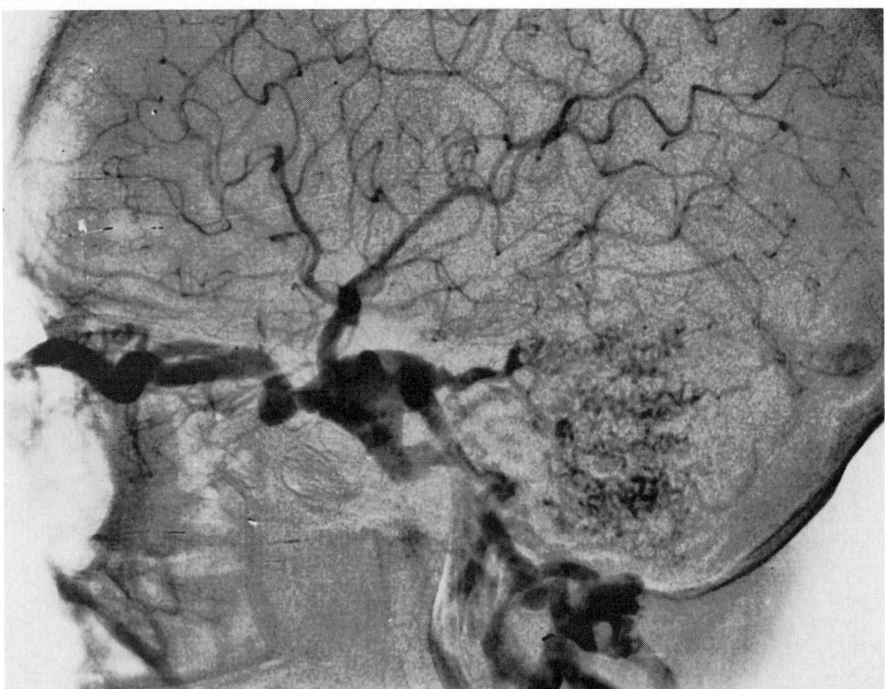

C

Figure 10.116. Carotid-cavernous fistulas. **A.** There is much more contrast material leaving the cranium by way of the ophthalmic veins than by way of perfusing the brain. Only the middle cerebral vessels are outlined by the opaque substance, because hypotension on the side of the fistula causes both anterior cerebral arteries to fill from the opposite side. **B.** The patient had a left-sided proptosis, and the left carotid angiogram was normal. A right angiogram was then performed, and the base view demonstrates the filling across the anterior intracavernous (circular) sinus and drainage by way of the ophthalmic veins on the side of the proptosis (arrows). **C.** In a third patient, a large carotid-cavernous shunt is present, but there is still good middle cerebral perfusion on the ipsilateral side. The ipsilateral superior ophthalmic vein is greatly dilated from retrograde flow under arterial pressure; there was also cross flow through the anterior intercavernous sinus with opacification of the contralateral cavernous sinus and superior ophthalmic veins. There was prominent opacification of the superior and inferior petrosal sinuses with unusual backflow into many tortuous veins on the surface of the cerebellum. Further retrograde opacification of the rectus (straight) sinus and other dural sinuses was observed. The cavernous sinus also emptied caudally by way of the pterygoid plexus, and there was very early opacification of the jugular, vertebral, and deep cervical veins.

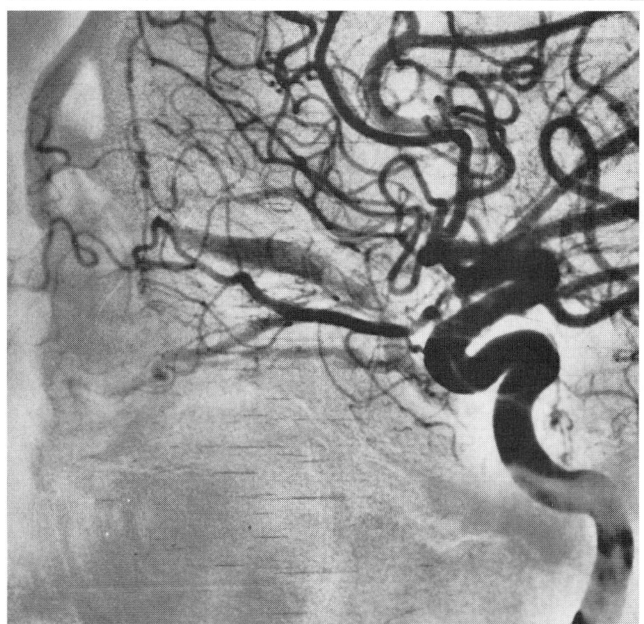
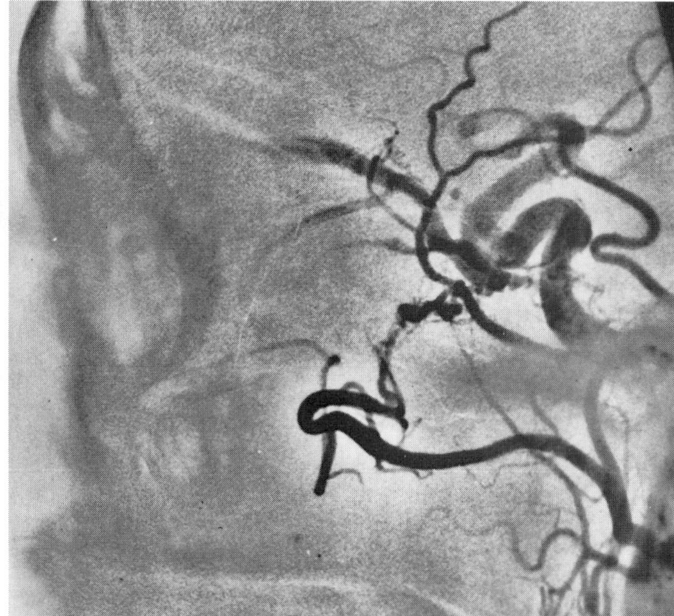

A B

Figure 10.117. Indirect carotid-cavernous communication. **A.** The selective internal carotid angiogram reveals enlarged intracavernous branches supplying a malformation in the wall of the cavernous sinus. There is opacification of the anterior part of the sinus and retrograde flow of contrast material into the superior and inferior ophthalmic veins. **B.** The external carotid injection, with some internal carotid reflux, shows that there are also numerous branches of the external system supplying the dural arteriovenous malformation, causing opacification of the cavernous sinus and ophthalmic veins.

some cases, other veins and sinuses are seen to participate in the runoff of arterial flow through the fistula.

The internal carotid artery frequently fills poorly distal to the fistula; there must be a relative ischemia of the corresponding hemisphere unless the opposite carotid is able to carry the entire load. Some blood from the opposite hemisphere also may be shunted through the fistula. Injection of a greater amount of contrast substance in any case suspected of having a carotid-cavernous fistula is advantageous since sometimes the ophthalmic veins are not well shown with the amount usually injected. The anatomic detail of the actual fistula may be best shown on rapid serialograms, particularly when the films are made at four per second during the injection and immediately afterward.

Full axial (basal) views may be useful in studying some carotid-cavernous fistulas to demonstrate the anastomotic channels between the two cavernous sinuses. A basal view permitted a diagnosis of the correct side of the fistula in one angiogram, shown in Figure 10.116*B*, while a pulsating exophthalmos clinically indicated the opposite side (Table 10.23).

The management of carotid-cavernous fistulas is discussed in Chapter 18. Other arteriovenous fistulas, such as between the carotid artery and jugular vein in the neck and between the vertebral arteries and the veins that surround it, are the result of puncture wounds or of spinal fractures. These are also discussed in Chapter 18.

Table 10.23.
Carotid-Cavernous Fistulas

- Etiologies
  - Penetrating or nonpenetrating trauma
  - Aneurysmal rupture
  - Development of communication between small arteries and veins of cavernous sinus
- Types
  - High-flow (direct) fistula
  - Low-flow (indirect) fistula
- Clinical findings
  - Proptosis
  - Chemosis
  - Orbital bruit
- Angiographic findings
  - Early opacification of veins draining cavernous sinus, including superior ophthalmic vein, inferior and superior petrosal sinuses, or contralateral cavernous sinus
- CT and MRI findings
  - Proptosis
  - Widened cavernous sinus with lateral convex borders
  - Dilated superior or inferior ophthalmic vein
  - Enlarged vascular flow void channels in cavernous sinus on MRI

Vascular Malformations

ARTERIOVENOUS MALFORMATIONS

The term *arteriovenous malformation* (AVM) implies the existence of abnormal communications between arteries and veins in the brain. They are congenital but tend to become

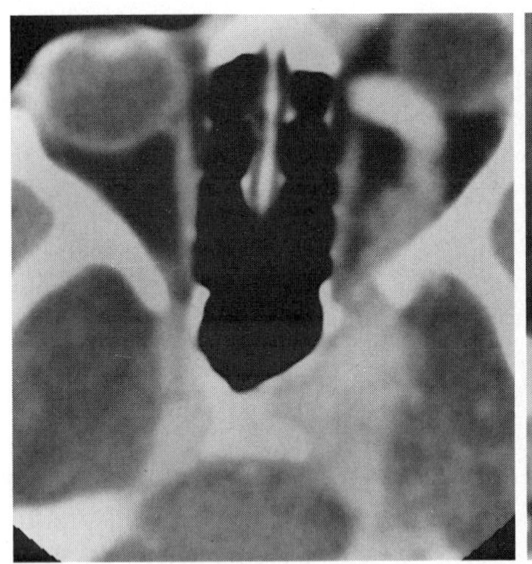

A

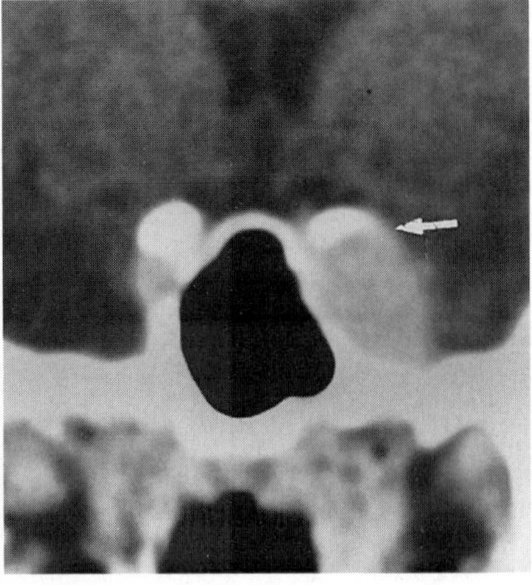

B

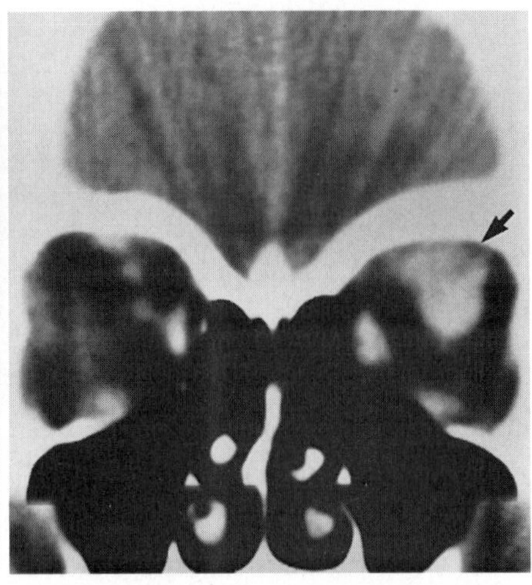

C

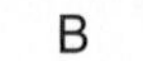

Figure 10.118. Carotid cavernous fistula shown by CT and angiography. **A.** Axial CT image with contrast shows enlargement and increased opacity in left cavernous sinus. The opacification extends directly into the orbit, which shows marked enlargement of the superior ophthalmic vein. **B** and **C.** Coronal views show the enlarged left cavernous sinus and the ophthalmic veins. The left internal carotid artery is displaced upward and flattened (arrow). **D.** Angiography shows the rapid filling of the cavernous sinus (arrow) and the superior ophthalmic vein, which drains into the facial vein (curved arrows). **E.** Vertebral angiography shows retrograde flow into the internal carotid artery via the posterior communicating artery (arrow), filling the cavernous sinus and allowing much better definition. **F.** Left carotid angiography following installation of a balloon through the fistulous connection shows preservation of the carotid lumen. The intracavernous carotid is compressed but patent and yields good intracranial arterial filling.

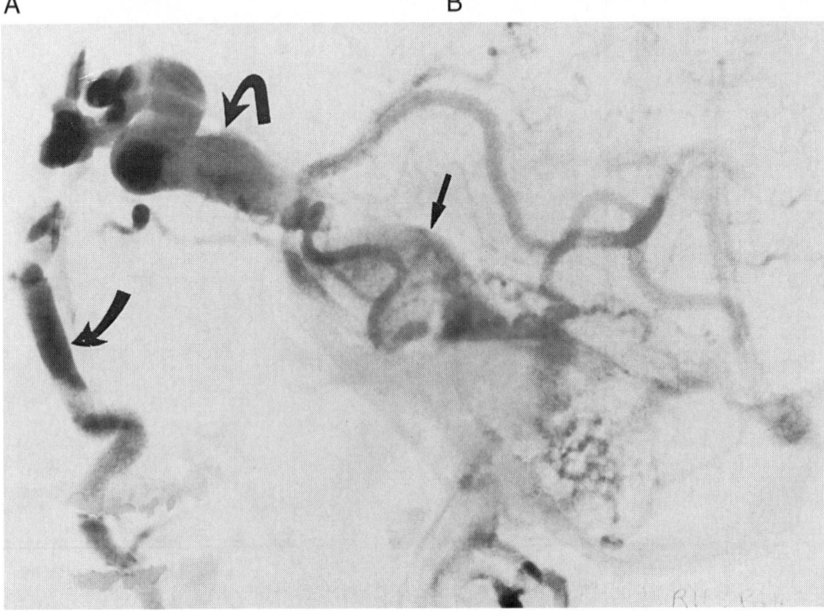

D

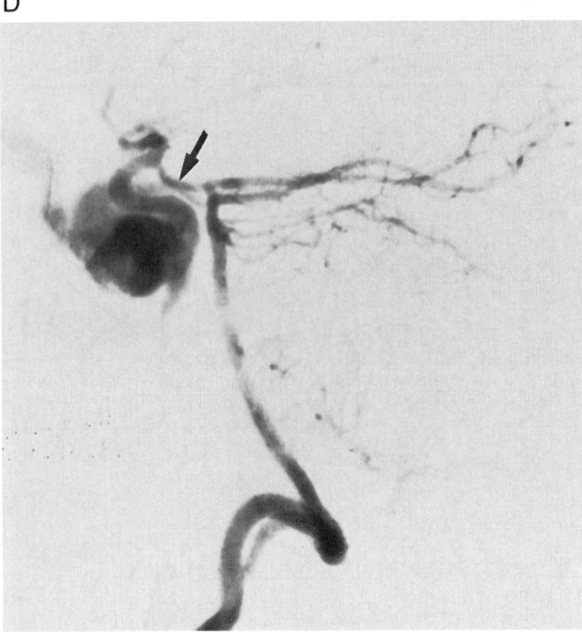

E

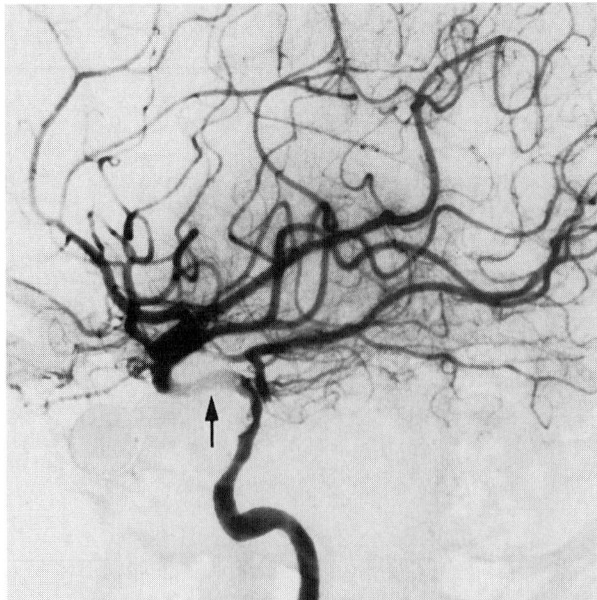

F

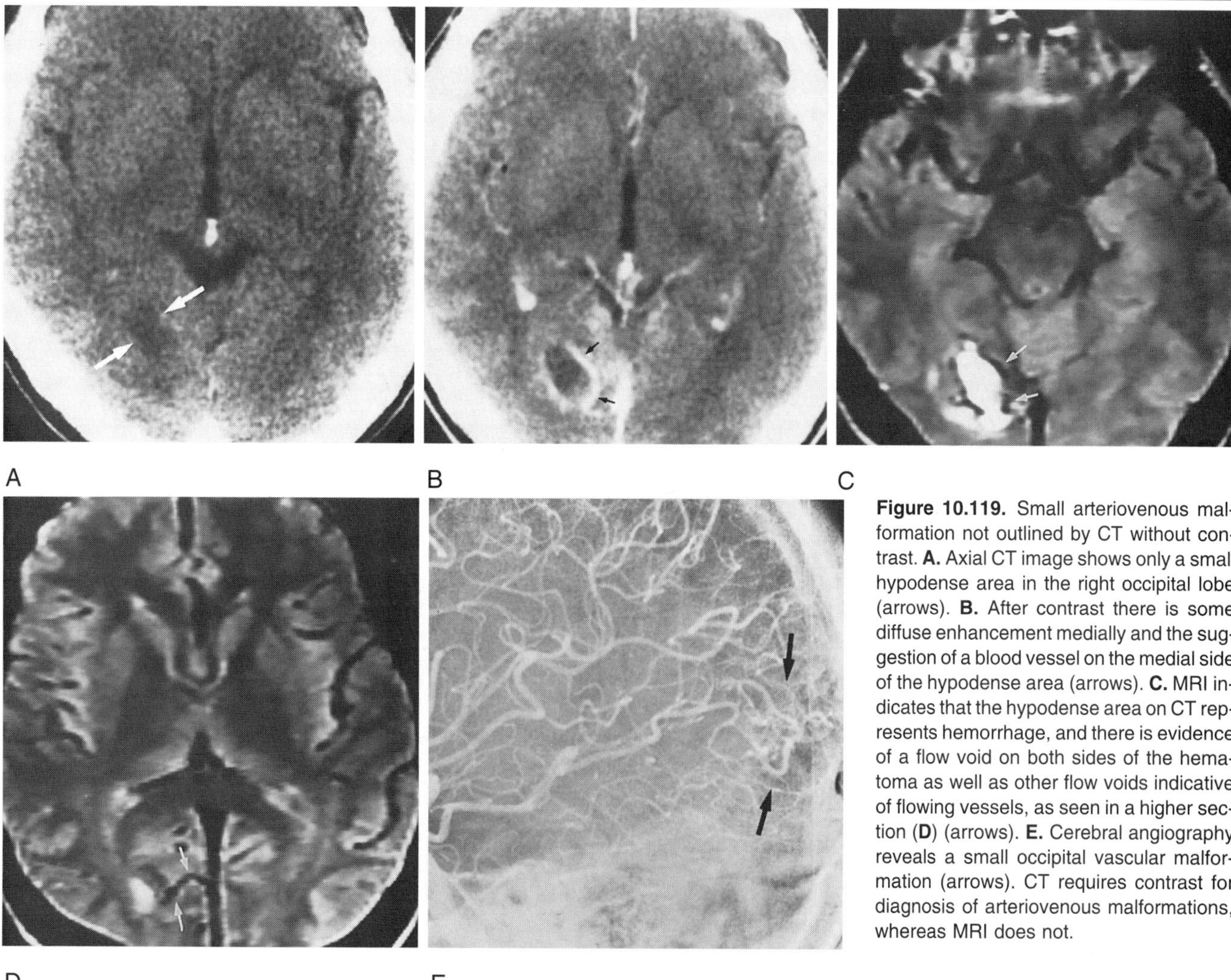

Figure 10.119. Small arteriovenous malformation not outlined by CT without contrast. **A.** Axial CT image shows only a small hypodense area in the right occipital lobe (arrows). **B.** After contrast there is some diffuse enhancement medially and the suggestion of a blood vessel on the medial side of the hypodense area (arrows). **C.** MRI indicates that the hypodense area on CT represents hemorrhage, and there is evidence of a flow void on both sides of the hematoma as well as other flow voids indicative of flowing vessels, as seen in a higher section (**D**) (arrows). **E.** Cerebral angiography reveals a small occipital vascular malformation (arrows). CT requires contrast for diagnosis of arteriovenous malformations, whereas MRI does not.

larger with the passage of time because of the recruiting of adjacent small arteries and veins by the initial focus or nidus where the primary abnormality existed. However, the growth is not like that of a neoplasm, and the term *angioma* should not be used to denominate these lesions.

The patient may present with convulsive seizures, headaches, weakness, or sensory manifestations, but often no symptoms are present and the lesion may be detected on a CT or MRI examination performed for entirely unrelated reasons. Hemorrhage of AVMs occurs less commonly than with saccular aneurysms, but AVMs are also relatively uncommon lesions. It is said that there is a 4 percent chance of bleeding per year, so that eventually about 50 to 70 percent bleed. The smaller malformations seem to have a greater chance of bleeding (235).

CT examination with contrast enhancement usually makes the diagnosis, and *if contrast is not given the diagnosis will probably be overlooked.* The appearance is that of a cluster of enhanced vessels that do not have the appearance of a neoplasm and which usually produce no mass effect (Fig. 10.119). Some AVMs are extremely large and involve a large portion of a hemisphere; they do interfere with the blood supply of the normal brain tissue because flowing blood tends to follow the path of least resistance through the malformation. MRI is superior to CT in diagnosing AVMs (Fig. 10.120). It also demonstrates old bleeding, which CT may not. In addition, MRI does not require contrast for diagnosis, whereas CT requires contrast injection.

Blood usually drains rapidly into veins either on the brain surface or deep in the brain (Fig. 10.121). This can usually be detected by MRI without contrast. The presence of deep venous drainage may lead, over a period of time, to thrombosis of the straight sinus or the vein of Galen and the internal cerebral veins. This thrombosis is caused by a high-flow angiopathy in which the endothelium becomes thickened and narrows the lumen, followed later by more changes in the wall of the vessel that may terminate in complete occlusion (236). In addition to a clumped endothelium, denuded in some area with adherent platelets, an irregular duplicated and thinned internal elastic mem-

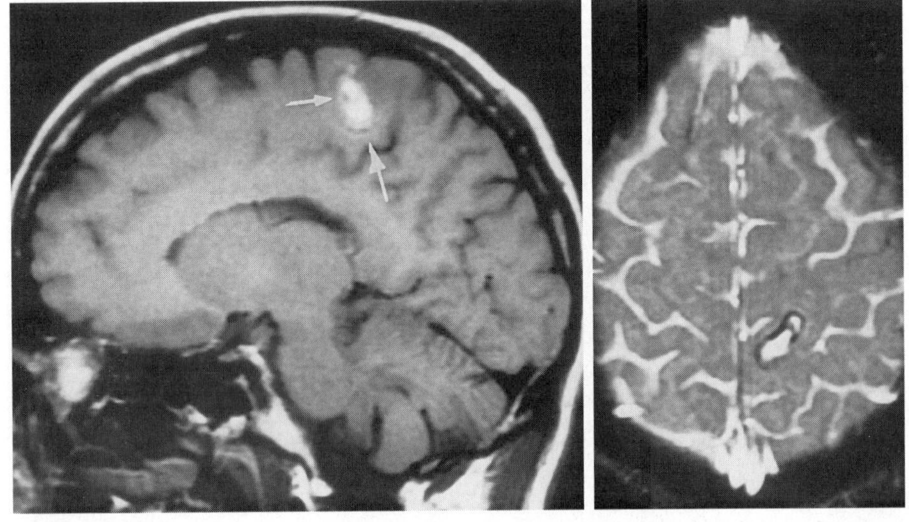

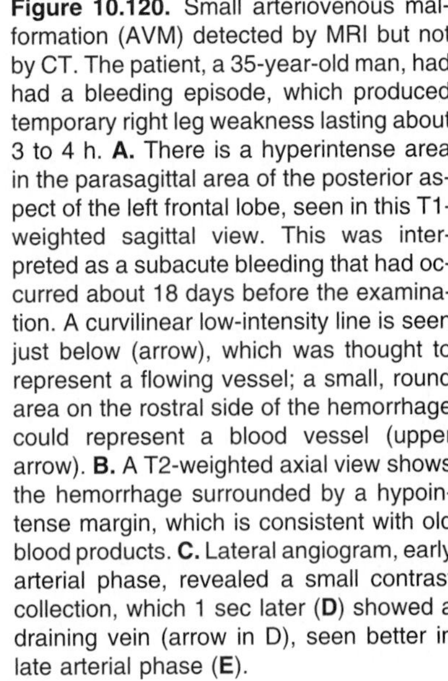

A B

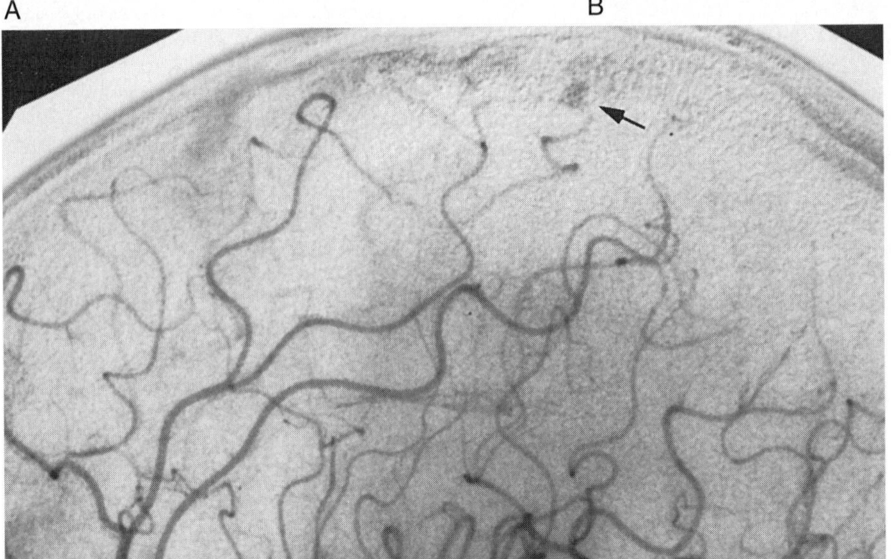

C

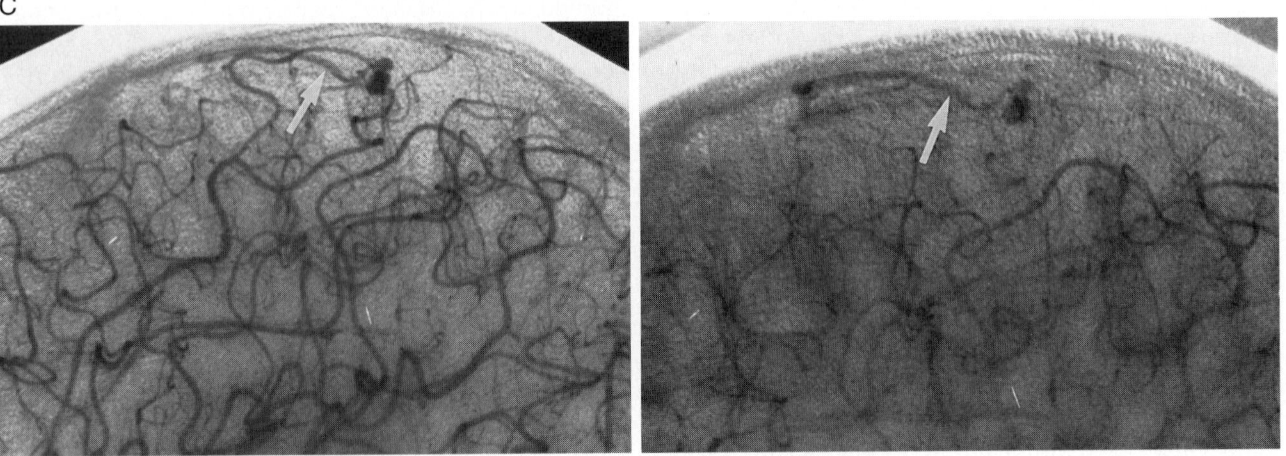

D E

Figure 10.120. Small arteriovenous malformation (AVM) detected by MRI but not by CT. The patient, a 35-year-old man, had had a bleeding episode, which produced temporary right leg weakness lasting about 3 to 4 h. **A.** There is a hyperintense area in the parasagittal area of the posterior aspect of the left frontal lobe, seen in this T1-weighted sagittal view. This was interpreted as a subacute bleeding that had occurred about 18 days before the examination. A curvilinear low-intensity line is seen just below (arrow), which was thought to represent a flowing vessel; a small, round area on the rostral side of the hemorrhage could represent a blood vessel (upper arrow). **B.** A T2-weighted axial view shows the hemorrhage surrounded by a hypointense margin, which is consistent with old blood products. **C.** Lateral angiogram, early arterial phase, revealed a small contrast collection, which 1 sec later (**D**) showed a draining vein (arrow in D), seen better in late arterial phase (**E**).

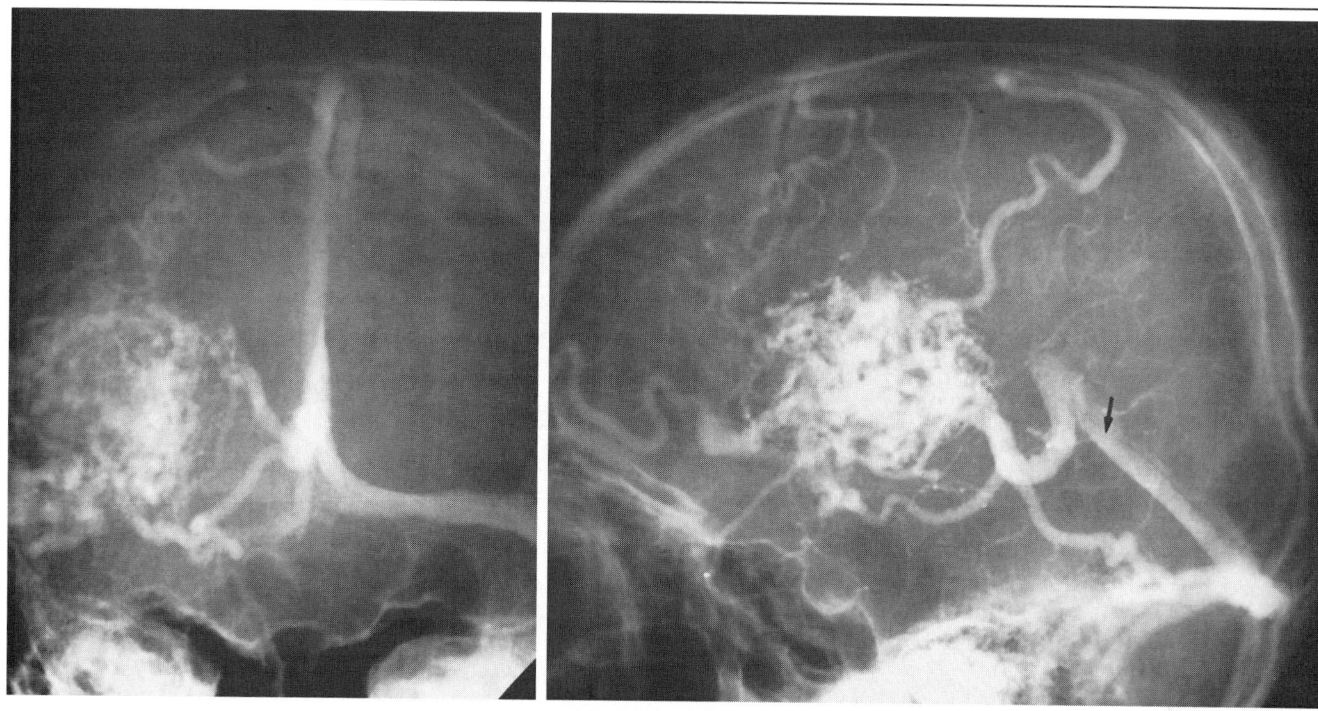

Figure 10.121. High-flow, deep arteriovenous malformation (AVM) draining mostly by way of the deep veins but also through some superficial veins. **A.** Frontal angiographic view shows deep venous drainage. The right lateral sinus is not seen because it is most probably occluded. The left lateral sinus is well seen. **B.** Lateral view shows the large, elongated internal cerebral vein and the vein of Galen, as well as the straight sinus. The anterior aspect of the straight sinus (arrow) may be narrower than the rest of it, possibly because of high-flow angiopathy. However, the difference could also be due to some contrast dilution from the internal cerebral vein from the opposite nonopacified side. This is unlikely in view of the high flow and the fact that the internal cerebral vein drains into the vein of Galen, which seems fully opacified.

brane, with invasion of the intima by mesenchymal cells, may be found. The occurrence of veins and venous sinus occlusions is more common in high-flow AVMs; arteries, as well as veins and dural sinuses, may become occluded (237,238).

The deeply situated AVMs are more likely to produce thrombosis of the deep veins and straight sinus because of their flow through these vessels (Fig. 10.122). Venous dilatation also occurs, sometimes leading to the formation of venous "aneurysm" or varix formation that may show calcification in its wall (Fig. 10.122).

Perhaps the most significant of these saccular venous dilatations is the so-called vein of Galen aneurysm in which the vein of Galen becomes markedly dilated, sometimes enormously so (239) (Fig. 10.123). The blood supply of these malformations is usually through various arterial territories (bilateral carotid, basilar artery), and the lesion may be fully formed in the newborn. The blood flow may be so large that the infant may go into high-output cardiac failure. The diagnosis may be suggested by CT or MR examination.

Saccular aneurysms may be seen in the same arterial system supplying the AVM, but they may also be found in other vascular territories (240) (Figs. 10.124 and 10.125). Their development may be related to increased flow through the vessel feeding the AVM, as in the two cases shown in Figure 10.125, but not always.

DURAL ARTERIOVENOUS COMMUNICATIONS

There are two types of dural arteriovenous communications deserving description in this section; both types are dealt with more extensively in the section "Endovascular Therapeutic Neuroradiology" in Chapter 18.

The first one is the dural fistula involving the cavernous sinus, which was described in text preceding together with the other type of carotid-cavernous fistula. In these cases there is no evidence of thrombosis of the cavernous sinus preceding the appearance of symptoms. One wonders, however, about the relatively sudden occurrence of signs of an arteriovenous communication in this location in a previously asymptomatic patient, usually a woman.

The second type involves the dural arteriovenous communications involving the transverse and sigmoid sinuses, which were identified by Houser et al. (241) and Chandhary et al. (242) as an acquired condition resulting from prior thrombosis of the dural venous sinuses that could be

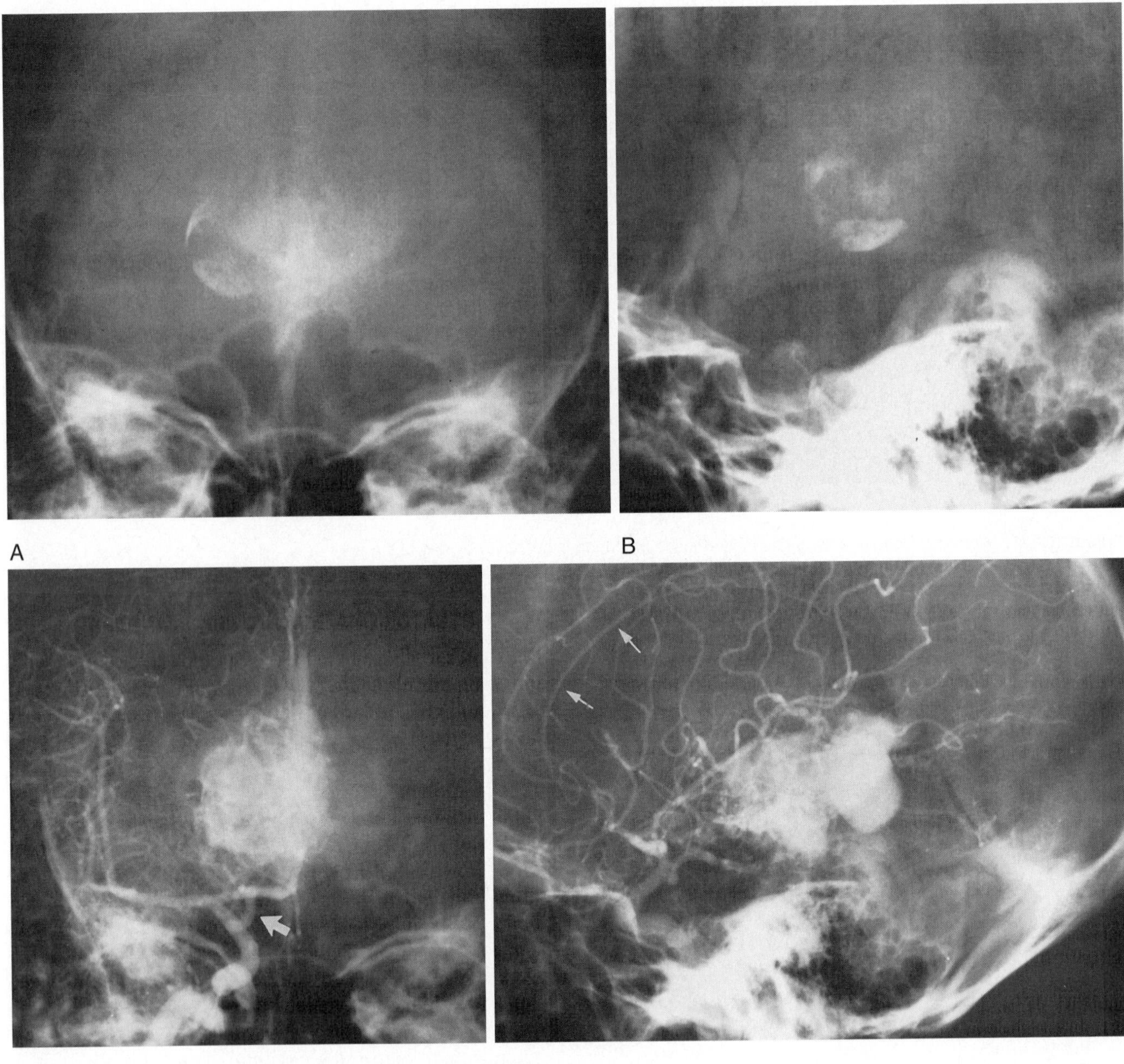

Figure 10.122. Calcification in arteriovenous malformation. **A.** The frontal skull film reveals a 2 × 3 cm oval shell-like calcification located centrally, at and to the right of the midline. **B.** The lateral view shows the shadow to still have a rounded exterior, but at the upper and lower poles there are thick, irregular layers of calcium, suggesting thrombosis in an aneurysmal sac. **C.** The frontal angiogram discloses an arteriovenous malformation fed principally by lenticulostriate vessels and a huge anterior choroidal artery (arrow). One of the large venous sacculations appears to correspond to the residual lumen in the partially thrombosed, calcified mass. **D.** Hydrocephalus is present, apparently caused by third-ventricular obstruction. Note marked elevation of the pericallosal artery (arrows).

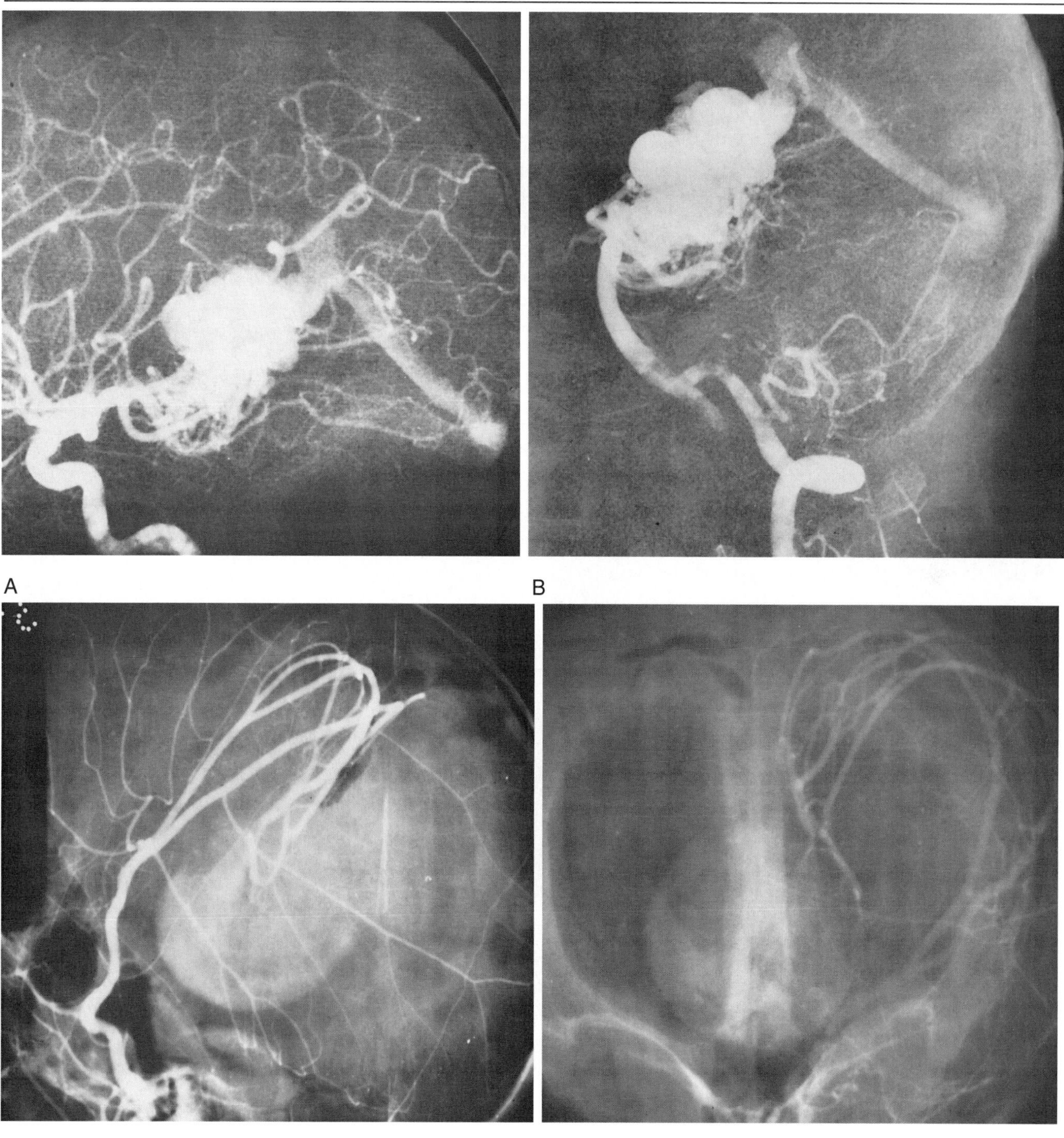

Figure 10.123. Vein of Galen aneurysms. A larger venous aneurysm of the vein of Galen and its tributaries fills almost as well from the carotid (**A**) as from the vertebral-basilar system (**B**). The actual arteriovenous shunts, fed principally by the posterior choroidal and other posterior cerebral branches and superior cerebellar branches, were better seen on earlier frames of the serialogram. Marked enlargement of the afferent internal carotid and posterior communicating arteries, the vertebral and basilar arteries, and anastomotic branches of the anterior and posterior interior cerebellar arteries is shown. There is premature filling of the straight and transverse sinuses. Hydrocephalus was not present in this patient, who was admitted because of seizures. **C.** In another case, the lateral view of the cerebral angiogram shows the filling of the vein of Galen by way of branches of the middle cerebral artery. **D.** The anteroposterior projection demonstrates the partially filled aneurysmal dilatation of the vein of Galen. The course of the feeding middle cerebral vessels is clear on this film. The anterior cerebral artery is not filled from this side.

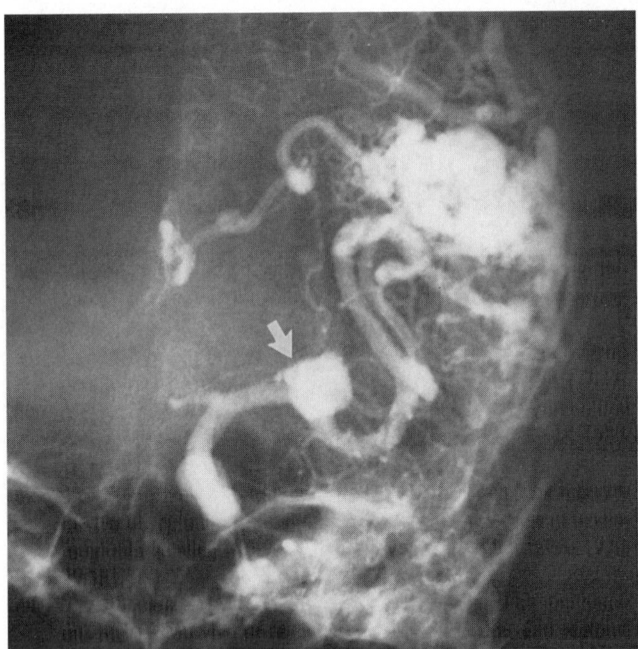

Figure 10.124. Arteriovenous malformation (AVM) and arterial aneurysm in same arterial system. **A.** There is a large saccular aneurysm arising from the region of the trifurcation of the middle cerebral artery trunk (arrow) in addition to the AVM more distally. When an AVM is found in addition to a saccular aneurysm, the saccular aneurysm is most frequently the cause of bleeding. **B** and **C.** AVM causing great aneurysmal dilatation of the vein of Galen. **B.** CT scan. **C.** Lateral angiogram, venous phase.

A

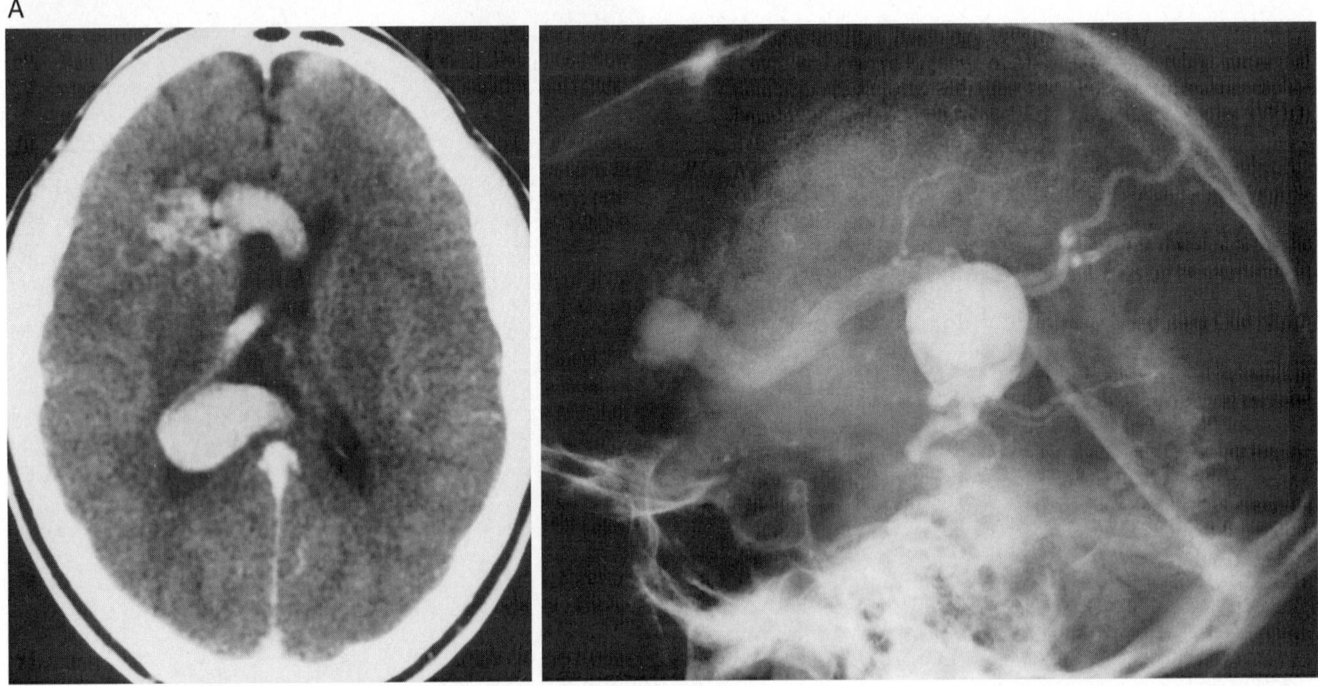

B C

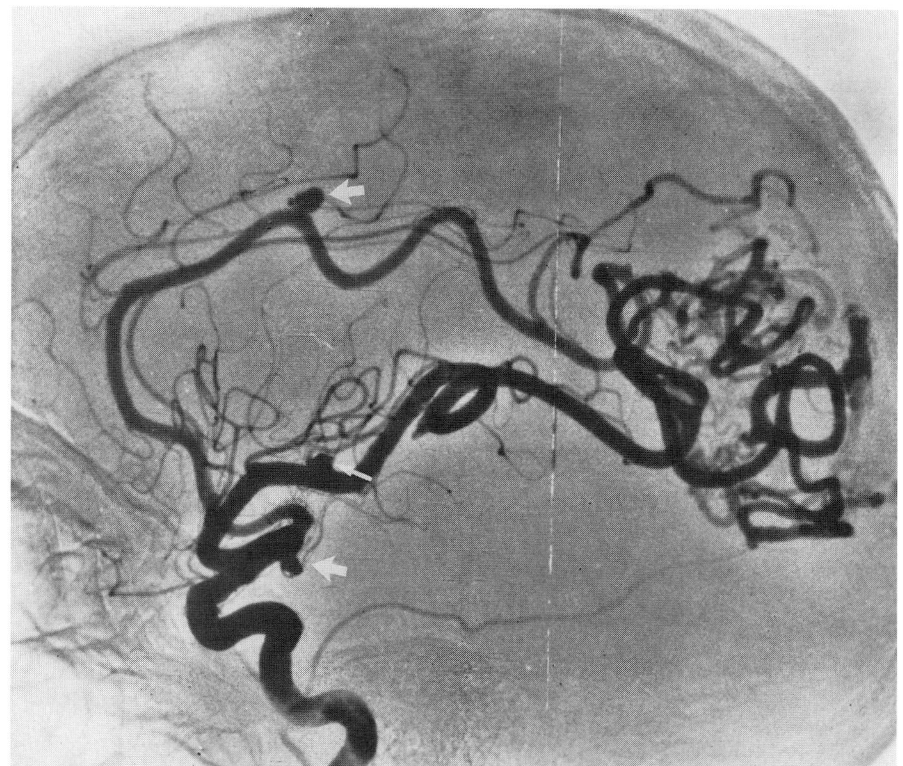

Figure 10.125. Multiple aneurysms in a patient with an occipital AVM. There is an aneurysm arising from the internal carotid artery at or just above the origin of the anterior choroidal artery. In addition, there is a saccular aneurysm arising from the middle cerebral artery in the sylvian fissure and another originating from the pericallosal artery (arrows).

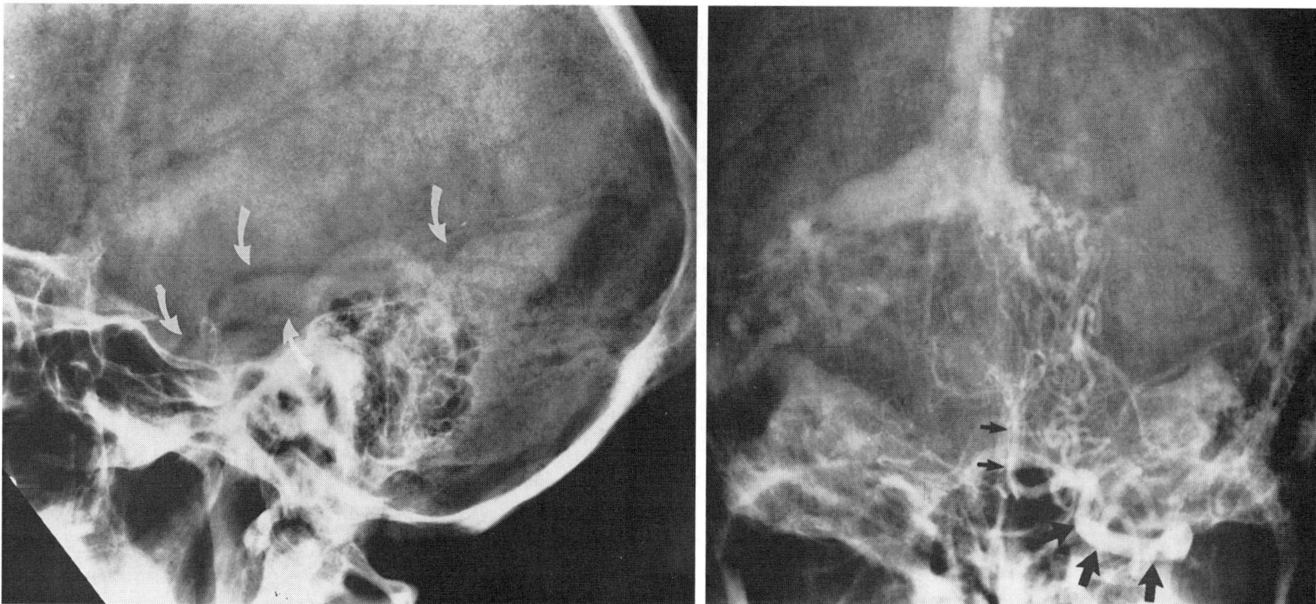

A B

Figure 10.126. Dural arteriovenous fistulas with thrombosis of both lateral sinuses and enlarged meningeal artery channels in the skull. **A.** Lateral view demonstrates enlarged meningeal artery grooves on the inner table of the skull in the posterior temporal and occipital regions (arrows). **B.** Vertebral angiography reveals numerous extracranial and meningeal branches of the vertebral arteries going directly to the stump of the occluded left lateral sinus. The branches are filling the torcular and from there the superior sagittal sinus. On the right, the occluded lateral sinus seems to be partly draining via enlarged tortuous veins. The basilar artery (arrows) and its branches are very thin, probably because of stealing off the major flow by the fistula. Other venous channels are seen faintly to the left of the torcular and the posterior sagittal sinus. There were numerous large dilated veins over the brain surface (not shown).

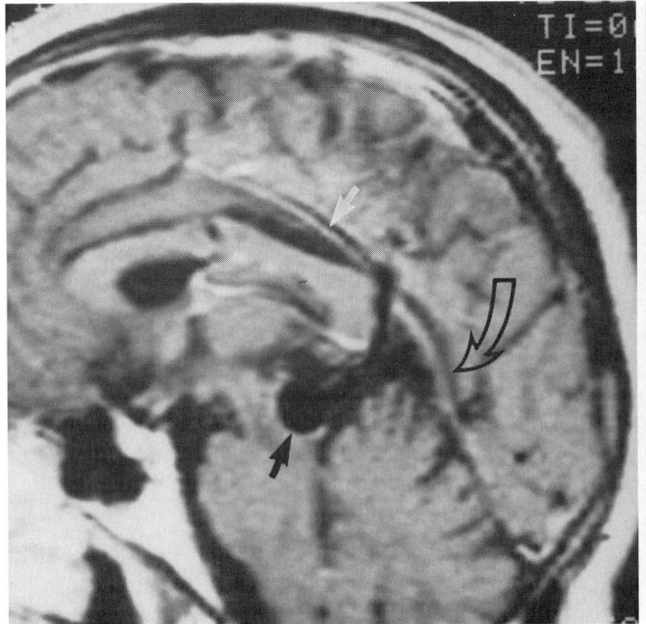

A

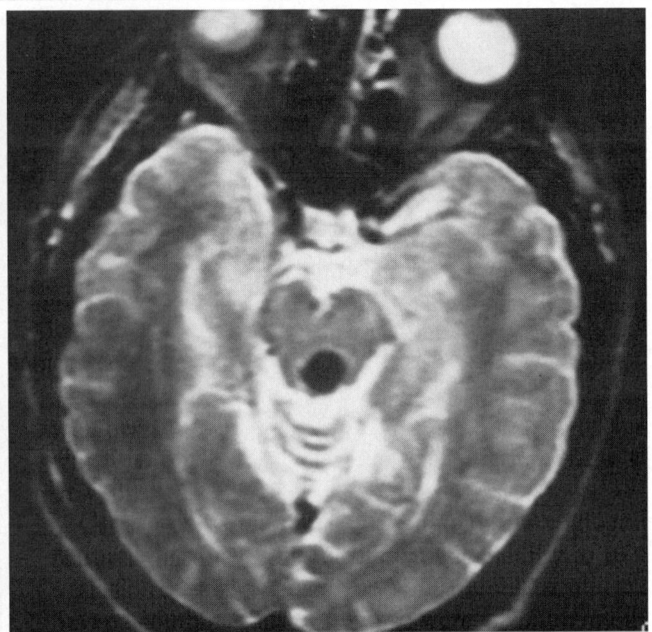

B

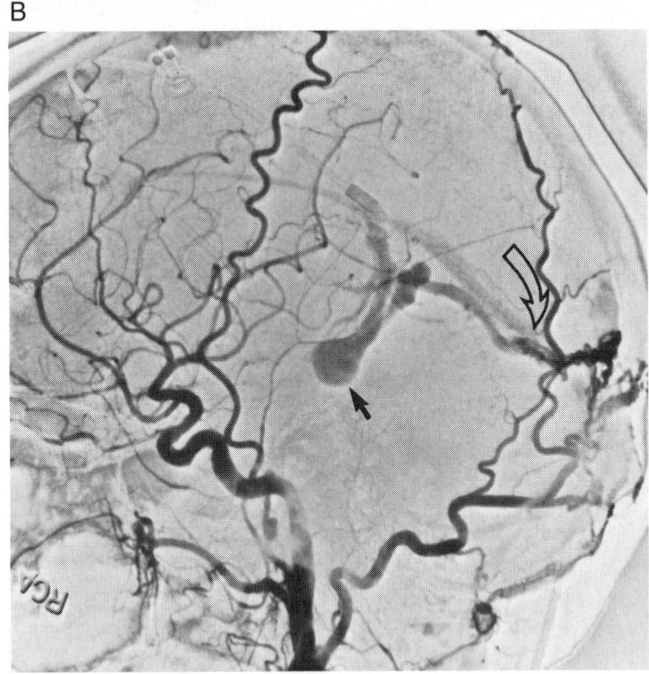

C

Figure 10.127. Dural AVM. **A.** MR postcontrast sagittal image shows a sharp, low-intensity, rounded area in the region of the quadrigeminal plate (arrow). The sinus rectus (open arrow) has slow flow, as do the inferior sagittal sinus (white arrow) and the internal cerebral vein. **B.** T2-weighted axial image shows a large flow void overlying the tectum of the midbrain. This was later shown to represent a venous aneurysm. **C.** Common carotid angiography shows the dural AVM supplied by the occipital artery. There is a venous aneurysm filling from a dilated midline vein (arrow). The straight sinus seems to be occluded posteriorly (curved open arrow). The venous aneurysm is seen in the MR images.

posttraumatic or postinfectious. The probable mechanism involves organization of the thrombus and subsequent recanalization of the lumen of the sinus, resulting in the formation of direct arteriovenous communications. With the passage of time, more vessels are recruited into the area, and the abnormality increases in size. The blood supply usually comes from several external carotid artery branches, but there is also a supply from the dural or radicular branches of the vertebral arteries and/or from dural branches of the internal carotid arteries (243).

The diagnosis is made by angiography; it can be suspected by CT or MRI, particularly the latter, if flow voids are observed in the brain surface near the dural sinuses, particularly if there is apparent occlusion of one of the lateral sinuses. If plain films of the skull are made, there is usually evidence of dilatation of the grooves of the meningeal arteries on the inner table of the skull (Fig. 10.126). Diagnosis can be made by MRA (Fig. 10.127) (Table 10.24).

It should be mentioned here that although dural arteriovenous fistulas usually involve the lateral and sigmoid si-

Table 10.24.
Dural Arteriovenous Communications Involving the Dural Sinuses

May result from previous dural sinus thrombosis and subsequent recanalization
Most commonly supplied by external carotid artery branches, but may also be supplied by dural or radicular branches of vertebral and internal carotid arteries
Contrast angiography findings include opacification of conglomeration of vessels near a dural sinus with early-draining veins
CT or MRI findings may include increased numbers of small vessels on brain surface adjacent to an occluded dural sinus

nuses and the cavernous sinuses, deep dural fistulas involving the deep cerebral venous system also occur, although less frequently (244). It may be difficult to diagnose these and to distinguish them from deep cerebral arteriovenous malformations. The principal diagnostic characteristic is their blood supply, as shown by serial angiography primarily by dural vessels, as against, for instance, an aneurysm of the vein of Galen, in which the supply is via arterial branches from the carotid and basilar artery systems.

CAVERNOUS ANGIOMAS

These lesions have been well known pathologically for a long time, but until the advent of cross-sectional imaging by CT and MRI, the diagnosis could not be made in vivo because they are not visible by angiography and so were called *occult* vascular malformations (245, 246). They are considered vascular hematomas and have clinical importance because they can bleed, sometimes producing large hematomas and death. In addition, they are most frequently located in the cerebral hemisphere and can cause seizures; if they are situated in the brainstem (most frequently in the pons), they can produce long tract involvement as well as cranial nerve dysfunction, even before bleeding.

They are usually composed of a honeycomb of small spaces filled with blood and separated by fibrous walls rich in collagen. Areas of thrombosis are common, and calcification may occur. The size varies from a pinhead to several centimeters in diameter. The great majority are about 1.0 cm in diameter. On the fresh specimen, the surrounding brain tissue may show discoloration owing to old blood products from previous hemorrhage. They can be multiple and have a higher incidence in some families. In the cases reported by Rigamonti et al., in several members of a family multiple lesions were found in 11 out of 14 family members (247). MRI is much more likely to reveal multiple cavernous angiomas than CT. The lesions can also occur in the spinal cord.

The angiomas can be detected at any age; some report a higher incidence in males, but others deny this. Gomori et al. reported 46 angiomas demonstrated by MRI (only 24 were seen by CT) in 19 patients, of whom only 8 were male (248). Of the 46 angiomas, 34 were supratentorial and 12 were infratentorial, all in the brainstem.

Table 10.25.
Cavernous Angiomas

Consist of dilated, blood-filled sinusoids without intervening brain parenchyma
Most common presentations include headache and seizures, but are often asymptomatic
May occur in brain (most commonly in the supratentorial compartment), brainstem, or spinal cord
Often multiple and may have a familial basis
MRI is more sensitive than CT for diagnosis
CT imaging appearance can include foci of calcification that may contrast enhance
MRI findings typically consist of heterogeneous foci of hypointense and hyperintense signal on T2 images, often with a surrounding region of hypointense signal

CT will demonstrate calcification, and contrast administration may reveal areas of enhancement (Fig. 10.128). MRI is the diagnostic procedure of choice because it will not only demonstrate evidence of bleeding at various stages of evolution but will also show evidence of hemosiderin indicative of old hemorrhage, which is not seen at all with CT (Fig. 10.128) (Table 10.25). Histologically there is evidence of septation demarcating the cavernous spaces, but there is no capsule around the lesion. The absence of a capsule produces an irregular border on the lesions in most instances (Figs. 10.128 to 10.130). The T1-weighted images often do not show a typical appearance of methemoglobin. Only slight hyperintensity may be seen, whereas the T2-weighted images usually show hyperintensity (Figs. 10.128 to 10.130). This indicates that there must be another factor, possibly slow blood flow through the malformation, responsible for some of the changes. The association of venous angioma with cavernous angiomas has been emphasized by Atlas (249) and Zimmerman et al. (250) (Fig. 10.131).

If the patient presents with an acute hemorrhage, the typical configuration of a cavernous angioma may not be apparent, and other possibilities, such as neoplasm or hemorrhage from other causes, must be considered. Some days or weeks later the usual appearance will return, and the diagnosis can be suggested.

Superficially located angiomas can be resected surgically and are sometimes associated with a seizure disorder (Fig. 10.130). About two-thirds to three-quarters of the occult angiomas are supratentorial and tend to occur either near the cerebral cortex or in the periventricular area. In the posterior fossa they occur in the brainstem and are rare in the cerebellum. Angiomas that bleed or are symptomatic may also be treated by radiosurgery. Surgical treatment of superficially located brainstem cavernous malformations has been suggested by Zimmerman et al. (250).

Ojemann et al. have suggested the following useful guidelines for therapy (251):

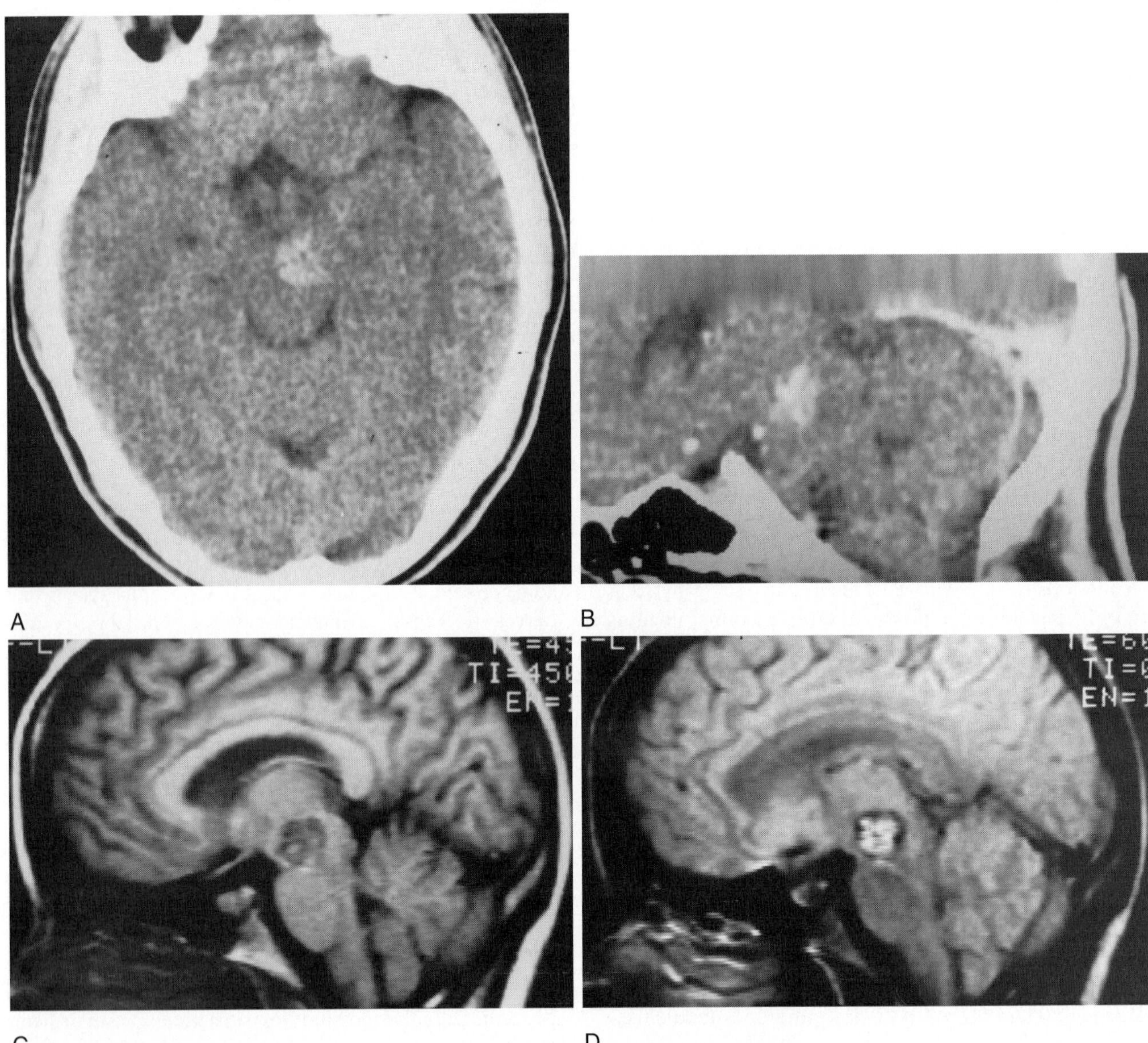

Figure 10.128. Midbrain cavernous angioma. Axial CT image without contrast (**A**) and reformatted sagittal view with contrast (**B**) reveal an area of hyperdensity mostly due to calcification. The area enhances slightly with contrast and is somewhat irregular in shape, measuring about 12 mm in diameter. **C.** Sagittal T1-weighted MR image shows a well-circumscribed, mostly hypointense lesion with a few small areas of isointensity or hyperintensity. **D.** Proton density image reveals hyperintensity surrounded by a well-developed hypointense rim representing old blood products. The hyperintensity may be produced by slow flow, with some areas containing methemoglobin (those that are brighter on C). Calcification can also appear bright on T2-weighted images; at other times it is bright on T1-weighted images.

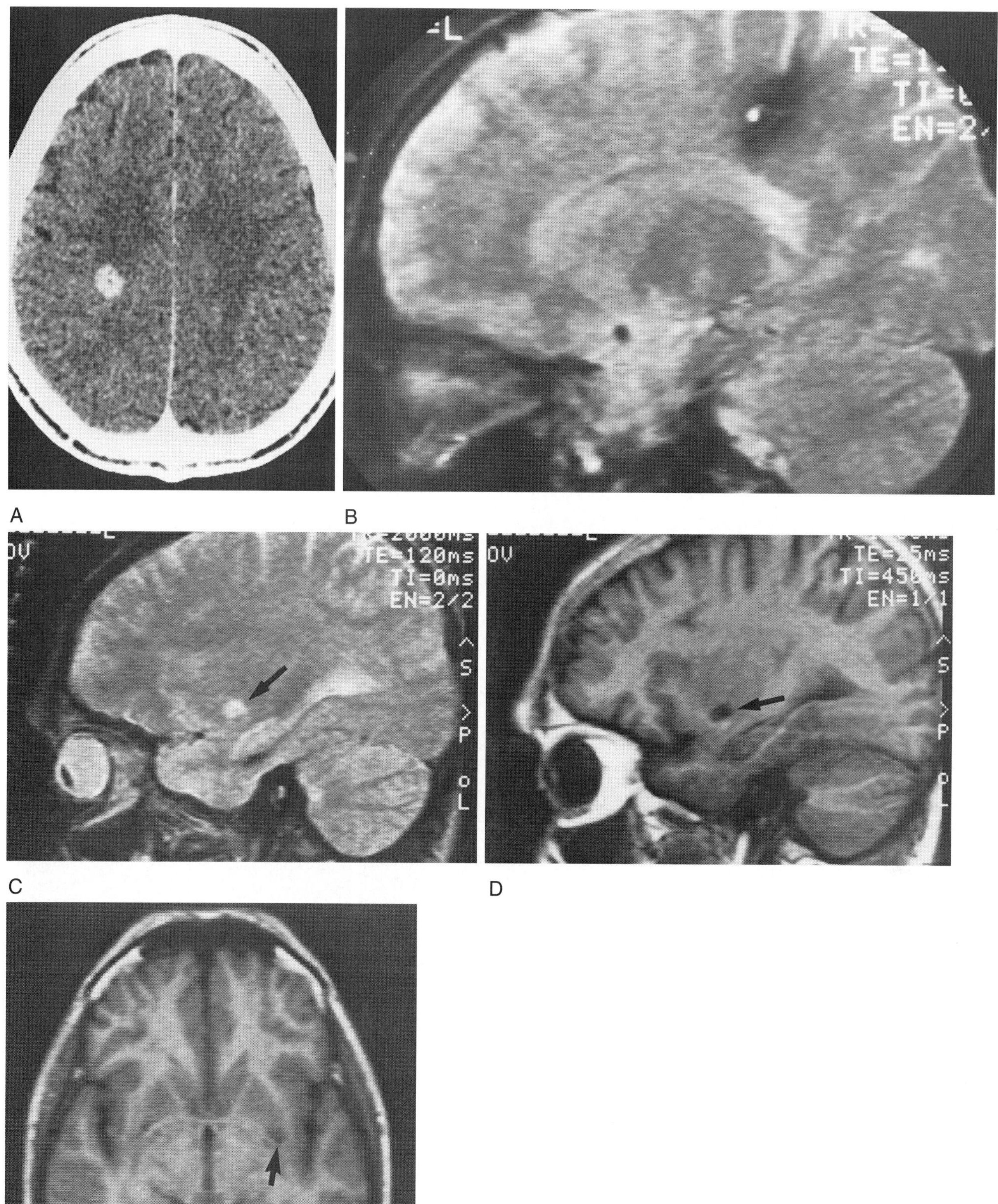

Figure 10.129. Cavernous angioma showing calcification and old blood products. **A.** CT image of partly calcified cavernous angioma in the right frontoparietal junction. **B.** Sagittal T2-weighted MR image reveals only one area of brightness, probably methemoglobin, surrounded by a large area of magnetic susceptibility due to old hemorrhage. Some of the hypointensity may be due to the calcification. **C.** Another lesion was seen in the left frontal operculum with no sign of prior hemorrhage (arrow). **D.** On a T1-weighted image this area was hypointense, similar to CSF. **E.** On an axial T1-weighted image it was located adjacent to the anterior commissure along with other smaller hypointense dots. The area was felt to represent an enlarged Virchow-Robin space.

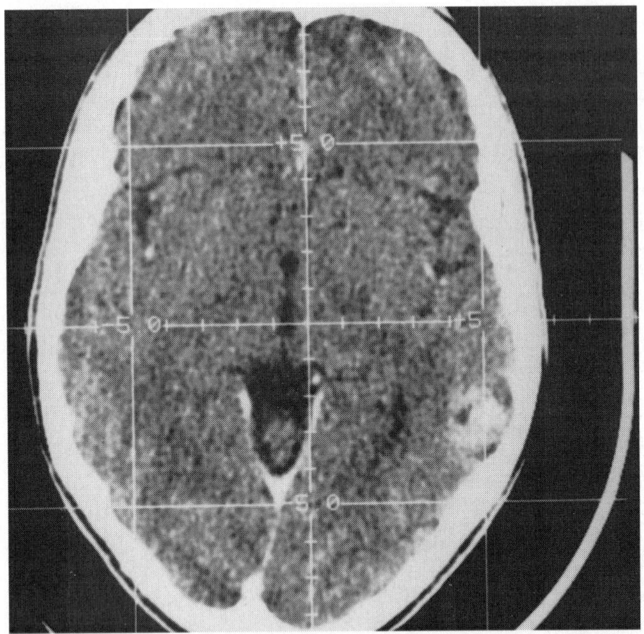

Figure 10.130. Occult vascular malformation (cavernous angioma). **A.** CT with contrast shows some enhancement of the lesion in the left temporal cortex. **B.** T1-weighted axial MR image shows a slightly hyperintense area surrounded by a markedly hypointense halo (arrows). Axial (**C**) and sagittal (**D**) T2-weighted images show marked hyperintensity with an irregular border surrounded by a markedly hypointense halo consistent with hemosiderin (arrows).

A

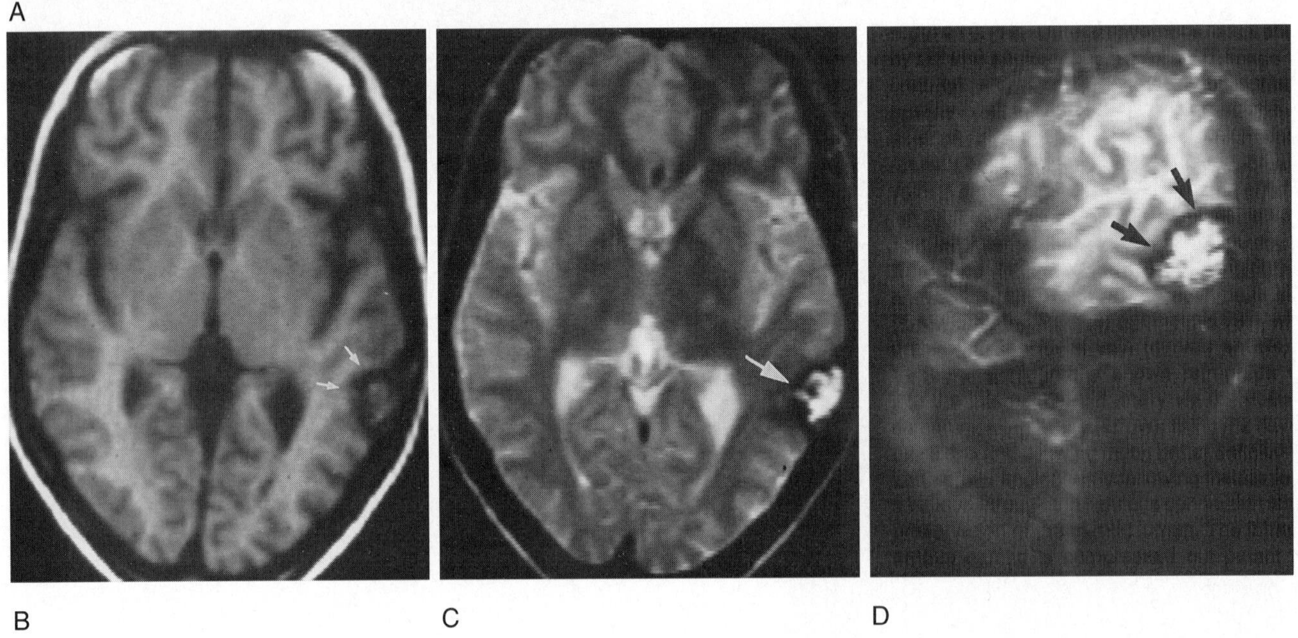

B C D

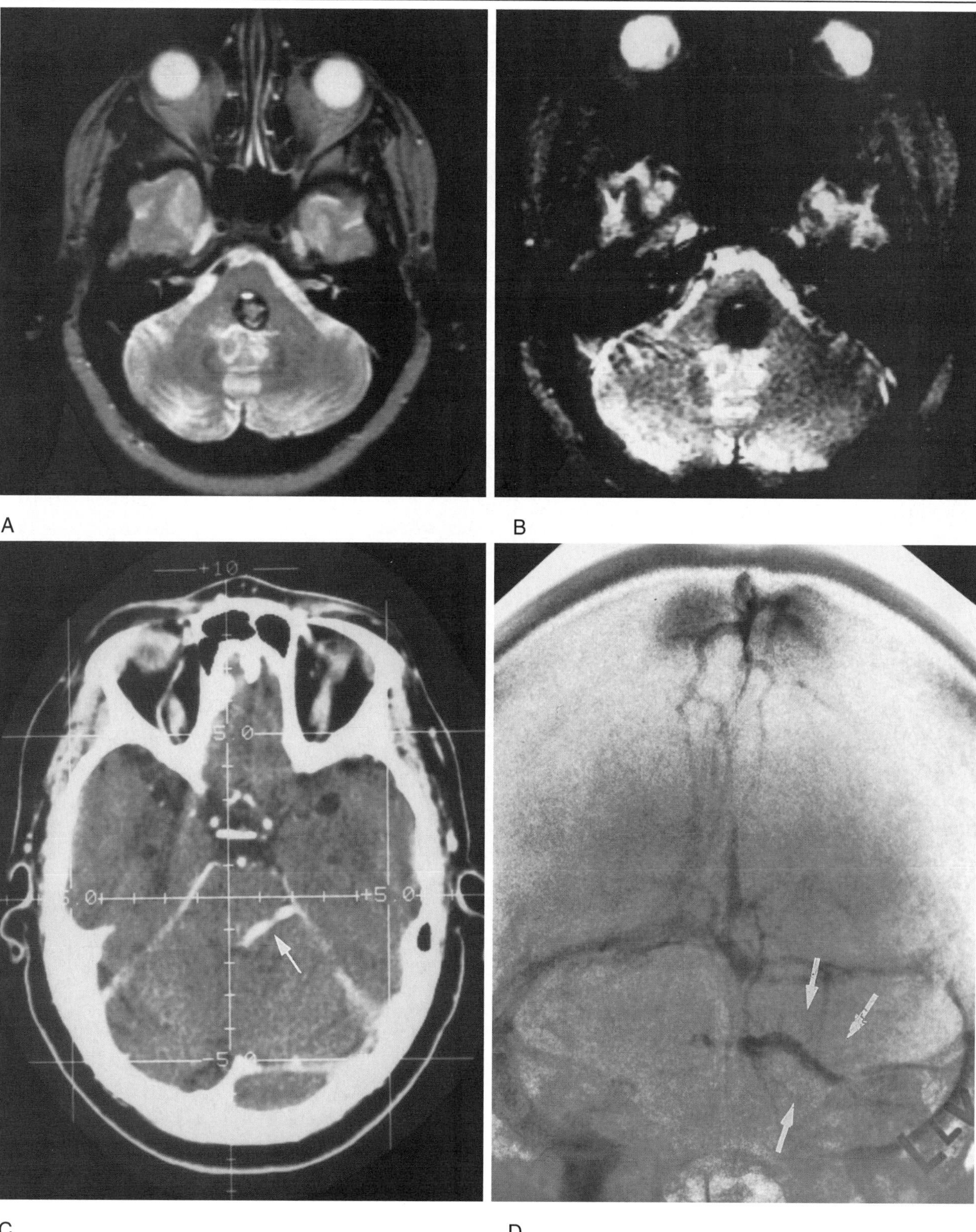

Figure 10.131. "Cavernous angioma" found to be associated with a "venous angioma" (venous malformation). **A.** There is a typical cavernous angioma appearance in the posterior aspect of the pons in this T2-weighted axial image. **B.** A gradient-echo image shows considerable susceptibility with blooming of the susceptibility area, which appears larger than in A. **C.** Postcontrast CT shows what appears to be a blood vessel going into or coming out of the area. For this reason, an angiogram was carried out (**D**) that revealed a typical appearance of a large venous channel filling late, receiving a number of fine veins, and draining into the superior petrosal sinus (arrows). These lesions should be called not venous angiomas but venous malformations.

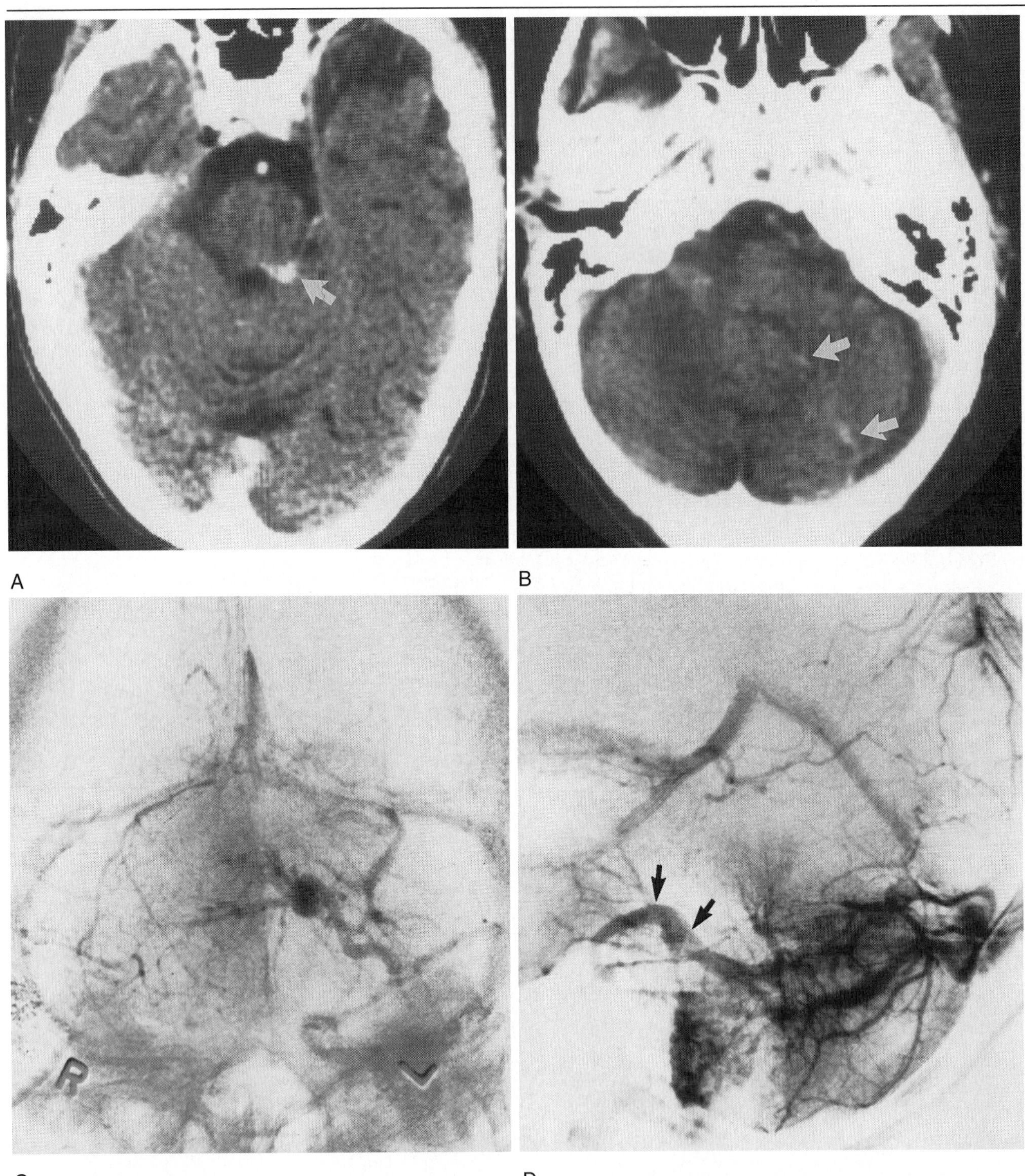

Figure 10.132. Venous angioma in cerebellum. **A.** CT with contrast reveals a hyperdense area adjacent to the fourth ventricle (arrow). **B.** A long venous channel is seen draining into the lateral sinus (arrows). **C.** Vertebral angiography (frontal view) shows many radiating small veins draining into a large venous channel that is seen only in the venous phase. No arterial feeders were identified. This lesion had bled. **D.** In this lateral view, the large vein is shown draining into the lateral sinus (arrows).

Figure 10.133. Venous angioma (venous malformation) **A.** CT with contrast shows a vein in the white matter. This is always abnormal. **B.** CT coronal view shows that the vein drains into the lateral sinus. **C.** Angiography demonstrates a normal arterial phase. There is a fetal-type carotid origin of the right posterior cerebral artery. **D.** The intermediate phase shows a conglomerate of fine vessels in the occipital lobe (arrows). **E.** The venous phase shows a large vein draining into the lateral venous sinus (arrows). **F.** The frontal view demonstrates the vein draining into the lateral sinus as seen in the later venous phase and on the coronal CT (B). An MRI examination was not done.

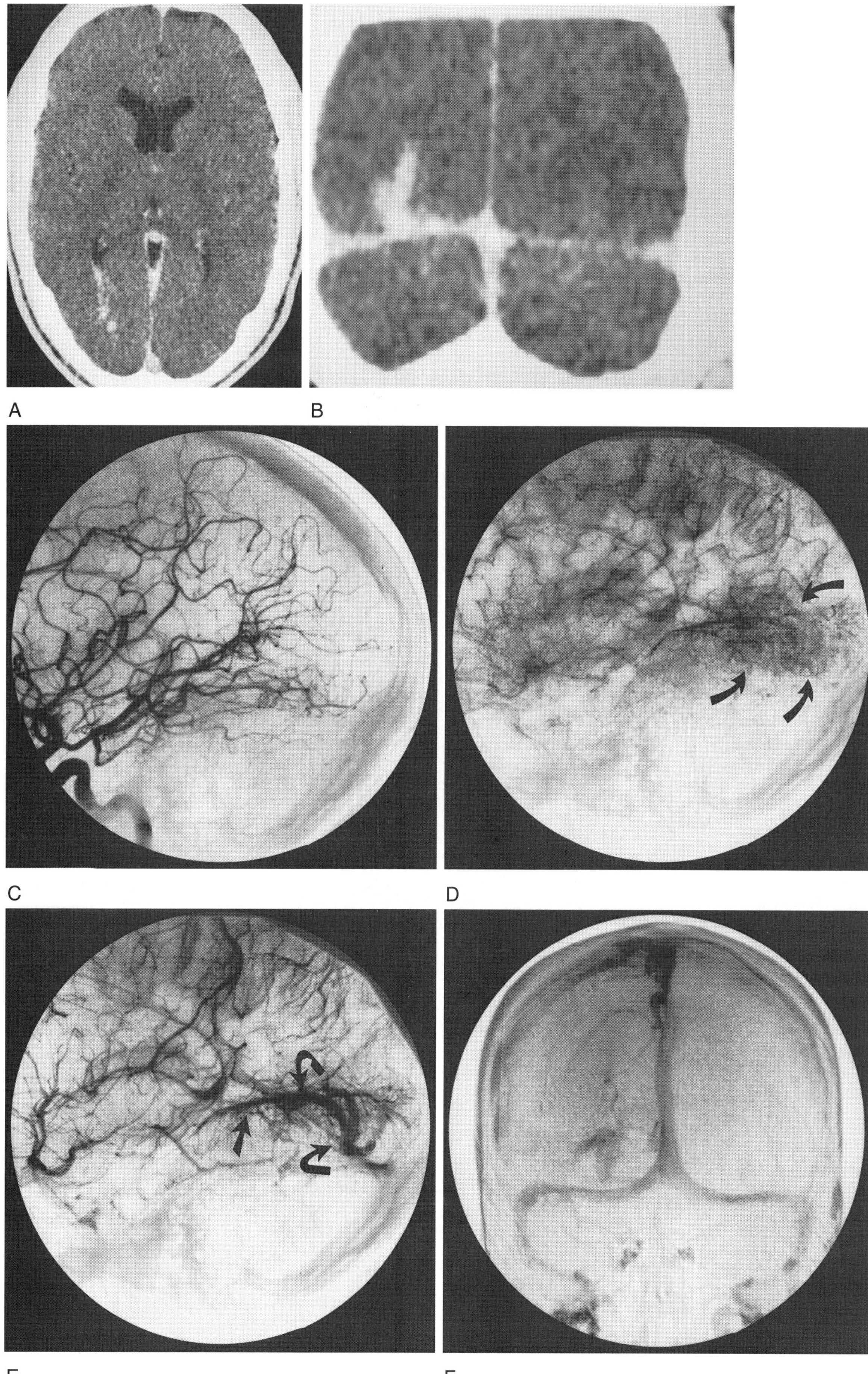
A
B
C
D
E
F

1. Asymptomatic individuals are observed.
2. When there is an acute or progressive neurologic deficit, surgery is advised if the lesion is surgically accessible.
3. The presence of seizures is an indication for surgical removal of the lesion if the patient has had a hemorrhage or if the lesion is in an accessible area.
4. After a single hemorrhage, surgical removal is recommended if the lesion is in an area where surgery would carry less hazard. Hemorrhage in the brainstem, thalamus, or basal ganglia is usually observed.
5. Patients with multiple hemorrhages should be strong candidates for surgery unless the surgical risks are deemed too high.

CEREBRAL CAPILLARY TELANGIECTASES

These are lesions composed of dilated capillaries in a local area of the brain. They are most frequent in the pons, but also may occur supratentorially and in the cerebellum. Histologically, "the dilated capillaries are everywhere separated by neural tissue," which, according to Russell and Rubinstein, is not the case in cavernous angiomas (252). They rarely bleed, and this is another important distinction from cavernous angiomas. On MRI examination there would be no evidence of hemosiderin indicative of prior bleeding, and this fact could be used in the differential diagnosis between the two. They also tend to be single. They may be the lesion that produces temporal lobe epilepsy in some cases, according to Vaquero et al. (253). These lesions may calcify. It is likely that capillary telangiectasis does not evolve into a cavernous angioma. The two types of hamartomas occasionally coexist in the same patient.

VENOUS ANGIOMAS (VENOUS MALFORMATIONS)

This type of lesion is usually clinically silent. Although Malik et al. reported on bleeding venous angiomas in 9 of 21 cases, the collective experience is that bleeding of pure venous angiomas is very uncommon (254). The author has seen some cases where bleeding occurred.

Typically the venous angioma is composed of a three-dimensional star arrangement of small venous channels that drain into a larger vein. This vein drains into other veins in the periphery of the brain, or into a deep vein or venous sinus. The vein itself is usually in the substance of the brain or in the cerebellum, and this location distinguishes it from normal veins, which are never normally in the brain substance but on the external or internal surface of the hemisphere or in the internal cerebral vein and vein of Galen (also extracerebral). The visualization of a sizable vascular channel in the brain white matter *should always be considered abnormal,* and in the absence of other findings the diagnosis of venous angioma or venous malformation should be considered. If a star-shaped arrangement of tiny veins is seen at one end of the channel, venous angioma is the most likely explanation.

The diagnosis can be suggested by CT or MRI, but final diagnosis is made by cerebral angiography, which shows the radiating veins draining into a larger venous channel in the venous phase, without increase in the local speed of circulation. In the late venous phase the venous channel usually remains open (Figs. 10.132 and 10.133). The association with cavernous angiomas has just been mentioned and illustrated (Fig. 10.131).

REFERENCES

1. Pullicino P, Kendall BE: Contrast enhancement in ischemic lesions: I. Relationship to progress. Neuroradiology 1980;19: 235–240.
2. Whisson CC, Wilson AJ, Evill CA, et al: The effect of intracarotid nonionic contrast media on the blood-brain barrier in acute hypertension. AJNR 1994;15:95–100.
3. Schwartz RB, Jones KM, Chernoff DM, et al: Common carotid artery bifurcation: Evaluation with spiral CT. Radiology 1992;185: 513–519.
4. Marks MR, Napel S, Jordan JE, et al: Diagnosis of carotid artery disease: Preliminary experience with maximum-intensity-projection spiral CT angiography. AJR 1993;160:1267–1271.
5. Dillon EH, van Leeuwen MS, Fernandez MA, et al: Spiral CT angiography. Pictorial essay. AJR 1993;160:1273–1278.
6. Schwartz RB, Tice HM, Hooten SM, et al: Evaluation of cerebral angiograms with helical CT: Correlation with conventional angiography and MR angiography. Radiology 1994;192:717–722.
7. Dorch NWC, Young N, Kingston RJ, Compton JS: Early experience with spiral CT in the diagnosis of intracranial aneurysms. Neurosurgery 1995;36:230–236.
8. Aoki S, Sasaki Y, Machida T, et al: Cerebral aneurysms: Detection and delineation using 3-D-CT angiography. AJNR 1992;13: 1115–1120.
9. Mosely ME, Kucharczyk J, Mintoravitch J, et al: Diffusion weighted MR imaging of acute stroke: Correlations with T2-weighted and magnetic susceptibility-enhanced MR imaging in cats. AJNR 1990;11:423–429.
10. Kucharczyk J, Vexler ZS, Roberts TP, et al: Echo-planar perfusion-sensitive MR imaging of acute cerebral ischemia. Radiology 1993; 188:711–717.
11. Lewin JS, Laub G: Intracranial MR angiography: A direct comparison of three time-of-flight techniques. AJNR 1992;12:1133–1139.
12. Blatter DD, Parker DL, Ahn SS, et al: Cerebral MR angiography with multiple overlapping thin slab acquisition: II. Early clinical experience. Radiology 1992;183:379–389.
13. Nishimura DG, Macovski A, Jackson JI, et al: Magnetic resonance angiography by selective recovery using a compact gradient echo sequence. Magn Reson Med 1988;8:96–103.
14. Wagle WA, Dumoulin CL, Souza SP, et al: 3DFT MR angiography of carotid and basilar arteries. AJNR 1989;10:911–919.
15. Dumoulin CL, Cline HE, Souza SP, et al: Three-dimensional time of flight magnetic resonance angiography using spin saturation. Magn Reson Med 1989;11:35–46.
16. Ruggieri PM, Laug GA, Masaryk TJ, et al: Intracranial circulation: Pulse-sequence considerations in three-dimensional (volume) MR angiography. Radiology 1989;171:785–791.
17. Wehrli FW, Shimakawa A, Gullberg CT, et al: Time-of-flight MR flow imaging: Selective saturation recovery with gradient refocusing. Radiology 1986;160:781–785.
18. Atlas SW: MR angiography in neurologic disease. Radiology 1994; 193:1–16.
19. Korogi Y, Takahashi M, Mabuchi N, et al: Intracranial aneurysms: Diagnostic accuracy of three-dimensional, Fourier transform, time-of-flight MR angiography. Radiology 1994;193:181–186.
20. Huston J, Rufenacht DA, Ehman RL, Wiebers DO: Intracranial aneurysms and vascular malformations: Comparison of time-of-

flight and phase-contrast MR angiography. Radiology 1991;181: 721–730.

21. Huston J III, Lewis BD, Wiebers DO, et al: Carotid artery: Prospective blind comparison of two-dimensional time-of-flight MR angiography with conventional angiography and duplex US. Radiology 1993;186:339–344.
22. Applegate BR, Talagala SL, Applegate LJ: MR angiography of the head and neck: Value of two-dimensional phase contrast projection technique. AJR 1992;159:369–374.
23. Lin W, Tkach JA, Haacke EM, Masaryk TJ: Intracranial MR angiography: Application of magnetization transfer contrast and fat saturation to short gradient-echo, velocity-compensated sequences. Radiology 1993;186:753–761.
24. Edelman RR, Ahn SS, Chien D, et al: Improved time-of-flight MR angiography of the brain with magnetization transfer contrast. Radiology 1992;184:395–399.
25. Tsuruda JS, Sevich RJ, Hallbach Van V: Three dimensional time-of-flight MR angiography in the evaluation of intracranial aneurysms treated by endovascular balloon occlusion. AJNR 1992;13: 1129–1136.
26. Wright GA, Nishimura DG, Macouski A: Flow-independent magnetic resonance projection angiography. Magn Reson Med 1991; 17:126–140.
27. Polak JF, Kalina P, Magruder CD, et al: Carotid endarterectomy: Preoperative evaluation of candidates with combined Doppler sonography and MR angiography. Radiology 1993;186:333–338.
28. Ackerman RH, Candia MR: Identifying clinically relevant carotid disease. Stroke 1994;25:1–3.
29. Barnett HJM, Peerless SJ, Fox AJ, et al: North American symptomatic carotid endarterectomy trial: Methods, patient characteristic, and progress. Stroke 1991;22:711–720.
30. Fox AJ: How to measure carotid stenosis. Radiology 1993;186: 316–318.
31. Polak JF, Bajakian RL, O'Leary DH, et al: Detection of internal carotid artery stenosis: Comparison of MR angiography, color Doppler sonography and arteriography. Radiology 1982;182: 35–40.
32. Anderson CM, Saloner D, Lee RE, et al: Assessment of carotid artery stenosis by MR angiography: Comparison with x-ray angiography and color-coded Doppler ultrasound. AJNR 1992;13: 989–1003.
33. Heiserman JE, Drayer BP, Keller PJ, et al: Intracranial vascular stenosis and occlusion: Evaluation with three-dimensional time-of-flight MR angiography. Radiology 1992;185:667–673.
34. Ross MR, Pelc NJ, Enzman DR: Qualitative phase contrast MRA in the normal and abnormal circle of Willis. AJNR 1993;14:19–25.
35. Mattle HP, Edelman RR, Wentz KU, et al: Middle cerebral artery: Determination of flow velocities with MR angiography. Radiology 1991;181:527–530.
36. Chakeres DW, Schmalbrock P, Brogan M, et al: Normal venous anatomy of the brain: Demonstration with gadopentetate dimeglumine in enhanced 3-D MR angiography. AJNR 1990;11: 1107–1108.
37. Ackerman RH, Candia MR: Assessment of carotid artery stenosis by MR angiography. Commentary. AJNR 1992;13:1005–1008.
38. Barnett GO: Cerebral blood flow: Factors influencing pulsatile flow in individual vessels. In Fourth Princeton Conference on Cerebral Vascular Disease. New York: Grune and Stratton, 1965.
39. Knisely MH, Warner L, Harding F: Antemortem settling. Microscopic observations and analyses of the settling of agglutinated blood cell masses to the lower sides of vessels during life: A contribution to the biophysics of disease. Angiology 1960;11:535.
40. Schechter MM, Elkin M: Layering effect in cerebral angiography. Acta Radiol 1963;1:427.
41. Greitz T: Dilatation of cerebral veins during cerebral angiography with water-soluble contrast media. Acta Radiol 1966;4:625.
42. Huber P, Handa J: Effect of contrast material, hypercapnia, hyperventilation, hypertonic glucose and papaverine on the diameter of the cerebral arteries: Angiographic demonstration in man. Invest Radiol 1967;2:17.
43. Moniz E: L'Angiographie Cerebrale. Paris: Masson et Cie., 1934.
44. Leeds NE, Taveras JM: Dynamic factors in diagnosis of supratentorial brain tumor by cerebral angiography. Philadelphia: Saunders, 1969.
45. Ingvar DH, Risberg J: Increase of regional cerebral blood flow during mental effort in normals and in patients with focal brain disorders. Exp Brain Res 1967;3:195.
46. Ingvar DH, Rosen T, Elnqvist D: Effects of sensory stimulation upon RCBF. Presented at the Seventh International Symposium on Cerebral Circulation and Metabolism, Aviemore, Scotland, 1975.
47. Blauenstein UW, Halsey JH, Wilson EM, et al: The xenon-133 inhalation method: Analysis of reproducibility. Presented at the Seventh International Symposium on Cerebral Circulation and Metabolism, Aviemore, Scotland, 1975.
48. Nylin G: Application of blood flow measurements to future investigation. In Cerebral Vascular Diseases. Third Princeton Conference, CH Millikan (Chairman). New York: Grune and Stratton, 1961, p 67.
49. Greitz T: A radiologic study of the brain circulation by rapid serial angiography of the carotid artery. Acta Radiol 1956;suppl 140.
50. Taveras JM, Poser CM: Roentgenologic aspects of cerebral angiography in children. Am J Roentgenol 1959;82:371.
51. White E, Greitz T: Subependymal venous filling sequence at cerebral angiography: Influence of grey and white matter distribution. Acta Radiol (Diag) 1972;13:272.
52. Farrell FW, Davis DO: The correlation of cerebral angiography circulation times with arterial PCO_2 levels. Acta Radiol Diag 1972; 13:86.
53. Amundsen P, Malm OJ, Poole GJ: Cerebral angiography in the diagnosis of brain death. Paper presented at Ninth Symposium Neuroradiologicum, Goethenburg, 1970.
54. Sokoloff L: Aspects of cerebral circulator physiology of relevance to cerebrovascular disease. Proceedings of International Conference on Vascular Diseases of the Brain. Neurology 1961;11:34.
55. Tachibana H, Meyer JS, Okayasu H, Kandula P: Changing topographic patterns of human cerebral blood flow with age measured by xenon CT. AJNR 1984;5:139–146.
56. Pribram HFW: Angiographic appearances in acute intracranial hypertension. Neurology 1961;11:10.
57. Horwitz NH, Dunsmore RH: Some factors influencing the non-visualization of the internal carotid artery by angiography. J Neurosurg 1956;13:155.
58. Greitz T, Gordon E, Kolmodin G, et al: Aortocranial and carotid angiography in determination of brain death. Neuroradiology 1973;5:13.
59. Lassen NA: The luxury perfusion syndrome and its possible relation to acute metabolic acidosis localized within the brain. Lancet 1966;2:1113–1115.
60. Farrell FW, Taveras JM. Angiographic stain produced by seizures: A case report. Neuroradiology 1974;8:49–53.
61. Krueger TP, Rockoff SD, Thomas J, et al: The effect of changes of end expiratory carbon dioxide tension on the normal cerebral angiogram. Am J Roentgenol 1963;90:56.
62. Du Boulay G, Edmunds-Seal J, Bostick T: Effect of intermittent positive pressure ventilation upon cerebral angiography: Clarity of films and diameter of vessels including those in spasm. In J Taveras, H Fischgold, D Dilenge (eds), Recent Advances in the Study of Cerebral Circulation. Springfield, IL: Charles C. Thomas, 1970, p 59.
63. Samuel R, Grange RA, Hawkins TD: Anaesthetic technique for carotid angiography: The use of hyperventilation to improve the angiographic demonstration of intracranial tumours. Anaesthesia 1968;23:543.

64. Kety SS, Schmidt CF: The nitrous oxide method for the quantitative determination of cerebral blood flow in man: Theory, procedure, and normal values. J Clin Invest 1948;27:476.
65. Lassen NA, Ingvar DH: The blood flow of the cerebral cortex determined by radioactive krypton-85. Experimentia 1961;17:42.
66. Meyer JS, Hayman LA, Yamamoto M, et al: Local cerebral blood flow measured by CT after stable xenon inhalation. AJNR 1980; 1:213–225. Also in AJR 1980;135:239–251.
67. Ter-Pogossian MM, Eichling JO, Davis DO, et al: The measure in vivo of regional cerebral oxygen utilization by means of oxyhemoglobin labelled with radioactive oxygen-15. J Clin Invest 1970; 49:381.
68. Ter-Pogossian MM, Eichling JO, Davis DO, et al: The simultaneous measure in vivo of regional cerebral blood flow and regional cerebral oxygen utilization by means of oxyhemoglobin labelled with radioactive oxygen-15. In C Fieschi, DH Ingvar, NA Lassen, K Chiroman (eds), Cerebral Blood Flow. Berlin: Springer, 1969.
69. Raichle ME, Martin WRW, Herscovitch P, et al: Brain blood flow measured with intravenous H2 15 O.II: Implementation and validation. J Nucl Med 1983;24:790–798.
70. Frackowiak RSJ, Lenzi GL, Jones T, et al: Quantitative measurement of regional cerebral blood flow and oxygen metabolism in man using 15 O and positron emission tomography: Theory, procedure, and normal values. J Comput Assist Tomogr 1980;4: 727–736.
71. Buxton RG, Wechsler LR, Alpert NM, et al: Measurement of brain pH using 11 CO_2 and positron emission tomography. J Cereb Blood Flow Metab 1984;4:8–16.
72. Buxton RB, Alpert NM, Wechsler RH, et al: Kinetic model for the measurement of brain pH with 11 CO_2 and emission computed tomography. In T Greitz, DH Ingvar, L Widen (eds), The Metabolism of Human Brain Studies with Positron Emission Tomography. New York: Raven, 1985, pp 273–278.
73. Rempp KA, Brix G, Wenz F, et al: Quantification of cerebral blood flow and volume with dynamic susceptibility contrast-enhanced MR imaging. Radiology 1994;193:637–641.
74. Bloor BM, Aslei RP, Nugent GR, et al: Relationship of cerebrovascular reactivity to degree of extracranial vascular occlusion. Circulation 1966;33, 34(suppl 2):28.
75. Burt RW, Witt RM, Cikrit DF, et al: Carotid artery disease: Evaluation with acetazolamide-enhanced Tc-99m HMPAO SPECT. Radiology 1992;182:461–466.
76. Yamashita T, Hayashi M, Kashiwagi S, et al: Cerebrovascular reserve capacity in ischemia due to occlusion of a major arterial trunk: Studies by Xe-CT and the acetazolamide test. J Comput Assist Tomogr 1992;16:750–755.
77. Rogg J, Rutigliano M, Yonas H, et al: The acetazolamide challenge: Imaging techniques designed to evaluate cerebral blood flow reserve. AJNR 1989;10:803–810.
78. Lassen NA. Autoregulation of cerebral blood flow. Circ Res 1964; 15(suppl 1).
79. Hoedt-Rassmussen K, Skinhoj E, Paulson E, et al: Regional cerebral blood flow in acute apoplexy; "Luxury perfusion syndrome" of brain tissue. Arch Neurol 1967;17:271.
80. Taveras JM, Wood EH: Diagnostic Neuroradiology, ed 1. Baltimore: Williams and Wilkins, 1964.
81. Cronqvist S, Laroche F: Transitory hyperaemia in focal cerebral vascular lesions: Studies by angiography and regional cerebral blood flow measurements. Br J Radiol 1967;40:270.
82. Taveras JM, Gilson JM, Davis DO, et al: Angiography in cerebral infarction. Radiology 1969;93:549.
83. Brock M, Beck J, Markasis E, et al: Intracranial pressure gradients, local tissue perfusion pressure and regional cerebral blood flow. In Cerebral Blood Flow and Intracranial Pressure. Proceedings of the Fifth International Symposium, Roma-Siena 1971, p 74.
84. Heiskanen I: Cerebral circulatory arrest caused by acute increase of intracranial pressure. Acta Neurol Scand 1963;40(suppl 7).
85. Braunstein P, Korein J, II Kricheff, et al: A simple bedside evaluation for cerebral blood flow in the study of cerebral death: A prospective study on 34 deeply comatose patients. Am J Roentgenol 1973;18:757.
86. DeWitt LD, Caplan LR: Antiphospholipid antibodies and stroke. Commentary. AJNR 1991;12:454–456.
87. Pulpeiro JR, Cortes JA, Macarron J, et al: MR findings in primary antiphospholipid syndrome. AJNR 1991;12:452–453.
88. Brey L, Hart RC, Sherman DG, et al: Antiphospholipid antibodies and cerebral ischemia in young people. Neurology 1990;40: 1190–1195.
89. Kushner MJ: Prospective study of anticardiolipin antibodies in stroke. Stroke 1990;21:295–298.
90. Provenzale JM, Heinz ER, Ortel TL, et al: Antiphospholipid antibodies in patients without systemic lupus erythematosus: Neuroradiologic findings. Radiology 1994;192:531–537.
91. Tournier-Lasserve E, Joutel A, Melki J, et al: Cerebral autosomal dominant arteriopathy with subcortical infarcts and leukoencephalopathy maps to chromosome 19 q 12. Nature Genetics 1993;3: 256–259.
92. Mas JL, Dilouya A, de Recondo JA: Familial disorder with subcortical ischemic strokes, dementia and leukoencephalopathy. Neurology 1992;42:1015–1019.
93. Bell BA, Symon L, Branston NM: CBF and time thresholds for the formation of ischemic cerebral edema, and effect of neoperfusion in baboons. J Neurosurg 1985;62:31–41.
94. Ter Penning B: Pathophysiology of stroke. Neuroimag Clin North Am 1992;2:389–408.
95. Garcia JH, Mitchen HL, Briggs L, et al: Transient focal ischemia in subhuman primates: Neuronal injury as a function of local cerebral blood flow. J Neuropathol Exp Neurol 1983;42:44–60.
96. Sage MR: Blood-brain barrier: Phenomenon of increasing importance to the imaging clinician. AJR 1982;138:887–898.
97. DiChiro G, Timins EL, Jones AE, et al: Radionuclide scanning and microangiography of evolving and complete brain infarction. Neurology 1974;24:418–423.
98. Whisnant JP, et al: Classification of cerebrovascular disease III. Stroke 1990;21:637–676.
99. Siekert, RG: Diagnosis and classification of focal ischemic cerebrovascular disease. Proc Staff Meet Mayo Clin 1960;35:473.
100. Wisoff HS, Rothballer AB: Cerebral arterial thrombosis in children. Review of literature and addition of two cases in apparently healthy children. Arch Neurol 1961;4:258.
101. Martin MJ, Sayre GP, Whisnant JP: Incidence of occlusive vascular disease in the extracranial arteries contributing to the cerebral circulation. Trans Am Neurol Assoc 1960;85:103.
102. Fisher CM: Occlusion of the carotid arteries: Further experiences. Arch Neural Psychiatry 1954;72:187.
103. Martin MJ, Whisnant JP, Sayre GP: Occlusive vascular disease in the extracranial cerebral circulation. Arch Neurol 1960;3:530.
104. Stein BM, McCormick WF, Rodriguez JN, Taveras JM: Postmortem angiography of cerebral vascular system. Arch Neurol 1962; 7:545.
105. Fisher CM: Observation of the fundus oculi in transient monocular blindness. Neurology 1959;9:333.
106. Truwit CL, Barkovich AJ, Gean-Marton A, et al: Loss of the insular ribbon: Another early CT sign of acute middle cerebral artery infarction. Radiology 1990;176:801–806.
107. Bryan RN, Levy LM, Whitlow WD, et al: Diagnosis of acute cerebral infarction: Comparison of CT and MR imaging. AJNR 1991; 12:611–620.
108. Yuh WTC, Crain MR, Loes DJ, et al: MR imaging of cerebral ischemia: Findings in the first 24 hours. AJNR 1991;12:621–629.
109. Crain MR, Yuh WTC, Greene GM, et al: Cerebral ischemia: Evaluation with contrast-enhanced MR imaging. AJNR 1991;12: 631–639.

110. Shimosegawa E, Inugami A, Ikudera T, et al: Embolic cerebral infarction: MR findings in the first 3 hours after onset. AJR 1993; 160:1077–1082.
111. Kummer R von, Meyding-Lamadé U, Forsting M, et al: Sensitivity and prognostic value of early CT in occlusion of the middle cerebral artery trunk. AJNR 1994;15:9–15.
112. Elster AD: MR contrast enhancement in brainstem and deep cerebral infarction. AJNR 1992;12:1127–1132.
113. Kendall BE, Pullicino P: Intravascular contrast injection in ischemic lesions: II. Effect on prognosis. Neuroradiology 1980;19: 241–243.
114. Herderschel D, Hijdra A, Algra A, et al: Silent stroke in patients with transient ischemic attack or minor ischemic stroke. Stroke 1992;23:1220–1224.
115. Percheron G: The anatomy of the arterial supply of the human thalamus and its use for the interpretation of the thalamic vascular pathology. J Neurol 1973;20:1–13.
116. Fisher CM: Lacunes: Small, deep cerebral infarcts. Neurology 1965;15:774–784.
117. Nabatame H, Fujimoto N, Nakamura K: High intensity areas on noncontrast T1-weighted MR images in cerebral infarction. J Comput Assist Tomogr 1990;14(4):521–526.
118. Boyko OB, Burger PC, Shelburne JD, et al: Non-heme mechanisms for T1 shortening: Pathologic, CT, and MR elucidation. AJNR 1992;13:1439–1445.
119. Araki Y, Furukaya T, Tsuruda K, et al: High field MR imaging of the brain in pseudohypoparathyroidism. Neuroradiology 1990;32: 325–327.
120. Henkelman RM, Watts JF, Kucharczyk W: High signal intensity in MR images of calcified brain tissue. Radiology 1991;179:199–206.
121. Roda JM, Carceller F, Perez-Higueras A, et al: Encapsulated intracerebral hematomas: A defined entity. J Neurosurg 1993;78: 829–833.
122. Gomori JM, Grossman RI, Goldberg HI, et al: Intracranial hematomas: Imaging by high field MR. Radiology 1985;157:87–93.
123. Gomori JM, Grossman RI, Hackney DB, et al: Variable appearance of subacute intracranial hematomas on high-field spin-echo MR. AJNR 1987;8:1019–1026.
124. Grossman RI: Magnetic resonance imaging of hemorrhage. In JM Taveras, JT Ferrucci (eds), Radiology: Diagnosis/Imaging/Intervention. Philadelphia: Lippincott, 1990.
125. Levy DE: Medical treatment of acute ischemic stroke. Neuroimag Clin North Am 1992;2:597–605.
126. Zoppo GJ del: An open, multicenter trial of recombinant tissue plasminogen activator in acute stroke. A progress report. Stroke 1990;21(suppl 4):174–175.
127. Barnett HJM, the North American Symptomatic Carotid Endarterectomy Trial Collaboration: Beneficial effects of carotid endarterectomy in symptomatic patients with high-grade carotid stenosis. N Engl J Med 1991;325:445–453.
128. Taveras JM, Mount LA, Friendenberg RM: Arteriographic demonstration of external-internal carotid anastomosis through the ophthalmic arteries. Radiology 1954;63:525.
129. Bossi R, Pisani C: Collateral cerebral circulation through the ophthalmic artery and its efficiency in internal carotid occlusion. Br J Radiol 1955;28:462.
130. Ackerman RH: Cerebrovascular noninvasive evaluation. In JM Taveras, JT Ferrucci (eds), Radiology: Diagnosis/Imaging/Intervention. Philadelphia: Lippincott, 1995.
131. Mount LA, Taveras JM: Arteriographic demonstration of the collateral circulation of the cerebral hemisphere. Arch Neurol Psychiatry 1957;78:235.
132. Taveras JM: Multiple progressive intracranial arterial occlusions: A syndrome of children and young adults. Am J Roentgenol Radium Ther Nucl Med 1969;106:235.
133. Lyons C: Progress report of the joint study on extracranial arterial occlusion. In CH Millikan, RG Siekert, JP Whisnant (eds), Cerebral Vascular Diseases, Fourth Conference. New York: Grune and Stratton, 1965.
134. Rob CG: Operation for acute completed stroke due to thrombosis of internal carotid artery. Surgery 1969;65:862.
135. Wood EH, Correll JW, Boschenstein Fk, et al: Neurologic evaluation of results of surgical treatment of extracranial atherosclerotic disease. Acta Radiol 1969;9:537.
136. Ojemann RG, Austen WG: Surgical treatment of extracranial occlusive vascular disease. In JL Smith (ed), Neuro-ophthalmology, Vol 4, Symposium of the University of Miami and the Bascom Palmer Eye Institute. St. Louis: Mosby, 1968, p 388.
137. Gurdjian ES, Lindner DW, Hardy WG, et al: Arteriography. In Cerebral Vascular Diseases. Third Princeton Conference, CH Millikan (Chairman). New York: Grune and Stratton, 1961, p 200.
138. Crawford ES, De Baley ME, et al: Surgical treatment of atherosclerotic occlusive lesions in patients with cerebral arterial insufficiency. Circulation 1959;20:168.
139. Moossy J: Cerebral infarcts and the lesions of intracranial and extracranial atherosclerosis. Arch Neurol 1966;14:124.
140. Hunt JR: The role of the carotid arteries in the causation of vascular lesions of the brain, with remarks on certain special features of the symptomatology. Am J Med Sci 1914;704.
141. Denny-Brown D, Meyer JS: Cerebral collateral circulation: II. Production of cerebral infarction by ischemic anoxia and its reversibility in early stages. Neurology 1957;7:567.
142. Wood EH, Correll JW: Atheromatous ulceration in major neck vessels as a cause of cerebral embolism. Acta Radiol (Diagn) 1969; 9:520.
143. Kishore PRS, Chase NE, Krisheff II: Carotid stenosis and intracranial emboli. Radiology 1971;100:351.
144. Barton JW, Margolis MT: Rotational obstruction of the vertebral artery at the atlantoaxial joint. Neuroradiology 1975;9:117.
145. Fields WS, Crawford ES, DeBakey ME: Surgical considerations in cerebral arterial insufficiency. Neurology 1958;8:801.
146. Metz H, Murray-Leslie RM, Bannister RG, et al: Kinking of the internal carotid artery. Lancet 1961;1:424.
147. Hauser OW, Mokri B, Sundt TM Jr, et al: Spontaneous cervical cephalic arterial dissection and its residium: Angiographic spectrum. AJNR 1984;5:27–34.
148. Petro GR, Witwer GA, Cacayorin ED, et al: Spontaneous dissection of the cervical internal carotid artery: Correlation of arteriography, CT, and pathology. AJNR 1986;7:1053–1058.
149. Castillo M, Kramer L: Raeder sydrome: MR appearance. AJNR 1992;13:1121–1123.
150. Milandre L, Perot S, Khalil R: Spontaneous dissection of both extracranial internal carotid arteries. Neuroradiology 1989;31: 435–439.
151. Riggs HE: Anomalies of circle of Willis. Transactions of the Philadelphia Neurological Society, December 1937.
152. Webster JE, Gurdjian ES, Lindner DW, et al: Proximal occlusion of the anterior cerebral artery. Arch Neurol 1960;2:19.
153. Kudo T: Spontaneous occlusion of circle of Willis: Disease apparently confined to Japanese. Neurology 1968;18:485–496.
154. Nishimoto A, Takeuchi S: Abnormal cerebrovascular network to internal carotid arteries. J Neurosurg 1968;29:255.
155. Maki Y, Nakata Y: Autopsy case of hemangiomatous malformation of bilateral internal carotid artery at the base of brain. Brain 1965; 17:764.
156. Prensky AL, Davis DO: Obstruction of major cerebral vessels in early childhood without neurological signs. Neurology 1970;20: 945.
157. Kudo K: A disease with abnormal intracranial vascular network: Spontaneous occlusion of the circle of Willis. In Proceedings of Symposium of 25th Congress of Japan. Neurosurgical Society. Tokyo: Igaku Shoin, 1966.

158. El Gammal T, Adams RJ, Nichols FT, et al: MR and CT investigation of cerebrovascular disease in sickle cell patients. AJNR 1986; 7:1043–1049.
159. Stockman JA, Nigro MA, Mishkin MM, et al: Occlusion of large cerebral vessels in sickle cell anemia. N Engl J Med 1972;287: 846–849.
160. Wood DH: Cerebrovascular complications of sickle cell anemia. Stroke 1977;12:73–76.
161. Rebollo M, Val JF, Garijo F, et al: Livedo reticularis and cerebrovascular lesions (Sneddon's syndrome). Brain 1983;106:965–979.
162. Blom RJ: Sneddon syndrome: CT, angiography, and MR imaging. J Comput Assist Tomogr 1989;13:119–122.
163. Rumple E, Neuhofer J, Pallua A, et al: Cerebrovascular lesions and livedo reticularis (Sneddon's syndrome): A progressive cerebrovascular disorder? J Neurol 1985;231:324–330.
164. Jonas J, Kolble K, Volckor HE, et al: Central retinal artery occlusion in Sneddon's disease associated with antiphospholipid antibodies. Am J Ophthalmol 1986;14:37–40.
165. Pauranik A, Parwani S, Jain S: Simultaneous bilateral central retinal artery occlusion in a patient with Sneddon syndrome. Angiology 1987;38:158–163.
166. Ring BA: Angiographic recognition of occlusion of isolated branches of the middle cerebral artery. Am J Roentgenol 1963;89: 391.
167. Wollschlaeger F, Wollschlaeger PB: Arterial anastomosis of the human brain: A radiographic anatomic study. Acta Radiol (Diagn) 1966;5:604.
168. Gannon WE, Chait A: Occlusion of middle cerebral artery with recanalization. Am J Roentgenol 1962;88:24.
169. Allcock JM: Occlusion of the middle cerebral artery: Serial angiography as a guide to conservative therapy. J Neurosurg 1967;27:353.
170. Solis OJ, Roberson GR, Taveras JM, et al: Cerebral angiography in acute cerebral infarction. Revist Interam Radiol 1977;2:19–25.
171. Hoedt-Rasmussen K, Skinhoj E: Transneural depression of the cerebral hemispheric metabolism in man. Acta Neurol Scand 1964; 40:41.
172. Yarnell PR, Burdick D, Sanders B, et al: Focal seizures, early veins, and increased flow: A clinical angiographic and radioscopic correlation. Neurology 1974;24:512.
173. Jannetta PJ, Abbasy LM, Maroon JC, et al: Etiology and definitive microsurgical treatment of hemifacial spasm: Operative techniques and results in 47 patients. J Neurosurg 1977;47:321–328.
174. Wilkins RH: Hemifacial spasm: A review. Surg Neurol 1991;36: 251–277.
175. Tash R, De Merritt J, Sze G, et al: Hemifacial spasm: MR imaging features. AJNR 1991;12:839–842.
176. Tien RD, Wilkins RH: MRA delineation of the vertebral-basilar system in patients with hemifacial spasm and trigeminal neuralgia. AJNR 1993;14:34–36.
177. Esfahani F, Dolan KD: Air CT cisternography in diagnosis of vascular loop causing vestibular dysfunction. AJNR 1989;10: 1045–1049.
178. Bergeron RT, Wood EH: Oral contraceptives and cerebrovascular complications. Radiology 1969;92:231.
179. Goldberg AI, Rosenbaum AE, Wang H, et al: Computed tomography of dural sinus thrombosis. J Comput Assist Tomogr 1986;10: 16–20.
180. Ulmer JL, Elster AD: Physiologic mechanisms underlying the delayed delta sign. AJNR 1991;12:647–650.
181. Maachi PJ, Grossman RI, Gomori JM, et al: High field MRI of cerebral venous thrombosis. J Comput Assist Tomogr 1986;10: 10–15.
182. Bauer WM, Einhäupl K, Heywang SH, et al: MR of venous sinus thrombosis: A case report. AJNR 1987;8:713–715.
183. Sze G, Simmons B, Krol G, et al: Dural sinus thrombosis: Verification with spin-echo techniques. AJNR 1988;9:679–686.
184. Edwards MK, Kuharik MA, Cohen MD, et al: Sonographic demonstration of cerebral sinus thrombosis. AJNR 1987;8:1153–1154.
185. Brisman R, Hilal SK, Tenner M: Doppler ultrasound measurements of superior sagittal sinus blood velocity. J Neurosurg 1972; 37:312.
186. Scotti LN, Goldman RL, Hardman DR, et al: Venous thrombosis in infants and children. Radiology 1974;112:393–399.
187. Massachusetts General Hospital—Case Records. Case 20-1988. N Engl J Med 1988;318:1322–1328.
188. Crompton MR: Cranial nervous lesions consequent upon ruptured cerebral berry aneurysms. Thesis, University of London, and personal communications, 1963.
189. Riggs HE, Rupp C: Miliary aneurysms: Relation of anomalies of the circle of Willis to formation of aneurysms. Arch Neurol Psychiatry 1943;49:615.
190. Housepian EM, Pool JL: A systematic analysis of intracranial aneurysms from the autopsy file of the Presbyterian Hospital, 1914 to 1956. J Neuropathol Exp Neurol 1958;17:409.
191. Sorek DA, Silbergleit R: Multiple asymptomatic cervical cephalic aneurysms. AJNR 1993;14:31–33.
192. Blane G: History of some cases of disease in the brain, with an account of the appearances upon examination after death, and some general observations on complaints of the head. Trans Soc Improv Med Chir Knowl 1800;2:192.
193. Morgagni CB: De sedibus et causis morborum. Venetiis ex. typog. Remondiniana, Book 1, letter 4, case 19, 1761.
194. Blackall J: Observations on the Nature and Cure of Dropsies. London, 1813, case IV, p 126.
195. Bull J: A short history of intracranial aneurysms. London Clin Med J 1962;3:984.
196. Forbus WD: On the origin of miliary aneurysms of the superficial cerebral arteries. Bull Johns Hopkins Hosp 1930;47:239.
197. Padget DH: The circle of Willis, its embryology and anatomy. In WE Dandy (ed), Intracranial Arterial Aneurysms. Ithaca, NY: Comstock, 1944, p 67.
198. Padget DH: The development of the cranial arteries in the human embryo. Contrib Embyol Carnegie Inst 1948;32:205.
199. Sahs AL: Intracranial aneurysms and polycystic kidney. Arch Neurol Psychiatry 1950;63:524.
200. Baker TW, Shelden WD: Coarctation of the aorta with intermittent leakage of congenital cerebral aneurysm. Am J Med Sci 1936; 191:626.
201. Crompton MR: The comparative pathology of cerebral aneurysms. Brain 1966;89:789.
202. Stehbens WE: Cerebral aneurysms of animals other than man. J Pathol Bacteriol 1963;86:160.
203. Campos J, Fox AJ, Vinuela F, et al: Saccular aneurysms in basilar artery fenestration. AJNR 1987;8:233–236.
204. Sanders WP, Sorek PA, Mehta BA: Fenestration of intracranial arteries with special attention to associated aneurysms and other anomalies. AJNR 1993;14:675–680.
205. Heinz ER: Aneurysms and MR angiography. AJNR 1993;14: 974–977.
206. Friedman A: Subarachnoid hemorrhage of unknown etiology. In RH Wilkins, SS Rangachary (eds), Neurosurgery, update 2. New York: McGraw-Hill, 1991, pp 73–77.
207. Rinkel GJ, Wijdicks EF, Vermeulen LM, et al: Nonaneurysmal perimesencephalic hemorrhage: CT and MR patterns that differ from aneurysmal rupture. AJNR 1991;12:829–834.
208. Van Gijn J, van Dongen KJ, Vermeulen M, et al: Perimesencephalic hemorrhage: A nonaneurysmal and benign form of subarachnoid hemorrhage. Neurology 1985;35:493–497.
209. LeBlanc R: The minor leak preceding subarachnoid hemorrhage. J Neurosurg 1987;66:35–39.
210. McKissock W, Paine KWE, Walsh LS: An analysis of the results of treatment of ruptured intracranial aneurysms, report of 772 consecutive cases. J Neurosurg 1960;17:762.

211. Pakarinen S: Incidence, etiology, and prognosis of primary subarachnoid hemorrhage: A study based on 589 cases diagnosed in a defined urban population during a defined period. Acta Neurol Scand 1967;43(Suppl 29):1–128.
212. Wiebers DO, Whisnant JP, Sundt TM, et al: The significance of unruptured intracranial saccular aneurysms. J Neurosurg 1987;66: 23–29.
213. Fisher CM, Kistler JP, Davis JM: Relation of cerebral vasospasm to subarachnoid hemorrhage visualized by computerized tomography scanning. Neurosurgery 1980;6:1–9.
214. Bergvall U, Galera R: Time relationship between subarachnoid haemorrhage, arterial spasm, changes in cerebral circulation and posthaemorrhagic hydrocephalus. Acta Radiol 1969;9:229.
215. Fletcher TM, Taveras JM, Pool JL: Cerebral vasospasm in angiography for intracranial aneurysms: Incidence and significance in one hundred consecutive angiograms. Arch Neurol 1959;1:38.
216. Heros RC, Zervas NT: Cerebral vasospasm after subarachnoid hemorrhage: An update. Ann Neurol 1983;14:599–608.
217. Wilkins RH: Attempts at prevention or treatment of intracranial arterial spasm: An update. Neurosurgery 1986;18:808–825.
218. Haley EC, Kassell NF, Torner JC, et al: A randomized control trial of high-dose intravenous nicardipine with aneurysmal subarachnoid hemorrhage. J Neurosurg 1993;78:537–547.
219. New PFJ, Price DL, Carter B: Cerebral angiography in cardiac myxomas: Correlation of angiographic and histopathological findings. Radiology 1970;96:335.
220. Michael AS, Mikhael MA, Christ M: Myxoma of the heart presenting with recurrent episodes of hemorrhagic cerebral infarction: MR findings. J Comput Assist Tomogr 1989;13:123–125.
221. Thomson AT: A case of aneurisms within the skull, terminating in apoplexy and paralysis, with clinical remarks. Lond Edinb Mon J Med Sci 1842;2:557.
222. Wood EH: Angiographic identification of the ruptured lesion in patients with multiple cerebral aneurysms. J Neurosurg 1964;21: 182.
223. Jain KK: Mechanism of rupture of intracranial saccular aneurysms. Surgery 1963;54:347.
224. Curnes JT, Shogry MEC, Clark DC, et al: MR angiographic demonstration of an intracranial aneurysm not seen by conventional angiography. AJNR 1993;14:974–977.
225. Perret LV, Bull JWD: The accuracy of radiology in demonstrating ruptured intracranial aneurysms. Br J Radiol 1959;32:85.
226. Huston J III, Nichols DA, Luetmer PH, et al: Blinded prospective evaluation of sensitivity of MR angiography to known intracranial aneurysms: Importance of aneurysm size. AJNR 1994;15: 1607–1614.
227. Araki Y, Kohmura E, Tsukaguchi I: A pitfall in detection of intracranial aneurysms on three-dimensional phase-contrast MR angiography. AJNR 1994;15:1618–1623.
228. Crompton MR: Cerebral infarction following the rupture of cerebral berry aneurysms. Brain 1964;87:263.
229. Wijdicks EFM, Verneulen M, ten Haff JA, et al: Volume depletion and natriuresis in patients with a ruptured intracranial aneurysm. Ann Neurol 1985;18:211–216.
230. Graff-Radford NR, Torner J, Adams HP, et al: Factors associated with hydrocephalus after subarachnoid hemorrhage: A report of the cooperative aneurysm study. Arch Neurol 1989;46:744–752.
231. Galera R, Greitz T: Hydrocephalus in the adult secondary to the rupture of intracranial arterial aneurysms. J Neurosurg 1970;23: 634.
232. Hodes PJ, et al: Cerebral angiography: Fundamentals in anatomy and physiology. Am J Roentgenol 1953;70:61–82.
233. Mount LA, Taveras JM: Further observations of the significance of the collateral circulation of the brain as demonstrated arteriographically. Trans Am Neurol Assoc 1960:109.
234. Newton TH, Hoyt WF: Dural arteriovenous shunts in the region of the cavernous sinus. Neuroradiology 1970;1:71.
235. Perret G, Nishioka H: Report on the cooperative study of intracranial aneurysms and subarachnoid hemorrhage: Section VI. Arteriovenous malformations. J Neurosurg 1966;25:467–490.
236. Pile-Spellman JM, Baker KF, Lisczak TM, et al: High flow angiopathy: Cerebral blood vessel changes in experimental chronic arterio-venous fistula. AJNR 1986;7:811–815.
237. Viñuela F, Nombela L, Roach MR, et al: Stenotic and occlusive disease of the venous drainage system of deep brain AVM's. J Neurosurg 1985;63:180–184.
238. Mawad ME, Hilal SK, Michelsen WJ, et al: Occlusive vascular disease associated with cerebral arteriovenous malformations. Radiology 1984;153:401–408.
239. Horowitz MB, Jungreis CA, Quisling RG, et al: Vein of Galen aneurysms: A review and current perspective. AJNR 1994;15: 1486–1496.
240. Turjman F, Massoud TF, Viñuela F, et al: Aneurysms related to cerebral arteriovenous malformations: Superselective angiographic assessment in 58 patients. AJNR 1994;15:1601–1605.
241. Houser OW, Campbell JK, Cambell RJ, et al: Arteriovenous malformations affecting the thrombosed dural venous sinus: An acquired lesion. Mayo Clin Proc 1979;54:651–661.
242. Chandhary MY, Sachdev VP, Cho SH, et al: Dural arteriovenous malformations of the major venous sinuses: An acquired lesion. AJNR 1982;3:13–19.
243. Willinsky R, Terbrugge K, Montanera W, et al: Venous congestion: An MR finding in dural arteriovenous malformations with cortical venous drainage. AJNR 1994;15:1501–1507.
244. Hallbach UV, Higashida RT, Hieshima SB, et al: Treatment of dural fistulas involving the deep cerebral venous system. AJNR 1989;10:393–399.
245. Dandy WE: Venous abnormalities and angiomas of the brain. Arch Surg 1928;17:715.
246. Becker DH, Townsend JJ, Kramer RA, Newton TH: Occult cerebrovascular malformations: A series of 18 histologically verified cases with negative angiography. Brain 1979;102:249.
247. Rigamonti D, Hadley MN, Drayer BP, et al: Cerebral cavernous malformations: Incidence and familial occurrence. N Engl J Med 1988;319:343–347.
248. Gomori JM, Grossman RI, Goldberg HI, et al: Occult cerebral vascular malformations: High field MR imaging. Radiology 1986; 158:707–713.
249. Atlas SW: Intracranial vascular malformations and aneurysms. In SW Atlas (ed), Magnetic Resonance Imaging of the Brain and Spine. New York: Raven, 1991, pp 379–409.
250. Zimmerman RS, Spetzler RF, Lee KS, et al: Cavernous malformations of the brain stem. J Neurosurg 1991;75:32–39.
251. Ojemann RG, Crowell RM, Ogilvy CS: Management of cranial and spinal cavernous angiomas. Clin Neurosurg 1993;40:98–123.
252. Russell DS, Rubinstein LJ: Pathology of tumors of the nervous system. Baltimore: Williams and Wilkins, 1989.
253. Vaquero J, Manrique M, Oya S, et al: Calcified telangiectatic hamartomas of the brain. Surg Neurol 1980;13:453.
254. Malik GH, Morgan JK, Boulos RS, et al: Venous angiomas: An underestimated cause of intracranial hemorrhage. Surg Neurol 1988;30:350–358.

SELECTED READINGS

Ackerman RH: Noninvasive diagnosis of carotid disease in the era of digital subtraction angiography. Neurol Clin 1983;1:263–277.

Anderson CM, Saloner D, Lee RE, et al: Assessment of carotid artery stenosis by MR angiography: Comparison with x-ray angiography and color-coded Doppler ultrasound. AJNR 1992;13:909–1003.

Banach MJ, Flamm ES: Supraclinoid internal carotid artery fenestration with an associated aneurysm. J Neurosurg 1993;79:438–441.

Barnett GO: Cerebral blood flow: Factors influencing pulsatile flow in individual vessels. In Fourth Princeton Conference on Cerebral Vascular Disease. New York: Grune and Stratton, 1965.

Baron JC, Bausser MG, Rex A, et al: Reversal of focal "misery perfusion syndrome" by extra-intracranial arterial bypass in hemodynamic cerebral ischemia: A case study with O-15 positron emission tomography. Stroke 1981;12:454–459.

Bergeron RT: Radiographic demonstration of cortical heteropia. Acta Radiol 1969;9:135.

Broderick JP, Brott T, Tomsick T, et al: Intracerebral hemorrhage more than twice as common as subarachnoid hemorrhage. J Neurosurg 1993; 78:188–191.

Brugieres P, Castrec-Carpo A, Heran F, et al: Magnetic resonance imaging in the exploration of dissection of the internal carotid arteries. J Neuroradiol 1989;16:1–10.

Brunberg JA, Papdopoulos SM: Technical note. Device to facilitate MR imaging of patients in skeletal traction. AJNR 1991;12:746–747.

Bull JWD, Nixon WLB, Pratt RTC, et al: Paget's disease of the skull and secondary basilar impression. Brain 1959;82:10. (Abstract: Radiology 1960;75:654.)

Casasco AE, Aymard A, Gobin YP, et al: Selective endovascular treatment of 71 intracranial aneurysms with platinum coils. J Neurosurg 1993; 79:3–10.

Chappell PM, Steinberg GK, Marks MI: Clinically documented hemorrhage in cerebral arteriovenous malformation: MR characteristics. Radiology 1992;183:719–724.

Chiari, H.: Uber veranderungen des klienherns, des pons und der medulla oblongata in folge von congenitaler hydrocephalic des grosshirns. Dtsch. Med. Wochenschr., 27:1172, 1891.

Chien D, Kwong KK, Gress DR: MR diffusion imaging of cerebral infarction in humans. AJNR 1992;13:1097–1102.

Dean BL, Lee C, Kirsch JE, et al: Cerebral hemodynamics and cerebral blood volume: MR assessment using gadolinium contrast agents and T1-weighted turbo-flash imaging. AJNR 1992;13:39–48.

Du Bouley GH, Trickey S: The sella in aqueduct stenosis and communicating hydrocephalus. Br J Radiol 1970;43:319.

Enzmann DR, Pelc NJ: Normal flow patterns of intracranial and spinal cerebrospinal fluid defined with phase-contrast cine MR imaging. Radiology 1991;178:467–474.

Fisher CM: Early-life carotid-artery occlusion associated with late intracranial hemorrhage. Lab Invest 1959;8:680.

Fujita N, Harada K, Hirabuki N, et al: Asymmetric appearance of intracranial vessels on routine spin-echo MR images: A pulse sequence-dependent phenomenon. AJNR 1992;13:1153–1159.

Gibby WA, Stecker MM, Goldberg HI, et al: Reversal of white matter edema in hypertensive encephalopathy. AJNR 1989;10:S78.

Gopinath SP, Robertson SC, Grossman RG, et al: Near-infrared spectroscopic localization of intracranial hematomas. J Neurosurg 1993;79: 43–47.

Goraj B, Rifkinson-Mann S, Leslie DR, et al: Cerebral blood flow velocity after head injury: Transcranial Doppler evaluation. Radiology 1993; 188:137–141.

Gurdjian ES, Lindner DW, Hardy WG, et al: Incidence of surgically treatable lesions in case studies angiographically. Proceedings of International Conference on Vascular Disease of the Brain. Neurology 1961; 11:150.

Hasuo K, Yasumori K, Yoshida K, et al: Magnetic resonance imaging compared with computed tomography and angiography in Moyamoya disease. Acta Radiol 1990;31:191–195.

Ida M, Mizunuma K, Hata Y, et al: Subcortical low intensity in early cortical ischemia. AJNR 1994;15:1387–1393.

Johnson DW, Hogg JP, Dasheiff R, et al: Xenon/CT cerebral blood flow studies during continuous depth electrode monitoring in epilepsy patients. AJNR 1993;14:245–252.

Jones KM, Barnes PD: MR diagnosis of brain death. AJNR 1992;13: 65–66.

Kashiwagi S, Yamashita T, Nakano S, et al: The wash-in/washout protocol in stable xenon CT cerebral blood flow studies. AJNR 1992;13: 49–53.

Keeney G, Gebarski SS, Brunberg JA: CT of severe inner ear anomalies, including aplasia, in a case of Wildervanck syndrome. AJNR 1992;13: 201–202.

Kestle JRW, Hoffman HJ, Mock AR: Moyamoya phenomenon after radiation for optic glioma. J Neurosurg 1993;79:32–35.

Kuhn MJ, Johnson KA, Davis KR: Wallerian degeneration: Evaluation with MR imaging 1. Radiology 1988;168:199–202.

Lalwani AK, Dowd CF, Halbach VV: Grading venous restrictive disease in patient with dural arteriovenous fistulas of the transverse/sigmoid sinus. J Neurosurg 1993;79:11–15.

Larson TC III, Kelly WM, Ehman RL, et al: Spatial misregistration of vascular flow during MR imaging of the CNS: Cause and clinical significance. AJNR 1990;11:1041–1048.

Lebrun-Grandie P, Baron JC, Soussaline F, et al: Coupling between regional blood flow and oxygen utilization in the normal human brain: A study with positron tomography and oxygen-15. Arch Neurol 1986; 4:230–236.

Lenzi GL, Frakowiak RS, Jones T: Cerebral oxygen metabolism and blood flow in human cerebral ischemic infarction. J Cereb Blood Flow Metab 1982;2:321–335.

Mattle HP, Wentz KU, Edelman RR, et al: Cerebral venography with MR. Radiology 1991;178:453–458.

Pierot L, Chiras J, Debussche-Depriester C, et al: Intracerebral stenosing arteriopathies. Serv de Neuroradiologie Charcot, Hopital de la Salpetriere, Paris.

Reivich M: Crossed cerebellar diaschisis. AJNR 1992;13:62–64.

Rokitansky, C. von: Handbuch der pathologischen Anatomie, Vols. 1, 2, and 3. Vienna: Braumüller und Seidel, 1842–1846.

Schechter MM: Percutaneous carotid catheterization. Acta Radiol 1963; 1:417.

Stringer WA, Hasso AN, Thompson JR, et al: Hyperventilation-induced cerebral ischemia in patients with acute brain lesions: Demonstration by xenon-enhanced CT. AJNR 1993;14:475–484.

Sullivan HG, Kingsbury TB, Morgan MS, et al: The rCBF response to Diamox in normal subjects and cerebrovascular disease patients. J Neurosurg 1987;67:525–534.

Takikawa S, Dhawan V, Spetsieris P, et al: Noninvasive quantitative fluorodeoxyglucose PET studies with an estimated input function derived from a population-based arterial blood curve. Radiology 1993;188: 131–136.

Titelbaum DS, Frazier JL, Grossman RI, et al: Wallerian degeneration and inflammation in rat peripheral nerve detected by in vivo MR imaging. AJNR 1989;10:741–746.

Tzika AA, Massoth RJ, Ball WS, et al: Cerebral perfusion in children: Detection with dynamic contrast-enhanced T2-weighted MR images. Radiology 1993;187:449–458.

Wessbecher FW, Maravilla KR, Dalley RW: Optimizing brain MR imaging protocols with gadopentetate dimeglumine: Enhancement of intracranial lesions on spin-density and T2-weighted images. AJNR 1991; 12:675–679.

Wood EH: Thermography in the diagnosis of cerebrovascular disease: Preliminary report. Radiology 1964;83:540.

Vogl TJ, Bergman C, Villringer A, et al: Dural sinus thrombosis: Value of venous MR angiography for diagnosis and follow-up. AJR 1994;162: 1191–1198.

11

Intracranial Neoplasms

PATHOLOGIC CONSIDERATIONS

Intracranial neoplasms present a remarkable variety of histologic appearances and growth characteristics. The distinction between benign and malignant characteristics is often difficult but may be made by considering the tumor's histology and location. A tumor may be relatively benign in its growth characteristics but may be malignant because of its location, producing neurologic disability by invading important functional areas (such as the brainstem or the hypothalamus and optic chiasm) or by seeding through the cerebrospinal fluid (CSF). Seeding produces distant metastases within the central nervous system (CNS), usually on meningeal or ependymal surfaces. The majority of brain tumors are neuroepithelial in origin.

An important characteristic of brain tumors is that they are not composed of a single cell type, and thus they present a rather heterogeneous morphology and frequently unpredictable growth characteristics. Although the tumor classification may be based on the predominant cell type, such as astrocytoma or oligodendroglioma, usually more than one type of cell is present. More recently, this feature of astrocytomas has received attention in regard to chemotherapeutic management because of the variable responses of the histologic types, for instance, a mixed oligodendroglioma and astrocytoma versus an astrocytoma. The published incidence of brain tumor histologic types varies according to whether the investigation used surgical or autopsy data. Tables 11.1 to 11.6 present various aspects of the incidence of intracranial tumors.

The histologic classification that is most widely accepted is that proposed by the World Health Organization (WHO) (1). The classification used here also partly follows one used by Bonnin and Garcia (2).

Brain tumors are among the more frequent neoplasms of humans. Patients tend to concentrate in the institutions where diagnostic and therapeutic services are available (3).

Table 11.1.
Reported Incidence of Intracranial Tumors by Histopathologic Type (6803 cases)

Type of tumor	Zimmerman (1971) %	Courville (1950) %	Baker (1943) %
Glioma	31	34	50
Metastatic	23	26	15
Meningioma	15	12	16
Inflammatory masses	6	14	4
Vascular masses	6	2	5
Pituitary	4	5	4
Sarcoma	4	3	1
Craniopharyngioma	2	2	3
Medulloblastoma	2	—	—
Neurinoma	2	—	—
Pinealoma	1	—	—
All others	4	2	2

Source: Taveras JM, Wood EH: Diagnostic Neuroradiology. Baltimore: Williams & Wilkins, 1976, p 399.

Table 11.2.
Incidence of Intracranial Gliomas

Intracranial Gliomas	All Ages* (%)	Children† (%)
Glioblastoma	55	
Astrocytoma	20.5	48.0
Ependymoma	6.	8.
Medulloblastoma	6.	44.0
Oliogodendroglioma	5.	
Choroid plexus papilloma	2.	?
Colloid cyst	2.	

* Rubinstein LJ: Tumors of the Central Nervous System, 1972: Armed Forces Institute of Pathology (AFIP).
† Bodian M, Lawson D: The intracranial neoplastic diseases of childhood: A description of their natural history based on a clinico-pathological study of 129 cases. Br J Surg 1953;40:368–392.

Table 11.3.
Brain Tumors in Children

Supratentorial	1347
infratentorial	1423
Spinal	160
Multiple compartments	
Supratentorial and infratentorial	99
Infratentorial and spinal	199
Supratentorial, infratentorial, and spinal	32
Total	3260

Source: Childhood Brain Tumor Consortium. J Neurooncol 1988;6:9–23.

Gliomas

The term *glioma* is usually applied to a variety of astrocytoma because of its frequency, but it also includes the oligodendrogliomas. The notable characteristic of the gliomas is that they are poorly circumscribed, and even if apparently distinct borders are seen microscopically, close scrutiny may show that tumor cells extend beyond the apparent margins that represent part of the neoplasm. Even small gliomas are already poorly circumscribed. The metastatic carcinomas tend to be well circumscribed and actually displace brain tissue rather than invade it. Ependymomas and

Table 11.4.
Incidence of Cerebellar and Fourth Ventricle Tumors by Histology

	Percentage
Astrocytoma	29.0
Medulloblastoma	24.8
Ependymoma	11.1
Hemangioblastoma	11.6
Meningioma	5.3
Choroid plexus papilloma	2.0
Metastatic neoplasm	2.5

Source: Zülch KJ: Brain Tumors: Their Biology and Pathology. New York: Springer, 1965, p 78.

Table 11.5.
Diagnoses of 3291 Tumors and Their Distributions Across Anatomic Compartments in Children*

Diagnosis	Overall		Proportion *in* each compartment† (% *within* compartment)		
	N	*% of all tumors*	*Supratentorial*	*Infratentorial*	*Spinal*
Astrocytoma, nos	153	4.7	35.9 (3.7)	50.4 (3.7)	9.4 (9.6)
Fibrillary astrocytoma	214	6.5	57.1 (8.9)	35.0 (3.8)	5.1 (7.8)
Protoplasmic astrocytoma	80	2.4	31.4 (1.9)	57.1 (2.5)	7.1 (4.4)
Gemistocytic astrocytoma	2	0.1	100.0 (0.1)	0.0 (0.0)	0.0 (0.0)
Pilocytic astrocytoma	622	18.9	22.5 (12.2)	74.0 (28.3)	2.4 (13.0)
Subependymal giant cell astrocytoma	31	0.9	93.6 (2.6)	0.0 (0.0)	0.0 (0.0)
Anaplastic astrocytoma	194	5.9	74.0 (12.5)	19.8 (2.4)	3.7 (6.1)
Glioblastoma	11	0.3	70.0 (0.6)	20.0 (0.1)	0.0 (0.0)
Giant cell glioblastoma	18	0.6	88.9 (1.4)	0.0 (0.0)	0.0 (0.0)
Oligodendroglioma	40	1.2	71.8 (2.5)	20.5 (0.5)	2.6 (0.9)
Mixed oligo-astrocytoma	29	0.9	82.8 (2.1)	10.3 (0.2)	0.0 (0.0)
Anaplastic oligodendroglioma	4	0.1	100.0 (0.4)	0.0 (0.0)	0.0 (0.0)
Ependymoma	273	8.3	21.1 (5.0)	71.9 (12.0)	3.0 (7.0)
Myxopapillary ependymoma	13	0.4	0.0 (0.0)	7.7 (0.1)	92.3 (10.0)
Papillary ependymoma	11	0.3	30.0 (0.3)	40.0 (0.3)	30.0 (2.6)
Subependymoma	6	0.2	0.0 (0.0)	100.0 (0.4)	0.0 (0.0)
Anaplastic ependymoma	57	1.7	48.2 (2.3)	50.0 (1.7)	0.0 (0.0)
Choroid plexus papilloma	60	1.8	75.0 (4.0)	15.0 (0.6)	1.7 (0.9)
Anaplastic choroid plexus papilloma	6	0.2	66.7 (0.4)	16.7 (0.1)	0.0 (0.0)
Gangliocytoma	1	0.0	0.0 (0.0)	100.0 (0.1)	0.0 (0.0)
Ganglioglioma	36	1.1	82.9 (2.6)	5.7 (0.1)	11.4 (3.5)
Ganglioneuroblastoma	2	0.1	50.0 (0.1)	0.0 (0.0)	0.0 (0.0)
Neuroblastoma	7	0.2	85.7 (0.5)	14.3 (0.1)	0.0 (0.0)
Medulloblastoma	565	17.2	4.1 (2.0)	93.7 (32.4)	0.9 (4.4)
Desmoplastic medulloblastoma	93	2.8	1.1 (0.1)	93.6 (5.4)	3.2 (2.6)
Medulloepithelioma	3	0.1	66.7 (0.2)	33.3 (0.1)	0.0 (0.0)
Pineocytoma	9	0.3	33.3 (0.2)	33.3 (0.1)	16.7 (0.9)
Pineoblastoma	25	0.8	31.8 (0.6)	50.0 (0.7)	9.1 (1.7)
Germinoma	44	1.3	84.1 (3.3)	6.8 (0.2)	0.0 (0.0)
Embryonal carcinoma	11	0.3	72.7 (0.7)	0.0 (0.0)	0.0 (0.0)
Choriocarcinoma	2	0.1	50.0 (0.1)	50.0 (0.1)	0.0 (0.0)
Teratoma	20	0.6	70.0 (1.2)	10.0 (0.1)	5.0 (0.9)
Neurilemmoma	24	0.7	13.0 (0.3)	39.1 (0.6)	47.8 (9.6)
Neurofibroma	3	0.1	0.0 (0.0)	0.0 (0.0)	33.3 (0.9)
Anaplastic neurofibroma	1	0.0	0.0 (0.0)	0.0 (0.0)	100.0 (0.9)
Meningioma, nos	25	0.8	85.0 (1.5)	10.0 (0.1)	0.0 (0.0)
Meningotheliomatous meningioma	2	0.1	100.0 (0.1)	0.0 (0.0)	0.0 (0.0)
Fibroblastic meningioma	3	0.1	100.0 (0.1)	0.0 (0.0)	0.0 (0.0)
Transitional (mixed) meningioma	8	0.2	75.0 (0.5)	0.0 (0.0)	0.0 (0.0)
Psammomatous meningioma	4	0.1	33.3 (0.1)	0.0 (0.0)	66.7 (1.7)
Haemangiopericytic meningioma	4	0.1	25.0 (0.1)	25.0 (0.1)	50.0 (1.7)
Primary lymphoma	3	0.1	66.7 (0.2)	33.3 (0.1)	0.0 (0.0)
Haemangioblastoma	6	0.2	0.0 (0.0)	100.0 (0.4)	0.0 (0.0)
Craniopharyngioma	225	6.8	74.1 (14.9)	11.4 (1.6)	0.0 (0.0)
Epidermoid cyst	9	0.3	50.0 (0.4)	20.0 (0.1)	20.0 (1.7)
Dermoid cyst	1	0.0	100.0 (0.1)	0.0 (0.0)	0.0 (0.0)
Colloid cyst	2	0.1	100.0 (0.2)	0.0 (0.0)	0.0 (0.0)
Vascular malformation	2	0.1	0.0 (0.0)	0.0 (0.0)	100.0 (0.9)
Pituitary adenoma	8	0.2	100.0 (0.7)	0.0 (0.0)	0.0 (0.0)
Chondrosarcoma	1	0.0	0.0 (0.0)	0.0 (0.0)	100.0 (0.9)
Unclassified or unknown	230	7.0	73.3 (8.5)	16.8 (1.4)	4.6 (5.2)
Disagreement between slide reviewers	88	2.7			

* Column or row % may sum to less than 100% or appear inconsistent because some tumors involved multiple compartments, did not have location information, or fell into the last two categories in the table.

† The following WHO categories were not present in this group: anaplastic gangliocytoma, anaplastic ganglioglioma, angiomatous meningioma, anaplastic neurilemmoma, astroblastoma, chondroma, chordoma, choristoma (pituicytoma, granular cell), enterogenous cyst, esthesioneuroblastoma, fibroxanthoma, gliomatosis cerebri, glomus jugulare tumor, haemangioblastic meningioma, medullomyoblastoma, melanoma, meningeal melanomatosis, metastatic, mixed glioblastoma and sarcoma, monstrocellular sarcoma, pituitary adenocarcinoma, primitive polar spongioblastoma, xanthosarcoma.

Source: Childhood Brain Tumor Consortium. J Neurooncol 1988;6:9–23.

Table 11.6.
Origin of Metastatic Brain Tumors

Primary	Percentage
Sarcomas	5
Melanoblastic	12
Carcinomas:	
Lung	40
Breast	11
Gastrointestinal tract	8
Retroperitoneal	7
Female genital	4
Eyes and nose	3
Other head and neck	3
Male genital	2
Primary not discovered	5

Source: Taveras JM, Wood EH, Diagnostic Neuroradiology. Baltimore; Williams & Wilkins, 1976, p 399.

choroid plexus papillomas are predominantly expansive and displace brain tissue but do not invade it directly.

Tumors of the brain do not metastasize outside the CNS. However, when they reach the ependymal surface of the ventricles or the meningeal surface on either the medial or lateral aspects of the structure in which they are contained, they tend to seed through the CSF. In this way the tumors may spread into the spinal subarachnoid space, producing tumors over the surface of the spinal cord as well as over the surface of the brain and of the ventricles. This type of spread is much more common in certain tumors such as medulloblastomas, ependymomas, and malignant choroid plexus tumors. Glioblastomas and high-grade astrocytomas may also seed but do so far less frequently.

ASTROCYTOMAS AND GLIOBLASTOMA MULTIFORME

The astrocytomas are by far the most common primary intrinsic neoplasms of the brain and can be graded by how rapidly they grow. In grade I the cells are spread relatively far apart and look somewhat normal but are more numerous than the usual astrocytes in a given area of the brain. These tumors contain increased water or edema, which produces a mass effect. However, some of the tumors do not produce an appreciable mass and do not appear to displace the adjacent structures, such as the lateral ventricles or the surface sulci and convolutions of the brain.

This type of astrocytoma is easily overlooked on computed tomography (CT) examinations because there is no mass effect and no evidence of enhancement after intravenous iodine compound administration. Magnetic resonance imaging (MRI) seems to demonstrate the abnormal tissue and water present in the area of the tumor and thus, on T2 imaging, reveals an increased intensity (Fig. 11.1).

A grade II astrocytoma contains more cells and produces more of a mass lesion but still may not enhance on CT or MRI. However, it is easily recognizable because of the mass effect, which is usually caused by the increased number of cells and primarily by a greater degree of edema (Fig. 11.2).

A grade III astrocytoma is usually malignant and contains many more cells (histologically more abnormal-looking cells) and some necrosis. Frank disruption of the blood-

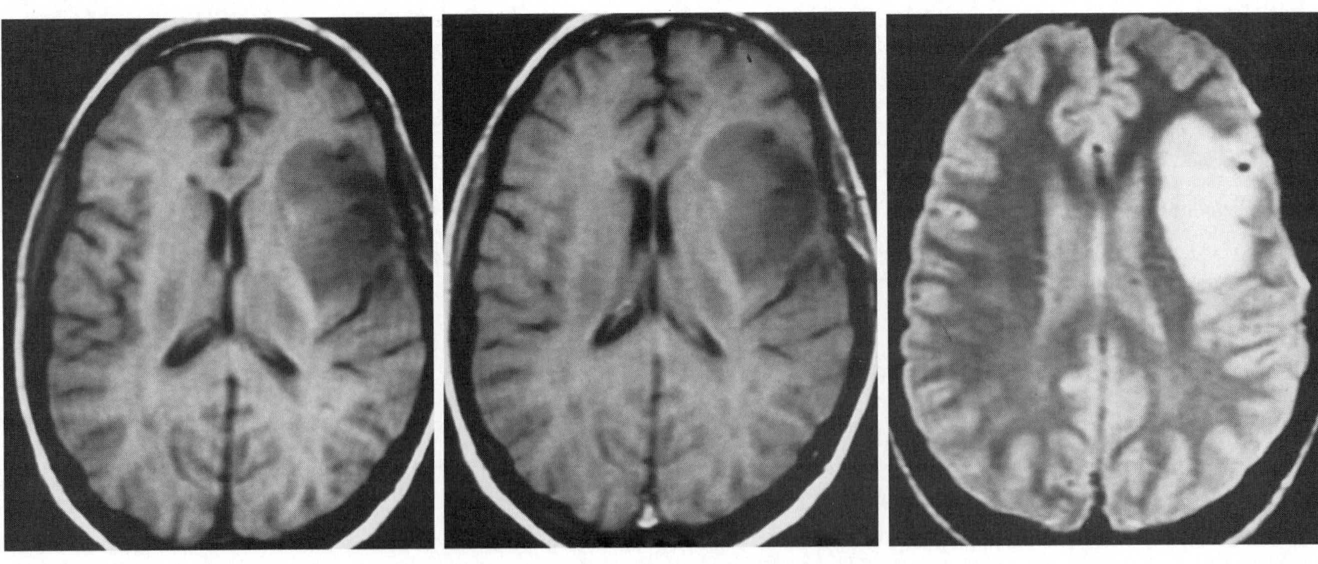

Figure 11.1. Left frontal glioma, slowly growing, not showing enhancement after contrast. **A.** Preenhancement T1-weighted image shows a well-circumscribed low-intensity area. The midline shift is minimal, indicating that there is only a small amount of edema; the tumor is mostly infiltrative. **B.** Postcontrast image shows no enhancement. **C.** T2-weighted image shows a hyperintense lesion about the same size as that shown on the T1-weighted images. The appearance does not suggest surrounding edema because of its homogeneity.

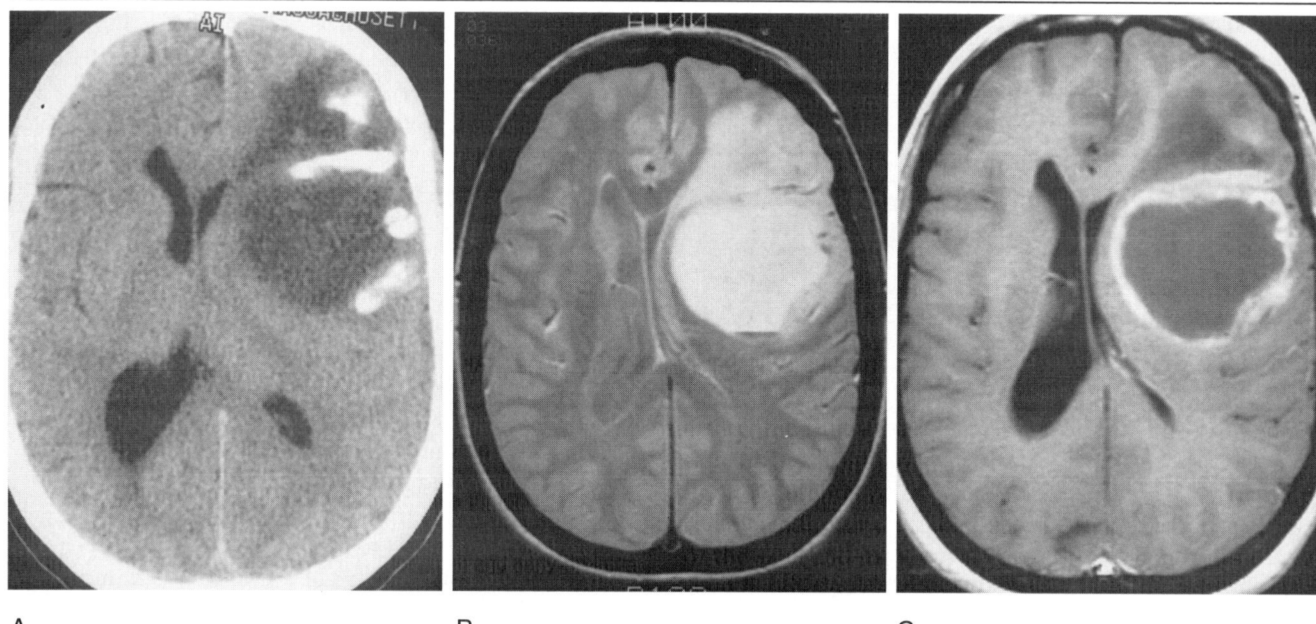

A B C

Figure 11.2. Edema in a more rapidly growing glioma. **A.** CT shows low attenuation probably due to tumor and edema. There is extensive, chunky calcification suggestive of oligodendroglioma, possibly associated with astrocytoma. **B.** T2-weighted axial image demonstrates the surrounding tumor edema anteriorly. The calcifications cannot be seen. **C.** A T1-weighted postcontrast axial image shows enhancement of the wall of the neoplasm, which has an irregular inner surface, probably indicating that it is a cystic space caused by necrosis. The edema does not enhance anteriorly. There is no hint of calcifications.

brain barrier allows enhancement of the mass on CT or MRI scans. The glioblastoma multiforme is the most malignant of the group. In addition to the abnormal astrocytic cells, there is intense proliferation of mesenchymal elements arising from the walls of the blood vessels, giving the tumor a sarcomatous growth pattern. If there is a predominance of mesenchymal elements, the term *gliosarcoma* is used. This kind of tumor frequently grows to the meninges or the ependymal surface; it may then spread within the CSF, but only rarely spreads outside the nervous system. At the site of surgery, tumor cells may spread into the soft tissues if the dural covering is not replaced. Hemorrhage in the tumor may sometimes occur. It should be mentioned that a more benign astrocytoma may degenerate into a glioblastoma with the passage of time. Sometimes an oligodendroglioma or ependymoma may start to grow rapidly and present a histologic appearance like that of a glioblastoma, with nuclear pleomorphism, necrosis, and hypertrophy of the vascular endothelium.

Multicentric malignant astrocytomas or frank glioblastomas are not rare. The majority occur in the same hemisphere but occasionally may be observed in both hemispheres. Glioblastomas do not occur in the cerebellum, although an astrocytoma may secondarily degenerate and begin rapidly growing in this location.

The more benign astrocytomas may occur at any age. Characteristically they occur in the cerebellum in children or in the brainstem. In the brain the more slowly growing astrocytomas occur in younger individuals in the second and third decades. The glioblastomas, on the other hand, tend to occur in the fifties and sixties.

A number of different histologic types of astrocytomas have been described.

1. *Protoplasmic astrocytomas,* as a pure form, are rare, but these cells may form part of the histologic picture.
2. *Fibrillary astrocytomas.* The diffuse form occurs in the cerebral hemispheres, in the brainstem in children, and sometimes in the cerebellum in young adults. The circumscribed form occurs in the cerebellum and in the diencephalon region of young adults (4).
3. *Gemistocytic astrocytomas.* Again, these are rare as a pure form. This variety is a premalignant tumor; according to Russell and Rubinstein, about 80 percent convert to glioblastomas (4).
4. *Subependymal giant cell astrocytomas* tend to occur in the region of the foramen of Monro. They are seen particularly in patients with tuberous sclerosis but may be seen in those who do not have the stigmata of tuberous sclerosis. The tumors have a mixed appearance: some cells look like neuronal cells and others look like astrocytes.
5. *Astroblastomas* are rare tumors encountered in the supratentorial region. They may be solid or cavitary and are well circumscribed from the surrounding brain tissue. These masses usually remain within the brain

tissue and do not invade the ventricular surface, but their behavior cannot be predicted from the histologic appearance. They may grow rapidly or may remain relatively benign and not recur after removal.

6. *Pleomorphic xanthoastrocytomas* are a recently recognized type of tumor. They are usually located in the brain, may or may not show cystic necrotic areas, and tend to reach the surface of the brain or the ventricular wall. The tumor cells may be pleomorphic, as indicated by the name of the neoplasm, and many contain large amounts of lipid in their cytoplasm. Reticulin fibers surrounding the cells suggest a mesenchymal tumor. They tend to occur in young individuals, and the prognosis is quite good, certainly much better than the histologic appearance might suggest.
7. *Pilocytic astrocytomas* are composed of elongated cells that usually are found in the floor of the third ventricle, the hypothalamus, and the optic chiasm and optic nerves, that is, in areas where there may be tight nerve bundles and the cells tend to attain an elongated appearance.

GLIOMATOSIS CEREBRI

This is a type of spread by a diffuse astrocytoma. Practically the entire cerebral hemisphere is infiltrated by an astrocytic tumor, which may cross the midline and involve both sides almost equally. Sometimes there is no mass visible. One question is whether the tumor started as a focal lesion or whether it started widely. Some cases of gliomatosis cerebri show areas typical of oligodendrogliomas.

OLIGODENDROGLIOMAS AND MIXED GLIOMAS

These usually well-circumscribed tumors of the cerebral hemispheres are composed of small cells of a rather uniform size that often calcify in various locations within the tumor. The relatively monotonous histologic appearance of many of these tumors does not necessarily predict their behavior, for some of them may grow more rapidly than others and may invade the brain surface and leptomeninges. They are frequently not pure but mixed with astrocytes. The terms *mixed glioma* or *mixed oligodendroglioma and astrocytoma* are fairly common. Sometimes the classification of a tumor may depend on which cells predominate in the area where the biopsy was taken. The oligodendrogliomas usually do not enhance on CT or MRI; enhancement may indicate malignant degeneration or at least a more aggressive oligodendroglioma. Degeneration of an oligodendroglioma into a glioblastoma, a rare occurrence, may be related to the astrocytic component of the neoplasm.

EPENDYMOMAS

The ependymoma is a neoplasm arising from cells lining the ventricular walls. The tumors may well protrude into the ventricular cavity and may grow as much or more into the surrounding brain tissue. Sometimes there is very little intraventricular tissue, and practically all of it is outside the ventricles. Ependymomas do not have large areas of necrosis. The cells tend to surround small blood vessels, giving the typical appearance of perivascular pseudorosettes. Unlike the astrocytomas, the ependymomas are quite variable in their configuration, and grading is not possible. Ependymomas can metastasize within the subarachnoid space and seed on the surface of the spinal cord or elsewhere in the intracranial areas. Supratentorial ependymomas appear to be more malignant in their behavior than infratentorial ones. They calcify much more frequently than astrocytomas (Table 11.7).

Table 11.7.
Ependymomas

Usually occur in fourth ventricle in childhood
Supratentorial ependymomas are frequently extraventricular, but often close to ventricular surface
Often calcified, with large cystic components

SUBEPENDYMOMAS

These tumors, also called *subependymal glomerate astrocytomas*, are composed of cells that normally lie beneath the surface of the ependyma, the subependymal glial plate. The tumors are small and can occur anywhere in the ventricular system, supratentorially or around the fourth ventricle. They may occur on the floor of the fourth ventricle, where surgical removal is sometimes possible in spite of their location because they do not invade the surrounding brain parenchyma. When totally removed they do not tend to recur (Table 11.8).

Table 11.8.
Subependymomas

Usually found as a small, incidental intraventricular tumor at autopsy in elderly individuals
Frequently located in fourth ventricle
Rarely may have aggressive characteristics

Choroid Plexus Papillomas

These tumors occur in childhood in the lateral ventricles or in the fourth ventricle. Occasionally they occur in the third ventricle. They are usually benign and are composed of normal-appearing cells similar to those of the choroid plexus, but sometimes they may be pleomorphic, and in this case malignancy may be present. The term *choroid plexus carcinoma* or *malignant choroid plexus papilloma* may be used. Seeding of the subarachnoid space is common in the malignant variety but much less common in the other. They tend to invade the adjacent brain. In the adult it may be difficult to differentiate histologically between a choroid plexus carcinoma and a metastatic papillary carcinoma to the choroid plexus. (Table 11.9).

Table 11.9.
Choroid Plexus Papillomas

Typically occur in lateral ventricles in children and fourth ventricle in adults
Usually benign but about 2% are malignant (choroid plexus carcinoma)
Choroid plexus carcinomas may locally invade adjacent brain and much more commonly disseminate along CSF pathways than choroid plexus papillomas

Table 11.10.
Ganglion Cell Tumors

Comprises gangliogliomas and ganglioneuromas
Usually well circumscribed and slow growing
Usually located in the temporal lobe
Typically found in children and young adults
Occasionally undergo malignant transformation

Tumors of the Neuron Series

Included here are the ganglioneuromas (or gangliocytomas) and gangliogliomas. These tumors are rare, usually occurring in children and young adults. They may occur in the temporal lobe or in the hypothalamic region and are usually fairly well circumscribed. The ganglioneuromas are composed of a relatively pure population of dysplastic or neoplastic neuronal elements, and the gangliogliomas contain astrocytic elements mixed with the ganglion cells. Although the tumors may be slowly growing and relatively benign, the astrocytic component may undergo malignant transformation. In that case, the ganglion cells would be mixed with an appearance suggesting glioblastoma (Table 11.10).

Embryonal Tumors of the Neuroectoderm

These include the *neuroblastoma*, the *pineoblastoma*, the *ependymoblastoma*, the *polar spongioblastoma*, and, in the posterior fossa, the *medulloblastoma*. Another designation is *primitive neuroectodermal tumor (PNET)*, which may well be applied to a tumor that cannot be sharply differentiated from other embryonal cell types.

All these tumors have a tendency to seed via the CSF. They tend to occur in children and young adults. Microscopically they may be quite similar in appearance but are partly differentiated because of their location; for example, the pineoblastoma and medulloblastoma occur in the region of the pineal gland and in the cerebellum, respectively. The diagnosis may be suggested on the basis of the gross appearance. All of these tumors are composed of very immature cells. They frequently have areas of focal maturation with development of ganglion cells and sometimes glial elements. The cerebral neuroblastomas tend to occur in the frontal and parietal lobes and often undergo cavitary degeneration, hemorrhage, and necrosis. The polar spongioblastoma tends to grow in close proximity to the ventricular system, and the same may be true of the ependymoblastoma. Because of their tendency to seed via the CSF, radiation therapy must include the entire neuraxis. Metastases outside the CNS occur at times but rarely before surgical intervention (5) (Table 11.11).

Table 11.11.
Embryonal Tumors of Neuroectoderm

Primitive neuroectodermal tumors consisting of small, round cells
Comprises medulloblastoma, neuroblastoma, pineoblastoma, ependymoblastoma, and polar spongioblastoma
Usually seen in children and young adults
Tendency to disseminate along CSF pathways
Medulloblastomas are primitive neuroectodermal tumors of the posterior fossa

Primary Brain Lymphomas

Brain lymphomas may occur in the absence of systemic lymphoma. They may occur spontaneously but are much more common in patients who are immunocompromised because of either organ transplantation or acquired immune deficiency syndrome (AIDS). They may be single or multiple. They frequently involve the corpus callosum, hypothalamus, brainstem, and cerebellum. Although the gray matter may be involved, the tendency is for tumor development to be particularly pronounced in the white matter of the brain (6).

Histologically, brain lymphomas do not differ from those found elsewhere in the body. The large-cell variant of the T-cell type is the most common (about 70 percent of patients).

Primary brain lymphomas are different from secondary involvement of the brain by systemic lymphoma or Hodgkin disease. In Hodgkin disease the intracranial involvement would be on the dura or on the surface of the brain, and there may be invasion of the brain along the perivascular spaces (Table 11.12).

Tumors of the Pineal Region

A frequent tumor type arising from the pineal region is the germ cell tumor—the germinoma. The cellular component of the germinoma is quite similar to that found at other sites, such as the ovaries and testicles. Germinomas may occur in the floor of the third ventricle as well as in the pineal region, or they may seed from the pineal region

Table 11.12.
Primary CNS Lymphomas

Brain involvement without extra-CNS involvement
Usually occur in immunocompromised hosts, especially in AIDS patients or organ transplant recipients
Often multiple lesions involving periventricular regions of white matter and corpus callosum

elsewhere, such as the floor of the third ventricle and other surfaces in contact with CSF. Although the tumor is often made up exclusively of germ cells, it may also present a differentiation toward embryonal cell lines (embryonal carcinoma) or extraembryonal structures (yolk-sac tumor or choriocarcinoma) (2). Germinomas may also differentiate into all three germ cell lines, producing pineal teratomas. The pineal region may be the site of quite a variety of histologic types: the pineocytomas, the pineoblastomas, which are more cellular than the pineocytomas, astrocytomas, glial cysts, ganglioneuromas, gangliogliomas, epidermoid cysts, and even metastatic tumors. See text following under "Midline Extracerebral Lesions."

Posterior Fossa Tumors

MEDULLOBLASTOMAS

The medulloblastoma has already been mentioned as a component of the group of embryonal neuroectodermal tumors. These tumors tend to occur in the vermis of the cerebellum and also have a tendency to invade and grow into the fourth ventricle, in which case they may be difficult to differentiate from ependymomas. However, ependymomas often present areas of calcification, whereas medulloblastomas tend to produce areas of necrosis without calcification. They may also occur in the cerebellar hemispheres, more commonly in adolescents and young adults.

In addition to seeding via the CSF, the medulloblastomas have a tendency to invade adjacent structures. They do this fairly rapidly, for they grow rapidly. In addition to metastases within the neuraxis, distant metastases may occur, most commonly in bone but also in the peritoneum and lymph nodes (7). Some medulloblastomas, especially those occurring in the cerebellar hemispheres of adolescents and adults, have a remarkable capacity to induce an exuberant proliferation of mesenchymal elements when they infiltrate the ieptomeninges (2). These desmoplastic features presumably indicate a less aggressive tumor than the classic medulloblastoma. (Table 11.13).

HEMANGIOBLASTOMAS

Hemangioblastomas typically occur in the cerebellum but may also occur in the spinal cord and sometimes in the medulla oblongata. They are histologically composed of a meshwork of capillaries and small vessels that frequently present sclerotic walls; the intervascular spaces are filled with large polyhedral cells with clear, sometimes foamy, cytoplasm. Hemangioblastomas may present as single or multiple nodules with or without a cystic component. Frequently the nodule is present in one wall of the cyst, which is considerably larger than the solid nodule. Removal of a nodule by surgical methods results in a cure. Unfortunately, other nodules may be present, and these will later grow. For that reason, a thorough investigation with cross-sectional imaging and contrast enhancement as well as angiography is required prior to surgical treatment. Hemangioblastomas are sometimes associated with other manifestations of von Hippel-Lindau syndrome, in which there is retinal angioma and spinal cord hemangioblastoma as well as tumors in the kidney (clear cell carcinoma). Although supratentorial hemangioblastomas are supposed to occur, this point is controversial because these tumors are usually on the surface of the brain and resemble angioblastic meningiomas (see text following) (8) (Table 11.14).

Table 11.13.
Medulloblastomas

Usually occur in the midline and involve the cerebellar vermis
Those occurring in adolescents and adults are frequently in the cerebellar hemisphere
Much less frequently calcified than ependymoma, another typically midline posterior fossa tumor
CSF dissemination is common; Distant metastases can rarely be seen

Table 11.14.
Hemangioblastomas

Most common primary posterior fossa tumor in adults
May also occur in the spinal cord (especially in von Hippel-Lindau syndrome)
Variety of appearances, but usually a cyst with a single mural nodule or a solid mass
Solid components are densely contrast enhancing and highly vascular
A component of von Hippel-Lindau syndrome (renal cell cysts or carcinomas, retinal angiomas, pancreatic or epididymal cysts, pheochromocytomas)

Metastatic Neoplasms

As is well known, secondary deposits of tumors in the cranial cavity are a common occurrence and require an evaluation prior to surgical therapy on the primary neoplasm.

Practically any tumor can occasionally metastasize to the brain, but by far the most common sources are carcinomas of the lung, the breast, the genitourinary tract and the gastrointestinal tract and the malignant melanoma (Table 11.15). Systemic lymphomas may invade the leptomeninges; tumors of the paranasal sinuses may invade the intracranial structures by direct invasion rather than metastatic spread. Some sarcomas may metastasize to the brain, including soft-tissue and bone sarcomas. Metastases usually occur at the junction between the gray and white matter but may occur anywhere and may also primarily involve

Table 11.15.
Metastases

Most common primary tumors are lung or breast carcinomas, malignant melanomas, and gastrointestinal or genitourinary tract carcinomas
Most frequently occur at gray/white junction
Solitary metastases may be treated by surgical excision followed by radiation therapy

Table 11.16.
Meningiomas

Most common locations include parasagittal regions, convexities, sphenoid wing, planum sphenoidale, and perisellar region
Almost always benign but occasionally malignant, and may invade brain or bone
Frequently calcified, resulting in hyperdense appearance on CT and occasionally hypointense appearance on T2-weighted MR images

Table 11.17.
Nerve Sheath Tumors

Include schwannomas and neurofibromas
Schwannomas most commonly involve the eighth cranial nerve, but may involve other cranial nerves or spinal nerve roots
Neurofibromas often occur at the base of skull and face
Schwannomas are often seen in neurofibromatosis type II, whereas neurofibromas occur in neurofibromatosis type I

the cortex and sometimes the leptomeninges or the dura mater. Such is the case with breast carcinomas, lymphomas, and sarcomas. Solitary metastases are not uncommon, and surgical removal followed by radiation therapy is being utilized with increasing frequency, sometimes with rewarding results in terms of survival with good function (Table 11.15).

Tumors of the Meninges

Meningiomas are some of the most frequent brain tumors and occur on the surface of the brain. In order of distribution, they are most common in the parasagittal regions, followed by the basal areas of the brain, including the sellar region, the perisellar region, the olfactory area, and the region of the clivus down to the foramen magnum. They may occur inside the ventricles, in which case they probably originated from cells related to the choroid plexus. Although meningiomas are well-circumscribed and surgically resectable tumors, recurrence is common if a small fragment of tumor is not resected. This is sometimes the case in locations such as those associated with the superior sagittal sinus or in the cavernous sinus region, as well as in other basal locations. In general, however, the results of surgical removal are excellent. The rate of tumor growth varies considerably, and meningiomas can grow very slowly in some instances (Fig. 11.123). Psammomatous calcifications within meningiomas are common and may be seen as a diffuse increase in density on CT scans and sometimes as decreased intensity on MR T1 or T2 images.

Angioblastic meningiomas are important to recognize histologically because of the frequency with which they may recur. They are apparently related to hemangiopericytomas, which may be more invasive. More recently, angioblastic meningiomas have been classified as hemangiopericytomas. The histologic similarities of meningiomas with hemangioblastomas have led to controversy on whether the latter do occur in the supratentorial space (8).

Malignant meningiomas do occur and tend to invade the brain, provoking an intense glial reaction that may cause the tumor to be classified as a gliosarcoma.

It is important to mention here that meningiomas frequently invade adjacent structures (such as the paranasal sinuses, the orbital contents, and the mastoid area) while preserving their relatively benign histologic appearance. Invasion, therefore, is not necessarily an indication of malignant degeneration. In the base of the brain they may surround or encase the internal carotid artery or the basilar artery, producing narrowing of the artery. The term *encasement* implies actual involvement of the arterial wall, and arteriography shows that the arterial wall does become irregular (Table 11.16).

Nerve-Sheath Tumors

The term *neuroma* is commonly employed in the description of these tumors, but they are not really composed of neural tissue.

The *schwannoma* is a well-known tumor that occurs most frequently in the vestibular portion of the acoustic nerve (cranial nerve 8) but may also occur in nerve 5 and occasionally in nerve 7 (facial) and other cranial nerves (nerves 9, 10, 11). These tumors are composed of tightly packed spindle-shaped cells that sometimes show cellular pleomorphism, which is usually interpreted as a sign of degeneration rather than malignant transformation of the neoplasm. They may show cystic components, sometimes they calcify, and occasionally they show hemorrhage. They occur bilaterally rather frequently and are associated with type II neurofibromatosis.

The *neurofibromas* occur in type I neurofibromatosis and may involve nerves at the base of the skull or in the facial areas, where they are usually referred to as *plexiform neurofibromas*, sometimes forming large, deforming masses. In the schwannomas, the tumors adhere to the nerve fibers rather than infiltrate them, whereas in the neurofibromas they grow within the nerve, leading to a dissociation of the nerve fibers. The optic nerve gliomas occur in patients with neurofibromatosis type I but are not neurofibromas; rather, they are pilocytic astrocytomas. For further details, see Chapter 5 and also under "Perisellar Lesions" later in this chapter (Table 11.17).

Other Intracranial Tumors

EPIDERMOID TUMORS

Epidermoid tumors are also known by the terms *epidermoidoma*, *congenital* or *primary cholesteatoma*, and *pearly tumor*. They are slow-growing, usually extra-axial masses. The tumors are thought to arise from epithelial inclusions formed at the time of closure of the neural tube between the third and fifth week of fetal life (9). They may occur in the posterior fossa, in the region of the cerebellopontine angle, in the parasellar region, and occasionally in the

Table 11.18.
Epidermoid Tumors

Also known as epidermoidomas, congenital/primary cholesteatomas, or pearly tumors
Extra-axial masses consisting of epithial cells and their desquamation products
Most common locations are cerebellopontine angle and parasellar region
May also occur within the calvarium

brain, usually in the frontal lobe or inside the ventricles. They sometimes occur in the bones of the calvarium, the orbital area, or the skull base. They contain high concentrations of lipid and cholesterol, and are composed of an outer layer of stratified squamous epithelium with variable degrees of keratinization. The inner component is produced by a desquamation of the cells of the squamous epithelium. They may grow outside the brain and insinuate themselves along spaces in the base of the brain, or they may grow in the choroidal fissure and thus are extracerebral, even though they may be imaged inside the brain. The intraventricular location is also related to their origin in the choroidal fissure (Table 11.18).

The dermoid cysts differ from the epidermoid cysts in that they contain skin appendages such as sebaceous glands, sweat glands, apocrine glands, and hair. The presence of hair or any fragment of hair would classify the lesion as a dermoid cyst.

Epidermoid and dermoid cysts can be congenital or acquired. Congenital cysts are related to the trapping of dermal elements at the time of closure of the neural tube. Acquired cysts may follow multiple punctures and even a single puncture, and may follow gunshot wounds (Table 11.19).

TERATOMAS

Teratomas contain cells from all three germ cell lines and usually occur in the midline: the pineal gland and peripineal region, the third ventricle, the pituitary fossa, and the fourth ventricle region. They contain elements of fat, skin, glandular structures, cartilage, and bone.

CRANIOPHARYNGIOMAS

These tumors arise from remnants of squamous cells found in the distal portion of the pituitary stalk. They mostly lie in the junction of the stalk with the pars distalis (anterior lobe). (See Figure 11.49*A*.) The tumors are usually cystic

Table 11.19.
Dermoid Cysts

Contain skin elements, e.g., sebaceous glands, hair, sweat glands
May occur within the intracranial compartment as well as the orbit
May rupture, producing a chemical meningitis due to the irritating nature of their contents

and occur most frequently in children (over 50 percent of cases), but they are also found in adults and in that case tend to be solid. Stratified squamous epithelium surrounds the cyst. The solid tumors and the solid portions of cystic tumors are composed of strands of squamous cells supported by a hypovascular stroma of connective tissue. The solid craniopharyngiomas are often referred to as *adamantinomas.*

Craniopharyngiomas tend to become adherent to adjacent structures, particularly the hypothalamus, making total surgical removal difficult or impossible. They may also infiltrate farther. Only about 30 percent of the craniopharyngiomas can be completely removed, but even in these there is about a 20 percent recurrence rate (10,11) (Table 11.20).

Table 11.20.
Craniopharyngiomas

Usually cystic tumors with solid components composed of stratified squamous epithelium
Frequently calcified
May be completely solid
Typical location is at the junction of the pituitary gland and infundibulum
Frequently tightly adherent to adjacent structures, making total resection difficult

RATHKE CLEFT CYSTS

These tumors are mentioned here because they must be differentiated from craniopharyngiomas. They arise from the residual cleft remaining between the anterior and posterior lobes of the pituitary gland, and are lined with cuboidal epithelium, as against the squamous epithelium that surrounds craniopharyngioma cysts (see text following under "Perisellar Lesions").

INTRACRANIAL LIPOMAS

These are uncommon and usually small, except for the lipomas associated with partial agenesis of the corpus callosum. They may be formed as a single mass, or they may be spread around the adjacent sulci in the midline (see under "Congenital Anomalies," Chapter 5, and Figs. 5.33 and 5.34). Lipomas may also occur in the quadrigeminal plate region, sometimes extending caudally behind the fourth ventricle; they may also occur in the region of the tuber cinereum. Sometimes they may produce obstructive hydrocephalus. The author has seen a case of precocious puberty associated with a small lipoma in the tuber cinereum. The lipomas are usually midline, but a cerebellopontine angle location has been reported (12). The lipomas are composed of adult-type adipose cells but also contain a variable amount of collagen, which may penetrate the adjacent brain tissue along the perivascular spaces. In the spinal cord, the lipomas are intimately intertwined with the neural tissue, making total removal impossible.

HAMARTOMAS

These are masses composed of heterotopic neuroepithelial tissue and usually have no capacity for growth. Some well-circumscribed masses of gray matter within the centrum semiovale would qualify as hamartomas, but because they can be diagnosed by CT and MRI and may be associated with epileptic seizures, they should be considered anomalies of neuronal migration. Hypothalamic hamartomas are an important type that is usually associated with precocious puberty, usually occurring in males. They are composed of neurons varying in size and shape, and resemble the cerebral gray matter. Myelinated and nonmyelinated fibers are found in bundles. Some of these hamartomas may be large, displacing and compressing the hypothalamus and the upper brainstem. The precocious puberty is probably produced as a result of the mechanical effect, which leads to hypothalamic hyperactivity.

Hamartomas can be found within the brain tissue, in which case they could qualify histologically as gliomas, but the lack of growth would make one consider them more appropriately as hamartomas. This is particularly true in the temporal lobes in children and young adults with a long history of temporal lobe–type epilepsy (13). Occasionally a glioma that seems to remain stationary over a period of years is seen and can be followed by CT and MRI, which suggests that they are hamartomas. However, when followed long enough, they all seem to enter a period of rapid growth that denies their hamartomatous nature, although it could be theorized that a true neoplasm arose within a hamartoma.

The most common hamartomas are the vascular hamartomas (cavernous angiomas and capillary telangiectases), which are described in Chapter 10.

Cysts of Neuroepithelial Origin

COLLOID CYSTS OF THE THIRD VENTRICLE

This is a cystic tumor occurring in the roof of the third ventricle in the region of the foramen of Monro, between the columns of the fornix. It occurs predominantly in young adults. It is composed of a thin, fibrous capsule and a lining epithelium. The epithelium is usually composed of ciliated columnar or mucin-secreting cells with occasional areas of squamous cells. The material within the cysts usually contains a high percentage of protein, which may affect their appearance on CT and MRI (Table 11.21).

EXTRAVENTRICULAR EPENDYMAL CYSTS

These are ependyma-lined cysts occasionally encountered in the frontal lobes and other locations. Gherardi et al. reported cases in the brainstem and cerebellum (14).

CHOROID PLEXUS CYSTS

These are not uncommon and are usually asymptomatic. They may occur in the lateral ventricles, most frequently in the region of the glomus of the choroid plexus and in the fourth ventricle.

Table 11.21.
Colloid Cysts of the Third Ventricle

Typically found in young adults
Occur in anterosuperior portion of third ventricle, often obstructing the foramen of Monro
Can produce intermittent or persistent symptoms/signs due to obstructive hydrocephalus
Cyst usually contains highly proteinaceous material that can result in a variety of appearances on CT and MRI

GLIAL CYSTS OF THE PINEAL GLAND

These are found more frequently now with the use of MRI and are best seen in sagittal T1-weighted images. They are rarely greater than 14 mm in diameter and cause no symptoms. If they become larger, a therapeutic decision may have to be made, particularly if they are causing ventricular dilatation.

ARACHNOID CYSTS

Arachnoid cysts that occur in the subarachnoid space have been described in Chapter 5. Apparently intracerebral arachnoid cysts are also seen: that is, cystic lesions that, from the imaging point of view and also on surgical intervention, seem to be located under the pia mater. These are usually found in the frontal region in a parasagittal location and may grow to a large size, necessitating surgical exploration (Fig. 11.26). Although various etiologies, such as trauma and inflammation, have been mentioned as possible causes of arachnoid cysts, careful histologic studies demonstrate that the cyst is between the two layers of the arachnoid membrane instead of in the subarachnoid space; a congenital origin is most likely (15). The pia mater is found surrounding the deep portion of the cysts, attesting to their extracerebral origin (Fig. 11.26; see also Figs. 5.38 to 5.40).

Primary Melanomas of the Brain and Meninges

It is always possible that a metastatic melanoma may occur from an unknown focus of malignant melanoma elsewhere in the body. However, there are a sufficient number of documented examples in which no melanoma ever developed elsewhere in a patient who had a melanoma removed from the CNS, and of others who have come to autopsy and a careful search failed to reveal one. For that reason the existence of this condition in the CNS is accepted.

Pigmentation of the meninges in patches is sometimes seen, as well as melanosis of the meninges in association with melanotic pigmentation of various areas of the skull. The base of the brain and the cerebellum are favorite sites (17).

Primary meningeal melanomas may occur as well as intraparenchymal lesions, particularly in the cerebellum. The pituitary gland may also sometimes harbor a primary melanoma.

GENERAL DIAGNOSTIC CONSIDERATIONS

Clinically, a brain tumor may present with a rather wide variety of symptoms and signs. The patient may seek the doctor's opinion because of headache, seizures, or weakness of one or both extremities on one side that develops slowly and progressively. Changes in mentation or personality may be the first manifestation; the patient may not be aware of these, and the family may be the first to notice. Neurologic examination may be entirely negative, particularly in patients who present only with persistent headache. Papilledema may be present in some of these cases.

In general it may be said that any patient who presents with slowly progressive symptoms as against a sudden onset should be suspected of harboring a brain tumor. Late onset of seizures should always raise the question of intracranial tumor.

Brain tumors have a number of features not commonly found with neoplasms growing elsewhere. First, they are encountered at all ages and they are not predominantly associated with degenerative changes of later life. Second, gliomas, in particular, often change their biologic nature and cellular type with the passage of time. Many astrocytomas, beginning as benign, well-differentiated lesions, become malignant glioblastomas spontaneously or undergo malignant metaplasia when they recur after treatment. Third, for all practical purposes, brain tumors do not metastasize outside of the CNS.

The etiology of primary brain tumors is still poorly understood. Heredity is a factor in some cases, and brain tumors in multiple members of a family are not infrequently observed. Neurofibromatosis and tuberous sclerosis, for example, have a familial occurrence, and brain tumors are often found in these conditions. Recently, it has been possible to separate neurofibromatosis into two definite groups: neurofibromatosis I (NFI, von Recklinghausen disease) and neurofibromatosis II (NFII, bilateral acoustic neurofibromatosis). The groups appear to be genetically distinct. NFI has an abnormal chromosome 17, and NFII has an abnormal long arm of chromosome 22.

The tumors found in NFI are numerous and include optic pathway gliomas, other varieties of astrocytomas, CNS dysplasia, gliomas of the spinal cord, syringomyelia, and neurofibromas of peripheral nerves or plexiform neurofibromas. Pigmented hamartomas of the iris (Lisch nodules) are also found in patients with NFI (Table 11.22).

Table 11.22.
Neurofibromatosis I

Also known as von Recklinghausen's disease
Optic pathway gliomas
Astrocytomas
Dysplastic lesions ("hamartomas") of the CNS
Spinal cord gliomas
Peripheral nerve neurofibromas
Pigmented hamartomas of the iris (Lisch nodules)

Table 11.23.
Neurofibromatosis II

Bilateral acoustic neuromas
Meningiomas of brain or spine
Schwannomas of cranial nerves or peripheral nerves
Unlike neurofibromatosis I, parenchymal gliomas are not a characteristic feature

The neoplasms in NFII are bilateral acoustic neuromas, multiple intracranial meningiomas, and schwannomas of other cranial nerves; spinal meningiomas and schwannomas; and occasional peripheral nerve tumors. No parenchymal gliomas are found in NFII (18–22) (Table 11.23).

The majority of these lesions are described in various locations in text following: optic gliomas (described with suprasellar lesions), the eighth nerve (acoustic) neuromas (described with posterior fossa tumors), and cerebellopontine angle lesions and meningiomas (described in text following). For further details on neurofibromatosis see Chapter 5.

In some cases of tuberous sclerosis, benign gangliogliomas develop. Another etiologic factor appears to be viral infections, which are considered by increasing numbers of investigators to be important in neoplasia. In some cases trauma may be a causative factor. Cushing and Eisenhardt found some meningiomas at the sites of cranial injury (23). In a few cases radiation therapy may be a causative factor.

The general incidence of brain tumors, and particularly of specific cellular types, depends in large measure on the institution where statistics are gathered. It is well established, however, that throughout the United States approximately 2 percent of patients coming to necropsy have a brain tumor. On an average neurologic service, brain tumors rank only third in frequency behind cerebrovascular disease and infectious diseases of the nervous system.

Brain neoplasms are seen at any age, as noted in text preceding, and are common in infants and children. In many series, gliomas are second only to leukemia among the malignant lesions affecting young patients. A rather significant percentage of intracranial mass lesions arise from congenital rests or the inclusion of cellular elements not normally resident in the CNS.

Table 11.1 shows the incidence of various types of brain tumors in the experience of three investigators with large series of cases. It is of interest to see the similarities and some differences in the incidence of various mass lesions in these three series. Primary tumors, or gliomas, are by far the most common lesions encountered by all. The relative frequency of gliomas arising from astrocytes, both benign and malignant, is shown in Table 11.2. It is important to appreciate the shift in incidence of various types of brain tumors with advancing age, not shown in the tables. Although the percentage of all gliomas in relation to other brain tumors may even be reduced beyond the age of 60 years, according to some reports, there is a distinct shift toward malignancy in older persons. Thus, although approximately 35 percent of brain tumors beyond the sixth decade are gliomas, practically all are glioblastomas; the incidence of benign atrocytomas (1 to 2 percent), oligodendrogliomas (1 percent), and other well-differentiated cell types is drastically reduced. The frequency of occurrence of meningiomas (28 percent), acoustic neurinomas (12 percent), and metastatic carcinomas is high. More than 90 percent of brain tumors in elderly patients fall into one of four categories: glioblastoma, meningioma, metastatic carcinoma, and acoustic neurinoma.

With increasing longevity, the number of metastatic tumors of the CNS that are observed has been steadily increasing. The most common source, by far, is carcinoma of the lung (Table 11.6). The spread of melanotic tumors to the brain is a particularly common occurrence.

Approximately 75 percent of all brain tumors are hemispheric in location or originate in sites from which they affect the lateral and third ventricles. The frontal lobes are the largest portions of the cerebrum, and 50 percent of cerebral lobar tumors, or one-fourth of all brain tumors, are located in the frontal lobe areas. The next most frequent site of origin of glial tumors is the cerebellum. This is not too surprising when it is appreciated that the metencephalon constitutes 13 percent of the total brain tissue. The temporal lobes are third with regard to the location of glial tumors. It must be realized that the temporal lobes are more difficult to define than some other segments of the brain. Many tumors arising in the infrasylvian region are central in location and originate in the insular or limbic lobes or in the diencephalon. Nevertheless, one-fourth of all supratentorial tumors originate in the temporal areas. Parietal tumors form one-sixth of cerebral lesions; this means that three out of every four supratentorial tumors will be situated in the frontal, temporal, or parietal regions. One tumor in four is then to be found in the occipital lobes, the thalamic and hypothalamic (including suprasellar) regions, the ventricles, and other special structures of the supratentorial portion of the brain.

IMAGING APPROACHES

Plain Films of the Skull

The plain film examination of the skull is omitted in any institution where cross-sectional imaging devices are available (CT, MRI). The findings on skull films in intracerebral tumors are calcification in cases where such is present, and evidence of demineralization of the sella turcica as a manifestation of increased intracranial pressure. In extracerebral tumors such as meningiomas, there may be changes in the bone (hyperostosis on the inner table, hyperdensity of the bone, and sometimes hyperostosis on the outer table). In schwannomas of the acoustic nerve and other nerves and in gliomas of the optic nerve, enlargement of the osseous conduits is found. In adenomas of the pituitary gland and in craniopharyngiomas, enlargement of the sella turcica may be found.

All these findings, however, can usually be seen on CT examination more clearly. For instance, the presence of calcium is seen considerably earlier on CT than on plain films. Bone erosions are usually seen more clearly on the bone window images of CT. In addition, CT and MRI will demonstrate the intracranial soft-tissue structures and will show a tumor with an accuracy that approaches 100 percent. When brain tumor is clinically suspected, it is always necessary to carry out an examination without and with contrast material in both CT or MRI. The latter is considered a more sensitive and more noninvasive examination, both because it does not use ionizing radiation and because the contrast material used causes fewer reactions.

Radionuclide Examination

Radionuclide (RN) examinations are not performed to detect brain tumors unless CT or MRI is unavailable. The RN examination reveals an abnormal uptake of the radionuclide in a fairly high percentage of neoplasms (about 70 percent), particularly in primary malignant and metastatic tumors as well as in meningiomas (24). It is superior to plain films of the skull in diagnosing intracerebral tumors; in these cases skull films usually show no abnormality, except in some cases that may show calcifications or evidence of increased intracranial pressure.

Computed Tomography

CT is usually the first examination carried out in patients who are suspected of having a brain tumor. This is partly because CT is more widely available and partly because there are no contraindications to the use of this technique. As already indicated, it is necessary to plan on a noncontrast examination followed by contrast unless there is a contraindication to the use of contrast, such as an elevated serum creatinine level of 2.0 mg/100 ml or higher. A prior reaction to intravenous contrast material is not a contraindication. If the reaction was mild, the chances are that it may not occur again; also, a low-ionic contrast may be used if the hyperosmolar variety was used previously. If the reaction was considered more severe or if the patient is asthmatic or has some other manifestation of severe allergy, pretreatment with steroids and Benadryl may be advisable.

Brain tumor findings are extremely variable, depending on the type of lesion. On preenhancement images perhaps the most frequent finding is an area of *low density* that partly represents the tumor. This area normally contains less protein and more fluid (edema) than the adjacent brain. The area surrounding the tumor contains some edema fluid in nearly all cases. The edema is a reaction of the brain to any foreign material. In low-grade infiltrating tumors, the degree of edema may be very slight, to the point where it may not be visible by CT; that is, the neoplasm is isodense, and unless there are other findings, such as a mass effect, it may be overlooked. In the great majority of cases, however, the edema is sufficient to produce a low-density effect (Fig. 11.1). Rapidly growing tumors and particularly metastatic tumors usually produce more edema. In general, the presence of a large amount of edema usually reflects the reaction of the brain to the neoplasm. This reaction is probably related to the individual, but it is also related to the type of neoplasm. For instance, a glioblastoma usually presents more surrounding edema than other gliomas, and the same is true of a rapidly growing astrocytoma or any other rapidly growing glioma (Fig. 11.2). Metastatic tumors usually generate proportionately more edema than neoplasms derived from brain tissue, but some metastatic neoplasms produce no brain edema, at least while they are small.

The *mass effect* produced by the tumor and the edema is manifested by a shift of the midline structures to the opposite side (the midline shift). A larger midline shift usually means more tumor cells, but also mass generated by the surrounding edema.

When measuring the degree of midline shift, it seems most useful to use the posterior aspect of the septum pellucidum on axial views as the point of reference. Any difference between the right and the left side, measured from the inner table to the middle of the posterior septum pellucidum and from there to the opposite side divided in half, represents the midline shift, as corrected by the usual minification noted in the scale. This subject and the secondary effects and possible complications (particularly hippocampal herniations) are described in detail in Chapter 4 under the discussion of edema (Fig. 11.3).

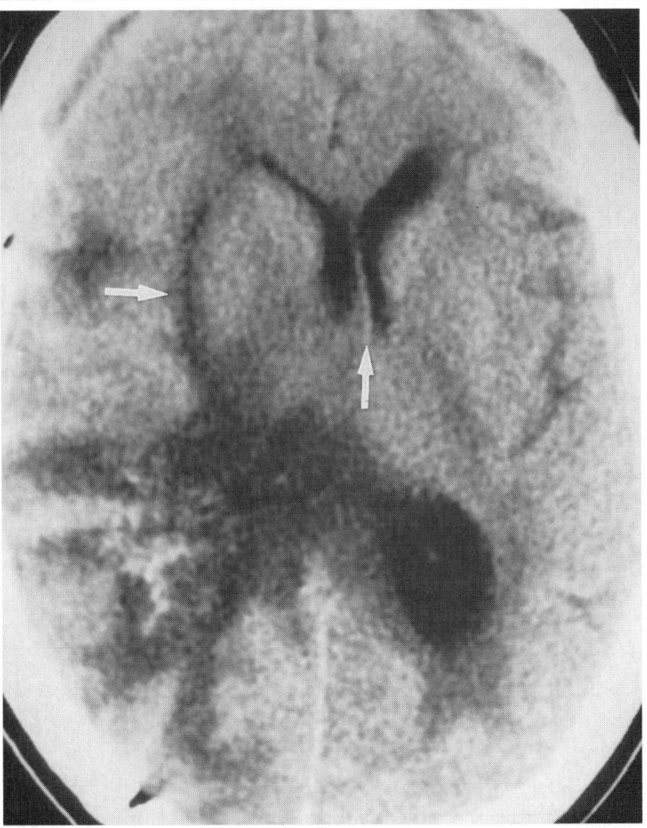

Figure 11.3. Right parietal glioblastoma with calcification and midline shift. There is low attenuation and spotty calcification, and the lesion is either surrounding or invading the atrium of the lateral ventricle. The edema extends forward along the external capsule (arrow). The best method of measuring the midline shift is to use the posterior aspect of the septum pellucidum in the region of the foramen of Monro (vertical arrow). The distance between the inner tables on both sides is measured; in this case it was 9.0 cm in the original photographic image. One half is 4.5 cm, and the midline shift is 8.0 mm, which corrected for minification was about a 10.0-mm midline shift. The maximum allowable is less than 3.0 mm. The displacement from the midline is greater posteriorly than anteriorly because the tumor is located in the parietal lobe.

Slowly growing astrocytomas and oligodendrogliomas usually do not enhance because the blood-brain barrier is preserved (Figs. 11.1, 11.6). When considering brain neoplasms, perhaps we should speak of a blood-tumor barrier instead. The *blood-brain barrier* is based on the existence of *tight junctions* between the cells of the capillary endothelium in the brain, which regulates capillary permeability. Furthermore, brain capillaries have a continuous basement membrane, whereas in other tissues the capillaries have a discontinuous one. Another important feature distinguishing brain tissue from nonneural tissue is the nearly complete absence of pinocytosis across the normal brain capillaries (25). Pinocytosis is a method of transporting macromolecules across the capillary wall; its absence means that no large molecules can pass out of the blood vessels and into the extravascular space in the brain.

Contrast media molecules are large enough so that they remain within the normal brain capillaries, whereas in other tissues they readily leave the capillaries, and equilibrium between the intra- and extravascular spaces occurs within a short period of time (26). It is also known that astrocytic foot plates surround the brain capillaries, but not completely, and their function is not well understood. There are a few areas in the brain that have no blood-brain barrier: the pineal, the choroid plexus, the area postrema, the tuber cinereum, the paraphysis (27), and the pituitary gland. In addition, the dura mater and the pia have no capillary tight junctions. For this reason, the pineal is bright on CT and on T1-weighted images following iodide or gadolinium contrast, as is the choroid plexus. The contrast uptake in the pituitary gland is used to diagnose solid tumors or cysts within the pituitary fossa. The smaller structures, such as the tuber cinereum and the area postrema, can sometimes be seen if looked for carefully in postcontrast sagittal images on MRI; they cannot be seen on postcontrast CT images. The dura mater enhances readily and is seen better on delayed images on both CT and MRI, but the pial enhancement cannot usually be discerned by either method (Table 11.24).

The lack of enhancement of many gliomas is probably owing to the fact that their capillaries possess the usual qualities of normal brain tissue capillaries. The more ma-

Table 11.24.
Blood-Brain Barrier

Formed by tight junctions between capillary endothelial cells
Absence of pinocytosis further prevents transport of large molecules across capillary walls
Blood-brain barrier is absent at the pineal gland, area postrema, tuber cinereum, choroid plexus, and paraphysis

lignant gliomas and glioblastomas possess an active angiogenesis factor that forms dysmorphic capillaries. The metastatic neoplasms would have the type of capillary bed of their tissue of origin and thus would allow the passage of contrast.

The effect of *corticosteroid therapy* is important. Steroids are used in the management of brain tumors (and other conditions) when there is clinical evidence of increased intracranial pressure associated with edema. The mechanism of edema reduction is purported to be at the capillary wall. Corticosteroids act to tighten the capillary cell junctions, thus reducing the edema (28). By the same mechanism, a previously enhancing tumor may not enhance after the administration of corticosteroids. This is particularly well shown in primary brain lymphomas, where rapid clinical improvement is often observed following corticosteroid therapy. If repeat CT or MRI with contrast is carried out, there may be a marked "improvement" or at times complete disappearance of the enhancement 24 to 48 h after the start of corticosteroid therapy. It is important to keep this possibility in mind particularly at the first examination, when diagnosis is dependent on imaging, for patients may be started on corticosteroid therapy, if clinically indicated, before they are referred for CT or MRI examination.

From the point of view of enhancement, the behavior of iodide- or gadolinium-based contrast media is similar (29). That is, if the lesion enhances on CT, it will also enhance on MRI and vice versa. However, cases are seen in which enhancement on MRI is found but not on CT. Possibly the T1 shortening effect of gadolinium is more sensitive than the increased density of the extravascular space by CT, and may be seen when a lesser amount of the contrast has left the vascular system. This is an uncommon occurrence, however.

On precontrast images it is often not possible to visualize the tumor. The hyperintensity seen following intravenous contrast injection is based on a breakdown of the blood-brain barrier or, better, on the absence of a blood-brain barrier in the neoplasm, which allows extravasation of contrast out of the blood vessels.

Perineoplastic edema does not enhance because the blood-brain barrier is intact in these areas. The same is true of edema from other causes, such as abscess, inflammation, or trauma (unless there is accompanying brain contusion) (Figs. 11.2 and 11.15).

Neoplasms may be solid or partly cystic. In the latter case the density on CT may be similar to that of CSF. If the fluid contains a moderate amount of protein, however, the density is higher than that of CSF, a fact that can be easily ascertained as the two are compared.

If the protein content is higher, the density will be higher. This is part of the reason why colloid cysts of the third ventricle may be very hyperdense on CT (Fig. 11.38).

As already indicated, solid tumors are usually less dense than the surrounding brain because of their increased water content. If the tumor is rich in cells, however, the density (and the intensity on T1-weighted MRI) increases or surpasses that of the surrounding brain, and this difference becomes more conspicuous if the tumor is surrounded by edema (Fig. 11.4). The types of neoplasms that are likely to be hyperdense are the medulloblastomas, the neuroblas-

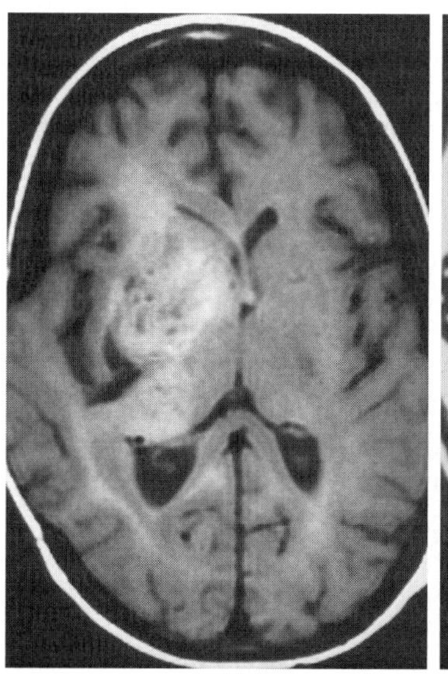

A

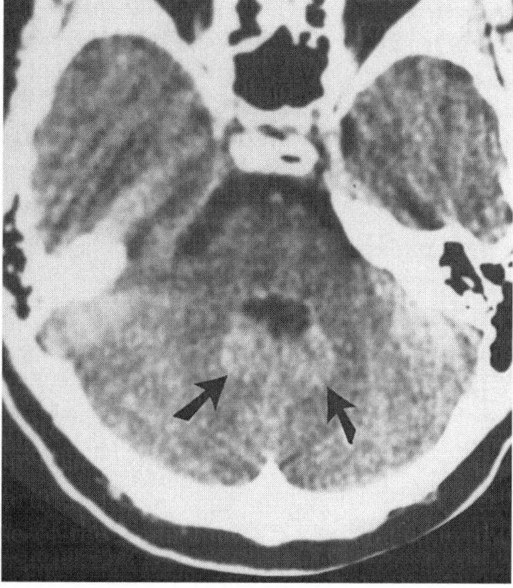

B

Figure 11.4. Neuroblastoma, primitive neuroectodermal tumor (PNET), in a 21-year-old woman showing hyperintensity on T1 images. **A.** This T1-weighted nonenhanced axial image shows hyperintensity probably indicative of high cellularity. **B.** Another patient, a child with a pineoblastoma that had seeded extensively (arrows). All the metastatic seeding was hyperdense on CT without contrast owing to high cellularity (see also Fig. 11.45).

Table 11.25.
Tumors That Are Often Hyperdense on Noncontrast CT

Medulloblastomas
Pineoblastomas
Lymphomas
Many meningiomas

tomas, the pineoblastomas (which fall into the category of PNET), and the lymphomas (Table 11.25). Meningiomas are usually denser than brain because many of them are cellular and contain a compact stroma, but also because some contain calcified psammoma bodies. The presence of hemorrhage is another reason for hyperdensity on CT, but the hemorrhage is likely to be very hyperdense and also occupies only part of the area of the mass.

Calcification is very well demonstrated by CT and may be diffuse, as in psammomatous meningioma, or may be in a fine stippled pattern or in heavier chunks. The chunky type is typical of oligodendrogliomas (Fig. 11.24).

The tumor mass and the accompanying edema may form a large mass that provokes not only displacement of the midline structures toward the opposite side but also displacement of the medial, temporal lobe toward the midline, which may lead to downward transtentorial hippocampal herniation. If the neoplasm is in the cerebellum, it may produce an upward transtentorial herniation. These changes have been described in Chapter 4, "Cerebral Edema." See under "Meningioma" in text following for further details.

Magnetic Resonance Imaging

MRI yields more overall information about the shape of the neoplasm and its relationship to the surrounding structures. It does not show calcification within the tumor reliably, and probably it is not superior to CT in helping us determine, prior to biopsy, the probable histology of the lesion. As already expressed, it is slightly better than CT in its overall detection rate, particularly in metastatic tumors. In this group, MRI will show tumors that are not seen clearly by CT, and it will demonstrate more lesions than CT in a given case. For this reason MRI without and with contrast is the examination of choice when looking for metastases. In some cases the presence of multiple T2-weighted hyperintense white matter foci prior to contrast may make it difficult to differentiate between these and multiple metastases. However, the postcontrast examination clarifies the problem because the white matter foci do not enhance, and any area of enhancement should be considered a neoplasm or an inflammatory process.

The majority of neoplasms are hypointense on T1-weighted images and hyperintense on T2-weighted images (first and second echoes) (Fig. 11.1).

Slowly growing gliomas (astrocytomas and oligodendrogliomas) may not enhance after contrast administration in the same manner as with CT, presumably because these tumors possess a capillary structure with tight junctions between the endothelial cells similar to that seen in normal brain tissue. The more malignant tumors almost always enhance, at least the portion that is growing more rapidly (Figs. 11.14 and 11.15). The preceding discussion concerning contrast enhancement with CT applies to MRI as well.

Cystic tumors may be isointense with CSF, or, if the cystic portion contains protein, it may be hyperintense in relation to CSF. If the protein content is very high, the intensity on T1-weighted images may be high, whereas on T2-weighted images it may be isointense or even hypointense, as in some colloid cysts (Fig. 11.38). Contrast enhancement may show an enhanced nodule or an entire enhanced wall, as on CT.

The presence of hemorrhage may be evaluated more completely with MRI than with CT. This is because CT shows the blood only in the acute stage and rapidly loses its density (within about 8 to 12 days), whereas on MRI the subacute blood is dense on T1- and T2-weighted images. Furthermore, old blood will show magnetic susceptibility on T2-weighted images on a gradient echo, which is an indication that the tumor bled in the past. The presence of old or new blood is an indication of tumor malignancy, although some tumors, like choroid plexus papillomas, may bleed without showing malignant degeneration. Some tumors, like metastatic melanomas, may be hyperdense on CT and hyperintense in T1-weighted images but on T2-weighted images are usually hypointense (T2 dark), which is fairly specific for melanoma (Fig. 11.93). The hyperintensity on T1-weighted images (and the hyperdensity on CT) is not due to blood but to melanin.

The presence of hippocampal herniation can be better demonstrated with MRI than with CT because sagittal as well as coronal images may be added to the axial images.

Cerebral Angiography

This was the primary diagnostic method before the advent of cross-sectional imaging by CT and MRI, and its use in the diagnosis and management of intracerebral tumors has continued to decrease. It may be requested by the neurosurgeon when a biopsy procedure is being planned and it becomes necessary to ascertain the degree of vascularity.

There are three main findings in cerebral angiography of brain tumors (Table 11.26):

1. Local displacement and deformity of the arteries and veins adjacent to the mass.
2. Displacement of midline vessels (anterior cerebral arteries and internal cerebral veins)—the *midline shift*—and sometimes evidence of transtentorial hippocampal herniation when the mass effect is large.
3. Abnormal vascularity of tumors (*tumor stain*) and early filling of veins due to increased speed of circulation through the tumor.

Local displacement and deformity of the arteries vary with the location of the tumor mass. In the suprasylvian area

Table 11.26.
Angiographic Findings of Intracranial Neoplasms

Displacement/deformity of vessels adjacent to the tumor
Shift of midline vessels due to mass effect
Abnormal vascularity of the tumor itself (tumor blush and early-draining veins)

(mid and posterior frontal and frontoparietal operculum), the arteries are spread out (Fig. 11.5). In a parasagittal tumor, the anterior cerebral artery branches may be buckled (Fig. 11.14); in an extracerebral subfrontal tumor, such as a meningioma, the branches of the anterior and middle cerebral arteries may be elevated. In a temporal tumor the finding would be medial displacement and elevation of the branches of the middle cerebral artery situated within the sylvian fissure, and if the mass involves the posterior portion of the temporal lobe, elevation and medial displacement of the *angiographic sylvian point.* The latter is defined as the last vessel emerging from the sylvian fissure to reach the surface of the brain (Fig. 11.18).

In our present practice these findings would only correlate with what may already have been seen by CT or MRI.

Displacement of midline vessels (midline shift) is the result of the mass effect and is related both to the size of the tumor and to the amount of accompanying reactive edema of the adjacent brain. The edema can occupy significantly more space than the tumor. The vessels that are shifted are the anterior cerebral artery, particularly the pericallosal artery, the callosomarginal branch, and the proximal portion of the frontopolar artery. The other vessels are the internal cerebral veins. The internal cerebral vein is a more reliable indicator of midline shift because it is in the center of the skull and its position in relation to both sides of the skull is not significantly affected by rotation. Also, it may be shifted when the anterior cerebral artery is not (Fig. 11.6). The anterior cerebral artery and its branches are more conspicuous, and in spite of their being affected by rotation of the head during filming, good information is derived from their position because the configuration of the shift varies with the position of the tumor. For instance, if the tumor is anterior frontal, the arterial shift will be round. If the tumor is high, the superior portion will be more displaced, and vice versa if it is lower. If the tumor is temporal or posterior, the chances are that the shift will be square; that is, the subfalcial portion and the inferior aspects will be displaced to the same extent, although the central portion may not be because of the influence of the falx cerebri and its relationship to the anterior cerebral artery (Figs. 11.7 to 11.9).

Transtentorial herniation may also be shown by angiography. Downward hippocampal herniation in its anterior portion may be shown by the medial displacement of the anterior choroidal artery, which is normally wrapped around the uncus. An anterior, middle, and posterior (unilateral total) transtentorial herniation produces medial and downward displacement of the posterior cerebral arteries. The angiogram demonstrates why a middle and posterior transtentorial downward herniation can produce an occipi-

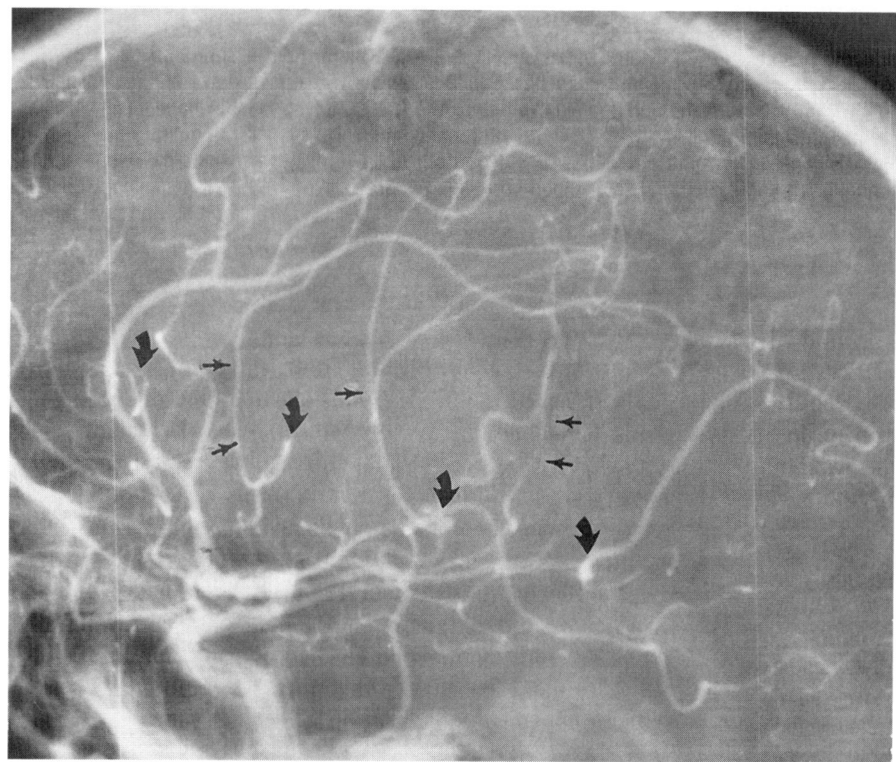

Figure 11.5. Local spreading of arteries over suprasylvian area and operculum. There is marked spreading and some bowing of arteries and of branches of the middle cerebral artery in the region above the sylvian triangle (arrow), causing disruption and downward displacement of the angiographic sylvian triangle (outlined by short, curved, black arrows). The last two loops of the sylvian triangle are more downwardly displaced, indicating that the center of the tumor mass is farther back. This is confirmed by the bowing of the more anterior vessels (marked by two arrows and one small horizontal arrow). The vessel situated near or at the equator of the mass is likely to be straight (two posterior small arrows).

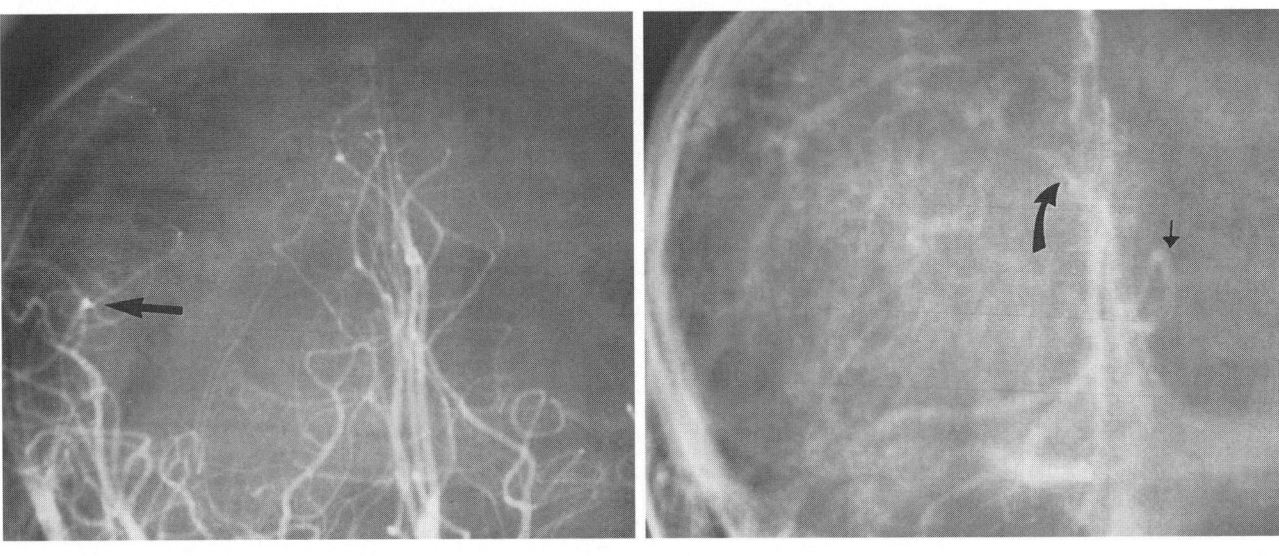

A B

Figure 11.6. Midline shift in which there was displacement of the internal cerebral vein but not of the anterior cerebral artery. **A.** Carotid angiography performed with compression of the opposite carotid artery during the injection of contrast shows excellent bilateral filling. The anterior cerebral arteries are in the midline. Note that there is lateral displacement of the right angiographic sylvian point (arrow) as compared to the other side. The space between the midline and the point is larger on the right than on the left. This appearance suggests the presence of a mass in the basal ganglia–thalamic area. **B.** In the venous phase the internal cerebral vein is markedly shifted to the left (arrow). Also, there is elevation and medial displacement of the thalamostriate vein, a typical appearance for a thalamic tumor (curved arrow).

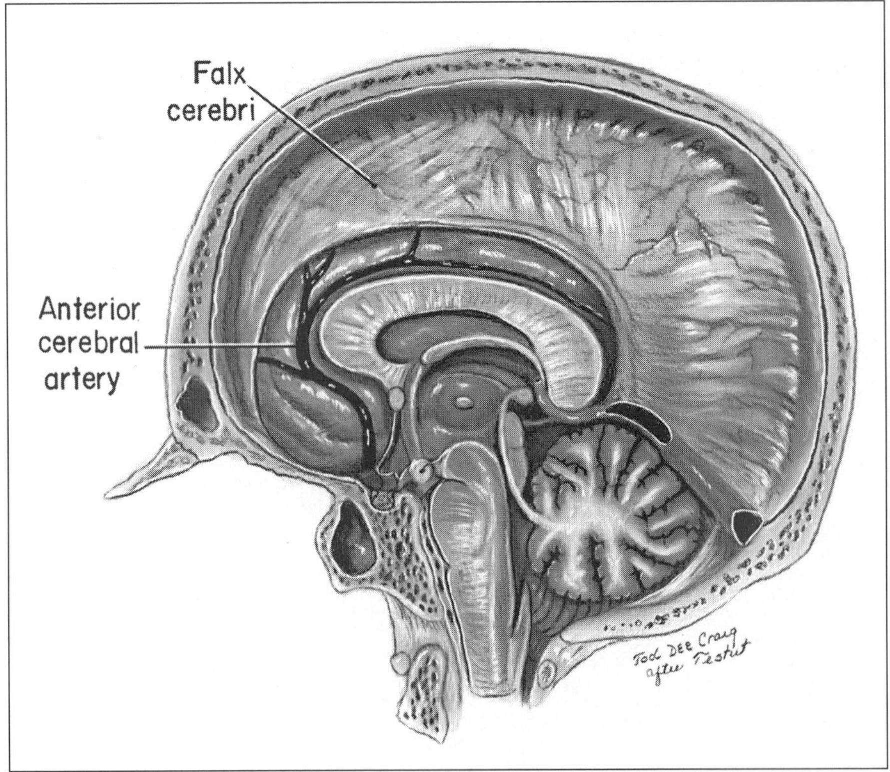

Figure 11.7. The relationship of the pericallosal artery and other branches of the anterior cerebral artery to the edge of the falx cerebri.This diagram explains the midline shift of the anterior cerebral vessels. The only portions of the vessels that shift are those situated in the window. The vessels return to the midline as they move peripherally and reach the edge of the relatively rigid falx.

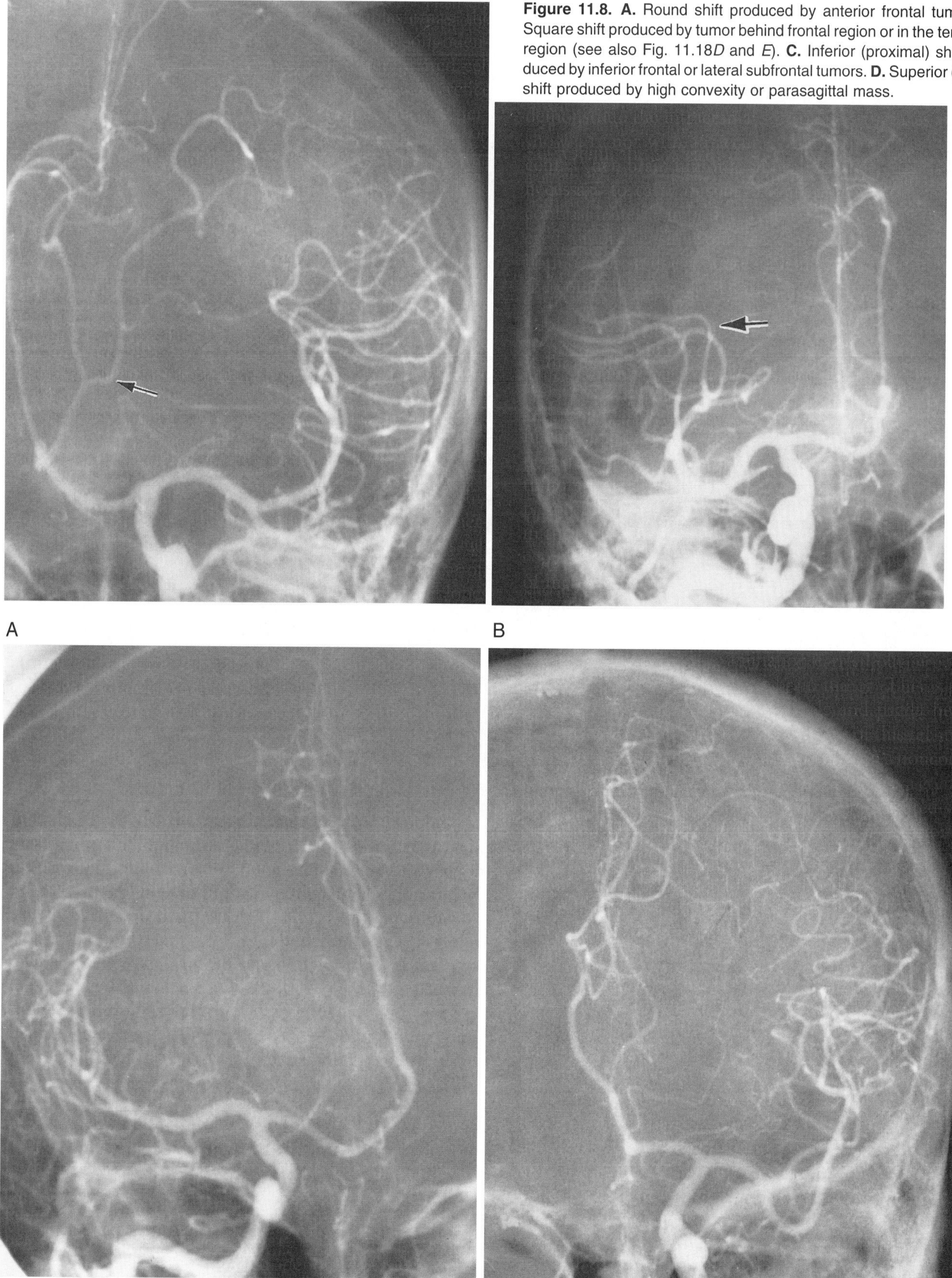

Figure 11.8. **A.** Round shift produced by anterior frontal tumor. **B.** Square shift produced by tumor behind frontal region or in the temporal region (see also Fig. 11.18*D* and *E*). **C.** Inferior (proximal) shift produced by inferior frontal or lateral subfrontal tumors. **D.** Superior (distal) shift produced by high convexity or parasagittal mass.

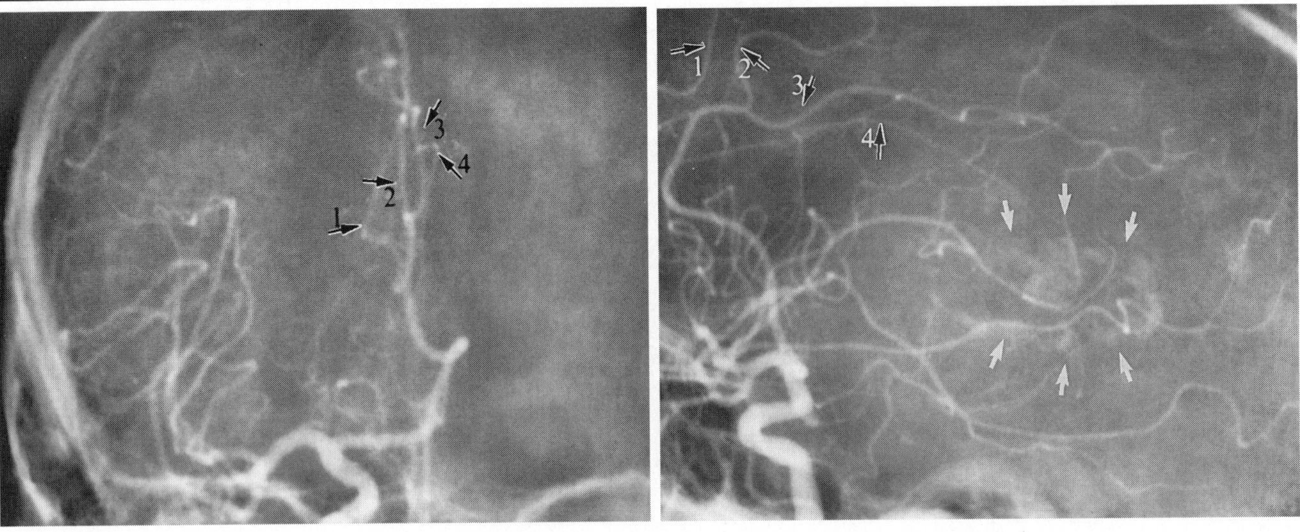

A B

Figure 11.9. Square midline shift of the branches of the anterior cerebral artery. **A.** Frontal view. **B.** Lateral view. The position of the tumor blush is seen (white arrow). The anterior curve of the pericallosal artery goes far anteriorly and therefore returns to the midline because, it reaches the edge of the semirigid falx; the subfalcial and proximal portions are displaced approximately to the same degree. The relations of the arterial segments in the frontal and lateral views are indicated with corresponding numbers.

tal infarction by compression of the posterior cerebral artery at the edge of the tentorium (Fig. 11.10).

The *tumor vascularity* is usually related to the histology of the tumor. Slowly growing gliomas are usually avascular (Fig. 11.11), and malignant gliomas, particularly glioblastomas, are usually hypervascular, showing both a tumor blush and large veins; furthermore, there is commonly early filling of veins, indicating increased speed of circulation through the tumor. For these reasons it is usually advisable to carry out the conventional angiogram if a needle biopsy, steriotactically performed, is contemplated. If the tumor is very vascular, an open biopsy may be preferred (Fig. 11.12).

About a quarter of *oligodendrogliomas* show hypervascularity (30). This feature usually indicates a more aggressive tumor. Some mixed gliomas (mixed oligo- and astrocytomas) present interesting patterns of vascularity, such as slow-flowing vascular malformations, with venous lakes and dilated veins (Fig. 11.12*D* to *F*). Practically all malignant tumors present tumor vascularity on angiography. *Meningiomas* also present a tumor blush that tends to be homogeneous and persistent, but some meningiomas may present rapid circulation or early venous filling. The latter tumors were once called *angioblastic meningiomas*, but the classification of some of these has been changed to *hemangiopericytomas*. See under "Meningiomas" for further detail.

SUPRATENTORIAL INTRACEREBRAL TUMORS

These may be divided into hemispheric, midline, and intraventricular tumors. The various histologic types are described under "Pathologic Considerations" in text preceding.

Hemispheric Tumors

Hemispheric intracerebral tumors probably occur with equal frequency in the various lobes of the brain, depending on the amount of brain tissue present. For instance, gliomas are most common in the frontal lobes, but the frontal lobes are by far the largest of the lobes of the brain. The majority are *astrocytomas* (20 percent) or *glioblastomas* (55 percent). The rest are oligodendrogliomas, ependymomas, and lymphomas, as well as metastatic tumors (Table 11.27).

The more slowly growing tumors may produce minor neurologic findings such as headache, seizures, or some focal findings such as weakness of one or both extremities on the contralateral side. This leads to a neurologic consultation and referral for a CT or MRI examination. The examination is carried out first without contrast and then with contrast. As already discussed, some tumors may not enhance on CT or MRI; in these cases the tumor is probably a slowly growing glioma (Fig. 11.1). Some may be cys-

Table 11.27.
Hemispheric Tumors

Major primary tumors include glioblastomas (55%), astrocytomas (20%), oligodendrogliomas, ependymomas, and lymphomas
Glioblastomas frequently have a region of cystic necrosis with irregular inner margins
Frontal glioblastomas frequently extend across the genu or body of the corpus callosum ("butterfly" pattern)
About 5% of glioblastomas are multicentric
A diffuse infiltrating form of glioma ("gliomatosis cerebri") that does not form a dominant mass is seen in a small minority of cases

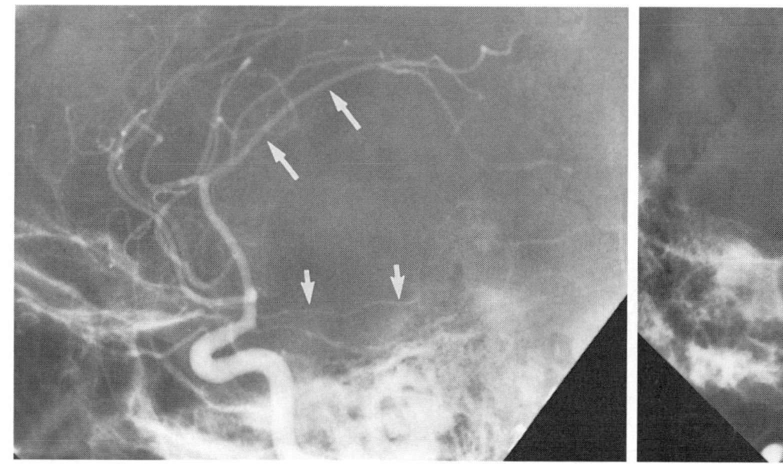

A

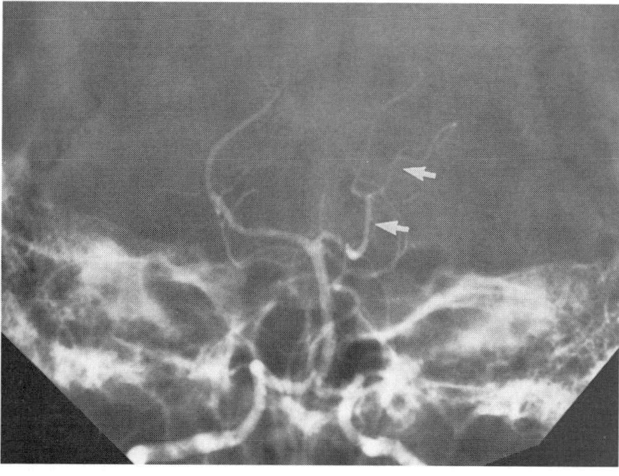

B

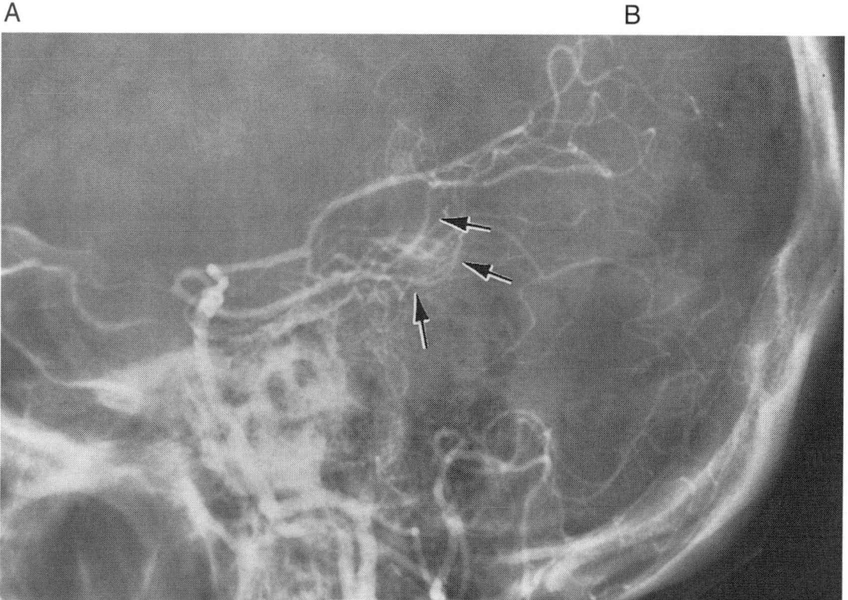

C

Figure 11.10. Complete unilateral downward transtentorial herniation in a patient with a temporal lobe mass. **A.** Lateral view shows marked elevation of the middle cerebral artery and branches (arrows). There is filling of the anterior choroidal artery, which is displaced downward (two lower arrows). Below it is the posterior cerebral artery, markedly displaced downward. **B.** Frontal view of vertebral angiogram reveals the marked medial displacement of the posterior cerebral artery (two arrows). **C.** Lateral vertebral angiogram. There is downward displacement of the posterior cerebral artery on one side. The two lower arrows show the large step that a main branch of the posterior cerebral artery has to take to go to the upper surface of the tentorium at the tentorial edge. The upper arrow shows another branch stepping up. Ischemia of the occipital lobe may result, particularly if the posterior downward herniation occurs rapidly.

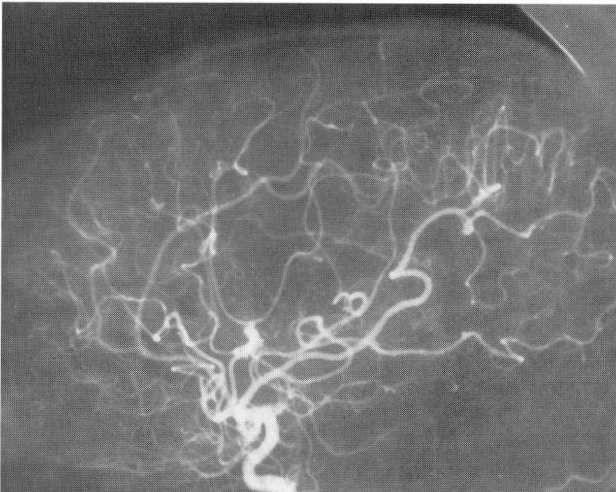

A

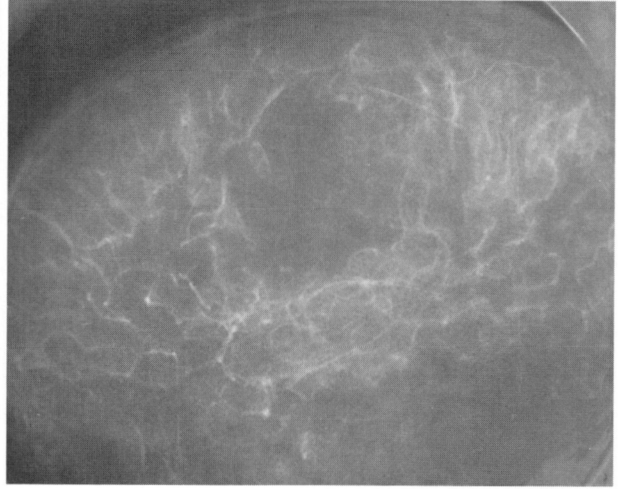

B

Figure 11.11. Low-grade avascular glioma. **A.** Lateral angiogram in arterial phase shows some spreading of the lateral suprasylvian branches and downward displacement of the sylvian triangle. **B.** The avascular tumor produces a "hole in the brain" that becomes evident in the intermediate phase of the angiogram.

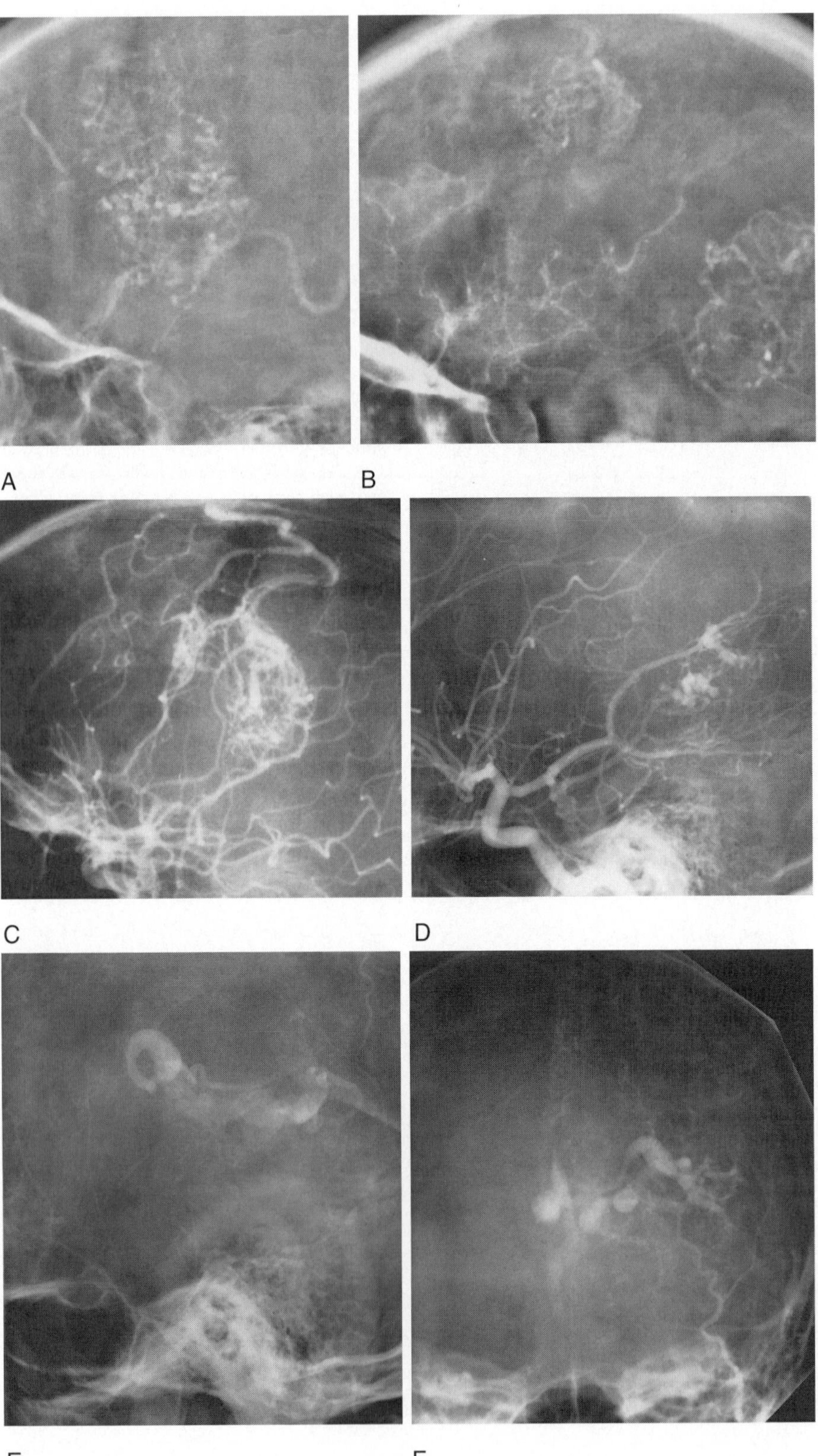

Figure 11.12. Three examples of vascularity of intracerebral malignant tumors. **A.** Large vascularity with many small venous lakes and early drainage by way of the internal cerebral vein and vein of Galen. Malignant glioma. **B.** Another patient. Two vascular metastatic lesions with much vascularity and early venous filling. **C.** The venous filling and large irregular veins occur much earlier in this glioblastoma. Stereotactically guided needle biopsy in any of these cases could lead to uncontrollable bleeding. **D** to **F.** Another patient. Partly intraventricular mixed glioma (oligo and astrocytoma) growing mostly in the periatrial region. **D.** The arterial phase reveals marked vascularity. **E** and **F.** In the venous phase there are large venous channels that resemble those seen in slowly flowing arteriovenous malformations.

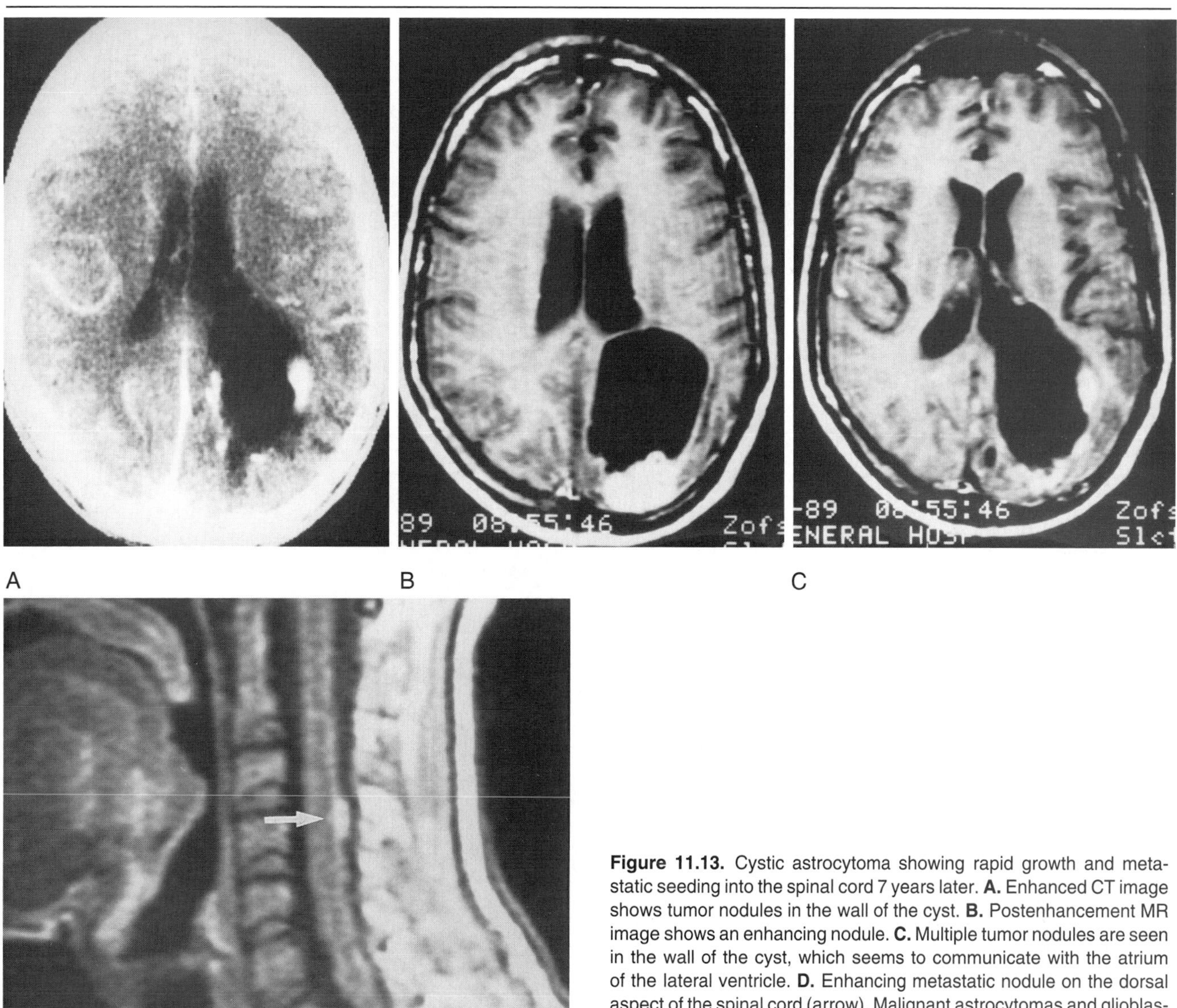

Figure 11.13. Cystic astrocytoma showing rapid growth and metastatic seeding into the spinal cord 7 years later. **A.** Enhanced CT image shows tumor nodules in the wall of the cyst. **B.** Postenhancement MR image shows an enhancing nodule. **C.** Multiple tumor nodules are seen in the wall of the cyst, which seems to communicate with the atrium of the lateral ventricle. **D.** Enhancing metastatic nodule on the dorsal aspect of the spinal cord (arrow). Malignant astrocytomas and glioblastomas may seed via the CSF if they communicate with the ventricles, as in this case. They may also invade over the surface if the meningeal covering is defective, which may occur occasionally following surgery.

tic. Cystic astrocytomas usually present an enhancing nodule. The nodule may be solitary and well circumscribed, or it may be somewhat more diffuse, with some signs of infiltration beyond the wall of the cyst. Some of these tumors can be followed for a number of years without much change. However, eventually they reach a size that may require intervention, or else they may enter a phase of rapid growth, which usually indicates malignant degeneration. Practically all slowly growing gliomas may behave in this manner (Fig. 11.13).

More rapidly growing astrocytomas may enhance only partially. This is usually interpreted as a malignant degeneration of that portion of the tumor (Fig. 11.14).

The typical picture of a glioblastoma on CT or MRI is that of an irregular mass with much surrounding edema that enhances on intravenous contrast injection and that presents zones of necrosis that do not enhance. The surrounding edema does not enhance. There is nearly always a well-developed mass effect with a shift of the midline structures to the opposite side. The "cystic" (necrotic) cavity presents an irregular margin. This irregularity is typical for a necrotizing tumor as against an abscess or a benign cyst, which usually presents a smooth cystic cavity (Fig. 11.15). The tumor may involve the ventricular wall, thus increasing the chances for seeding via the CSF. The tumor may also invade the brain surface and the pia mater and can grow exophytically in the subarachnoid space. Unless there is a surgical defect in the dura, however, the tumor will not grow outside the dura, with rare exceptions. Once the neoplasm invades outside the dura, it can rapidly in-

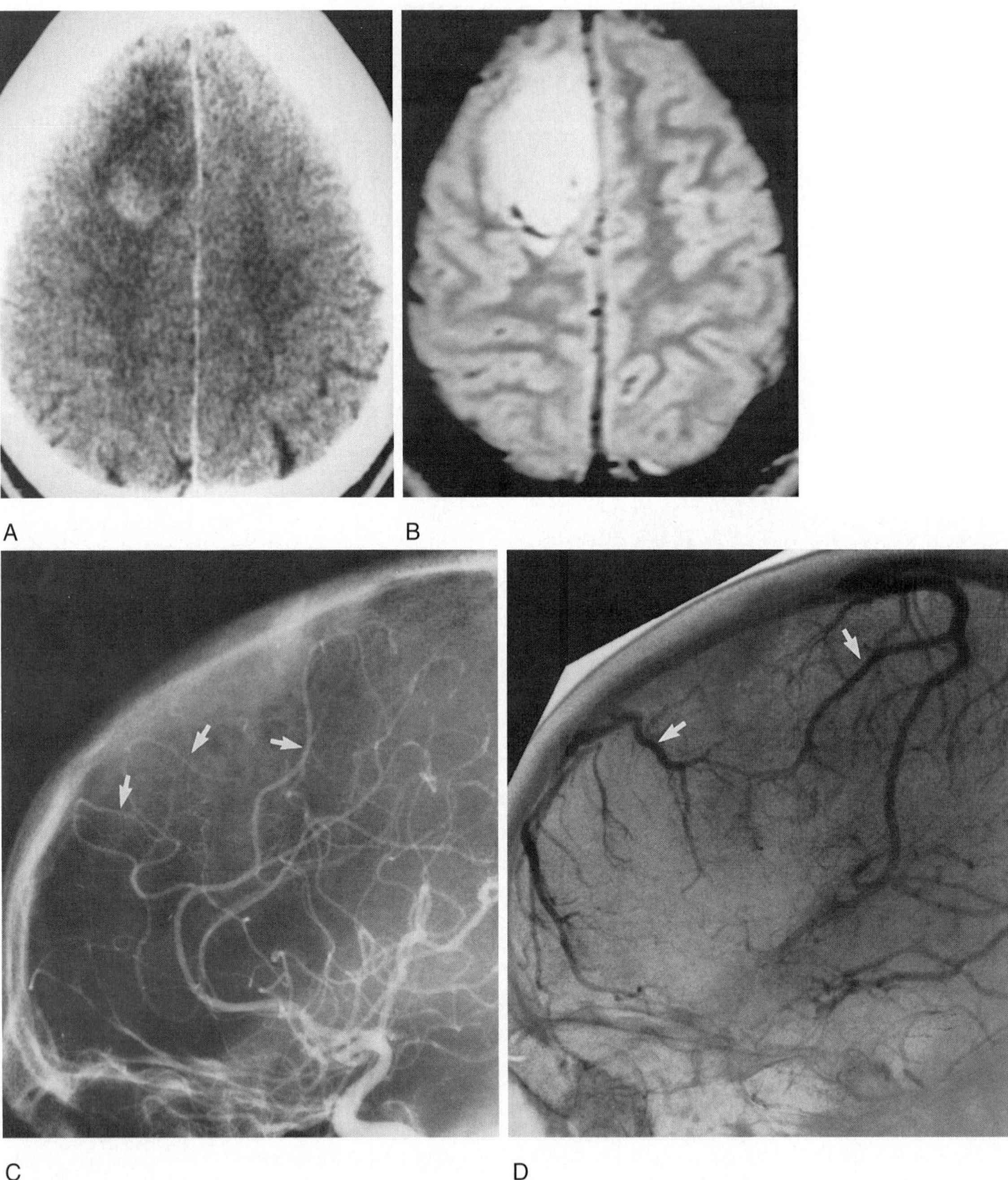

Figure 11.14. Right frontal, parasagittal glioma with partial enhancement indicating a zone of malignant degeneration. **A.** Axial CT postintravenous contrast image shows a low-attenuation area with enhancement of an area on the dorsal side. **B.** Proton density MR axial image shows a well-circumscribed hyperintense frontal mass. A flow void is seen on the dorsal aspect that may indicate hypervascularity of this portion of the tumor. **C** and **D.** An angiogram was carried out to determine tumor vascularity, and it demonstrated a vascular configuration very suggestive of an extracerebral mass (arrows) in the arterial (C) as well as in the venous phase (D); no tumor vascularity was seen. Surgical intervention revealed an intracerebral tumor, an astrocytoma with malignant changes.

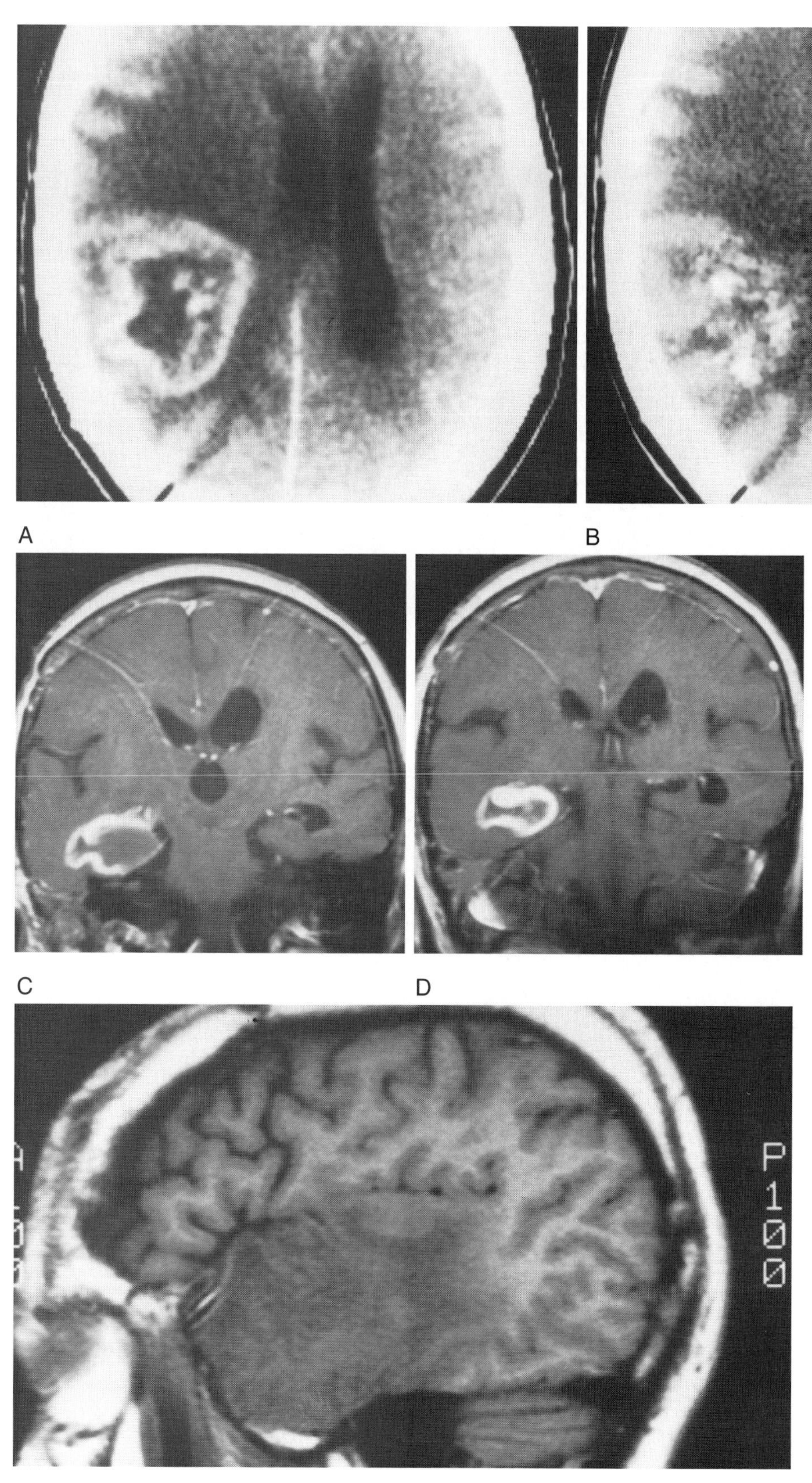

Figure 11.15. Glioblastoma. **A.** There is enhancement of a lesion in the right fronto-parietal region. The lesion is fairly well circumscribed and presents a central necrotic area with an irregular inner contour. The densities within the necrotic cavities represent calcification. There is considerable edema, involving about two-thirds of the hemisphere, and a midline shift to the opposite side. The septum pellucidum is well across the midline (about 12 mm). **B.** An image taken prior to contrast shows spotty calcifications in the tumor. Calcification can occur spontaneously in glioblastomas but occurs more frequently following radiation therapy. Note than in A there is an apparent hyperintensity of the gray matter gyri that may be due to the pronounced white matter edema, which increases the contrast between the two. This might have been attributed to hypervascularity or to relative loss of the blood-brain barrier related to the edema and the chronic compression of the convolutions. However, it is also seen in the noncontrast image (B). **C** and **D.** Another example of a glioblastoma in the parahippocampal gyrus–medial temporal lobe. Post-contrast MRI anterior (C) and more posterior (D) coronal views show the typically peripheral enhancement with the necrotic center containing high protein. Compare the hypointensity of the "cystic" space with the CSF in the ventricles. There is considerable edema of the temporal lobe with elevation of the sylvian fissure, less conspicuous in these T1-weighted images. **E.** Temporal malignant astrocytoma in another case. Non-contrast-enhanced sagittal T1-weighted MR image shows enlargement of the temporal lobe and elevation of the sylvian fissure.

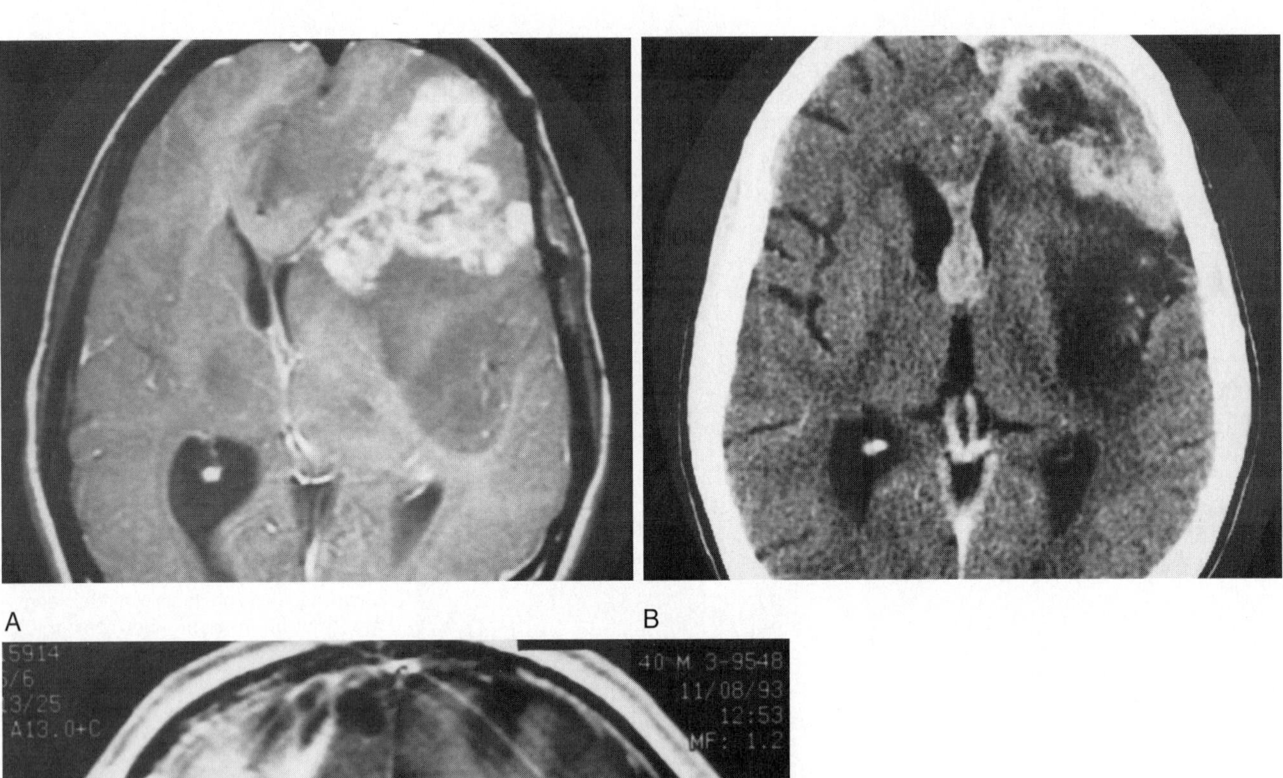

A

B

C

Figure 11.16. Frontal glioblastoma growing into the corpus callosum and septum pellucidum. **A.** Postcontrast T1-weighted axial MR image shows a large enhancing tumor with edema. There is some enhancement on the lateral aspect of the rostrum of the corpus callosum. The septum pellucidum is markedly shifted but thin. **B.** Three months later a CT postcontrast image shows an enhancing tumor and edema. There is also enhancement in the region of the septum pellucidum, a sure indication of corpus callosum involvement, not well shown at this time. The patient had received radiation therapy after A. **C.** Glioblastoma involving the corpus callosum and extending to the opposite medial frontal lobe (bifrontal tumor) in another patient. T1-weighted postcontrast image shows thickening of the septum pellucidum indicative of early involvement by tumor extension.

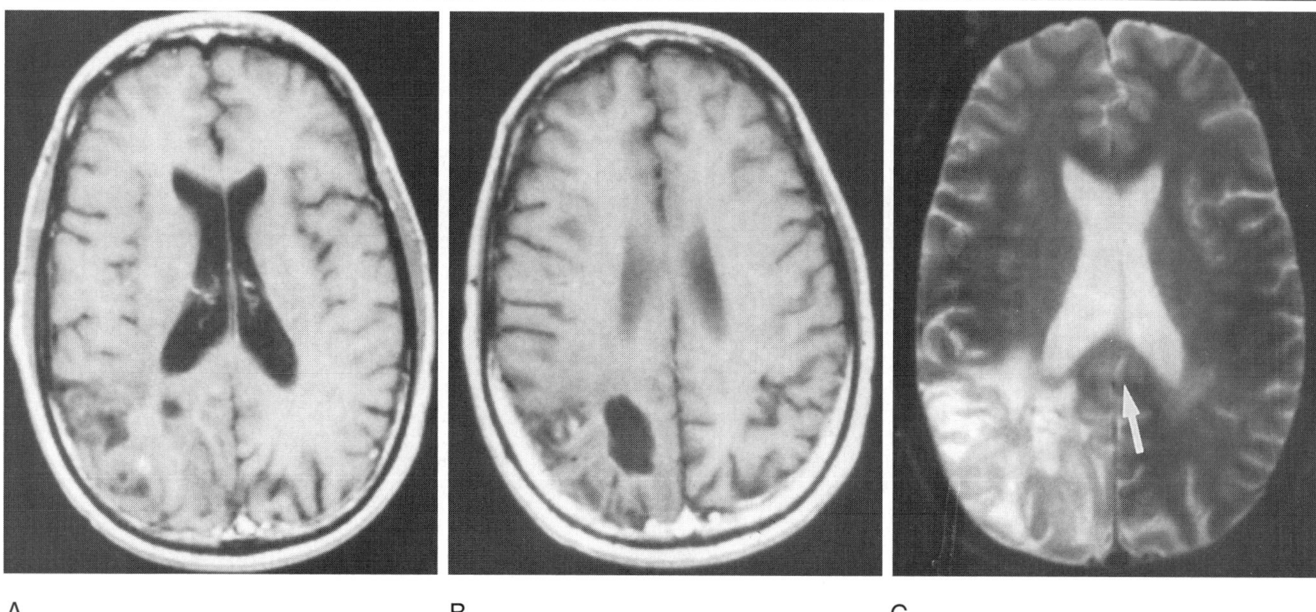

Figure 11.17. Malignant astrocytoma nonenhancing on MRI but involving the splenium of the corpus callosum. **A** and **B.** Postcontrast T1-weighted MR axial view shows no significant enhancement of this partly cystic parieto-occipital tumor. There is no midline shift, partly because of the far posterior location. The patient had previously undergone a partial resection, and this accounts for the marked enhancement of the dura on both sides in the posterior half of the brain. **C.** T2-weighted axial image shows the edema in the right parieto-occipital region. There is hyperintensity in the region of the splenium of the corpus callosum, which most likely represents early involvement by the tumor. Simple edema is not usually seen in the corpus callosum because of the closely packed myelinated nerve fibers. Thus the presence of hyperintensity (or hypodensity on CT) on proton density or T2-weighted images suggests actual involvement of the corpus callosum by the neoplasm (arrow).

volve the scalp and can metastasize to the lungs. This occurrence is very rare.

One of the most common paths of growth of malignant astrocytomas or glioblastomas is through the corpus callosum, most frequently in the frontal region following the forceps minor. This generates what is usually known as a *bifrontal tumor*. Less frequently a deep parietal glioblastoma will grow through the splenium of the corpus callosum (Figs. 11.16 and 11.17).

Glioblastomas may bleed spontaneously, and on MRI it is not uncommon to see foci of magnetic susceptibility compatible with old blood products. Sometimes the hemorrhage may be large, but usually it is focal and multicentric. Fluid levels may be seen in the cystic necrotic areas, which are partly composed of cell debris.

Glioblastomas may be multicentric (about 5 percent of cases, according to Russell and Rubinstein [4]). In the majority of examples the multiple tumors, usually two, are adjacent to each other, but sometimes they may be far apart and occasionally in opposite hemispheres (Figs. 11.18 and 11.19). From the point of view of imaging characteristics, the multicentric malignant gliomas are identical to the solitary ones.

Calcification is frequently seen on CT images of glioblastomas, particularly if they have been treated with radiation therapy (Fig. 11.15). The calcification may be heavy at times. MRI does not usually reveal the calcification, and sometimes the tumor enhancement seems to fall right in the area of calcification (Fig. 11.20). The calcification is probably occurring in a necrotic area of the tumor and probably does not have any prognostic significance.

Gliomas usually start in the white matter and tend to grow in the same area, later pushing and finally invading the gray matter. Sometimes, however, a glioma will start in the gyri. Under these circumstances it may be difficult to decide, on imaging alone, whether one is dealing with a tumor or another lesion, usually inflammatory, such as a focal viral encephalitis. Two such examples have come to the author's attention within the last 18 months, and both were initially diagnosed by MRI. In both cases there was enhancement of the involved cortical area (Figs. 11.21 and 11.22).

Sometimes astrocytomas can grow to a very large size before producing noticeable symptoms and signs. This is particularly true with children (Fig. 11.23).

Diffuse glioma (*gliomatosis cerebri*) represents a type of astrocytoma, not necessarily anaplastic, that does not produce a mass but infiltrates the entire brain. CT may be entirely negative or may show minor areas of edema with or without enhancement. MRI has a better chance of showing

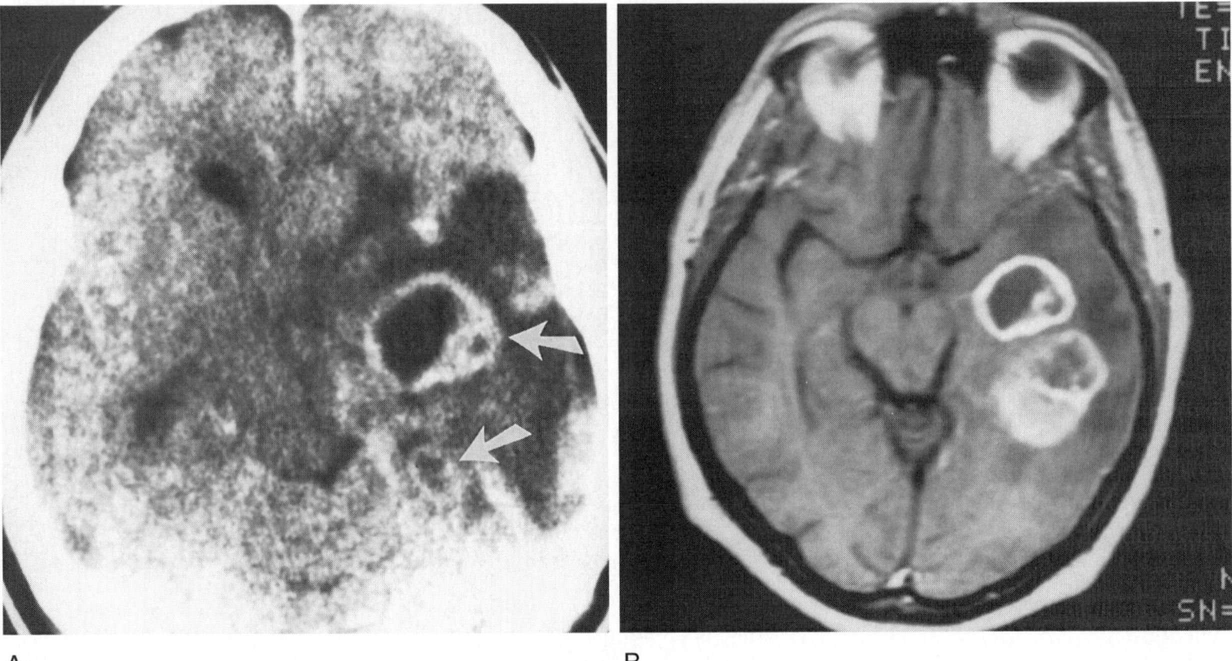

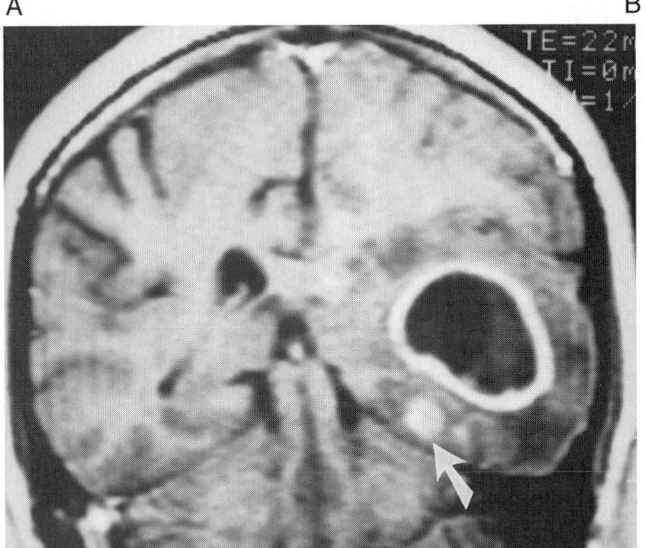

Figure 11.18. Multicentric glioblastomas. **A.** CT image after contrast demonstrates at least two foci of necrotic tumor in the mid and posterior left temporal lobe (arrow). There is considerable edema present. **B.** Postcontrast MR image shows the two nodules of tumor, which individually have the usual characteristics of a glioblastoma but may also be compatible with metastases. **C.** Coronal postcontrast MR image shows a third smaller nodule in the vicinity and below the larger tumor nodules (arrow). The very small hyperintense spot to the right of the nodule may be another small nodule of tumor. **D.** Cerebral angiography, performed to determine the degree of vascularity prior to surgery, revealed the expected elevation of the middle cerebral artery branches, deformation of the sylvian triangle, and elevation of the angiographic sylvian point. In addition, it demonstrated abnormal vascularity involving both larger nodular tumor areas, but they are not separated (arrows). **E.** Frontal view of left carotid angiogram demonstrates medial displacement of the middle cerebral branches in the sylvian fissure and elevation of the sylvian point (arrow), as well as a square midline shift of the anterior cerebral artery (arrows).

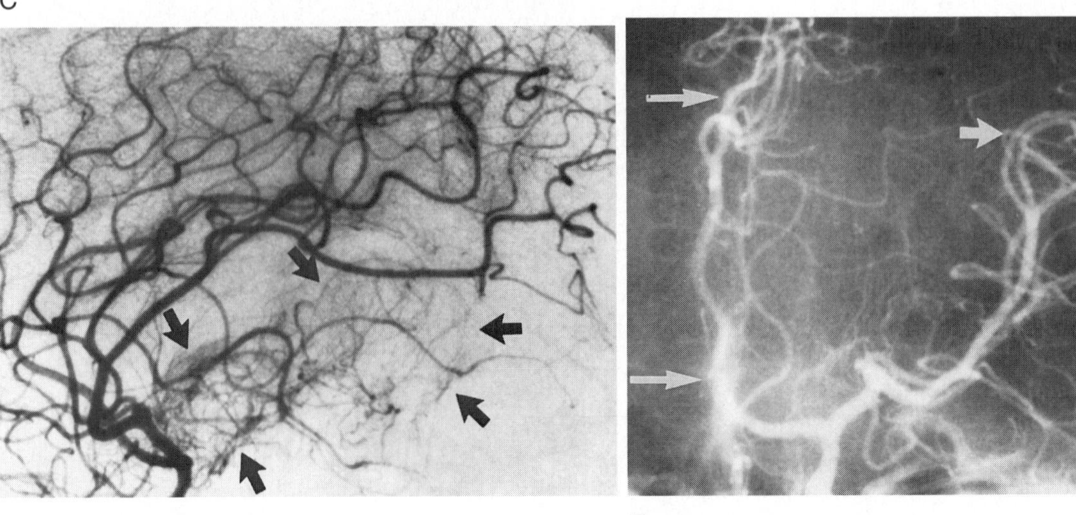

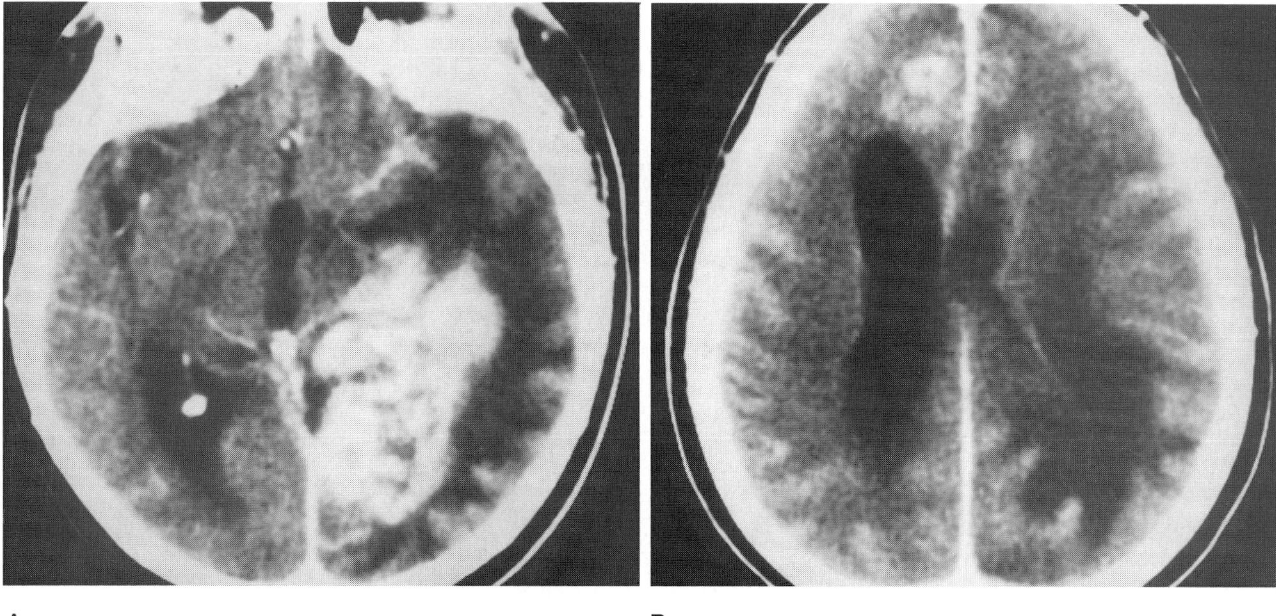

A B

Figure 11.19. Widely separated multicentric malignant astrocytomas (grade IV). **A** and **B.** Two large foci of high-grade glioma: one in the left temporo-occipital area, large, markedly enhancing, and deeply placed; and the other in the right anterior frontal area. This represents the exception in that the lesions are situated in both hemispheres, and multicentric malignant gliomas tend to be in the same hemisphere. There is also considerable edema around the larger lesion, as well as marked ventriculomegaly.

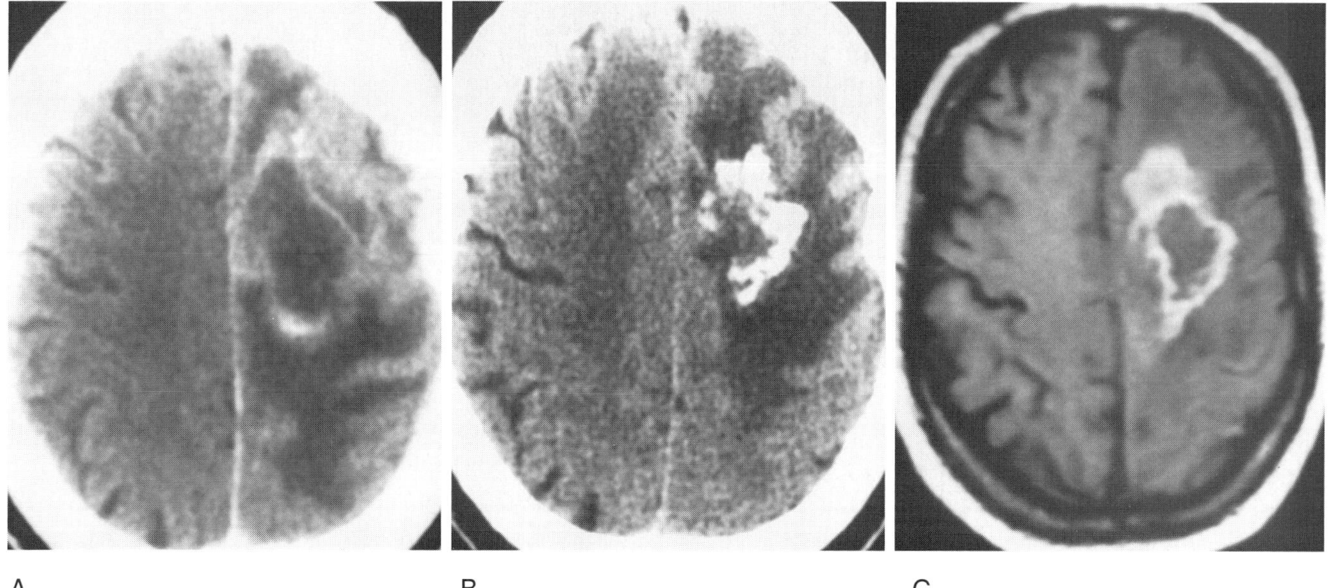

A B C

Figure 11.20. Calcified glioblastoma seen on CT but showing no calcium on MRI. **A.** Axial enhanced CT scan shows a large tumor with an irregular necrotic area. **B.** Nine months later, following treatment, a large area of calcification is seen presenting a shape that suggests that the calcium is located around a cavity. **C.** Postcontrast MR image shows that the extensive calcification is not seen; on the contrary, the area of enhancement seems to follow the calcified irregular, elliptical area. B and C were done within a day of each other.

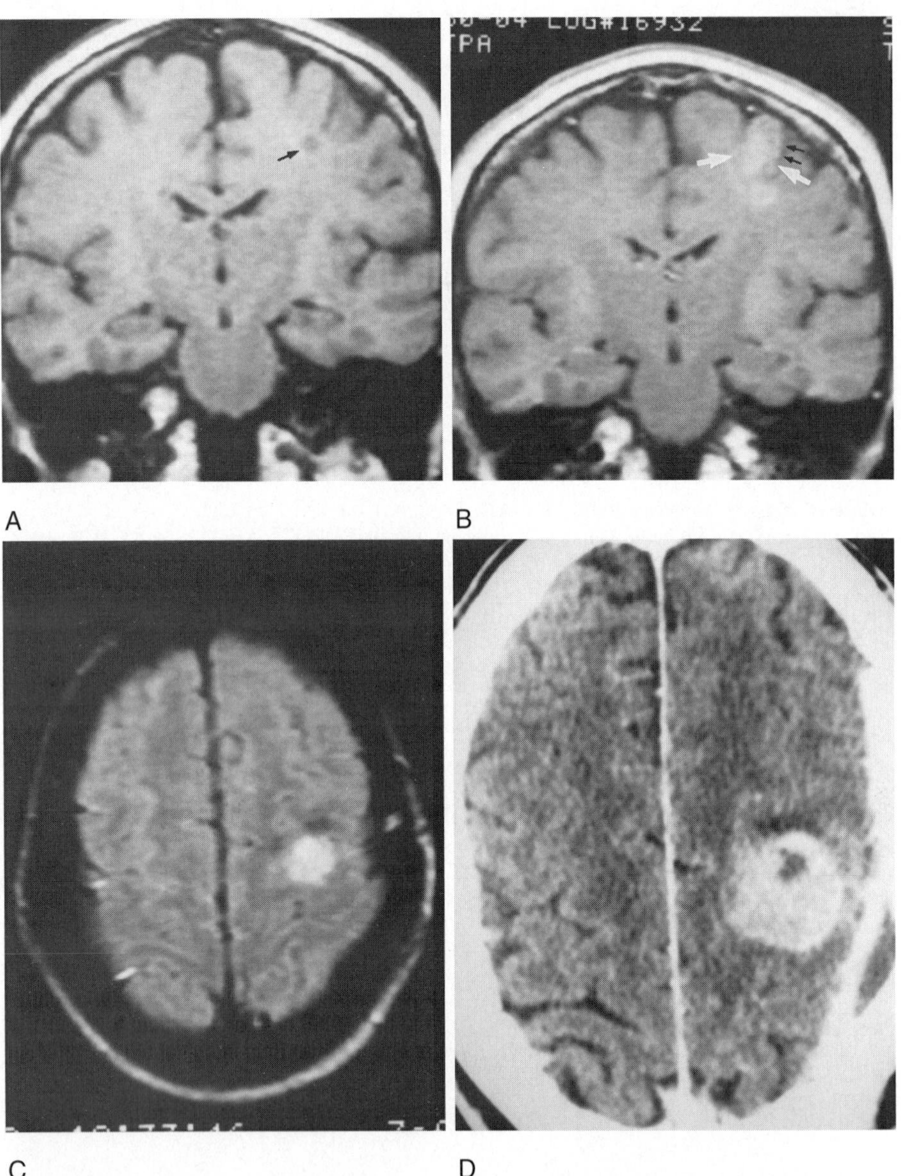

Figure 11.21. Malignant glioma starting in the gray matter in a 68-year-old woman presenting with seizures. **A** and **B.** T1-weighted coronal images. Precontrast image (A) shows only a rounded area of hypointensity (arrow). Postcontrast image (B) shows enhancement of the adjacent gyrus. **C.** Axial proton density image shows a hyperintense cortical lesion. **D.** CT scan with contrast performed 3 months later reveals a larger lesion with a necrotic area. Biopsy at this time showed a malignant glioma. Previously a possible inflammatory process was considered.

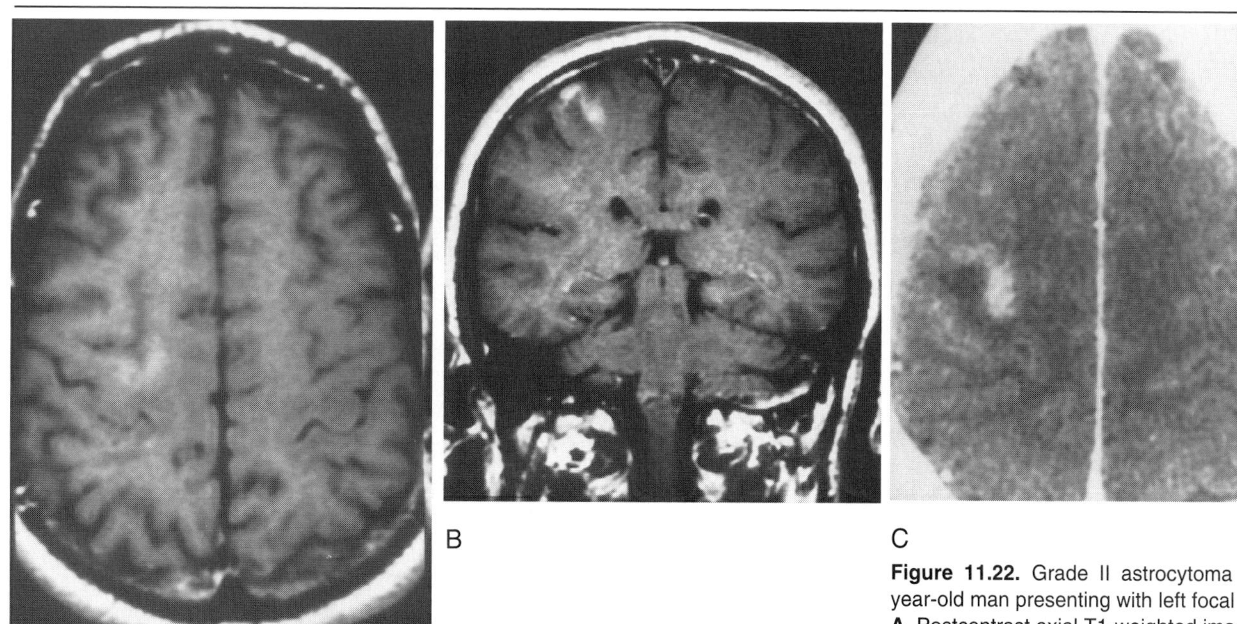

Figure 11.22. Grade II astrocytoma in a 45-year-old man presenting with left focal seizures. **A.** Postcontrast axial T1-weighted image shows an area of gyral enhancement in the right posterior frontal lobe in the precentral gyrus. **B.** Coronal T1-weighted postcontrast image confirms the cortical location of the gyral enhancement. **C.** CT postcontrast image also reveals the area of enhancement. Although a focal viral encephalitis could produce such a finding, it was decided to biopsy the lesion, which was classified histologically as a grade II astrocytoma.

changes consistent with edema because edema shows as hyperintensity (which is more conspicuous than hypointensity) on proton density and T2-weighted images. But even when changes are observed, the degree of involvement is underestimated when compared with the findings at postmortem examinations. The case shown in Figure 11.23 may represent the first variety of gliomatosis cerebri described by Russell and Rubinstein (4), in which the infiltrative tumor grows along the convolutions around the hemispheres without forming a mass. The second variety would be one in which there is pial and ependymal infiltration, giving rise to meningeal and ventricular gliomatosis. Gliomatosis cerebri is more common in younger adults and children.

Oligodendrogliomas are a relatively frequent hemispheric tumor. They usually grow slowly but can be more aggressive (survival with treatment is about 6 years from onset). They occur primarily in adults, with a peak incidence between 25 and 50 years of age. They are more frequent in males (about a 3:2 ratio). Of 6180 intracranial tumors of all types reported by Mǫrk et al. (30), 208 were oligodendrogliomas, an incidence of 3.4 percent, but if only intracerebral neoplasms are considered, the incidence approaches 5 percent. The majority occur in the frontal lobes (50 percent) and the rest in other lobes of the brain. Only a very small percentage occur within the ventricles or are primarily intraventricular (6 of 208) (Table 11.28).

The most important imaging characteristic of oligodendrogliomas is their tendency to calcify, and the calcium deposits are frequently heavy (Fig. 11.24). CT is usually necessary to suggest the diagnosis, for MRI may not show the calcium deposits. Only about 25 to 30 percent will show calcification on plain skull films (see Fig. 4.12); CT shows calcification much more commonly. If the patient survives long enough, calcification will probably develop in almost every instance.

The majority of oligodendrogliomas do not enhance (about 75 percent). The tumors that do enhance, as well as those that present a tumor blush on cerebral angiography, are usually more aggressive and indicate a shorter survival time. Of 181 tumors in the Mǫrk et al. series (30), 42

Table 11.28.
Oligodendrogliomas

Approximately 5% of intracerebral tumors
Peak age is the third to sixth decade
Frequently are seen to contain calcification on CT imaging
Often do not contrast-enhance

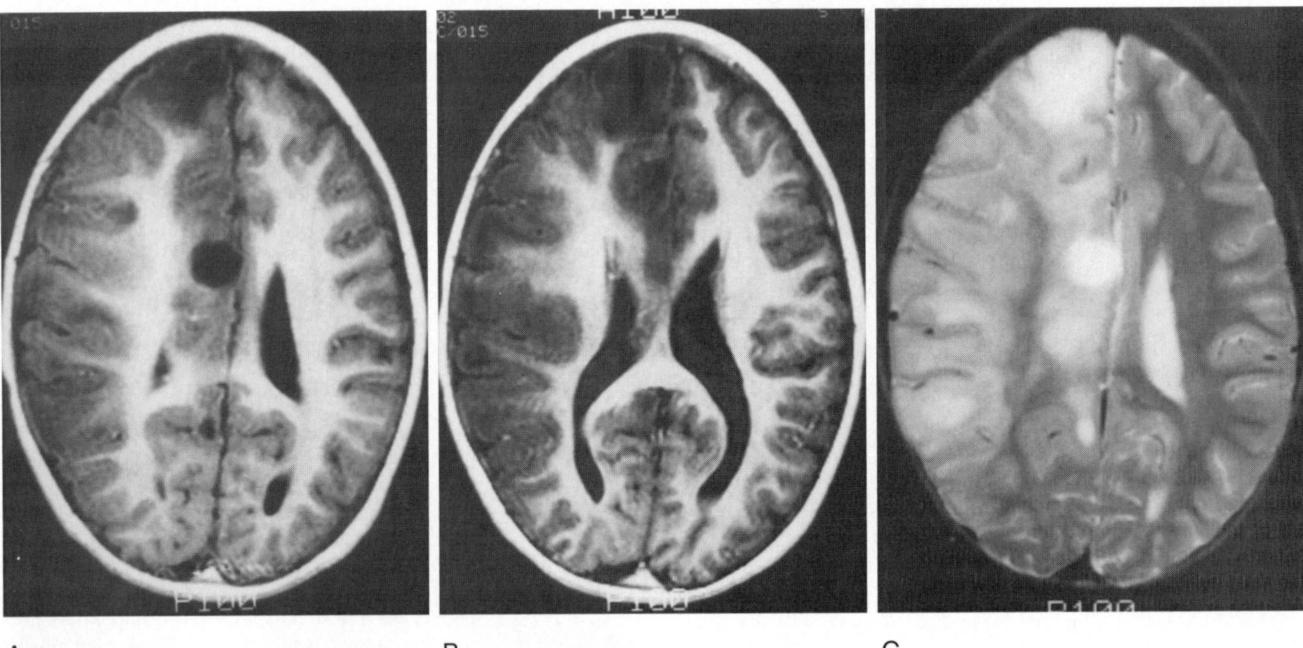

A B C

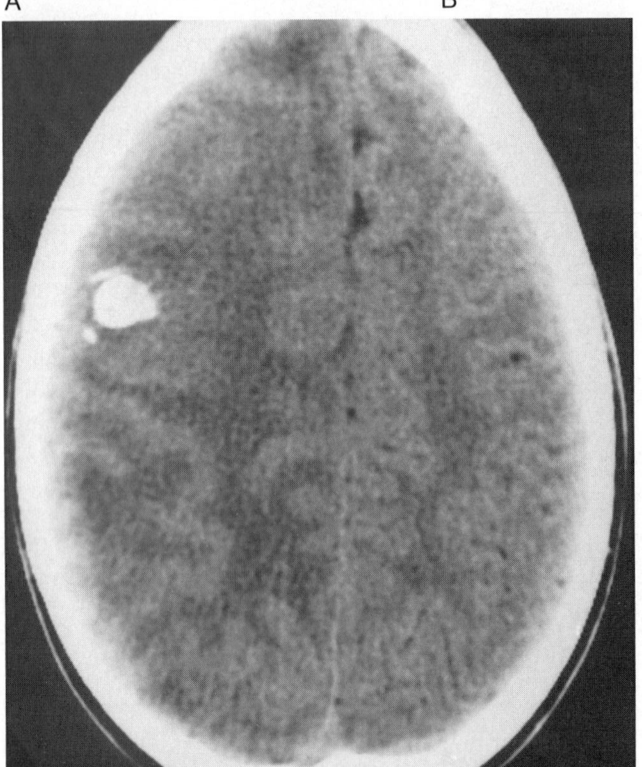

D

Figure 11.23. Astrocytoma involving practically the whole hemisphere in a 10-year-old girl presenting after a few episodes of facial twitching and a negative neurologic examination. **A** and **B.** MR axial T1-weighted (inversion recovery) image reveals an appearance that was at first glance thought to be congenital because of the pachygyric appearance of the cortex on the right side. There are two cystic areas in the frontal pole and in the parasagittal region. **C.** T2-weighted axial image shows white matter diffuse hyperintensity, which favored an active process, most probably diffuse neoplasm. **D.** CT examination was then performed. It confirmed the findings and also demonstrated a zone of heavy calcification unsuspected in the MRI examination. In spite of the enormous size of the abnormality, there was no midline shift. Biopsy demonstrated a grade II astrocytoma. A diagnosis of pachygyria was entertained on the basis of the MRI, the absence of midline shift, and the essentially negative neurologic examination, but the calcified portion seen on CT more strongly suggested a diagnosis of neoplasm.

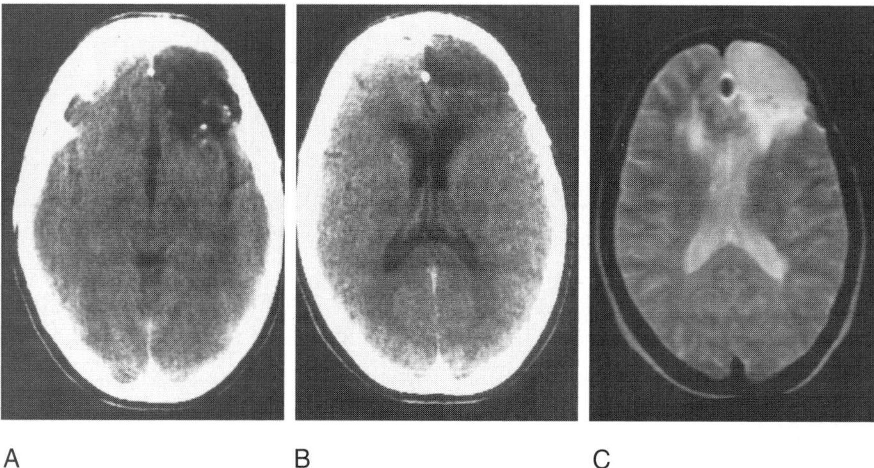

Figure 11.24. Oligodendroglioma showing postoperative changes. **A** and **B.** CT image shows a low-density left frontal area consistent with fluid density and several areas of calcification on the medial and posterior aspects. **C.** T2-weighted image shows the medial calcified area as a hypointense area, consistent with calcium, surrounded by a hyperintense, thin halo. The residual tumor on the dorsal side is more hyperintense than the cystic fluid, which is situated anteriorly.

were hypervascular and had a shorter survival time (3.5 years as against 7 years for the nonvascular group).

Neuroblastomas occur in the cerebral hemispheres, usually in children or adolescents and occasionally in young adults. They are included in the group of PNETs. They grow rapidly and often acquire a large size. Calcification is common (probably over 50 percent of cases) and sometimes heavy; they enhance with contrast on CT or MRI (Fig. 11.25). They may seed via the CSF, particularly if they invade the ventricles. Distant metastases can occur (31) (Table 11.29).

A variety of neuroblastoma occurs in the ventricles that has received the name of *central neurocytoma* (see text following). *Gangliogliomas* are also hemispheric tumors that occur usually in children and young adults (60 percent of the cases). They are composed of well-differentiated but

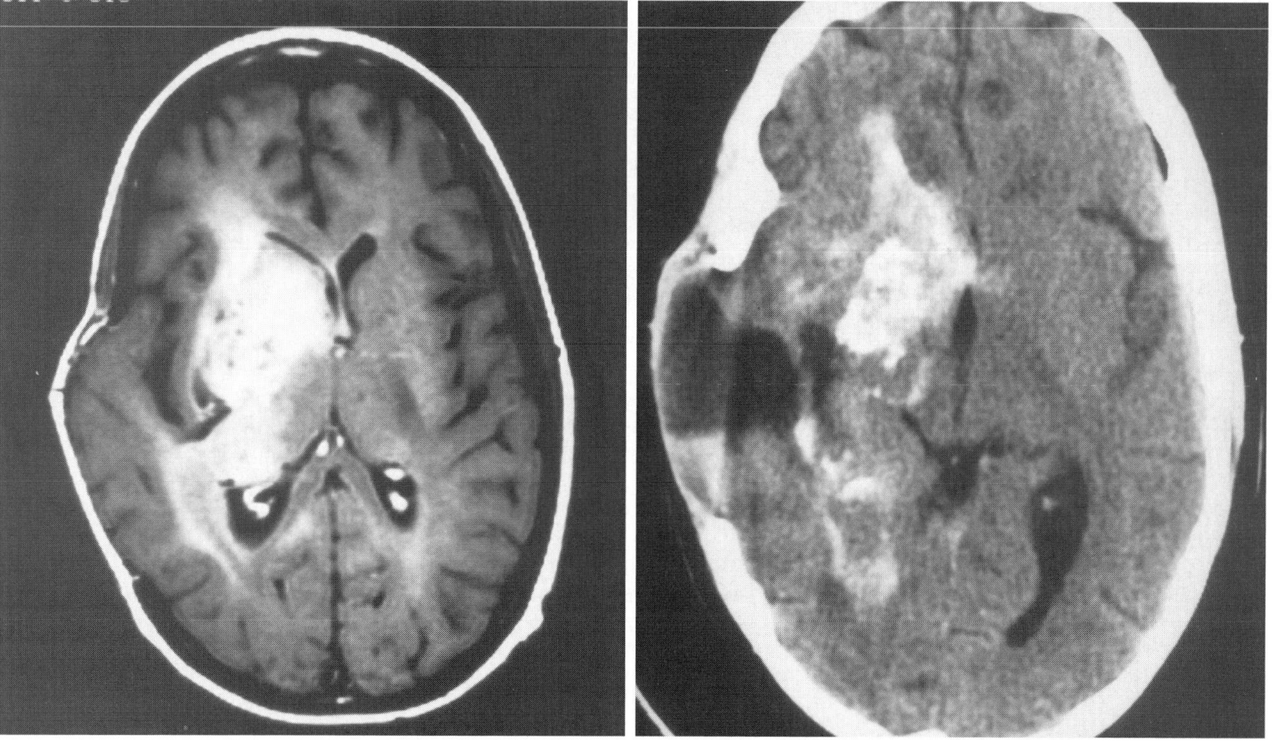

Figure 11.25. Neuroblastoma, primitive neuroectodermal tumor (PNET), in a 21-year-old woman. **A.** Postcontrast image shows marked enhancement of the lesion. **B.** CT examination performed 6 months later following radiation and chemotherapy shows extensive calcification in the tumor, postoperative atrophic changes, and some residual mass effect. Most PNETs will show calcification.

Table 11.29.
Neuroblastomas

Usually occur in children and adolescents
One form of primitive neuroectodermal tumor
Often very large in size and frequently calcified
One form (central neurocytoma) occurs within cerebral ventricle

Table 11.30.
Gangliogliomas

Majority occur in children and young adults
Typically well differentiated and slow growing
Usually very little or no edema and little mass effect
Many do not contrast-enhance

atypical neuronal elements and glial cells. They are slowly growing and often present with seizures and no focal signs (Table 11.30). Of the four cases reported by Benitez et al. (32), two were in the temporal lobe and two in the parietal lobe, but they may also occur in the cerebellum, brainstem, and spinal cord, as well as in any of the lobes of the brain, in the thalamus, and in the third-ventricular wall (33). They often calcify (three of the four cases of Benitez et al.) and usually present no (or little) edema around the tumor. They may not enhance with contrast. The terms *ganglioneuroma*, *gangliocytoma*, and *ganglioneuroblastoma* have been applied to histologic variants of this tumor, but the original description and terminology of Perkins (34) and Courville (35) still remain the most appropriate.

A rare tumor is the *melanotic neuroectodermal tumor of infancy*, a rapidly growing tumor that most frequently involves facial structures, including the mandible. It can also occur intracranially. One of the six cases reported by Mirich et al. occurred in the posterior fossa and produced a hyperdense tumor on nonenhanced CT; it also inhanced markedly (36). Another case involved the parietal bone and the cerebral hemisphere. Clinically, the tumor is dark be-

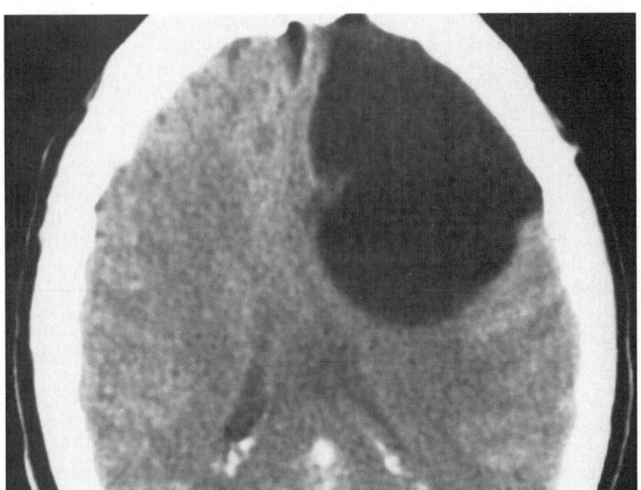

A

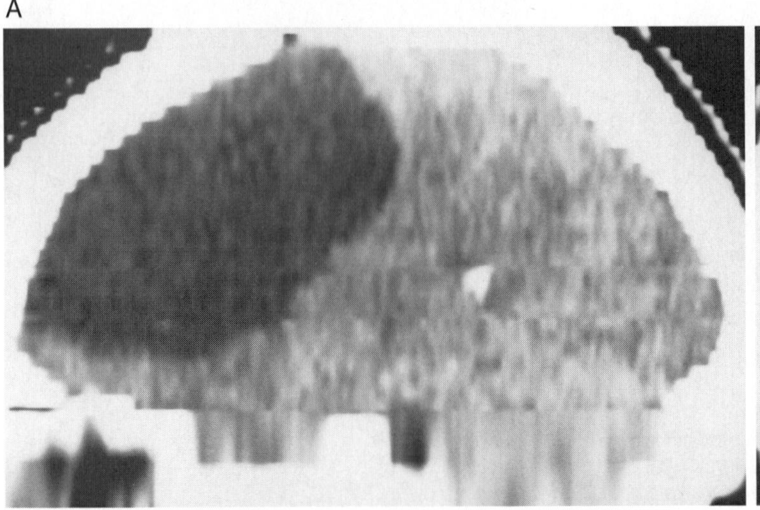

B

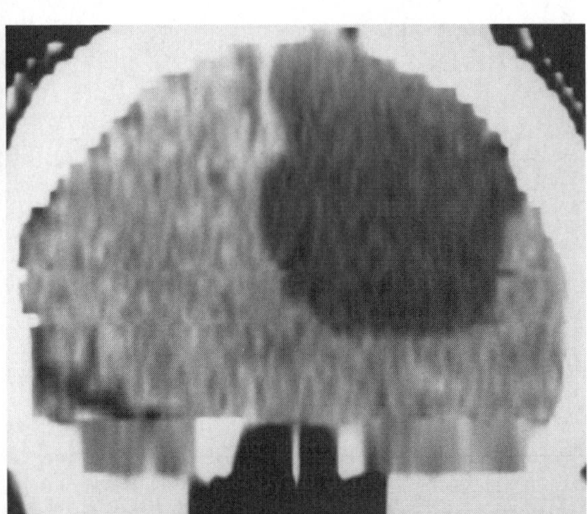

C

Figure 11.26. Hemispheric arachnoid cyst. **A.** Axial CT image shows a CSF-type density compressing and displacing the lateral ventricles to the opposite side; there is also posterior displacement of the brain cortex. The outline is sharp, and there is nothing to suggest tumor nodules. Sagittal (**B**) and coronal (**C**) reformatted images reveal no evidence of tumor nodules, and there is no enhancement. In addition, the external surface is against the inner skull table, with no suggestion of intervening soft tissue.

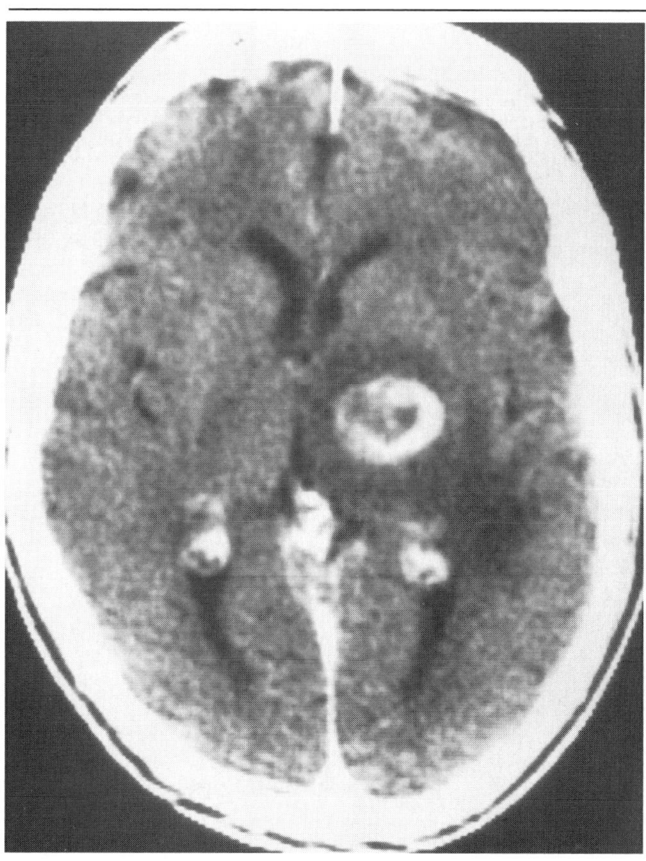

Figure 11.27. Thalamic tumor. CT postcontrast axial image shows a hyperdense mass in the left thalamic region surrounded by a hypointense halo. There is compression of the third ventricle, which is displaced to the opposite side.

cause it is rich in melanin. If it is diagnosed and treated early, a cure is possible.

Other solid hemispheric lesions may suggest neoplasm and must be differentiated. Among these are granulomatous lesions such as tuberculomas, chronic fungal infections, syphilitic gumma, and parasitic infestations. A rare mass effect may be produced by an amyloidoma (37).

Arachnoid cysts can produce hemispheric masses, sometimes large. They must be differentiated from cystic tumors. The most important characteristics of the arachnoid cysts are that their contents are identical to CSF, there is no enhancement of the cyst wall, there is no tumor nodule around the wall, and the mass effect is proportionately less than its size would suggest (Fig. 11.26; see also Figs. 5.38 to 5.40).

Metastatic neoplasms represent a large group of hemispheric tumors and are discussed in text following under "Multiple Intracerebral Tumors" along with primary brain lymphomas.

Thalamic Tumors

The thalamic location represents an area of transition between what we are classifying as hemispheric and midline locations. The tumors appear to arise from the thalamus rather than from the adjacent corpus striatum because of the relationship of the mass to the posterior portion of the third ventricle and the posterior limb of the internal capsule, as seen on CT or MRI (Figs. 11.27 to 11.29). The majority of these tumors are high-grade astrocytomas, and the life expectancy is relatively short (6 to 24 months), with some patients living several years. Quite commonly they extend to the opposite side via the massa intermedia (adhesio interthalamica) without violating the ependymal lining (Fig. 11.29). Thalamic tumors tend to grow toward the brainstem, and it is important to look at the cerebral peduncles in the midbrain sections to ascertain whether downward growth has already occurred. Brainstem tumors may extend into the thalamus. Partlow et al. emphasize the frequency of personality change or dementia in patients with bithalamic tumors (38).

Corpus Callosum Tumors

These tumors are usually gliomas starting in the corpus callosum and growing within it. They may stay mostly in the corpus callosum or may grow into the adjacent hemisphere. Most of them are high-grade gliomas and have a poor prognosis (Fig. 11.30). More frequently, the tumor is a hemispheric glioma, usually frontal, that grows into the rostrum of the corpus callosum. It often traverses the corpus callosum and grows on the other side, following the forceps minor fibers to become a *bifrontal glioma.* This feature is taken as a sign of poor prognosis (Fig. 11.30).

Lymphomas may also occur in the corpus callosum, along with other areas of the brain.

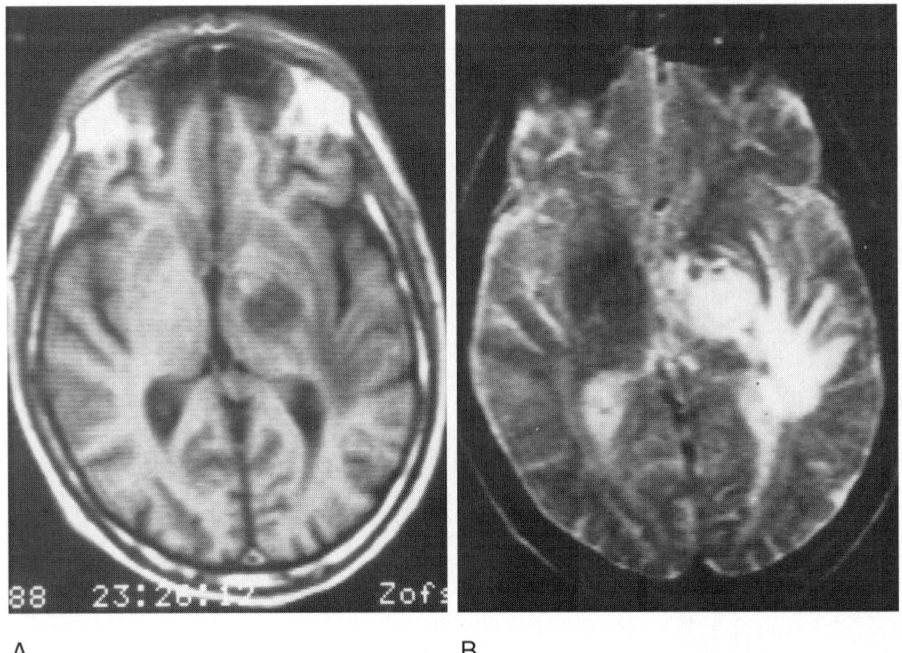

Figure 11.28. Thalamic tumor. **A.** Axial T1-weighted image reveals a hypointense area in the left thalamus. There is evidence of mild mass effect, and there is moderate edema around the low-intensity area lateral to it. The edema is much more conspicuous in the T2-weighted image (**B**). Note the fingerlike extension of edema following the external capsule and the gyral white matter. Same case as Figure 11.27.

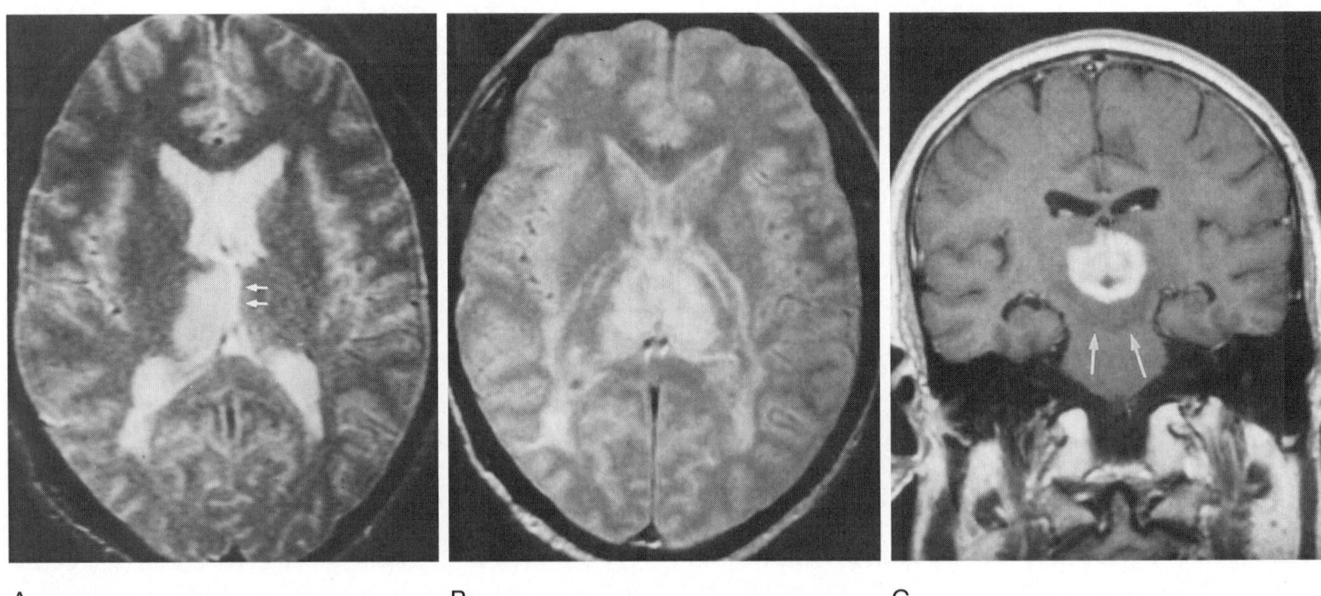

A B C

Figure 11.29. Thalamic tumor later extending to the opposite side in a 38-year-old man. **A.** T2-weighted axial MR image reveals a hyperintense bright thalamic mass. There is very little edema present in this instance. The third ventricle is flattened and displaced to the opposite side (arrows). **B.** Reexamination 9 months later shows that the tumor has extended to the other side. **C.** Coronal postcontrast T1-weighted image shows marked enhancement of tumor and some surrounding edema extending to the midbrain (arrows).

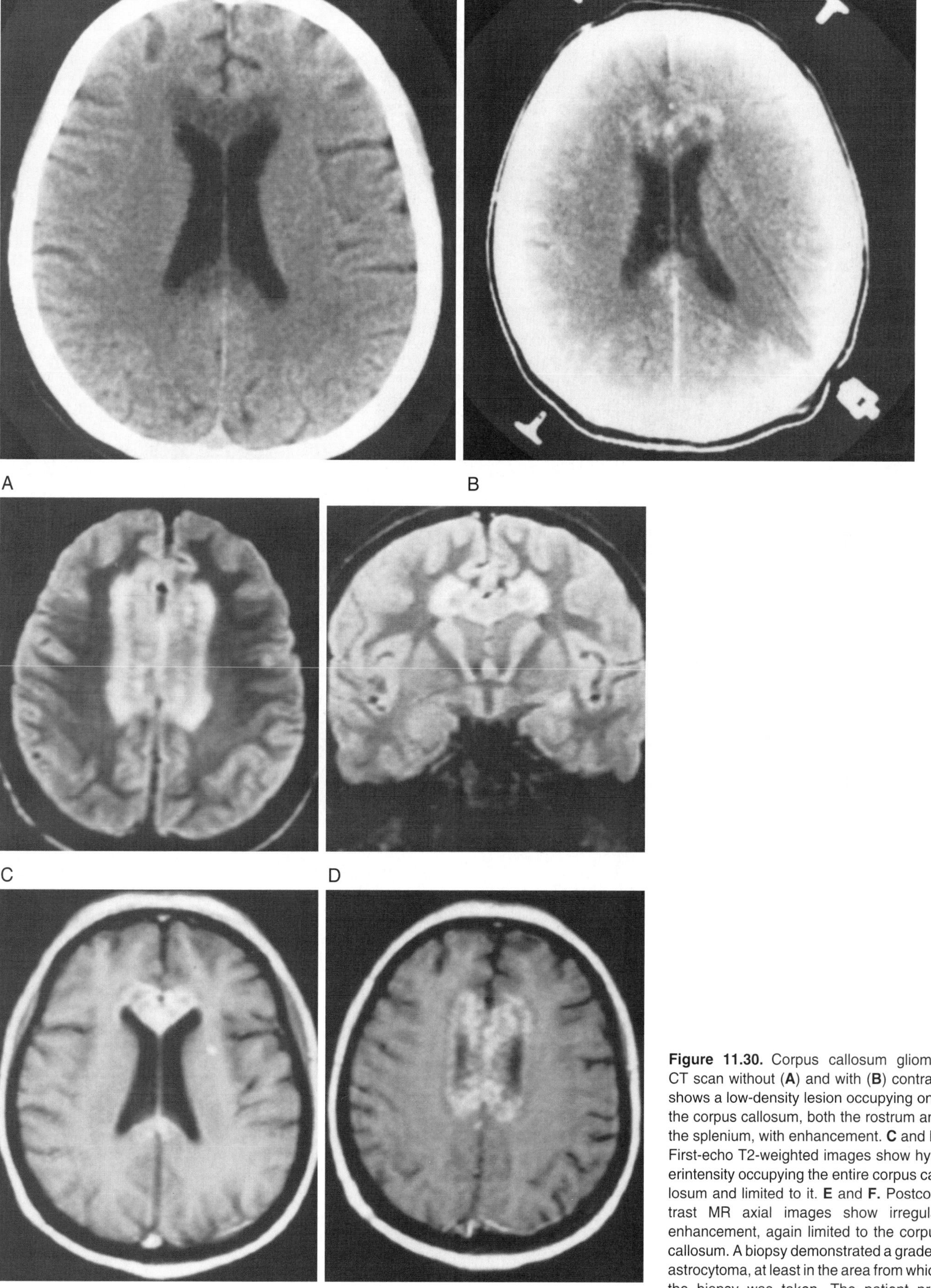

Figure 11.30. Corpus callosum glioma. CT scan without (**A**) and with (**B**) contrast shows a low-density lesion occupying only the corpus callosum, both the rostrum and the splenium, with enhancement. **C** and **D**. First-echo T2-weighted images show hyperintensity occupying the entire corpus callosum and limited to it. **E** and **F.** Postcontrast MR axial images show irregular enhancement, again limited to the corpus callosum. A biopsy demonstrated a grade II astrocytoma, at least in the area from which the biopsy was taken. The patient progressed rapidly to severe disability.

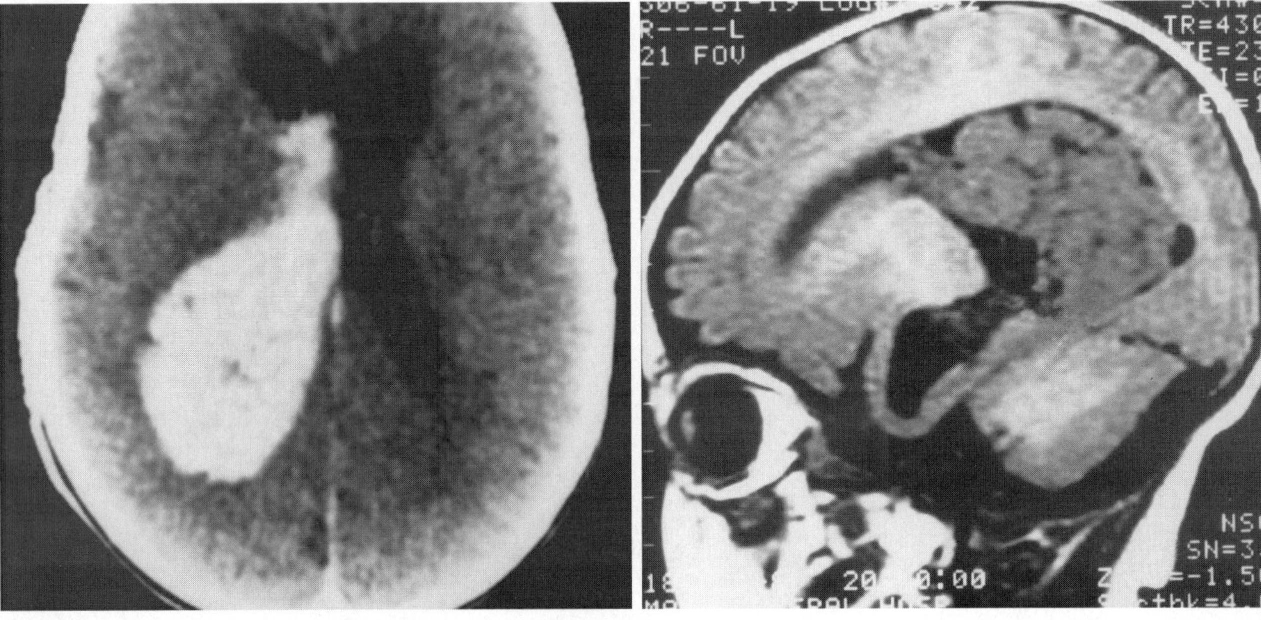

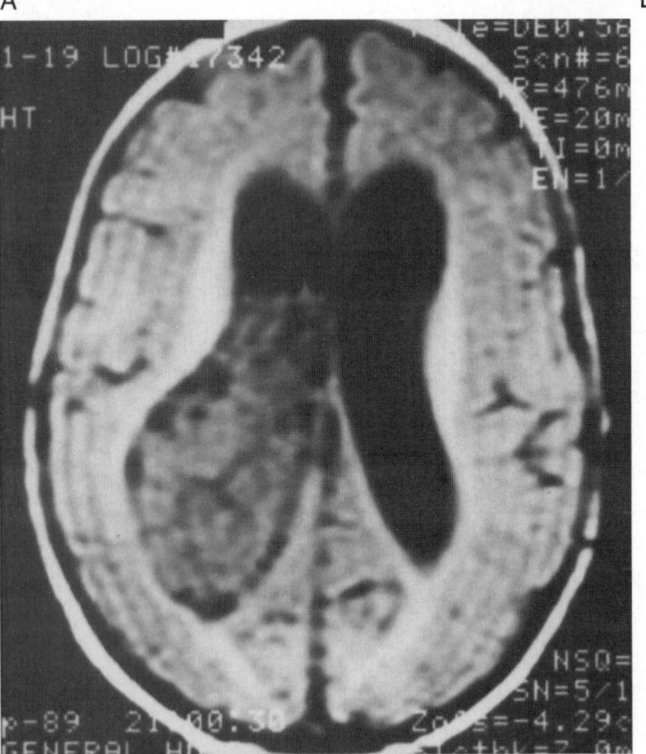

Figure 11.31. Choroid plexus papilloma in 3-month-old male infant. **A.** CT scan after contrast shows a strongly enhancing intraventricular mass in the atrium of the right lateral ventricle. **B.** T1-weighted sagittal view shows the position of the irregular, cauliflowerlike mass. **C.** Axial T1-weighted image shows a similar configuration to that shown on CT. Most choroid plexus papillomas in young children arise from the region of the choroid plexus glomus in the lateral ventricles.

SUPRATENTORIAL INTRAVENTRICULAR TUMORS

Histologically these tumors arise from the ependyma, the choroid plexus, and the pineal, from neuropithelial cells, and from cell nests of embryologic origin.

Intraventricular tumors are more common in children and young adults. The tumors may be primary, originating entirely within the ventricle, or may result from invasion of a neoplasm that arose outside the ventricles. In the supratentorial region the ependymal lining acts as a deterrent to tumor invasion, and even glioblastomas do not grow into the cavity of the lateral or third ventricles as frequently as one might expect in such a malignant tumor. In the posterior fossa, invasion of the fourth ventricle by medulloblastomas is more common (Table 11.31).

Choroid plexus papillomas usually arise from the glomus of the choroid plexus but occasionally may arise from the plexus more anteriorly or from the choroid plexus of the third-ventricular roof. They occur primarily in children and are rare at a more advanced age. They are most frequently histologically benign, and for that reason the term

Table 11.31.
Intraventricular Tumors

Choroid plexus papillomas: Often associated with hydrocephalus and grow to a large size
Ependymomas: Usually in the fourth ventricle and in children; Supratentorial intraventricular ependymomas frequently also involve adjacent brain
Subependymomas: Usually seen in the fourth ventricle in elderly males
Meningiomas: A small minority are intraventricular, usually in the atrium of the lateral ventricle
Oligodendrogliomas: Approximately 2 to 3% are intraventricular
Subependymal giant cell tumors: Occur at foramen of Monro in tuberous sclerosis patients

choroid plexus papilloma is ordinarily applied to them. They usually present an irregular contour within the enlarged ventricle containing the neoplasm. Characteristically, a tumor within a ventricle causes enlargement of that ventricle, usually a local enlargement. In the case of choroid papilloma, however, there appears to be overproduction of CSF. This leads to generalized dilatation of the ventricles, a communicating type of hydrocephalus (Fig. 11.31).

Cells from a choroid papilloma may seed elsewhere in the subarachnoid space of the neuraxis even though they are not malignant.

The tumor can grow to a rather large size. It may present hemorrhagic areas, and in fact red blood cells are frequently detected by lumbar puncture. Spotty calcifications occur at times. In a child the typical location of the tumor in the atrium of the lateral ventricle, along with communicating

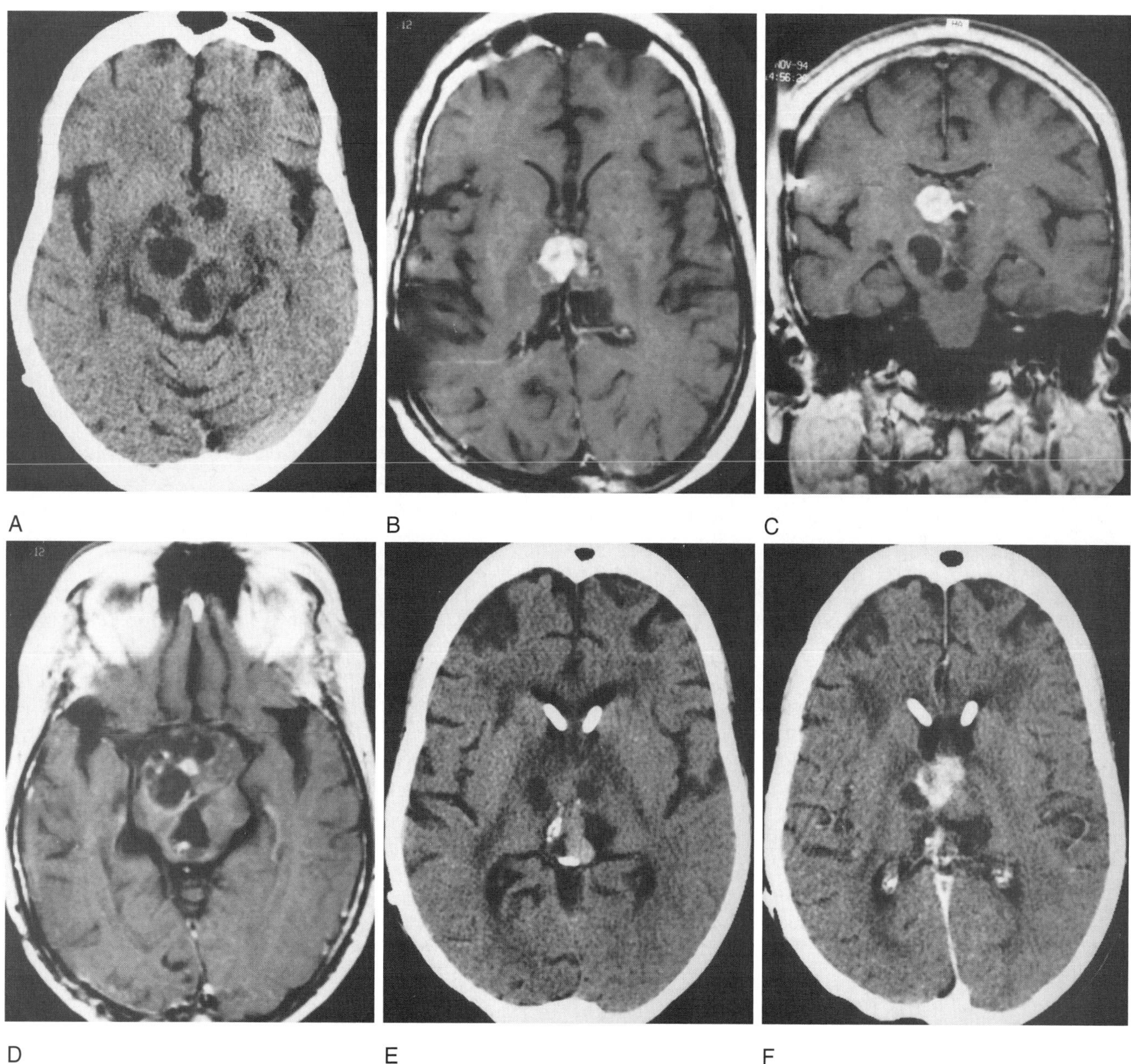

Figure 11.32. Third ventricle ependymoma with cystic changes extending into the brainstem. **A.** CT without contrast enhancement reveals irregular cystic spaces in the midbrain and in the lower aspect of the third ventricle. **B** and **C.** Axial MRI after contrast reveals an enhancing mass in the midline in the region of the third ventricle but extending toward the right side outside the ventricle. **D.** Enhanced axial image reveals small nodules in the walls of the cysts. Bilateral ventricular shunts were installed to correct the ventricular obstruction. **E.** and **F.** CT reexamination 4 months later shows calcification in areas of the tumor and tumor enhancement after contrast.

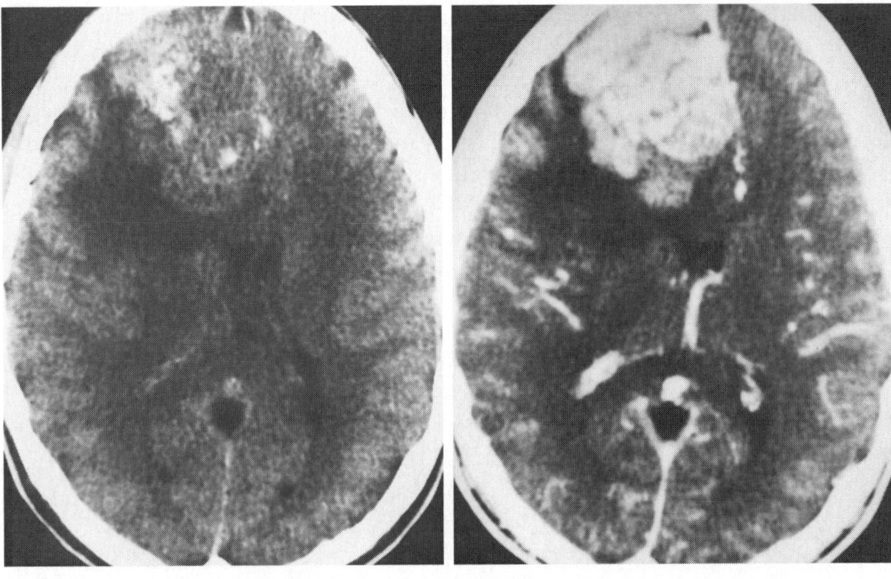

Figure 11.33. Extraventricular ependymoma in a 25-year-old man complaining of 3 months of headaches and 3 to 4 weeks of blurred vision and neck stiffness. **A.** Nonenhanced CT shows a tumor with irregular calcifications extending to the ventricular wall. **B.** Postcontrast CT shows a nodular enhancing lesion, which flattens the frontal horn of the lateral ventricle and is surrounded by edema. There is moderate midline shift to the left, and the shift is more pronounced anteriorly. The falx is also shifted. The tumor probably arose from the frontal horn but was almost totally extraventricular.

hydrocephalus, is almost diagnostic of choroid plexus papilloma. Malignant choroid tumors (choroid carcinoma) also occur, and these are more likely to seed via the CSF (Fig. 11.106).

Ependymomas are much less common in the lateral and third ventricles than in the fourth ventricle. Although they may grow directly into the ventricular cavity, they commonly grow out from the ventricular wall into the adjacent brain tissue (39). Ependymomas tend to calcify in an irregular manner (about 50 percent of the supratentorial group), and this is a good differential diagnostic point. Some are partly cystic. Ependymomas usually enhance after contrast (Figs. 11.32 and 11.33). See text following on posterior fossa tumors for further details.

Subependymomas occur mostly in the fourth ventricle (about 70 percent of cases), grow intraventricularly, and tend to have an extraventricular component but are noninvasive and can be completely removed. They occur more frequently in males from the fifth to the eighth decade. They may demonstrate minimal enhancement after contrast (40).

Choroid plexus cysts are not rare; they occur in the glomus of the choroid plexus and occupy the atrium of the ventricle, which always enlarges to accommodate the cyst. The appearance can be disturbing, particularly in a child, because the ventricle on the same side may be larger, more so in the atrial region, and if the child complains of headache it may be difficult to deny a possible relationship. Typically, the choroid plexus cyst is partly surrounded by choroid plexus (Fig. 11.34). The density of the fluid is identical to CSF on CT and MRI. MRI is a more useful examination because of the possibility of obtaining images in several planes (41). Czervionke et al. reported some cases of neuroepithelial cysts of the lateral ventricles, one of which was proven surgically, that on the published MRI and CT images have a similar appearance to that shown on Figure 11.34 (42). They are probably the same entity.

Meningiomas occur within the ventricles, most commonly in the lateral ventricles but also occasionally in the third and fourth ventricles. They arise either from the tela choroidea or from the stroma of the choroid plexus and tend to grow to a fairly large size before they are discovered.

Intraventricular meningiomas may show psammomatous calcification in a homogeneous manner or in spotty and granular depositions. Although they tend to occur in the region of the atrium of the lateral ventricles, they may be found elsewhere in the lateral ventricles as well as in the third and fourth ventricles. Intraventricular meningiomas enhance following contrast administration, and the enhancement tends to be fairly homogeneous. They may occur in children as well as in adults, and the diagnosis can be suggested if the above features are encountered in an intraventricular mass that is usually smoothly lobulated (Fig. 11.35).

Oligodendrogliomas can occur in the ventricles (6 of the Mørk et al. 208 cases [30]). They tend to occur in the anterior half of the lateral ventricles. The imaging characteristics are similar to those of the hemispheric oligodendrogliomas, but in the cases reported by Ribeiro et al. the tumors were hyperdense on CT images in relation to brain density (43); calcification may be seen (about 50 percent) (Fig. 11.36). Three of the 4 cases of Ribeiro et al. enhanced with contrast.

Histologically, the tumor has an appearance very similar to the recently recognized *central neurocytoma*, which is a variant of the neuroblastoma that may occur within the ventricles. Electron microscopy to detect neuronal differ-

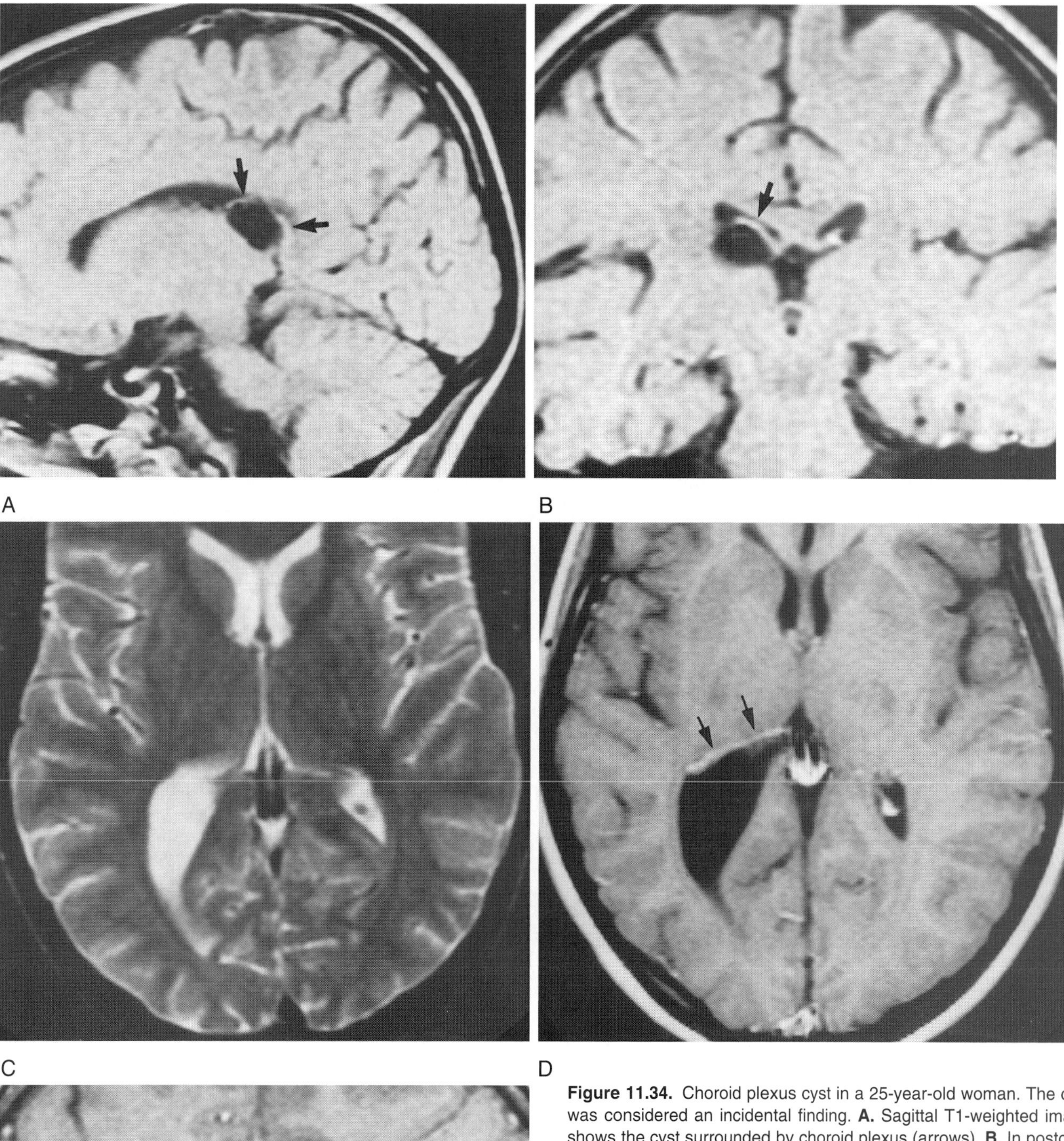

Figure 11.34. Choroid plexus cyst in a 25-year-old woman. The cyst was considered an incidental finding. **A.** Sagittal T1-weighted image shows the cyst surrounded by choroid plexus (arrows). **B.** In postcontrast coronal T1-weighted images, the enhanced choroid plexus is again seen surrounding the upper margin of the cyst (arrow). Another incidental finding is a partially empty sella in A. **C.** T2-weighted axial image demonstrates the enlargement of the atrium and occipital horn. The right frontal ventricular area is slightly larger than the left. (Courtesy of Dr. Eugenio Suran, Boston, Mass.) **D.** Another choroid plexus cyst in a 13-year-old girl. The displaced choroid plexus is evident (arrows). Postcontrast T1-weighted image. **E.** Postcontrast coronal view shows the glomus of the choroid plexus displaced laterally. The wall of the cyst is seen separate from the ventricular cavity, slightly enhanced with contrast (arrow). The girl was complaining of intermittent headaches. Follow-up examination 9 months later showed no change. The cyst contents are identical to the CSF in the ventricles. In this instance the ventricle over the cyst is significantly enlarged and raises the question of a surgical intervention, but this would not be considered unless there were evidence of growth.

E

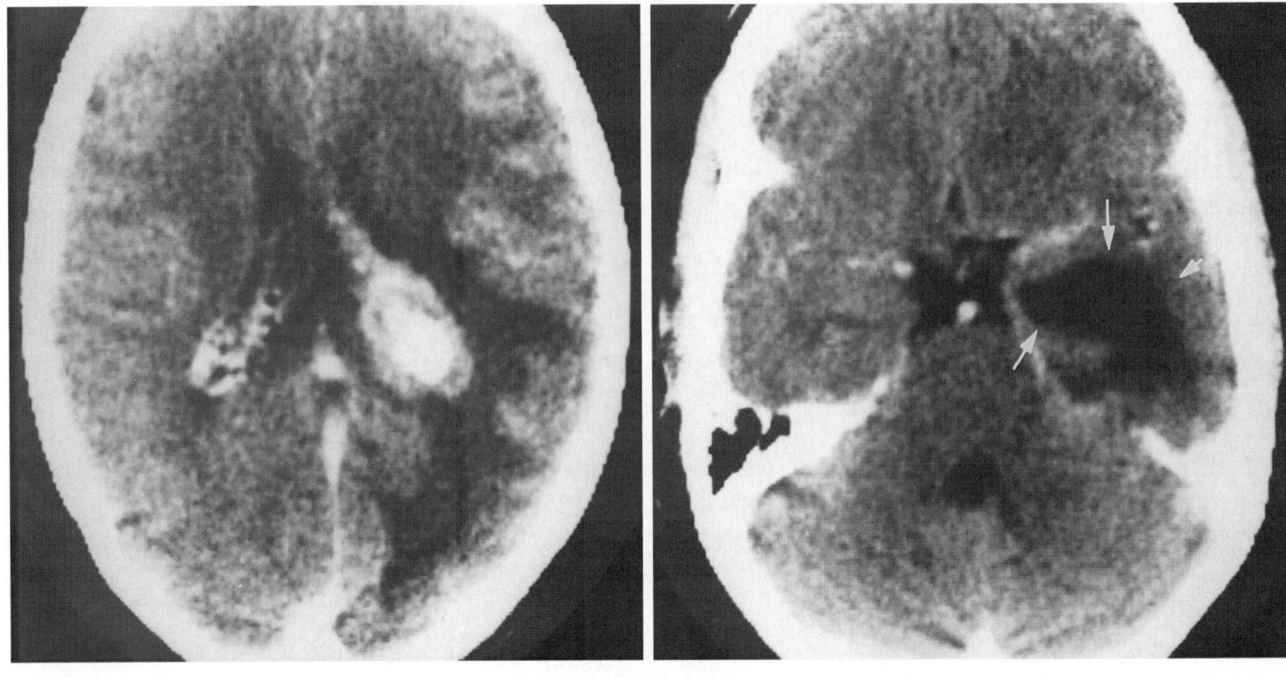

A B

Figure 11.35. Intraventricular meningioma in a 61-year-old woman complaining of headaches. **A.** There is a lobulated mass in the region of the left atrium. **B.** A section lower down shows a markedly dilated temporal horn (arrows) due to obstruction in the atrial region.

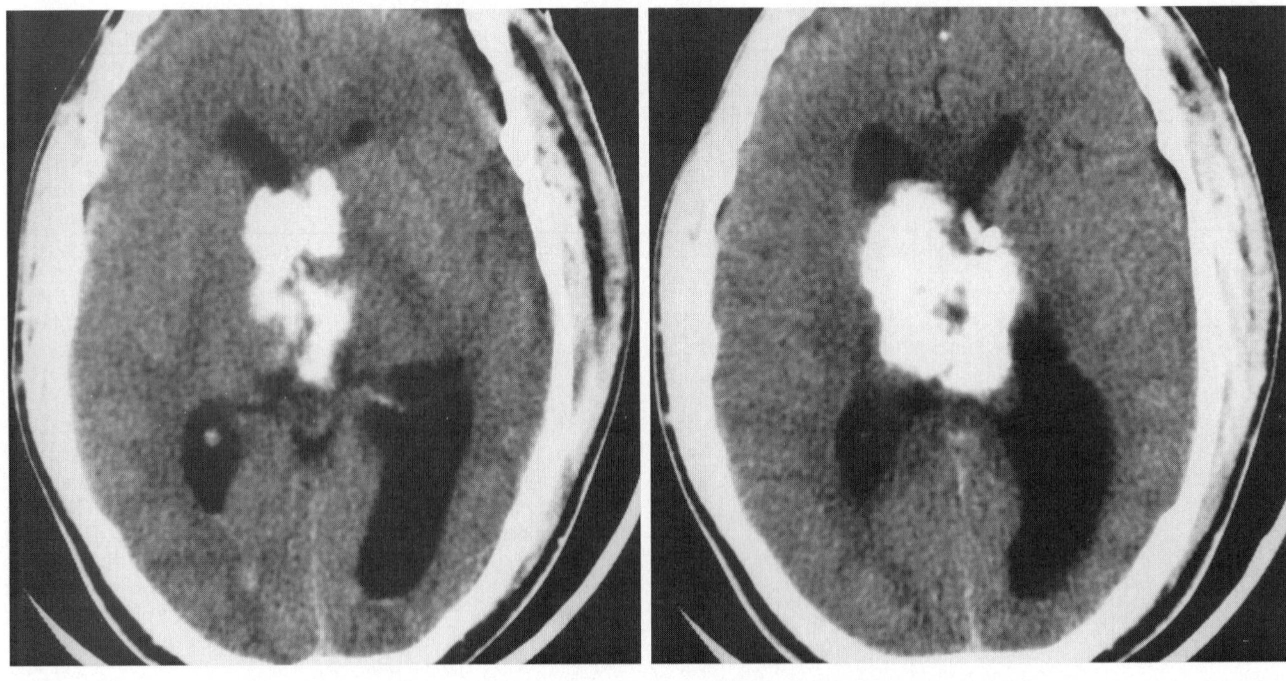

A B

Figure 11.36. Heavily calcified midline oligodendroglioma in patient with a 1-year history of headaches. **A.** There is extensive calcification seen on this CT axial view, with some moderate ventricular dilatation. **B.** The mass was larger in a section above A.

entiation, possibly including the presence of synapses, is needed to differentiate oligodendrogliomas from neurocytomas because they are both made up of small cells. Immunocytochemistry may also be used for differentiation. The prognosis of neurocytomas is much better than that of neuroblastomas, and complete removal may result in a cure. Neurocytomas tend to calcify (about 50 percent) and usually enhance. The case reported by Smoker et al. presented with a localized intraventricular hematoma (44).

Subependymal giant cell astrocytomas are the typical tumors that occur in patients affected with tuberous sclerosis. They usually occur in the region of the foramen of Monro and grow slowly. Because of their strategic location, however, they produce hydrocephalus as a result of obstruction at the junction of the lateral and third ventricles (Fig. 11.37).

Epidermoid cysts as well as *dermoid cysts* can occur in the lateral ventricles, usually in the frontal region, but they are very rare. More often they occur in the posterior fossa. They can rupture, and when they do, a chemical meningitis is produced that can lead to adhesion and hydrocephalus. The epidermoid cyst grows by desquamation of its lining into the cavity. It has a pearly white appearance that has yielded the term *pearly tumor*. The dermoid cyst contains other elements of the skin, such as hair and sebaceous glands, that lead to the production of fatty material. Malignant intraventricular gliomas are sometimes seen.

Metastasis or CSF seeding from other intracranial tumors is seen, most frequently from medulloblastomas, pineal germinomas or pineoblastomas, and choroid plexus carcinomas.

Nonneoplastic masses can also occur in the ventricles. The most frequent of these is cysticercosis, but possibly other parasitic cysts may occur within the ventricles, such as paragonimiasis and echinococcosis.

The third ventricle intraventricular masses have been included with the next group, midline masses.

MIDLINE MASSES AND OTHER LESIONS

These could be extraventricular or intraventricular within the third ventricle. The midline lesions are numerous and represent a great variety of pathological processes. The histologic types of tumors found here are also extensive. In addition to the masses arising from the walls of the third ventricle, the midline masses arising under the third ventricle are included: the sellar, suprasellar, and parasellar masses.

Midline Intraventricular Masses

These are contained within the third ventricle and may arise from the wall of the third ventricle, the choroid plexus, the pineal gland, or the vascular system.

COLLOID CYSTS OF THE THIRD VENTRICLE

These are special tumors arising at the roof and located just at and behind the foramen of Monro, between the columns of the fornix. They arise in the primitive neuroepithelium that forms the roof plate of the tela choroidea. Because of their location, they tend to produce dilatation of the lateral ventricles due to obstruction of the foramen of Monro. For this reason the presenting symptoms may be headaches, which can be intermittent, fainting spells, and behavioral changes, usually in young adults (mean age about 30). The cysts are usually 1.5 to 2.0 cm in diameter when discovered, but some are larger.

On CT examination the cysts are most frequently hyperdense on precontrast images, most probably because of the high protein content of the cyst fluid. On MRI the cysts are more frequently hyperintense on T1-weighted images and hypointense on T2-weighted images. This could again be due to the high protein content. However, the brightness on T1 may present an area of low intensity, and the same may be true on T2-weighted images. It has been postulated that the low-intensity area may be due to the high concentration of ions of sodium, calcium, magnesium, copper, and iron (Fig. 11.38) (45). Some of the cysts are isodense or hypodense on CT and usually do not contain calcification. The presence of solid calcification should suggest another histology. One case reported by Waggenspack and Guinto presenting such calcification turned out to be an astrocytoma, and yet the appearance and location were typical for colloid cyst (46).

The cysts may be surgically removed or aspirated with stereotactic guidance. Kondziolka and Lunsford reported their experience with 22 patients and found that an isodense or hypodense cyst on CT is suitable for aspiration (8 of 22 cases, with complete success in 6), whereas a hyperdense cyst usually indicates that the contents are thick and not suitable for aspiration (14 of 22 cases, subtotal aspiration only, in 13) (47). Surgery may be required after an attempted aspiration. The same authors believe that MRI is less useful for deciding on the suitability of aspiration. Smaller cysts may move away as they are approached by the needle.

Choroid plexus papillomas and meningiomas arising from the roof of the third ventricle are reported from time to time, but they are rare. Colloid-type neuroepithelial cysts are sometimes reported in other locations, the most frequent being the posterior fossa and the fourth ventricle (48). The association of colloid cyst with xanthogranuloma as a mixed tumor is not too rare (49).

OTHER THIRD VENTRICLE TUMORS

Ependymomas should also be considered in any primarily intraventricular tumor within the third ventricle, particularly in the anterior third-ventricular cavity. *Craniopharyngiomas* may be found within the third ventricle (see text following). A rare tumor occasionally reported in the third ventricle is the *hemangioblastoma*, which may be associated with von Hippel-Lindau syndrome (50). Another infrequently reported lesion is *xanthogranuloma* arising from the

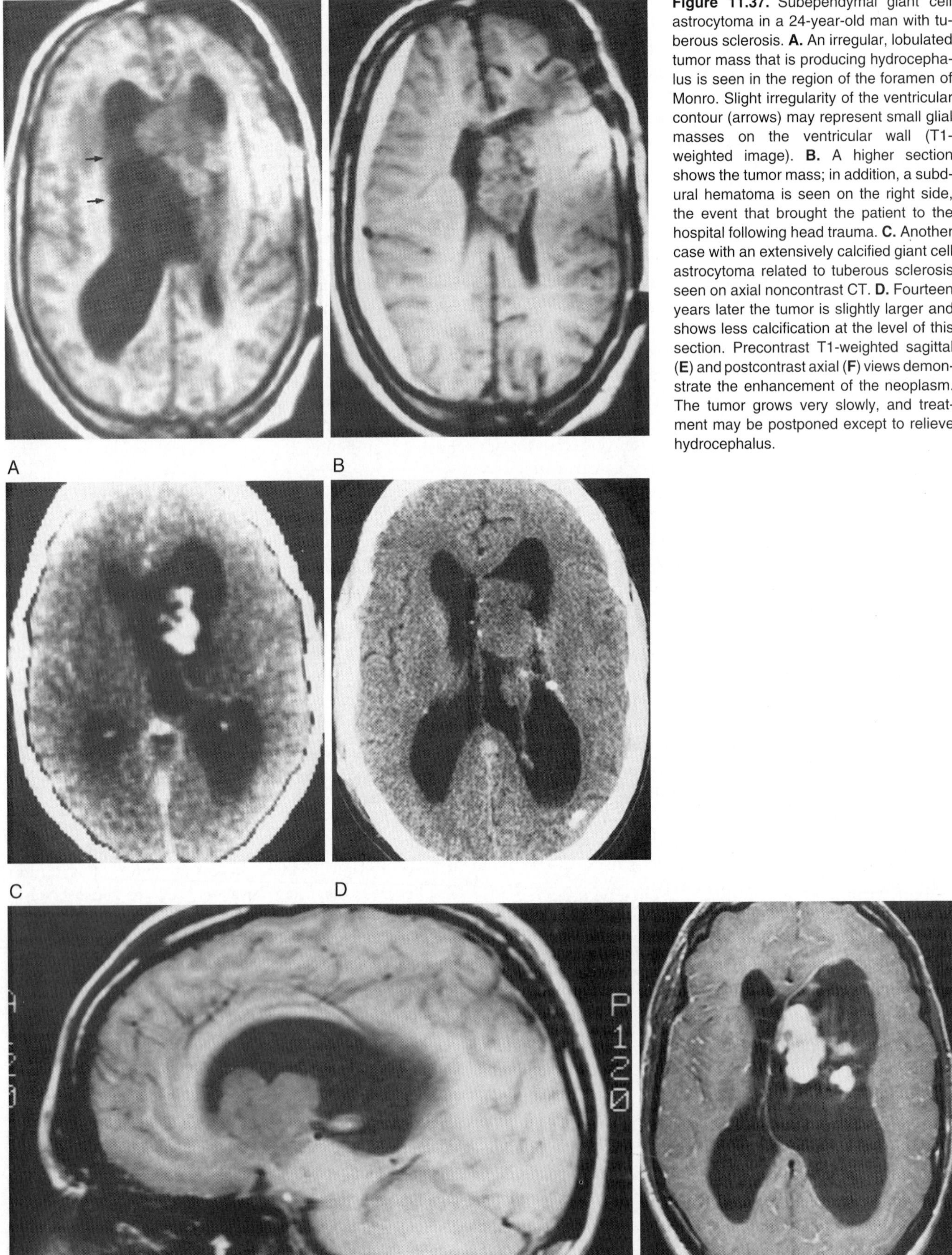

Figure 11.37. Subependymal giant cell astrocytoma in a 24-year-old man with tuberous sclerosis. **A.** An irregular, lobulated tumor mass that is producing hydrocephalus is seen in the region of the foramen of Monro. Slight irregularity of the ventricular contour (arrows) may represent small glial masses on the ventricular wall (T1-weighted image). **B.** A higher section shows the tumor mass; in addition, a subdural hematoma is seen on the right side, the event that brought the patient to the hospital following head trauma. **C.** Another case with an extensively calcified giant cell astrocytoma related to tuberous sclerosis seen on axial noncontrast CT. **D.** Fourteen years later the tumor is slightly larger and shows less calcification at the level of this section. Precontrast T1-weighted sagittal (**E**) and postcontrast axial (**F**) views demonstrate the enhancement of the neoplasm. The tumor grows very slowly, and treatment may be postponed except to relieve hydrocephalus.

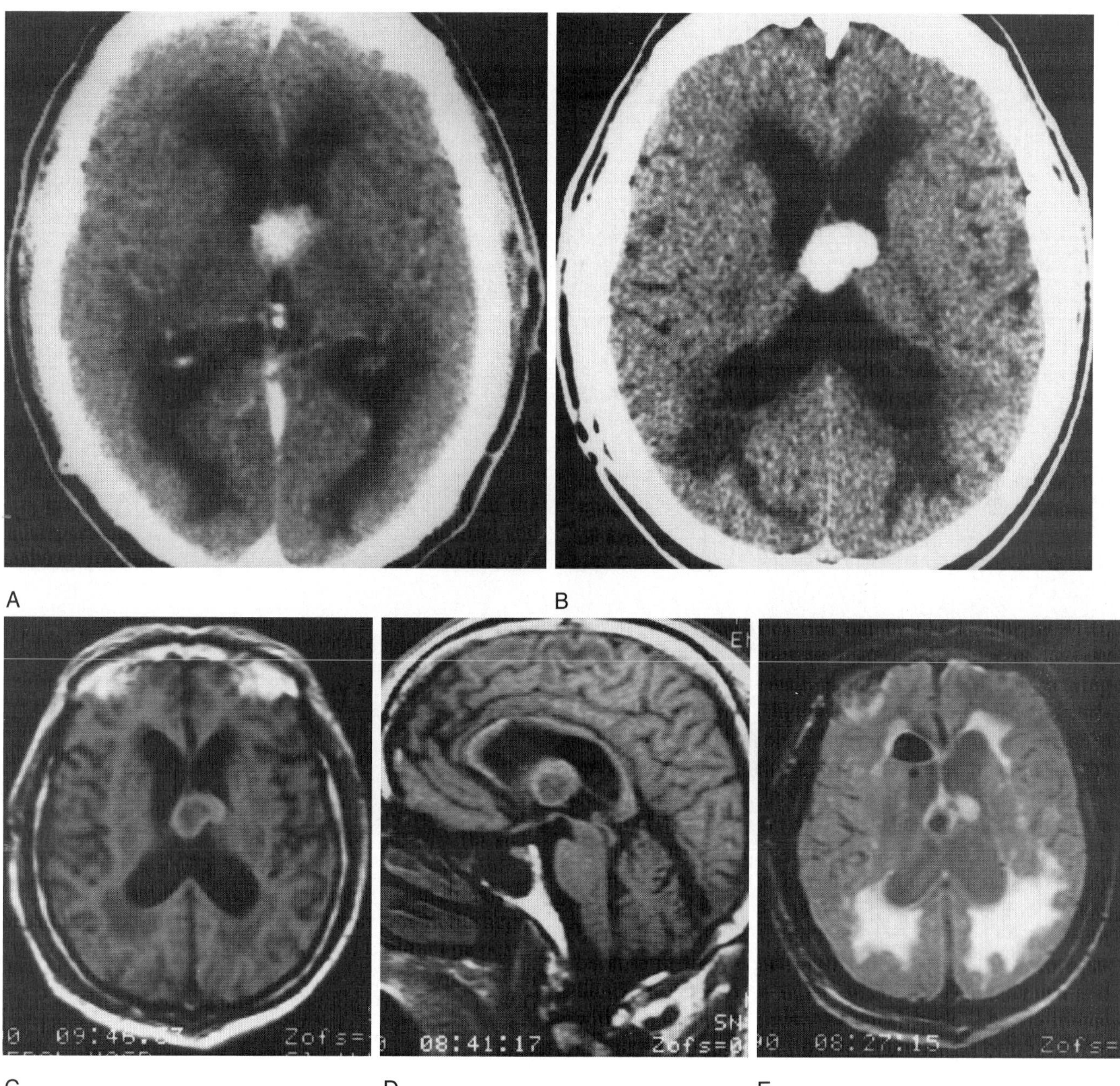

Figure 11.38. Colloid cyst. **A.** CT shows a hyperdense oval mass in the region behind the foramen of Monro. **B.** Reexamination 2 years later shows an increase in size and also a marked increase in density in a noncontrast CT image. T1-weighted axial (**C**) and lateral (**D**) images reveal a slightly hyperintense mass with a central portion that is hypointense. **E.** Proton density axial image (puncture of cyst had been attempted) shows hyperintensity in the cyst with a hypointense area that is relatively more hypointense than on C and D. There is air in the right frontal horn secondary to the attempted surgical tapping of the cyst. There is marked bioccipital, and some bifrontal, hyperintensity, which is most likely due to ventricular obstruction and transependymal passage of CSF.

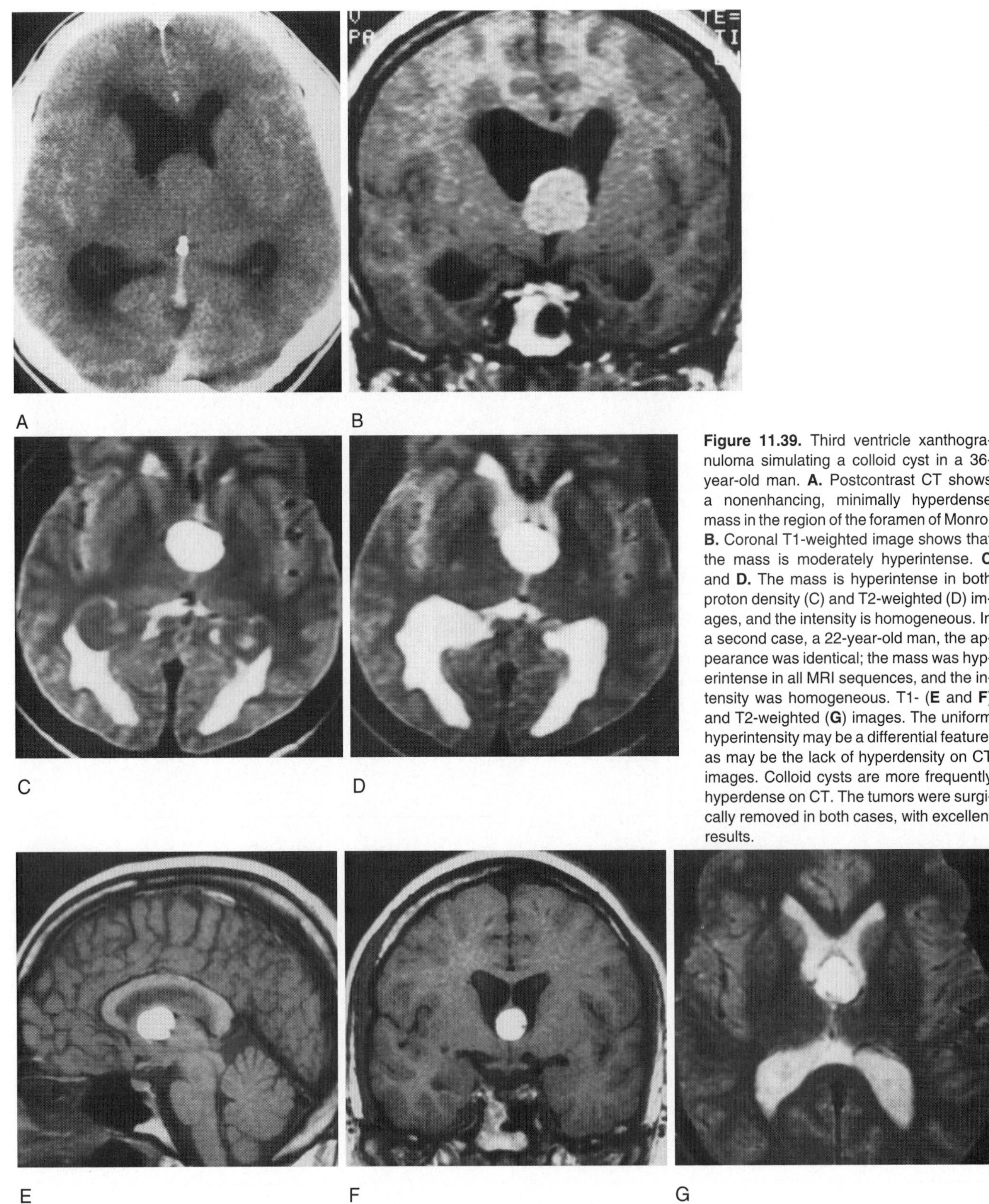

Figure 11.39. Third ventricle xanthogranuloma simulating a colloid cyst in a 36-year-old man. **A.** Postcontrast CT shows a nonenhancing, minimally hyperdense mass in the region of the foramen of Monro. **B.** Coronal T1-weighted image shows that the mass is moderately hyperintense. **C** and **D.** The mass is hyperintense in both proton density (C) and T2-weighted (D) images, and the intensity is homogeneous. In a second case, a 22-year-old man, the appearance was identical; the mass was hyperintense in all MRI sequences, and the intensity was homogeneous. T1- (**E** and **F**) and T2-weighted (**G**) images. The uniform hyperintensity may be a differential feature, as may be the lack of hyperdensity on CT images. Colloid cysts are more frequently hyperdense on CT. The tumors were surgically removed in both cases, with excellent results.

choroid plexus of the third ventricle. It is hyperintense on T2-weighted images and presents calcification on CT (51). Xanthogranulomas tend to occur in the region of the foramen of Monro and produce hydrocephalus. They may be included in the differential diagnosis of colloid cyst. Pathologically they show innumerable cholesterol clefts and may present microscopic foci of colloid cyst-like strucures. In the two cases reported by Tatter et al. (52) the clinical presentation was similar to that of colloid cysts; imaging was also similar to that of classical colloid cysts (Fig. 11.39). Xanthogranulomas are perhaps differentiated from colloid cysts by a lack of hyperdensity on CT and the rather uniform hyperintensity seen on all MRI sequences.

PINEAL REGION MASSES

Tumors arising from the pineal gland and its surroundings are usually included with intraventricular tumors of the third ventricle. The pineal, however, is really outside the ventricle, but when it increases in size as the mass grows, it projects into the posterior third ventricle and looks like an intraventricular mass. In reality, the masses, unless they violate the ependymal lining, push this membrane forward and separate the leaves of the velum interpositum, pushing the choroid plexus down and forward.

Most of the pineal region tumors are malignant germ cell neoplasms that occur in young male patients. However, there is a great variety to the type of histology that may be encountered, which includes teratoma, choriocarcinoma, endodermal sinus tumor, embryonal cell carcinoma, pineocytoma, and pineoblastoma. In addition, some of the tumors that occur in this area include astrocytomas, choroid plexus papillomas, hemangioblastomas (the latter two are very rare), glial cysts, ganglioneuromas, gangliogliomas, epidermoid cysts, and metastatic tumors (see also "Pathologic Considerations") (Table 11.32).

Pineal cysts are fairly common and are of no clinical significance in the immense majority of cases. In general, if the cyst is 14 mm in diameter or less, it is not necessary to recommend a follow-up, but if it is larger it may be advisable to follow it to determine possible growth. Some pineal cysts may grow to a sufficiently large size that they produce symptoms (mostly visual disturbance, Parinaud syndrome) when they compress the quadrigeminal plate, the aqueduct, and the vein of Galen (53). Although pineal cysts may arise from incomplete fusion of the third ventricle diverticulum that gives rise to the pineal gland, in which case they may have an ependymal lining, the majority of the cysts are surrounded by residual pineal tissue and dense neuroglial fibers closely matted. The cyst is best demonstrated on sagittal and coronal MR images. The cyst contents are like CSF, low intensity on T1-weighted images and high intensity on T2-weighted images, but may be brighter because of some protein content in the fluid. The pineal calcification is usually to one side of the cyst (Fig. 11.40). The wall or a portion of it may enhance after contrast because pineal tissue has no blood-brain barrier (54).

Germinomas are the most common tumors of the pineal (40 percent of all tumors and about 65 percent of germ cell tumors) (55). Most frequent in males from 10 to 20 years of age, the masses are usually in the pineal region (80 percent) or in the anterior third ventricle or suprasellar cistern (20 percent). They are 10 to 15 times more common in males than in females. Because they are not encapsulated tumors, they tend to grow over the surface as well as to invade adjacent structures, and they also may seed via CSF (about a third of cases). The tumor surrounds the pineal calcification; its density on CT is higher than that of the white matter and about equal to that of gray matter. The tumors enhance on CT or MRI (Fig. 11.41). Calcification, in addition to what may be called the pineal, may also occur (56). The calcium deposits tend to assume a coarse, stippled appearance (Table 11.33).

The most common seeding sites are the anterior third ventricle and the suprasellar cistern, and some tumors may be found here without a visible mass in the region of the pineal (Fig. 11.42). Seeding at a distance, particularly to the dorsal aspect of the spinal cord, is also found, and sometimes wide dissemination may be found when the patient is first seen. Seeding may sometimes be provoked by the biopsy (57–59).

The tumors are radiosensitive and also respond to tumor chemotherapy. Very long survivals compatible with cure are often seen.

Histologically as well as in their response to therapy, the pineal germinomas are identical to testicular and ovarian germinomas.

Teratomas are composed of all three embryonic tissue components (ectoderm, mesoderm, and endoderm) and thus have a more complex appearance than epidermoid or

Table 11.32.
Pineal Region Tumors

Germ cell tumors are usually seen in young males
Tumors composed of primitive elements: teratoma, choriocarcinoma, embryonal cell carcinoma, choriocarcinoma
Pineal tissue tumors: pineoblastoma and pineocytoma
Tumors arising from adjacent tissues: thalamic astrocytoma and meningioma
Pineal cysts: usually small, incidental findings but may be large and symptomatic
Vein of Galen aneurysm is a vascular lesion, usually seen in early infancy, that may mimic a tumor

Table 11.33.
Pineal Region Germinomas

Identical to testicular and ovarian germinomas
Vast majority occur in young males
Frequently disseminate in CSF pathways
Very radiosensitive

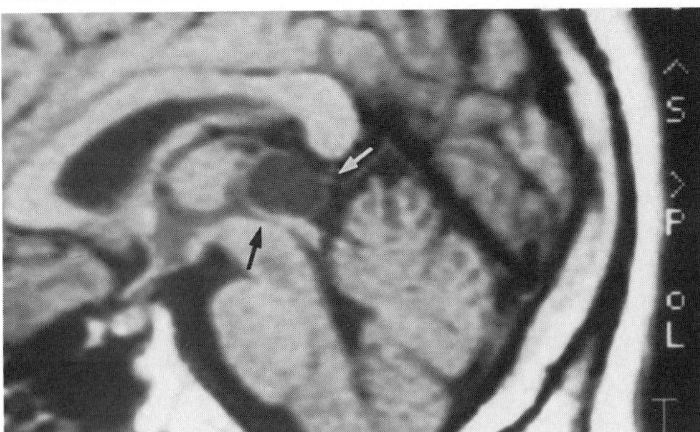

Figure 11.40. Glial pineal cyst with follow-up showing no change. **A.** A T1-weighted sagittal image reveals a cystic lesion in the region of the pineal that was considered asymptomatic, although there is a slight compression of the aqueduct (arrow). The cyst contents are slightly brighter than the ventricular CSF. **B.** Reexamination 4 years later reveals no significant increase in size. This T1 postcontrast image shows enhancement of the posterior wall of the cyst (arrow), which may be residual pineal tissue. Again the cyst is slightly brighter than CSF, probably indicative of higher protein content. **C.** Proton density image also shows the cyst to be hyperintense in relation to CSF (arrow).

A

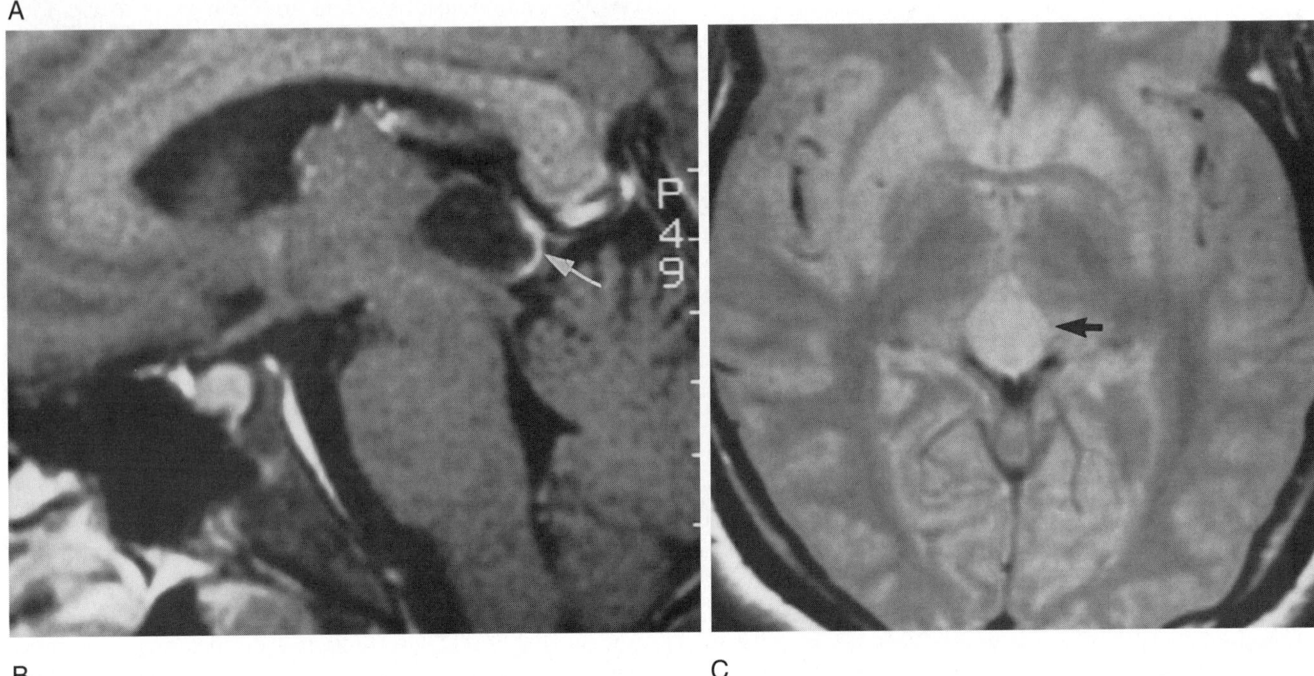

B C

dermoid cysts, which are composed of squamous epithelium (epidermoids) or of all component skin elements, including hair follicles and sweat glands (dermoids). Nevertheless, one or another of the elements may predominate in teratomas. Epidermoid cysts occur when there is ectodermal infolding into the developing head of the embryo at 3 to 5 weeks. They are usually unilocular, although they may grow around the cerebellopontine angle and the perimesencephalic space into the choroidal fissure (see text following) (60) (Table 11.34).

Table 11.34.
Teratomas

Composed of all three embryonic tissue components
Often have elements of fat, bone, cartilage
Variable degrees of contrast enhancement

As mentioned, teratomas are likely to be much more complex, containing areas of fat, cartilage and even bone, and soft-tissue and fluid cysts (Figs. 11.43 and 11.44). When this complexity is appreciated on CT and MRI, the appearance is diagnostic. Because of the calcium present, CT is more useful for final diagnosis. The lipid contents of a teratoma forming a cystic space may be prominent in some cases, and rupture of the cysts may take place, as with dermoid cysts. The tissue within a teratoma may enhance with contrast or the enhancement may occur only along the capsule. Islands of neuroectodermal tissue are often present, and somewhat mature neural elements may be found. Some teratomas contain a large amount of immature tissue and may metastasize (Fig. 11.44).

The *choriocarcinomas*, *endodermal sinus (yolk sac) tumors*, and *embryonal carcinomas* occur in the pineal region but are rare and possess no specific imaging characteristics that would allow us to suggest the diagnosis. Serum and CSF

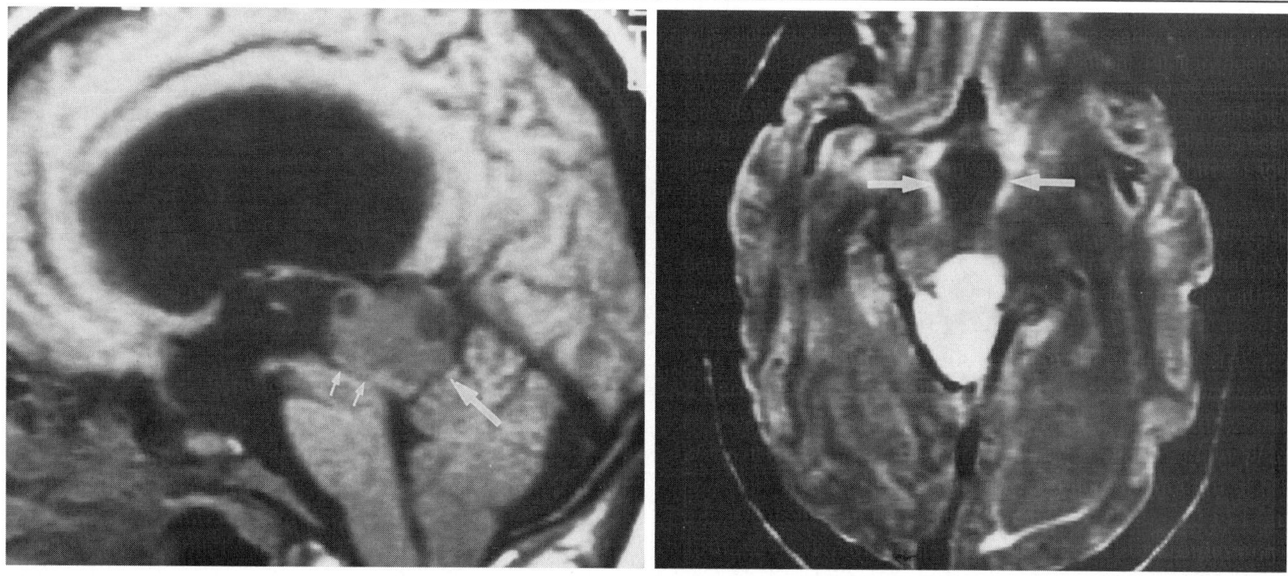

Figure 11.41. Pineal germinoma in a 25-year-old man. **A.** Sagittal T1-weighted view reveals an irregularly rounded mass in the region of the pineal gland containing two low-intensity areas representing calcification (arrow); the anterior one is evidently completely surrounded by tumor, which is typical of germinoma. The mass is producing ventricular dilatation of the lateral and anterior third ventricles, producing flattening and downward displacement of the quadrigeminal plate with narrowing of the aqueduct (double arrows) and posterior displacement of the cerebellar culmen. **B.** Proton density weighted axial image shows a hyperintense lesion in the posterior third ventricle that is markedly dilated anteriorly (arrows) and that presents periventricular hyperintensity consistent with obstructive hydrocephalus. The lesion enhanced with gadolinium contrast (not shown).

examination may show elevated chorionic gonadotropin levels, in which case the histologic type (choriocarcinoma or embryonal carcinoma) may be suspected clinically prior to biopsy. Mixed histology may also be found.

The *pineal parenchymal tumors* represent the minority (15 percent) of tumors in the pineal area. The two main types are the *pineocytoma* and the *pineoblastoma.* They tend to occur in either sex and usually at a more advanced age (after 20). The pineocytoma has a better prognosis than the pineoblastoma, which is a much more aggressive tumor. The latter is included in the PNET group. The diagnosis can be suggested in the presence of a tumor in the pineal region that enhances brightly and may contain calcification. In this case the pineal calcification may not be seen within the tumor but may be diffuse, in what Smirniotopoulos et al. called the "exploded pineal pattern" (55). Like the germinomas, the pineoblastoma can grow in the third-ventricular wall and seed via the CSF (Fig. 11.45).

Some pineal region tumors are *astrocytomas,* and these can be differentiated because of their tendency to grow transversely across the midline and to have more poorly defined margins. They may actually involve the splenium of the corpus callosum rather than the spineal area. They may also grow into the quadrigeminal plate and around the aqueduct.

Lipomas tend to occur in this region. The great majority are small, but some may acquire a larger size. Usually they are an incidental finding and are more frequently observed now on MRI because they are bright on T1-weighted images. On CT they are inconspicuous because they usually project partly into CSF-containing spaces, whether in the quadrigeminal cistern, the suprasellar and interpenduncular cisterns, or the perimesencephalic cisterns. For further detail see text preceding under "Pathologic Considerations," and Chapter 5; see also Figs. 5.33 and 5.34). A small lipoma has been seen in the tuber cinereum in a boy with precocious puberty (Fig. 11.48).

The typical vascular lesion occurring in this area is the *aneurysm of the vein of Galen.* The dilatation of this vein is associated with an arteriovenous malformation draining by way of the vein of Galen. It may become apparent in early infancy because of high-output cardiac failure, but it is usually discovered somewhat later because of hydrocephalus, failure to thrive, or the presence of a bruit (see Figs. 10.123 and 10.124).

ANTERIOR THIRD VENTRICLE TUMORS

These can be contained within the cavity of the ventricle (see text preceding) or may primarily involve the wall of the hypothalamus. In this case they are most frequently gliomas, usually astrocytomas, growing in the wall and

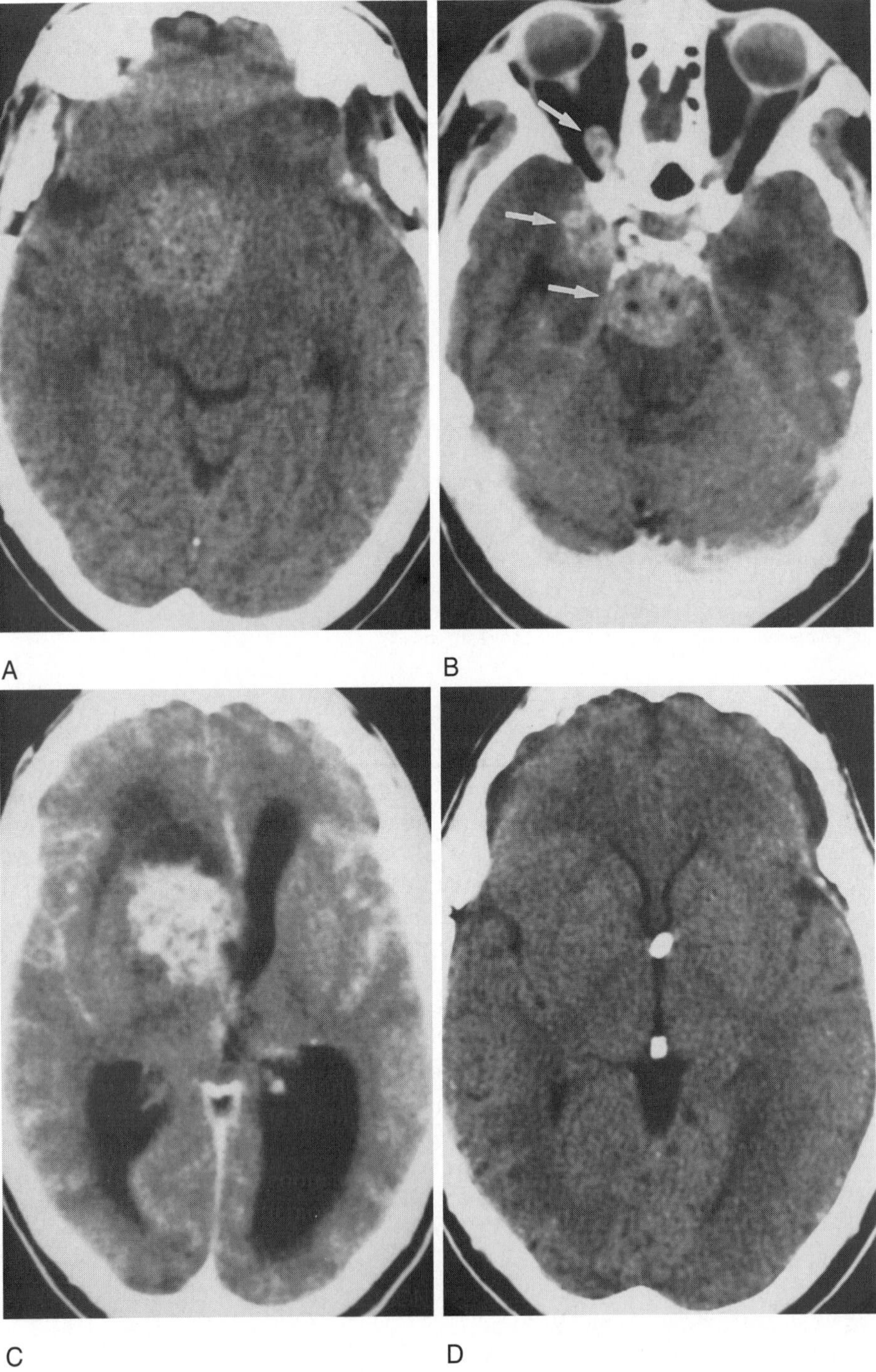

Figure 11.42. Perisellar germinoma in a 25-year-old man. **A.** Precontrast CT scan shows a hyperdense suprasellar mass off the midline. The hyperdensity is not related to calcium, and one would suspect a lesion with a high nuclear-cytoplasmic ratio. **B.** After contrast there is enhancement of the mass, which also extends into the interpeduncular fossa and indents the anterior aspect of the brainstem. It also extends into the right parasellar region and into the orbit (arrows). **C.** The suprasellar portion grows into the anterior aspect of the third-ventricular wall and obstructs the foramen of Monro, producing hydrocephalus. **D.** One year later, following partial removal, ventricular shunting, and radiation therapy, the tumor has completely disappeared.

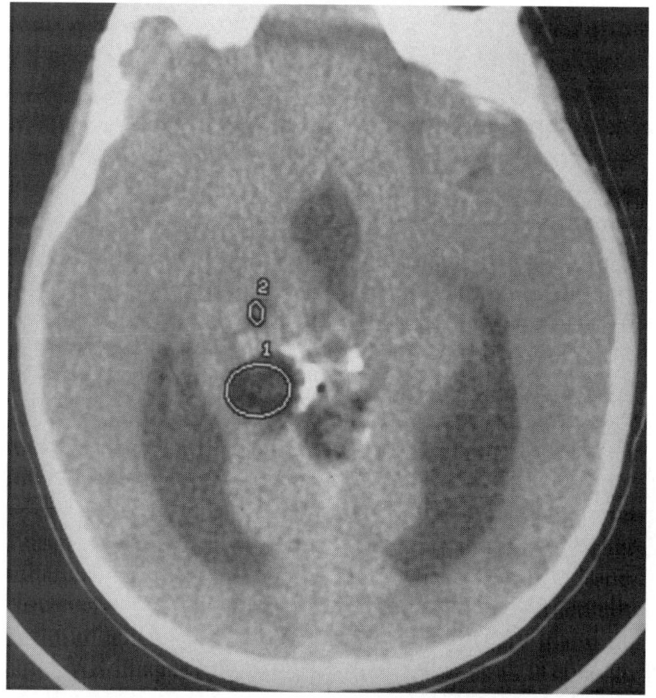

A

Figure 11.43. Pineal teratoma in a 7-year-old boy. **A.** CT axial view shows a mass in the region of the pineal, with calcification and hypodense areas (area 1 measures 10 Hounsfield units [HU]; area 2 measures 3 HU). Small fatty areas are dark. The tumor is growing eccentrically, which is common. **B.** Sagittal reformatting reveals more hypodense areas consistent with fat (arrow). **C.** Axial T2-weighted MR image reveals the heterogeneity of the mass.

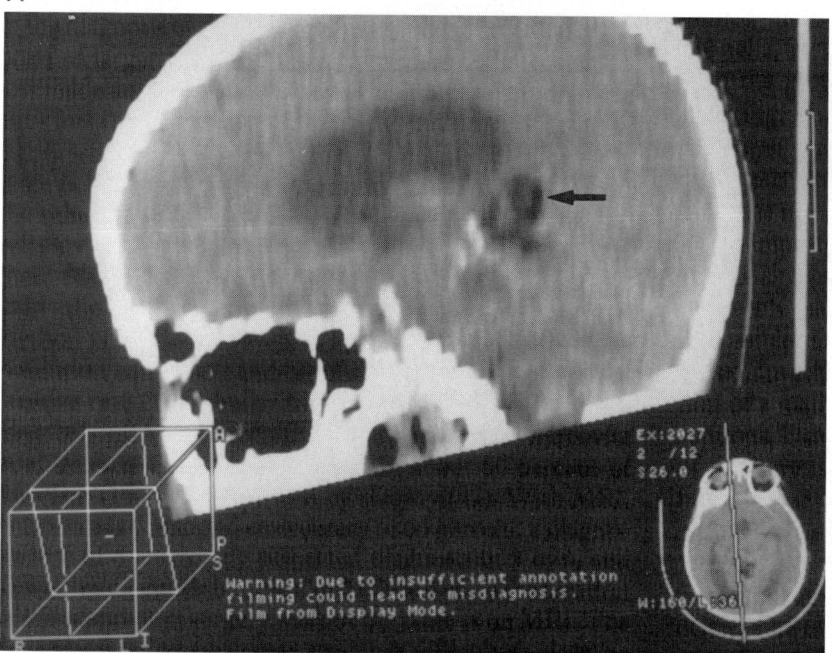

B

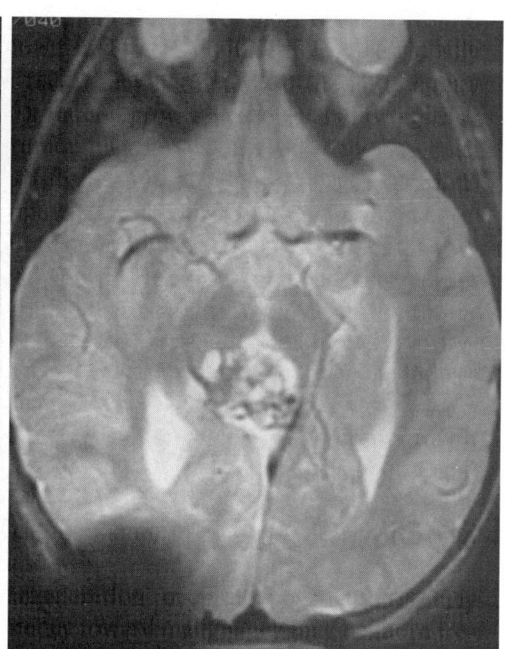

C

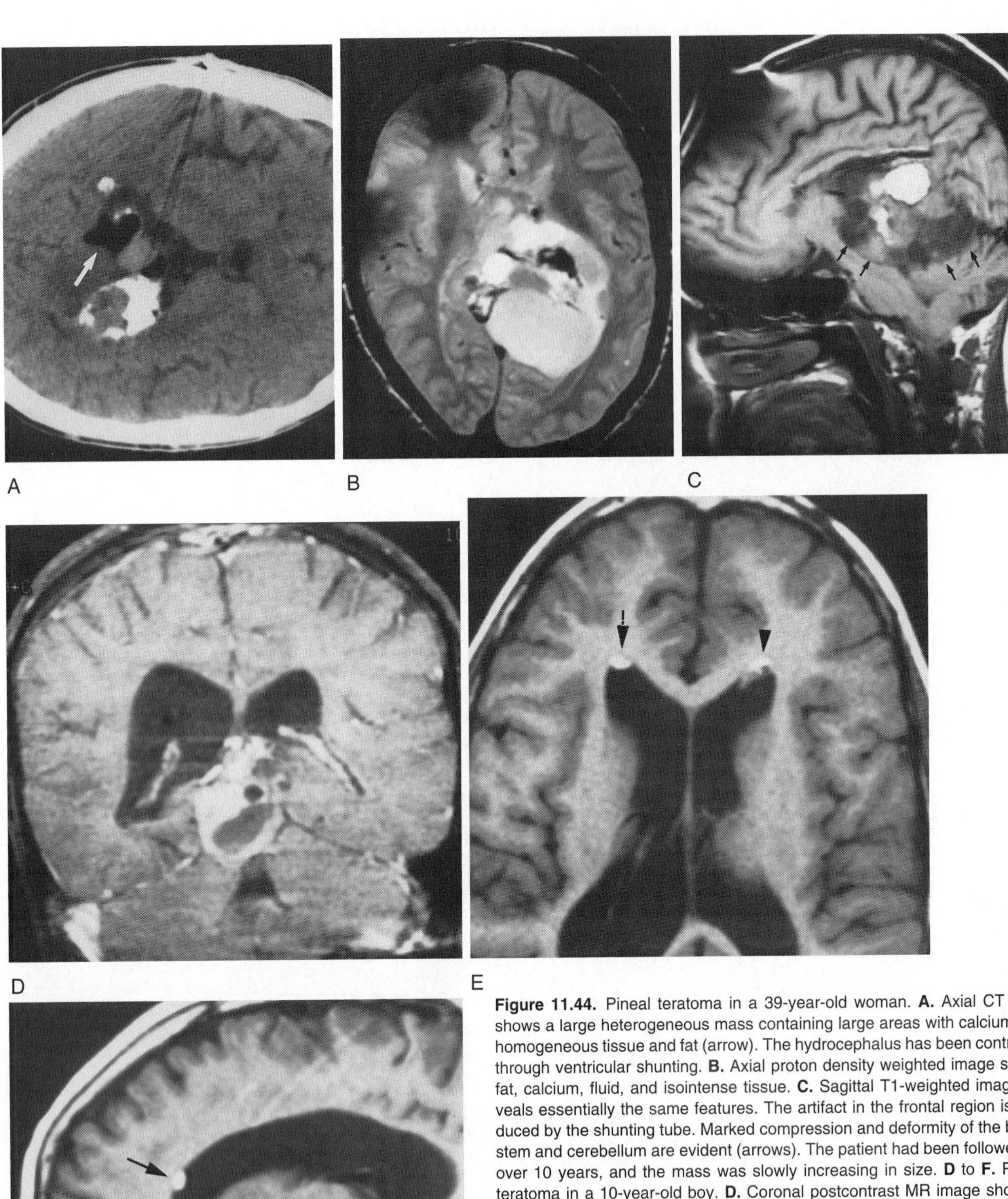

Figure 11.44. Pineal teratoma in a 39-year-old woman. **A.** Axial CT scan shows a large heterogeneous mass containing large areas with calcium and homogeneous tissue and fat (arrow). The hydrocephalus has been controlled through ventricular shunting. **B.** Axial proton density weighted image shows fat, calcium, fluid, and isointense tissue. **C.** Sagittal T1-weighted image reveals essentially the same features. The artifact in the frontal region is produced by the shunting tube. Marked compression and deformity of the brainstem and cerebellum are evident (arrows). The patient had been followed for over 10 years, and the mass was slowly increasing in size. **D** to **F.** Pineal teratoma in a 10-year-old boy. **D.** Coronal postcontrast MR image shows a hyperintense mass with low-intensity areas representing cysts or calcification obliterating the third ventricle. The axial view at a higher level (**E**) as well as the sagittal passing through the right lateral ventricle (**F**) show seeding, enhancing nodules in the frontal horns of the lateral ventricles (arrows).

Figure 11.45. Pineoblastoma in a child producing diffuse seeding periventricularly and in the subarachnoid space. **A.** CT image without contrast shows hyperdense irregular periventricular involvement. The pineal is particularly hyperdense. **B.** Postcontrast sagittal view shows a hyperintense rounded mass surrounding the pineal calcification (low-intensity area) (arrows). The mass is compressing and displacing the aqueduct. There is a large nodule in the hypothalamus (lower arrow).

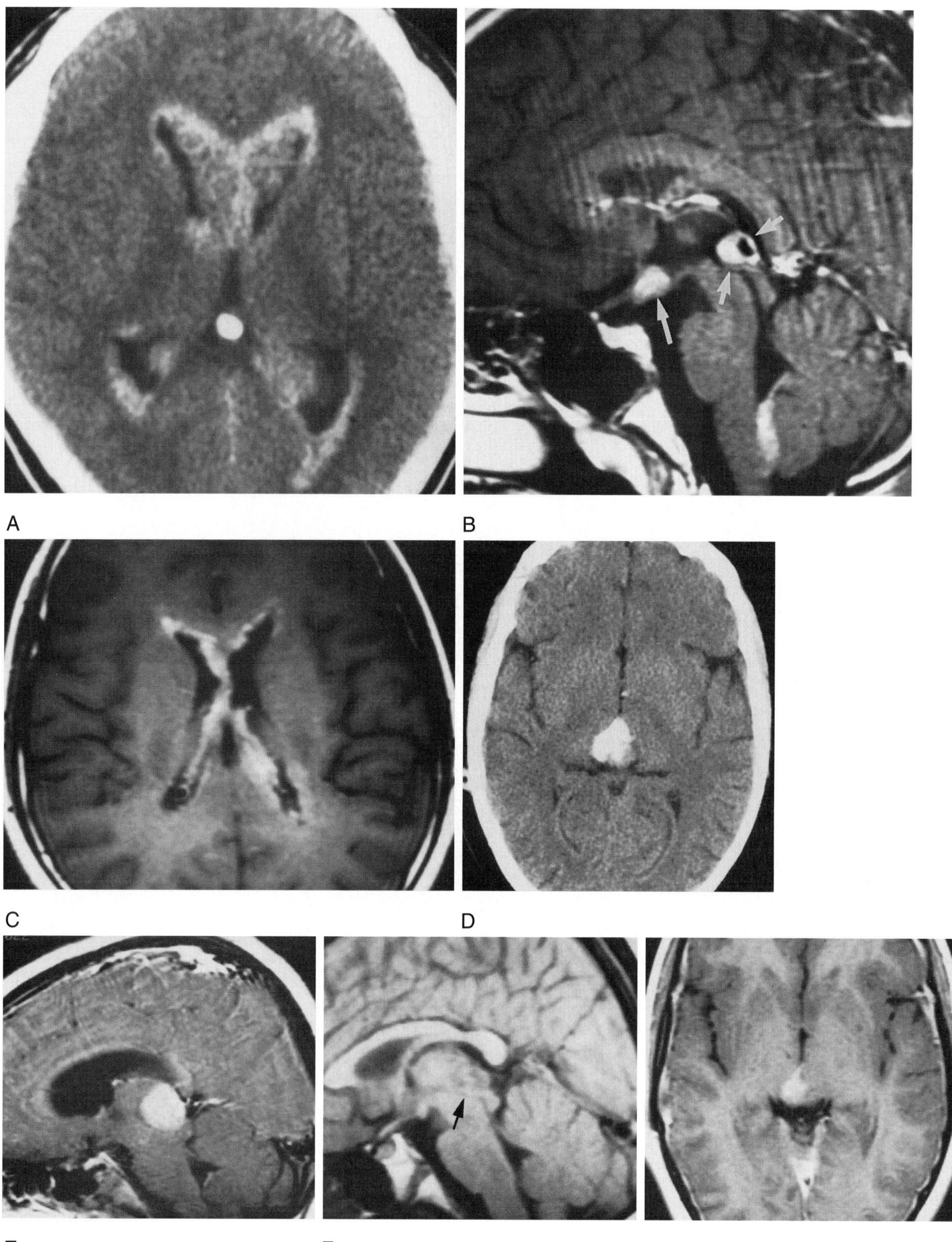

Figure 11.45. *(continued)* **C.** Postcontrast axial view shows the growth of the tumor on the ependymal surface. The configuration of the tumor surrounding the pineal calcification is typical of a germinoma and is also seen in pineoblastomas. **D.** Pineoblastoma in a 12-year-old girl showing marked enhancement on CT. **E.** MR sagittal postcontrast image reveals the position of the mass. **F.** Precontrast sagittal image shows the downward displacement of the aqueduct (arrow). The mass is partly isointense and partly hypointense. **G.** An axial postcontrast view made 6 months after D and after surgery and radiation shows the pineal region mass as much smaller. The enhancement of the dura all around the brain represents postoperative change and is not due to meningeal invasion by tumor.

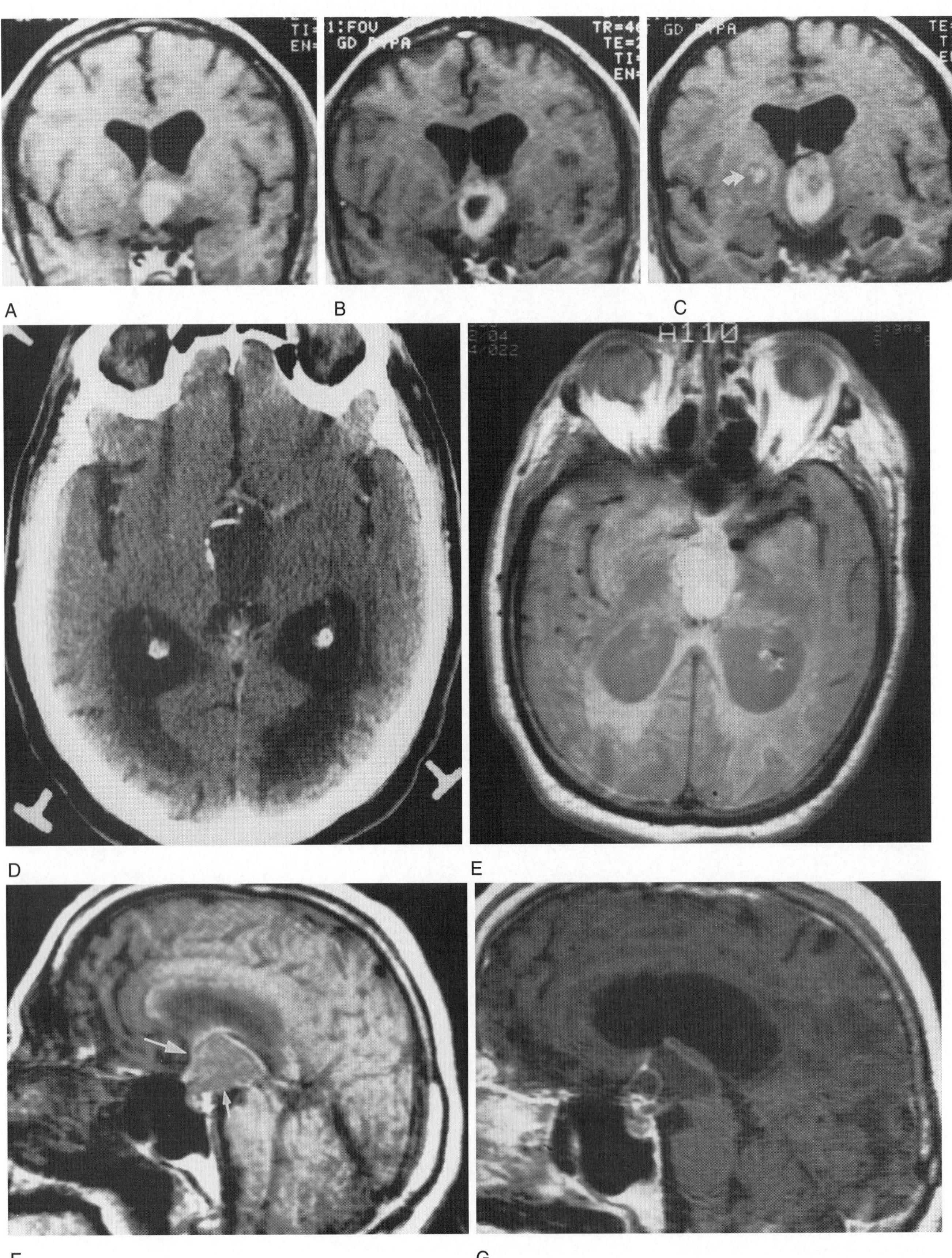
A
B
C
D
E
F
G

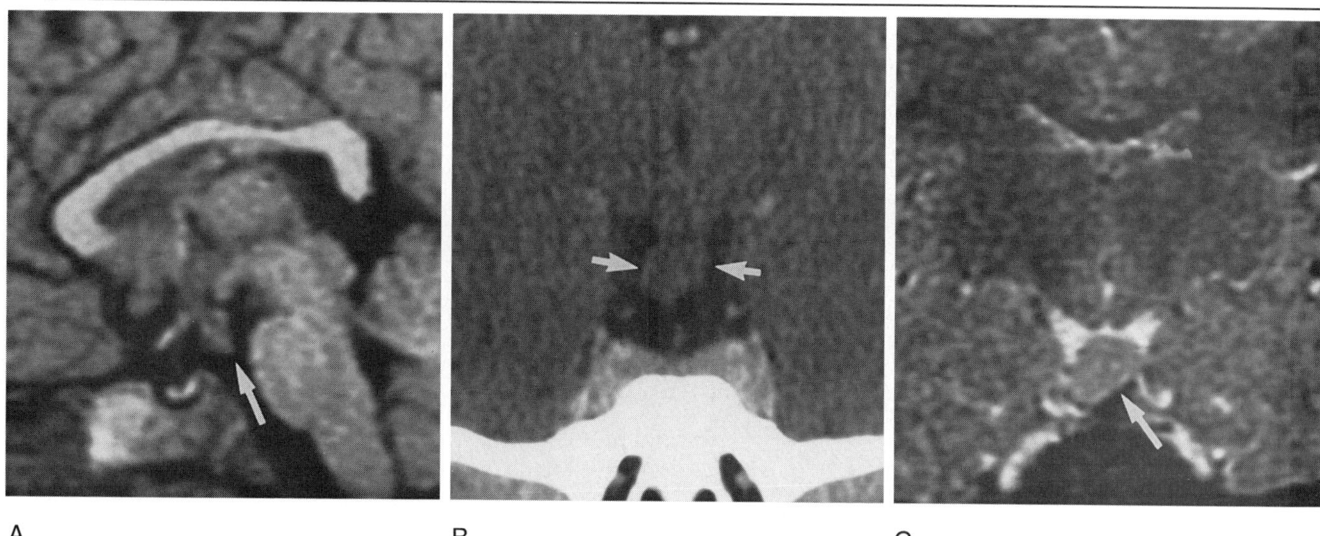

A B C

Figure 11.47. Hypothalamic hamartoma in a 16-month-old female with precocious puberty. **A.** T1-weighted sagittal view. There is a small hypothalamic mass projecting into the suprasellar cistern, isodense with gray matter (arrow). **B.** Coronal CT postcontrast view. The mass is oval and hangs down from the hypothalamus (arrows). There is no enhancement. **C.** On a coronal T2-weighted image, the mass is isodense with gray matter (arrow). (Courtesy of Dr. John Crawford, Massachusetts General Hospital, Boston.)

Table 11.35. Anterior Third Ventricle Tumors

Colloid cysts
Craniopharyngiomas
Gliomas arising from adjacent structures, e.g., hypothalamus
Meningiomas (rare)

causing a mass without any intraventricular growth but obstructing the third-ventricular cavity (Fig. 11.46). Some of these tumors may be associated with precocious puberty (Table 11.35).

Intraventricular craniopharyngiomas are found not too rarely within the cavity of the third ventricle. They probably originate from squamous cell rests in the region of the lamina terminalis and grow intraventricularly, producing hydrocephalus. In a group of 73 intraventricular tumors, Morrison et al. found 5 cases, of which 3 presented calcification on CT, 3 were low density, and 1 was classified as high density (40). In the case reported by Mathews, the tumor enhanced, was noncalcified, and was attached to the inferior lateral wall of the third ventricle in a 65-year-old woman (61). The age range is higher than that seen in the usual suprasellar craniopharyngioma (Fig. 11.46*D* to *G*). For further details see under "Perisellar Lesions" in text following.

◄

Figure 11.46. Hypothalamic glioma. **A.** Enhanced coronal MRI view shows a hyperintense mass involving the walls of the third ventricle primarily in the anterior inferior region. **B.** The hyperintensity extends to the upper aspect of the wall of the third ventricle and presents a small cystic area. The tumor proved to be an astrocytoma. **C.** A section farther posteriorly shows that the ventricular cavity is obliterated and there is some ventricular dilatation. A hyperintense area in the right anterior thalamic region (arrow) probably represents growth of neoplasm (also suggested in A). **D** to **G.** Another patient, a 71-year-old man with intraventricular craniopharyngioma. **D.** CT shows slight hyperdensity in the third ventricle as compared to the CSF in the enlarged lateral ventricle. **E.** Proton density T2-weighted axial view shows hyperintensity in the third ventricle compared to the lateral ventricles. **F.** T1 sagittal precontrast view shows relative hyperintensity in the third ventricle (arrows). **G.** Postcontrast view shows a small solid portion inferiorly, and the rest appears to be cystic.

HAMARTOMAS OF THE HYPOTHALAMUS

Hamartomas of the hypothalamus are an important tumor because they are frequently associated with precocious puberty (35 to 70 percent of cases). They may be small, measuring only 5 to 10 mm in size, but may acquire a large size, compressing and elevating the hypothalamus and posteriorly displacing the upper brainstem (Figs. 11.47 and 11.48). The mechanism by which the tumor produces precocious puberty is not well understood. Possibly it may be related to direct hormonal secretory activity by the hamartoma. The precocious puberty results from the premature disappearance of the normal inhibitory factors on the hypothalamus. The luteinizing hormone–releasing hormone (LHRH) is released prematurely and activates the pituitary-gonadal axis. A test can be performed to determine the response to intravenous LHRH administration: the follicle-stimulating hormone (FSH) and luteinizing hormone (LH) will show marked elevation in precocious puberty.

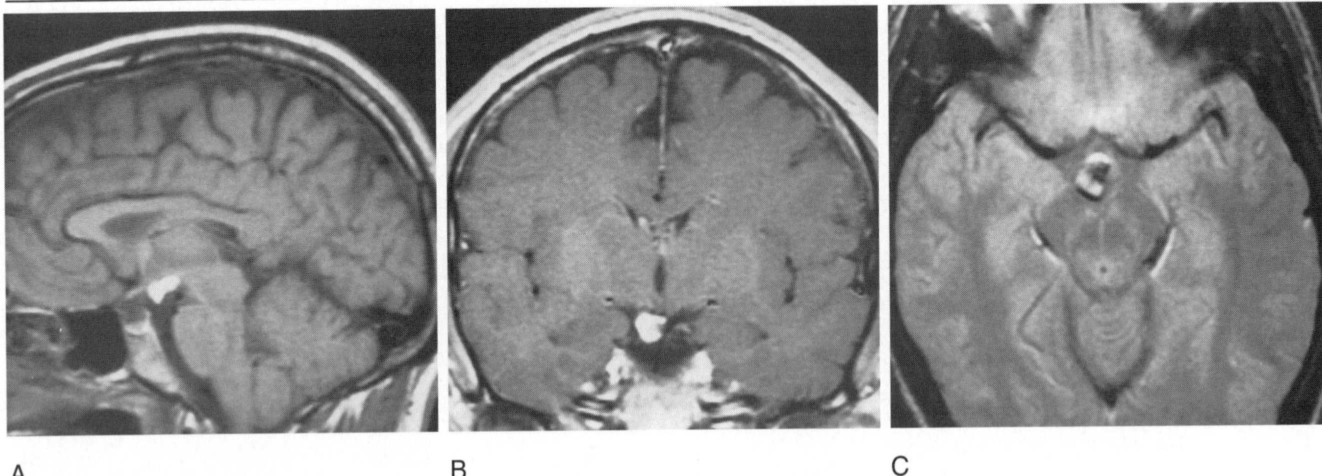

Figure 11.48. Hypothalamic lipoma in a male patient with precocious puberty. **A.** Sagittal T1-weighted image reveals a bright, sharply circumscribed lesion in the inferior hypothalamus. **B.** In a coronal image the lipoma is slightly eccentric. **C.** Axial view showing the distribution of the bright fatty elements. The patient was 25 years old at the time of this examination and was entirely normal. At age 5 to 6 he developed precocious puberty. The lipoma had not changed in several years of follow-up. (Courtesy of Dr. John Crawford, Massachusetts General Hospital, Boston.)

Table 11.36.
Hypothalamic Hamartomas

Associated with precocious puberty
Typically attached to the tuber cinereum
Similar in intensity to gray matter on CT and MRI
Unlike other masses occurring at this site (e.g., optic gliomas, hypothalamic gliomas, craniopharyngiomas), these lesions do not contrast-enhance

The mass is usually attached to the tuber cinereum of the hypothalamus, but cases have been reported in which the mass did not seem to have an attachment and yet produced precocious puberty (62–64). The larger hamartomas are less likely to produce precocious puberty (65). (Table 11.36).

On imaging, hamartomas are characteristic in that they produce, on CT or MRI, images that are similar to brain tissue gray matter in all sequences, and they do not enhance. Calcification sometimes occurs (66,67). Fat is sometimes demonstrated and was seen in one of the author's cases (Fig. 11.48).

If all children with precocious puberty were examined, a lesion might be demonstrated in at least one-third. However, the lesions are not all hamartomas. In the report of Rieth et al. (66), out of a total of 90 cases (73 girls and 17 boys), a lesion was demonstrated by CT in 32, consisting of hamartomas, 17; hypothalamic astrocytoma, 1; optic chiasm lesion, 6; arachnoid cyst, 1; teratoma, 1; and ventricular abnormalities, 8. The report was based on CT images only, and it is known that MRI is superior to CT for masses in this area, partly because of the possibility of obtaining high-resolution sagittal and coronal images. Some small lesions may be overlooked with CT (62). In the differential diagnosis we must consider craniopharyngiomas, optic gliomas, hypothalamic gliomas, and gangliogliomas, but all these tumors usually enhance after contrast on CT or MRI and some present calcification, like the craniopharyngioma or some optic gliomas. The hypothalamic gliomas are usually inhomogeneous and enhance (Fig. 11.46). Enhancement of hamartomas has rarely been reported in patients with neurofibromatosis (66). It appears that a fairly secure imaging diagnosis can be reached in order to avoid surgical exploration or biopsy, which present potential complications. Furthermore, in the patients who present precocious puberty, hormonal investigations would support the diagnosis, and this is sufficient in the majority of instances to decide on medical treatment. Moreover, the result of surgical treatment is not always favorable. In patients under medical management, relatively frequent follow-up examinations, preferably with MRI, are recommended, possibly every 6 to 12 months in order to demonstrate lack of growth, since lack of growth is a typical behavior of hamartomas.

A special hamartoma has been described under the name of *congenital hypothalamic hamartoblastoma syndrome* (Pallister-Hall syndrome). It occurs in infancy and is associated with congenital anomalies in other systems (polydactyly, nail dysplasia, congenital heart defects, inperforate anus, and micropenis with hypoplastic testes in males). Pituitary aplasia may be present, as well as craniofacial anomalies (68).

Midline Extracerebral Lesions

As part of the discussion of midline tumors it is logical to continue with extracerebral midline lesions, most of which are neoplasms, because of their intimate relationship with the adjacent brain structures and because some of them, such as optic gliomas, may grow directly into the hypothalamus. Moreover, one must include a large number of them in the differential diagnosis. For practical reasons, other lesions besides neoplasms will be included in the discussion, since all types of pathologic processes must be included in a diagnosis.

A great variety of pathologies are encountered in the sellar-perisellar area, most of which can be visualized and analyzed by neuroradiologic approaches: CT, MRI, MR angiography, and conventional angiography. Hence a detailed discussion is warranted, for the therapeutic decision is based in large part on the neuroradiologic findings.

THE NORMAL PITUITARY GLAND

The pituitary gland is composed of four parts; the anterior lobe (about 75 percent of the gland mass), the pars intermedia, the posterior lobe, and the pituitary stalk. The pars intermedia is usually quite small and represents no more than a cleft. The posterior lobe is continuous with the stalk and hypothalamus (Fig. 11.49*A*).

The blood supply of the anterior lobe is indirectly by way of the superior hypophyseal arteries through the hypothalamic-pituitary portal system (Fig. 11.49*B*). The posterior lobe blood supply is through the inferior hypophyseal arteries arising from the internal carotid artery (Fig. 11.49*C* and *D*).

The anterior lobe produces and secretes growth hormone (GH), prolactin, thyroid-stimulating hormone (TSH), luteinizing hormone (LH), adrenocorticotropic hormone (ACTH), and melanophore-stimulating hormone, which are mediated and released through the hypothalamus. The posterior lobe, the infundibular stalk, and the supraoptic and paraventricular hypothalamic nuclei form the neurohypophysis. The hypothalamus synthesizes vasopressin and oxytocin, which are coupled to carrier proteins (neurophysins) to form crystal aggregates that are enveloped in a phospholipid membrane and carried via unmyelinated fibers down the pituitary stalk to be stored in the posterior pituitary lobe (69). These vesicles probably account for the brightness of the posterior lobe on T1-weighted images.

The pituitary stalk is somewhat variable in its thickness; Simmons et al. indicate that the dimensions as measured on coronal MR images are 1.56 to 4.58 mm at the level of the optic chiasm and 1.04 to 2.93 mm at the insertion of the stalk on the posterior lobe of the gland (70). The stalk is seen best after contrast enhancement because it always enhances.

INTRASELLAR LESIONS

The soft-tissue pathology of the sella turcica is described in this section as a part of the discussion of midline extracerebral lesions encountered in the supratentorial space.

The greatest proportion of these masses arise from the pituitary gland. Some of the lesions are found incidentally when they are not suspected clinically. In general, however, some type of clinical manifestation makes the primary physician, neurologist, or endocrinologist suspect a pituitary abnomality. The symptoms may be related to endocrine function or to a mass effect. In either case a primary tumor of the gland would be considered a probable cause, but instead a cyst, granuloma, abscess, aneurysm, or metastatic or extrasellar lesion may be found.

Examination Techniques

The examination is carried out by CT and/or by MRI, without and with contrast material. Because of its easy availability, CT is usually done first, but MRI is proving to be superior to CT in the investigation of sellar and perisellar lesions unless one wishes to determine the presence or absence of calcification or one needs to evaluate the surrounding bones, in which case CT is necessary.

On CT examination the preenhancement axial views are carried out first. If a small pituitary tumor is suspected, then coronal views of the sellar region are done. Preferably these should be 1 to 2 mm thick. The coronal views may be difficult to obtain, and it is necessary to avoid the teeth because of the frequent artifacts they produce. Most patients are able to lie supine with the head extended and with large pillows under the upper back. The additional angulation of the gantry in the equipment is helpful. Some patients may prefer a prone position with the head extended, which makes the intravenous injection of contrast rather awkward, although this could be prepared prior to turning the patient prone.

Once the precontrast coronal views are made, the injection of iodide contrast is started, and after half of the 300 ml of the 30 percent solution has been injected, the exposures can be started. These exposures should preferably be made as a *dynamic set* of images (1 to 2 mm thick) centered over the pituitary gland *anterior to the pituitary stalk.* Most microadenomas occur in the anterior portion of the anterior lobe of the gland.

After the dynamic set of images is done, one should *proceed immediately* to taking a set of thin coronal slices of the pituitary from front to back. This should be done as quickly as possible to avoid accumulation of contrast material in an adenoma, which diminishes the density difference between the unenhanced tumor and the surrounding enhanced gland. Once this is completed, the patient is relieved from his or her uncomfortable position and a set of postcontrast axial views are made.

From thin axial views it is also possible to reformat coronal and sagittal images. If this is carefully done, the detail is quite satisfactory.

MRI is the method of choice for examining the intrasellar and perisellar area, unless one needs to determine

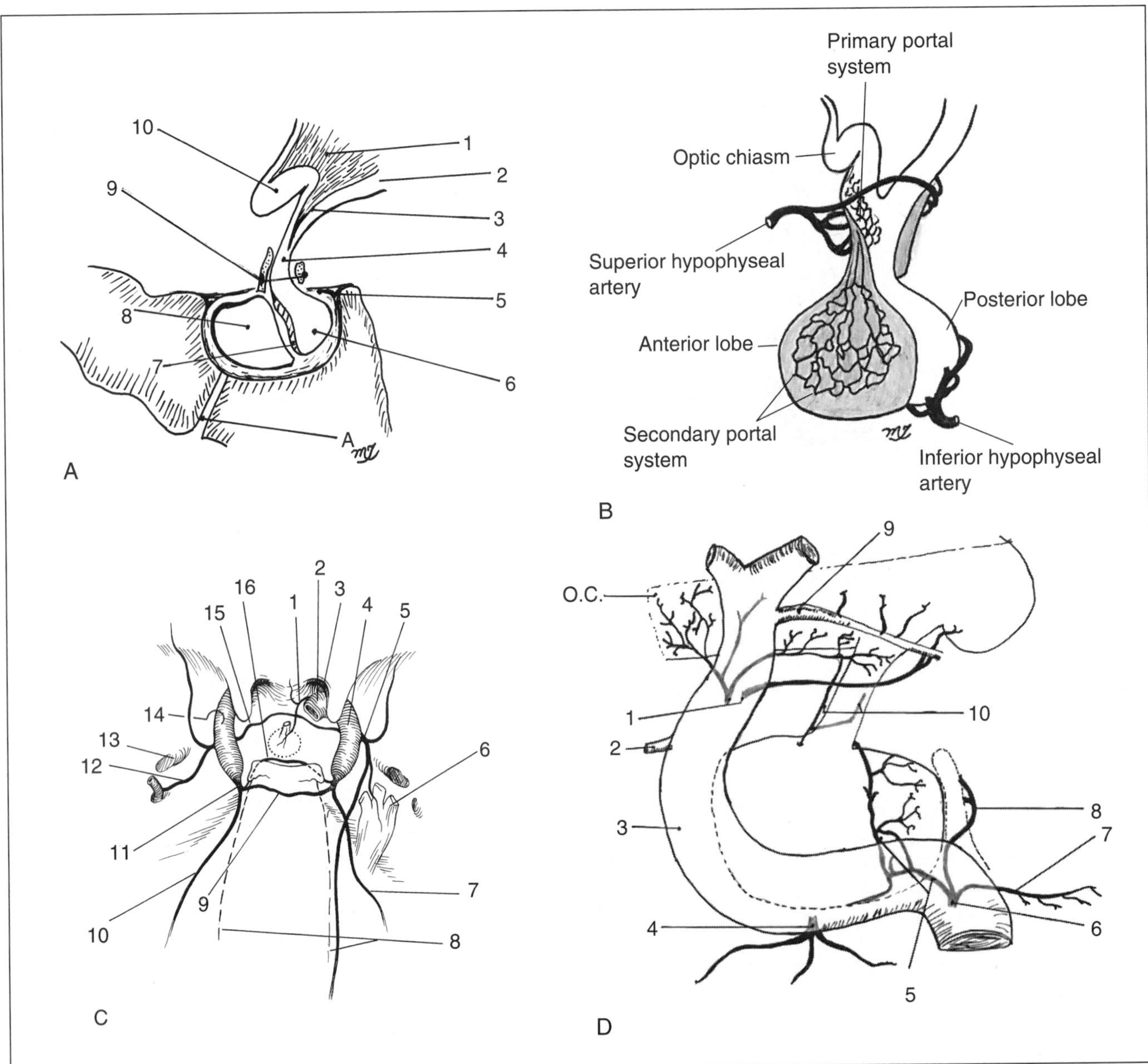

Figure 11.49. A. Diagram of sagittal section of hypophyseal region of embryo at approximately 3 months: (1) third ventricle, (2) wall of hypothalamus, (3) infundibular recess, (4) infundibular stalk, (5) diaphragma sellae, (6) pars neuralis, (7) pars intermedia; Rathke cleft, (8) pars distalis (anterior lobe), (9) pars tuberalis, (10) optic chiasm, (A) craniopharyngeal duct. **B.** Circulation of pituitary gland showing arterial branches and hypothalamic pituitary portal system. The posterior lobe is supplied directly by the inferior hypophyseal artery; the anterior lobe blood supply is indirect via the portal system, as shown. (Modified from Sakamoto et al: Radiology 1991;178:441–445.) **C.** Diagrammatic representation of arterial branches from the intracavernous portion of the internal carotid and blood supply to the hypophysis and parahypophyseal area. Superior view: (1) superior hypophyseal artery, (2) internal carotid artery, (3) optic foramen, (4) carotid intracavernous portion, (5) inferior cavernous artery, (6) gasserian ganglion, (7) medial artery of the tentorium, (8) tentorial edge, (9) dorsal meningeal artery, (10) lateral artery of the tentorium, (11) meningohypophyseal trunk, (12) branch from inferior cavernous artery anastomosing with middle meningeal artery, (13) foramen ovale, (14) internal carotid artery, (15) anterior capsular artery anastomosing with opposite side, (16) inferior hypophyseal artery anastomosing with opposite side and forming circle around dorsum. The dotted circle represents the opening of the diaphragma sellae for the passage of the pituitary stalk. **D.** Lateral view: (O.C.) optic chiasm, (1) superior hypophyseal group, (2) ophthalmic artery, (3) internal carotid artery, (4) inferior cavernous artery, (5) inferior hypophyseal artery and interlobar artery, (6) meningohypophyseal trunk, (7) artery of the tentorium, (8) dorsal meningeal artery, (9) posterior communicating artery, (10) local arteries. (Modified from McConnell: Anat Rec 1953;15:175, and Parkinson: Can J Surg 1964;7:251.)

the presence or absence of calcifications or to diagnose certain lesions involving the bones, such as with chondromas and chondrosarcomas or destructive bone lesions. As with CT, the MRI examination is carried out without and with contrast. When looking for a microadenoma, it is important to image as soon as possible after the contrast injection to avoid slowly increased concentration of contrast material in the microadenoma, which would eliminate the difference between the adenoma and the enhanced surrounding gland (the pituitary gland has no blood-brain barrier). It is best to begin with coronal views, but sagittal views should also be made. These are followed by a routine postcontrast axial T1-weighted series. If the microadenoma is seen without contrast, the contrast injection can be eliminated.

In relation to the pulse sequences used in coronal and sagittal planes, T1-weighted images are superior because in the T2-weighted images the CSF isodensity or hyperdensity obscures the anatomy.

Pathologic Conditions

Hypoplasia of the pituitary gland is not too rare, but congenital absence of the pituitary gland is very unusual. When there is a basal transsphenoidal encephalocele, the gland may be ectopically found and may be deformed. Hypoplasia of the gland may occur but is difficult to diagnose and may not be clinically significant. In *pituitary dwarfism* (GH deficiency) the posterior lobe of the gland is *not* usually found within the sella but may be located in the inferior hypothalamus next to the tuber cinereum. In this case the pituitary stalk is absent (71,72). It is theorized that the absent pituitary stalk may be related to birth trauma in a difficult delivery, which produces rupture of the structure. Kuroiwa et al. found an ectopic posterior pituitary lobe in 7 of 18 patients (73). In 11 patients with pituitary dwarfism the posterior lobe was intrasellar and the stalk was seen on MRI, but the pituitary gland was small. An absent pituitary stalk correlated with brain trauma.

In *transsphenoidal encephalocele* there is an extension of the midline structures through a midline defect. Although these encephaloceles are usually associated with other anomalies, in some cases they seem to represent the only abnormality. (See Fig. 5.14 and Chapter 5 for further discussion.)

The "Empty Sella"

This is defined as a sella turcica that is larger than seems necessary to contain the pituitary gland. The gland is usually flattened against the inferior aspect of the sella, and the pituitary stalk may be longer than usual in order to reach the atrophic gland (Fig. 11.50). The clinical significance is questionable. Patients are frequently encountered who are referred for an MRI examination for persistent headaches and the only finding is that of an "empty sella" or, much more frequently, a partially empty sella. It is difficult, however, to conclude that there is any relationship between the two. A partially empty sella may result from a previous pituitary adenoma that was treated. The previously enlarged sella would be filled with CSF as the tumor shrinks. Sometimes the optic chiasm and the hypothalamus are pulled down into the sella (see Fig. 11.50). This may sometimes produce symptoms such as headaches and visual disturbances (74). In one case the posterior aspect of the gyrus rectus on both sides was pulled down into the anterior aspect of the sella (Fig. 11.55).

Tumors

The most frequent intrasellar tumors are the pituitary adenomas that arise from the anterior lobe of the gland, the adenohypophysis. The posterior lobe, the neurohypophysis, is an outgrowth of the hypothalamus and remains connected with it via the infundibulum or pituitary stalk. It rarely gives rise to tumors. The anterior lobe is of ectodermal origin and results from an invagination of the Rathke pouch from the nasopharynx, although this origin is being challenged (75). Between the two lobes is the intermediate portion, which is nonfunctional but may be the site where small and sometimes large cysts occur.

On T1-weighted images of the normal pituitary, the posterior lobe is hyperintense and the anterior lobe is isointense to gray matter. The hyperintensity is not due to fat but possibly to some phospholipidlike vesicles within the gland (69). The brightness of the posterior lobe does not change when a fat-suppression T1-weighted image is obtained. The hyperintensity disappears in patients affected by diabetes insipidus.

The brightness of the posterior lobe is quite variable; its frequency decreases with age, and it may be seen in one examination and not in another done at a later time (76). The entire gland is bright during the first year of life and the changed intensity between the posterior and the anterior lobes develops gradually (77), particularly after 2 months (78). The increased brightness is probably related to higher protein synthesis in the gland owing to greater metabolic activity in the early postnatal period.

The anterior lobe occupies 80 percent of the volume of the gland and projects on both sides of the much smaller posterior lobe, sometimes surrounding it completely.

The pituitary gland is 12 mm wide, 8 mm in its anteroposterior diameter, and up to 8 mm in height. The height is the most important dimension clinically. The size of the sella turcica is determined by the size of the gland; if the gland grows, the sella enlarges, and vice versa: if the gland shrinks, the sella decreases in size, particularly in children and young adults. The gland increases in size in adolescents and also in young women before menstruation. The most important increase in size occurs during pregnancy, and this increase can be fairly pronounced, sometimes causing

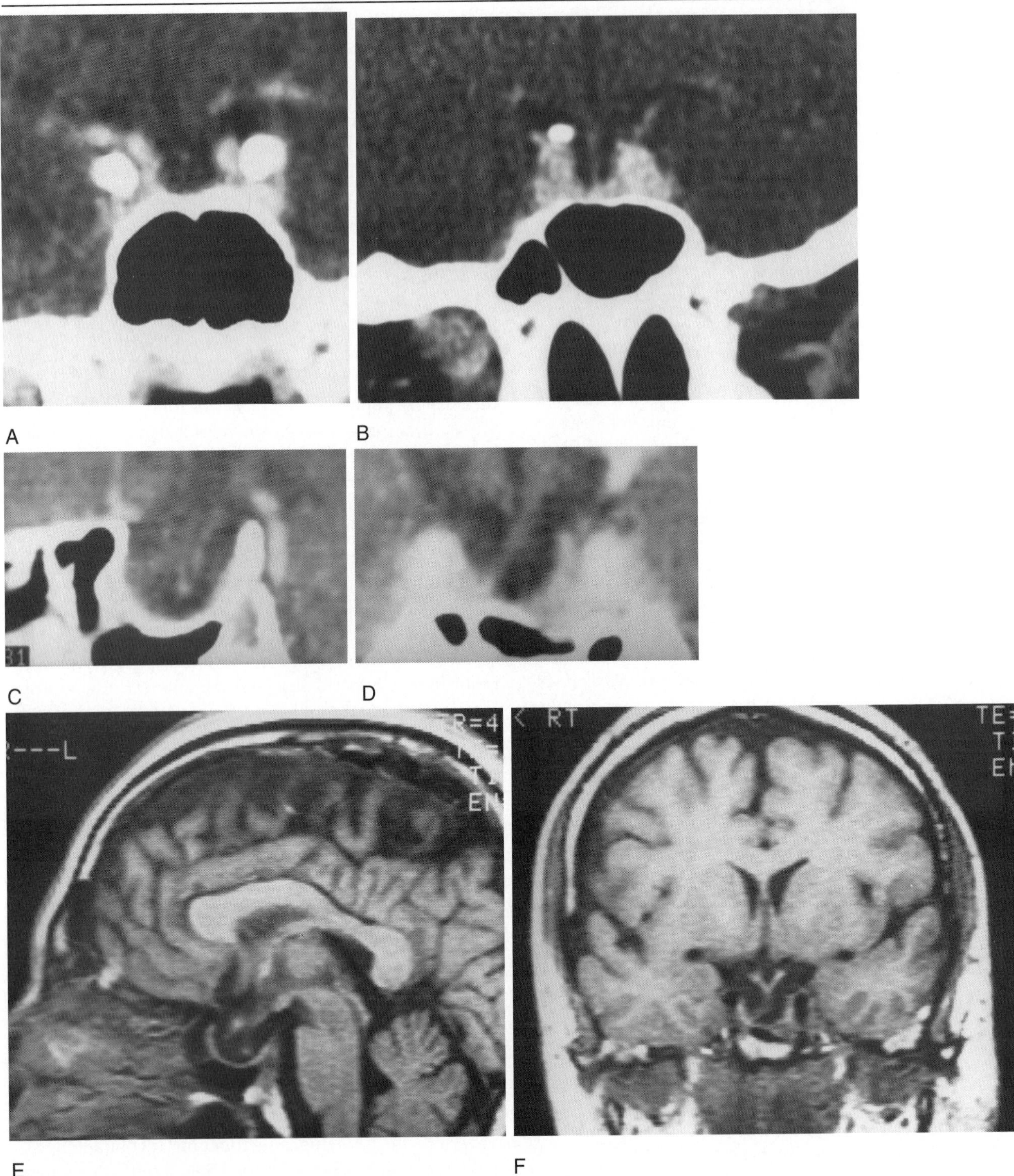

Figure 11.50. A. Empty sella. There is no pituitary gland seen along the floor of the sella, but a thin rim of tissue was seen behind this section. **B.** The pituitary stalk is midline. **C** to **F.** Empty sella with retraction of chiasm and hypothalamus into enlarged sella. The patient had a large prolactinoma with a suprasellar extension that was treated with bromocriptine. The tumor shrunk and brought down the optic chiasm and hypothalamus because it was adherent to it. **C.** Reformatted sagittal CT image shows an enlarged sella and chiasmal and hypothalamic structures. **D.** Coronal reformation shows the stalk attached to the right side of the floor of the sella. **E.** Sagittal T1-weighted image shows essentially the same findings as B but more clearly. **F.** Coronal MR image shows a V-shaped chiasm. This is typical for this condition because the chiasm is pulled down with the floor of the third ventricle, to which it is attached.

enlargement of the sella that persists after the gland shrinks back to normal size. This is one of the mechanisms responsible for the "partially empty sella," which is much more frequently encountered in women.

The pituitary gland is covered by the diaphragma sellae, which usually has a small opening for the passage of the pituitary stalk. The opening, however, can be larger, and sometimes it is much larger, allowing free communication with the CSF in the suprasellar cistern. According to some authors, this is the cause of many cases of empty sella (79).

When the gland enlarges, the upper margin becomes convex, whereas normally it is flat. Slight upward convexity may be encountered in young women before menstruation, and if a young woman is examined at this time, the increased height of the gland should not be considered pathologic unless it is associated with other findings, described in text following.

A *microadenoma* is defined as a pituitary tumor smaller than 10 mm in diameter, and *macroadenoma* one that is larger than 10 mm in size.

The tumors of the pituitary may be divided according to functional or endocrinologic aspects, and also according to histologic characteristics. The endocrinologically active adenomas are the most common (three-quarters of the cases). There are three basic types:

1. *Prolactinomas.* These are by far the most common. They occur most often in women (4:1 ratio) and are found most frequently in menstruating women because the most common manifestation is amenorrhea. The women are usually referred for diagnosis when the tumor is still small. An elevated prolactin level is usually found (above 25 ng/ml in females and above 15 ng/ml in males, and up to 7000 ng/ml), and it is necessary to exclude other causes of this finding, such as pregnancy, some medications, or primary hypothyroidism. In men and postmenopausal women the tumor is silent and can be much larger when it is discovered, which probably occurs because of headaches or visual difficulties due to compression of the optic nerves or chiasm. The tumor frequently invades the wall of the cavernous sinus and may grow into it; this is not an indication of malignant growth.
2. *Growth hormone (somatotrophic) adenomas* are associated with acromegaly in the adult and gigantism in children. They constitute about 20 percent of pituitary adenomas. They are more frequent in males (2:1 ratio). The majority are about 1.0 cm in diameter or larger when first seen and may or may not compress the optic chiasm. They may be pure GH–secreting adenomas, or they may be mixed somatotrophic- and prolactin-secreting adenomas, and occur in about 20 percent of acromegalic patients (80).
3. *Adrenal corticotropic hormone–secreting adenomas.* These occur in patients with Cushing disease and can also be associated with Nelson syndrome (accelerated growth of an ACTH-secreting pituitary adenoma in a patient previously adrenalectomized for Cushing syndrome). A small percentage of these tumors are asymptomatic.

Thyrotrophic (secreting thyroid-stimulating hormone [TSH]) and *gonadotrophic* (secreting follicle-stimulating hormone [FSH]) pituitary adenomas are rare: less than 1 percent of cases (81,82) (Table 11.37).

The *endocrinologically inactive* pituitary adenomas constitute one-quarter of the tumors. The old term, *chromophobic pituitary adenomas*, is not appropriate because many of the tumors were prolactinomas that were not recognized. Because of the lack of function, they are likely to grow to a large size and are revealed only by signs of chiasmal compression or hypopituitarism, or are incidentally discovered in a patient being investigated for headaches. The term *oncocytoma* is applied to a subset of these tumors because their cytoplasm is packed with mitochondria (83). Some pituitary oncocytomas may be endocrinologically active (4).

Tumors arising from the neurohypophysis are rare. There are two types: the *gliomas*, also known as *pilocytic astrocytomas* or *pituicytomas;* and the *granular cell tumors*, also known as *choristomas*, *myoblastomas* or *granular cell myoblastomas* (84). Most of these are discovered as an incidental finding at autopsy, but some may grow to a large size and cause compression of the optic pathways. The choristomas may be very vascular and may be composed of a tough tissue that is difficult to remove at surgery (Fig 11.54*E* and *F*).

Imaging Diagnosis

Microadenomas are typically hypodense on CT in relation to the pituitary gland. This appearance can be brought out further by intravenous contrast injection, as explained in text preceding. The pituitary gland enhances rapidly and the adenoma enhances more slowly, and if the examination is carried out within 15 min, the adenoma may not have enhanced sufficiently to reach the level of the pituitary tissue. However, Sakamoto et al. have shown that enhancement of the entire normal pituitary occurs within 80 sec after the end of a rapid bolus injection of gadolinium (85). Furthermore, they have shown that maximum differential enhancement between the adenoma and the gland is seen at 60 sec on a dynamic scan. Unfortunately, it is difficult to obtain such rapid imaging on a routine basis, although single images using a spin-echo technique can be obtained rapidly on a 1.5-Tesla magnet. MRI is the preferred diagnostic modality because of the ease of obtaining multiple

Table 11.37.
Pituitary Adenomas

Prolactinomas: Usually small at time of discovery; Frequently present with amenorrhea
Somatotrophic (growth hormone secreting): Produce acromegaly in adulthood, gigantism in children; Usually larger than 1 cm (macroadenomas)
Adrenocorticotrophic hormone–secreting tumors: Cushing disease
About 25% of adenomas are endocrinologically inactive
Thyrotrophic and gonadotrophic adenomas are rare

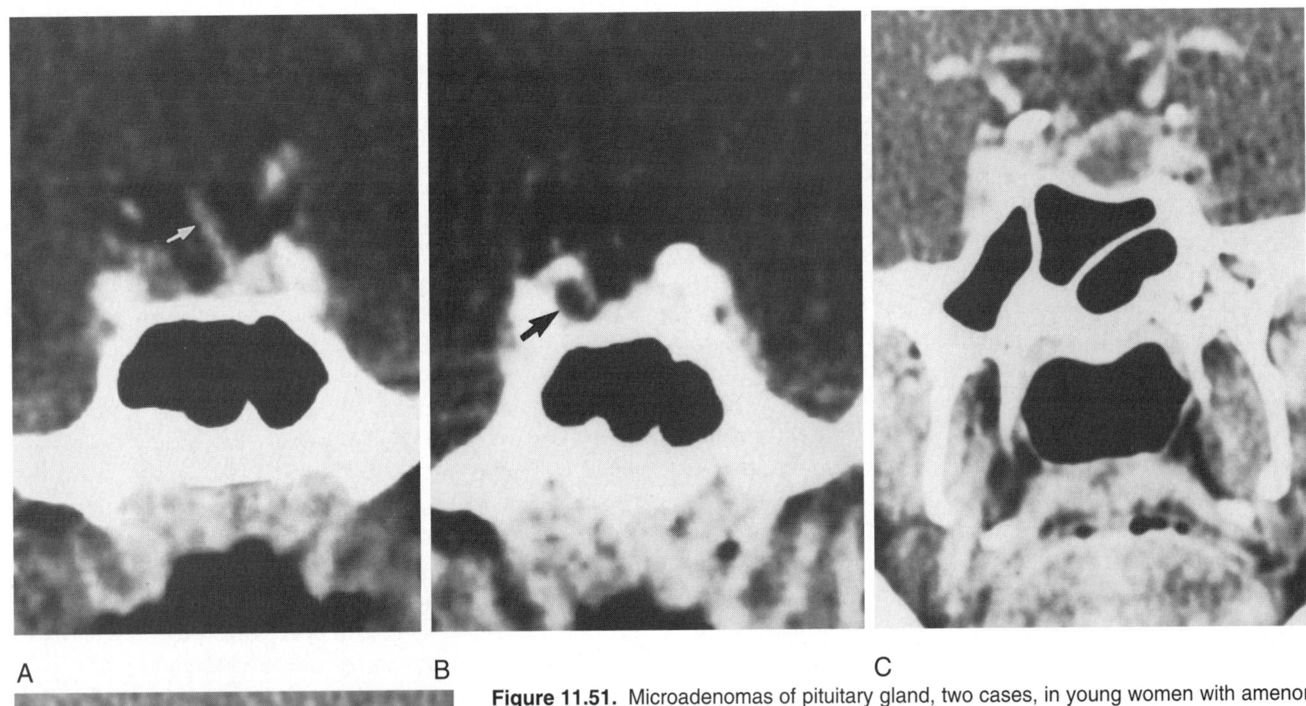

Figure 11.51. Microadenomas of pituitary gland, two cases, in young women with amenorrhea and elevated prolactin. **A** and **B.** Enhanced CT coronal images show an unenhanced, low-density, slightly oval, anteriorly placed lesion consistent with a microadenoma (black arrow). The stalk is deviated to the left (white arrow), and the sella turcica is partially empty. **C** and **D.** Enhanced CT scan shows a microadenoma larger than the one in A and B that is also situated anteriorly in the sella and to the left of the midline. The anterior clinoid process on the left is seen (arrow).

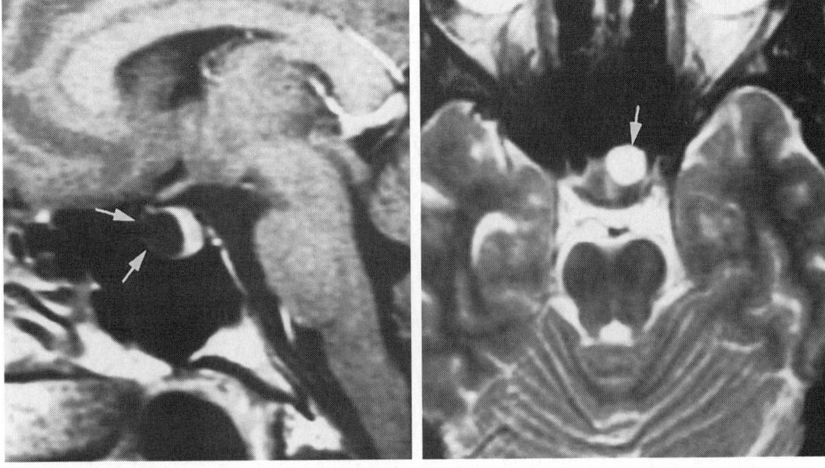

Figure 11.52. Pituitary microadenoma, cystic. **A.** Sagittal view (T1-weighted) shows a hypointense, sharply circumscribed area (arrows) in the sella turcica, which on a T2-weighted axial image (**B**) is bright and slightly brighter than CSF (arrow).

views and because the contrast media, namely, gadolinium compounds, are less likely to produce even minor intolerance effects. The microadenomas are hypointense on T1-weighted images (long T1) in relation to the surrounding pituitary gland and hyperintense on T2-weighted images (long T2). As in CT, contrast enhancement causes greater contrast between the adenoma and the gland (Figs. 11.51 and 11.52).

The lower-intensity adenoma seems to become even more so momentarily. This has been attributed to earlier enhancement of the remaining normal pituitary tissue. However, Yuh et al. have shown that the adenomas actually begin enhancement before the normal pituitary gland on rapid MR images (86). If the study by Yuh et al. is correct, contrast enhancement does not really add any information, and one wonders about the value of this added procedure in the diagnosis of microadenomas. In the differential diagnosis of larger lesions, however, contrast enhancement is justifiable and necessary. The prolactinomas tend to occur anteriorly and on either side of the gland because the prolactin-secreting cells are more abundant laterally. The same is true of the growth hormone cells (Fig. 11.51); on the other hand, the ACTH-, TSH-, and FSH-producing cells are more numerous in the center of the gland, and these adenomas tend to occur centrally.

In the diagnosis of microadenomas, the preferred method is MRI. However, CT, if performed with high-resolution equipment and carefully monitored, will yield a positive rate quite similar to that of MRI (87–89). In the diagnosis of ACTH-secreting microadenomas Marcovitz et al. reported a correct diagnosis in about 60 percent of the cases (14 of 24) as proven by surgery (87). With MRI, Newton et al. reported an accuracy of 66 percent, a diagnosis in 2 of 6, a strongly suspected diagnosis in 3 of 6, and a negative diagnosis in 1 (90). In 1 of the 6 cases the location of the adenoma at surgery was not the same as on MRI. The ACTH-secreting adenomas are more difficult to visualize than the prolactinomas, which are seen on CT and particularly on MRI in a high percentage of cases (about 90 percent). The exact percentage is difficult to assess because an elevated serum prolactin level may be found in the absence of a prolactinoma. Such a case is illustrated in Figure 11.53, that of a young woman with hypermenorrhea and elevated prolactin level in whom an intrasellar arterial anomaly was found. In the ACTH-secreting adenomas a diagnosis is important because surgery is usually necessary for cure. Surgery is often performed even if a microadenoma is not shown on CT or MRI. Proton beam or cobalt radiosurgery are also possible choices, but conventional radiation therapy is not effective on a long-term basis.

Secondary signs of microadenomas are sometimes helpful. If the microadenomas reach sufficient size—6 to 8 mm in diameter—and are situated on one side or the other, as is most frequently found, the pituitary stalk is displaced to the opposite side. A lateral stalk position, however, is not a very reliable sign, for it is sometimes seen in the absence of a tumor, and occasionally the stalk may be displaced to the same side. Another secondary sign of adenoma is a downward concavity of the floor of the sella under the small tumor. This was considered a very important sign of adenoma on coronal bone tomograms of the sellar floor prior to the advent of CT, but is less frequently relied upon today.

The larger pituitary adenomas are diagnosed by CT or MR in 100 percent of cases. Most cases show growth in a superior direction, encroaching on the suprasellar cisternal space. If the tumors grow sufficiently upward, they bend and elevate the optic chiasm, producing visual disturbances, usually bitemporal hemianopia (Fig. 11.54). Sometimes the mass is very large and lifts the third-ventricular floor sufficiently to cause partial blockage of the foramen of Monro and hydrocephalus. Following surgery in these large adenomas, the shrinkage of the tissues pulls the chiasm into the sella, as shown in Figure 11.50*C* to *E*. Occasionally even the gyrus rectus may herniate into the large empty sella (Fig. 11.55). Lateral growth takes place in two different ways: the tumor may invade the wall and the actual cavernous sinus (Fig. 11.56), or it may displace the sinus but does not appear to invade it.

It is important to determine whether invasion of the cavernous sinus wall and of the sinus itself has occurred because this makes complete surgical removal of the tumor impossible, and in these cases radiation therapy is preferred. Invasion of the cavernous sinus wall is not an indication of a malignant tumor; they remain, with very few exceptions, histologically benign tumors. Downward growth of pituitary macroadenomas occurs not infrequently, and in these cases bone invasion and erosion at the floor of the pituitary fossa can be demonstrated by CT or MRI (Fig. 11.57).

Malignant degeneration of pituitary adenomas may occur. The tendency toward malignancy may be more frequently seen in the GH- and the ACTH-secreting adenomas. Metastases may occur via the CSF or at a distance, particularly to the liver, but sometimes to the lungs and the skeleton (91).

Hemorrhage

Hemorrhage into pituitary adenomas is common and usually asymptomatic. It was thought that when hemorrhage occurred, it led frequently to the clinical syndrome referred to as *pituitary apoplexy*. However, with the advent of MRI, signs of hemorrhage in smaller and larger pituitary adenomas are frequently seen. An acute hemorrhage will be bright on T2-weighted images and isodense on T1-weighted images; a subacute hemorrhage will be bright on T1- and T2-weighted images; and an older hemorrhage will show signs of magnetic susceptibility and will appear dark on T2-weighted images (Figs. 11.58 to 11.60) (92).

In the case of an acute severe hemorrhage, CT examination is superior to MRI because it will usually show hyperdensity. In a clinical pituitary apoplexy syndrome, however,

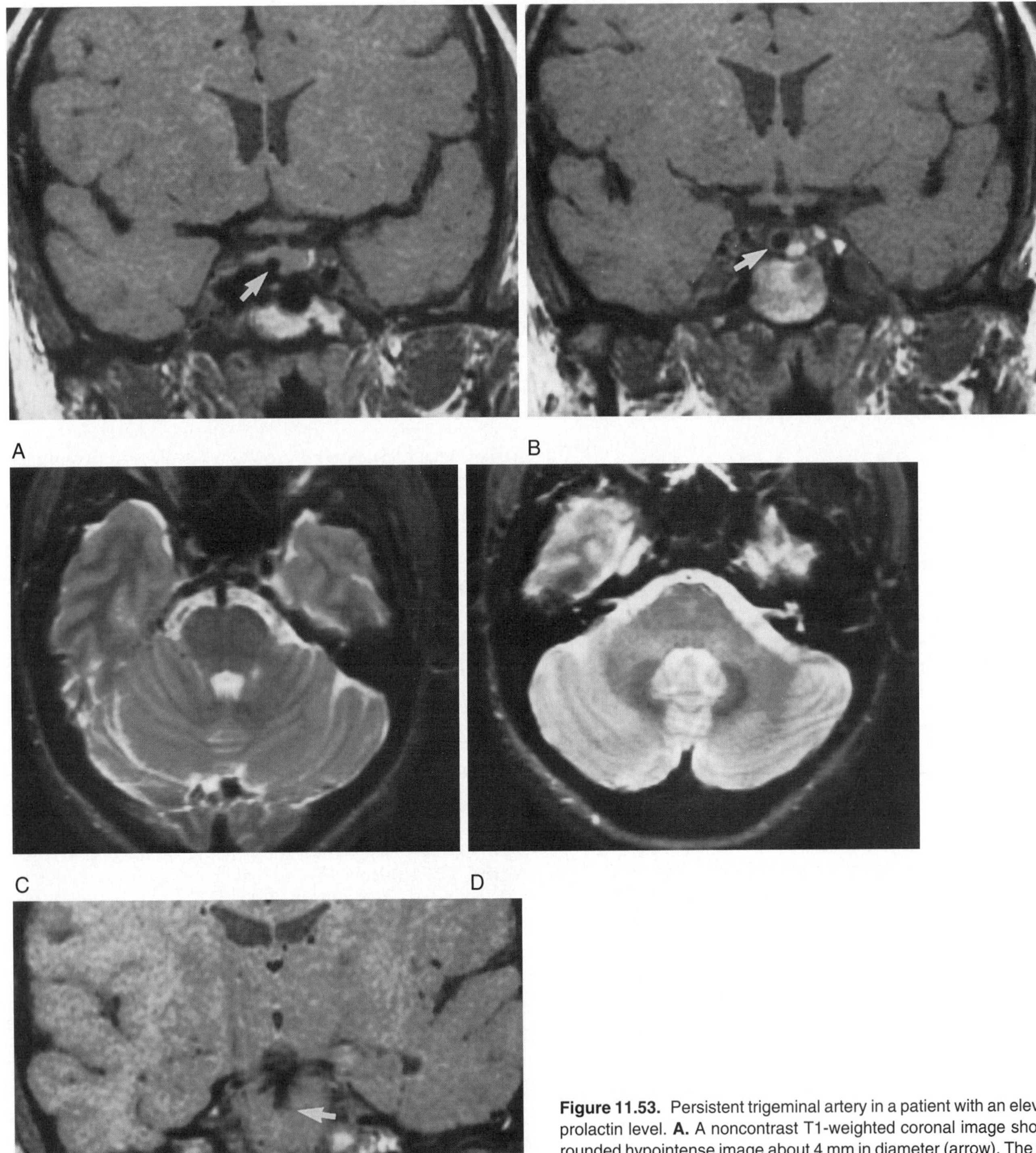

Figure 11.53. Persistent trigeminal artery in a patient with an elevated prolactin level. **A.** A noncontrast T1-weighted coronal image shows a rounded hypointense image about 4 mm in diameter (arrow). The pituitary gland is isointense; the pituitary stalk is slightly deviated to the other side. **B.** A section posterior to A shows the rounded hypointense image to have an appearance compatible with a flow void (arrow). The bright area below and to the left of it is a bright posterior lobe. The bright spots to the left represent some fat in the cavernous sinus. **C.** Axial T2-weighted image reveals a flow void crossing the prepontine cisternal space. **D.** An axial T2-weighted image below C shows absence of flow void for the basilar artery. **E.** A coronal view shows that the basilar artery stops abruptly at the upper pons (arrow).

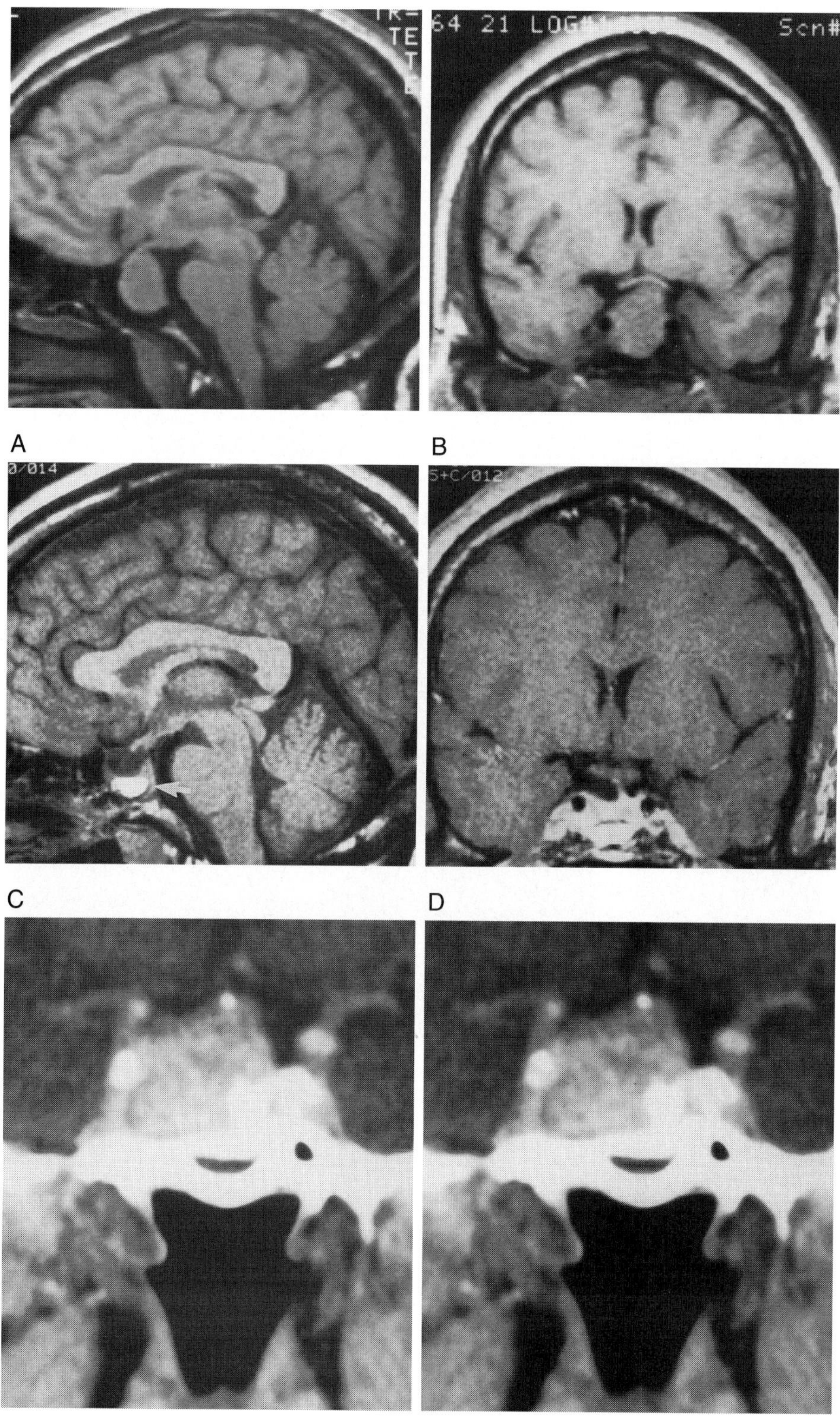

Figure 11.54. Large pituitary prolactinoma in a 40-year-old woman. **A.** Sagittal noncontrast T1-weighted view. The tumor enlarges the sella and is growing above it, elevating the optic chiasm and the lower third ventricle. **B.** Coronal T1-weighted image shows the elevated chiasm bowed over the dome of the tumor. The tumor is isointense with cerebral gray matter. **C.** Reexamination 9 months later following transsphenoidal hypophysectomy. T1-weighted sagittal image shows a partially empty sella and slight depression of the hypothalamus and optic chiasm in the suprasellar cistern. There is an oval hyperintense area within the sella representing fat placed there at the time of surgery (arrow). **D.** Coronal postcontrast T1-weighted image shows the pituitary stalk deviated to the left. The residual pituitary tissue enhances and obscures the fatty mass within the sella. No residual tumor is seen. **E.** Granular cell tumor (granular cell myoblastoma, choristoma) of the pituitary. Surgical removal had been performed, but the tumor was found to be tough and bloody. There is suprasellar extension, and the tumor enhanced, as shown in this coronal postcontrast CT image. **F.** Reexamination 2 years later shows no change at all in the size, configuration, or enhancing characteristics of the tumor. This is typical for granular cell tumors, which enhance and grow very slowly or remain stationary.

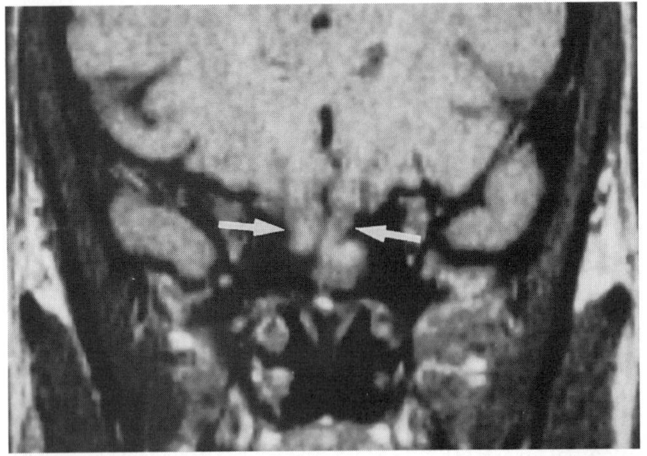

A

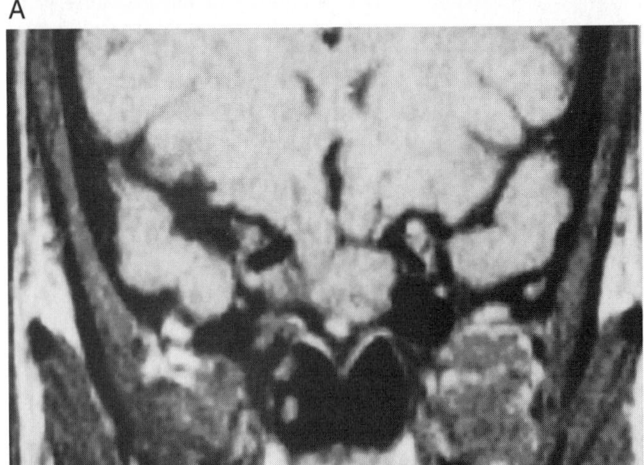

B

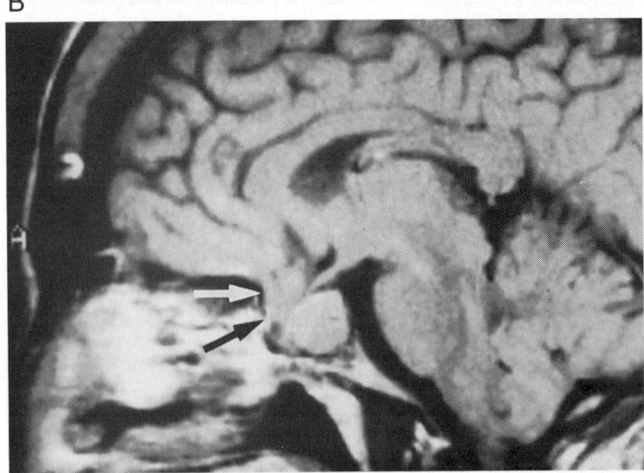

C

Figure 11.55. Pituitary adenoma. Postoperative herniation of gyrus rectus into anterior aspect of sella turcica. **A.** Coronal T1-weighted noncontrast image shows that both gyri recti are elongated and extending downward. **B.** The section posterior to it shows that the right gyrus rectus extends down into the sella alongside the isointense, operatively placed mass of muscle in the sella. Surgery had been performed several years previously. **C.** Sagittal T1-weighted postcontrast image shows the tongue of the gyrus rectus extending down into the anterior sella (arrows). There is no enhancement of the soft tissues.

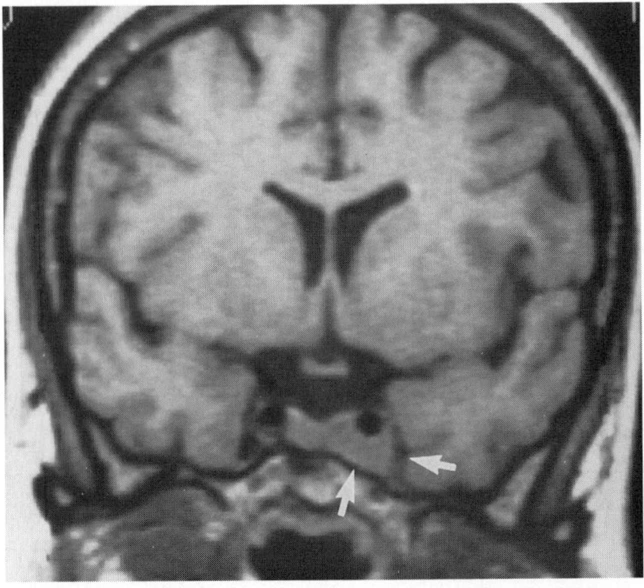

A

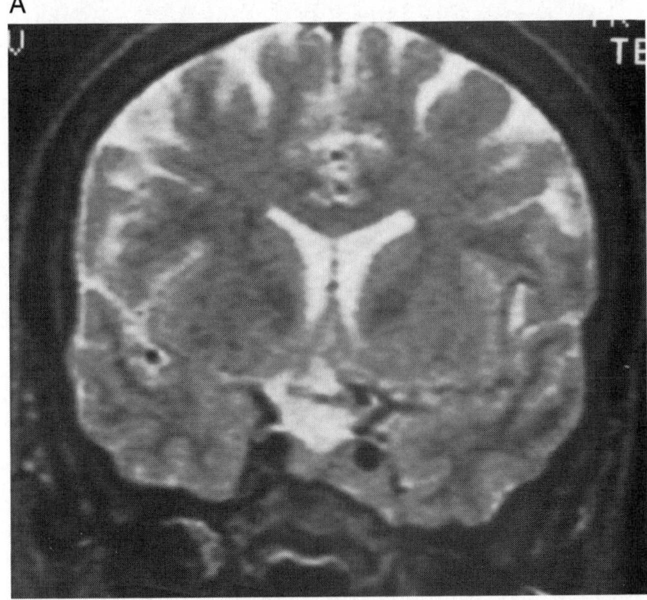

B

Figure 11.56. Pituitary growth hormone–secreting adenoma invading the cavernous sinus. **A.** Coronal view without contrast shows direct involvement of the left cavernous sinus by the isointense adenoma (arrows). The internal carotid artery is surrounded by tumor laterally, medially, and inferiorly but is not narrowed. The lateral margin of the cavernous sinus is seen separating the sinus contents from the medial temporal lobe (lateral arrow). **B.** T2-weighted coronal view shows the tumor and its intracavernous portion to be isointense compared with brain tissue gray matter. The tumor does not project into the suprasellar space, and the suprasellar cistern is bright, like CSF. The patient had had two surgical procedures but had persistent elevated growth hormone serum levels. Because of invasion of the cavernous sinus, surgery was ineffective, and it was decided to treat with proton beam "radiosurgery," because conventional radiation therapy would control the tumor only temporarily.

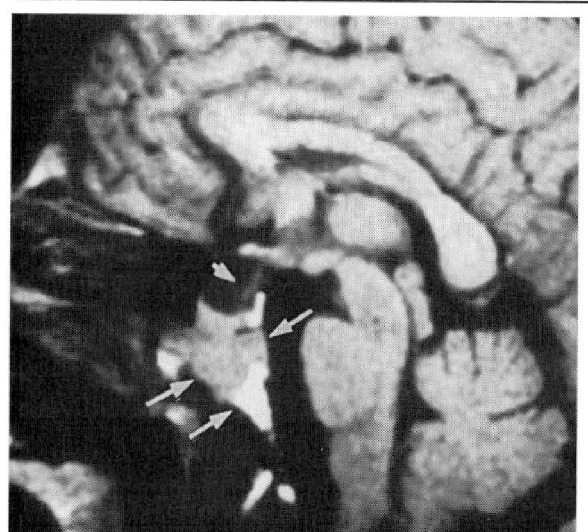

A

Figure 11.57. Invasion of the clivus by a pituitary adenoma in a 48-year-old man. The patient had a surgically treated pituitary adenoma. **A.** The T1-weighted sagittal view reveals loss of the bone marrow hyperintensity in most of the clivus (arrows); only the lower portion remains normal (lower arrow). The enlarged sella and the pituitary stalk are seen above (arrowhead). Invasion of the cavernous sinus and even of the bone is not necessarily an indication of malignant degeneration of a pituitary adenoma. **B** and **C.** Another patient. Pituitary adenoma extending into the cavernous sinus and involving the clivus. **B.** Precontrast sagittal image shows a fairly large macroadenoma extending into the suprasellar region and growing down into the sphenoid sinus and clivus (arrows). The hyperintense area in the middle represents a large fat pad surgically inserted following prior surgical resection. **C.** Postcontrast sagittal image reveals moderate enhancement of the neoplasm.

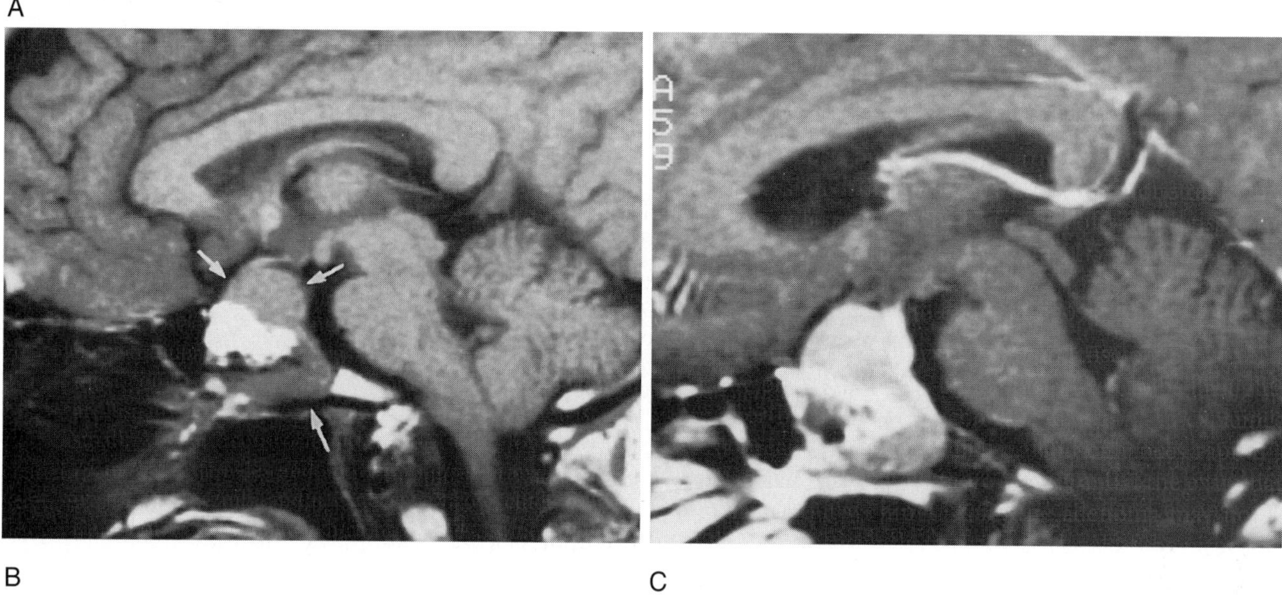

B C

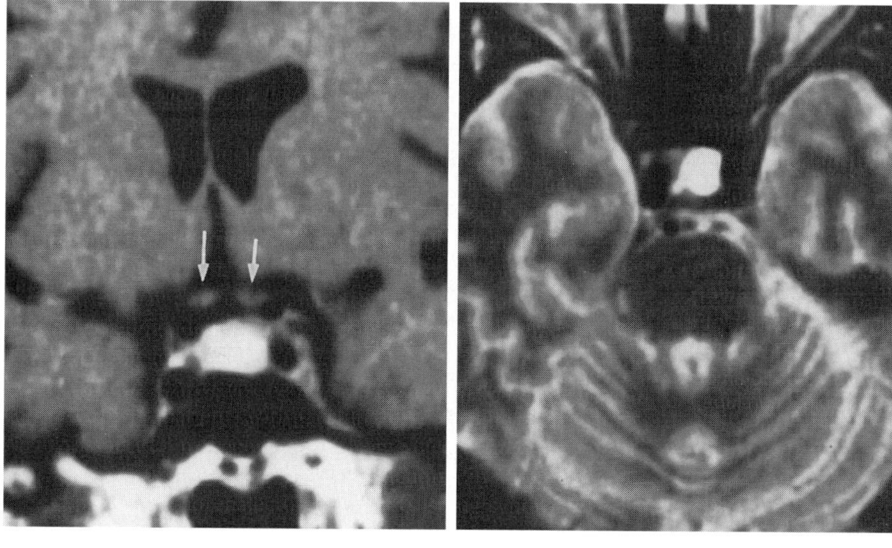

A B

Figure 11.58. Postpartum pituitary hemorrhage. **A.** Coronal T1-weighted image shows a bright, moderately bulging pituitary gland that does not reach the optic chiasm situated above (arrows). **B.** T2-weighted axial image shows a very bright pituitary gland that remains confined within the sella turcica.

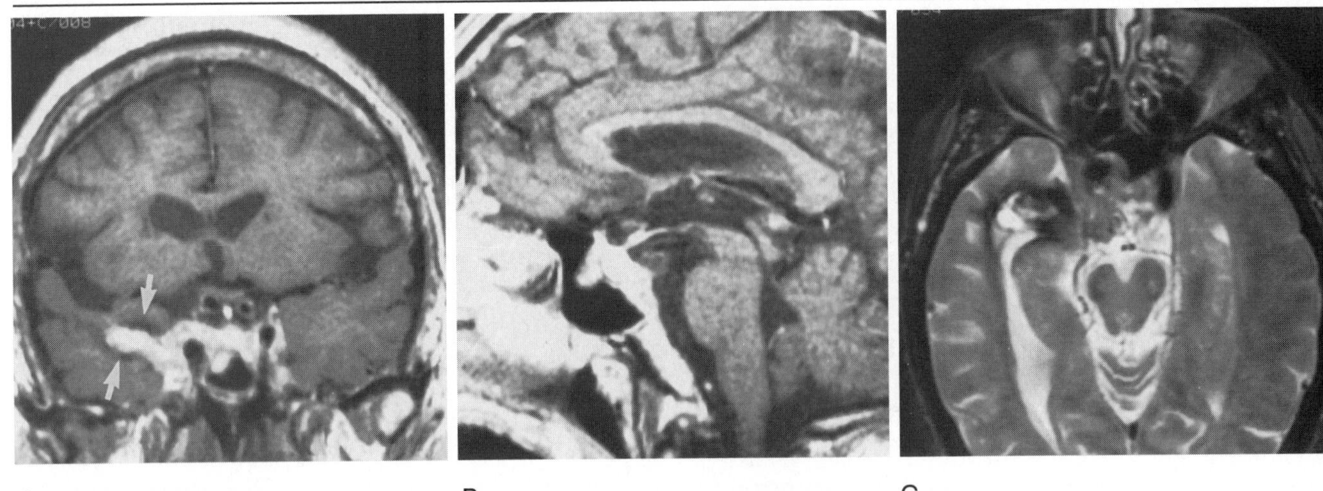

A B C

Figure 11.59. Pituitary adenoma extending laterally and showing signs of previous bleeding. **A.** Postcontrast T1-weighted coronal image shows enhancement of the pituitary gland and enhancement of the right lateral extension of the tumor, which goes beyond the cavernous sinus wall. The lateral hyperintense portion is surrounded by a hypointense halo (arrows). There is no suprasellar extension and the pituitary stalk is enhancing normally. The right internal carotid intracavernous portion is displaced slightly downward compared to the left. **B.** Midline lateral view. **C.** Axial T2-weighted image shows magnetic susceptibility in the right anterior temporal region consistent with prior hemorrhage. The patient was under treatment with bromocriptine, which accounts for the disappearance of the suprasellar extension of the tumor. The hemorrhage is probably unrelated to the therapy and was an incidental finding.

CT may sometimes show a hypodense image that may indicate acute necrosis of the gland with swelling (92). Reformatting can be used to obtain sagittal and coronal images on CT in orter to appreciate the size of the mass more completely.

Emergency surgical decompression may be needed, and CT and MRI demonstration are very important for deciding on the approach. The decompression can be done with stereotactically directed needling, which allows for drainage of the liquid component. Sometimes the adenoma may completely disappear after the hemorrhage (1 out of 12 cases of Ostrov et al., surgically proved [92]). In one of the author's cases, a 12-month follow-up revealed a partially empty sella that did not seem to contain a tumor (Fig. 11.60). The same case also presented carotid artery dissection, an unusual occurrence that was felt to have been provoked by the pituitary hemorrhage (93). A case was reported by Momose and New in which the gland increased in size so rapidly that it compressed the internal carotid artery against the anterior clinoid process, leading to hemiparesis (94).

A T1-bright microadenoma is sometimes found that is probably produced by hemorrhage into the adenoma. At surgery a cyst containing brown blood may be found (95).

PERISELLAR LESIONS

Rathke Cleft Cysts

Small intrasellar cysts are commonly found at autopsy. They are situated between the two lobes of the pituitary and are of no clinical significance. They arise from remnants of Rathke pouch, the cephalic end of which terminates normally between the anterior and posterior lobes. The cysts are lined by cuboidal or columnar epithelium, sometimes ciliated, and not by squamous epithelium, as in the craniopharyngiomas. These cysts can be large and can grow into the suprasellar space, sometimes compressing the optic chiasm. Their content is fluid or viscid, mucoid, and sometimes brown from old hemorrhage.

When the cyst is large, it may be difficult to differentiate from a noncalcified craniopharyngioma. The arachnoid cysts are likely to be clearly suprasellar in location and produce flattening of the pituitary gland from above. Their contents are like CSF on all pulse sequences on MRI. The diagnosis of a Rathke cleft cyst may be suggested when a cystic mass has a clearly intrasellar location with variable suprasellar extension. If the contents are hyperintense on T1-weighted images, they are usually also hyperintense on T2-weighted sequences, indicating the presence of high protein. Some can be hypointense on T2-weighted images, possibly from old blood products (Fig. 11.61). If the fluid content is like CSF, it will follow the CSF density on CT or MRI. Rathke cleft cysts do not enhance.

Craniopharyngiomas

The frequency of craniopharyngiomas is usually quoted as 3 percent of all intracranial tumors. More than 50 percent occur in children or adolescents, and there is no sex predilection. A second peak occurs around the fourth and fifth

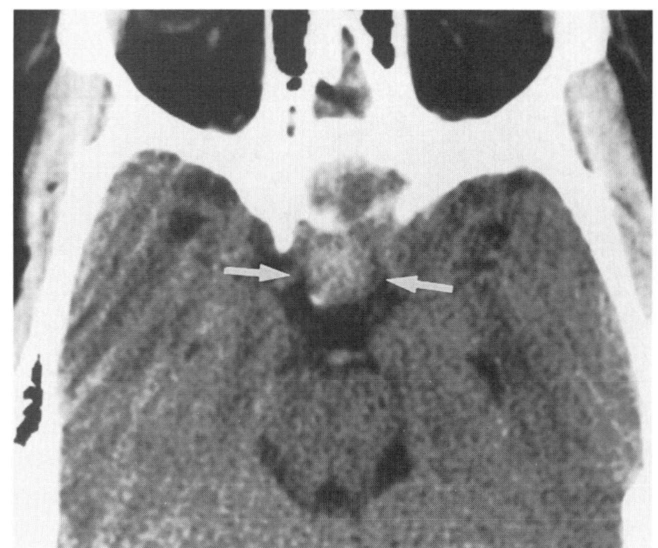

Figure 11.60. Pituitary hemorrhage. **A.** CT shows a hyperdense area in the suprasellar region (arrows). **B** and **C.** Coronal and sagittal T1-weighted images show a hyperintense large mass upwardly displacing the optic chiasm. There is evidence of isodense soft tissue in the inferior aspect. **D.** The intrapetrosal portion of the internal carotid artery in the carotid canal shows hyperintensity in this T1-weighted image consistent with dissection of the internal carotid artery (arrows). **E.** A higher section reveals the left internal carotid artery lumen surrounded by a bright halo. The flow void shows a narrower lumen on the left side (horizontal arrow) as compared to the right (vertical arrow). (Courtesy of Dr. James Provenzale, Duke University Medical Center, Durham, NC.) **F.** Sagittal postcontrast T1-weighted image 12 months later shows shrinkage of the sellar and suprasellar mass and a concave residual soft-tissue component in a partially empty sella. There was no surgical proof that the tumor had self-destructed, and the residual tissue is inhomogeneous, which may indicate that there is some tumor remaining. It is felt that the pituitary hemorrhage provoked internal carotid dissection in this patient.

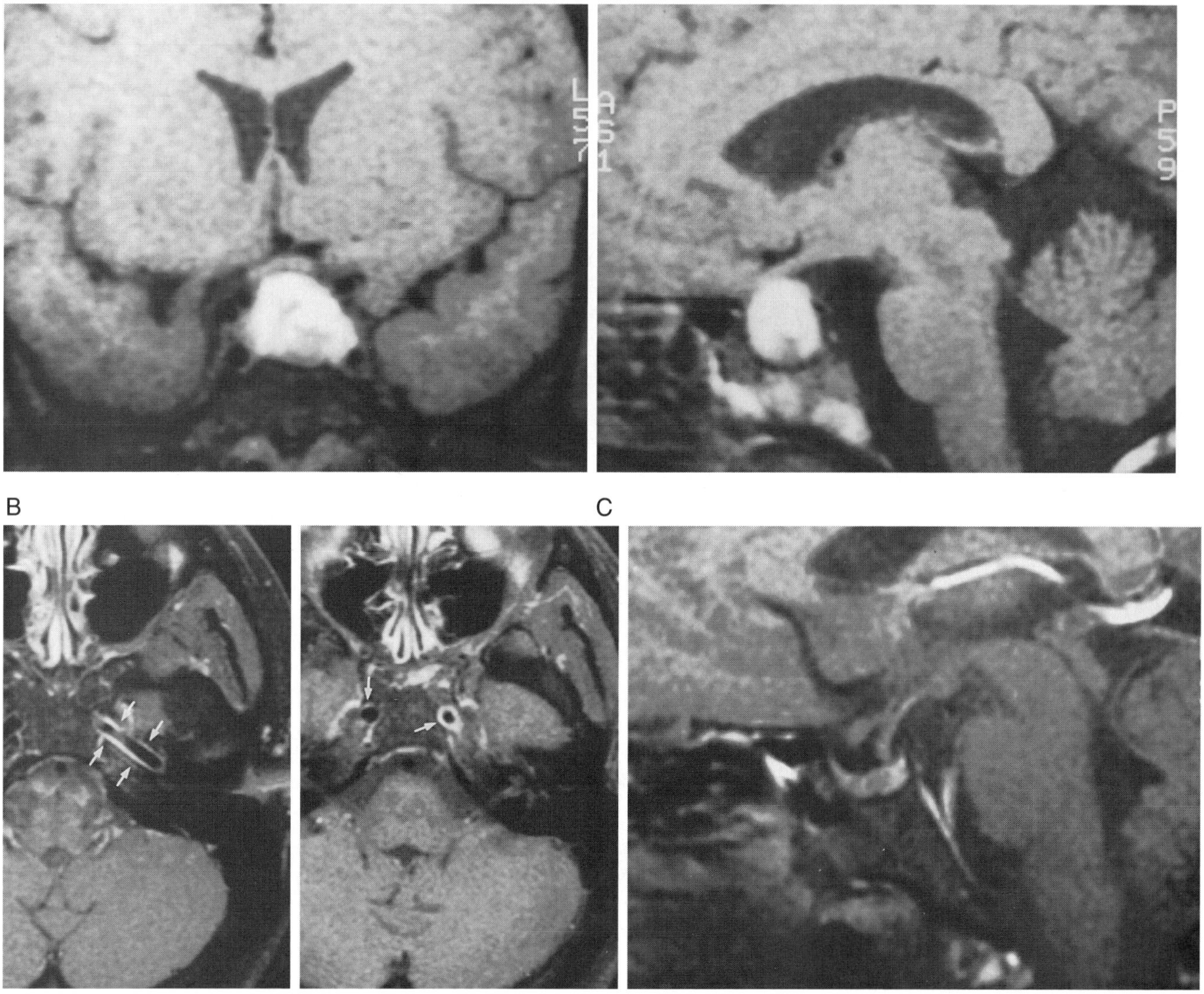

A

B C

D E F

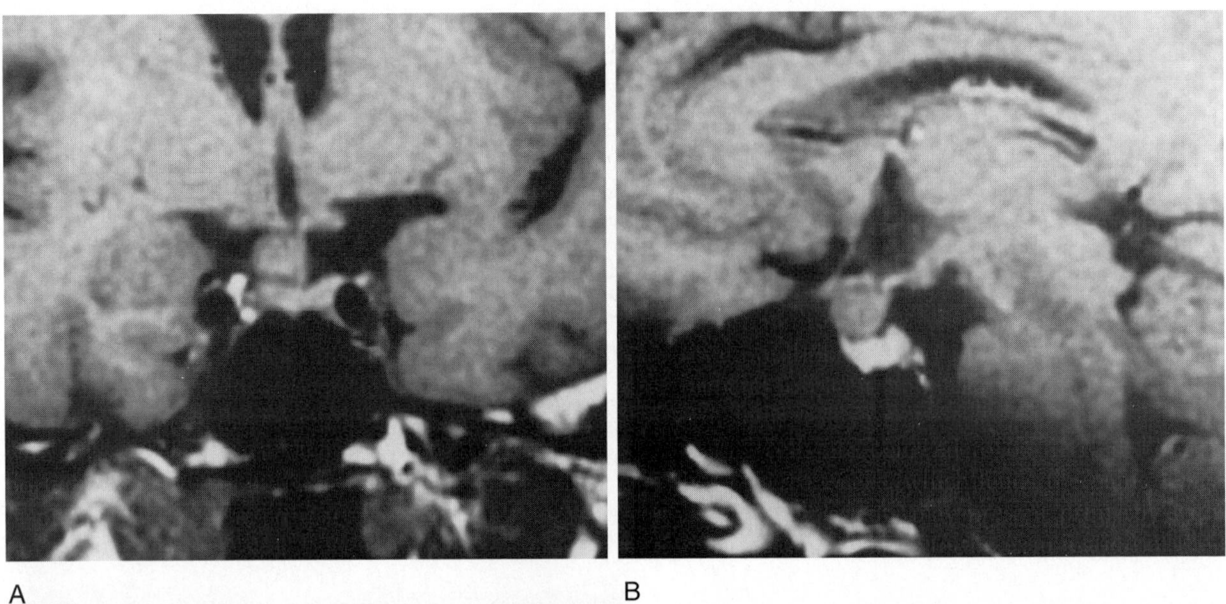

Figure 11.61. Rathke cleft cyst. **A.** There is a suprasellar cyst isodense on T1-weighted image. **B.** Sagittal T1-weighted image. It is moderately hyperintense on proton density axial image (**C**). **D** and **E.** Sagittal and coronal T1-weighted images done 2 years later showing no change.

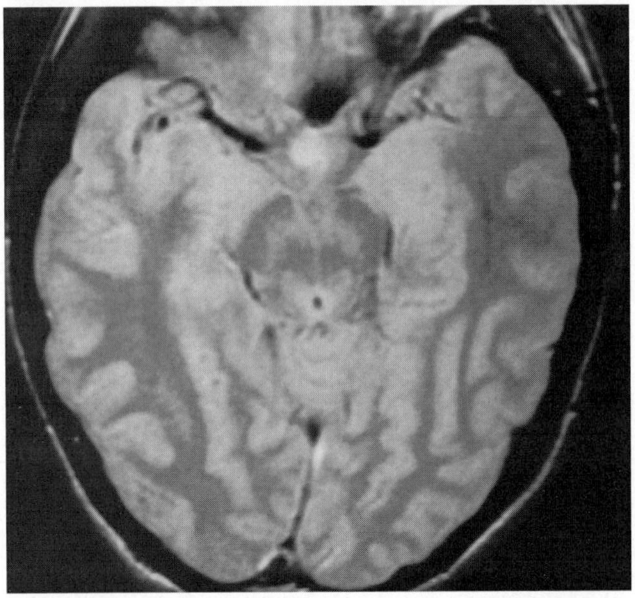

C

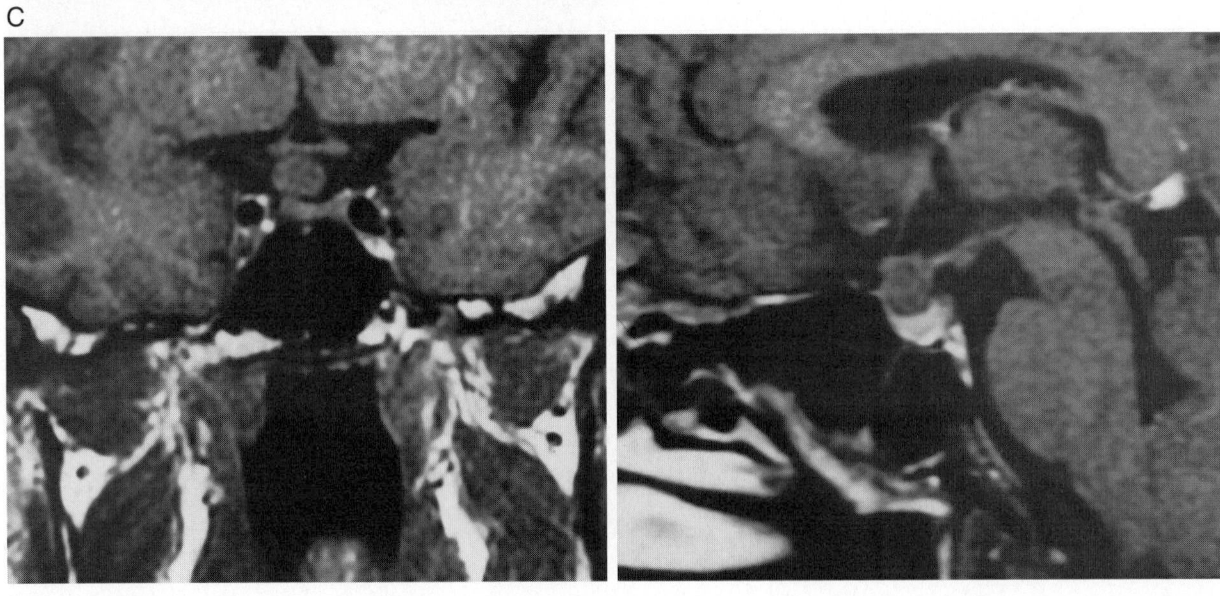

decades. They usually present a cystic component lined by a simple stratified squamous epithelium. Solid components are often present, and at times the entire tumor is solid or nearly so. The name *adamantinoma* has been applied to some craniopharyngiomas because they look microscopically like these tumors, but the term is somewhat confusing and should not be used.

It is widely accepted that craniopharyngiomas arise from remnants of the Rathke pouch and particularly from remnants in the region of the pars tuberalis around the pituitary stalk (Fig. 11.49*A*); as can be seen in the diagram, the pars tuberalis is in the suprasellar region, and most craniopharyngiomas arise above the sella. Some arise inside the sella and grow out of it.

Calcification is present in about 70 percent of craniopharyngiomas and is somewhat less frequent in the adult type (Fig. 11.62). The tumors are usually in the midline and grow in the suprasellar region, compressing the third ventricle and producing hydrocephalus. They tend to extend backward and downward behind the sella, producing posterior displacement of the brainstem (Fig. 11.63). Some grow to a very large size, and the cysts can extend laterally and forward, markedly displacing the brain. Some craniopharyngiomas can be entirely intraventricular and remain within the third ventricle (40,61). See text preceding under "Anterior Third Ventricle Tumors."

The content of the cysts is classically described as "machine oil" and contains remnants of cells, cholesterol crystals (which vary in abundance from case to case), and a variable amount of protein. These combinations tend to modify the imaging characteristics on MRI. On CT the most characteristic features in a child are a partly calcified cystic tumor in the suprasellar region. Hydrocephalus may or may not be present (Fig. 11.62). The solid components of the cyst wall usually enhance with contrast.

On MRI the calcification is not usually seen, although it may be suspected in the T2-weighted images where the suprasellar CSF should be bright; the cyst fluid will be hyperintense on T1- and T2-weighted images if it is rich in cholesterol (96,97) (Fig. 11.64). Five of the 15 cases of Price et al. were intrasellar (97). Enhancement is common.

Suprasellar Arachnoid Cysts

Arachnoid cysts are considered congenital anomalies and are described in Chapter 5. These cysts occur in various locations. The most common location is the anterior temporal fossa, but they may also be found elsewhere (perimesencephalic, interhemispheric, velum interpositum, hemispheric, and suprasellar regions). Pathologically the cyst is located between two membranes that are continuous at the margin of the cyst with the arachnoid membrane (98,99). Thus the cysts could be called intra-arachnoid cysts. A theory was proposed by Fox and Al-Mefty concerning the origin of the suprasellar arachnoid cysts from the membrane of Liliequist, in which the membrane is considered to split into two leaves with the cyst forming in the middle (100). The theory is disputed by some, but it remains as a possibility.

On CT and MRI the cysts are CSF density or intensity in all images, their wall does not enhance, and there are no nodules or irregularities in the wall (Fig. 11.65). They can become very large, compressing the third ventricle, elevating the floor up to the foramen of Monro, and producing hydrocephalus. Hoffman et al. indicate that as they grow upward, they seem to split the septum pellucidum, and the dome of the cyst in these cases will be found immediately below the corpus callosum as this structure is sectioned for the preferred surgical transcallosal approach of these cysts (98).

NONNEOPLASTIC LESIONS OF THE PITUITARY AND PERISELLAR REGION

Pituitary Abscess

Pituitary abscess is rare, and when it occurs the diagnosis is made upon transsphenoidal surgical intervention. The abscess can occur spontaneously and not be associated with any known condition, such as sinusitis, meningitis, or intrasellar tumor, or it may be seen with a preexisting pathologic process. There are two interesting aspects of pituitary abscesses: (a) the lesions usually do not produce systemic signs of infection, and (b) they develop slowly enough so that they appear to be a chronic condition, similar to tumor.

Deossification of the sellar contour is common, as is enlargement of the sella (101). On CT or MRI there is enlargement of the sellar contents with suprasellar and/or parasellar extension. Contrast enhancement of the abscess wall occurs, but on CT this resembles an ordinary cystic or old hemorrhagic pituitary adenoma (102). On MRI, however an old hemorrhagic pituitary adenoma is diagnosable because there are signs of old blood.

Pituitary abscess may be found in patients with meningitis or sinusitis and may also be seen with pituitary adenomas, craniopharyngiomas, or other intrasellar lesions. In the latter cases it is impossible to make a diagnosis, but abscess should be listed in any case presenting peripheral enhancement of a cystic mass around the sella. This may be crucial in terms of management because the treatment is transsphenoidal surgery and drainage. The subfrontal approach may lead to spread of infection. The usual bacterium is staphylococcus or pneumococcus.

Other inflammatory or parasitic conditions in or around the sella include those described in the following paragraphs.

Cysticercosis

One or multiple cysts may occur in the supra- and parasellar area, and other cystic lesions may be identified that would make diagnosis possible. If the lesion is multilocular, suggesting multiple cysts, the diagnosis should be sug-

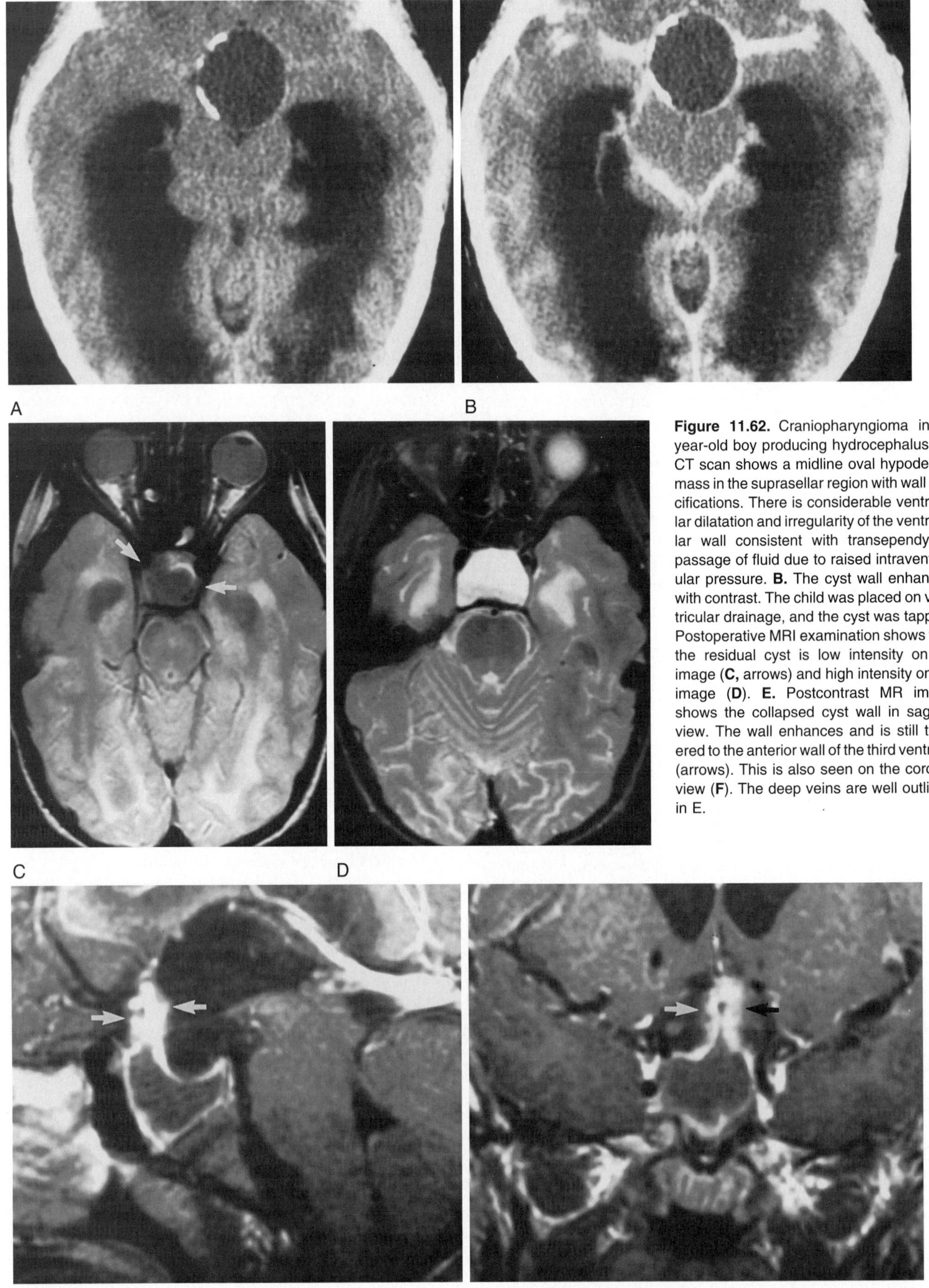

Figure 11.62. Craniopharyngioma in 9-year-old boy producing hydrocephalus. **A.** CT scan shows a midline oval hypodense mass in the suprasellar region with wall calcifications. There is considerable ventricular dilatation and irregularity of the ventricular wall consistent with transependymal passage of fluid due to raised intraventricular pressure. **B.** The cyst wall enhanced with contrast. The child was placed on ventricular drainage, and the cyst was tapped. Postoperative MRI examination shows that the residual cyst is low intensity on T1 image (**C,** arrows) and high intensity on T2 image (**D**). **E.** Postcontrast MR image shows the collapsed cyst wall in sagittal view. The wall enhances and is still tethered to the anterior wall of the third ventricle (arrows). This is also seen on the coronal view (**F**). The deep veins are well outlined in E.

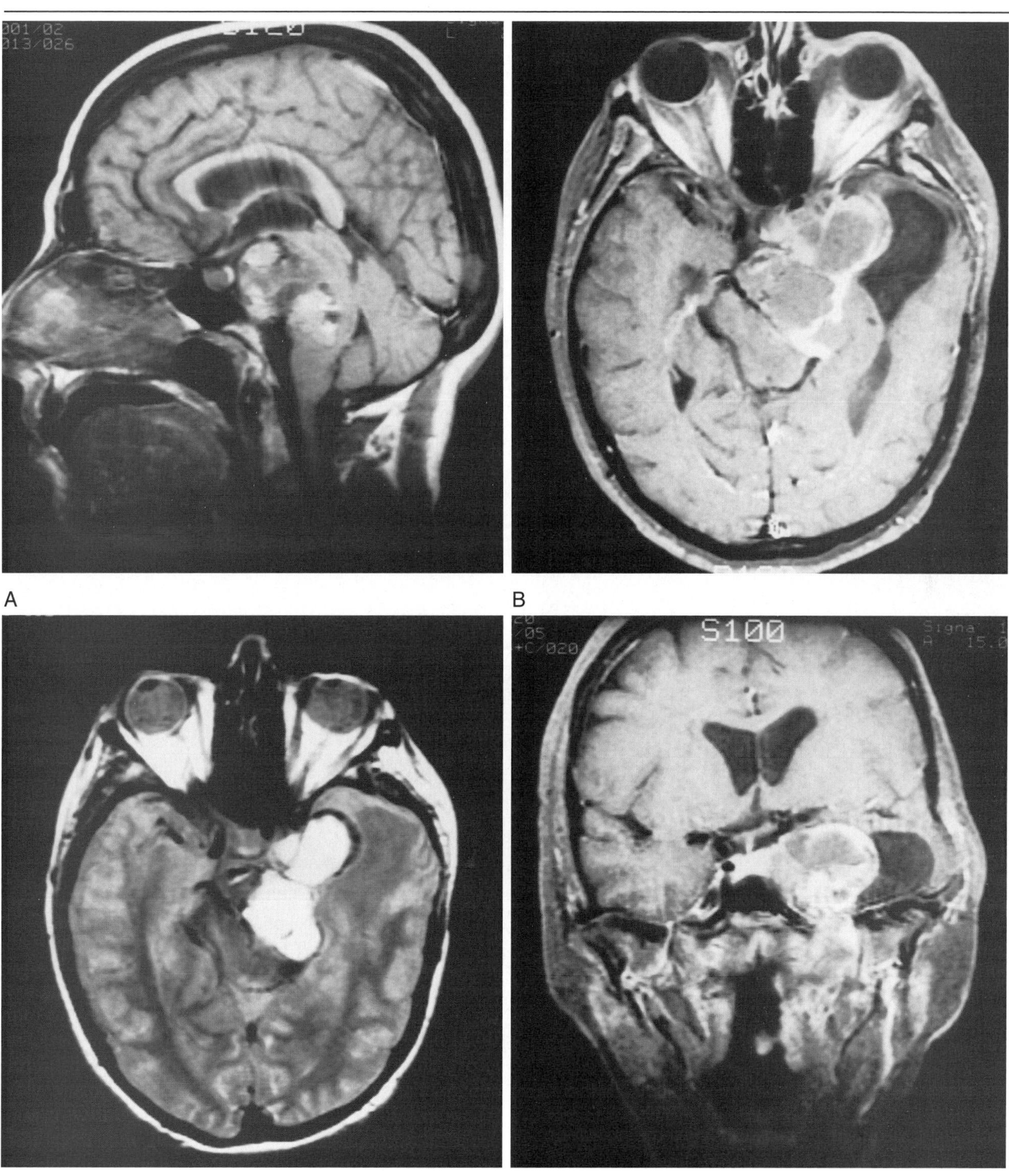

Figure 11.63. Craniopharyngioma extending laterally and dorsally behind the sella turcica. **A.** T1 sagittal precontrast image shows a large retrosellar mass that markedly displaces the brainstem backward, elevates the horn of the third ventricle, and contains isointense and hyperintense areas. **B.** After contrast, the mass shows peripheral enhancement and is multiloculated. The loculi remain isointense. The left temporal horn is enlarged. **C.** On a proton density axial image, the tumor is hyperintense except for portions of the capsule that showed enhancement with gadolinium in B. There is hypodensity in the left temporal lobe due to a dilated and displaced temporal horn. **D.** Coronal T1-weighted postcontrast image shows the lateral position of the mass, somewhat unusual for craniopharyngioma. The pituitary stalk is displaced to the right and appears uninvolved. The position and shape of the lesion are of an epidermoid tumor, but the enhancing characteristics do not correspond.

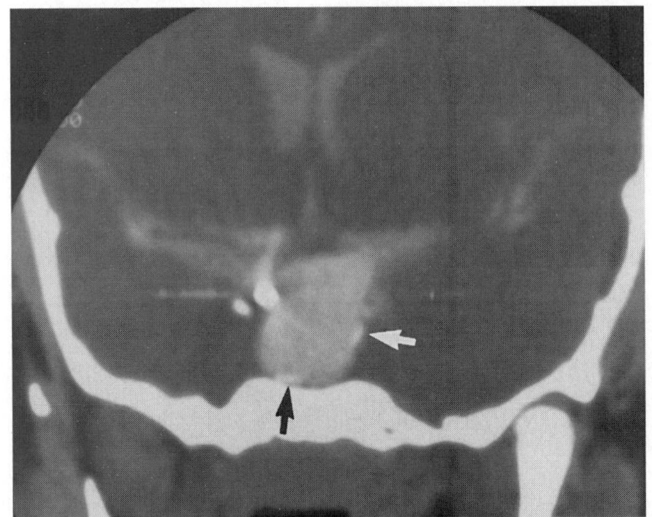

Figure 11.64. Craniopharyngioma in a 6-year-old girl. **A.** CT scan made after intrathecal injection of metrizamide contrast shows some contrast in the ventricles and in the sylvian fissures. There is a midline dense suprasellar mass with some calcification in its wall (arrows) consistent with craniopharyngioma. **B.** T1-weighted axial image shows a hyperintense midline mass that is also bright on a T2-weighted image (**C**). **D.** Coronal view shows the suprasellar extension and elevation of the structures in the region of the third ventricle.

A

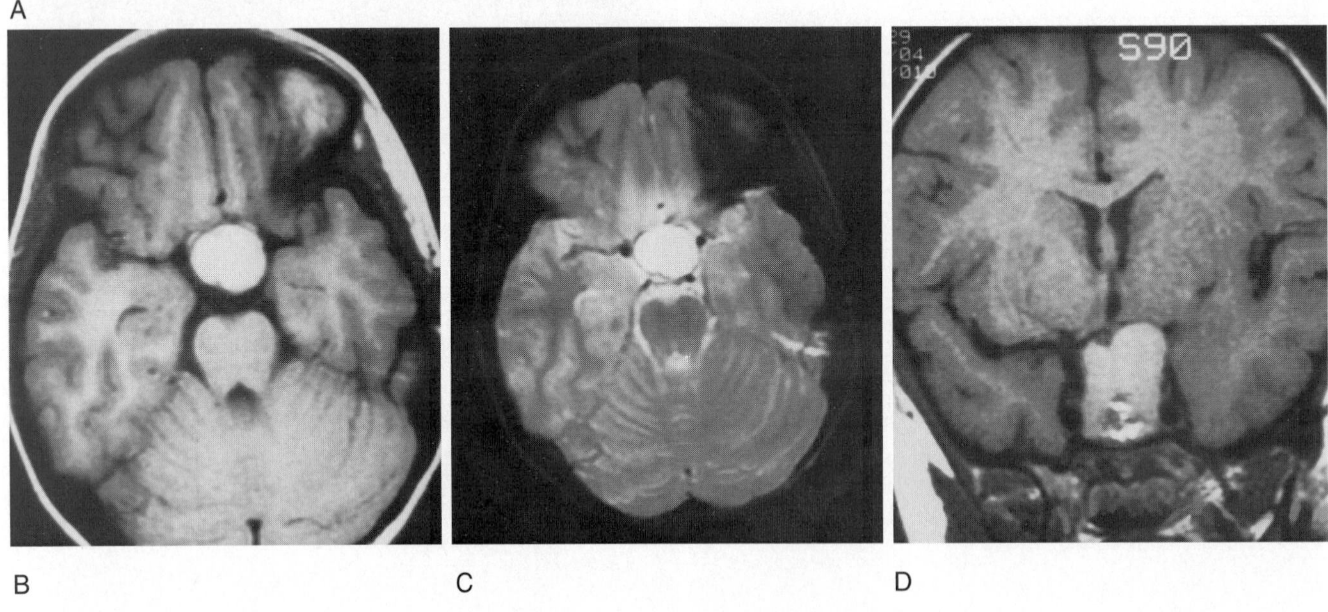

B C D

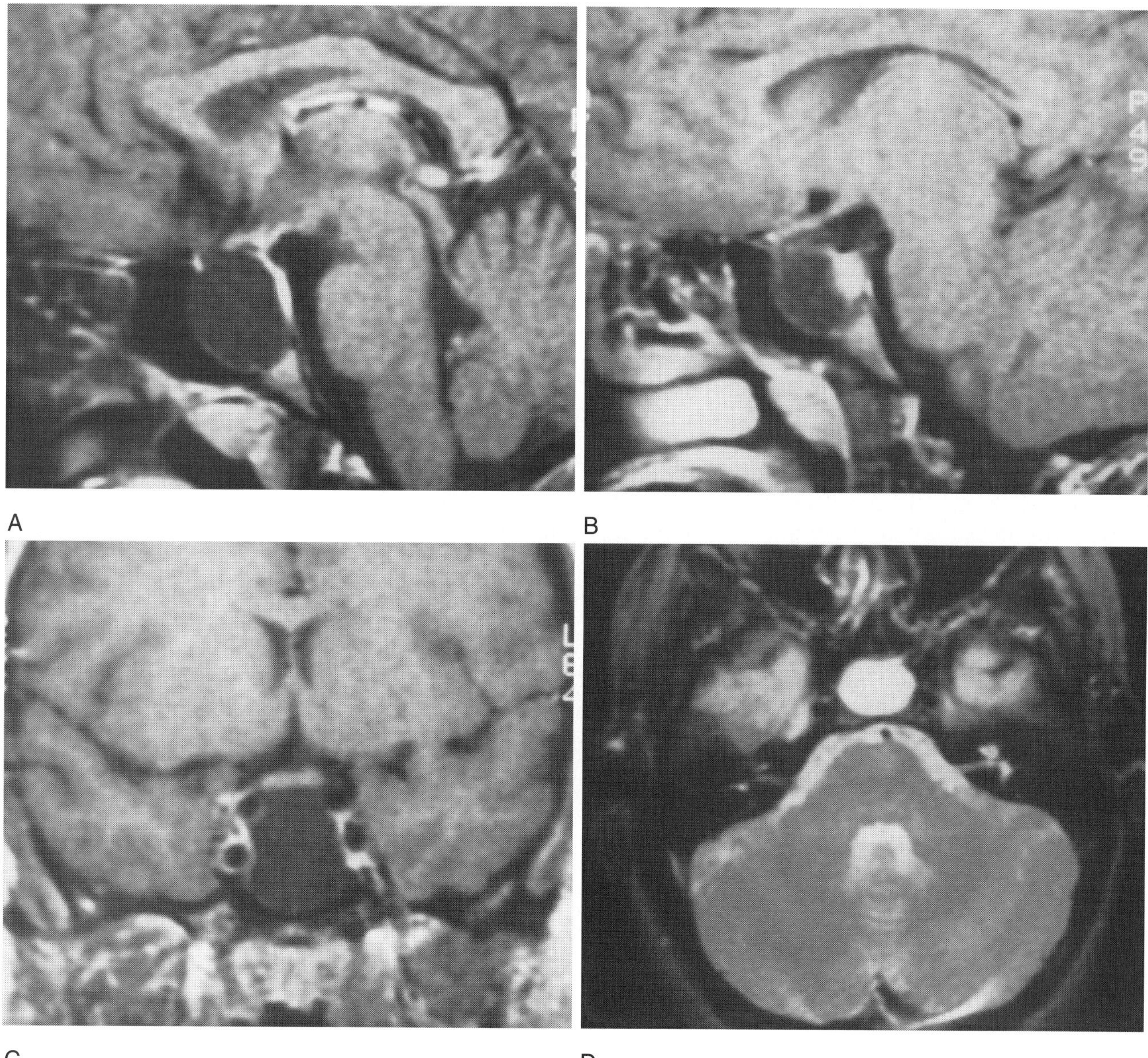

Figure 11.65. Intra- and suprasellar arachnoid cyst in a 16-year-old girl. **A.** Postcontrast sagittal T1-weighted image shows that the sella is distended with a homogeneously hypointense mass. **B.** A sagittal section 7 mm lateral to the midline shows a bright small mass representing displaced enhanced pituitary tissue. **C.** A coronal T1-weighted image shows elevation of the optic chiasm by this cystic mass. **D.** Axial T2-weighted image shows that the mass is hyperintense. The signal characteristics are consistent with CSF. Surgical intervention revealed an arachnoid cyst.

gested, particularly in the population groups where cysticercosis is common.

Lymphocytic Adenohypophysitis

This is a rare, probably autoimmune, disorder occurring mainly in women that is related to pregnancy (late pregnancy and postpartum). The anterior lobe of the pituitary gland does not contain lymphocytes, and in this condition there is diffuse infiltration of the adenohypophysis by lymphocytes accompanied by destruction of the pituitary tissue. There may be elevation of prolactin, and the pituitary is increased in size, so that differentiation from a pituitary tumor is difficult. The sella turcica enlarges, and CT and MRI reveal suprasellar extension of the enlarged pituitary with chiasmal elevation and compression (103,104). An important differential point is the occurrence toward the end of pregnancy or in the postpartum period. In the case reported by Quencer (103), the patient was 5 months postpartum, and in the Hungerford et al. case (104) visual problems began in the last month of pregnancy; hemianopia was discovered 3 weeks postpartum.

The pituitary gland increases in size during pregnancy because of prolactin cell hyperplasia. The growth of the gland sometimes leads to slight enlargement of the sella turcica. Following delivery the gland may undergo rapid changes, and, particularly after difficult, complicated deliveries, pituitary hemorrhage and necrosis may occur (*Sheehan syndrome*). As mentioned, it is felt that the enlargement of the gland in pregnancy is often followed by a significant postpartum decrease in the size of the gland, leading to the *partially empty sella*, which is much more frequent in women than in men (10:1 ratio). Pituitary infarction can lead to acute swelling, causing compression of the internal carotid arteries (Fig. 11.66).

Langerhans Cell Histiocytosis

This is also called *eosinophilic granulomatosis* or *histiocytosis X*. The term *histiocytosis X* is now considered obsolete. This is a group of conditions that includes eosinophilic granuloma and Hand-Schüller-Christian disease. Letterer-Siwe disease is a malignant form occurring in children and probably belongs among the lymphomas. Eosinophilic granuloma is often a single benign lesion of bone that is now referred to as Langerhans cell (eosinophilic) granulomatosis. Twenty-five percent of cases of Hand-Schüller-Christian disease are cases of eosinophilic granulomatosis (multifocal), but many with the same triad (exophthalmos, diabetes insipidus, and destructive bone lesions) may have a malignant disease.

The cells are believed to be derived from specialized bone marrow cells, which lends the name *Langerhans cell histiocytosis*. Patients may present primarily with diabetes insipidus, which leads to the examination of the hypothalamic-pituitary axis. Thickening of the pituitary stalk is the most important finding. Diabetes insipidus may be the result of deficient secretion of the antidiuretic hormone by the hypothalamus, or it may be due to an inadequate response at the level of the renal tubules (nephrogenic diabetes insipidus). Diagnosis is sometimes made by biopsy of the thickened pituitary infundibulum if there are no other accessible lesions for biopsy. The other finding in this condition is disappearance of the high signal of the posterior pituitary lobe on T1-weighted MR images (105). The thickening of the stalk may diminish following radiation therapy (106), but the diabetes insipidus may remain and did so in 3 of the 4 cases reported by Tien et al. (105).

Eosinophilic granuloma commonly occurs as a single lesion of bone, and the skull is a frequent site. For that reason skull examination should be carried out in any patient with

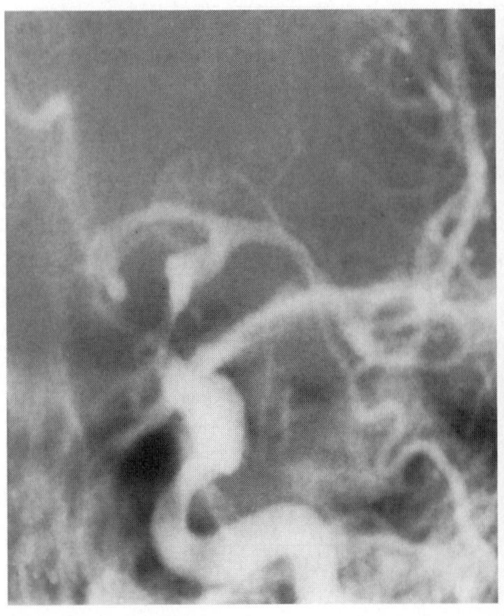

A

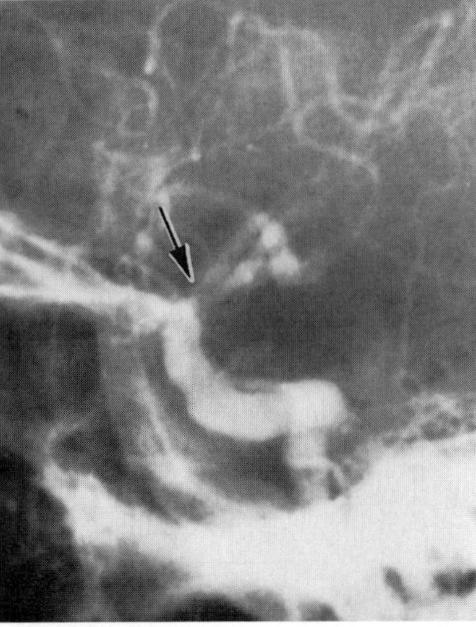

B

Figure 11.66. Pituitary adenoma, undergoing acute swelling due to infarction, compressing the internal carotid artery against the clinoid process. **A.** The frontal view demonstrates marked narrowing of the clinoid portion of the internal carotid artery. **B.** Lateral view. The arrow points to the anterior clinoid process. The patient, a 67-year-old woman, had rapid appearance of compression of the optic nerves and chiasm, progressing almost to blindness, and developed a right hemiplegia. Surgical intervention revealed a pituitary infarct without a hematoma. The hemiplegia improved and vision returned (Momose and New: AJR 1973;118:550–566).

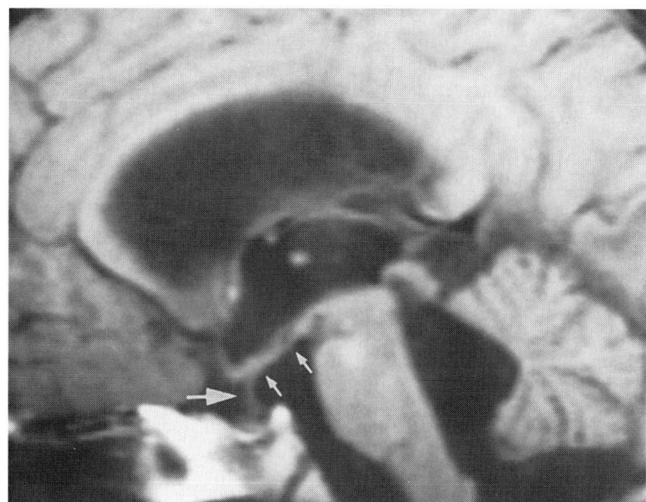

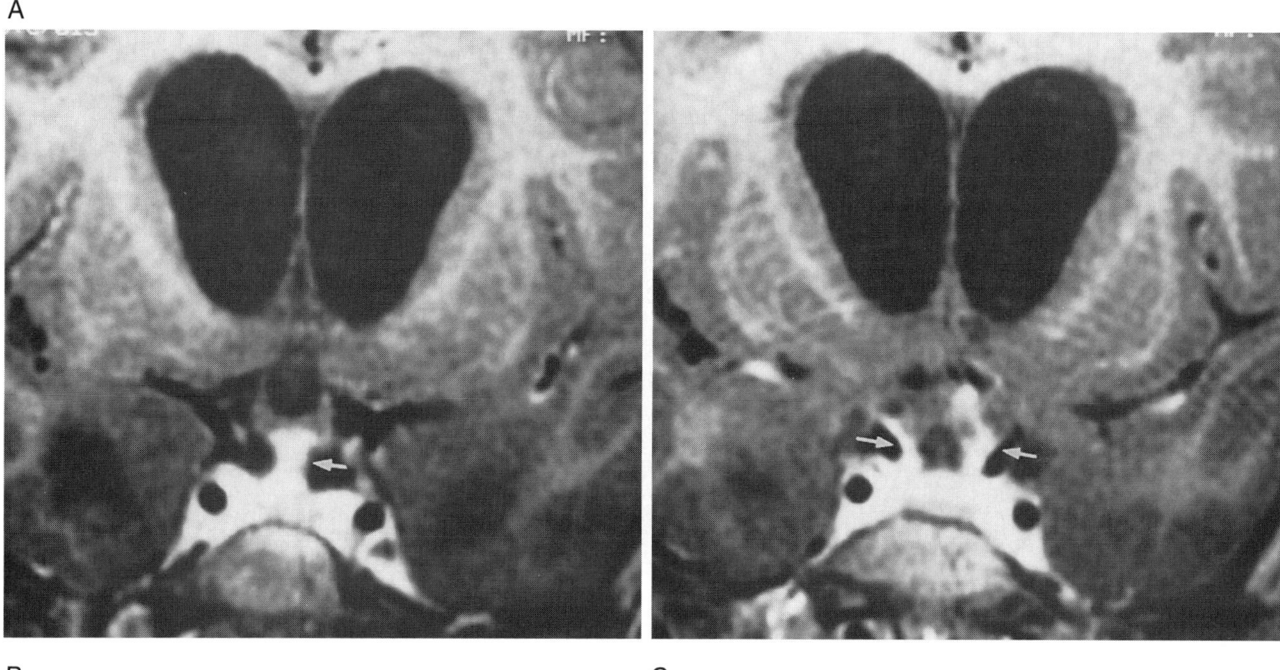

Figure 11.67. Thickening of the pituitary stalk in a child with eosinophilic granulomatosis. **A.** Sagittal T1 precontrast image shows a prominent pituitary stalk (arrow) and thickening of the inferior wall of the third ventricle (small arrows). **B.** After contrast, the coronal view shows a markedly thickened pituitary stalk. **C.** A coronal view posterior to B shows invasion along the walls of the third ventricle (arrows). Hydrocephalus was present due to ventricular obstruction that necessitated a shunt.

diabetes insipidus. MRI will demonstrate the thickening of the pituitary stalk (Fig. 11.67). It also will show absence of the normal bright posterior pituitary on T1-weighted sagittal images.

The involvement of the hypothalamus may not be apparent at the time of examination in patients (children or adults) with diabetes insipidus, and follow-up examination is recommended. In a recent report, Appignani et al. included two cases of "idiopathic" central diabetes insipidus who within 13 to 24 months later showed a positive lesion in the hypothalamus on follow-up MRI. In both cases the final diagnosis was germinoma, although in one the diagnosis was based on response to therapy without a biopsy (107). Both cases showed absence of posterior pituitary brightness on T1-weighted images on the initial examination. The pineal area was not involved.

Tolosa-Hunt Syndrome

This is a condition characterized by painful ophthalmoplegia caused by cavernous sinus inflammation, usually unilateral. Yousem et al. found abnormalities on MRI examination in 9 of 11 patients (108). There was enlargement of a sinus by a mass lesion (6 of 10) and in 2 there was no enlargement. One patient had a thrombosed cavernous sinus and superior ophthalmic vein. CT may also demonstrate the bulging cavernous sinus, convex laterally (109). The lesion may enhance with contrast, and Yousem et al. emphasize the fact that on MRI it is isointense with muscle on T1-weighted images and isointense with fat on T2-weighted images (108). The orbital apex is frequently involved and was found so in 8 of 11 cases by MRI. The combination of an enlarged cavernous sinus with the signal characteristics just described and involvement of the orbital apex should be considered al-

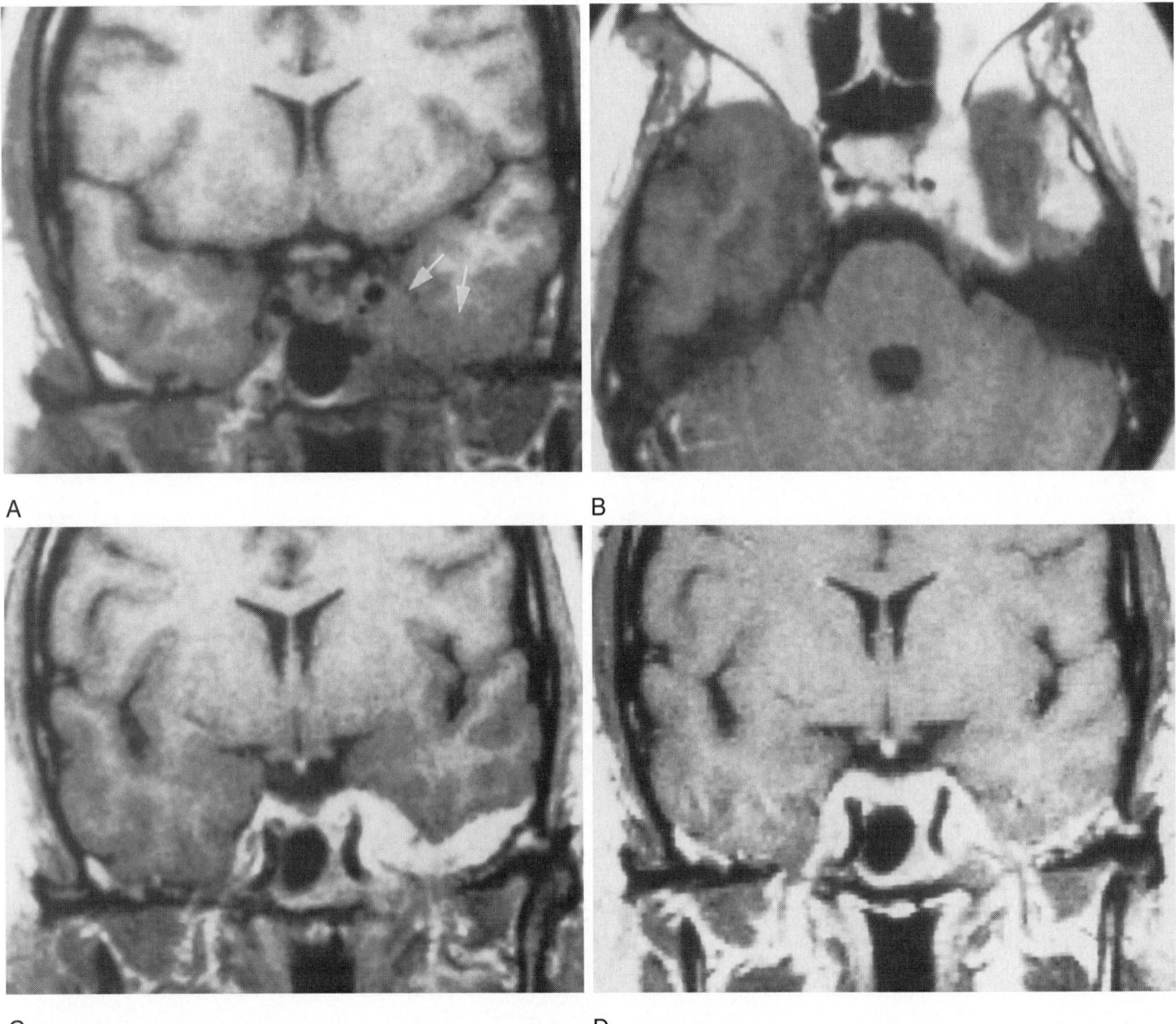

Figure 11.68. Tolosa-Hunt syndrome in a 25-year-old woman complaining of painful ophthalmoplegia and a sixth nerve palsy. **A.** Precontrast T1-weighted coronal image shows thickening of tissues in left cavernous sinus region and loss of definition of lower margin of left temporal lobe (arrows). **B.** Axial postcontrast T1-weighted image shows enlargement and hyperintensity of left cavernous sinus, also involving the middle fossa. **C.** Coronal postcontrast image reveals the extensive enhancement along the floor of the middle fossa as well as the left cavernous sinus. The internal carotid artery is displaced medially. **D.** Coronal postcontrast images after 3 weeks of steroid therapy reveal considerable decrease in the size of the enlarged left cavernous sinus and of the dural enhancement along the floor of the middle fossa. The patient's symptoms had disappeared. (Courtesy of Dr. Ann C. Price, Massachusetts General Hospital, Boston, Mass.)

most diagnostic of Tolosa-Hunt syndrome (Fig. 11.68). The symptoms, in addition to retro-orbital pain, consist of involvement to a variable degree of the first, third, fourth, sixth division of the fifth nerves, and sometimes the sympathetic fibers around the internal carotid artery, leading to a Horner syndrome. The dura may enhance after contrast and may be thickened. The lesion responds to steroid therapy and does so fairly rapidly.

Orbital inflammatory pseudotumor may extend intracranially (110). In these cases the patient presents with the usual symptoms of orbital pseudotumor (proptosis and ophthalmoplegia). The endocranial extension may be discovered on CT or MRI examination, and there may not be additional clinical findings. The proptosis should be a differential point with the Tolosa-Hunt syndrome.

Sarcoidosis

A frequent area of CNS involvement by a sarcoid is the hypothalamus. The lesions enhance with contrast and characteristically are dark on T2-weighted images (see Figs.

Table 11.38.
Suprasellar Masses

Anterior: meningiomas arising from the planum sphenoidale or tuberculum sella, optic nerve/chiasm glioma, olfactory neuroblastoma, mucocele arising within posterior ethmoid air cells (rare)
Directly suprasellar: upward extension of pituitary macroadenoma, suprasellar cysts, optic chiasm gliomas, hypothalamic tumors, aneurysms, germinomas
Posterior suprasellar: craniopharyngioma, hypothalamic hamartoma, basilar artery aneurysm, clivus meningioma, chordoma, chondrosarcoma

6.28 and 6.29). Also see under "Inflammatory Diseases," Chapter 6.

Tuberculous Meningitis

Tuberculous meningitis has a predilection for the suprasellar region. Thick, heavy exudate may form, leading to narrowing of arteries in this region (supraclinoid carotid artery and anterior and middle cerebral artery trunks [111]). Enhancement of the meninges with contrast on CT or MRI will be found, which is much better demonstrated by MRI with contrast.

SUPRASELLAR MASSES

Suprasellar masses (Table 11.38) typically indent the lower aspect of the third ventricle. If they are below the optic chiasm, they first elevate this structure (pituitary adenomas, meningiomas, suprasellar cysts); if they arise above the chiasm, they will depress and distort this structure. In either case the anterior third ventricle will be involved. The mass may arise directly from the optic chiasm. The lesions arising above the optic chiasm are described in text preceding with the hypothalamus and third ventricle lesions.

Optic Chiasm Gliomas

These tumors are found primarily in young patients, mostly children. There is a relationship to neurofibromatosis type I, but only in about one-quarter of the cases can a definite relationship be established (112). The tumor can involve one or both optic nerves and may not extend into the chiasm, being entirely within the orbit, or it may involve primarily the optic chiasm (Figs. 11.69 and 11.70). From the chiasm the tumor may grow posteriorly to involve the optic tracts (Fig. 11.71). Some optic chiasm gliomas grow directly into the hypothalamus or vice versa. The biology of optic gliomas is very interesting. In general they are slowly growing tumors, usually pilocytic astrocytomas. The growth is sometimes extremely slow and sometimes more rapid; the period of rapid growth may be interrupted by radiation therapy or sometimes by a surgical biopsy or partial removal (113–115). Some optic gliomas may present calcifications; the mass can achieve a fairly large size. CT and MRI are usually diagnostic, and the tumor frequently enhances after intravenous contrast (Fig. 11.70). It is usually isointense on T1-weighted images and hyperintense on T2-weighted images, and MRI is the preferable imaging procedure.

In the intraorbital optic gliomas the differential diagnosis includes *optic sheath meningioma*, in which there is usually calcification in the optic nerve sheath. The calcification sometimes assumes the so-called train track sign because of the parallel lines. Growth can be quite indolent over a long period of time. Sometimes more of a mass is encountered and will enhance with contrast (Fig. 11.69*D* to *F*). The train track type of calcification is typical for optic sheath meningioma.

Meningiomas

These tumors arise from the tuberculum sellae, the diaphragma sellae, or the wall of the cavernous sinus. In the last case they may be called *parasellar* (arising and growing on the side instead of at the top of the sella). The tuberculum sellae origin may be accompanied by bony changes in this structure (hyperostosis, or "blistering effect" due to growth of the underlying paranasal sinuses as the bone is invaded and weakened by the meningioma). The sagittal views, either reformatted CT or MRI, are usually diagnostic, and there is usually strong postcontrast enhancement (Fig. 11.72).

Other Suprasellar Lesions

Other suprasellar masses may be the following:

1. *Anterior suprasellar.* Most of these are meningiomas arising from the tuberculum sellae or planum sphenoidale. Some are olfactory neuroblastomas growing posteriorly, and an occasional case may be a mucocele of the posterior ethmoid cells projecting intracranially.
2. *Straight suprasellar.* Pituitary adenomas are by far the most frequent (Fig. 11.54), followed by meningiomas, suprasellar cysts, craniopharyngiomas, optic gliomas, hypothalamic tumors, germinomas (primary or seeding), sarcoids, metastatic neoplasms, and aneurysm.
3. *Posterior suprasellar.* Craniopharyngioma is the most frequent, followed by hamartoma of the hypothalamus, aneurysm of the basilar artery, meningioma arising from the upper portion of the clivus–dorsum sellae, chordoma, chondrosarcoma, and metastasis.

Each one of these will have some imaging characteristics, and combining CT with MRI without and with contrast allows one to suggest a specific diagnosis. Plain films are often useful, and angiography is needed to diagnose aneurysms. MR angiography may be diagnostic before conventional angiography.

Craniopharyngiomas, suprasellar extensions of the pituitary adenomas, hypothalamic gliomas, hypothalamic hamartomas, intrasellar arachnoid cysts, Rathke cleft cysts, and sarcoidosis are described in text preceding.

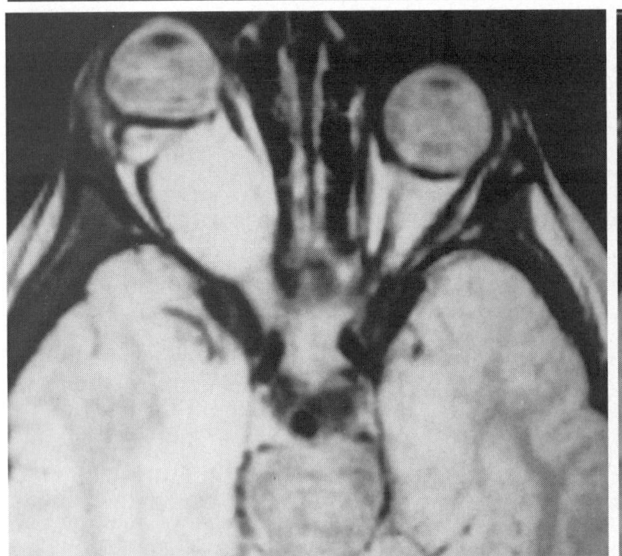

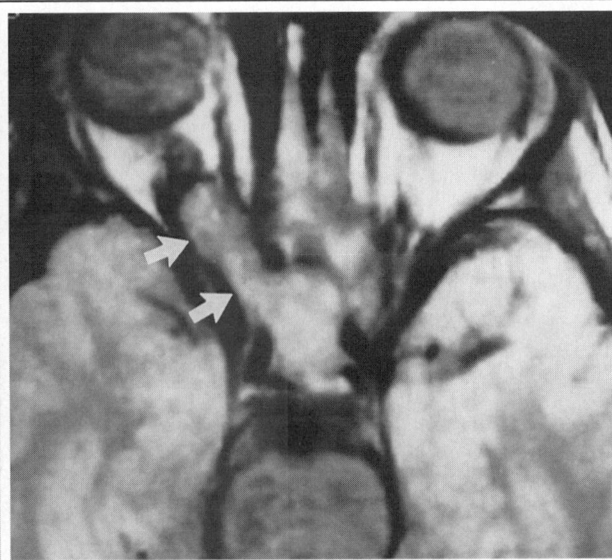

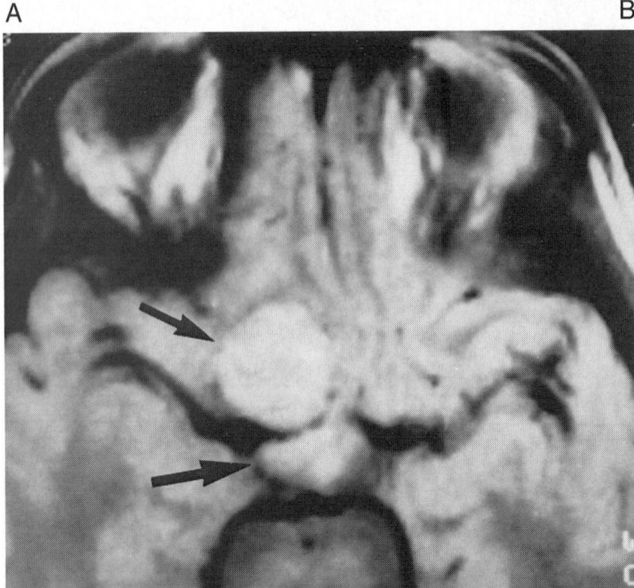

Figure 11.69. Optic glioma, intraorbital, extending into the chiasm. **A.** Large intraorbital oval mass extending into the optic nerve posteriorly. **B.** There is direct extension of the enlarged optic nerve into the chiasm (arrows). **C.** A rounded off-lateral suprasellar mass is present, and the displaced chiasm is thickened posteriorly (arrows). **D** to **F.** Meningioma of the optic nerve sheath. **D.** There is an enhancing mass at the apex of the orbit. **E.** A higher slice on soft tissue window and a bone window (**F**) demonstrate the mass and the presence of a small calcium deposit at the optic foramen. There was no train-track-type calcification in this case.

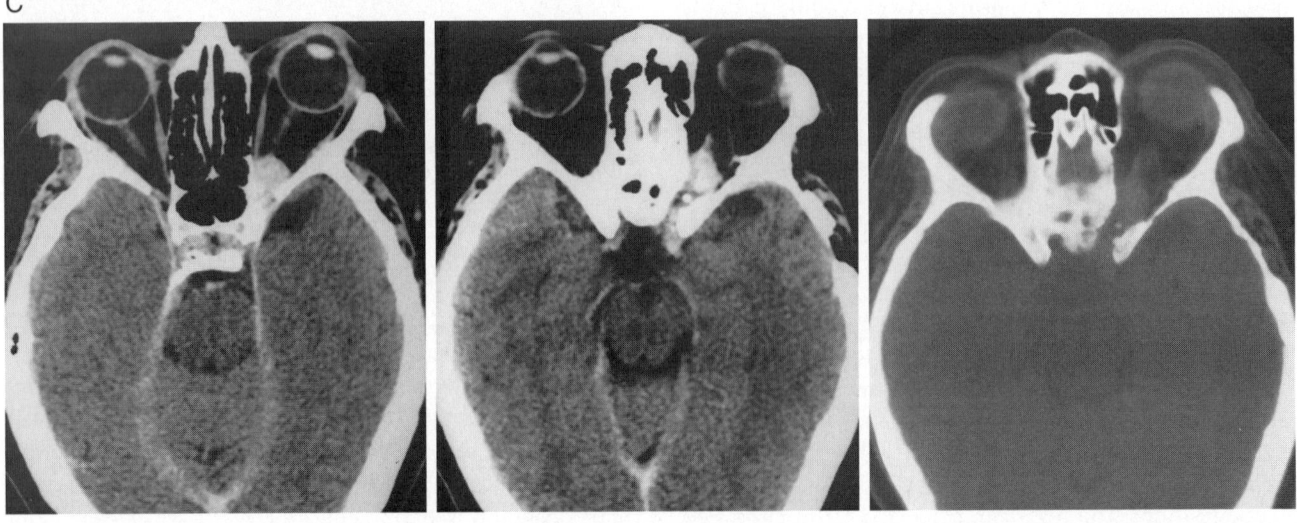

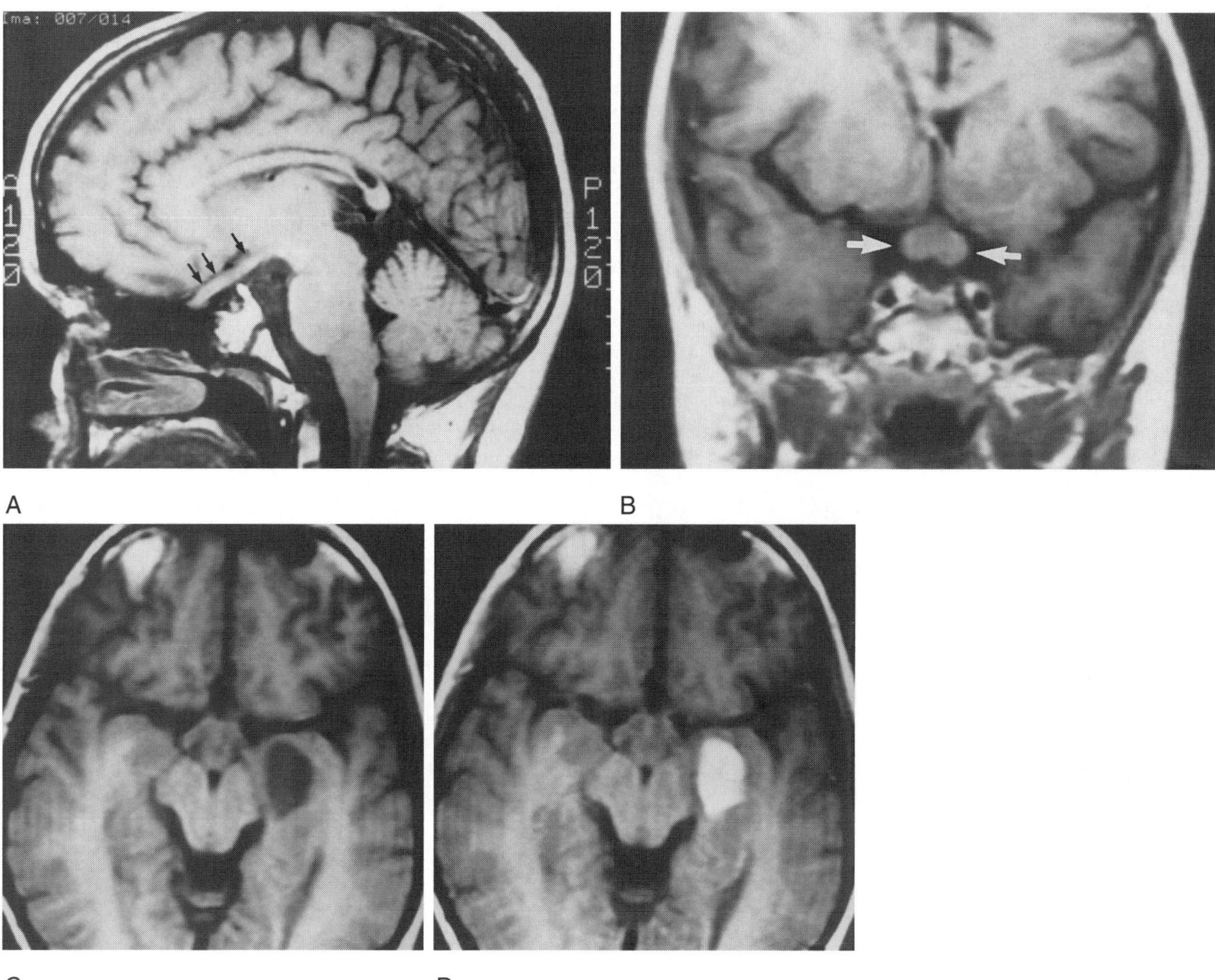

Figure 11.70. Optic glioma in a 10-year-old boy with neurofibromatosis type I. **A.** Precontrast T1-weighted sagittal view shows the enlargement of the optic chiasm, nerve, and optic track (arrows). **B.** In a coronal T1 noncontrast image, the chiasm is enlarged (arrows). **C.** A T1-weighted axial image shows an oval low-intensity lesion in the left anterior temporal lobe. **D.** After contrast there is enhancement of the lesion, indicating that it is most probably a glioma. The child had other bright patches on T2-weighted images in the cerebellum.

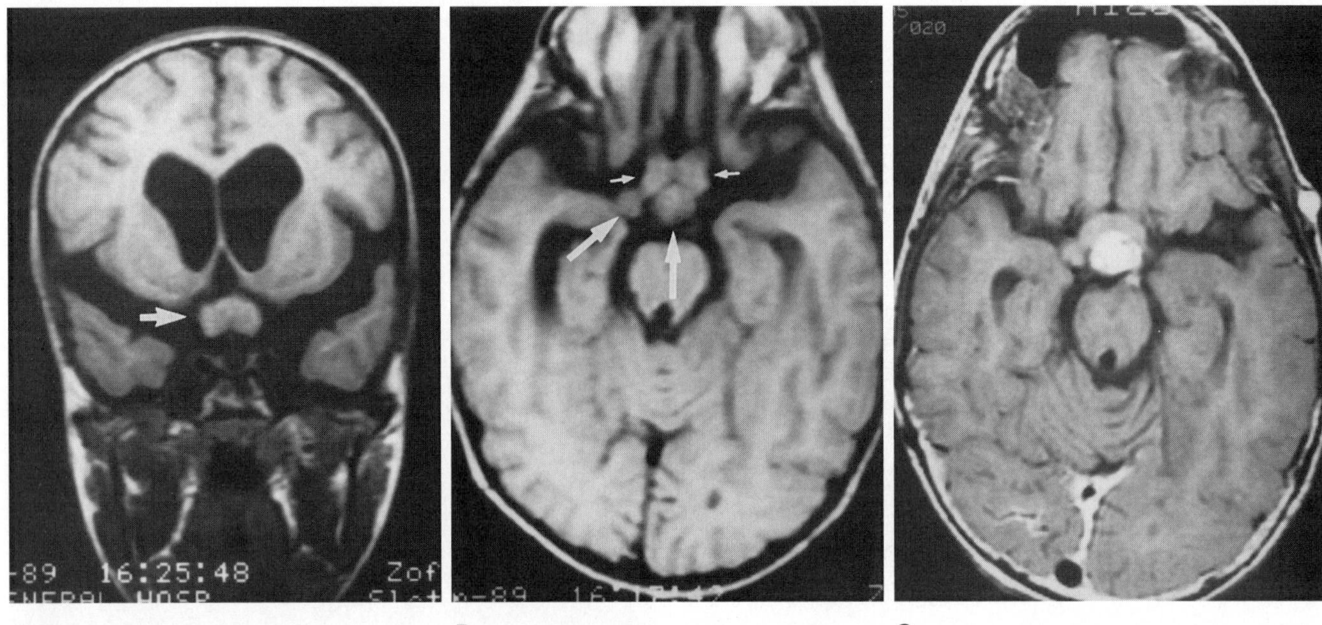

A B C

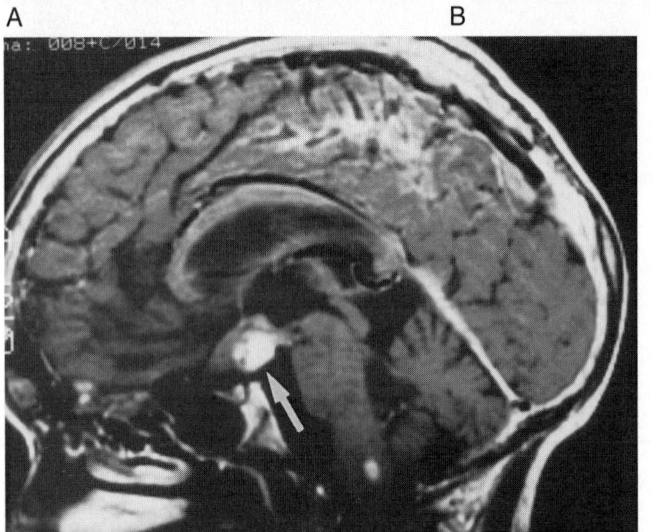

D

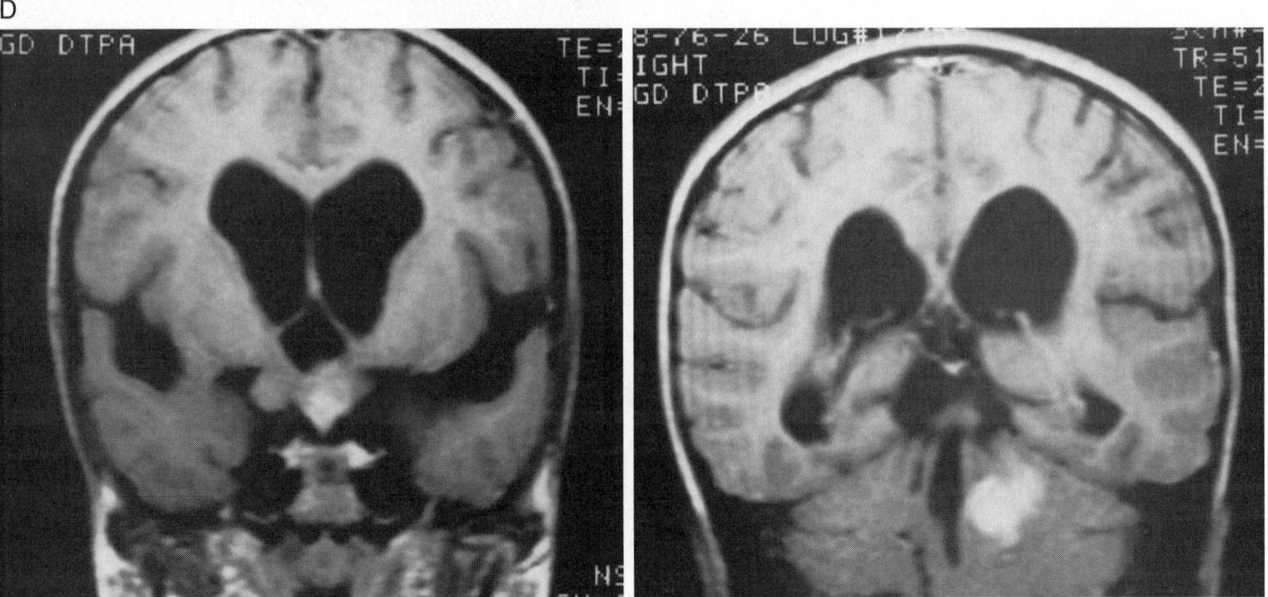

E F

Figure 11.71. Optic glioma growing into optic tracts in a 12-year-old boy with neurofibromatosis. **A.** Coronal noncontrast T1 image shows a large chiasm (arrow). **B.** Noncontrast T1-weighted axial image shows enlargement of the optic chiasm (small arrows) and small masses behind the chiasm: one in the midline, one in the hypothalamus, and another to the right (right-sided arrow). **C.** The hypothalamic mass enhances after contrast in this sagittal view. **D.** The dura enhances brightly in some areas because of previous shunting procedures. **E.** Coronal postcontrast image shows the enhanced hypothalamic mass, (arrow) most probably a glioma, and to the right of it a nonenhancing enlarged optic tract. **F.** A bright enhancing lesion is seen in the cerebellum that was regarded as a glioma because of enhancement and a slight mass effect. On proton density and T2-weighted images, it looked like a white matter patch (compare with Figs. 5.41 and 5.43).

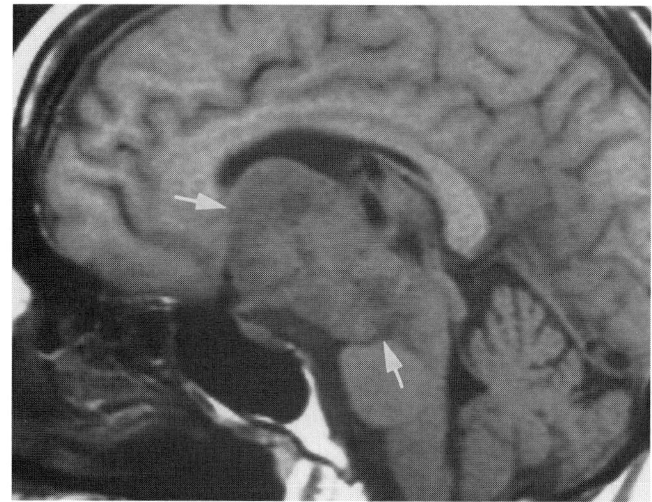

A

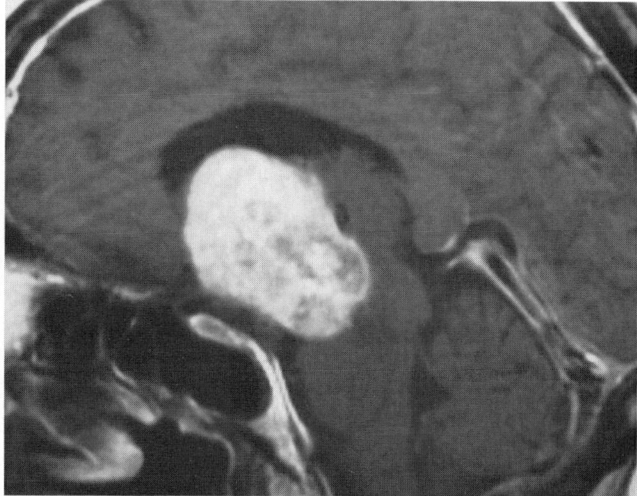

B

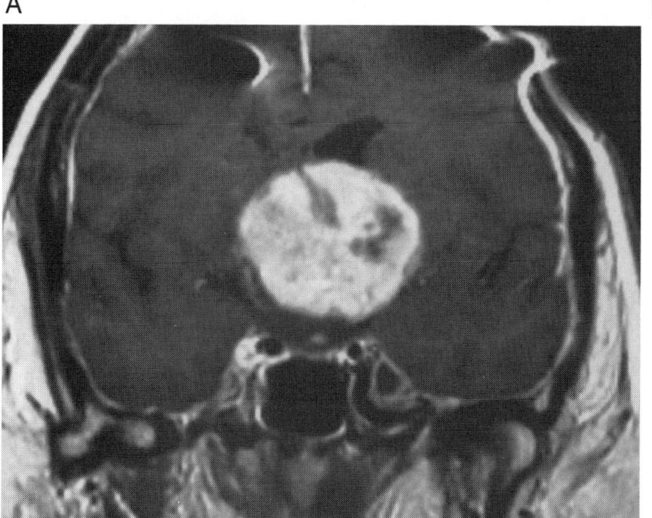

C

Figure 11.72. Suprasellar meningioma. **A.** T1-weighted sagittal image shows an isointense mass above the sella turcica producing obstruction at the foramen of Monro and compressing the midbrain (arrows). **B.** Postcontrast T1-weighted sagittal image shows extensive enhancement of this sharply circumscribed mass. The dorsum sellae seems to be bent downward. **C.** Coronal postcontrast image demonstrates the central location of the mass. Bilateral shunts had been performed, causing artifacts. Upon transcallosal surgical removal, the mass was adherent to the third-ventricular wall. The histology revealed an atypical histologic picture of meningioma.

PARASELLAR LESIONS

These arise from structures within the cavernous sinus on each side of the sella turcica or from the wall of the sinus, as well as from embryonic nests. The most frequent are the meningiomas, followed by aneurysms arising from the intracavernous portion of the internal carotid artery, the carotid-cavernous fistulas, neuromas of the fifth nerve and rarely of other nerves in the cavernous sinus, lymphomas, metastatic tumors, chordomas and chondrosarcomas, thrombosis of the cavernous sinus, and inflammatory lesions such as the Tolosa-Hunt syndrome (Table 11.39).

Meningiomas

The meningiomas typically enhance after contrast. They may invade the wall and lumen of the cavernous sinus, surrounding the internal carotid artery and sometimes encasing it, in which case angiography shows narrowing of the arterial lumen. In coronal views their probable site of origin is well seen (Figs. 11.73 and 11.74). In addition to the cavernous sinus wall, they may arise from the medial portion of the sphenoid ridge (medial lesser wing of the sphenoid bone). Tumors arising from the medial temporal lobe are not included in the parasellar category. Because these meningiomas are usually attached to the wall of the cavernous sinus, they cannot be totally removed surgically.

A rare lesion, parasellar cavernous hemangioma, occurs in this location and may be confused with meningioma (Fig. 11.75).

Table 11.39.
Parasellar Masses

Tumors: meningiomas, epidermoids, chordomas, chondrosarcomas, metastases, lymphomas, fifth-nerve schwannomas
Vascular lesions: internal carotid artery aneurysms, carotid-cavernous fistulas
Inflammatory: e.g., Tolosa-Hunt syndrome

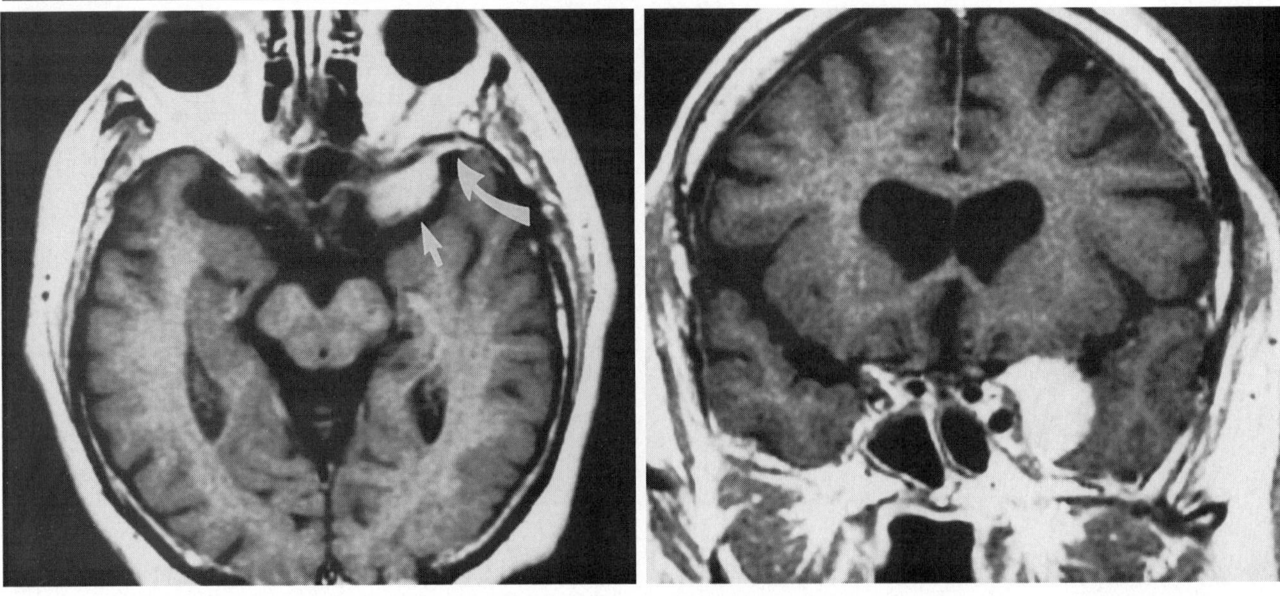

Figure 11.73. Parasellar meningioma probably arising from the wall of the cavernous sinus or from the medial portion of the sphenoid ridge. **A.** Postcontrast axial T1 image shows a hyperintense lesion against the medial aspect of the left sphenoid ridge (arrow). There is dural enhancement lateral to and continuous with the tumor, usually referred to as the "dural tail" (curved arrow). **B.** Coronal postcontrast image shows apparent attachment to the wall of the left cavernous sinus.

Fifth-Nerve Schwannomas

These are rare tumors arising from the fifth nerve that may present with signs of involvement of the fifth nerve such as pain and numbness. The symptoms can be rather mild, and the patient may not be referred for examination by cross-sectional imaging until the tumor is fairly large. CT or plain skull films may reveal evidence of erosion of the base of the skull at the middle fossa. Enlargement of the foramen ovale is common. The mass is typically located in the middle fossa and in the posterior fossa, and is a classical incisural-type mass that straddles the incisural edge and may be referred to as a *saddle tumor* (Fig. 11.76). It usually enhances on CT or MRI similar to schwannomas in the posterior fossa. On plain films and on CT there may be erosion of the petrous tip, which is typical of these tumors. Enlargement of the foramen ovale may be seen, as well as extension of the tumor through this foramen, producing a mass extracranially.

Epidermoid Tumors

These tumors may grow forward across the incisura from the anterolateral aspect of the posterior fossa, or they may occur primarily in the temporal hippocampal portion of the choroidal fissure. They grow by desquamation of cells from the squamous epithelial lining. On CT they are low density, almost like CSF or slightly denser, and on MRI they are also hypointense on T1-weighted images like CSF and hyperintense on T2-weighted images (Fig. 11.77). They may also occur intraventricularly.

Other Parasellar Lesions

Other tumors that may occur in the parasellar–cavernous sinus region include *lymphomas* and *metastatic* tumors. They enhance after contrast on CT or MRI and should be listed in the differential diagnosis. It may be difficult to differentiate between this type of tumor and cavernous sinus thrombosis by CT or MRI alone, and the clinical history may help in achieving a more accurate diagnosis. Chordomas may grow eccentrically on one side of the sella and act like parasellar lesions. They may invade the cavernous sinus, displacing the internal carotid artery and sometimes surrounding and obstructing the artery.

Cavernous Sinus Thrombosis is discussed in Chapter 10 under "Dural Sinus Thrombosis." Also see Figure 10.83.

Aneurysms of the intracavernous portion of the internal carotid artery can be quite large and are sometimes bilateral (10 percent of cases). The plain films of the skull may present erosion of the anterior clinoid process as well as depression of one side of the floor of the sella turcica. But this is also shown by axial and coronal CT images, well demonstrated on the bone windows. MR angiography is diagnostic and can be confirmed by conventional angiography (see Fig. 10.90). Giant basilar artery aneurysms may present as posterior suprasellar masses and sometimes as a straight suprasellar mass (Fig. 11.78).

ANGIOGRAPHIC FINDINGS IN PERISELLAR AND INTRAVENTRICULAR TUMORS

Angiography is not used as a primary diagnostic procedure to study perisellar lesions. Nevertheless, it is often carried

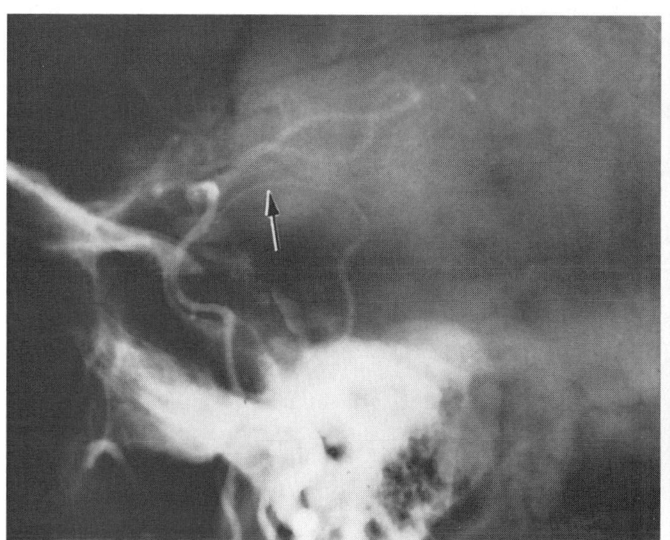

A

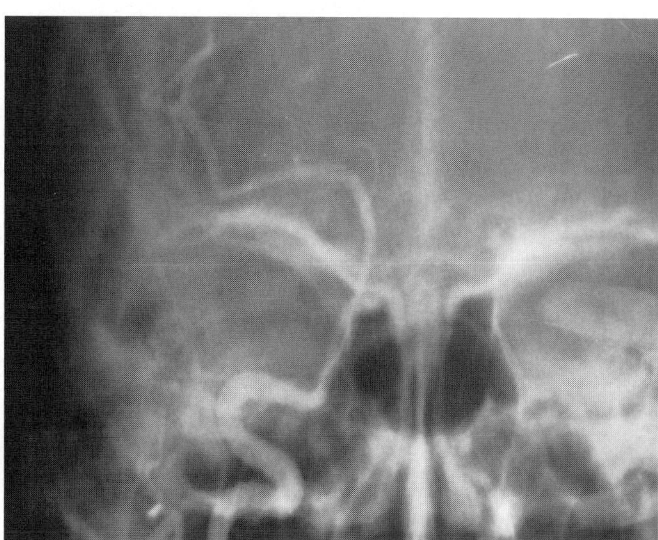

B

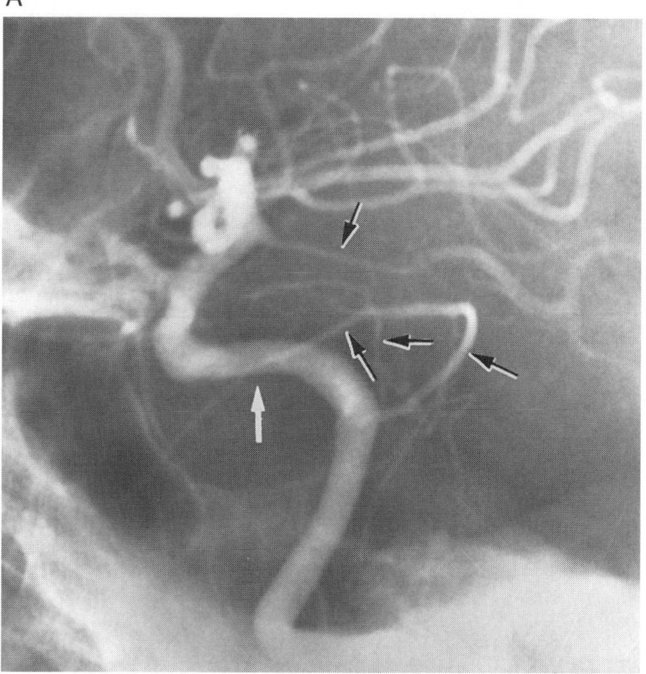

C

Figure 11.74. Parasellar meningioma: Angiographic findings in two cases. Narrowing of intracavernous portion of internal carotid artery due to extradural growth of meningioma. **A.** Lateral view. The elevation of the anterior choroidal artery is an indication of an intracranial subtemporal mass (arrow). **B.** The frontal film confirms the marked narrowing of the internal carotid artery, which extends to involve a portion of the supraclinoid segment as well. The meningioma is wrapped around the internal carotid artery, and in these cases complete removal is not possible without sacrificing the artery. **C.** Angiogram of another case: Lateral view of the carotid artery. The carotid siphon is open because of the elevation of the supraclinoid carotid artery. There is also elevation of the intracavernous segment of the internal carotid artery (vertical white arrow), as well as marked enlargement of the posterior meningohypophyseal trunk, which produces other branches supplying the tumor (three arrows). The posterior communicating artery (upper arrow) is stretched. A large tumor stain was seen in later serial films (not shown).

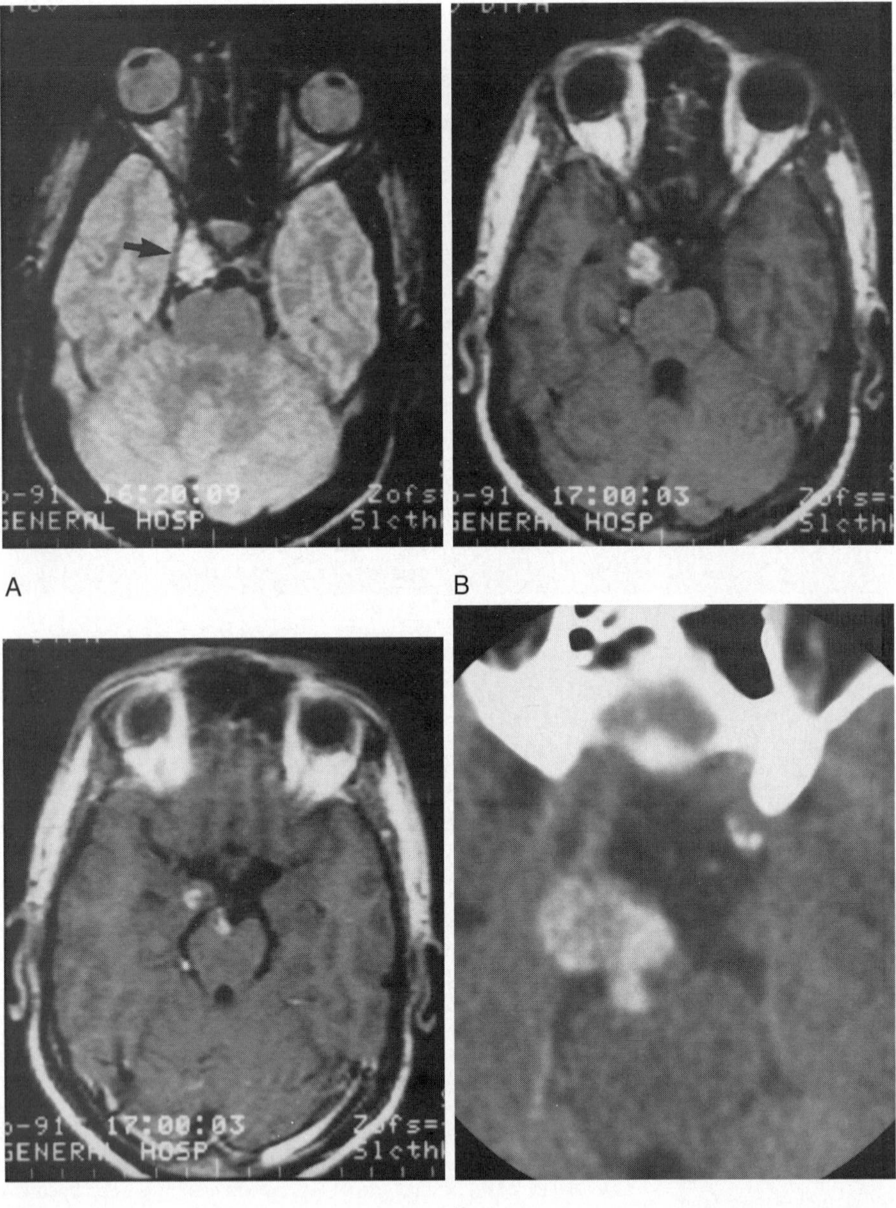

Figure 11.75. Parasellar cavernous hemangioma in a 28-year-old man who came in complaining of double vision and was found to have right third-nerve palsy. **A.** An axial proton density image shows a bright right parasellar lesion (arrow). **B** and **C.** T1 axial postcontrast MR images show enhancement of the lesion, which extends back to the interpeduncular fossa. **D.** An enhanced axial CT image shows the enhanced mass to extend to the site of origin of the third nerve, lateral to the interpeduncular fossa. This lesion would qualify as an incisural mass because of its position. On surgical intervention it was found to arise in the third nerve.

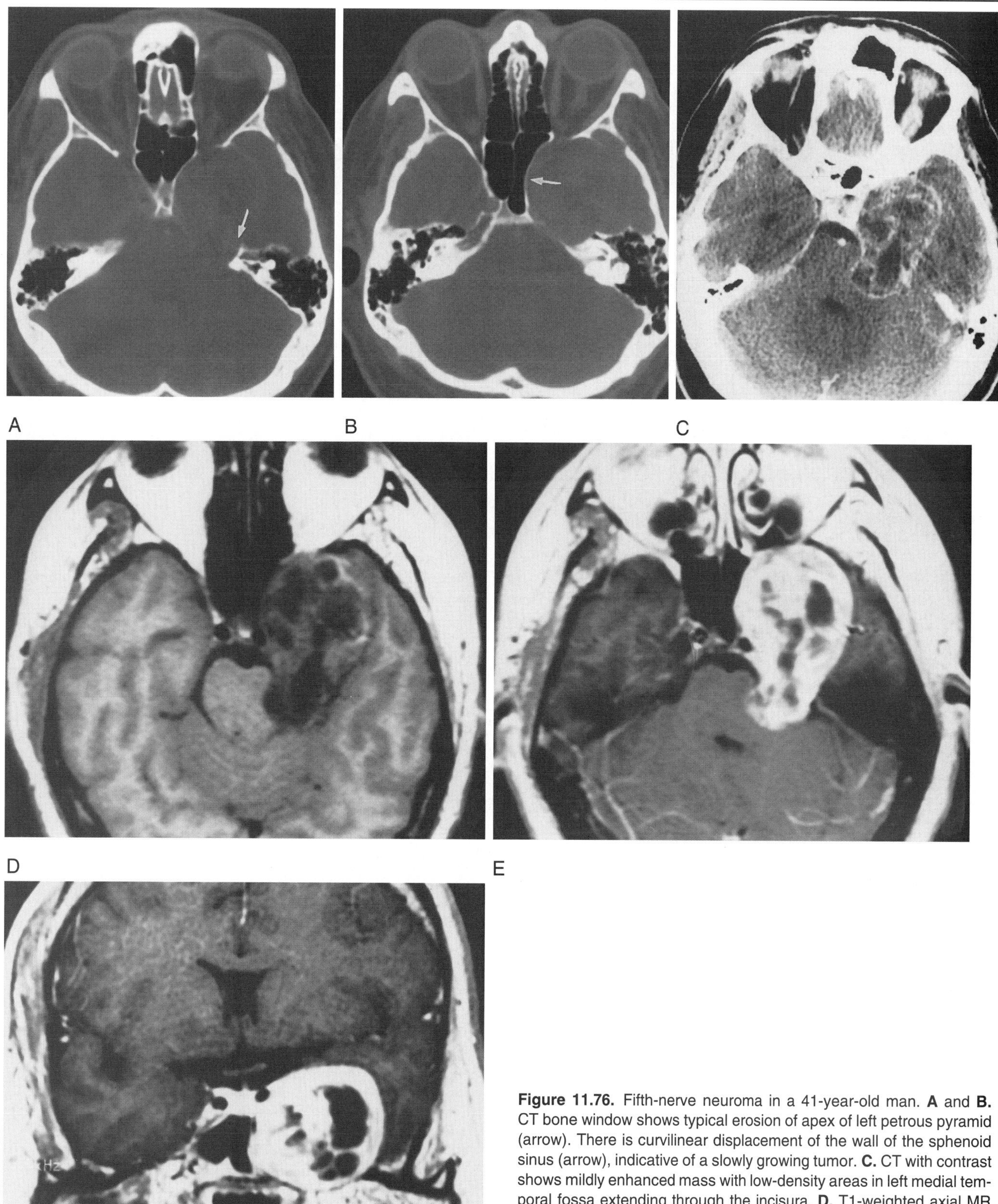

Figure 11.76. Fifth-nerve neuroma in a 41-year-old man. **A** and **B.** CT bone window shows typical erosion of apex of left petrous pyramid (arrow). There is curvilinear displacement of the wall of the sphenoid sinus (arrow), indicative of a slowly growing tumor. **C.** CT with contrast shows mildly enhanced mass with low-density areas in left medial temporal fossa extending through the incisura. **D.** T1-weighted axial MR image shows the same multicystic lesion, which enhances markedly (**E** and **F**). The indentation on the structures in the cerebellopontine angle is evident. The anteromedian posterior fossa and the medial middle fossa, or parasellar, locations are typical for fifth-nerve neuromas.

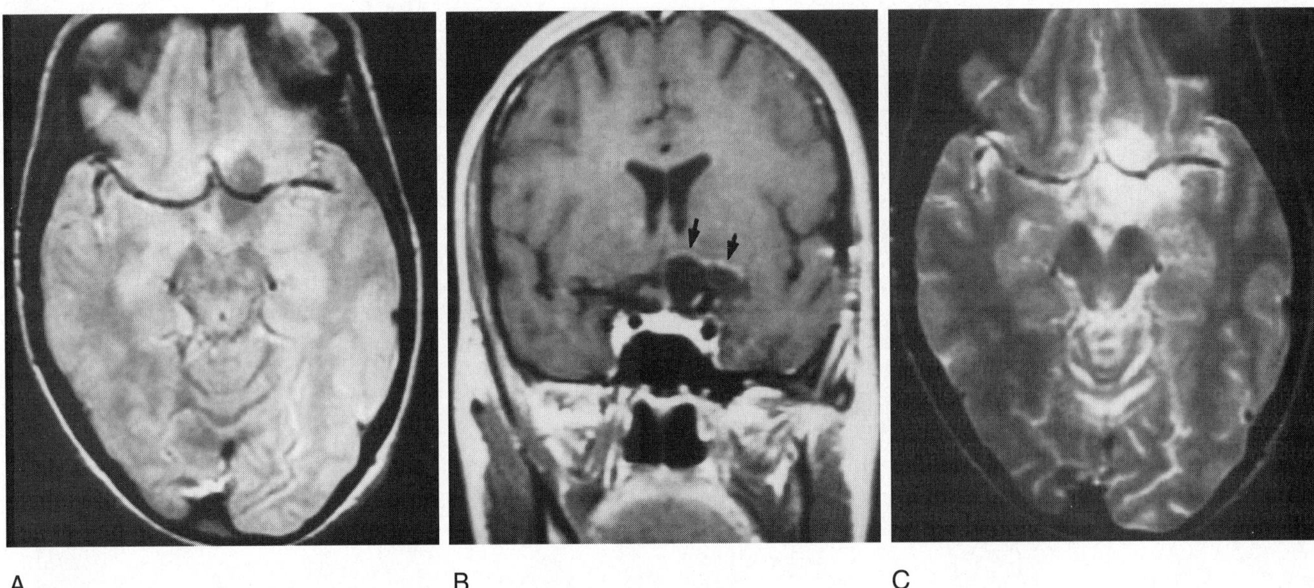

A B C

Figure 11.77. Parasellar epidermoid. **A.** T1-weighted coronal image shows a low-intensity lesion after contrast. Enhancement in the upper margin of the lesion is produced by upwardly displaced arteries (arrow). **B.** Proton density axial image shows that the lesion is slightly hypointense, similar to CSF. **C.** On a T2-weighted axial image the lesion is hyperintense. At surgery the lesion was totally removed.

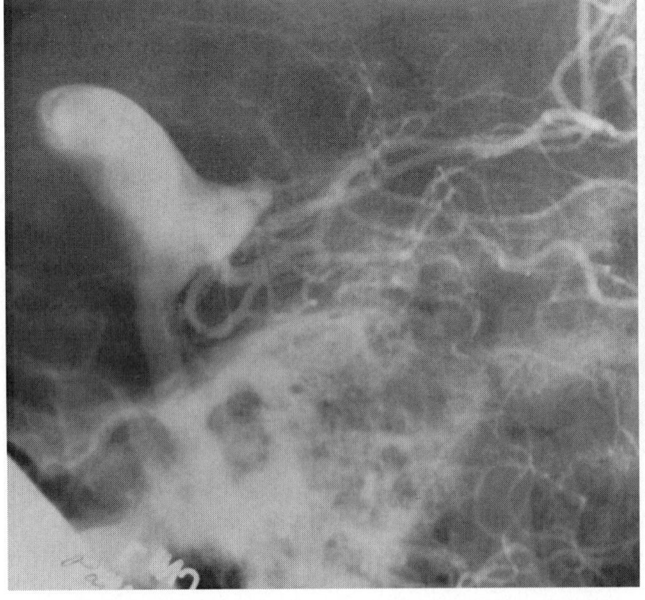

A

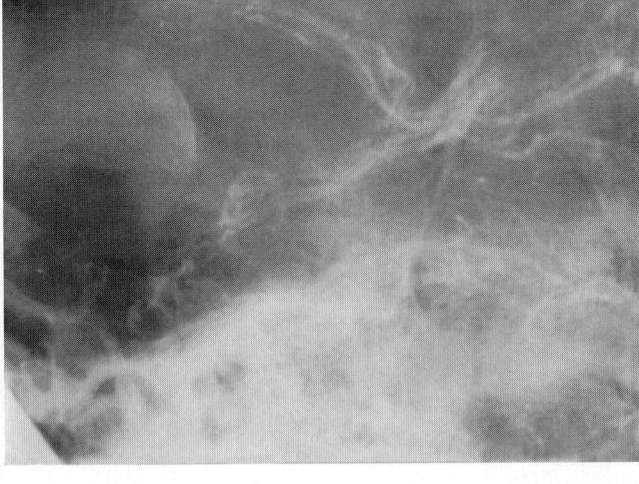

B

Figure 11.78. Suprasellar mass, aneurysm of top of basilar artery. **A.** The patient had signs of chiasmal compression with a bitemporal hemanopia. Angiography of the basilar artery demonstrates a large aneurysm, partly thombosed, at the top of the artery. **B.** In the venous phase, the full size and the position of the mass above the sella turcica can be appreciated.

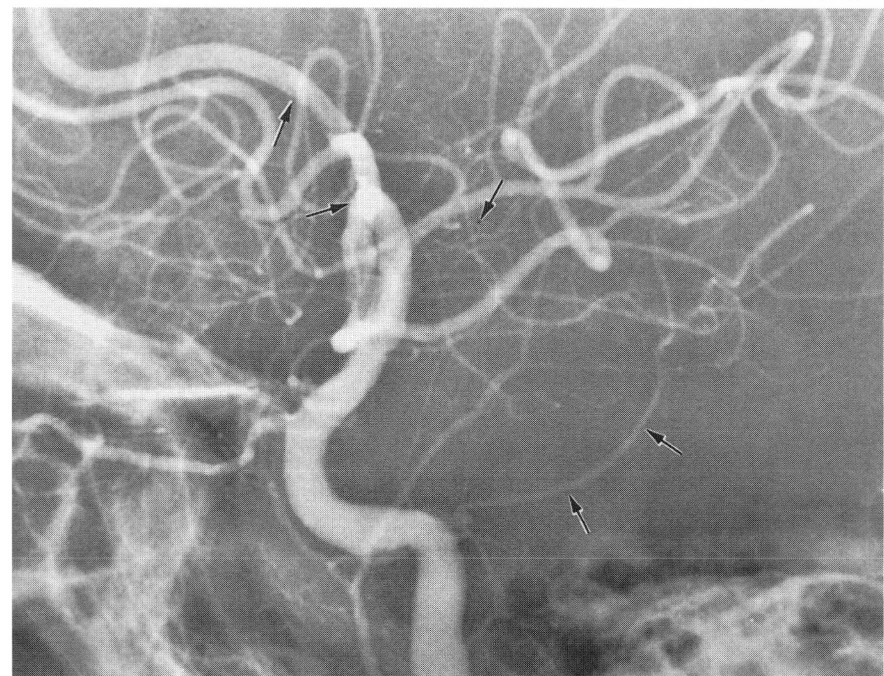

A

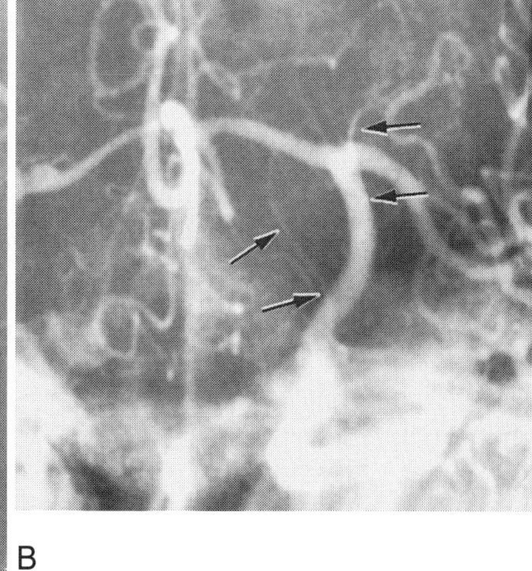

B

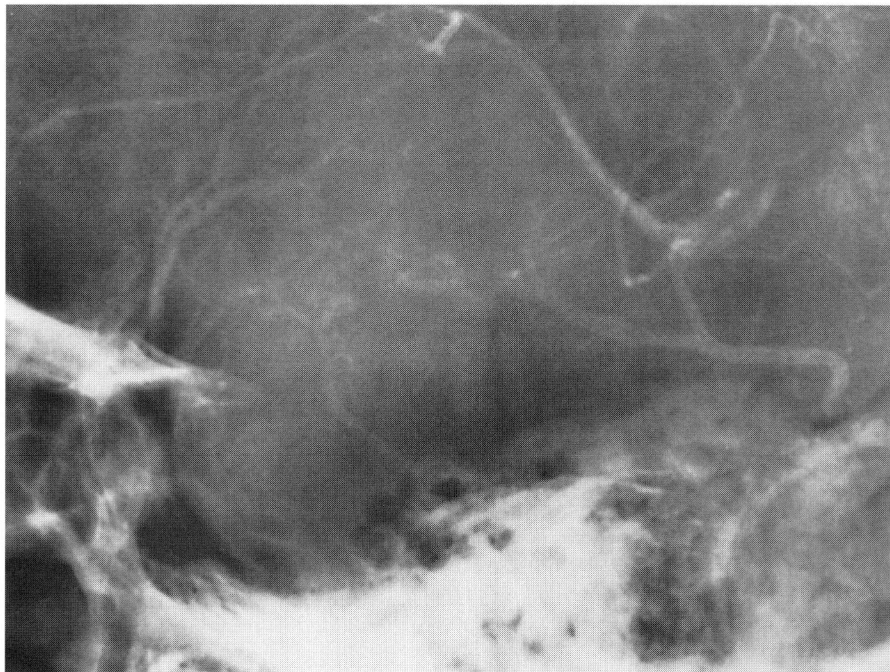

C

Figure 11.79. Large pituitary adenoma. **A.** The lateral arterial phase shows opening of the siphon, elevation of the bifurcation of the internal carotid artery (lower anterior arrow), and elevation of the proximal portion of the anterior cerebral artery (upper anterior arrow). There is an enlarged inferior hypophyseal artery that is displaced posteriorly and stretched (double posterior arrow). The other fine vessels, seen just behind the elevated bifurcation of the internal carotid, represent part of the circuminfundibular plexus pushed upward (posterior arrow). **B.** The frontal projection demonstrates lateral displacement of the supraclinoid portion of the carotid artery (lateral arrow) and elevation of the bifurcation of the internal carotid and of the horizontal portion of the anterior cerebral artery. The enlarged inferior hypophyseal artery again is well seen (lower arrows). The anterior choroidal artery is displaced laterally (upper arrows). **C.** There are bumping and elevation of the internal cerebral and septal veins. The long subependymal veins are evidence of ventricular dilatation, caused by obstruction at the foramen of Monro.

out to diagnose or to exclude an aneurysm, and also to determine the blood supply and the degree of vascularity of the lesion. Also, at times, the artery may be narrowed and occasionally occluded. The anatomy and technique are described elsewhere.

Suprasellar and perisellar masses produce displacement of the carotid artery and its branches, depending on their site of origin.

Pituitary adenomas extending above the sella produce (a) elevation of the supraclinoid carotid (opening of the carotid siphon); (b) elevation of the bifurcation of the carotid artery; (c) elevation of the anterior cerebral arteries; and (d) lateral displacement of the intracavernous portion of the carotid arteries due to lateral displacement of the cavernous sinuses, which is shown best by venography of the cavernous sinuses (Figs. 11.79 and 11.80). If large, the

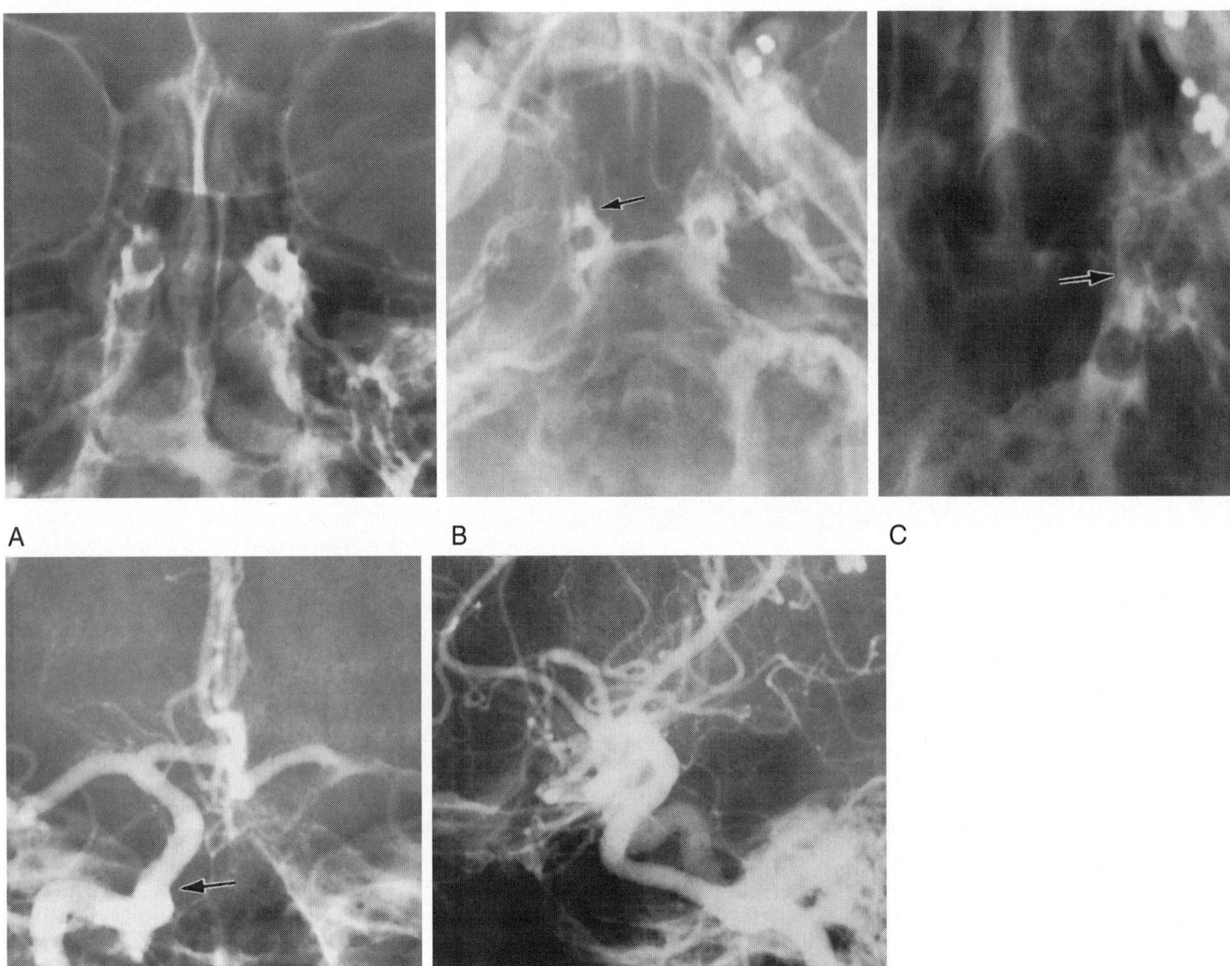

Figure 11.80. Cavernous sinogram. **A.** The injection was made into the inferior petrosal sinus. Frontal film demonstrates bilateral filling. The radiolucency of the internal carotid artery is seen within the opacity of the cavernous sinus. The width of the pituitary fossa contents can be estimated with ease. **B.** Base view. The posterior portion of the sinus is well filled bilaterally, and the internal carotid radiolucency is well shown. There is a posterior communicating channel filled; the anterior communicating channel is not filled. A slight indentation is present on the right side owing to lateral bulging of an eosinophilic pituitary adenoma (arrow) pressing on the cavernous sinus. **C** to **E.** Deformity of the cavernous sinus and the cavernous segment of the carotid artery by a pituitary adenoma. **C.** The base view demonstrates the medial indentation of the left cavernous sinus (arrow). The injection was made via a catheter advanced into the inferior petrosal sinus on the right side, but the right cavernous sinus did not fill. This usually indicates occlusion or compression of the sinus. **D.** The frontal projection of the right carotid angiogram demonstrates lateral displacement of the intracavernous segment (arrow). **E.** The lateral view of the right brachial angiogram demonstrates flattening of the siphon on the right side but not on the left (which filled by regurgitation), indicating greater lateral extension of the tumor on the right side.

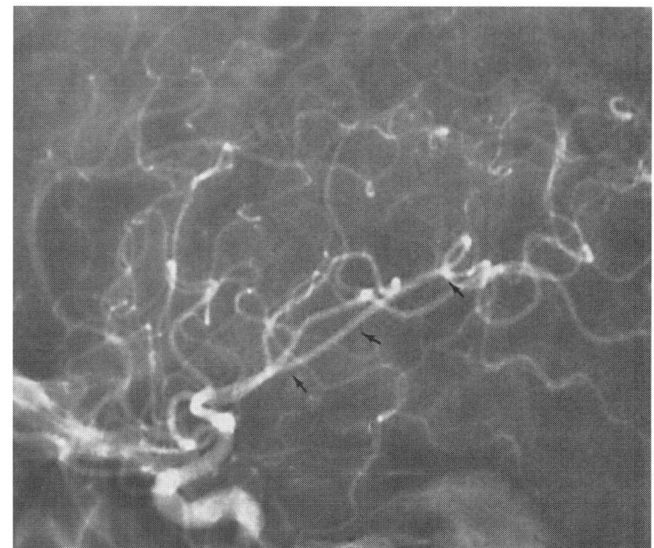

A

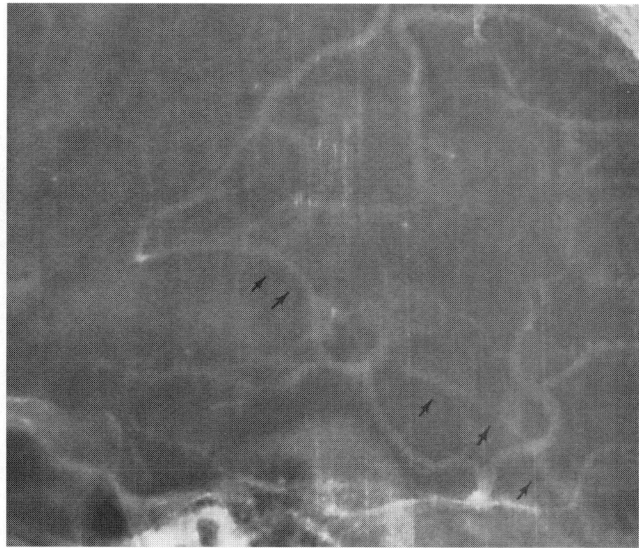

B

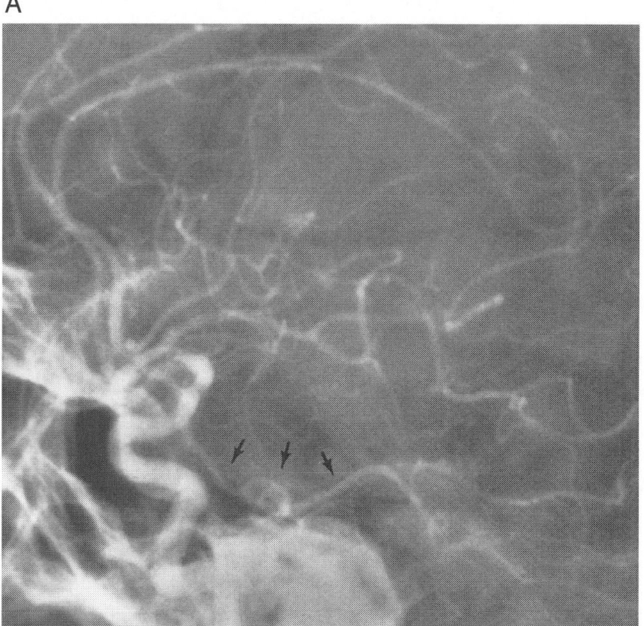

C

Figure 11.81. Tumor of the posterior part of the third ventricle (Pinealoma). **A.** The lateral view in the arterial phase shows no significant elevation of the pericallosal artery, but there is moderate elevation of the lower boundary of the sylvian triangle (arrows). The elevation of the middle cerebral branches is straight and uniform due to the dilatation of the temporal horn. **B.** The lateral venogram discloses elevation of the posterior portion of the internal cerebral vein (arrows) without any deformity of the basal vein. The straight sinus is curved in this instance (posterior arrows) as a normal variant. **C.** Large third-ventricular tumor (intraventricular craniopharyngioma). The lateral arterial phase shows lateral ventricular dilatation shown by the wide sweep of the pericallosal artery and elevation of the inferior side of the sylvian triangle. As often occurs with such large midline masses, there is not only obstruction at the foramen of Monro but a complete downward transtentorial herniation, manifested by marked downward displacement of the posterior communicating artery and the anterior portion of the posterior cerebral artery (arrows). In addition, there is slight regurgitation into the basilar artery, which discloses downward displacement of this artery as well. Similar changes were found on the opposite side, indicating that a central (bilateral complete) herniation existed.

tumor elevates the foramen of Monro and the internal cerebral vein.

Other suprasellar tumors, such as craniopharyngiomas, do not usually produce elevation of the carotid bifurcation or opening of the siphon; on the contrary, depression and closing of the siphon may be seen.

Laterally placed tumors (parasellar) may elevate the supraclinoid carotid segment, but they also will elevate the intracavernous portion of the carotid artery (Fig. 11.74*C*). In addition, they may surround the carotid artery and produce narrowing (Fig. 11.74*A* and *B*) and sometimes true encasing.

Tumors in the anterior third ventricle may elevate the internal cerebral veins anteriorly and may cause depression of the posterior communicating artery (Fig. 11.81). Posterior third ventricle tumors may elevate the posterior portion of the internal cerebral veins. They also produce ventricular dilatation (Fig. 11.82).

Thalamic tumors produce elevation of the thalamostriate vein, lateral displacement of the angiographic sylvian point and sylvian vessels, and midline shift of the internal cerebral vein. Elevation of the posterior choroidal vessels and enlargement and stretching of the thalamoperforating branches of the posterior communicating and posterior cerebral arteries are important features (Fig. 11.82).

Intraventricular meningiomas and choroid plexus papillomas produce enlargement of the choroidal vessels and a

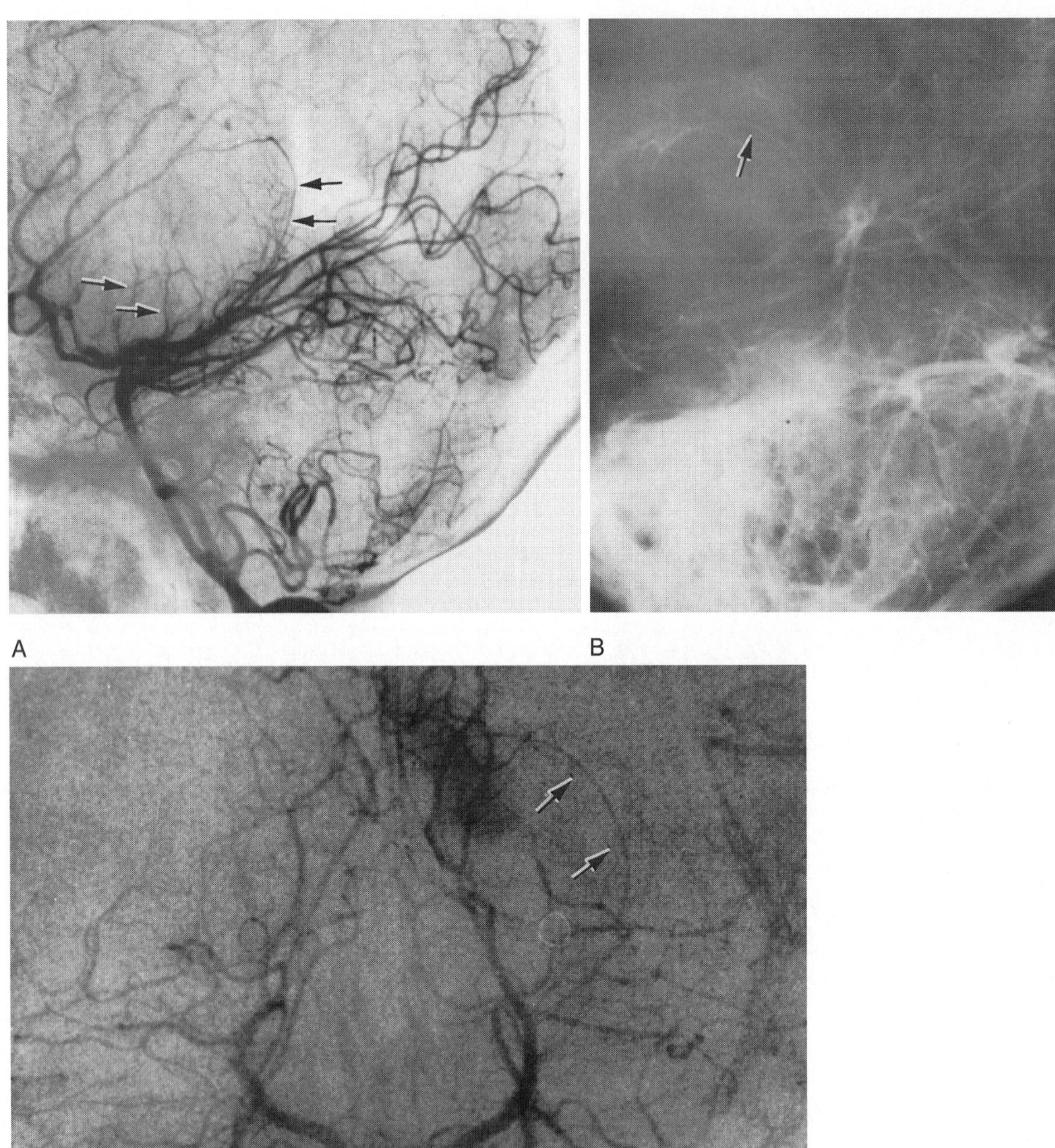

A B

C

Figure 11.82. Thalamic tumor shown by vertebral angiography. **A.** The lateral arterial phase shows enlargement of the thalamoperforating arteries (anterior arrows) and widening of the curvature of the lateral posterior choroidal artery (posterior arrows). **B.** The venous phase shows upward displacement of the internal cerebral vein (arrow). **C.** The frontal projection demonstrates lateral bowing of an enlarged lateral posterior choroidal artery (arrows).

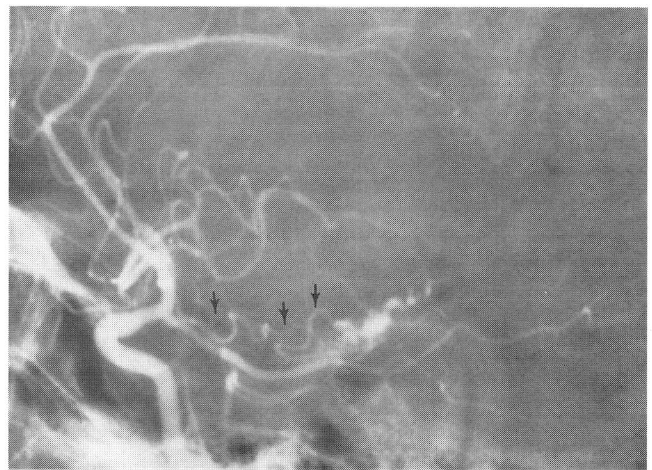

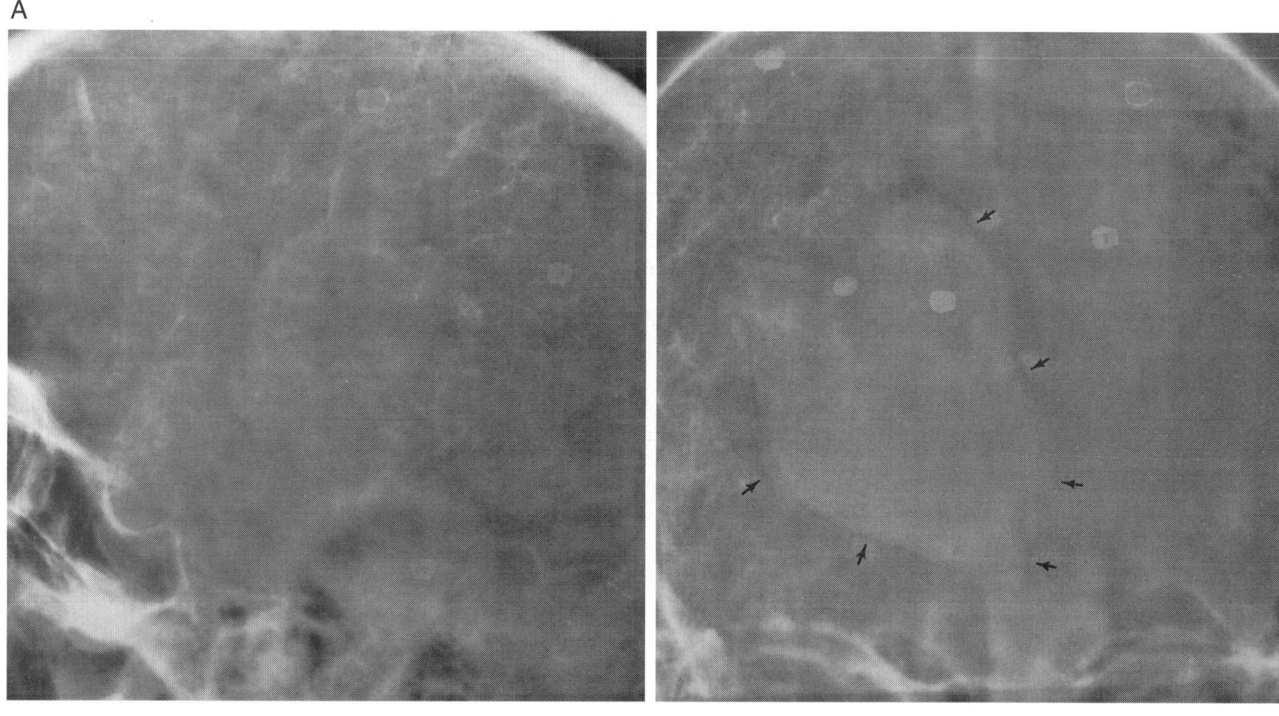

Figure 11.83. Intraventricular meningioma with abnormal blood supply. **A.** In the arterial phase there is enlargement and considerable tortuosity of the anterior choroidal artery (anterior and middle arrows). There is enlargement of the posterior choroidal arteries arising from the posterior cerebral artery as well (posterior arrow). **B.** The film made at 3.5 sec shows a homogeneous, almost perfectly round, radiopacity in the center of the skull that has an appearance consistent with the cloud of a meningioma. **C.** The frontal film made at the same time (3.5 sec) shows the position of the homogeneous cloud to the right of the midline and partly beyond the midline. The position of the collection of contrast material would place the tumor most likely within the ventricle, and therefore a diagnosis of intraventricular meningioma was justified on the basis of the angiogram alone.

tumor blush that, when homogeneous and persistent, favor meningioma (Fig. 11.83), and when more intense and irregular, favor a choroid plexus papilloma. Other types of circulation are shown in Figure 11.12.

MULTIPLE INTRACEREBRAL TUMORS

Two types of tumors are described in more detail here: the primary brain lymphoma and the metastatic tumors. Other tumors can be multiple and will be or have been mentioned at the time they are described. These include multiple meningiomas, which may be seen in patients with a history of neurofibromatosis type II; multiple cranial nerve tumors, also seen in patients with a history of neurofibromatosis type II; and multicentric glioblastomas.

Primary Brain Lymphomas

These tumors are included under the group of multiple intracerebral tumors because the great majority will be multiple if they are followed for a period of time, although early on they may be single (about 60 percent). They occur much more frequently in immunocompromised patients, and undoubtedly the marked increase in incidence of primary CNS lymphoma noted in the last decade is related to AIDS and the extensive use of immunosuppressive drugs with organ transplantation and in the treatment of some malignant lesions. However, primary brain lymphoma, which represents only 1 percent of all lymphomas, also seems to be increasing in frequency in nonimmunocompromised patients (116) (Table 11.40).

Table 11.40.
Primary CNS Lymphomas

Vast majority are B-cell lymphomas
About 60% are a solitary mass at time of discovery
Rapid growth and rapid initial (but temporary) response to steroids and radiation therapy
Typically periventricular and often involve the corpus callosum
Usually a homogeneous mass in non-AIDS patients
Frequently ring-enhancing masses in AIDS patients, simulating toxoplasmosis

The tumors grow rapidly and may also disappear rapidly under therapy (steroids, radiation therapy, chemotherapy) (Fig. 11.85*H* to *J*). The majority of CNS lymphomas are of the B-cell type similar to the systemic lymphomas. Burkitt lymphoma and T-cell lymphoma are seen occasionally (117). Although they are primary CNS lymphomas, at autopsy some cell infiltrations may be found in other tissues as small, incidental, often microscopic deposits in various organs (lung, myocardium, intestinal tract, adrenals, kidney) (4). The tumors are often well circumscribed but more commonly are poorly delineated. They occur in the subcortical white matter; the periventricular white matter is commonly involved, as well as the ventricular wall (Fig. 11.85). Meningeal involvement is sometimes seen but is more common in secondary involvement from systemic lymphoma. The latter also tends to involve the CNS by perivascular infiltration along the Virchow-Robin spaces (Fig. 11.88). Involvement of the spinal cord is not uncommon (Fig. 11.86). Imaging diagnosis is best done by MRI, but CT with contrast is also satisfactory. The tumor may be hyperintense on CT prior to enhancement, probably due to its high cellularity (Fig. 11.84*D*). The lesions enhance with contrast on CT or MRI (Figs. 11.84 to 11.88). An occasional case may show no enhancement, but then one should carefully determine whether steroids have been administered, for steroids close the intercellular spaces in the capillary endothelium and tend to correct the blood-brain barrier disruption. Some lymphoma masses are T2-dark (Fig. 11.87), which may be related to old blood products from previous hemorrhage or to high cellularity; also, some may be rich in collagens (118). Brain lymphoma masses only show evidence of necrosis in cases associated with immunodeficiency, particularly in AIDS (Fig. 11.87).

The corpus callosum is frequently involved. Third ventricular involvement sometimes requires differentiation from germinoma (Fig. 11.85*E*,*F* and *H* to *J*), but the presence of a parenchymal lesion would argue against the diagnosis of germinoma. The differential diagnosis includes glioma, metastatic tumor, toxoplasmosis, progressive multifocal leukoencephalopathy (PML), and other CNS infections, such as viral encephalitis. The most important differential is that of toxoplasmosis in patients who are HIV positive. Antitoxoplasmosis therapy is usually instituted, and if the lesion does not improve in about 2 weeks, a biopsy may be carried out. Under these circumstances Chappell et al. reported an incidence of 36 percent lymphoma, 24 percent PML, and 8 percent toxoplasmosis, but this study included only the patients who did not respond to anti-inflammatory therapy (119). Lymphoma in AIDS patients may coexist with an inflammatory lesion, and some lesions may respond and others would not.

Metastatic Tumors

Brain metastases are among the most common intracranial tumors. The great majority involve the brain, but as is well known, metastases occur also in the surrounding bone and occasionally in the meninges, the pituitary gland, and the cavernous sinus.

The skull metastases occur in conjunction with other skeletal metastases and are best investigated first by radionuclide bone scans and later by plan film examination. Interestingly, a tumor that produces skull metastases very rarely also produces brain metastases. The author has searched for a case showing both types of lesions for some years, without success. Bone metastases are particularly common in lung, breast, and renal metastases. However, almost any malignant tumor can metatasize to the skull.

Pure meningeal metastases are uncommon. A tumor that typically metastasizes to the dura is the neuroblastoma. The majority of cases of neuroblastoma, however, represent metastases to the skull bones that are growing inwardly, leading to brain edema and increased intracranial pressure. Leptomeningeal metastases are sometimes extensive. The seeding can be localized in one area or sometimes may cover most of the leptomeninges. It may produce small masses projecting into the subarachnoid space and growing into the adjacent brain. MRI with contrast enhancement is the best diagnostic approach (Fig. 11.96).

The relative incidence of metastatic brain lesions from primary sites is listed in Table 11.6. The most common origin is the lung, followed by melanomas and breast tumors. The percentages vary by institution (Table 11.41).

When a search for metastases is being made, it is essential to carry out the examination without and with contrast. On CT examination the pathology may be missed altogether unless there is some edema surrounding the lesion or lesions (Fig. 11.89*E* and *F*). Edema may be present but may be slight, and thus not conspicuous on the examination. On MRI the lesion and the edema are usually well seen on T2-weighted and proton density images, and thus the chances of overlooking a lesion are lessened.

The brain reacts strongly to metastatic lesions by producing vasogenic edema in the great majority of cases. However, there are many tumors that the brain seems to tolerate, and the nodules are surrounded by very little or no edema (Fig. 11.91). Sometimes edema may not be apparent if the lesion is very small. These cases can be totally overlooked on nonenhanced CT or MRI examinations.

The great majority of lesions occur subcortically near or at the corticomedullary junction (Figs. 11.89 and 11.92). An occasional tumor is seen that seems to metastasize exclusively within the gray matter (Fig. 11.90). The majority

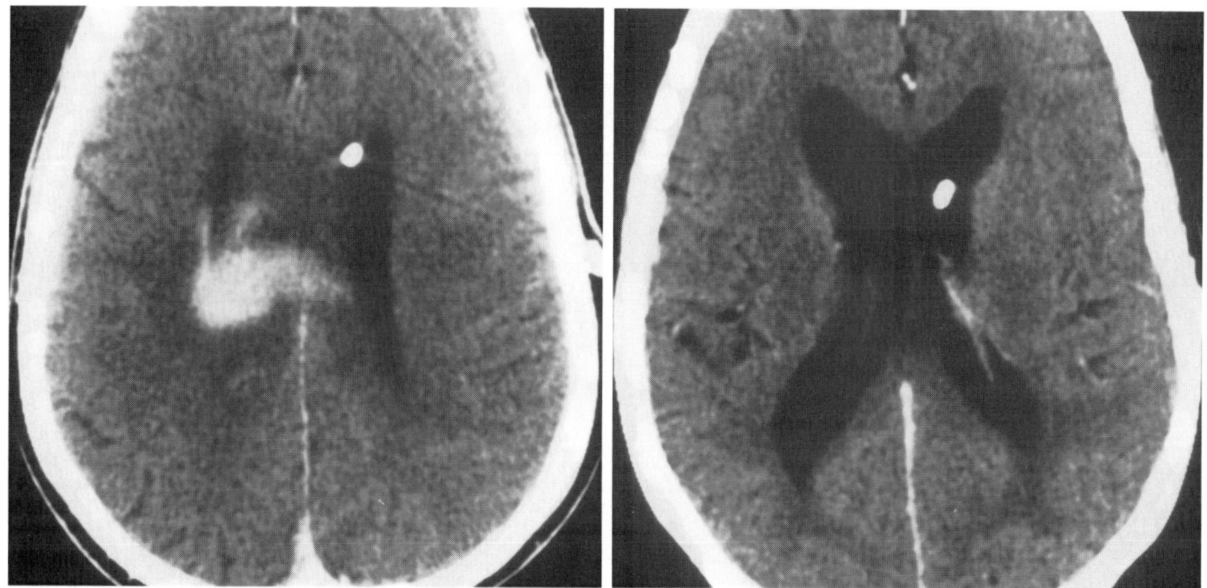

A B C

Figure 11.84. Lymphoma involving primarily the corpus callosum and also the lateral ventricle. **A.** Enhanced axial CT scan shows an irregular area of enhancement in the corpus callosum on the right side extending to the left. **B.** An elongated area of enhancement is seen in the wall of the left lateral ventricle. **C.** On a T1-weighted postcontrast axial MR image there is intraventricular hyperintensity in the left atrium and adjacent occipital horn. **D.** Another case of lymphoma. Preenhanced CT scan shows marked surrounding edema. **E.** After contrast there is uniform enhancement of the tumor, which is sharply circumscribed. Uniform enhancement is typical of primary lymphomas not associated with AIDS.

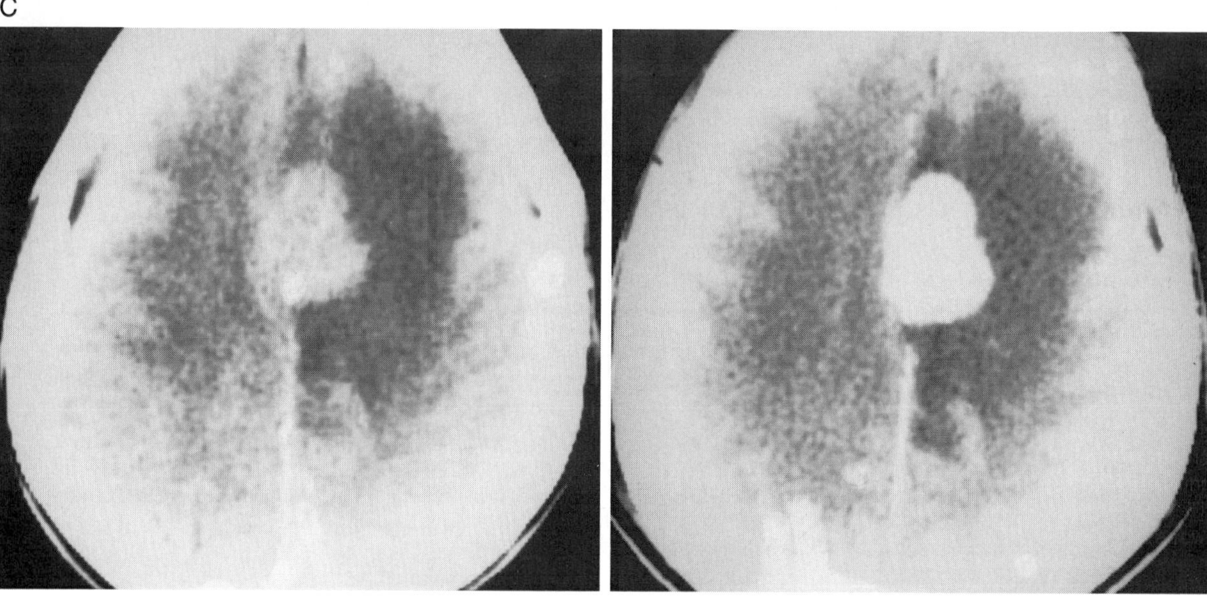

D E

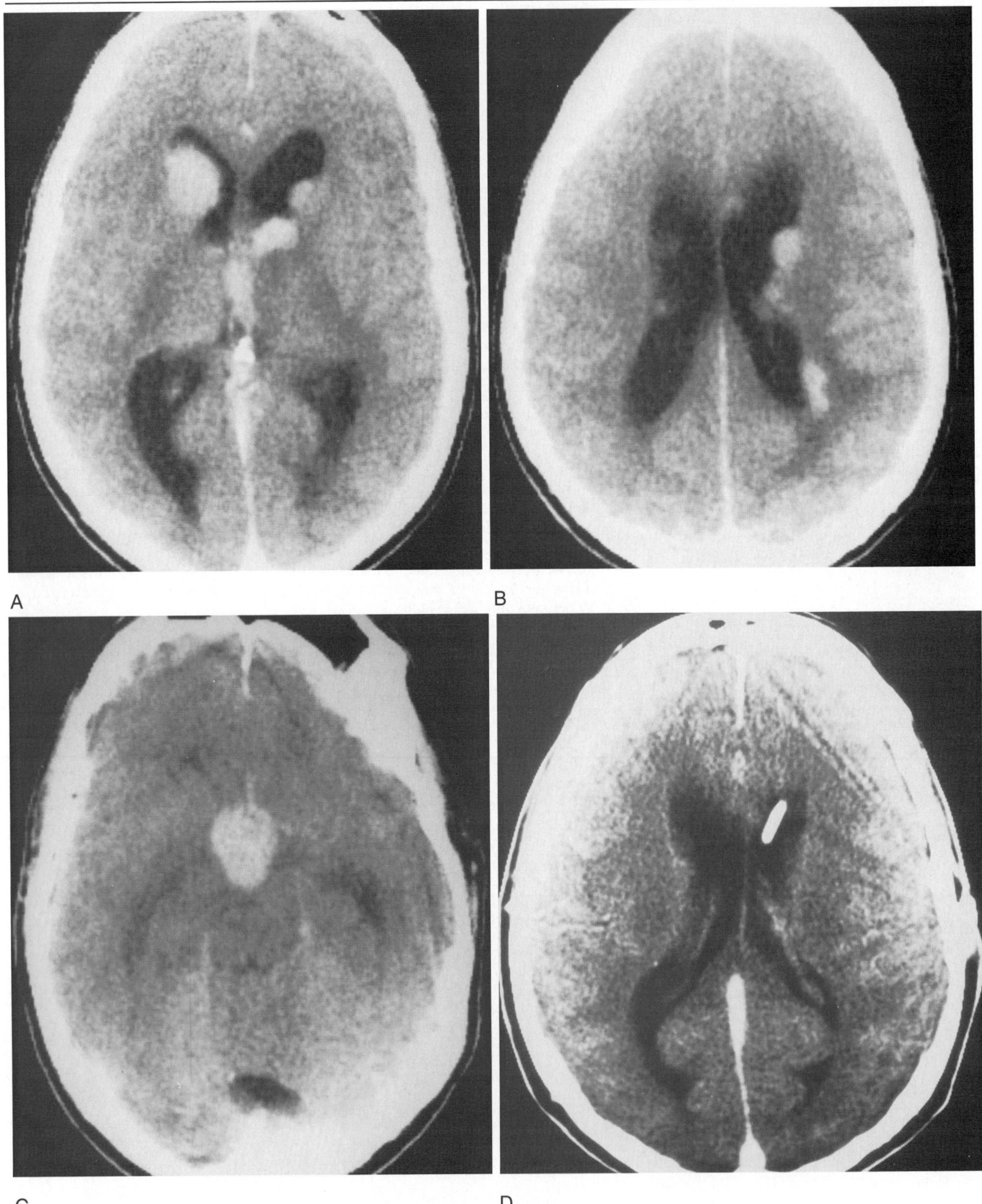

Figure 11.85. A to **D.** Primary brain lymphoma in a 42-year-old man brought in complaining of somnolence but no focal neurologic findings. On admission spinal tap showed increased protein (126 mg) and 57 white cells (49 lymphocytes). The biopsy showed lymphoma, large-cell type. **A** to **C.** Scans showing multinodular, subependymal, uniformly enhancing tumor nodules. The ventricular dilatation required a shunting procedure. The patient improved with radiation therapy, and reexamination 2 months later (**D**) showed disappearance of the masses on postcontrast CT.

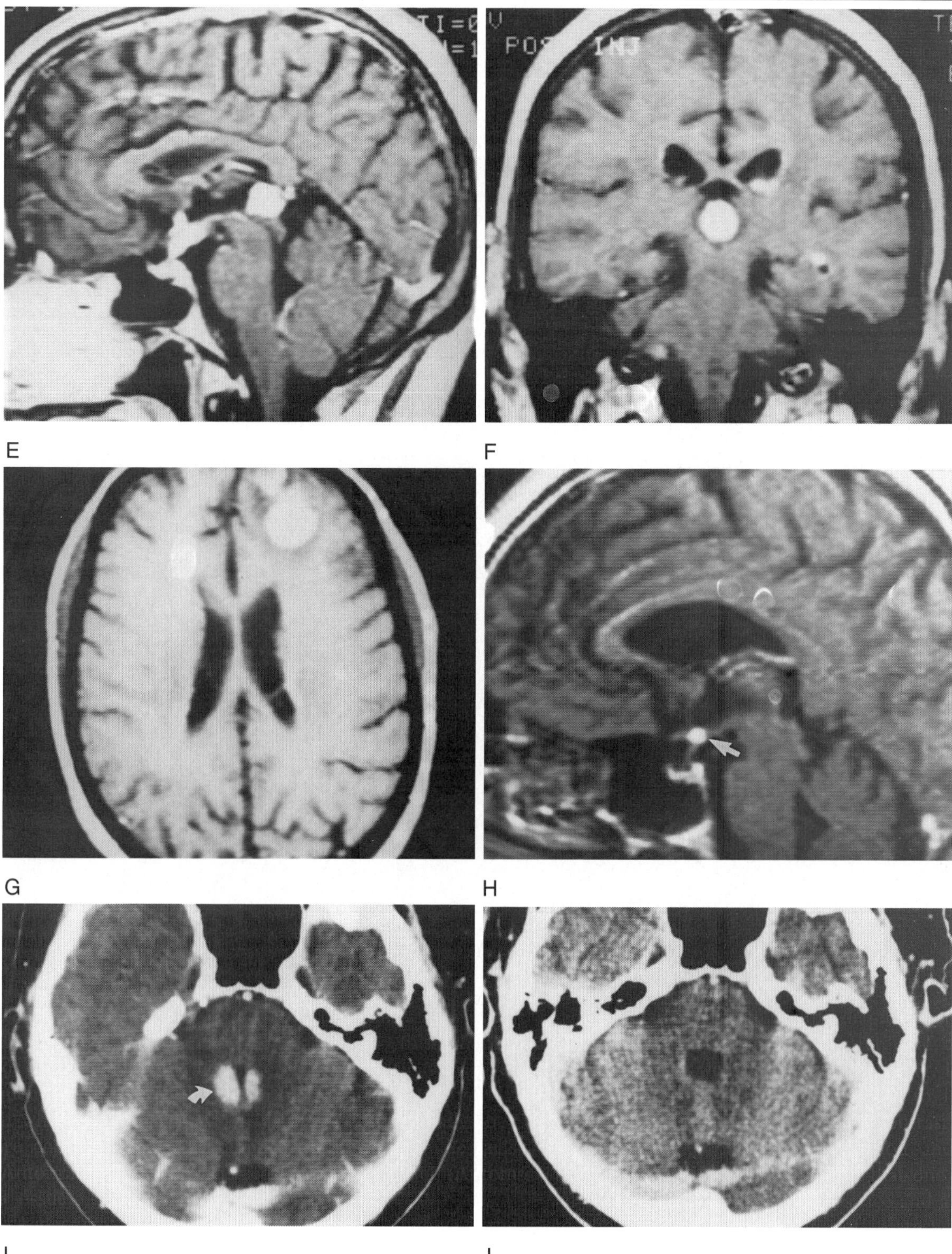

Figure 11.85. *(continued)* **E** and **F.** Another case of lymphoma in a location that would be considered typical of a pineal-origin tumor. Postcontrast T1-weighted image. **G.** In the same case, another enhancing lesion is shown in the left frontal region. **H** to **J.** A third case of lymphoma presenting periventricular lesions. **H.** One was located in the hypothalamus, in the tuber cinereum region (arrow). **I.** Another, not seen in H, was seen on an enhanced CT scan 3 weeks later in the fourth ventricle (arrow). **J.** The fourth ventricle lesion had totally disappeared with treatment and was not seen 6 days later. The possibility that this represents lack of enhancement due to high-dosage steroid therapy should be considered, but is not felt to be likely because there was a mass effect in the fourth ventricle previously. The author has seen virtual disappearance of a mass within 48 h.

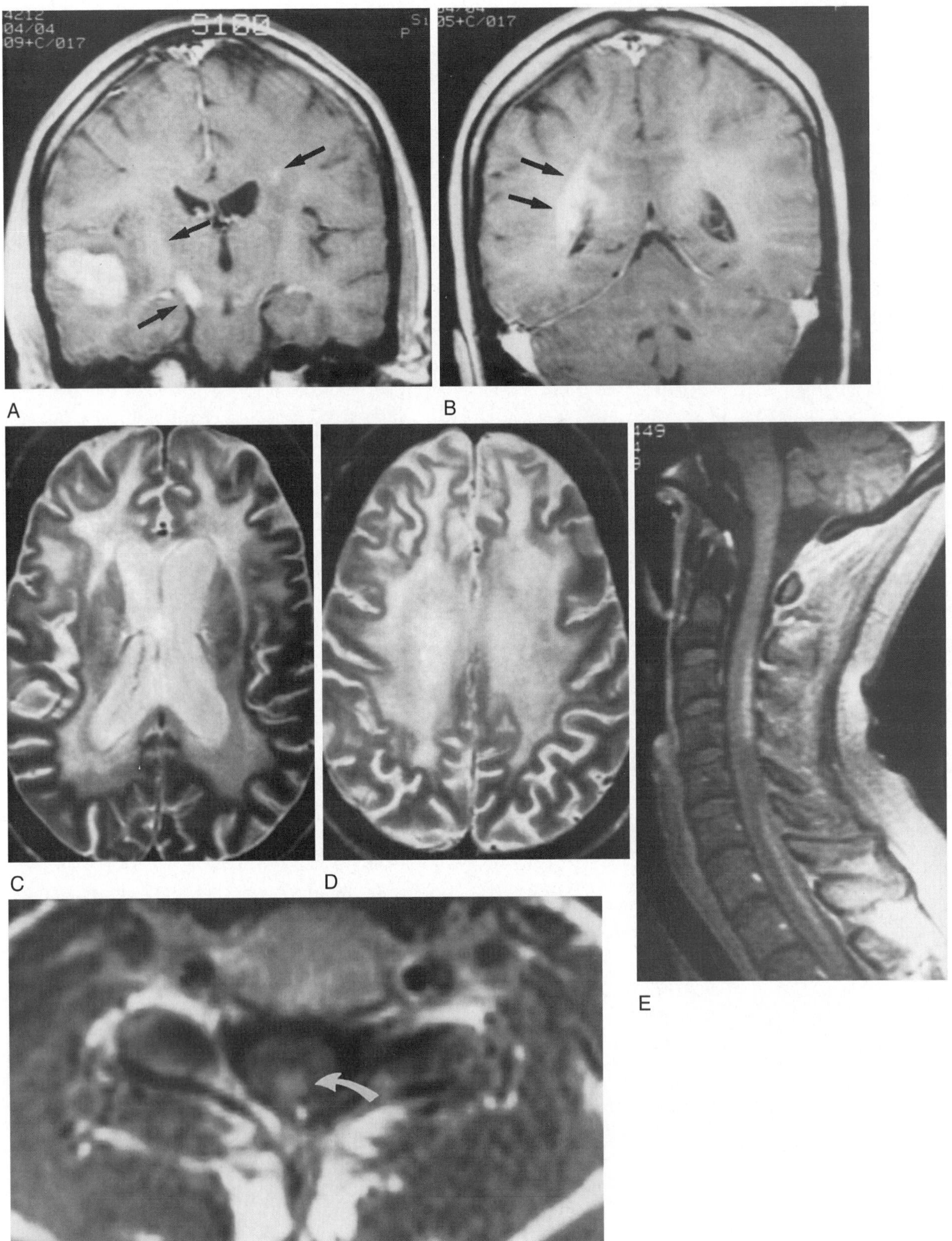

Figure 11.86. Lymphoma in a 37-year-old woman. **A.** Postcontrast T1-weighted coronal image shows a homogeneously enhancing tumor in the right temporal and right internal capsule and pyramidal tract, and another small lesion in the left paraventricular area (arrows). **B.** Coronal T1-weighted postcontrast image shows a large right-sided periventricular lesion (arrows). **C** and **D.** A year later, after the patient received whole-brain radiation therapy and presented a long period of remission, the patient returned, and repeat MRI examination showed extensive diffuse white matter disease on T2-weighted images. CT scanning (not shown) showed similar diffuse low-density white matter changes. The differential diagnosis was between diffuse postradiation cerebritis and lymphoma. The fact that the spinal cord presented enhancing lesions on the postcontrast images (**E,** sagittal; **F,** axial [arrow]) favored lymphoma because the cord had not received radiation therapy. At the autopsy there was diffuse lymphoma.

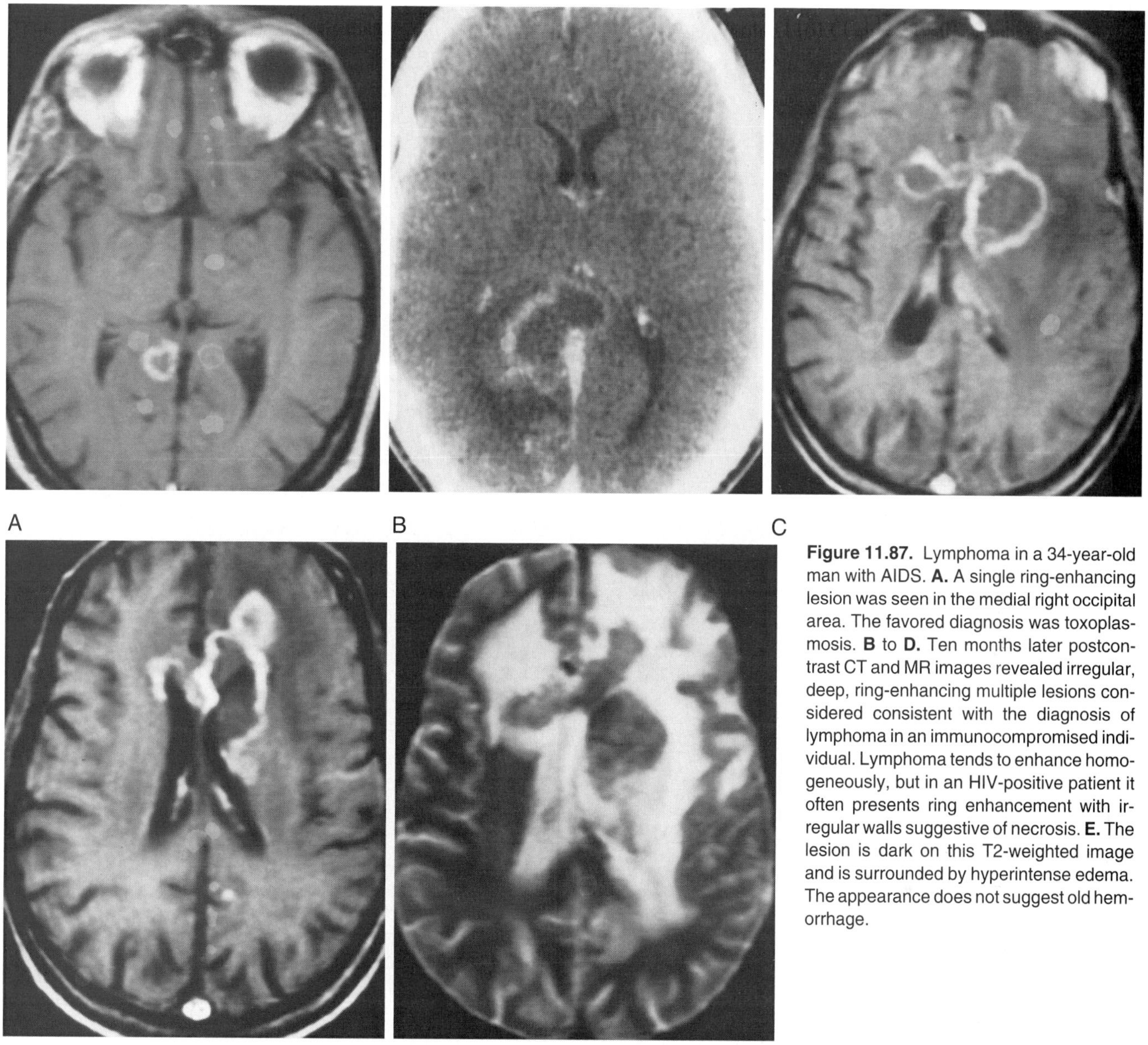

A

B

C

D

E

Figure 11.87. Lymphoma in a 34-year-old man with AIDS. **A.** A single ring-enhancing lesion was seen in the medial right occipital area. The favored diagnosis was toxoplasmosis. **B** to **D.** Ten months later postcontrast CT and MR images revealed irregular, deep, ring-enhancing multiple lesions considered consistent with the diagnosis of lymphoma in an immunocompromised individual. Lymphoma tends to enhance homogeneously, but in an HIV-positive patient it often presents ring enhancement with irregular walls suggestive of necrosis. **E.** The lesion is dark on this T2-weighted image and is surrounded by hyperintense edema. The appearance does not suggest old hemorrhage.

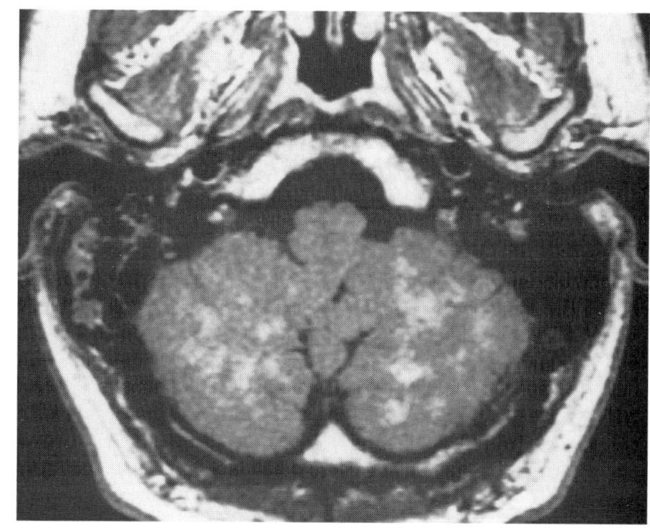

Figure 11.88. Perivascular lymphomatous infiltration in a 35-year-old man with systemic lymphoblastic lymphoma. Postcontrast T1-weighted axial image shows patchy areas of enhancement in both cerebellar hemispheres felt to represent conglomerations of perivascular cerebellar infiltration, the type that may be seen in systemic lymphoma. There was no meningeal involvement. It is possible that this represents the first manifestation of a primary brain lymphoma in a patient who has been immunosuppressed in the treatment of systemic lymphoma, but the appearance is somewhat unusual for primary brain lymphoma.

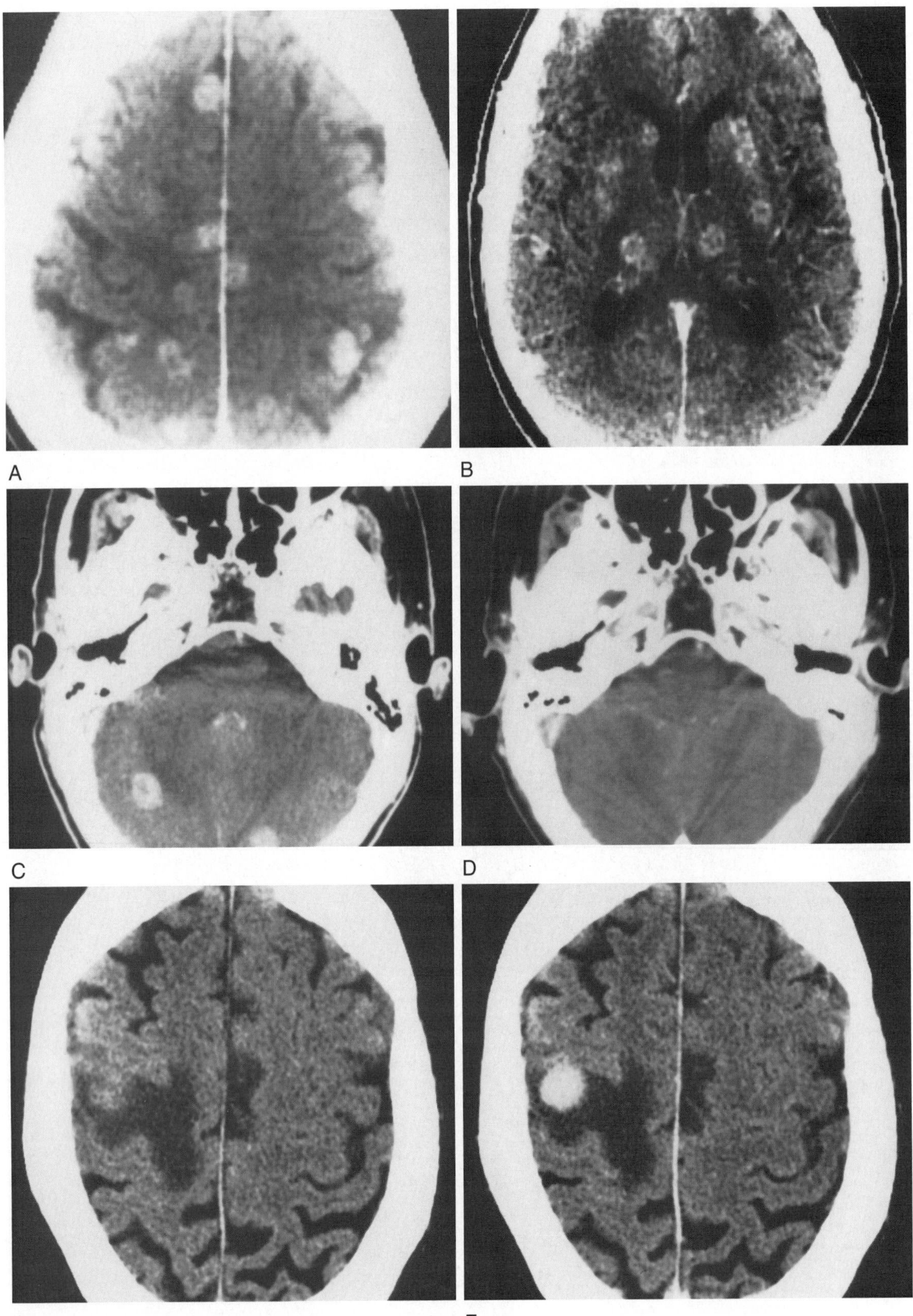

Figure 11.89. Metastases from a small-cell carcinoma of the lung. **A.** Postcontrast CT scan shows multiple enhancing nodules. **B.** An image with different windowing shows that each lesion seems to be excavated, giving a multiple ring–enhancing pattern. There is little edema around the masses. **C.** Another patient with small-cell cancer of the lung showing cerebellar metastases, again with little edema around the lesions. **D.** Reexamination 2 months later shows disappearance of the lesions after chemotherapy; no radiation therapy was given. A few supratentorial metastases also had disapppeared.

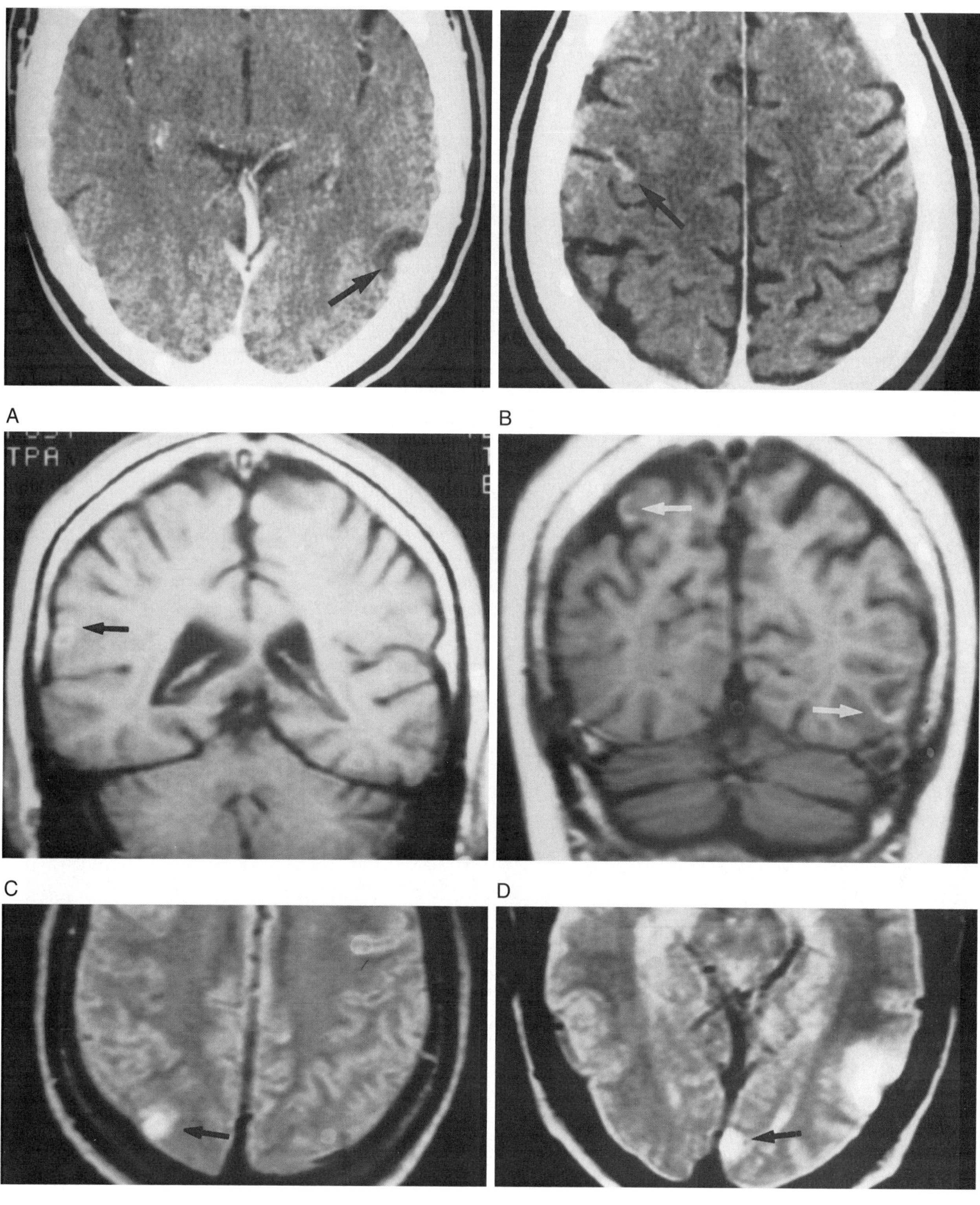

Figure 11.90. Metastases from a lung carcinoma, all in cortical gray matter. **A** and **B.** CT shows two cortical lesions (arrows). There is some surrounding edema. **C** and **D.** Coronal postcontrast T1-weighted image shows three cortical lesions (arrows). **E** and **F.** Proton density axial images show at least two more images—one left occipital, the other right parietal. The larger edematous lesion is the same as that shown in A.

Figure 11.89. *(continued)* **E.** Another metastatic lesion from squamous cell cancer of the lung. The lesion shows considerable edema, and it might have been called an ischemic infarction on the noncontrast examination, but the postcontrast image (**F**) shows a tumor nodule. In retrospect, the rounded lesion was isointense to gray matter and resembled a part of the gyrus.

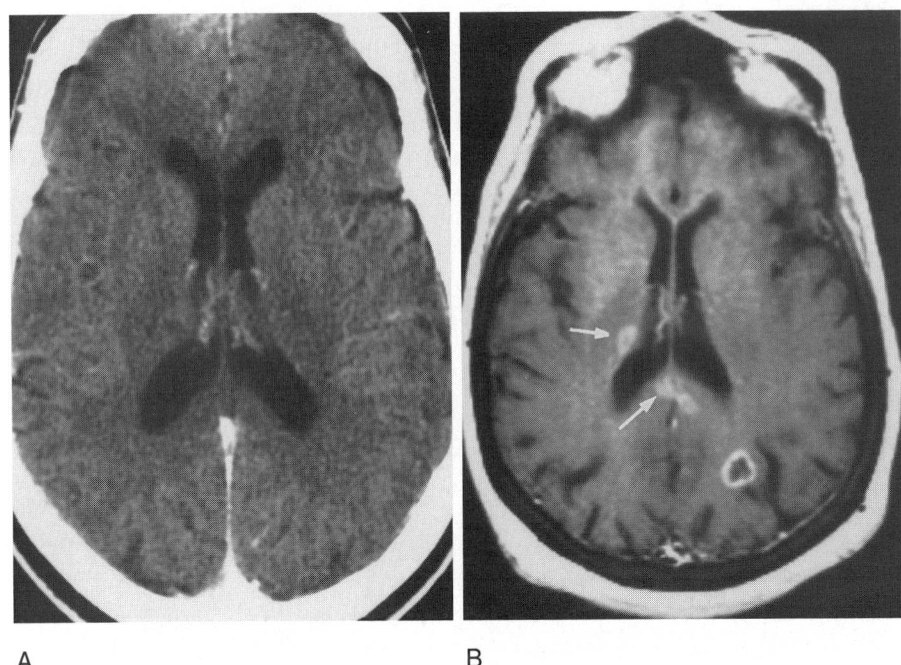

Figure 11.91. Metastases from breast cancer not seen on enhanced CT but seen on MRI. **A.** An enhanced CT examination showed no clear metastatic lesion. **B.** MRI done on the following day showed three lesions: one in the corona radiata, one in the splenium of the corpus callosum (arrow), and one in the left parieto-occipital region, seen on a postcontrast T1-weighted image. In retrospect, the right thalamic lesion might have been suspected on the CT examination. These were the only metastatic lesions discovered.

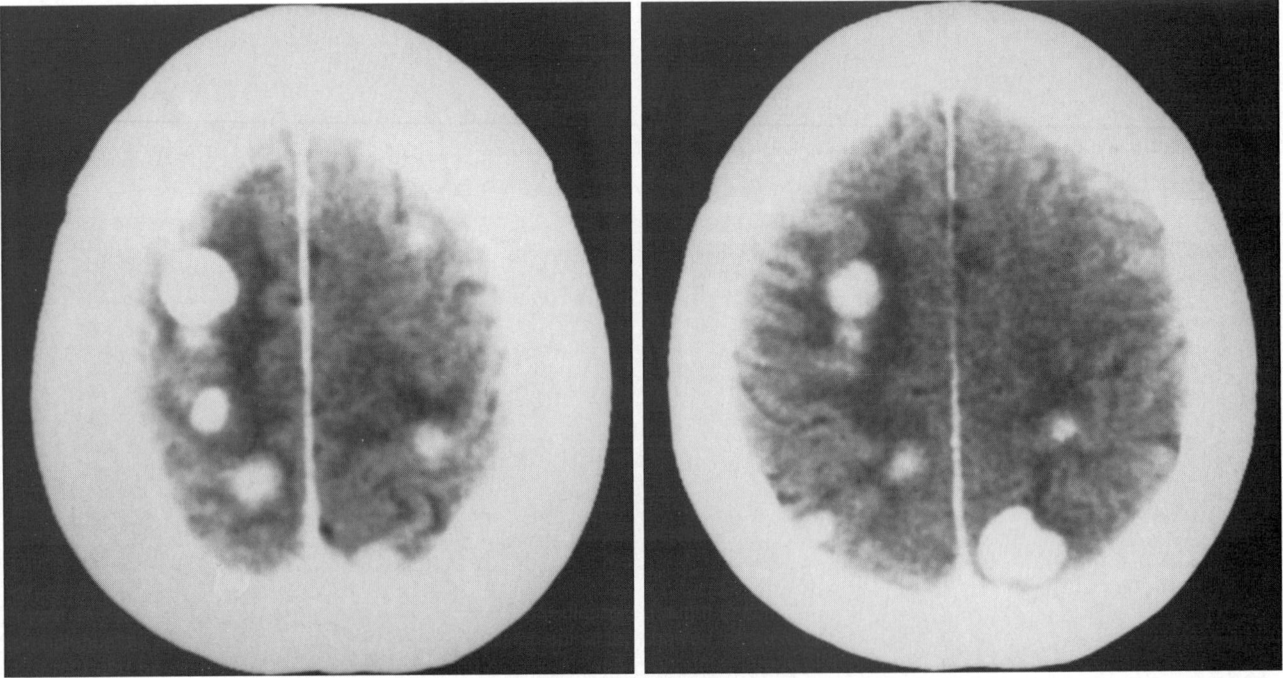

Figure 11.92. Multiple enhancing metastases from atrial myxoma shown on postenhanced CT.

Table 11.41.
Metastases

Lung and breast carcinomas and malignant melanoma are the most common primary tumors
Frequently surrounded by large amounts of vasogenic edema
Majority occur at gray/white junction
Vast majority contrast-enhance
The most common metastases to hemorrhage are lung, melanoma, breast, renal cell, and choriocarcinoma

of the tumors are hypodense on CT and hypointense on T1-weighted images. They enhance in a high percentage of cases, probably well above 90 percent. The lesions may be single or multiple. If multiple, the differential diagnosis with a primary tumor is relatively easy. In a single lesion one must consider other possibilities, mainly a primary brain tumor. In the management of metastatic brain lesions, it is essential to carry out a thorough examination without and with contrast material when only a single lesion is found in a patient who is known to have a malignant neoplasm elsewhere. This is particularly important because the tendency today, with the development of the subspecialty of neurooncology, is to treat the single lesion rather aggressively (surgical resection followed by chemotherapy and radiation therapy), but the therapy would be different if other lesions were found (Fig. 11.89*C* and *D*).

Some metastatic lesions are hemorrhagic. Melanomas are often hemorrhagic but not necessarily so. They are often hyperdense on CT (Fig. 11.93*A*); this may be due to the richness in melanin or to a combination of hemorrhage and melanin. The same lesion may be hyperintense on T1-weighted images and hypointense on T2-weighted images (Fig. 11.93). The lesions enhance after contrast. Hemorrhagic metastases are sometimes encountered from certain types of tumors (most frequently lung, breast, renal, and

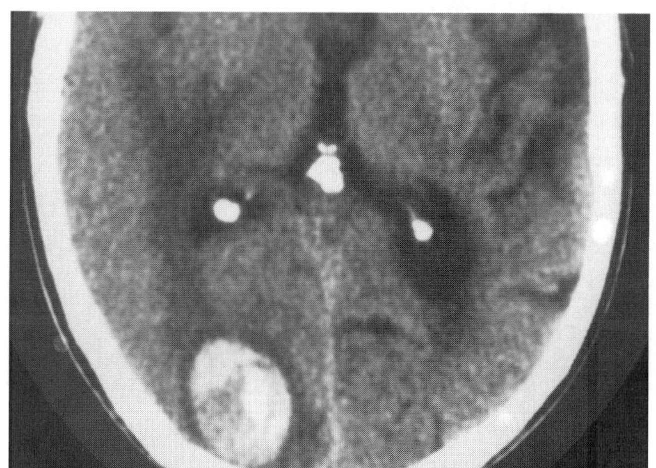

A

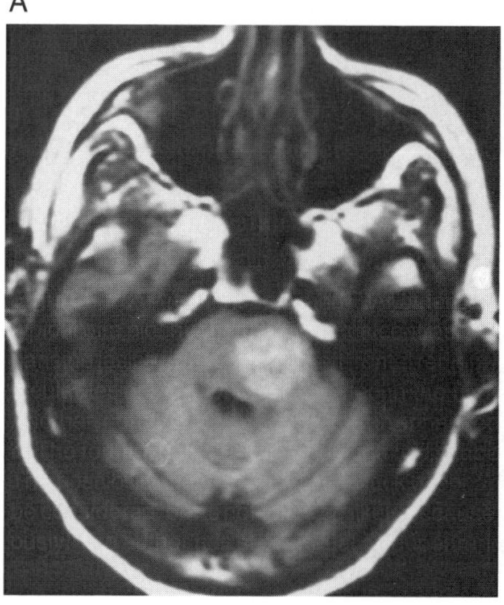

B

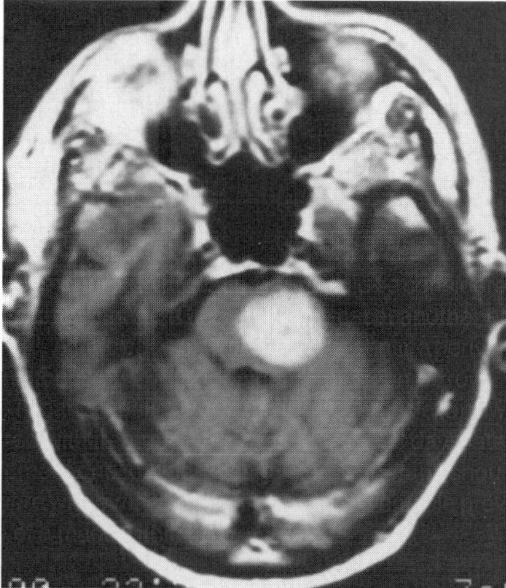

C

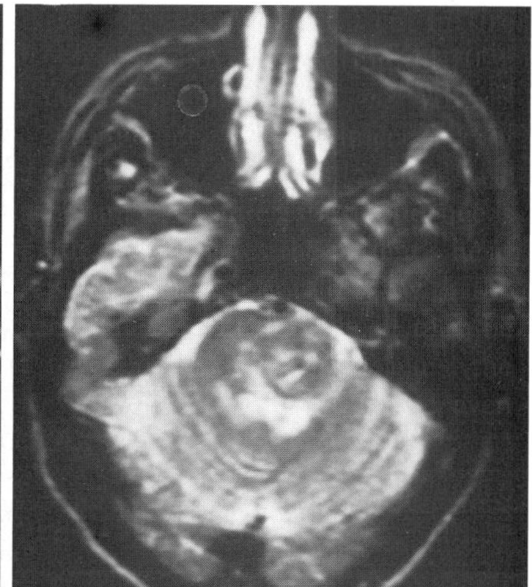

D

Figure 11.93. Metastatic melanoma, hyperdense on CT without contrast enhancement. The hyperdensity may be due to hemorrhage or to the melanoma itself. **A.** Nonenhanced CT shows occipital hyperdense mass that may be hemorrhagic. **B** to **D.** Another case of metastatic melanoma. **B.** MR T1-weighted noncontrast image. **C.** After contrast there is increase in the brightness, indicating contrast uptake. **D.** On a T2-weighted image, the metastatic nodule is isodense, whereas the surrounding edema is bright. The hyperdensity on T1 is due to the melanin and not to methemoglobin in the tumor. On T2-weighted images the melanin shows susceptibility effects and produces shortening of T2.

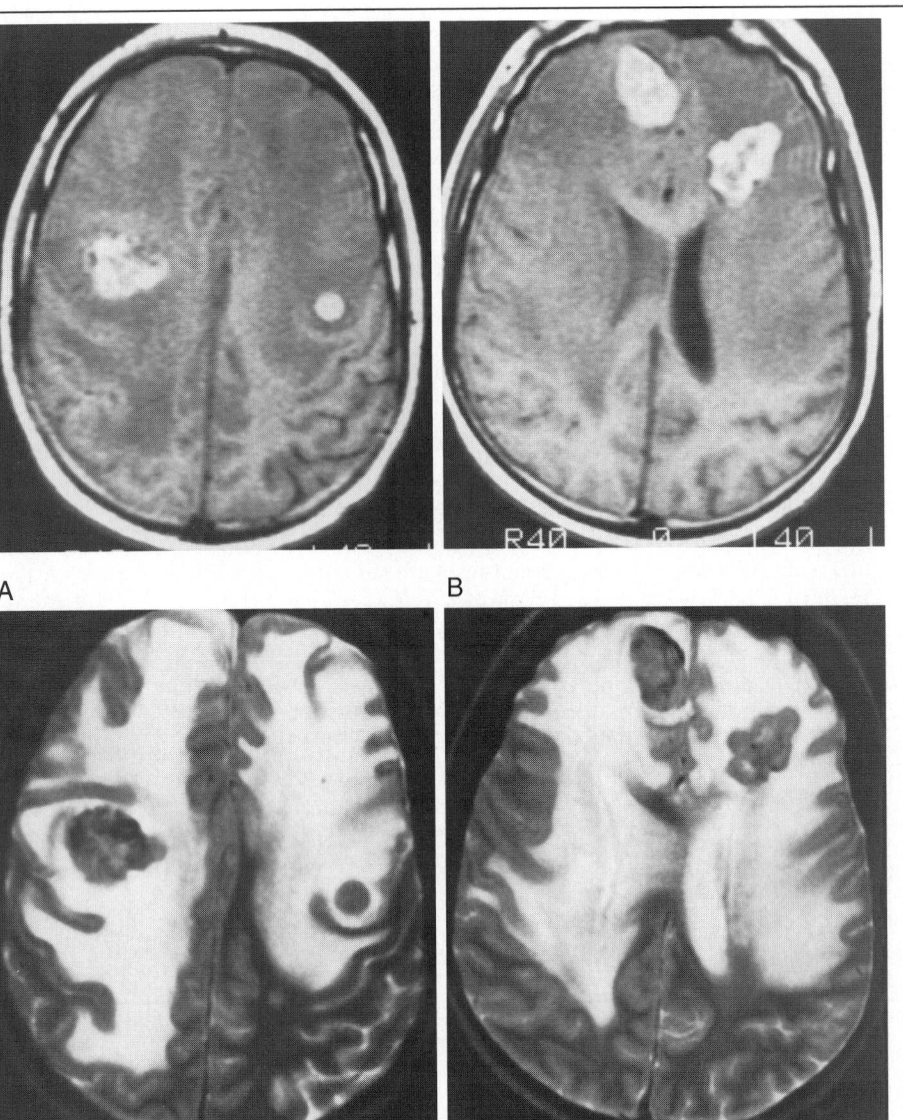

Figure 11.94. Hemorrhagic metastases from malignant fibrous hystiocytoma. **A** and **B.** The lesions were bright on nonenhanced T1-weighted images and enhanced after contrast (not shown). There is much edema. **C** and **D.** T2-weighted images show a marked degree of edema. There were bifrontal metastases as well, and the lesions are all T2-dark. One wonders whether hemorrhage appeared simultaneously in all lesions after they acquired a certain size. If this is only hemorrhage, why are they all at this stage T1-bright and T2-dark? The lesions were also hyperdense on precontrast CT (not shown).

choriocarcinoma), but almost any tumor metastasis can bleed (Fig. 11.94).

Solitary cystic metastases may sometimes suggest a cystic astrocytoma. Usually they produce more surrounding edema than a cystic primary glioma (Fig. 11.95). The history of a known malignancy elsewhere would help in the diagnosis.

Some metastases calcify, sometimes after treatment, sometimes spontaneously. The most frequent metastases to calcify appear to be lung, but also breast and gastrointestinal tract metastases. At autopsy the deposits are found mostly in areas of necrosis in larger tumor nodules. The calcium deposits are usually small and granular sometimes coalescing to form larger deposits (120) (Fig. 11.95*D* to *G*). At autopsy they were identified in 7 percent of specimens. Meningeal carcinomatosis is not rare. The tumors usually originate from the lung and the breast (Fig. 11.96).

Other Multiple Tumors

These include meningiomas (described in text following); multiple schwannomas and neurofibromas related to neurofibromatosis types I and II; multiple gliomas, also related to neurofibromatosis type I; and multiple hemangioblastomas in the cerebellum and spinal cord with or without other features of von Hippel-Lindau syndrome (described in text following). Seeding of intracranial tumors is a feature of CNS tumors that differentiates them from metastases arising from neoplasms outside the CNS. This subject has been mentioned in text preceding; see also spinal cord seeding described in text following.

PARANEOPLASTIC SYNDROMES

These are discussed under systemic disorders affecting the nervous system (Chapter 13).

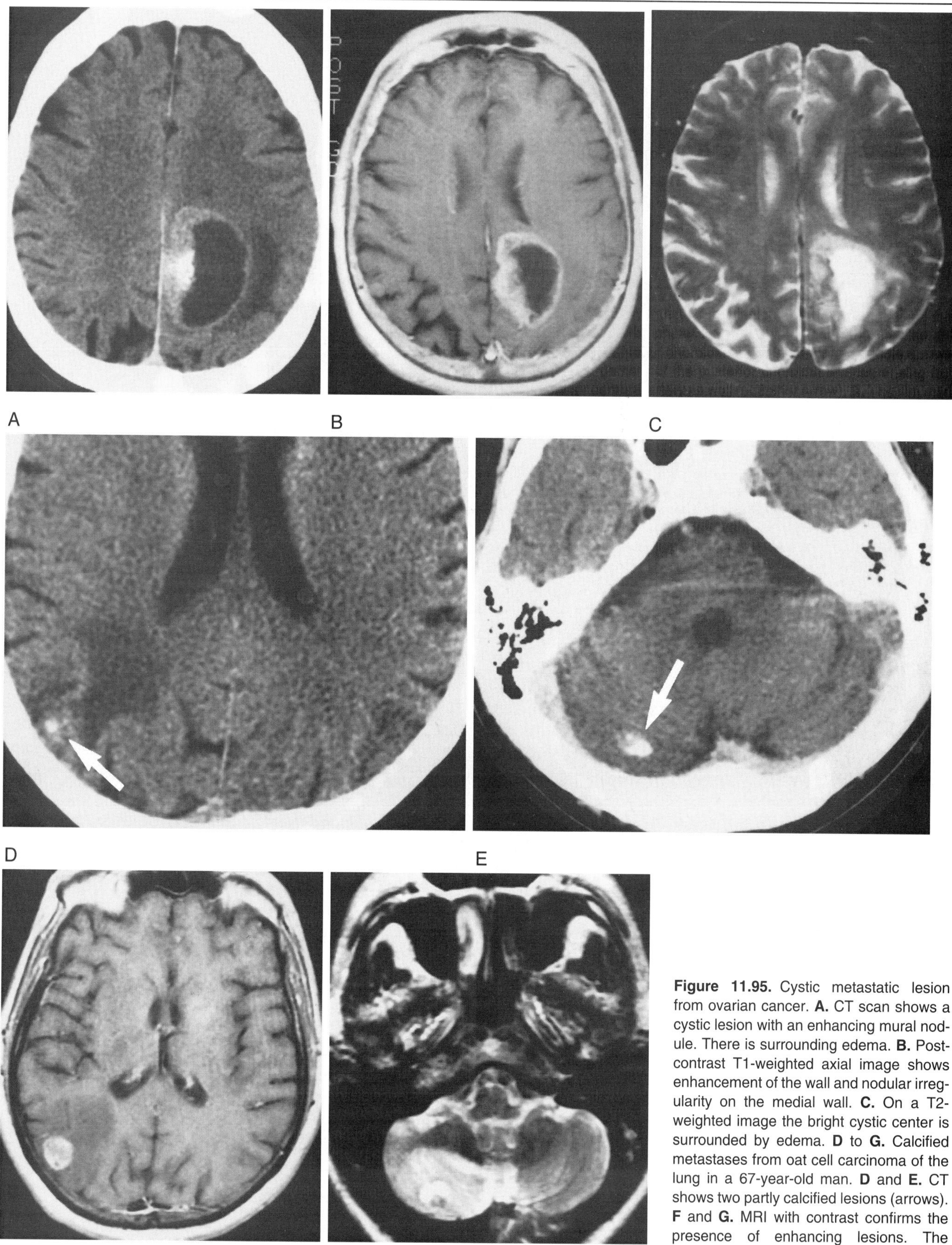

Figure 11.95. Cystic metastatic lesion from ovarian cancer. **A.** CT scan shows a cystic lesion with an enhancing mural nodule. There is surrounding edema. **B.** Postcontrast T1-weighted axial image shows enhancement of the wall and nodular irregularity on the medial wall. **C.** On a T2-weighted image the bright cystic center is surrounded by edema. **D** to **G.** Calcified metastases from oat cell carcinoma of the lung in a 67-year-old man. **D** and **E.** CT shows two partly calcified lesions (arrows). **F** and **G.** MRI with contrast confirms the presence of enhancing lesions. The calcified portion is partly seen as low-intensity areas.

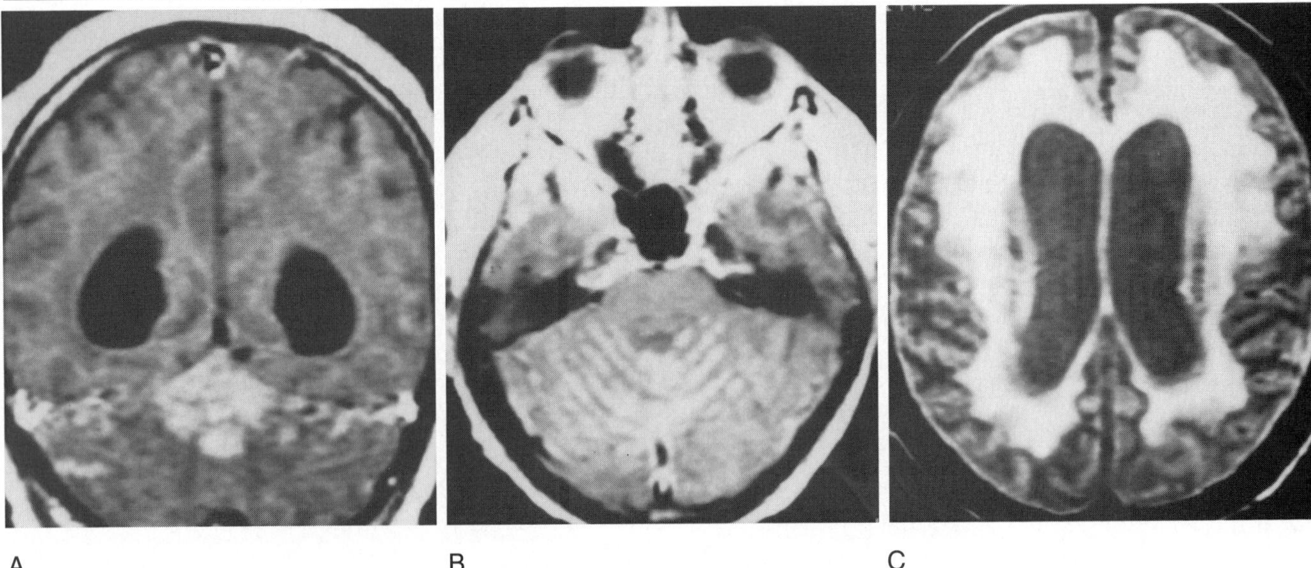

Figure 11.96. Extensive leptomeningeal metastases from a poorly differentiated breast adenocarcinoma. **A.** Numerous enhancing nodules are seen in this postcontrast T1 image. **B.** The extension and diffuse involvement are well shown over the cerebellar folia. **C.** Proton density axial image. There was considerable ventricular enlargement and white matter edema, probably secondary to transependymal CSF extravasation, but no metastases were seen in the supratentorial leptomeninges.

POSTERIOR FOSSA TUMORS

The tumors of the posterior fossa represent a special group because their histology tends to be different from that of neoplasms occurring in the supratentorial space, although sometimes it is similar. Among the gliomas, astrocytomas occur in the cerebellum and brainstem. They may range from slowly growing, such as in the cerebellum, to malignant, particularly in the brainstem. Interestingly enough, the glioblastoma, the most common malignant brain tumor, does not usually occur in the cerebellum, although a rare one may be found. Some special intra-axial neoplasms include the hemangioblastoma, which occurs primarily in the cerebellum but does not occur supratentorially. The medulloblastoma is also a special tumor of the cerebellum (Table 11.42).

The intraventricular tumors are of the same histologic classification as found elsewhere and include the ependymoma, the choroid plexus papilloma, and the meningioma.

In the posterior fossa are located most of the cranial nerves, and for that reason the schwannomas of these nerves occur mostly in the posterior fossa, another important difference between the posterior fossa and the supratentorial compartment.

In the following discussion, the tumors will be divided according to location: brainstem tumors, cerebellar tumors, intraventricular tumors, and extra-axial posterior fossa tumors.

Table 11.42.
Posterior Fossa Tumors

Parenchymal: brainstem—gliomas; cerebellum—astrocytomas, medulloblastoma, hemangioblastomas, metastases
Intraventricular: ependymomas and choroid plexus papillomas
Extra-axial: schwannomas (especially acoustic schwannomas), meningiomas, epidermoids

Brainstem Tumors

These are usually gliomas and tend to occur more frequently in children, constituting about 15 percent of CNS tumors in children. They are usually astrocytomas, and their rate of growth is variable, but because of their location, brainstem gliomas are usually regarded as malignant. They grow up and down from their most common site of origin, the pons, invading the midbrain and the medulla. If the tumor starts in the midbrain, it may grow into the thalamus.

The tumor mass produces enlargement of the brainstem and usually deforms the brainstem shape as it grows eccentrically. The tumor frequently grows exophytically (nearly two-thirds of the cases), and this growth can be (a) forward, sometimes surrounding the basilar artery or having the artery remain in a groove; the tumor may fill the interpeduncular cistern; (b) posteroinferiorly toward the perimedullary cistern; (c) laterally toward the cerebellopontine angle cisterns; or (d) posteriorly toward the fourth ventricle (Table 11.43).

CT usually provides a diagnosis, particularly in a patient, possibly a child 3 to 10 years of age, who presents with

Table 11.43.
Brainstem Tumors

Vast majority are gliomas
Approximately 15% of childhood tumors
Expand and deform brainstem and frequently extend exophytically
MRI is optimal imaging examination due to absence of CT artifact and multiplanar capability

cranial nerve findings and/or pyramidal tract signs. The tumors are most frequently located in the pons, and enlargement occurs mostly in a forward direction, increasing the curvature and the prominence of the belly of the pons. The tumor also stretches the floor of the fourth ventricle and may produce a decrease in the anteroposterior diameter of this structure as a result of both a backward bulge of the pons and stretching of the floor of the ventricle. The fourth ventricle is almost always displaced dorsad.

MRI is preferred for diagnosis because CT may present artifacts in the region of the tumor, depending on its location (Fig. 11.97). The multiplanar capability and the absence of artifacts in the posterior fossa make MRI superior to CT in the majority of posterior fossa tumors (Fig. 11.98).

If the glioma occurs in the quadrigeminal plate, it will produce hydrocephalus early (see Fig. 4.49); otherwise hydrocephalus is a late manifestation of brainstem tumors.

Tumors may invade the brainstem from the cerebellum or from the fourth ventricle. Care should be taken not to overinterpret deformities of the pons and medulla produced by widened and elongated vertebral and basilar arteries (Fig. 11.99).

Cerebellar Tumors

Primary cerebellar neoplasms occur more frequently in children. They may be more benign, such as astrocytomas, or more malignant, the classic type being medulloblastomas. The astrocytoma is often cystic and if completely removed will not usually recur. Some astrocytomas may calcify; they occur in the cerebellar hemispheres and may enhance on CT or MRI after contrast.

Medulloblastomas are included in the group of PNETs. Another PNET type is the medulloepithelioma, but this is a rare tumor. The medulloblastoma is probably the most common cerebellar tumor in children, although it may vary among institutions, with astrocytoma sometimes being equally common (see Table 11.4). It occurs primarily in the cerebellar vermis but may also be found in the hemi-

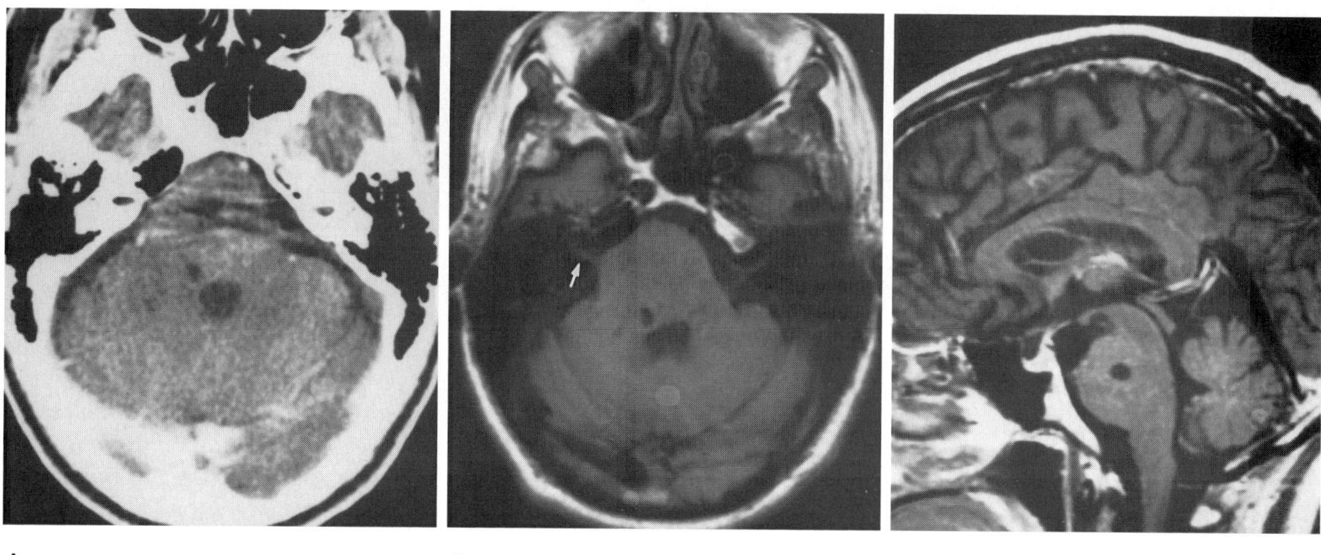

A B C

Figure 11.97. Brainstem glioma in a 51-year-old man. **A.** CT axial view after contrast shows an abnormal pons, no prepontine cistern, and poorly outlined cerebellopontine angle cisterns, particularly on the right; no clear enhancement was seen. The fourth ventricle seems to lie more posteriorly than usual. There is a hypodense spot anterior and to the right of the fourth ventricle, which is slightly deformed. **B.** Axial T1-weighted MR image shows definite enlargement of the pons with an irregular contour mostly toward the right. The seventh and eighth nerves are seen (small arrow). The cystic space near the fourth ventricle is visible, and the anterior wall of the fourth ventricle is deformed. **C.** Sagittal T1-weighted postcontrast image shows increased curvature of the belly of the pons; another cystic space is seen farther forward than that seen on A and B. The lesion is isodense and did not enhance with contrast. It was a slowly growing lesion that had remained stationary for several years. The slow growth is not uncommon in brainstem tumors in adults.

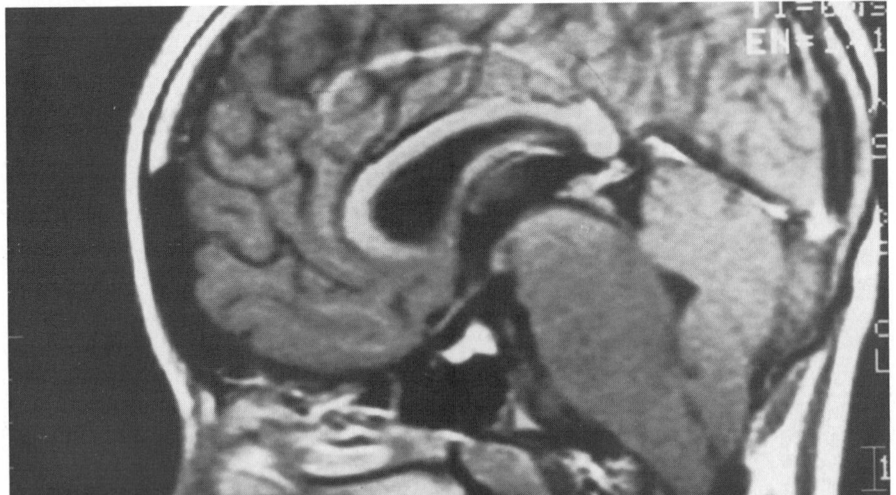

A

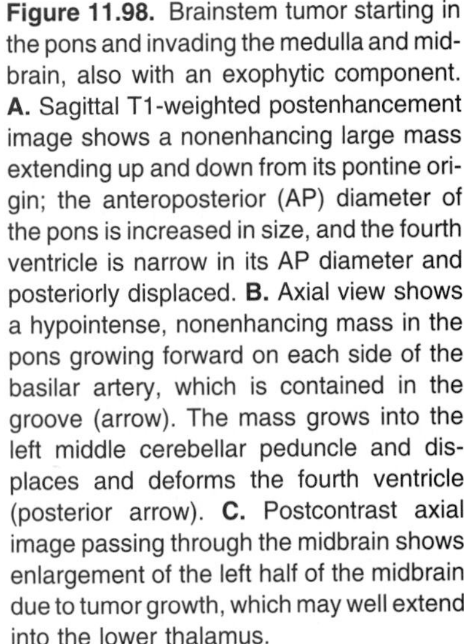

Figure 11.98. Brainstem tumor starting in the pons and invading the medulla and midbrain, also with an exophytic component. **A.** Sagittal T1-weighted postenhancement image shows a nonenhancing large mass extending up and down from its pontine origin; the anteroposterior (AP) diameter of the pons is increased in size, and the fourth ventricle is narrow in its AP diameter and posteriorly displaced. **B.** Axial view shows a hypointense, nonenhancing mass in the pons growing forward on each side of the basilar artery, which is contained in the groove (arrow). The mass grows into the left middle cerebellar peduncle and displaces and deforms the fourth ventricle (posterior arrow). **C.** Postcontrast axial image passing through the midbrain shows enlargement of the left half of the midbrain due to tumor growth, which may well extend into the lower thalamus.

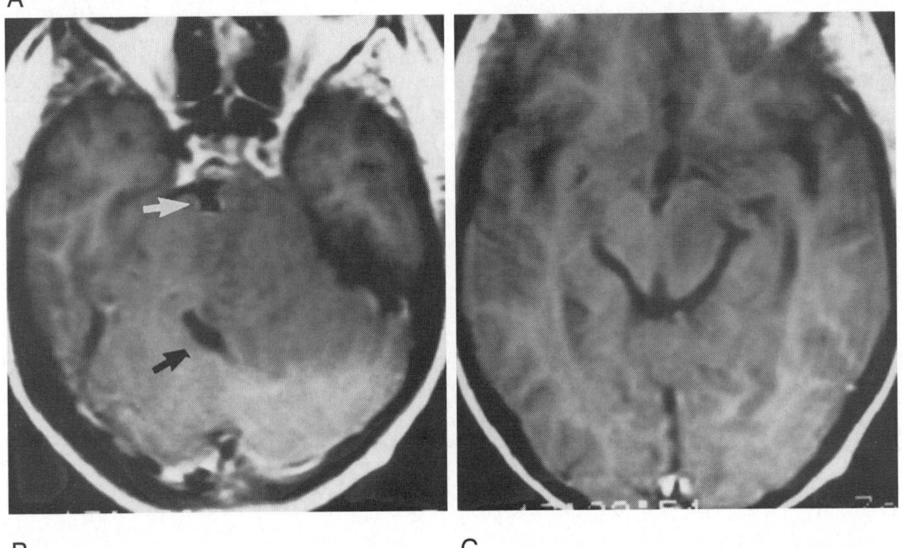

B C

sphere. It frequently invades the fourth ventricle; it may grow into the subarachnoid space and may infiltrate throughout the middle cerebellar penduncle and into the pons. It only rarely calcifies, whereas ependymomas do so frequently, and this point may be used in the differential diagnosis when a medulloblastoma is found to invade the fourth ventricle (Table 11.44).

CT may show a mass that is slightly hyperdense in relation to the surrounding cerebellum because the tumor is quite cellular and may have a high nuclear-cytoplasmic ratio. It may present hemorrhage, and it enhances after contrast. MRI may show an isointense or hypointense mass on T1-weighted images and a slightly hyperintense mass on first- and second-echo T2-weighted images. Because the tumors arise most frequently in the vermis, they often invade the fourth ventricle (Fig. 11.100). It is well known that the medulloblastoma is one of the most frequent tumors to seed via the CSF, both into the spinal canal and into the supratentorial subarachnoid space and meninges (Fig. 11.101). In adults, the cerebellar hemisphere location is more common.

Table 11.44.
Medulloblastomas

Usually involve cerebellar vermis in children, may originate in the cerebellar hemisphere in adults
Often slightly hyperdense on noncontrast CT
Calcification is usually mild or absent (unlike ependymoma)

The *hemangioblastoma* is another tumor of the cerebellum that does not usually occur in the supratentorial space. The tumor may be associated with von Hippel-Lindau disease (retinal angiomatosis, cerebellar and spinal cord hemangioblastoma, and cysts in the pancreas, kidneys, and liver) (Fig. 11.102), but the majority are found without other manifestations of the disease. Typically, a hemangioblastoma has a vascular nodule and a cystic component.

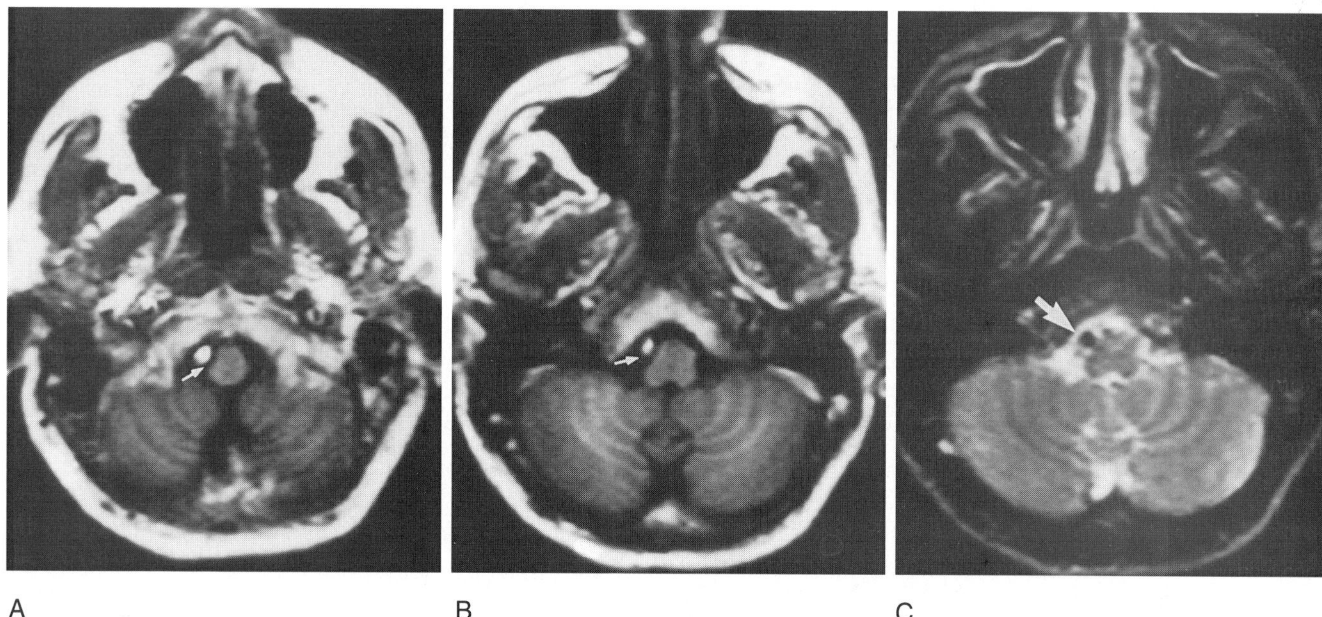

A B C

Figure 11.99. Indentation and flattening of the medulla produced by a large, dominant, right vertebral artery. T1-weighted inversion recovery images show entry phenomenon bright vertebral in the first and second slices (**A** and **B**) (small arrows). **C**. T2-weighted axial image shows a normal flow void at the right vertebral artery (arrow).

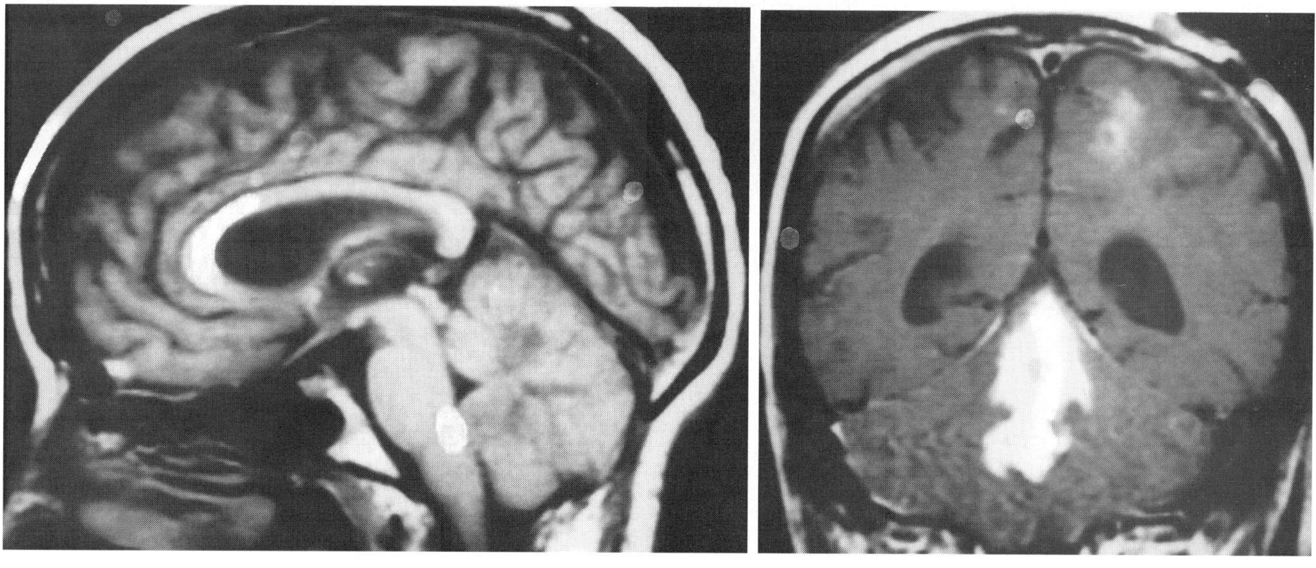

A B

Figure 11.100. Medulloblastoma in a 27-year-old woman. **A.** Nonenhanced T1-weighted sagittal image shows some hyperintensity in the region of the vermis in the upper half of the cerebellum. **B.** Enhanced coronal view shows marked uptake of contrast in the region of the vermis extending from the culmen to the mid vermis. There is also evidence of hyperintensity in the upper hemisphere bilaterally, which probably represents meningeal seeding.

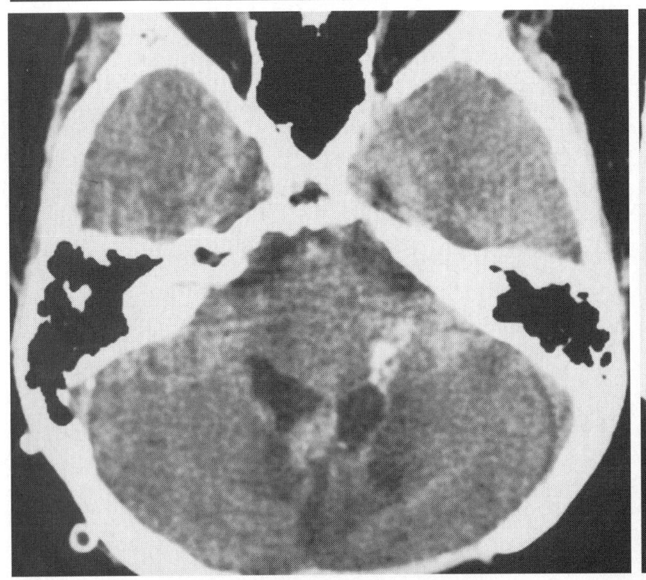

A

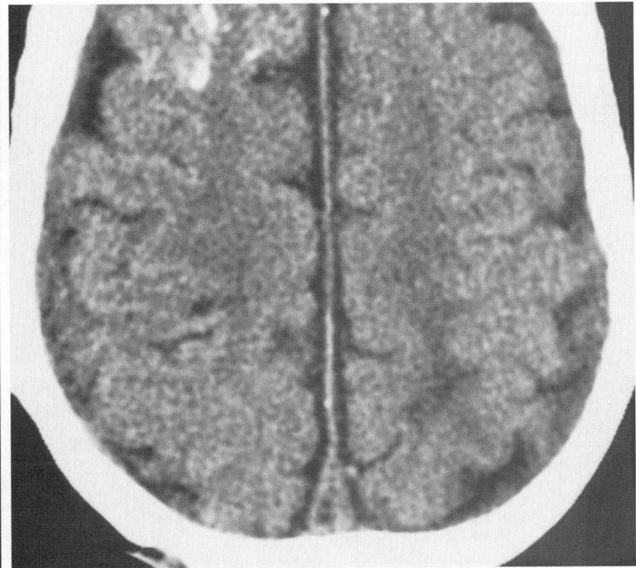

B

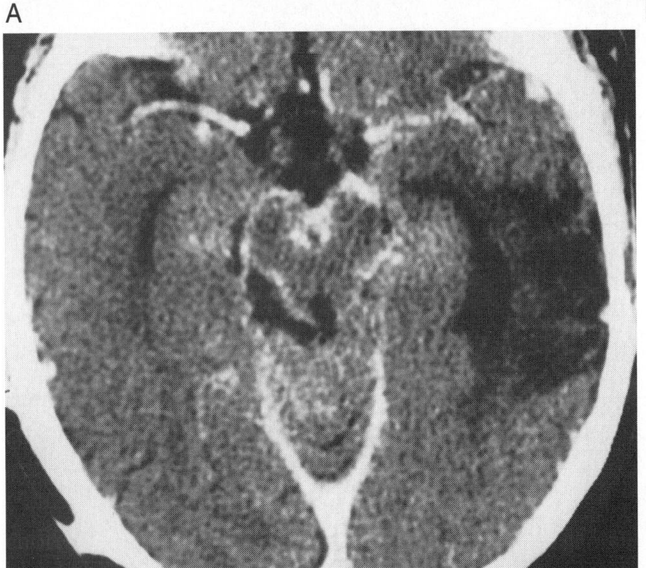

C

Figure 11.101. Medulloblastoma (postoperative) with meningeal seeding. **A.** CT scan of the cerebellum shows an enhancing midline tumor and irregular cystic spaces, and probably an enlarged fourth ventricle. **B.** Supratentorially there is an area of dystrophic calcification in the right frontal region. **C.** An enhanced image at the level of the incisura reveals enhancement around the midbrain and in the interpeduncular fossa due to meningeal seeding. **D** and **E.** Enhanced coronal MR images reveal leptomeningeal enhancement due to metastatic involvement, as well as extensive dural enhancement, believed to be due to previous surgical procedures. The dura is thickened in the falx, in the tentorium, and over the cerebral convexities, but it is smooth. The marked thickening of the dura has also been reported in patients with long-standing shunts, which this patient had.

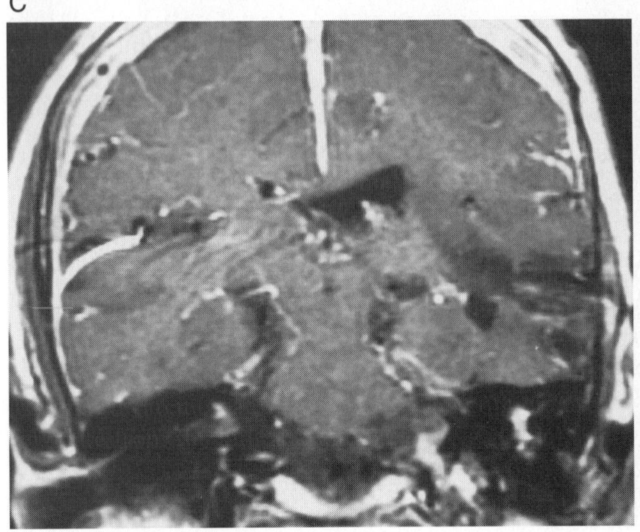

D

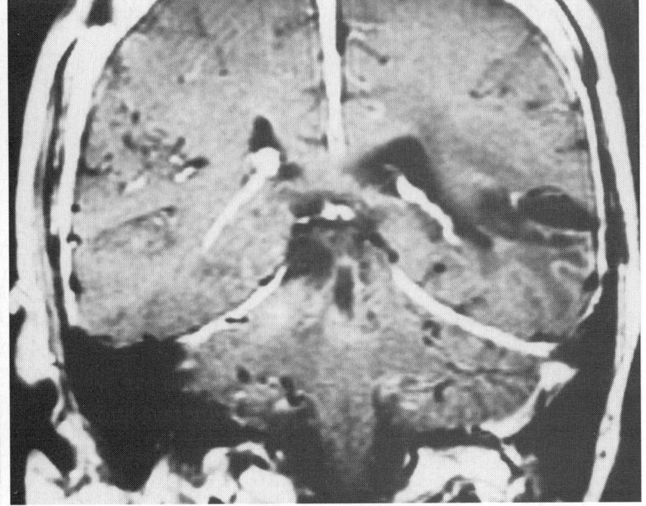

E

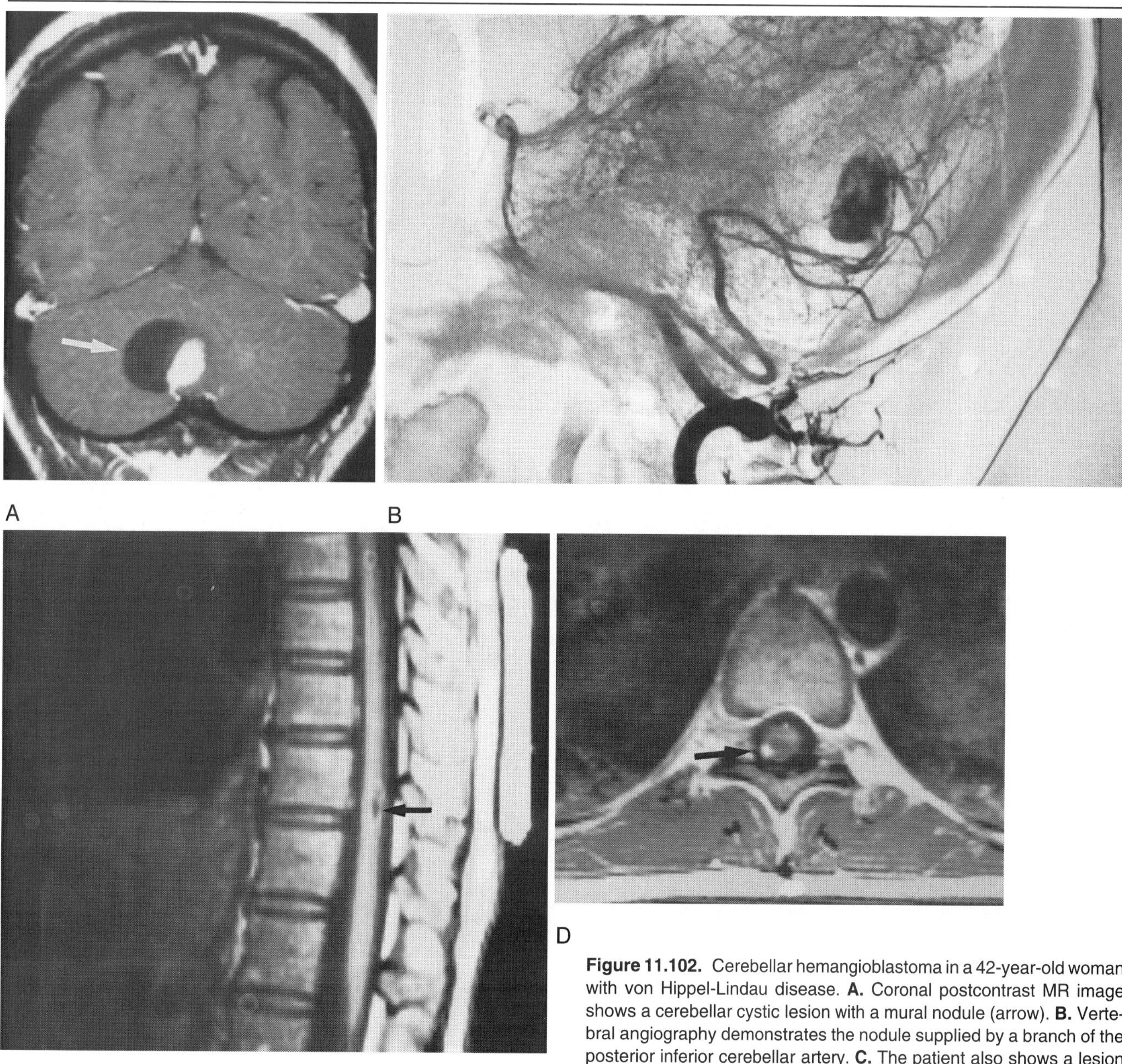

Figure 11.102. Cerebellar hemangioblastoma in a 42-year-old woman with von Hippel-Lindau disease. **A.** Coronal postcontrast MR image shows a cerebellar cystic lesion with a mural nodule (arrow). **B.** Vertebral angiography demonstrates the nodule supplied by a branch of the posterior inferior cerebellar artery. **C.** The patient also shows a lesion in the spinal cord as a hypointense area in a T1-weighted sagittal view (arrow). **D.** The lesion enhances with contrast (arrow) on this T1-weighted axial image and has a cystic component.

The nodule may be shown with enhanced CT or MRI (Fig. 11.103). Vertebral angiography usually demonstrates the nodule, which usually exhibits increased speed of circulation with an early-filling vein, a fairly typical feature of hemangioblastomas (Fig. 11.103*D* and *E*). The nodules in the spinal cord are usually associated with a cyst that may extend up and down the spinal cord for some distance, suggesting a syringomyelia. However, the demonstration of a nodule on enhanced MRI makes the diagnosis of hemangioblastoma more likely. Gliomas may also produce syringomyelia, but these tumors tend to grow up and down the cord rather than as a single nodule (Table 11.45).

Table 11.45.
Hemangioblastomas

Usually cystic with a mural nodule
May be completely solid
Densely enhance with contrast material
Often multiple in von Hippel-Lindau syndrome

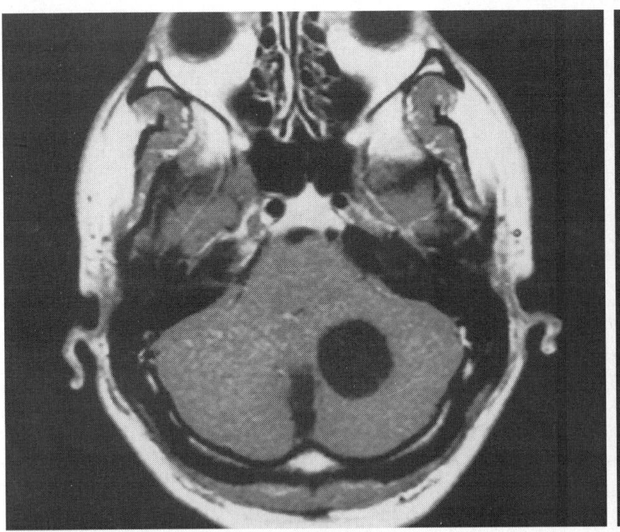

A

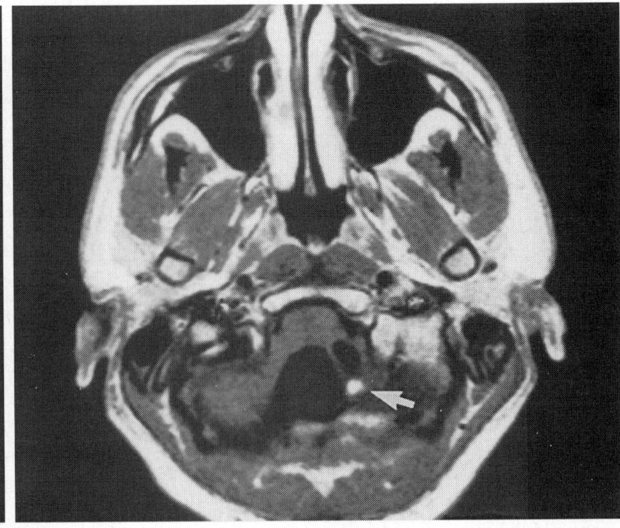

B

Figure 11.103. Cystic hemangioblastoma of the cerebellum with a wall nodule. **A.** A section through the cerebellum shows a clean wall cyst. Postcontrast T1-weighted image. **B.** A lower section shows that there is an enhanced small nodule (arrow), demonstrated better on sagittal view (**C**). **D** and **E.** Vertebral angiography in early arterial (D) and late arterial (E) phases shows the nodule and an early-draining vein in the arterial phase (arrows). The early-filling vein is typical of hemangioblastoma.

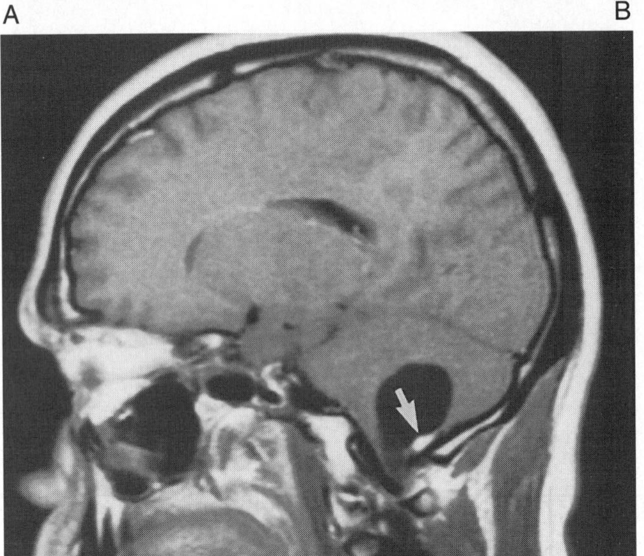

C

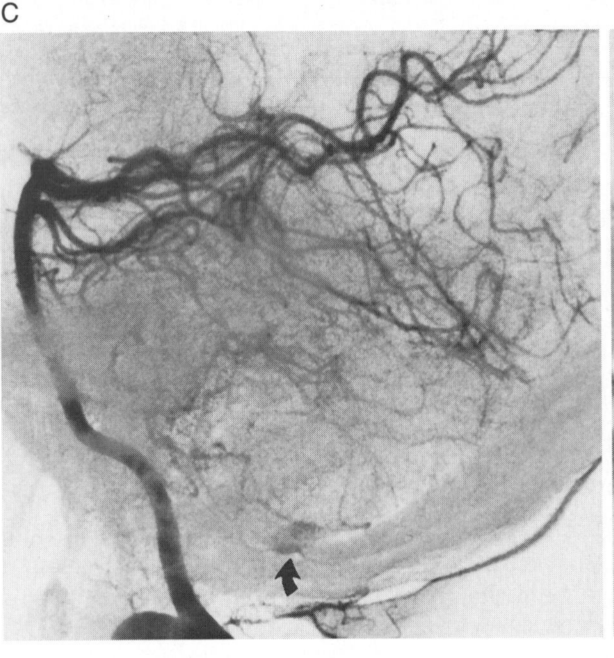

D

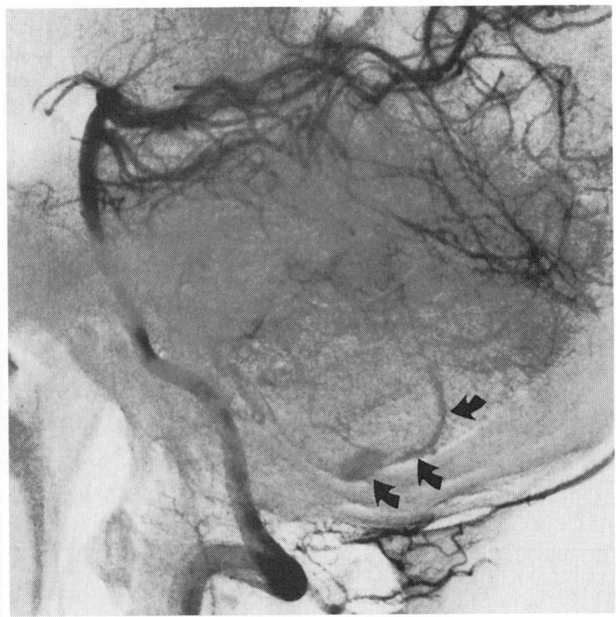

E

Cerebellar dysplastic gangliocytoma (Lhermitte-Duclos disease) is a condition that could be classified as congenital, but it is usually found in the second or third decade. The CT or MRI appearance is of a cerebellar lesion that disrupts the cerebellar hemisphere anatomy with or without a significant mass effect. The lesion does not enhance with contrast on CT or MRI. Serpiginous areas that suggest cerebellar folia were well seen in the case described by Smith et al. (121). At surgery the cerebellar surface involved by the tumor is difficult to differentiate from the adjacent normal cerebellum. Microscopically the thickened folia are composed of an inner layer containing many abnormal neurons, some of which resemble Purkinje cells, and an outer layer containing many myelinated fibers (4).

Intraventricular Posterior Fossa Tumors

The most frequent primarily intraventricular tumor in the posterior fossa is the ependymoma (Fig. 104); other tumors occur less frequently, such as choroid plexus papillomas and an occasional meningioma. Also, medulloblastomas frequently invade the fourth ventricle, and sometimes it is necessary to differentiate them from ependymomas because ependymomas may have an intraventricular component but may grow mostly outward into the cerebellum.

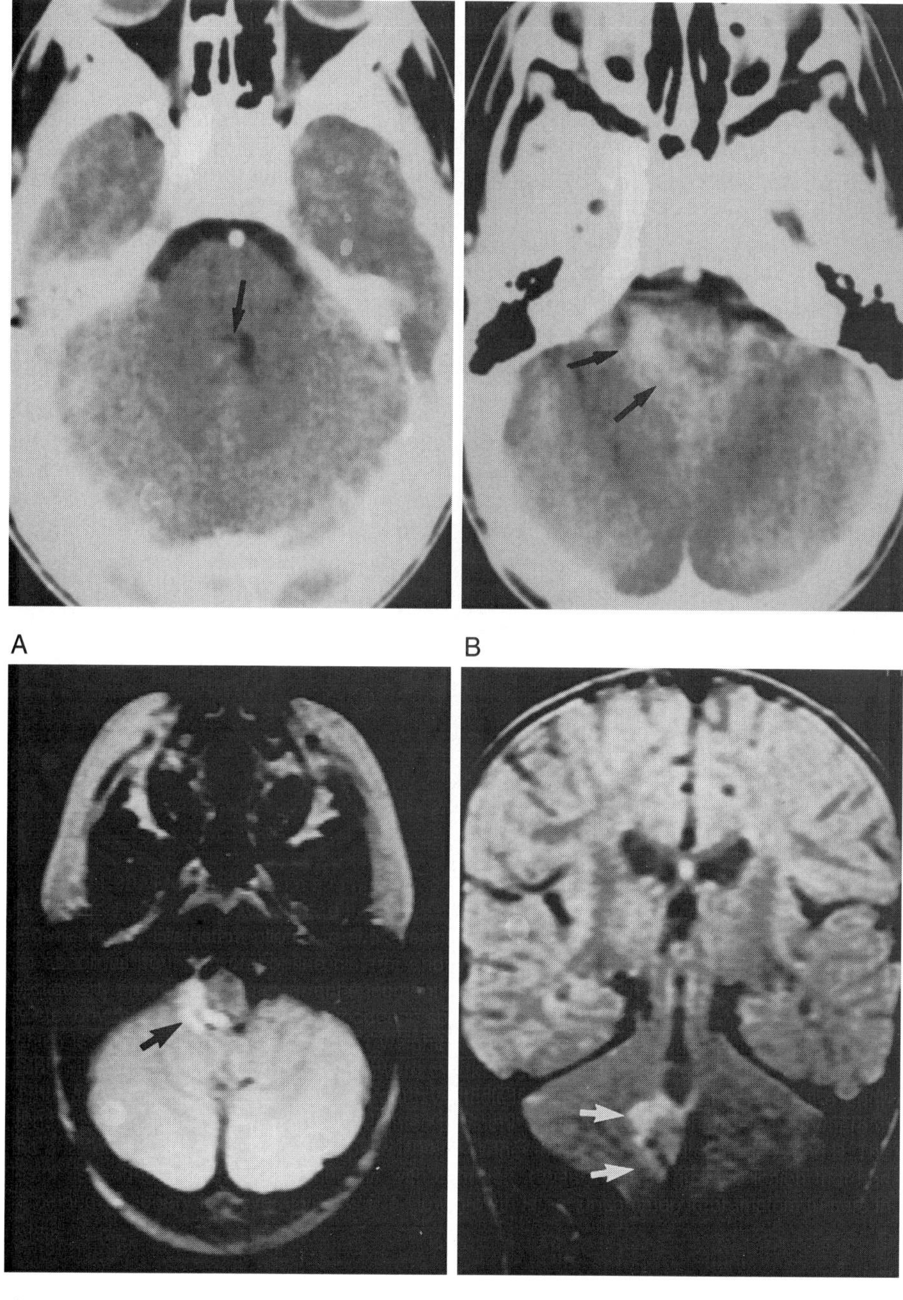

Figure 11.104. Ependymoma. **A.** CT examination shows a mass within the fourth ventricle containing a small hyperdense area consistent with calcification (arrow). **B.** A lower postcontrast section shows deformity of the medulla and hyperdensity surrounding it, particularly on the right side (arrows), representing a poorly defined tumor. **C.** Proton density axial image shows the hyperintense tumor surrounding a deformed brainstem (arrow). **D.** This is also well seen in coronal view (arrows).

Table 11.46.
Ependymomas

Posterior fossa ependymomas are found in the fourth ventricle, often extending out through the foramina of Magendie or Luschka
May encircle the brainstem/spinal cord ("plastic ependymoma")
Frequently found to be calcified on CT imaging
Often heterogeneous on T2-weighted MR images due to foci of calcification, necrosis, and hemorrhage

More frequently, however, they grow out of the ventricular foramina (foramen of Magendie and foramina of Luschka) and into the subarachnoid space, forming masses around the brainstem and surrounding the blood vessels (Fig. 11.104) (Table 11.46).

Ependymomas frequently present calcifications on CT examinations. This is an important diagnostic point because medulloblastomas rarely present calcifications, except possibly after therapy (Fig. 11.101).

Ependymomas may seed into the subarachnoid space, but this is more likely to occur with ependymoblastomas, a much less differentiated type that may be included with the PNETs.

On MRI, ependymomas tend to be iso- or hypointense in relation to white matter on T1-weighted images, and hyperintense on proton density and T2-weighted images. They tend to enhance after contrast and often present a heterogeneous appearance due to methemoglobin and hemosiderin from focal hemorrhage, necrosis, and calcification (39) (Fig. 11.105). Cystic areas may be present.

Subependymomas tend to be well-defined intraventricular masses that enhance after contrast and that are hyperintense on proton density and T2-weighted images.

Choroid plexus papillomas arise more frequently in the lateral ventricles, but they may be seen in the fourth ventricle. The lesion may arise from the choroid plexus within the fourth ventricle main cavity, or it may arise from the choroid plexus in the foramina of Luschka (Fig. 11.106). Choroid plexus papillomas and carcinomas may seed via the CSF into the spinal canal and into the ventricles and cranial subarachnoid space, as shown in Figure 11.106. The imaging and angiographic characteristics are similar to those described under supratentorial intraventricular tumors (122).

Meningiomas of the fourth ventricle probably arise from the choroid plexus and are rare (5 percent of intraventricular meningiomas), according to Criscuolo and Symon (123). Meningioma may be suggested as a diagnostic possibility if the tumor has a smooth contour, enhances brightly, and contains fine calcifications.

Extra-axial Posterior Fossa Tumors

Whereas in children the cerebellar, intraventricular, and brainstem tumors are much more common, in adults the extra-axial tumors predominate. These may arise from four sources: (a) the cranial nerves; (b) the meninges; (c) cell rests (epidermoid, dermoid); and (d) osseous structures of the posterior fossa. In addition, the glomus jugulare tumors may bulge into the posterior fossa, particularly when they are large.

TUMORS ARISING FROM CRANIAL NERVES

The tumors arising from the nerves are usually schwannomas (neurinomas) or neurofibromas (in patients with neurofibromatosis). The most common are the *eighth-nerve schwannomas* (acoustic neuromas), which usually *arise from*

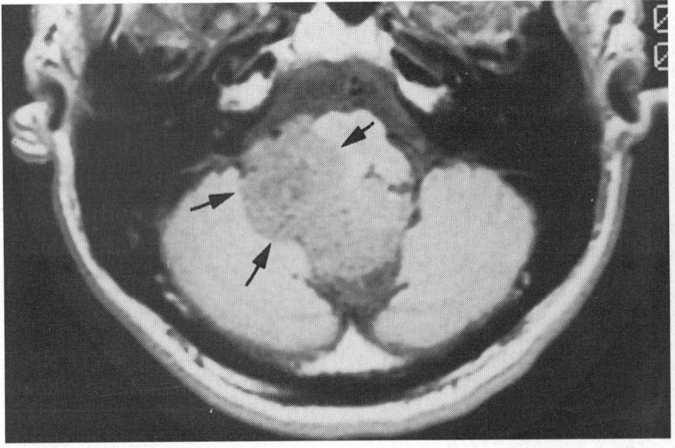

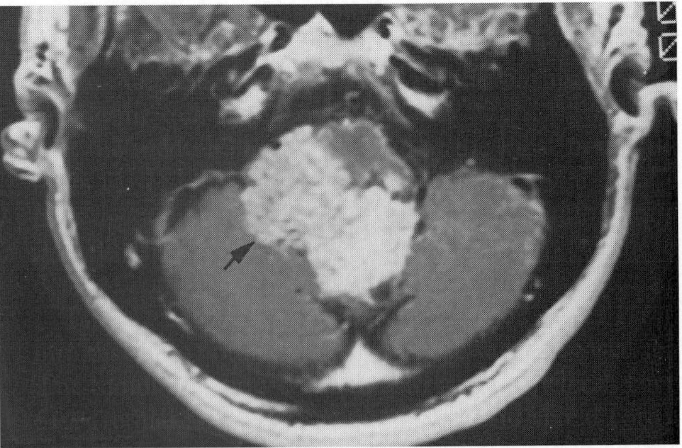

A B

Figure 11.105. Fourth-ventricle ependymoma in a 51-year-old man. MRI. **A.** There is an intraventricular mass in the fourth ventricle, which seems to extend out through the foramen of Luschka (arrows). **B.** The tumor shows marked enhancement after contrast. The tumor is not homogeneous, which may be due to deposits of calcium. The extension out through the foramen of Luschka usually leads to extension over the meninges, which makes the tumor surgically nonresectable. The tumor presented low-grade intermittent bleeding, which led to chronic meningeal siderosis (see Fig. 6.56, same patient).

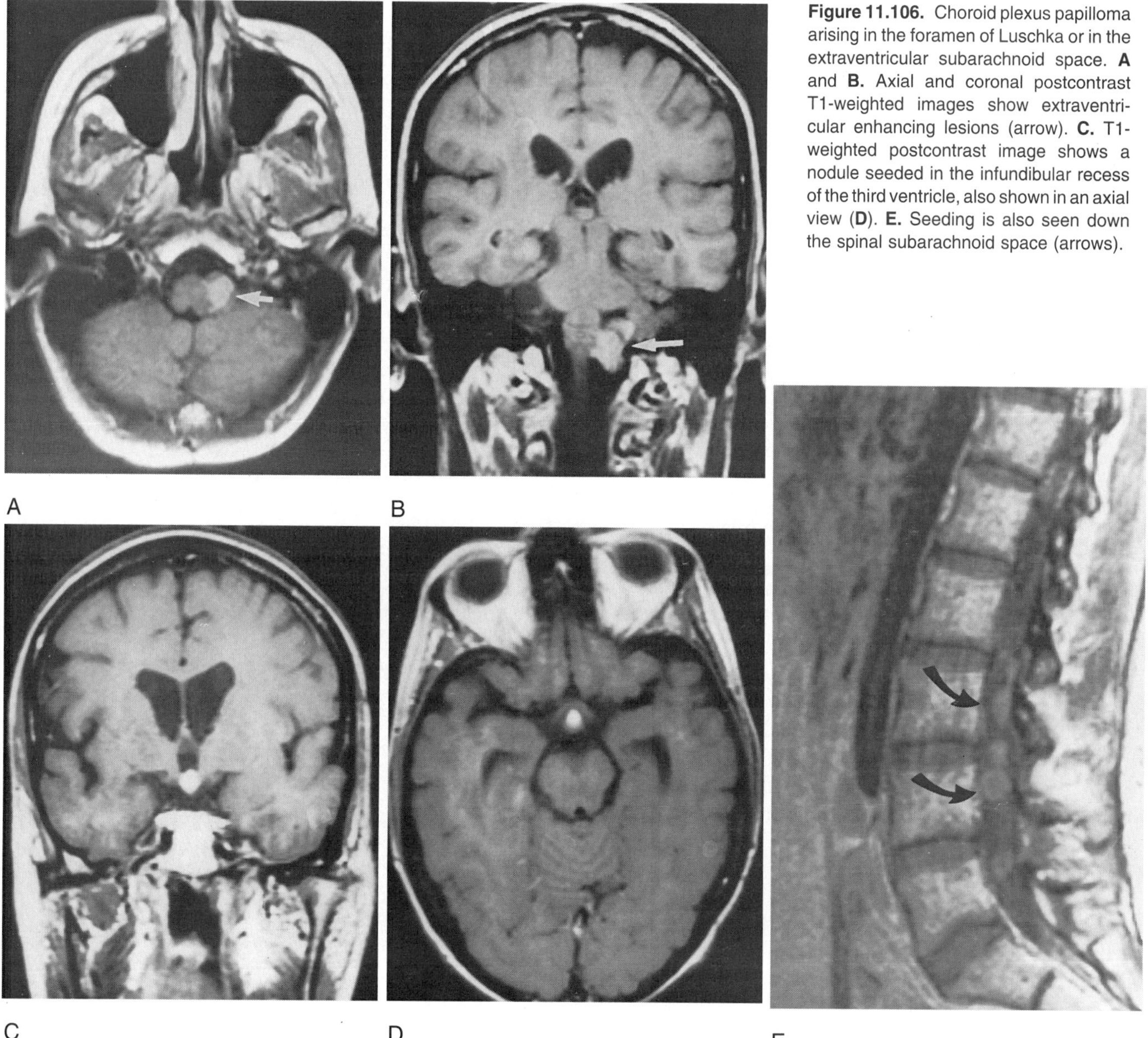

Figure 11.106. Choroid plexus papilloma arising in the foramen of Luschka or in the extraventricular subarachnoid space. **A** and **B.** Axial and coronal postcontrast T1-weighted images show extraventricular enhancing lesions (arrow). **C.** T1-weighted postcontrast image shows a nodule seeded in the infundibular recess of the third ventricle, also shown in an axial view (**D**). **E.** Seeding is also seen down the spinal subarachnoid space (arrows).

the vestibular division of the acoustic nerve. See under "Pathologic Considerations" earlier in this chapter for their histology. Eighth-nerve schwannomas are frequently found in patients with neurofibromatosis type II, in which case they may be bilateral. Histologically they are composed of tight bundles of bipolar spindle cells (Antoni A tissue), interspersed with looser tissue (Antoni B tissue).

Acoustic schwannomas frequently involve the intracanalicular portion of the nerve, producing enlargement and erosion of the internal acoustic canal. Sometimes they seem to be limited to the extracanalicular portion of the nerve and produce no enlargement of the internal acoustic canal and only a mass in the cerebellopontine cistern.

CT is fairly accurate in the diagnosis of eighth-nerve tumors because it will demonstrate the acoustic canal enlargement as well as the mass itself (Fig. 11.107). However, a tumor that is less than 9 mm to 1.0 cm in size can go undetected by CT even with contrast (Fig. 11.107). If there is a good clinical suspicion and no MRI is available, the author recommends that one inject 5 cc of air in the lumbar subarachnoid space and allow it to rise to the cerebellopontine angle of interest. If one needs to examine the right side, one elevates the patient's head to entice the air to rise to the posterior fossa, with the right side held higher than the left. The head may be flexed at this point to keep the air from leaving the posterior fossa. CT examination will demonstrate even very small tumors (124).

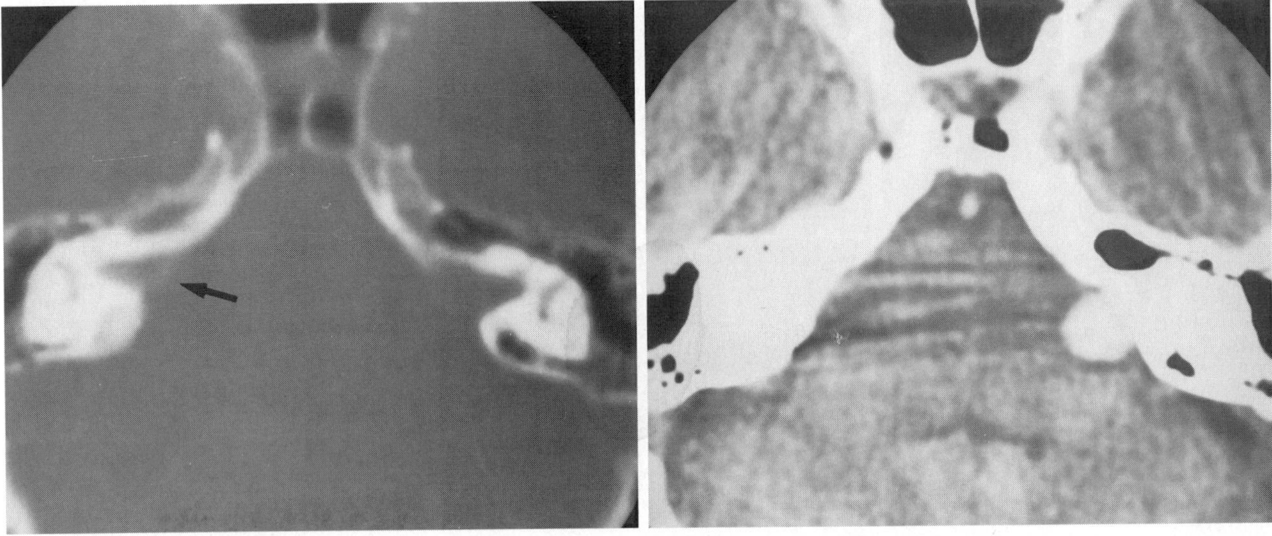

Figure 11.107. Bilateral eighth-nerve tumors. **A.** A bone window CT image shows funnel enlargement and erosion of the internal acoustic canal on the left. On the right side there is funneling of the canal and a slight soft-tissue hyperdensity in this postcontrast image (arrow). **B.** An enhanced soft-tissue window reveals a rounded mass in the region of the cerebellopontine angle. The tumor on the right side does not bulge sufficiently into the cerebellopontine cistern and is not seen, although it is suspected in the bone window image.

If MRI is available, however, examination without contrast followed by contrast demonstrates these tumors in practically every instance, even when they are very small and intracanalicular in location (Fig. 11.108) (125,126).

Some acoustic tumors develop cystic changes. The cyst may be within the tumor or it may be surrounding parts of it, that is, in the subarachnoid space, and formed by adhesions around the neoplasm (Fig. 11.109).

Bilateral acoustic schwannomas are usually related to neurofibromatosis type II, and may be the only manifestation of neurofibromatosis. They are inherited in an autosomal dominant pattern with 95 percent penetrance (22). However, other manifestations may also be present, such as multiple meningiomas, spinal nerve tumors usually arising from the dorsal root, gliomas (usually slowly growing), and juvenile posterior subcapsular lenticular opacity. A child of an affected parent with bilateral acoustic schwannomas has a 50 percent chance of inheriting the disease. Halliday et al. reported that dorsal root spinal tumors are usually neurofibromas in neurofibromatosis I and schwannomas in neurofibromatosis II (127). See also neurofibromatosis, Chapter 5, "Congenital Anomalies" (Table 11.47).

In addition to an acoustic nerve origin, the schwannomas may originate from the fifth nerve, the facial (seventh) nerve, the nerves in the jugular foramen (ninth, tenth, and eleventh nerves), and the hypoglossal (twelfth) nerve. When the tumor arises in the jugular fossa region, it is often difficult to determine precisely whether it arose from the glossopharyngeal (ninth), the vagus (tenth), or the spinal (eleventh) nerve.

Table 11.47.
Acoustic Schwannomas

Bilateral in neurofibromatosis II
Found within cerebellopontine angle, centered at the internal auditory canal (which is frequently widened)
May be located solely within the internal auditory canal or, alternatively, only in the cerebellopontine cistern
Can grow to large size and may contain cysts of various sizes

Fifth-nerve schwannomas typically produce saddle-shaped tumors with a component in the posterior fossa anterolaterally and another in the posterior parasellar region. The relative size of the two components varies, and the mass adjacent to the sella may be larger than the posterior fossa component (Figs. 11.110 and 11.76). See text preceding under "Parasellar Lesions." Erosion of the petrous tip may be demonstrated by CT, as well as erosion and enlargement of the foramen ovale.

Facial nerve schwannomas are rare. They may occur in the horizontal portion beyond the acoustic canal fundus, in which case they may erode through the roof of the petrous pyramid and project into the posterior aspect of the middle fossa, lifting the temporal lobe. In these cases CT will demonstrate the petrous pyramid erosion, particularly if coronal views are taken, and sagittal MR images with contrast enhancment may demonstrate the position of the tumor. If the seventh-nerve tumor arises elsewhere, the bone erosion along its course may be diagnostic (see Fig. 12.10).

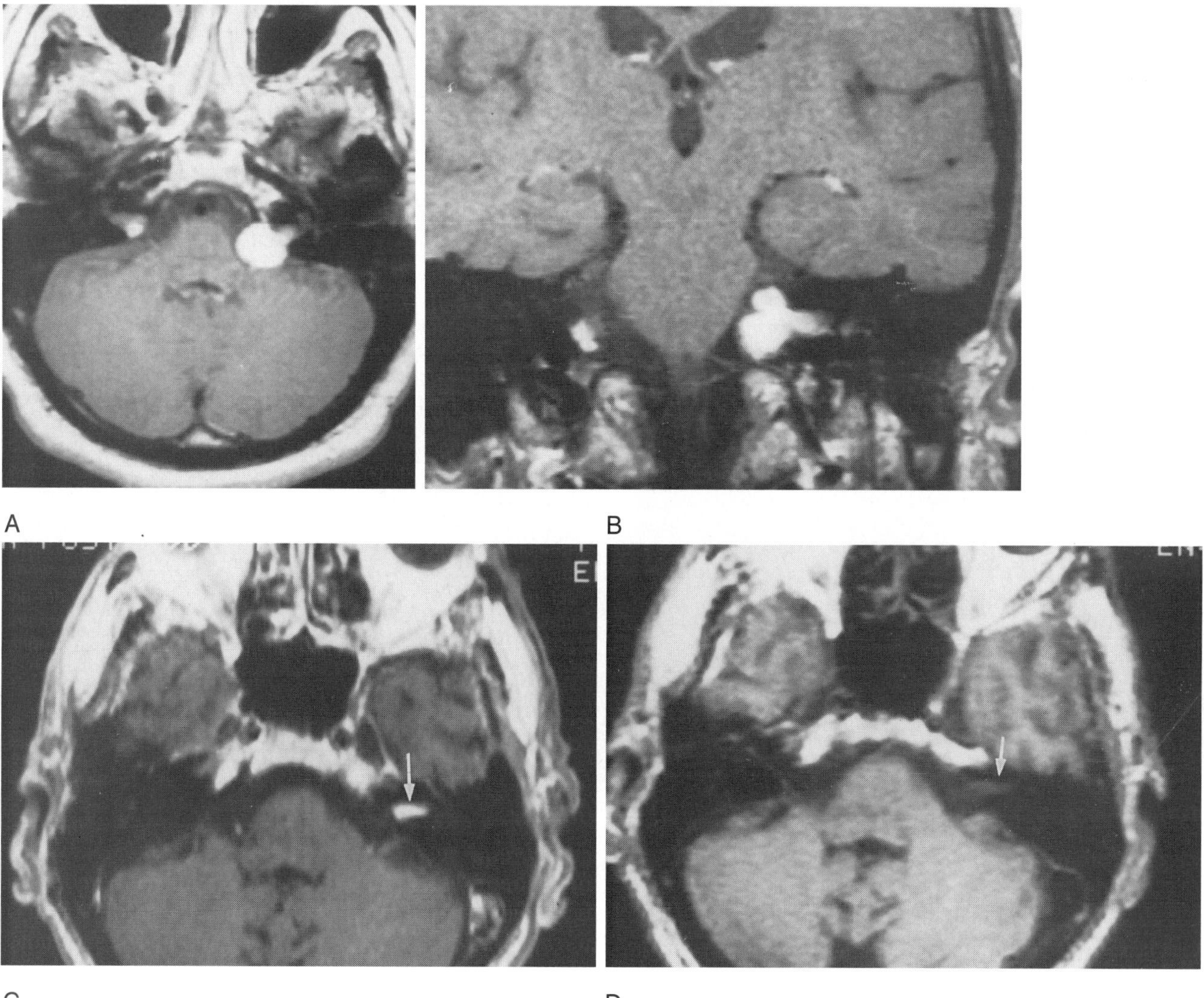

Figure 11.108. Bilateral acoustic neuromas showing typical extension of enhancement into the internal acoustic canal. **A.** Postcontrast MR axial view shows a larger tumor on the left. **B.** Coronal cuts reveal the same information. **C** and **D.** Another case. **C.** Intracanalicular small acoustic schwannoma seen on a postcontrast MR axial image (arrow). **D.** In the precontrast T1-weighted axial image, the nerve is minimally hyperintense (arrow).

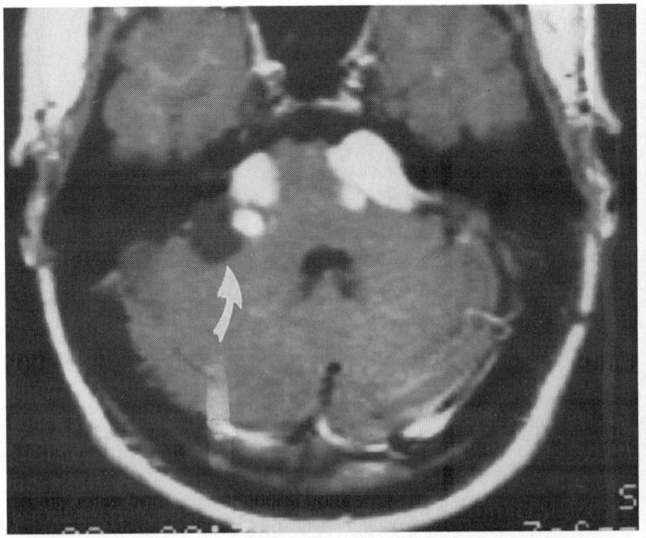

A

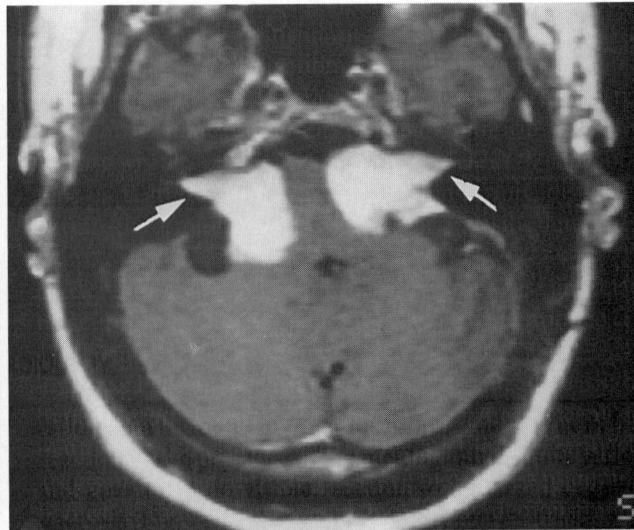

B

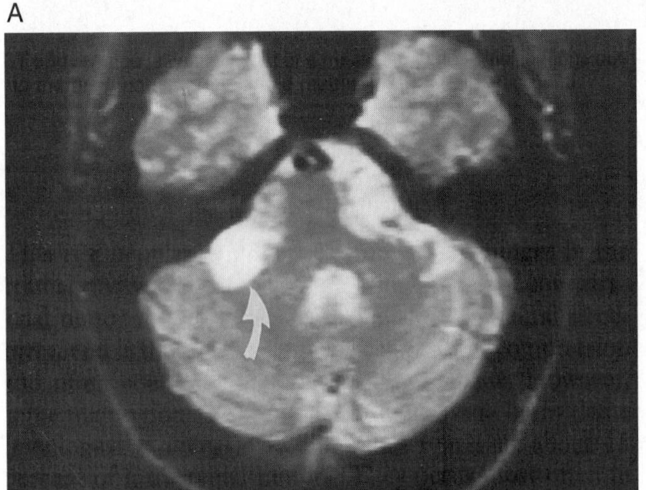

C

Figure 11.109. Bilateral acoustic schwannomas, with cystic component. **A** and **B.** Postcontrast axial T1-weighted views show large bilateral tumors producing compression and deformity of the pons. A cystic component is seen, particularly on the right side (arrow). The separate nodule seen on both sides in A probably indicates some lobulation of the tumor and artifact of the slice. In B there is no separate nodule. The tumor is seen to grow into the internal acoustic canal on both sides (arrows). **C.** On a T2-weighted axial image the cystic space is slightly brighter than CSF (arrow).

Schwannomas of the ninth, tenth, or eleventh nerves produce erosion of the jugular fossa. This is demonstrable on plain films or tomograms of the skull but is much more easily demonstrated on CT. The tumors enhance after contrast on CT or MRI, and their typical location should suggest the diagnosis (Fig. 11.111). The accompanying mass bulges into the anterolateral aspect of the posterior fossa, suggesting a typical cerebellopontine angle mass. However, careful inspection should show that it is situated lower than the cerebellopontine angle as compared to the opposite side on axial views.

Neuromas (schwannomas) of the twelfth nerve produce erosion of the hypoglossal canal in the occipital condyle, which should be detectable by CT axial images but can also be shown by plain films and tomography. The mass of the tumor may be shown in an anterolateral location but lower than the preceding group and perhaps more laterally (Fig. 11.112). Unilateral tongue atrophy may be seen. The presence of erosion of the condyle should suggest the diagnosis.

Schwannomas of the third and fourth cranial nerves are extremely rare, but neurofibromas may be seen in patients with type I or II neurofibromatosis.

Glomus jugulare tumors also occur and must be differentiated from schwannomas. They may produce erosion of the jugular fossa. Some clinical features (such as a bruit heard by the patient) may be helpful. Sometimes spontaneous bleeding from the ear may occur. Angiography shows a well-developed tumor stain with early-filling veins, which is not seen in schwannomas. Jugular venography may show an obstruction or tumor nodule in the jugular vein (Fig. 11.113). The larger tumors bulge into the inferior aspect of the posterior fossa more caudally than the acoustic schwannomas, in the same manner as the schwannomas of the ninth, tenth, and eleventh nerves (Table 11.48).

The glomus jugulare tumors (*paragangliomas*) may arise from various sites: (a) the glomus jugulare, a small group of cells situated in the adventitia of the jugular bulb; (b)

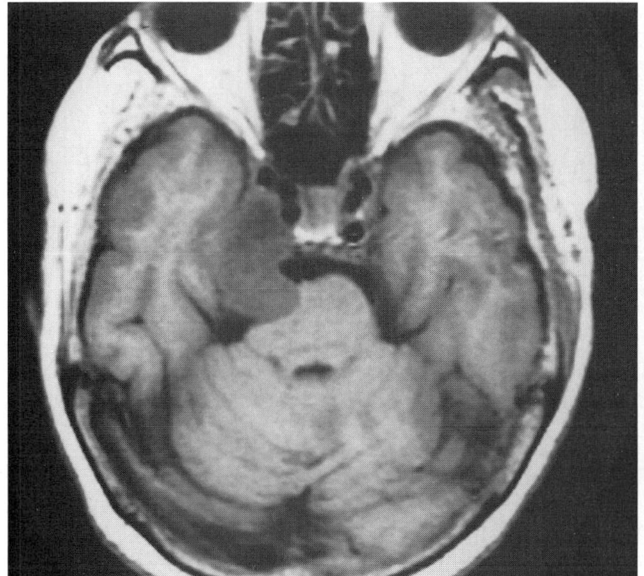

A

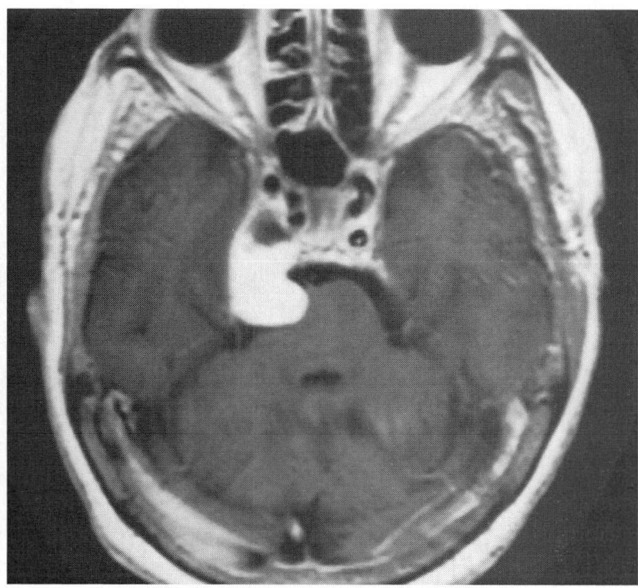

B

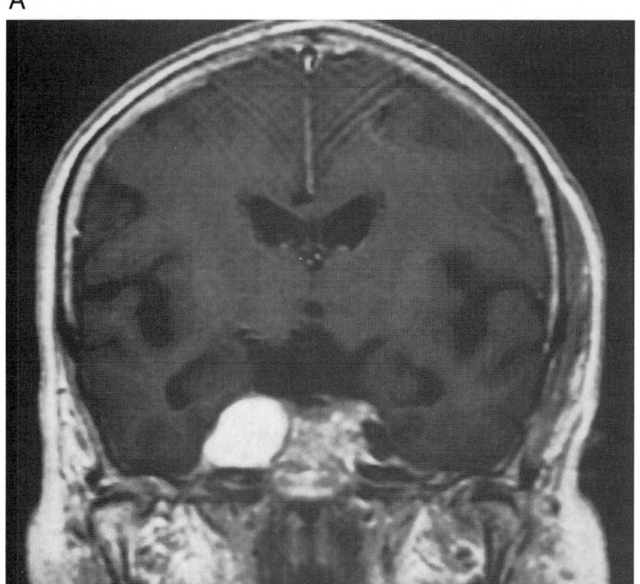

C

Figure 11.110. Fifth-nerve schwannoma with a component in the posterior fossa and another in the middle fossa (saddle incisural tumor) in a 69-year-old woman. Nonenhanced T1-weighted axial (**A**) and postenhanced axial (**B**) images show a typical configuration of fifth-nerve neuroma. Note the direct involvement of the cavernous sinus. **C.** Coronal postenhanced view showing the relationship of the tumor to the dorsum sellae, which is eroded on the right side.

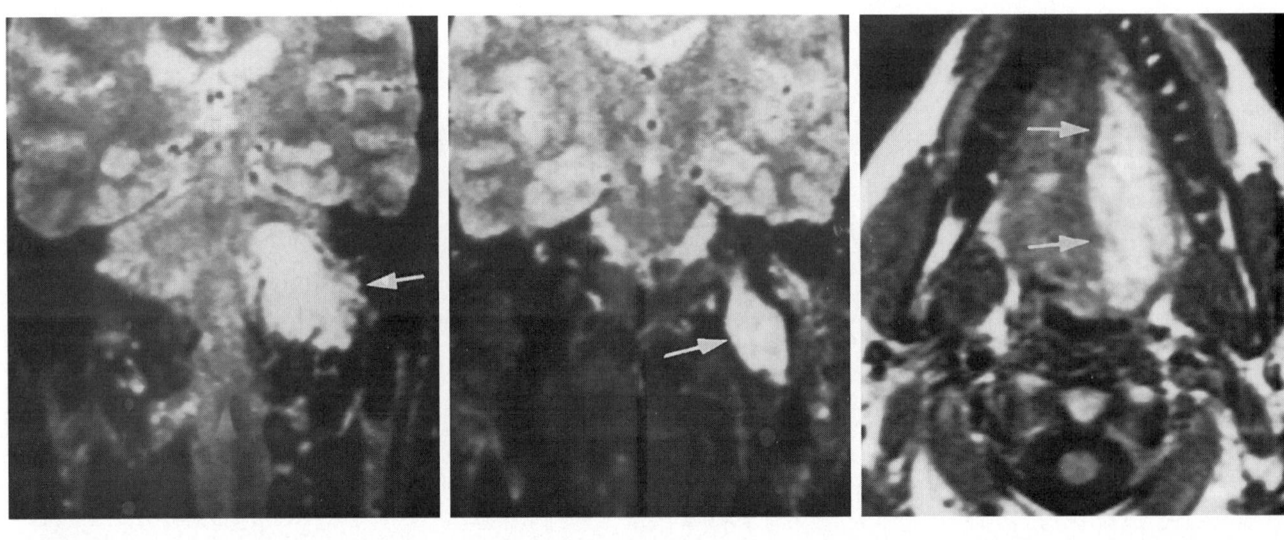

Figure 11.111. Schwannoma of ninth, tenth, and eleventh cranial nerves. **A** and **B.** Coronal postcontrast views show a large hyperintense mass on the left side bulging into the posterior fossa and projecting downward below the base of the skull (arrows). **C.** An axial T1-weighted view taken 11 months later shows a bright left side of the tongue indicative of tongue atrophy and fatty infiltration (arrows). This is indicative of ninth or twelfth nerve involvement.

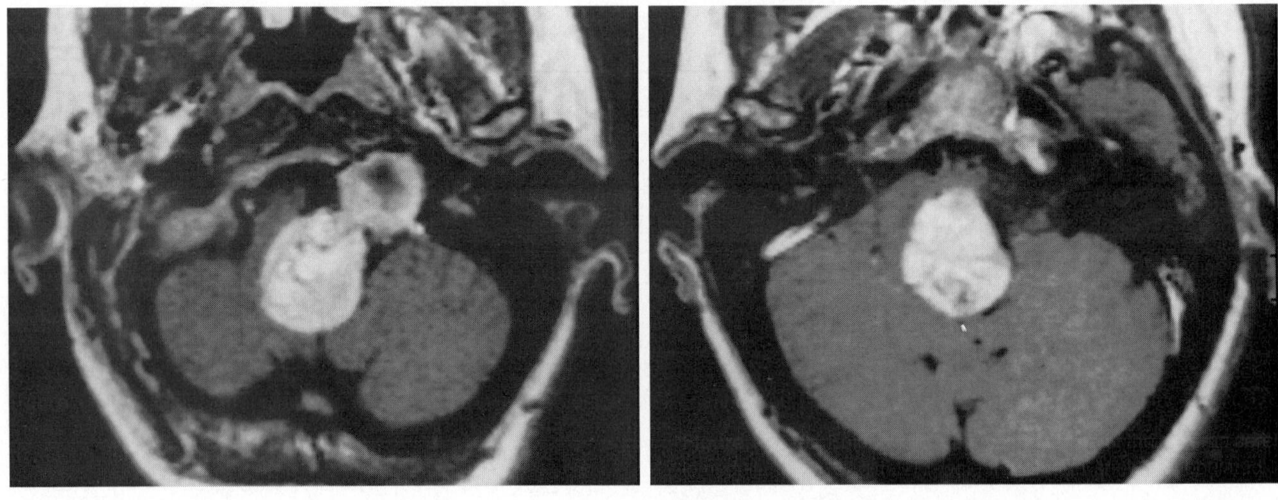

Figure 11.112. A and **B.** Hypoglossal (twelfth-nerve) neuroma. **A.** There is a bilobed, markedly enhancing mass in the left anterolateral aspect of the posterior fossa. There is erosion of the bone anteriorly (no bone marrow is seen). The medulla is flattened, and the cisternal space is enlarged. **B.** A section higher up shows that the mass appears to be intra-axial, indicating a slowly growing mass that slowly compresses the structures without producing neurologic signs.

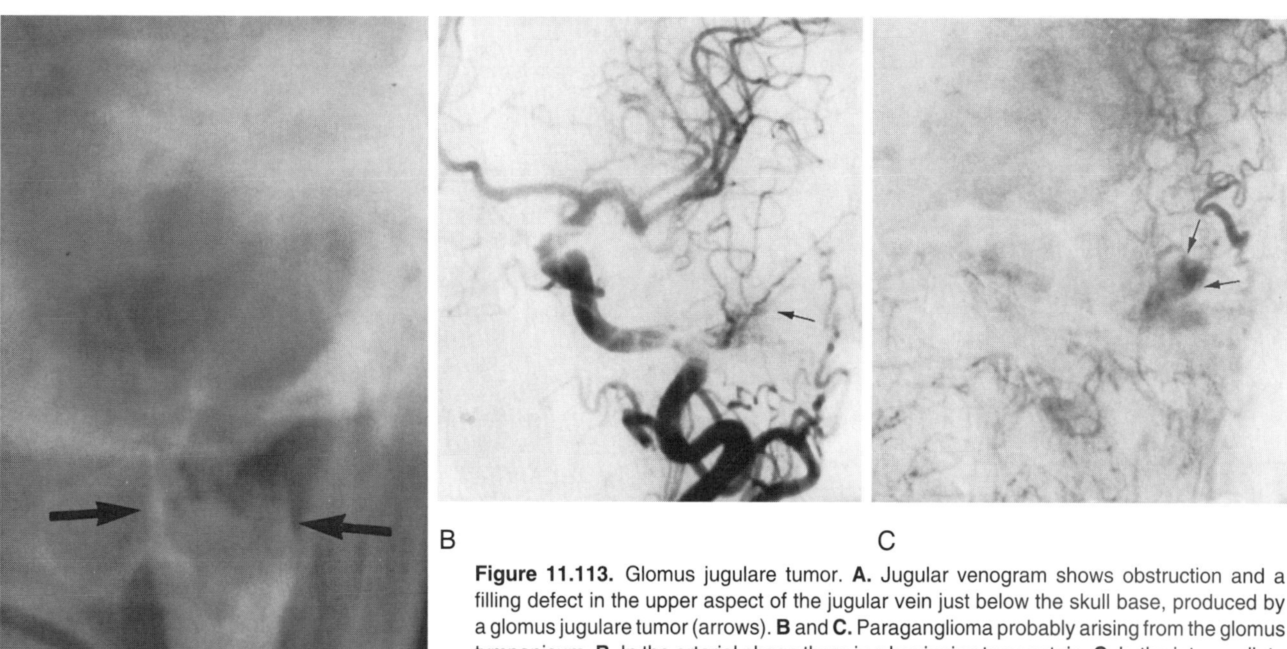

Figure 11.113. Glomus jugulare tumor. **A.** Jugular venogram shows obstruction and a filling defect in the upper aspect of the jugular vein just below the skull base, produced by a glomus jugulare tumor (arrows). **B** and **C.** Paraganglioma probably arising from the glomus tympanicum. **B.** In the arterial phase there is a beginning tumor stain. **C.** In the intermediate phase there is a well-developed tumor blush (arrows). The patient was a 66-year-old woman who complained of loss of hearing and an episode of brisk bleeding from the ear. **D.** CT scan (in a similar case) shows a mass in the middle ear cavity (arrow). **E.** Coronal CT scan shows some bone erosion on the inferior aspect of the middle ear cavity (arrow).

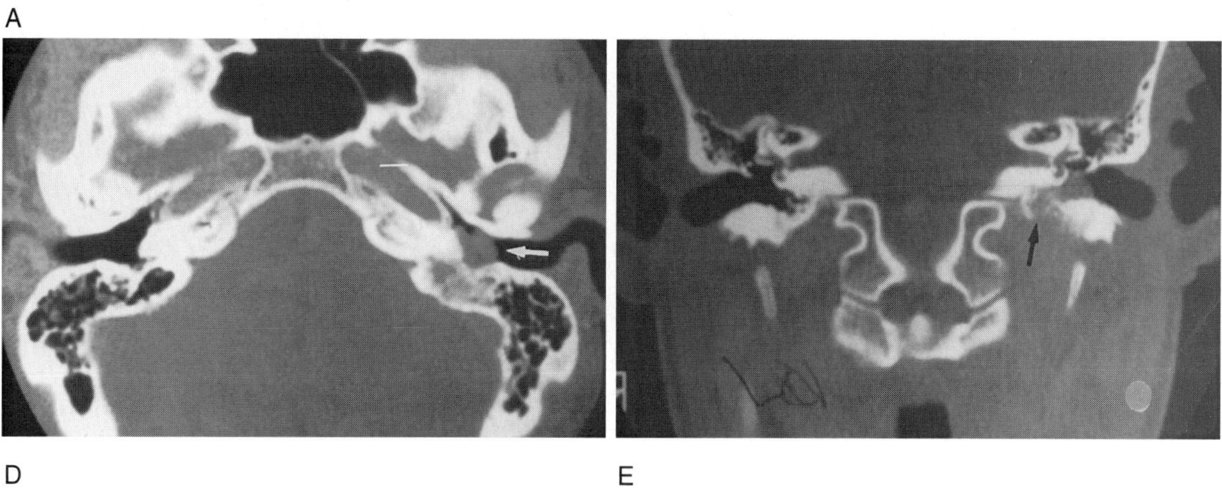

Figure 11.114. Cerebellopontine-angle meningioma showing adjacent meningeal enhancement (dural tail). The postcontrast MR axial view reveals a smooth half-moon-shaped mass in the cerebellopontine angle with a tail projecting forward (arrow). The tumor does not enter into the internal acoustic canal.

Table 11.48.
Glomus Jugulare Tumors

Vascular tumors arising within (and often eroding) the jugular fossa
Presenting symptoms/signs may include a bruit and bleeding from the ear
Dense vascular blush seen on angiography
CT demonstrates a densely enhancing mass often accompanied by bone erosion
On MRI, alternating regions of hypointense and hyperintense signal ("salt and pepper appearance") are seen on T2-weighted images

the glomus tympanicum, related to the tympanic branch of the glossopharyngeal nerve in the middle ear; (c) the vagal body, found within the perineurium of the vagus nerve; or (d) the carotid bodies, situated at the bifurcation of the common carotid artery on each side (4) (Fig. 11.113).

TUMORS ARISING FROM THE MENINGES

Meningiomas arising in the cerebellopontine angle and prepontine area usually have a broader base than acoustic neuromas and do not usually grow into the internal acoustic canal. In addition, on contrast MRI examination they may present enhancement of the adjacent dura mater, usually called *dural tail enhancement* (Fig. 11.114). Meningiomas

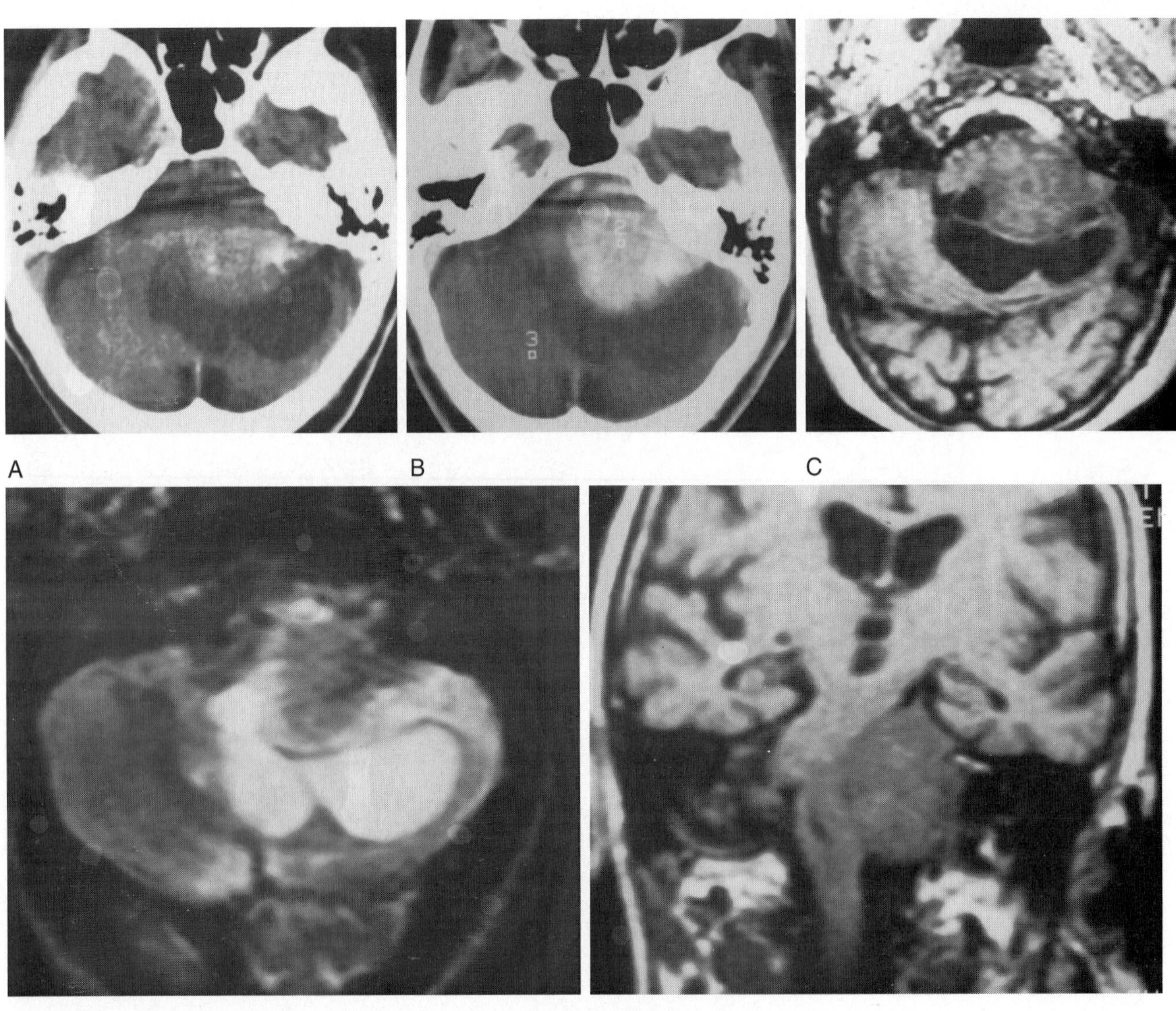

Figure 11.115. Posterior fossa meningioma showing a large surrounding arachnoidal cyst. **A** and **B.** CT without and with contrast shows areas of calcification in A and enhancement in B. There is a large, loculated, surrounding cystic space presenting a density similar to that of CSF. T1-weighted axial MR image without contrast (**C**) and T2-weighted axial image (**D**) show the multiloculated cystic space. **E.** Coronal T1-weighted MR image shows the marked distortion and displacement of the brainstem produced by the tumor, better appreciated than in axial views.

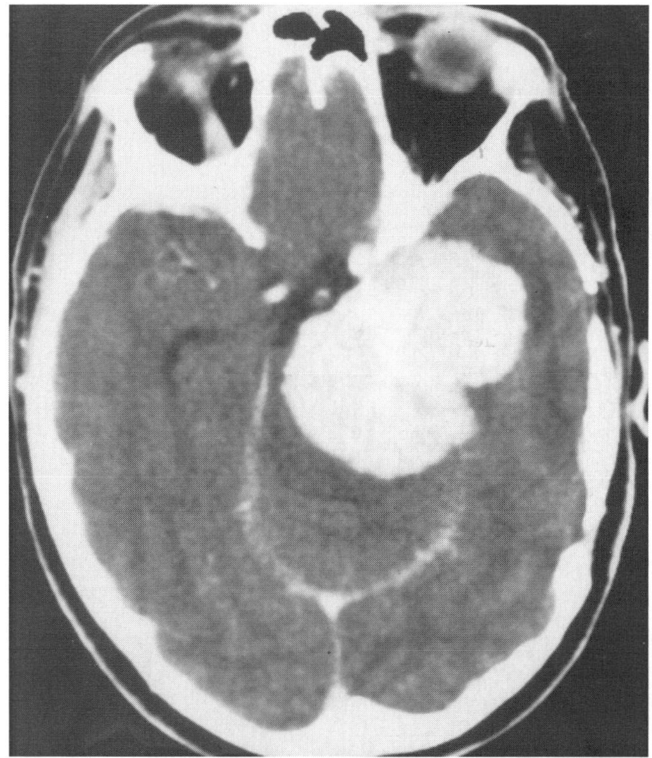

A

B

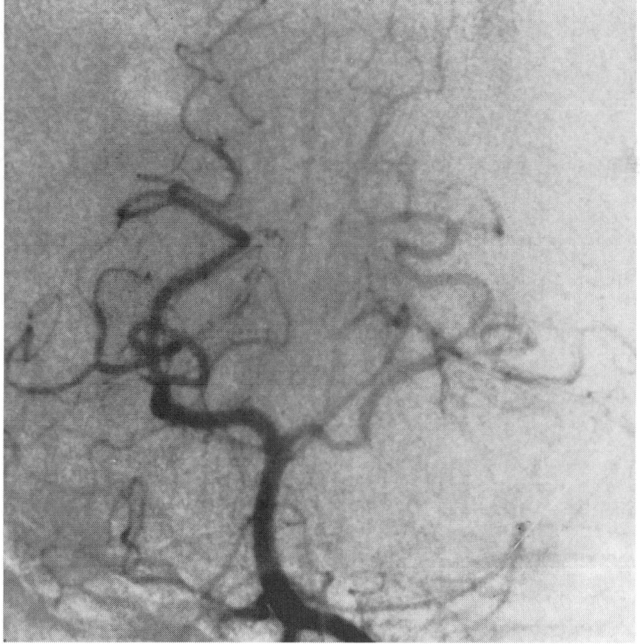

C

Figure 11.116. Saddle-shaped incisural meningioma. **A.** CT after contrast shows an anterolateral tumor in the region of the incisura with a posterior fossa and a middle fossa component and a narrow segment in the middle. The lesion could be a meningioma or a fifth-nerve neuroma, but meningioma is more common. **B.** Angiography was carried out to study the blood supply. The left carotid angiogram shows supply via the meningohypophyseal trunk (lower arrow) and via the posterior cerebral artery, which in this case arises from the internal carotid artery (upper arrow). **C.** Vertebral angiography demonstrates vascular displacements but no blood supply.

may sometimes form large arachnoidal cysts around them (Fig. 11.115), and this is a good differential point, although acoustic schwannomas sometimes form cysts, as shown in Fig. 11.109. See text following for further details on meningiomas. Meningiomas form typical saddle-shaped incisural tumors similar to the fifth-nerve neuromas and should be differentiated from them (Fig. 11.116). The exact location of the tumor is extremely important for appropriate surgical removal, which may require a dual surgical approach (temporal and posterior fossa) and most often results in incomplete removal of the lesion (Fig. 11.117) (Table 11.49).

Table 11.49.
Cerebellopontine Angle Meningiomas

Broader base than acoustic schwannomas
Usually centered anterior or posterior to (rather than at) the internal auditory canal
Often associated with large arachnoidal cysts (more than acoustic schwannomas)

TUMORS ARISING FROM CELL RESTS

Epidermoid and dermoid tumors are considered to be derived from epithelial inclusions within the neural canal during its closure. They are not true neoplasms but grow because the cells continue to divide and desquamate like epidermal tissue, and the desquamation over a period of time becomes bulky. They have a stratified epithelial lining and a fibrous connective tissue capsule. Eighty percent are intradural (128). The term *epidermoid cysts* is appropriate, and neuro-

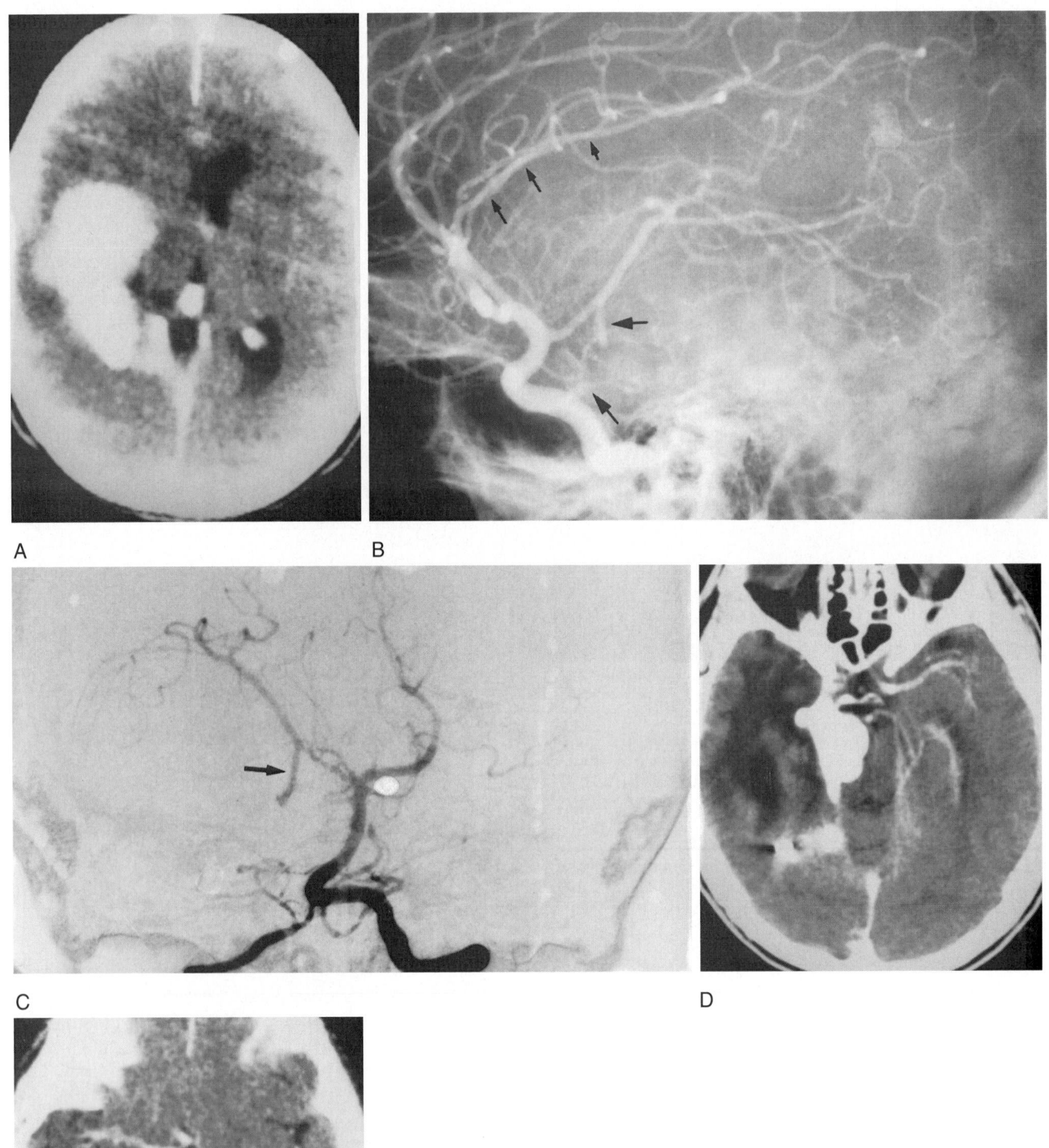

Figure 11.117. Large incisural, saddle meningioma before and after partial surgical removal. **A.** Postcontrast CT scan shows a large mass in the middle fossa, as well as enhancement on the right side of the tentorium. A lower section (not shown) revealed tumor off the anterolateral aspect of the incisura. **B.** Right carotid angiography demonstrates marked elevation of the sylvian triangle (arrows) typical of a temporal mass. There is also filling of the posterior communicating and posterior cerebral arteries. The vessel directed caudally (posterior arrow) is the proximal portion of the posterior cerebral artery. Some blood supply of the meningioma is seen arising from the intracavernous carotid artery (lower arrow). **C.** Vertebral angiography demonstrates the dislocation of the posterior cerebral artery and branches. The posterior communicating artery fills in retrograde fashion (arrow). **D** and **E.** Following partial surgical removal via a temporal approach, the posterior fossa component could not be removed. The postcontrast CT scan shows the residual mass and the postoperative changes in the right temporal region. E is a higher section than D.

Table 11.50.
Epidermoid Tumors

Derived from epidermal inclusions during closure of the neural plate
80% are intradural
Nearly isointense with CSF on CT imaging
Do not contrast-enhance on CT or MRI
On MRI can usually be distinguished from CSF by slightly different signal characteristics or inhomogeneity on at least one pulse sequence

surgeons use the term *pearly tumors* because of the shiny white appearance of their usually multinodular surface.

In the posterior fossa the epidermoids tend to occur near the midline anteriorly or anterolaterally. From there they may extend through the incisura into the parasellar region medial to the temporal lobe. They may also occur in the region of the cisterna cerebellomedullaris (Fig. 11.118). In some cases a sinus tract can be seen in the occipital bone leading to an epidermoid cyst in the posterior fossa. These dermal sinuses can be very subtle (Table 11.50).

On CT an epidermoid cyst is low density, similar to CSF. Contrast enhancement does not occur except in the extradural epidermoids, where enhancement of the capsule may take place. The extradural epidermoids arise in the bone, usually the petrous pyramid and most frequently near the tip. These are congenital tumors and should not be confused with the postinflammatory cholesteatomas seen at the base of the petrous pyramid, which are associated with drum perforations and chronic mastoid disease.

On MR T1-weighted images the tumor may show low intensity like CSF (Fig. 11.118), or it may show inhomogeneity. On T2-weighted images it is usually bright, similar to CSF. The tumors do not enhance after contrast. Those epidermoid cysts that have intensities similar to CSF and that do not enhance after contrast should be considered typical. The inhomogeneous density on T1 and proton density weighted images is less typical, for these tumors present an appearance similar to a glioma. Their lack of enhancement and extra-axial location, however, should be a differential point. Dermoid tumors or cysts have an origin similar to that of epidermoids, but they contain fatty elements and thus are bright on T1-weighted images. The CT appearance is similar to that of epidermoids except that the density is lower than CSF if the Hounsfield units are measured. They occur essentially in the same locations as epidermoids. They may rupture and form fluid levels that can be detected by CT or MRI (129). Like epidermoids, they tend to occur at or near the midline, sometimes within the ventricles. The contents of dermoid and epidermoid tumors or cysts can be very irritating and produce a chemical meningitis, sometimes severe. Great care must be taken to avoid spilling the contents of the cysts (130,131).

The differential diagnosis includes arachnoid cysts, cystic astrocytomas and hemangioblastomas, and ependymomas.

Epidermoids may also occur in the bones of the skull, in the vault as well as in the periorbital area.

TUMORS ARISING FROM OSSEOUS STRUCTURES

Tumors arising from the bone include chordomas and chondrosarcomas, nasopharyngeal carcinomas that directly invade the bone, and metastatic tumors. Primary bone tumors such as osteogenic sarcomas and giant cell tumors are extremely rare. Fibrous displasia may occasionally produce cranial nerve compression but usually does not produce a mass effect. These usually remain within the bone, but may bulge toward the posterior fossa.

Chordomas are tumors composed of cells derived from notochordal rests, which are most frequent in the sacrum and in the clivus but may also be found in other regions of the spine. The tumors may occur at any age but are most frequent in the third and fourth decades, and there is a male predominance (2:1). The tumors may produce bulky masses in the prepontine space, displacing the brainstem dorsally. Although they tend to be midline, they often occur to the right or left of the midline and may grow in the parasellar region, sometimes extending to the apex of the orbit. In doing so they displace the intracavernous portion of the carotid artery laterally and/or forward, sometimes surrounding or encasing it and occasionally producing obstruction of the vessel. The tumors displace the basilar artery dorsally and to the side if they are situated off the midline. It is important to determine the position of the vessels if a surgical approach is planned (Table 11.51).

On CT there is usually bone destruction. Calcification is usually present, some of it possibly due to residual undestroyed bone. The tumor enhances after contrast. On MRI the soft-tissue components can be outlined much more clearly, and the multiple projections are very advantageous when one is outlining the size and scope of the tumor mass (Fig. 11.119).

Considerable progress in the surgical treatment of these lesions has taken place in the last 10 years. This, combined with proton beam radiation therapy, which delivers a high dose of radiation with sharp margins and minimal radiation

Table 11.51.
Chordomas

Composed of cells derived from notochordal rests
Most commonly found at level of clivus and sacrum
Usually found in young adults
Found in a midline or near-midline location, producing mass effect on the brainstem, cranial nerves, or adjacent arteries
CT appearance is that of a hypodense destructive mass that is calcified or contains osseous fragments
The MRI appearance is typically that of an often multilobulated inhomogeneous clival mass that contrast-enhances

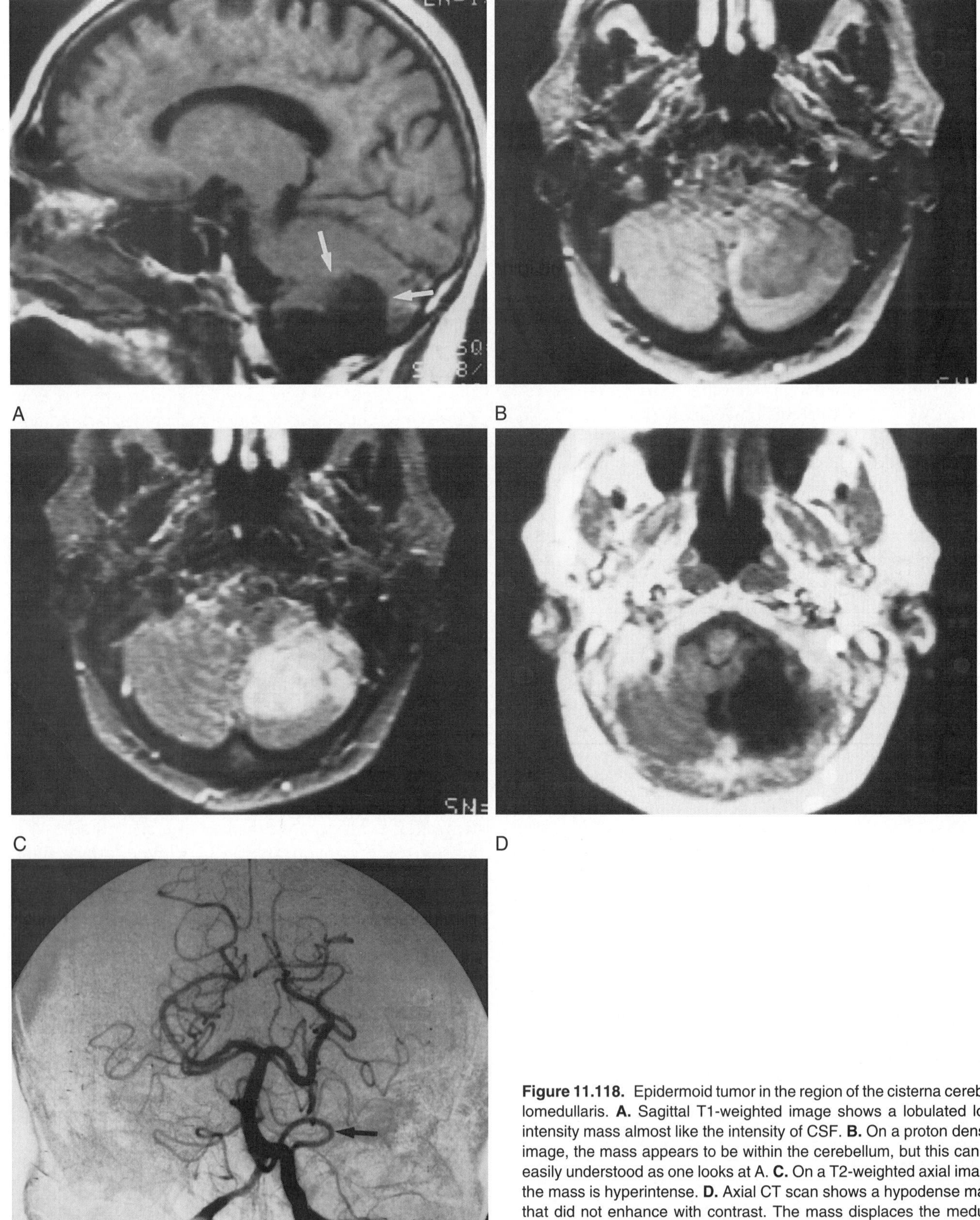

Figure 11.118. Epidermoid tumor in the region of the cisterna cerebellomedullaris. **A.** Sagittal T1-weighted image shows a lobulated low-intensity mass almost like the intensity of CSF. **B.** On a proton density image, the mass appears to be within the cerebellum, but this can be easily understood as one looks at A. **C.** On a T2-weighted axial image, the mass is hyperintense. **D.** Axial CT scan shows a hypodense mass that did not enhance with contrast. The mass displaces the medulla toward the opposite side and flattens it. **E.** A left vertebral angiogram reveals an avascular mass that displaces the posterior inferior cerebellar artery toward the left (arrow), indicating that it is an extracerebellar mass growing in the intertonsillar area and displacing the artery away from the midline.

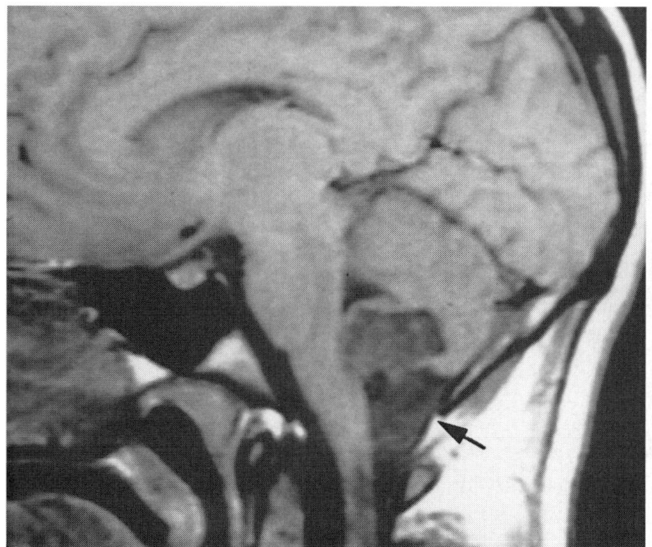

F

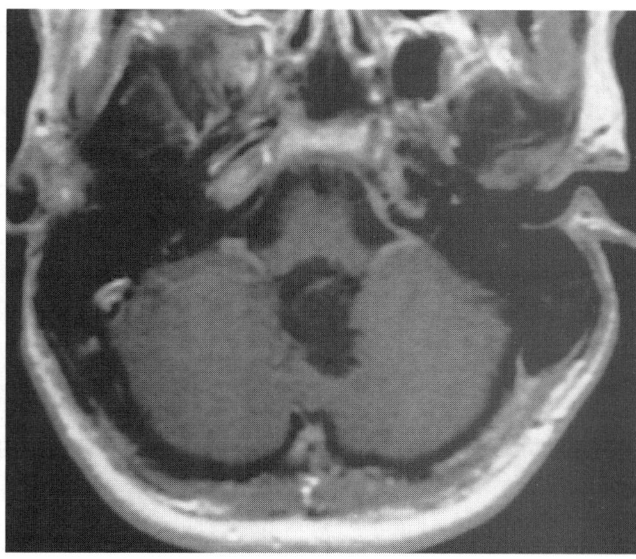

G

Figure 11.118. *(continued)* **F** to **J.** Epidermoid tumor attached to inferior medullary velum in a 22-year-old man. **F.** The sagittal T1-weighted image reveals a hypointense mass pressing on the caudal portion of the fourth ventricle and occupying also the posterior portion of the cerebellomedullary cistern. **G.** Axial T1-weighted postcontrast image shows no enhancement. **H.** Axial CT image shows a low-density mass. **I.** Proton density image shows that the mass is isointense in relation to the cerebellar tissue. **J.** T2 axial image reveals that the mass is hyperintense. These findings are consistent with a diagnosis of an epidermoid tumor. A cyst could produce identical findings but would not have a component with slightly irregular intensities in the cistern (arrow in F).

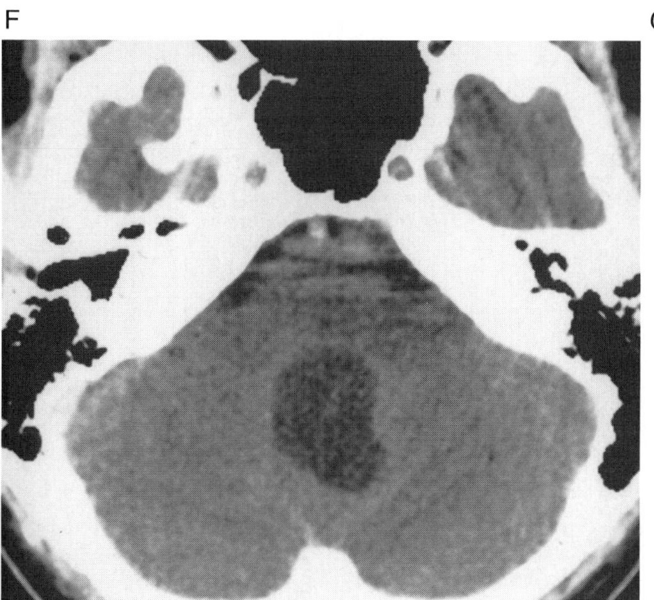

H

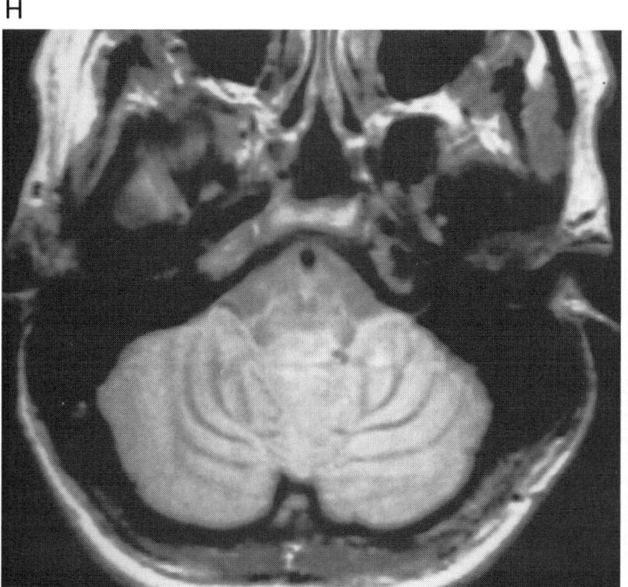

I

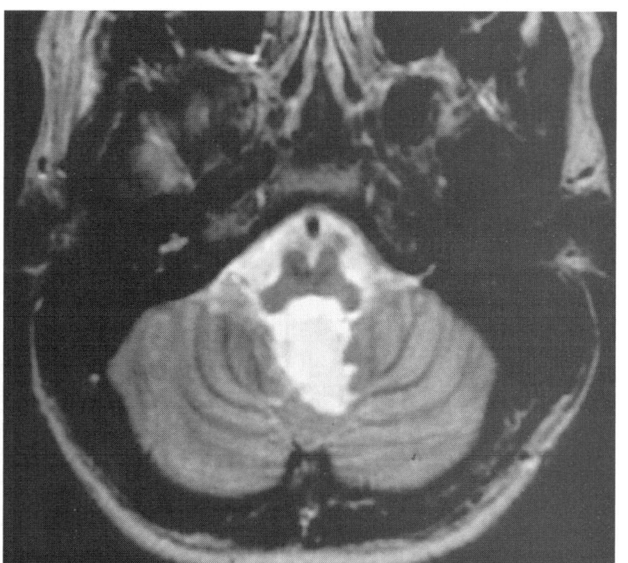

J

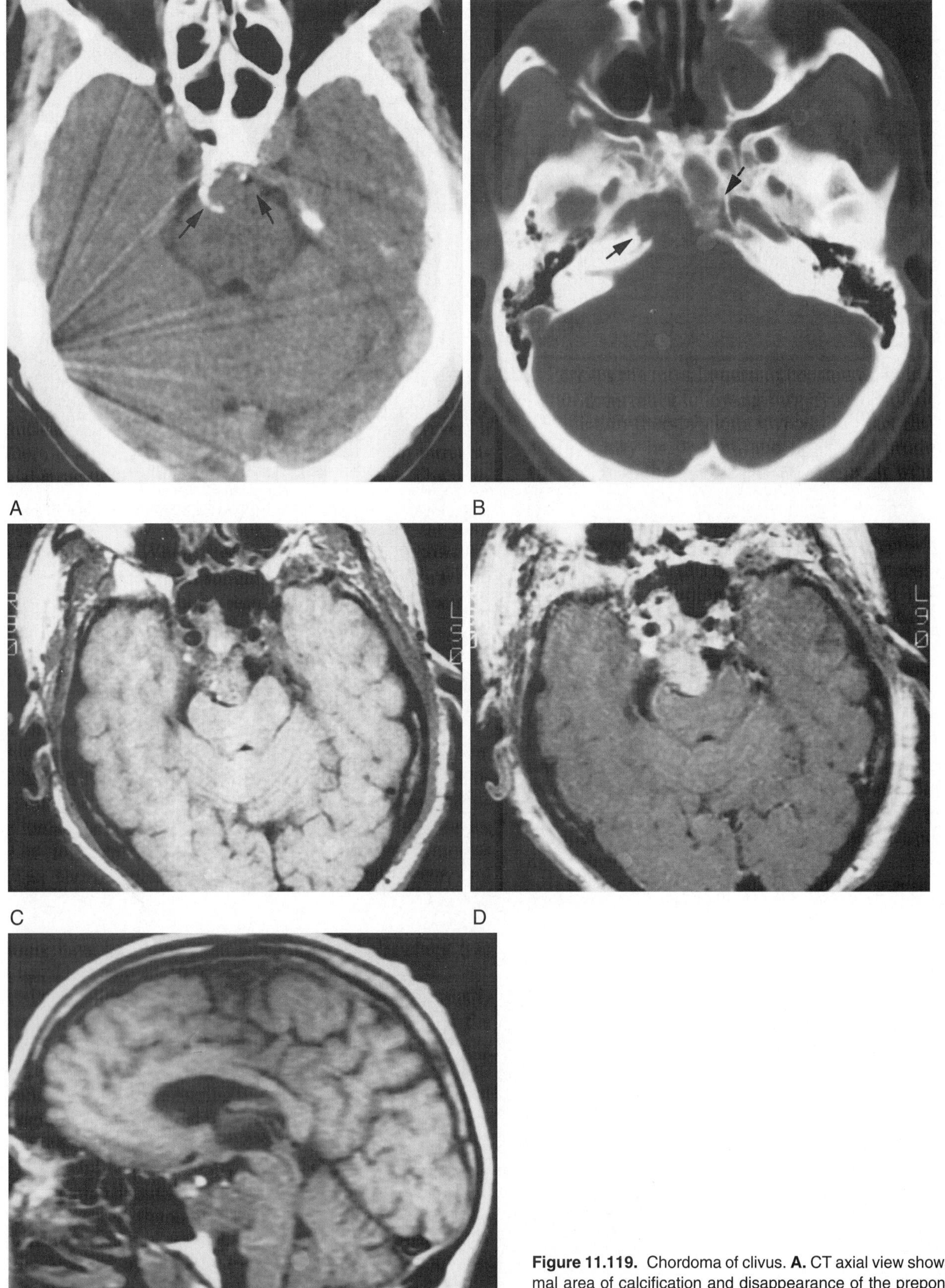

Figure 11.119. Chordoma of clivus. **A.** CT axial view shows an abnormal area of calcification and disappearance of the prepontine cistern in the midline (arrows). **B.** CT bone window image shows destruction of the right side of the clivus and the adjacent petrous tip (arrows). **C.** Axial T1-weighted MR image shows the mass and the indentation of the pons caused by it. **D.** The mass enhances after contrast. **E.** Sagittal noncontrast T1-weighted view demonstrates the posterior displacement of the brainstem.

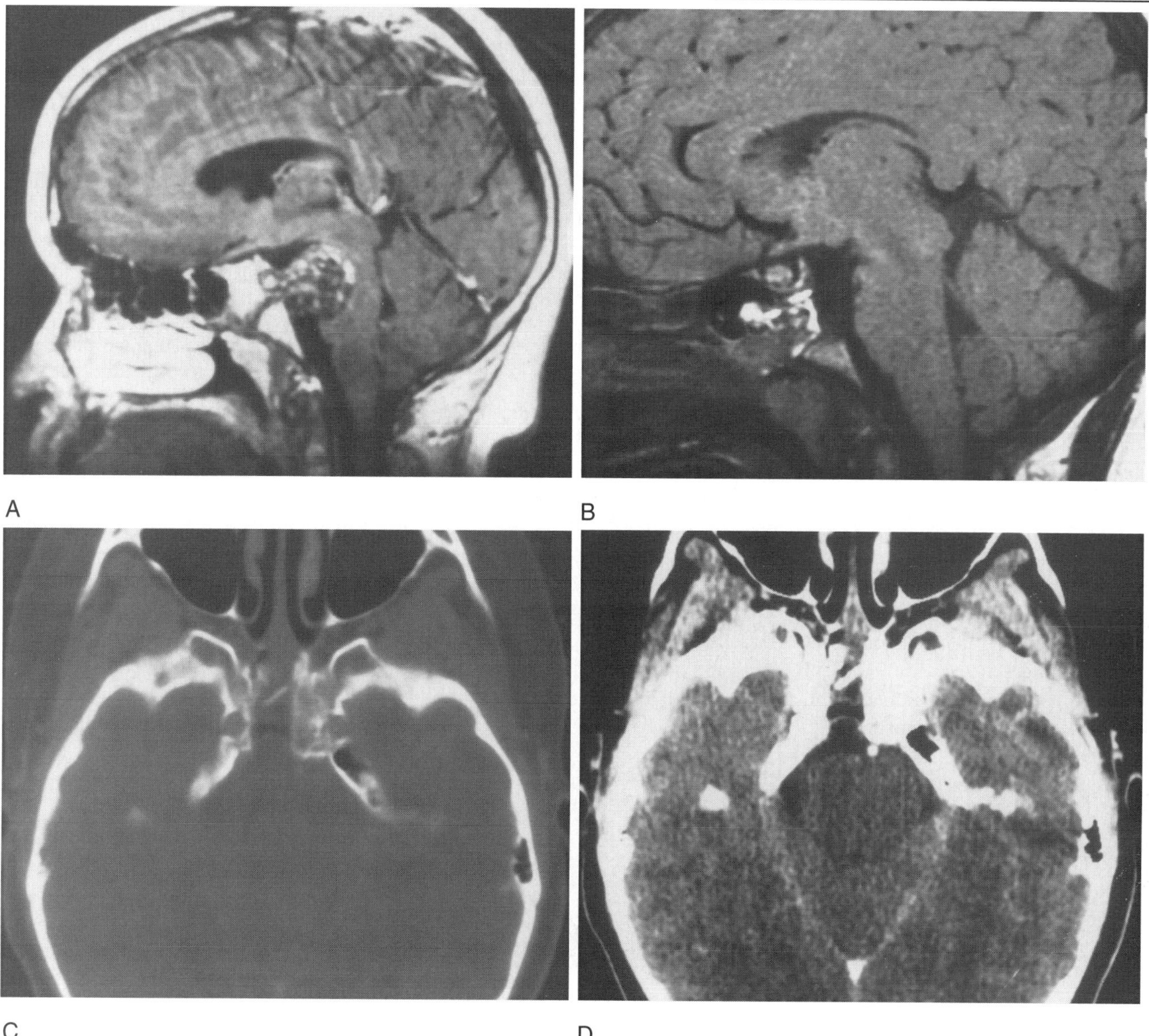

Figure 11.120. Clivus chondrosarcoma totally surgically removed. **A.** The tumor arises from the clivus, has a thick "pedicle," and enlarges dorsally, burrowing into the pons. Sagittal T1-weighted MR image. **B.** Postoperative T1-weighted sagittal view shows disappearance of the tumor. **C.** CT axial bone window scan reveals the transoral surgical approach with removal of a segment of the clivus. **D.** Postcontrast CT scan shows the basilar artery to the left of the surgically resected bone.

to the brainstem, has resulted in considerable improvement in survival with normal function, frequently with total cures. Proton beam radiation was pioneered at the Massachusetts General Hospital.

The just-mentioned treatment approach is particularly applicable to *chondrosarcomas*, which often may have a better-defined site of attachment to the clivus (Fig. 11.120). The tumors may occur in the posterior fossa, arising from the sphenoid bone at the clivus, or from the sphenoid bone in the parasellar region. An occasional case is found arising from the falx, possibly from primitive mesenchymal totipotential cells found in the meninges. The great majority arise from the base of the skull, which has an enchondral type of ossification, as against the skull vault, which does not (132) (Table 11.52).

The lesion can be quite bulky and remain extracerebral, producing displacement and compression of brain structures. Thus complete removal can often be accomplished.

On CT there are usually calcifications within the tumor and bone erosion rather than bone destruction at the site of origin. The tumors enhance on CT and MRI. On MRI they are hypointense on T1-weighted images and hyperintense on T2-weighted images. The calcifications are not usually visible.

Table 11.52.
Chondrosarcomas

Usually arise from endochondral bone
Frequently located at central skull base
May grow to large size and displace brain, cranial nerves, and blood vessels
CT appearance is typically that of a mass containing calcifications due to the presence of a chondroid matrix or from destroyed bone

MENINGIOMAS

This is a neoplasm that arises from the meninges in the cranial cavity or in the spine. It is the most frequent extra-axial tumor that usually remains outside the neural structures, and it then produces displacement and compression and often edema of the adjacent brain tissue. However, some meningiomas are malignant and invade brain tissue (meningeal sarcomas). Meningiomas represent about 15 percent of intracranial tumors. They occur most often in the skull convexity, in the parasagittal region and falx (about 50 percent) or in the parasellar, subfrontal (olfactory groove) sphenoid ridge and clivus (40 percent). The remaining 10 percent occur in the foramen magnum, the tentorium, and the optic nerves. They are more frequent in women (about 2:1). The usual locations of meningiomas are shown in the diagram of Figure 11.121.

Histologically, Russell and Rubinstein (4) consider three groups, but the great variation in the histologic appearance of meningiomas has led authors to describe many more varieties. Cushing and Eisenhardt described 9 types and 22 subtypes (23). Zülch of the World Health Organization described 9 types (1). Although the basic histologic appearance is variable, the relationship to prognoses does not usually follow, with a few exceptions. Thus a simpler classification is preferred. As mentioned, Russell and Rubinstein propose three groups. Group 1 is the classical type, which comprises the meningothelial (or syncytial) type, the transition type, and the fibroblastic type. Group 2 is the angioblastic type, which is now more frequently regarded as hemangiopericytomas. Group 3 is the malignant meningioma, which may be an angioblastic or other type of meningioma but which may end as a frank meningeal sarcoma (spindle cell sarcoma) (4).

Meningiomas tend to grow slowly and at varying rates. Some remain stationary for a number of years, but some growth can be expected in the great majority. Obviously, some meningiomas grow more rapidly and also tend to recur more rapidly, and this can usually be predicted on the basis of the histologic appearance.

The shape of meningiomas is quite variable and partly depends on their location. Over the cavity of the skull they tend to assume a globoid appearance, often lobulated (Fig. 11.122). In the sphenoid ridge they often grow alongside the bone and present a flat configuration usually referred to as *meningioma en plaque* (Fig. 11.123). The same configurations can be found in other locations. The degree of bone reaction to the presence of the meningioma is quite variable and goes from no visible reaction to a marked degree of sclerosis (Fig. 11.123), and sometimes bone destruction due to invasion by tumor (Table 11.53).

Calcifications in meningiomas are basically of two types from the imaging point of view. The classical type is the psammomatous calcification, in which there are myriads of tiny calcifications called *psammoma bodies* uniformly distributed throughout the tumor, causing a uniform increase in density visible on plain films (Fig. 11.122*D*). The other type is scattered calcifications nonuniformly distributed within the tumor. Both types are very easily detected by CT.

Meningiomas can be multiple and in this case are related to neurofibromatosis type II, as previously mentioned (Fig. 11.124).

On CT meningiomas are easily visualized as slightly hyperdense masses, usually denser than the adjacent gray matter. The density is partly due to the cellularity, but also is often related to the presence of calcified psammoma bodies. If the tumor is near bone, it may demonstrate increased density and/or increased thickness of the bone due to hyperostosis at the site of attachment to the bone (Figs. 11.122 and 11.123). Meningiomas enhance after intravenous contrast administration, and the enhancement tends to be uniform. Ninety-five percent of meningiomas enhance, and those that do not probably present some histologic characteristics. For example, the lipomatous meningiomas contain large amounts of fatty tissue. However, the tissue is dark on CT and bright on noncontrast T1-weighted images, like fat, and this would permit a differentiation.

On MRI, meningiomas tend to be isodense with gray matter, and if they are small they can be overlooked without contrast because the calcifications that may be present, as well as any bone hyperostosis, would not usually be imaged.

Table 11.53.
Meningiomas

Shape: Frequently either globoid or en plaque
Location: Most common locations include along the greater sphenoid wing, falx, convexities, parasellar region, planum sphenoidale, and clivus
Calcifications: Psammomatous (homogeneous distribution of fine calcifications) or nonuniform distribution of slightly larger calcifications
Bone reaction: Frequently some reactive sclerosis and hyperostosis can be seen in adjacent bone
Noncontrast CT appearance: Often slightly hyperdense due to calcification or dense cellularity
Contrast CT appearance: Usually densely enhance in a relatively homogeneous manner
Noncontrast MRI appearance: Usually relatively isointense with gray matter on T1-weighted images; may have variable signal intensity
Contrast MRI appearance: Typically densely enhance and often are seen to have a "dural tail," probably due to dural reaction

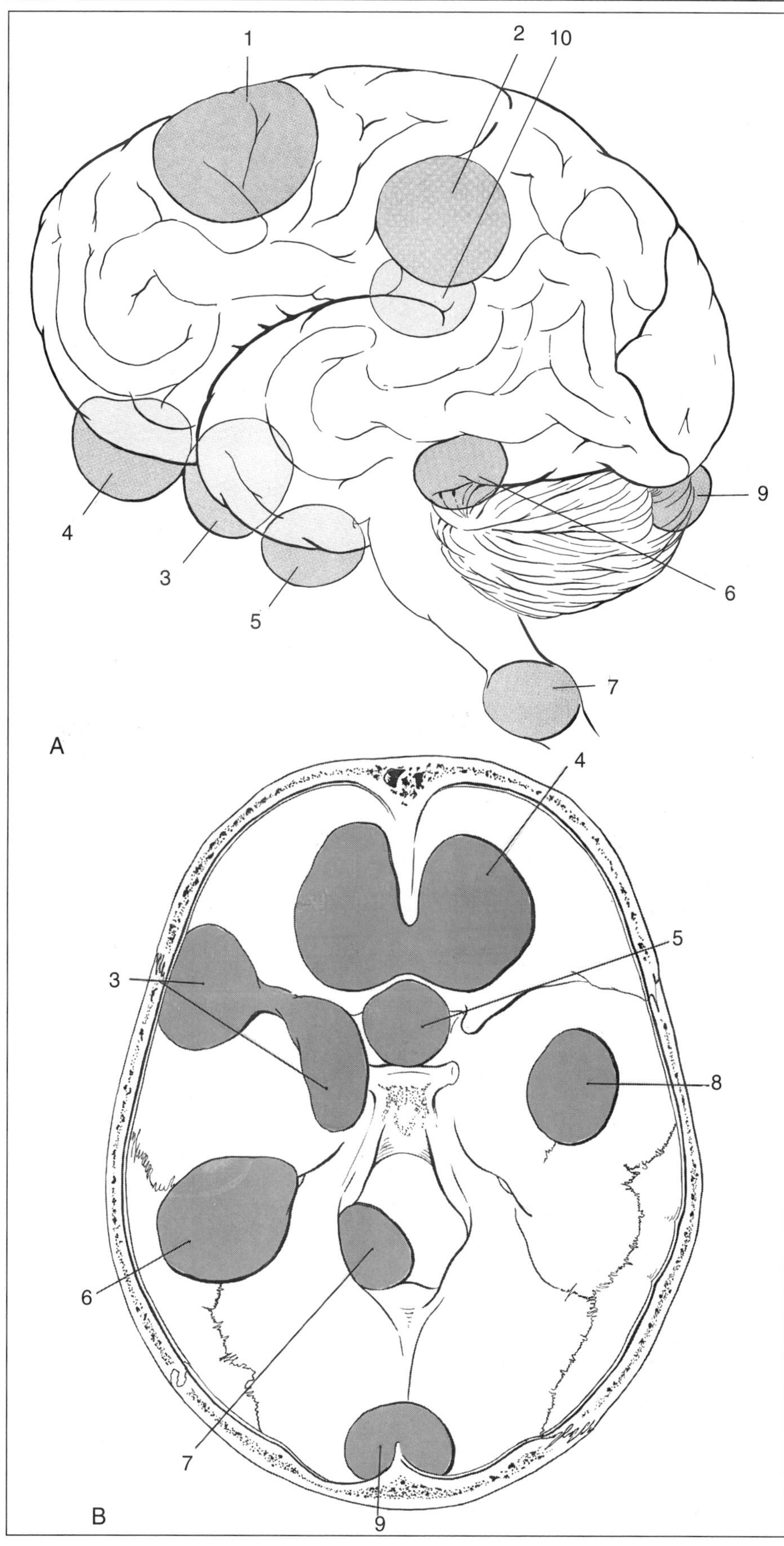

Figure 11.121. Common sites of occurrence of meningiomas of the central nervous system. **A** and **B.** The 10 most common locations in which meningiomas are found, in order of frequency, are parasagittal (1), cerebral convexity (2), sphenoid ridge (3), olfactory groove (4), suprasellar (5), cerebellopontine angle (6), spinal (7), floor of middle fossa (8), torcular (9), and intraventricular (10).

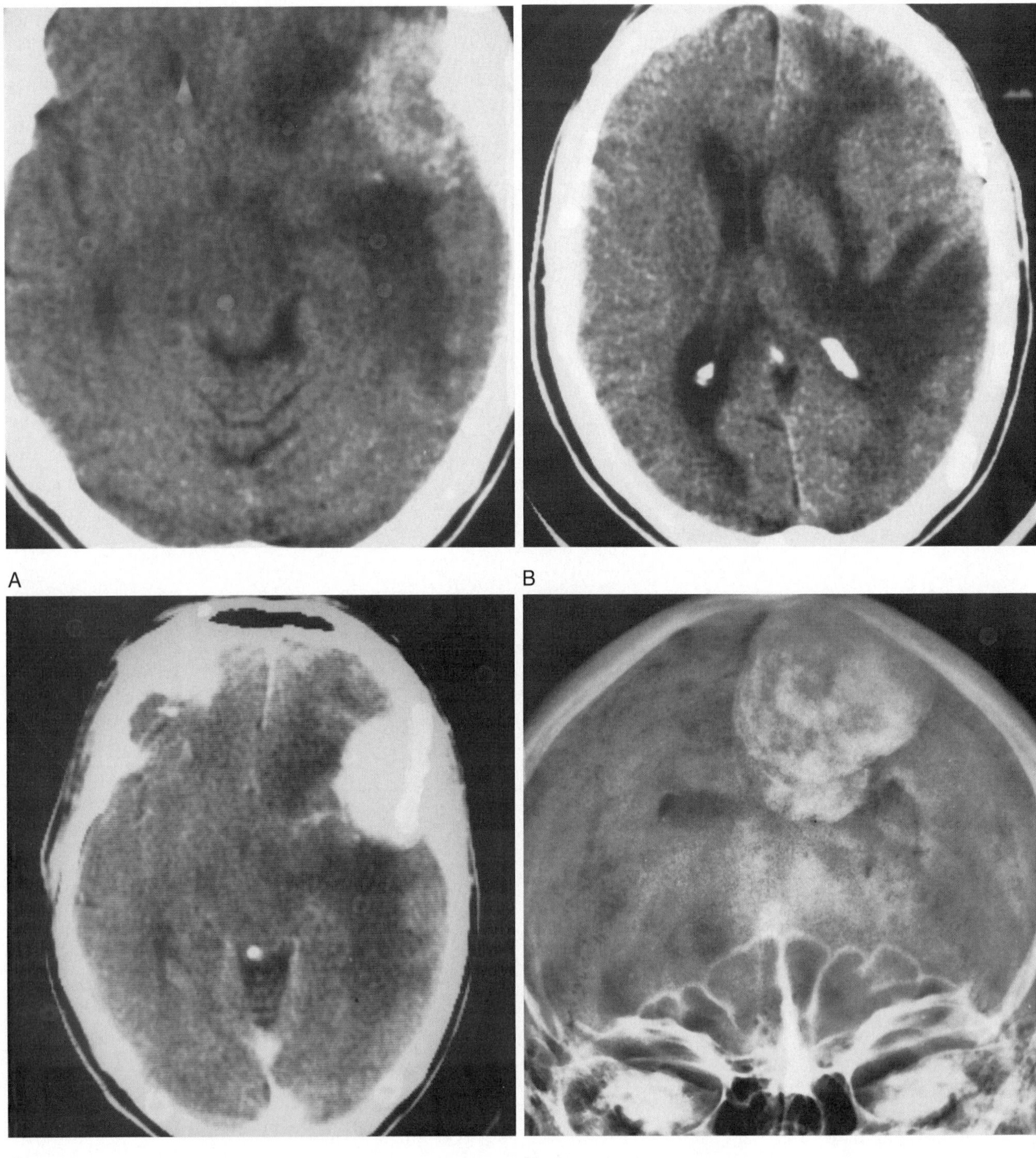

Figure 11.122. Globoid meningioma arising in the pterional region. **A.** Nonenhanced CT scan shows a hyperdense lesion over the lower convexity of the hemisphere. The spotty areas of increased density represent calcium deposits. There is also hypodensity surrounding the lesion, indicative of edema and thickening of the adjacent bone. **B.** A higher section demonstrates considerable edema and a midline shift. Some meningiomas produce a marked edematous reaction, whereas others do not. **C.** Postcontrast CT scan shows homogeneous enhancement of the tumor. **D.** Parasagittal meningioma showing the typical cloudlike appearance of a meningioma on a plain film of the skull due to diffuse psammomatous calcification.

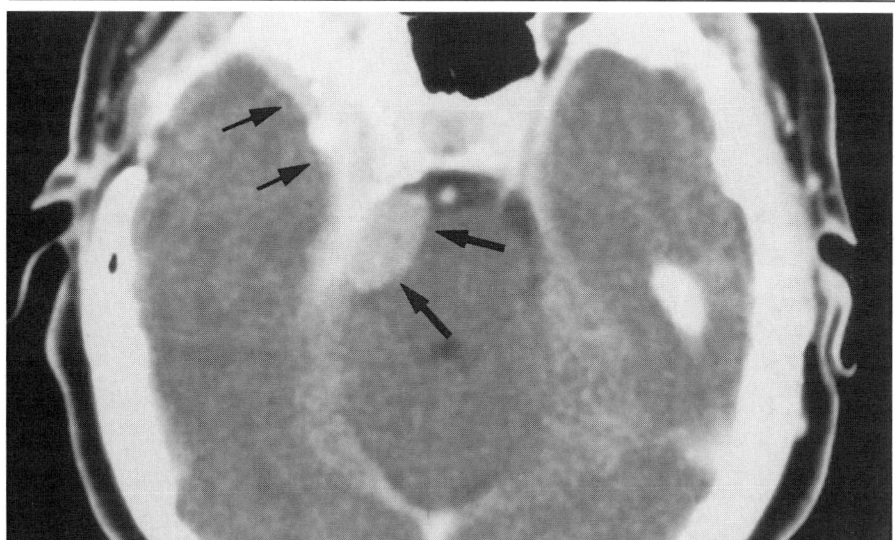

Figure 11.123. Meningioma en plaque in the sphenoid ridge and parasellar region. There is only a relatively thin soft-tissue component and a marked degree of hyperdense bone reaction involving the right sphenoid ridge and the adjacent portion of the body of the sphenoid. The neoplasm extends posteriorly to form a nodule projecting medially from the edge of the tentorium, compressing and deforming the brainstem (arrows). There is no surrounding edema. These meningiomas often grow very slowly, and this patient showed almost no growth on follow-up for several years.

Thus contrast enhancement is needed. As in CT, contrast enhancement usually yields a homogeneous mass. Inhomogeneity may be due to calcifications, cystic areas, blood vessels, or histologic variables within the tumor. As demonstrated in Figure 11.125, the dura immediately adjacent to the neoplasm enhances (enhanced "dural tail"). The enhancement and thickening of the dura are probably not due to tumor infiltration but to reactive proliferation of loose connective tissue in the dura (133,134).

Edema in association with meningiomas is quite variable. Some very large meningiomas present no edema in spite of their large size, whereas others, even when they are small, present edema that sometimes is very pronounced (Fig. 11.122). Figure 11.126*A* and *B* shows a meningioma of the falx posteriorly at the junction with the tentorium without edema, whereas an anterior falx meningioma (Fig. 11.126*C* to *E*) presents considerable edema. Venous thromboses or interference with venous circulation has been suggested as a possible mechanism, but this is unlikely. It is more plausible that the edema represents a reaction of the individual's brain tissue to the presence of the neoplasm, even though the tumor is extracerebral. It does not seem to be related to the histology of the neoplasm; that is, the tumors with edema are not more malignant histologically. Thus, at present we must accept that the reaction may be on an individual basis.

Cyst formation around meningiomas is not uncommon and may be related to the formation of adhesions with loculation of CSF that sometimes forms a large cystic space; the cystic spaces are usually small (Fig. 11.115).

The blood supply of meningiomas is of interest, and before the age of CT and MRI, the angiographically demonstrated blood supply had great diagnostic importance in differentiating meningiomas from a glioma or another type of tumor. Currently, the blood supply is important for determining the degree of vascularity and for deciding whether preoperative embolization to decrease the tumor vascularity is advisable. In the tumors over the convexity, the blood supply usually stems from the middle meningeal artery or its branches or from other meningeal arteries (accessory meningeal artery, anterior meningeal artery, branches of occipital artery, and posterior auricular artery) (Figs. 11.127 and 11.128). Additional branches from the intracavernous portion of the internal carotid artery (meningohypophyseal, inferior trunk) would supply blood to meningiomas arising in the parasellar region and tentorium. However, a fairly high proportion of meningiomas receive their supply also from branches of the internal carotid or vertebral-basilar system. This implies a violation of the leptomeningeal brain cover. It means that the meningioma is heavily adherent to the leptomeninges, but does not mean that the meningioma is malignant or particularly invasive. In separate external and internal carotid artery injections, it is possible to determine the portions of the tumor supplied by the external and the internal carotid artery branches. Intraventricular meningiomas are usually supplied by the anterior and posterior choroidal arteries.

The so-called angioblastic meningiomas, which now are felt to represent hemangiopericytomas, have a rich blood supply and rapid circulation with large draining veins. On MRI these tumors will show flow voids within them due to rapid-flowing veins (Fig. 11.129).

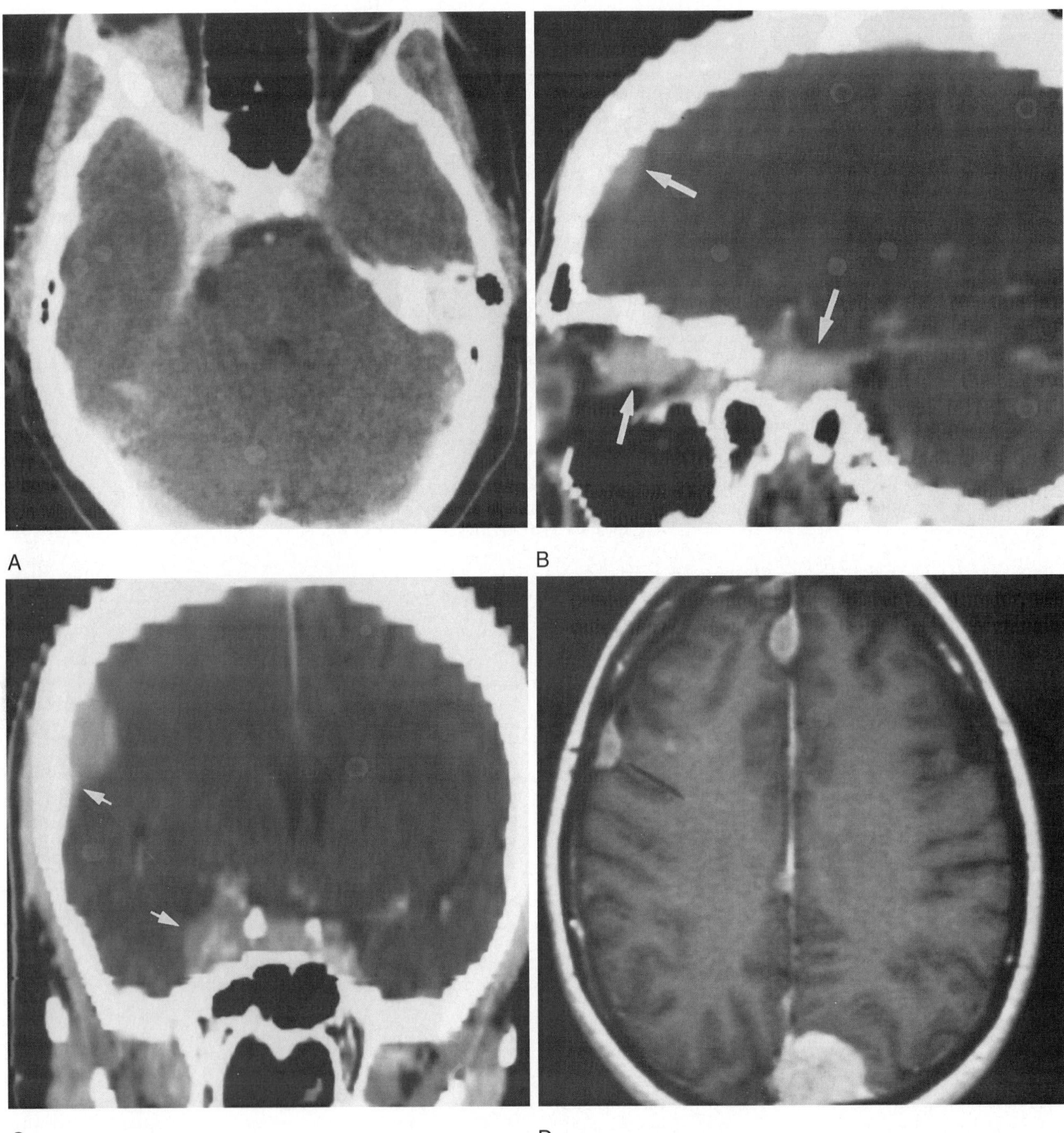

Figure 11.124. Multiple meningiomas in a patient with neurofibromatosis II. **A.** There is a right parasellar meningioma and either a separate orbital meningioma or extension of the parasellar lesion into the orbit through the superior orbital fissure. **B.** Sagittal reformatting shows the two components well (arrows). There is also a small meningioma off the frontal inner table (upper arrow). **C.** A coronal reformatted image shows the right parasellar tumor (arrow) and another convexity tumor showing a dural enhancing tail on its lower aspect (arrow). Dural tails are best seen on MRI. The image in A was taken 4 years prior to B, and there was no increase in the size of the parasellar and orbital masses.

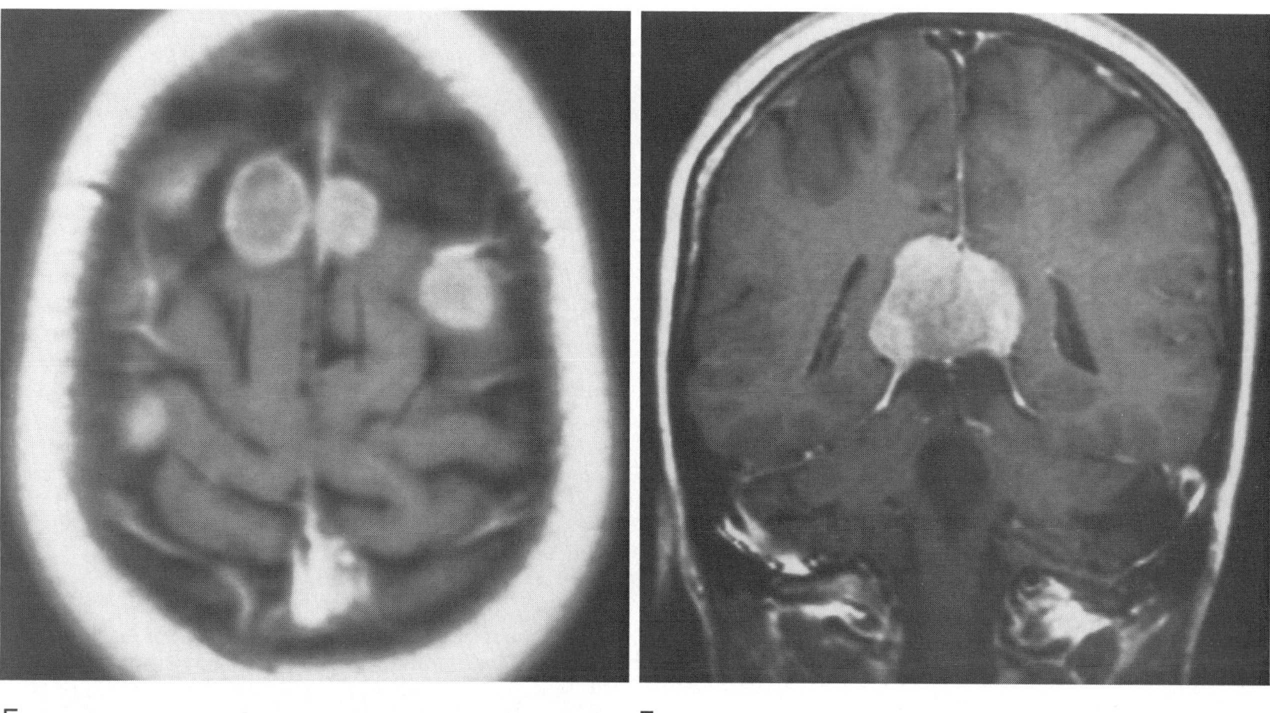

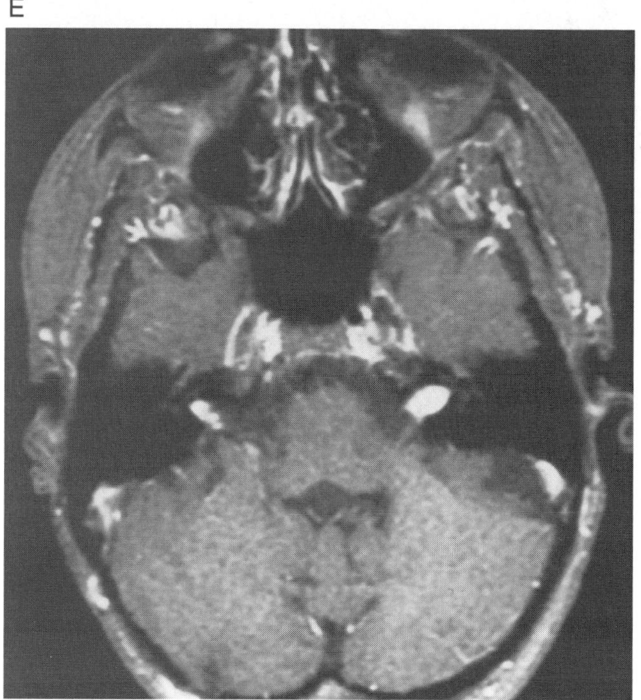

Figure 11.124. *(continued)* **D** to **F**. The postcontrast images reveal eight or nine tumors. There is a tumor arising at the apex of the tentorium at the junction with the falx. **G.** Bilateral enhancing small acoustic neuromas are seen.

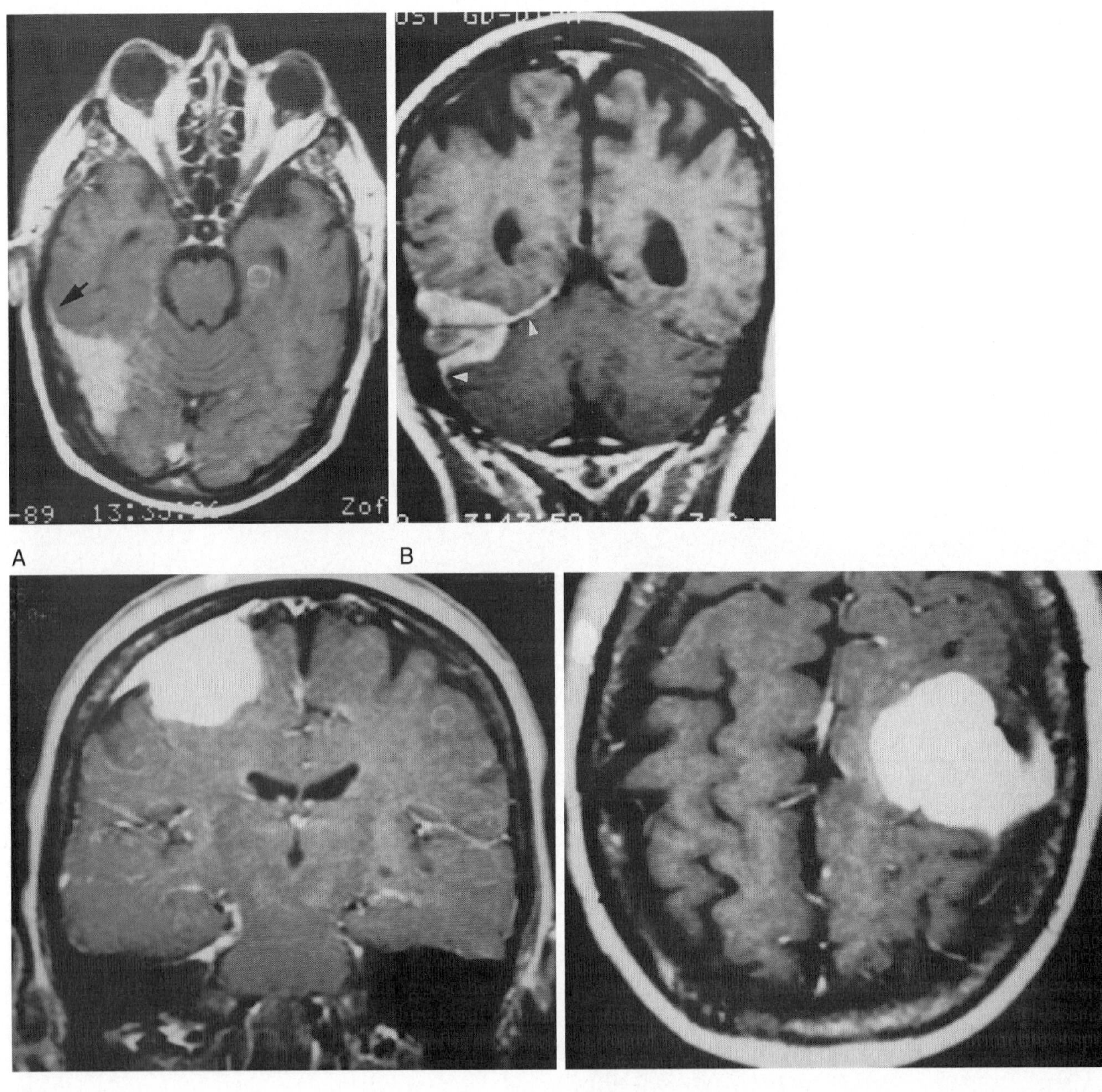

Figure 11.125. Meningioma of the lateral aspect of the tentorium showing an enhanced dural tail and no edema. **A.** Axial T1 postcontrast view shows the enhanced tumor and a long dural tail (arrow). **B.** Coronal postcontrast image shows the enhanced dural tail extending along the tentorium and caudally along the posterior fossa dura (arrowhead). The tumor is on both sides of the tentorium. The total absence of edema is interesting; compare with Figure 11.122. Postcontrast coronal (**C**) and axial (**D**) views of another meningioma, fairly large in size, presenting a dural tail on both its superior and inferior aspects, and presenting no edematous reaction by the brain.

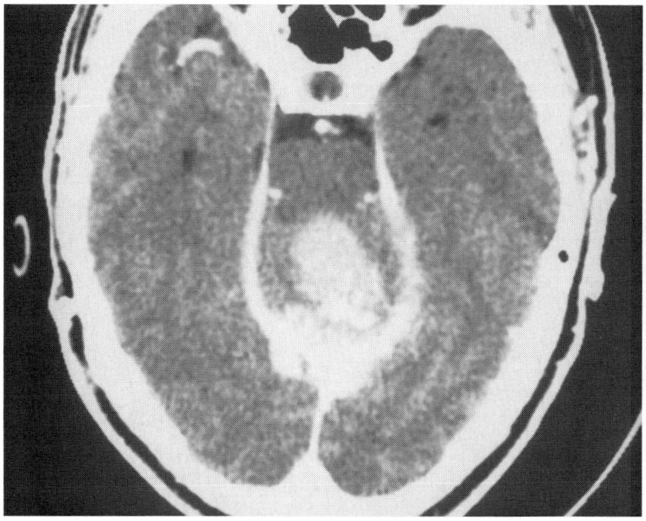

A

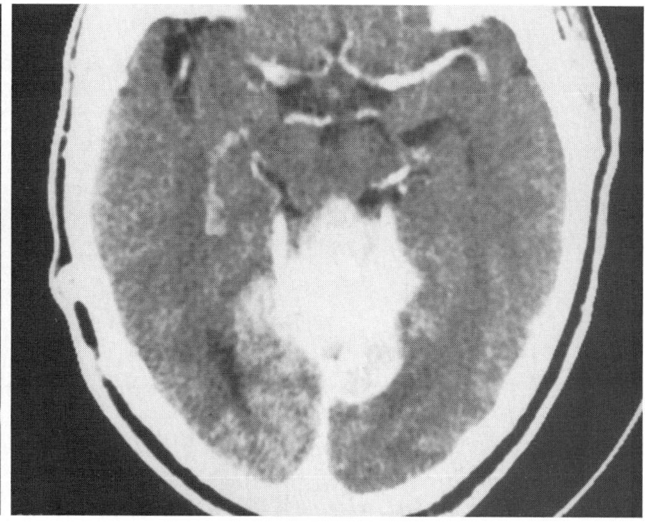

B

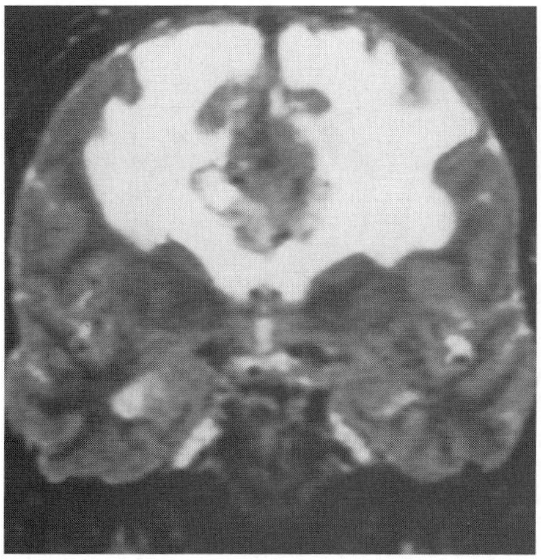

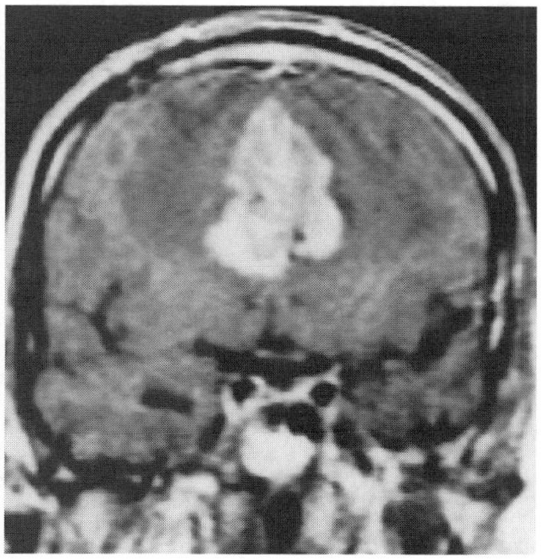

C

D

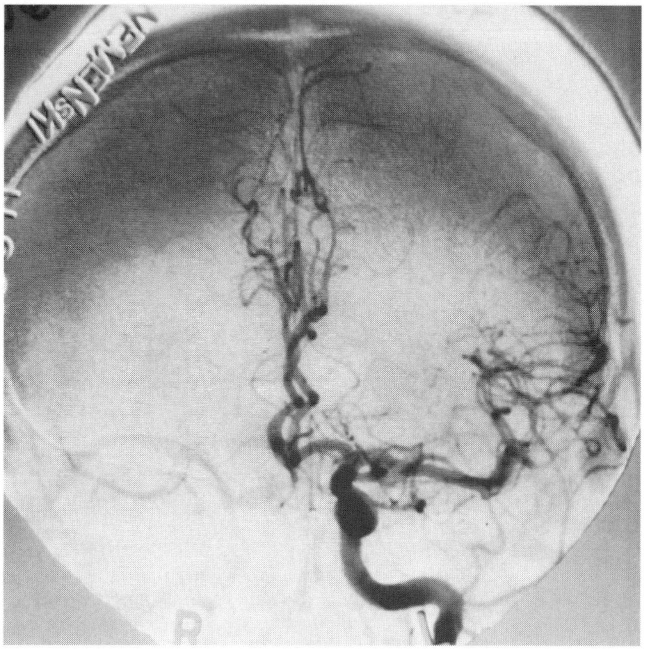

E

Figure 11.126. Meningiomas arising at the junction of the tentorium and falx and on another patient arising from the falx anteriorly. **A** and **B.** Typical appearance of a meningioma arising from the tentorial-falx junction. The meningioma grows in the midline, displaces the cerebellum downward, and indents the brainstem. There is no edema around this tumor, which is growing on both sides of the falx. **C.** Anterior falx meningioma. T2-weighted image shows considerable edema around the mass, which is isodense with gray matter. **D.** Postcontrast T1 image shows the shape of the tumor. **E.** Left carotid angiogram showing the separation of the right and left anterior cerebral arteries, which is typical of meningiomas arising from the falx in this area.

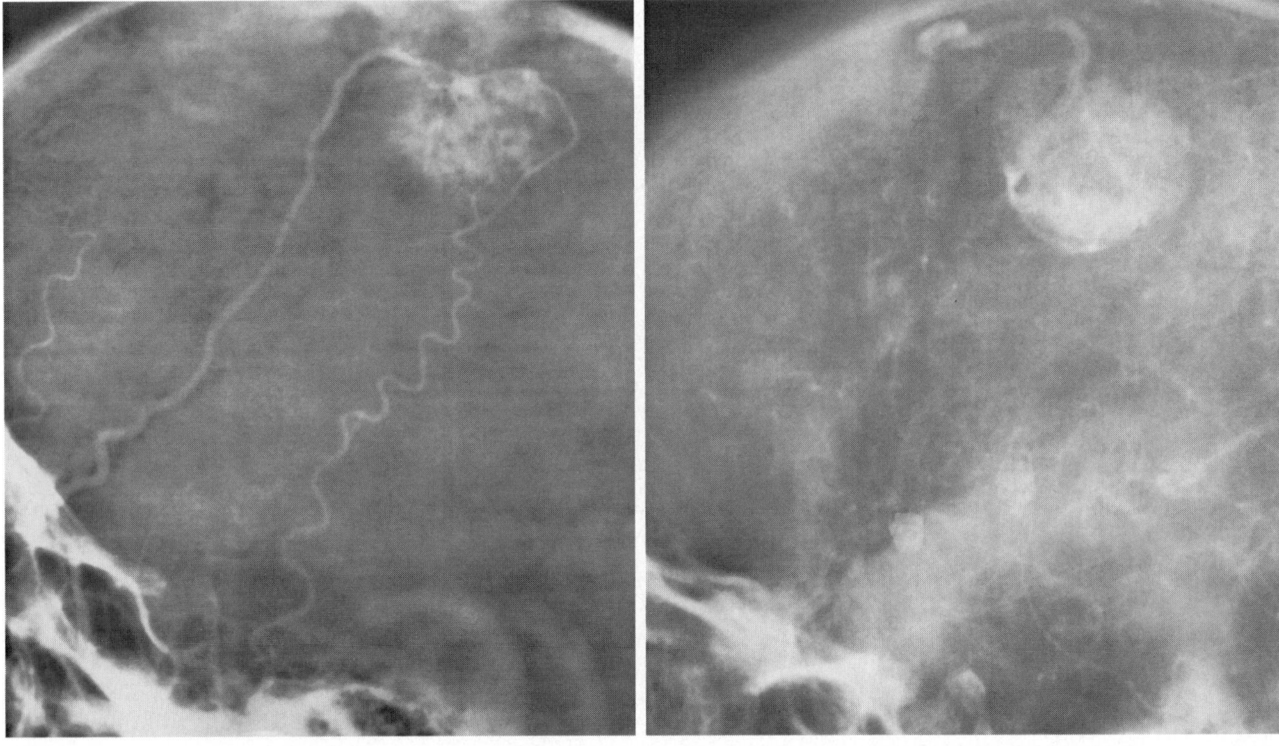

A B

Figure 11.127. A. External carotid angiogram of a parasagittal meningioma. The middle meningeal artery divides into two branches, both of which enter the meningioma to supply it. What may be called the hilum of the tumor is seen where the major branch seems to enter the tumor. However, the radial distribution of vessels from the hilum of the tumor ("sunburst" appearance) is not shown in this instance. The tumor blush was homogeneous from the start. The superficial temporal artery overlies the tumor but is not supplying it. The tumor blush is fairly homogeneous, and it persisted into the later venous phase. **B.** Another parasagittal meningioma with a homogeneous tumor blush after internal carotid injection, indicating supply via this route. Note also that there is an early-filling vein at this time (late arterial phase). No veins are filled anywhere in the brain. This appearance indicates a more rapid circulation through the meningioma, which usually correlates with a more rapidly growing tumor.

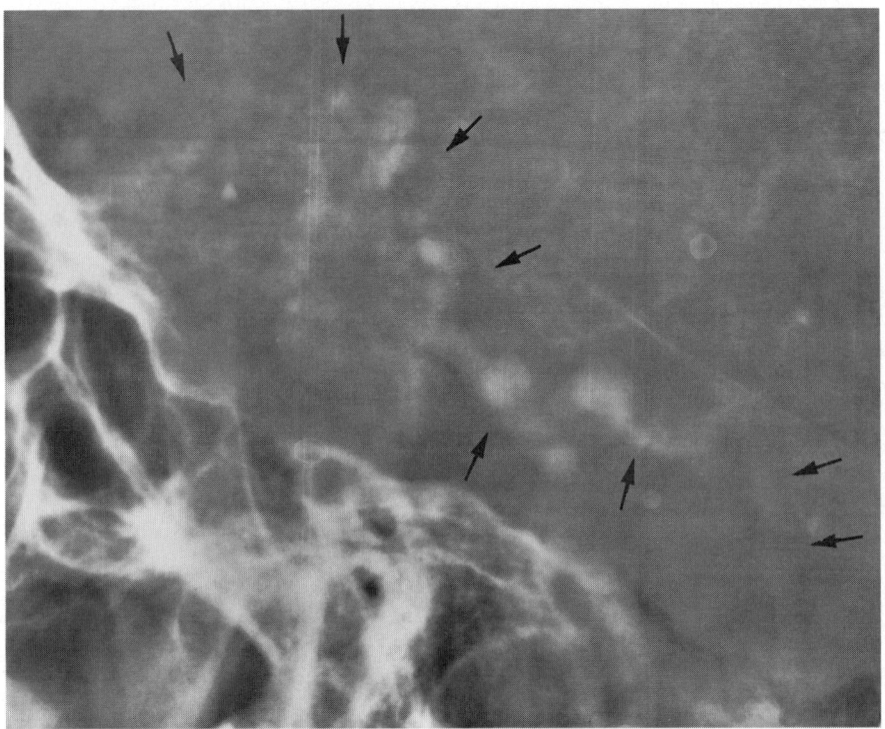

Figure 11.128. Meningioma, angioblastic variety (hemangiopericytoma?), with increased speed of circulation and drainage by way of the basal vein. The tumor blush is well circumscribed (anterior arrows). This film, made at 3.5 sec, shows irregular distribution of densities within the tumor due to the presence of large draining veins, indicating a very vascular tumor. The tumor drains by way of the basal vein, which is extremely tortuous and enlarged (lower arrows), and thence into the straight sinus (posterior arrows). Such drainage indicates invasion of the brain.

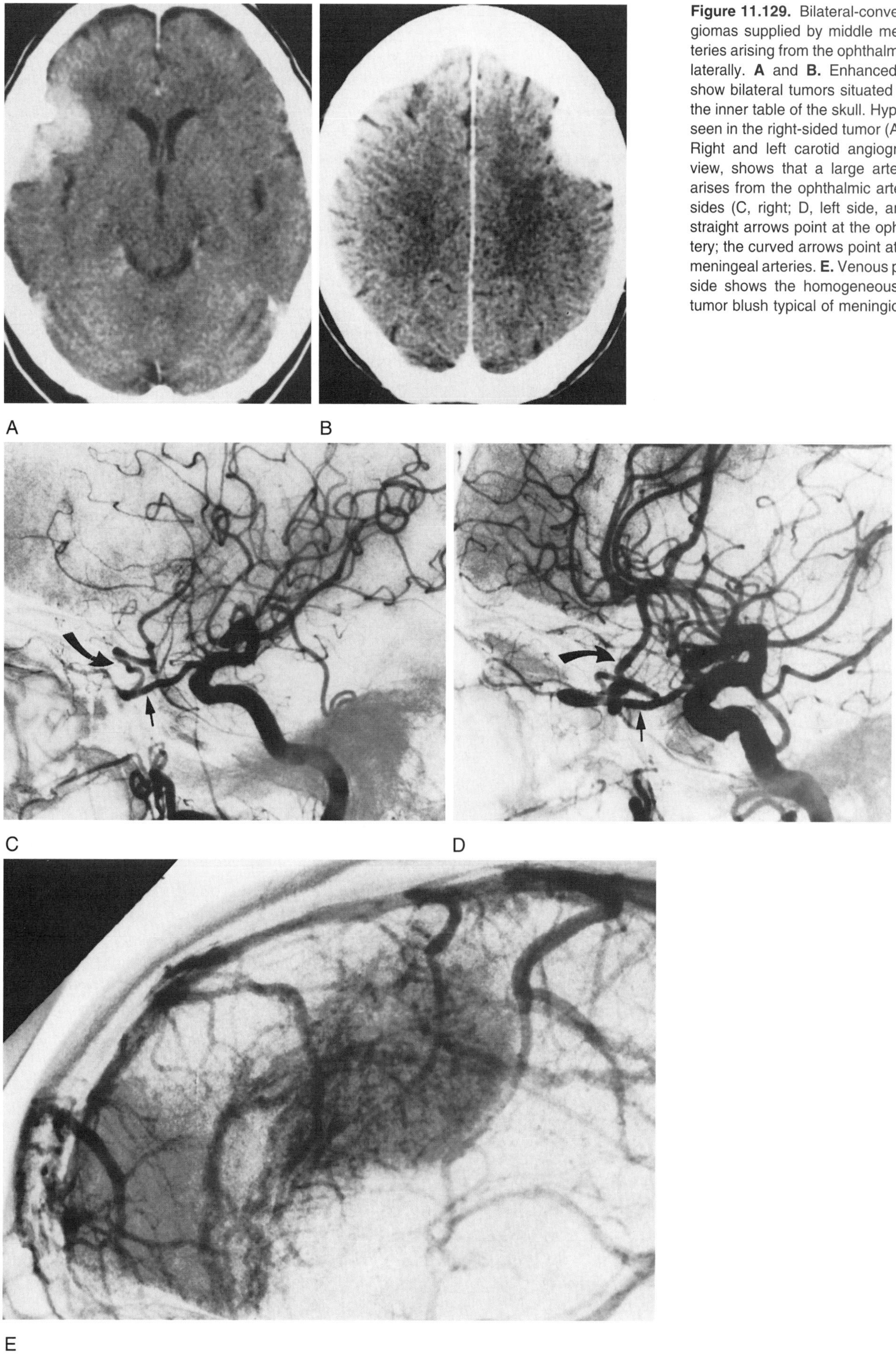

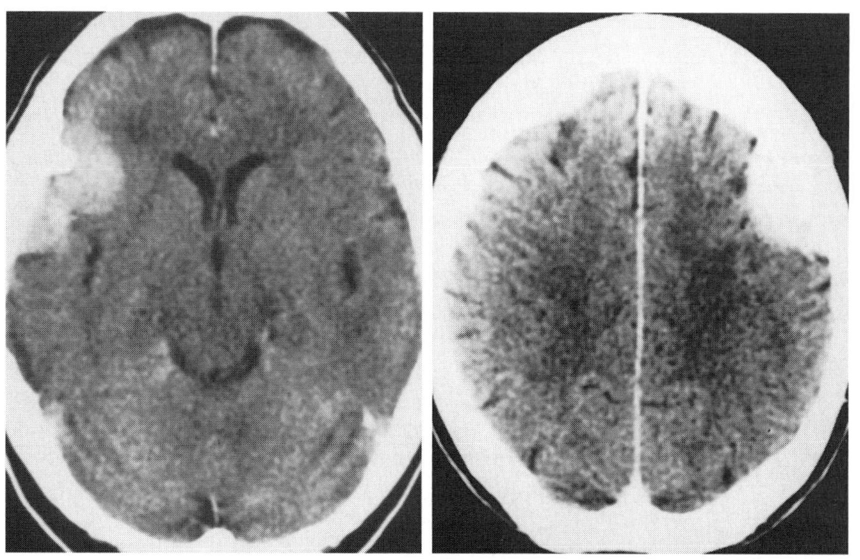

A B C D E

Figure 11.129. Bilateral-convexity meningiomas supplied by middle meningeal arteries arising from the ophthalmic artery bilaterally. **A** and **B.** Enhanced CT scans show bilateral tumors situated flat against the inner table of the skull. Hyperostosis is seen in the right-sided tumor (A). **C** and **D.** Right and left carotid angiogram, lateral view, shows that a large arterial branch arises from the ophthalmic artery on both sides (C, right; D, left side, arrows). The straight arrows point at the ophthalmic artery; the curved arrows point at the middle meningeal arteries. **E.** Venous phase of left side shows the homogeneous persistent tumor blush typical of meningiomas.

SKULL METASTATIC TUMORS

These are best studied by plain films of the skull or by nuclear medicine procedures for detection. However, if there is any question concerning their effect on intracranial structures, CT or MRI becomes necessary. The digital lateral view made prior to CT cross sections is often useful. It is easy to overlook skull metastases on both CT and MRI. When these are being sought, however, the rest of the skeleton should also be examined, in which case a radionuclide bone scan is most useful as a survey examination.

RECURRENCE OF MALIGNANT INTRACEREBRAL TUMORS

Tumor recurrence following either partial or "complete" surgical removal of intracerebral neoplasms is common. This is particularly true when dealing with malignant astrocytomas and glioblastoma multiforme. The oligodendrogliomas also recur, and the same is true of ependymomas. The intraventricular tumors other than ependymomas (e.g., choroid plexus papillomas) also usually recur, and they may also seed through the CSF. Medulloblastomas recur and, in addition, frequently seed through the CSF; some have been discussed and illustrated elsewhere (see Figs. 11.45 and 11.102).

The malignant astrocytomas and glioblastomas usually recur locally, but they can occasionally seed through the CSF. When they recur locally, the changes are usually fairly obvious; there is increased edema and contrast enhancement in the recurring tumor. In fact, the postcontrast examination is essential to determine whether a recurrence has taken place.

In the initial postoperative period, the surgeons are often interested in determining how much tumor was left behind. In these cases, the administration of contrast may give a false impression of residual tumor because the adjacent tissues affected by the surgical intervention and tumor removal may take up the contrast, particularly on MRI, indicating that there is a change in the blood-brain barrier. This finding can be seen in the first 2 to 12 weeks following the surgical intervention and disappear after that. Thus, if contrast uptake is seen after about 12 weeks, it can be taken as a sure indication of residual tumor. Forsting et al. (135) indicate that contrast enhancement in first 3 days after surgery, particularly as seen on MRI, is usually indicative of residual tumor. After that the contrast uptake cannot be attributed to residual tumor. Sometimes it is difficult to decide whether a residual postoperative cystic space found following the surgical removal contains any neoplastic cells around the wall. Usually the cystic space is peripheral and involves the meninges. The meninges usually take up contrast on MRI examination following a surgical intervention, as explained elsewhere, and the meningeal enhancement is considered as a postoperative change rather than a tumor effect around the postoperative cyst, unless the contrast uptake is on the brain side of the cyst.

Perhaps the most important consideration in diagnosing tumor recurrence following surgery and radiation therapy or radiation therapy alone involves the fact that radiation necrosis may be present, and this could produce a mass effect due to the accompanying edema; it would take up contrast material on both CT and MRI. Under these circumstances, it is usually necessary to try to determine which is present: recurrence or radiation necrosis. The best way to determine this is through positron emission tomography (PET) scanning. The tumor would usually show hypermetabolism as determined by either oxygen consumption or via fluorodeoxyglucose (Figs. 11.130 and 11.131). Lacking PET scanning, it may be possible to attempt single photon emission computed tomography (SPECT) examination for blood flow determination. The radiation necrosis will have very low blood flow, whereas a recurrent neoplasm would have increased blood flow through the area. In the future, it may be possible to accomplish this with MR functional imaging (local cerebral blood volume), but the reliability of this method has not yet been determined.

If none of these methods is available, a surgical biopsy is the only way to determine whether radiation necrosis or tumor occurrence is present. Usually radiation necrosis can be surgically resected with improvement of the patient's clinical condition.

EPILEPSY

The primary manifestations of epilepsy are paroxsymal changes in behavior caused by abnormalities in the electric activity of the brain. Each event is usually called a seizure, and there is a great variability in seizures, ranging from repetitive movements to a brief lapse in attention or a change of the individual's interaction with the environment. An epileptic seizure is due to a hypersynchronous and repetitive activation of neurons within the brain. A relatively small group of neurons on one side may have little behavior change whereas bilateral cortical discharges may produce an abrupt and prolonged loss of consciousness (136).

Epilepsy is a symptom of neurologic dysfunction. It may occur in some individuals with no apparent cause, whereas in others it may be attributable to an underlying structural or biochemical lesion in the CNS. Thus, a tumor, traumatic brain damage, a stroke, or cortical dysplasia due to abnormal cell migration may cause seizures.

The function of diagnostic imaging is to assist in the identification and localization of a lesion or lesions capable of causing epileptic seizures. Some areas of the cerebral cortex are more epileptogenic than others. The frontal and especially the temporal areas are usually considered to be particularly epileptogenic. Complex partial seizures usually originate in the temporal region. Any lesion of the brain that affects the cortical area may produce a focus of abnormal electric activity, which could cause a seizure to occur. The lesion may be posttraumatic, postinflammatory, vascular occlusive, an arteriovenous malformation, a neoplasm,

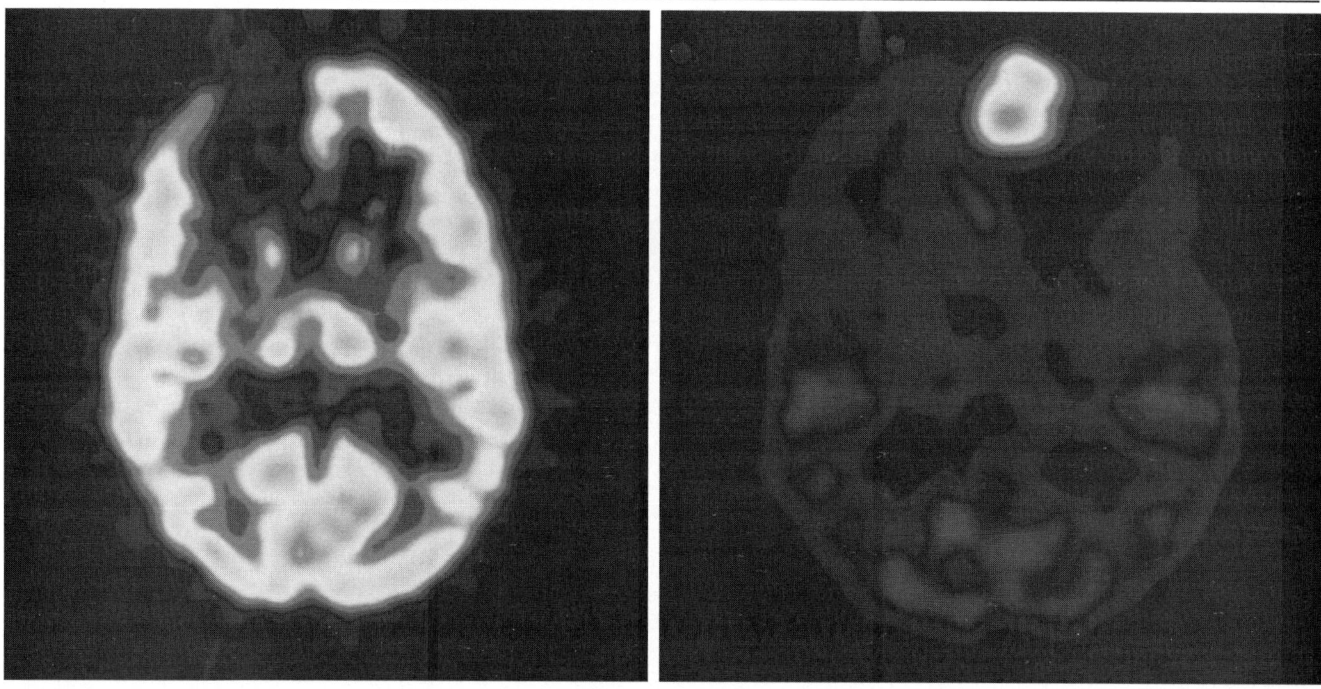

A B

Figure 11.130. Radionecrosis versus recurrent tumor evaluated by PET in two patients. The left image shows a lesion on the right frontal region (**A**) diagnosed as radionecrosis because it shows no metabolic activity. CT and MRI (not shown) revealed contrast enhancement indicating blood-brain barrier breakdown; tumor recurrence could not be excluded. **B.** The image on the right is from another patient, who presented essentially the same findings on CT and MRI (an enhancing lesion consistent with tumor recurrence). Fluorodeoxyglucose PET examination reveals high metabolic activity indicative of tumor recurrence.

hemorrhage, or a focus of demyelination that affects a cortical area. Ischemic lesions of the brain are very common, but they seldom produce seizures. Toxic agents often produce seizures; alcohol in excess or alcohol withdrawal after chronic abuse may lead to seizures.

In the great majority of seizure disorders no organic lesion is detectable, and they are likely to be controllable by medication; when there is an organic lesion, medication frequently fails to control the seizures completely. It is in this type of case that investigation with special variations of electroencephalography (EEG) and imaging techniques is needed. The majority of cases are generalized, and in about a third the seizures are classified as partial; among this group we consider simple partial and complex partial. Partial, secondarily generalized seizures are another group.

The complex partial seizures are quite variable. They usually present some impairment of consciousness, such as a vacant or glazed look, chewing, swallowing, singing, laughing, featuring, expressing fear or anger, or walking in circles. It was thought that they were all of temporal origin, so they were referred to as temporal lobe seizures, but it has been proven that they may also occur with frontal lobe lesions.

The location of the temporal focus varies and has been divided into opercular, temporal polar, basal or limbic, and mesial limbic types. In the frontal region, several recognized areas include the rolandic, supplementary motor, frontal polar, adversive, and pseudogeneralized areas.

In addition to EEG, with surface as well as deep electrodes, as needed, it is possible today to utilize a number of approaches to detect a possible focus. The primary approaches are CT, before and after contrast material; MRI, also without and with contrast; single photon emission tomography; and PET. CT and/or MRI may show a lesion that can be detected by these methods, such as neoplasm (Fig. 11.132). CT may demonstrate a calcification that is part of a neoplasm, or simply a decrease in the size of the temporal horn (Fig. 11.132), or the calcification may be an old inflammatory process. If it is neoplastic, MRI would reveal other abnormalities, such as T2 hyperintensity, but if it is a residual calcification from other causes, it may be overlooked by MRI. On the other hand, MRI will demonstrate many more deviations from normal than CT, such as medial temporal sclerosis, focal atrophy, and small neoplasms.

Mamourian and Brown suggest, on the basis of three cases, that the mammillary bodies may be related to the problem of seizures (137). They report three cases of partial complex or generalized seizures; these cases were not typical of partial complex seizures in all respects (138), but do raise the question of whether the mammillary system can

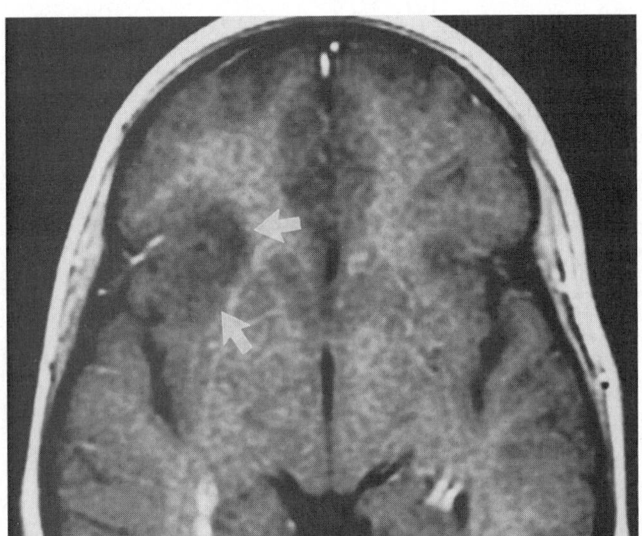

A

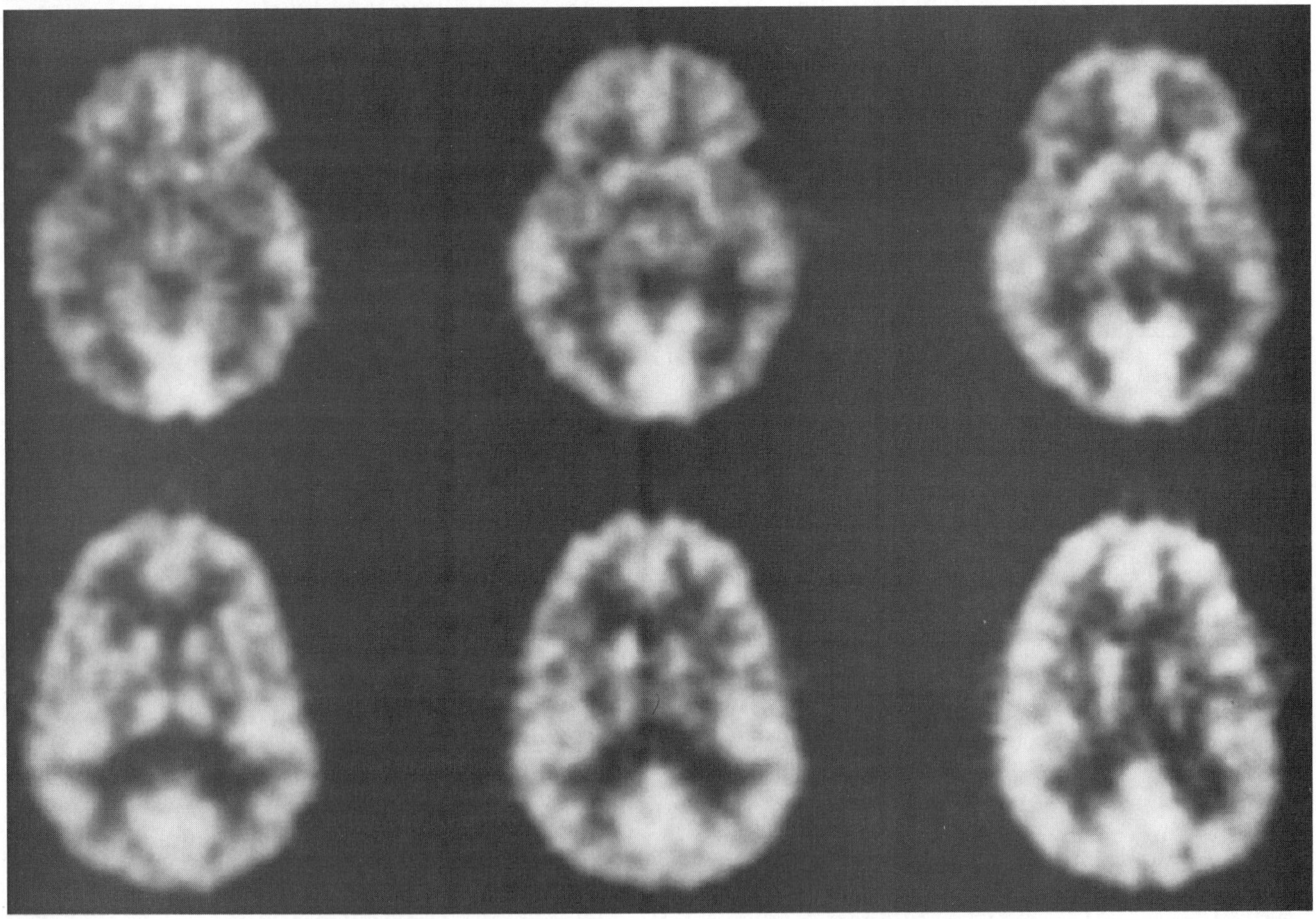

B

Figure 11.131. PET scan in a patient with a slowly growing astrocytoma. **A.** Postcontrast axial image reveals a nonenhancing low-intensity lesion in the right frontal operculum and insular regions with slight mass effect. **B.** A PET scan with fluorodeoxyglucose showed no increased metabolism in the area of the tumor.

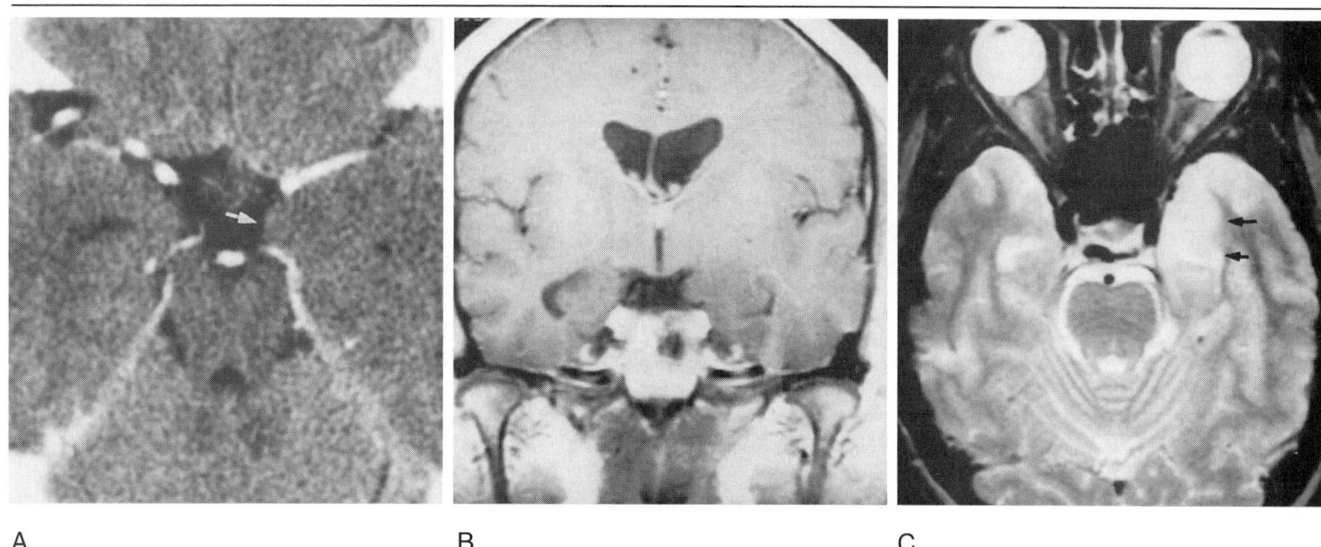

Figure 11.132. Temporal lobe tumor in a 26-year-old man with partial complex seizures. **A.** Contrast-enhanced CT axial image shows that the left temporal horn is small compared to the right. The medial margin of the hippocampus is sharper and slightly more medial than the right (arrow). **B.** Coronal postcontrast T1-weighted MR image shows no enhancement of the left temporal lobe. The temporal horn on the left is smaller, and again there is a slight suggestion of a mass effect; the medial hippocampal margin is more rounded on the left side. **C.** T2-weighted axial image shows hyperintensity in the medial temporal lobe due either to edema or infiltrating tumor (arrows). Low-grade astrocytoma.

serve as an important link mediating paroxysmal activity between the brainstem and forebrain in generalized epilepsy. It may also be involved in partial seizures, due to the close association with the hippocampus (Fig. 11.133).

Positron Emission Tomography

PET scanning may show increased blood flow and metabolism in focal areas of the brain during a seizure. The blood flow may also be measured with single photon emission tomography, or with xenon/CT (139). The metabolism, using PET, employs fluorine 18 deoxyglucose. The hypermetabolic rate may be seen well during the attacks, while in the interictal phase the same area may be hypometabolic. The latter may be more difficult to ascertain if the hypometabolic rate is slight compared with the other side (Fig. 11.134) (140,141).

Magnetic Resonance Imaging

On the other hand, MRI may show permanent changes that can be analyzed at any time, and comparison between MRI and CT shows that MRI is superior (142,143). The MRI findings, however, can be slight and must be interpreted with care. The anatomy of the hippocampus is best studied in coronal images and should be imaged without contrast and after contrast enhancement. T2-weighted images in the coronal plane are also needed. CT with xenon enhancement has also been suggested (144).

Hippocampal sclerosis appears to be by far the most common pathologic finding in patients with intractable temporal partial complex seizures (15 out of 21). Heinz et al. describe three findings: (a) decrease in size of the hippocampus as compared to the other side; (b) hyperintensity seen on proton density and on T2-weighted images; (c) loss of the sharp margin between the cortex of the parahippocampal complex and the subjacent collateral white matter, increased signal intensity in the white matter on T2, and decreased volumes of white matter (Heinz, 1993, personal communication) (145). Jack et al. (146), Ashtari et al. (147), and Free et al. (148) propose a method for determining the volume of the temporal lobe by MRI, but its accuracy in determining significant differences between the two sides in clinical cases requires more data.

Enlargement of the temporal horn as a sign of atrophy has been used since the advent of pneumoencephalography as an indication of the probable pathologic temporal lobe; this is often correct but is also frequently wrong. Enlargement of the anterior aspect of the temporal horn is commonly the only finding visible on CT, while MRI will demonstrate the enlargement of the horn, but also may show a decrease in size of the hippocampus and hyperintensity on T2-weighted images believed due to gliosis.

Bronen et al. (149) indicate that the best coronal image for comparison between the two sides is the one passing through the red nucleus of the midbrain or one passing through the immediate area (Fig. 11.135), because it shows more details of the hippocampal body. They also used the height multiplied by the width to compare the two sides. In order to obtain the product of two comparable measurements, they corrected for angulation of the coronal plane

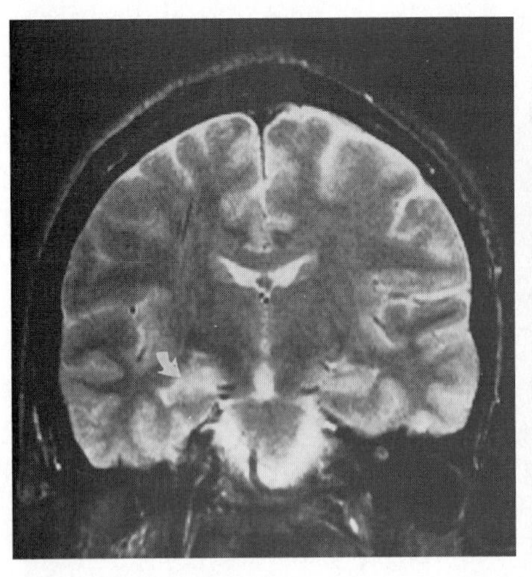

A

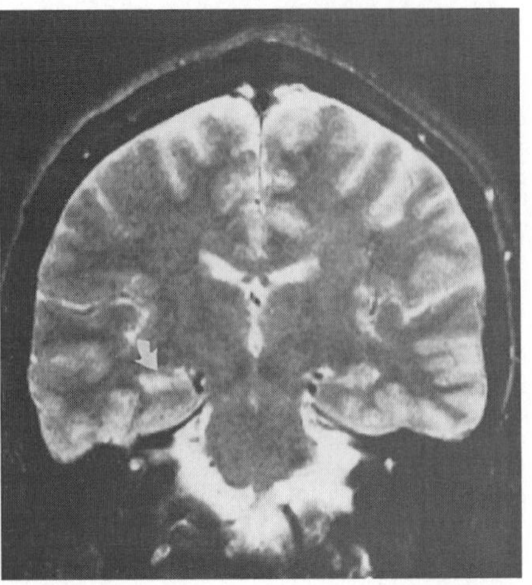

B

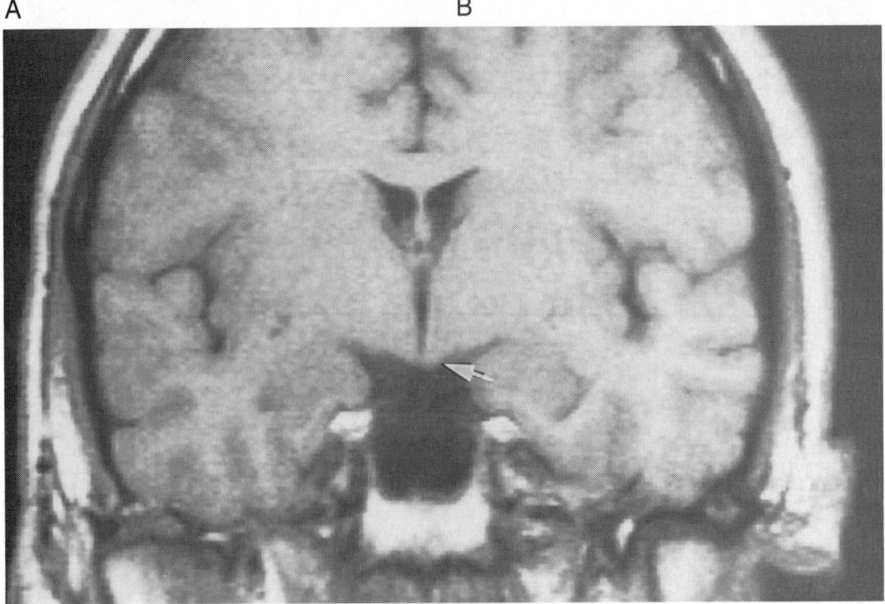

C

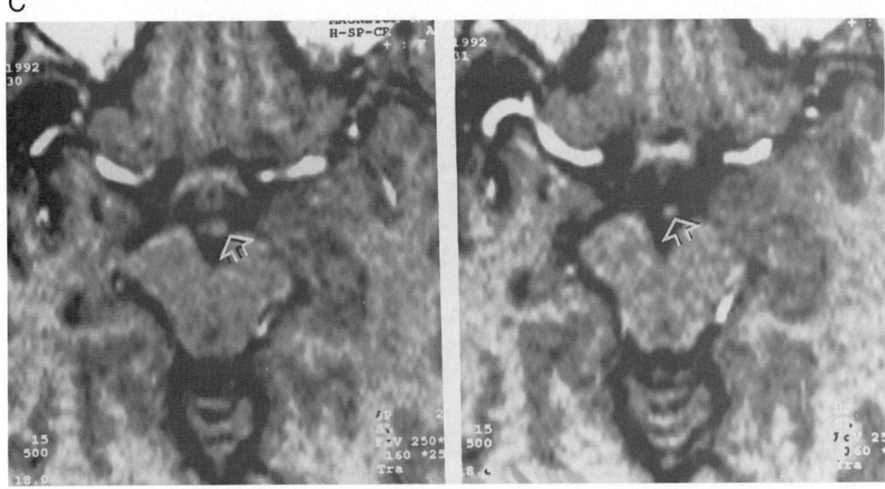

D E

Figure 11.133. A 33-year-old man with intractable epilepsy. **A** and **B.** The coronal MR scan (2500/90) demonstrated increased signal in the right hippocampus (arrow) compared with the left, consistent with hippocampal sclerosis. **C.** The coronal scan (600/15) through the mamillary bodies revealed a smaller mamillary body on the side of the hippocampal sclerosis. The left mamillary body appeared normal (arrow). **D** and **E.** The axial reformation of 1.0-mm sections from a magnitude preparation–rapid acquisition gradient-echo sequence demonstrated a smaller right than left mamillary body (arrow). (Courtesy of Dr. A Mamourian, Dartmouth, NH. AJNR 1993;14:1332–1335.)

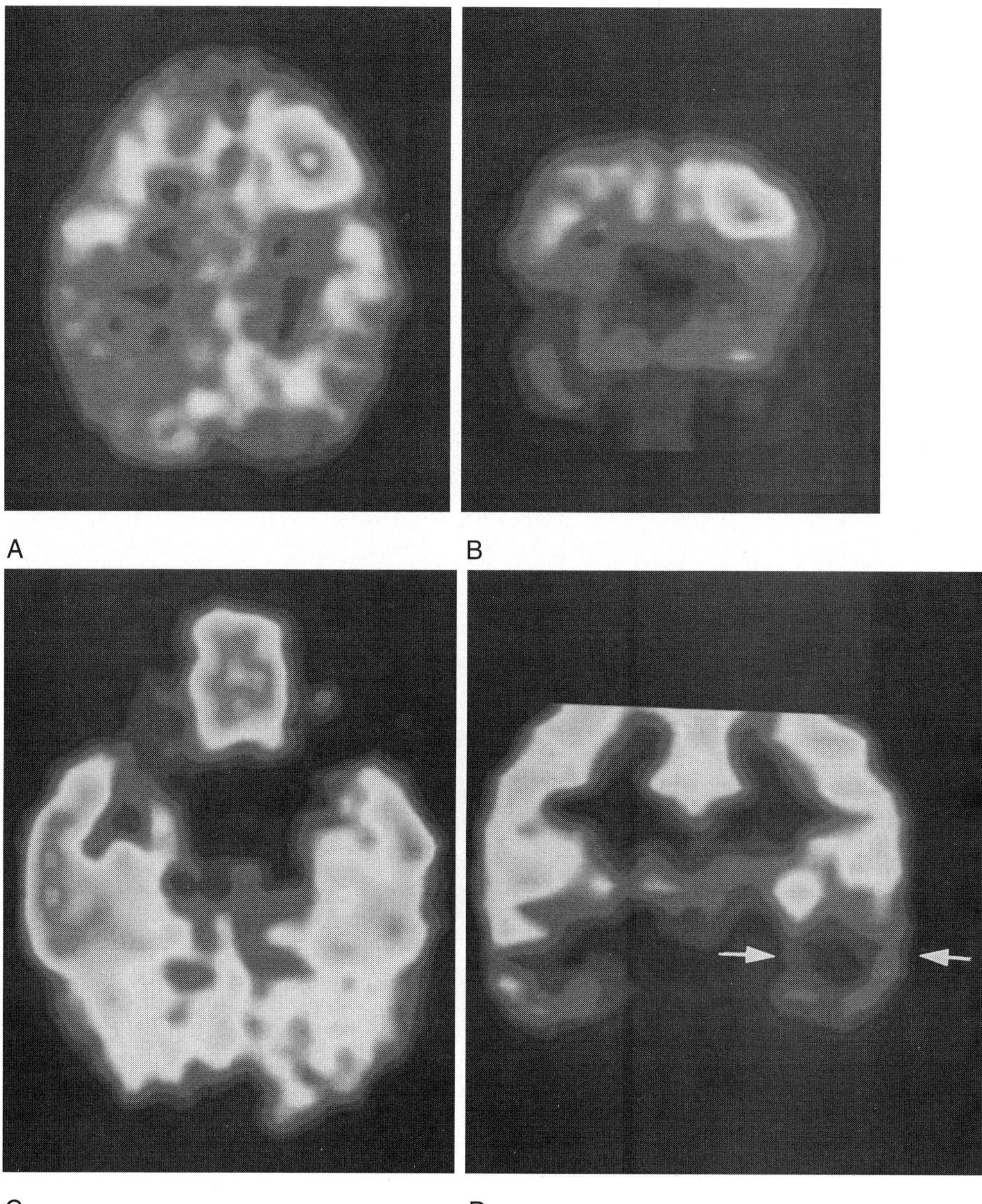

Figure 11.134. PET scans in patients with partial complex epilepsy. **A** and **B.** In a child shortly after attack there is a marked increase in activity in the left frontal region, shown in axial (A) and coronal (B) views. **C** and **D.** On another patient in the interictal stage a decrease in activity on the pathologic left temporal region as compared to the opposite, normal, side is more apparent in the coronal plane (arrows). (Courtesy of Dr. Allen Fischman, Massachusetts General Hospital, Boston, Mass.)

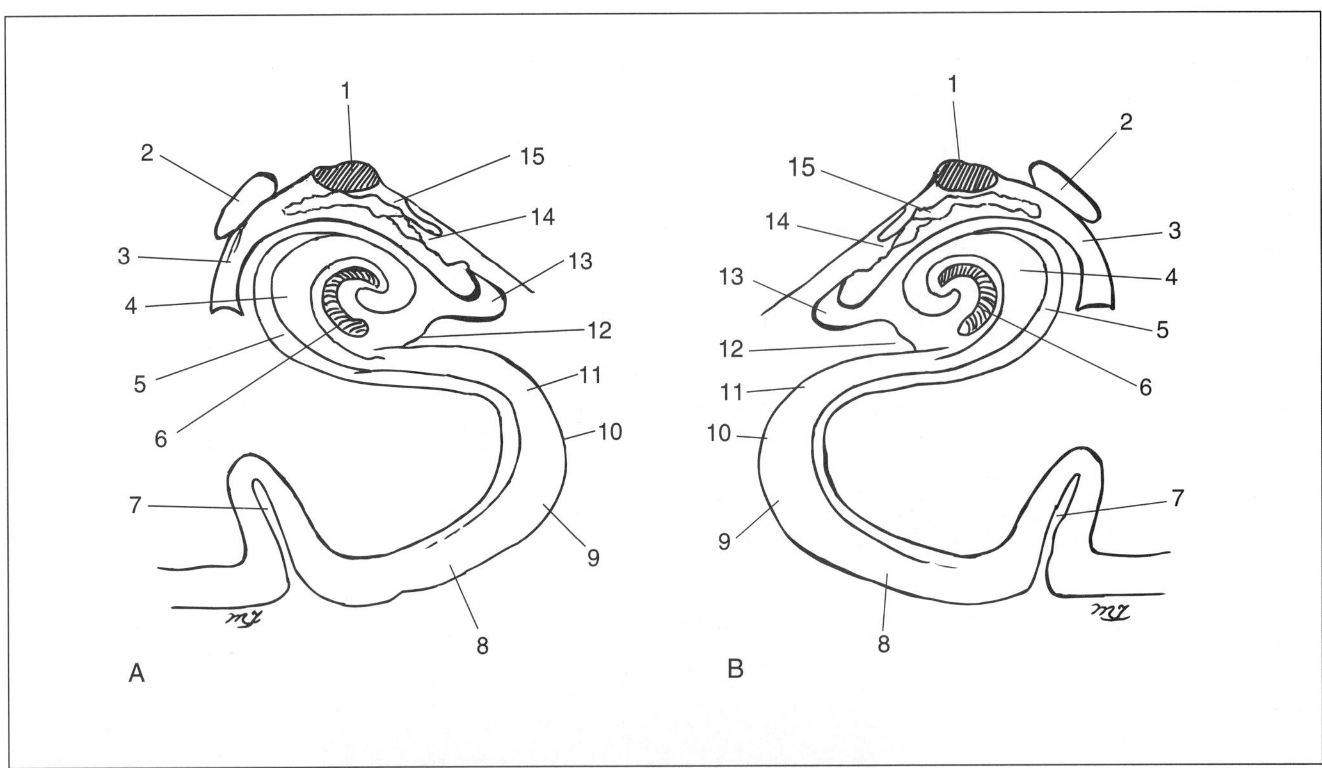

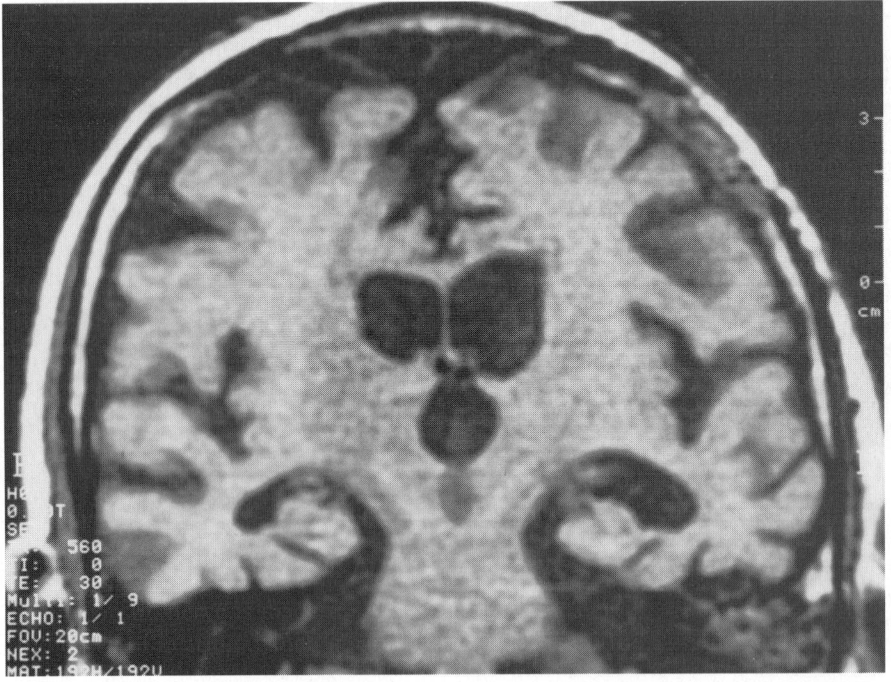

C

Figure 11.135. A and **B.** Diagram of a cross section of the hippocampus, right and left sides. (1) Optic tract; (2) caudate nucleus; (3) temporal horn of lateral ventricle; (4) hippocampal formation; (5) alveus; (6) dentate gyrus; (7) collateral sulcus; (8) parahippocampal gyrus; (9) presubiculum; (10) subiculum; (11) prosubiculum; (12) hippocampal fissure; (13) fimbria; (14) choroid fissure; (15) choroid plexus. **C.** Coronal section passing through the anterior hippocampus in a patient with moderate cerebral atrophy. The section passes through the anterior pons, the preferred level to visualize hippocampal sclerosis (see also Fig. 3.26).

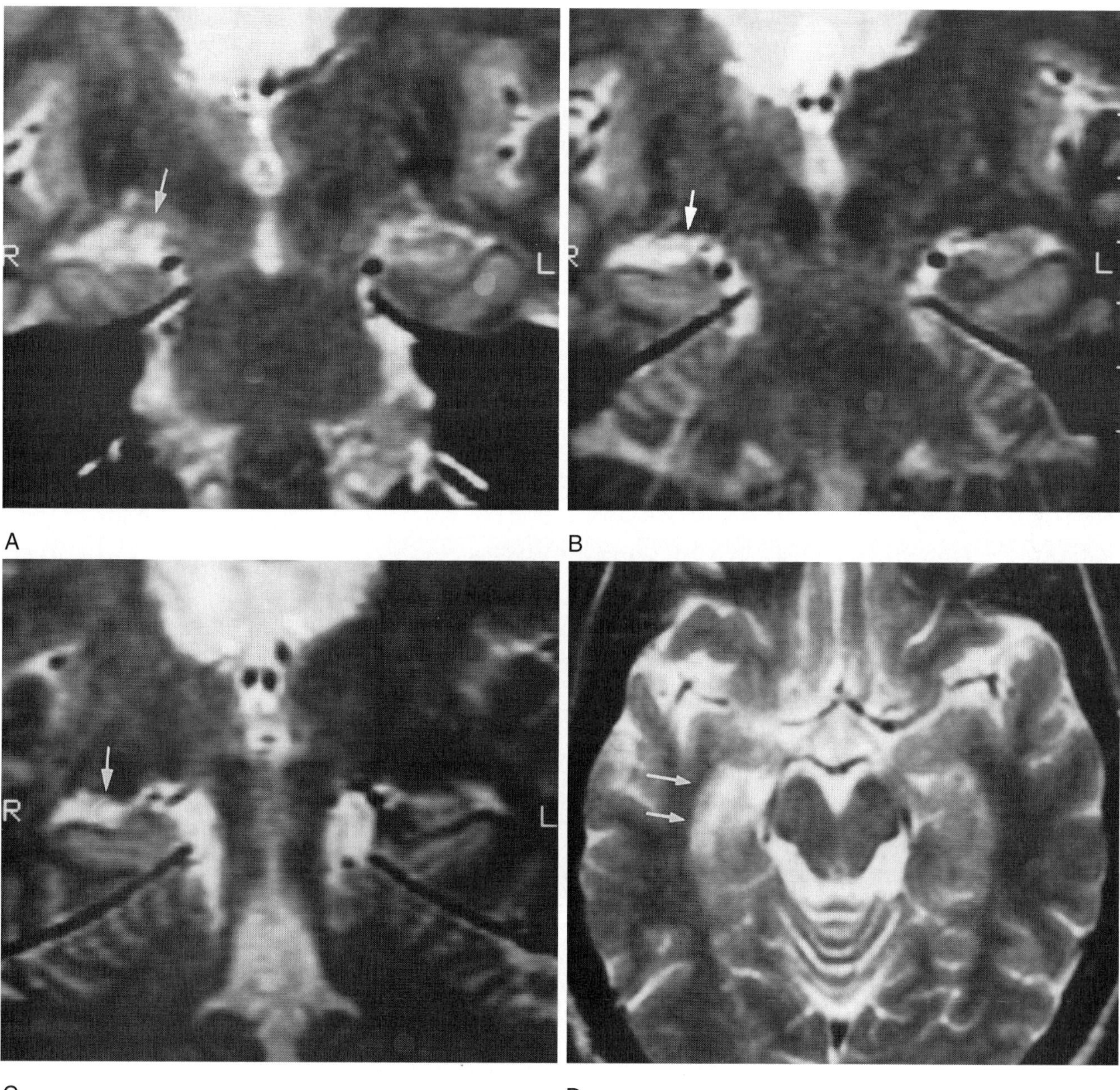

Figure 11.136. Forty-year-old man with chronic partial complex seizures due to hippocampal sclerosis. **A** to **C.** Coronal T2-weighted sections passing through the anterior hippocampus 6 mm apart. There is hyperintensity in the right hippocampus (arrow) as compared with the left due to hippocampal sclerosis. Below the hippocampus is the parahippocampal gyrus, which is smaller than the one on the other side. The temporal horn, which surrounds the superior aspect of the hippocampus, is often enlarged. There is usually a decrease in the vertical diameter of the hippocampus, often also involving the parahippocampal gyrus in cases of medial temporal sclerosis. The coronal T1-weighted images serve to separate the enlarged temporal horn from the sclerotic hippocampus. **D.** Axial T2-weighted image demonstrates the T2 hyperintensity on the right hippocampus (arrows).

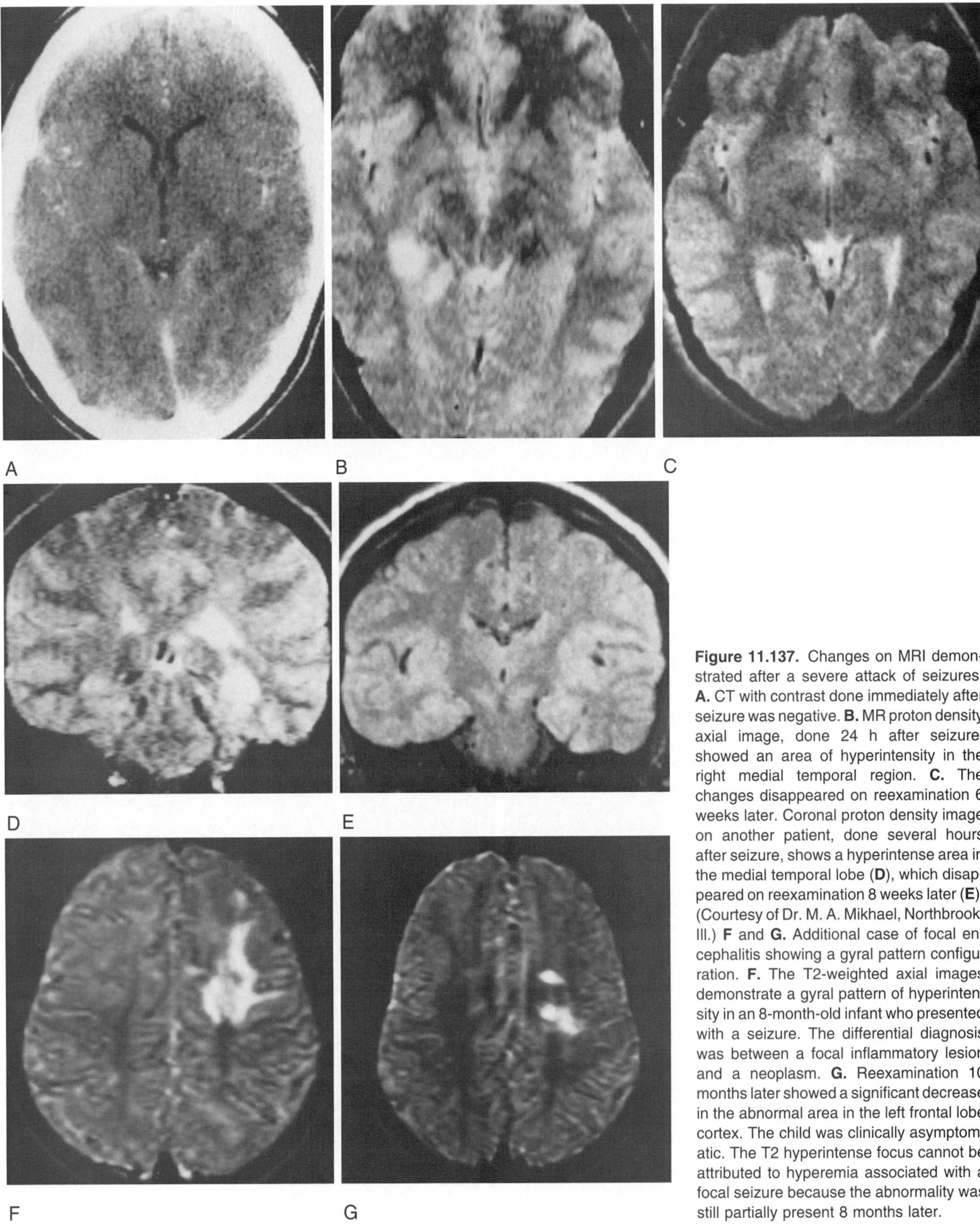

Figure 11.137. Changes on MRI demonstrated after a severe attack of seizures. **A.** CT with contrast done immediately after seizure was negative. **B.** MR proton density axial image, done 24 h after seizure, showed an area of hyperintensity in the right medial temporal region. **C.** The changes disappeared on reexamination 6 weeks later. Coronal proton density image on another patient, done several hours after seizure, shows a hyperintense area in the medial temporal lobe (**D**), which disappeared on reexamination 8 weeks later (**E**). (Courtesy of Dr. M. A. Mikhael, Northbrook, Ill.) **F** and **G.** Additional case of focal encephalitis showing a gyral pattern configuration. **F.** The T2-weighted axial images demonstrate a gyral pattern of hyperintensity in an 8-month-old infant who presented with a seizure. The differential diagnosis was between a focal inflammatory lesion and a neoplasm. **G.** Reexamination 10 months later showed a significant decrease in the abnormal area in the left frontal lobe cortex. The child was clinically asymptomatic. The T2 hyperintense focus cannot be attributed to hyperemia associated with a focal seizure because the abnormality was still partially present 8 months later.

with the angle of the temporal horn as seen on sagittal views. The assumption is that the vertical diameter of the hippocampus is shortest if measured along a line perpendicular to the direction of the hippocampus. This is more important when comparing sizes in a group of cases, but if one only needs to compare the right with the left side, both sides are presumably cut at the same oblique angle (Figs. 11.135 and 11.136; see also Fig. 3.26).

CT as well as MRI will demonstrate many other larger lesions encountered in patients with intractable seizures resulting from trauma, cerebral infarction, and severe inflammatory lesions. Some may require hemispherectomy for control (150).

Other uses for MRI in patients with epilepsy include the possibility of determining the relationship of an epileptic focus, detected by CT, MRI, and possibly by PET scanning, to the elocuent (motor, speech, and sensory) areas of the brain prior to surgical intervention (also see under "Functional Neuroimaging," Chapter 14).

Concerning the relative accuracy of the three principal diagnostic methods, EEG is still the most important, since it has the highest percentage of positive findings. MRI and PET are about equal, and it is advisable to do both prior to surgical intervention, particularly in cases of partial complex seizure with temporal lobe localization. The results of surgery in these cases are good if the correct side was operated on (151). The chronically implanted electrodes for depth EEG recording may have some complications (152).

Finally it must be stated that MRI may demonstrate an abnormality, hyperintensity on T2-weighted images in a focal area in the postictal period. The abnormality may last for a few days, and will disappear in a few weeks. Thus reexamination is recommended in cases where MRI examination soon after a seizure shows changes without a mass effect, in order to exclude the possibility of postictal change (153) (Fig. 11.137). In addition to glioma and hippocampal sclerosis Lehericy et al. report some significant minor abnormalities in the hippocampus that can be detected on MRI (154). Among these they list focal gray matter heterotopia, focal cortical dysgeneses such as cortical thickening, poor gray/white demarcation, and abnormal gyration.

REFERENCES

1. Zülch KJ: Histological typing of tumors of the central nervous system. International Histologic Classification of Tumors, No. 21. Geneva: World Health Organization, 1979.
2. Bonnin JM, Garcia JH: Histology and growth characteristics of brain neoplasms. In JM Taveras, J Ferrucci (eds), Radiology: Diagnosis/Imaging/Intervention. Philadelphia: Lippincott, 1986, vol 3, chap 52.
3. Berens ME, Rutka JT, Rosenblum ML: Brain tumor epidemiology, growth, and invasion. Neurosurg Clin N Am 1990;1:1–18.
4. Russell DS, Rubinstein LJ: Pathology of Tumors of the Nervous System, ed 5. Baltimore: Williams and Wilkins, 1989.
5. Takeuchi J, Handa H: Spontaneous extracranial metastasis of cerebral neuroblastoma. Surg Neurol 1979;12:337.
6. Jack CR, O'Neill BP, Banks PM, et al: Central nervous system lymphoma: Histologic types and CT appearance. Radiology 1988; 167:211–215.
7. Kleinman GM, Hochberg FH, Richardson EP: Systemic metastases from medulloblastoma: Report of two cases and review of the literature. Cancer 1981;48:2296.
8. Horton BC, Ulrich H, Rubinstein LJ, et al: The angioblastic meningioma: A reappraisal of a nosological problem. J Neurol Sci 1977; 31:387.
9. Horowitz BL, Chari MV, James R, Bryan RN: MR of intracranial epidermoid tumor: Correlations of in vivo imaging with in vitro 13C spectroscopy. AJNR 1990;11:299–302.
10. Sweet WH: Radical surgical treatment of craniopharyngioma. Clin Neurosurg 1976;23:52.
11. Humphreys RP, Hoffman HJ, Hendrick EB: A long term postoperative follow-up in craniopharyngioma. Childs Brain 1979;5:530.
12. Christensen WN, Long DM, Epstein JI: Cerebellopontine angle lipoma. Hum Pathol 1986;17:739.
13. Cavanaugh JB: On certain small tumors encountered in the temporal lobe. Brain 1958;81:389–405.
14. Gherardi R, Lacombe MJ, Poirer J, et al: Asymptomatic encephalic intraparenchymatous neuroepithelial cysts. Acta Neuropathol 1984;63:264.
15. Ghatak NR, Mushrush GJ: Supratentorial intra-arachnoid cyst. J Neurosurg 1971;35:477–482.
16. Brooks BS, El Gammal T, Allison ID, et al: Frequency and variation of the posterior pituitary bright signal on MR images. AJNR 1989;10:943–948.
17. Humes RA, Roskamp K, Eisenbrey AB: Melanosis and hydrocephalus: Report of four cases. J Neurosurg 1984;61:365.
18. Aoki S, Barkovich AJ, Nishimura K, et al: Neurofibromatosis types 1 and 2: Cranial MR findings. Radiology 1989;172:527–534.
19. National Institutes of Health Consensus Development: Neurofibromatosis. Arch Neurol 1988;45:575–578.
20. Riccardi VM: Von Recklinghausen neurofibromatosis. N Engl J Med 1981;305:1617–1627.
21. Mirowitz S, Sartor K, Gado M: High intensity basal ganglia lesions on T1-weighted MR images in neurofibromatosis. AJNR 1989;10: 1159–1163.
22. Martuza RL, Eldridge R: Neurofibromatosis 2 (bilateral acoustic neurofibromatosis). N Engl J Med 1988;318:684–688.
23. Cushing H, Eisenhardt L: Meningiomas. Springfield: Thomas, 1938, p 76.
24. Fischman AJ, McKusick KA: Single photon radionuclide imaging of the brain. In JM Taveras, J Ferrucci (eds), Radiology: Diagnosis/Imaging/Intervention. Philadelphia: Lippincott, 1995, vol 3, chap 27A, pp 1–12.
25. Sage MR: Review. Blood-brain barrier: Phenomenon of increasing importance to the imaging clinician. AJNR 1982;138:887–898.
26. Newhouse JH: Fluid compartment distribution of intravenous Iothalamate on the dog. Invest Radiol 1974;9:241.
27. Putnam TJ: The intercolumnar tubercle, an undescribed area in the anterior wall of the third ventricle. Johns Hopkins Med Bull 1922;33:181–182.
28. Blomstand C, Johansson B, Rosengren B: Dexamethasone effect on blood-brain damage caused by acute hypertension in x-irradiated rabbits. Acta Neurol Scand 1975;52:331–334.
29. Haustein J, Laniado M, Niendorf H-P, et al: Administration of gadopentetate dimeglumine in MR imaging of intracranial tumors: Dosage and field strength. AJNR 1992;13:1199–1206.
30. Mørk SJ, Lindegaard K-F, Halvorsen TB, et al: Oligodendrogliomas: Incidence and biological behaviour in a defined population. J Neurosurg 1985;63:881–889.
31. Wiegel B, Harris TM, Edwards MK, et al: MR of intracranial neuroblastoma with dural sinus invasion and distant metastases. AJNR 1991;12:1198–1200.
32. Benitez WI, Glasier CM, Husain M, et al: MR findings in childhood ganglioglioma. J Comput Assist Tomogr 1990;14:712–716.
33. Johannsson JH, Rekate HL, Roessmann U: Gangliogliomas: Pathological and clinical correlation. J Neurosurg 1981;54:58–63.

34. Perkins OC: Ganglioglioma. Arch Pathol 1926;2:11–17.
35. Courville CB: Ganglioglioma: Tumor of the central nervous system. Review of the literature and report of two cases. Arch Neurol Psychiatry 1930;24:439–491.
36. Mirich DR, Blaser SI, Harwood-Nash DC, et al: Melanotic neuroectodermal tumor of infancy: Clinical, radiologic, and pathologic findings in five cases. AJNR 1991;12:689–697.
37. Lee J, Krol G, Rosenblum M: Primary amyloidoma of the brain: CT and MR presentation. AJNR 1995;16:712–714.
38. Partlow GD, del Carpio-O'Donovan R, Melanson D, et al: Bilateral thalamic glioma: Review of eight cases with personality change and mental deterioration. AJNR 1992;13:1225–1230.
39. Spoto GP, Press GA, Hesselink JR, et al: Intracranial ependymoma and subependymoma: MR manifestations. AJNR 1990;13:83–91.
40. Morrison G, Sobel DF, Kelley WM, et al: Intraventricular mass lesions. Radiology 1984;153:435–442.
41. Nakase H, Marimoto T, Sakaku T: Bilateral choroid plexus cysts in the lateral ventricles. AJNR 1991;12:1204.
42. Czervionke LF, Daniels DL, Meyer GA, et al: Neuroepithelial cysts of the lateral ventricles: MR appearance. AJNR 1987;8:609–613.
43. Ribeiro C, Medeiros E, Ferreira F, et al: Oligodendrogliomas intraventriculares. Acta Radiol Portuguesa 1992;4:39–42.
44. Smoker WRK, Townsend JJ, Reichman ML: Neurocytoma accompanied by intraventricular hemorrhage: Case report and literature review. AJNR 1991;12:765–770.
45. Wilms G, Marchal G, Van Hecke P, et al: Colloid cysts of the third ventricle: MR findings. J Comput Assist Tomogr 1990;14(4):527–531.
46. Waggenspack GA, Guinto FC: MR and CT of masses of the anterosuperior third ventricle. AJNR 1989;10:105–110.
47. Kondziolka D, Lunsford LD: Stereotactic management of colloid cysts: Factors predicting success. J Neurosurg 1991;75:45–51.
48. Tada M, Koiwa M, Chono Y, et al: Neuroepithelial (colloid) cyst of the cerebellar vermis containing a xanthogranuloma. AJNR 1993;14:951–953.
49. Shuangshoti S, Phonprasert C, Suwanuela N, et al: Combined neuroepithelial (colloid) cyst and xanthogranuloma (xanthoma) in the third ventricle. Neurology 1975;25:547–552.
50. Black ML, Tien RD, Hesselink JR: Third ventricular hemangioblastoma: MR appearance. AJNR 1991;12:553.
51. Wiot JG, Lukin RR, Tomsick TA: Xanthogranuloma of the third ventricle. AJNR 1989;10:S57.
52. Tatter SB, Ogilvy CS, Golden JA, et al: Third ventricular xanthogranulomas clinically and radiologically mimicking colloid cysts: Report of two cases. J Neurosurg 1994;81:605–609.
53. Vaquero J, Martinez R, Escandron J, et al: Symptomatic glial cysts of the pineal gland. Surg Neurol 1988;30:468–470.
54. Mamourian AC, Yarnell T: Enhancement of pineal cysts on MR images. AJNR 1991;12:773–774.
55. Smirniotopoulos JG, Rushing EJ, Mena H: Pineal region masses: Differential diagnosis. Radiographics 1992;12:577–596.
56. Ganti SR, Hilal SK, Stein BM, et al: CT of pineal region tumors. AJNR 1986;7:97–104.
57. Mathews VP, Broome DR, Smith RR, et al: Neuroimaging of disseminated germ cell neoplasms. AJNR 1990;11:319–324.
58. Berger MS, Baumeiser B, Geyer JR, et al: The risks of metastases from shunting in children with primary central nervous system tumors. J Neurosurg 1991;74:872–877.
59. Rosenfeld JV, Murphy MA, Chow CW: Implantation metastasis of pineoblastoma after stereotactic biopsy—case report. J Neurosurg 1990;73:287–290.
60. Tien RD, Barkovich AJ, Edwards MSB: MR imaging of pineal tumors. AJNR 1990;11:557–565.
61. Mathews FD: Intraventricular craniopharyngioma. AJNR 1983;4:984–985.
62. Burton EM, Ball WS, Crone K, et al: Hamartoma of the tuber cinereum: A comparison of MR and CT findings in four cases. AJNR 1989;10:497–501.
63. Culler FL, James HE, Simon ML, et al: Identification of gonadotropin-releasing hormone in neurons of a hypothalamic hamartoma in a boy with precocious puberty. Neurosurgery 1985;17:408.
64. Albright L, Lee PA: Neurosurgical treatment of hypothalamic hamartomas causing precocious puberty. J Neurosurg 1993;78:77–82.
65. Hubbard AM, Egelhoff JC: MR imaging of large hypothalamic hamartomas in two infants. AJNR 1989;10:1277–1279.
66. Rieth KG, Comite F, Dwyer AJ, et al: CT of cerebral abnormalities in precocious puberty. AJNR 1987;8:283–290.
67. Lin SR, Bryson MM, Goblen RP, et al: Radiologic findings of hamartomas of the tuber cinereum and hypothalamus. Radiology 1987;127:697–703.
68. Iafolla K, Fratkin JD, Spiegel PK, et al: Case report and delineation of the congenital hypothalamic hamartoblastoma syndrome (Pallister-Hall syndrome). Am J Med Gene 1989;33:489–499.
69. Kucharczyk W, Lenkinski RE, Kucharczyk J, et al: The effect of phospholipid vesicles on the NMR relaxation of water: An explanation for the appearance of the neurohypophysis? AJNR 1990;11:693–700.
70. Simmons GE, Suchnicki JE, Rakk M, et al: MR imaging of the pituitary stalk: Size, shape, and enhancement pattern. AJR 1992;159:375–377.
71. Kelly WM, Kucharczyk W, Kucharczyk J, et al: Posterior pituitary ectopia: An MR feature of pituitary dwarfism. AJNR 1988;9:453–450.
72. Abrahms JJ, Trefelner E, Boulware SD: Idiopathic growth hormone deficiency: MR findings in 35 patients. AJNR 1991;12:155–160.
73. Kuroiwa T, Okabe Y, Hasuo K, et al: MR imaging of pituitary dwarfism. AJNR 1991;12:161–164.
74. Kaufman B, Tumsak RL, Kaufman BA, et al: Herniation of suprasellar visual system and third ventricle into empty sellae: Morphologic and clinical considerations. AJNR 1989;10:65–76.
75. Elster AD: Modern imaging of the pituitary. Radiology 1993;189:1–14.
76. Krawchenko J, Collins GH: Pathology of an arachnoid cyst. J Neurosurg 1979;50:224–228.
77. Wolpert SM, Osborne M, Anderson M, et al: The bright pituitary gland: A normal MR appearance in infancy. AJNR 1988;9:1–3.
78. Cox TD, Elster AD: Normal pituitary gland: Changes in shape, size, and signal intensity during the 1st year of life at MR imaging. Radiology 1991;179:721–724.
79. Kaufman B: The "empty" sella turcica: A manifestation of the intrasellar subarachnoid space. Radiology 1968;90:931–941.
80. Scheithauer BW: Surgical pathology of the pituitary: The adenomas. Pathology Annual 1984;19(2):269.
81. Saeger W, Lüdecke DK: Pituitary adenoma with hyperfunction of TSH. Frequency, histological classification, immunohistochemistry and ultrastructure. Virchows Archive A (Pathological Anatomy and Histology) 1982;394:255.
82. Kovacs K, Horvath E, Rewcastle NB, et al: Gonadotroph cell adenoma of the pituitary in a woman with longstanding hypogonadism. Arch Gynecol 1980;229:57.
83. Kovacs K, Horvath E: Pituitary chromophobe adenoma composed of oncocytes: A light and electron microscopic study. Arch Pathol 1973;95:235.
84. Cone L, Srinivasan M, Flaviu C, et al: Granular cell tumor (choristoma) of the neurohypophysis: Two cases and a review of the literature. AJNR 1990;11:403–406.
85. Sakamoto Y, Takahashi M, Korogi Y, et al: Normal and abnormal pituitary glands: Gadopentate dimeglumine-enhanced MR imaging. Radiology 1991;178:441–445.

86. Yuh WT, Fisher DJ, Nguyen HD, et al: Sequential MR enhancement pattern in normal pituitary gland and in pituitary adenoma. AJNR 1994;15:101–108.
87. Marcovitz S, Wee R, Chan J, et al: The diagnostic accuracy of preoperative CT scanning in the evaluation of pituitary ACTH-secreting adenomas. AJR 1987;149:803–806.
88. Marcovitz S, Wee R, Chan J, et al: Diagnostic accuracy of preoperative CT scanning of pituitary prolactinomas. AJNR 1988;9:13–17.
89. Marcovitz S, Wee R, Chan JD, et al: Diagnostic accuracy of preoperative CT scanning of pituitary somatotroph adenomas. AJNR 1988;9:19–22.
90. Newton DR, Dillon WP, Norman D, et al: Gd-DTPA-enhanced MR imaging of pituitary adenomas. AJNR 1989;10:949–954.
91. Scheithauer BW, Kovacs DT, Lows ER, et al: Pathology of invasive pituitary tumors with special reference to functional classification. J Neurosurg 1986;65:733–744.
92. Ostrov SG, Quencer RM, Hoffman JC, et al: Hemorrhage within pituitary adenomas: How often associated with pituitary apoplexy syndrome? AJNR 1989;10:503.
93. Provenzale JM, Hacein-Bey L, Taveras JM: Pituitary apoplexy associated with carotid dissection: MR findings. J Comput Assist Tomogr 1995;19:150–152.
94. Momose JK, New PFJ: Non-atheromatous stenosis and occlusion of the internal carotid artery and its main branches. Am J Roentgenol 1973;118:550–566.
95. Kucharczyk W, Montanera WJ: The sella and parasellar region. In SW Atlas (ed), Magnetic Resonance Imaging of the Brain and Spine. New York: Raven, 1991, p 625.
96. Pusey E, Kortman KE, Flannigan BD, et al: MR of craniophyngioma: Tumor delineation and characterization. AJNR 1987;8: 439–444.
97. Price AC, Runge V, Allen JH, et al: Craniopharyngioma: Correlation of high resolution CT and MRI. AJNR 1985;6:465.
98. Hoffman HJ, Hendricks B, Humphries RP, et al: Investigation and management of suprasellar arachnoid cysts. J Neurosurg 1982;57: 597–602.
99. Starkman SP, Brown TC, Linell EA: Cerebral arachnoid cysts. J Neuropath Exp Neurol 1958;17:484–500.
100. Fox JL, Al-Mefty O: Suprasellar arachnoid cysts: An extension of the membrane of Liliequist. Neurosurgery 1980;7:615–618.
101. Domingue JN, Wilson CB: Pituitary abscesses. J Neurosurg 1977; 46:601–608.
102. Enzman DR, Sieling RJ: CT of pituitary abscess. AJNR 1983;4: 79–80.
103. Quencer RM: Lymphocytic adenohypophysitis: Autoimmune disorder of the pituitary gland. AJNR 1989;1:343–345.
104. Hungerford GD, Biggs PJ, Levine JH, et al: Lymphoid adenohypophysitis with radiologic and clinical findings resembling a pituitary tumor. AJNR 1982;3:444–446.
105. Tien RD, Newton TH, McDermott MW, et al: Thickened pituitary stalk on MR images in patients with diabetes insipidus and Langerhans cell histiocytosis. AJNR 1990;11:703–708.
106. Greenberger JS, Cassady JR, Jaffe N, et al: Radiation therapy in patients with histiocytosis-X: Management of diabetes insipidus and bone lesions. Int J Radiat Oncol Biol Phys 1975;5:1749–1755.
107. Appignani B, Landy H, Barnes P: MR in idiopathic central diabetes insipidus in childhood. AJNR 1993;14:1407–1410.
108. Yousem DM, Atlas SW, Grossman RI, et al: MR imaging of Tolosa-Hunt syndrome. AJNR 1989;10:1181–1184.
109. Kwan ESK, Wolpert SM, Hedges TR III, et al: Tolosa-Hunt syndrome revisited: Not necessarily a diagnosis of exclusion. AJNR 1987;8:1067–1072; AJR 1988;150:413–418.
110. Bencherif B, Zouaoui A, Chedid G, et al: Intracranial extension of an idiopathic orbital inflammatory pseudotumor. AJNR 1993;14: 181–184.
111. Greitz T: Angiography in tuberculous meningitis. Acta Radiol (Diagn) 1964;2:369.
112. Pont MS, Elster AD: Lesions of skin and brain: Modern imaging of the neurocutaneous syndromes. AJR 1992;158:1193–1203.
113. Taveras JM, Mount LA, Wood EH: The value of radiation therapy in the management of glioma of the optic nerves and chiasm. Radiology 1956;66:518.
114. Hoyt WF, Baghdasarian SA: Optic glioma of childhood: Natural history and rationale for conservative management. Br J Ophthalmol 1969;53:793–798.
115. Sweet W, Taveras JM: Radical surgical approach to optic glioma: Their diagnosis and capacity for spontaneous regression. In HH Schmidek, WH Sweet (eds), Operative Neurosurgical Techniques: Indications, Methods and Results, ed 3. Philadelphia: Saunders, 1995, pp 253–288.
116. Roman-Goldstein SM, Goldman DL, Howieson J, et al: MR of primary CNS lymphoma in immunologically normal patients. AJNR 1992;13:1207–1213.
117. Dumas JL, Visy JM, Lhote F, et al: MRI and neurological complications of adult T-cell leukemia lymphoma. J Comput Assist Tomogr 1992;16:820–823.
118. Kalimo H, Lehto M, Nanto-Salenenk, et al: Characterization of the perivascular reticulin network in a case of primary brain lymphoma: Immunohistochemical demonstration of collagen types I, III, IV and V; laminin; and fibronectin. Acta Neuropathol 1985;66:299.
119. Chappell ET, Guthrie BL, Orenstein J: The role of stereotactic biopsy in the management of HIV-related focal brain lesions. Neurosurgery 1992;30:825–829.
120. Potts DG, Svare GT: Calcification in intracranial metastases. AJR 1964;92:1249.
121. Smith RR, Grossman RI, Goldberg HI, et al: MR imaging of Lhermitte-Duclos disease: A case report. AJNR 1989;10:187–189.
122. Domingues RC, Taveras JM, Reimer P, et al: Foramen magnum choroid plexus papilloma with drop metastases to the lumbar spine. AJNR 1991;12:564–565.
123. Criscuolo GR, Symon L: Intraventricular meningioma: A review of 10 cases of the National Hospital, Queen Square (1974–1985) with reference to the literature. Acta Neuropathol 1986;83:83–91.
124. Kricheff II, Pinto RS, Bergeron RT, et al: Air-CT cisternography and canalography for small acoustic neuromas. AJNR 1980;1: 57–63.
125. Press GA, Hesselink JR: MR imaging of cerebellopontine angle and internal auditory canal lesions at 1.5 T. AJNR 1988;9:241–251.
126. Daniels DL, Millen SJ, Meyer GA, et al: MR detection of tumor in the internal auditory canal. AJNR 1987;8:249–252.
127. Halliday AL, Sobel RA, Martuza RL: Benign spinal nerve sheath tumors: Their occurrence sporadically and in neurofibromatosis 1 and 2. J Neurosurg 1991;74:248–253.
128. Tampieri D, Melanson D, Ethier R: MR imaging of epidermoid cysts. AJNR 1989;10:351–356.
129. Smith AS, Benson JE, Blaser SI, et al: Diagnosis of ruptured intracranial dermoid cyst: Value of MR over CT. AJNR 1991;12: 175–180.
130. Shijman E, Mongos J, Cragnaz R: Congenital dermal sinus: Dermoid and epidermoid cysts of the posterior fossa. Childs Nerv Syst 1986;2:83–89.
131. Yasargil MG, Abernathy CD, Sarioglu AC: Microneurosurgical treatment of intracranial dermoid and epidermoid tumors. Neurosurgery 1989;24:561–567.
132. Lee YY, Tassel PV, Raymond AK: Intracranial dural chondrosarcoma. AJNR 1988;9:1189–1193.
133. Wilms G, Lammens M, Marchal G, et al: Thickening of dura surrounding meningiomas: MR features. J Comput Assist Tomogr 1989;13:763–768.
134. Tien RD, Yang PJ, Chu PK: "Dural tail sign": A specific MR sign for meningioma? J Comput Assist Tomogr 1991;15:64–66.
135. Forsting M, Albert FK, Kunze S, et al: Extirpation of glioblastomas: MR and CT follow-up of residual tumor and regrowth patterns. AJNR 1993;14:77–87.

136. Selzer ME, Dichter MA: Cellular pathophysiology and pharmacology of epilepsy. In AK Asbury, GM McKhann, WI McDonald (eds), Diseases of the Nervous System: Clinical Neurobiology. Philadelphia: Saunders, 1992, chap 70, pp. 916–935.
137. Mamourian AC, Brown DB: Asymmetric mammillary bodies: MR identification. AJNR 1993;14:1332–1335.
138. Mirski MA: Unraveling the neuroanatomy of epilepsy. AJNR 1993; 14:1336–1342.
139. Johnson DW, Hogg JP, Dasheiff R, et al: Xenon/CT cerebral blood flow during continuous depth electrode monitoring in epilepsy patients. AJNR 1993;14:245–252.
140. Kuhl DE, Engel J Jr, Phelps ME, et al: Epileptic patterns of local cerebral metabolism and perfusion in humans determined by emission computed tomography of 18 FDG and 13 NH 3. Ann Neurol 1980;8:348–360.
141. Engel J Jr, Kuhl DE, Phelps ME, et al: Comparative localization of epileptic foci of partial epilepsy by PET and EEG. Ann Neurol 1982;12:529–537.
142. Heinz ER, Crain BJ, Radtke RA, et al: MR imaging in patients with temporal lobe seizures: Correlation of results with pathologic findings. AJNR 1990;11:827–832.
143. Heinz ER, Heinz TR, Radtke R, et al: Efficacy of MR vs. CT in epilepsy. AJNR 1988;9:1123–1128.
144. Patil A-A, McConnel JR, Torkelson RD: Stereotactic location and excision of seizure focus with xenon-enhanced CT. AJNR 1995; 16:637–643.
145. Kim JK, Tien RD, Felsberg GJ, Osumi AK, Lee N, Friedman AH: Fast spin-echo MR in hippocampal sclerosis: Correlation with pathology and surgery. AJNR 1995;16:644–646.
146. Jack CR, Twomey CK, Zinsmeister AR, et al: Anterior temporal lobes and hippocampal formations: Normative volumetric measurements from MR images in young adults. Radiology 1989;172: 549–554.
147. Ashtari M, Barr WB, Schaul N, et al: Three-dimensional fast low-angle shot imaging and computerized volume measurement of the hippocampus in patients with chronic epilepsy of the temporal lobe. AJNR 1991;12:941–947.
148. Free SL, Bergin PS, Fish DR, Cook MJ, Shorvon SD, Stevens JM: Methods for normalization of hippocampal volumes measured with MR. AJNR 1995;16:627–636.
149. Bronen RA, Cheung G, Charles JT, et al: Imaging findings in hippocampal sclerosis: Correlation with pathology. AJNR 1991; 12:933–940.
150. Dietrich BR, Saden SE, Chugani HT, et al: Resective surgery for intractable epilepsy in children: Radiologic evaluation. AJNR 1991; 12:1149–1158.
151. Ojemann GA: Surgical therapy for medically intractable epilepsy. J Neurosurg 1987;66:489–499.
152. Merriam MA, Bronen RA, Spencer DD, et al: MR findings after depth electrode implantation for medically refractory epilepsy. AJNR 1993;14:1343–1346.
153. Mikhael MA, Trommer BL: Relative accuracy of MRI and CT in radiological evaluation of patients with seizures. Scientific exhibit presented at the annual meeting of the American Society of Neuroradiology, 1990.
154. Lehericy S, Dormont D, Sémah F, et al: Developmental abnormalities of the medial temporal lobe in patients with temporal lobe epilepsy. AJNR 1995;16:617–626.

SELECTED READINGS

Angeid-Backman E, Wuiny DJ: CNS non-Hodgkin lymphoma in a patient previously treated for systemic Hodgkin disease. AJNR 1990;11: 1254–1256.

Baker AB: An Outline of Neuropathology, ed 3. Minneapolis: University of Minnesota Press, 1943.

Berens ME, Rutka JT, Rosenblum ML: Brain tumor epidemiology, growth, and invasion. Neurosurg Clin North Am 1990;1(1).

Bodian M, Lawson D: The intracranial neoplastic diseases of childhood. A description of their natural history based on a clinico-pathological study of 129 cases. Br J Surg 1953;40:368–392.

Chambers EF, Turski PA, Sobel D, et al: Radiologic characteristics of primary cerebral neuroblastoma. Radiology 1981;139:101–104.

Childhood Brain Tumor Consortium. A study of childhood brain tumors based on surgical biopsies from ten North American institutions: Sample description. J Neurooncol 1988;6:9–23.

Courville CB: Pathology of the Central Nervous System, ed 2. Mountain View, CA: Pacific Press Publishing Association, 1945.

Courville CB: Pathology of the Central Nervous System, ed 3. Mountain View, CA: Pacific Press Publishing Association, 1950.

De Groen PC, Aksamit AJ, Rakela J, et al: Central nervous system toxicity after liver transplantation: The role of cyclosporine and cholesterol. N Engl J Med 1987;317:861–866.

Delgado-Escueta AV, Baesal FE, Treiman DM, et al: Complex partial seizures on closed circuit television and EEG: A study of 691 attacks in 79 patients. Ann Neurol 1982;11:292–300.

Dina TS: Primary central nervous system lymphoma versus toxoplasmosis in AIDS 1. Radiology 1991;179:823–828.

Eby NL, Grufferman S, Flannelly CM, et al: Increasing incidence of primary lymphoma in the US. Cancer 1988;62:2461–2465.

Fain JS, Tomlinson FH, Scheithauer BW, et al: Symptomatic glial cysts of the pineal gland. J Neurosurg 1994;80:454–560.

Hassoun J. Gambarelli D, Grisoli F, et al: Central neurocytoma: An electron microscopic study of two cases. Acta Neuropathol (Berl) 1982;56: 151–156.

McConnell EM: The arterial blood supply to the human hypophysis cerebri. Anat Rec 1953;115:175.

Parkinson D: Collateral circulation of cavernous carotid artery: Anatomy. Can J Surg 1964;7:251.

Poon T, Matoso I, Tchertkoff V, et al: CT features of primary cerebral lymphoma in AIDS and non-AIDS patients. J Comput Assist Tomogr 1989;13(1):6–9.

Provenzale JM, Taveras JM: Clinical Cases in Neuroradiology. Malvern, PA: Lea and Febiger, 1994, case 48.

Queimadelos V, Paz FJ, Campos JM, et al: El "signo meningeo" en un linfoma meningocraneal primario. NRX Revista Espanola de Neuroimagen 1991;1:155–165.

Schwaighofer BW, Hesselink JR, Press GA, et al: Primary intracranial CNS lymphoma: MR manifestations. AJNR 1989;10:725–729.

Silver AJ, Ganti SR, Hilal SK: Computed tomography of tumors involving the atria of the lateral ventricles. Radiology 1982;145:71–78.

Ward AA Jr: Perspectives for surgical therapy of epilepsy. In AA Ward Jr, SK Penry, D Purpura (eds), Epilepsy. New York: Raven Press, 1983.

Welton PL, Reicher MA, Kellerhouse LE, et al: MR of benign pineal cyst. AJNR 1988;9:612.

Zimmerman HM: The ten most common types of brain tumor. Semin Roentgenol 1971;6:48.

12

Cranial Nerves: Anatomy and Pathology

The new imaging methods, particularly magnetic resonance imaging (MRI), provide visualization of a number of the cranial nerves (II, III, V, VII, and VIII) and, in combination with computed tomography (CT), allow us to examine the osseous canals through which they pass. Thus it was felt that presentation of a relatively brief discussion of the anatomy and pathology of the cranial nerves would be a useful addition to this work.

CRANIAL NERVE I: OLFACTORY NERVE

The first cranial nerve originates in the upper nasal mucosa, from nerve cells distributed in the nasal lining. The fibers generated penetrate through the cribriform plate of the ethmoid and join the inferior aspect of the olfactory bulb (Fig. 12.5). The cribriform plate can be seen on lateral tomograms of the skull; CT will show the cribriform plate and adjacent bone structures on coronal sections, and MRI may show the olfactory bulb as well as the olfactory tract in coronal images (Figs. 12.1 and 12.2).

Lesions that affect the olfactory nerve are esthesioneuroblastoma, which usually produces bone destruction in the cribriform plate region, and a subfrontal mass (Fig. 12.3). More extensive involvement may be seen in these tumors, which can be very aggressive. Subfrontal olfactory groove meningiomas affect the olfactory nerves by compression. They may be attached to the planum sphenoidale or arise more anteriorly. These tumors are easily diagnosed by CT or MRI with contrast, and angiography would reveal their blood supply, which may involve branches of the middle meningeal and anterior meningeal arteries, as well as the ophthalmic arteries (Fig. 12.4). Also, the meningioma may involve the bone and extend below it (Fig. 12.4) (Table 12.1).

The olfactory nerves may also be affected by trauma involving the anterior skull base, and chronic inflammatory conditions involving the nasal mucosa may blunt the ability to perceive odors. Lesions such as Wegener granulomatosis may present with anosmia due to involvement of the upper nasal mucosa (Fig. 12.2).

The anatomy is demonstrated in Fig. 3.6.

CRANIAL NERVE II: OPTIC NERVE

The optic nerve has an intraorbital portion, a foraminal portion where it passes through the optic canal (or foramen), and an intracranial prechiasmal portion where the nerves join to form the optic chiasm. They reemerge posterior to the chiasm and form the optic tracts. The tracts contain half of the fibers of the right and left eyes, as shown in Figure 3.27*B*. They are directed to the geniculate bodies, from where they swing around the temporal horn, pass on each side of the atrium of the lateral ventricle (optic radiations), and end at the medial occipital cortex in the region of the calcarine fissure. A lesion of the chiasm usually produces a bitemporal hemianopia, whereas a lesion in the postchiasmal tracts or optic radiations produces a homonymous visual defect.

In the orbits, the nerves are surrounded by the meninges (dura and pia-arachnoid).

The optic chiasm and nerves can be shown on MRI, preferably with T1-weighted images and fat-suppression technique (Fig. 12.4*C* and *D*).

In the presence of papilledema, enlargement of the meningeal sleeve may be visible on MRI; this space may be filled with opaque material and shown by CT on radiopaque cisternography.

Meningiomas of the meningeal coverings can occur in the orbital portion. Optic nerve gliomas are seen in patients with neurofibromatosis type I and sometimes may be seen in patients without a clear-cut history of neurofibromatosis. The tumor may arise from any portion of the optic nerves, chiasm, or tracts (Table 12.1).

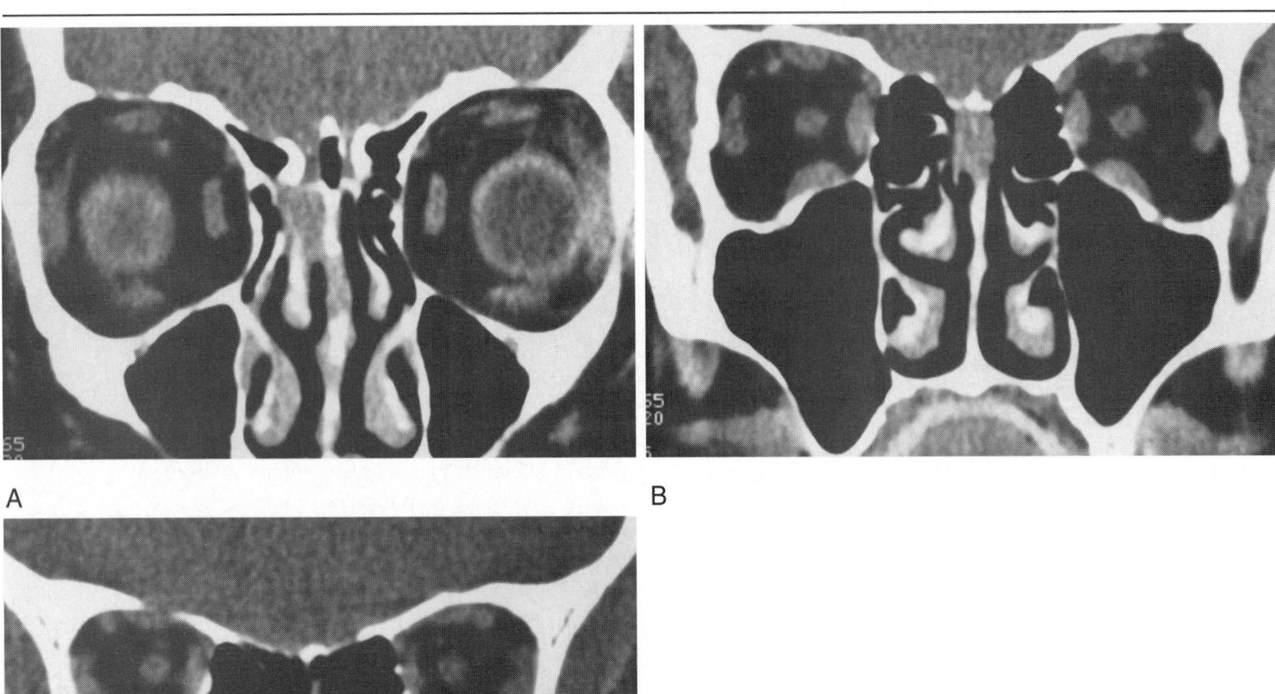

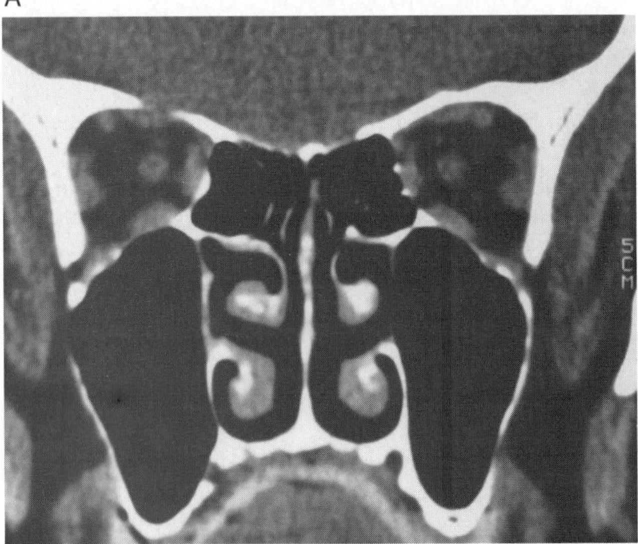

Figure 12.1. Coronal CT of crista galli, cribriform plate, and planum sphenoidale. **A.** Partially pneumatized crista galli. On each side there is a deep groove, at the bottom of which is the cribriform plate. There is evidence of involvement of the superior ethmoid cells on the right. **B.** Section behind A as the crista galli tapers down. **C.** Section behind B at the level of the planum sphenoidale.

Compression, invasion, or destruction of the optic pathways may be produced by tumor, vascular ischemia, hemorrhagic lesions, trauma, infection, or demyelination. Demyelination may be the earliest lesion demonstrated in multiple sclerosis (see Fig. 4.63). Radiation-induced optic neuropathy will enhance and can be shown by MRI (1). For further details see under "Sellar and Perisellar Lesions," Chapter 11.

CRANIAL NERVE III: OCULOMOTOR NERVE

This nerve is particularly important because it innervates all the muscles of the orbit except the external rectus and the superior oblique muscles. It has a fairly long course and can be affected by pathology in several locations.

The third nerve originates in the midbrain just anterior to the periaqueductal gray matter and just behind and medial to the medial longitudinal fasciculus (see Fig. 3.19*A* and *B*). From there, the fibers pass around the red nucleus as they move rostrally to emerge on each side of the interpeduncular fossa (see Figs. 3.15 and 3.18). At this point the two (right and left) nerves move forward and laterally, pass between the posterior cerebral and the superior cerebellar arteries, and cross the perimesencephalic cistern.

As it crosses the posterior aspect of the perimesencephalic cistern, the third nerve is parallel to the posterior communicating artery, where it can be affected by saccular aneurysms of this artery (Fig. 12.5; see Fig. 10.93). The nerve passes on one side of the dorsum sella, where it pierces the dura, passing between the free and attached borders of the tentorium cerebelli, to reach the lateral wall of the cavernous sinus. It continues in the wall of the cavernous sinus (it is the highest of the four nerves on the lateral cavernous sinus wall) (Fig. 12.6; see Fig. 10.89), passes just under and slightly lateral to the anterior clinoid process, and enters the orbit via the superior orbital fissure to become intraorbital.

The third nerve can be affected at its origin in the midbrain or in the midbrain more anteriorly before emerging from the anterior surface of the brainstem. Third-nerve palsy may result from involvement at these levels. The syndrome of internuclear ophthalmoplegia (failure of adduc-

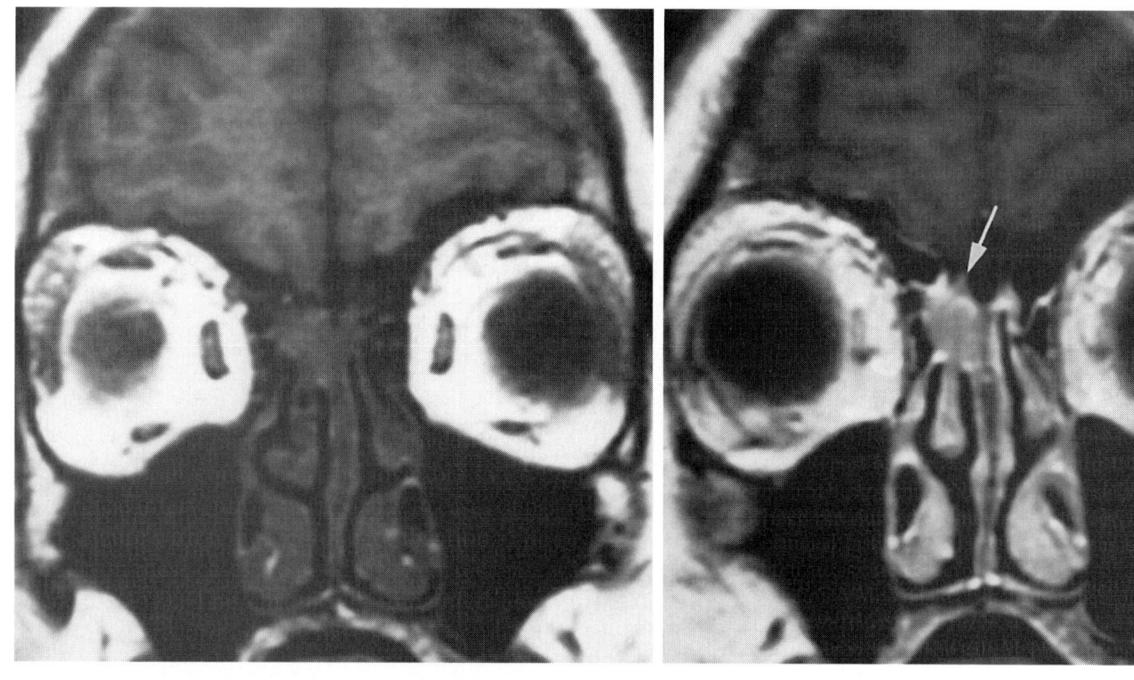

A B

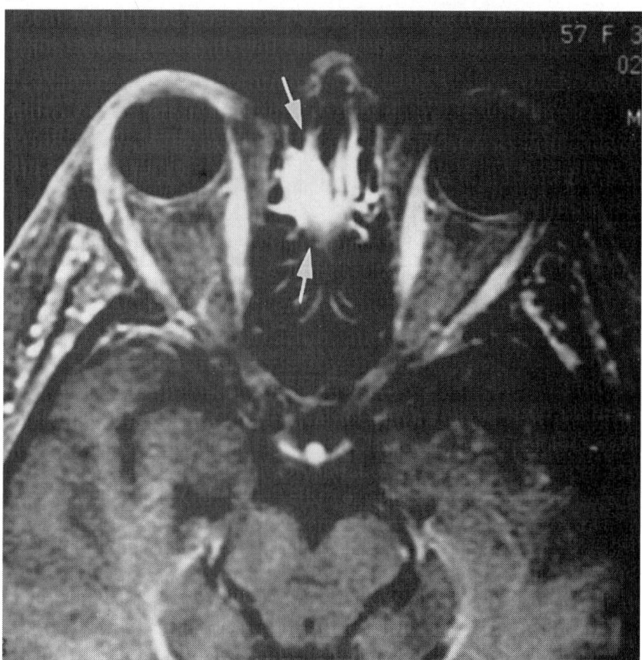

C

Figure 12.2. Wegener granulomatosis in a 57-year-old woman complaining of anosmia. **A.** Noncontrast coronal T1-weighted MRI and (**B**) following contrast. There is an enhancing lesion extending up to the cribriform plate on the right (same patient as the CT of Figure 12.1). Slight enhancement may be present intracranially (arrow). **C.** Axial postcontrast fat-suppressed image shows the enhancement on the right side (arrows). In A there is some asymmetry of the gyri recti; the right is larger than the left. On each side of the gyrus rectus is the olfactory sulcus.

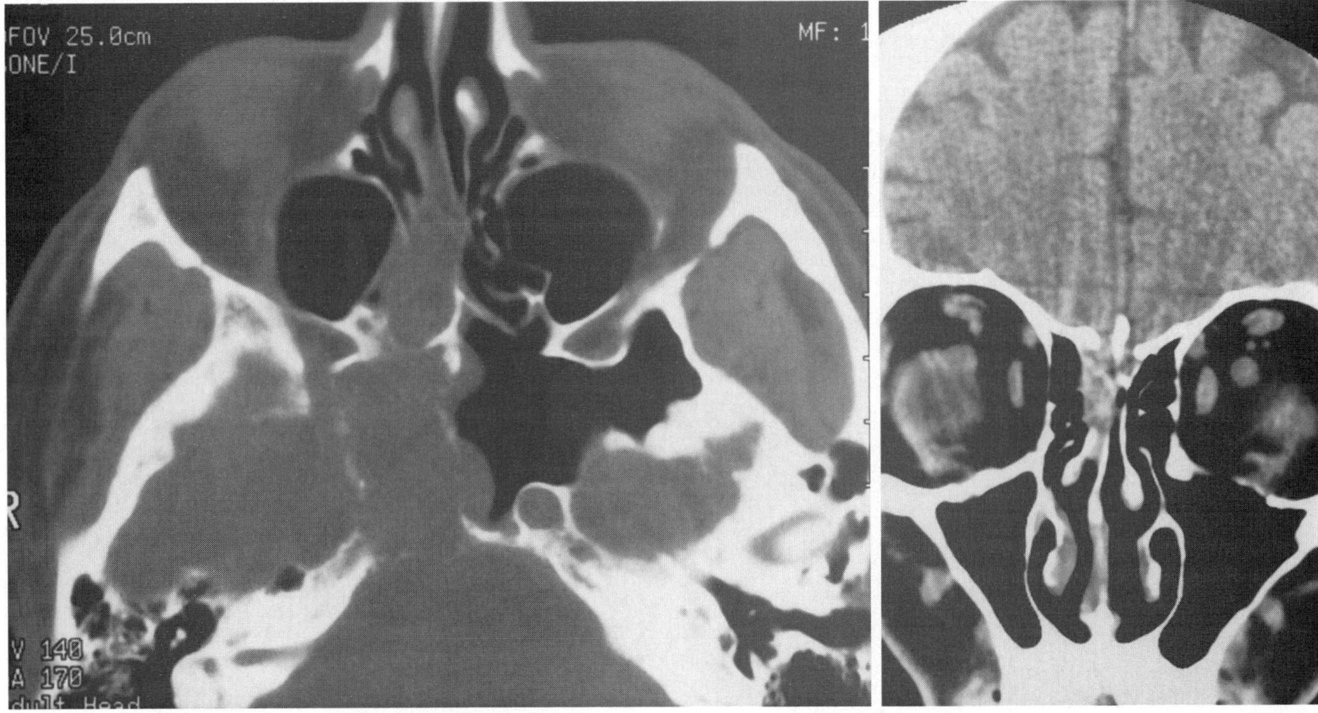

A B

Figure 12.3. Esthesioneuroblastoma involving the right ethmoidal area and destroying the sphenoid sinus. **A.** Axial CT. **B.** Coronal CT reveals destruction of the right side of the cribriform plate. This esthesioneuroblastoma also involves the upper aspect of the nasal septum; others invade the anterior fossa of the cranial cavity more extensively.

Table 12.1.
Major Pathologic Conditions Affecting the Cranial Nerves

- CN I (Olfactory nerve)
  - Nasal mass lesions (e.g., esthesioneuroblastoma)
  - Subfrontal masses: meningioma
  - Inflammatory: Wegener granulomatosis
- CN II (Optic nerve)
  - Mass involving nerve and nerve sheath: optic nerve glioma, meningioma
  - Demyelinating: multiple sclerosis
  - Inflammatory: optic neuritis
  - Compressive lesions
  - Ischemia
- CN III (Oculomotor nerve)
  - Intraparenchymal midbrain lesions: infarcts, neoplasms
  - Cisternal (e.g., compression by aneurysm, uncal herniation)
  - Cavernous sinus: meningiomas, aneurysms
  - Intraorbital: meningiomas, inflammatory processes (e.g., pseudotumor cerebri), metastases, cavernous angiomas
  - Within nerve itself: diabetes
- CN IV (Trochlear nerve)
  - Extrinsic mass lesions (e.g., pineal region tumors)
  - Nerve sheath tumors (e.g., schwannomas)
- CN V (Trigeminal nerve)
  - Infectious: herpes zoster
  - Neoplasms: extrinsic (e.g., perineural spread of tumor, meningioma) or nerve sheath (e.g., schwannomas)
  - Other compressive lesions (e.g., vascular compression)
- CN VI (Trochlear nerve)
  - In cavernous sinus: intracavernous aneurysm; sinus thrombosis
  - Extrinsic mass lesions: meningiomas, chordomas, epidermoids
  - Inflammatory (e.g., fungal infections); Tolosa-Hunt syndrome
  - Trauma
- CN VII (Facial nerve)
  - Cisternal: acoustic neuromas, epidermoids
  - Nerve sheath: schwannomas
  - Inflammatory (e.g., Ramsay Hunt syndrome)
  - Vascular compression
  - Postinfectious (e.g., many cases of Bell palsy)
- CN VIII (Acoustic nerve)
  - Neoplastic (e.g., acoustic schwannoma)
  - Inflammatory (e.g., Ramsay Hunt syndrome)
- CN IX–XI
  - Extrinsic masses (e.g., local extension of nasopharyngeal)
  - Nerve sheath: carcinoma, schwannomas
  - Jugular sheath masses (e.g., glomus jugulare tumor)
- CN XII (Hypoglossal nerve)
  - Nerve sheath tumors (e.g., schwannomas)
  - Extrinsic masses: meningioma
  - Brainstem processes (e.g., infarcts)

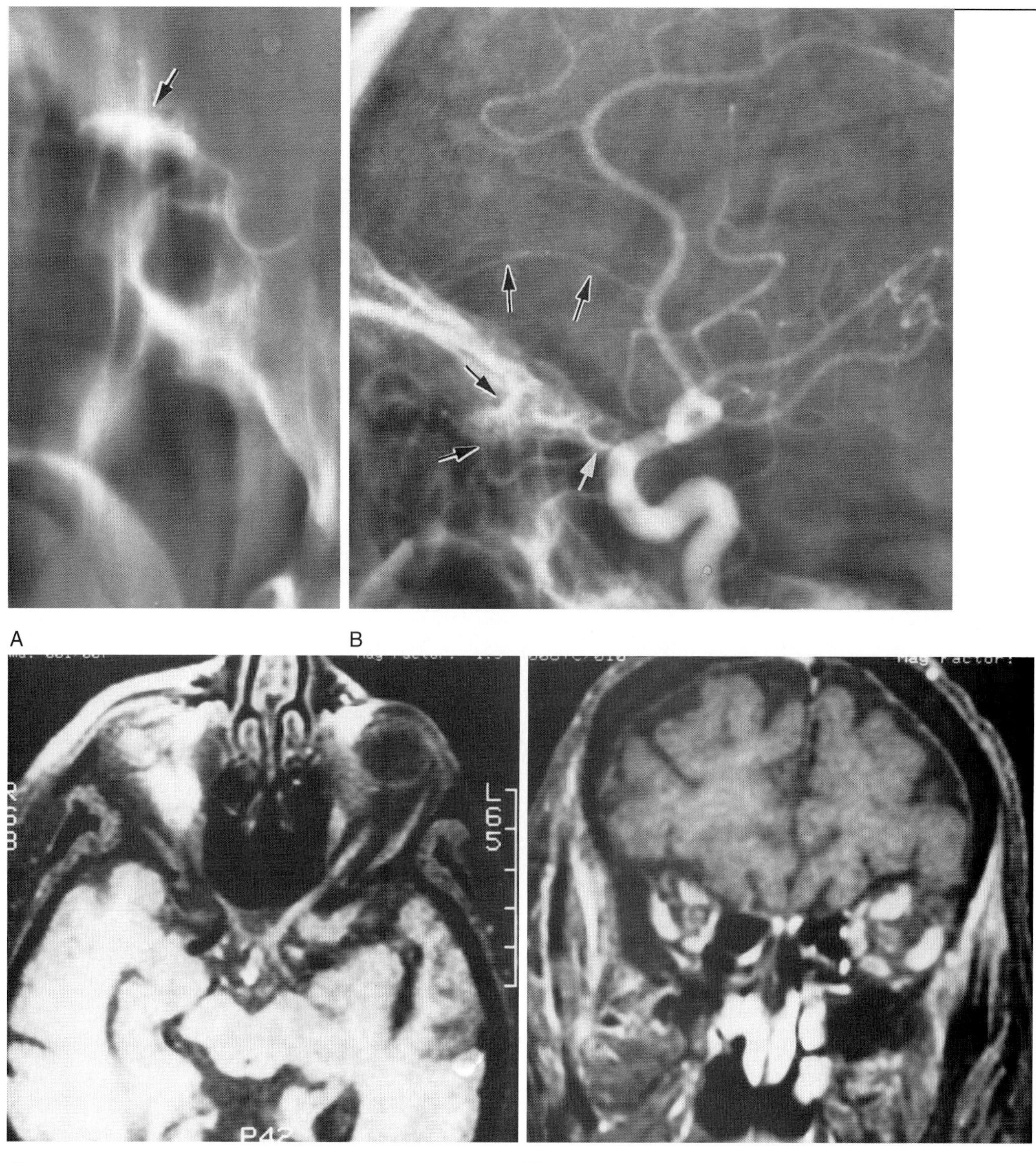

Figure 12.4. Midline subfrontal meningioma producing anosmia due to compression of the olfactory bulb and stretching of olfactory nerve fibers. **A.** Lateral tomogram shows thickening and sclerosis of planum sphenoidale. **B.** There is elevation of the branches of the anterior cerebral artery (upper arrows). The ophthalmic artery gives branches to the area of the tumor, which seems to extend just below the bone (lower arrows). **C.** Fat-suppressed T1-weighted axial image in another patient demonstrates the optic chiasm and nerves as they extend forward and enter the orbits. **D.** A postcontrast coronal view demonstrates the intraorbital optic nerves. The orbital muscles are bright because of contrast enhancement. The gyrus rectus is seen on each side of the midline; lateral to it is the olfactory sulcus, lateral to which is the medial orbital gyrus of the frontal lobe.

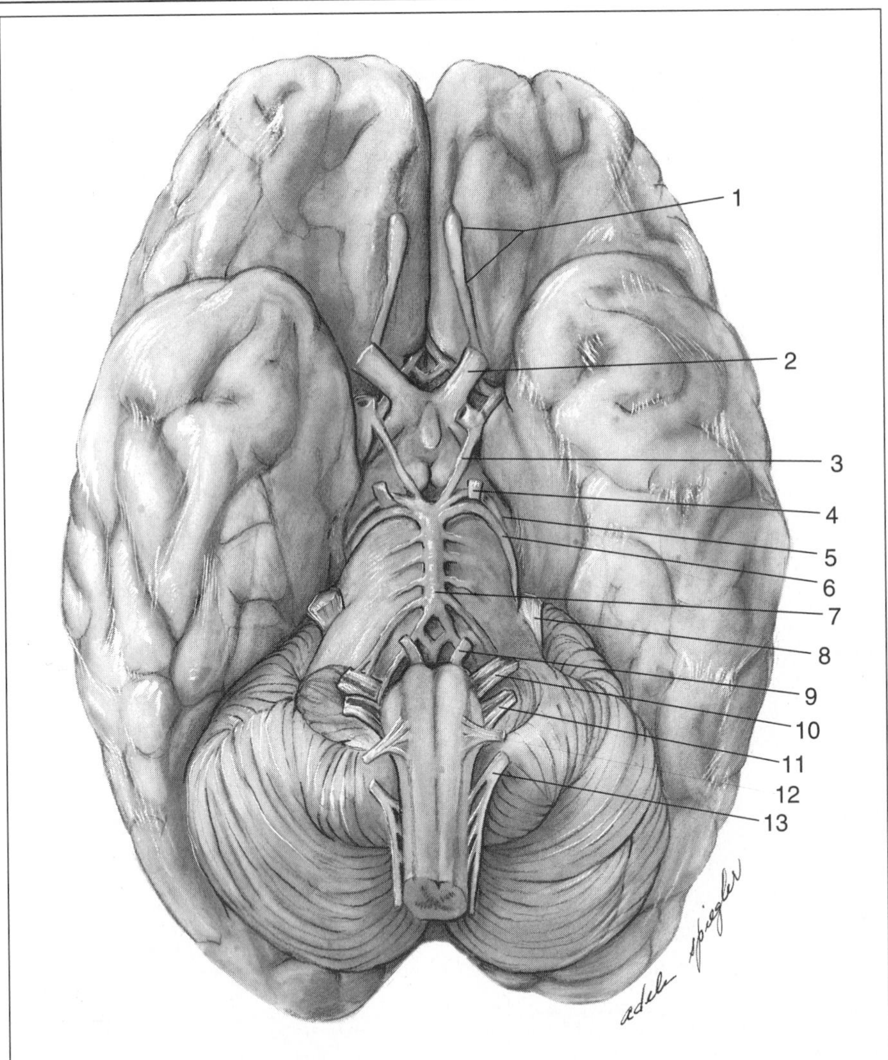

Figure 12.5. Base of brain. (1) Olfactory bulb and track; (2) optic nerve; (3) posterior communicating artery; (4) third nerve; (5) posterior cerebral artery; (6) superior cerebellar artery; (7) basilar artery; (8) trigeminal nerve; (9) sixth nerve; (10) seventh and eighth nerves; (11) ninth and tenth nerves (vagus and glossopharyngeus); (12) hypoglossal nerve; (13) spinal accessory nerve.

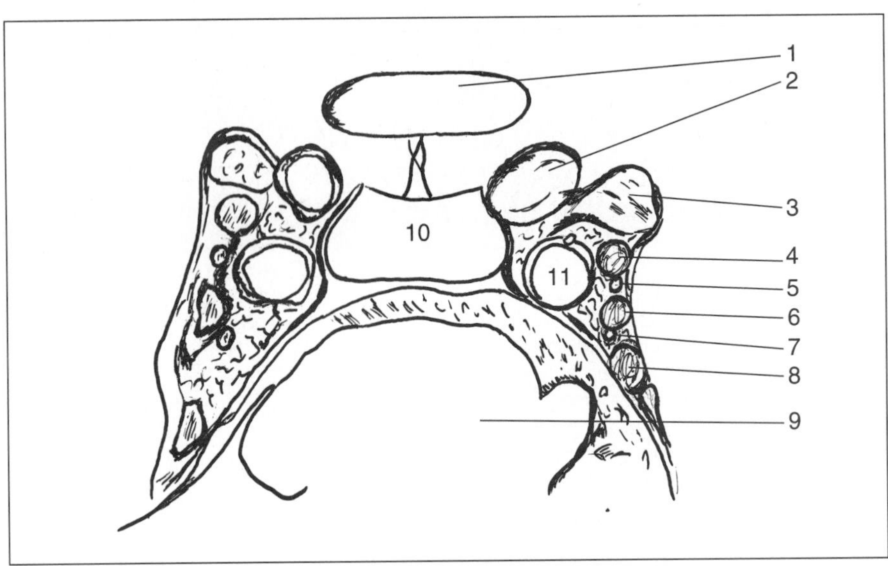

Figure 12.6. Coronal cross section of sella and cavernous sinuses. (1) Optic chiasm; (2) internal carotid upper part of carotid siphon; (3) anterior clinoid process; (4) third cranial nerve; (5) fourth cranial nerve; (6) ophthalmic division (V1) of fifth cranial nerve; (7) sixth cranial nerve (nerves III, IV, and V are in the wall of the cavernous sinus; the sixth nerve is inside the sinus [see Fig. 10.89]); (8) maxillary (V2) division of trigeminal nerve; (9) sphenoid sinus; (10) pituitary gland with pituitary stalk; (11) internal carotid artery inside cavernous sinus.

tion but preservation of convergence of the two eyes) results from involvement between the two nuclei, which are adjacent to the medial longitudinal fasciculi (see Fig. 3.19). Lesions in front of the nuclei of origin and the anterior aspect of the midbrain lead to some of the known crossed syndromes (Weber syndrome: ipsilateral complete third-nerve palsy and contralateral hemiplegia; Benedikt syndrome: ipsilateral third-nerve palsy and contralateral hemiparesis with tremor and hyperkinesia due to involvement of red nucleus and corticospinal tract). The evaluation of Kelly is particularly useful (2).

On MR images the third nerve can be seen on axial T1-weighted views and sometimes in sagittal views (Fig. 12.7).

Tumors of the third nerve are rare, which follows the rule that motor nerves have a much lower incidence of tumors than sensory nerves. Extra-axial as well as intrinsic brainstem tumors can secondarily compress and displace the third nerve. In one instance a patient presented with third-nerve palsy and turned out to have an angioma surrounding the nerve (see Fig. 11.75). Among the extra-axial tumors are meningioma, chordoma, chondrosarcoma, epidermoid tumors, and neuroma of the fifth cranial nerve. Neoplastic perineural infiltration can occur. Most of these cases turn out to be a nasopharyngeal carcinoma infiltrating through the base of the skull and in the epidural space. Other nerves in the wall of the cavernous sinus may also be involved, and the same is true of traumatic lesions involving the sphenoid bone.

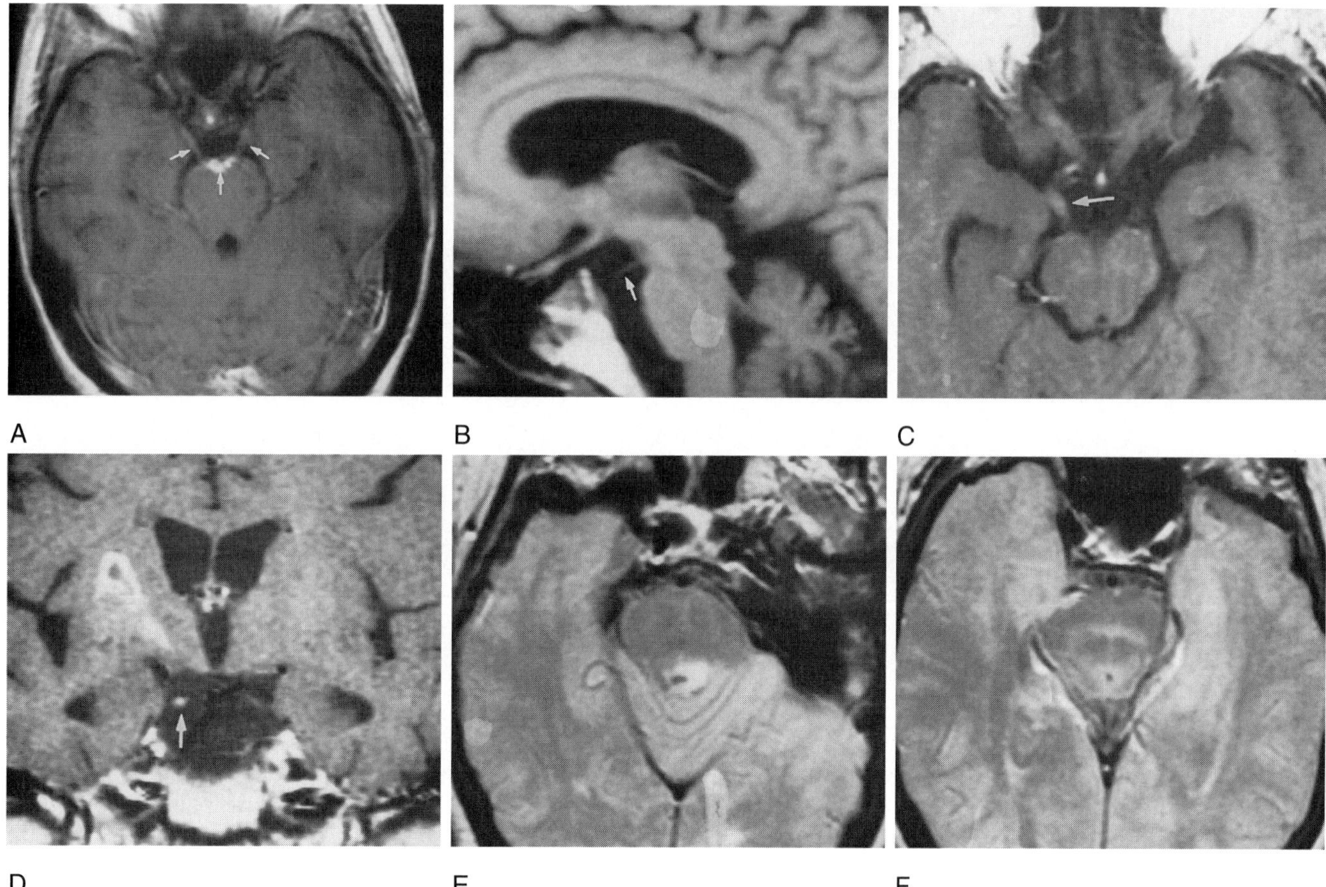

Figure 12.7. Images of third cranial nerve. **A.** Axial postcontrast image showing the third cranial nerves diverging as they move forward to reach the wall of the cavernous sinuses. The patient had meningitis, which explains the enhancement in the interpeduncular fossa (lower arrow). The third nerves are also brighter than usual, probably due to some degree of enhancement. **B.** Sagittal T1-weighted noncontrast MRI view in another patient demonstrating the third nerve in its cisternal portion as it moves forward and slightly downward to reach the wall of the cavernous sinus (arrow). **C.** In another patient who also had meningitis (HIV-positive), and a right third nerve palsy for a week, there is enhancement of the right third nerve (arrow). The patient also had enhancement of lumbar roots in the cauda equina. **D.** The nerve also can be seen in coronal postcontrast images. There is an enhancing inflammatory lesion in the basal ganglia region on the right. **E.** Proton density weighted axial image in a patient who presented an internuclear ophthalmoplegia reveals a small hyperintense area in the left periaqueductal region representing an ischemic lesion. **F.** A higher section reveals hyperintensity around the aqueduct, slightly more on the left side.

As mentioned earlier, an important, relatively frequent condition producing third-nerve palsy is an aneurysm of the posterior communicating artery (see Fig. 10.93). For this reason, magnetic resonance angiography (MRA) is indicated in those cases; if the MRA is negative, cerebral angiography is indicated.

The nerve can be affected farther forward by lesions that involve the wall of the cavernous sinus, such as meningiomas, aneurysm of the internal carotid artery in the cavernous sinus, cavernous sinus venous thrombosis, Tolosa-Hunt syndrome, and meningioma of the sphenoid ridge, and by inflammatory processes (fungus infection such as mucormycosis, aspergillosis). Vogl et al. reported a case of syphilitic gumma situated in the upper brainstem and third cranial nerve, which produced third-nerve palsy (3) (Table 12.1).

CRANIAL NERVE IV: TROCHLEAR NERVE

This is the smallest of the cranial nerves. It originates in the midbrain just anterior to the periaqueductal gray matter and adjacent to the medial longitudinal fasciculus (see Fig. 3.19*C*). From its origin the fibers run caudally for a small distance, decussate right to left with the opposite counterpart, and emerge below the inferior colliculus (see Fig. 3.16). The nerve turns around the brainstem just above the junction of the pons and midbrain and moves forward, crossing the premesencephalic space to pierce the dura below the third nerve to continue forward in the lateral wall of the cavernous sinus (Fig. 12.6; see Fig. 10.89). It enters the orbit through the superior orbital fissure, where it is the highest of the nerves. It innervates the superior oblique muscle.

In spite of its long course, it is not involved by adjacent pathologic processes as often as the third nerve. Similar conditions such as tumor of the pineal and quadrigeminal plate, vascular lesions, neoplasm involving the wall of the cavernous sinus, and trauma may affect the fourth nerve (Table 12.1). Primary tumors of this nerve are extremely rare (4).

CRANIAL NERVE V: TRIGEMINAL NERVE

This is the largest cranial nerve. It is the sensory nerve of the head and face, and the motor nerve of the muscles of mastication. It emerges from the pons at the level of the middle cerebellar peduncle (Fig. 12.5; see Figs. 3.15 and 3.17) The motor root is smaller and situated in front of and medial to the larger sensory root. The nerve moves forward, crossing the prepontine cisternal space, pierces the dura to the side of the clivus, and enters a space, the cavum meckelii (Meckel cave) (Figs. 12.8 and 12.9). The nerve, on its move forward, passes below the superior petrosal sinus and tentorium but above the apex of the petrous pyramid. Within the cavum is situated the gasserian ganglion (semilunar ganglion), which is fairly large, and which provides the sensory fibers of the fifth nerve. Within the Meckel cave the nerve divides into three main branches: the ophthalmic division, the maxillary division, and the mandibular division. The first and second divisions are sen-

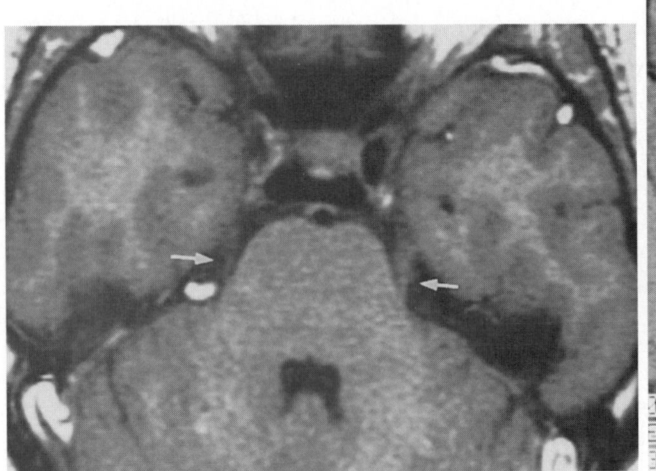

A

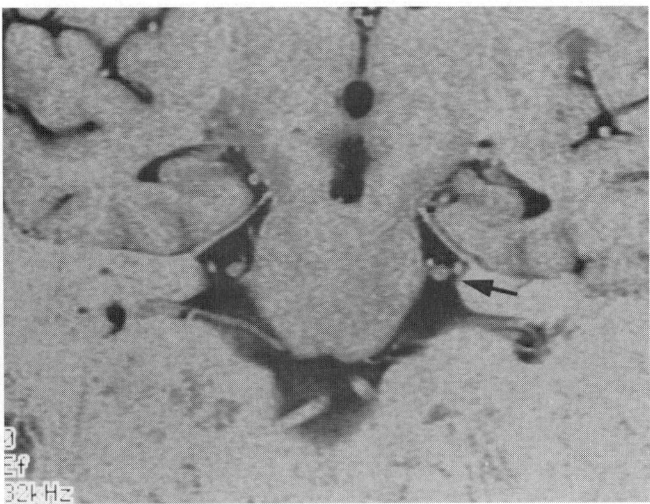

B

Figure 12.8. A. Axial view, T1-weighted, demonstrating the fifth nerves as they move forward from the pons to enter Meckel cave (arrows). **B.** Fifth cranial nerve demonstrated by the cerebrospinal fluid (CSF) cisternography technique. Coronal view (image is video reversed; the CSF is black) shows the trigeminal nerve and, on the left, on each side of the nerve is a blood vessel, artery, or vein (arrow); on the right side, one vessel is clearly seen, and another, medially and superior in relation to the nerve, is only faintly visualized. The cisternography brings out vessels in the cisternal spaces, including the cistern of the velum interpositum below the septum pellucidum. (Courtesy of Drs. T. El Gammal and B.S. Brooks, Birmingham [AJNR 1994;15:1647–1656].)

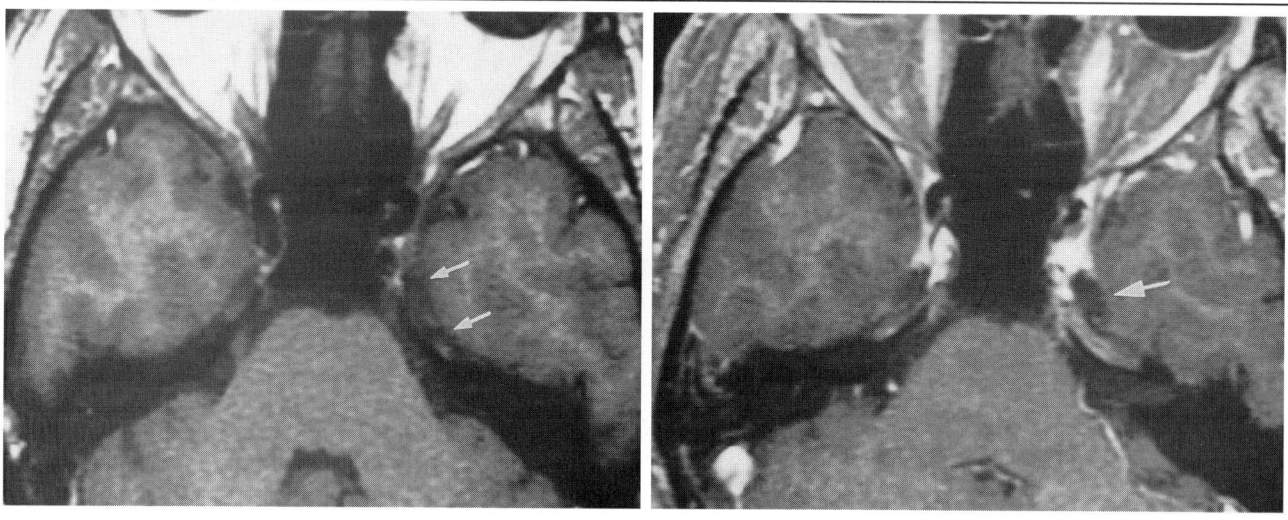

Figure 12.9. Meckel cave shown in pre- and postcontrast axial MR images. **A.** Precontrast. **B.** Postcontrast. The cavernous sinuses reveal the venous blood and behind it Meckel cave. The Gasserian ganglion (arrow) occupies a good portion of the cisternal space (two arrows in A). The fifth nerve is clearly seen on the right (A).

sory, and the third is both motor and sensory. The first division (sensory) innervates the cornea and iris, ciliary body, conjunctiva, and lacrimal gland; the mucous membrane of the nasal cavity; and the skin of the eyelids, the eyebrow, the forehead, and nose. The first division passes forward on the wall of the cavernous sinus below the third and fourth nerves, and enters the orbit through the superior orbital fissure. The second division, the maxillary division (sensory), is also in the lower aspect of the cavernous sinus wall but leaves the cranial cavity through the foramen rotundum (see Fig. 10.89). It passes forward, lateral to the sphenopalatine fossa, and bends laterally to enter the infraorbital canal. It emerges in the infraorbital foramen and innervates the side of the nose, the lower lid, and the upper lip.

The third division (mandibular division), the largest of the three, is a motor and sensory nerve. It leaves the cranial cavity through the foramen ovale and innervates the teeth and gums of the mandible, the skin of the temporal region, the auricula, the lower lip, the lower part of the face, and the mucous membrane of the anterior two-thirds of the tongue. It also provides motor innervation to the muscles of mastication.

The fifth nerve can be involved in inflammatory processes; herpes zoster is a typical example. It usually involves the ophthalmic division (20 times more frequently than the other two) (5). Two cases of mycotic aneurysm reported by Donohue and Enzmann (5) were thought to be secondary to a herpes zoster angiitis. Hyperintensity of the preganglionic segment of the fifth nerve may be demonstrated on contrast-enhanced MR images, presumably due to neuritis. Enhancement of the nerve may be considered as an indication of loss of blood–peripheral nerve barrier, but the mechanism is not clear; presumably it is similar to the blood-brain barrier as defined by Bradbury (6). In a reported case, the finding was associated with rhombencephalitis, all of which cleared in 6 to 8 weeks and was attributed to herpes simplex virus (7). As is well known, the herpesvirus lives in the gasserian ganglion, and there is transaxonal movement of the virus between the ganglion and the peripheral nerves, which accounts for the intermittent appearance of aphthous ulcers in the buccal mucosa and blistering in the lips (fever blisters) in many individuals (8).

Schwannomas of the fifth nerve are uncommon but sometimes are seen, not necessarily associated with neurofibromatosis. They may produce incisural saddle-shaped tumors with one portion in the anterolateral aspect of the posterior fossa and another in the middle fossa (see Figs. 11.76 and 11.111) (9–11).

These tumors may show erosion of the middle fossa (foramen ovale region) and erosion of the tip of the petrous pyramid on plain films and on CT. CT with contrast and MRI, particularly the latter, are usually diagnostic. The saddle-shaped configuration is typical but may also be seen in meningiomas. The presence of masseter muscle atrophy due to involvement of the third division is characteristic.

Lymphoma of the fifth nerve in patients with systemic lymphoma has been reported (12).

Perineural neoplastic involvement may be seen in carcinomas of the nasopharynx infiltrating upward. The presence of pain in the trigeminal distribution should make us suspect this possibility (Table 12.1).

Finally, it should be remembered that the trigeminal nerve has a descending sensory root that goes as far down as the fourth cervical vertebra, and that lesions in the appropriate areas of the cord, in the lateral region, may cause trigeminal symptoms such as facial pain; neurologic examination may reveal loss of sensation (pain, temperature, and touch) in the face and forehead. A herniated disc at C3–C4 may produce such findings (13).

Trigeminal neuralgia is an important medical entity. In the majority of cases no pathology can be found, but it is necessary to look carefully for a cause before considering it idiopathic; and CT and MRI examinations are essential to rule out a possible pathologic process (14). The treatment of trigeminal neuralgia is medical; if the condition does not respond to medication, injection of appropriate compounds or radiofrequency coagulation may be used. Ordinarily the injection procedure is controlled, preferably by a "C" arm fluoroscope with image intensification to ascertain the proper location of the needle.

Trigeminal neuralgia as well as hemifacial spasm may be produced by vascular loops as pointed out by Jeanetta (15) and by Jeanetta and coworkers (16). Subsequently, other workers have confirmed his findings, and there has been much further discussion of the subject (17, 18). The vascular loop compression may occur at the root exit zone of the fifth or seventh nerve, and the neuroimaging object would be to demonstrate the possible presence of such vascular compression. MRI may show a flow void near the exit of the nerve or may demonstrate a vascular loop. However, this is difficult to do in most instances, and a number of techniques have been suggested with CT and MRI besides cerebral vertebral angiography. The tortuosity of the compressing vessels may be congenital or associated with atherosclerosis. Nagaseki et al. have suggested a special sagittal oblique technique, which they claim to be useful by obtaining sagittal images parallel to the direction of the nerve of interest (19). Air CT cisternography has also been suggested as a slightly invasive method (20). Tash et al. indicate that the flow voids can be seen, if carefully looked for, on ordinary T1- and T2-weighted images in axial and coronal planes (21). In their cases all patients with hemifacial spasm showed a vascular loop in relation to the root zone of the seventh nerve, whereas only 21 percent of control patients had such apparent contact. If surgical therapy for intractable hemifacial spasm or trigeminal neuralgia is to be considered, visualization of nerve compression by tortuous arteries should be carefully attempted.

CRANIAL NERVE VI:—ABDUCENT NERVE

The abducent nerve supplies the lateral rectus muscle of the orbit. It originates in a small nucleus in the floor of the rhomboid fossa (floor of fourth ventricle) close to the midline (see Fig. 3.22). The fibers move forward, and the nerve emerges at the sulcus between the pons and the medulla, above the pyramid (Fig. 12.5; see Fig. 3.17). The nerve crosses the prepontine cistern and reaches the lateral dorsum sella, where it pierces the dura and enters the cavernous sinus. Before reaching the cavernous sinus, it passes over the tip of the petrous pyramid and lateral to the dorsum sella. In this area it is contained within an osteofibrous (semirigid) compartment known as *Dorello canal.* Because of this, the sixth nerve is more liable to injury by some conditions such as trauma or inflammatory lesions involving the petrous apex (22). In the cavernous sinus it lies lateral to the internal carotid artery. It actually runs through the sinus and not in the sinus wall (Fig. 12.6; see Fig. 10.89). For this reason, intracavernous aneurysms of the internal carotid artery may affect the sixth instead of the third nerve. It enters the orbit through the superior orbital fissure above the opthalmic vein, from which it is separated by a lamina of dura mater; it then passes between the two heads of the lateral rectus muscle and enters this muscle on the medial side.

The abducent nerve may be affected by essentially the same processes that affect the third nerve in its cisternal portion. Because of its lower position, however, it is not affected by posterior communicating artery aneurysms. Brainstem tumors and extra-axial tumors may compress and displace the nerve (meningiomas, chordomas, chondrosarcomas, epidermoid tumors, fifth-nerve neuromas). Inflammatory lesions involving the petrous tip may affect the sixth nerve (Gradenigo syndrome). Other processes affecting the medial petrous pyramid, such as cholesterol granuloma and cholesteatomas, as well as fractures, may produce abducent nerve palsy (23).

Within the cavernous sinus, intracavernous aneurysms of the internal carotid artery are an important consideration. Lateral cavernous sinus wall involvement (total ophthalmoplegia, Foix syndrome) is usually produced by malignant neoplasms, cavernous sinus thrombosis, or Tolosa-Hunt syndrome due to subacute granulomatous inflammation. At the superior orbital fissure, meningioma and inflammatory processes such as fungus infection would be most likely, whereas intraorbitally, pseudotumor, lymphoma, and invasion from periorbital neoplasms should be considered (Table 12.1).

CRANIAL NERVE VII: FACIAL NERVE

This nerve has a motor and a sensory root, the latter often described under the name *nervus intermedius* (Wrisberg nerve). The two portions emerge from the anterolateral aspect of the pontomedullary sulcus, lateral and posterior to the sixth nerve (see Figs. 3.15 and 3.17). The more medial part is the motor, the larger component, which supplies the muscles of the face, scalp, and auricle; the buccinator and platysma; the stapedius; the stylohyoideus; and the posterior belly of the digastric muscle. Also, through the chorda tympani nerve it supplies vasodilator sympathetic nerves to the submaxillary and sublingual glands. The sensory component supplies the taste fibers for the anterior two-thirds of the tongue. The motor root arises from a nucleus situated deeply in the reticular formation of the lower pons. The fibers swing medially and upward, passing around and behind the nucleus of the sixth nerve before emerging.

The nerves enter the internal acoustic canal together with the eighth nerve and are anterior to the acoustic. Upon reaching the fundus of the bony canal, they enter the facial canal.

The facial canal is first directed laterally between the cochlea and vestibule toward the medial wall of the tympanic cavity. Before reaching its wall, it bends sharply backward and bends downward behind the tympanic cavity to emerge at the stylomastoid foramen. The point where the nerve (and facial canal) suddenly changes direction is called the *geniculum*, and from that the ganglion of the facial nerve situated at this point takes the name of *geniculate ganglion*. The geniculate ganglion gives origin to the sensory fibers that travel in the opposite direction toward the pons, constituting the intermediate nerve.

After exiting from the stylomastoid foramen, the nerve runs forward through the parotid gland. It passes the gland and, just before reaching the posterior margin of the as-

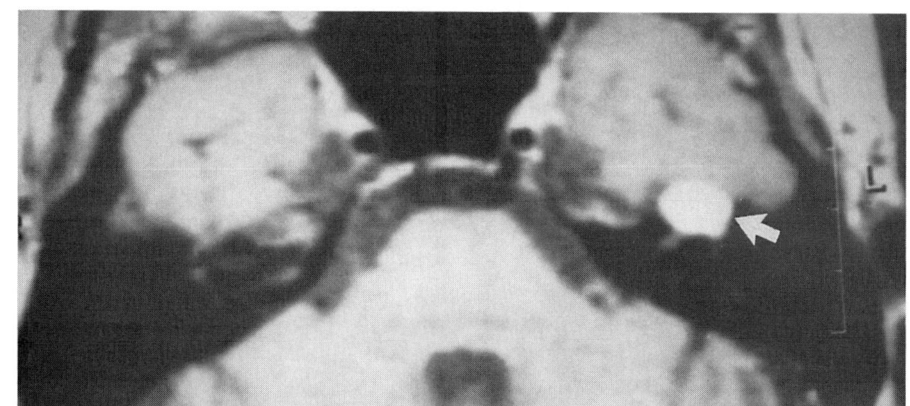

A

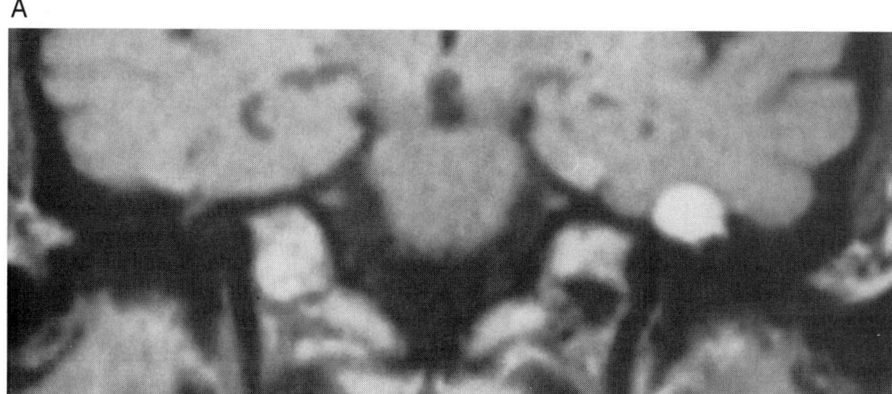

B

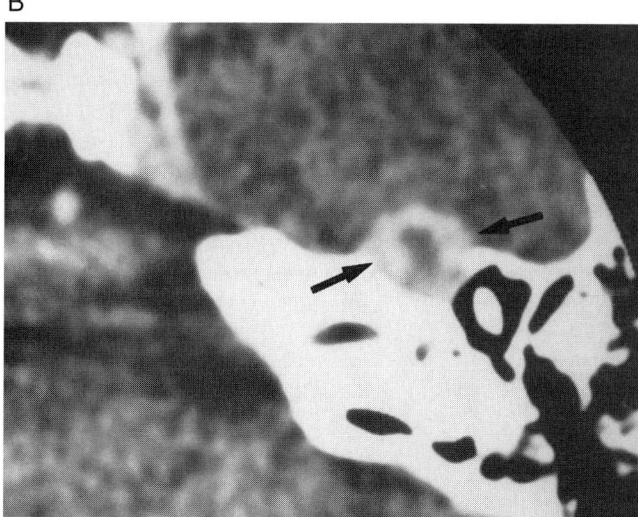

C

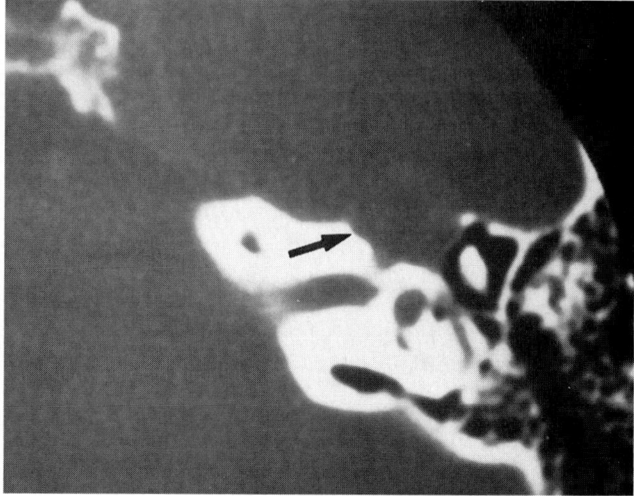

D

Figure 12.10. Neuroma of facial nerve (VII) arising at the first bend of the nerve. Postcontrast axial (**A**) and coronal (**B**) MRI revealed a 1.0-cm enhancing mass in the middle fossa adjacent to the petrous pyramid (arrow). **C.** A CT image shows an enhancing soft-tissue mass arising from the roof of the left petrous pyramid (arrows). **D.** The bone window of the same image reveals bone erosion of the root of the petrous bone (arrow).

cending ramus of the mandible, divides into a number of branches.

The facial nerve can be involved in a number of conditions along its complex course. In the cerebellopontine angle cistern, tumors of the acoustic nerve and cerebellopontine angle meningiomas are the most common.

Displacement and stretching of the facial nerve may lead to facial weakness. In the internal acoustic canal acoustic neuromas compress the facial nerve. Primary neuromas of the facial nerve are rare. They seem to occur around the first bend of the nerve at the geniculate ganglion and thus produce bone erosion of the roof of the petrous pyramid growing toward the middle fossa, giving the mass the appearance of a temporal fossa tumor. The presence of facial paresis should suggest the possible etiology. Bone destruction of the roof of the petrous pyramid may be demonstrable on CT or on plain films with tomography of the petrous pyramid (24,25) (Fig. 12.10). Otherwise they are like other neuromas from the imaging point of view. Facial nerve schwannomas may also occur in the descending segment of the facial nerve and produce typical bone erosion. Facial neuromas involving the cisternal and the intracarotid portions are even rarer.

The facial nerve may be affected by inflammatory processes; a typical example is the Ramsay Hunt syndrome (facial palsy, otalgia, vesicular eruption in external auditory canal), caused by herpes zoster virus. Facial nerve palsy (Bell palsy) is a common symptom, and in most cases no specific cause can be found. If symptoms are typical, there is no need to carry out detailed imaging examinations; if atypical signs are present, further investigation should be carried out. Some examples of atypical Bell palsy include slowly progressive palsy, facial spasms preceding the paralysis, recurrent palsies, excessive pain, involvement of other cranial nerves, and excessive duration of the palsy (longer than 2 months). Tien et al. carried out MRI examination with contrast in 11 patients with facial paralysis, and found that the nerve enhanced in 8 of the 11 patients; in 1 patient both sides enhanced (26). This raises a question regarding the significance of facial nerve enhancement. In the great majority of the patients studied, the enhancement was only on the affected side. The findings tend to suggest an inflammatory etiology for Bell palsy, possibly viral. The most marked enhancement in the series by Tien et al. was seen in the patient with herpes zoster virus infection (Ramsay Hunt syndrome) (26). Enhancement of the facial nerve is sometimes seen in normal cases.

Hemifacial spasm is important from the neuroimaging point of view (see under "Cranial Nerve V") (Table 12.1).

CRANIAL NERVE VIII: ACOUSTIC NERVE

The acoustic nerve is made up of (1) the cochlear nerve, the nerve of hearing, which goes from the cochlea to the pons, passing through the internal auditory canal and the cistern of the cerebellopontine angle; and (2) the vestibular division, the nerve of equilibrium. There is a nerve ganglion, the Scarpa ganglion, situated in the upper part of the internal auditory canal, at the fundus.

The vestibular portion gives origin to the rather frequent acoustic neuromas. When bilateral, the lesions are surely related to neurofibromatosis type II. See under "Posterior Fossa Tumors," Chapter 11; and under "Neurofibromatosis," Chapter 5, for further details (Table 12.1).

CRANIAL NERVE IX: GLOSSOPHARYNGEAL NERVE

The ninth cranial nerve has motor and sensory fibers and distributes itself to the tongue and pharynx. It provides sensory innervation to the pharynx and tonsillar area, and taste innervation to the posterior part of the tongue.

The nerve emerges from the medulla in the sulcus between the olive and the inferior peduncle (see Figs. 3.15 and 3.17). It is directed laterally and forward, passing through the anterior medial part of the jugular foramen slightly in front of the tenth and eleventh nerves. The superior ganglion of the glossopharyngeus is situated in the upper part of the groove in which it is lodged during its passage through the jugular foramen. The petrous ganglion is larger and situated below the other. Both supply the sensory fibers of the nerve.

It is mostly a sensory nerve, and connects with the vagus, the facial nerve, and the sympathetic nerve. The sensory distribution is as explained earlier; in addition, it supplies carotid branches that, together with the vagus and a sympathetic component, innervate the carotid sinus.

A muscular branch is distributed to the stylopharyngeus muscle.

The ninth nerve may be affected, along with the tenth and eleventh, by masses in the area, intrinsic or extrinsic, involving the medulla and perimedullary region. Further anterolaterally it may be involved in the jugular fossa region by bony destructive processes from malignant neoplasms due to direct invasion by nasopharyngeal carcinoma or metastatic disease.

Schwannomas in the region of the jugular fossa occur, and it is usually not possible to tell whether the lesion originated in a particular cranial nerve. For this reason we usually refer to jugular foramen schwannoma or schwannomas of the ninth, tenth, and eleventh nerves (see Fig. 11.112). The lesions usually produce erosion of the jugular foramen and must be differentiated from glomus jugulare tumors. Angiography may be required for this purpose. On angiography the glomus jugulare tumors are very vascular, have rapid circulation with early venous filling, and may invade and sometimes obstruct the jugular vein, which jugular foramen schwannomas do not usually do (Table 12.1).

CRANIAL NERVE X: VAGUS (PNEUMOGASTRIC) NERVE

The vagus is a complicated, extensively distributed nerve going down to the abdomen. It emerges from the medulla at the sulcus behind the olive, just below the ninth nerve (see Figs. 3.15 and 3.17). Like the glossopharyngeus, it is directed laterally and anteriorly beneath the cerebellar flocculus to the jugular fossa through which it passes, slightly behind and lateral to the ninth nerve and anteromedial to the jugular bulb, together with the posterior meningeal artery, a sympathetic branch, and a meningeal arterial branch.

The vagus has two ganglia. The *jugular ganglion* (in the jugular foramen region) is small and connects with the cranial portion of the eleventh, the seventh, and the ninth nerves. The inferior ganglion (*ganglion nodosum*) is about 2.5 cm in length and situated below the vagus nerve exit from the jugular foramen. At the ganglion the cranial portion of the eleventh (accessory) nerve joins the vagus.

The vagus descends within the carotid sheath behind and between the internal carotid artery and internal jugular vein and continues down with the common carotid artery to the root of the neck. The right nerve passes downward between the subclavian artery and innominate vein, parallel to the trachea, and behind the right main bronchus to reach the esophagus. Below the subclavian artery it gives off the recurrent laryngeal nerve that winds under and behind the artery to ascend parallel to the trachea to the larynx.

The left vagus descends in front of the subclavian artery, between it and the innominate vein, crosses the aortic arch, and descends behind the root of the left lung to the anterior surface of the esophagus. The vagus is composed of parasympathetic efferent fibers, and somatic motor and sensory fibers.

The nerve may be affected with the ninth and eleventh in the jugular fossa, or it may be involved above the jugular fossa, like the ninth nerve. Below the base of the skull, glomus intravagale tumors have been described (27). The glomus tumors (chemodectomas) arise from chemoreceptor tissue situated in the jugular fossa around the superior (jugular) ganglion of the vagus nerve and the tympanic branch of the glossopharyngeal nerve (see Figs. 10.121 and 11.113*D*, *E*, and *F*). In addition, chemoreceptor tissue can be found along the cervical portion of the vagus nerve, where tumors of this type can occasionally be found (vagus intravagale).

CRANIAL NERVE XI: SPINAL (ACCESSORY) NERVE

The eleventh nerve has two portions: the cranial portion, which emerges from the medulla caudal to the vagus and in the sulcus behind the olive (posterolateral sulcus), and the spinal portion, which originates from the upper cervical spinal cord, down to C4. The fibers of the nerve emerge from the cord at the posterolateral sulcus and join in a trunk, which ascends to enter the skull through the foramen magnum, only to join the cranial portion and exit the cranial cavity through the jugular fossa.

The cranial portion joins the vagus at the lower ganglion. The spinal portion innervates the sternocleidomastoid and the trapezius muscles, together with branches of the third and fourth cervical nerves.

The eleventh nerve may be affected by processes similar to those that affect the ninth and tenth nerves, except for the glomus tumor of the tenth nerve.

CRANIAL NERVE XII: HYPOGLOSSAL NERVE

The twelfth nerve is the motor nerve of the tongue. It originates in the medulla in the hypoglossal nucleus, which is a prolongation of the anterior column of gray substances of the spinal cord (see Fig. 3.22). It emerges from the medulla in the anterolateral sulcus between the pyramid and the olive (see Fig. 3.15). After emerging from the anterolateral sulcus, the various roots of the nerve perforate the dura mater separately and join together in the nerve trunk outside the dura as they pass through the hypoglossal canal (or foramen) (sometimes double) situated at the base of the occipital condyle on the endocranial surface. The vertebral artery swings under the lower roots of the hypoglossal nerve as it swings medially and forward to enter the skull through the foramen magnum.

After exiting the skull, the nerve descends almost vertically behind and between the internal carotid artery and the jugular vein (next to the vagus nerve) until about the level of the angle of the mandible, where it swings forward, passing lateral to the external carotid artery and under the occipital artery.

The nerve can be affected by primary schwannomas, which may produce erosion of the hypoglossal canal (see Fig. 11.113). Malignant tumors may destroy the occipital condyle region and compress the nerve. A fusiform aneurysm of the vertebral artery may compress the lower portion of the nerve, and intrinsic tumors as well as vascular ischemic lesions of the medulla may affect the nerve origins (Table 12.1).

REFERENCES

1. Hudgins PA, Newman NJ, Dillon WP, Hoffman JC Jr: Radiation-induced optic neuropathy: Characteristic appearances on gadolinium-enhanced MR. AJNR 1992;13:235–238.
2. Kelly WM: Functional anatomy and cranial neuropathy: Neuroimaging perspective. Neuroimag Clin North Am 1993;3:1–45.
3. Vogl T, Dresel S, Lockmüller H, et al: Third cranial nerve palsy caused by gummatous neurosyphilis: MR findings. AJNR 1993;14:1329–1331.
4. Gentry LR, Mehta RC, Appen RC, et al: MR imaging of primary trochlear nerve neoplasms. AJNR 1991;12:707–713.
5. Donohue JM, Enzmann DR: Mycotic aneurysm in angiitis associated with herpes zoster ophthalmicus. AJNR 1987;8:615–619.
6. Bradbury M: The Concept of the Blood-Brain Barrier. New York: Wiley, 1979.
7. Tien Rd, Dillon WP: Herpes trigeminalneuritis and rhombencephalitis on Gd-DTPA-enhanced MR imaging. AJNR 1990;11:413–414.
8. Croen KD, Ostrove JM, Dragovic LJ, et al: Latent herpes simplex virus in human trigeminal ganglia. N Engl J Med 1987;317:1427–1432.
9. Yamada K, Ohta T, Miyamoto T: Bilateral trigeminal schwannomas associated with von Recklinghausen disease. AJNR 1992;13:299–300.
10. Pollack IF, Sekhar LN, Jeanetta PJ, et al: Neurinomas of the trigeminal nerve. J Neurosurg 1989;70:737–745.

11. McCormack PC, Bello JA, Post KD: Trigeminal schwannoma. J Neurosurg 1988;69:850–860.
12. DePena CA, Lee YY, Van Tassel P: Lymphomatous involvement of the trigeminal nerve and Mekel cave: CT and MR appearance. AJNR 1989;10:S15–S17.
13. Barakos JA, D'Amour PG, Dillon WP, et al: Trigeminal sensory neuropathy caused by cervical disk herniation. AJNR 1990;11:609.
14. Tash RR, Sze G, Leslie DR: Trigeminal neuralgia: MR imaging features. Radiology 1989;172:767–770.
15. Jeanetta PJ: Arterial compression of the trigeminal nerve at the pons in patients with trigeminal neuralgia. J Neurosurg 1967;26:159–162.
16. Jeanetta PJ, Abbasy M, Maroon JC, et al: Etiology and definitive microsurgical treatment of hemifacial spasm. Operative techniques and results in 47 patients. J Neurosurg 1977;47:321–328.
17. Bederson JB, Wilson CB: Evaluation of microvascular decompression and partial rhizotomy in 252 cases of trigeminal neuralgia. J Neurosurg 1989;71:359–367.
18. Nagahiro S, Takada A, Matsukado Y, et al: Microvascular decompression of hemifacial spasm: Patterns of vascular compression in unsuccessfully operated patients. J Neurosurg 1991;75:388–392.
19. Nagaseki Y, Horikoshi T, Omata T, et al: Oblique sagittal magnetic resonance imaging visualizing vascular compression of the trigeminal or facial nerve. J Neurosurg 1992;77:379–386.
20. Esfahani F, Dolan KD: Air CT cisternography in the diagnosis of vascular loop causing vestibular nerve dysfunction. AJNR 1989;10:1045–1049.
21. Tash R, De Merritt J, Sze G, et al: Hemifacial spasm: MR imaging features. AJNR 1991;12:839–842.
22. Umansky F, Elidan J, Valarezo A: Dorell's canal: A microanatomical study. J Neurosurg 1991;75:294–298.
23. Depper MH, Truwit CL, Dreisbach JN, Kelly WM: Isolated abducens nerve palsy: MR imaging findings. AJR 1993;160:837–841.
24. Lidov M, Som PM, Stacy C, et al: Eccentric cystic facial schwannoma: CT and MR features. J Comput Assist Tomogr 1991;15:1065–1067.
25. Martin N, Sterkers O, Mompoint D, et al: Facial nerve neuromas: MR imaging. Neuroradiology 1992;34:62–67.
26. Tien RD, Dillion WP, Jackler RK: Contrast-enhanced MR imaging of the facial nerve in 11 patients with Bell's palsy. AJNR 1990;11:735–741.
27. Berk ME: Chemodectoma of the glomus intravagale: A case report and review. Clin Radiol 1961;12:219.

13

Systemic Diseases Affecting the Central Nervous System

Because a number of systemic diseases affect the central nervous system (CNS) with varying frequency, it is worthwhile to include a discussion of the CNS involvement encountered in these conditions, as well as the type of computed tomography (CT) or magnetic resonance imaging (MRI) findings. Some, like malignant neoplastic disease, may involve the brain or spinal cord through metastases; these have been discussed earlier, together with neoplastic diseases of the brain and spine (Chapter 11); the same is true of most infectious disease (Chapter 6). The material will be divided into seven groups.

INFLAMMATORY CONDITIONS

Lymphomatoid Granulomatosis

This is a necrotizing pseudogranulomatous process characterized by a multifocal pleomorphic cellular infiltrate involving the blood vessels (1). It affects primarily the lungs, kidneys, and skin. The CNS is involved in 20 percent of cases and sometimes is the first to be affected. In the four patients reported by Kapila et al. the most frequent area involved was the cerebellum (2). The lesions were hemorrhagic in three of the four cases, and systemic involvement (particularly the lungs) was present in three cases and was suspected in one case. It is a severe illness with a high mortality rate if the CNS is involved. The lesions enhance with contrast and may or may not be hemorrhagic when the patient is first seen. Lymphomatoid granulomatosis may be related to lymphoma, but this seems unlikely in view of the fact that brain parenchymal involvement in systemic lymphoma is relatively infrequent. On the other hand, about half of patients later develop true malignant lymphoma. Lymphomatoid granulomatosis has been reported in patients with acquired immunodeficiency syndrome (AIDS) (3) (Table 13.1).

Wegener Granulomatosis

This is a chronic condition characterized by granulomatous vasculitis of the upper and lower respiratory tracts together with glomerulonephritis. Variable degrees of disseminated vasculitis involving arteries and veins may occur (4).

There is necrotizing vasculitis of small arteries and veins as well as granuloma formation, which may be extravascular

Table 13.1.
Lymphomatoid Granulomatosis

Necrotizing process affecting CNS and non-CNS blood vessels
Systemic process involving lungs, kidneys, and skin
CNS involvement in 20 percent of cases
Variety of CNS manifestations, including leptomeningeal infiltration, solid or necrotic masses, and intraparenchymal hemorrhages

or intravascular. The lungs are most frequently involved. The kidneys are also frequently involved, and a glomerulitis evolving to glomerulonephritis is typical of the disease. The paranasal sinus and nose are usually involved.

CNS involvement occurs in about one-quarter to one-fifth of patients. Yamashita et al. described three types of lesions: (*a*) direct intracranial involvement from nasal and paranasal sinus lesions; (*b*) remote intracranial involvement (intracerebral and meningeal granulomas), in patients presenting nasal and paranasal sinus lesions; and (*c*) vasculitic lesions (5) (Fig. 13.1; Table 13.2).

Whipple Disease (Intestinal Lipodystrophy)

This rare disease occurs mostly in white males. Arthritis, prolonged diarrhea, malabsorption, and weight loss are characteristic. Arthritis develops in 90 percent of patients (often prior to other symptoms); it usually is acute in onset, is migratory, lasts a few days, and is not chronic (6). Other symptoms include fever, edema, pleural effusion, pericardial effusion, hypotension, pneumonia, and lymphadenopathy. CNS involvement may appear with memory loss, confusion and depression, diplopia, papilledema, and headaches. Periodic acid–Schiff–staining bacilliform structures in the biopsy of small intestinal mucosa are diagnostic. We have recently seen a patient presenting diffuse thickening of the dura in the head and the spine. The lesions were extensive and long-standing, producing bone thinning in the adjacent skull bones and vertebrae (Fig. 13.2). The lesions enhanced with contrast and were markedly hyperintense on proton density and T2-weighted images. Occasionally parenchymal brain lesions may be found.

Lyme Disease

The CNS lesions have been described in Chapter 6. The spinal cord may also be involved.

Table 13.2.
Wegener Granulomatosis

Granulomatous vasculitis, primarily involving the upper and lower respiratory tracts and kidneys
CNS involvement in about 20 percent of cases
CNS findings include direct intracranial extension of nasal/paranasal disease, distant parenchymal and meningeal lesions, and vasculitis

Septicemia and Endocarditis

In addition to abscess, mycotic aneurysm is an important manifestation. This has been described in Chapter 6 (see Fig. 6.18). Brain hemorrhage, a frequent manifestation, may be the first evidence of the disease process.

Sarcoidosis

Sarcoidosis has also been discussed in Chapter 6. Involvement of the CNS occurs in about 5 percent of patients. It can affect the meninges; the dura may be locally thickened and would enhance with contrast. The hypothalamus, the optic chiasmal area, chronic meningitis and hydrocephalus, and sometimes a mass lesion suggesting tumor, usually on the meningeal surface, are seen (see Figs. 6.28 through 6.30). The sarcoid lesions enhance with contrast, and on MRI they are usually "T2 dark," which is a fairly characteristic feature, almost diagnostic in a patient who has sarcoid manifestations elsewhere (Table 13.3).

Table 13.3.
Neurosarcoidosis

Present in about 5 percent of patients with systemic sarcoidosis
Preferential involvement of optic chiasm, hypothalamus
Often manifested as a chronic meningitis
Parenchymal lesions often seen as hypointense regions on T2-weighted MR images

IMMUNOLOGIC CONDITIONS

Systemic Lupus Erythematosus

Systemic lupus erythematosus (SLE) is a disease of unknown etiology in which tissues and cells are damaged by deposition of immune complexes and pathogenic antibodies. It is seen particularly in young women and affects all races. The symptoms vary according to the affected organs; the disease may involve only one organ system. The joints are frequently involved; arthralgias and swelling at joints are frequent. Also common are erythematous rash in the face (butterfly distribution) and proteinuria due to renal involvement (in about 50 percent of patients). CNS involvement occurs in about one-third of cases.

Basically any portion of the brain or spinal cord can be involved, including the meninges. Psychoses are not uncommon, and grand mal seizures can occur. What we may see on imaging examinations are abnormalities that represent vascular lesions. We may see true infarcts at times, but also symptomatic "edematous" areas in the brain that seem to be migratory in that they disappear, only to reappear in other areas of the brain at a later date (7) (Figs. 13.3 and 13.4). Bell et al. found that in patients with focal lesions there were elevated levels of cardiolipin and lupus anticoagulant; they also found more diffuse subcortical involvement in some patients in whom there was elevation of the antineurofilament antibodies (8). These lesions re-

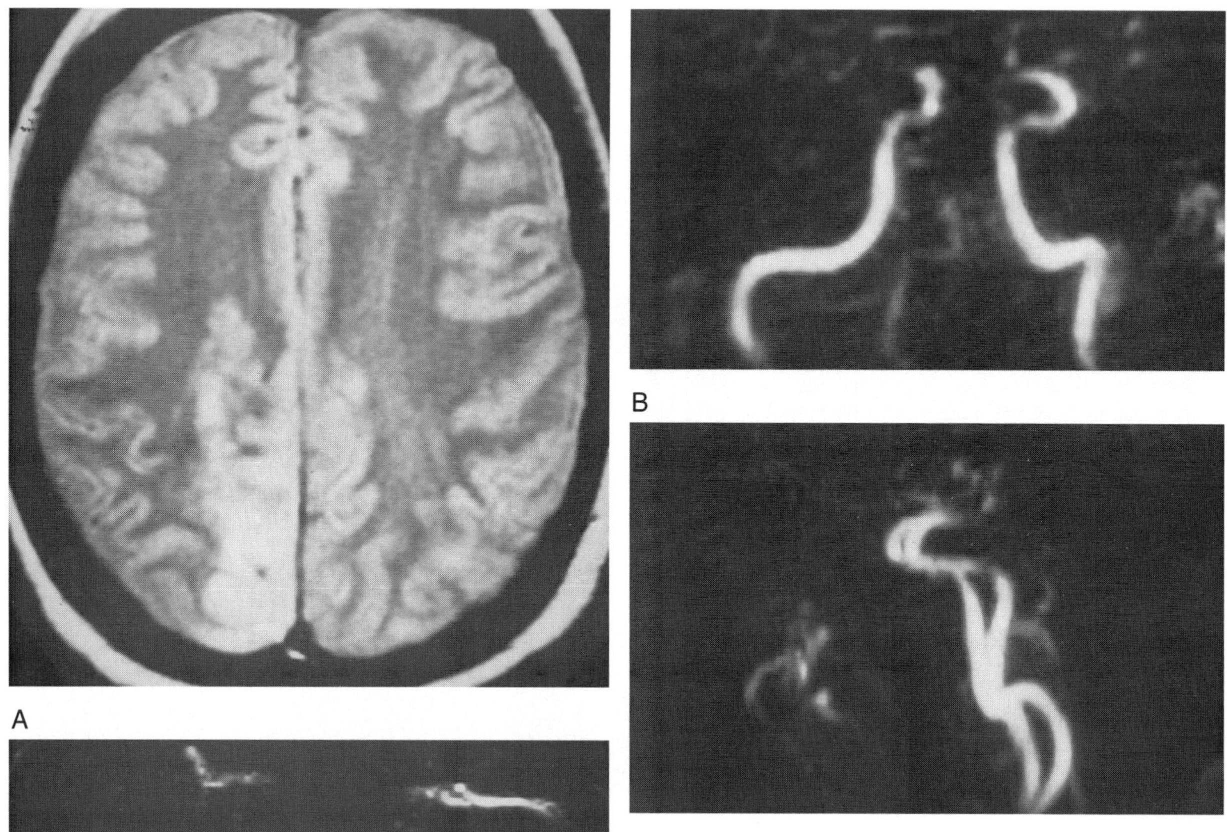

Figure 13.1. Wegener granulomatosis showing diffuse arteritis. **A.** There is a hyperintense area in the right occipital region, which was thought to represent an ischemic lesion. **B** and **C.** MRI angiography demonstrated flow in the internal carotid arteries and poor flow or no flow in the basilar artery. Also, the trunks of the middle and anterior cerebral arteries are not imaged normally. A diffuse arterial disease was suspected. (**B**) Frontal. (**C**) Sagittal. **D.** The collapse view shows the lack of normal flow in all major cerebral arteries. Only the internal carotid arteries are well seen. **E** and **F.** Vertebral angiography shows multiple narrow segments in the vertebral artery and the right and left posterior cerebral arteries (arrows). The basilar artery is fairly normal, and the lack of imaging on MRI must be interpreted as meaning slower flow due to diffuse arteritis of cerebral arteries.

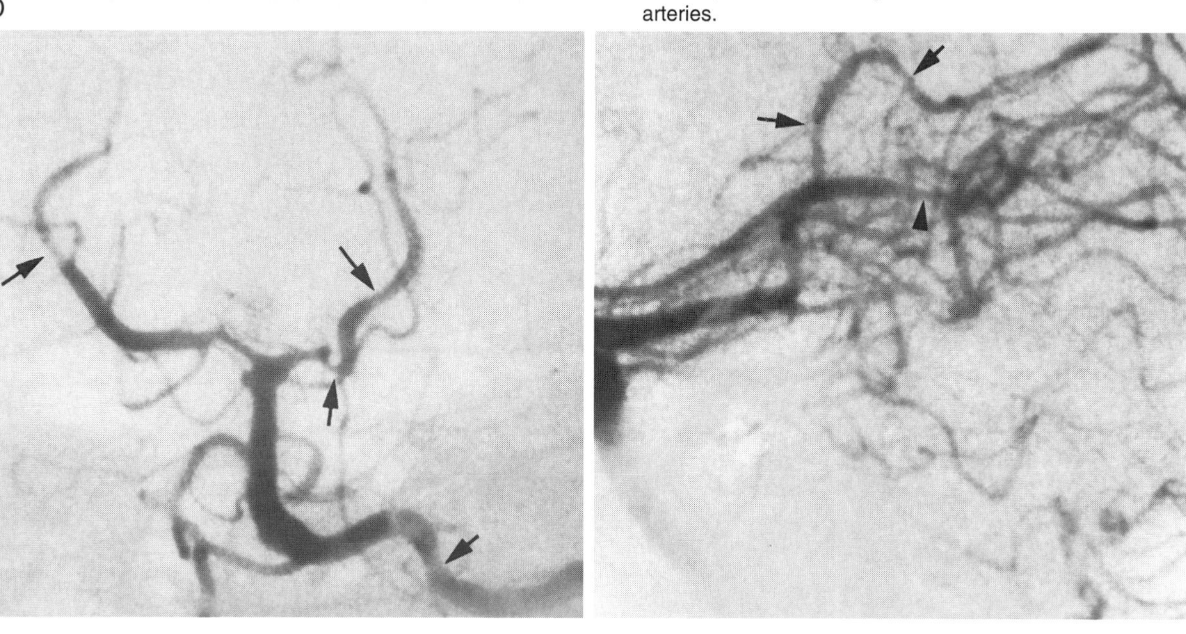

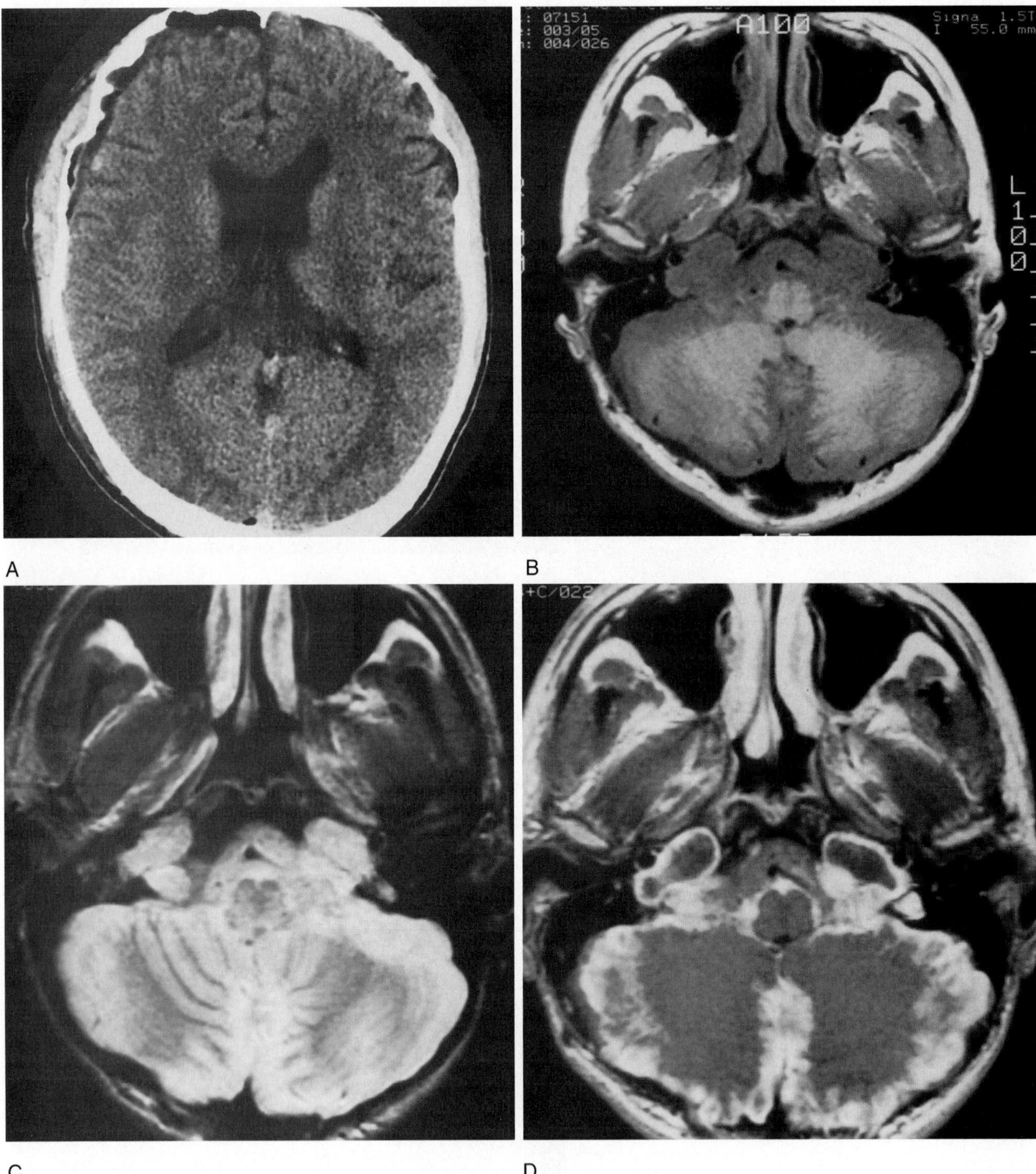

Figure 13.2. Whipple disease showing diffuse hypertrophic pachymeningitis. **A.** CT shows thickening of meninges in the right frontal area and erosion of the inner table of the skull with considerable thinning of the bone, mostly on the right side but also on the left. **B.** T1-weighted noncontrast axial shows a low-intensity area surrounding the cerebellum and medulla, seen on proton density to be moderately hyperintense (**C**). **D.** After contrast there is marked enhancement of the thickened meninges. The thickened meninges are seen to extend through the jugular foramen.

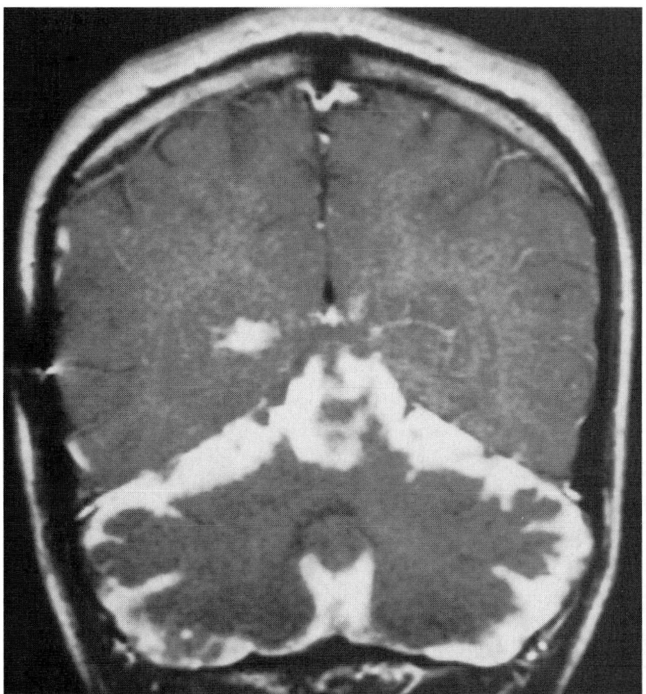

E

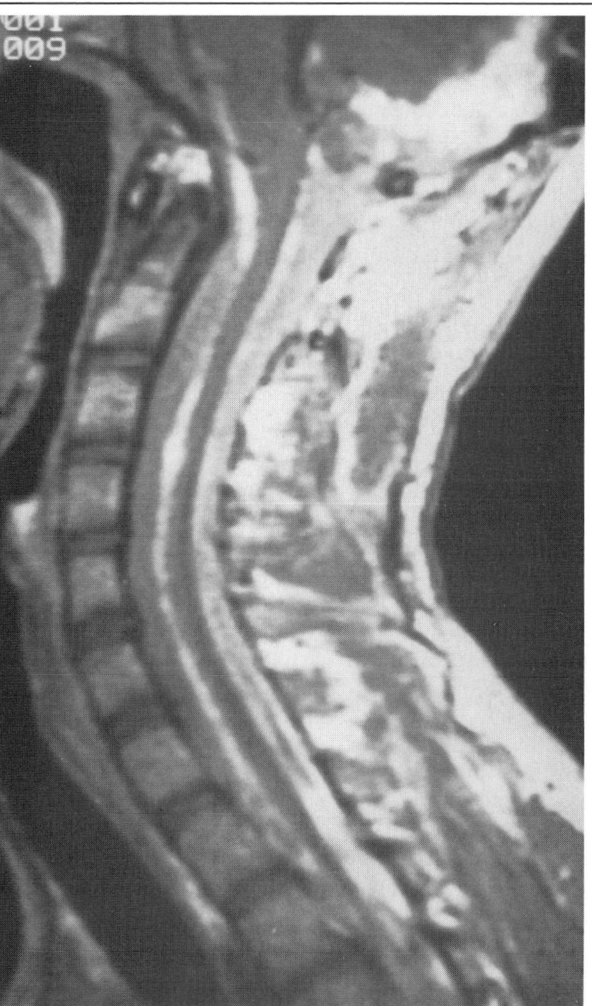

F

Figure 13.2. *(continued)* **E.** Coronal view following enhancement. **F.** Postcontrast sagittal cervical spine shows that only the deeper layers of the thickened meninges enhance. The spinal cord is uniformly narrow throughout, but as yet there were no neurologic signs of cord compression. The appearance is rather unusual. The relationship with Whipple disease is not proved, but meningeal biopsy showed an atypical histiocytic infiltrate with PAS-positive diastase-resistant coccobacilli consistent with Whipple disease.

sponded rapidly to high doses of methylprednisolone, whereas the focal lesions did not. Aisen et al. indicate that there are three patterns: (*a*) focal infarcts; (*b*) multiple hyperintense areas on T2-weighted images consistent with microinfarctions; and (*c*) focal areas of increased intensity, primarily in the gray matter (7) (Fig. 13.4). To these we add a fourth pattern consisting of diffuse subcortical changes, which rapidly respond to steroid therapy. The case reported by Marsteller et al. probably belongs in this group (9) (Table 13.4).

Table 13.4.
Systemic Lupus Erythematosus (SLE)

CNS involvement seen in about one-third of cases
Symptomatic manifestations can include psychosis, strokes, cranial neuropathies, and transverse myelitis
Cross-sectional imaging findings can include arteritis, infarcts of various sizes, cortical signal changes on MRI, and subcortical regions of signal abnormality, which may respond to steroids

Calcification in the lesions of SLE has been reported (10).

Aneurysms are seen in patients with lupus; they may be fusiform in shape and may be associated with cerebral arteritis (11).

Cerebral hemorrhage is seen with relative frequency in lupus; it may consist of multiple small hemorrhages or larger ones.

Antiphospholipid Syndrome

Antiphospholipid antibodies (APLA) are immunoglobulins (IgG, IgM, and IgA) with activity against negatively charged phospholipids. In antiphospholipid syndrome lupus anticoagulant and anticardiolipin antibodies, false-positive VDRL, and rapid plasma reagin (RPR) may be found (12). The syndrome has been associated with an increased frequency of venous and arterial thrombosis, spontaneous abortions, thrombocytopenia, cardiac valve vegetations, strokes in the young, and livedo reticularis and other

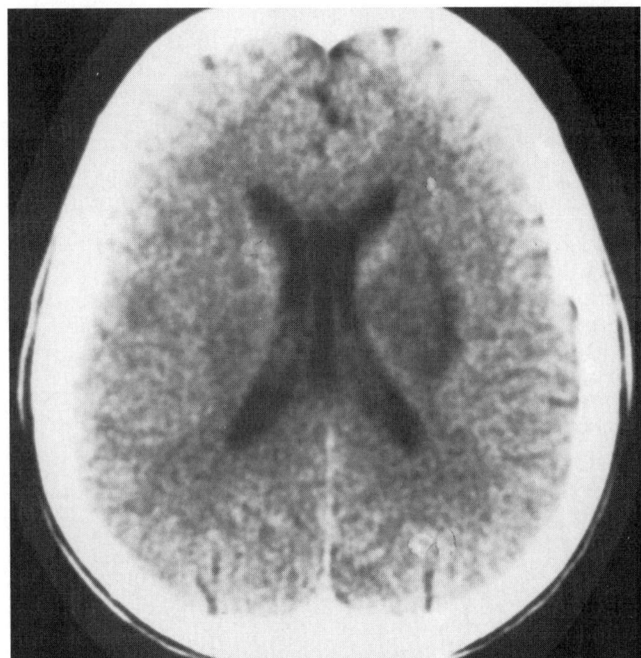

Figure 13.3. Lupus erythematosus in a 55-year-old woman. **A** and **B.** CT and T2-weighted MRI show a large lesion involving the left lenticular nucleus and adjacent portion of the external capsule, and also the posterior limb of the internal capsule, causing some right-sided weakness. **C.** When the patient was reexamined eight months later, the previous lesion had totally disappeared, but she now presented a lesion on the other side (arrow) in approximately the same area. Another lesion was present in the left periventricular region around the frontal horn and foramen of Monro (**D**).

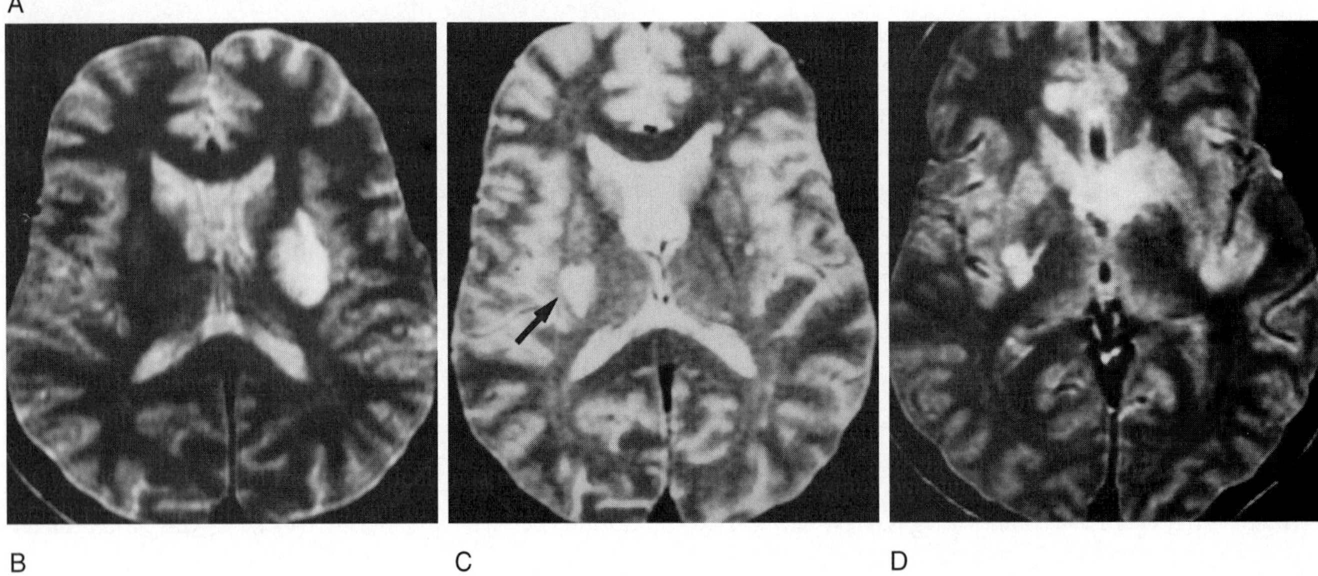

skin manifestations. Neurologic manifestations include strokes and transient ischemic attacks, multi-infarct dementia, and ischemic encephalopathy (13). In the case reported by Pulpeiro et al., the history resembled multiple sclerosis, there were a number of bright white matter patches in T2-weighted images, and the patient did not have SLE (14).

Perhaps the most important concept to keep in mind is the possible association of the antiphospolipid syndrome with stroke in the young (Table 13.5). See also Chapter 10.

The term *lupus anticoagulant* is misleading because what is found is venous and arterial thrombosis, not bleeding.

Table 13.5.
Antiphospholipid Antibody Syndrome

Venous and arterial thromboses, recurrent abortions, strokes, and livedo reticularis
Major antibodies include the lupus anticoagulant and anticardiolipin antibody
CNS manifestations can include larger artery thromboses, diffuse white matter MRI signal abnormalities, cortical atrophy, and dural sinus thrombosis

Rheumatoid Arthritis

Neurologic manifestations are uncommon in rheumatoid arthritis. The most common finding, which may or may

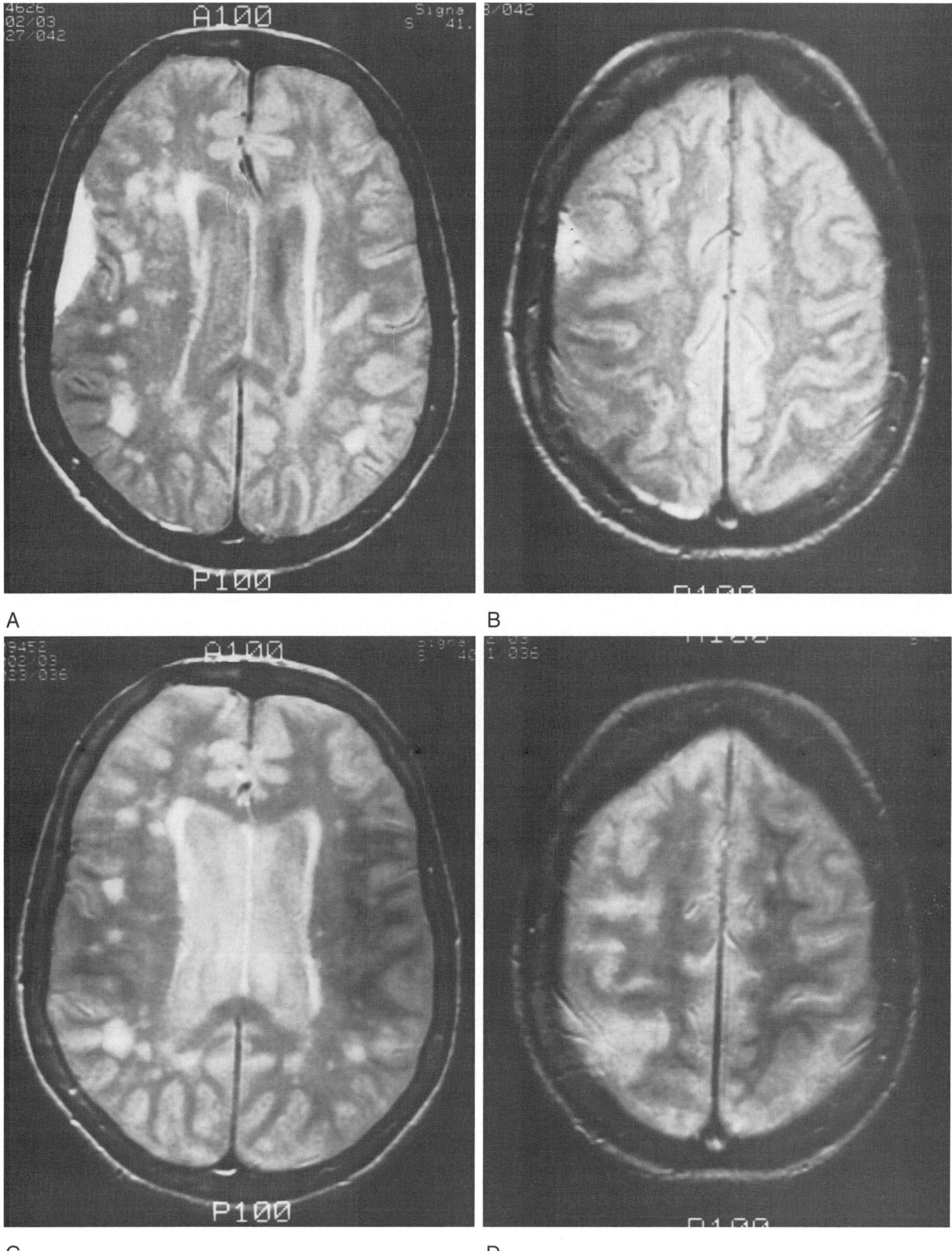

Figure 13.4. Lupus erythematosus in a 71-year-old woman with spontaneous intracranial hemorrhage. The patient had prolonged prothrombin time but a tendency to thromboses. **A** and **B.** There is periventricular hyperintensity on proton density axial. There are a number of white matter hyperintense foci, mostly in the region of the U fibers. There is a right subdural hematoma. **C.** Reexamination several months later showed disappearance of the subdural collection but no change in the hyperintense white matter U fiber lesions, the nature of which is not clear. **D.** Proton density image higher in the hemisphere revealed a white and gray matter lesion. Bleeding as well as thromboses (mostly the latter) are seen in lupus patients related to the lupus anticoagulant and anticardiolipin antibodies.

not be associated with neurologic symptoms, is rheumatoid arthritis of the atlantoaxial joint. It may be associated with large panus formation, which may compress the cervicomedullary junction, sometimes combined with subluxation, leading to neurologic findings (see Fig. 15.8). See also Chapter 15.

Other neurologic manifestations are related to rheumatoid nodules in the brain, but these are very rare and are not necessarily symptomatic (15). Rheumatoid nodules have also been described pathologically within the choroid plexus (16). Hypertrophic pachymeningitis associated with rheumatoid arthritis has been reported and is also rare, judging by the scarcity of reports. The patient may present with headaches not responding to usual medications. In the case reported by Yuh et al. there was marked enhancement with gadolinium (17).

Vasculitis

Arteritis and related diagnoses are described and illustrated in Chapter 6.

Behçet Disease

This is a multisystem immune-related vasculitis characterized by oral and genital ulcers, ocular inflammation, pulmonary infarctions, a fluctuating course, and sometimes skin lesions, arthritis, and ulcerative colitis. Neurologic manifestations, which occur in 10 to 25 percent of cases, consist of loss of vision, diplopia, nystagmus, cranial nerve palsies, speech disorders, cerebellar signs, and cerebral and spinal sensory and motor disturbances. Three patterns have been described: a brainstem syndrome, a meningoencephalitic syndrome, and an organic confusion syndrome (18).

The imaging findings, as reported by Banna and El-Ramahi, include high-intensity foci in the white matter *not* showing predilection for the periventricular area like multiple sclerosis (19). They may occur in the brain or in the brainstem. Banna and El-Ramahi's reported cases were all from Saudi Arabia; Behçet disease is more common in Mediterranean countries, Middle Eastern countries, and Japan (19). In the series by Banna and El-Ramahi, four patients had cerebral angiography and two showed venous thrombosis (19). Venous thromboses occur in about one-third of patients. Arterial involvement has rarely been reported, but one case of multiple aneurysms has been reported (20).

Table 13.6.
Behçet Disease

Immune-related vasculitis characterized by oral and genital ulcers, ocular inflammation, and occasionally skin lesions
Most commonly seen in the Middle East, Mediterranean countries, and Japan
MRI findings: Hyperintense foci on T2-weighted images in brainstem, thalamus, and hemispheric white matter

The white matter patches seen on T2-weighted images are most common in the brainstem, followed by the thalamus and the cerebral hemisphere white matter (Fig. 13.5). They probably represent inflammatory cellular infiltrate, demyelinations, and edema, which may improve with corticosteriod therapy alone or in combination with immunosupressive drugs. The differential diagnosis includes multiple sclerosis, brainstem encephalitis, and infarction (Table 13.6).

Lymphomatoid Granulomatosis

This rare condition is described briefly earlier under "Inflammatory Conditions."

Chronic Fatigue Syndrome

Chronic fatigue syndrome has been placed among the immunologic conditions for lack of a more definite known etiology. It may be a chronic viral encephalitis (21).

This is a debilitating multisystem condition of unknown origin manifested by fatigue, flulike complaints, and neurologic signs and symptoms, including persistent headaches, impaired cognitive abilities, mood disorders, and sensorimotor disturbances. The diagnosis is difficult to make clinically or by usual tests. The hallmark of the disease is the disabling fatique, which may be accompanied by low-grade fever, myalgia, pharyngitis, and adenopathy. The patients are usually young adults, more frequently females (2:1 ratio with males) (21).

The imaging in patients who fit the clinical criteria for chronic fatigue syndrome is as follows: CT is usually negative; MRI will show bright foci on T2-weighted images in the centrum semiovale, corona radiata, internal capsule, periventricular region, or the subcortical white matter (U fibers). The abnormal foci were found in about 50 percent of patients (22). The significance of the foci is always open to question because of the frequency with which they are encountered in practice, particularly in subjects over 65 years of age. However, the disease tends to affect younger subjects (average 42 years), and it is known that the number and size of these foci in subjects under 50 years are rather slight.

Schwartz et al. carried out single photon emission computed tomography (SPECT) examinations as well as MRI in 16 patients who fit the criteria of chronic fatigue syndrome (23). They found perfusion defects in the cerebral cortex and basal nuclei on SPECT in 80 percent of the patients, whereas only 50 percent presented white matter foci on MRI. The combination of the two procedures may be of help in arriving at a diagnosis of chronic fatigue syndrome, which may be a chronic viral encephalitis. Further studies are needed. The cortical perfusion defects can be studied with MRI using echoplanar techniques to compare with the SPECT findings, and confirmation with positron emission tomography would be very valuable.

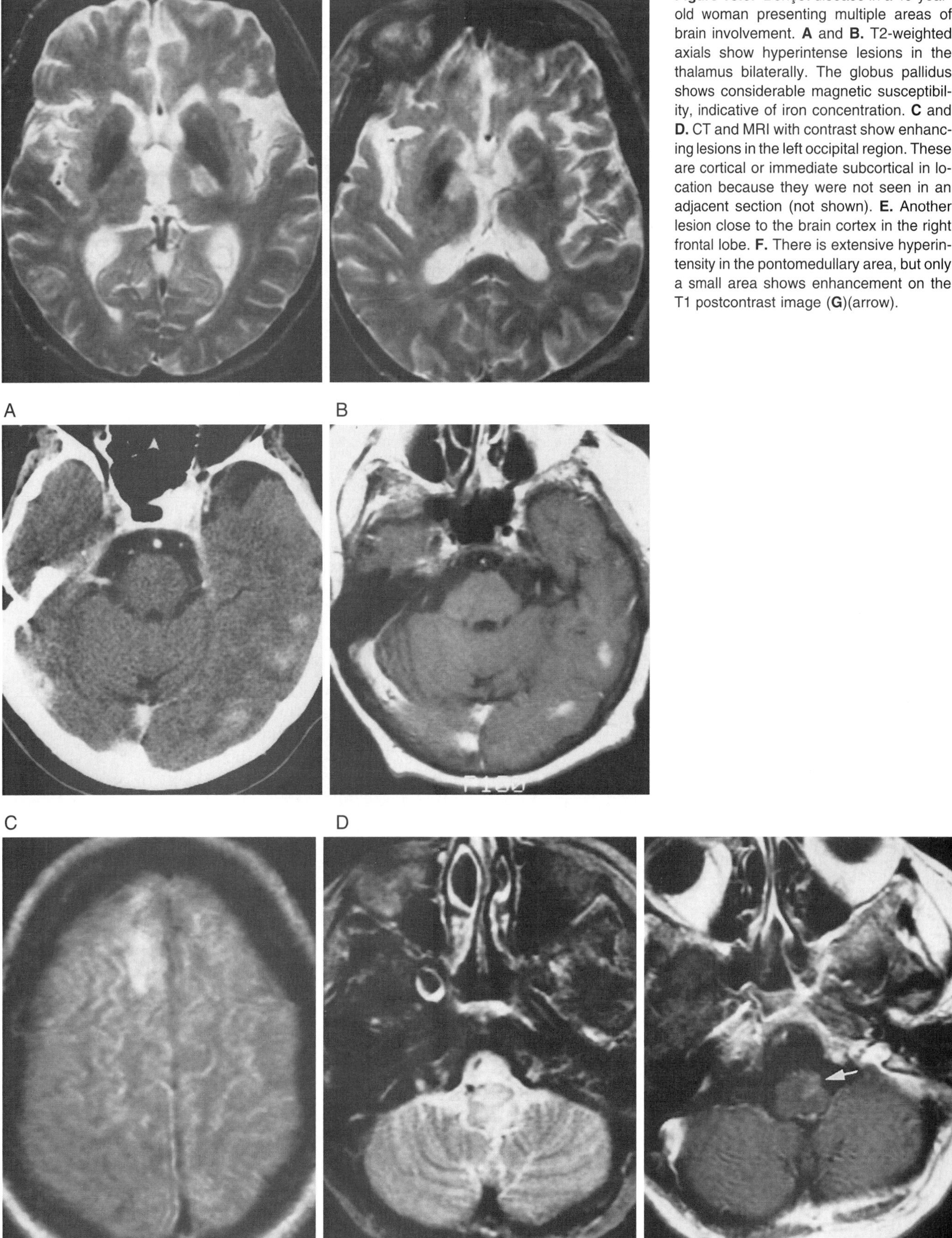

Figure 13.5. Behçet disease in a 49-year-old woman presenting multiple areas of brain involvement. **A** and **B.** T2-weighted axials show hyperintense lesions in the thalamus bilaterally. The globus pallidus shows considerable magnetic susceptibility, indicative of iron concentration. **C** and **D.** CT and MRI with contrast show enhancing lesions in the left occipital region. These are cortical or immediate subcortical in location because they were not seen in an adjacent section (not shown). **E.** Another lesion close to the brain cortex in the right frontal lobe. **F.** There is extensive hyperintensity in the pontomedullary area, but only a small area shows enhancement on the T1 postcontrast image (**G**)(arrow).

BLOOD DISORDERS

Anemias

Anemia per se does not cause any neurologic problems unless the hemoglobin concentration falls below 50 percent of normal. In these cases retinal pallor may be observed ophthalmoscopically, and flame-shaped hemorrhage with edema may occur. Signs of brain involvement are usually lacking.

Among the anemias, however, there are some with specific neurologic manifestations.

VITAMIN B_{12} DEFICIENCY LEADING TO PERNICIOUS ANEMIA

The classic picture is that of subacute combined degeneration of the spinal cord, optic neuropathy, and mental changes. None of these has been described as producing findings detectable by imaging methods. Possibly MRI of the spinal cord could demonstrate changes in the white matter. But, with very few exceptions in which an extreme degree of neglected, prolonged nutritional deficiency state was allowed to persist, treatment would probably arrest the condition before it could become visible by MRI.

FOLIC ACID DEFICIENCY

Folic acid deficiency often accompanies vitamin B_{12} deficiency but is much more common (24). It produces a polyneuropathy and, again, no detectable imaging findings.

SICKLE CELL ANEMIA

This disease principally affects blacks. Most of the manifestations of sickle cell anemia (hemoglobin S disease) are related to the characteristic tendency of hemoglobin S to crystallize under conditions of reduced oxygen tension. Because of this, sickled erythrocytes become trapped in terminal arterioles and capillaries, which produces more hypoxia and increases sickling, thrombosis, and infarction. The sickled erythrocytes are mechanically rigid and less flexible than normal erythrocytes.

Tiny local ischemic lesions may not be visible on CT or MRI, but larger lesions, produced by vascular occlusions, are seen. Larger vessels may be affected and become occluded. It is possible that the occlusion may be produced by an effect on the vasa vasorum, but high flow angiopathy resulting from the anemia has also been suggested as a mechanism (see Chapter 10, and Fig. 10.74*D* to *F*). The prevalence of strokes is around 20 percent in patients with sickle cell anemia. Most of the strokes are due to small arterial occlusions. The presence of a number of arterial occlusions may lead to development of collaterals, sometimes quite pronounced, suggestive of moya-moya on angiography. Hemorrhage may also be seen. Seventy-five percent of strokes are infarcts; the remainder are hemorrhages (25). Fat embolism is not uncommon in sickle cell anemia and is another cause of arterial occlusions. Infections, leading most commonly to meningitis, are the most common cause of death, and children, particularly those younger than 3 years, are particularly susceptible (Table 13.7).

Table 13.7.
Sickle Cell Anemia

Vascular manifestations due to sickling of red blood cells within terminal arterioles and capillaries
End result is cerebral infarctions of various sizes, hemorrhagic, in about 20 percent of patients
Moya-moya–type appearance may be seen on cerebral angiography due to larger artery occlusions and development of collateral pathways

THALASSEMIA

This is a microcytic and hypochromic anemia resulting from a diverse group of congenital disorders in which there is a defect in the synthesis of one or more of the subunits of hemoglobin. The abnormalities can lead to very mild to severe disease. The two major varieties are produced by a defective α chain synthesis, and the other involving β chain synthesis; the latter is the most common (Cooley anemia, Mediterranean anemia, thalassemia major). There are three different neurologic manifestations: meningitis after splenectomy to control hemolysis; neuromuscular disorders; and, most important, compression of the spinal cord due to extramedullary hematopoiesis. The skull bone thickening is a classic radiographic picture due to enlargement of the diploic spaces associated with bone marrow hypertrophy, but brain compression as a result is rare unless there is extramedullary hematopoiesis in the epidural and subdural space. On the other hand, in the spine, particularly the thoracic spine, where the spinal canal is narrower, the enlargement of the bone leads to compression of the cord (26,27). MRI is particularly useful for visualizing the bone marrow changes and the extramedullary hematopoiesis (27) (Table 13.8).

Myeloproliferative Disorders

These include polycythemia vera, myelofibrosis with myeloid metaplasia, acute and chronic myelogenous leukemia, essential thrombocytopemia, and the Di Guglielmo syndrome. The neurologic manifestations in these conditions may be related to hyperviscosity of the blood, the tendency to thrombosis, or extramedullary hematopoiesis.

Table 13.8.
Thalassemia

Microcytic anemia due to defective synthesis of hemoglobin subunits
Three major neurologic manifestations
Spinal cord compression due to extramedullary hematopoiesis
Depressed immune status following splenectomy, leading to increased risk of CNS infections
Neuromuscular disorders
Radiologic findings: enlargement of the diploic space in skull and vertebrae due; epidural masses to extramedullary hematopoiesis

In polycythmia vera, strokes are a frequent complication; 15 to 30 percent of patients will present strokes, and about 10 to 15 percent will die of strokes. These may be visible as ischemic areas in the brain or cerebellum. Secondary polycythemia may be seen as a manifestation of cardiac anomalies such as tetralogy of Fallot and other cyanotic cardiac anomalies, and prolonged exposure to high altitudes. Some tumors produce hematopoietin and lead to secondary polycythemia (erythrocytosis); among these are the cerebellar hemangioblastoma and some renal tumors (renal cell carcinoma, adenoma, and sarcoma). Usually no symptoms result, but a high-altitude disease has been described, and there may be a tendency to thromboses due to the increased blood viscosity. The slowing of the pulmonary circulation provoked by the increased viscosity may lead to further interference with oxygenation and an increase in erythocytosis. Aside from possible thrombosis and strokes, no other serious neurologic complications are seen.

Involvement of the subthalamic nuclei and the corpus striatum bilaterally has been reported in patients in this group who develop sudden chorea.

Blood rheology is significantly affected by viscosity, and a steep rise in viscosity occurs when the hematocrit rises above 50 (28).

Hemorrhagic Conditions

HEMOPHILIA

The main complication of hemophilia affecting the nervous system is hemorrhage, which may be intracerebral, subarachnoid, subdural, or epidural, resulting from mild to moderate trauma depending on the severity of the hemophilic disease. No direct involvement of the CNS occurs in hemophilia (29). Cerebral hemorrhage remains as an important cause of death in hemophiliacs. A hyperviscosity syndrome has been described as producing inattention, drowsiness, stupor, delirium, coma, venous engorgement in the eye fundus, retinal hemorrhages, blurred vision, and headache. In addition to an increased hematocrit, hyperviscosity of the blood may be produced by an abnormal protein, a macroglobulin in large amounts (24).

THROMBOCYTOPENIA

This condition results from either diminished production or increased destruction of platelets, which results in an abnormally low platelet count. Diminished production may be seen in drug effects on the bone marrow, myelophthisic phenomena, and ineffective thrombopoiesis. Increased destruction of platelets may be due to mechanical factors such as hypersplenism, disseminated intravascular coagulation (DIC), and thrombotic thrombocytopenic purpura.

The neurologic complications consist of bleeding, usually intracerebral, of varied severity. Purpuric petechial hemorrhage occurs with some frequency and seems to involve the gray matter frequently; usually no direct neurologic manifestations can be detected because the hemorrhagic spots are small, although they can be numerous. The CT is negative unless accompanied by larger hemorrhages. Larger parenchymal hemorrhages are easily detectable by CT in spite of lack of clot retraction, characteristic of thrombocytopenic states (30).

The neurologic picture may be only that related to the hemorrhage, but when underlying the thrombocytopenia there is lupus erythematosus, thrombotic thrombocytopenic purpura, or leukemia, other neurologic manifestations may be added.

In *thrombotic thrombocytopenic purpura* the changes in the brain arterioles and capillaries are much more extensive (widespread hyaline occlusion of terminal arterioles and capillaries) (31). There is an increase in the cellularity of the walls of arterioles and capillaries, and platelet thrombi, multiple foci of parenchymal necrosis, and petechial hemorrhages similar to those seen in other organs. Neurologic manifestations include headache, agitation and confusion, delirium aphasia, visual changes, seizures, cranial nerve palsies, altered state of consciousness, and coma.

CT and MRI findings would reveal hemorrhage and ischemic changes in the gray and white matter, depending on the predominant pathologic change. Tardy et al. reported many bright T2 foci in subcortical white matter (32). The *hemolytic uremic syndrome* in children is similar to thrombotic thrombocytopenic purpura and is usually triggered by immunologic factors. Sherwood and Wagle reported a case in which there was hyperintensity in the putamen, globus pallidus, and head of caudate nucleus bilaterally seen on both T1- and T2-weighted images, and also a nonhemorrhagic infarct (33). The child recovered, but some persistent neurologic deficit remained. Hemorrhagic infarction as well as lacunar infarcts have also been described (34,35) (Table 13.9).

Disseminated Intravascular Coagulation

DIC is a relatively common hemorrhagic thrombotic syndrome associated with or following other conditions such as trauma, head trauma, bacterial and viral infections, obstetric and surgical complications, neoplasms, and diabetic ketoacidosis. CT and MRI findings may represent hemorrhage and/or ischemic lesions. Angiography may demonstrate intravascular clotting in the major vessels (internal carotid and middle cerebral arteries, basilar arteries). It is

Table 13.9.
Thrombotic Thrombocytopenic Purpura

Widespread hyalinization and occlusion of terminal arterioles and capillaries
Development of multiple foci of petechial hemorrhage and parenchymal necrosis
Neurologic features include encephalopathy, seizures, visual changes, and focal motor/sensory deficits
CT and MRI findings of multifocal regions of infarction and/or hemorrhage within gray and white matter

a severe complication that, unless recognized and treated early, results in severe disability or death. CT-visible blood-fluid levels in hemorrhagic brain lesions should suggest the possibility of a treatable blood coagulation defect (36).

Leukemias

In acute lymphatic and acute myelogenous leukemia (ALL and AML) the neoplastic cells may infiltrate into the subarachnoid space (leukemic meningitis) or directly into the brain parenchyma. While CNS involvement may not be apparent early, it is more frequently seen at the time of recurrence, particularly of ALL. The symptoms may be recurrent headache, nausea, and, as the disease progresses, cranial nerve palsies, seizures, papilledema, and reduced mentation. Leukemia cells may be seen in the cerebrospinal fluid (CSF), along with elevated protein and low glucose concentration.

In the treatment of ALL and AML methotrexate may be employed as a prophylactic treatment as well as radiation (37). See under "Toxic and Iatrogenic Conditions," Chapter 9.

Chloroma, a green tumor seen in patients with myelogenous leukemia, may occasionally occur in the brain but is more frequent elsewhere. In addition to meningeal involvement, which may be demonstrable on gadolinium-enhanced MR images, and a rare chloroma, hemorrhages are the most important complication.

In the review of 245 patients reported by Pagani et al., there were six enhancing masses in various locations in ALL (out of 150 patients) and two masses in AML (out of 57 patients) (38). Out of 38 cases of chronic leukemia there were only 2 cases of cerebral hemorrhage, whereas there were 7 instances of cerebral hemorrhage in the 207 cases of acute leukemia. The masses enhanced with contrast on CT, and the enhancement was greater in the 1-hour delayed images following contrast administration. Some of the lesions enhanced only in the periphery. Abscess must be differentiated; there were two abscesses in the entire series.

Cytologic evidence of meningeal leukemia was found in a high percentage of cases (148 out of 156). The hemorrhage may be intracerebral or subarachnoid (also subdural), related to thrombocytopenia. The CSF may show signs of mild subarachnoid hemorrhage due to cortical small purpuric lesions, which may not be visible on CT or MRI, associated with the thrombocythemia. The hemorrhages can be severe and multiple, resulting in death (39).

The leukemic meningitis may also involve the spinal meninges, and it may be possible to demonstrate enlargement of the roots by myelography (40) or by CT-myelography (41). The enlarged roots, better demonstrated by CT-myelography, may extend beyond the thecal sac. All or most of the roots of the cauda equina may be involved, filling the thecal sac and producing a block on myelography (Table 13.10).

Table 13.10.
Leukemia

- CNS manifestations are due to infiltration of tumor cells into the subarachnoid space or brain parenchyma
- CNS involvement usually seen at time of disease recurrence
- Parenchymal involvement can be due to metastatic mass lesions or hemorrhages
- Subarachnoid or parenchymal hemorrhages may be seen due to thrombocytopenia
- Leukemic meningitis can be seen as enhancing lesions involving subarachnoid space or enlargement of spinal nerve roots

Hypercoagulable States

There are a number of conditions in which arterial, dural venous sinus thrombosis, and superficial and deep venous thrombosis may be observed. Patients are considered to have a hypercoagulable state if they have laboratory abnormalities or clinical conditions that are associated with an increased risk of thrombosis, or if they have recurrrent thrombosis without recognizable predisposing factors (42).

In this group are included a number of well-known conditions such as those promoting venous stasis (immobilization, obesity, advancing age, postoperative state); hyperviscosity (polycythemia, sickle cell disease); abnormalities of coagulation and fibrinolysis (pregnancy and delivery, malignant neoplastic disease, use of oral contraceptives, nephrotic syndromes); and abnormalities of platelets or platelet concentration (essential thrombocytoses, myeloproliferative disorders, paroxysmal nocturnal hemoglobinuria, hyperlipidemia, diabetes mellitus). Other prethrombotic states have been mentioned earlier, such as antiphospholipid syndromes (lupus anticoagulant, anticardiolipin), which may be seen in lupus erythematosus but are also encountered in some normal individuals. DIC and thrombocytopenic purpura have also been mentioned previously.

A series of primary hypercoagulable states may also be listed; they include antithrombin III deficiency, protein C deficiency, protein S deficiency, fibrinolytic disorders, dysfibrinogenemia, and factor XII deficiency (24) (Table 13.11).

Any of these states may be in the background of patients presenting with arterial as well as venous or dural venous sinus thrombosis, which frequently is evaluated or diagnosed by both CT and MRI. See under "Dural Venous Sinus Thrombosis," Chapter 10.

Table 13.11.
Hypercoagulable States

- Primary hypercoagulable states:
  - Deficiencies of protein C, protein S, antithrombin III
- Hyperviscosity states (e.g., polycythemia)
- Antiphospholipid antibodies
- Enhanced venous stasis (e.g., postoperative state, obesity)

CHRONIC LIVER FAILURE

Histologic alterations in the CNS of patients with chronic hepatocellular dysfunction have been well described (43). The pathologic findings include nerve cell degeneration or loss, the presence of laminar or pseudolaminar necrosis of the cerebral cortex with polymicrocavitation at the gray-white matter junction, as well as the appearance of type II Alzheimer astrocytes within the gray matter of the cerebral cortex and basal ganglia.

Cerebral atrophy and mild cerebral edema may be seen on CT. Brunberg et al. (44), Kulisevsky et al. (45), and Inoue et al. (46) described findings seen only on MRI in the basal ganglia. These consist of hyperintensity in T1-weighted images, involving the globus pallidus in 30 and the putamen in 21 out of 42 patients in the Brunberg et al. series (44). The T2-weighted images did not demonstrate the hyperintensity. T1 hyperintensity was also noted in the midbrain surrounding the red nucleus (17 of 42) and in the quadrigeminal plate (4 instances). Three presented T2 hyperintensity in the pons. Noncontrast T1 hyperintensity in the anterior lobe of the pituitary was found in 28 of 35 patients.

Other T2-hyperintense areas may be seen in the periventricular white matter (Fig. 13.6). The basal ganglia changes may develop within a relatively short period of time. For instance, in the patient shown in Figure 13.6 no T1 hyperintensity in the globus pallidus was seen initially, whereas 1 month and 3 months later progressive hyperintensity was developing. In the same patient there was marked enlargement of Virchow-Robin spaces around both atria, probably not related to the condition (Table 13.12).

Hepatic encephalopathy may manifest as altered mental status, or it may present with tremor, incoordination, asterixis (flapping tremor), rigidity, or myoclonic seizures.

The cause of the T1 hyperintensity remains undetermined. Presumably there is deposition of a paramagnetic substance that has bypassed the detoxification mechanism of the liver due to portacaval shunting, or hepatocyte dysfunction can be postulated. CT is usually negative, which tends to rule out calcification as a possible cause; and tiny petechial hemorrhages in the globus pallidus, bright on T1 because of methemoglobin, are not acceptable as an explanation because, on follow-up examinations, there is no transition to magnetic susceptibility due to hemosiderin on T2-weighted images.

Some cerebral cortical atrophy was demonstrated in 19 of 42 patients, and cerebellar cortical volume loss was present in 9 (44) (Fig. 13.7). Cerebral hemorrhage may be seen in the posttransplantation stage (Fig. 13.7).

RENAL FAILURE

There are two possible imaging findings: (*a*) cerebral atrophy, cortical atrophy, and some ventricular dilatation in patients with chronic renal disease, particularly if they are on hemodialysis (Fig. 13.8); or (*b*) hypertensive encephalopathy in acute renal failure.

Uremia is usually associated with neurologic manifestations, including inability to concentrate, drowsiness and insomnia, mild behavior changes, loss of memory, errors in judgment, hiccups, cramps, and fasciculations. More severe neurologic manifestations include asterixis, chorea, stupor, seizures, and coma. No specific imaging findings are associated with uremia alone.

Hypertensive encephalopathy may also be seen in preeclampsia and eclampsia, essential hypertension, pheochromocytoma, Cushing syndrome, or adrenocorticotropic hormone (ACTH) toxicity.

In hypertensive encephalopathy, the CT and/or MRI may demonstrate the presence of findings, particularly in the bioccipital region. On CT, hypodensity, and on MRI, hyperintensity, on T2-weighted images may be found, involving the cortical and subcortical area (47). In the series by Weingarten et al. more scattered areas of edema were found in subcortical areas and in the basal ganglia (48). In addition, petechial hemorrhages may be seen, showing slight hyperdensity on CT if they are confluent enough, and hyperintensity on T1-weighted images followed at a later date by hypointensity on T2-weighted images as a long-term marker of the episode of hypertensive encephalopathy. It is important to recognize the entity because there is a high mortality rate unless appropriate treatment is applied (Fig. 13.9). The edematous areas disappear as the patient recovers, but some of the areas may represent ischemic lesions, and those would remain, while the areas of cofluent petechial hemorrhages would also remain as areas of magnetic susceptibility shown on T2-weighted images on high-field MR instruments or on gradient-echo images (Table 13.13).

The changes may develop and disappear in a relatively short period of time, owing to the rapidly changing state

Table 13.12.
CNS Manifestations of Chronic Liver Failure

Histologic changes include neuronal degeneration, laminar or pseudolaminar cortical necrosis, and development of type II Alzheimer cells
MRI findings may include hyperintensity of basal ganglia and regions of the midbrain on T1-weighted images, areas of hyperintense signal on T2-weighted images in the pons and cerebral white matter, and cortical atrophy

Table 13.13.
Hypertensive Encephalopathy

Due to loss of autoregulation when blood pressure reaches high levels
Cortical and subcortical regions, which are hypodense on CT and hyperintense on T2-weighted MR images
Reversible regions of hyperintensity within basal ganglia and white matter on T2-weighted images due to edema
Foci of petechial hemorrhage

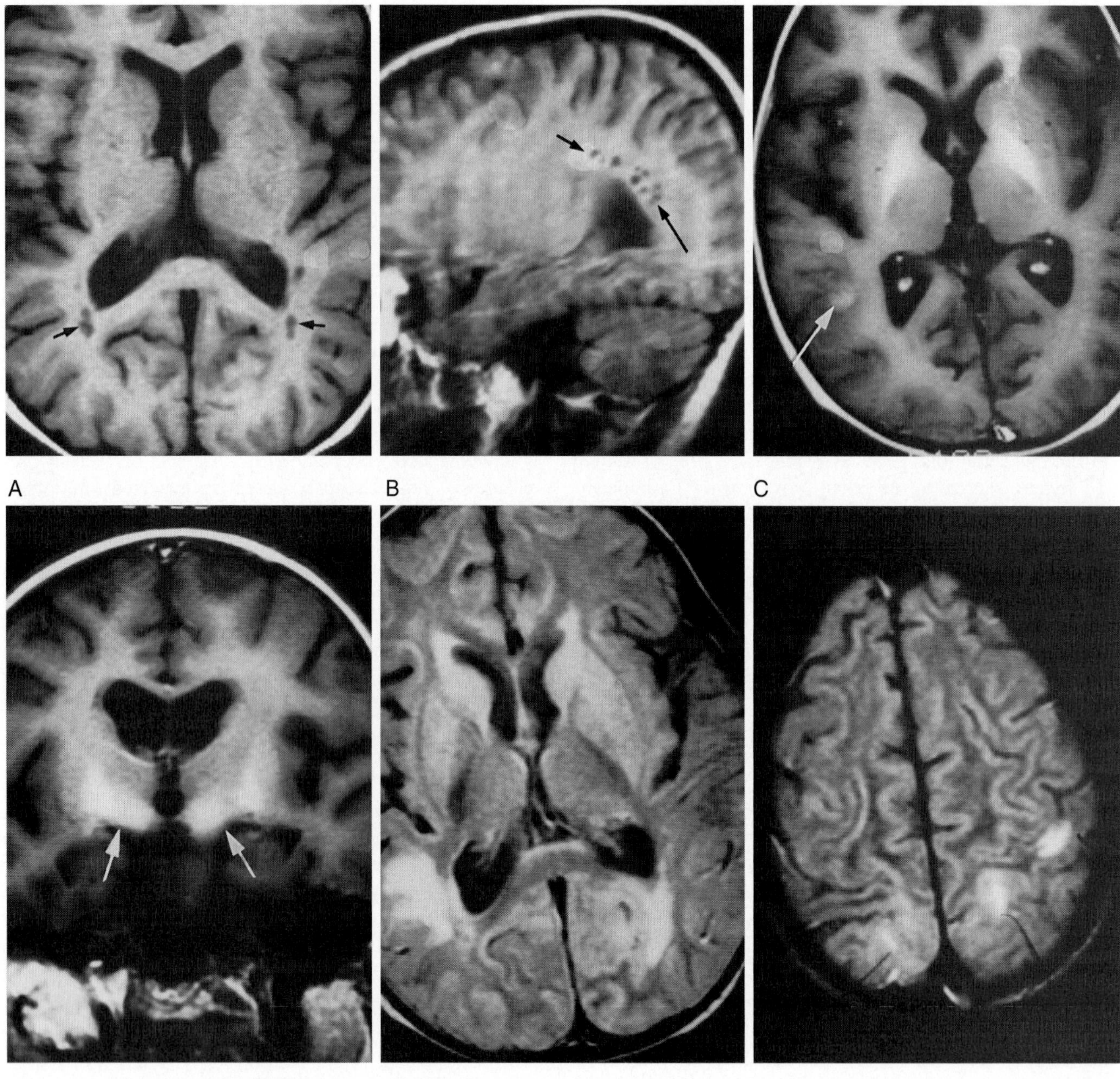

Figure 13.6. Cerebral imaging changes in hepatic failure in an 8-year-old boy. **A.** Initial T1-weighted axial shows no abnormalities. There are large Virchow-Robin spaces in the periatrial area (arrows). The sagittal (**B**) demonstrates these better (arrows). **C.** T1-weighted axial made 4 months later reveals hyperintensity in the globus pallidus bilaterally. A small, round, hyperintense area is also seen in the cortex of the right parietal area (arrow), which could represent a small hemorrhagic lesion. CT was negative. **D.** T1-weighted coronal demonstrates the bright globus pallidus (arrows). **E.** Proton density axial shows other bright areas in the periventricular white matter. However, the globus pallidus is not hyperintense. The caudate nuclei are bright. **F.** There are other bright patches remote from the ventricular wall. CT did not demonstrate these changes. The child underwent a liver and small bowel transplant.

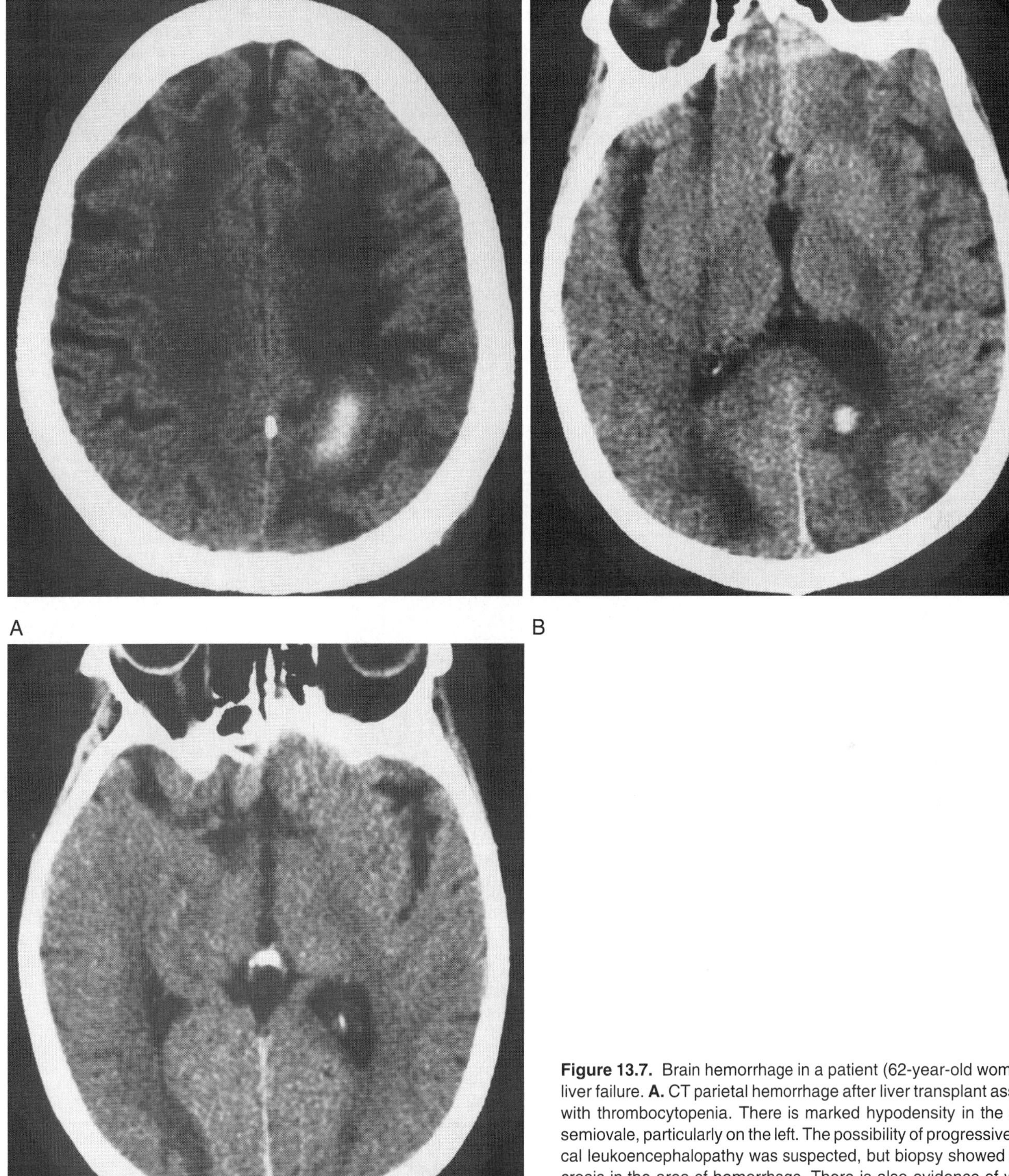

Figure 13.7. Brain hemorrhage in a patient (62-year-old woman) with liver failure. **A.** CT parietal hemorrhage after liver transplant associated with thrombocytopenia. There is marked hypodensity in the centrum semiovale, particularly on the left. The possibility of progressive multifocal leukoencephalopathy was suspected, but biopsy showed only necrosis in the area of hemorrhage. There is also evidence of widening of the cerebral sulci consistent with tissue loss. **B** and **C.** Another patient (a 67-year-old woman), also after liver transplant with thrombocytopenia, showing multiple sites of hemorrhage in the left occipital and the right basal ganglia. There was another small hemorrhage in the left basal ganglia lower down (not shown).

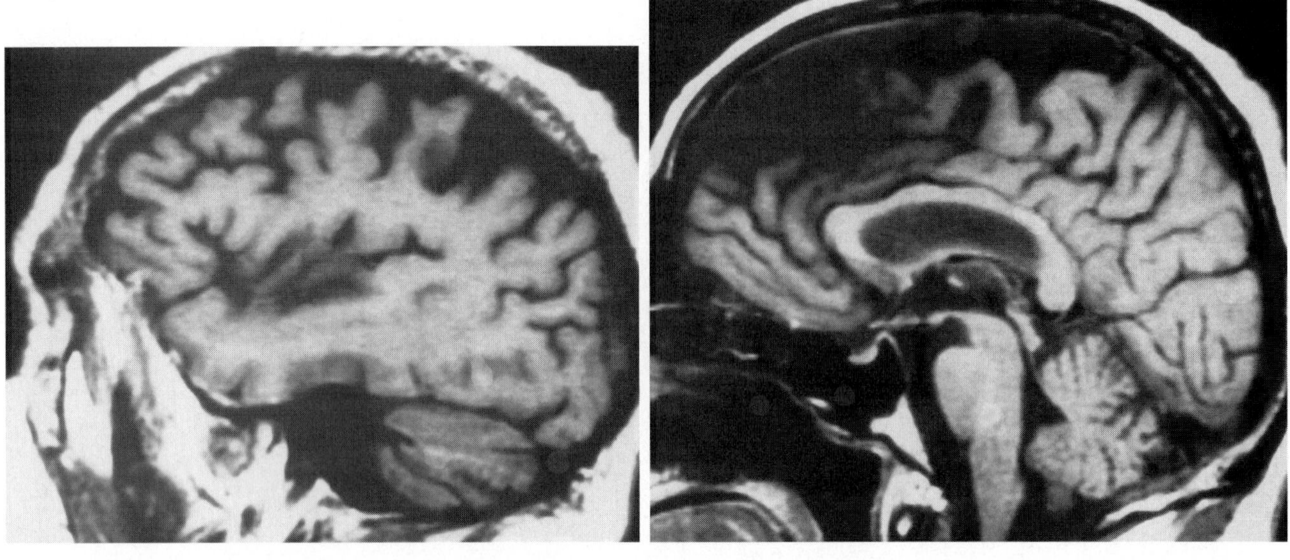

A B

Figure 13.8. Cerebral cortical atrophy in a 64-year-old man with chronic renal failure. **A** and **B.** There is considerable widening of the surface sulci and around the sylvian fissure area. Other structures are normal.

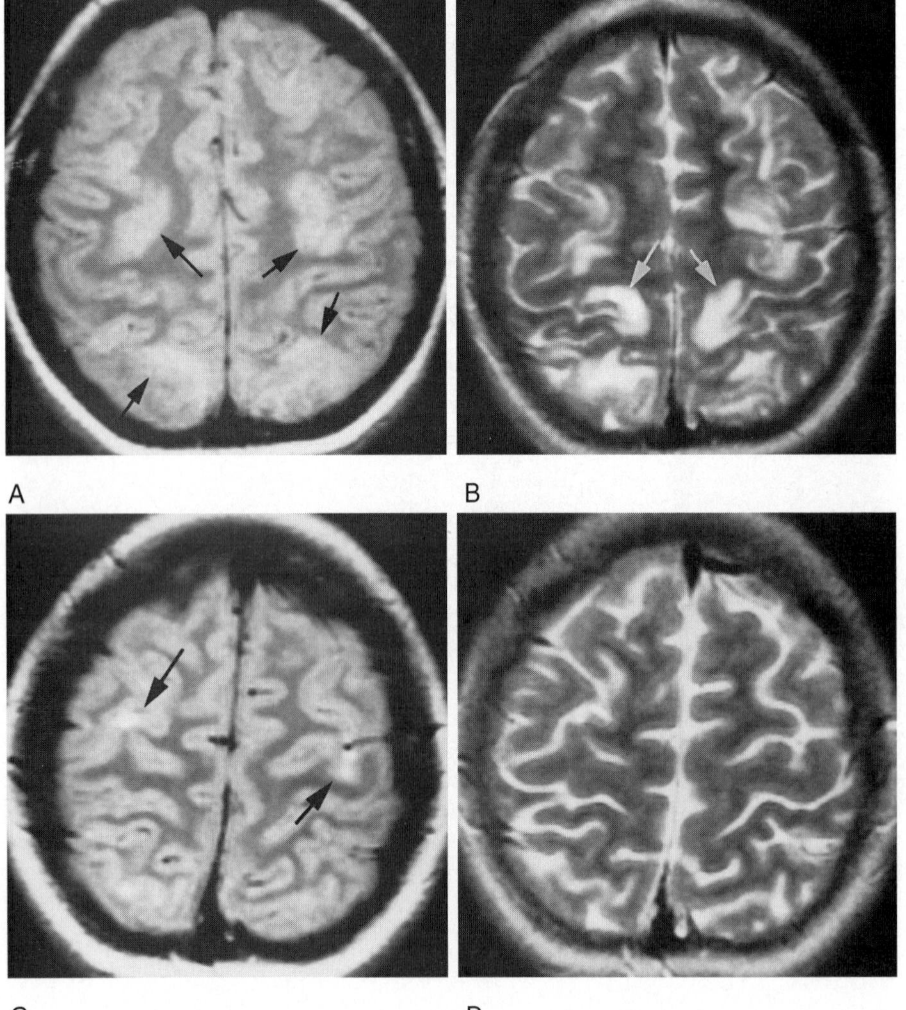

A B C D

Figure 13.9. Hypertensive encephalopathy in a 16-year-old girl with chronic renal disease (patient had Wegener granulomatosis). **A** and **B.** Proton density and T2-weighted images showing multiple hyperintense areas involving cortex and adjacent subcortical areas as hyperintense, poorly circumscribed areas. **C** and **D.** Proton density and T2-weighted images made 10 days later show almost total disappearance of the edematous areas. The smaller area remains. The hyperintense lesions are probably secondary to edema. There are more in the occipital and parietal areas than elsewhere, but the distribution was not as clearly localized in the occipital region as reported by Schwartz et al. (47) in patients with eclampsia (see text).

of the cerebral circulation in this condition, but it may take from 1 to 10 days to reach full development. Patients usually complain of increasing headache.

The pathogenesis of hypertensive encephalopathy is probably related to the loss of autoregulation that occurs when the blood pressure rises to higher limits (e.g., 240 systolic over 150 diastolic). This causes brain hyperperfusion, which leads to diffuse cerebral edema due to increased vascular permeability; focal areas of disruption of the blood-brain barrier lead to greater focal edema in scattered areas. There is a tendency for these changes to occur earlier in the occipital region, the brainstem, and the cerebellum, supplied primarily by the posterior circulation, where there is less sympathetic control of autoregulation (49,50). Other theories have been proposed.

In more acute hypertensive crises caused by cocaine or other sympathomimetic agents, abrupt and marked elevations of systemic blood pressure occur, which may lead to hemorrhage or infarction due to vessel rupture, again presumably due to failure of autoregulatory mechanisms in the brain. In the case of cocaine, vasoconstriction may also be induced by the effect on the sympathetic nervous system surrounding intracranial arteries (51).

PARANEOPLASTIC DISORDERS

It is not the intention here to describe metastatic disease of the brain or spinal cord; rather, it is to discuss some aspects of malignant disease that have not been dealt with in relation to the CNS. These include a number of conditions involving the brain, the spinal cord, or the peripheral nervous system in many patients with manifested malignant disease, but sometimes as the first manifestation and other times preceding the development of the cancer by months or even years. Usually there are no specific imaging findings, but sometimes changes are seen that require a differential diagnosis.

Paraneoplastic Syndromes

The paraneoplastic syndromes may be anatomically divided into three groups for descriptive purposes: brain, spinal cord, and peripheral nervous system. The paraneoplastic syndromes are relatively common in patients with malignant disease if one includes minor neurologic symptoms or mild peripheral neuropathy (possibly 6 percent of cancer patients) but are much less common if we consider only patients with moderately severe neurologic involvement (less than 1 percent incidence) (52).

The tumors most often associated with paraneoplastic neurologic manifestations are small-cell cancer of the lung and ovarian cancers. The pathogenesis is not clear, but it may be via an autoimmune reaction or possibly an opportunistic viral infection. Evidence for both mechanisms has been reported (53,54).

CEREBELLAR DEGENERATION

In paraneoplastic cerebellar degeneration, the more common of the paraneoplastic syndromes involving the brain, the only observable imaging finding is cerebellar atrophy, which may not be apparent early but develops later. There is widening of the sulci due to thinning of the cerebellar folia, and enlargment of the fourth ventricle (55) (Table 13.14).

Table 13.14.
Paraneoplastic Syndromes

Most often associated with small-cell carcinoma of lung and ovarian carcinoma
Cerebellar degeneration—most common CNS paraneoplastic syndrome
Limbic encephalitis—encephalopathy and seizures; particularly associated with oat cell carcinoma of the lung
Myelitis—upper and motor neuron findings involving extremities

LIMBIC ENCEPHALITIS

Most commonly associated with oat cell carcinoma of the lung, but also with other types of malignancy, limbic encephalitis, a rare disease, may accompany or precede the discovery of a malignant lesion. Clinically it consists of a profound recent memory loss, anxiety, depression, hallucinations, seizures, and dementia. Usually CSF examination shows elevated protein and lymphocytosis. Some patients may also show involvement of the brainstem, spinal cord, cerebellum, and autonomic neurons. On MRI may be seen hyperintensity in the medial temporal lobe, the amigdaloid nucleus, and the hypothalamus on T2-weighted images (56,57). Biopsy of the temporal lobe may show extensive loss of neurons, reactive gliosis, and perivascular cuffing. The changes affect the gray matter of the hippocampus, cingulate gyrus, pyriform cortex, orbital frontal lobes, insula, and amygdaloid nuclei (Fig. 13.10).

BRAINSTEM ENCEPHALITIS

Brainstem encephalitis also occurs, with pathologic changes similar to those seen in limbic encephalitis. In the literature are found reports of encephalitis syndromes, which are not really those of paraneoplastic CNS involvement but represent diffuse invasion of the nervous system (58). The term *encephalitis* should not be applied to this type of malignant spread.

MYELITIS

Myelitis is usually part of the paraneoplastic encephalitis syndrome, clinically presenting muscle weakness and wasting, and sometimes fasciculation. Imaging findings have not been described, but one possibly might expect spinal cord atrophy seen on MR images. Necrotizing myelopathy has also been described in association with cancer, but it is questionable whether it is cancer because of its rarity.

Motor neuronopathy occurs, usually associated with Hodgkin disease or other malignant lymphomas. Only motor weakness (mostly the legs) without sensory findings

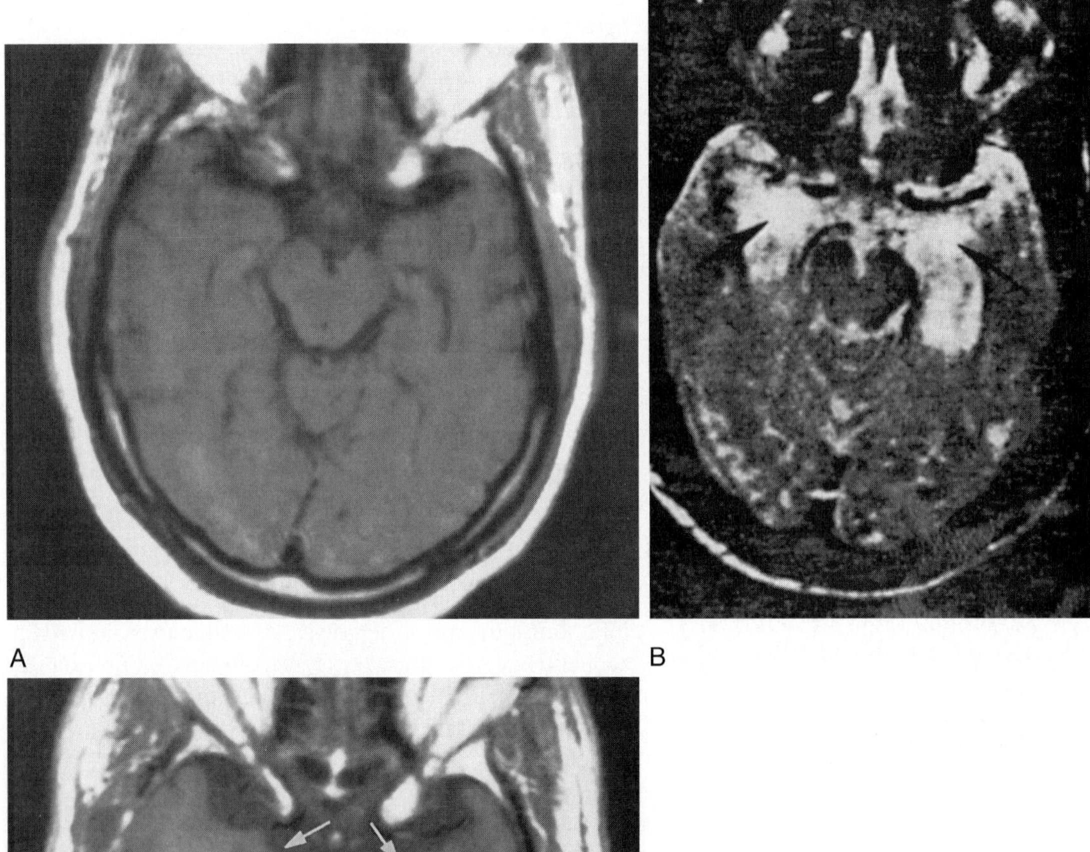

Figure 13.10. Paraneoplastic limbic encephalopathy in a 46-year-old man with mixed oat cell and large-cell carcinoma of the lung metastatic to paratracheal lymph nodes. **A.** T1-weighted axial shows a normal appearance of both medial temporal lobes. **B.** T2-weighted image shows marked hyperintensity in the medial temporal lobes bilaterally. Postcontrast T1 images showed no change from before contrast. **C.** Reexamination 10 months later showed bilateral atrophy of the temporal lobes with enlargement of the temporal horns (arrows). Compare with A. T2-weighted images did not show hyperintensity at this time. The patient presented with a dementia picture (disorientation, memory difficulties, difficulty with name and facial recognition). Biopsy showed no neoplastic cells, but lymphocytic infiltration of the perivascular region and leptomeninges and several glial nodules. (Courtesy of Dr. Allen D. Elster, Winston-Salem, N.C.)

is found, and the course is variable; it usually does not progress, and sometimes remissions occur. In this, in paraneoplastic sensory neuropathy, and in the distal sensory neuropathies that are fairly common in patients with cancer, no imaging findings have been described.

In a number of neurologic manifestations associated with malignant disease, no imaging findings related to the brain or spinal cord have been described, and usually none can be expected except possibly for white matter T2 bright foci, brain atrophy, and ventricular dilatation, which for the most part cannot be separated from age-related phenomena. Among these are peripheral neuropathies, myasthenic syndromes, myasthenia gravis (30 percent of patients with thymomas), dermatomyositis and polymyositis, carcinoid myopathy, myotonia, and neuromyotonia.

Systemic Lymphoma

Systemic lymphoma usually involves meninges and may involve the brain through spread along the perivascular (Virchow-Robin) spaces. Thus, if any masses are seen, they are usually peripherally situated (38) (Fig. 13.11).

The lesions enhance with contrast, and the involved meninges will show enhancement (Fig. 13.12). Cisternal and sulcal enhancement, irregular tentorial enhancement, and hydrocephalus may be demonstrated (59,60) (Table 13.15).

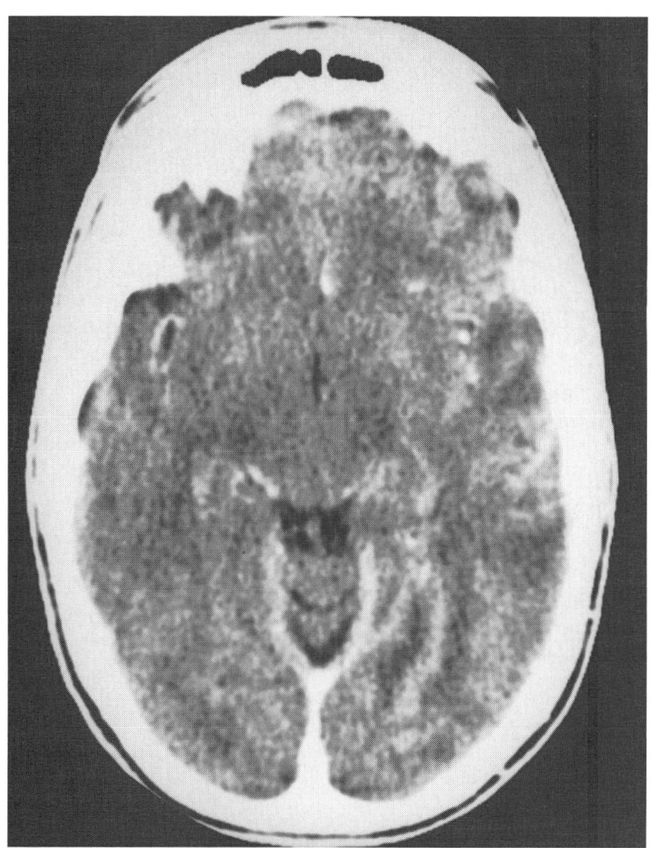

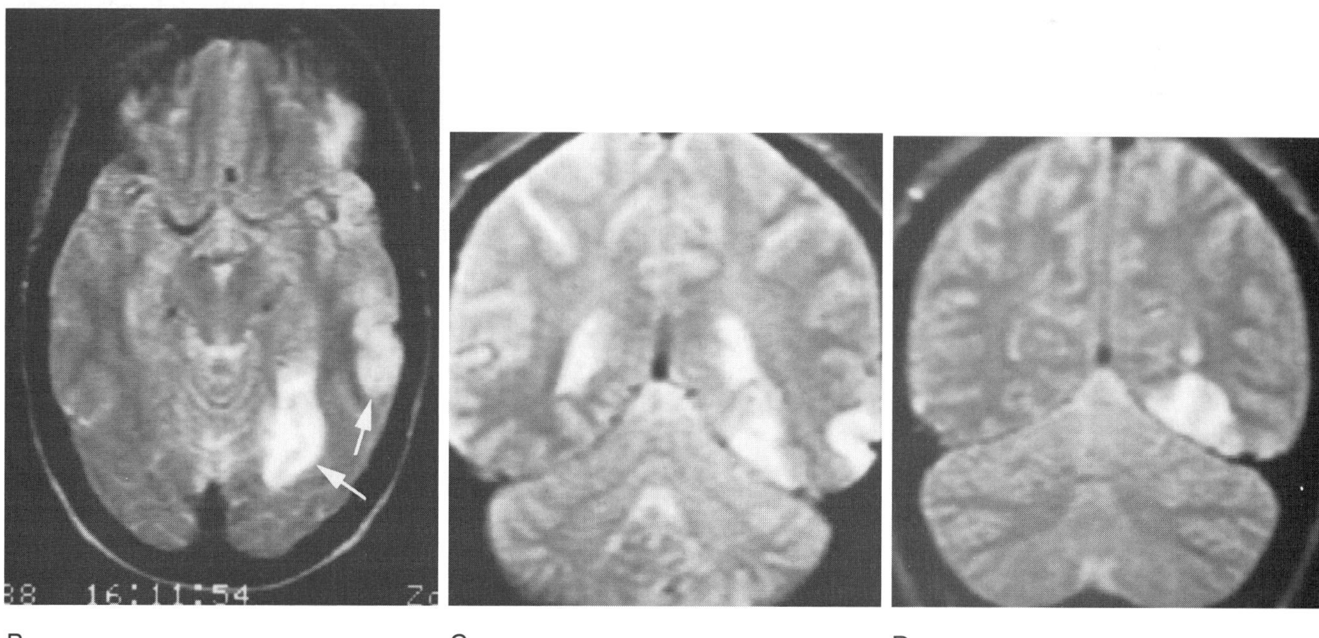

Figure 13.11. Brain involvement in a patient with Hodgkin disease. **A.** The axial CT after contrast shows some irregular hyperintensity in the left occipital region due to cortical enhancement. **B.** MRI T2-weighted axial shows the same lesion in the left occipital region (arrow); in addition, it reveals a hyperintense area on the left posterior temporal cortex (anterior arrow). **C** and **D.** Coronal T2-weighted images show that the abnormalities are cortical in location, probably due to extension from meningeal involvement. Intracerebral isolated lesions in the brain are unusual as a manifestation of systemic lymphoma. However, patients who are immunosuppressed as part of the treatment may develop primary CNS lymphoma.

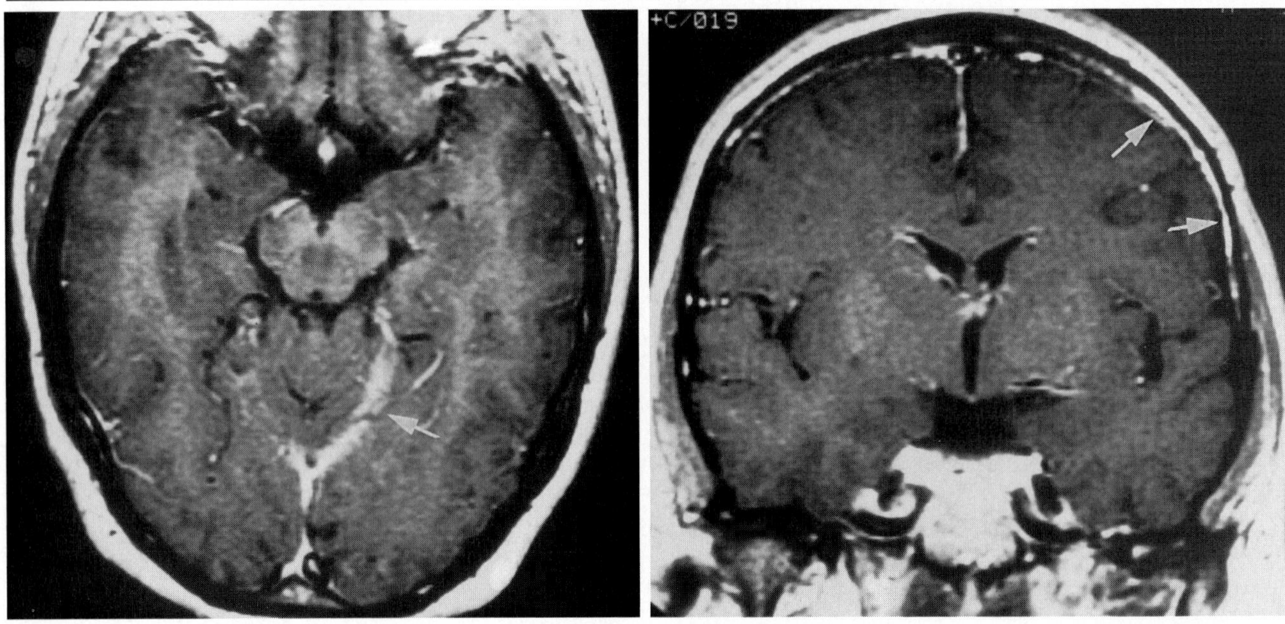

A B

Figure 13.12. Meningeal involvement in a patient with non-Hodgkin systemic lymphoma. **A** and **B.** Postcontrast axial and coronal views show enhancement of the tentorium, more on the left side, and over the convexity on the left (arrow). There are no parenchymal areas of involvement, which is the case in the nonprimary CNS lymphoma.

Table 13.15.
CNS Manifestations of Systemic Lymphoma

Usually involves meninges or extends along perivascular spaces; occasionally involves brain parenchyma
Usually seen as leptomeningeal enhancement, cranial nerve masses, and hydrocephalus

The most frequent presenting symptoms in secondary CNS lymphoma usually refer to the cranial nerves, especially the facial, third, and six nerves (61,62). For further details, see Chapter 11.

INBORN METABOLIC ERRORS

Many of these fall into the category of systemic conditions that affect the nervous system; they have been described in Chapter 5. One deserves specific mention here because the diagnosis may not be made until the second or third decades of life.

Porphyric Encephalopathy

Porphyria is a multisystem disease, an inborn metabolic error characterized by specific inherited enzyme defects in heme biosynthesis, which leads to overproduction of intermediate compounds, called porphyrins. Abdominal pain, limb weakness, constipation, vomiting, tachycardia, photosensitive skin changes, and neuropsychiatric manifestations all fit into the clinical picture of porphyria. The attacks are intermittent, and the neurologic manifestations may be related to vascular spasm, leading to cerebral cortical changes (63,64). In the case reported by Aggarwal et al., there was cortical uptake of gadolinium, producing a gyriform pattern in two or three areas in the brain cortex, which resolved in about 2 to 3 months (64). Clearance also occurred in the case reported by King and Bragdon (63).

REFERENCES

1. Liebow AA, Carrington CRB, Feldman PJ: Lymphomatoid granulomatosis. Hum Pathol 1972;3:457–458.
2. Kapila A, Gupta KL, Garcia JH: CT and MR of lymphomatoid granulomatosis of the CNS: Report of four cases and review of the literature. Am J Neuroradiol 1988;9:1139–1146.
3. George JC, Caldemeyer KS, Smith RR, et al: CNS lymphomatoid granulomatosis in AIDS: CT and MR appearance. AJR 1993;161: 381–383.
4. Fauci AS, Haynes BF, Katz P, et al: Wegener's granulomatosis: Prospective clinical and therapeutic experience with 85 patients for 21 years. Ann Intern Med 1983;98:76–85.
5. Yamashita Y, Takahashi M, Brussaka H, et al: Cerebral vasculitis secondary to Wegener's granulomotosis: Computed tomography and angiographic findings. J Comput Assist Tomogr 1986;10: 119–120.
6. Fleming JL, et al: Whipple's disease: Clinical, biochemical and histopathologic features and assessment of treatment in 29 patients. Mayo Clin Proc 1988;63:539.
7. Aisen AM, Gabrielsen TO, McCune WJ: MR imaging of systemic lupus erythematosus involving the brain. AJNR 1985;6:197–201.
8. Bell CL, Partington C, Robbins M, et al: Magnetic resonance imaging of central nervous system lesions in patients with lupus erythematosus: Correlation with clinical remission and antineurofilament and anticardiolipin antibody titers. Arthritis Rheum 1991;34: 432–441.

9. Marsteller LP, Marsteller HB, Braun A, et al: An unusual CT appearance of lupus cerebritis. AJNR 1987;8:737–739.
10. Yamamoto K, Nogaki H, Takase V, et al: Systemic lupus erythematosus associated with marked intracranial calcification. AJNR 1992; 13:1340–1345.
11. Kelley RE, Stokes N, Reyes P, et al: Cerebral transmural angeitis and ruptured aneurysm (a complication of systemic lupus erythematosus). Arch Neurol 1980;37:526–527.
12. Asherson RA, Khamashta MA, Ordi-Ros J, et al: The primary antiphospholipid syndrome: Major clinical and serological features. Medicine 1989;68:366–374.
13. Briley DP, Coull BM, Goodnight SH Jr: Neurological disease associated with antiphospholipid antibodies. Ann Neurol 1989;25: 221–227.
14. Pulpeiro JR, Cortés JA, Macarron J, et al: MR findings in primary antiphospholipid syndrome. AJNR 1991;12:452–453.
15. Jackson CG, Chess RL, Ward JR: A case of rheumatoid nodule formation within the central nervous system and review of the literature. J Rheumatol 1984;11:237–240.
16. Kim RC, Collins GH, Parisi JE: Rheumatoid nodule formation within the choroid plexus. Arch Pathol Lab Med 1982;106:83–84.
17. Yuh WTC, Drew JM, Rizzo M, et al: Evaluation of pachymeningitis by contrast-enhanced MR imaging in a patient with rheumatoid disease. AJNR 1990;11:1247–1248.
18. Serdaroglu P, Yazici H, Ozdermir C, et al: Neurologic involvement in Behcet's syndrome: A prospective study. Arch Neurol 1989;46: 265–269.
19. Banna M, El-Ramahi K: Neurologic involvement in Behcet disease: Imaging findings in 16 patients. AJNR 1991;12:791–796.
20. Bartlett ST, McCarthy WJ III, Palmer AS, et al: Multiple aneurysms in Behcet's disease. Arch Surg 1988;123:1004–1008.
21. Buchwald D, Cheney PR, Peterson DL, et al: A chronic illness characterized by fatigue, neurologic and immunologic disorders, and active human herpesvirus-6 infection. Ann Intern Med 1992;116: 102–113.
22. Schwartz RB, Garada BM, Kormaoff AL, et al: Detection of intracranial abnormalities in patients with chronic fatigue syndrome: Comparison of MR imaging and SPECT. AJR 1994;162:935–941.
23. Schwartz RB, Komaroff AL, Garada BM, et al: SPECT imaging of the brain: Comparison of findings in patients with chronic fatigue syndrome, AIDS dementia complex, and major unipolar depression. AJR 1994;162:943–951.
24. Samuels MA: Neurologic manifestations of hematologic diseases. In AK Asbury, GM McKahnn, WI McDonald (eds), Disease of the Nervous System: Clinical Neurobiology. Philadelphia: Saunders, 1992, pp 1510–1521.
25. Grotta JC, Manner C, Pettigrew LC, et al: Red blood cell disorders and stroke. Stroke 1986;17:811–817.
26. Logethetis J, Constantoulakis M, Economidau J, et al: Thalassemia major: A survey of 138 cases with emphasis on neurologic and muscular aspects. Neurology 1972;22:294–304.
27. Ziegler L, Lange M, Feiden W, et al: Spinal cord compression in thalassemia major: Value of MR imaging. Eur J Radiol 1992;1:81.
28. Wood MH, Kee DB Jr: Hemorrheology of the cerebral circulation in stroke. Stroke 1985;16:765–772.
29. Silverstein A: Intracranial bleeding in hemophilia. Arch Neurol 1960;3:141–157.
30. Pierce JN, Taber KH, Hayman LA: Acute intracranial hemorrhage secondary to thrombocytopenia: CT appearances unaffected by absence of clot retraction. AJNR 1994;15:213–215.
31. Moschcowitz E: An acute febrile pleiochromic anemia with hyaline thrombosis of the terminal arterioles and capillaries: An undescribed disease. Arch Intern Med 1975;35:89–95.
32. Tardy B, Page Y, Convers P, et al: Thrombotic thrombocytopenic purpura: MR findings. AJNR 1993;14:489–490.
33. Sherwood JW, Wagle WA: Hemolytic uremic syndrome: MR findings of CNS complications. AJNR 1991;12:703–704.
34. Crisp DE, Siegleo RL, Bale JF, et al: Hemorrhagic cerebral infarction in the hemolytic uremic syndrome. J Pediatr 1981;99:273–276.
35. Di Mario FJ, Brone-Stewart H, Sherbotie J, et al: Lacunar infarction of the basal ganglia as a complication of hemolytic uremic syndrome. Clin Pediatr 1987;26:586–590.
36. Pfleger MJ, Hardee EP, Contant CF, et al: Sensitivity and specificity of fluid-blood levels for coagulopathy in acute intracerebral hematomas. AJNR 1994;15:217–223.
37. Robain O, Dulac O, Dommerges JP, et al: Necrotizing leukoencephalopathy complicating treatment of childhood leukemia. J Neurol Neurosurg Psychiatry 1984;47:65–72.
38. Pagani JJ, Libshitz Hi, Wallace S: Central nervous system leukemia and lymphoma: Computed tomography manifestations. AJNR 1981; 2:397–403.
39. Kelly JK, Laxo A, Metes J, et al: Intracerebral hemorrhagic dissemination of acute myelocytic leukemia. AJNR 1985;6:113–114.
40. Mirvis S, Stewart M, Raok CVG: Myelographic demonstration of "nodular radiculopathy" in acute myelogenous leukemia. AJNR 1984;5:641–643.
41. McAllister MD, O'Leary DH: CT myelography of subarachnoid leukemic infiltration of the lumbar thecal sac and lumbar roots. AJNR 1987;8:568–569.
42. Schafer AI: The hypercoagulable states. Ann Intern Med 1985;102: 814–828.
43. Finlayson MH, Superville B: Distribution of cerebral lesions in acquired hepatocerebral degeneration. Brain 1981;104:79–95.
44. Brunberg JA, Kanal E, Hirsch W, et al: Chronic acquired hepatic failure: MR imaging of the brain at 1.5 T. AJNR 1991;12:909–914.
45. Kulisevsky J, Ruscalleda J, Gran JM: MR imaging of acquired hepatocerebral degeneration. AJNR 1991;12:527–528.
46. Inoue E, Shinichi H, Narumi Y, et al: Portal-systemic encephalopathy: Presence of basal ganglia lesions with high signal intensity on MR images. Radiology 1991;179:551–555.
47. Schwartz RB, Jones KM, Kalina RL, et al: Hypertensive encephalopathy: Findings on CT, MR imaging, and SPECT imaging in 14 cases. AJR 1992;159:379–383.
48. Weingarten K, Barbut D, Filippi C, et al: Acute hypertensive encephalopathy: Findings on spin-echo and gradient-echo MR imaging. AJR 1994;162:665–670.
49. Hauser RA, Lacey DM, Knight MR: Hypertensive encephalopathy. Arch Neurol 1988;45:1078–1083.
50. Beausang-Linder M, Bill A: Cerebral circulation in acute arterial hypertension: Protective effects of sympathetic nervous activity. Acta Physiol Scand 1981;111:193–199.
51. Jacobs IG, Roszler MH, Kelly JK, et al: Cocaine abuse: Neurovascular complications. Radiology 1989;170:223–227.
52. Posner JB: Paraneoplastic syndromes. In AK Asbury, GM McKahnn, WI McDonald (eds), Diseases of the Nervous System: Clinical Neurobiology. Philadelphia: Saunders, 1992, pp 82–1104.
53. Anderson NE, Cunningham JM, Posner JB: Autoimmune pathogenesis of paraneoplastic neurological syndromes. Crit Rev Neurobiol 1987;3:245–299.
54. Furneaux HM, Reich L, Posner JB: Autoantibody synthesis in the central nevous system of patients with paraneoplastic syndrome. Neurology 1990;40:1085–1091.
55. Greenberg HS: Paraneoplastic cerebellar degeneration: A clinical and CT study. J Neurooncol 1984;2:377–382.
56. Lacomis D, Khoshbin S, Schick RM: MR imaging of paraneoplastic limbic encephalitis. J Comput Assist Tomogr 1990;14:115–117.
57. Dirr LY, Elster AD, Donofrio PD, et al: Evaluation of brain MRI abnormalities in limbic encephalitis. Neurology 1990;40: 1304–1306.
58. Olsen WL, Winkler ML, Ross DA: Carcinomatous encephalitis: CT and MR findings. AJNR 1987;8:553–555.
59. Lee YY, Glass JP, Geoffray A, et al: Cranial computed tomographic abnormalities in leptomeningeal metastasis. AJNR 1984;5:559–563.
60. Palacios E, Gorelick CF, Gonzales SF, et al: Malignant lymphoma of the nervous system. J Comput Assist Tomogr 1982;6:689–701.
61. Herman TS, Hammond N, Jones SE, et al: Involvement of the

central nervous system by non-Hodgkin's lymphoma. Cancer 1979; 43:390–397.

62. DePina CA, Lee YY, Tassel PV: Lymphomatous involvement of the trigeminal nerve and Meckel cave: CT and MR appearance. AJNR 1989;10:S15-S17.
63. King PH, Bragdon AC: MRI reveals multiple reversible cerebral lesions in an attack of acute intermittent porphyria. Neurology 1991; 41:1300–1302.
64. Aggarwal A, Quint DJ, Lynch JP III: MR imaging of porphyric encephalopathy. AJR 1994;162:1219–1220.

SELECTED READINGS

Anderson NE, Rosenblum MK, Posner JB: Paraneoplastic cerebellar degeneration: Clinical-immunologic correlation. Ann Neurol 1988;24: 559–567.

Eaton WA, Hofrichter J: Hemoglobin S gelatin and sickle cell disease. Blood 1987;70:1245.

Embury S: The clinical pathophysiology of sickle cell disease. Ann Rev Med 1986;37:36.

Okada J, Yoshikawa K, Matsuo H, et al: Reversible MRI and CT findings in uremic encephalopathy. Neuroradiology 1991;33:524–526.

14

Selection of CT Versus MRI and Functional Neuroimaging

SELECTION OF CT AND MRI

Computed tomography (CT) utilizes only one parameter in the generation of images: absorption of photons by the tissues. This makes CT scanning a relatively simple procedure. There are no known contraindications to a CT examination; it can be carried out in all patients under any circumstances. A number of situations may affect the quality of the images, such as a patient who moves and cannot be sedated or a patient who may have a metallic object for immobilization or for bone fixation, such as a halo in the cervical region or metallic fixation devices in the spine. These affect the quality of the images by the production of artifacts but represent no contraindication to the CT examination.

Magnetic resonance imaging (MRI) images via a much more complex set of magnetic and radiofrequency interactions, as described in Chapter 2. It does have the advantage of generating considerably more contrast in many circumstances than is possible with CT scanning. For instance, the contrast between gray and white matter is rather slight with CT, whereas MR is capable of generating more contrast between the two, owing to the MR sensitivity to the difference between the water content of the gray and white matter. Gray matter contains more water than white matter and thus is brighter on T2-weighted images than white matter, and vice versa on T1-weighted images. Also, in the presence of any increased water in the white or gray matter, it is possible to see a rather bright image on T2-weighted images that sometimes is not visible by CT scanning and, when visible, is likely to be only a slightly decreased density in relation to the surrounding tissues. Blood and blood products offer special opportunities for comparison between CT and MR. CT is excellent for demonstrating acute bleeding in the brain. However, with the passage of days or weeks the blood loses the initial increased density, becomes isodense, and later becomes hypodense. On the other hand, MR will show the blood in the acute stage, but will also continue to show the blood throughout all the stages, as explained in Chapter 10. Later it will show the effects of old blood products related to the retention of iron molecules in the tissues, which is not seen by CT.

On the other hand, MRI is contraindicated in certain circumstances, such as in the presence of any metallic objects in the head (except on the surface of the head), for example, aneurysm clips in the arteries of the brain, the presence of any metallic object within the brain, or the presence of a cardiac pacemaker. Even situations where there may be no contraindication to the examination because of the presence of metallic objects, the images would be so full of artifacts that they would be useless.

Another important problem with MRI is that the exposure times are longer than those used in CT scanning and thus are unsatisfactory if the patient is uncooperative and cannot remain still for some minutes. This may change somewhat in the future with the availability of such improved techniques as echoplanar and other variations of gradient echos.

Thus, in the usual clinical situations the relative indications and diagnostic value of CT and MR might be considered as follows.

Head Trauma

ACUTE

CT scanning is by far the preferred method of examination in the acute stage. This is due to the fact that intracerebral hemorrhage can be shown extremely well in the acute stage, and fractures of the skull and the surrounding facial and paranasal structures can be studied. Such a complete evaluation would not be possible with MRI. In addition, patients with acute head trauma are usually uncooperative and cannot hold still for the time required to do a satisfactory MR examination.

SUBACUTE

The MRI examination is far superior to CT subacutely because it would show a subdural hematoma, even though extremely thin and in a situation that makes it difficult to visualize, such as around the base of the skull. MRI will show focal brain edema or small hemorrhage associated with shear axonal injury extremely well, often when nothing can be seen by CT. In the chronic stage, MRI will show evidence of old small or large hemorrhage within the brain, which, again, could not be evaluated by CT scanning. The latter will show only evidence of tissue loss as a hypodensity in areas of the brain. Thus, if the patient is able to cooperate and there is no contraindication to MRI, the latter should be the procedure of choice in examining patients with head trauma in the subacute or chronic stages.

Inflammatory Conditions

In this type of clinical condition CT with contrast may be satisfactory. It will show edema as well as the presence of contrast uptake in an abscess. However, MRI is capable of providing a more complete evaluation in that changes in the brainstem may be poorly visualized by CT whereas they are ideally well shown by MRI. Also, CT scanning is particularly poor in the diagnosis of meningitis. Even after contrast, unless there is involvement of the tentorial region, CT could be negative because the enhanced meninges under the bones cannot be differentiated from the inner table of the skull. On the other hand, MRI is particularly good at showing peripheral meningeal enhancement as well as enhancement of the affected meninges in any location, including the spine. Thus, in the presence of a suspected inflammatory process, MRI is the procedure of choice.

Demyelinating Conditions

This is one of the areas where MRI is far superior to CT scanning, and in general in the presence of suspected multiple sclerosis, CT can be considered as an unsatisfactory examination. It does not show the lesions in a high proportion of the cases, whereas MRI is likely to show the lesions extremely well. In fact, a patient with symptoms involving the cerebral structures suspected for multiple sclerosis would be placed in the doubtful category for this diagnosis if the MRI examination is negative. The same may apply to some inborn metabolic errors in the newborn and childhood periods. Many of these are visible by CT, but MRI provides a much more complete examination.

Hydrocephalus

Both CT and MRI are satisfactory in the study of hydrocephalus, but MRI may show more detail—for instance, in the diagnosis of aqueductal stenosis or insufficiency, in the demonstration of cerebrospinal fluid (CSF) flow via a special flow technique, and possibly in the demonstration of meningeal changes in the patient with basal arachnoiditis.

Cerebral Vascular Disease

When the patient is brought in at the acute stage, CT is preferred because at first we are trying to determine whether the patient has a hemorrhage or an ischemic lesion, and this is easily done by CT. In addition, patients are often uncooperative, and CT scanning allows for single exposures of 1 to 2 sec, whereas MRI may require several minutes for an examination. As indicated earlier, this may change in the future as rapid exposure times are developed for MRI. Also, there are other considerations that may tip the balance toward MRI for the indications in acute stroke. These include the functional neuroimaging investigations, such as diffusion imaging and blood volume determinations, and possibly oxygen consumption, as determined by the change of oxyhemoglobin to deoxyhemoglobin. In the study of chronic strokes, MRI is preferred because it will show the amount of tissue loss and will also show whether there was an old hemorrhage in the area because of the retained hemosiderin.

Subarachnoid Hemorrhage

CT is the procedure of choice. MRI does not show acute subarachnoid hemorrhage because the blood signal changes cannot be separated from the CSF in which it is mixed. The blood is initially in the oxyhemoglobin stage, and remains so because the CSF is partially saturated with oxygen. Thus, the T2-weighted images will not demonstrate any difference between CSF and blood with oxyhemoglobin, and nothing would be seen unless there is clot formation. The effect of old blood products in the meninges, such as may be seen after repeated subarachnoid hemorrhage (meningeal siderosis), can be seen by MRI and is not visible by CT.

Brain Tumors

In the study of brain tumors we may differentiate between intracerebral and extracerebral neoplasms. In the study of extracerebral neoplasms, mostly meningiomas, CT is preferable because it shows 100 percent of these lesions and may also demonstrate the presence of bone involvement, which might not be visible by MRI. Both CT and MRI require contrast in the examination of all brain tumors, including extracerebral tumors.

In the intracerebral tumors, MRI is preferable. CT is capable of showing an extremely high percentage of intracerebral brain tumors, probably around 98 percent, but can miss some lesions if they do not take up the contrast and do not produce sufficient edema to be visible by CT. This includes slowly growing astrocytomas and some metastatic tumors. For this reason, in view of the frequent clinical search for intracerebral neoplasms associated with cancer, MRI is the procedure of choice and should be carried out without and with contrast enhancement.

Epilepsy

When examining a patient who presents an epileptic condition MRI is the procedure of choice, not only because it will show a neoplasm, if one is present, but it also may show such lesions as hippocampal sclerosis, which may not be seen by CT. Also, if carried out 6 to 24 h after the last seizure, MRI may show hyperintensity on T2-weighted images, which may disappear later, indicating the presence of a focus in that area, as discussed in Chapter 11.

Posterior Fossa Lesions

MRI is superior to CT in the study of posterior fossa lesions of all types. The only exception is represented by a bone lesion, which might be more clearly shown by CT than by MRI if it presents calcifications projecting into the posterior fossa, such as may be the case in a chordoma or a chondrosarcoma.

Calcifications

Calcifications anywhere in the brain, due mostly to neoplasms but sometimes the result of a vascular condition, are shown much better by CT and may not be shown at all on MRI examinations even in retrospect. While calcification is supposed to show up as a hypointensity on MR images, the opposite can be true or the lesions may simply be isodense around the surrounding pathology and thus not visible by MRI. The detection of possible calcification remains one of the important indications for CT examinations in addition to MRI studies when one is trying to arrive at a differential diagnosis of a visible lesion. The presence of calcification in a neoplasm or in any lesion represents an important differential diagnostic factor that should not be forgotten.

Craniovertebral Junction

MRI again turns out to be far superior to CT in most aspects in the study of lesions in this area. However, there is a need for a CT examination to visualize the bones, particularly in posttraumatic conditions, in order to see fractures, which are not seen by MRI.

Spine and Spinal Cord

MRI has been an extremely important advance in the examination of the spine and spinal cord. This is so in the study of metastatic disease to the spine, a very common clinical problem, as well as in studies of herniated cervical, thoracic, and lumbar intervertebral discs. In the lumbar region, CT scanning is an excellent method to look for a possible herniated intervertebral disc, and it would also show the bony structures and the articulations, as well as the presence of degenerative osteophytic changes, somewhat better than MRI. Thus, in the lumbar region one might consider CT as the first examination to perform, to be followed by MRI to complete the examination. In the cervical region, on the other hand, MRI is preferable as it will show not only the disc but also its relation to the spinal cord and the roots, something that is usually not possible by CT.

In the study of a patient who has a possible spinal cord lesion MRI is the procedure of choice.

Progressive Paraparesis or Paraplegia

Emergency MRI examination is the procedure of choice not only because it will show the presence of vertebral involvement but because it will demonstrate the relationship of vertebral involvement to the spinal cord and will clearly outline the site as well as the degree of cord compression. MRI has completely replaced myelography for this purpose. At present, a rapidly progressing paraparesis is the only MRI emergency the author accepts.

MRI, therefore, is the procedure of choice for examining the spinal cord. This has resulted in a considerable decrease, almost a disappearance, of myelography as a test to study the spinal cord in the cervical and thoracic regions. However, CT-myelography is sometimes indicated in the study of certain conditions such as a suspected vascular malformation of the cord, where MRI without and with contrast does not reveal clear evidence of abnormal vessels. The myelogram will usually show the enlarged serpentine veins associated with vascular anomalies of the cord. Another indication for CT-myelography would be those cases in which there is a contraindication to the use of MRI or where the artifacts produced by metallic objects may obscure the anatomy in the area, such as may be the case in some postoperative conditions.

The relative indications of CT and MRI are summarized in Tables 14.1 and 14.2.

FUNCTIONAL NEUROIMAGING

MR Functional Imaging

This is one of the more interesting developments in MRI in the last few years, first introduced by the investigative group at the Massachusetts General Hospital. Perhaps the first step in this area was introduced by Wedeen et al. with

Table 14.1.
General Considerations in Cross-Sectional Imaging

MRI Advantages
Multiplanar imaging capability
Superior gray matter/white matter contrast
Generally superior lesion definition
Patency of blood vessels can usually be easily determined
Sensitive for detection of white matter disorders (e.g., multiple sclerosis)
MRI Disadvantages
Contraindicated in certain patients (e.g., those with cardiac pacemaker)
Close patient monitoring is generally more difficult
Low sensitivity for detection of subarachnoid hemorrhage
Poor bone detail
Typically longer examination time than CT
Image quality is sensitive to patient motion
CT Advantages
No patient contraindications
Sensitive for detection of acute hemorrhage, including subarachnoid hemorrhage
Good image quality can often be obtained even in the presence of patient motion
Good bone detail
Short examination time
Is typically able to quickly provide necessary information for evaluation of trauma patients
CT Disadvantages
Predominantly axial imaging only
Less sensitive for detection of small lesions and lesion extent
Detail of posterior fossa anatomy/pathology is less than for MRI
Spinal anatomy/pathology detail is poor without introduction of intrathecal contrast material
MR Functional Imaging
Two major methods
Measurement of susceptibility effect generated by passage of contrast material through regon of interest
Noncontrast method measuring susceptibility effect of deoxyhemoglobin through region of interest
Diffusion techniques
Potential applications of greatest interest
Preoperative functional mapping prior to tumor resection
Localization of language function prior to epilepsy surgery
Early diagnosis of ischemic infarction

their first report on imaging of pulsatile flow, which rapidly led to the development of MR angiography (1). Later, the development of rapid imaging utilizing the echoplanar approach allowed Rosen et al. and Belliveau et al. to image the rapid passage of contrast (e.g., gadolinium-DTPA) through the brain blood vessels (2–4). The rapid passage of this paramagnetic substance generates a susceptibility effect (T2 shortening) instead of the T1 shortening seen when the contrast agent reaches the tissues. The T2 effects predominate with gadolinium at higher concentrations. This only records the local cerebral blood volume and the rapid passage of contrast and may show delayed passage in ischemic areas, or in contrast, increased speed such as may be seen in an arteriovenous malformation. MR demonstration of cerebral blood volume is based on the ability of MR to rapidly image the susceptibility effect (T2 signal loss) provoked by the passage of gadolinium. The first passage of the gadolinium compound produces the maximum susceptibility effect, followed by recirculation, which produces a minor decrease in T2 signal in tissue, followed by a gradually decreasing susceptibility effect on second and subsequent passages until the effect almost disappears.

The signal loss is proportional to the blood volume in each voxel and is similar to standard trace measuring techniques frequently employed in nuclear medicine. Relative cerebral blood volume maps can therefore be generated. Cerebral blood volume decreases in the acute stage of cerebral infarction, increases during the hyperemic state (the stage often called *luxury perfusion*), and would decrease again in the chronic stage.

The data obtained with MRI utilizing echoplanar techniques indicate that it will be possible in the foreseeable future to obtain physiologic information as well as clinically applicable pathophysiologic data of brain tissue function. At present it is possible to record visual cortex activity, which normally works bilaterally in the full visual field but shows activation in the occipital visual cortex unilaterally if only half of the visual field (right or left) is illuminated.

Progress continues in this area, and recent publications indicate the possibility of performing these tasks with a normally equipped 1.5- or 2.0-T unit (5–7). It was thought that echoplanar techniques or 4.0-T units might be indispensable (8), and it is evident that increased resolution is obtained with these units. But as time goes on, the possibility of modifying techniques in the clinical instruments to acquire data without contrast media is yielding progressively more promising results.

Essentially there are two approaches to obtaining data with MR. The first is information on circulation obtained rapidly based on the passage of a bolus of a paramagnetic agent (e.g., gadolinium) through the cerebral circulation

Table 14.2.
Relative Indications for CT and MRI

	Preferred Examination
1. Head trauma	
Acute	CT
Subacute	MRI
2. Vascular: stroke	
Acute stroke	CT
Subacute	MRI
Subarachnoid hemorrhage	CT
3. Neoplasm	
Extracerebal	CT or MRI
Intracerebral	MRI or CT
4. Convulsive disorder	MRI
5. Headaches: vague symptoms	MRI
6. Suspected multiple sclerosis	MRI
7. Degenerative diseases	MRI
8. Posterior fossa lesions	MRI
9. Craniovertebral junction (C-V)	MRI
10. Suspected saccular aneurysm	MRA
11. Suspected arteriovenous malformation	MRI or (CT + contrast)
12. Spine:	
Spinal cord	MRI
Spinal trauma	CT and MRI
13. Emergencies	CT
In rapid progressive paraparesis	MRI

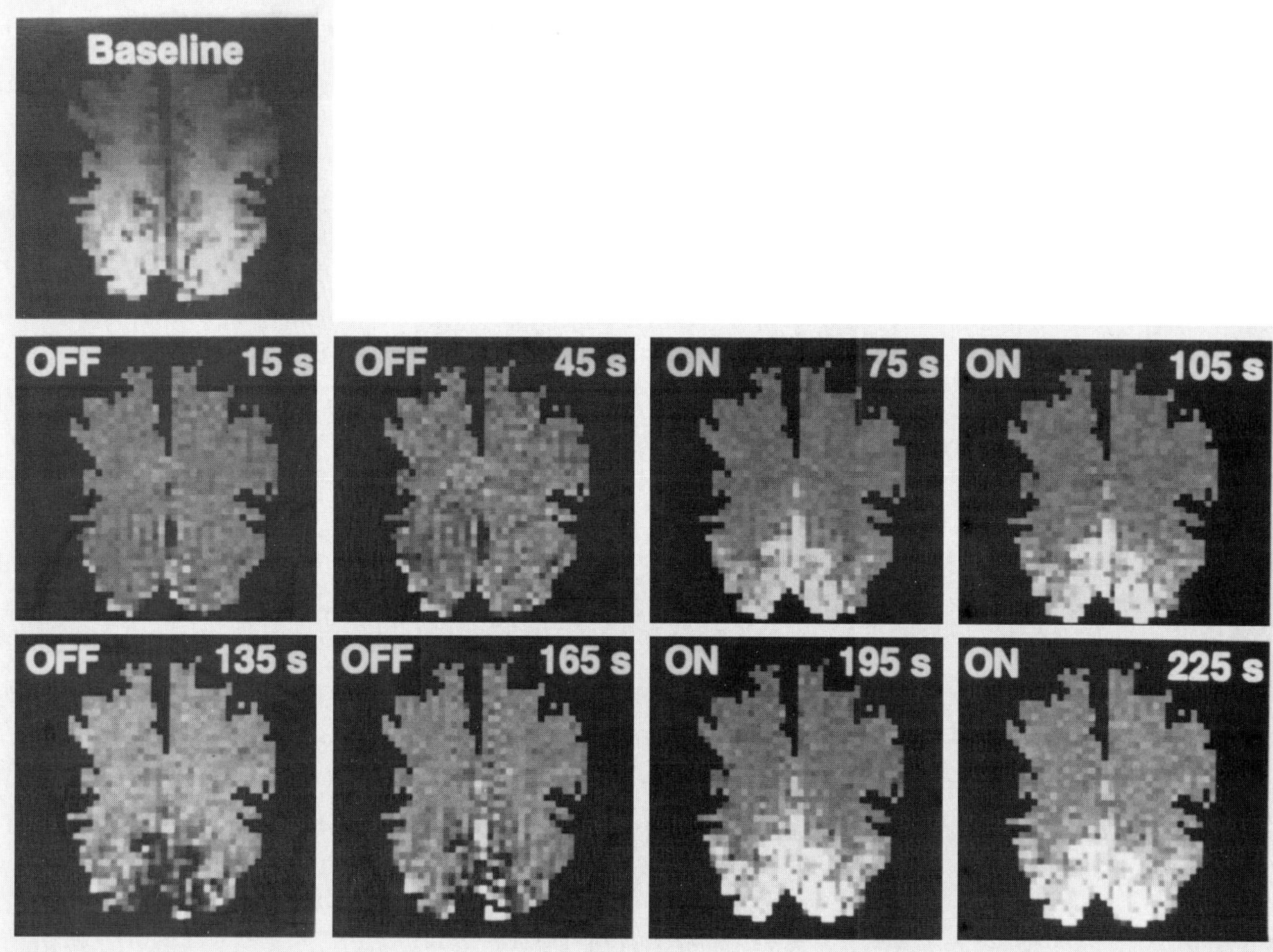

Figure 14.1. Visual stimulation. It is possible to show increased circulatory activity in the visual cortex by turning light on and off as shown every 30 sec. When the lights are on, there is increased brightness in both occipital regions.

following intravenous (IV) injection. This requires the availability of rapid imaging, such as echoplanar techniques, in order to record the arrival, short stay, and departure of the agent, a total of about 10 to 20 sec. There is a susceptibility effect created by the gadolinium, which produces a drop in signal. The drop in signal is proportional to the amount of blood passing through a specific area of the brain. A blood volume map is produced (see Fig. 14.9).

The second method does not utilize any contrast but depends on the varying magnetic susceptibility of hemoglobin as it changes from oxyhemoglobin to deoxyhemoglobin following its passage through the brain tissue capillary bed. Oxyhemoglobin has no unpaired electrons and is not paramagnetic, whereas deoxyhemoglobin has four unpaired electrons and is paramagnetic (9). This effect causes a heterogeneous shortening of T2 relaxation time in the area. The effect probably comes almost entirely from the veins, mostly the surface veins, which have the greatest concentration of deoxyhemoglobin. While the effect is very slight, almost imperceptible, it can be magnified by repeated sequences and by subtracting data. For example, the data from the resting state are subtracted from the activation state (visual stimulation, hand movements, language, hearing) (10–13). More recently the subtraction approach has been replaced by a more sophisticated statistical approach.

The images obtained are low in resolution (64 × 128 matrix) but have sufficient topographic accuracy so that they can be placed over a detailed three-dimensional brain image (Figs. 14.1 through 14.3).

The possibility of applying these techniques clinically is of great importance. Perhaps the main immediate application is that of brain mapping of surgically resectable lesions in relation to the eloquent areas of the brain (e.g., motor cortex, sensory cortex, speech, visual cortex). This is important because there is a variability in the position of these functions between individuals, and because a lesion may displace a function sufficiently so that surgical removal can be accomplished without producing permanent damage

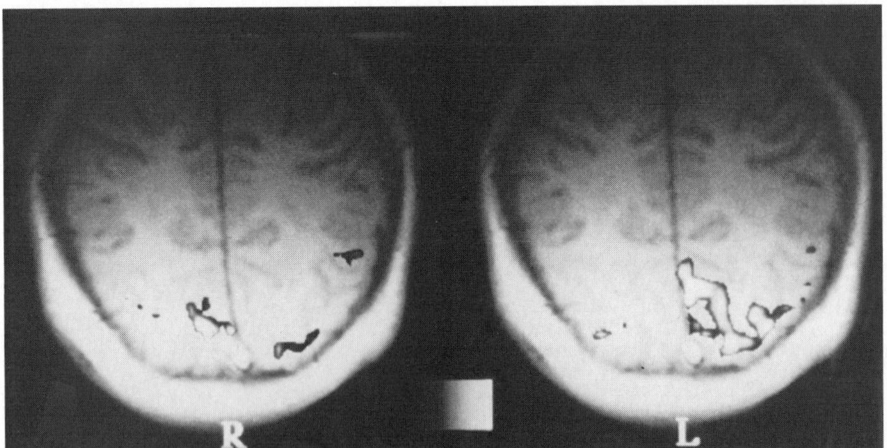

Figure 14.2. Visual hemifield stimulation. By stimulating only one-half of the visual field, it is possible to cause circulatory changes in only one occipital area, with very little activity on the other side. Stimulation of the right visual field caused circulatory changes in the left occipital area (L).

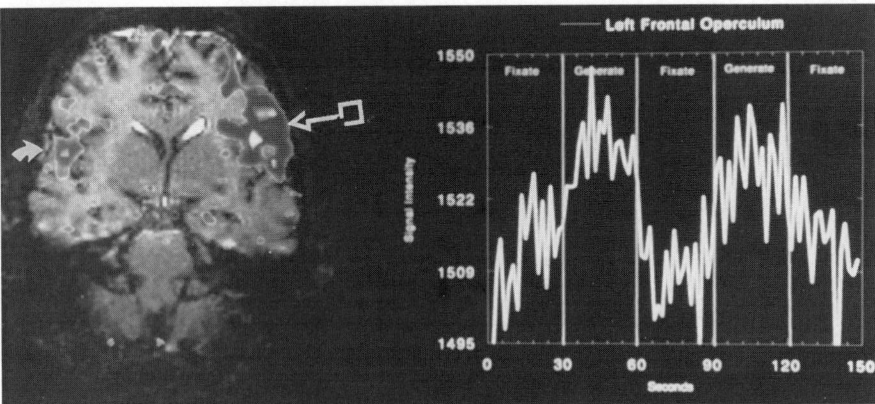

Figure 14.3. Covert verb generation. The language localization was done by using a covert verbal technique in order to avoid confusion produced by tongue movement and other associated movements. The main location is in Broca's area in the left frontal operculum (open arrow), but there is some activation of the opposite hemisphere (curved arrow). (Courtesy of Dr. Bradley Buchbinder, Massachusetts General Hospital, Boston.)

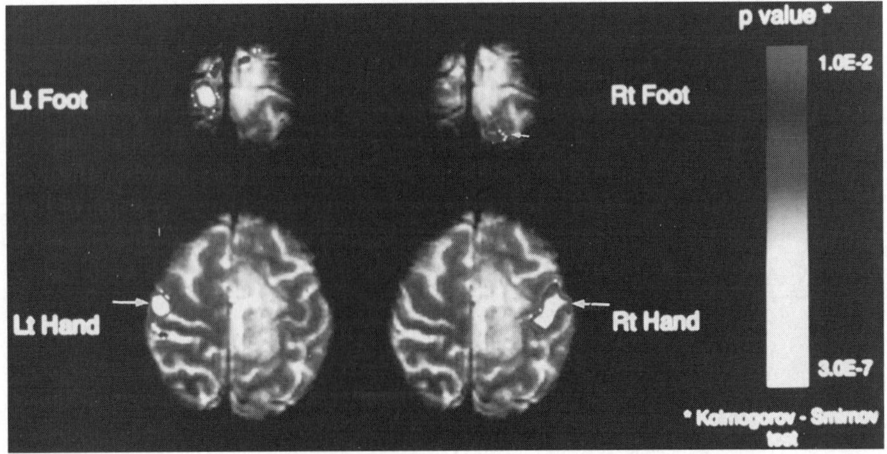

Figure 14.4. fMR sensorimotor activation. Determination of the position of hand and foot motion areas in a patient with a tumor in the left parasagittal region. Upper images. The right foot area (arrow) is displaced posteriorly but is separated from the margin of the tumor. The original color did not reproduce in the black and white print. Lower images. The hand activation areas are clearly shown, and the right hand area is clearly separated from the tumor.

(Figs. 14.4 to 14.7). The method is sufficiently sensitive so that changes in a patient with homonymous hemianopia can be shown as compared with the normal (Fig. 14.8) (14).

The calculation of cerebral blood volume may be a useful procedure in dealing with cerebral vascular disease in order to evaluate brain tissue perfusion. Regional cerebral blood flow (not tissue perfusion) may be calculated using the gadolinium IV injection technique. The method may be useful clinically if it can be simplified, but it would not give information on brain tissue viability because it gives no information on regional oxygen consumption by the brain. Theoretically, it should be possible to determine

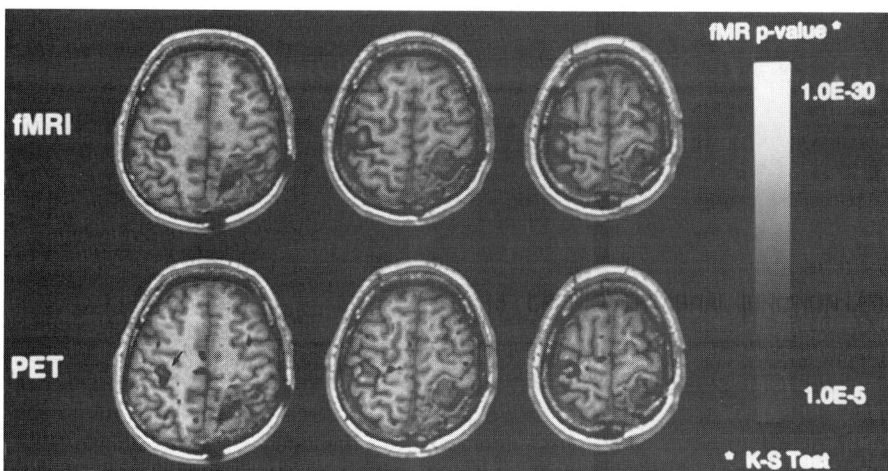

A

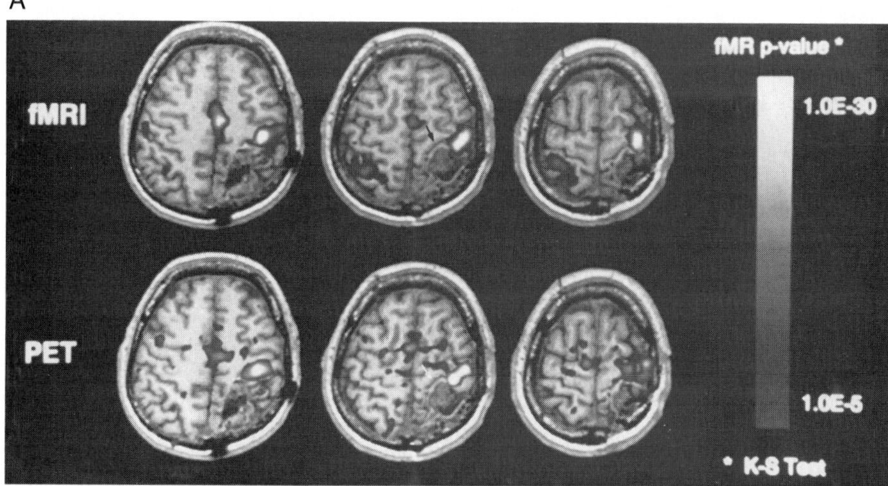

B

Figure 14.5. Determination of the location of right and left hand activation areas in a patient with arteriovenous malformation (AVM) in the left frontoparietal area. **A.** AVM: Left hand activation. The images show the position of the left hand activation area (arrow). **B.** AVM: Right hand activation. The images show the right hand activation area (bright area) to be very close to the lesion. The AVM is apparently located just behind the central sulcus.

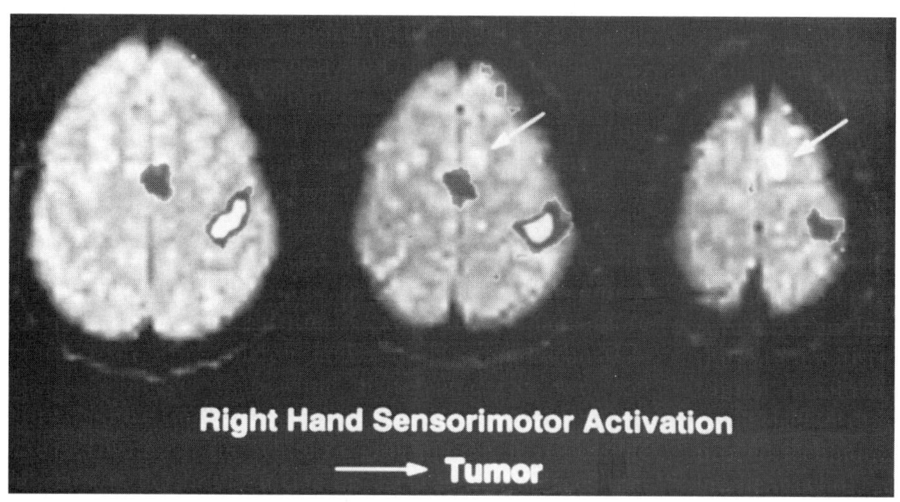

Figure 14.6. SMA seizures. Demonstration of activation in supplemental motor areas in a patient with seizures associated with an intracerebral tumor. The hand area is in its usual location, and there is an active area behind and adjacent to the tumor (arrow). Removal of the tumor should not affect the primary motor cortex.

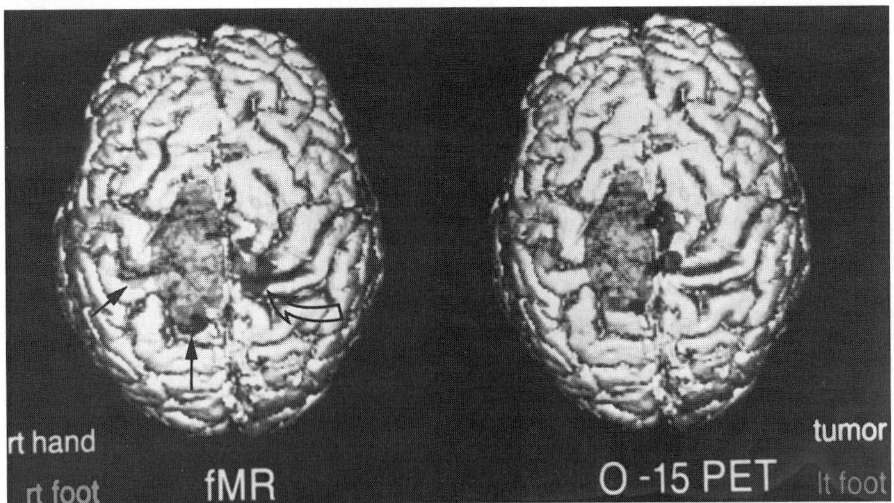

Figure 14.7. Sensorimotor mapping. Forty-nine-year-old male three weeks s/p stroke. The surface three-dimensional images are helpful to the surgeon and are quite similar to what is seen after craniotomy. On the side of the tumor, the hand activation area is in normal position (left arrow), while the right foot area is displaced dorsally (posterior arrow). On the opposite hemisphere the position of the foot activation area is farther forward, in normal position. The tumor has displaced the right foot activation area. The image on the right was obtained with PET, and the location of the activated areas is essentially the same. Note: The image is reversed for the surgeon; it is presented as if seen from above, and the tumor is in the left hemisphere. (Courtesy of Dr. Bradley Buchbinder, Massachusetts General Hospital, Boston.)

lack of oxygen consumption in the presence of luxury hyperperfusion. It is doubtful, however, whether an increase in oxygen extraction fraction by viable tissue in a hypoperfused area, affected by low blood flow, could be imaged; the sensitivity of the method is probably not sufficient at 1.5 or 2.0 T. However, as shown in the example in Figure 14.8, the conversion of hemoglobin to deoxyhemoglobin may be quantitated, and this should be an indicator of oxygen utilization.

Positron emission tomography (PET) scanning, on the other hand, has these capabilities. At present the two are being combined at our institution, both to develop the MR methodology and to expand its capabilities (Table 14.1). For further details see under "Measurement of Cerebral Blood Flow," Chapter 10.

MR Diffusion Imaging

An extremely important development in functional neuroimaging is represented by diffusion imaging, which consists of the ability to image proton motion at the microscopic level. The movement of water molecules from and into capillaries is a most important phenomenon of biologic life. As the molecules move within a magnetic gradient, the frequency changes, and thus the received signal changes, because some protons would have moved out of their initial position in space. See under "Magnetic Resonance," Chapter 2.

The most important application of diffusion imaging will undoubtedly be in the early diagnosis of strokes in order to determine that we are in fact dealing with an ischemic stroke and not with a transient ischemic attack or a reversible neurologic deficit in order to decide on management. Diffusion imaging should allow us to make the diagnosis within 2 h or less by detecting early edema in the ischemic area. At present this requires very rapid imaging, such as is possible with echoplanar techniques, because the diffusion weighted imaging techniques are extremely sensitive to even the slightest motion. We are trying to image proton motion of less than 1 mm. There is decreased diffusion in the acute stage of infarction. At this stage the Brownian motion that induces this diffusion change is mostly intracellular. An intermediate stage follows, in which diffusion is increased but is not particularly noticeable because it approaches that of the surrounding normal brain. In the chronic stage there is a better-defined diffusion increase following cell death and replacement by gliosis and microcystic changes. The blood volume is decreased except possibly in the luxury perfusion stage. The functional imaging at present is done utilizing the perfusion technique (Fig. 14.9), and the diffusion sequence is carried out as well (15) (see Figs. 10.20 and 10.21).

Diffusion imaging is an important technical development which has revolutionized the early diagnosis of ischemic stroke. At the Massachusetts General Hospital it is being used routinely and is available 24 hours a day. It is quite accurate in the diagnosis of early ischemic infarction. Moreover, it can differentiate between a transient ischemic attack (TIA) or a reversible ischemic neurologic deficit (RIND), and an early stroke. This is extremely important if active treatment of a stroke is to be applied. A TIA or RIND will present a negative diffusion sequence. The presence of a positive diffusion test indicates the presence of a persistent ischemic deficit and if this is accompanied by a perfusion defect it indicates there are persistent occluded vessels and that fibrinolytic therapy may be valuable. On the other hand, if there is no perfusion defect fibrinolysis is not indicated. Thus, both diffusion and perfusion sequences must be used if we are going to improve our management of strokes through the use of fibrinolysis which requires early diagnosis (6–8 hours) and immediate treatment.

MR Spectroscopy

MR spectroscopy (MRS) was the first application of magnetic resonance in chemistry and thus still continues. From

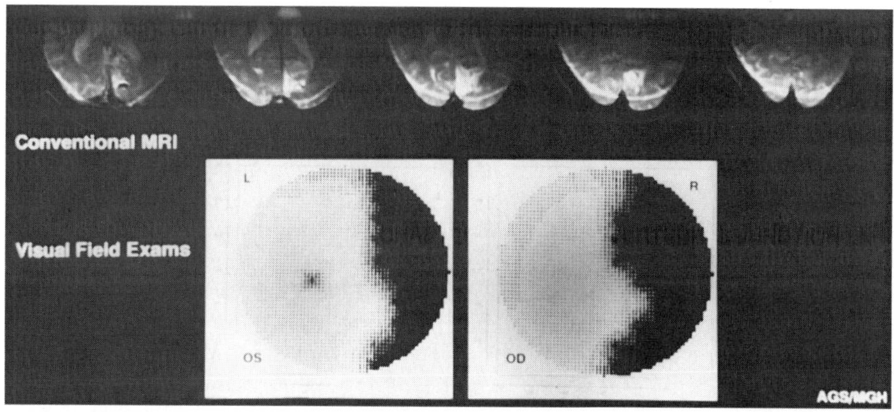

A

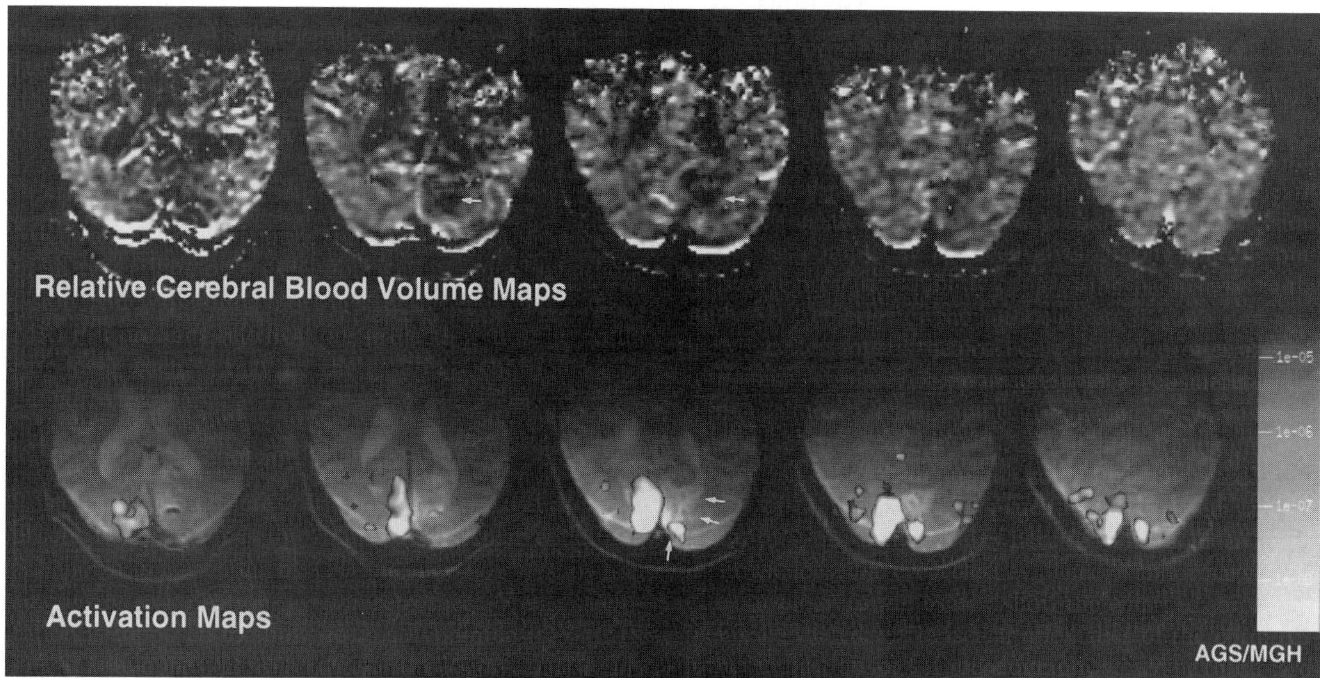

B

Figure 14.8. Functional neuroimaging in patient with homonymous hemianopia due to ischemic lesion in the occipital area. **A.** Forty-nine-year-old male three weeks s/p stroke. The upper row indicates the position of the infarct in the visual area (medial occipital lobe). The lower row shows a right homonymous hemianopia (dark portion of field) with sparing of central vision accounting for the rounded projection into the dark area. **B.** Forty-nine-year-old male three weeks s/p stroke. The upper row shows the blood volume maps demonstrated by gadolinium passage. There is decreased blood volume in the infarcted area (arrow). The lower row is an activation map obtained with full-field visual stimulation. Only the right occipital area shows activation. The central visual sparing is represented by a small activated area on the left occipital cortex (lower arrow). Note that hyperintensity of the infarct is seen above the functionally active portion (arrows). (Courtesy of Gregory Sorenson, Massachusetts General Hospital, Boston.)

its beginning in the middle 1940s until 1973, when Lauterbur published a paper that suggested the possibility of localizing the nuclear spins in space, only spectroscopy was used (16). Once clinical MRI began, the possibility of using spectroscopy was considered, both to carry out biological research in vivo and to apply it clinically.

MRS requires a much more homogeneous magnetic field and a stronger magnetic field than MRI for satisfactory results. Although at present 1.5 T is being utilized, stronger fields are being used for research in animals (4.7 T). Nevertheless, it seems that a 1.5-T magnet is capable of producing satisfactory spectra for clinical purposes. Although a few 4.0-T installations for human use are now available in the United States and abroad, it is very doubtful that in the future these will be found in more than a few scattered institutions, even as the technology for manufacturing stronger magnets improves.

The principal difficulties relate to the relatively small concentration of the chemical element being detected. For instance, phosphorus 31 could be an excellent element to detect by spectroscopy in the brain; it also is extremely important in energy metabolism. Unfortunately, the concentration is very low, and it takes a relatively long time and a large volume of brain tissue to produce a poor spectrum at 1.5 T. Thus, proton spectroscopy has received considerably more attention, and efforts are being made to uncover clinically useful data.

Typically, the phosphorus 31 spectrum is composed of seven peaks: phosphomonoesters, phosphodiesters, inorganic phosphate, phosphocreatine, and the three peaks of adenosine triphosphate (ATP) (Fig. 14.10).

Proton spectroscopy is more promising. The technical problems associated with the large pool of protons in brain water have been mostly resolved, and it is now possible to obtain hydrogen 1 spectra on relatively small brain volumes (as little as 2 to 4 cubic ml), whereas phosphorus 31 spectroscopy requires much larger volumes, about 10 times larger. In practice, 10 to 30 ml^3 are used for proton spectroscopy in humans with a 1.5-T magnet.

Some of the clinical problems that have been studied are stroke, neonatal asphyxia, brain tumors, and concentration of certain pharmacologic agents in brain tissue. Although phosphorus 31 spectroscopy would appear to be extremely useful in the study of stroke, it turns out that in cerebral infarction there is a rapid depletion of organic phosphate (less than 10 min) and conversion to inorganic phosphates, and later, diffusion of the inorganic phosphates into the interstitial space. This is rather disappointing, although possibly the penumbra area surrounding the ischemic core does offer some interest. Unfortunately, the resolution is insufficient because of the requirement for a large volume of tissue for phosphorus 31 spectroscopy.

In hydrogen1 spectroscopy smaller volumes can yield satisfactory results, and the variety of compounds that can be recognized in the spectrum is greater (17). A typical hydrogen spectrum is shown in Figure 14.11*B*. Highest peaks are creatine/phosphocreatine, *N*-acetylaspartate (NAA), and choline. Lactate and lipids also may be detected in abnormal cases. The spectrum may change as a response to disease (e.g., ischemic lesions) or owing to the presence of a neoplasm (18); an infarct (19,20); or edema around neoplasms (21); or in inherited metabolic errors (22).

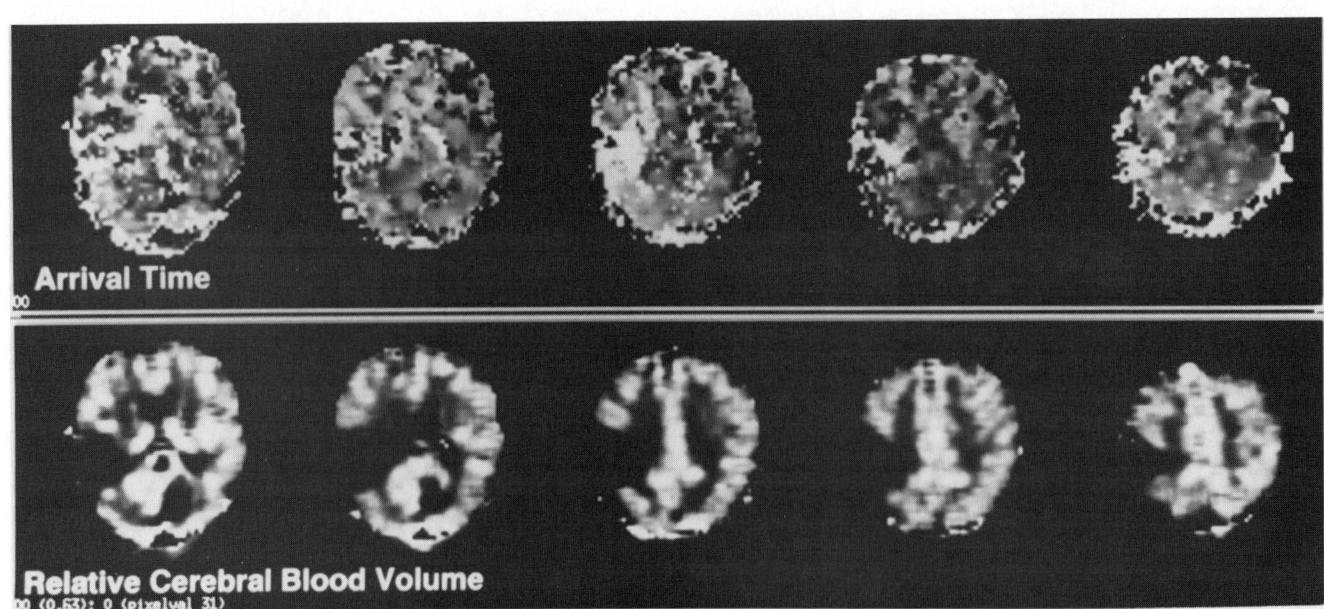

Figure 14.9. Perfusion imaging with contrast. Perfusion imaging in a patient with a right frontoparietal infarct. The top row shows the rapid passage of gadolinium. The images are video-reversed so that the infarcted area is brighter at the peak time during the passage of the contrast (about 18 sec). The bottom row reveals a markedly decreased cerebral blood volume in the infarcted area.

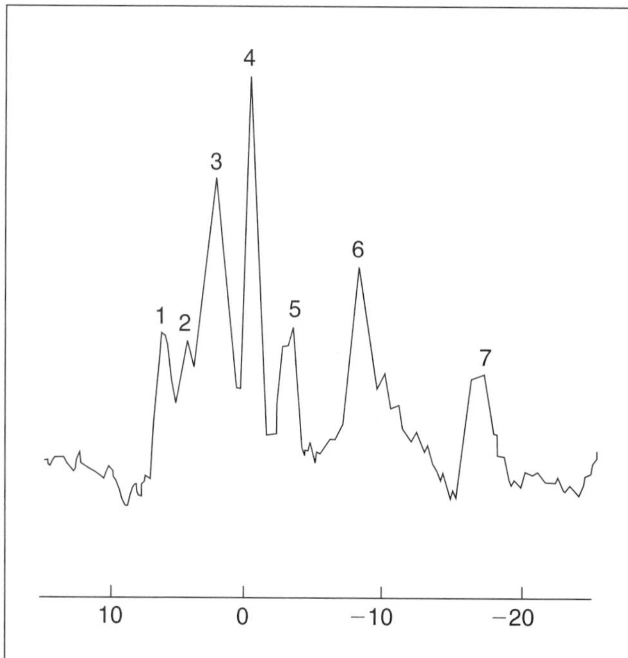

Figure 14.10. Typical local normal brain phosphorus 31 spectrum obtained with 1.5-T magnet. The numbers present the peaks of (1) phosphomonoesters; (2) inorganic phosphorus; (3) phosphodiesters; (4) phosphocreatine; (5, 6, 7) three peaks of adenosine triphosphate (ATP), gamma, beta, alpha.

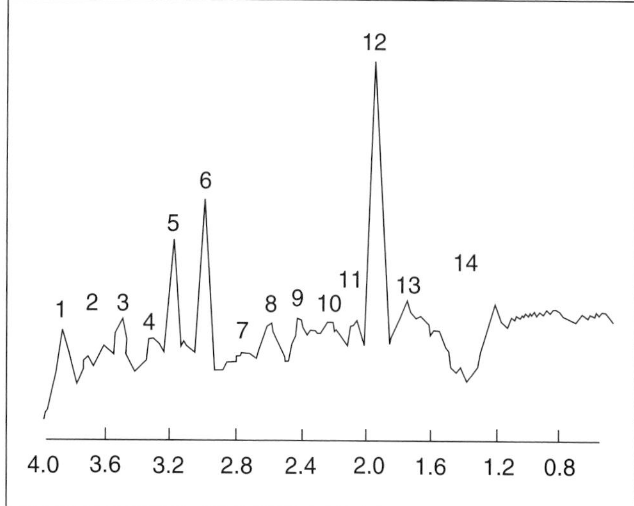

Figure 14.11. Human normal water-suppressed proton spectroscopy spectrum at 64 MHz with a TR of 6000 ms and a TE of 50 ms. The resonances are (1) creatine/phosphocreatine; (2) glutamate-glutamine; (3) inositol phosphates; (4) taurine; (5) choline-containing compounds; (6) creatine/phosphocreatine; (7) aspartate; (8) *N*-acetylaspartate; (9) glutamine; (10) gamma-aminobutiric acid (GABA); (11) glutamate; (12) *N*-acetylaspartate (NAA); (13) acetate; (14) lipids. (Modified from Frahm et al. [Magn Reson Med 1989;9:79–93].)

The basic components that are affected by the various pathologic processes are *N*-acetylaspartate, choline, creatine/phosphocreatine, and the inositols. Lactate may appear in stroke, tumors, and tumor edema. In a reported case of a large gray matter hamartoma in a newborn the MR–hydrogen 1 spectrum was essentially like that of gray matter, which obviated the need for an open biopsy (23).

Another important area in MRS is that involving the detection and determination of the concentration of certain drugs in the brain. Lithium MRS is an example. Gonzalez et al. (24) found that the serum concentration of lithium does not necessarily mirror the brain concentration in patients maintained on this medication for bipolar disorders. For instance, two patients on the same daily dose of lithium carbonate may have similar serum levels but vastly different brain levels, thus accounting for different responses. Other drugs, such as those containing fluorine (19F), may likewise be detected and their concentration in the brain estimated. Most drugs do not have a handle such as fluorine 19 for MRS and have to be studied through hydrogen 1 or perhaps through carbon 13 MRS (25). Recent reports indicate the decrease in *N*-acetylaspartate, which is a neuronal marker, in conditions in which there is neuronal loss such as Alzheimer disease. The results are promising and may be used to differentiate Alzheimer disease from other conditions (26).

Positron Emission Tomography

This refers to the production of images using isotopes that emit a pair of photons at 180° from each other (Table 14.3). These isotopes are usually produced by a cyclotron and have a relatively short half-life: oxygen 15, 2 min; carbon 11, 20 min; nitrogen 13, 10 min; fluorine 18, about 2 h. Because of their short half-life it is difficult to work with them. In the first place, they must be used either immediately, such as oxygen 15, or within an hour (such as carbon 11, which has three half-lives in one hour). The most satisfactory isotope turns out to be fluorine 18; its 2 h half-life permits us to prepare compounds such as fluorodeoxyglucose in order to study glucose metabolism in the brain. Deoxyglucose can be made with carbon 11, but the short half-life (20 min) requires a fast production time. It takes nearly 1 h to produce carbon 11 glucose, and the activity will have gone down considerably. Deoxyglucose is used because this compound behaves like glucose but stops at the stage of glucose-6-phosphate; it can be detected where

Table 14.3.
Positron Emission Tomography (PET)

Image production by emission of pairs of photons at 180° to one another
Important use in distinguishing tumor from radiation necrosis using 18-fluorodeoxyglucose
Other important uses include preoperative evaluation for epilepsy surgery and for evaluation of cognitive and psychiatric disorders
Limitations include necessity of a cyclotron for generation of isotopes and short half-life of isotopes

it was taken up in the tissues and metabolized to that point. This can be accomplished well within the times using fluorodeoxyglucose. Fluorine can be transported for as long as 2 h or more if there is sufficient activity.

The first functional studies were carried out with fluorodeoxyglucose. The regional brain glucose metabolism using light stimulation, movement stimulation, and hearing was carried out (27–30). The localization of these functions was found to be fairly consistent but quite variable, depending on other added factors and combination of stimuli (e.g., visual with language and/or with music).

One of the most important applications of PET scanning is the determination of the fluorodeoxyglucose uptake by a tumor, or the absence thereof. It may be a hypermetabolic tumor (i.e., malignant), or a hypometabolic tumor, which is usually associated with a more benign course. There is one exception to this rule: a recent report indicates that piloid astrocytomas are hypermetabolic, but their clinical behavior is that of a more benign lesion (31). The hypermetabolic area in a tumor is often seen to extend significantly beyond the tumor margin shown by enhanced CT or MRI, and histology usually shows tumor cells in the presumably edematous area surrounding the tumor (32).

The hypermetabolism of malignant tumors, as shown by fluorodeoxyglucose, is used to differentiate between neoplasm recurrence and radiation necrosis, which cannot be differentiated on MRI or CT with contrast. The tumor and the necrotic area both would take up contrast, but the metabolic rate would be high in tumor recurrence and very low in radionecrosis (33) (see Fig. 11.135). The possibility that the same difference in blood flow exists (higher flow in tumor) may make it possible to accomplish the same with the MRI tissue blood volume technique mentioned previously. Single photon emission tomography (SPECT) could also be used if this were the case. The circulatory changes, however, do not seem to be high enough, and for that reason, with the lower-resolution SPECT system one could not rely on the results.

The use of PET scanning in the study of epilepsy is discussed in Chapter 11 (see Fig. 11.133). The use of PET scanning in the study of cerebral circulation in stroke has been discussed in Chapter 10.

In the study of degenerative diseases the most important is Alzheimer-type dementia, where PET deoxyglucose or oxygen 15 scans demonstrate hypometabolism in the biparietal areas, also involving the posterior bitemporal areas. These appear to be areas physiologically affected in Alzheimer's disease; they are the parietal association areas believed to mediate integration of somatosensory, visual, and auditory inputs to the cortex (34). Decreased circulatory rate in the same areas, in some cases also involving the bifrontal region, has been recorded with SPECT (35).

It is possible to tag a number of pharmaceutical compounds with carbon 11 and also amino acids (methionine and others) (32). This has the advantage of yielding a short-lived radioactive compound that does not change the original molecule, contrary to the immense majority of compounds that have been tagged with other elements, in which a change of the original molecule may occur that changes the intended distribution in the human body, sometimes drastically.

Psychiatric conditions such as schizophrenia have been studied with PET to determine whether any metabolic changes can be demonstrated. For this, glucose tagged with carbon 11 as well as fluorodeoxyglucose has been utilized. The results appear to be similar. Brodie et al. found a decreased activity in the left frontal area, which became less pronounced after and during neuroleptic drug treatment but did not disappear (36). Widen et al. reported some asymmetry also in schizophrenias consisting in higher glucose uptake in the left basal ganglia area (37). The lower carbon 11 glucose uptake in the left frontal region was also found by Wiesel et al. (38).

In depression no cerebral blood flow, blood volume, and metabolic rate of oxygen differences with the normal were found by Raichle et al. (39). The bipolar illness (manic-depressive) may reveal observable reduction in glucose metabolism during the depressed phase; the same is true of unipolar depression (40,41).

In the manic phase some changes take place, but it does not seem to change to a hypermetabolic state (Table 14.3).

An ability to superimpose images obtained with different technologies such as CT, MRI, PET, and SPECT is very useful (42). In this way any local pathologic process can be analyzed and compared. The aim is to make the method sufficiently accurate that it can be used for a stereotactic approach.

REFERENCES

1. Wedeen VJ, Meuli RA, Edelman RR, et al: Projective imaging of pulsatile flow with magnetic resonance. Science 1985;230:946–949.
2. Rosen BR, Belliveau JW, Vevea JM, et al: Perfusion imaging with NMR contrast agents. Magn Reson Med 1990;14:249–265.
3. Belliveau JW, Rosen BR, Kantor HL, et al: Functional cerebral imaging by susceptibility-contrast NMR. Magn Reson Med. 1990; 14:538–546.
4. Belliveau JW, Kennedy DN, McKinstry RC, et al: Functional mapping of the human cortex by magnetic resonance imaging. Science 1991;254:716–719.
5. Connelly A, Jackson GD, Frackowiak RSJ, et al: Functional mapping of activated human primary cortex with a clinical MR imaging system. Radiology 1993;188:125–130.
6. Thompson RM, Jack CR, Butts K, et al: Imaging of cerebral activation at 1.5 T: Optimizing a technique for conventional hardware. Radiology 1994;190:873–877.
7. Yousry TA, Schmid UD, Jassoy AG, et al: Topography of the cortical mater hand area: Prospective study with functional MR imaging and direct mater mapping at surgery. Radiology 1995;195:23–29.
8. Menon RS, Ogawa S, Tank DW, et al: 4 Tesla gradient recalled echo characteristics of photic stimulation-induced signal changes in the human primary visual cortex. Magn Reson Med 1993;30: 380–386.
9. Pauling L, Coryell C: The magnetic properties and structure of hemoglobin, oxyhemoglobin and carboxyhemoglobin. Proc Natl Acad Sci USA 1936;22:210–216.
10. Kwong KK, Belliveau JW, Chesler DA, et al: Dynamic magnetic resonance imaging of human brain activity during primary sensory stimulation. Proc Natl Acad Sci USA 1992;89:5675–5679.

11. Frahm J, Bruhn H, Merbolt K, et al: Dynamic MR imaging of human brain oxygenation during rest and photic stimulation. J Magn Reson Imaging 1992;2:501–505.
12. Turner R, Jezzard P, Wen H, et al: Functional mapping of the human visual cortex at 4 and 1.5 Tesla using deoxygenation contrast EPI. Magn Reson Med 1993;29:277–279.
13. Ogawa S, Tank DW, Menon R, et al: Intrinsic signal changes accompanying sensory stimulation: Functional brain mapping with magnetic resonance imaging. Proc Natl Acad Sci USA 1992;89: 5951–5955.
14. Sorensen AG, Caramia F: Extrastriate activation in patients with visual field deficits. Presented at meeting of Society of Magnetic Resonance in Medicine, New York, 1993.
15. Sorensen A, Buonanno F, Schwamm I, et al: Accuracy of diffusion and perfusion-weighted MR imaging in diagnosis of acute stroke. Presented at the American Society of Neuroradiology, Chicago, 1995.
16. Lauterbur P: Image formation by induced local interactions: Examples employing nuclear magnetic resonance. Nature 1973;242: 190–191.
17. Frahm J, Bruhn H, Gyngell ML, et al: Localized high resolution proton NMR spectroscopy using stimulated echos: Initial applications to human brain in-vivo. Magn Reson Med 1989;9:79–93.
18. Bruhn H, Frahm J, Gyngell ML, et al: Noninvasive differentiation of tumors with use of localized H-1 MR spectroscopy in-vivo: Initial experience in patients with cerebral tumors. Radiology 1989;172: 541–548.
19. Fernstermacher MJ, Narayana PA: Serial proton magnetic resonance spectroscopy of ischemic brain injury in humans. Invest Radiol 1990;25:1034–1039.
20. Graham GD, Blamire AM, Howseman AM, et al: Proton magnetic resonance spectroscopy of cerebral lactate and other metabolites in stroke patients. Stroke 1992;23:333–340.
21. Kamada K, Kiyohiro H, Kazloshi H, et al: Localized proton spectroscopy of focal brain pathology in humans: Significant effects of edema on spin-spin relaxation time. Magn Reson Med 1994;31: 537–540.
22. Johannik K, VanHecke P, Francois B, et al: Localized brain proton spectroscopy in young adult phenylketonuria patients. Magn Reson Med 1994;31:53–57.
23. Castillo M, Kwock L, Scatliff J, et al: Proton MR spectroscopy characteristics of a presumed giant subcortical heterotopia. AJNR 1993; 14:426–429.
24. Gonzalez RG, Guimaraos AR, Sachs GS, et al: Measurement of human brain lithium in-vivo by MR spectroscopy. AJNR 1993;14: 1027–1037.
25. Komoroski RA: Measurement of psychoactive drugs in the human brain in-vivo by MR spectroscopy. AJNR 1993;14:1038–1042.
26. MacKay S, Ezekiel F, DiSclafani V, et al: Alzheimer disease and subcortical ischemic vascular dementia: Evaluation by combining MR imaging segmentation and H-1 MR spectroscopic imaging. Radiology 1996; 198:537–545.
27. Phelps ME, Kuhl DE, Mazziotta JC: Metabolic mapping of the brain's response to visual stimulation: Studies in humans. Science 1981;211:1445–1448.
28. Mazziotta JC, Phelps ME, Miller J, et al: Tomographic mapping of human cerebral metabolism: Normal unstimulated state. Neurology 1981;31:503–516.
29. Mazziotta JC, Phelps ME, Carson RE, et al: Tomographic mapping of human cerebral metabolism: Auditory stimulation. Neurology 1982;32:921–937.
30. Mazziotta JC, Phelps ME, Carson RE, et al: Tomographic mapping of human cerebral metabolism: Subcortical responses to auditory and visual stimulation. Neurology 1984;34:825–828.
31. Fulham MJ, Melisi JW, Nishimiya J, et al: Neuroimaging of juvenile pilocytic astrocytoma: An enigma. Radiology 1993;189:221–225.
32. Ogawa T, Shishido F, Kanno I, et al: Cerebral glioma: Evaluation with methionine PET. Radiology 1993;186:45–53.
33. Patronas NJ, DiChiro G, Brooks RA, et al: (18F) fluorodeoxyglucose and positron emission tomography in the evaluation of radiation necrosis of the brain. Radiology 1982;144:885–889.
34. Chase TN, Brooks RA, DiChiro G, et al: Focal cortical abnormalities in Alzheimer's disease. In H Ingvar, L Widen, T Greitz (eds), The Metabolism of the Human Brain Studied with Positron Emission Tomography. New York: Raven Press, 1985, pp 433–440.
35. Onishi T, Hoski H, Nagamach S, et al: Regional cerebral blood flow study with 1131-IMP in patients with degenerative dementia. AJNR 1991;12:513–520.
36. Brodie JD, Gomez-Mont F, Volkow ND, et al: Analysis of positron emission transaxial tomography images in psychiatric disorders. In T Greitz, H Inguar, L Widen (eds), The Metabolism of the Human Brain Studied with Positron Emission Tomography. New York: Raven Press, 1985, pp. 441–451.
37. Widen L, Blomqvist G, Greitz T, et al: PET studies of glucose metabolism in patients with schizophrenia. AJNR 1983;4:550–552.
38. Wiesel FA, Blomquist G, Ehrin E, et al: Brain every metabolism in schizophrenia studied with 11C-glucose. In T Greitz, H Inguar, L Widen (eds), The Metabolism of the Human Brain Studied with Positron Emission Tomography. New York: Raven Press, 1985, pp 485–493.
39. Raichle ME, Taylor JR, Herscovitch P, et al: Brain circulation and metabolism in depression. In T Greitz, H Inguar, L Widen (eds), The Metabolism of the Human Brain Studied with Positron Emission Tomography. New York: Raven Press, 1985, pp 453–456.
40. Phelps ME, Mazziotta JC, Baxter L, et al: Study design in the investigation of affective disorders: Problems and strategies. In T Greitz, H Inguar, L Widen (eds), The Metabolism of the Human Brain Studied with Positron Emission Tomography. New York: Raven Press, 1985, pp 457–470.
41. Phelps ME, Mazziotta JC, Gerner R, et al: Human cerebral glucose metabolism in affective disorders: Drug-free states and pharmacologic effects. J Cereb Blood Flow Metab 1983;3(suppl 1): S7–S8.
42. Greitz T, Bergstrom M, Boethius J, et al: A method for reproducible position alignment in transmission CT and positron emission tomography. J Cereb Blood Flow Metab 1981(suppl 1):48–49.

15

Craniovertebral Junction Lesions

ANATOMIC CONSIDERATIONS

The craniovertebral junction is important from many points of view. It represents the area of the body that possesses a considerable variety and extent of motion while at the same time providing for the passage of the lower aspect of the brainstem, the medulla, and the upper spinal cord. Thus, it has two major components: (*a*) the osteoarticular component and (*b*) the spinal canal, which contains the spinal cord and medulla. The anatomic structures to consider are demonstrated in Figures 15.1 through 15.5.

The ligaments involved in the articulations between the occipital bone, the atlas, and the axis are demonstrated in Figures 15.1 through 15.4. The joint margins of the atlanto-occipital joints and of the atlantoaxial joints can be well demonstrated on x-ray lateral and frontal tomograms. However, if the patient cannot cooperate, computed tomography (CT) scans made without turning the patient, in the supine position, can be reformatted with satisfactory results, provided that the slice thickness is thin enough: 1 or 2 mm (see text following).

Examination

The plain films in frontal and lateral projection are still basic in the evaluation of the craniovertebral junction. In addition to ordinary frontal views, open mouth frontal views may be made to demonstrate the odontoid process and the anterior arch of the atlas. It is well known, however, that pathology can be overlooked even in the osseous part. For that reason, tomography in frontal and lateral projections may be obtained. Ordinary tomography has been mostly replaced by CT, which allows for the taking of axial views from which coronal and sagittal images can be reformatted. In order to visualize the soft tissues satisfactorily, magnetic resonance imaging (MRI) is usually necessary; if no MRI is available, a myelogram followed by CT-myelography is the procedure of choice in any case where neurologic manifestations are encountered. In the last several years no CT-myelography to examine this area has been necessary because MRI yields all the needed information about the spinal canal and its contents, while CT has demonstrated the bones and joints.

PATHOLOGY

Congenital, traumatic, inflammatory, degenerative, metabolic, vascular, and neoplastic conditions involving the skeletal and neural components can occur in this region.

Congenital

SKELETAL

Fusion of the atlas with the occipital bone can occur (atlanto-occipital assimilation). The atlas may present an ununited posterior arch, which is a relatively frequent finding, usually of no clinical significance. The anterior arch is sometimes deficient, but this is a much more uncommon occurrence (1). The odontoid process may be hypoplastic; it may be congenitally separated from the body due to failure of fusion of the centers of ossification. The etiology of this condition, however, can be controversial because the center of ossification extends farther down into the body of C2, and the usual defect is at the base of the odontoid process (Fig. 15.6). The separate odontoid may be fused to the occipital bone.

A separate odontoid process moves with the anterior arch of the atlas. Head flexion may produce sufficient narrowing of the space between the upper posterior margin of the body of C2 and the posterior arch of the atlas so that compression of the cord can occur (Fig. 15.6).

The foramen magnum itself may be too narrow, such as is seen in achondroplasia.

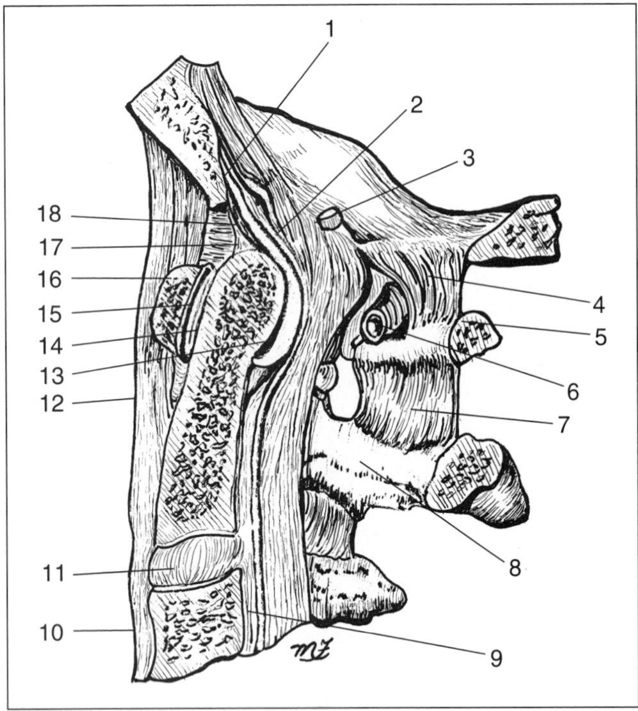

Figure 15.1. Midline sagittal cross section through the craniocervical junction. (1) Membrana tectoria; the superficial and deep layers have been slightly separated by a retractor; (2) membrana tectoria superficial layer; (3) hypoglossal foramen and nerve; (4) posterior atlanto-occipital ligament; (5) posterior arch of atlas; (6) vertebral artery; (7) posterior atlantoaxial ligament; (8) arch of axis; (9) posterior longitudinal ligament; (10) anterior longitudinal ligament; (11) intervertebral disc; (12) anterior atlantoaxial ligament; (13) transverse ligament; (14) odontoid process; (15) anterior articular cavity of atlantoaxial joint; (16) anterior arch of atlas; (17) apical odontoid ligament; (18) crus superior of transverse ligament.

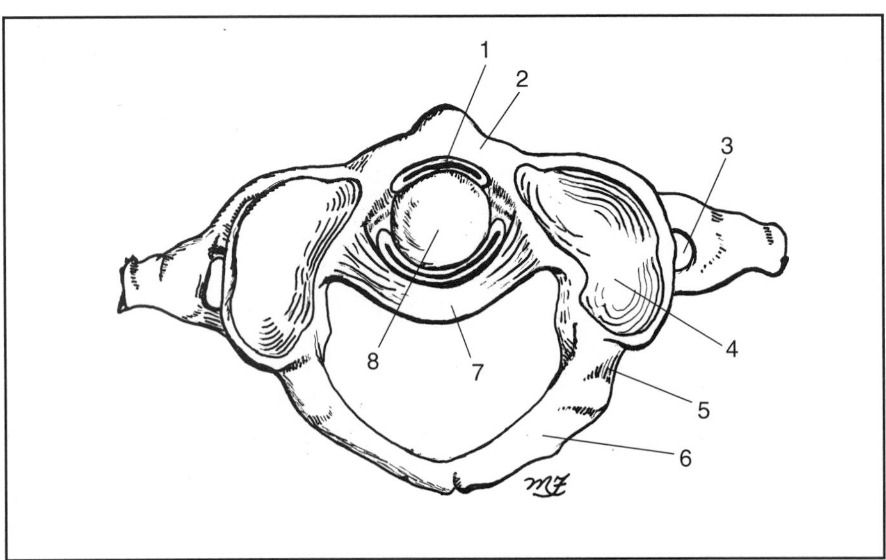

Figure 15.2. Atlas seen from above to demonstrate articulations between odontoid process and atlas. (1) Anterior articulation between atlas arch and odontoid process; (2) anterior arch of atlas; (3) orifice for vertebral artery; (4) lateral mass and superior articulating surface; (5) groove for vertebral artery as it swings behind lateral mass; (6) posterior arch of atlas; (7) transverse ligament; (8) odontoid process; the posterior articulation between the odontoid and the transverse ligament is shown.

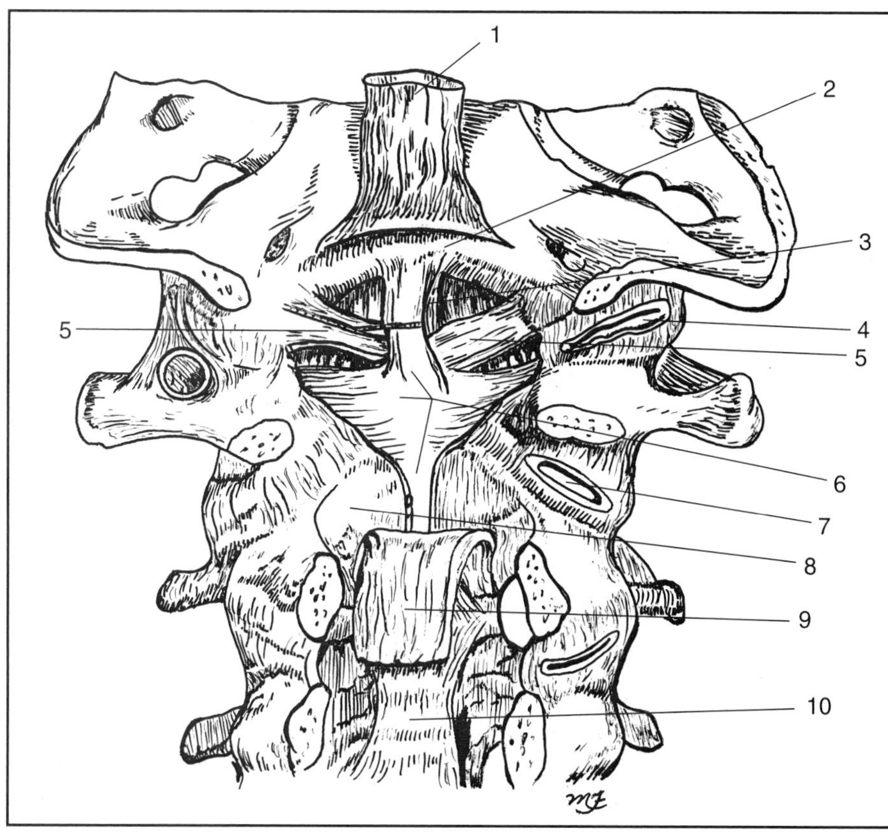

Figure 15.3. Anterior aspect of spinal canal at the craniovertebral junction demonstrating the membrana tectoria and the transverse and alar ligaments. (1) Membrana tectoria sectioned and retracted upward; (2) foramen magnum, anterior border; (3) apical odontoid ligament; (4) atlanto-occipital articulation; (5) odontoid or alar ligament; (6) transverse ligament with vertical portion (the upper part is retracted to the left to reveal the apical odontoid ligament); (7) atlantoaxial joint; (8) body of axis; (9) membrana tectoria sectioned and swung down; (10) posterior longitudinal ligament.

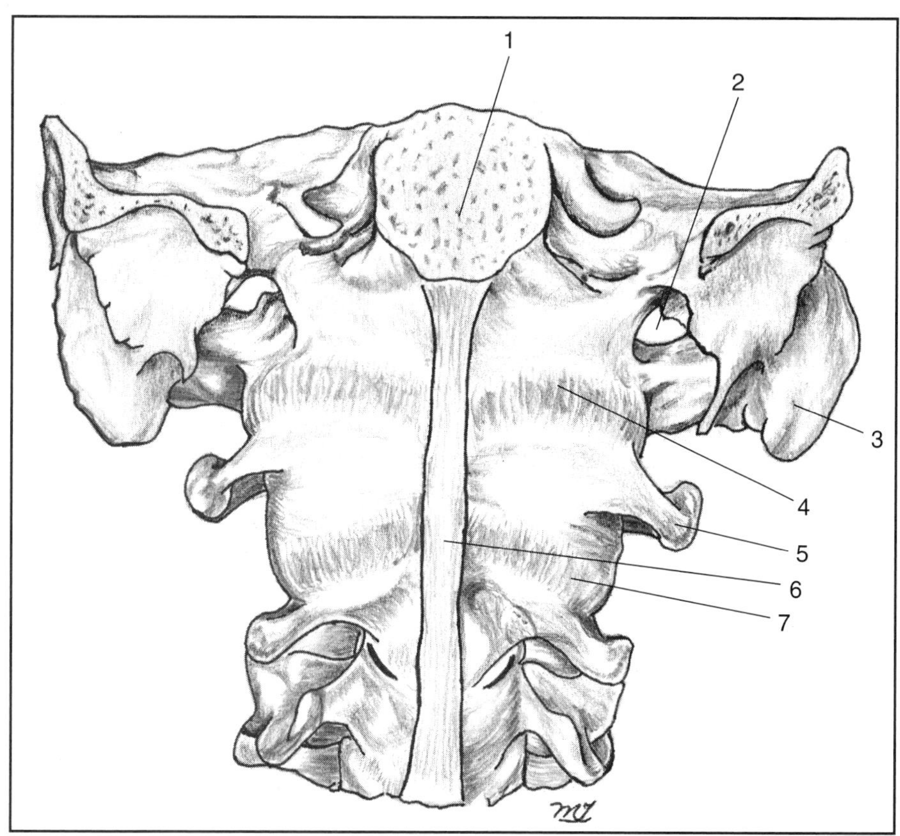

Figure 15.4. Anterior view of craniovertebral junction. (1) Basilar part of occipital bone; (2) jugular foramen; (3) mastoid process; (4) articular capsule of atlanto-occipital joint; (5) transverse process of atlas; (6) anterior longitudinal ligament (attached to anterior tubercle of atlas); (7) articular capsule of atlantoaxial joint.

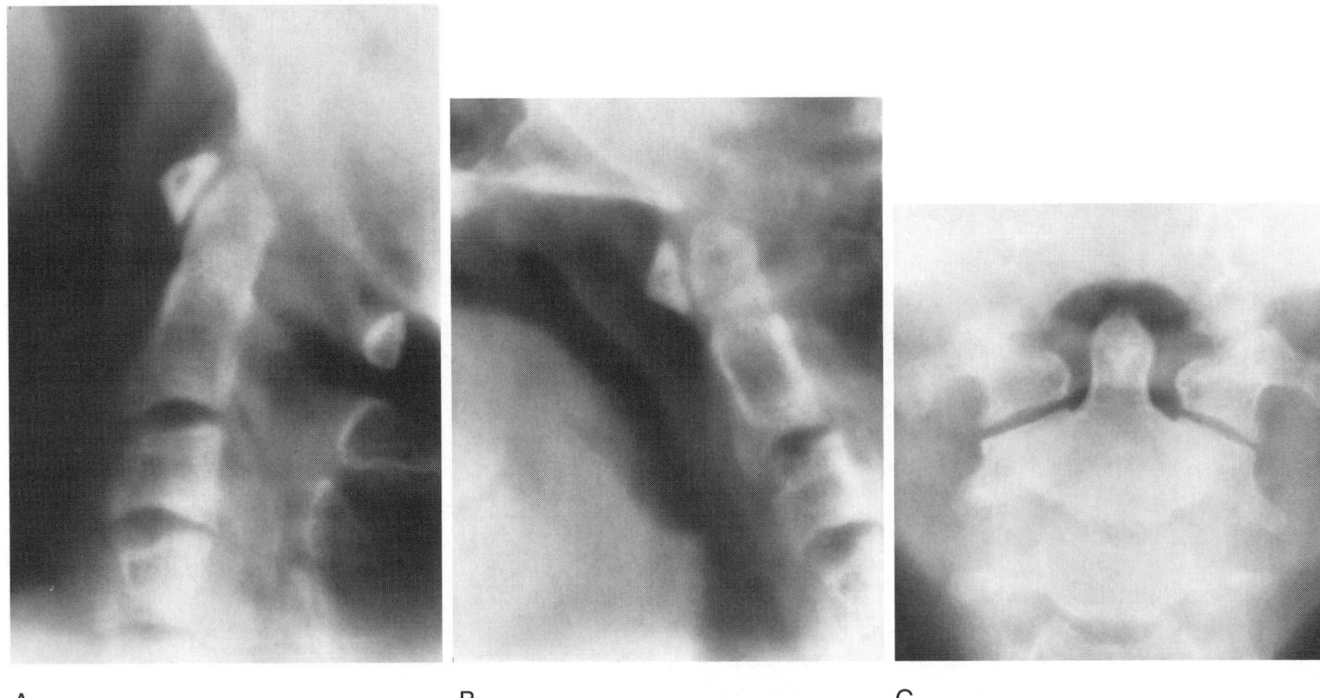

A B C

Figure 15.5. Frontal and midline sagittal tomogram of craniovertebral junction in extension and flexion. **A.** Tomograms in extension. **B.** In flexion the anterior arch of the atlas moves down and the angle of the clivus with the odontoid narrows. **C.** Open mouth tomogram. The odontoid is slightly off center, but this is commonly seen in these coronal tomograms or in open mouth views in normal individuals.

CEREBELLAR AND SPINAL CORD ANOMALIES

Anomalies of the cerebellum and spinal cord are described in Chapter 5.

Trauma

Subluxation and dislocation of the atlas on the occipital bone may occur. Much more common than this is fracture of the odontoid. Fractures usually occur at the base or a little below the base of the odontoid process; they usually present a ragged appearance (Fig. 15.6).

Rupture of the transverse ligament of the atlas may occur and can be suspected whenever an increase is seen in the space between the anterior arch of the atlas and the odontoid process (2). An increase in the space between the anterior arch of the atlas and the anterior odontoid surface is a contraindication to the taking of films in flexion. It may indicate either a tear of the transverse ligament of the atlas or a luxation of the odontoid (usually a relatively hypoplastic odontoid) under the lower margin of the ligament. In either case, flexion of the head may cause compression of the cord-medulla between the posterior arch of the atlas and the odontoid.

In young children (aged 3 to 5), fractures of the odontoid usually occur at the normal synchondrosis. Frontal and lateral views are usually sufficient to demonstrate them, but CT with reformatting may be required (3,4).

An important group of fractures includes the Jefferson fracture of the atlas, which consists of an injury to the top of the head, causing the laterally and downwardly slanting C1–C2 joints to spread the atlas, fracturing the arches of the atlas in four places, two anteriorly and two posteriorly next to the junction with the articular pillar. Diagnosis is made in the frontal view because the articular pillars of the atlas slide out symmetrically so that the joint surfaces of C1 and C2 in frontal projection do not meet properly; the superior surface has slid laterally.

Variants of atlas fractures may occur and are important to recognize from the management point of view (5).

Combinations of subluxation and fractures often occur, and CT axials and reformatted images are essential to understand the pathology present (6) (Fig. 15.7).

On plain films it may be necessary to take flexion and extension films in the lateral projection in order to demonstrate an increase in the atlas-odontoid distance. A lateral view made in the supine position may serve the same purpose if the occiput is elevated with a pad. It should be remembered that flexion and extension films should not be made until it has been determined that it is safe to do so from the preliminary films.

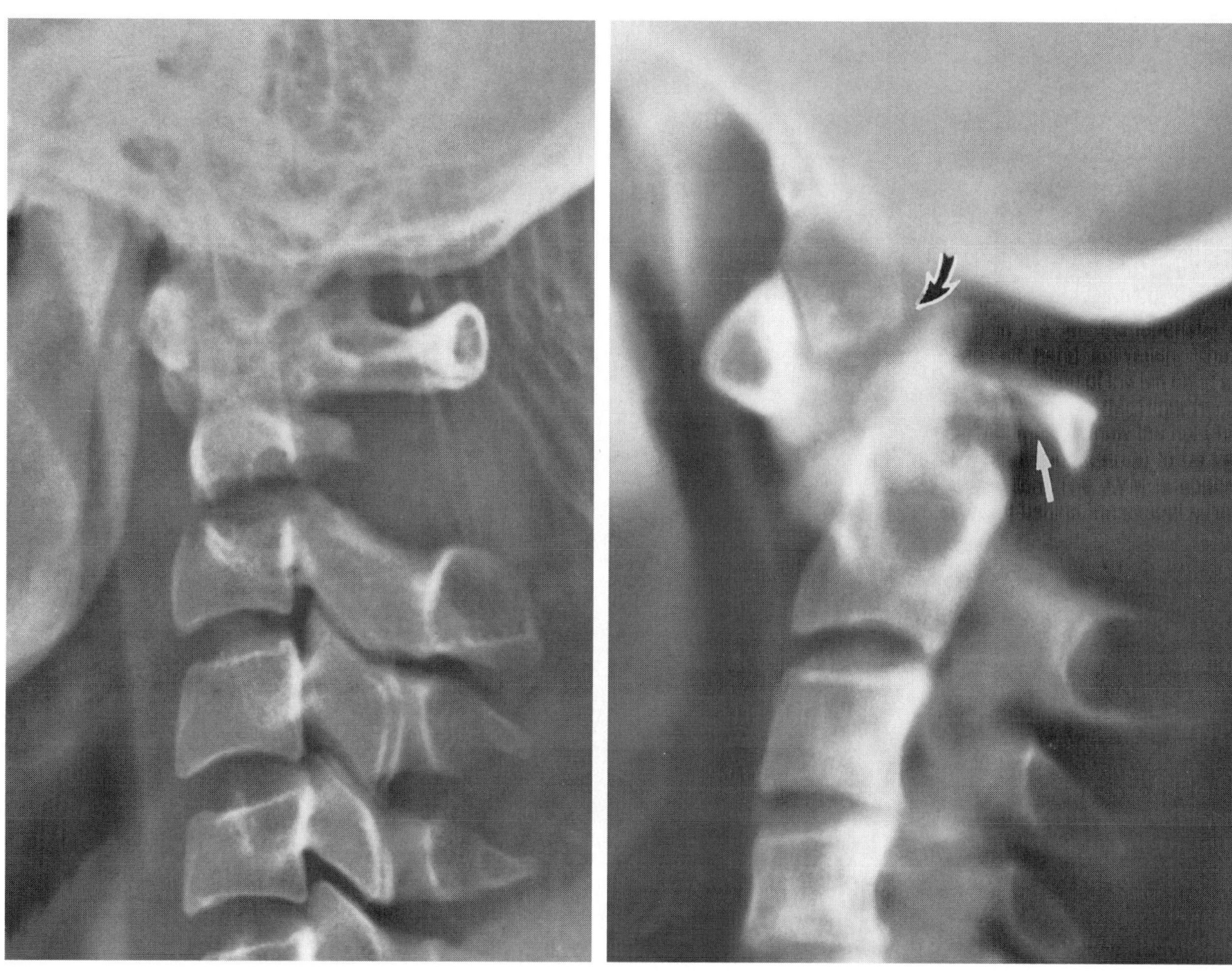

Figure 15.6. Fracture and congenital anomaly of odontoid process. **A.** Fracture of the odontoid occurs just below the base of the structure. The edges are ragged. **B.** Separated odontoid process, which shows a smooth upper margin of C2 and occurs at the base of the dens (open arrow). The margins tend to be smoother. In flexion, the space between the posterior arch of the atlas and the body of the axis can be even narrower than it is in this case, and compression of the spinal cord may occur (solid arrow). Usually the cord may move to either side, thus avoiding frank compression; if this does not occur, cord compression would definitely happen when the head is flexed.

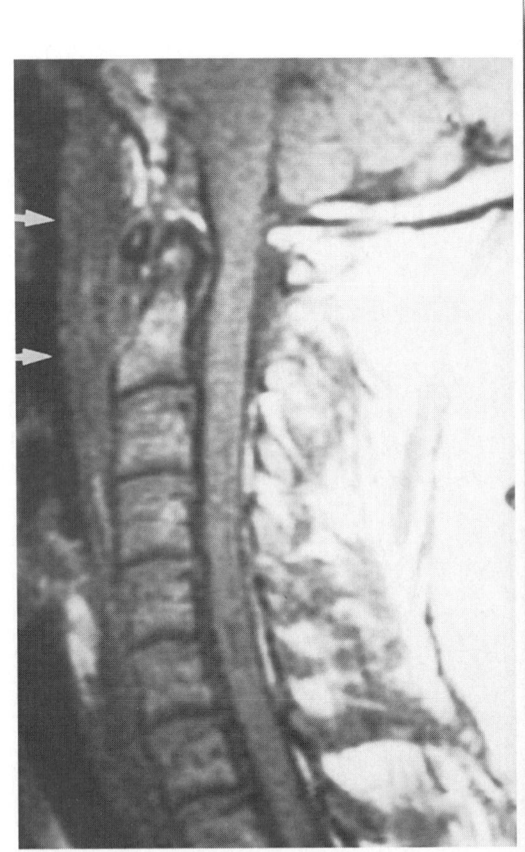

A

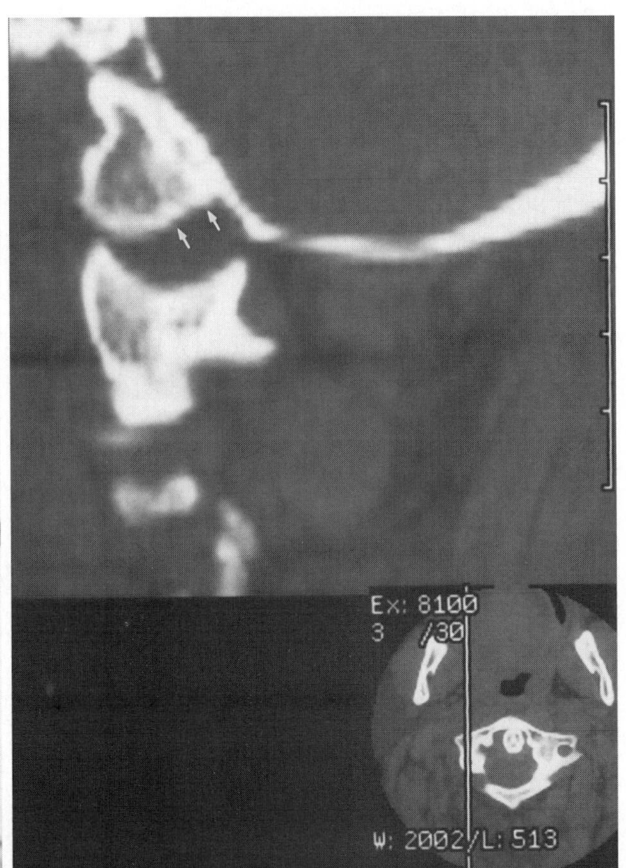
Ex: 8100
3 /30
W: 2002/L: 513

B

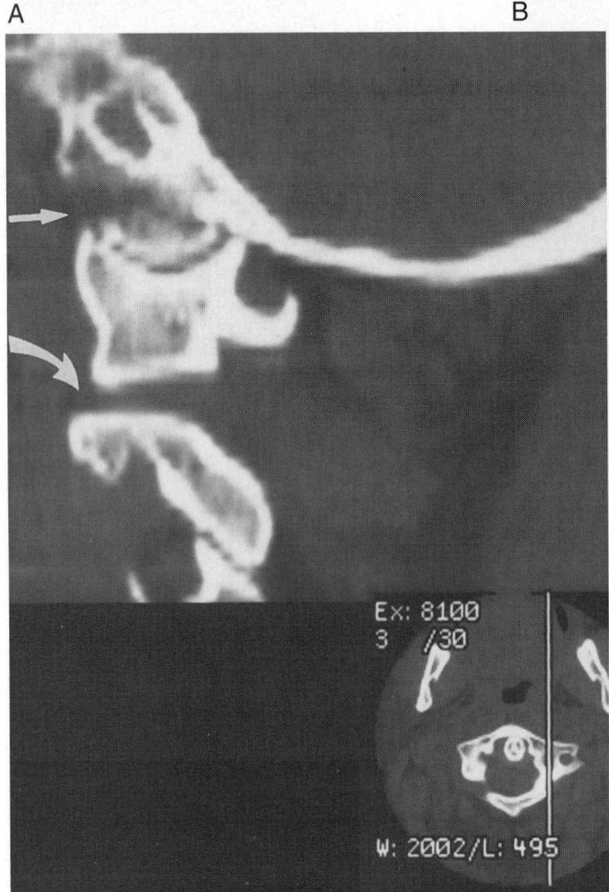
Ex: 8100
3 /30
W: 2002/L: 495

C

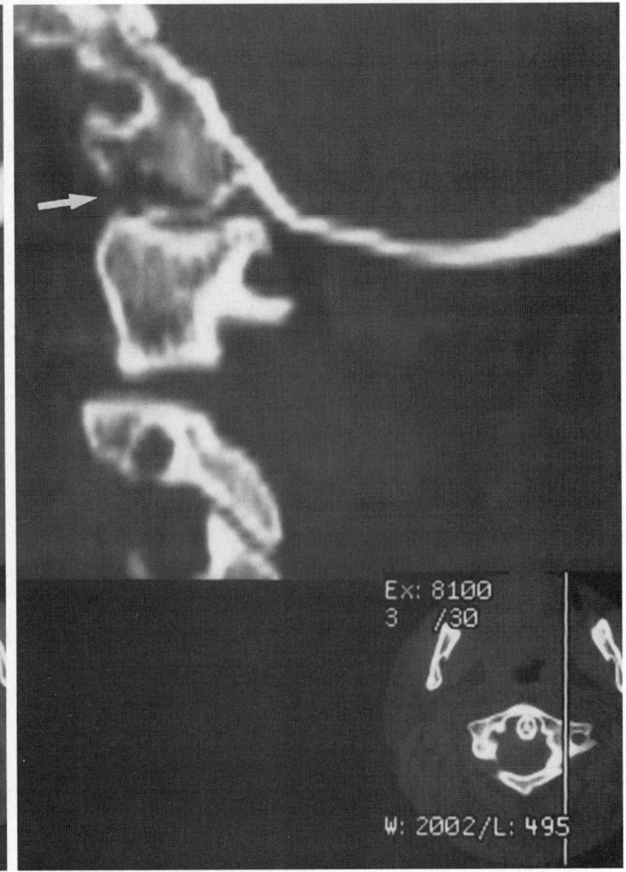
Ex: 8100
3 /30
W: 2002/L: 495

D

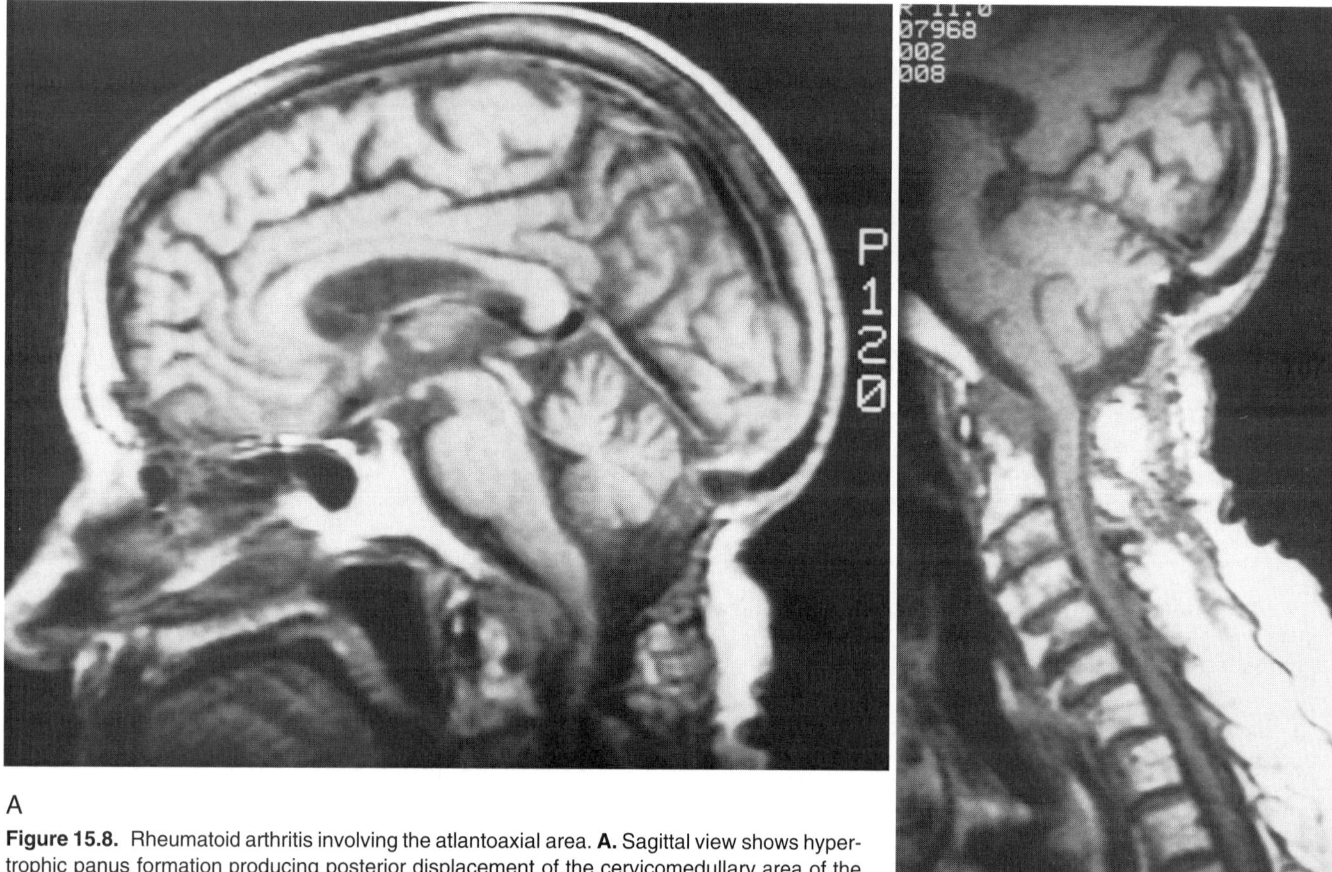

Figure 15.8. Rheumatoid arthritis involving the atlantoaxial area. **A.** Sagittal view shows hypertrophic panus formation producing posterior displacement of the cervicomedullary area of the cord. There is erosion of the odontoid process by soft tissue, seen also in sections slightly off the midline (B). In **B**, the cord displacement is less pronounced, indicating that the cord is slightly displaced to one side. The patient was an elderly woman with no prior history of rheumatoid arthritis who was experiencing extreme weakness.

Inflammatory

EPIDURAL ABSCESS

Epidural abscess may extend up to the craniovertebral junction but usually would compress the spinal cord below this area (see Fig. 16.77).

RHEUMATOID ARTHRITIS

Involvement of the synovial articulations around the odontoid process (Fig. 15.2) tends to occur in rheumatoid arthritis. Sometimes the panus formation is large (Fig. 15.8). Subluxation and luxation may occur, as may involvement of other cervical levels.

PACHYMENINGITIS

Pachymeningitis may affect the cervical spinal cord medullary junction by diminishing the available spinal canal space. Hypertrophic pachymeningitis has been seen in Whipple disease (see Fig. 13.2) and has been reported of unknown etiology (7). Sarcoid may produce focal meningeal dural masses or more diffuse changes. Syphilis, once a common etiology, is now rare. Among the causes of hypertrophic dural thicken-

Figure 15.7. Multiple traumatic abnormalities at the foramen magnum demonstrated by CT with reformatting. Insert shows position of reformatted slice. **A.** Sagittal MRI shows a normal odontoid, but there is questionable bulging of the membrane or ligaments behind the odontoid. Some narrowing at the foramen magnum appears to be present, but there is no significant compression of the spinal cord. There is some prevertebral soft tissue swelling (arrow). **B.** Reformatted sagittal CT passing through the right occipital condyle shows a distraction (with forward movement of the condyle) of the condyle and atlas articular surfaces. **C.** Reformatted sagittal passing through left atlanto-occipital joint shows there is a fracture through the occipital condyle, but the atlantoaxial joint is preserved at this point, although a little more laterally (**D**) the fracture is reaching the articular surface (arrow). There is rotary subluxation of the atlas on the axis, and the inferior articular facet is posteriorly situated on the left in relation to the superior facet of the axis (curved arrow). This example emphasizes the importance of obtaining reformatted CT images in the craniovertebral junction.

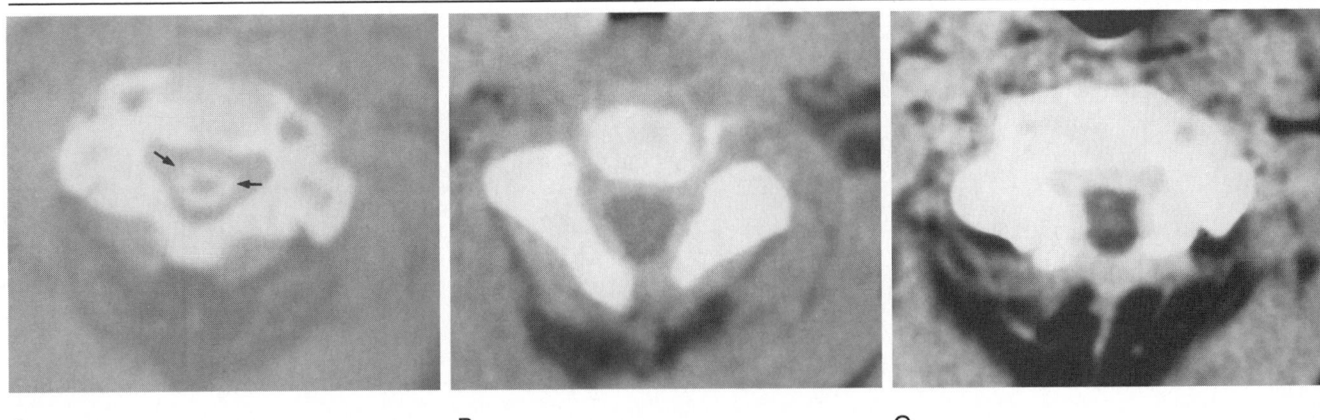

A B C

Figure 15.9. Hypertrophic thickening of the dura in a patient with mucopolysaccharidosis type VIA, B (Maroteaux-Lamy syndrome). **A.** The axial view (upper cervical), following myelography, shows the contrast material in the thecal sac constricted by a thick, soft tissue space surrounding it (arrows). The spinal cord is very thin and is seen in the center of the opacified thecal sac. The patient underwent a laminectomy and medical treatment, which resulted in clinical improvement. **B** and **C.** Repeat examination without myelography performed 2 years later. (B) Without contrast. (C) After intravenous contrast enhancement. The spinal cord appears to be of normal width, and there is less tissue around the thecal sac.

ing should be included the Maroteaux-Lamy variety of mucopolysaccharidosis (type VIA, B) (Fig. 15.9).

Neoplasms

The neoplasms in this region may arise (*a*) from the surrounding osseous structures; (*b*) from the meningeal structures; or (*c*) from the neural elements, nerves, and brainstem-cervical cord. The tumors arising from the surrounding osseous structures (extradural) include the chordoma, the metastatic tumors, and the chondromas-chondrosarcomas. The chordoma may arise from the clivus on the vertebral body of C2. The chondromas-chondrosarcomas usually arise from the clivus and adjacent base of the skull.

The tumors arising from the meninges are usually meningiomas. They tend to arise at the anterolateral aspect of the foramen magnum and are in an ideal location to show by myelography (Fig. 15.10). MRI with contrast is the procedure of choice, however. In the extramedullary intradural group

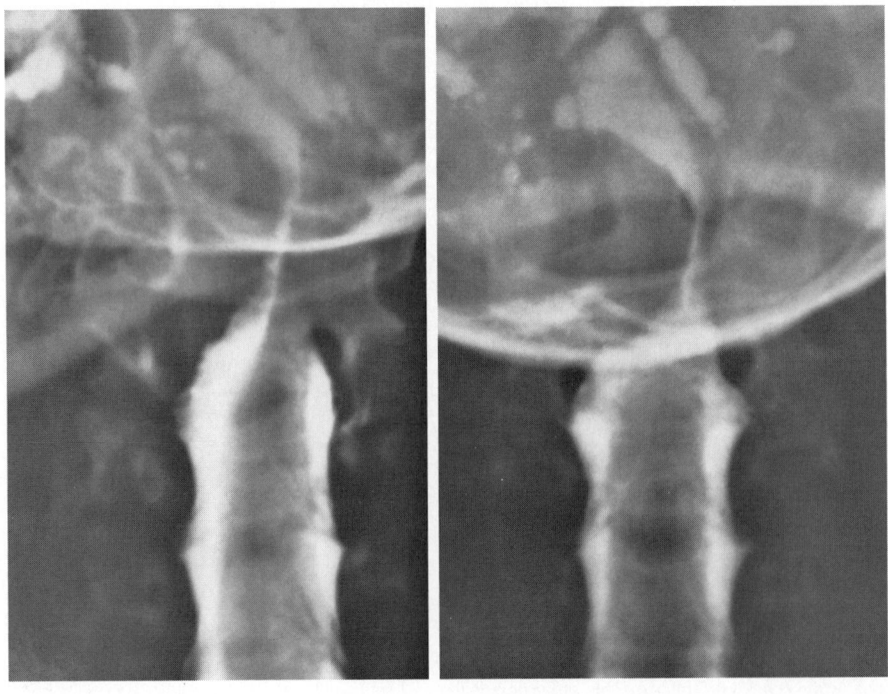

A B

Figure 15.10. Meningioma of anterolateral aspect of foramen magnum. The location is typical, and the myelogram shows it well because the patient is lying prone. **A.** Head turned to right. **B.** Head straight.

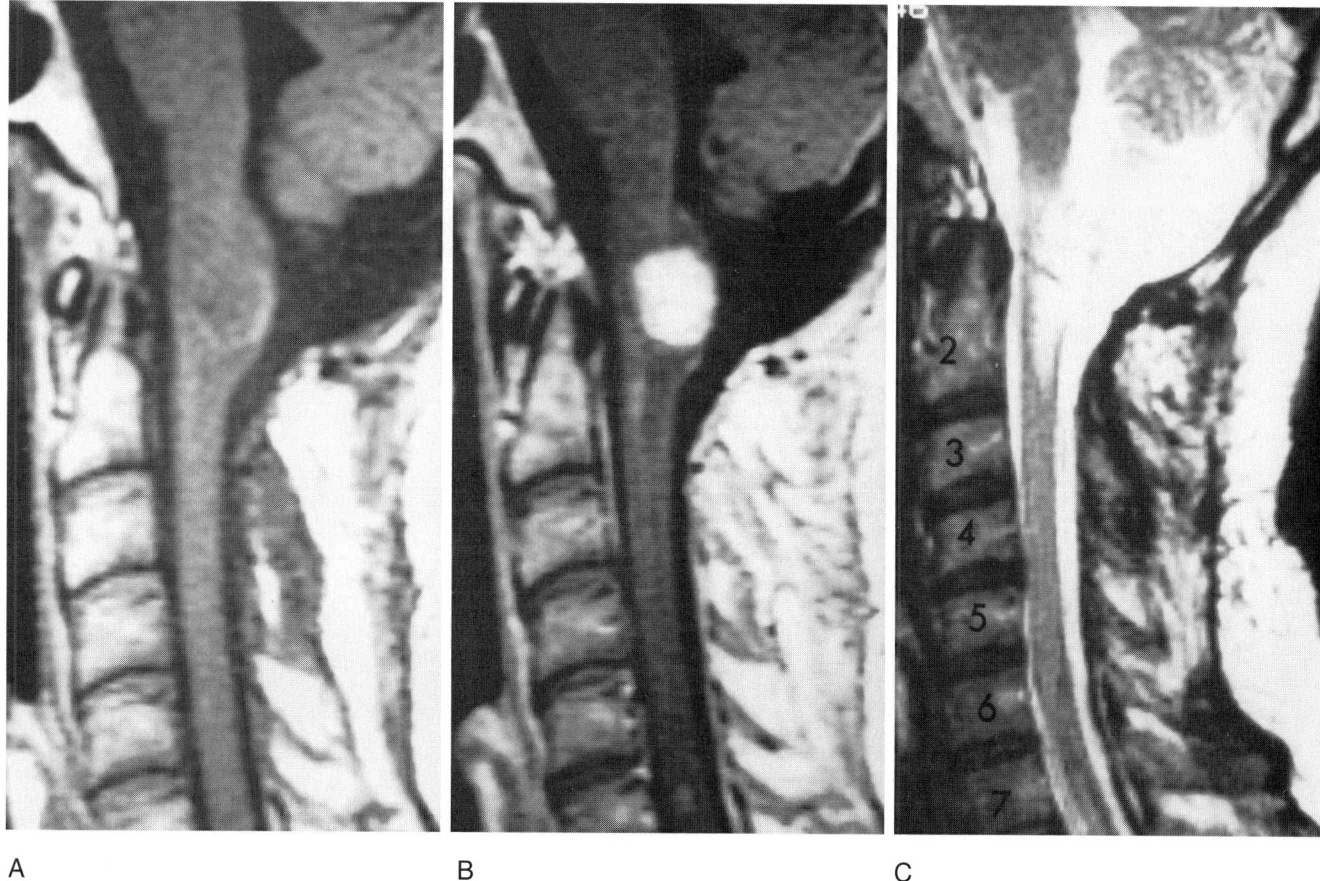

Figure 15.11. Ependymoma of cervical cord at junction with medulla in patient with neurofibromatosis II. **A.** Noncontrast T1-weighted image shows the intrinsic mass, slightly heterogeneous. **B.** After contrast there is marked uptake and a homogeneous hyperintensity. **C.** T2-weighted sagittal view shows edema in the center of the cord extending caudally from the main mass.

we should include the aneurysms of the vertebral artery or of the posterior inferior cerebellar artery, and also fusiform aneurysms as well as very dolichoectatic vertebral and basilar arteries. In the same group, the tumor masses arising from the nerves must be considered. This includes the schwannomas or neurofibromas arising from the ninth, tenth, and eleventh nerves (see Fig. 11.112), and those arising from the twelfth nerve (see Fig. 11.113). Glomus jugulare tumors may be situated in the same area (See Fig. 11.113). Neurofibromas arising from the upper cervical nerves may be seen in patients with neurofibromatosis type I.

Intra-axial masses include the astrocytomas and ependymomas (Fig. 15.11). Syringo hydromyelia can produce enlargement of the cord, which would be homogeneous (see Fig. 16.94). Hemorrhage can be focal and possibly associated with an arteriovenous malformation. Venous malformations would produce cerebral hemorrhage, which can be focal and suggest a neoplasm (see Chapter 16, "Intramedullary Lesions," for further detail).

Lesions of multiple sclerosis may produce focal cord swelling; the same is true of myelitis (see Figs. 4.64 and 16.82). However, in these cases, the increase in cord size is rather small.

REFERENCES

1. Chambers AA, Gaskill MF: Midline anterior atlas clefts: CT findings. J Comput Assist Tomogr 1992;16:868–870.
2. Fielding JW, Cochran GVB, Lawsing JF, et al: Tear of the transverse ligament of the atlas: A clinical and biomedical study. J Bone Joint Surg Am 1974;56A:1683–1691.
3. Bulas DI, Fitz CR, Johnson DI: Traumatic atlanto-occipital dislocation in children. Radiology 1993;188:155–158.
4. Lee C, Woodring JH, Goldstein SJ, et al: Evaluation of traumatic altantooccipital dislocations. AJNR 1987;8:19–26.
5. Lee C, Woodring JH: Unstable Jefferson variant atlas fractures: An unrecognized cervical injury. AJNR 1991;12:1105–1110.
6. Fielding JW, Hensinger RN, Bjorkengren AG, et al: "Cranioatlantoaxial injuries." In JM Taveras, JT Ferrucci (eds), Radiology: Diagnosis/Imaging/Intervention, vol 5. Philadelphia: Lippincott, 1994, ch 141.
7. Martin N, Masson C, Henin D, et al: Hypertrophic cranial pachymeningitis: Assessment with CT and MR imaging. AJNR 1989;10: 477–484.

SELECTED READINGS

Effendi B, Roy D, Cornish B, et al: Fractures of the ring of the axis: A classification based on the analysis of 131 cases. J Bone Joint Surg Am 1981;63B:319.

Smoker WRK, Dolan KD: The "fat" C2: A sign of fracture. AJNR 1987; 8:33–38.

16

Spine and Spinal Canal

GENERAL CONSIDERATIONS

The examination of the spine included only plain films until 1922, when Sicard and Forestier demonstrated the possibility of injecting an iodized oil (Lipiodol) into the spinal canal to demonstrate pathology, originally only to demonstrate the presence and level of a spinal block. These remained as the only two possibilities for visualizing pathology. Two decades later Lipiodol was replaced by iodophenylundecanoate (Pantopaque; Miodil). Air myelography was also developed around 1921, and its use was continued, particularly in Scandinavia, for four decades until the development of water-soluble contrast media for myelography. Air myelography was first performed by Jacobaeus in Stockholm.

Spinal angiography was introduced by the French school of neuroradiology in the early 1960s, when it became possible to demonstrate arteriovenous malformations involving the spinal cord by angiography. Until then the diagnosis was made by myelography, and usually no further attempt at visualization of these malformations was made. Their demonstration by angiography allowed surgeons to approach the lesions and revolutionized the management of vascular malformations in the spinal canal.

In 1972, computed tomography (CT) was developed for examinations of the skull; several years later, a body scanner was available commercially. Following the introduction of the body CT scanners, examination of the spine began to improve considerably. At about the same time, the newly developed water-soluble contrast media began to be slowly accepted by the medical profession, although there were still too many side effects, which held up the final universal acceptance of these contrast media for a number of years.

The advent of magnetic resonance imaging (MRI) was a revolutionary step in the diagnosis of spinal and spinal cord pathology. For the first time it became possible to examine the spinal canal contents without any contrast media and with considerable detail. Finally, the introduction of contrast media for MRI (gadolinium-DTPA) was another important step that allowed us to demonstrate neoplasms much more clearly and also to better study postoperative changes following surgery for disc disease.

At present MRI is the principal examination for studying the spinal cord and is preferred for survey examinations of the spine when looking for pathology of the intervertebral discs. However, the latter preference is shared with CT, and sometimes CT and myelography combined and utilized to better define the intervertebral disc pathology particularly in postoperative cases. One wonders whether myelography may not disappear altogether in the future. I had thought that with the combination of CT and MRI examinations it was going to be possible to eliminate myelography altogether. However, we find ourselves at the Massachusetts General Hospital still doing a rather large number of myelograms for lumbar spinal pathology, always followed by CT examination, particularly in the evaluation of postoperative spinal problems and spinal canal stenosis, and also in preoperative cases where the clinical findings are atypical and the CT and MRI do not allow a clear localization. Myelography is still useful in the preliminary diagnosis of vascular malformations of the spinal cord.

This rather large chapter will attempt to cover all aspects of the spine and the spinal cord, including anatomy; technical considerations; intervertebral disc disease and osteoarthrosis; the postoperative spine; stenosis of the spinal canal; congenital, inflammatory, and traumatic conditions; vascular disorders; and neoplastic diseases. The discussion will concentrate on those aspects affecting the spinal canal that may cause compression of the spinal cord or of the emerging nerves.

TECHNICAL CONSIDERATIONS AND ANATOMY

Vertebral Column

Ordinarily a vertebra can be identified by palpation of landmarks on the back, within an allowable error of one segment. Topographically, the L4-L5 intervertebral space is situated at the level of the iliac crest; the twelfth thoracic vertebra can be identified by palpation of the lowest ribs; the angle of the scapula ordinarily falls at the level of T7; and C7 is the highest segment to have a large and prominent spinous process. With the body flexed, persons of average build will exhibit sessile midline prominences of the back over each vertebral spine. Identification of vertebral levels in individuals who are excessively corpulent may be extremely difficult.

A double curvature of the vertebral column in the sagittal plane is characteristic of animals that occupy the upright posture, and, in the absence of disease or injury, these curves are maintained throughout life. In the cervical and lumbar areas, there is a ventral convexity, while in the thoracic and sacrococcygeal areas, a dorsal convexity is presented. The cervical and lumbar curves are produced by variations in thickness of the intervertebral discs, the discs being thicker in front than behind in these regions. The intervertebral fibrocartilages are nearly of uniform thickness in the thoracic region, and the anterior concavity is dependent almost entirely on the slightly wedged shape of the vertebral bodies.

The *intervertebral discs* are composed, at their circumference, of laminae of fibrous tissue and fibrocartilage, forming the annulus fibrosus. The center of each disc is composed of a soft, pulpy, elastic substance, which bulges out when the disc is divided horizontally. The latter is called the *nucleus pulposus.* The nucleus pulposus is a remnant of the notochord and is particularly well developed in the lumbar region. The sizes of the intervertebral discs correspond to the sizes of the two adjacent vertebrae that they separate except in the cervical region, where they are slightly smaller in a transverse direction than the corresponding vertebral bodies. This is not strictly true, however, because there is a lateral extension of the intervertebral fibrocartilage extending into the articulation formed by the articular lip of the cervical vertebra below and the lateral aspect of the vertebra above, the so-called uncovertebral joints. Separating the intervertebral fibrocartilages from the upper and lower surfaces of the vertebral bodies is a layer of hyaline cartilage. The intervertebral discs are closely connected to the anterior and posterior longitudinal ligaments, and in the thoracic region they are joined, by means of the interarticular ligaments, to those ribs that articulate with two adjacent vertebrae.

A summation of the thickness of all of the intervertebral discs discloses that the fibrocartilaginous elements separating the vertebrae account for approximately one-fourth of the entire length of the vertebral column. The length of the vertebral column is greatest in the maturely developed young adult. Dehydration, loss of elasticity, and varying degrees of degeneration in the intervertebral discs occur with advancing age and result in an actual reduction in the individual's height.

The vertebral arches are joined by the ligamenta flava, which are present from the second cervical vertebrae to the sacrum. One is present on each side, commencing on either side at the base of the articular process and extending dorsally to the point where the two laminae meet to form the spinous process. There is usually a small interval present between the right and the left yellow ligaments for the passage of blood vessels and sometimes a little areolar tissue.

An adequate knowledge of the radiologic anatomy of all of the components of the vertebrae, which are often distorted by the radiologic projection and by disease, is indispensable. The reader is referred to the standard texts. However, some reference to certain anatomic structures will be made in the section on intervertebral disc disease and osteoarthritis.

Spinal Canal

The vertebral canal, in schematic cross section, has its contents arranged in a laminated manner (Fig. 16.1). The various components, which may be considered as a series of cylinders one within another, are designated by their relationship to the meninges. The outermost tubular compartment, between the bony structures and the dura mater, is usually referred to as the *epidural or extradural space.* In this space are located spinal ligaments, connective tissue, areolar tissue, the epidural venous plexus, lymphatic channels, and supporting elements. The thickness of the epidural space varies considerably in different individuals, chiefly with the quantity of epidural fat that is present and, also in the same individual, depending on the amount of blood in the epidural plexus.

Between the dura mater and the arachnoid membrane is the *subdural space.* Classically this compartment is regarded more often as a potential rather than an actual cavity. Not-

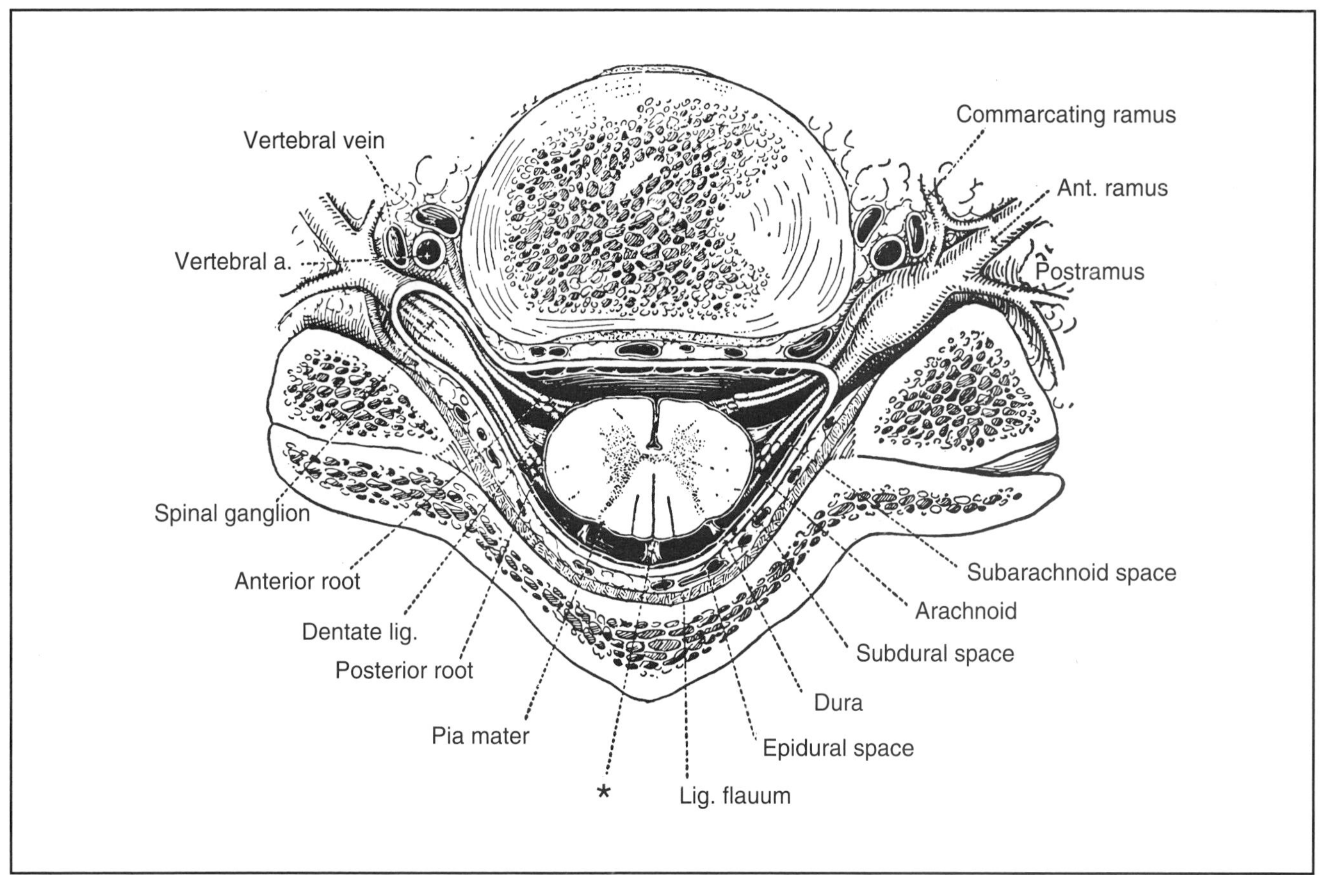

Figure 16.1. Vertebral canal and its contents. A transverse section at the level of C4 provides an axial view of the extradural, subdural, subarachnoid, and subpial compartments. The spinal cord, at the cervical enlargement, fills the greater portion of the vertebral canal. The relation of the spinal nerve roots and ganglia to the meningeal sheaths and the intervertebral foramina is depicted. The asterisk indicates the posterior longitudinal subarachnoid septum. (From The Manual of Surgical Anatomy, U.S. Army Medical Department, 1918.)

withstanding the fact that the subdural space usually is very small when identified at the operating table or in the anatomy laboratory, studies in radiologic anatomy made after the injection of contrast media disclose that in some patients the subdural space is relatively wide or at least distensible. Defects, presumably developmental, may be present in the leptomeninges, which allow a free passage of cerebrospinal fluid (CSF) from the subarachnoid space to the subdural space, but this is debatable. Traumatic perforations of the delicate arachnoid, which are produced by piercing the meninges with a needle, frequently result in large subdural collections of CSF that may persist for many days or weeks following a diagnostic lumbar puncture.

The middle meningeal layer is the *arachnoid*, which ordinarily bounds circumferentially the compartment in which the major portion of the CSF is contained. The most common anatomic variation of the arachnoid sac is in its length. At the caudal end, a tapering cul-de-sac is formed, which usually terminates at the level of S2, but variations in length of as much as one vertebral segment are common. The subarachnoid space is partially divided by the *posterior longitudinal subarachnoid septum* (denoted by an asterisk in Fig. 16.1), which connects the arachnoid with the pia mater and forms a partition, most complete in the thoracic region, along the dorsal aspect of the spinal cord. It should be mentioned that this subarachnoid septum is composed of only a few discontinuous fibers in the cervical region. It is best developed in the thoracic region, but here also it is discontinuous and does not form a true septum. A surgeon who opens the dura in the thoracic region will often describe some "adhesions," which usually represent the dorsal subarachnoid septum. In the cervical region, it is very poorly developed.

The *dentate ligaments*, which incompletely subdivide the subarachnoid cavity into ventral and dorsal compartments, extend in the coronal plane on each side of the spinal cord. These ligaments are a series of narrow, bandlike structures that extend between the pia and arachnoid and at intervals are fixed to the dura mater. The function of the dentate ligaments presumably is to suspend the spinal cord in the central portion of the subarachnoid CSF space. However, the spinal cord does move transversely as well as dorsally and ventrally with changes in position. This is well demonstrated in air myelography.

The *spinal pia mater* covers the entire surface of the spinal cord and is intimately adherent to it. The pia forms sheaths for the spinal nerves, which are closely applied to the nerves and blend with their membranous investments.

The pia mater is a vascular membrane between and beneath the layers of which are carried the nutrient vessels of the spinal cord.

The arachnoid forms a sheath around spinal roots as far as the point of exit from the vertebral canal. The arachnoidal sheath around the root is sometimes quite loose and sometimes shows cystic dilatation, commonly encountered in the lumbar region (Fig. 16.17).

The *spinal cord* forms the cylindrical core of the laminated tubular divisions of the vertebral canal. In adult life, the spinal cord extends from the margin of the foramen magnum to the level of the lower part of the body of the first lumbar segment. On the average, the spinal cord is about 45 cm in length. The spinal cord is almost circular in shape, but it is expanded transversely to an oval contour at its cervical and lumbar enlargements, which are maximum at C5 and T12 vertebral levels. The spinal cord, in the adult, tapers conically (conus medullaris) at its lower end to terminate in a filament (filum terminale) that is composed chiefly of pia mater invested by dura but contains remnants of a few neural elements. The filum terminale is a delicate strand of tissue, measuring approximately 20 cm in length, which extends caudad from the conus through the lumbosacral canal to attach to the first segment of the coccyx. In early fetal life, the spinal cord itself extends the entire length of the vertebral canal, but in the second and third trimesters the vertebral column grows in length more rapidly than the spinal cord. At birth, the tip of the conus lies at the level of the third lumbar vertebra. The greater lengthening of the vertebral column in comparison to the growth of the spinal cord results in a special relationship between the spinal cord segments, the intradural arrangement of the spinal nerve roots, and the vertebrae; this relationship must be borne in mind during radiologic examination.

The spinal cord is divided into segments that are separated by imaginary lines drawn through the spinal cord in the transverse plane, midway between the points of origin of two adjacent nerve roots. There are 31 pairs of spinal nerves, the roots of which emerge from the vertebral canal at each intervertebral level from the occipitoatlantal to the sacrococcygeal articulation. There is a marked difference between the intradural course of the nerve roots at different levels. In the cervical region the roots pass out of the dural sac at almost right angles to the cord. In the thoracic region each successive root has a slightly greater inclination caudad from the transverse plane of its origin. The lumbar and sacral nerve roots descend in almost parallel bundles to form the cauda equina surrounding the centrally located filum terminale. The fifth lumbar nerve roots emerge from the vertebral canal six vertebrae caudad to the level of their origin from the spinal cord.

The special relations of the segments of the spinal cord and the spinal nerve roots to each other and to the vertebral column are portrayed in a clearly understandable composite diagram (Fig. 16.2). It is seen that the fourth cervical spinal cord segment lies approximately opposite the third cervical vertebra, and the twelfth thoracic spinal cord segment lies opposite the ninth thoracic vertebra, with the result that, between these levels, vertebral localization of lesions is approximately two segments higher than neurologic localization. The arrangement of the roots of the cauda equina is such that the nerve roots that originate

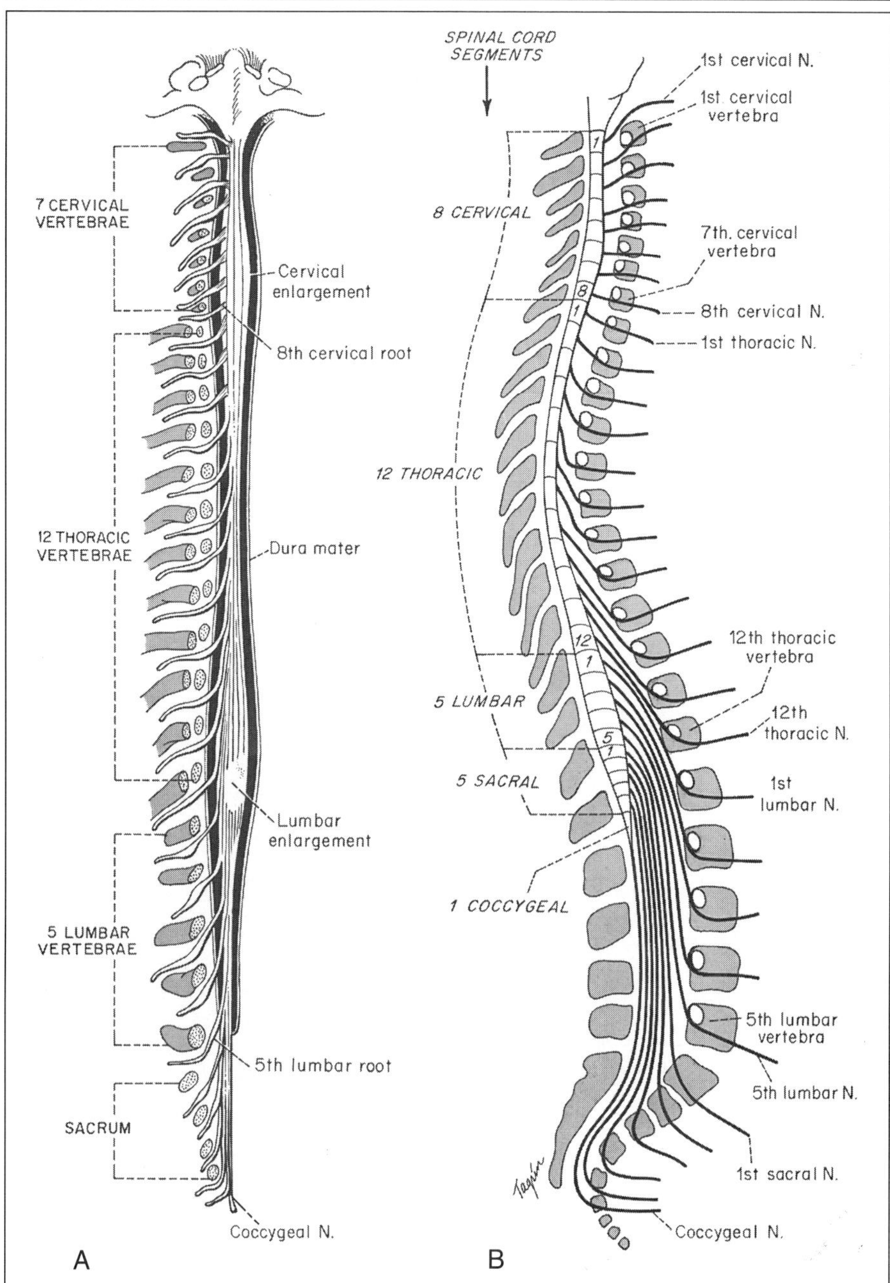

Figure 16.2. Relation of segments of spinal cord and nerve roots to vertebrae in frontal and lateral projection.

more cephalad from the spinal cord and exit higher from the dural sac occupy the outermost position in the bundle.

The vertebral canal is thus seen to be filled by four tubular compartments separated by the three meningeal layers. The outer and innermost sections are filled with soft tissue. The two intermediate compartments are formed by membranes that are not adherent to each other. The innermost of these two compartments is the subarachnoid space, which contains the CSF. The outer of these two compartments is the subdural space, which ordinarily is a potential space but can become enlarged by separating the two membranes with the formation of a subdural hygroma following spinal tap.

TECHNICAL CONSIDERATIONS

Plain-Film Examination

The careful study of plain roentgenograms of the spine is the first step for the proper evaluation of diseases of the spinal cord. Not only the bone and joint structures of the vertebral column are important from the neurologic standpoint but also the contour and caliber of the vertebral canal and the foramina of exit of the spinal nerve roots. An attempt should be made to correlate structural abnormalities with the patient's neurologic disturbances.

Examination of the cervical spine should include films in frontal, lateral, and each oblique projection. The frontal film may be made with the patient supine on the radiographic table, but the erect position is preferred to avoid having to place the patient in the recumbent position and then having him or her sit up for the remainder of the examination. A posteroanterior instead of an anteroposterior film may be preferable. With the patient in the upright position, not only is the appearance of the spine with weight bearing depicted, but the lower cervical segments are better visualized because the shoulders are lower. In the upright position, it is much easier to take the oblique projections, which can be made by rotating the patient in a swivel chair or stool.

In taking the oblique views, best results are obtained when the patient's body is rotated approximately 55 to 60°, and the head is turned to a true lateral position (Fig. 16.3). In a properly taken oblique view, therefore, the sella turcica is easily visible in a true lateral position. Additional special views may occasionally yield valuable information. Ordinarily, the upper cervical vertebrae cannot be satisfactorily visualized in the frontal projection because of superimposition of the facial bones. The atlas and axis can be satisfactorily visualized in films made through the open mouth, especially when the patient is edentulous. Films made in subaxial projection frequently depict the odontoid process to good advantage. Tomography in either coronal or sagittal plane is a satisfactory way of visualizing the upper cervical area.

Because of the inclination of the articular surfaces of the apophyseal joints, the latter are not visible in frontal films. Partial visualization of the joint spaces and of the shape of the articular pillars can be obtained in frontal films by angling the tube 30° caudad with the patient lying supine.

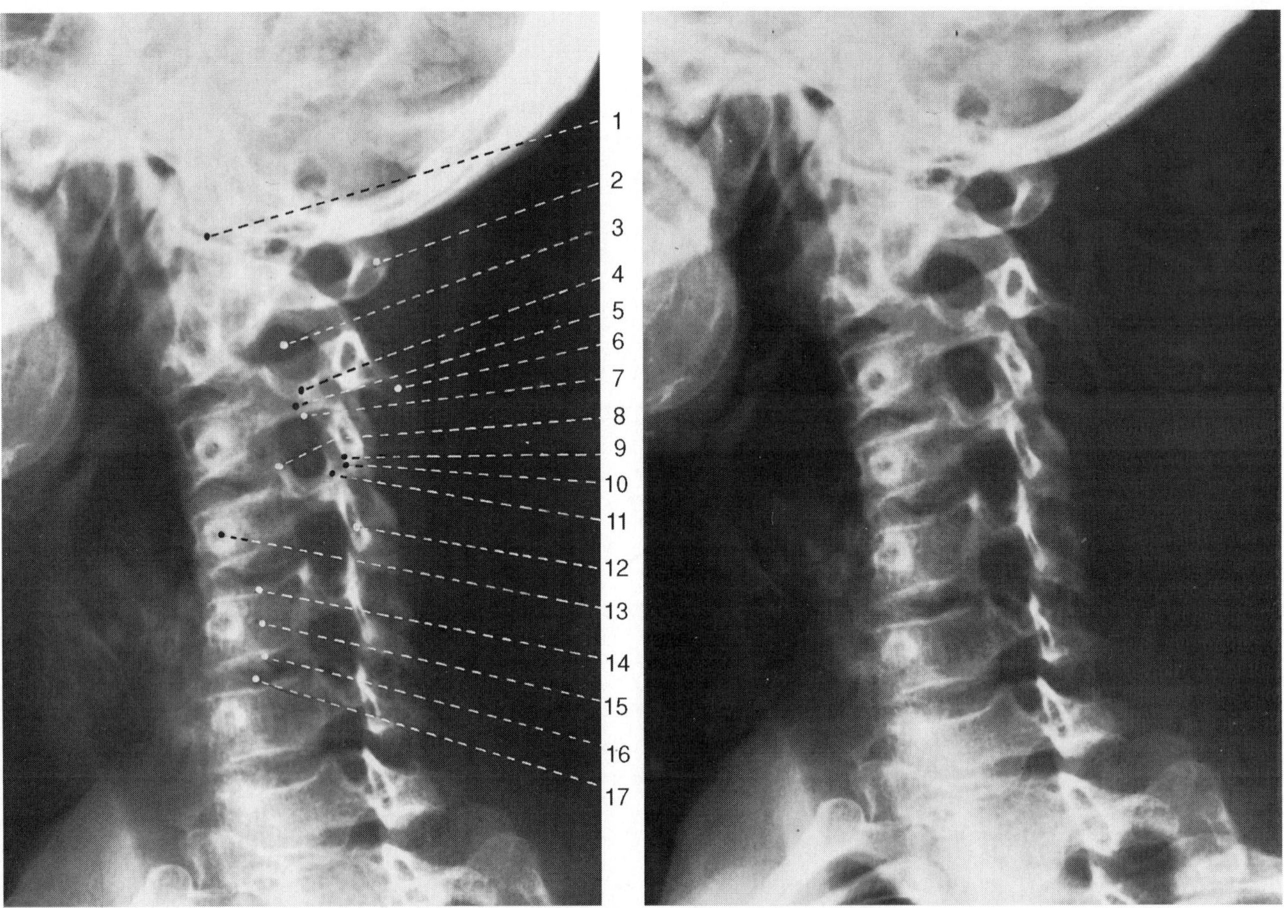

Figure 16.3. Oblique view of cervical spine. To obtain a good oblique view, the body is rotated (patient sitting) a little more than 45° and the head is rotated to a straight lateral position. The numbers indicate structures as follows: (1) atlantooccipital articulation; (2) posterior arch of atlas; (3) intervertebral (neural) foramen; (4) sulcus in transverse process for the third cervical nerve root; (5) pedicle; (6) spinous process; (7) inferior surface of pedicle; (8) uncovertebral joint, anterior margin of neural foramen; (9) inferior articular process; (10) apophyseal joint, the joint surface not well seen on oblique views, best seen in straight lateral; (11) superior articular surface; (12) homolateral lamina in cross section; (13) contralateral pedicle; (14) superior surface of vertebral body of C5; (15) vertebral body; (16) inferior surface of vertebral body of C5; and (17) C5-C6 intervertebral disc.

Slight asymmetry in the shape of the articular pillars between the right and left side may be observed in the absence of a compression fracture. Thus, care should be taken not to overread these asymmetries if they are slight.

Lateral films of the cervical spine with the neck in flexion and extension serve as an adjunct to examination of this area. Any time that it is desired to determine whether a reduction of the lordotic curve of the cervical spine is less than normal or has disappeared altogether, films in extension in the lateral projection should be obtained. Many subjects, particularly women with relatively long necks, will tend to reverse their normal curve when they are asked to assume the erect position for filming, and this may give a false impression. For this reason, it may be advisable, routinely, to instruct the technicians to take the film of the lateral cervical spine with the chin moderately elevated.

A special effort needs to be made to demonstrate the disc space between C7 and T1, particularly in cases of trauma, for subluxation or complete luxation occurs at this level. Lateral views may be made while applying traction to the arms if the examination is made in the supine position. *No examination of the cervical spine can be considered complete unless the C7-T1 disc space is demonstrated.*

Fractures of the lateral and posterior elements of the cervical vertebrae often are not demonstrated and cannot be seen even retrospectively on plain films. For this reason, tomography in frontal and lateral projection should be performed when the plain films are negative and fracture is suspected. It is often surprising to see several unsuspected fractures when the plain-film examination showed only one or none. In general, compression fractures of the vertebral bodies are easily shown by plain-film examination.

In *examining the thoracic spine*, single frontal and lateral films are usually sufficient. A film large enough to include all of the thoracic segments and, in addition, the lowermost cervical and uppermost lumbar vertebrae for orientation should be used. Usually the thoracic vertebrae can be properly identified in the lateral projection by the attached ribs. In heavyset individuals, a lead marker affixed to the skin of the back, lateral to the spine in the thoracic area, may be helpful in identifying thoracic segments in the lateral films by comparing the position of the marker in the frontal views. This should be done routinely when doing thoracic myelograms in which spot films are to be used. Stereoscopic films in frontal projection are of value when detailed examination of the component parts of certain vertebrae is desired. The highest thoracic vertebrae usually are not well visualized in the lateral view and, in selected cases, oblique films or tomograms in the sagittal plane may give the desired visualization of this area.

A routine *lumbosacral examination* includes films in frontal and lateral projection, and a film of the sacrum made with the x-ray beam angled 30° cephalad. Films in each posterior oblique projection are desirable to complete the examination. The routine views ordinarily are made with the patient recumbent on a horizontal x-ray table.

In selected cases, examination of the lumbosacral area under conditions of stress or weight bearing may be desirable. Thus, upright frontal films with lateral bending and upright lateral films in flexion and extension give a radiographic record of the continuity and extent of movement of the vertebrae. Bending films are usually made to test the postoperative status of a spinal fusion. Cinefluorography is a promising method of evaluating preoperative mobility, as well as stability following fusion. Frequently, films made with an extension cone centered over the lumbosacral junction are necessary for clear visualization of this usually very thick area. A true lateral view of the lumbosacral area may be obtained with the patient in prone position, using a horizontal x-ray beam and a grid cassette, when satisfactory lateral views cannot be obtained by other methods. This means of examination is frequently employed in all portions of the vertebral column in the event of spinal injury where it is desirable for the patient to remain in prone or supine position until the extent of vertebral deformity has been determined.

The examination should begin by counting the vertebrae to determine whether the usual number is shown. Supernumerary or infranumerary vertebrae are rare in the cervical region, although failure of segmentation in this region is a fairly frequent occurrence. An odd number of fully formed thoracic vertebrae with attached ribs is occasionally observed. Eleven thoracic vertebrae associated with six vertebrae of the lumbar type, with or without articulating transverse processes on the highest lumbar segment, is a common occurrence. Sacralization of L5 and lumbarization of S1 or a transitional vertebra is seen frequently at the lumbosacral junction. By sacralization it is usually meant that one or both transverse processes of L5 have become much thicker than normal and actually articulate with the sacrum. Bilateral sacralization is a stable condition, but unilateral sacralization is less stable. Lumbarization of the first sacral segment is present when a well-formed disc space is present between S1 and S2, or when one transverse process is similar to that of the lumbar vertebrae or both. Such variations are usually designated *transitional segments. Herniations of the intervertebral discs between the transitional segment and the sacrum are very rare or do not occur.* The author has never seen a case of herniation under these conditions at this level.

An indication of normal or abnormal mineral content of the vertebrae may be made from the apparent density of the vertebral bodies. The exact character of the various components of each vertebral segment should be determined, and especially the appearance of the pedicles of the vertebrae should be noted. A change in the normal oval contour of the pedicles in the interpediculate distances, as shown in frontal films, may indicate the presence of an expanding lesion within the vertebral canal. The upper limits of normal separation of the pedicles in frontal view were recorded by Elsberg and Dyke and are reproduced in Table 16.1 (1). The measurements can be applied to films made

Table 16.1.
Upper Limit of Normal Interpediculate Measurement of Each Vertebra in Millimeters

Usual upper limits (cm)	Cervical	Extreme upper limits (cm)
3.0	2	3.1
3.0	3	3.2
3.2	4	3.4
3.2	5	3.3
3.2	6	3.4
3.1	7	3.3
	Thoracic	
2.7	1	3.0
2.3	2	2.5
2.2	3	2.2
2.0	4	2.0
2.0	5	2.1
2.0	6	2.1
2.0	7	2.1
2.0	8	2.2
2.2	9	2.2
2.1	10	2.3
2.3	11	2.7
2.6	12	3.0
	Lumbar	
2.8	1	3.0
2.9	2	3.2
3.0	3	3.5
3.1	4	3.5
3.3	5	3.9

Source: Elsberg and Dyke: Bull Neuro/Inst New York 1934;34:359.

with the Potter-Bucky diaphragm and a target-film distance of 40 in. Occasionally, in individuals of large stature or where there is excessive magnification of the spine in the radiograph, the interpediculate measurements may be slightly above the upper limits of normal given. The object-film distance is increased by exaggeration of the ventral cervical and lumbar curves and reduction of the dorsal thoracic curve. An abrupt change from a normal to an abnormal measurement at successive vertebral levels, however, is of great significance. In certain areas of the spine, such as the upper lumbar region, *it is not uncommon to find flat pedicles in normal cases.* This usually involves the first and second lumbar, and sometimes the twelfth thoracic vertebrae and is more common in women. Sometimes the appearance is so exaggerated that it is difficult to be sure whether this is a normal variation, and in these cases it is necessary to look at the lateral projection. In normal cases, the lateral projection will reveal a normal appearance at the posterior margin of the vertebral bodies, whereas if the erosion of the pedicles is due to expansion of the intraspinal contents, the posterior margin of the vertebral bodies will be also excavated (Fig. 16.95).

The alignment of the vertebrae in both frontal and lateral projections is noteworthy. Altered alignment of the vertebrae may result from muscle spasm associated with spinal cord lesions as well as from structural deformities of the vertebrae and intervertebral discs. The articulations of the vertebral column consist of a series of slightly movable joints between the vertebral bodies and a series of mobile joints between the vertebral arches. *Normally the thickness of the intervertebral disc space gradually increases from C2-C3 to C6-C7 and from L1-L2 to L4-L5.* In the thoracic region, all of the intervertebral spaces are thin. The thickness of the intervertebral disc space at L5-S1 is subject to considerable normal variation and may be entirely absent with asymptomatic sacralization of L5.

The size of the intervertebral foramina can be observed in the oblique films of the cervical spine (Fig. 16.3) and in the lateral films of the thoracic and lumbar area. It should be determined whether the intervertebral foramen is narrowed by hypertrophic spurs, by collapse or herniation, or by enlargement of portions of the vertebral bodies and vertebral arches that form the boundaries of the foramina. Localized enlargement of one foramen denotes an expanding lesion in the canal. There is variation in the appearance of the intervertebral foramina in the cervical region. The C2-C3 intervertebral foramen is often larger than the lower foramina. The appearance of enlargement of a foramen, therefore, should be accompanied by a careful examination of the adjacent bony margins to determine whether erosion actually exists. In the oblique projections, the pedicles of the side against the film in the anteroposterior oblique views are seen on end, overlying the lateral aspect of the vertebral bodies, and usually are rounded in configuration. This results from the fact that the pedicles in the cervical vertebrae are directed posteriorly and laterally from the vertebral bodies at an angle of approximately 45°, and, therefore, when the patient is rotated as to take an oblique view, the corresponding pedicle would be seen on end. On the other hand, the pedicle on the opposite side will be seen in profile, forming the upper and lower margins of the intervertebral foramina that are situated immediately above and below each pedicle. Immediately lateral to the intervertebral foramina are the laminae, which in the oblique projection are seen on end, on the same side as the foramina. The lamina on the other side (the side against the film) is seen *en face* and overlies not only the vertebral bodies but also part of the intervertebral foramina and pedicles (Fig. 16.3). The lamina seen *en face* will be much more clearly distinguishable in stereoscopic oblique views.

Continuing with the oblique cervical spine view, the articular pillar is seen in an oblique projection, but the joint space between two articular pillars is usually not shown on the oblique views but on the lateral views. Unfortunately, in the lateral projection, the right and left joint spaces between two articular pillars (apophyseal joints) are either completely or partly superimposed and cannot be separated unless stereoscopic views are made. On an ordinary film in the lateral projection, the overlap of these joints can be avoided by rotating the patient into an off-lateral projection. If the direction of the rotation is known (i.e., the side away from the film is rotated either forward or backward), it is possible to determine which joint space is the right or the left without the need for steroscopic lateral views.

The soft tissue shadows adjacent to the spine should be carefully examined. Small paraspinal masses are best visualized in the thoracic region where convex lateral bulges are well delineated by air-containing lung. The shadow of a tortuous aorta may make it difficult for one to be certain of the presence of a paraspinal mass on the left side of the thoracic spine. Any lateral enlargement of the retropleural space on the right is almost surely indicative of a paraspinal mass. The prevertebral soft tissue shadow in the cervical region should always be carefully analyzed.

Computed Tomography and Magnetic Resonance Imaging

Spinal examination by CT has become nearly routine in any case in which there are local findings in the spinal column or focal neurologic findings pointing to an area of the spine. Most frequently specific findings point to either the cervical or the lumbar spine, more frequently the latter, but the thoracic region is also frequently examined. Plain films of the spine are usually performed first, but once this has been done the desire is to obtain information about the soft tissues, which can only be obtained by other methods. In addition to CT, MRI may be needed. In many cases, such as when the referring physician suspects intervertebral disc pathology, the plain-film examination is omitted in favor of CT or MRI. Whether this is wise is debatable from the medical point of view, but there is no question that it saves some time in patient evaluation and has a moderate economic benefit. As time goes on, we become more aware of the economic aspects of medicine, and we must frequently decide in a given situation which examination is likely to yield more valuable information in order to decide which one to perform first.

In a patient with a history suggestive of "radicular" compression, CT yields more information than MRI on the bones and joints in relation to osteoarthritic changes. It also demonstrates the intervertebral discs satisfactorily, particularly in the lumbar region. However, it does not demonstrate the spinal canal contents well. MRI shows the vertebral bodies best in sagittal or in frontal projection, but its main strength is demonstrating the soft tissues of the spinal canal, spinal cord, and roots, which cannot be seen well enough by CT unless one were to add contrast media for myelography. For that reason MRI is best to study the cervical region in order to visualize the spinal cord and roots as well as the intervertebral discs (Fig. 6.4). In the lumbar region CT yields considerable information about the bones and joints and about the presence or absence of a herniated disc. However, the soft tissues within the canal

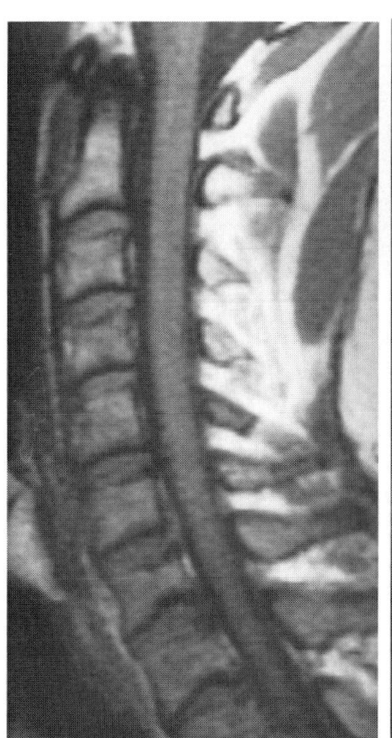

A

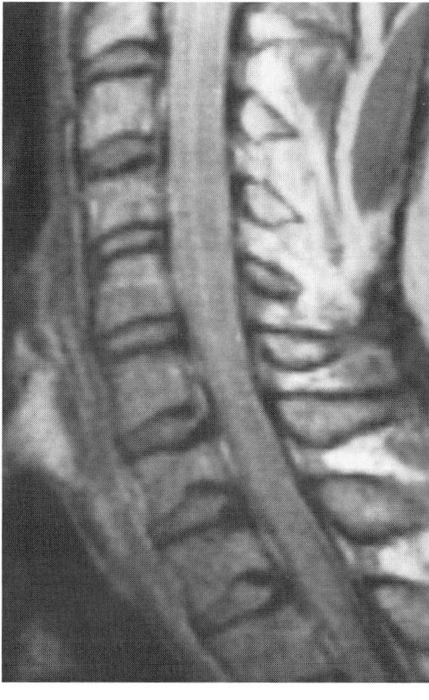

B

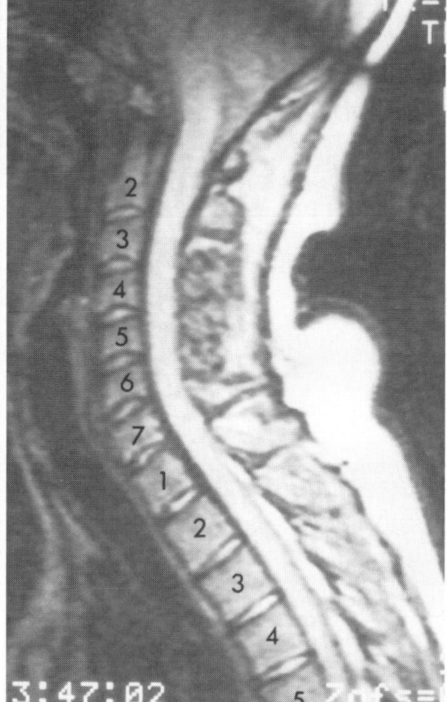

C

Figure 16.4. Normal cervical spine MRI. **A.** Sagittal T1-weighted image. **B.** Proton density image. The vertebral bodies of C7 and T1 show some flattening posteriorly, due to old injury. The intervertebral discs are normal. **C.** Lateral T2-weighted image on another patient. The intervertebral discs are normally bright on T2-weighted images and do not protrude dorsally in the normal patient. The low-intensity band anteriorly on the T2-weighted image represents the posterior longitudinal ligament and the vertebral venous plexus.

cannot be seen sufficiently well so that another type of lesion, such as a neoplasm, can be excluded. For that reason, if the patient requires surgery to relieve symptoms, surgeons worry about missing an intraspinal lesion and opt for an MRI examination. Undoubtedly, the combination of the two examinations yields sufficient information, in the great majority of cases, so that a decision can be made as to the appropriate therapy to follow. There are clinical situations, however, in which more information is needed based on the clinical history and neurologic findings; in such situations myelography may be necessary. This is often the case in patients with a history of prior spinal surgery.

In patients with a history suggesting a myelopathy, CT examination does not usually contribute much, and MRI is far superior. It shows not only the spinal cord but also the spine in long segments (which CT cannot do except with reformatted images). Also the possibility, routinely utilized, of obtaining T1- and T2-weighted sagittal images allows us to analyze the data with respect to the changing response of various types of lesions to the imaging sequences. The same can be done selectively in axial projec-

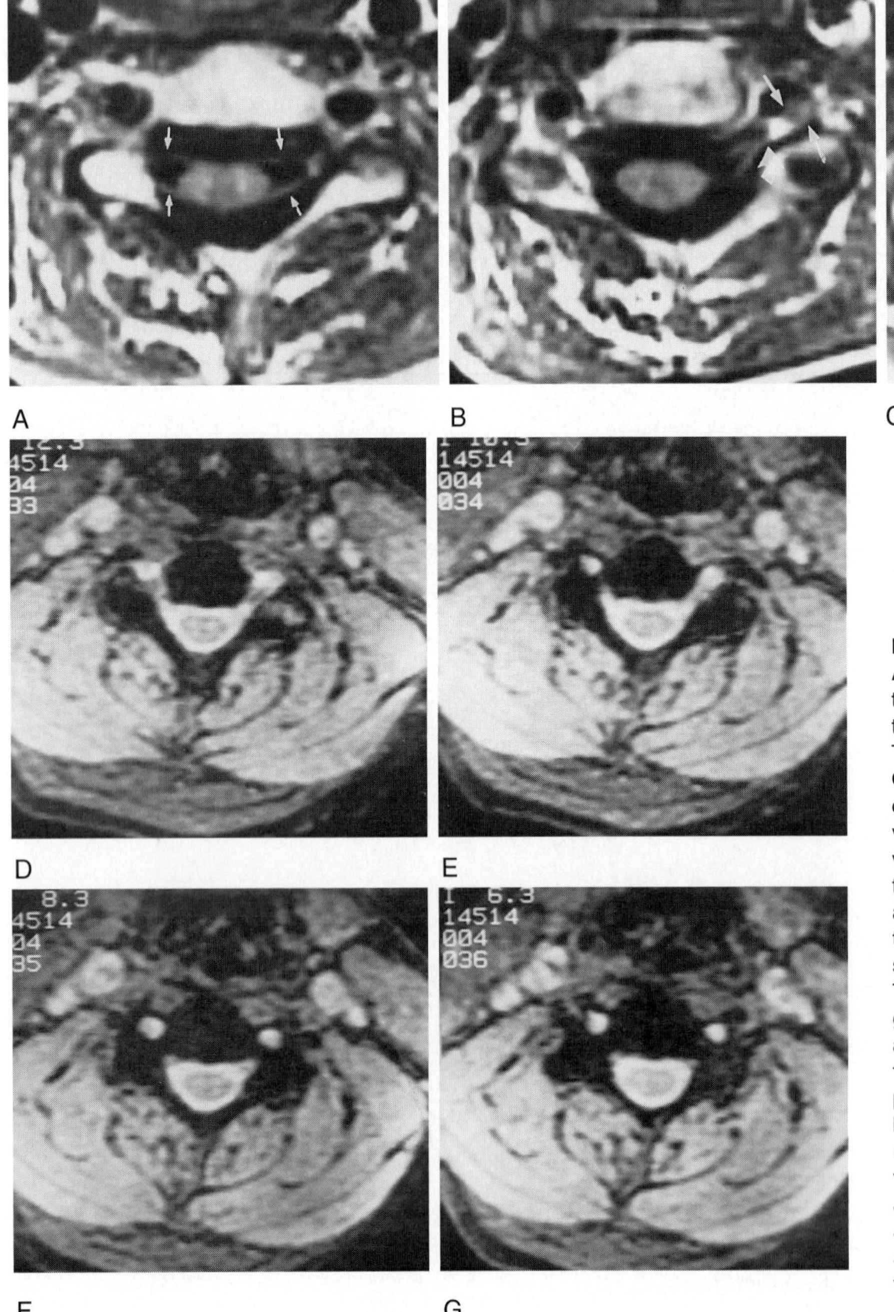

Figure 16.5. Axial MR images of cervical spine. **A.** T1-weighted axial MR images passing through upper body. The spinal cord and the anterior and posterior roots are well seen (arrows). The cut is just above the intervertebral foramina. On the right side the bright area next to the spinal canal is a segment of the articular pillar. The vertebral artery flow voids and accompanying veins are well seen anterior to the intervertebral foramina. **B.** A slice through midbody shows the anterior and posterior roots entering the intervertebral foramen as they approach each other. A small amount of epidural fat is present (arrows). The lower right arrow points at the dorsal root ganglion behind the ventral root (anterior arrow) and behind the vertebral artery (flow void partially covered by arrow). **C.** Slice lower than B passing through intervertebral disc. The two bright half-moon-shaped areas on each side represent the marrow containing articular lips of the vertebra below. The spin-echo T1-weighted axial images show the anatomy very well and are made when it is desired to visualize the spinal cord well; also after IV contrast administration. Compare with gradient-echo T2* thin axial images in **D** to **K**.

tions. On CT one can only analyze one factor, the absorption of the x-rays by the tissues. Contrast media add further information, but this is again much more valuable on MRI than on CT.

TECHNIQUE OF EXAMINATION FOR COMPUTED TOMOGRAPHY

Cervical Spine

With the patient supine, 3.0-mm slices are usually made. If the level of a lesion is known, 1.0- or 1.5-mm sections should be made for more detail. Also, reformatting of the latter images shows better detail, if needed. The orientation of the plane of section is preferably made parallel to the intervertebral disc axes. This limits reformatting but reveals the anatomy more clearly in axial projections.

In each image it is necessary to photograph the soft tissue window and the bone windows. This can be done in a number of ways: alternating soft tissue and bone; photographing 6 soft tissue followed by 6 bone windows in a 14 × 17 in film; or simply photographing one entire film of soft tissue and the following film (usually 12 images) all bone windows. The method selected may be the one that would save time.

Thoracic Spine

The patient is supine. For a survey examination 1-cm sections are used. If the approximate level of the probable pathology is known, 3-mm sections of that area are obtained. Reformatted sagittals or coronals can be made if needed. CT examinations of the thoracic spine are limited to visualizing bone problems such as metastases, trauma, or other pathology, provided the level is known. A patient with a myelopathic history should be examined by MRI because CT is likely to yield no information of value. Again, soft tissue and bone window settings should be recorded.

Lumbar Spine

This is the most frequent examination carried out because of the frequency of low back pain and sciatica as a symptom complex. It is our approach to take 3- or 5-mm sections from L2 to S1, aiming to be parallel to the corresponding intervertebral disc unless the referring physician requests a higher level. The slice thickness is usually 3- or 5-mm in a survey examination. Ten millimeters is not recommended because a herniated disc, the pathology most frequently investigated, may be overlooked if it happens to be small and falls between the centers of two adjacent slices.

The soft tissue and bone windows are important for visualizing the vertebral bodies, the posterior arches and apophyseal joints, the neural foramina, and the intervertebral discs. Sagittal and coronal reformatting can be used only for small areas, usually just above and below the intervertebral discs. If longer segments are desired, parallel slices of the entire lumbar spine would be necessary.

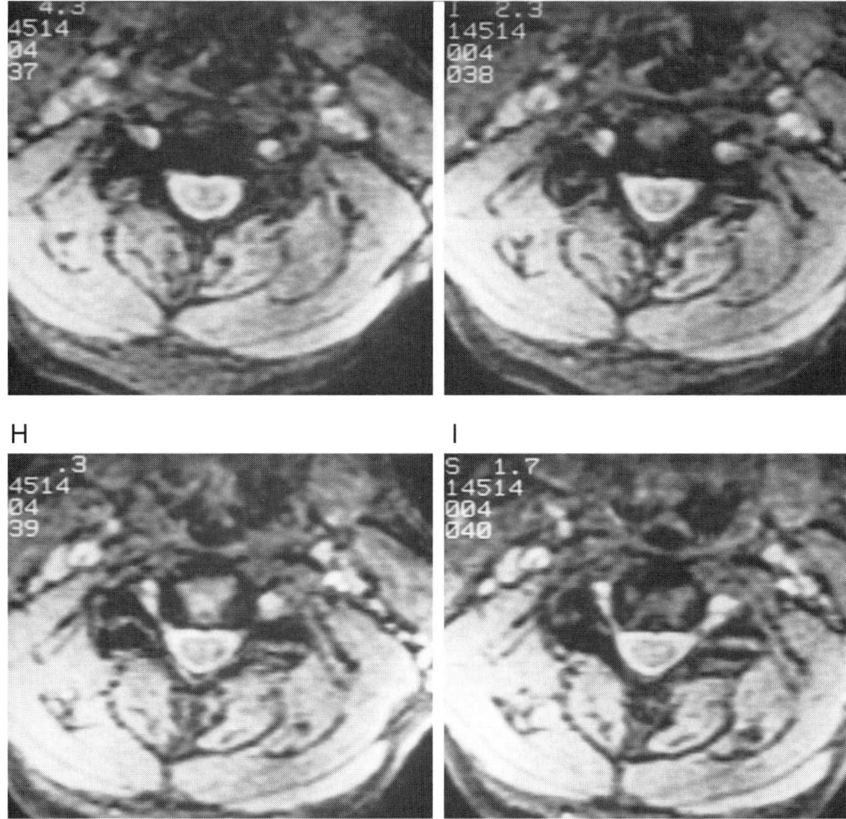

Figure 16.5. *(continued)* **D** to **K.** Gradient-echo axial images taken every 2.0 min. The CSF is white and the CSF accompanying the roots through the root canal is also bright. **D.** Both roots are emerging. The section passes through the vertebral body. The marrow in the body is dark. The disc is brighter when seen at **I, J,** and **K.** The presence of a hernia can easily be seen if one is present. Compression of the cord is easily visualized and can be readily compared with other levels.

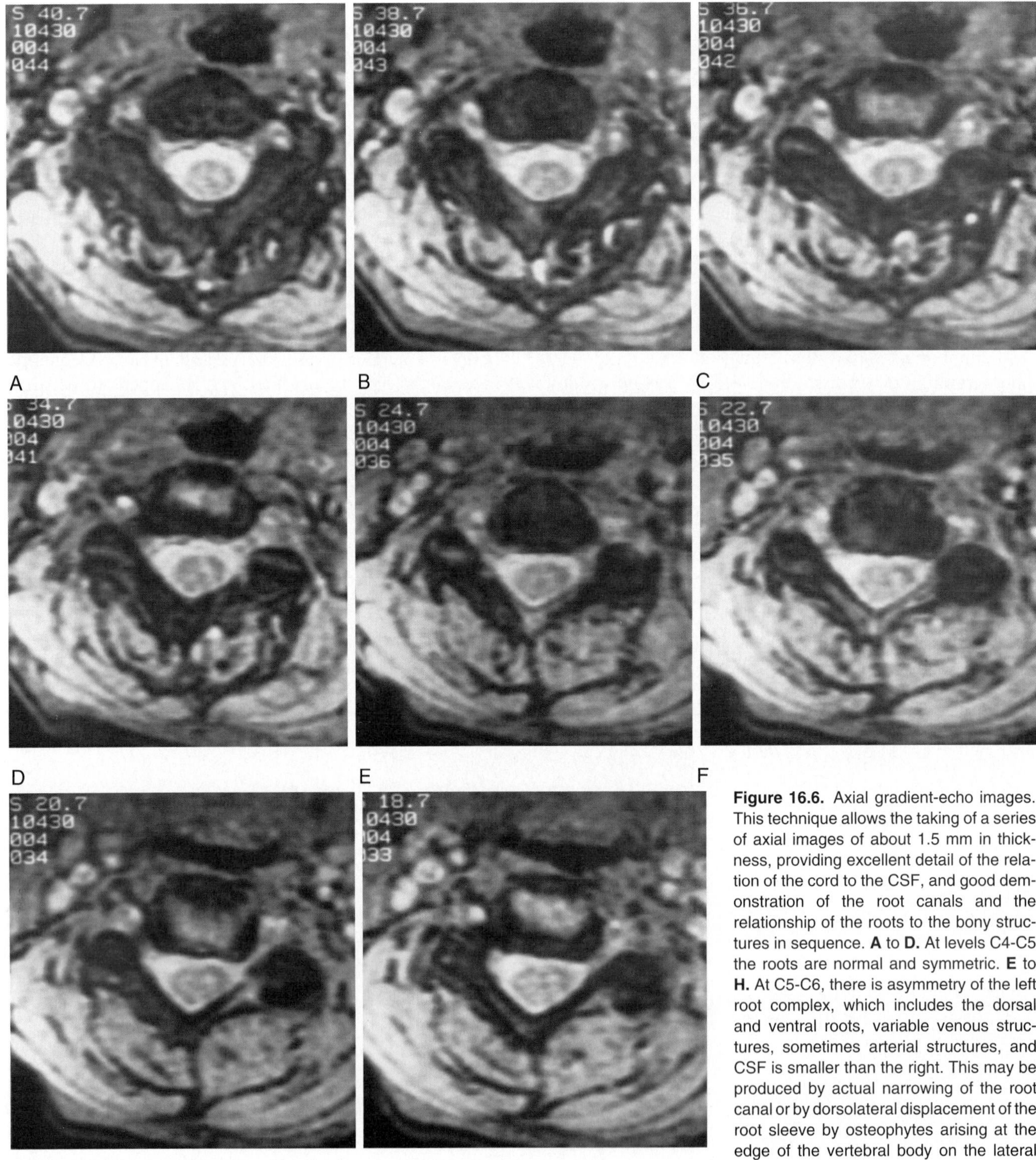

Figure 16.6. Axial gradient-echo images. This technique allows the taking of a series of axial images of about 1.5 mm in thickness, providing excellent detail of the relation of the cord to the CSF, and good demonstration of the root canals and the relationship of the roots to the bony structures in sequence. **A** to **D.** At levels C4-C5 the roots are normal and symmetric. **E** to **H.** At C5-C6, there is asymmetry of the left root complex, which includes the dorsal and ventral roots, variable venous structures, sometimes arterial structures, and CSF is smaller than the right. This may be produced by actual narrowing of the root canal or by dorsolateral displacement of the root sleeve by osteophytes arising at the edge of the vertebral body on the lateral corner at the joints of Luschka.

TECHNICAL EXAMINATION FOR MAGNETIC RESONANCE IMAGING

MRI is superior to CT examination in many respects, but the most important reason is that it shows the structures of the spinal canal in great detail and also the exiting roots through the intervertebral foramina in both sagittal and axial projections and, if desired, in the coronal projection.

Our technique in the cervical region consists of sagittal T1, proton density, and T2-weighted images (Fig. 16.4); and T2*-weighted gradient-echo 1.5- to 2.0-mm-thick axial slices, which yield excellent detail of the roots and the intervertebral discs of the entire cervical spine (Fig. 16.5*D* to *K*). These axial views do not yield reliable detail with respect to the spinal cord. If spinal cord detail is required, T1-weighted and spin-echo T2-weighted images are necessary (Figs. 16.5 and 16.6). Contrast enhancement is needed when one is looking for spinal cord disease (multiple sclerosis or neoplasm) and also in postoperative examinations.

In the *thoracic region* (Fig. 16.7) sagittal T1 and T2 images are made (Fig. 16.8), but the axials are usually T1-weighted and usually are localized to a selected area (Fig. 16.9). T2-weighted axial views are made if it is considered necessary, for instance, when looking for a demyelinating lesion that may show up more clearly on T2-weighted images. When searching for cord pathology, contrast should always be used.

In order to minimize the effect of cardiac and aortic pulsations, respiratory motions, and CSF pulsations, it is necessary to use certain technical variations such as cardiac gating, flow-compensation techniques, or gradient motion rephasing methods. Switching the phase- and frequency-encoding axes to orient the phase-encoding axis along the long axis of the spine reduces cardiac, respiratory, and swallowing, as well as CSF pulsation artifacts. This maneuver, however, increases the chemical shift artifacts along the posterior aspect of the vertebral bodies and disc margins.

The techniques in the *lumbar region* are similar. This is the most frequently performed MRI spine examination. It is our habit to use a spine surface coil covering the lumbar spine from T12-L1 to the first two sacral segments. It is important to see the conus medullaris in the sagittal T1-weighted images, which may require the use of a longer coil (24 cm).

Again, T1-weighted and first- and second-echo T2-weighted sagittal views are made, which yield excellent detail. The slice thickness is usually 5 mm with a gap of 1 mm (Fig. 16.10). More recently the fast spin-echo techniques have been used in order to increase throughput. They are somewhat less ideal than the standard spin-echo

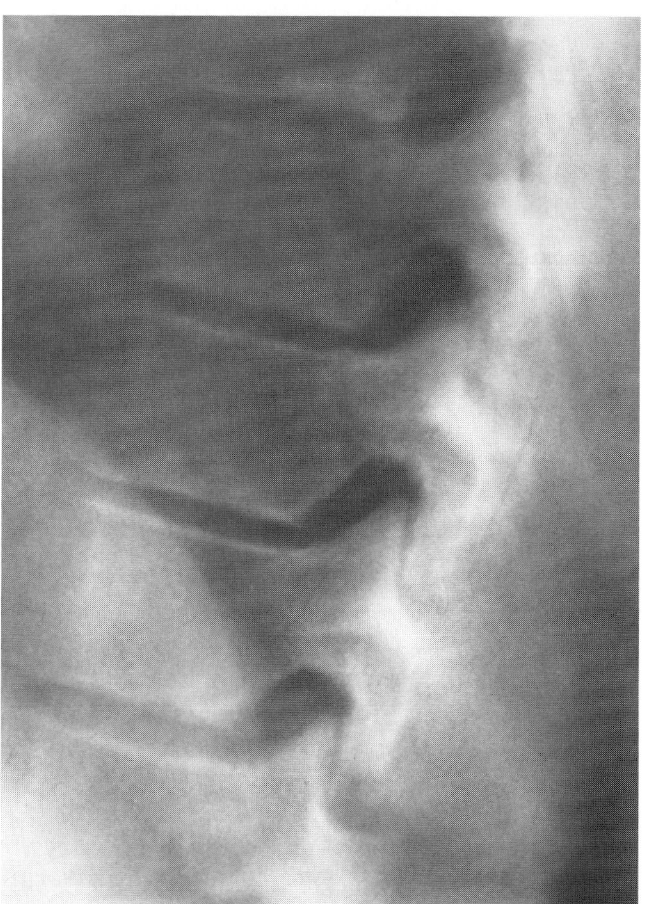

Figure 16.7. Sagittal tomogram of lower thoracic spine passing through the pedicles. In the thoracic region the pedicle takes off directly from the superior aspect of the vertebral body; the intervertebral foramen is straight lateral, and the joint surfaces of the superior and inferior articular facets are directed forward and backward, almost parallel to the frontal plane.

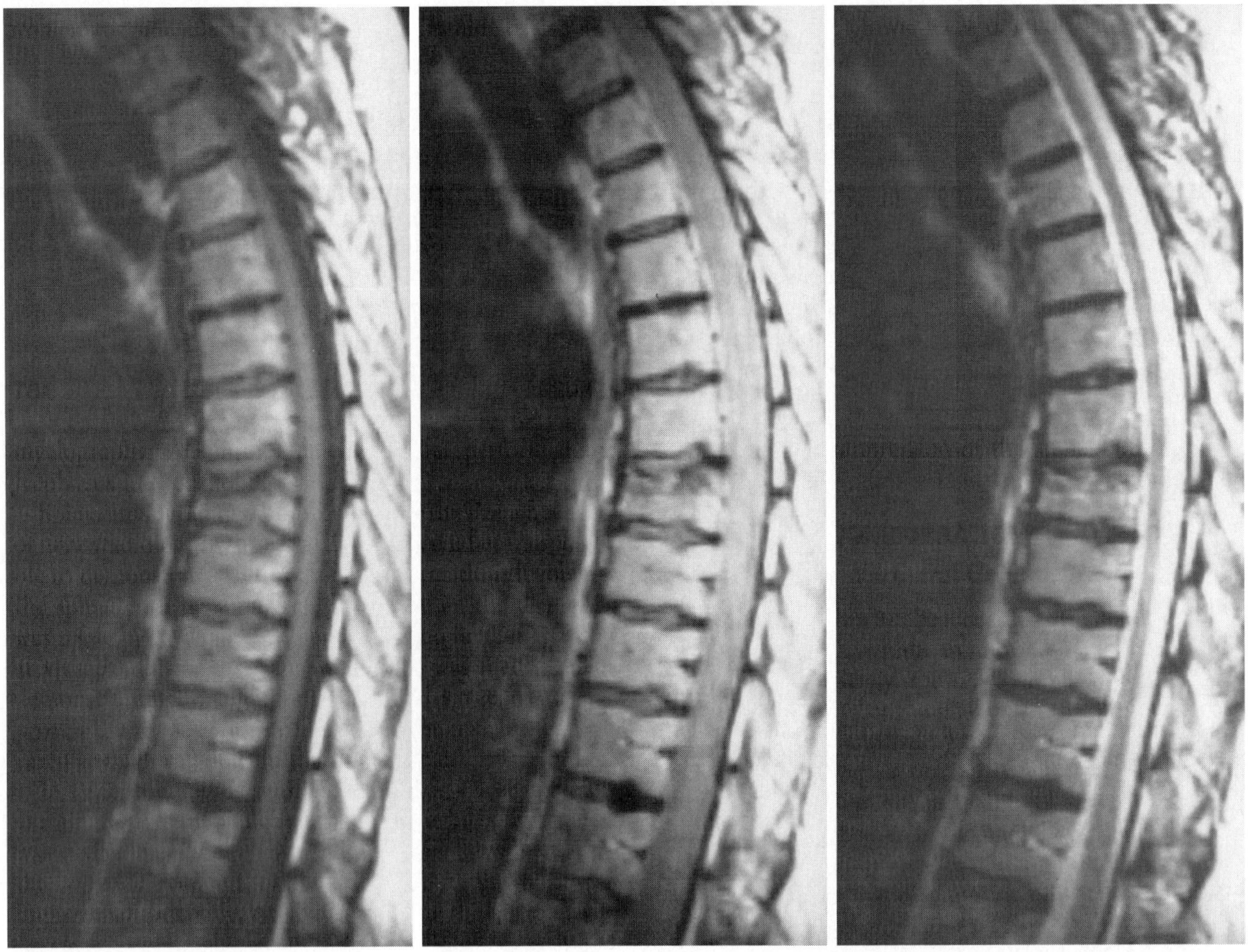

A B C

Figure 16.8. Sagittal MRI, thoracic spine. **A.** T1-weighted. The spinal cord always follows the shortest route and, thus, in the thoracic region, it is usually very close to the anterior margin of the canal. The CSF is dark. There is evidence of multiple Schmorl nodes involving the lower five thoracic vertebrae. The eighth vertebral body shows compression fracture. **B.** First-echo T2. The CSF is isodense with the spinal cord. **C.** T2-weighted. The CSF is bright; most of it is on the dorsal side of the spinal canal. Note that the spinal cord separates itself from the ventral surface and becomes closer to the dorsal surface as the kyphotic spinal curve reverses.

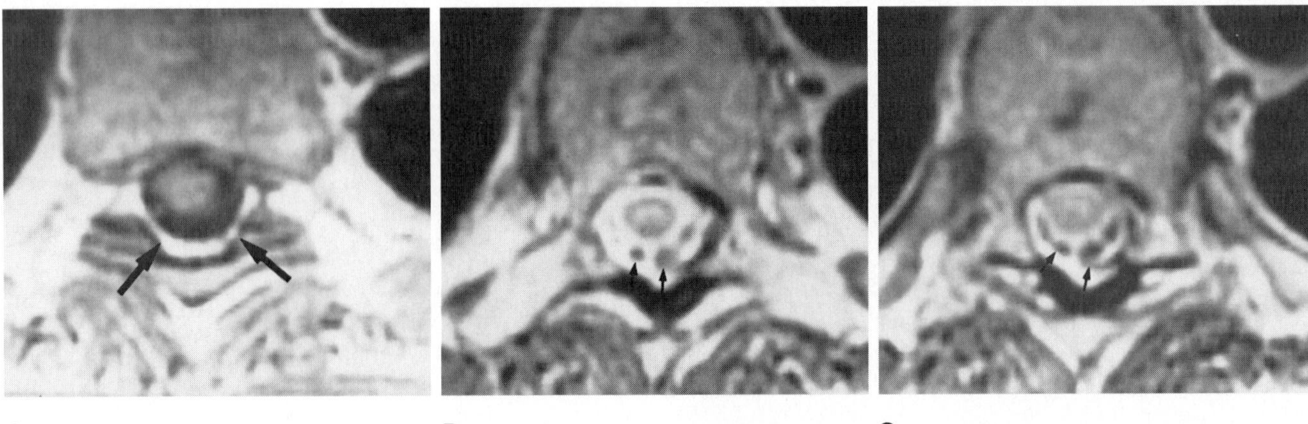

A B C

Figure 16.9. Axial T1- and T2-weighted images of thoracic spine demonstrating CSF flow artifacts on T2-weighted images. **A.** T1-weighted axials show a normal appearance. The slight off-center position of the spinal cord is probably caused by a minimal degree of scoliosis. The cord is isointense, the CSF is hypointense, and around the thecal sac there is fat, hyperintense on T1 (arrows). **B** and **C.** There are low-intensity spots on the dorsal side of the canal behind the cord, varying at adjacent levels thought to be due to CSF flow (arrows). These should not be confused with enlarged vessels such as may be seen on arteriovenous malformations of the cord. Same patient as in Figure 16.8.

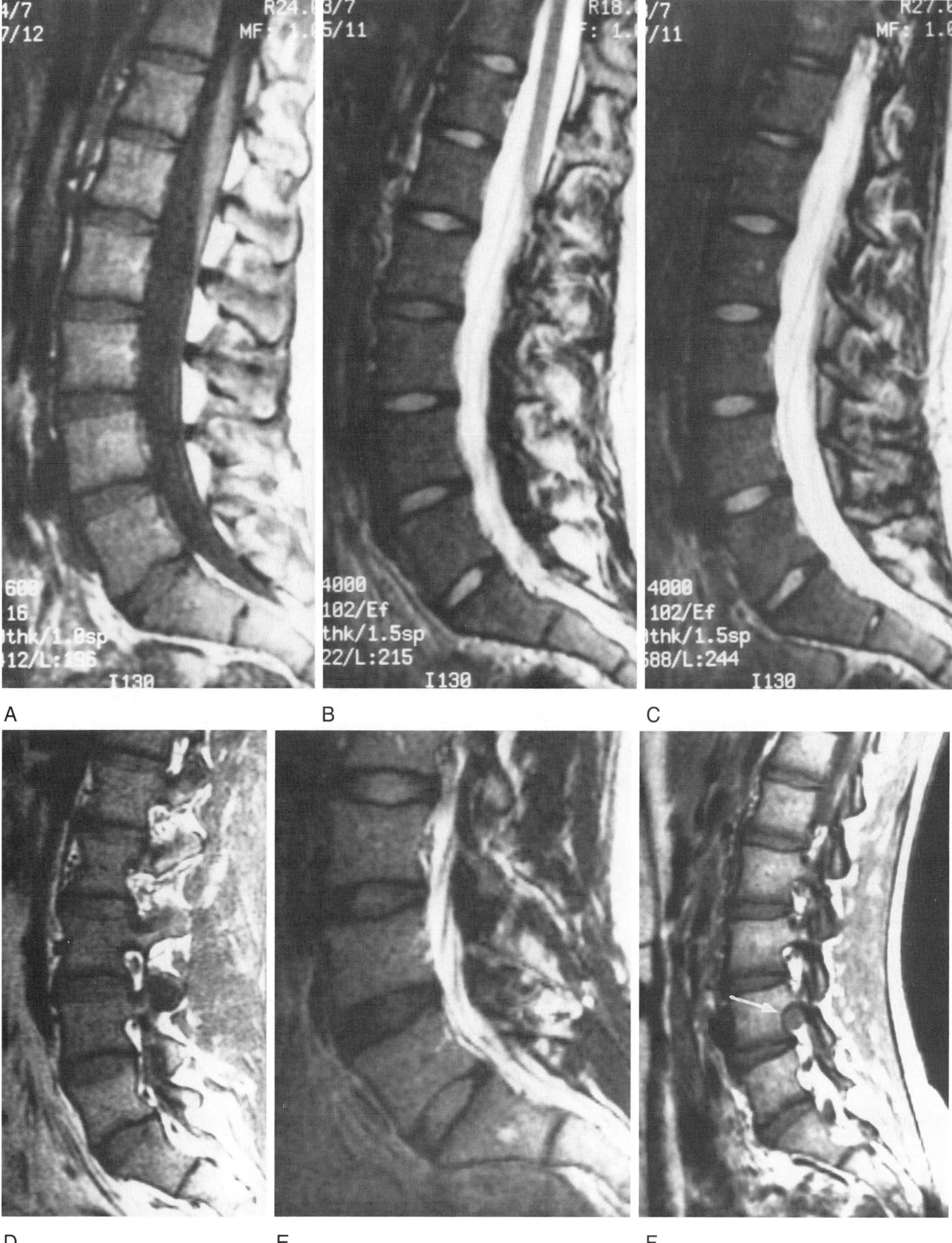

Figure 16.10. Normal sagittal lumbar spine images. **A.** T1-weighted image. The conus medullaris ends at L1; there is dorsal epidural fat at each level near the midline. The disc spaces are appropriate in width. **B.** T2-weighted image shows that the discs are all bright. The myelographic effect demonstrated on T2-weighted images is clearly seen. **C.** Slightly off the midline. Note that the dorsal fat is not bright. **D.** The intervertebral foramina are usually well imaged on T1-weighted sagittal images because in the lumbar region the foramina are directed straight laterally. They have the shape of a comma in most instances. The fat surrounds the root and the root ganglion, and there are epidural veins passing through the neural canal that communicate the inner venous epidural plexus with the external component. **E.** T2-weighted sagittal in another patient shows that the roots are located dorsally and move caudally and ventrally to approach the site where they will emerge. They also move laterally against the anterior lateral aspect of the thecal sac (neural canal recess) where they will emerge (see Fig. 16.11 and 16.13*A* to *D*.) **F.** Sagittal T1-weighted image in a case with a neurofibroma shows the enlarged root (arrow). There may be some enlargement of other roots as well in this patient with neurofibromatosis type I.

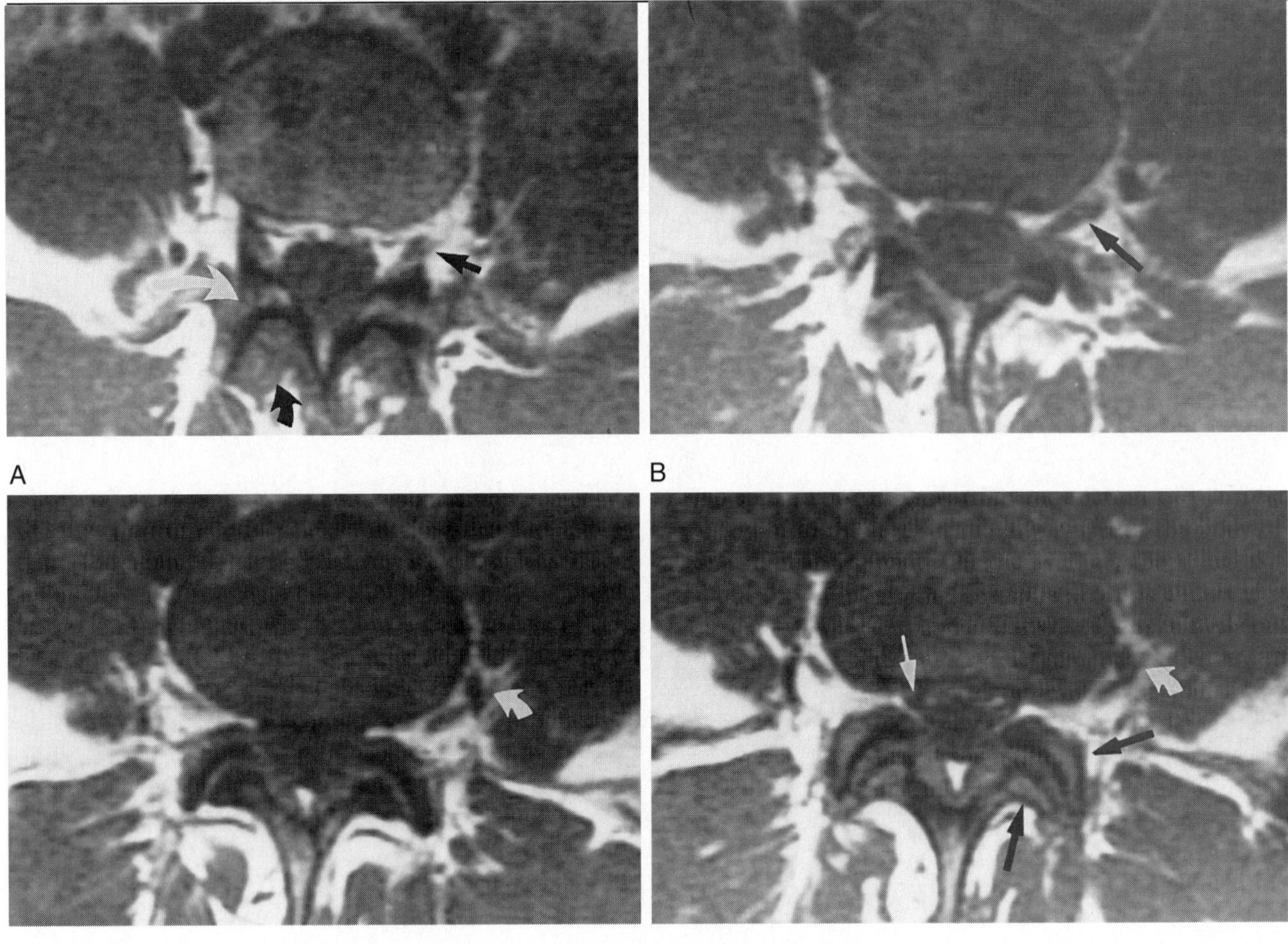

Figure 16.11. Normal T1-weighted lumbar axial views. **A.** Section passing through the lower aspect of the L4 vertebral body. The L4 root has separated itself from the thecal sac (arrow) and is at the neural canal recess. The apophyseal joint is seen: the superior articular facet of L4 is anterior (curved white arrow) and the inferior articular facet of L3 is posterior (curved black arrow). The apophyseal joint space is black because this is the bottom of the articulation. Only cortical bone is seen. **B.** Section 4 mm below A. The root is exiting under the pedicle in the intervertebral foramen (arrow). The thecal sac is normal in shape. **C.** Section 4 mm below B passing through the upper part of the L4-L5 intervertebral disc. The disc may be bulging slightly concentrically. The thecal sac is smaller at this level than it is at A or B. The apophyseal joint is well seen and because of the cephalad angulated plane of reconstruction it represents the L4-L5 apophyseal joint. The root is farther out, and the posterior root ganglion is partly seen (arrow). **D.** A section 4 mm below C, passing through inferior aspect of the L4-L5 intervertebral disc shows the inferior aspect of the L4 root laterally and the root ganglion (small curved arrow). The thecal sac is roughly triangular. The L4-L5 apophyseal joint is now seen completely: the two articular processes (superior L5 anteriorly and inferior L4 posteriorly, arrows). The joint space now shows the cartilage width, slightly bright between the compact bone of the joint surfaces. The next root to exit (fifth lumbar) is already at the anterior lateral corner of the thecal sac (anterior white arrow).

images but are helpful in obtaining images without motion because of the shorter exposure time.

The axial images are usually T1-weighted, and these are satisfactory in the majority of cases (Fig. 16.11), but sometimes T2-weighted images may be used, which may separate the CSF high intensity from that of ligaments that would normally be low intensity. In the last year we have been making T1 and second-echo T2 images in all lumbar spine MRI examinations.

Again, the axial views are oriented so that the plane of cut is parallel to the L2-L3, the L3-L4, the L4-L5, and the L5-S1 discs. It is our custom to take the upper vertebral levels down to L3-L4 with the slice parallel to the discs in one slice group, and the levels L4-L5 and L5-S1 together in a group (Fig. 16.12). This approach saves time. The thickness is usually 5 mm with a 1-mm interslice gap (Figs. 16.11 and 16.13).

Gadolinium enhancement is important in any case where cord pathology is suspected, although the T2-weighted im-

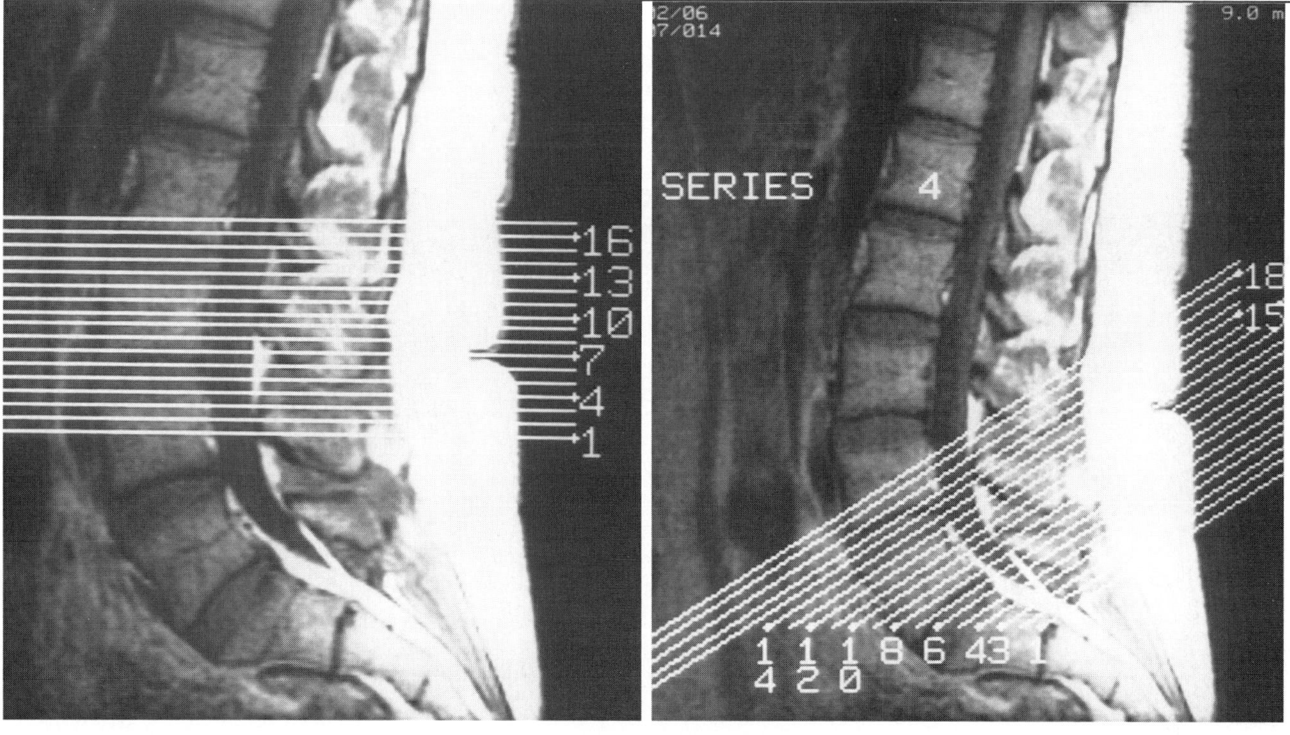

A B

Figure 16.12. Sagittal MR images to demonstrate the usual approach for orientation of angle of slices in axial projections. **A.** L1 to L3. **B.** L4 to S1. The slice may not be exactly parallel to some of the discs, but the continuity of the images to follow the roots from one slice to the next is advantageous.

ages will usually detect the pathology. However, the contrast enhancement will help characterize the lesion within the cord; that is, it will help separate an acute or subacute active lesion from an old lesion. Contrast enhancement is also important in examining the postoperative spine, particularly in the lumbar region. This is because epidural postoperative fibrosis enhances, whereas disc herniation does not. A small disc fragment can be surrounded by scar and somewhat obscured, so that thinner slices are required for visualization. See text following for further details.

Cervical Spine

As explained earlier, CT is satisfactory for showing the bones. In traumatic conditions of the cervical spine, for instance, CT will show fractures that may not be seen clearly on plain films even with tomography. It will show osteophytes from the vertebral bodies or the articular facets, which might only be presumed on MRI. If the patient presents with a myelopathic syndrome, CT alone is not very useful. If no MRI equipment is available or if MRI cannot be performed, a myelogram may complete the examination.

MRI shows the cervical spinal cord anatomy and the roots rather well (Figs. 16.4 to 16.6). For best results, the technique should employ technical refinements to minimize motion artifacts, which, in the cervical region, include swallowing, breathing, and arterial and CSF pulsations. The cervical intervertebral foramina are not directed laterally, as they are in the thoracic and lumbar regions. Rather, they point anterolaterally, as is shown in the oblique cervical spine view (Fig. 16.3). Therefore, the sagittal MRI view does not usually show the intervertebral foramina. The articular pillars are shown. However, the intervertebral foramina (also called the *neural canal* because it provides exit to the spinal nerve roots and has a certain dimension) are well seen in axial views. The sequence of axial slices in a cephalocaudal direction is pedicle-vertebral body, neural canal (foramen), vertebral body, disc (Fig. 16.14). In the neural canal or foramen the nerve root accompanied by a CSF-containing meningeal sleeve is seen. There are also some veins in the neural canal, as well as radicular arteries at certain levels.

As demonstrated in the diagrams in Figure 16.2, the exiting nerve root is the one corresponding to the lower of the two adjacent vertebrae forming the intervertebral or neural foramen down to T1. Thus, through the C5-C6 neural foramen exits the sixth nerve root; through the C6-C7 exits the seventh nerve root. Between the C7 and the T1 vertebrae exits the eighth cervical nerve root. At this point the arrangement changes, so that the first thoracic nerve root exits between T1 and T2; through the T12-L1 foramen exits the twelfth nerve root; between L4 and L5 exits the

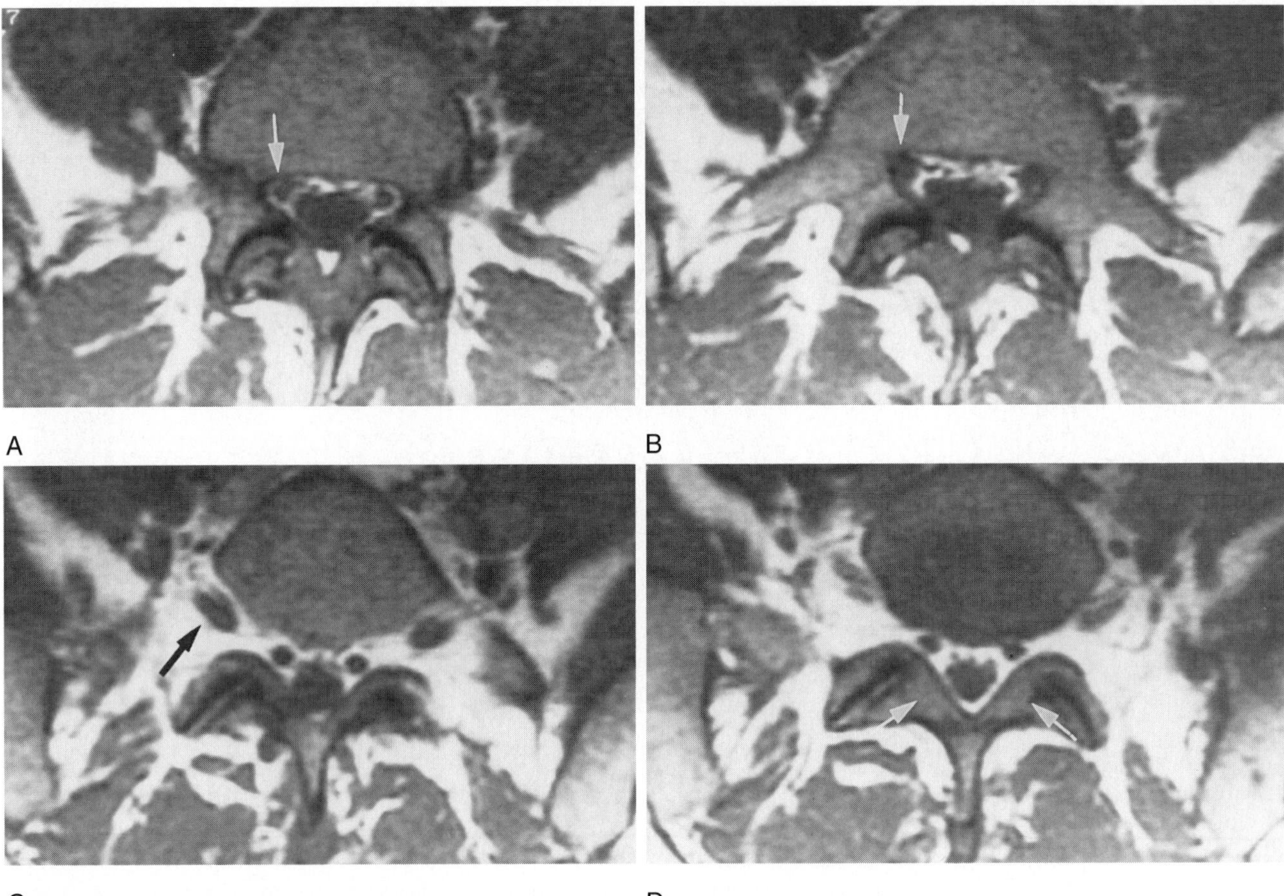

Figure 16.13. Normal T1-weighted axial views of lumbar region. **A.** Section 4 mm below that in Figure 16.11*D* passing just above the pedicles of L5. The L5 roots are still in the thecal sac and are in the process of emerging (arrow). Anterior to the thecal sac is a small amount of fat and flow voids related to flowing epidural veins. The triangular hyperintensity posterior to the sac marks the dorsal margin of the spinal canal or of the two ligamenta flava as they come together at this level. **B.** Section 4 mm below A is passing through the pedicles. The L5 roots are now separating from the thecal sac (arrow) and are in the lateral recess. **C.** Section passing through the lower part of L5. The L5 root has exited and the ganglion is in the foramen or canal (arrow). The S1 root has just separated from the thecal sac. The thecal sac is becoming smaller. The L5-S1 apophyseal joint is seen, and the cartilage is visible on the right. **D.** Section 4 mm below C shows the lower aspect of the root ganglion of the L5 root; the S1 root is slightly more separated from the thecal sac. The L5-S1 apophyseal joints are well seen, as well as the lamina of L5 (arrows). The thecal sac has a slightly triangular configuration, which is normal at this level. The posterior margin of the disc is seen bulging minimally between the two S1 roots.

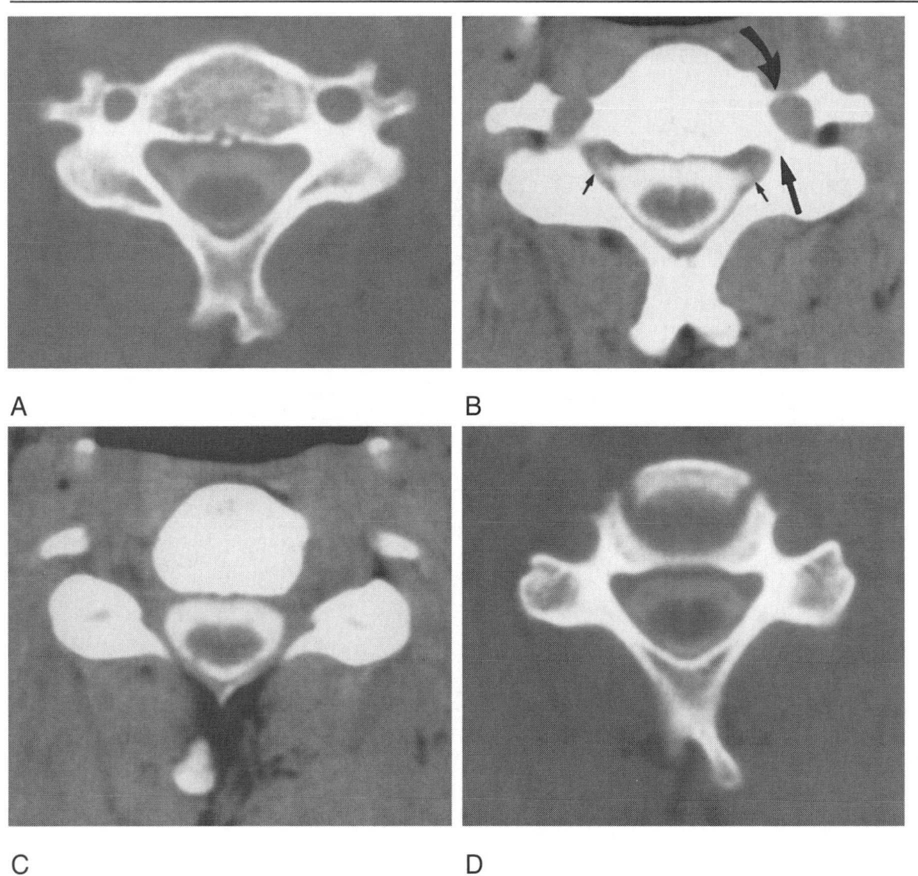

Figure 16.14. CT of cervical spine after myelography passing through the fourth cervical vertebra. **A.** Slice passing through vertebral upper body and pedicles of C4. **B.** Section 3 mm below A shows the C5 root sleeves on each side (small arrows). The section is through the lower aspect of the pedicles just above the intervertebral foramen or canal, midbody. Larger straight arrow, pedicle; curved arrow, foramen transversarium. **C.** Cut passing through neural canal, midbody. The root sleeves are actually just above this section because they exit just below the pedicle, in the cephalic aspect of the neural canal. This photograph was taken with a bone window, and the soft tissue is not as well shown as in B. **D.** The next section passes through the lower body and intervertebral disc. In the cervical spine the disc is less well defined because of the articular lips on each side of the vertebral body. These lips form the joints of Luschka with the vertebra above. For greater detail of the roots, 1- to 2-mm sections are needed. The anterior median sulcus of the spinal cord can usually be seen on CT-myelography; so can the roots, as they originate anteriorly and posteriorly from the spinal cord on each side.

fourth nerve root; and between L5-S1 vertebrae exits the L5 nerve root. The diagram and tomogram in Figure 16.15 are intended to show the relation of the pedicle attachment and the articular processes to the lumbar vertebral bodies and disc spaces, useful in the interpretation of axial images.

Myelography

Myelography with gases was speculated upon by Dandy in 1919 at the time of his description of the procedure for pneumoencephalography (2). Gas myelography, according to Bull, was probably first performed by Jacobaeus in Stockholm, Sweden, and was used fairly extensively in Scandinavia (3). It was also utilized, in combination with tomography, in many countries to investigate certain conditions and when there were considerations of allergies or sensitivities to contrast media. Today it has been totally eliminated, first by the introduction of water-soluble contrast media but particularly by the discovery of MRI.

Positive-contrast myelography utilizing iodized oil, first introduced by Sicard in 1922, was widely used all over the world, with the possible exception of Scandinavian countries, until 1944, when Pantopaque was introduced.

Pantopaque is a mixture of ethylesters of isomeric iodophenylundecyclic acids (4). It has a specific gravity of 1.26 at 20°C and contains 30.5 percent iodine. The radiopacity compared favorably with that of other contrast media and was quite adequate for demonstration of the spinal subarachnoid space, which is encased within the bones of the vertebral column.

Pantopaque (also Miodil) was widely used until the development of a safe water-soluble contrast media. In the United States and in many other countries it was customary to remove the Pantopaque following the myelographic examination. Occasionally the material could not be removed for technical reasons, and often a few drops of the contrast remained within the canal, but this was considered innocuous. The removal of the contrast was recommended because of the slight irritation that the iodized oily substance could produce and also because it remained as a foreign body within the spinal canal for a very long period of time. Pantopaque was absorbed about at the rate of 1 ml every 2 years. In most patients carrying any residual Pantopaque in the spinal canal, the contrast would remain mobile for years, but in some other patients portions would be fixed in the root sleeves in the lumbosacral region; in still other patients some droplets would be fixed in the subarachnoid space around the cauda equina. Presumably this is due to adhesions forming around the droplets of Pantopaque.

Starting in the late 1970s and up to the middle 1980s, Pantopaque myelography was essentially totally replaced by water-soluble contrast media, which had the advantages of not requiring removal and of slowly mixing with the

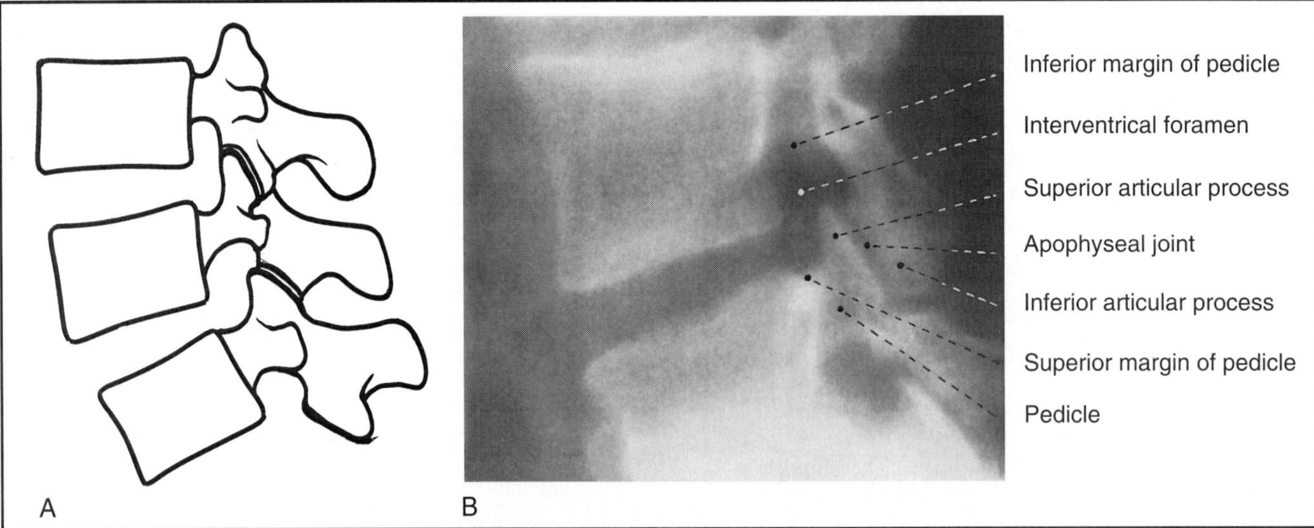

Figure 16.15. Lumbar spine. Diagram and sagittal tomogram to show the pedicles, the articular facets, and the superior and inferior articular processes. **A.** Diagram. **B.** Lateral tomogram. The pedicle in the lumbar region is attached slightly below the upper surface of the vertebral body.

CSF. In addition, the technique of myelography combined with CT was developed, and today this is commonly used in institutions where CT is available. At Massachusetts General Hospital, all myelograms are followed by a CT examination.

The first water-soluble contrast medium used was Abrodil in Sweden, but this was very irritating and required the use of spinal anesthesia (5). Following the development of the diatrizoate molecule for angiography, it was found to be toxic to the central nervous system and could not be injected intrathecally.

The iothalamate compound (Conray), developed later, was found to be nontoxic to the nervous system although poorly tolerated, attributed to its hyperosmolality. A dimer—two molecules of iothalamate bound with a bridge of adipic acid (iocarmate)—was tested because it reduces the hyperosmolar effect while maintaining adequate concentration. This reached the market after extensive testing, but was finally withdrawn.

In the early 1970s metrizamide, a nonionic compound, was tested and found superior to iocarmate. However, it was found to produce many side effects after intrathecal injection (headache, 50 percent; nausea and vomiting, 20 to 30 percent; behavior difficulties, 2 percent; epileptic seizures, 1 percent). While these side effects were considered severe at times, many investigators continued to use metrizamide because it was considered an improvement over Pantopaque, which required removal after the procedure.

Myelography, from its inception, has been a very important procedure in the diagnostic evaluation of a host of neurologic complaints related to the spinal cord and spinal nerves. When required, it had to be performed in order to decide on proper patient management. Perhaps the most problematic side effect in the early metrizamide trials was the behavior difficulties. Substances in the CSF tend to diffuse through the perivascular and intercellular spaces, and metrizamide or any other contrast dissolved in the CSF will do the same (6–8). The increase in density of the spinal cord a few to several hours after myelography can be measured with CT scanning; this is an indication of the penetration of the contrast into the substance of the spinal cord.

Later, new compounds representing variations or improvements on the metrizamide molecule have appeared (Amipaque, iopamidol, iohexol) with improved tolerance. The incidence of side effects is much lower (headaches, 15 to 20 percent; vomiting, 5 to 10 percent; no behavioral difficulties are usually observed) (9).

TECHNIQUE OF MYELOGRAPHY

With the patient prone on a tilting fluoroscopic table, a spinal puncture is performed under fluoroscopic control, usually at the L2-L3 level with a 22-gauge needle. The thin needle is strongly recommended in order to decrease the subsequent leakage of CSF through the needle hole into the subdural space, considered the principal cause of post–lumbar puncture headache. The fluoroscopic control is used in order to be sure that the needle is kept in the midline to avoid a faulty puncture. As the needle goes off to the side, the possibility of effecting an extra-arachnoidal injection is increased; the contrast goes into the subdural or the extradural space. In order to mark the interspinous space, a needle is placed transversely over the spine, and a film can be exposed in the posteroanterior projection (particularly if the fluoroscopic image is not clear enough), for, in general, the needle should go straight down the interspinous space in the midline. On occasions where there is calcification in the interspinous ligament, it may be necessary to use a lower level, or an off-lateral puncture can be made, inclining the needle just enough so that the tip reaches the midline at the thecal sac. Puncture at a high level is sometimes indicated, and occasionally an L1-L2 puncture is required, but this should be done with great caution because the tip of the conus medullaris usually ends at the caudal end of L1 and sometimes may be lower.

Once the needle is in place and CSF has been obtained (samples of CSF are usually obtained to measure cells and protein), the table is tilted upward to place the patient's head moderately higher than the feet. In this way when the contrast is injected, under fluoroscopic control, it can be seen to run caudally in the subarachnoid space. If it does not run freely, the injection should be stopped and a lateral prone film should be obtained to ascertain that the tip of the needle is in the correct position in the middle of the canal and that the injection is not being made in the subdural space. Sometimes the needle will push the arachnoid after piercing the dura and only half of the needle bevel is through, just enough to obtain CSF (which always runs slowly through a small-bore needle), giving the impression of being completely through the arachnoid. (Fig. 16.16). Under these circumstances, the injection would be made in the subdural space. If the injection is subdural, it will be held up in the dorsal side of the canal, and a lateral across-the-table view will demonstrate it. Also the contrast will not move freely, although it will move slowly.

Puncture between C1 and C2

This is performed when a lumbar puncture cannot be carried out or is contraindicated; also, some prefer to carry out a C1-C2 puncture for cervical myelography because a smaller amount of contrast is sufficient and the spot films made during fluoroscopy are superior. However, CT imaging to follow obviates the need for fluoroscopic spot filming and yields satisfactory images regardless of the amount of contrast present.

For myelography the C1-C2 puncture is carried out in the prone position, with the head straight and not overextended. The patient should be as comfortable as possible, and breathing should be checked carefully to avoid having the patient move at a crucial time later. The procedure should be carefully explained to the patient. Anteroposterior and lateral fluoroscopy are necessary, but if lateral fluoroscopy is not available lateral films made with the horizontal beam can be substituted. The level of the C1-C2 vertebral arch space should be indicated with a lead marker, in both the cephalocaudal and in the anteroposterior direction, and this should be recorded with films for greater accuracy. Prior to starting the puncture the hair may have to be shaved in a small area. A 20-gauge needle may be used, after adequate anesthesia, to be inserted and to extend horizontally, directed to the posterior aspect of the spinal canal. The needle stylet should be removed frequently as the thecal sac is being approached (checked fluoroscopically) in order to determine if CSF appears, at which time very little further insertion of the needle should be carried out.

The spinal cord falls forward in the prone position, and if the needle is directed posteriorly it will enter behind the posterior margin of the spinal cord. If there is any suspicion of the presence of an anomaly in the craniocervical junction, such as tonsillar ectopia, a high cervical spinal puncture should be avoided.

For lumbar myelography a dose of 10 ml of a 200 mg/ml of a nonionic compound is sufficient for the lumbar region. The filming procedure is carried out in frontal, oblique, and lateral projections. The oblique projections with the patient prone are done with the patient rotated about 30 to 45°, first in semierect position and later tilted as needed to visualize the L2-3 and L3-4 levels. Frontal and lateral projections are done to include all the interspaces from the first lumbar to the first sacral segment. It is our custom to always include the conus medullaris region in frontal views. When searching for a herniated intervertebral disc, semierect lateral as well as frontal and oblique views are useful because sometimes the deformity may become more obvious in the semierect or fully erect position (Fig. 16.16). The anatomy in myelography is illustrated in a normal myelogram in Figures 16.17 and 16.18.

The examination at our institution is always followed by CT carried out within 1 or 2 h. Immediately prior to CT, the patient is asked to turn around to the side, prone, and to the other side in order to mix the contrast with the CSF, particularly if he or she has been lying supine for some time prior to the CT examination. The levels to be examined are determined by the patient's history and physical examination as well as by the fluoroscopic data. The T12-L1 area is also included to visualize the conus medullaris.

Following the complete procedure, the patient is sent to a rest area or to his or her room and advised to remain in a position with the head elevated in order to decrease the amount of contrast that enters the head.

For *cervical myelography* the contrast injection may be made in the cervical region via a C1-C2 puncture. This would allow for the performance of the procedure utilizing a smaller amount of contrast while obtaining excellent contrast with very little manipulation. However, it has been our practice to perform the injection in the lumbar region using a maximum dose of 10 ml of a 300 mg/ml solution. The patient, in the prone position, is tilted head down (after securing to prevent the patient from sliding) somewhat slowly in order to keep the contrast together. With the patient's head well extended and straight, and with a small, thick pillow under the chin, the contrast will not enter the head. Once the contrast has accumulated in the upper cervical region, the table is brought back to a horizontal position; the head, maintained straight, is placed in the most advantageous position for filming under fluoroscopic control. Decreasing the extension diminishes the overlap of the occiput over the upper spine. Frontal and lateral views are most important and should include the

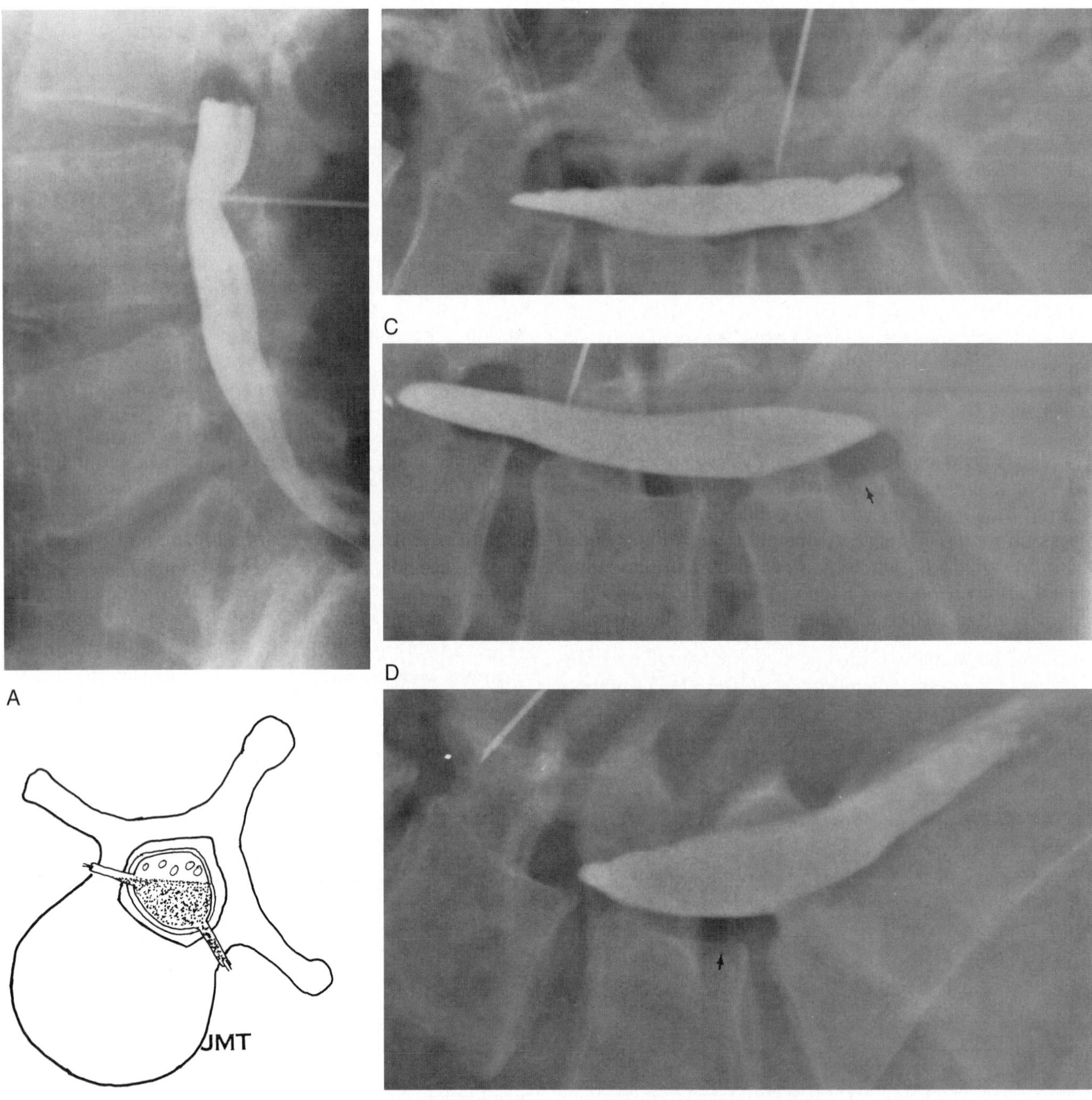

Figure 16.16. Lumbar myelography. **A.** Lateral, nearly erect view to demonstrate how the needle pushes the arachnoid membrane. In this case the injection seems to have entered the subarachnoid space, but part of it could have entered the subdural space. **B.** Diagram to illustrate better-filled dependent root in oblique position. When the patient is in the horizontal position or with the head above the horizontal but not in erect position, there may be incomplete filling of the subarachnoid space and a fluid level will be present separating the Pantopaque from the CSF. However, this fluid level is not seen because the fluoroscopic beam is directed across the fluid level. The lower root, which is covered by the main column of contrast, is completely filled, but the one on the lifted side is only partially filled. It should also be noted that the degree of rotation is important. In the illustration, the body is rotated about 30°. If the rotation were 45° or greater, the root sleeve would not be seen at all with this amount of contrast. The best way to assure complete filling is the erect position, which requires larger amounts of contrast material. **C** to **E.** Normal lumbar myelogram, variation of the epidural space. **C.** This patient has almost no epidural space. The venous plexus must be very small or collapsed. **D.** There is an epidural space, which increases behind L5 (arrow). **E.** Same patient as D, semierect postion. The epidural space behind L5 is smaller. When the epidural space is wide, the myelogram is insensitive for disc pathology, as shown in F and G. **F.** Another patient, large epidural space in horizontal position. **G.** In semierect position the epidural space is compressed and reveals a protruding disc at L4-L5. **H.** Lateral view in another patient to demonstrate a short cul-de-sac ending at the top of the sacrum. Note that the epidural space increases caudally in these cases, making the myelogram extremely insensitive to epidural pathology. **I** to **K.** Another patient. **I.** There is significant protrusion of the L4-L5 and particularly the L5-S1 discs. Film made in neutral position. **J.** Film made in hyperextended position reveals some exaggeration of the defects at L4-L5 and L5-S1; there is more bulging at L3-L4. **K.** In flexion the defects disappear.

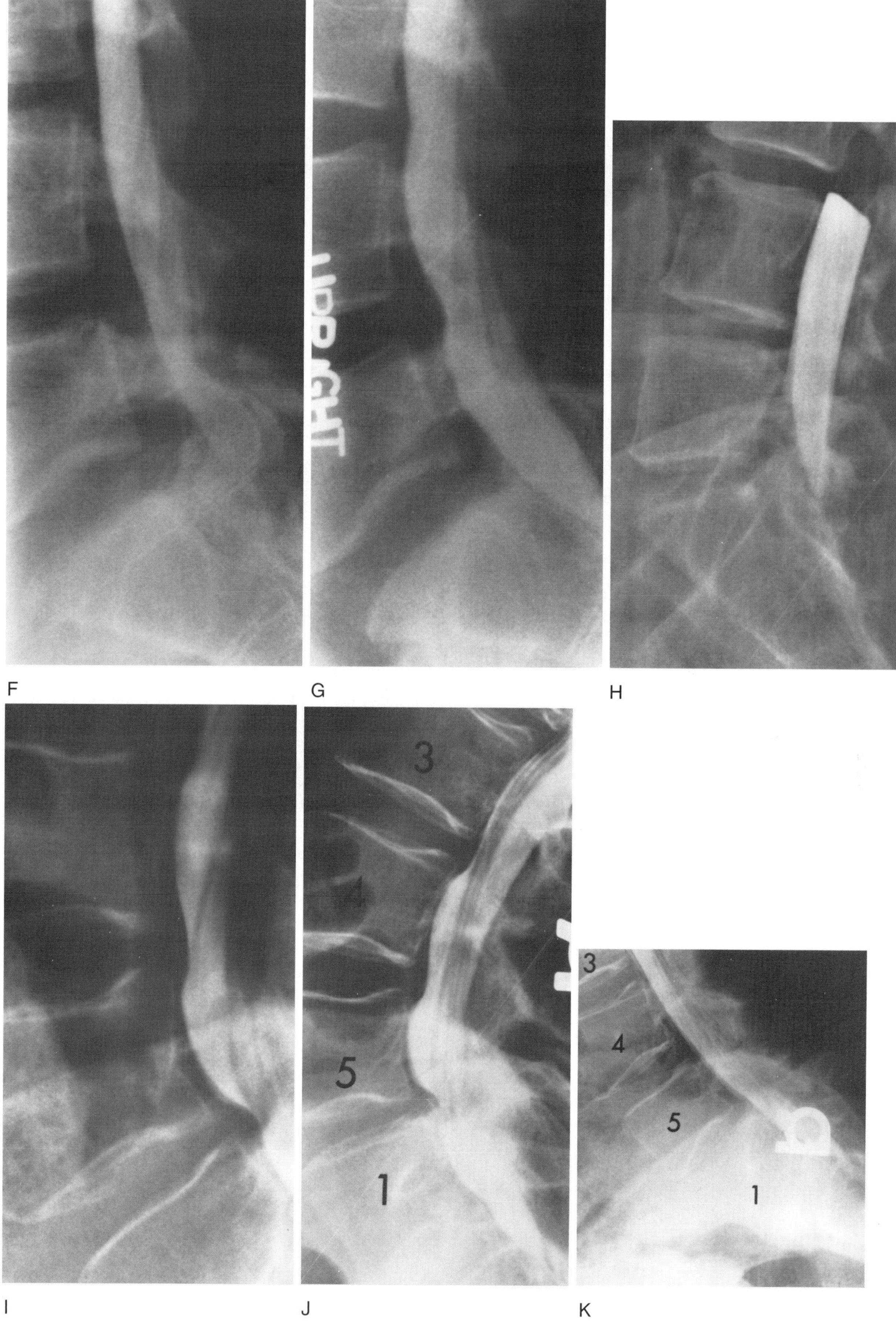
F
G
H
3
4
5
1
I
J
3
4
5
1
K

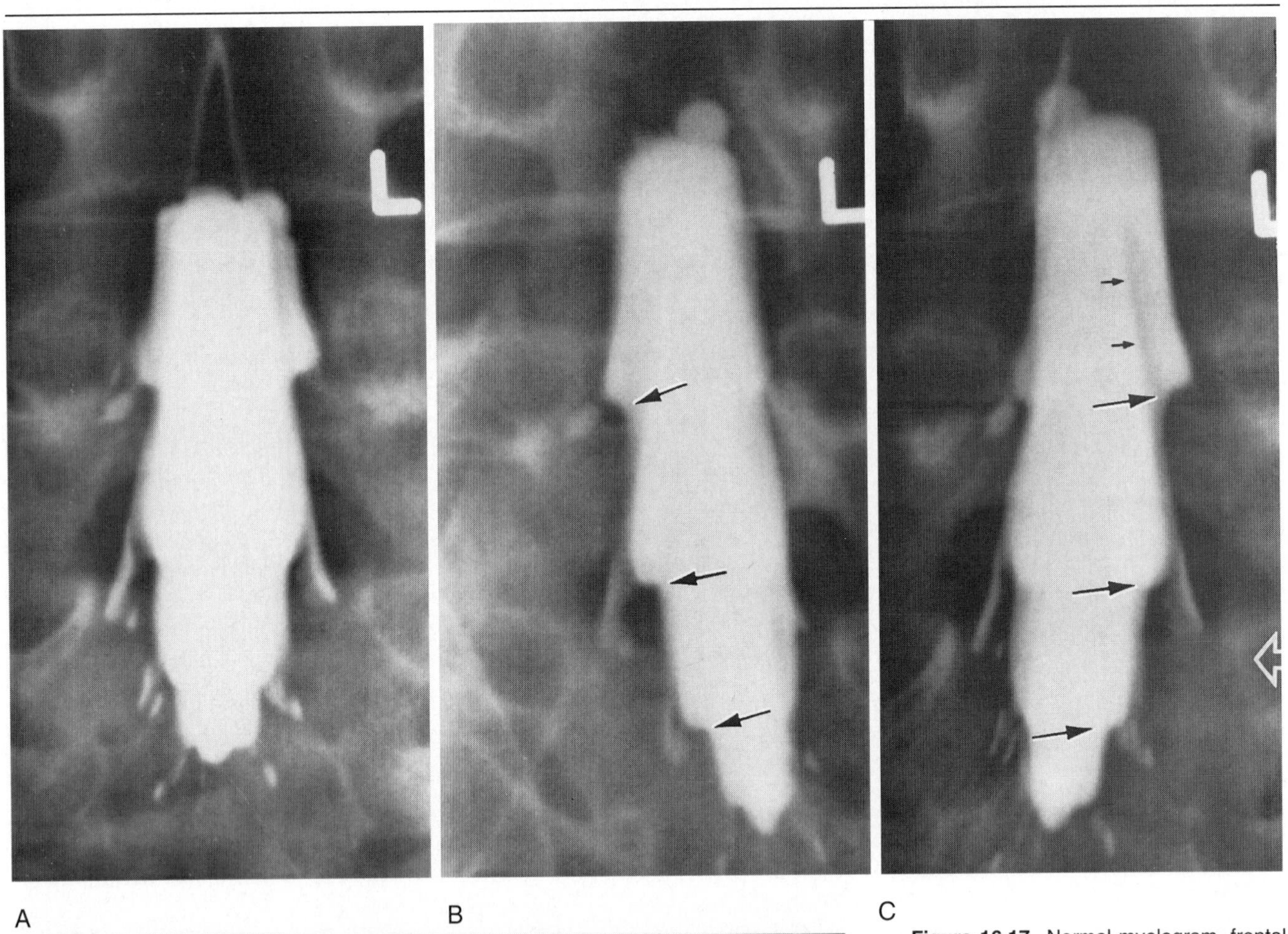

A B C

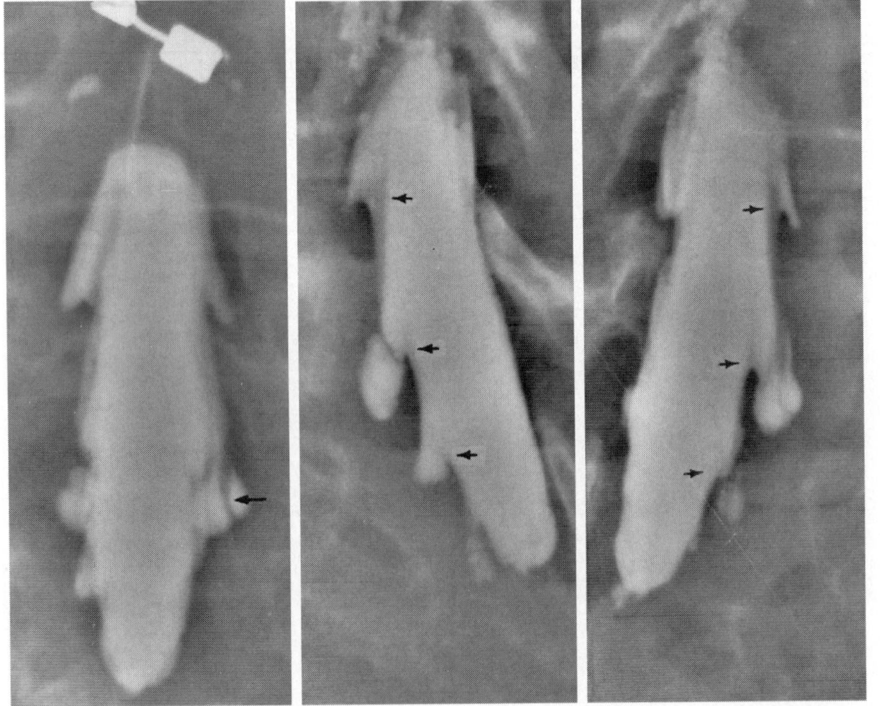

D E F

Figure 16.17. Normal myelogram, frontal and oblique views. **A.** The axillary pouches are usually fairly symmetric but often are not entirely symmetric in the frontal projection in normal cases. Whether these asymmetries are regarded as abnormal depends on factors, including the appearance in the oblique projections, and the distance from the column to the medial margins of the pedicles. **B** and **C.** The axillary branches of the nerve roots are visible in profile in oblique myelograms. If the patient is semi- or fully erect, the entire root sleeve is filled. If the film must be made recumbent, the root pouch in profile may not be filled (see Fig. 16.16*B* for explanation). The distance between two adjacent axillas (arrows) is almost exactly symmetric (with 1-mm allowable variation) when the right and left side are compared. **D** to **F.** Frontal and oblique views of another patient. In the frontal view apparent asymmetry is noted, which in the oblique projections is due to large root sleeves. The roots are surprisingly thin within the root pouch (arrow in **D**).

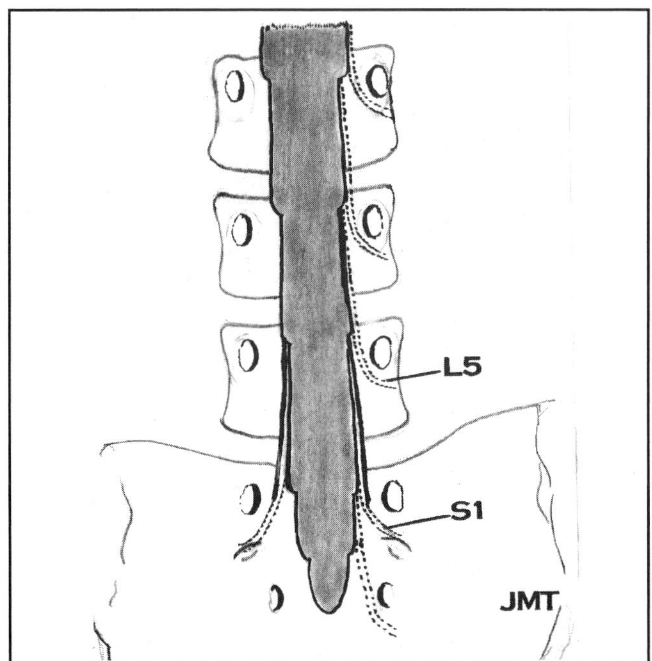

Figure 16.18. Normal lumbar myelography. The diagram indicates the appearance in frontal projection. The axillary pouch is the point of exit of the root that will run parallel to the thecal sac to emerge from the canal below the pedicle of the vertebra below. That is, the axillary pouch of the left fifth root is just above the pedicle of L4. A little contrast will run with the root for a variable distance, parallel to the thecal sac, and sometimes may be seen curving under the pedicle. The left S1 root on the oblique image of Figure 16.17*C* is seen as a radiolucent band through the contrast column as it descends approaching the lateral side of the thecal sac (two small arrows). It runs parallel to the sac with a small amount of contrast, and finally separates itself from the sac and runs down, still surrounded by contrast, to pass under the S1 pedicle (white open arrow).

lower, middle, and upper portions of the cervical spine. Oblique views are also useful and need only a slight lifting of each side for best results. Again, this is followed by CT scanning, which is a very useful addition. In institutions where MRI is available, myelography is not usually performed in search of a neoplasm or syringohydromyelia. If MRI is not available, however, CT will complement the filming sequence after determining the level to be scanned. In searching for syringomyelia, both a delayed scan and early scanning are recommended, up to 8 or even 12 h later (10).

To examine the thoracic region, CT is indispensable, and filming is often unsatisfactory. Fluoroscopic filming is employed, however, to determine the probably abnormal level to reduce the length of the area where detailed CT imaging is required. The contrast accumulates in the dorsal aspect of the canal with the patient supine, which facilitates the CT imaging procedure.

The use of an anticonvulsant prior to myelography is advisable, particularly if a higher dose is being given for cervical spine studies, and also if the patient has a history of seizures. The appearance of subdural contrast injection on CT was described by Dake et al. (11). Essentially, the contrast is outside the thecal sac. Partial extra-arachnoidal injection is more difficult to interpret; generally the thecal sac is not round, and there is a large space between the sac and the osseous canal.

DISCOGRAPHY

Radiography of the nucleus pulposus following its opacification with contrast substances has been advocated by Lindblom and has been practiced with enthusiasm in many localities (12). The procedure is used chiefly to study the lower lumbar region.

A preliminary lateral film of the lumbosacral spine is made with a metal marker attached to the midline of the lower back so that an accurate measurement of the distance from the skin to the center of the intervertebral disc in the midsagittal plane can be determined. Two needles of suitable length and caliber, usually an 18-gauge needle and a 26-gauge needle, are selected, and it is made certain that the smaller needle can pass through the lumen of the larger needle without difficulty. The inner needle must be at least 2 cm longer than the outer needle so that it can pass beyond the tip of the outer needle. Ordinary puncture of the subarachnoid space is then performed, with care taken to pass the needle as nearly in the midline as possible and to have the long axis of the needle directed toward the center of the intervertebral space. The insertion of the needle may be checked by fluoroscopic observation as desired at intervals during its passage. Ordinarily, both the L4-L5 and L5-S1 intervertebral spaces are investigated, and, if no abnormality is found, Lindblom recommends examination of the L3-L4 intervertebral space (12). When the dural and arachnoid sacs have been pierced, the stylet is withdrawn, and a small sample of CSF can be removed if desired. The needle is then passed as far as possible with ease toward the ventral aspect of the vertebral canal. The smaller needle is then passed through the lumen of the larger needle and advanced to a depth previously calculated to ensure the needle tip's being in the center of the intervertebral space, where the nucleus pulposus should be encountered.

Following nuclear puncture, the stylet of the smaller needle is withdrawn, and 1 to 2 ml of an opaque organic compound of iodine is injected into the nucleus pulposus. When a herniation is present, the patient's radicular pain may be reproduced or aggravated by injection of the opaque material under pressure into the diseased nucleus. The injection of radiopaque material, usually nonionic contrast medium, may be painful, and for this reason it might be desirable to mix it with small amounts of procaine. Radiographs should be made as soon as possible after the injection of the nucleus pulposus in frontal and lateral, and, if desired, in oblique projections. In the normal discogram, the nucleus pulposus is delineated as an oval space outlined with contrast material. The exact shape of the nucleus pulposus varies, but it usually does not reach the edge of the intervertebral disc. If the shadow reaches the edge of the intervertebral disc, a rupture of the annulus fibrosus may exist.

When a defect in the annulus fibrosus is present, varying quantities of the opaque material may be demonstrated passing from the intervertebral space into the ventral portion of the vertebral canal. The rupture is not necessarily toward the ventral side of the canal and may be lateral or even anterior. In some patients with disc protrusion, the lateral projection may demonstrate a semilunar collection of contrast medium directly behind the intervertebral space, which simulates calcification occurring in a degenerated herniated disc. With large disc extrusions, collections of the radiopaque material may be seen over a considerable area in the ventral part of the vertebral epidural space. A degenerated intervertebral disc that is not herniated will usually reveal an irregular cavity divided into two portions and with ragged margins instead of the usual oval, smooth, normal nucleus pulposus.

Discography has disadvantages. It requires multiple lumbar punctures and intermittent fluoroscopic control, although this may be done with films and, to increase speed, Polaroid films may be used. The possibility that needle puncture of the intervertebral disc, particularly of the nucleus pulposus, may induce degenerative changes leading to disc disease at a later date cannot be dismissed.

Although discography demonstrates very clearly the position and contour of the nucleus that is injected, it seems highly probable that the offending pathologic process will be overlooked in many instances when this method alone is employed, even in cases where abnormal nuclei are demonstrated at L4-L5 and L5-S1. The importance of thoroughly investigating the full length of the subarachnoid space with opaque material has been emphasized repeatedly by Camp (13,14).

Recently, in 1 year alone, three neoplasms of the cauda equina were disclosed by myelography in patients in whom the symptoms and neurologic findings were indistinguishable from those usually associated with intervertebral disc herniations.

Discography has the further disadvantage of not actually demonstrating the relationship of disc herniation to the nerve roots unless myelography is performed simultaneously. Horwitz has emphasized the frequent occurrence of herniated intervertebral discs as an incidental finding in anatomic material (15). Perhaps the greatest value of nuclear puncture is not the radiologic aspect at all but the reproduction of the patient's chief pain, which can be done by injecting the nucleus with saline. This is necessary in view of the frequent occurrence of asymptomatic degenerative disc disease.

It may be found desirable to restrict the use of discography to patients in whom anatomic variations, such as a subarachnoid space of small caliber associated with a large epidural fat space, make it impossible to determine from myelography whether herniation is present. The procedure may be of extraordinary value where technical errors of myelography occur with unsatisfactory examination by ordinary myelographic methods. Careful consideration of all of these factors has deterred most radiologists and neurosurgeons from the widespread use of discography.

In general, it may be said that if the procedure of discography is carried out, it indicates that the diagnosis of herniated intervertebral disc has already been made, and it is only a matter of localizing the offending herniated disc, whereas we look upon myelography as a procedure that not only will localize the herniated intervertebral discs but also will rule in or out the presence of a neoplasm in the subarachnoid space or in the epidural space, not only in the lumbar region but also in the lower thoracic region, which often gives a symptomatology indistinguishable from a lumbar root syndrome.

Discography may also be used in the cervical spine, and the same objections raised in the lumbar region may be raised in the cervical region. Degenerated intervertebral discs, particularly at C5-C6 and C6-C7 and also at C4-C5, are extremely common in the later decades of life, and a discogram will almost invariably show an abnormal disc at these levels. The advocates of this method in the cervical region argue that the reproduction of pain referable to the area at the time of the injection of the contrast material indicates that the correct intervertebral disc is being injected. However, if a complete examination were to be performed, it would be necessary to inject as many as five cervical intervertebral discs up to C3-C4, which is a frequent site of disc abnormality.

Discography is carried out as part of a therapeutic procedure, in the injection of a proteolytic enzyme (chymopapain) into the intervertebral disc. The lateral approach to disc puncture is recommended (16,17). The injection of the disc is always preceded by a myelogram to rule out other diseases and to localize the disc level. A discogram via the lateral approach is carried out prior to the injection of the enzyme in order to ascertain that the needle or needles are in an appropriate position for disc injection.

Chemonucleolysis became very popular following approval by the Food and Drug Administration, but due to the occurrence of many complications it rapidly lost followers. The complications can be classified as anaphylactic and infectious. Also, leakage of the material into the spinal canal was thought to be the cause of cases of bleeding and subarachnoid hemorrhage. The anaphylactic complications led to a number of deaths.

RADIONUCLIDE IMAGING

Radionuclide imaging is used to visualize the bones, not the intervertebral discs, and also in search of infection or neoplasm. The infection (acute or chronic) could be in the disc space and adjacent bones, and would usually reveal increased uptake of the radionuclide. Neoplasms, usually metastatic, would reveal an increased uptake in the involved bone. The finding of increased uptake in vertebrae, due to degenerative disease, is an incidental finding and must be differentiated from the other types of lesions mentioned previously. The examination is usually carried out with technetium 99m in diphosphonate compounds, and in degenerative disease may show moderately increased uptake on the upper and lower vertebral body margins on each side of the disc. The uptake is indicative of increased bone turnover related to osteophytes or discogenic sclerosis. In general, osteoarthritic changes around the intervertebral discs and in the apophyseal joints show a moderate uptake of the radiopharmaceutical. Increased uptake is also seen around the pars interarticularis defect in spondylolysis and in any acute or subacute traumatic injury to the bones.

SPINAL VENOGRAPHY

This is no longer used as a diagnostic procedure, although segments of veins are seen on MRI, particularly if gadolinium enhancement is used. Also, veins may be seen in spinal angiography, described in Chapter 17. The vertebral venous plexus (Batson plexus) is made up of two main portions: the external, around the vertebra, and the internal, situated in the epidural space of the spinal canal (Fig. 16.19). It is quite variable in size between subjects, but it also varies under various physiologic conditions. It often needs to be considered in the differential diagnosis of disc pathology, particularly in MRI examinations. Veins also cross the vertebral bodies, passing through canals within the cancellous bone, sometimes very conspicuous when they enhance after gadolinium.

INTERVERTEBRAL DISC DISEASE, SPINAL STENOSIS

Lumbar Region

Certain lesions of the vertebral column are of importance only, or primarily, because they involve the nervous system. Herniation of an intervertebral disc and osteoarthritis of the spine account for the majority of the complaints for which radiographic examination of this part of the body is carried out. A number of other lesions, belonging primarily in the category of diseases of the osseous system, such as osteitis deformans, hemangioma, and giant cell tumor, may have their chief clinical importance in neurologic involvement. Even malignant tumors that originate in vertebrae or extensively involve the spinal column by metastases may manifest themselves only by compression of the spinal cord. The latter group of lesions is discussed in the section dealing with metastatic tumors of the epidural space in text following. It is not the purpose of this chapter to describe individually each of the diseases of bone that may involve secondarily the spinal cord and spinal nerve roots. All of these lesions belong in the group of epidural lesions, which, by virtue of their frequency, constitute by far the most frequent type of lesion encountered in the spinal canal that causes compression of nerve structures. Benign tumors are much more frequently encountered proportionately in the intradural extramedullary group, whereas the malignant tumors occur much more frequently in the epidural space, and benign tumors are uncommon in this space. However, other types of epidural lesions that compress nerve tissue, which are not neoplastic, abound in the epidural space, as

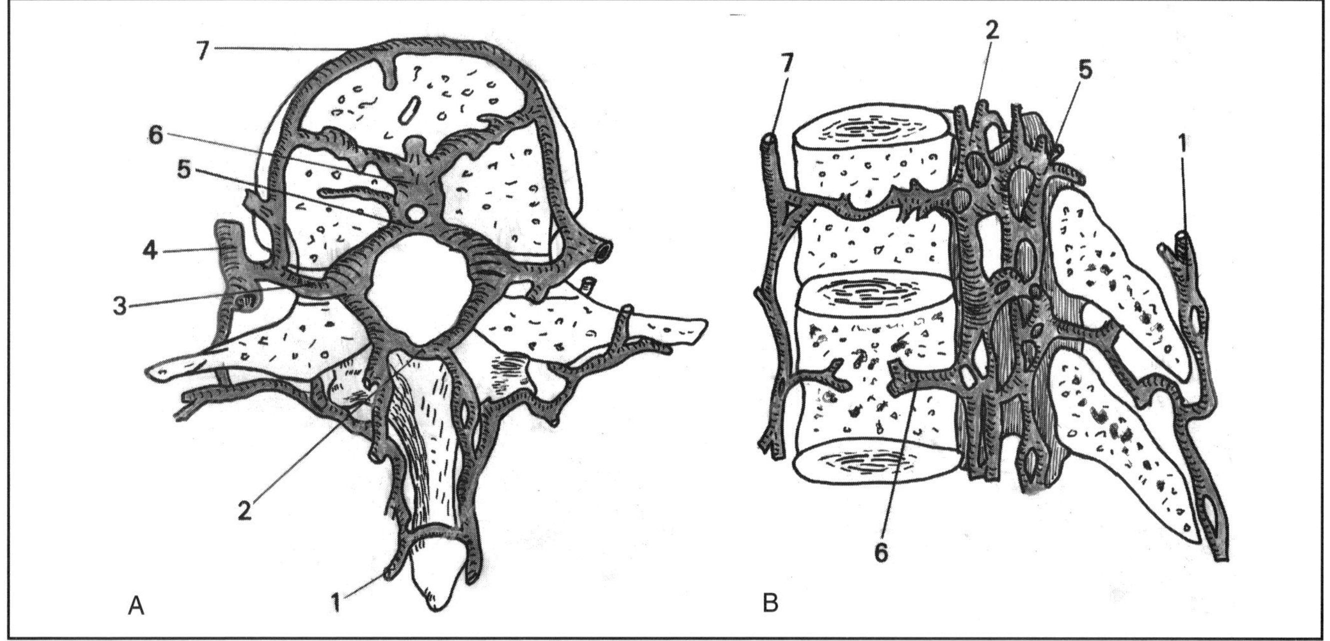

Figure 16.19. Vertebral venous plexus and epidural veins. **A.** Diagram of axial view. **B.** Diagram of lateral view. (1) Posterior external plexus; (2) posterior internal plexus; (3) intervertebral radicular vein; (4) intercostal vein; (5) posterior internal plexus; (6) basivertebral vein; (7) anterior external plexus.

attested by the great frequency of herniated and protruding intervertebral discs.

The intervertebral disc is composed of three distinct parts: the cartilaginous end plates, the annulus fibrosus, and the nucleus pulposus. The cartilaginous end plate is composed of hyaline cartilage covering the superior and inferior end plates of the adjacent vertebral bodies. It does not cover the outer ring made up by the epiphyseal ring observed during the secondary ossification period of the vertebral body. The annulus fibrosus, the limiting capsule of the nucleus pulposus, completely encircles the disc. It is made up of short, stout collagenous fibers, providing greater strength anteriorly than posteriorly. The fibers are thinner and fewer in number posteriorly. The annulus is firmly attached to the fused epiphyseal ring (by Sharpey fibers) and to the anterior and posterior longitudinal ligaments. It contains about 80 percent water in the young. Type I collagen fibers found in tendons elsewhere in the body are found in the periphery of the annulus fibrosus, whereas type II collagen fibers, of the type found in hyaline articular cartilage, make up the inner aspect where it is in continuity with the nucleus pulposus. The nucleus pulposus is an incompressible, gelatinous mass formed by delicate fibrous strands and containing a large amount of water—85 to 90 percent under normal conditions. The nucleus, more than the annulus, is rich in proteoglycans, and this molecule and collagen constitute the major macromolecular components of the disc. Other components are chondroitin 6-sulphate, chondroitin 4-sulfate, keratan sulfate, and hyaluronic acid.

When the disc degenerates it loses water (down to about 70 percent). This is associated with a loss of the water-binding capacity of the nucleus pulposus, possibly associated with a decrease in the molecular weight of the nuclear proteoglycan complexes. According to Lipson and Muir, there is an increase in the ratio of keratan sulfate to chondroitin sulfate and a decreased association with collagen (18).

As part of the degenerative aging process, the cartilaginous end plates become thinner and more hyalinized. This, in combination with the loss of water and elasticity in the nucleus pulposus and the annulus fibrosus, has the effect of decreasing the ability of the disc to respond to motion. The decrease in the height of the disc causes a caudal displacement of the apophyseal joint level, which produces other changes in the biomechanics of motion and may lead to degeneration of the cartilage in the apophyseal joints, elongation and thickening of some ligaments, and osteophyte formation.

The disc becomes progressively more fibrous, and at the end there is no clear distinction between the nucleus and the annulus. Fissuring and radial ruptures are often seen in the annulus at postmortem examination; this fissure allows for prolapse or herniation of the nucleus to occur.

Genetic predisposition to degenerative disc disease is a possibility. It is not uncommon to encounter patients with multiple disc problems developing at a young age and continuing later.

The degenerated disc may continue to become thinner with the passage of time, ending as a very thin intervertebral space. Granulation tissue may be found histologically in some areas, particularly close to necrotic degenerated portions (19). Protruded disc tissue can also disappear, as demonstrated by many examples (20). Now that CT and MRI are available, the disappearance or diminution in size of a herniated disc is more frequently observed. Is this due to the herniated portion returning home, so to speak, or is this reabsorption or "digestion" of the hernia by granulation tissue? The latter seems a more plausible explanation unless the disc herniation would disappear in a relatively short period of time.

RUPTURE OF INTERVERTEBRAL DISC

Although fibrocartilaginous masses in the ventral portion of the vertebral canal that compress the spinal cord or nerve roots were recognized and successfully removed by surgery as early as 1909, the true nature of the lesions was first explained by Mixter and Barr in 1934 (21). It is now generally agreed that trauma, single or repeated, exerted on a disc that has been weakened by degenerative changes, produces a rupture of the nucleus pulposus through the annulus fibrosus and protrusion or extrusion of intervertebral disc material into the vertebral canal.

Disc degeneration is a phenomenon of aging from normal wear and tear. It may occur in younger people who have instability of the vertebral column because of anatomic variations or congenital defects. The process is thought to begin with an exaggerated desiccation of the disc, which is a normal tendency with advancing age. The nucleus pulposus becomes inelastic, then soft, following which fissures and erosions of the cartilaginous plate of the vertebrae occur. Fibrous tissue and blood vessels extend through the bone plates from the vertebrae into the intervertebral disc, resulting in fibrosis, vascularization, and atrophy of the fibrocartilage. When the inelasticity of the disc is thus reduced by early or advanced degeneration, unusual forces applied to the spine may result in herniation of the intervertebral fibrocartilage into the vertebral canal. Occasionally, severe trauma will result in a rupture of an apparently healthy disc.

Herniation of the intervertebral disc may occur in any direction. Under pressure, the elastic nucleus pulposus becomes flattened and broadened, so that the resistant annulus fibrosus is displaced outward at the periphery. The lesions that are of clinical importance, however, are those that extend posteriorly or posterolaterally and compress the spinal cord or spinal nerve roots. Posterior ruptures most commonly result from force exerted on the spine in flexion (22).

LUMBAR DISC PROTRUSIONS AND HERNIATIONS

Disc herniations occur most frequently in the lower lumbar and lower cervical regions. The intervertebral discs at L4-

L5 and L5-S1 are involved with almost equal frequency, whereas the L3-L4 disc is less frequently subject to rupture. In the cervical region herniation of the disc at C5-C6 or C6-C7 most often is encountered. The more frequent occurrence of disc herniations at these levels is explained both by the strong force applied with the spine in flexion and by the anatomic size and shape of the discs in these areas. The nucleus pulposus is especially well developed in the lumbar region. The intervertebral fibrocartilages in the lumbar and cervical regions are thicker in front than behind, which contributes to the ventral convexity of these portions of the vertebral column. In the thoracic region, the discs are nearly uniform in thickness, and the dorsal convexity in this part of the spinal column results almost entirely from the shape of the vertebral bodies. Normally, the intervertebral discs increase progressively in thickness from T12 to L5, and to a less marked degree there is a relative increase in thickness of the cervical discs from C2 to C7. The lower cervical and lower lumbar portions of the spine have a relatively large proportion of the intervertebral disc material of the entire vertebral column, with the result that there is much greater freedom of movement here than elsewhere.

Plain spine roentgenograms may disclose few abnormalities as the result of a posterior intervertebral disc herniation. A common finding, however, is alteration of alignment of the vertebrae in the involved area. The ventral curve is usually reduced and may be absent in the cervical and lumbar region. Occasionally, the normal ventral curvature is reversed so that a slight dorsal angulation or convexity is present, usually maximum at the level of the lesion. Lateral angulation or scoliosis of the spine may be visible in frontal films. When lateral angulation is centered at one intervertebral level, it is strongly suggestive of intervertebral disc disease. This type of angulation should be differentiated from rotary scoliosis, which is common in the lumbar region and is usually not associated with local disc disease. Rotary scoliosis is commonly of unknown origin or may be associated with multiple disc disease.

The changes in vertebral curvature are the result of muscle spasm, which is an attempt, occurring by reflex, to shorten the course of the spinal nerve root involved and thereby reduce the tension on it.

Thinning of an intervertebral space is rarely present in acute disc herniation but is often observed as a result of degeneration of a disc without herniation. Since disc degeneration predisposes to rupture, however, narrowing of an intervertebral space may be interpreted as suggestive of a herniated disc if it is found at the appropriate level and when clinical examination discloses evidence of spinal cord or nerve root compression. The degree of disc thinning observed may be slight and may be detected only by comparison with the intervertebral spaces above and below. Marked narrowing of one disc space in the lumbar region is suggestive of herniation at that level but by itself does not justify a diagnosis of this condition because simple disc degeneration or other diseases (e.g., tuberculosis) may be responsible for the same appearance. It is also not rare to find that there is marked disc narrowing, whereas myelography reveals no evidence of disc protrusion. This might be the result of a primary degeneration of the disc without herniation or, perhaps, the herniation is entirely anterolateral in position where myelography would not show it. Anterolateral herniation would not compress the nerve roots, and therefore would produce no neurologic findings, but it may be a cause of back pain and even referred pain (23).

Calcification within the vertebral canal dorsal to an intervertebral space may be seen occasionally when advanced degenerative changes have occurred in the herniated portion of the disc. Ordinarily, the calcification is crescentic, concave ventrally with the greatest dorsal convexity behind the center of the intervertebral disc space. The calcification may extend 0.5 cm or more behind the posterior margin of the contiguous vertebral bodies at the level of the lesion. Although these calcium shadows are curvilinear, some calcifications may be rounded or oval in configuration, and occasionally lenticular, but almost always the center of the calcification is at the level of the middle of the intervertebral space. The size and shape of the calcification may suggest that the entire nucleus has been extruded and calcified. The undisplaced portion of the disc, which remains in the intervertebral space, frequently shows evidence of calcific degeneration when the herniated portion is calcified. Radiographically demonstrable (particularly with CT) calcium deposits in the intervertebral space are commonplace without disc herniation, especially in the thoracic region. Occasionally, the entire nucleus is calcified in a homogeneous manner, although more often linear and irregular scattered calcification in the fibrocartilage is demonstrated. Hypertrophic spurs projecting into the vertebral canal at the level of a herniated disc are the result of osteoarthritis associated with the disc degeneration rather than the result of the herniation per se. However, whenever osteophytes are seen arising from the margins of the vertebrae, it may be concluded that the disc extends to the level of the apex of the osteophyte. It is possible, however, with herniated discs of long standing, in which further thinning of the intervertebral disc occurs, that localized osteoarthritis may develop more rapidly and to a greater degree than in other portions of the same spine. Reversal of the cervical vertebral curve may make it difficult to obtain face-on views of the intervertebral foramina in oblique projection, with the result that several foramina may appear unduly narrowed in the routine oblique views, making it necessary to obtain additional oblique views using a greater and a lesser degree of rotation. The importance of osteoarthritis, either localized at the level of the lesion or diffuse, is of more prognostic than diagnostic significance. Hypertrophic changes denote degeneration and chronicity, and in such individuals, technical difficulties in surgical removal of the disc may be encountered, with incomplete relief or early recurrence of symptoms.

In some clinics, frontal films with the patient bending to the right and left and lateral views in flexion and extension are used in an attempt to detect and localize disc herniations. These maneuvers depend on muscle spasm (effects of which are often seen in ordinary radiographs) to prevent movement of the spine in a direction that increases the tension upon a compressed nerve root. There are other factors, both voluntary and involuntary, that affect the pliancy of the spine, and the results of the bending experiments frequently are inconclusive. Absence of compression of a disc with lateral bending is suggestive, however, of disc disease. Changes in width of the intervertebral space often may be demonstrated to best advantage in frontal films made with the patient prone.

The changes occurring in plain spine roentgenograms, aside from calcification within the vertebral canal, constitute indirect evidence of disc rupture since they do not depict the offending lesion. A diagnosis of posterior herniation of an intervertebral disc cannot be made justifiably unless a soft tissue mass in the vertebral canal continuous with the soft tissue shadow of the intervertebral space is demonstrated, which usually requires CT, MRI, or contrast methods. The actual demonstration of compression of the spinal cord or spinal nerve roots by the extraneous mass is a valuable part of any examination. Demonstration of disc protrusion alone is not enough, since the frequent occurrence of asymptomatic protruded discs is well known. For accurate diagnosis, it is essential that the morphologic changes present be depicted by the most accurate procedures available and that an objective correlation of the roentgen and clinical findings be made.

Following the technical improvements in body CT in the later 1970s and early 1980s, it became possible to diagnose disc herniations and protrusions noninvasively in the lumbar as well as the cervical and thoracic regions. Later, CT combined with myelography was introduced. One of the earliest reports of such combination was that of Sartor and Richter applied to the cervical region (24). Myelography with metrizamide became a much more acceptable procedure in the study of cervical herniated discs and degenerative osteoarthritis following the combination of the two. Until then, many workers preferred Pantopaque for cervical myelography.

In the lumbar region CT may show disc herniations and also will demonstrate calcification in the herniated portion or elsewhere in the disc. In addition, it will demonstrate degenerative osteoarthritic changes and osteophyte formation, which are not clearly seen with MRI.

It may be worth defining what is meant by the various terminologies used to describe the type of pathology present in the intervertebral disc. The term *ruptured intervertebral disc,* which was used by Mixter and Barr in their original description, is no longer used because it does not have a clear meaning (21).

The term *herniated intervertebral disc* implies that some of the nucleus pulposus has herniated through a rupture of the annulus fibrosus and there is a *focal bulge* in the contour of the disc margin, which can be posterior, posterolateral, extraforaminal, lateral, or anterior. The last two would not produce nerve compression; the extraforaminal may or may not produce nerve compression. The term *disc prolapse* has also been used, but the preferred term is *herniation* (Fig 16.20).

The term *bulging intervetebral disc* indicates that there is concentric enlargement or widening of the disc; if seen on the images, it should be so stated, indicating that this is a sign of disc degeneration. Bulging can be focal, in which case it is a herniation.

The term *disc protrusion* is interchangeable with *bulging,* although it is often used to mean a more important disc bulging. It should not be used to mean disc herniation unless it is qualified as a focal protrusion, in which case one may add "consistent—with disc herniation."

The generalized or concentric bulging or protrusion is associated with degenerative disc disease, and the disc space becomes thinner than it should be. The bulge or protrusion can be more pronounced dorsally or ventrally. The presence of scoliosis may lead to marked bulging or protrusion on one side or the other, always on the convex side of the scoliosis. This possibility must be excluded whenever a large extraforaminal bulge or protrusion is seen. As the degenerated widened disc bulges posteriorly, it may preserve its usual slight concavity in the center of the canal, or this normal concavity may disappear. In either case, it is referred to as a *concentric bulge.*

The term *herniated disc with a free fragment* means that a fragment of the herniation or the entire herniated portion has become totally free of the parent disc. In this case the free fragment may move cephalad or caudad, or dorsally outside the thecal space (Fig. 16.21). In some cases the free fragment may become intradural if an opening here occurred.

Extruded disk is a term applied to a large disc herniation. Sometimes the entire nucleus pulposus seems to have herniated, and in these cases a complete myelographic block may be found (Fig. 16.22). The terms *extruded* and *sequestered* (free fragment) have been used by others (25), giving them a different meaning than explained here, which can be somewhat confusing (26).

MRI has permitted an even clearer delineation of disc disease, and the two procedures (CT and MRI) are frequently performed in many cases, always in an effort to clarify the clinical problem in order to make the best decision for the patient. They are both noninvasive, and together they may work to avoid the use of myelography, an invasive procedure. Overall, MRI is more informative than CT because it provides sagittal as well as axial images and more than one sequence is usually obtained (T1- as well as T2-weighted). In addition, the spinal canal contents are evaluated, which is not possible by CT alone. A number of cases are illustrated utilizing one or both techniques with or without CT-myelography in Figures 16.20 to 16.24.

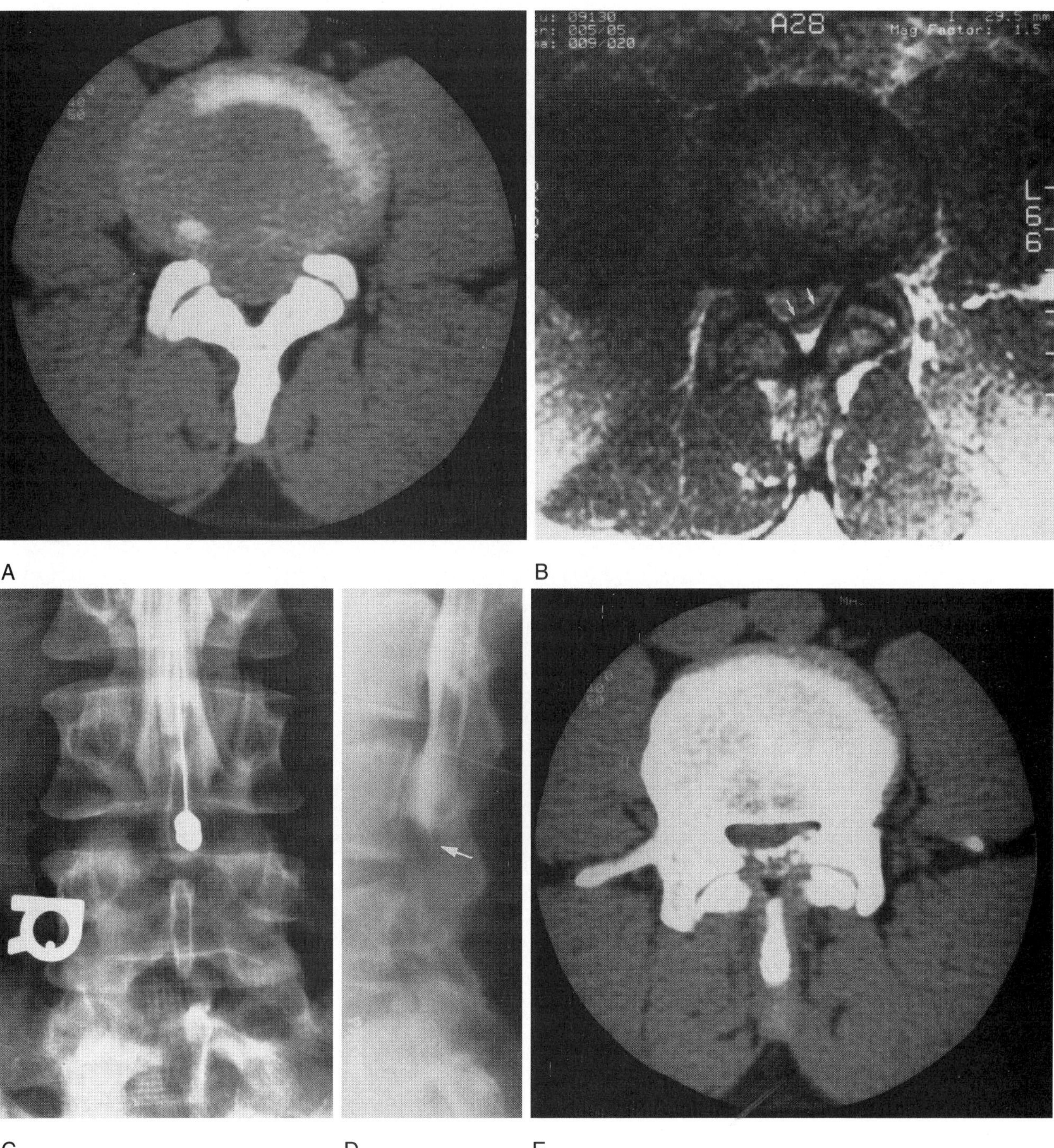

Figure 16.20. Large herniated intervertebral disc on CT, MRI, and CT-myelography. **A.** CT axial shows a uniform soft tissue mass in the spinal canal, and it is not possible to separate the thecal sac from the rest of the soft tissue. **B.** Proton density MR image shows what looks like a herniated disc flattening and displacing the thecal sac dorsally and to the left (arrows). **C.** Myelography was performed and demonstrated a complete block to the caudal flow of contrast. The needle was left in place in order to rule out a technical problem. The lateral view (**D**) shows dorsal displacement of the contrast away from the posterior margin of the vertebra just above the disc level (arrow). **E.** Repeat CT after myelography shows that some drops of contrast had passed down, and it confirms an appearance similar to that shown on the MR in B.

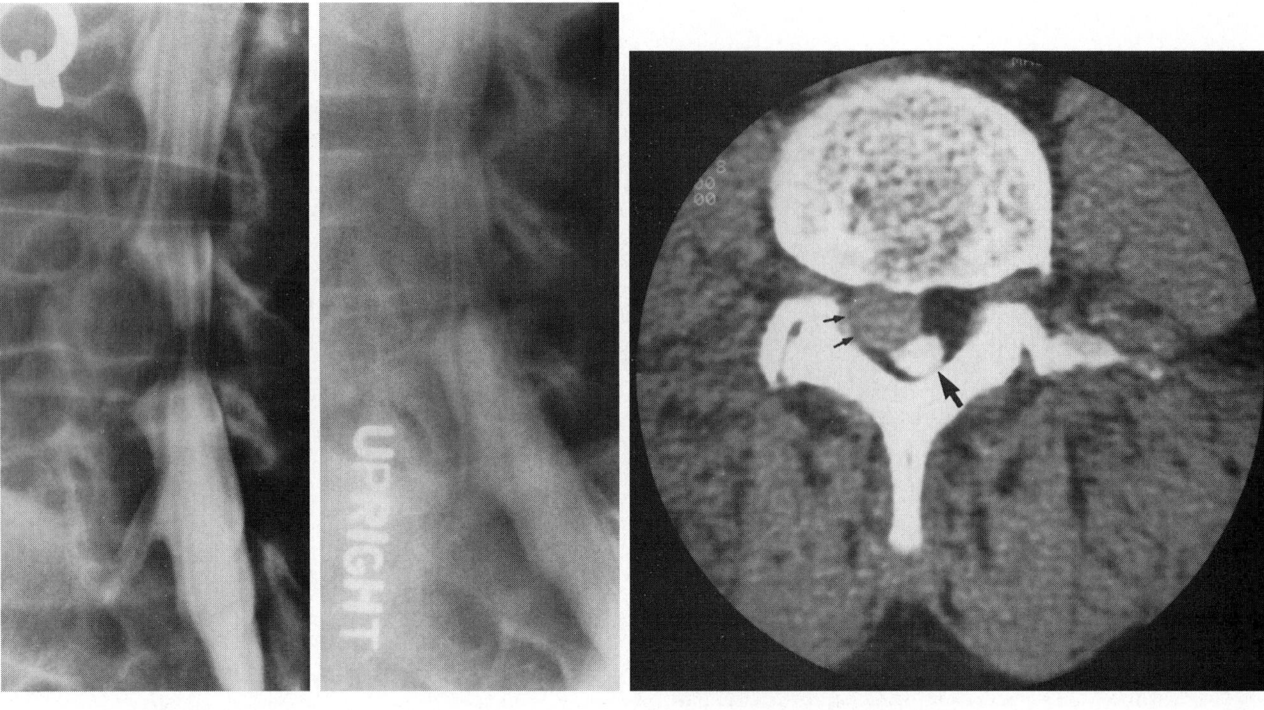

A B C

Figure 16.21. Herniated disc with a free fragment that moved cephalad. **A.** Semierect view. **B.** Erect oblique view. Both show marked displacement of the L4 root starting halfway up the vertebral body of L4. The root sleeve is not filled in A but seems to have filled with patient erect in B. **C.** The myelogram was followed by CT, which shows a small thecal sac posteriorly and displaced to the left (arrow) and a large soft tissue mass (small arrows) representing a free fragment as shown on the myelogram. The cross section is passing through the vertebral body and not through the disc. There is a fairly large fat collection to the left.

Gadolinium enhancement usually produces some increased intensity in the periphery of the herniated disc, which may facilitate interpretation. In general, we do not use contrast enhancement except in the postoperative spine, but one wonders whether the increased expense and examination time are warranted by the added information obtained in patients who have not had prior surgery. The affected roots may enhance after contrast (27–29). The root enhancement may extend intrathecally for several segments up to the conus.

As expressed earlier, narrowing of an interspace is an indication of a decrease in the height of the disc, a consequence of disc herniation or degeneration. The latter, however, is by far the most common, for herniation of a portion of the nucleus pulposus per se does not cause disc space narrowing unless it is a very large hernia. Calcification, visible on plain films and much more easily on CT images, is another sign.

MRI is better for visualizing disc degeneration. The accompanying loss of water decreases the brightness, particularly of the nucleus pulposus, on T2-weighted images (Fig. 16.25). This is particularly well seen on sagittal images. The degenerated discs may bulge anteriorly and/or posteriorly, or they may not. Axial views are needed to determine whether there is a focal bulge or protrusion in order to determine the possibilities of disc herniation (Fig. 16.26). Air can diffuse into large fissures in degenerated discs called "vacuum" discs; this is a fairly frequent finding. The gas is 90 to 92 percent nitrogen (30).

While sclerosis of the vertebral bodies adjacent to degenerated intervertebral discs (or, less frequently, secondary to disc infection) is a frequent finding on plain lumbar spine films (Figs. 16.27 and 16.29), it is not usually seen on CT because the axial images are not satisfactory to demonstrate it. If sagittal reformatting is done, however, the discogenic sclerosis becomes apparent.

The discogenic vertebral body changes can be seen on MR sagittal images, and the image will vary depending on the amount of fatty bone marrow present. Modic et al. describe three types of MR images (31). Type I shows low intensity on T1-weighted images. It is seen in patients who have been treated with chymopapain in the early period; presumably it is due to acute disc degeneration, but it can also be found in untreated patients (about 40 percent of referred cases for MR exam, according to Modic et al. (19,31). This may be a transient appearance, which will eventually convert to type II.

In type II there is hyperintensity on T1-weighted images and isointensity or slight hyperintensity on T2 (Fig 16.28). It is thought to be due to increased yellow bone marrow

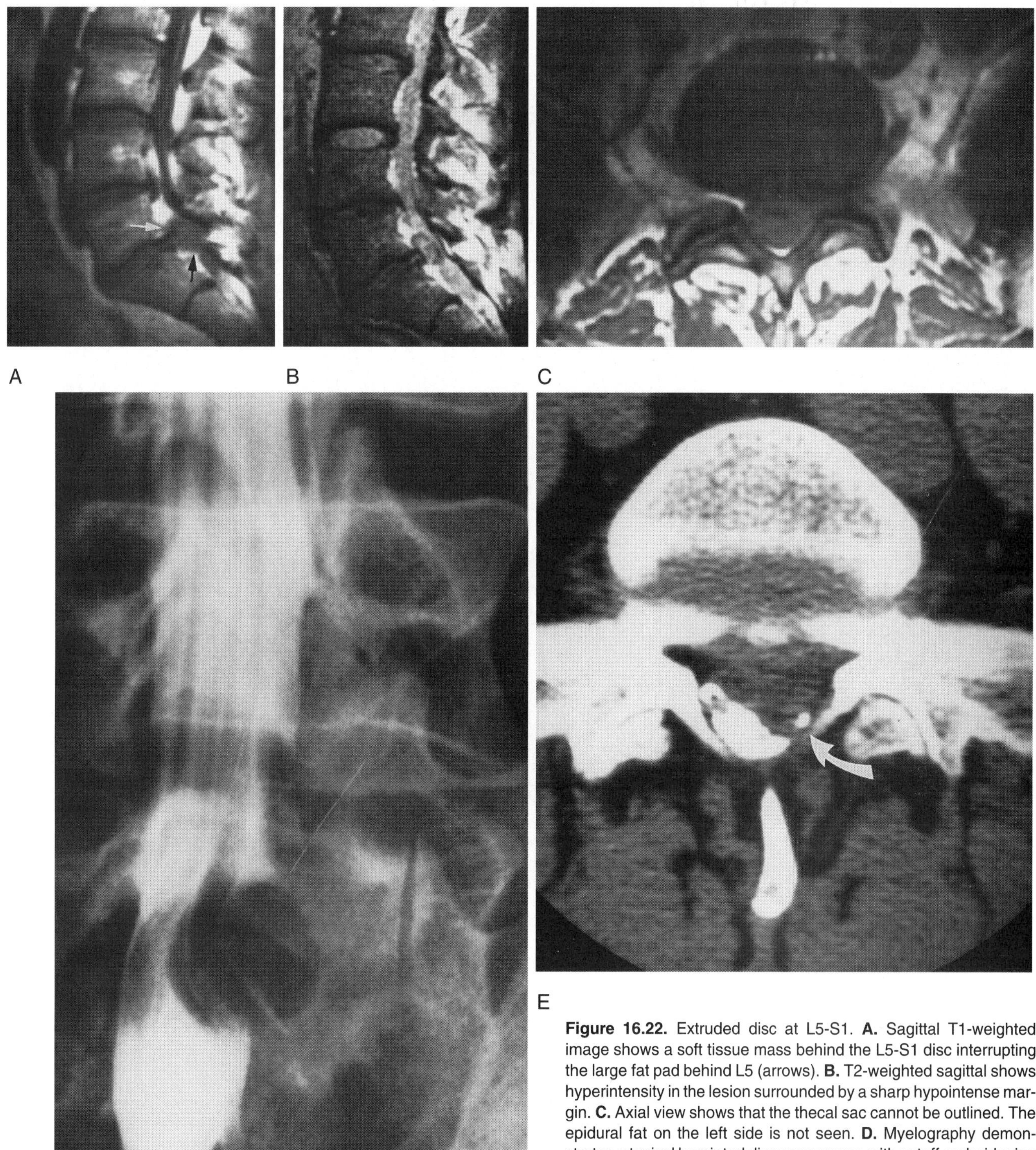

Figure 16.22. Extruded disc at L5-S1. **A.** Sagittal T1-weighted image shows a soft tissue mass behind the L5-S1 disc interrupting the large fat pad behind L5 (arrows). **B.** T2-weighted sagittal shows hyperintensity in the lesion surrounded by a sharp hypointense margin. **C.** Axial view shows that the thecal sac cannot be outlined. The epidural fat on the left side is not seen. **D.** Myelography demonstrates a typical herniated disc appearance with cutoff and widening of root. **E.** CT myelography shows a very large extruded disc on the left side producing marked flattening of the thecal sac, which is displaced dorsally and to the right. The left root sleeve is displaced dorsally and flattened (arrow); the right is also dorsally displaced or pulled by the displaced thecal sac. The hyperintensity noted on B is probably due to water diffusion into this extruded disc.

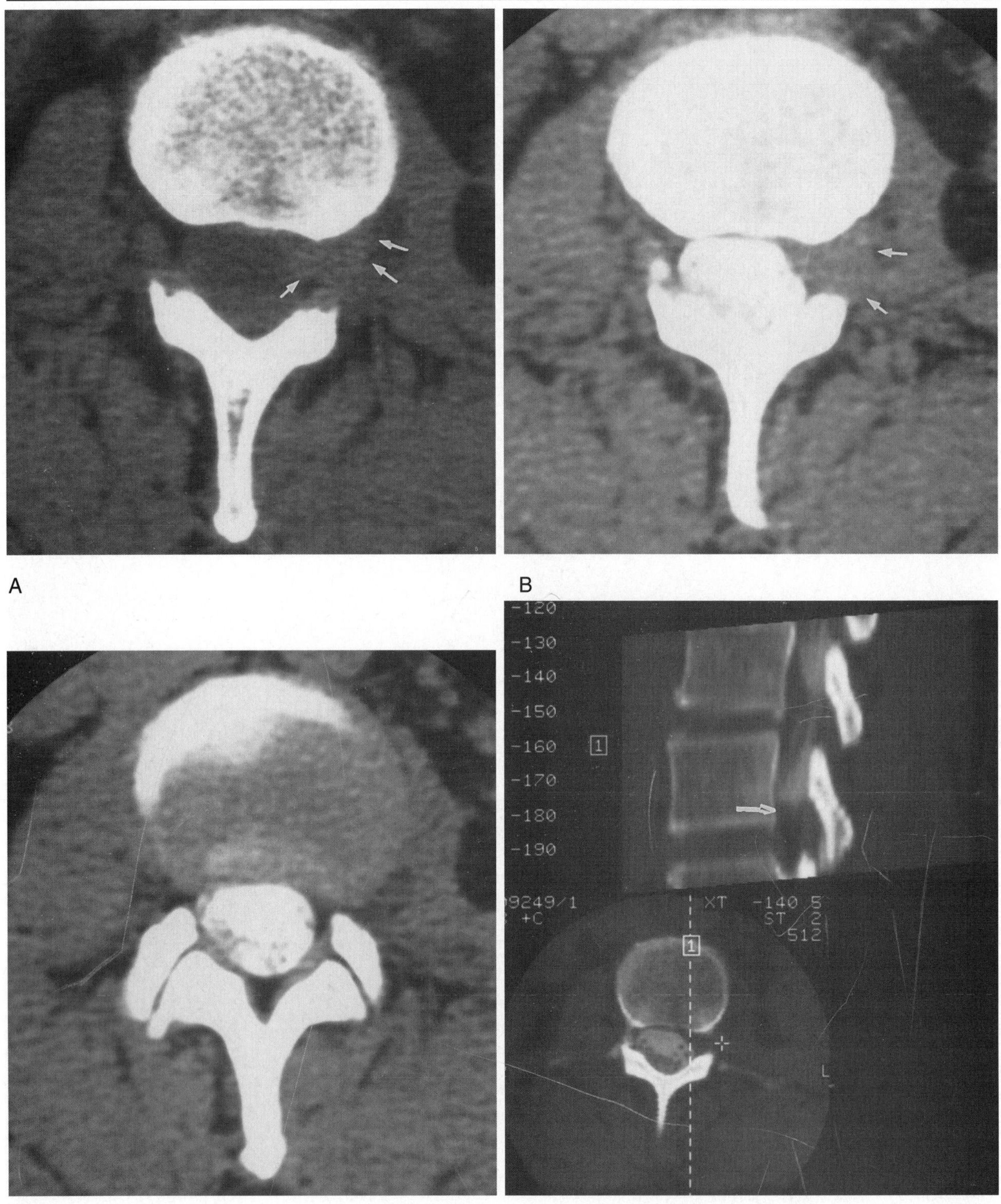

Figure 16.23. Foraminal and extraforaminal herniated disc shown by CT and CT myelography. **A.** CT prior to contrast shows a soft tissue mass partly occupying the intervertebral foramen and partly outside the foramen (arrow). **B.** CT after contrast shows flattening of the thecal sac and the soft tissue mass (arrows), projected over and outside the foramen. The section is passing at the level of the neural foramen, which is above the intervertebral disc. **C.** A section through the disc shows only a focal bulge, indicative of herniation on the left as well as lack of filling of the root sleeve as compared with the other side. **D.** Sagittal reformatting shows the interruption of the contrast on the left lateral aspect of the thecal sac (arrow).

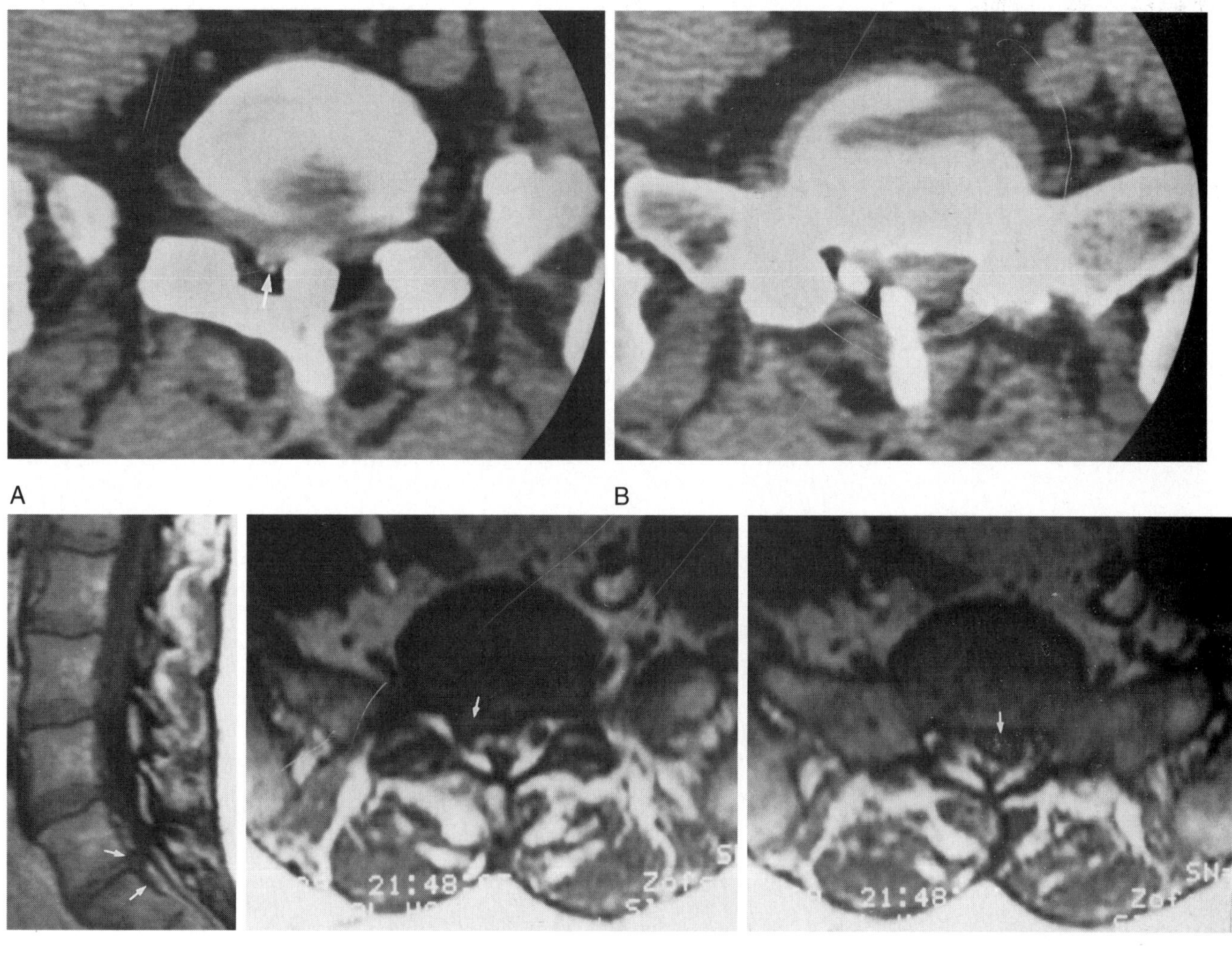

Figure 16.24. Bilateral herniation of intervertebral disc at the same level—CT and MRI. **A.** CT examination at the L5-S1 level reveals a herniated disc on the right side, which displaces the root dorsally (arrow). There is also an extraforaminal bulge of the disc. **B.** On the left side there is a larger disc hernia and the root does not fill. It was thought that the herniated portion moved caudally; the section is lower than A. **C.** Sagittal T1-weighted MRI shows a bulging L5-S1 disc (upper arrow). The caudal epidural fat is displaced away from the vertebral body of S1 (lower arrow). **D.** Axial T1-weighted MRI shows the right-sided herniation and the affected right root (arrow). The left root is in normal position. **E.** The lower section shows the hernia on the left, at the same level, similar to what was demonstrated in the CT. The unusual appearance was explained on the basis that the right herniated disc moved cephalad and the left moved caudad.

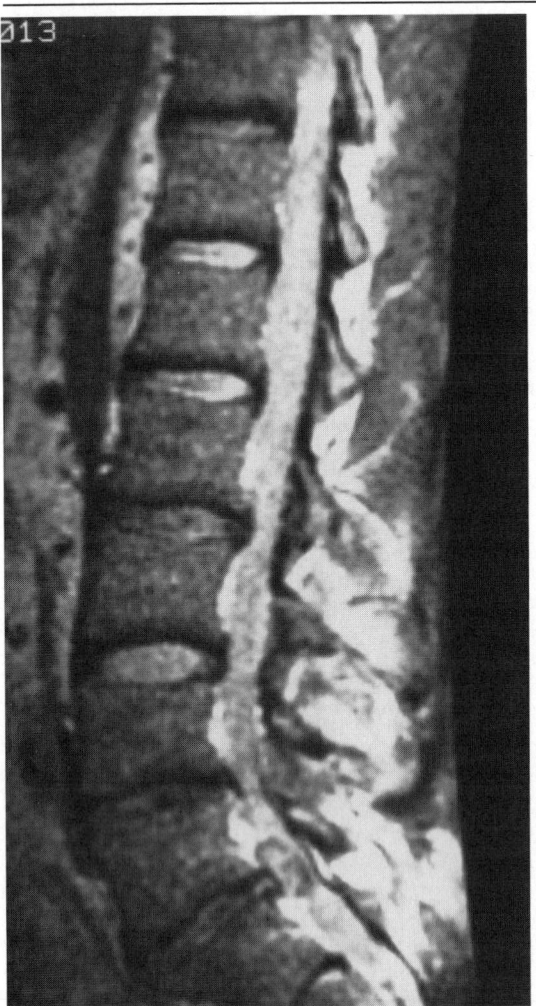

Figure 16.25. Disc degeneration. The sagittal T-2 weighted image reveals very low intensity in the L4-L5 and in the L5-S1 disc spaces. This means a loss of the normal amount of water present in the disc such as is demonstrated in the T12-L1, L1-C2 and L3-L4 interspaces. The T11-T12 and the L2-L3 discs show a decrease in brightness indicating an intermediate stage of water loss. The loss of water is representative of disc degeneration. There is usually a thinning of the disc space. The degree of loss of height (or thinning) of the disc space is related to the degree of degeneration. The loss of height may in part be due to herniation of the disc, anteriorly, posteriorly, or laterally, as well as to herniation into the body of the vertebra (Schmorl node). The degeneration can be associated with prior acute trauma but is not commonly a chronic condition.

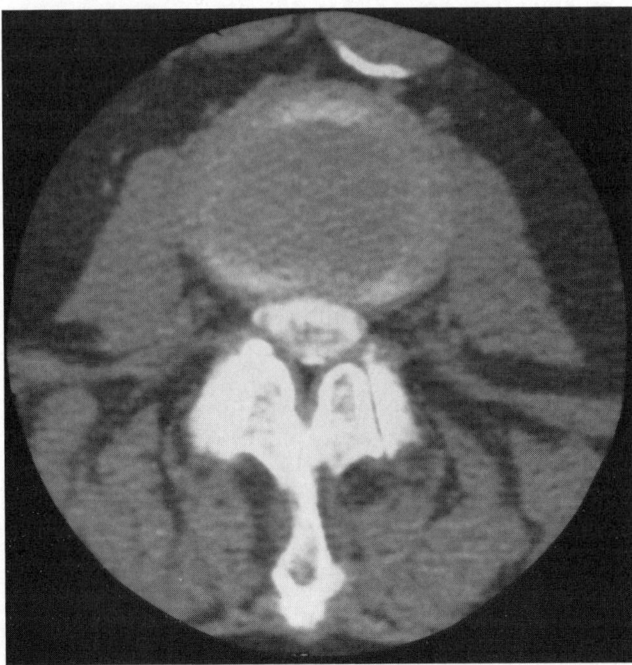

Figure 16.26. Lateral bulging of the intervertebral disc. Axial CT at L3-L4 shows that the intervertebral disc bulges slightly to the right. The patient also has evidence of spinal canal stenosis with hypertrophy of the articular facets and osteophyte formation. There is also a very acute posterior angle to the osseous canal, which is typical of canal stenosis.

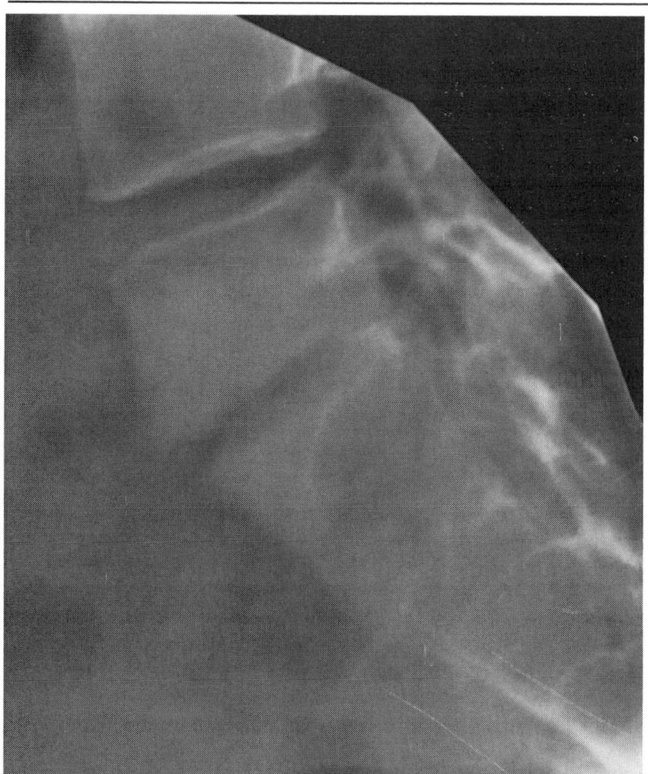

Figure 16.27. Discogenic sclerosis in 50-year-old woman. The L5-S1 disc space is not necessarily narrower than normal, but the changes in the vertebral body and sacrum indicate that there is a long-standing process involving this disc. There was no history of infection.

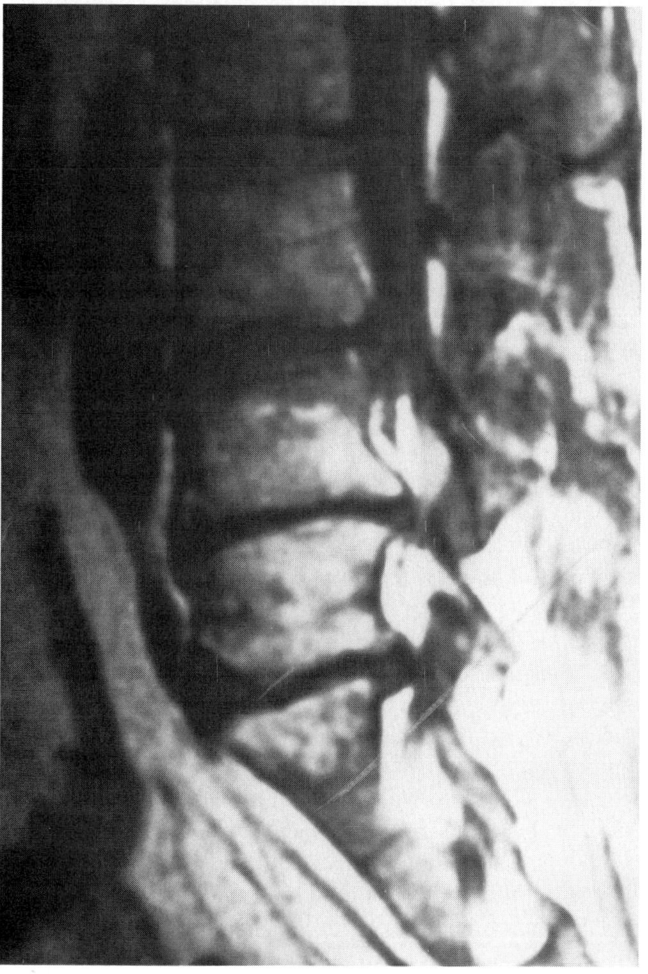

Figure 16.28. Type II (according to Modic et al.) changes in vertebral bodies. There is a hyperintensity in the L4, L5, and S1 vertebral bodies in this T1-weighted image. The changes are particularly well developed adjacent to the disc. The appearance was less pronounced on T2-weighted images (not shown) and is believed to be due to an increase in fatty marrow in the vertebral bodies. On plain films the bones may show some minor hyperdensity or be normal.

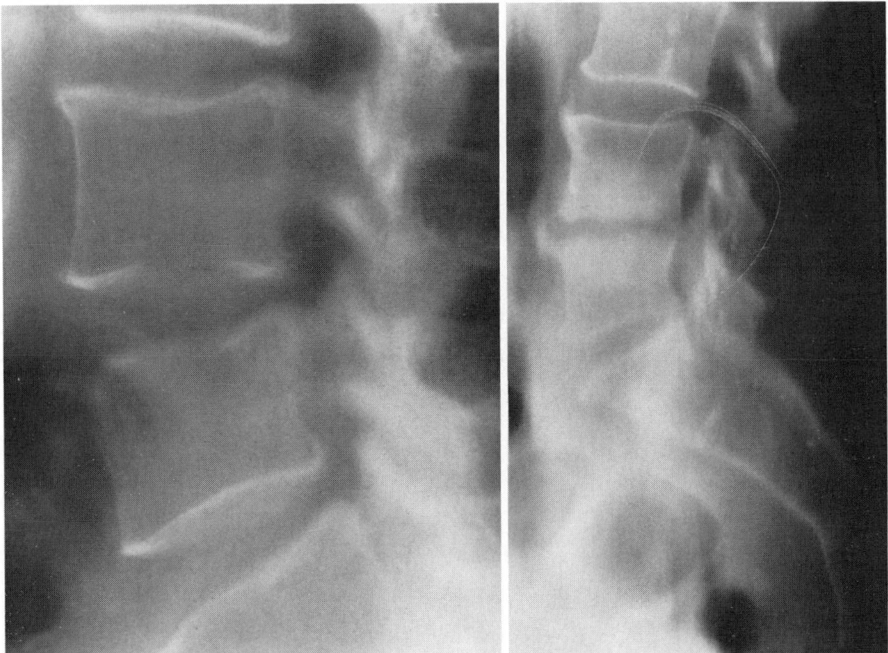

Figure 16.29. Postoperative disc infection (two cases). **A.** There is evidence of dissolution of the vertebral body plates and of the upper anterior margin of the vertebral body. This appearance is diagnostic of disc space infection. **B.** In another case, a more low-grade infection is present, and there is diffuse increase in density of the two vertebral bodies similar to that seen in discogenic sclerosis. The irregularity of contour of the vertebral bodies is helpful in the differential diagnosis; also, such factors as severe local back pain, elevated sedimentation rate, and history of relatively recent (2 to 4 months) surgery, at which time the vertebral bodies were not dense (see Figs. 16.72 and 16.73).

in the area, and it would behave like fat (bright on T1, less bright on T2, dark on gradient-echo images).

Type III has decreased signal intensity on both T1- and T2-weighted images. This appearance usually correlates with extensive bone sclerosis on plain films. Radiographic hyperdensity means dense woven bony trabeculae and decreased marrow spaces. What MR images is the soft tissue and the marrow, not the bone, and thus the low signal on T1 and T2.

The type I appearance may be seen in discitis with osteomyelitis, but in these cases the disc would be bright on T2-weighted images (Fig. 16.72). In this case also, contrast enhancement would be observed (Fig. 16.73). An important question is whether contrast enhancement can occur in degenerated intervertebral discs. The answer is that it can, but there is likely to be a preservation of thin cortical bone at the adjacent vertebral bodies, whereas in infectious discitis there is likely to be congestion and deossification of the bony margin, and disruption of the hyaline cartilage covering the vertebral body surface. Thus one would expect the enhanced degenerated disc to be fairly smooth, and to be separated from the vertebral bodies by a nonenhanced line. Enhancement of the adjacent degenerated vertebral bodies can also be observed (Fig. 16.30).

CT scanning is superior to MRI in demonstrating disease of the apophyseal joints; it also would demonstrate osteophyte formation at the edges of the vertebral bodies as well as calcified discs. The thickening of the ligamentum flavum is more clearly seen on CT but can also be observed on MR images. The cartilage of the apophyseal joints also can be seen by MRI, but in general CT is far superior for visualizing the changes in the articular facets, the osteophytosis, and the frequent disruption and marginal fragmentation occurring at L3 to L5-S1 (Figs. 16.31 and 16.32).

A frequent consequence of degenerative spinal disease involving both the discs and the apophyseal joints is the development of misalignment of the vertebrae. Retrolisthesis of the vertebral body above may be the direct result of disc collapse without apophyseal joint disease. This is because the apophyseal joints are inclined forward, and if the disc collapses the upper vertebral body would move back as it slides down. This may be a minor misalignment and may be of no clinical significance in itself. However, it is associated with narrowing of the neural foramen because the upper margin of the articular process moves up into the lower aspect of the foramen.

Much more important is the forward slippage of the vertebral body and arch as a result of degeneration and disruption of the apophyseal joint articular cartilage and the articular process itself (Fig. 16.33). The process usually occurs at the L4-L5 level and less frequently at L3-L4. Patients with the more severe degenerative spondylolisthesis may have sagittally oriented apophyseal joints or tropism of the facets, a term used to indicate that one facet may be oriented more sagittally whereas the other is more frontally oriented (Fig. 16.34). In this case, the forward slippage of the vertebra would be greater on one side than on the other, such as is shown in Figure 16.33; the right side of L4 is farther forward. In degenerative spondylolisthesis the entire vertebra moves forward. If there is sufficient displacement, the posterior arch, as it moves forward, would cause

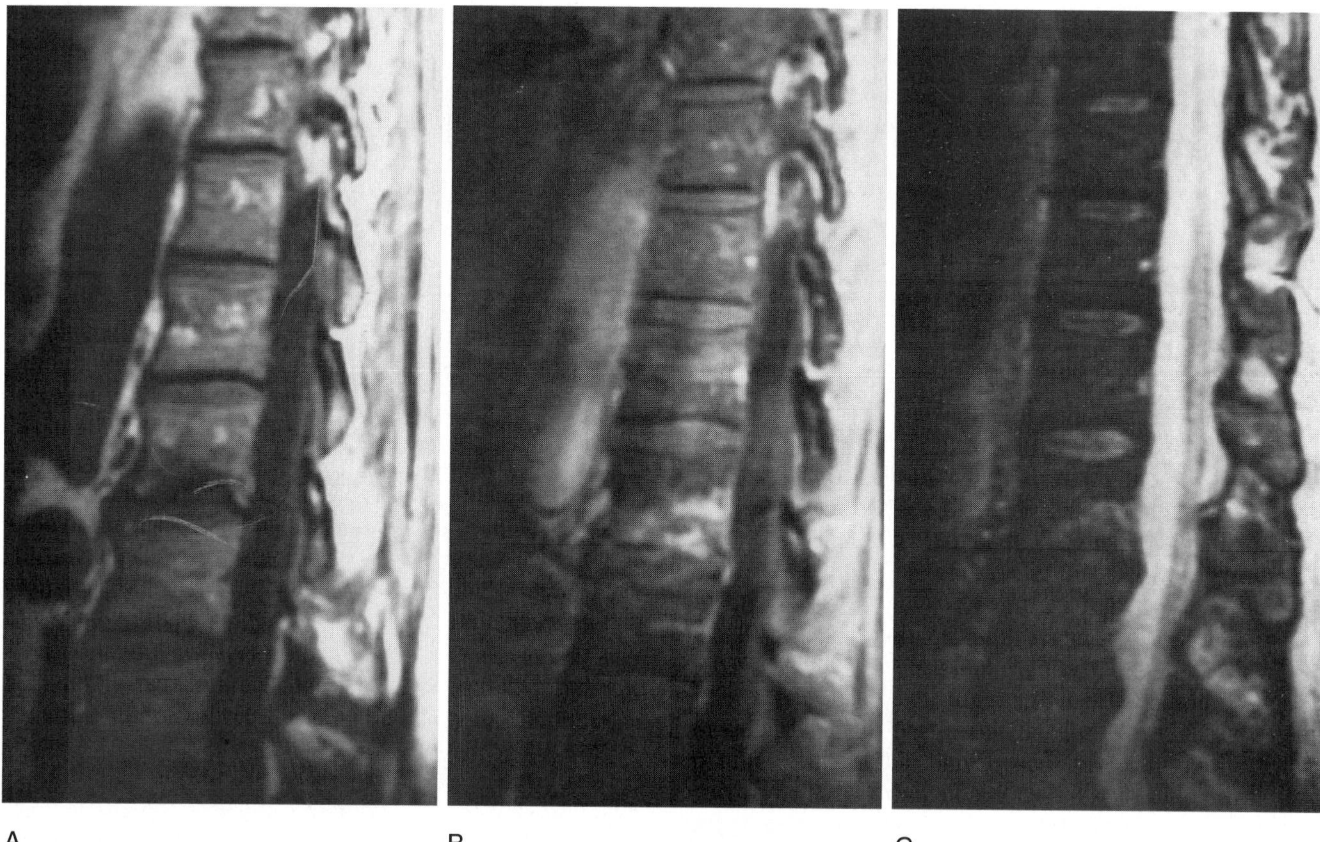

A B C

Figure 16.30. Contrast enhancement in degenerative disc. **A.** Precontrast sagittal view shows degenerative changes in the L2-L3 intervertebral disc region and adjacent vertebrae with Schmorl's node, particularly at L2. **B.** Postcontrast sagittal shows hyperintensity of lower aspect of L2 due to contrast enhancement. **C.** A T2-weighted sagittal shows only degenerative change.

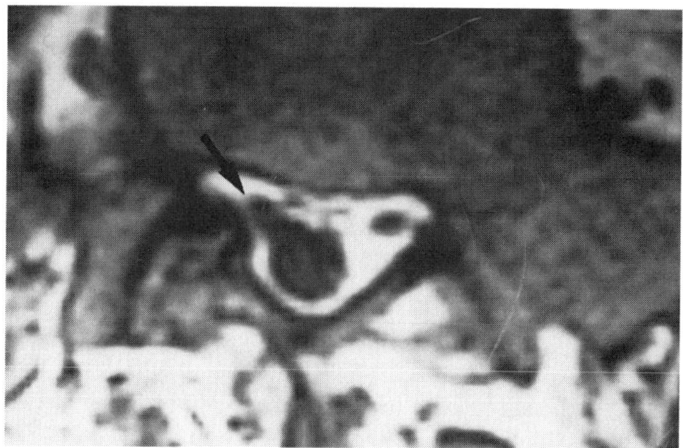

Figure 16.31. Hypertrophy of articular facets due to osteoarthritis seen in axial T1-weighted MRI. There is a typical dorsolateral deformity of the perithecal fat, and medial and slight forward displacement of the corresponding nerve root (arrow) on the right side. There is disruption of the right apophyseal joint.

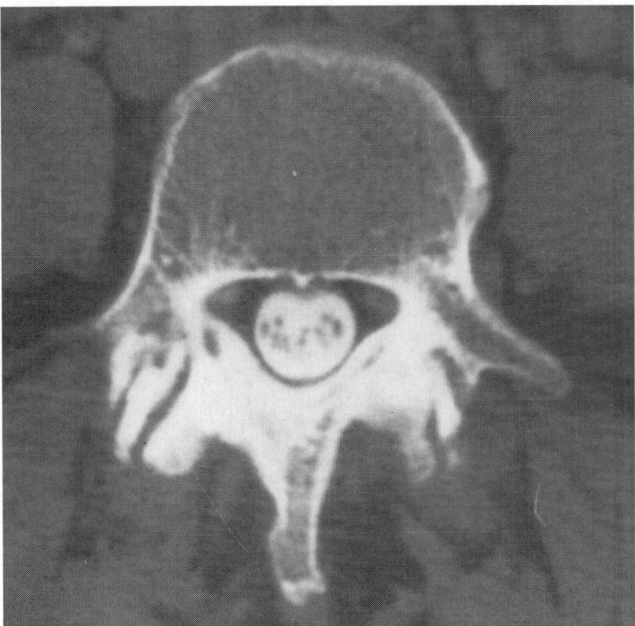

Figure 16.32. Degenerative disease of articular facets seen on CT-myelography. There is hyperdensity of the bones due to sclerosis, narrowing, and disruption of the articular facets with enlargement of the facets due to hypertrophic osteophyte formation. Also note that the direction of the articular surfaces is not the same on the two sides. This has been called "tropism" of the articular facets which often lead to instability and degenerative changes. The thecal sac is unaffected (see Fig. 16.34).

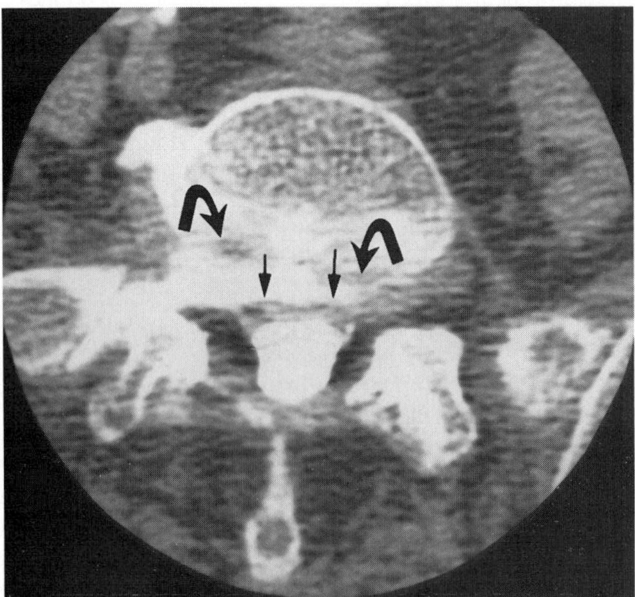

Figure 16.33. Degenerative disease of the lumbar spine, spondylolisthesis. The axial CT image shows a double contour to the posterior margin of the vertebral body. The posterior margin of L5 is seen close to the contrast-outlined thecal sac (arrows). Another posterior vertebral body contour is shown anterior to it (curved arrows). There is also evidence of soft tissue posterolaterally on both sides, representing a bulging disc. The forward slippage of the L4 or L5 vertebral body was not associated with a defect in the pars interarticularis but was due to degeneration and disruption of the apophyseal joints.

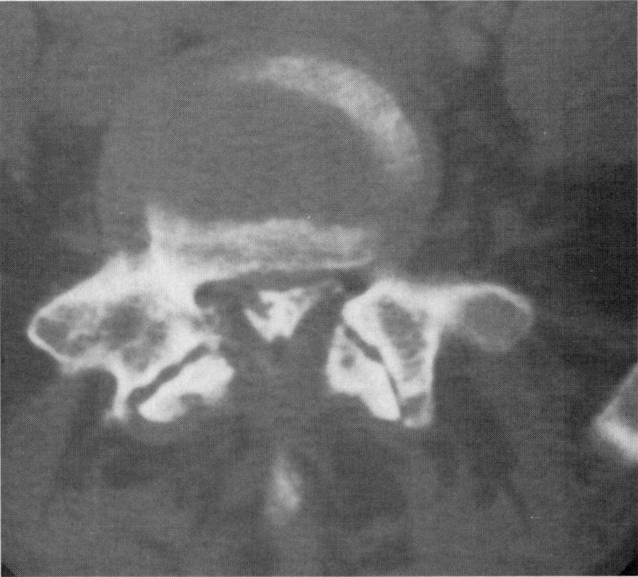

Figure 16.34. Tropism of articular facets. On the left side the joint is oriented obliquely, whereas on the right it is closer to parallel to the frontal plane. There is degeneration, narrowing of the joint space, irregularity of the joint margins, and sclerosis of the bones. In addition, there is evidence of thickening of the ligamentum flavum, causing the thecal sac, outlined with contrast, to acquire a triangular shape.

narrowing of the spinal canal between the anteriorly displaced arch and the posterior aspect of the vertebral body below, which leads to a syndrome of spinal stenosis (see text following). These findings can be seen on sagittal MRI but can also be demonstrated on reformatted CT images, as has been shown by Rothman and Glenn (32).

SPONDYLOLISTHESIS

The term *spondylolisthesis* is applied to a slippage of a vertebral body over another; usually the vertebra above slips forward, but sometimes backward slipping is observed, as explained earlier. The term *pseudospondylolisthesis* is confusing and probably should not be used.

The spondylolisthesis may be due to a defect in the neural arch, usually in the pars interarticularis, or, as shown previously, it may be the consequence of severe apophyseal joint disease (sometimes associated with anatomic variants in the orientation of the articular facets), usually referred to as *degenerative spondylolisthesis.*

The defect in the pars interarticularis (isthmus) is usually due to a fracture occurring early and usually not diagnosed because it may have occurred in the first decade of life. Sometimes no defect is found, but elongation and thinning of the isthmus or pars interarticularis can be shown. The most common defect is probably due to a fatigue fracture (33). Spondylolisthesis may also be the result of acute fracture, in which case it is an unstable injury. When only thinning and elongation of the isthmus is found, it may be due to an old healed fracture that occurred during childhood.

Plain films of the spine, including right and left oblique views and erect lateral views, are the classic way to diagnose spondylolisthesis. The diagnosis is also easy to make on MR sagittal images. If only axial views are available on CT, one must pay attention to the vertebral body relationship in successive slices. Also, because of the change of angulation to make the slices parallel to the intervertebral discs, the changing appearance makes it easy to misinterpret the anatomy and to overlook a spondylolisthesis. Most cases occur at L5-S1 when a pars interarticularis defect is present. On axial views the disc between L5 and S1 gives the appearance of marked protrusion. The spinal canal, at the same time, is larger than in the adjacent sections above. An appearance suggestive of a "double canal" is sometimes seen if the posterior arch of L5 is sectioned at the same level as the L5 vertebral body because of the reversing lordotic curve at L5-S1. The defect at the pars interarticularis is quite variable in its direction, but in general it can be seen well in the lateral views. The axial views may or may not show it clearly. Bone production at the defect is sometimes seen, particularly if the defect was the result of an old traumatic fracture rather than a fatigue fracture. The defect can be unilateral, and in these cases increased density of the intact isthmus may be seen, which has been attributed to a reaction to chronic strain.

In spondylolisthesis with a pars defect, the posterior portion of the neural arch stays behind, and only the body, pedicles, and upper articular processes move forward. For this reason symptoms of spinal stenosis with cauda equina compression do not occur as they do in degenerative spondylolisthesis, usually occurring at L4-L5 or sometimes at L3-L4. Also herniated disc does not usually accompany the forward slippage, but the disc, in its posterior portion, acquires a triangular configuration as seen in the sagittal view. Disc herniation in the presence of spondylolisthesis is diagnosed when a focal bulge in the disc is seen in axial images.

Pars interarticularis defects at L4 and L3 may look like osteoarthritis of the articular facets, and sagittal reformatting is needed to make a diagnosis (32). Most modern CT units allow for sagittal and coronal reformatting, although probably this capability is not used as frequently as it should. For best results, the axial slices (3 mm is usually sufficient) should all be made parallel. Angled axials, to make the planes parallel to the discs, allow for reformations of only small segments.

LUMBAR SPINAL STENOSIS

Some patients have a congenitally narrow spinal canal in both the anteroposterior and the transverse diameters. This is usually diagnosed from plain films of the spine by a short interpediculate distance. Often a narrow interpediculate width receives little attention when the spine films are examined, whereas an increase in the interpediculate

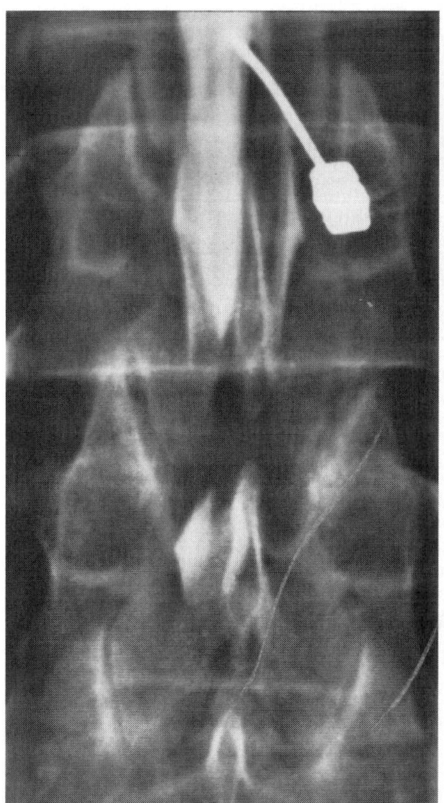

A

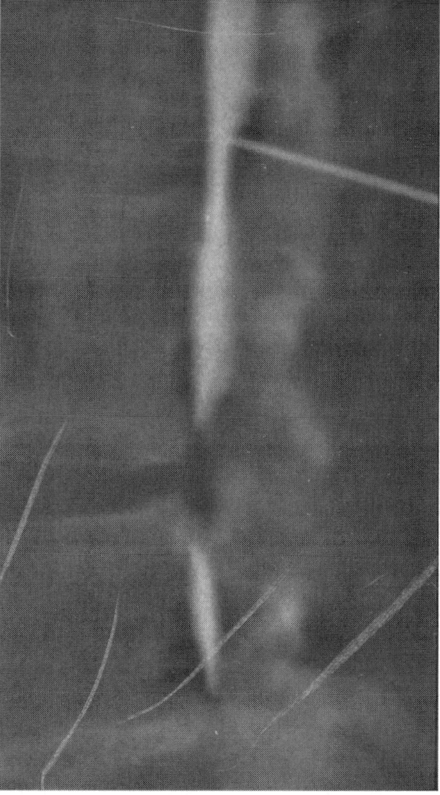

B

Figure 16.35. Partial and complete block in lumbar myelogram associated with congenitally narrow spinal canal. **A.** In the frontal projection, there is noted partial block at the level of L3-L4 and complete block at L4-L5. The contrast did not go down beyond this point in this erect view. **B.** In the lateral projection, there is only interruption of the contrast near the disc spaces with very little lifting away from the ventral surface of the canal. The interpediculate distance in this patient is of the order of 23 mm or less at L3, L4, and L5. The canal was very narrow in its anteroposterior diameter as well. There is no significant osteophyte formation around the margins of the vertebral bodies. The patient had a paraparesis secondary to multiple root involvement. Decompressive laminectomy resulted in improvement. Discs were not removed.

distance is usually observed and commented upon by the radiologist. In the cases that have a narrow spinal canal, a slight degree of protrusion or herniation of the intervertebral discs will produce signs of multiple root compression or severe signs of single root compression when the degree of protrusion into the spinal canal is rather small. This results from the fact that these patients have little available space (Fig. 16.35). The myelogram, not uncommonly, shows complete or incomplete block to the flow of contrast at more than one level, and the lateral myelogram films show only a slight degree of protrusion. In these cases, one is often puzzled to explain the large defects and the presence of a block in the presence of only minor dorsal deviation of the contrast column. The explanation lies in the congenital narrowing of the spinal canal, which causes a simple disc to produce multiple signs of root compression, often suggestive of a spinal cord tumor (34). The interpediculate distances at the levels of L3 and L4 will often fall at the 23- and 24-mm level instead of around 26 to 30 mm, which is a more common range. Less space is present for the roots to move within the dural sac.

The spinal canal should be measured in its anteroposterior (as well as in its transverse) diameter. Roberson et al. indicate that a corrected measurement of 16 to 17 mm is at the lowest limit of normal, and, when associated with narrowing of the interpediculate distance, it becomes more significant (35). In order to measure the anteroposterior diameter, a straight line is traced between the upper and lower margins of the vertebral body, and the distance is measured to the anterior margin of the spinous process (Fig. 16.36).

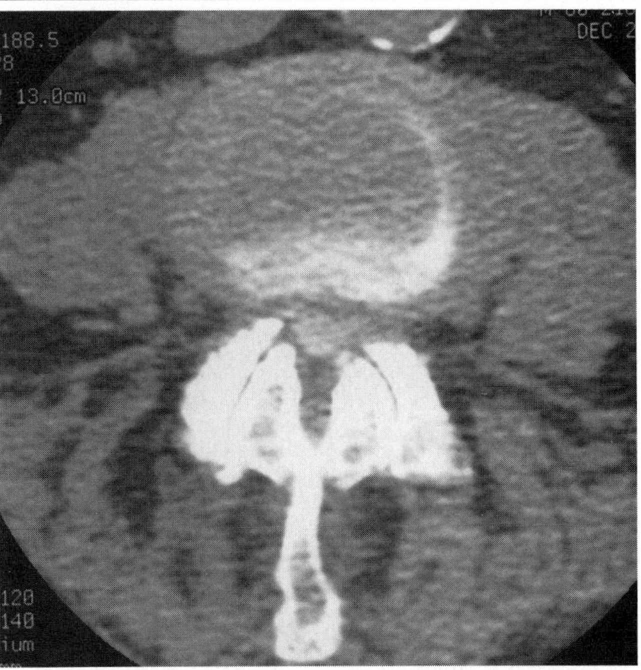

Figure 16.37. Markedly stenotic spinal canal. The articular processes are of a massive relative size bilaterally, and there is osteophyte production at the margins of the articular facets. The posterior angle of the spinal canal is so narrow that there is essentially no room for the thecal sac. Also, the hypertrophic facets are very close to the posterior margin of the vertebral body, which produces narrowing of the neural canal. The cross section is at the level of the disc, which is also bulging.

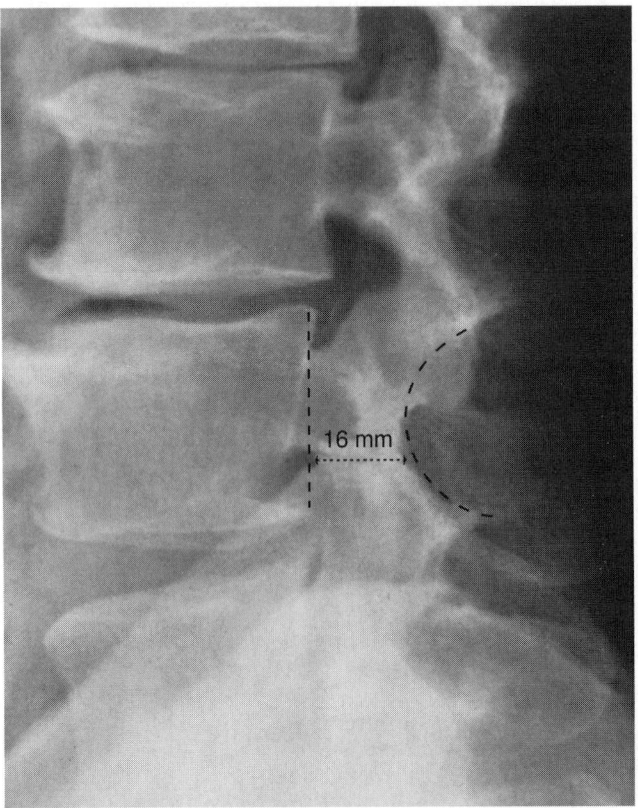

Figure 16.36. Method of measurement of spinal canal in lateral projection on plain films. The 16-mm anteroposterior diameter indicates the probable presence of a congenitally stenotic spinal canal. There is evidence of a narrow L3-L4 disc space with a vacuum phenomenon in the disc and discogenic sclerosis and osteophyte formation in the adjacent vertebrae.

The configuration of the spinal canal is important as seen in axial projections by CT or MRI; both methods can be used, but CT is preferable to evaluate the bony canal. There are essentially two types of configurations to stenotic canals: (*a*) The canal has a narrow posterior angle, usually associated with large, hypertrophic articular processes and facet joints with osteophytes. These cases also show narrowing of the medial aspect (lateral recess) of the neural canal on each side (trefoil configuration). The narrowing of the canal that this configuration produces can be extreme, leaving practically no room for the thecal sac (Fig. 16.37). (*b*) The spinal canal is of relatively normal size, but there is thickening of the ligamenta flava. This, combined with some concentric bulging (or protrusion) of the intervertebral disc, produces significant narrowing of the canal with compression of the thecal sac (Fig. 16.38). The short anteroposterior diameter of the spinal canal is not usually accompanied by narrowing of the posterior angle, but is felt to be produced by short pedicles, which are usually massive

(Fig. 16.38). The combination of the flat canal and the slight bulging of the intervertebral disc, as well as some degenerative osteoarthritic changes in the articular facets and thickening of the ligamentum flavum, lead to compression of all the roots of the cauda equina. The multiple foot compression produces a certain amount of weakness of the lower extremities, which causes the patient to slow down when walking or quit when going up a stairway. This neurologic claudication is different from the vascular insufficiency claudication in that there is no pain. Myelography usually demonstrates one or more areas of partial or complete myelographic block to the flow of contrast (Fig. 16.39).

The abnormality is more common in men (about 9 to 1) and manifests itself usually in the fifth or sixth decade of life, possibly due to the superimposition of a degenerative process upon the congenital narrowing of the canal.

The author has observed many instances of elongation and tortuosity of roots in association with a congenitally narrow lumbar canal. The appearance is suggestive of a vascular malformation because of the serpentine configuration of the elongated root (36). More than one root may be involved (Fig. 16.40).

THE POSTOPERATIVE LUMBAR SPINE

It is unfortunate that surgical treatment of herniated intervertebral disc and associated pathology is so frequently followed by either incomplete relief or by a recurrence of symptoms, at the same level or at a different level (37). It is said that about one-third of patients return for further diagnostic or therapeutic workup. The decision to apply surgical therapy must be made very carefully in the first place and should be preceded by a thorough investigation. But in the postoperative patient with recurrent symptoms, it is particularly important to carry out a thorough diagnostic investigation. Fortunately, we now have a number of ways to carry out a relatively noninvasive investigation of the lumbar spine, including plain films, CT without and with intravenous contrast, and MRI, also without and with contrast. These should be done prior to performing a more invasive procedure such as myelography, always followed by CT examination (CT-myelography), which usually is not performed unless the surgeon has decided that surgical treatment is probably necessary.

One of the more frequent reasons for recurrence of symptoms appears to be the formation of a fibrotic scar around the nerve root originally involved. The scar may be localized to the root area in the anterolateral aspect of the spinal canal where the surgical approach is concentrated to remove the intervertebral disc, but can extend along the lateral aspect of the thecal sac. The most important decision to be made on CT or MRI examination is therefore to differentiate fibrosis from recurrent disc herniation. MRI is superior to CT in this case, because gadolinium usually enhances the fibrotic mass, whereas the iodine compounds do not seem to do so as efficiently. This may have something to do with the presence of the surrounding bone, which may act to decrease the ability to appreciate small density differences by CT. MRI is therefore the procedure of choice, and this should always be carried out without contrast, followed immediately by contrast without moving the patient, in order to facilitate comparison. T1-weighted images are done, but the second-echo T2 images (long TR, long TE) are also routinely made. The T1-weighted postcontrast images are done using the fat saturation technique. Fibrosis would enhance, because it seems to contain sufficient vascularity to do so (38) (Fig. 16.41*F* and *G*). Herniated disc fragments would not enhance. Some herniated disc fragments could be T2 bright, because they seem to absorb some water, but they would not enhance with contrast, which would imply the presence of a significant amount of vascular supply (Fig. 16.41). In addition to differentiating fibrosis from recurrent herniated disc, there are other observations that can be made on postoperative cross section imaging (Fig. 16.41). These include postoperative pseudomeningoceles and artifacts produced by metal clips. The ability to differentiate fibrous scar from recurrent disc herniation is high (96 percent), according to Ross et al. (38), if contrast-enhanced MRI is carried out. Some of the patients in their series had both postoperative fibrosis and disc herniation, some had only a recurrent disc hernia, and others had only a fibrous scar.

Cervical Region

CERVICAL OSTEOARTHRITIS (SPONDYLOSIS) AND HERNIATED CERVICAL DISCS

Osteoarthritis of the vertebral column is commonly seen; it is a natural process of aging. Rarely is a patient beyond middle age seen in whom osteoarthritis of the vertebral column is not demonstrable. In the vast majority of instances, osteoarthritis of the spine does not give rise to neurologic symptoms. Occasionally, however, unusually large osteophytes project into the vertebral canal or narrow an intervertebral foramen to such a degree that spinal cord or nerve root compression occurs. Neurologic symptoms, which may be attributed to osteoarthritis, arise most frequently in the cervical area. Radicular pain, when present, may be severe, as exemplified by the patients in whom left arm pain may be misinterpreted as a manifestation of angina pectoris.

It is impossible from the radiologic examination of the vertebral column alone to evaluate the full significance of osteoarthritis. The lesions that encroach on the vertebral canal and narrow the intervertebral foramina, especially in the cervical region, are noteworthy, but the roentgen findings must be correlated closely with the patient's symptoms and neurologic disturbances. Osteoarthritis demonstrable in plain films of the spine is frequently used to explain a radicular syndrome, or even a simple neuralgia,

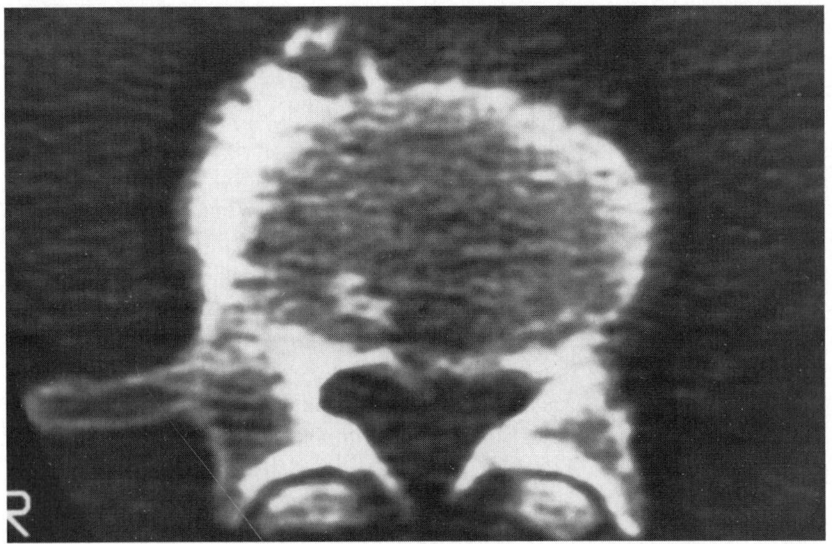

A

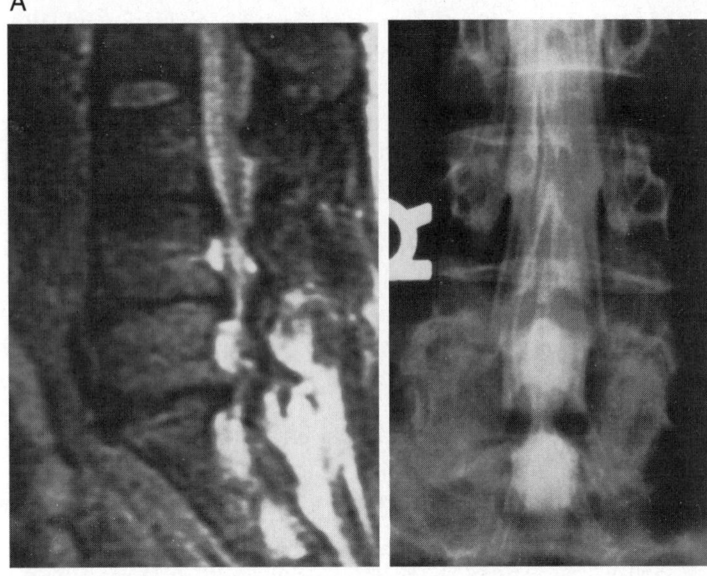

B C

Figure 16.38. Lumbar spinal canal stenosis—CT and MRI. **A.** Axial CT shows a triangular canal and massive short pedicles. **B.** On T2-weighted MRI sagittal view there is diffuse diminution of the anteroposterior diameter of the spinal canal from L2-L3 to L5-S1. At the disc levels there is greater narrowing, which is often due to a dorsal indentation produced by the laminae and ligamentum flavum, as well as a ventral indention produced by osteophytes and disc bulging. The T2-weighted myelographic effect is useful in estimating canal width by MRI. CT is usually preferred in the diagnosis of spinal stenosis. **C** to **E.** Acquired lumbar canal stenosis due to some disc bulging or protrusion and marked thickening of ligamentum flavum. **C.** Frontal myelogram shows bilateral narrowing at L5-S1. **D.** At L4-L5 there is a normal-sized spinal canal and a slightly triangular thecal sac due to thickening of the ligamentum flavum. **E.** At L5-S1 there is a pronounced thickening of the ligamentum flavum bilaterally, causing marked triangular narrowing of the thecal sac but only minor protrusion of the intervertebral disc.

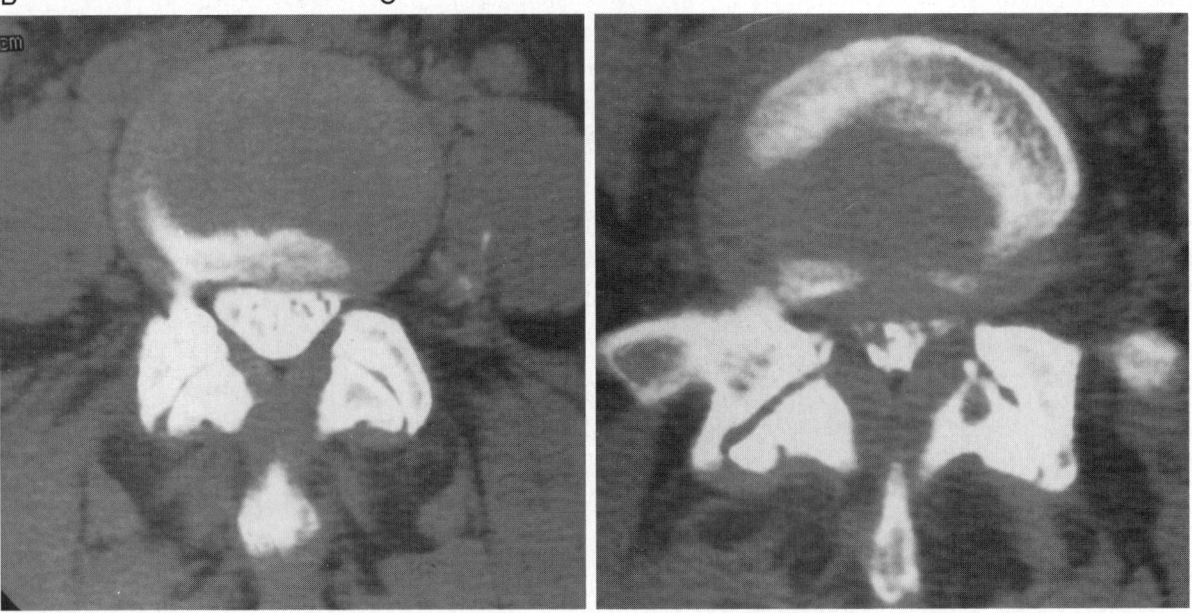

D E

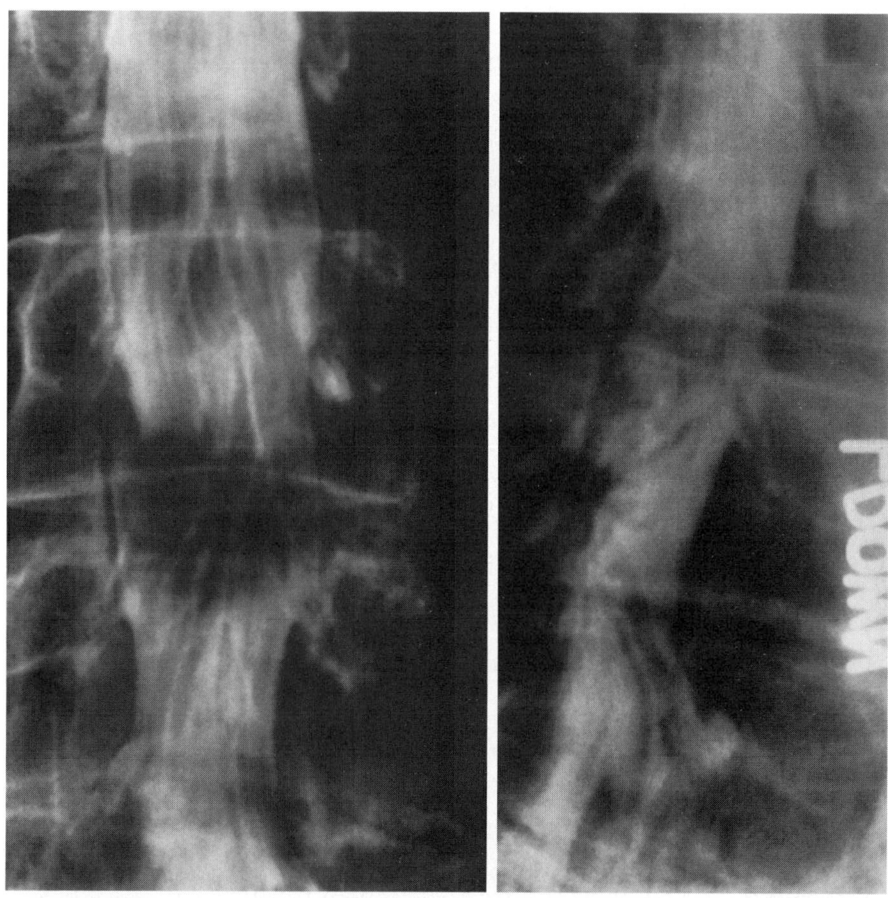

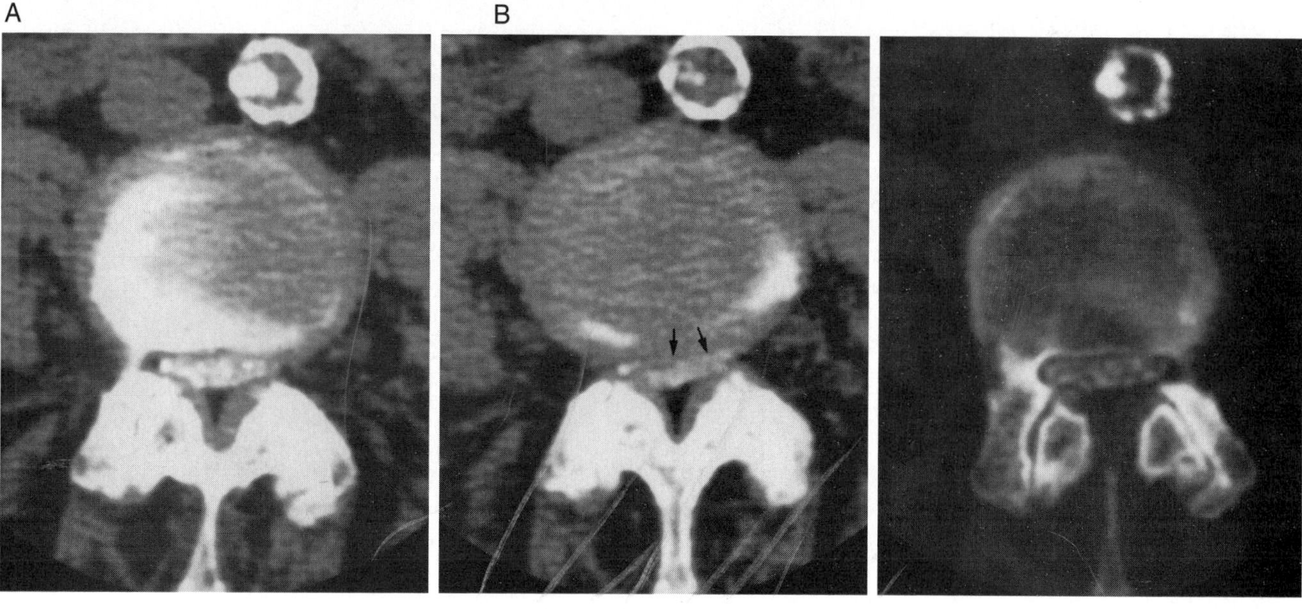

Figure 16.39. Lumbar canal stenosis. **A** and **B.** Myelography reveals a large filling defect at L3-L4. In B, an oblique view, there is elongation of a number of roots within the thecal sac. In A the canal is flattened and wide as shown in CT-myelography (**C**). The posterior angle between the laminae is narrow, and the narrowing is exaggerated by the marked thickening of the ligamentum flavum. There is also osteoarthritic hypertrophy of the apophyseal joints. **D.** Another section passing through the disc where the contrast was pressed out shows what might be interpreted as a centrally, broadly herniated intervertebral disc. However, there is enough contrast there, and the image in C indicates that this is a flattened, broadened thecal sac (arrows). There was no disc herniation, but the disc is broadened circumferentially, more so anterolaterally, as shown in C. **E.** The bone window demonstrates the hypertrophied apophyseal joints to better advantage.

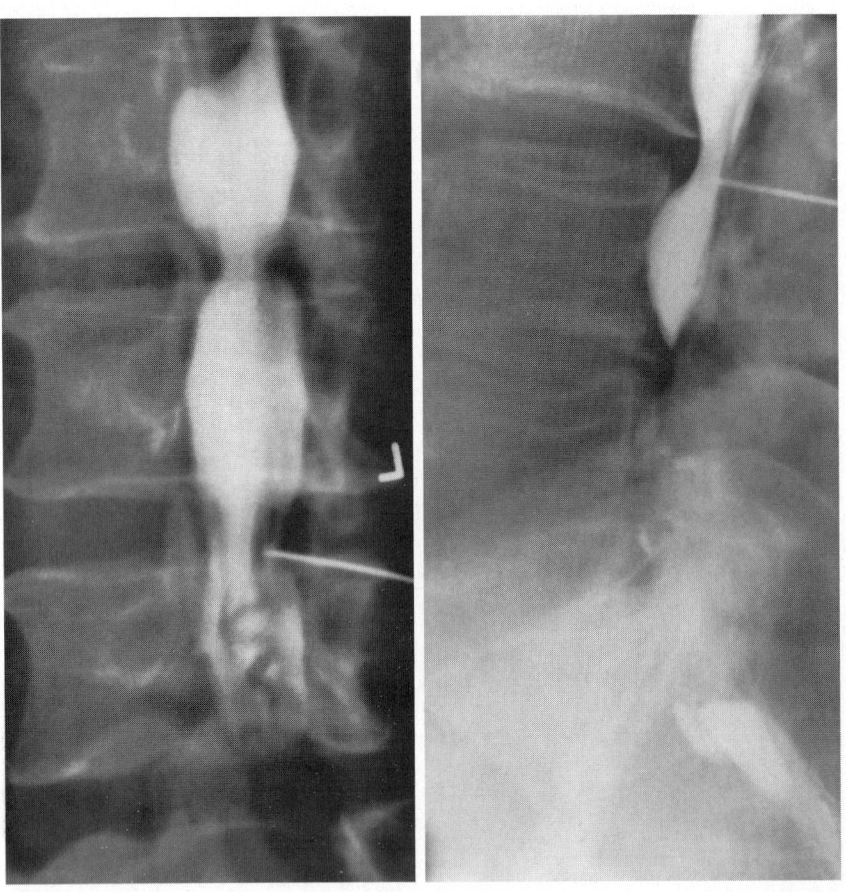

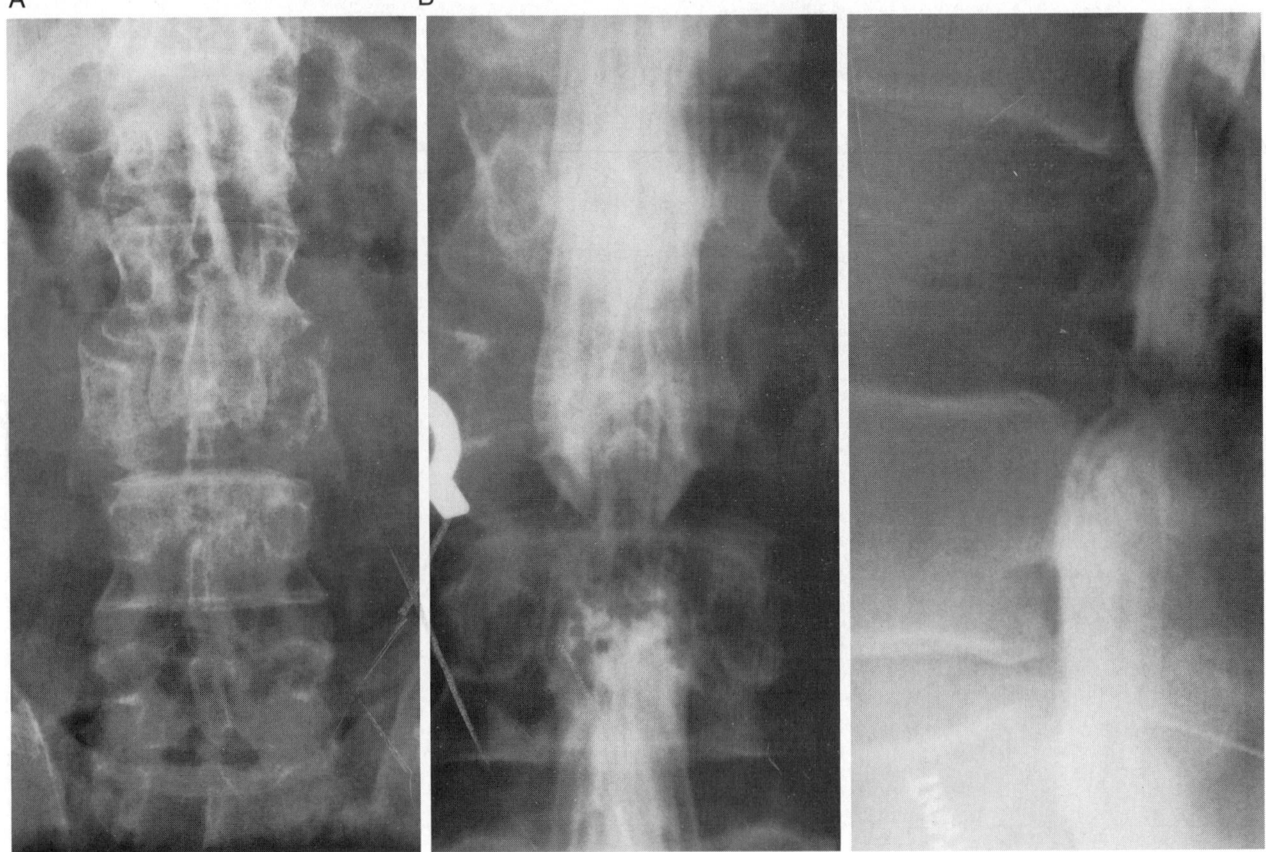

Figure 16.40. A and **B.** Elongated root simulating vascular anomaly in patient with spinal stenosis. **A.** The serpentine image is seen at the L4 level. **B.** There is an almost complete block at L4-L5, with only slight deviation of the opaque column. The dura mater was opened at the time of laminectomy, and the redundant root escaped and could not be replaced without adding a dural patch graft. **C** to **E.** Spinal stenosis associated with Paget disease. **C.** Frontal view showing widened L3 vertebral body. Frontal (**D**) and lateral (**E**) myelographic views demonstrate the dorsally compressed thecal sac. Note that there are serpentine images representing elongated roots in the immediate vicinity of the stenotic segment. This suggests that the elongation of the roots is a response to chronic diminished space for the roots of the cauda equina.

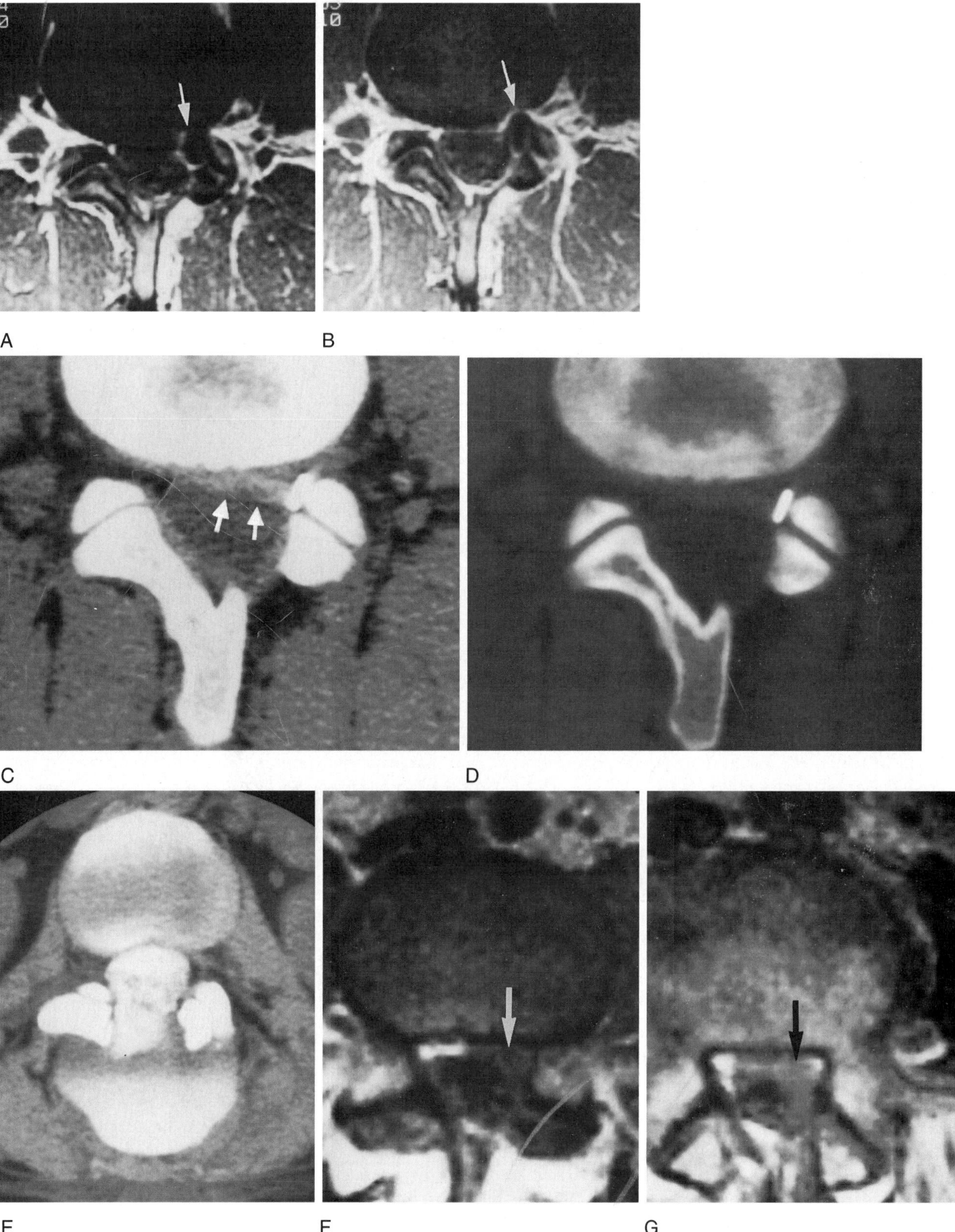

Figure 16.41. Postoperative spine—CT and MRI demonstrating a defect that simulated a recurrent disc but was an artifact on MR images. **A.** Precontrast T1-weighted image shows defect on left, the site of previous surgery (arrow). **B.** After contrast the defect is similar. There is virtually no evidence of postoperative fibrosis. **C.** CT shows focal protrusion in the areas of previous surgery suggestive of recurrent herniation (open arrows). There is no evidence of postoperative fibrosis on the dorsolateral side. There is a left laminectomy defect. **D.** A bone window reveals the metallic clip more clearly. Possibly the metal clip produced an artifact that made the protruding disc invisible. **E.** Postoperative pseudomeningocele (in another patient) shown by CT-myelography. There is a sac filled with contrast in the supine position. **F.** Another case of postoperative lumbar disc surgery. T1-weighted image shows suggestion of a recurrent disc hernia (arrow). **G.** Postcontrast axial image shows enhancement in the same area (arrow), indicating that this is most likely a fibrotic scar.

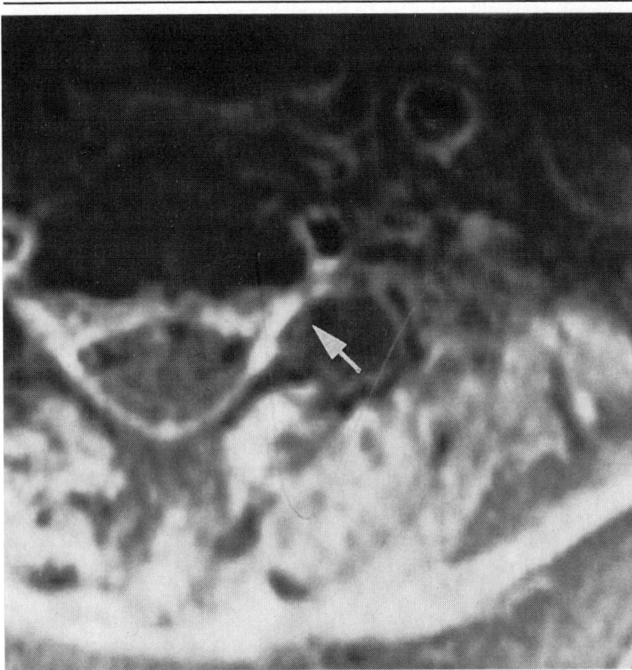

Figure 16.42. Narrowing of the cervical root canal produced by dorsolateral compression from osteophytes arising in the articular facets (arrow).

when actually a herniated intervertebral disc or spinal cord tumor is the cause of the patient's distress.

The osteophytes are actually preformed in cartilage and later ossify in three stages described by Hauser et al.: the cartilaginous stage; the intermediate stage, in which ossification begins at the base of the cartilaginous cap; and the final stage, in which the ossification is complete, often capped by a layer of cartilage (39).

An MRI or CT examination is advisable when an evaluation of the significance of osteoarthritic changes seen on plain radiographs is desired. MRI is preferable because it will clearly demonstrate the relationship of osteophytic ridges to the roots or to the spinal cord. The osteophytes may come from the vertebral bodies centrally or laterally, or they may arise from the apophyseal joints, in which case they will produce compression on the lateral aspect of the nerve root (Fig. 16.42). The osteophytes can usually be differentiated from a herniated disc on CT or on CT-myelography (Fig. 16.43 and 16.44). However, on MRI it may be difficult to differentiate between an osteophyte and a herniated calcified disc (Fig. 16.45). A herniated disc on MRI usually shows the hyperintensity of the disc (Fig. 16.50). Plain CT or MRI may provide a diagnosis without the need for an invasive procedure. As indicated previously, myelography is always followed by CT for best results. Sometimes the osteoarthritic changes are associated with a congenitally narrow cervical spinal canal. Under these circumstances, a smaller ridge may produce severe cord compression, and later cord degeneration and atrophy (Fig. 16.46).

Cervical canal stenosis is often unrecognized until it is too late, when cord atrophy has ensued. The treatment is surgical and requires extensive laminectomy to accomplish adequate decompression.

The most significant factor in the production of compression of the spinal cord by osteoarthritic ridges is perhaps the width of the spinal canal in its anteroposterior diameter. This is variable in normal individuals, and measurements of 13 to 20 mm in anteroposterior diameter are encountered in the cervical spine measured from the posterior margin of the vertebral bodies to the anterior margin of the spinous processes. Measurements under 13 mm are often encountered in patients who have neurologic signs secondary to spondylosis with compression of the spinal cord. In a survey of this subject performed by Pallis et al., it was found that the most significant factor that seemed to predispose the patient to the production of symptoms was the congenitally narrow spinal canal (40). Investigation of patients admitted to a general hospital to services other than neurology showed, on careful neurologic examination, the presence of frequent neurologic deficits of root compression in some cases, and cord compression in others, that were not sufficiently severe to bring the patients in this older age group to the neurologic service. It was found that the patients who presented signs of cord compression were those vertebral canals of a smaller anteroposterior diameter. It is still argued whether the symptoms are produced strictly by cord compression from the osteoarthritic ridges accompanied by the protruding disc that always accompanies the osteophytes, or whether the cord degenerates as a result of continued long-standing compression. It is felt that, in the initial stages, the symptoms are produced by cord compression and may not be too severe. In an older patient, symptoms may be disregarded as related to old age by the patient and the patient's family (Fig. 16.47). Later, when the symptoms become aggravated with the passage of time, the patient may seek

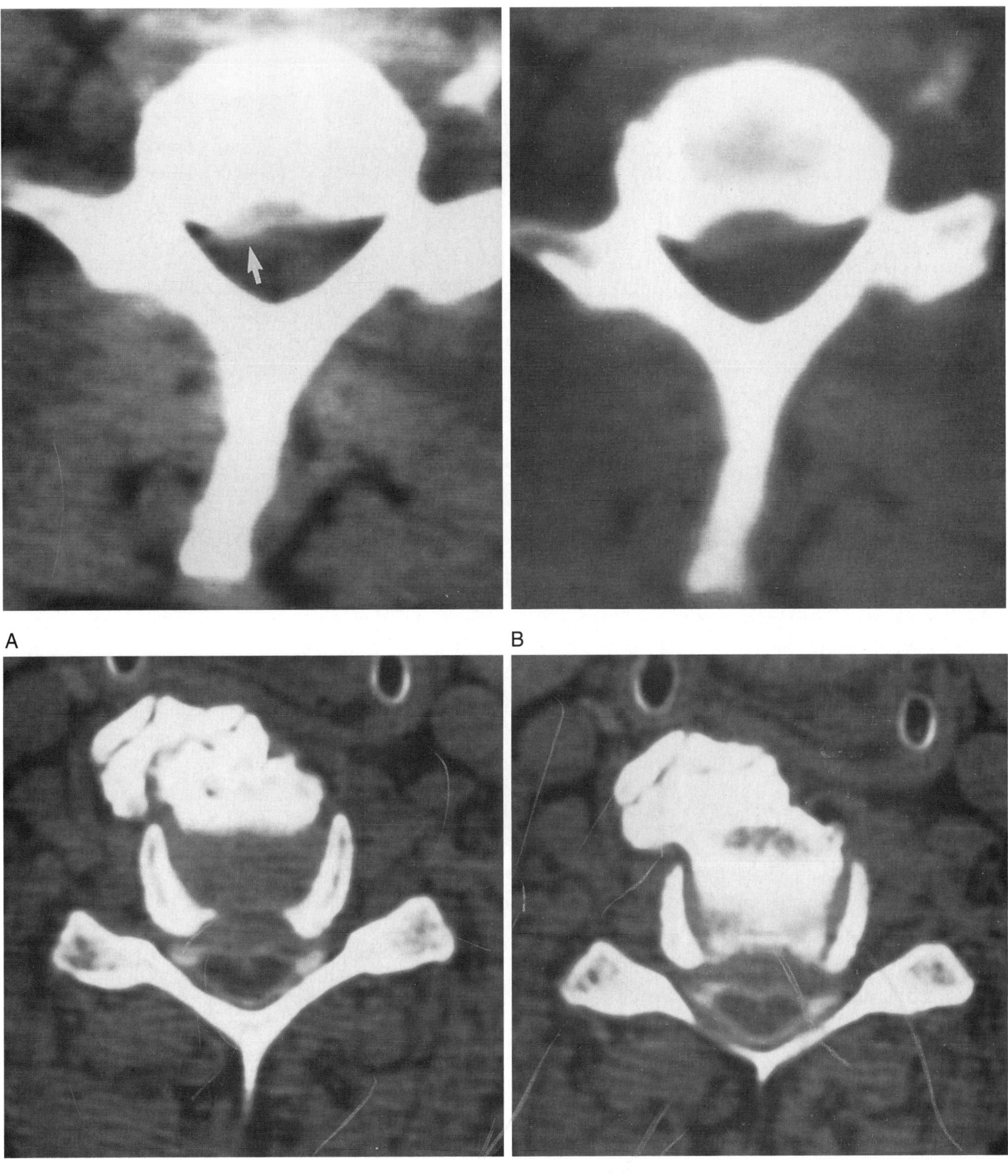

Figure 16.43. Cervical herniated intervertebral disc shown by CT. Soft tissue axial (**A**) and bone window (**B**) demonstrating a right-sided disc herniation (arrow). **C** and **D.** Very large anterior osteophytes arising from the vertebral bodies of C5-C6. There is also a large soft-tissue mass posteriorly, representing a disc herniation that is compressing the anterior subarachnoid space and flattening the spinal cord. No osteophytes are seen dorsally in this CT-myelogram.

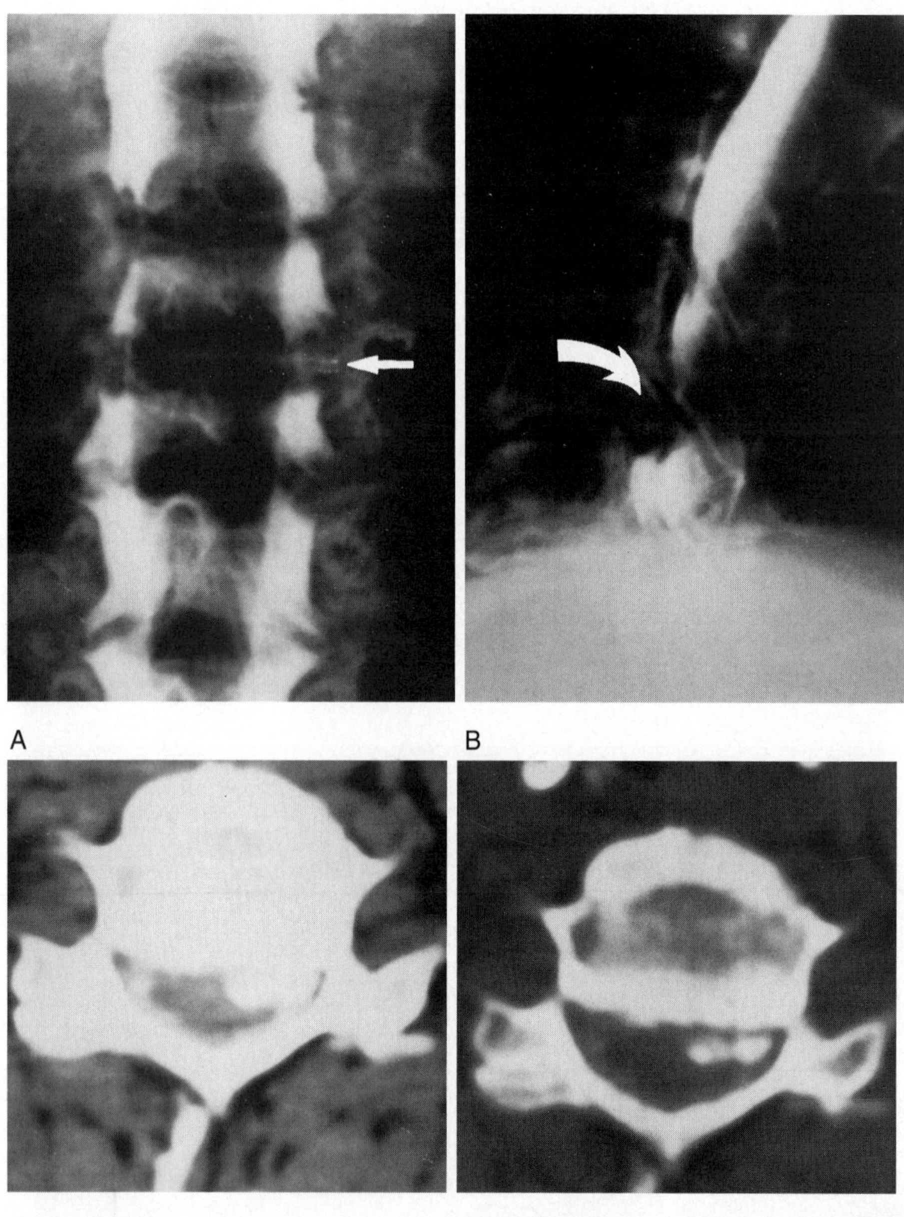

Figure 16.44. Calcified herniated cervical disc—CT-myelography. **A.** Frontal and lateral views made during myelography show multiple defects on the ventral surface and root widening at C4-C5 and C5-C6 on the right and at C5-C6 and C6-C7 on the left. At the level of the arrow the spinal cord shows slight widening due to flattening. **B.** Lateral prone view shows a large, slightly double-contoured ventral defect at C5-C6 (at arrow). **C.** CT soft tissue window shows a large, dense mass on the left side of the canal at C5-C6. **D.** The bone window shows that the mass is calcified and most likely represents a herniated disc. There is very little contrast at this level, as seen on the frontal myelographic view.

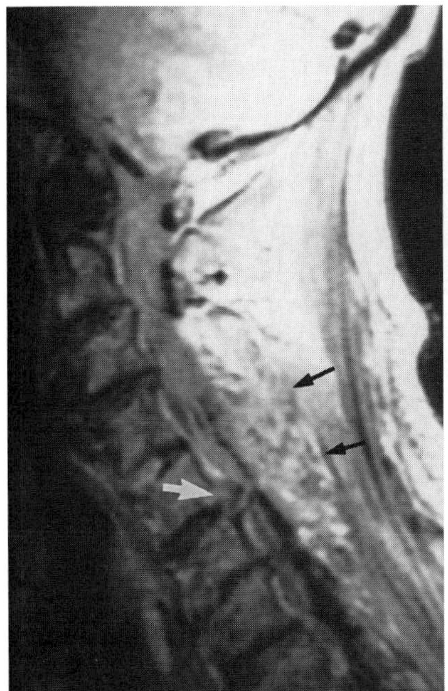

A

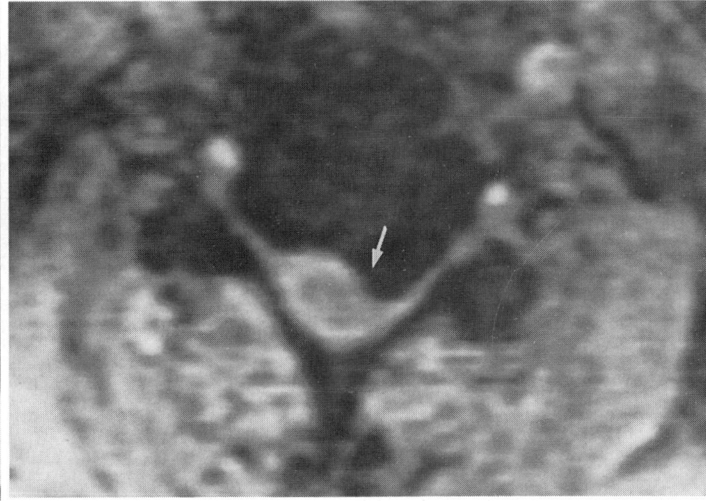

B

Figure 16.45. Large osteophyte, producing root displacement and compression. **A.** The patient had a previous surgical procedure at C3-C4 (arrows). There is a ventral indentation now at C5-C6, as is common following fixation at a higher level owing to stress at the level below (white arrow). The C4-C5 disc is light representing a bone graft. **B.** Axial view of C5-C6 demonstrates a hypointense mass displacing and deforming the left side of the thecal sac and root due to a large osteophyte (arrow). However, it is not possible to differentiate this from a herniated calcified disc by MRI alone (see Fig. 16.44).

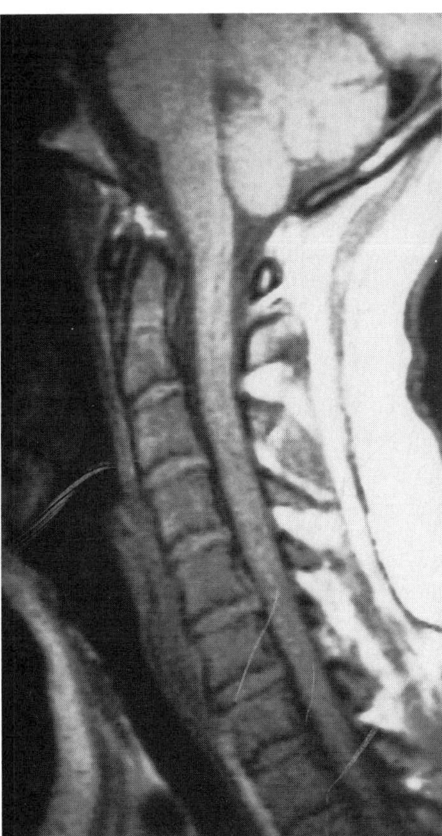

A

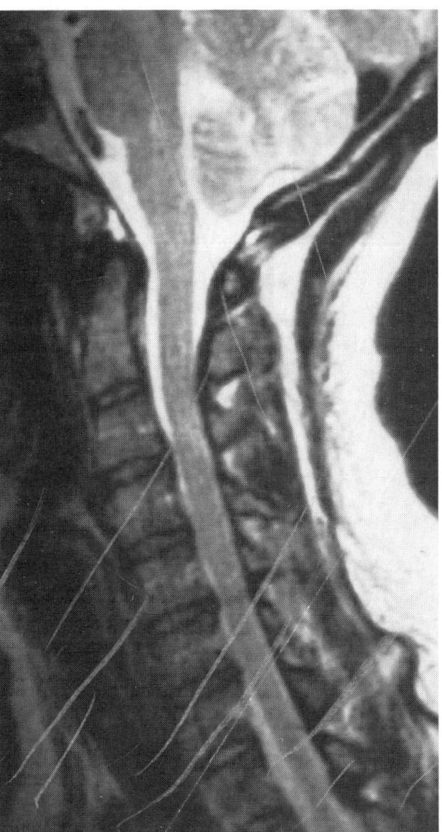

B

Figure 16.46. Borderline narrow cervical spinal canal in a 27-year-old woman. **A.** T1-weighted sagittal image shows that the cord seems to be touching the anterior and posterior margins of the canal. A slight bulge of the C5-C6 disc is producing minimal flattening of the cord. **B.** T2-weighted image confirms the almost complete absence of CSF anterior and posterior to the cord from C3-C4 to C6-C7. Under these circumstances, a moderate degree of osteophyte formation and thickening of ligamentum flavum dorsally would produce chronic spinal cord compression, which could lead to cord degeneration and atrophy.

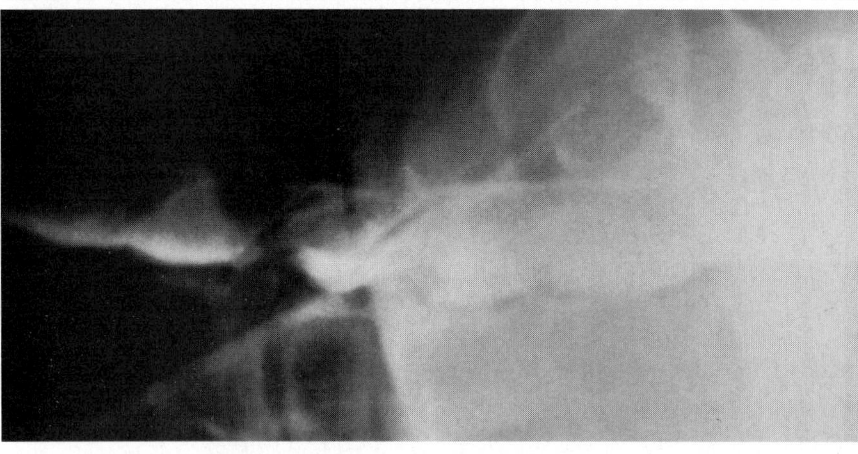

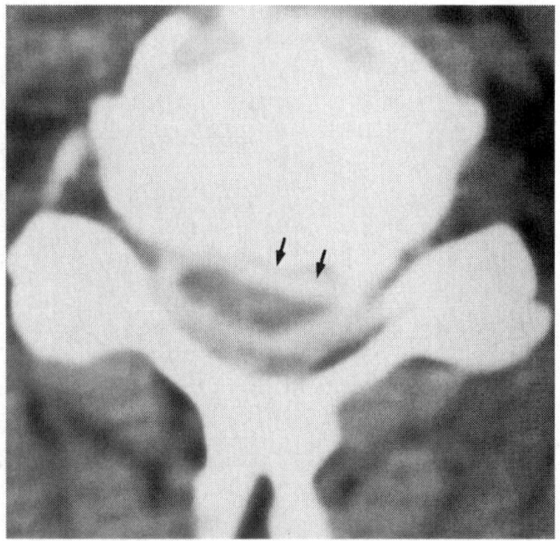

A B

Figure 16.47. Cervical osteoarthritis with cord compression—CT-myelography. **A.** The lateral myelogram reveals a large osteoarthritic ridge at C5-C6 reaching the spinal cord in this lateral view made in swimmer's position. **B.** The axial view reveals a wide vertebral body with large osteoarthritic ridge, larger on the left side, which is flattening and compressing the spinal cord (arrows).

medical help; when an imaging examination is performed, cord atrophy may be demonstrated. Under these circumstances, surgical intervention and decompression of the spinal cord would be foolish, inasmuch as the cord is no longer compressed. Surgical intervention is only advisable when compression of the spinal cord is actually demonstrated. The subject has been thoroughly reviewed in another publication (41).

On plain-film examinations, an osteoarthritic ridge may be considered as significant when it encroaches on 25 to 30 percent of the anteroposterior diameter of the vertebral canal at the same level. In a patient with a 13-mm or smaller anteroposterior spinal diameter, an osteoarthritic ridge measuring 3 mm is highly significant, whereas in a patient with an anteroposterior diameter of 18 mm, a ridge of this size may not be significant.

On plain films it is not possible to tell whether a visible ridge is in the center of the vertebral body without tomography. CT scanning is the procedure of choice to study osteoarthritis of the spine. But in the evaluation of the spinal cord and its relationship to the bony canal, the amount of CSF cushion in front and in back of the cord, MRI is far superior to CT without myelographic contrast (Fig. 16.46). It approaches CT-myelography in the evaluation of this condition. Myelography may show a block to the upward flow of contrast or a series of ridges producing complete or almost complete disappearance of the contrast at these levels (Figs. 16.44, 16.47, and 16.51).

Osteoarthritis involving the uncovertebral joints (joints of Luschka) is common. It may directly compress and displace the roots dorsally (Figs. 16.45). On the contrary, osteoarthritis involving the articular facets displaces the roots medially and forward (Fig. 16.42). On the myelogram uncovertebral joint osteoarthritis produces widening of the root shadow (see Fig. 16.44) and disappearance of the normal rootlets forming the anterior root (see Figs. 16.48*A* and 16.49). The apophyseal joint osteoarthritic spurs displace the contrast medially away from the pedicles and do not disturb the rootlets, which are still visible.

Synovial Cyst

In the cervical as well as in the lumbar region it is possible to encounter an occasional *synovial cyst* that will produce a deformity of the thecal sac. The lesion occurs on the lateral aspect of the canal and may compress the root as well as the adjacent thecal sac. It is more common in the lumbar region. The relationship of the mass to the apophyseal joint is usually clear on CT as well as on MR images, but CT is likely to be superior (Fig. 16.52 and 16.53), particularly if the cyst wall is calcified (42,43). Plain films and tomography may show erosion (44).

Vilonodular synovitis occurs rarely in the cervical region. It may produce an epidural defect associated with severe osteoarthritic changes (45,46).

Ossification of the posterior longitudinal ligament is well seen on plain lateral views of the cervical spine and also on CT axial views. On MR images it may be seen if this possibility is kept in mind; it is best seen on proton density images. If there is bone marrow in the ossified ligament, it is bright on T1-weighted images. The ossified ligaments, which may lead to radiculomyelopathy, are seen in about 2 percent of Japanese, and for this reason the condition is called the *Japanese disease*. It is very uncommon in the United States.

Thoracic Region

Osteoarthritis is not a problem in the thoracic spine. Most osteophyte formation takes place anteriorly and usually has

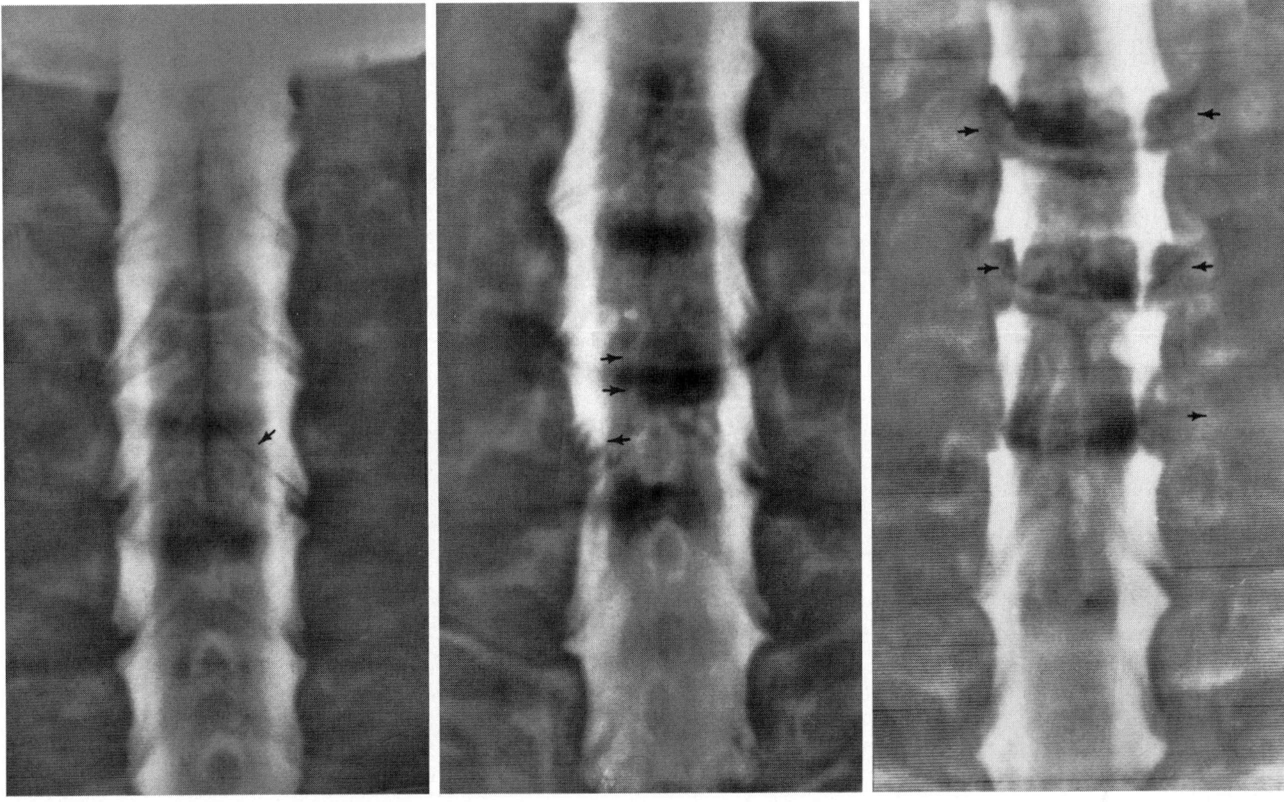

Figure 16.48. Three myelographic images to demonstrate normal, herniated disc, and osteoarthritis of the cervical spine. **A.** Normal. The radiolucent band of the cervical cord occupies approximately two-thirds of the diameter of the opaque column. The sites of exit of the roots are marked by slight protrusion of the lateral margin of the contrast column, and the ventral rootlets can be followed medially at most levels. A radiolucent line produced by the anterior spinal vessels is seen running up and down the center of the spinal cord. A radicular artery is seen to join the anterior spinal artery (arrow). **B.** Single root lesion at C6-C7 on right side due to herniated intervertebral disc. There is a gradual, tentlike displacement of the lateral margin of the contrast column away from the pedicles centered at the root shadow, which is itself slightly elevated (arrows). This is produced by tenting of the dura and is usually associated with acute disc herniation but is usually not present in osteoarthritic spurs because the dura has had time to accommodate to the deformity. In addition to the shadow of the anterior spinal artery, there are other vascular shadows on the cord (two arrows), which may represent engorged veins. Prominent vessels on the cord are often seen in association with acute disc herniations. **C.** Multiple root shadow widening associated with osteoarthritis. There is widening of the root shadow on both sides at the level indicated by arrows. Although this may indicate actual root compression at the time of the myelogram, it is not necessarily symptomatic, and the root may well have accommodated to the elevation of the ventral aspect of the root sleeve produced by osteoarthritic spurs. In this case there is also a ridge extending across the space and interrupting the opaque column. There is no tenting sign. At the lower involved level there is slight widening of the spinal cord due to a ventral bony ridge.

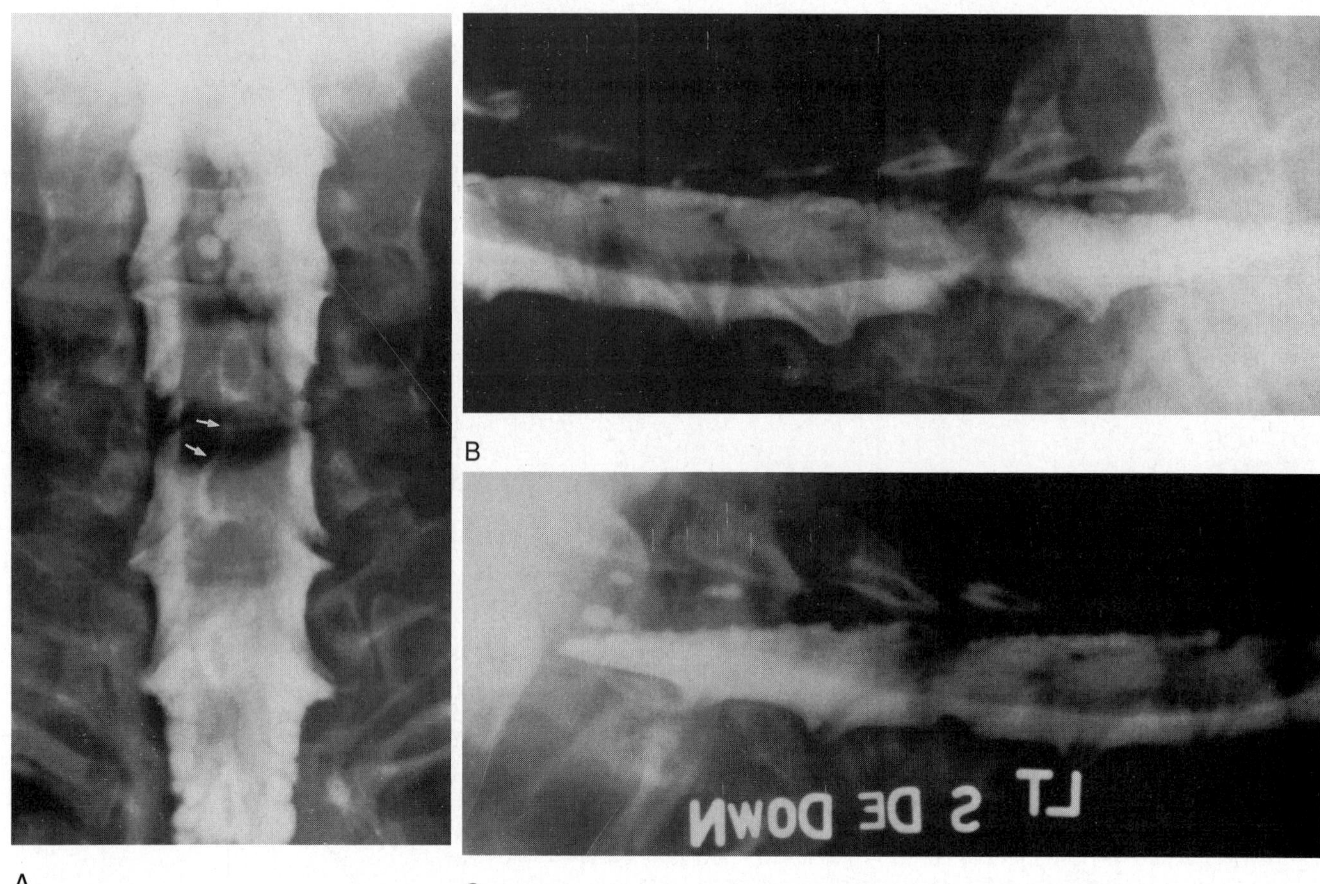

Figure 16.49. Cervical herniated disc and osteoarthritis at the same level on opposite sides seen on myelography. **A.** Frontal view of myelogram shows a bilateral defect. On the right side there is a ventral defect accounting for the low density; a contrast curvilinear contour is also seen (arrow), extending almost to the center of the canal representing the medial margin of a ventral mass effect. **B.** A horizontal beam right oblique view shows the lifting of the contrast produced by the herniated disc. **C.** On the left side oblique with horizontal ray the defect is minimal and confined to the root.

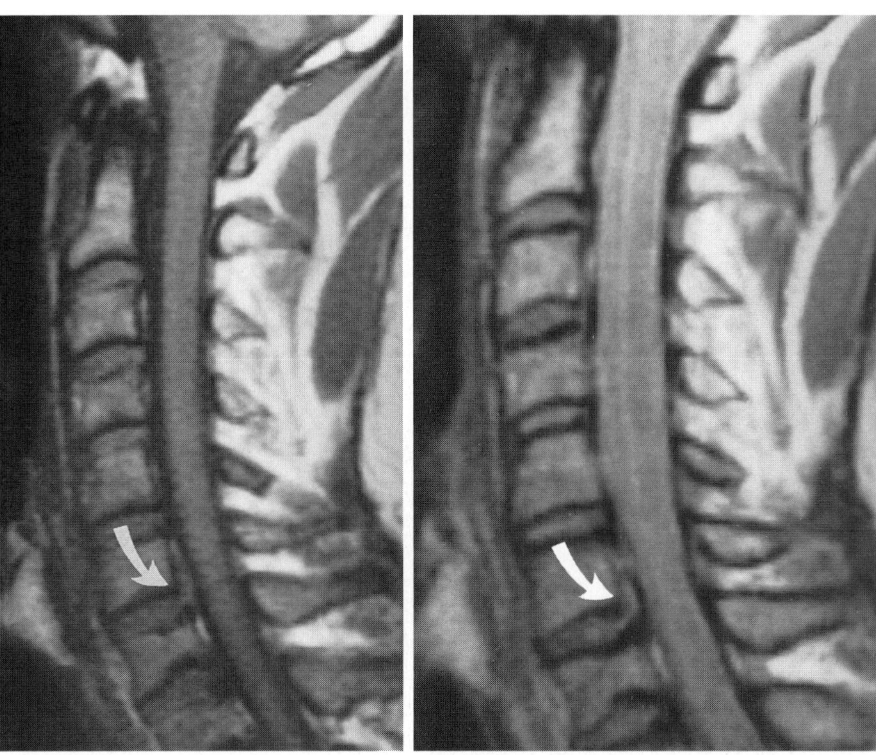

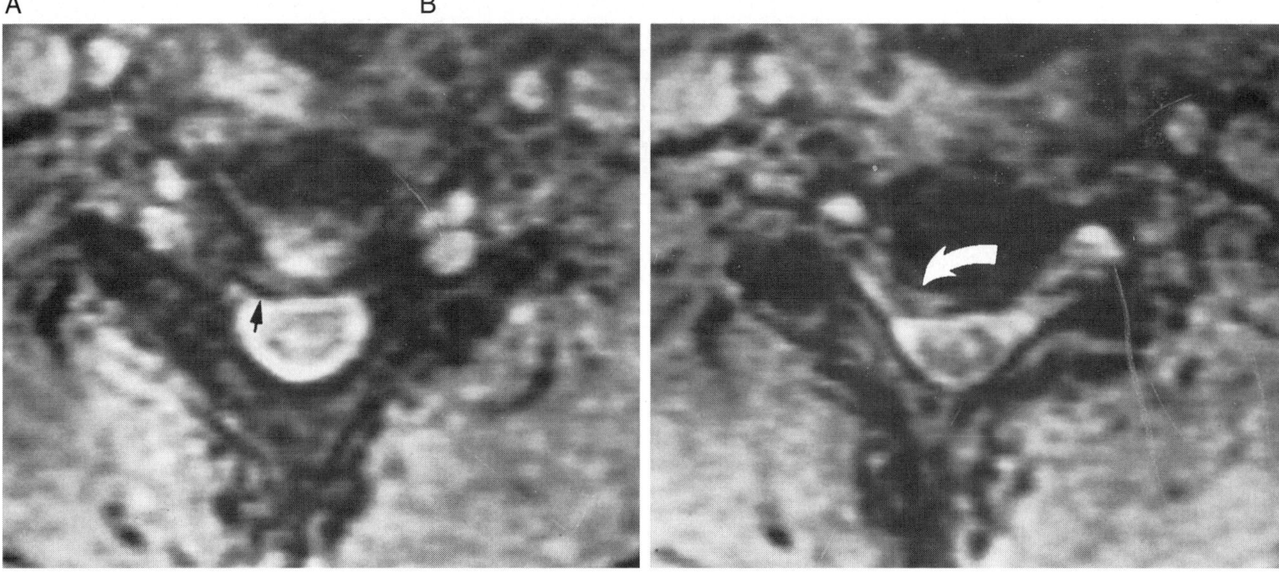

Figure 16.50. Herniated cervical disc demonstrated on MRI. **A.** Sagittal T1-weighted image shows a small area of hyperintensity in the ventral side of the canal starting at the C6-C7 intervertebral disc and extending cephalad (arrow). **B.** The proton density weighted image reveals the same abnormalities (arrow). **C.** Axial T2-weighted image reveals, at the disc level, a slight hyperintense area on the right side (arrow). **D.** A section just above C passing through the lower vertebral body of C6 demonstrates the herniation that has moved cephalad and is compressing the neural canal on the right (curved arrow).

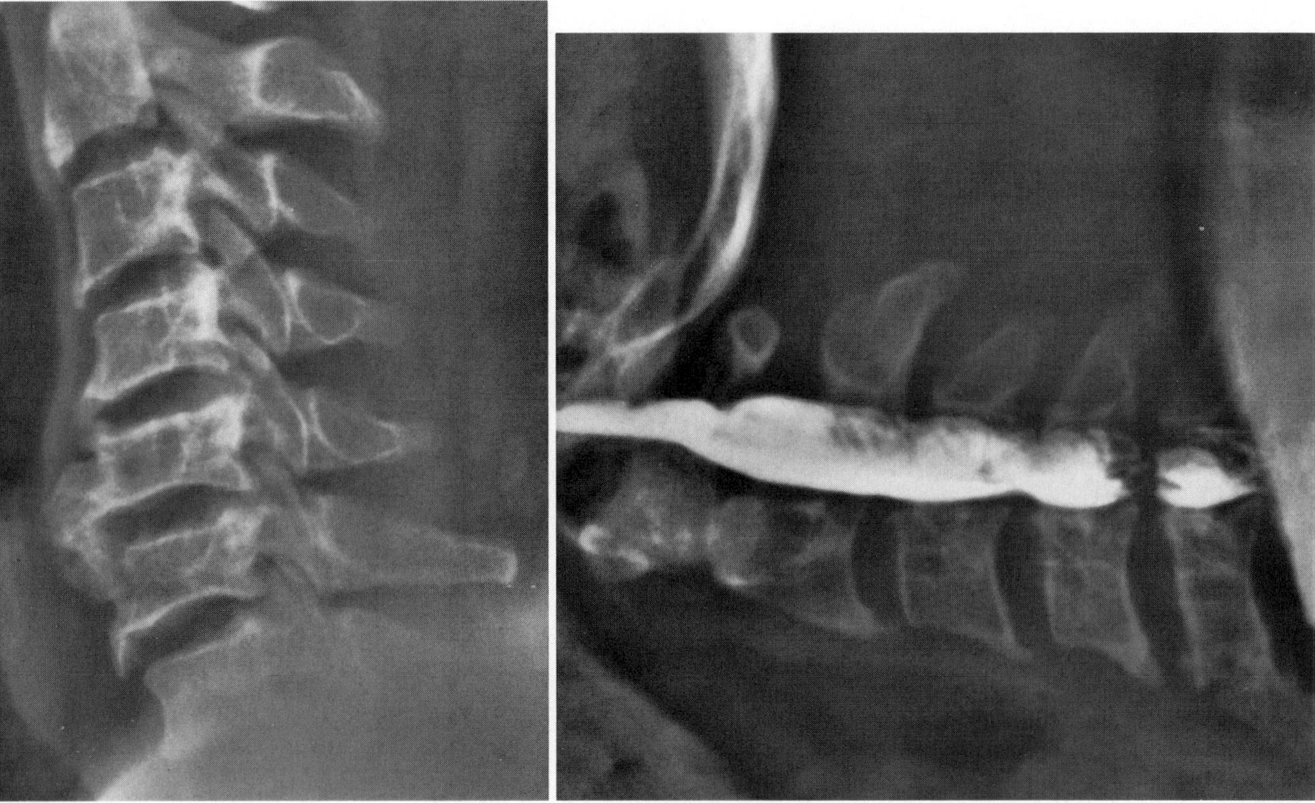

A B

Figure 16.51. Congenitally narrow spinal canal in cervical region with severe neurologic disturbances. **A.** The plain-film lateral view discloses a narrow spinal canal, which at C4, C5, and C6 measures only 11 to 12 mm in anteroposterior diameter. The posterior margin of the articular pillar almost overlies the anterior margin of the spinous process. When this is seen, it indicates a marginally narrow cervical canal. A mild degree of posterior osteophyte formation is present. **B.** In the prone lateral myelogram, only relatively small ventral indentations are present at C4-C5 and at C5-C6. The patient had a moderate paraparesis and, at the time of admission, was actually unable to walk. Following surgical decompression, the symptoms improved considerably.

no clinical significance. Osteophytic ridge formation is sometimes observed in the thoracic region, usually following trauma or infection, but usually the ridge does not produce neurologic findings.

The thoracic spine is examined by plain films, MRI, and CT. MRI is superior to CT, since CT requires localization of the area in question first, by other methods, before the appropriate level can be decided for axial images. MRI allows for sagittal as well as coronal and axial images (Fig. 16.53) and demonstrates the spinal cord with great clarity.

Thoracic myelography is always followed by CT, for it is usually difficult to obtain a complete visualization owing to the curve of the spine. Myelography is useful to visualize the surface vessels in order to rule out a vascular malformation (Fig. 16.54). In combination with CT it is also used in the diagnosis of thoracic herniated discs (Fig. 16.55). However, MRI turns out to be sufficient in most cases; CT-myelography is needed in only some cases (Fig. 16.56). Interestingly enough, some thoracic disc herniations are discovered accidentally in plain films or on CT examinations of the thorax (Fig. 16.57). A large percentage of herniated thoracic discs are calcified, and there is also calcification in the parent disc. Also it is most common in herniated thoracic discs to find irregularity of the surfaces of the vertebral bodies consistent with some degree of osteochondrosis of vertebral epiphyses (Scheuermann disease) (Figs. 16.55 and 16.56). The most common locations for thoracic herniation are the T10 to L1 levels, but they also occur at higher levels.

CONGENITAL ANOMALIES

Congenital anomalies, often referred to under the generic term *spinal dysraphism*, are divided into three groups:

1. *Open spina bifida*, neural tissue exposed. Includes myelocele and myelomeningocele. An occasional meningocele without skin cover may be encountered.
2. *Occult spina bifida*, a heterogeneous group that includes spinal lipoma, occult meningoceles, dorsal dermal sinus,

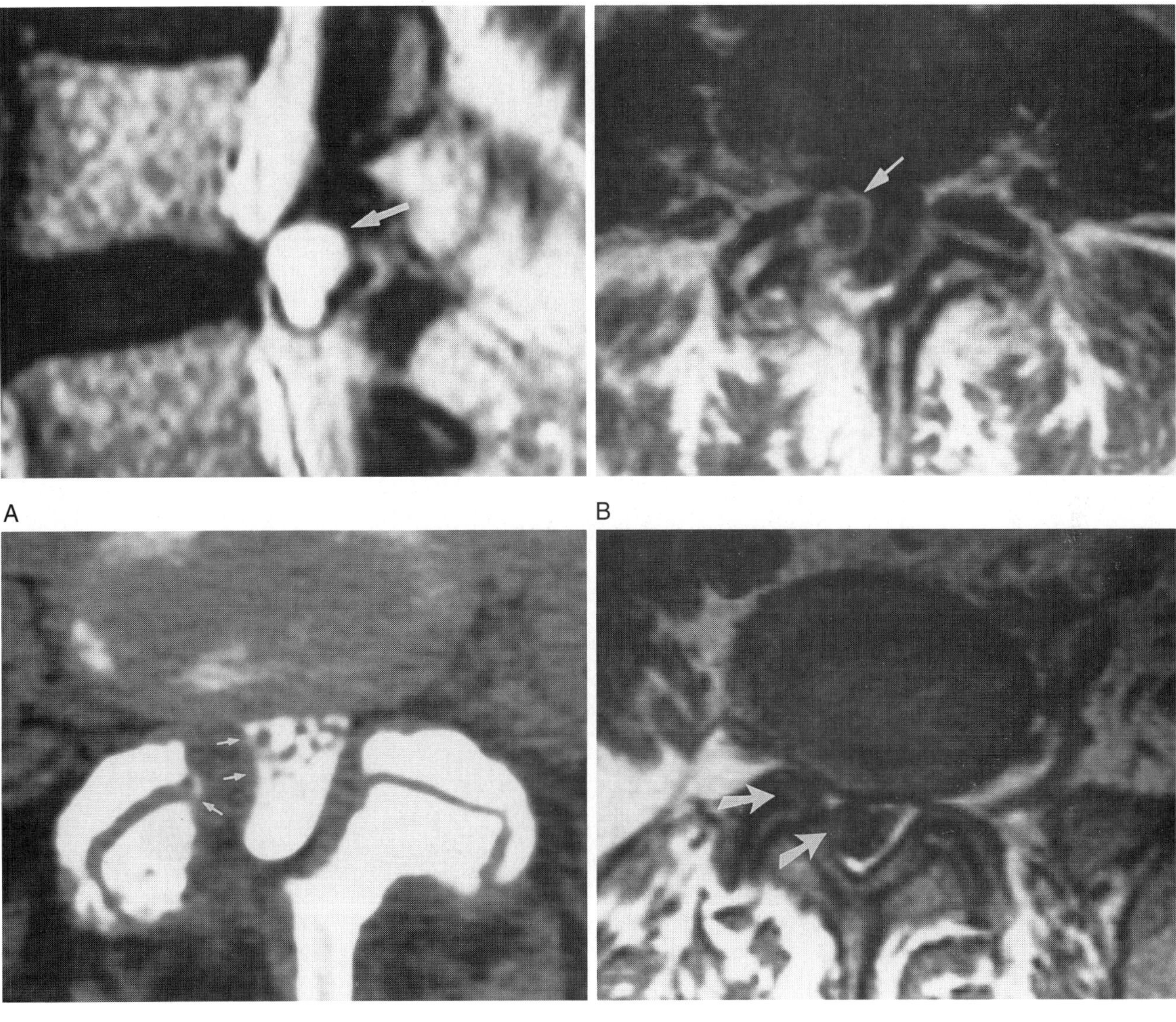

Figure 16.52. Lumbar synovial cyst in a 74-year-old woman complaining of low back pain radiating to the right leg. **A.** Sagittal T2-weighted image shows a cystlike area at the L4-L5 level (arrow). **B.** Axial T1-weighted image shows ring with low-intensity center representing the cystlike area (arrow). **C.** CT-myelography reveals a mild concentric bulge of the intervertebral disc. There is soft tissue mass with concentric margin, which appears to be centered at the apophyseal joint (arrows). Slight calcification is seen at the edge of the joint, and there is marked bilateral osteoarthritic change in the articular facets. There had been a prior laminectomy at the same level without relief of symptoms. The synovial cysts are more frequent in women, and right-sided lesions seem to be more common than left. **D.** Axial T1-weighted MR image in another patient showing disappearance of the fat rim on the right side of the canal and flattening of the lateral recess (arrows) due to osteoarthritis in the articular facets.

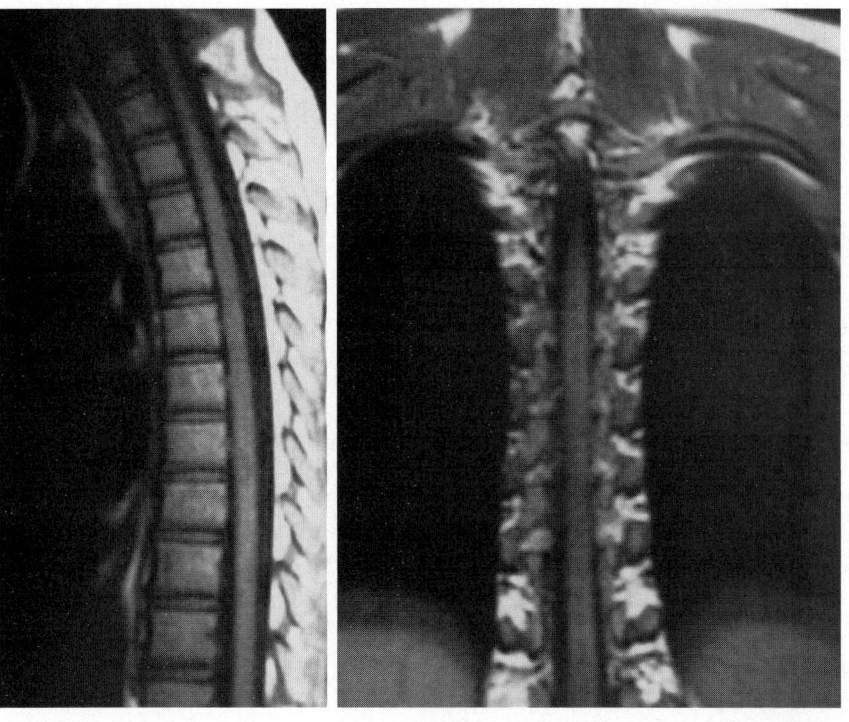

A B

Figure 16.53. Sagittal and coronal T1-weighted images in the thoracic region. **A.** Sagittal T1-weighted. **B.** Coronal T1-weighted. T2-weighted sagittals are shown in Figure 16.8.

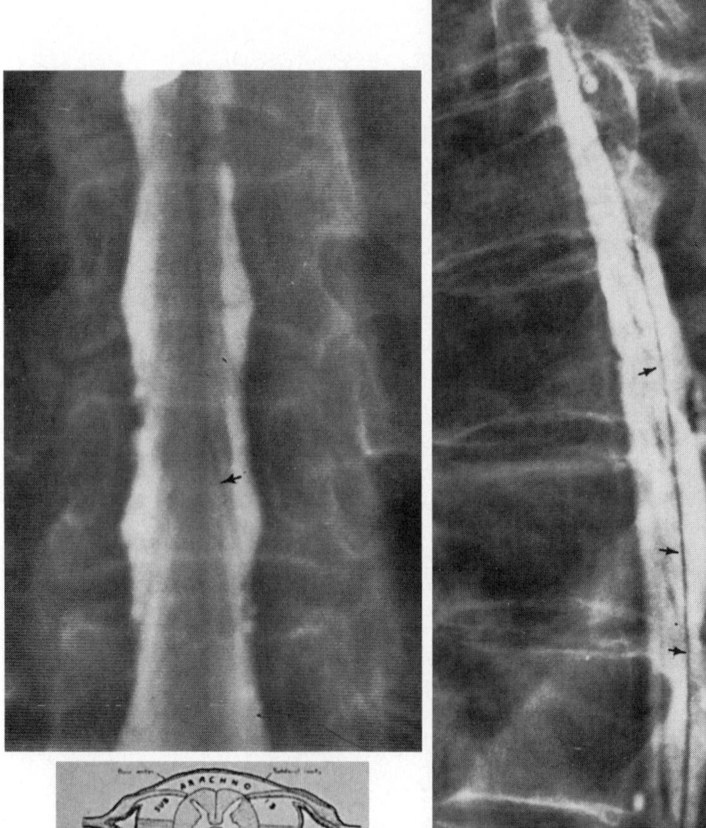

A B

Figure 16.54. Normal thoracic myelogram, patient prone. **A.** Frontal view showing the spinal cord. The anterior spinal artery is shown in the approximate center of the cord. A radicular artery (arrow) is seen joining the anterior spinal artery. Roots are seen on the right moving caudally from the anterolateral aspect of the cord. A diagram is shown at the bottom to indicate the contrast distribution and the absence of contrast on the dorsal surface. **B.** Lateral view taken with patient lying on right side. The contrast would pool on the right side and, if it is desired to show the margin, an across-the-table anteroposterior view can be made. The arrows point at the dentate ligaments, which sometimes form a continuous line, as shown.

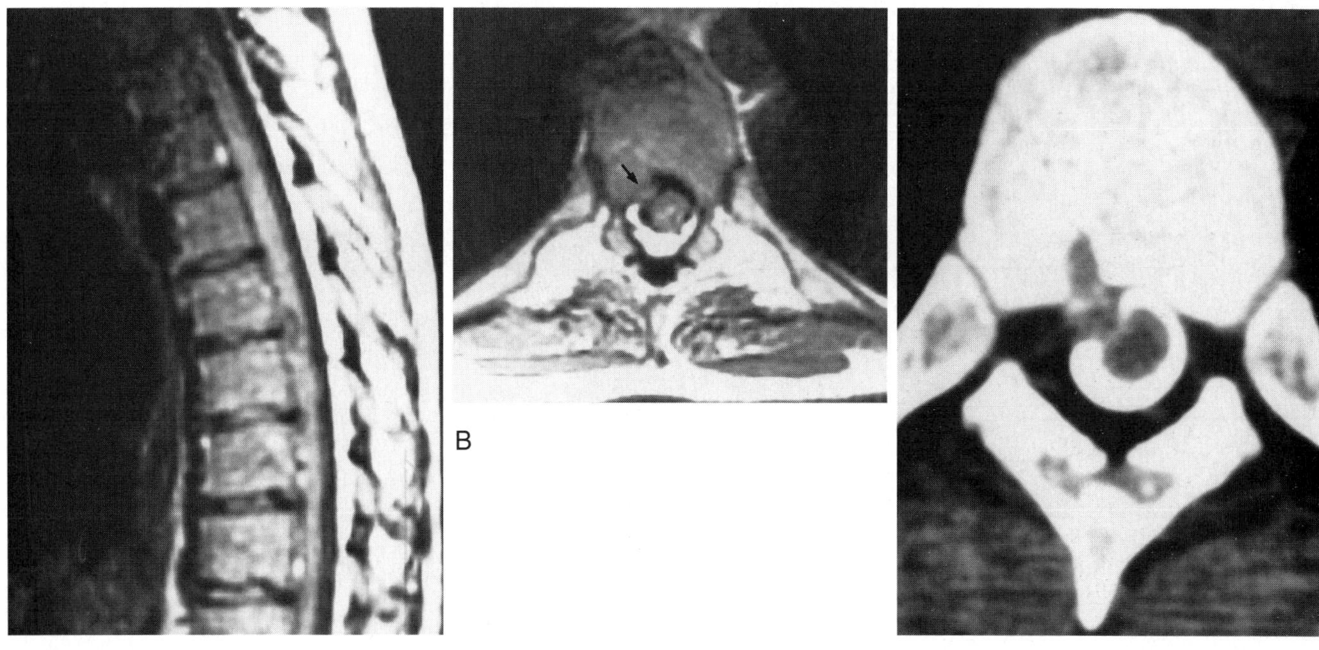

Figure 16.55. Herniated thoracic disc in a 53-year-old woman who complained of sudden onset of pain and a T6 sensory level sparing the posterior column. **A.** Sagittal view shows a ventral extramedullary hypointensity anterior to the cord, which after gadolinium revealed some enhancement (arrow)(**B**). There is irregularity of the vertebral bodies at the discs, which may be due to some degrees of osteochondrosis of the vertebral epiphyses, common in patients with herniated thoracic discs. **C.** CT-myelography shows a calcified herniated disc, as well as calcification in the main disc. The enhancing material on B is probably some granulation tissue in the epidural space. The calcification is represented by the low-intensity area. Calcification in the main disc as well as in the herniated portion is common in the thoracic region.

neurenteric cysts, diastematomyelia, tight filum terminale, and others. There may be external evidence pointing at possible occult pathology (e.g., subcutaneous lipoma, hypertrichosis in patches, skin dimples or tags).

3. *Caudal spinal anomalies*, which include sacral agenesis, anterior sacral meningocele, and terminal myelocystocele (47).

Embryologic Considerations

The spinal cord anomalies are based on disturbances during embryologic development. A short explanation and illustration follow.

NEURULATION

This term refers to the closure of the neural tube. Lack of closure is associated with anomalies. The development starts on the dorsal side of the embryo, going the entire length of it as the neural plate on the surface (the embryonic ectoderm). The development of the notochord slightly precedes that of the neural plate, all within the first 2 to 3 weeks of embryonic life.

The neural plate curves, becoming a groove, and then its edges close, becoming a closed tube. The neural tube then becomes separated from the embryonal skin (ectoderm) by a layer of mesoderm. Another component of the neural plate is the neural crest, which moves to each side as the neural plate closes and eventually will form the dorsal ganglia while the neural tube will form the spinal cord. This completes the initial process of neurulation explained in Figure 16.58.

Closure of the neural tube begins in the cervical portion and progresses caudally as well as rostrally. Interestingly, the lower end of the spinal cord, the conus medullaris, and the filum terminale form from a separate structure, the *caudal cell mass*, which later (around the sixth week) cavitates and forms a tube, covered by ependyma, which unites with the neural tube and forms the conus and filum (Fig. 16.58*F* to *I*). Thus, it is possible to have anomalies involving only the caudal end; indeed, these are much more frequent than those involving the higher levels.

Anomalies result from developmental arrests during the process of neurulation (closure of the neural tube). If the neural tube fails to close quickly or completely in an area, usually lumbar, it allows for growth of mesodermal elements inside the neural tube, as shown in Figure 16.59*A*. They would form lipomas if the lack of closure is protected by incompletely separated ectoderm, and if there is local lack of closure of the neural tube a sinus track forms, as shown in Figure 16.59*A* and *B*.

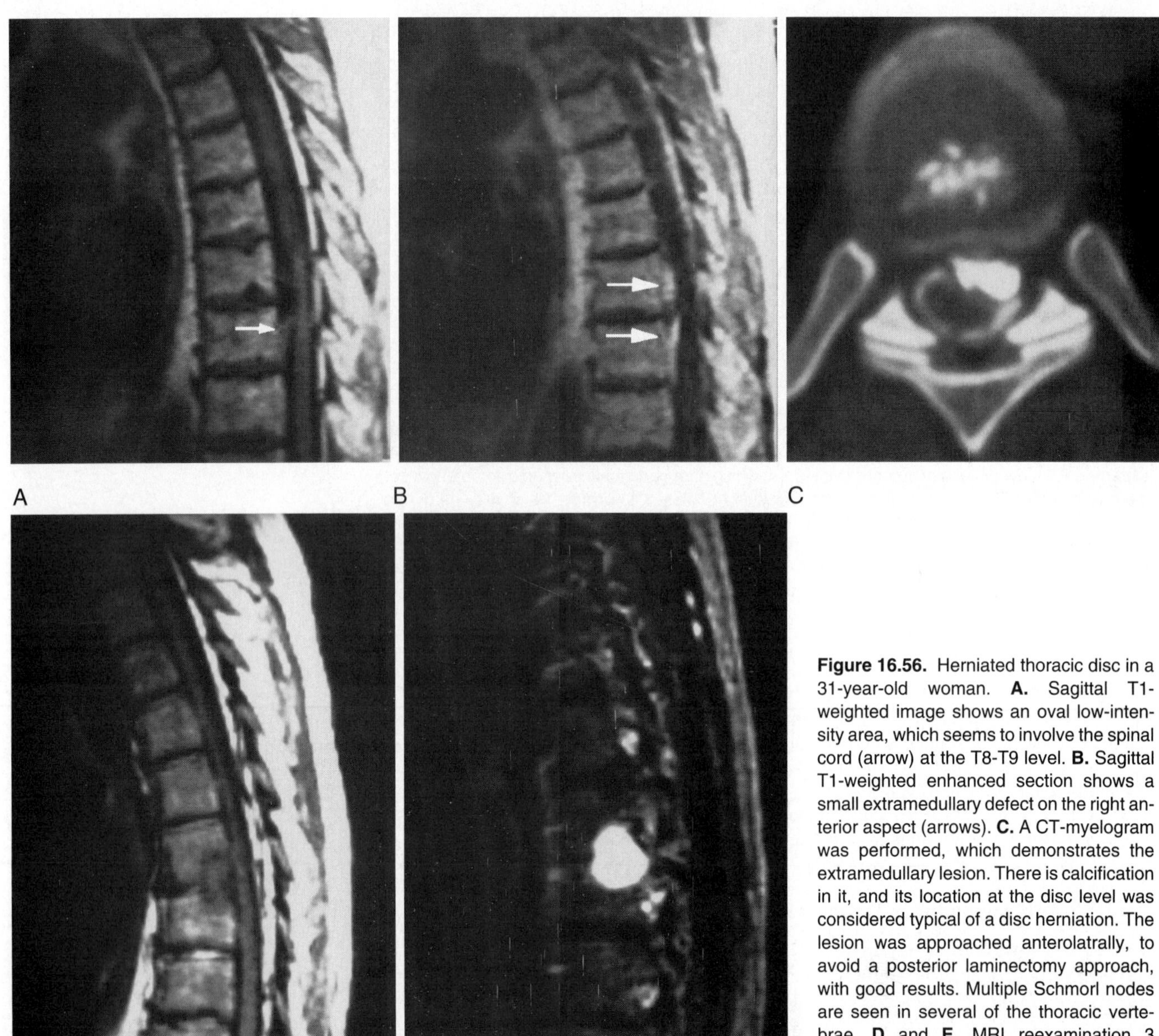

Figure 16.56. Herniated thoracic disc in a 31-year-old woman. **A.** Sagittal T1-weighted image shows an oval low-intensity area, which seems to involve the spinal cord (arrow) at the T8-T9 level. **B.** Sagittal T1-weighted enhanced section shows a small extramedullary defect on the right anterior aspect (arrows). **C.** A CT-myelogram was performed, which demonstrates the extramedullary lesion. There is calcification in it, and its location at the disc level was considered typical of a disc herniation. The lesion was approached anterolatrally, to avoid a posterior laminectomy approach, with good results. Multiple Schmorl nodes are seen in several of the thoracic vertebrae. **D** and **E.** MRI reexamination 3 months later shows a residual cystic space without hemorrhage on T1- and T2-weighted images.

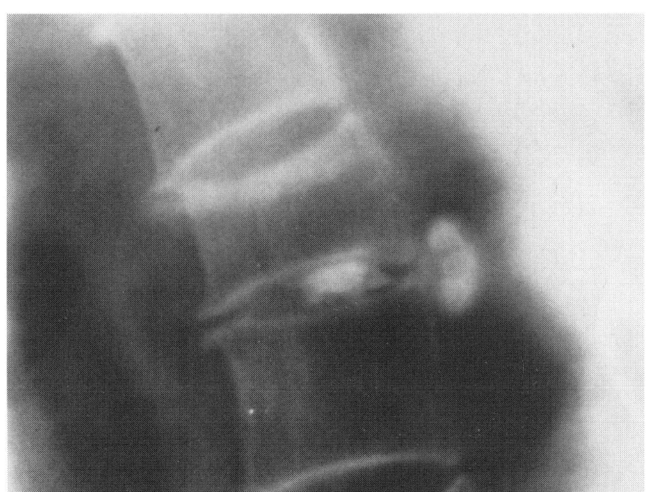

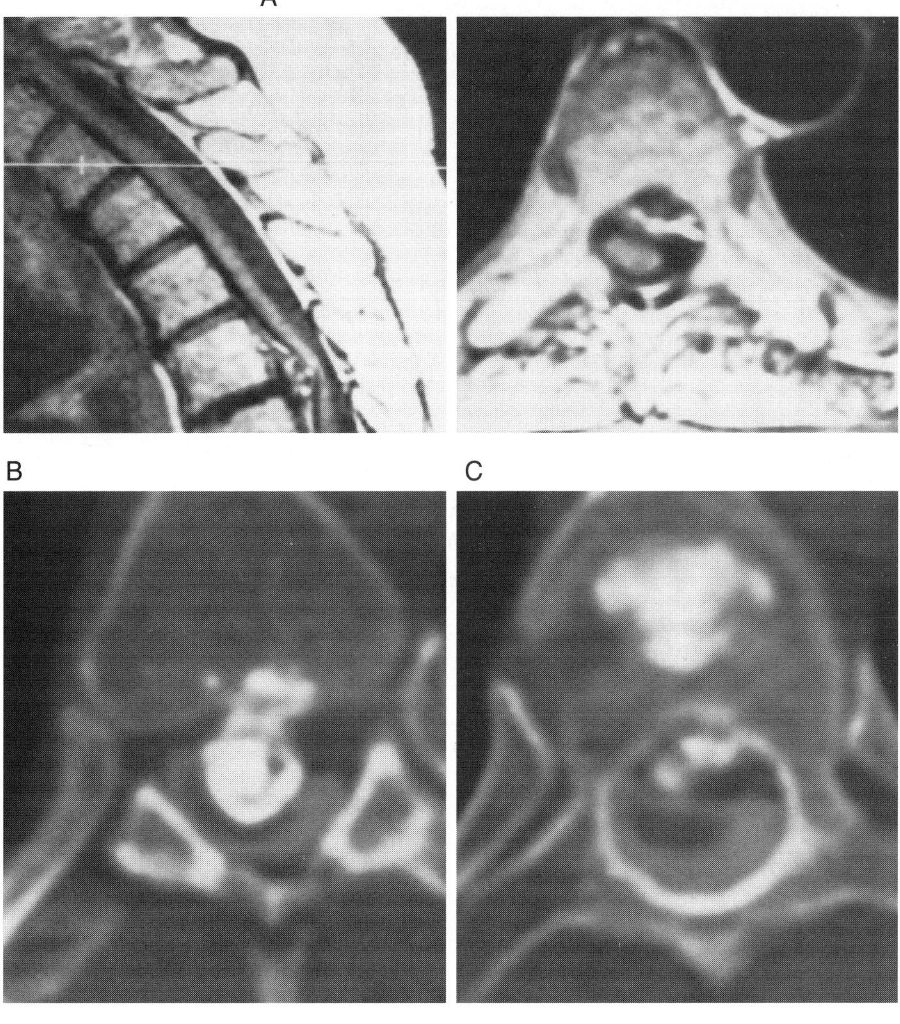

A B C D E

Figure 16.57. A. Asymptomatic large, calcified herniated thoracic intervertebral disc in 70-year-old patient examined for a pulmonary condition. There is a healing compression fracture of the vertebra above, probably related to osteoporosis. **B.** Asymptomatic large thoracic disc in a 68-year-old woman, at T7-T8. Sagittal T1-weighted view shows an irregular-density lesion displacing the spinal cord dorsally. **C.** Axial T1-weighted image shows hyperdensity in the periphery of the lesion. **D.** CT-myelography showed an extensively calcified herniated disc with calcification also in the parent disc (**E**). The T1 hyperintensity may be related to the calcification.

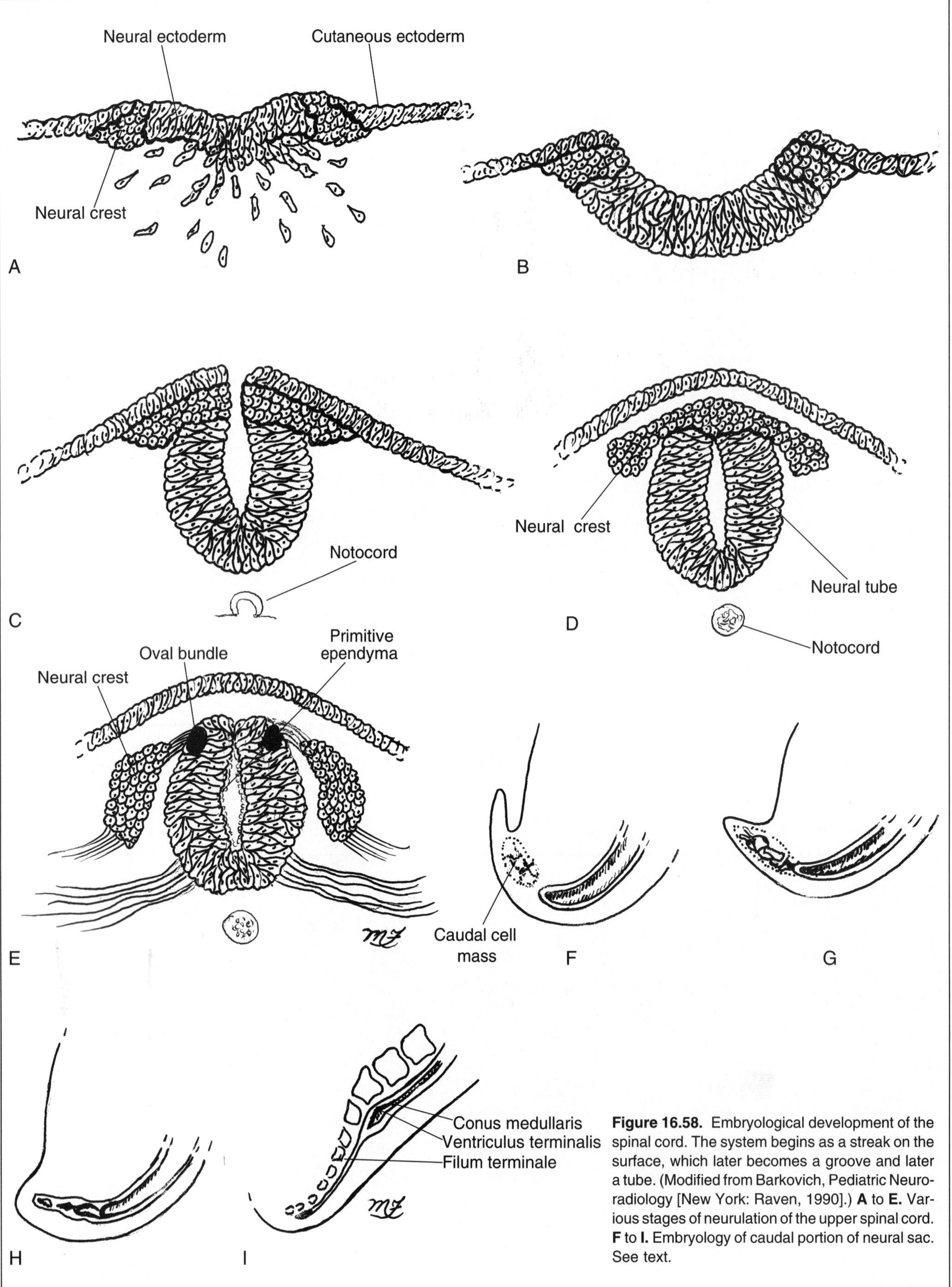

Figure 16.58. Embryological development of the spinal cord. The system begins as a streak on the surface, which later becomes a groove and later a tube. (Modified from Barkovich, Pediatric Neuroradiology [New York: Raven, 1990].) **A** to **E.** Various stages of neurulation of the upper spinal cord. **F** to **I.** Embryology of caudal portion of neural sac. See text.

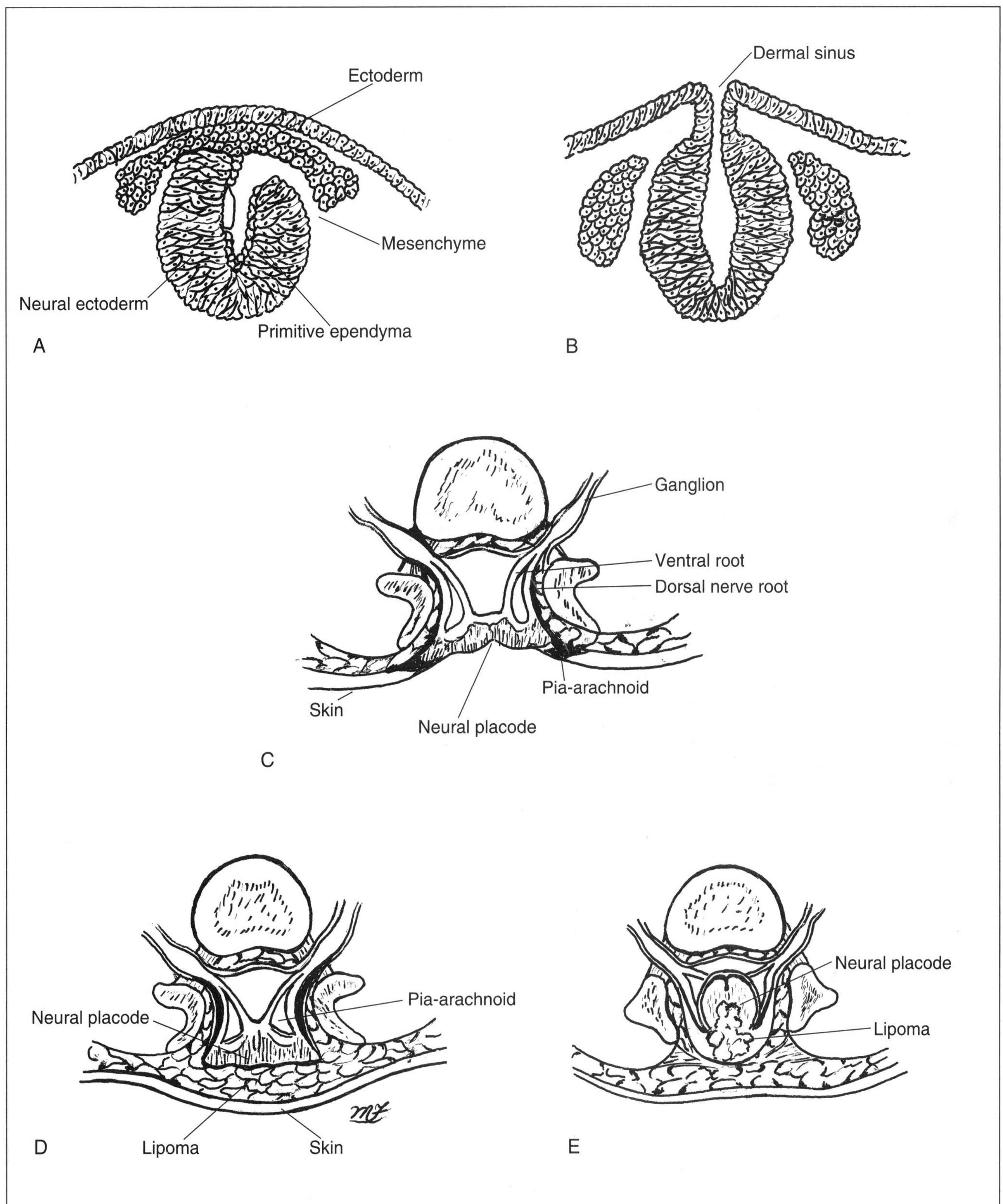

Figure 16.59. Anomalies related to incomplete closure of neural tube. **A.** A lipoma may form. **B.** Dermal sinus. **C.** Open myelocele, failure to form a groove. **D.** Failure to form a groove but the ectoderm covered the defect. **E.** Lipoma of the spinal cord. See text.

If the neural plate fails to form a groove in a given area (e.g., the lumbar area), it remains continuous with the skin (ectoderm) of the embryo (Fig. 16.59*C*). Under these circumstances the resulting myelocele would be exposed and the emerging nerves (Fig. 16.59*C*) would arise from the periphery of the open neural tube on the neutral aspect of the neural plate. The exposed neural plate in the myelocele is called the *neural placode* (Fig. 16.59*C*). The nerve roots would arise on the ventral surface of the neural placode and are directed ventrally. The outer surface would have been the ependymal canal of the neural tube if it had closed. The myelomeningocele is identical to the myelocele, but there is expansion of the subarachnoid space, which pushes the neural placode dorsally.

In a lipomyelomeningocele (Fig. 16.59*D*) the skin is intact. The anatomic configuration is similar to that in Figure 16.59*C*. The lipoma over the occult anomaly is continuous with the subcutaneous fat.

The myelocele and myelomeningoceles are often associated with Chiari II malformation, discussed in Chapter 5. Occasionally a Chiari II malformation is encountered without the lower spinal cord anomaly.

Spinal Lipomas

Lipomas are believed to occur as a result of premature separation of the ectoderm from the neuroectoderm, as shown in Figure 16.59*A*, before the neural tube closes completely. The surrounding mesenchyme then grows or is trapped in the groove and later is induced to become fat. Naidich et al. have theorized that the mesenchyme ventral to the neural plate is induced to form meninges, while the mesenchyme near the dorsal surface is induced to form fat (48,49). For this reason, spinal lipomas are always on the dorsal surface (Fig. 16.60*B*). They occur in the spinal cord (4 percent of cases) and may be found in the thoracic region and occasionally even in the cervical region, evidently representing a local premature dysjunction, as explained previously. These lipomas are usually covered by dura on the dorsolateral sides even though the dura may be very thin. The largest group of lipomas are those with deficient dura

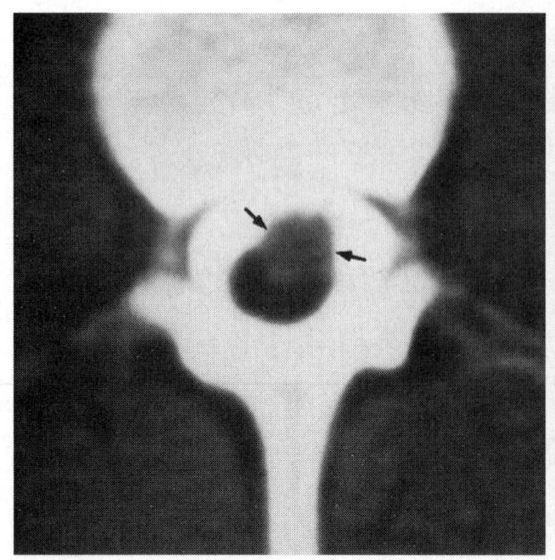

A

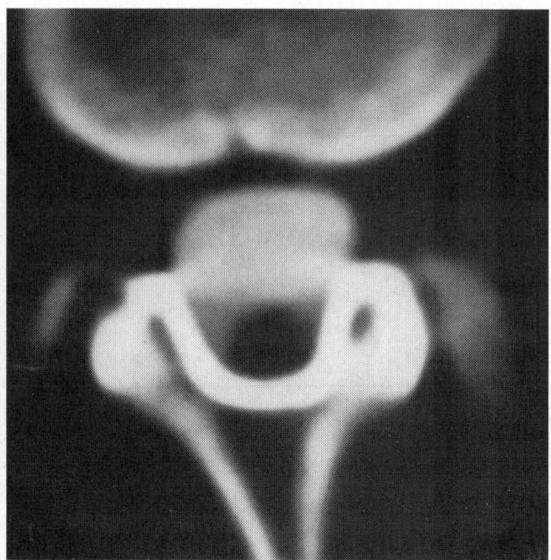

B

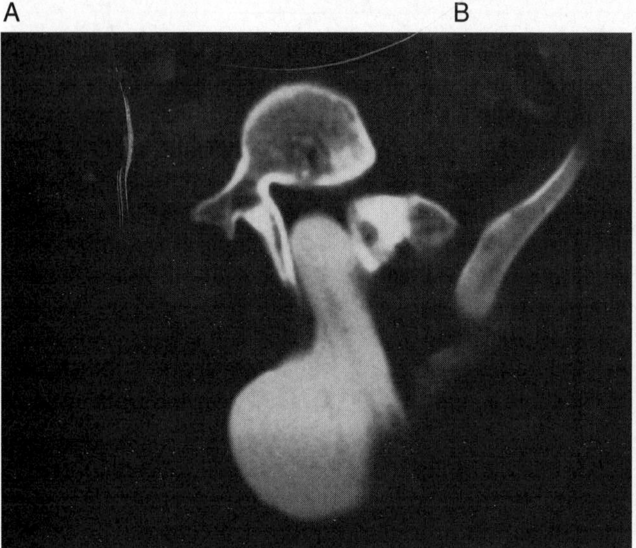

C

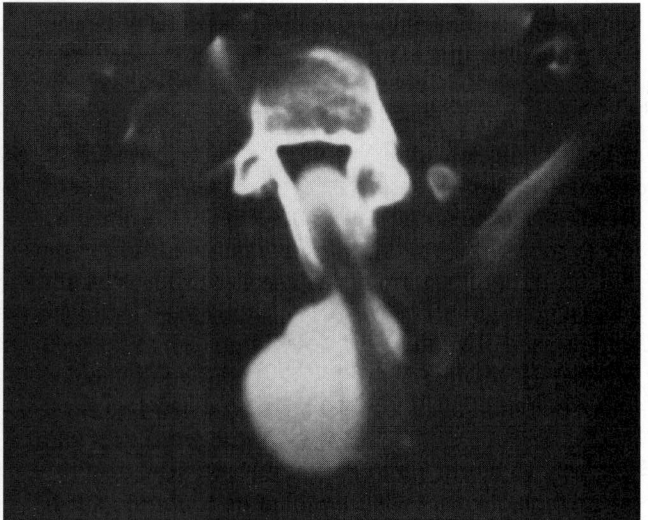

D

Figure 16.60. Lipoma of cord with tethered cord, myelomeningocele. **A.** CT-myelography at L3 shows the lipoma on the dorsolateral aspect of the canal and the cord in anterolateral aspect (less hypodense) (arrows). **B** to **D.** Lipoma and myelomeningocele. **B.** Lipoma in dorsal region at midlumbar area. The spine is well formed except for the spina bifida below. **C** and **D.** There is a large spina bifida in the lumbosacral region. Also note the large meningocele sac and neural tissue. Nerve roots are seen coursing in the anteroposterior direction as shown in the diagram in Figure 16.59*C* and *D*.

(four-fifths of the cases), most frequently found in the lower portions of the spine. Lipomas in the lumbar and lumbosacral regions are relatively common and in most cases are not associated with disabling neurologic deficit. When in the spinal cord, the lipoma cannot be totally removed surgically because of its association with a schismatic cord and the fact that the tissue is totally adherent to the inner cord (Fig. 16.59*E*). Lipomas can be associated with more severe anomalies, such as lipomyelocele and lipomyelomeningocele (Fig. 16.60).

Associated with lipomas, and other anomalies, there is always a spina bifida (failure of fusion) of the bony neural arch of the corresponding vertebrae or sacrum. The intra- and extradural lipomas communicate with the subcutaneous lipomas through the spina bifida defects; this can be demonstrated on sagittal MR images (Fig. 16.62). The lipoma can be attached to the filum terminale. Lipomas are easy to diagnose on MR images because of the T1 brightness of the fat (Fig. 16.61).

Tight Filum Terminale Syndrome (Tethered Cord)

This is believed to be due to a failure of involution of the lower aspect of the cord formed in the caudal cell mass (Fig. 16.58*F* to *I*). The filum normally has a thickness of 2 mm; in abnormal regression cases, it is thicker—sometimes the same thickness as the spinal cord (Fig. 16.62). The spinal cord normally ends between the first and second lumbar vertebrae. In the newborn it is at L2-L3, gradually moving up with the more rapid growth of the spinal column. The spinal cord extends down the coccygeal region when originally formed in the caudal cell mass, after which the lower portion becomes a glioependymal strand (filum terminale). By 3 months after birth the cord may have reached the L1-L2 level.

In cases of tight thickened filum, the spinal cord is usually lower than normal, sometimes very low. This may be associated with other anomalies such as lipoma, meningocele, or diastematomyelia (Fig. 16.63; see Figs. 16.70 and 16.71). It is important to make the diagnosis as early as possible, before 5 years of age, for best results of surgical correction. Neurologic manifestations include urinary bladder dysfunction, pes cavus, and pain and numbness in lower extremities. Developmental kyphoscoliosis is seen in about 25 percent of cases and in itself should be an indication for careful neurologic examination to rule out a tethered cord syndrome.

Lipoma of the filum terminale is seen as an isolated finding with no clinical significance in about 4 to 6 percent of adults. It is often associated with other anomalies, however. It can be diagnosed on MR sagittal images.

Caudal Spinal Anomalies

Caudal spinal anomalies can result when there is a derangement in the evolution of the caudal cell mass, which is closely related to the developing hindgut and mesonephros. The juxtaposition of developing hindgut, genitourinary, notochordal, and neural structures may be one reason for the occurrence of distal vertebral, neural, anorectal, renal, and genital anomalies (47). Among these anomalies are caudal regression syndrome and anterior sacral meningocele. Caudal regression syndrome may present sacral agenesis, which could exist without, or more frequently with, severe juxtaposed anomalies such as urogenital anomalies, anorectal stenosis or atresia, lipomas, elongated distal spinal cord, and others. The agenesis may be more extensive, extending up to T11 or T12, and may be unilateral. Isolated agenesis of the coccyx may be found and is not necessarily associated with other anomalies.

Anterior sacral meningocele is a meningocele passing forward into the pelvis through a defect in the sacrum or coccyx. It may be accompanied by other anomalies (tethered cord, spinal lipomas, sacral agenesis). The anterior sacral meningocele may be seen in patients with neurofibromatosis or Marfan syndrome (Fig. 16.63). The meningocele sac can be very large and may displace and compress the rectum, leading to constipation. The cyst becomes larger in the erect position and when bearing down, such as during defecation or vaginal child delivery. Surgical repair should be attempted.

TERMINAL (CAUDAL) MYELOCYSTOCELE

In this condition the spinal cord is tethered and the ventral ependymal canal widens considerably, forming a pouch, like a meningocele, except that the cord itself is the membrane around the cyst. It is a skin-covered anomaly and constitutes about 1 percent of skin-covered congenital masses (50). It may be associated with sacral agenesis and other anomalies.

VENTRICULUS TERMINALIS

This is an anatomic rest usually not seen by imaging methods, found at the level of the ependymal canal of the conus medullaris. Sometimes it may be visible or very large when there is cyst formation attributed to local dilatation of the ependymal canal (51).

OCCULT INTRASACRAL MENINGOCELES

Occult intrasacral meningoceles are common. They may be due to a defect in the dura, allowing for the herniation of arachnoid, or they may arise from one or more than one sacral root sleeve, leading to the entity usually referred to as *sacral cysts*. They usually produce considerable widening of the sacral canal due to erosion of its wall secondary to transmitted pulsations over a long period of time (Figs. 16.64 to 16.66). The meningoceles or cysts may communicate freely with the subarachnoid space, or the connecting neck may become narrow or even obstructed due to inflammation, in which case the cyst would not fill with contrast on myelography. The protein in these cysts may become elevated because of the narrow communicating neck, and this in itself would tend to provoke further growth of the cyst. On a T1-weighted MR image the elevated protein

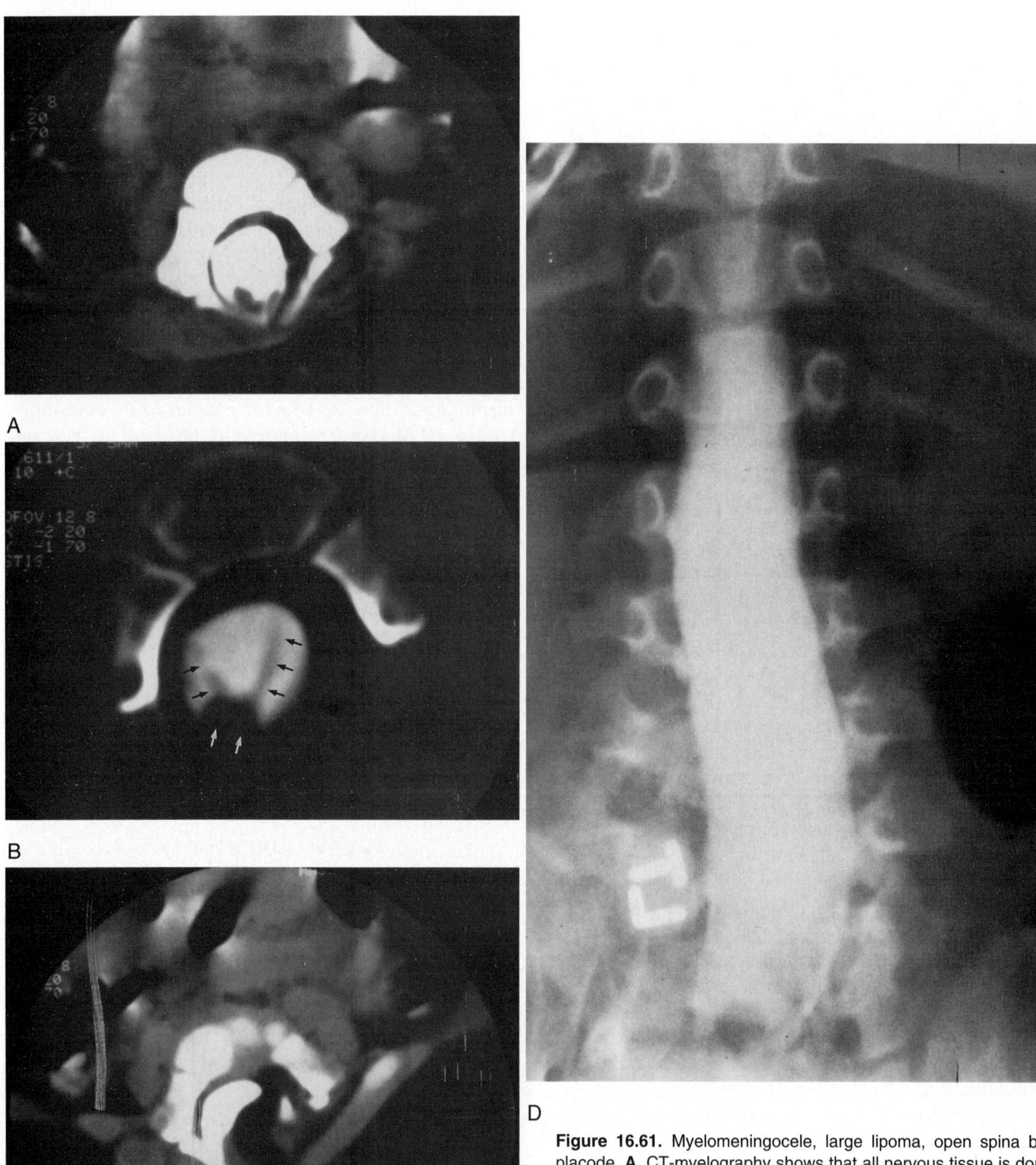

Figure 16.61. Myelomeningocele, large lipoma, open spina bifida, placode. **A.** CT-myelography shows that all nervous tissue is dorsally placed (upper lumbar). **B.** The neural arch is totally open. There is a placode on the dorsal aspect (white arrows), and the nerve roots are coursing forward (black arrows), third lumbar level. **C.** A lower section reveals the thecal sac with contrast, a large lipomatous mass in the canal extending out through the wide spina bifida to merge with subcutaneous tissue. The skin is intact at this level. **D.** Myelography, frontal view, reveals a dilated thecal sac, wide interpediculate distance, and filling defects in caudal portion due to lipoma, but there are no details in actual anatomy such as is shown in B and C.

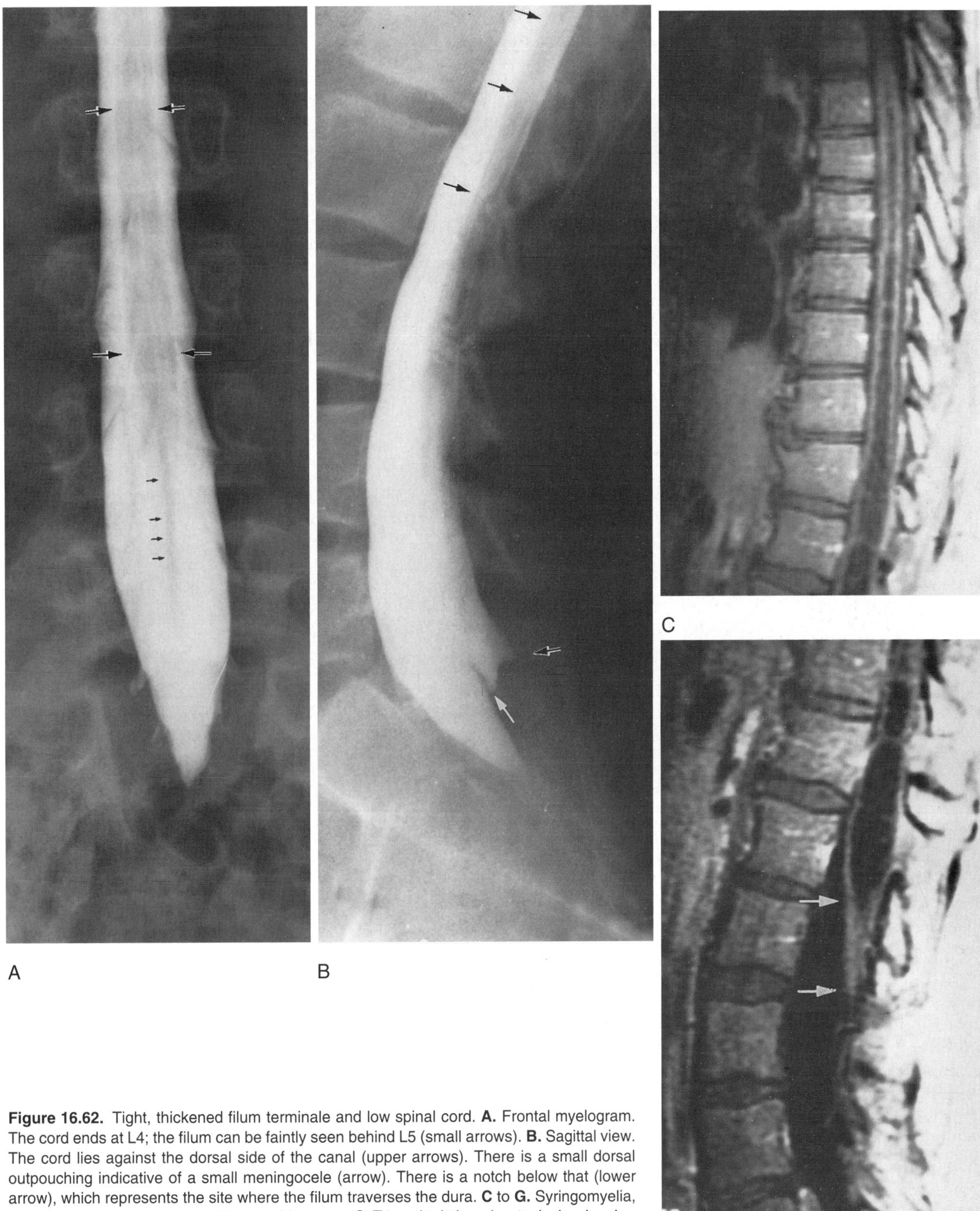

Figure 16.62. Tight, thickened filum terminale and low spinal cord. **A.** Frontal myelogram. The cord ends at L4; the filum can be faintly seen behind L5 (small arrows). **B.** Sagittal view. The cord lies against the dorsal side of the canal (upper arrows). There is a small dorsal outpouching indicative of a small meningocele (arrow). There is a notch below that (lower arrow), which represents the site where the filum traverses the dura. **C** to **G.** Syringomyelia, lipoma, and tethered cord in a 42-year-old woman. **C.** T1 sagittal; there is a typical syringohydromyelia present. **D.** The conus medullaris is too low (at L2-L3); the conus continues caudally to the level of L4, indicating a tethered cord (arrows).

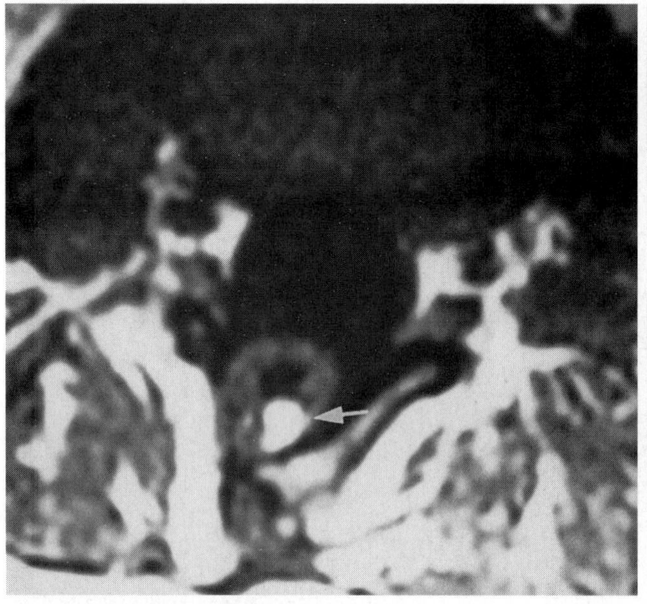

E

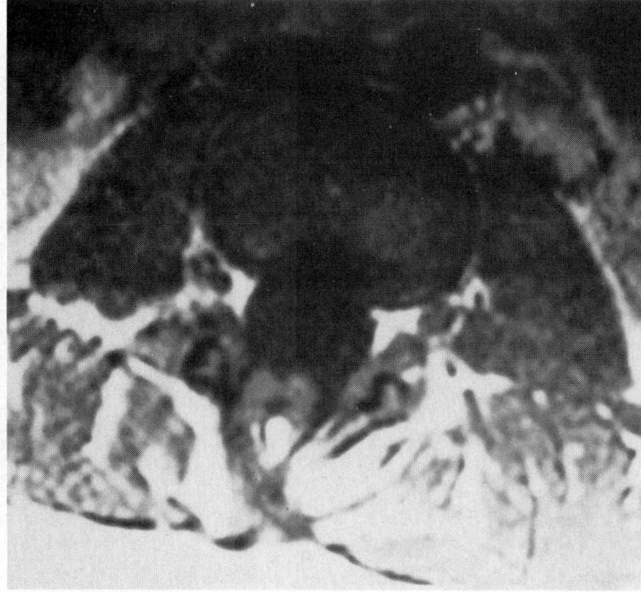

F

G

Figure 16.62. *(continued)* **E.** A T1 axial image shows the hydromyelic cord in cross section and a bright, partly intramedullary lipoma on the dorsal side of the cord (arrow). **F.** Lower down, the lipoma is seen to project dorsad due to the presence of a spina bifida. **G.** Sagittal T2 shows the bright syrinx cavity. The lower portion shows a nonuniform bright area probably due to CSF motion (arrows) at the bottom of the cavity.

may be sufficient to produce a slightly brighter image than the adjacent CSF.

The meningoceles or cysts may arise from the sacral roots or the lumbar roots. The sacral location is considerably more common than the lumbar. In addition to cysts, we most frequently see enlargement of the root sleeves around the nerve roots (Fig. 16.66). Some cysts do not seem to communicate with the subarachnoid space and do not fill with contrast (52), but the majority do.

Anomalies in the Thoracic Region

In the *thoracic region* there are three conditions worth discussing. The first is *dorsal arachnoid diverticula*—pockets on the dorsal side of the subarachnoid space that are freely open on the cephalic end. They can fill during contrast myelography if the patient is placed in the supine position. With the patient erect, the contrast remains in the pockets (Fig. 16.67). The pockets would empty in Trendelenburg position. It is possible to have some of these pockets develop a narrow neck and communicate poorly with the rest of the subarachnoid space, in which case they may grow in size, producing compression of the spinal cord and erosion of the adjacent lamina, but this is a rare occurrence. Other complications such as intracranial hypotension due to CSF "leak" through the diverticulum have been reported (53).

The second thoracic lesion is the *dorsal intrathoracic meningocele* (intraspinal extradural meningeal cyst), an entity described by Elsberg et al. (54). It is a true meningocele produced by a herniation of arachnoid through the dorsal dura. A pocket forms and grows in size, possibly via a flap-valve effect, leading to gradual increase in size of the thoracic spinal canal by erosion of its bony walls, owing to transmitted pulsations and mild compression of the spinal cord. It is usually discovered in the second decade of life, most frequently in boys, from whom the name applied by Elsberg comes (juvenile dorsal epidural cyst) (Fig. 16.68). MRI may be diagnostic (55,56). The cyst usually fills partially with contrast myelography.

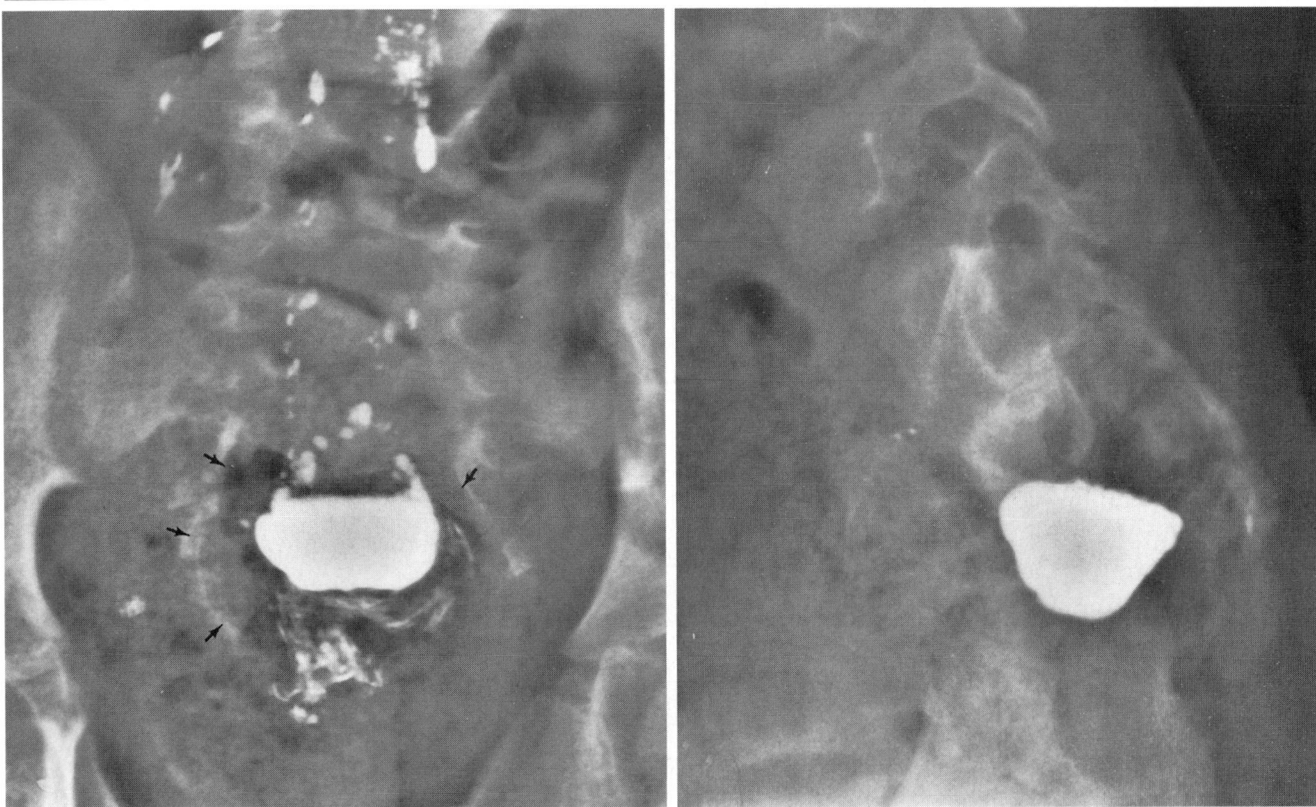

A B

Figure 16.63. Anterior sacral meningocele in a child with constipation. **A.** The contrast myelogram shows a large meningocele sac, which in the lateral projection (**B**) is seen to be anterior to the sacrum. The spinal canal in the lower lumbar and sacral region is widened. Also there is a spina bifida of L4, L5, and of the sacrum.

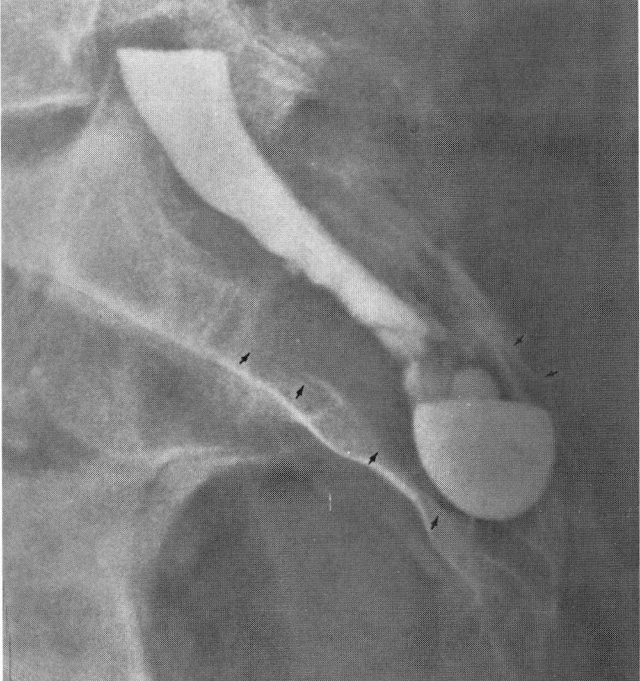

Figure 16.64. Occult sacral meningocele producing erosion of sacral canal associated with lipoma, which accounts for the low-density area above the sac with erosion of the sacrum (arrows).

The third lesion is the *lateral thoracic meningocele*, usually seen in patients with neurofibromatosis secondary to dural ectasia. These meningoceles are visible on chest radiographs and usually fill during myelography. Bone erosion may occur around the intervertebral foramen of exit (Fig. 16.69). In patients with neurofibromatosis dural ectasia may occur, which allows for widening of the dural sac, causing enlargement of the spinal canal. Herniation of the dural sac through the intervertebral foramina occurs at various levels. The widening of the dural sac produces a scalloped configuration of the vertebral bodies as well as widening of the interpediculate distance.

Diastematomyelia

Diastemalomyelia is a sagittal division or pseudoduplication of a segment of the spinal cord, which may be associated with a congenital anomaly of the vertebral column in which an osseous or fibrocartilaginous septum transfixes the spinal cord at the point of diastasis. The septum, which is attached anteriorly to one or more vertebral bodies and posteriorly to the dura, passes through the spinal cord and fixes it in low anatomic position, so that Arnold-Chiari deformity may result. Diastematomyelia most frequently

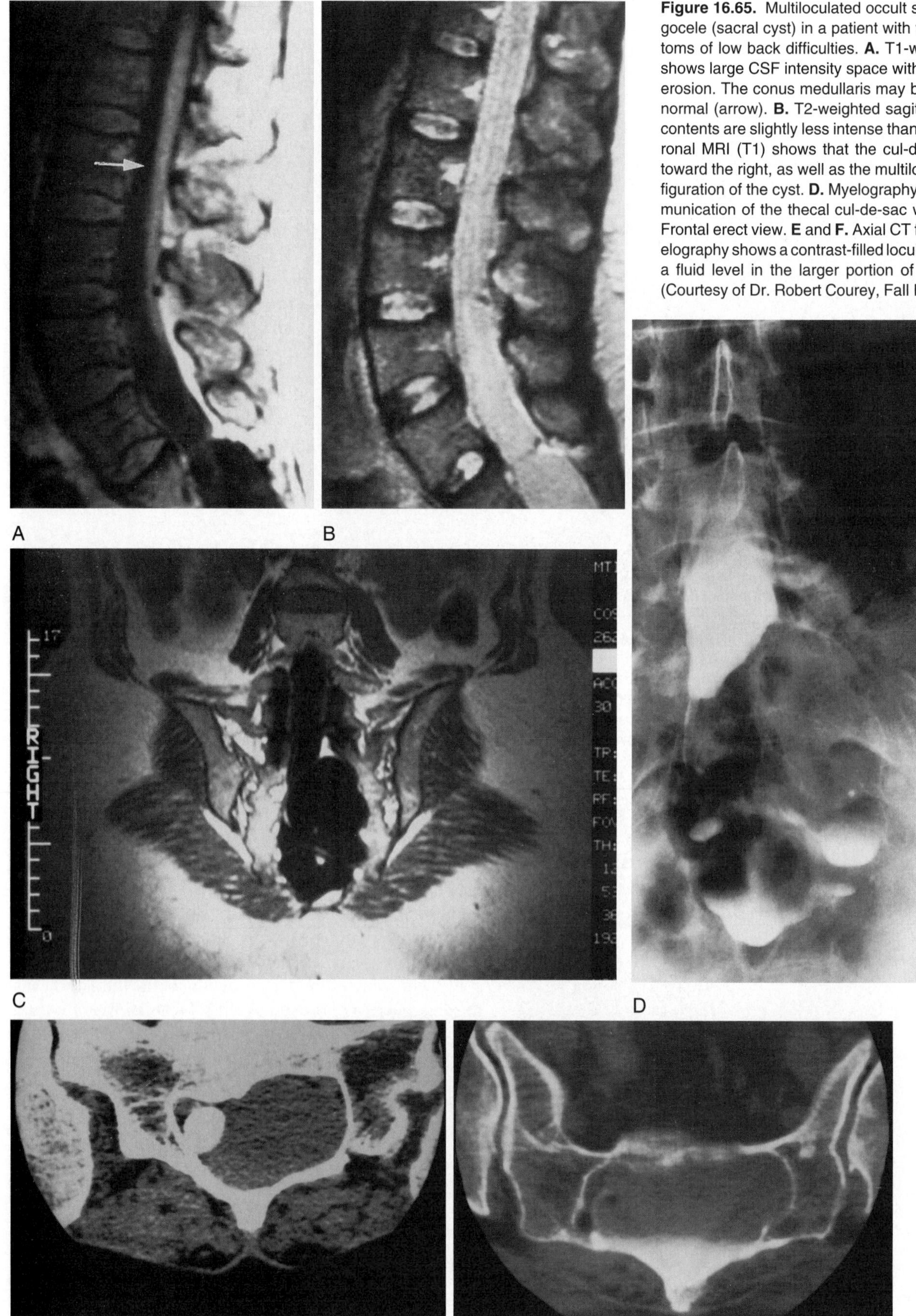

Figure 16.65. Multiloculated occult sacral meningocele (sacral cyst) in a patient with vague symptoms of low back difficulties. **A.** T1-weighted MRI shows large CSF intensity space with sacral bone erosion. The conus medullaris may be lower than normal (arrow). **B.** T2-weighted sagittal. The cyst contents are slightly less intense than CSF. **C.** Coronal MRI (T1) shows that the cul-de-sac tapers toward the right, as well as the multiloculated configuration of the cyst. **D.** Myelography shows communication of the thecal cul-de-sac with the cyst. Frontal erect view. **E** and **F.** Axial CT following myelography shows a contrast-filled loculation (**E**) and a fluid level in the larger portion of the sac (**F**). (Courtesy of Dr. Robert Courey, Fall River, Mass.)

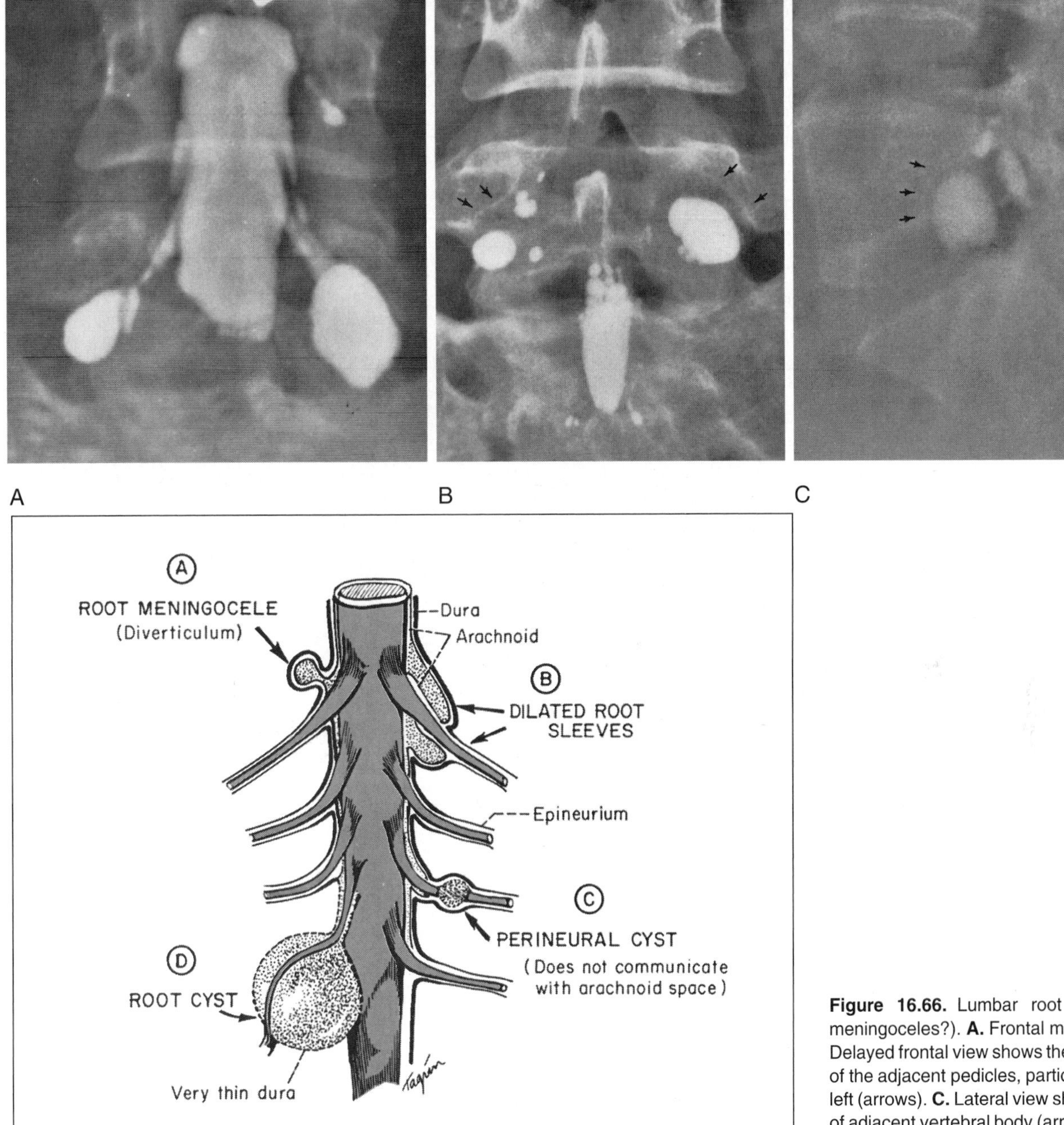

Figure 16.66. Lumbar root cysts (root meningoceles?). **A.** Frontal myelogram. **B.** Delayed frontal view shows there is erosion of the adjacent pedicles, particularly on the left (arrows). **C.** Lateral view shows erosion of adjacent vertebral body (arrows). **D.** Diagram to illustrate usual variations of arachnoid membrane around spinal roots.

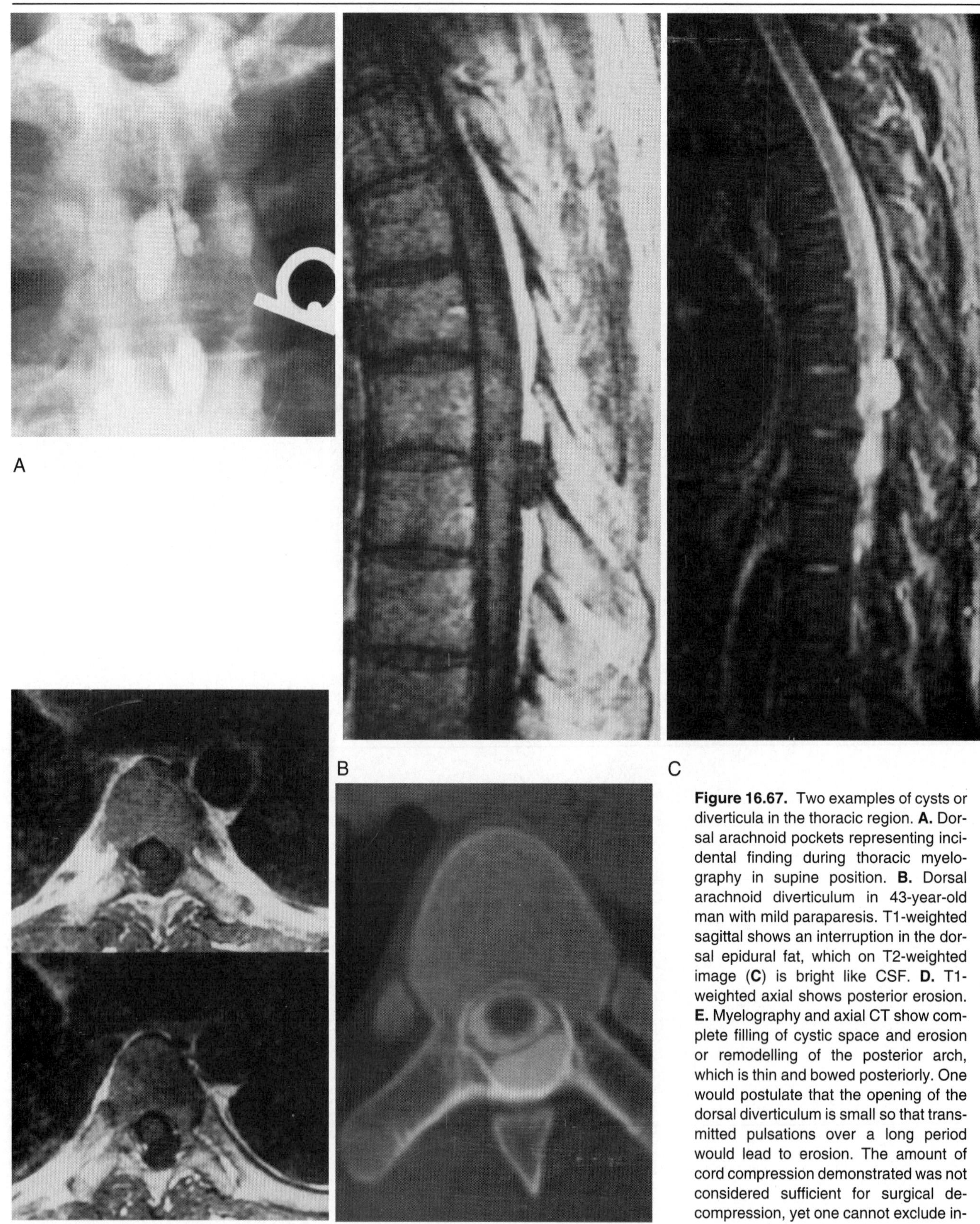

Figure 16.67. Two examples of cysts or diverticula in the thoracic region. **A.** Dorsal arachnoid pockets representing incidental finding during thoracic myelography in supine position. **B.** Dorsal arachnoid diverticulum in 43-year-old man with mild paraparesis. T1-weighted sagittal shows an interruption in the dorsal epidural fat, which on T2-weighted image (**C**) is bright like CSF. **D.** T1-weighted axial shows posterior erosion. **E.** Myelography and axial CT show complete filling of cystic space and erosion or remodelling of the posterior arch, which is thin and bowed posteriorly. One would postulate that the opening of the dorsal diverticulum is small so that transmitted pulsations over a long period would lead to erosion. The amount of cord compression demonstrated was not considered sufficient for surgical decompression, yet one cannot exclude intermittent increases and decreases in size.

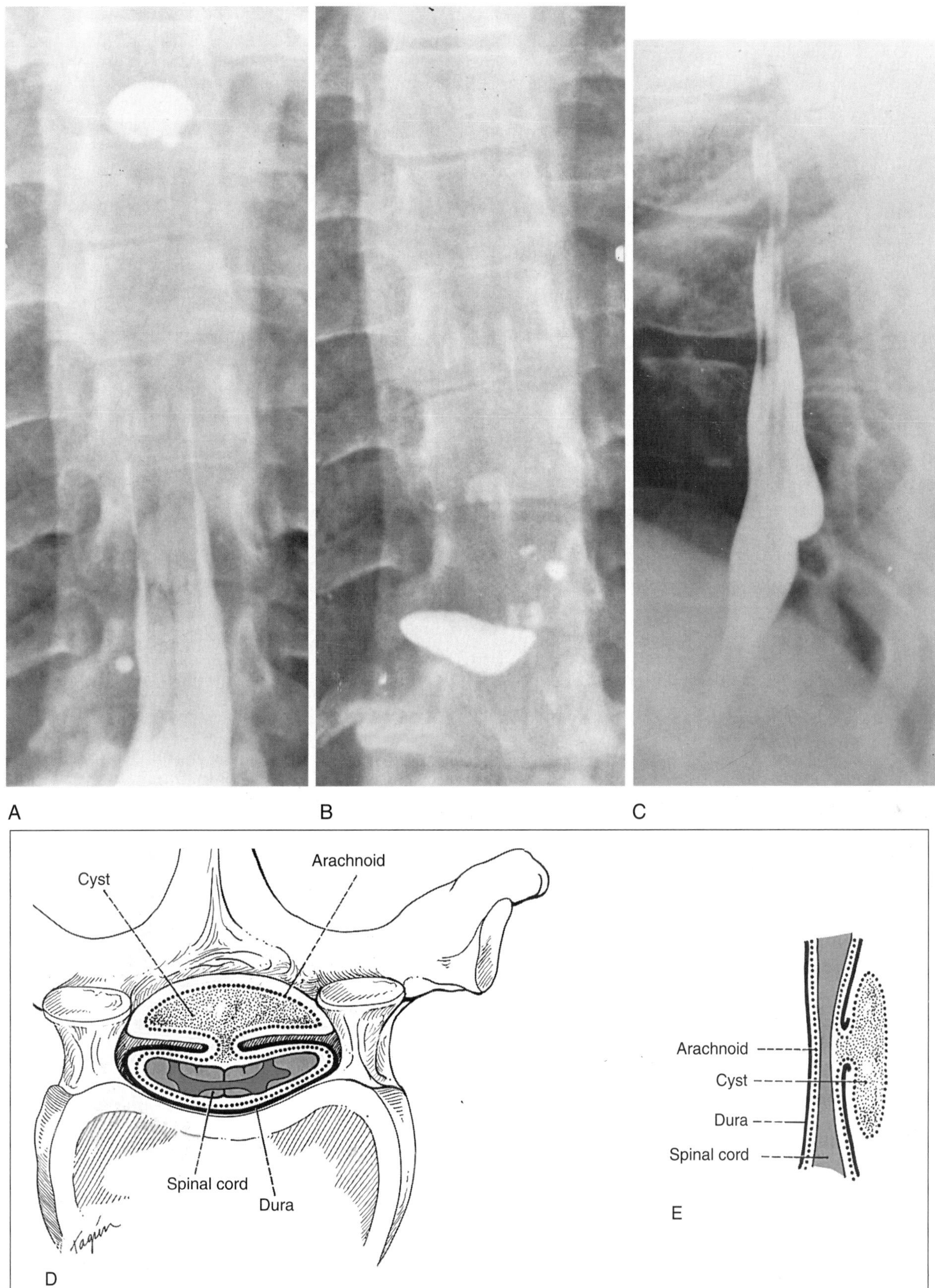

Figure 16.68. Thoracic occult meningocele in a 16-year-old boy complaining of leg weakness. **A.** Frontal myelogram in Trendelenburg position shows a flattened spinal cord; the upper limit of the large cyst is shown. **B.** Erect frontal view shows the contrast in dependent portion of cyst just below T9. **C.** Lateral myelogram shows forward displacement and flattening of the subarachnoid space. There is enlargement of the spinal canal in both anteroposterior and transverse directions; there is flattening of the pedicles bilaterally from T6 to T9. (Courtesy of Dr. James M. Martin, St. Louis, Mo.) The pathologic anatomy of this condition is explained in the diagram shown in (**D**) and the lateral diagram (**E**).

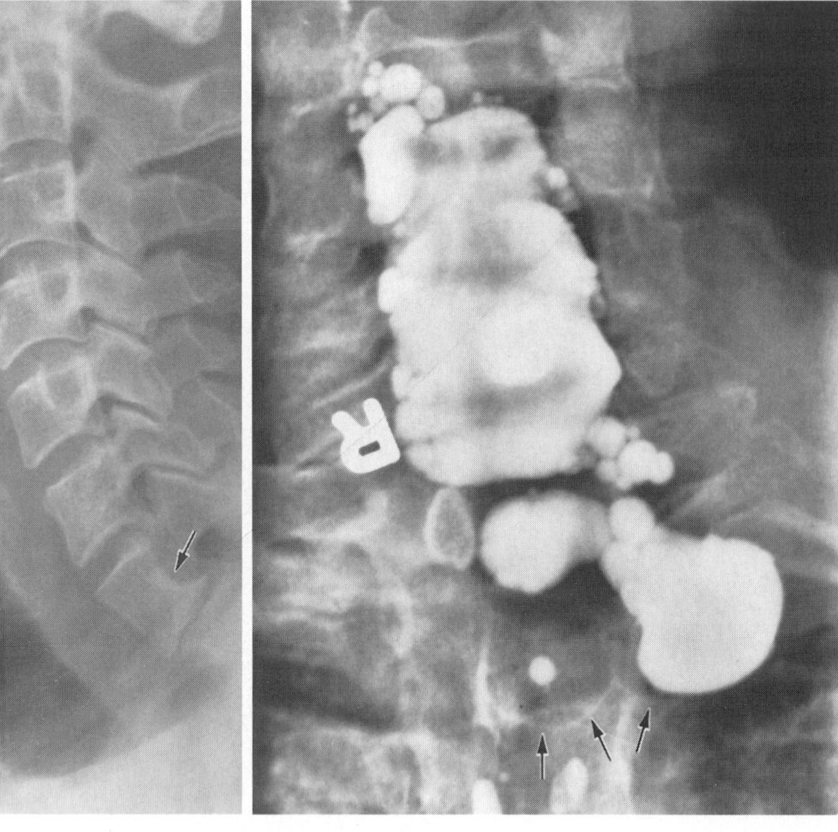

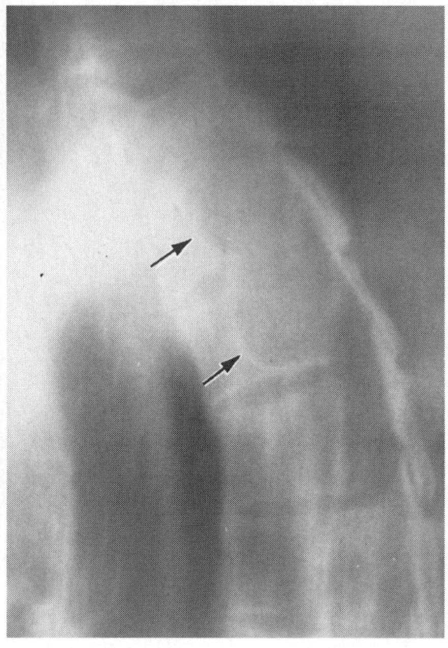

A B C

Figure 16.69. Dural ectasia and intrathoracic meningocele in patient with neurofibromatosis. **A.** Cervical tomography shows erosion with concavity in the posterior aspect of the C7 vertebral body (arrow). **B.** Pantopaque myelography reveals large outpouching of subarachnoid space in the left upper chest. The arrows point at erosion of the T1 vertebral body, which is shown in sagittal tomogram (**C**) (arrow).

occurs in the lower thoracic and upper lumbar regions. Characteristic roentgenographic changes have been described by Neuhauser et al. (57). Plain spine roentgenograms often show, in frontal projection, widening of the vertebral canal, which may extend longitudinally for as many as six vertebral segments. The interpediculate distance is increased in a fusiform manner over these segments. Numerous developmental abnormalities of the vertebral bodies and arches may be present in association with the widening of the vertebral canal (58). The pedicles, bodies, and laminae of the vertebrae show no evidence of bone atrophy, such as is usually present when the canal is enlarged as the result of an expanding lesion; that is, the pedicles are round although the interpediculate distance is widened and the posterior aspect of the vertebral bodies is not excavated. When the septum dividing the spinal cord is ossified, roentgenograms in the frontal projection may demonstrate a linear shadow of calcium density of approximately 1.0 to 1.5 cm in size in the midsagittal plane of the vertebral canal. This may be best demonstrated by tomography. In lateral view, calcification may be seen in the anterior portion of the septum behind the vertebral bodies or, occasionally, in the posterior portion of the septum near the laminae. Here again, tomography may be of use.

Myelography will demonstrate the cleft in the spinal cord and its relationship to the septum, even in those instances where the septum is cartilaginous or insufficiently ossified to be visible in plain spine roentgenograms. The septum produces an elongated filling defect in the central portion of the radiopaque column, or, when the septum is small, only a tiny rounded filling defect may be demonstrable (Fig. 16.70). In the case in which an ossified spicule is present, a linear calcium shadow may be demonstrated within the central zone of defective filling in the myelogram.

The neurologic findings are often surprisingly mild. Surgical intervention is recommended, particularly to prevent further damage to the cord caused by longitudinal growth. Surgical exploration usually reveals a complete double-barrel meningeal tube split by the central spicule (59).

It is probable that diastematomyelia represents a remnant of a connection between the primitive neural and enteric tubes.

CT and MRI permit the diagnosis without myelography. The cord splitting is particularly well demonstrated on axial MR images (Fig. 16.71). There are complete dural and pia-arachnoid coverings of the split cord, but sometimes there is a single covering subarachnoid. Diplomyelia can be found without diastematomyelia. The bridge is usually bony, but it may be only partly bony and fibrous, and other

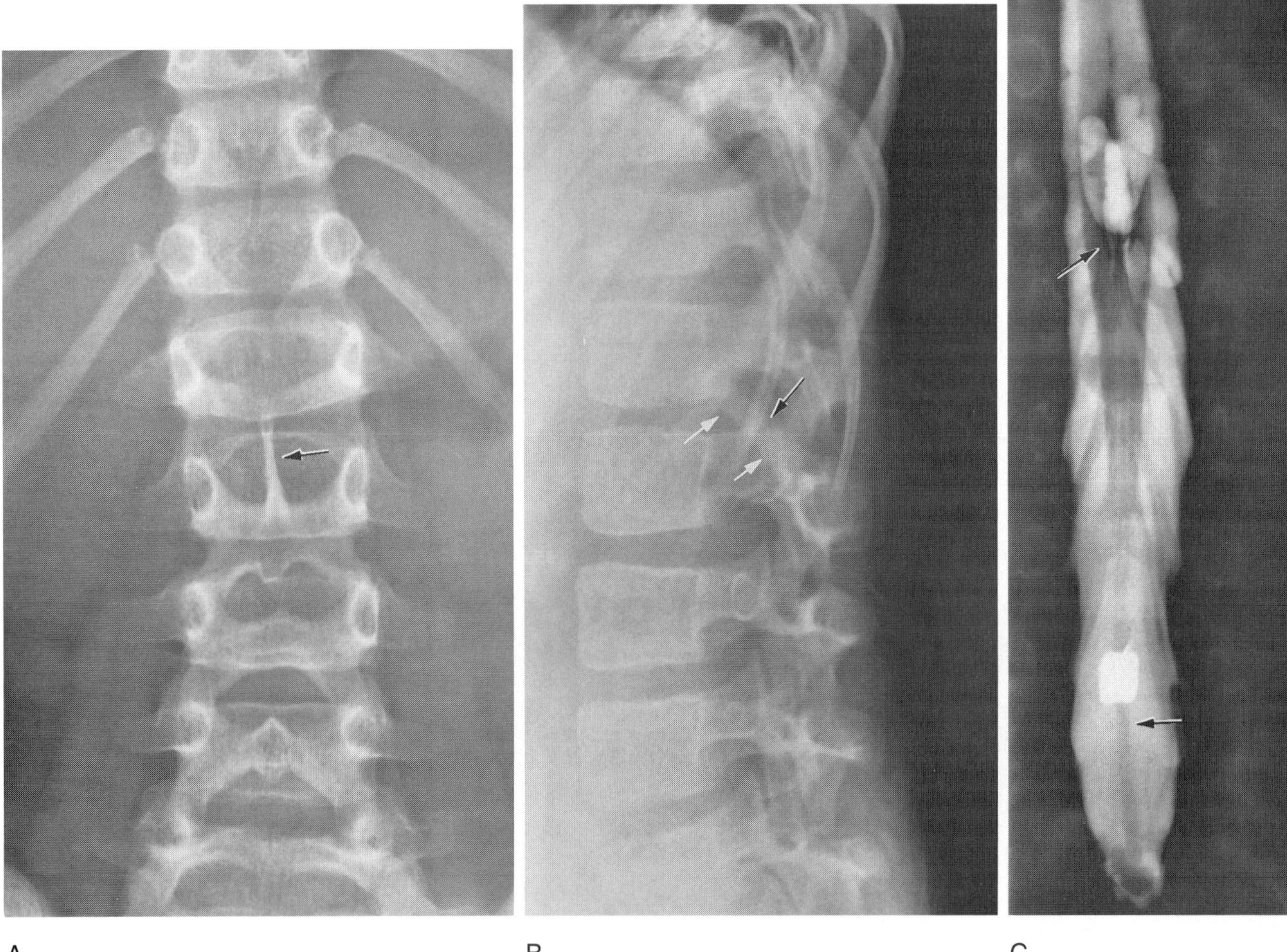

A B C

Figure 16.70. Diastematomyelia. **A.** There is a long spicule of bone between the lamina of L2 and the body of L1 (arrow), which in the lateral view (**B**) is seen to cross the canal (arrows) obliquely. There is focal widening of the spinal canal. **C.** On myelography the bony spicule is partly obscured (arrows). The spinal cord is too low, down to L3; the filum terminale is thick (lower arrow). The fusiform widening of the cord is indicative of the cord splitting due to the midline bony bridge, which splits the cord into two complete channels, both covered by dura and arachnoid. In some cases there is no dural covering of both cord segments with a single subarachnoid space.

times it may all be fibrocartilaginous, in which case it would not be visible by CT. The cord is usually split at the level of the bridge and extending cephalad for a variable distance, presumably indicating growth of the vertebral column and consequent elevation of the caudal end of the cord. The length of the cord split is best shown by cross-sectional MR images.

In addition to some neurologic changes, sometimes extremely mild, there may be external markers on the skin, the most frequent of which is a patch of hair. Diastematomyelia is much more common in females (80 to 90 percent of cases).

In true diplomyelia there may be two symmetric spinal cords with a central canal and gray and white matter. However, no clear reports of such condition are found. The split cord of diastematomyelia consists of two hemicords, each half containing a central canal but only one anterior and one posterior gray matter horn.

Neurenteric Cyst

Neurenteric cysts and anterior spina bifida result when the primitive neural tube (ectodermal) connects with the enteric tube (entodermal) at any area above the posterior neuropore (sacrococcygeal area). They are usually associated with anterior spina bifida and may be an isolated cyst or a tract situated in the epidural, subdural, or intra-arachnoid space. It may be associated with a mediastinal or a retroperitoneal cyst or duplication (60–64). The most common location is the upper thoracic and lower cervical area, followed in frequency by the sacral region. They may occur in craniocerebral junction and as high as the cerebellopontine angle (64). The cysts are lined by a single layer of cuboidal

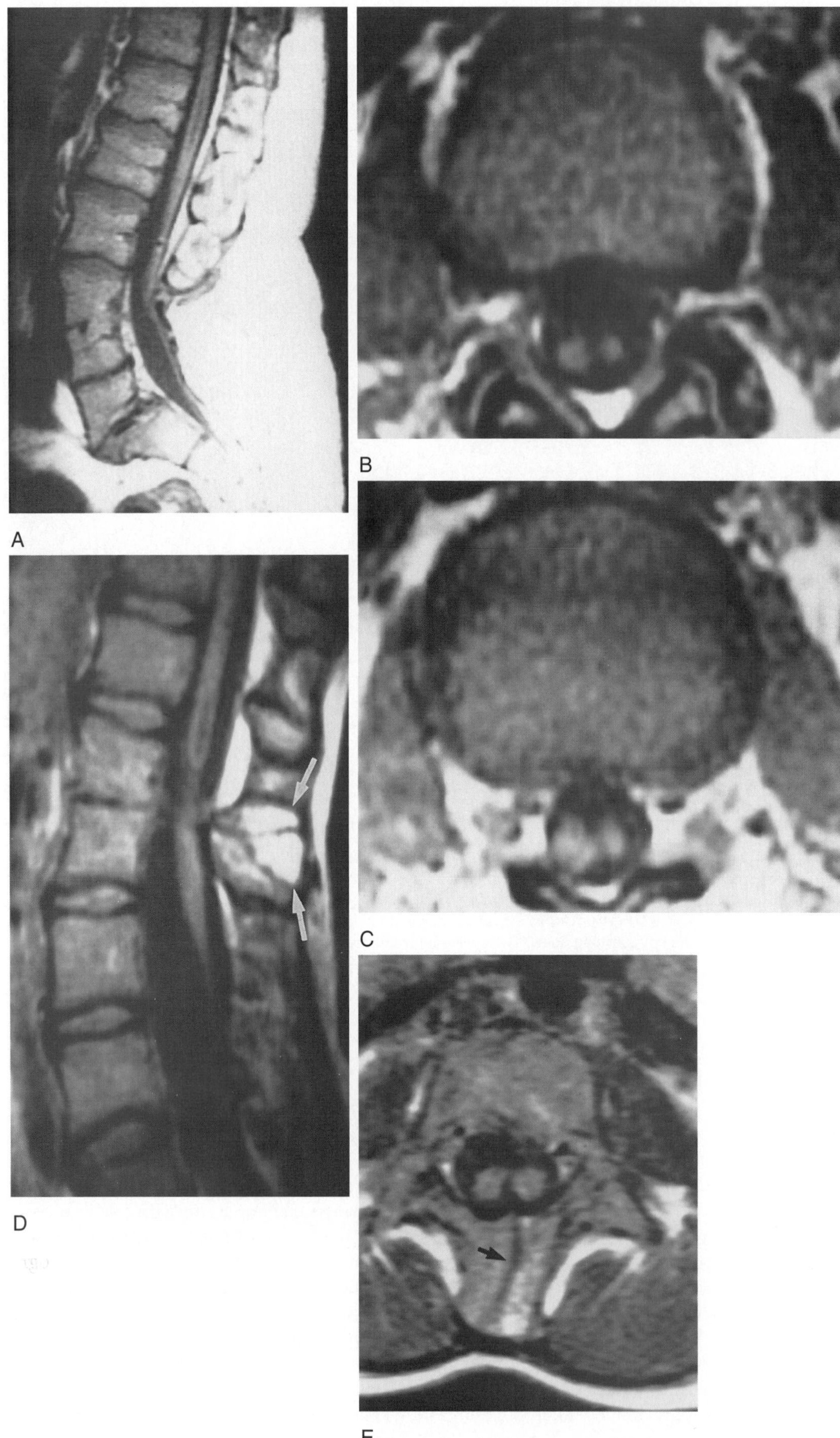
A
B
C
D
E

or columnar epithelium and may be intramedullary in location. It is probable that isolated cysts of this type without any spinal or other anomaly represent variants of enterogenous cysts. A round defect in the vertebral body as seen in the frontal projection is virtually characteristic of a neurenteric cyst. Neurentic cysts and diastematomyelia are components of what is known as the split notochord syndrome. The cyst could be anterior to the cord, between the two sides of a split cord, or dorsal to the cord. On MRI they are usually slightly hyperintense on T1 images because of protein content.

INFLAMMATORY CONDITIONS

Under this heading will be considered osteomyelitis and discitis, epidural abscess, subdural infections, meningitis, and myelitis.

Osteomyelitis and Discitis

In the United States the most frequent pathogens are the pyogenic bacteria (*Staphylococcus aureus*, 60 percent; *Enterobacter*, 30 percent; *Escherichia coli*, *Salmonella*, *Pseudomonas*, *Klebsiella pneumoniae*). Tuberculosis is common in many countries, and occasionally a fungus infection may be encountered. The infection usually starts in the vertebral body; intervertebral disc and disc involvement are to be expected. A hematogenous spread is most common. Puncture wounds or adjacent soft tissue infections are other possible causes. In the lumbar region disc infection may follow disc-removal surgery.

Most frequently the presenting symptom is focal back pain; fever is common but may be slight, and neurologic findings do not occur unless there is nerve or spinal cord compression. An elevated erythrosedimentation rate is frequently encountered.

IMAGING FINDINGS

Plain films may be diagnostic. They may show disc space narrowing, and density loss and/or erosion of the cortical bone of the adjacent vertebral bodies. However, the examination is most frequently negative in the first 8 to 10 days to 2 weeks, depending on how active the infection is. In low-grade infections it may take several weeks before changes are clearly visible. This is sometimes the case in postdiscectomy infection, often low-grade, in which 8 weeks or longer may pass before suspicious changes are seen on plain radiography.

CT may be helpful, but MRI is superior because it will demonstrate early changes in the vertebral bodies (loss of the normal marrow brightness); this would be low intensity on T1-weighted and high intensity on T2-weighted images. The corresponding affected disc is bright on T2-weighted and dark on T1-weighted images, but it would enhance after gadolinium, usually brightly. The adjacent affected bone may or may not enhance (Figs. 16.72 and 16.73) (65,66).

LOW-GRADE AND CHRONIC OSTEOMYELITIS AND DISCITIS

This may be the result of a low-grade bacterial infection such as is seen sometimes following spinal disc surgery, or it may be due to tuberculosis as well as other agents (fungus such as *Aspergillus*, *Actinomyces*, *Blastomyces*, *Coccidioides*, *Cryptococcus;* and *Brucella*, particularly seen in some countries). The disc infection may also be a complication of discography and chemonucleolysis.

Tuberculosis may involve the vertebral body primarily, followed by disc involvement, and the fibrocartilage may survive for some time, while in the pyogenic infections disc dissolution (digestion) occurs early. Typically, there is a spinal abscess, which is often large and dissects up and down the spine, sometimes for a long distance. The abscess may also extend back under the dura, producing a chronic epidural abscess (Figs. 16.74 and 16.75).

MRI is the diagnostic procedure of choice to ascertain the degree of involvement, the presence and extent of compromise of the spinal canal with cord compression, and the size of the perispinal abscess. A fungus infection may produce bone involvement similar to tuberculosis and may produce a perispinal abscess, but this is rare.

Epidural Abscess

Usually resulting from hematogenous spread, epidural abscess is probably increasing in frequency. This has been attributed to various causes, including immunodeficiency states, intravenous (IV) drug abuse, and diabetes mellitus. An epidural abscess is a severe infection that requires prompt attention and treatment, for it usually progresses rapidly. It compresses the spinal cord, leading to paraparesis or quadriparesis, depending on location, and may lead to vascular thrombosis and permanent cord damage.

While the diagnosis may be made by CT and myelography, MRI without and with contrast is the procedure of choice. Plain films of the spine are usually normal or noncontributory to the diagnosis. Patients usually present elevated temperatures and local pain, but the latter is quite variable.

MRI examination would show, on T1-weighted imaging, an increase in the epidural space with narrowing of

Figure 16.71. Diastematomyelia in 40-year-old woman with minor neurologic symptoms. **A.** T1-weighted sagittal shows congenital fusion of L3, L4, and L5 vertebrae; the spinal cord shows tethering; the conus ends at the upper aspect of L3; and the cord presents a small syringomyelic cavity behind the T12 vertebral body. **B.** Axial view reveals a split cord; the right hemicord is slightly larger than the left. **C.** A higher section than B shows that the two hemicords are coming together. The bony or fibrous spicule cannot be seen. **D** and **E.** Another similar case at a higher level (T12-L1). The sagittal T1-weighted image shows partial segmentation failure of the T12-L1 vertebral bodies with a rudimentary disc and the abnormal soft tissue. A lipomatous mass is seen dorsally (arrows). The axial view (**E**) shows the cord splitting and a sinus tract extending dorsally, which does not seem to reach the skin at this level (arrow).

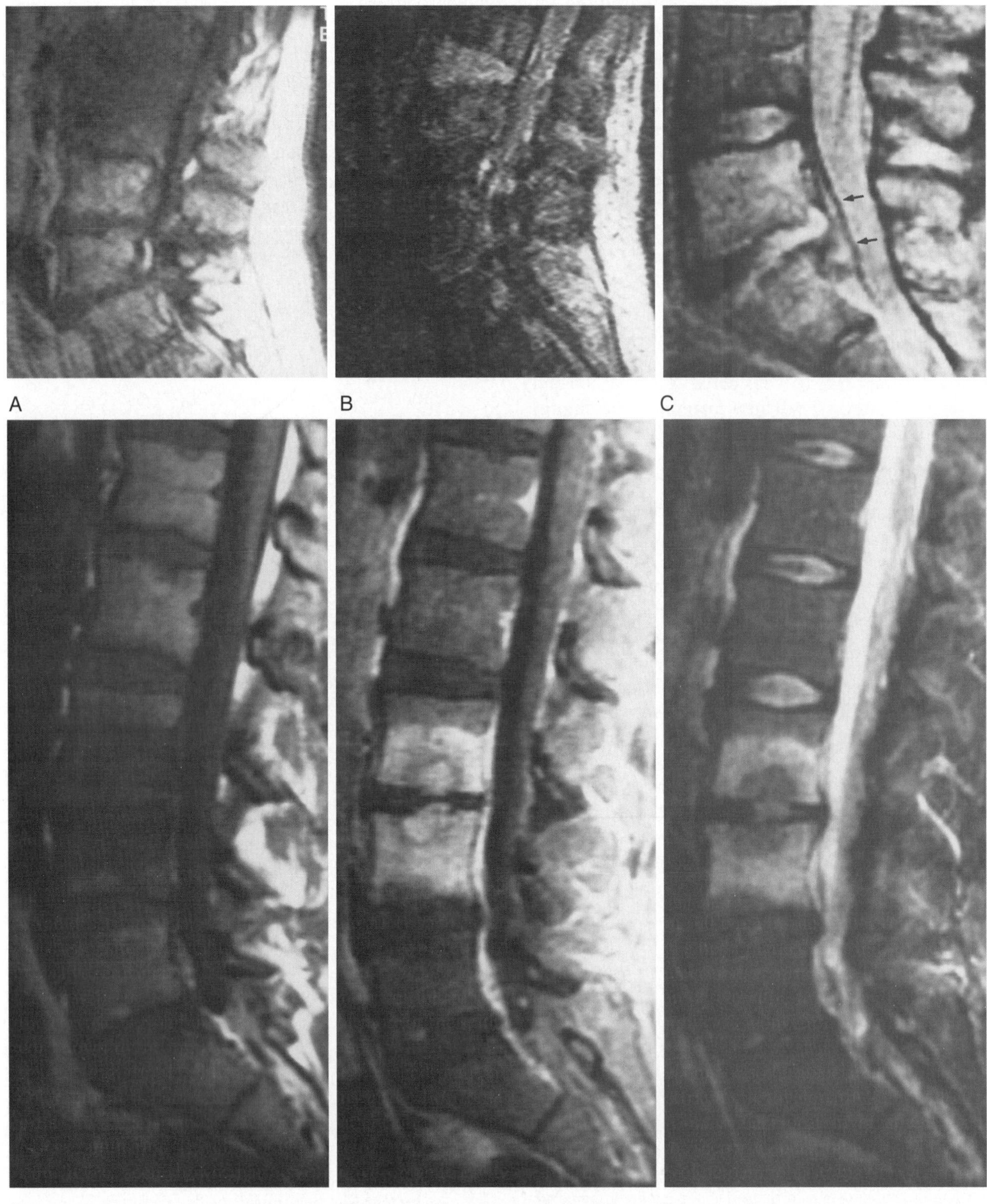

Figure 16.72. Lumbar osteomyelitis and discitis. **A.** T1-weighted image shows loss of bone marrow in the L1 and L2 vertebral bodies. **B.** T2-weighted image shows a bright intervertebral disc and moderate increase in intensity of L1-L2 vertebral bodies. **C.** Another case demonstrating the T2 increased intensity of the L5-S1 disc and of the L5 and S1 vertebral bodies. In addition, there is increased intensity behind L5-S1. The dura is displaced back (arrows), indicative of an epidural abscess. **D** to **F.** Another patient, a 28-year-old woman who underwent a tooth extraction and also had an abortion 6 weeks previously. **D.** T1 without contrast. There is total loss of bone marrow at L3-L4, and the disc is not seen. **E.** After contrast there is enhancement of two adjacent areas in the L4 and L5 vertebral bodies as well as the vertebral bodies. There is little enhancement of the disc. **F.** On T2 there is hyperintensity in the disc and hyperintensity involving both vertebral bodies.

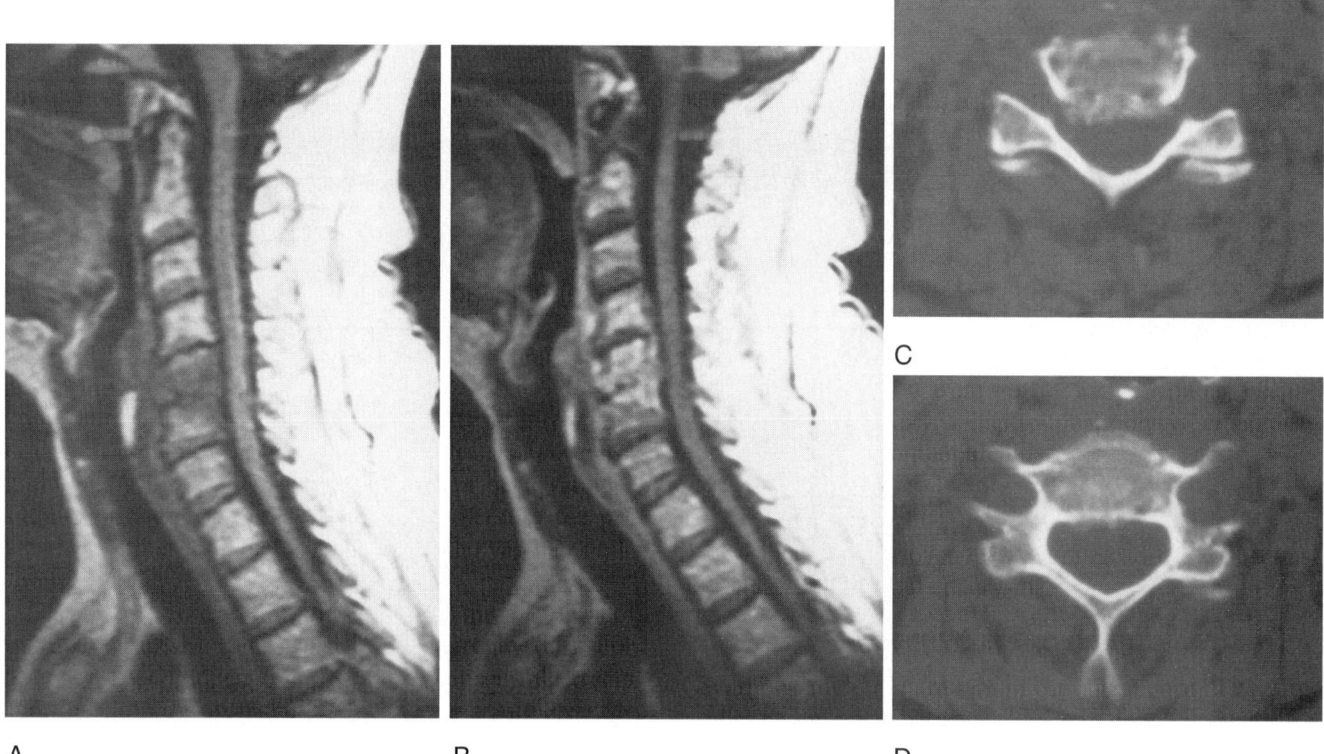

Figure 16.73. Osteomyelitis and discitis of cervical region shown by MRI and not really demonstrated by CT. **A.** T1-weighted sagittal precontrast and postcontrast (**B**) views show disappearance of the bone marrow of C5 and C6, and hyperintensity after contrast also involving the intervertebral disc, consistent with osteomyelitis with disc involvement. There may be some prevertebral soft tissue swelling. **C** and **D.** Two adjacent axial CT slices show nothing that would permit a diagnosis of osteomyelitis.

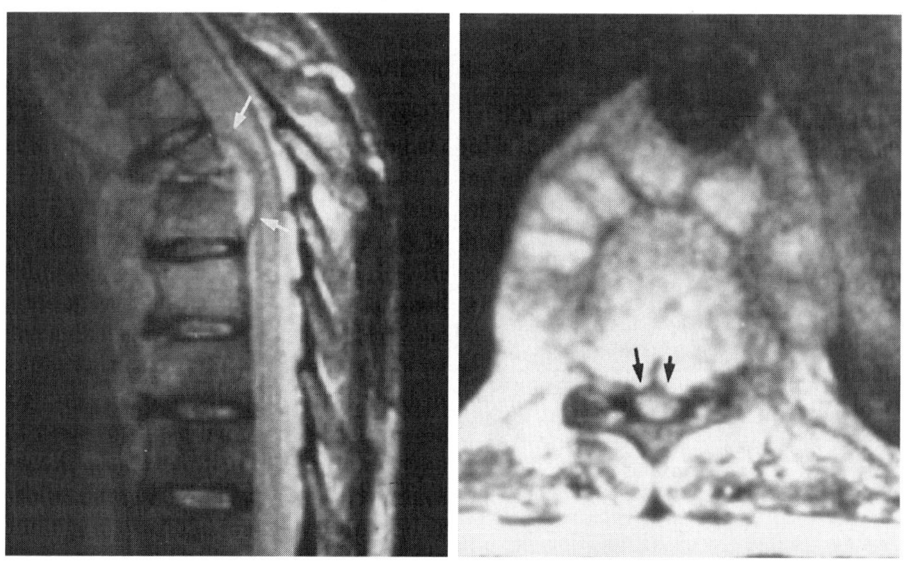

Figure 16.74. Tuberculous osteomyelitis-discitis with epidural and paraspinal abscess. **A.** There is bone destruction. The T2-weighted sagittal reveals wedge deformity of the body of T6, low intensity of the upper half of the body of T7, and partial destruction of the intervertebral disc, which has some bright area. There is an epidural collection compressing the spinal cord (arrow). **B.** Axial T2 shows the epidural collection flattening the cord (arrows). There is a larger paraspinal abscess typical of tuberculous spondylitis. (Courtesy of Dr. Erfan Hospital, Saudi Arabia.)

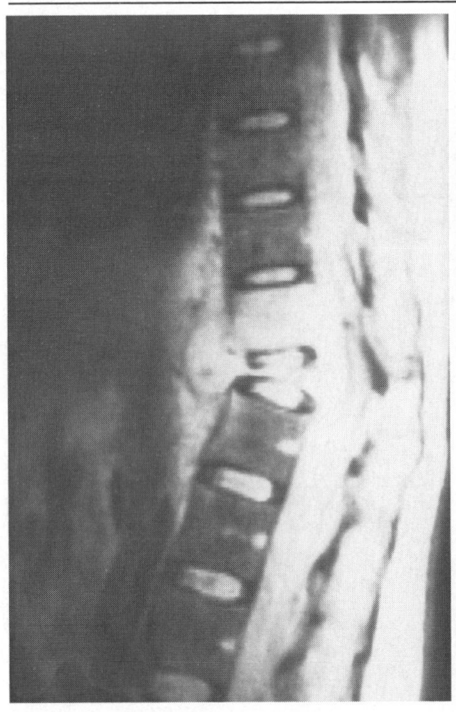

A

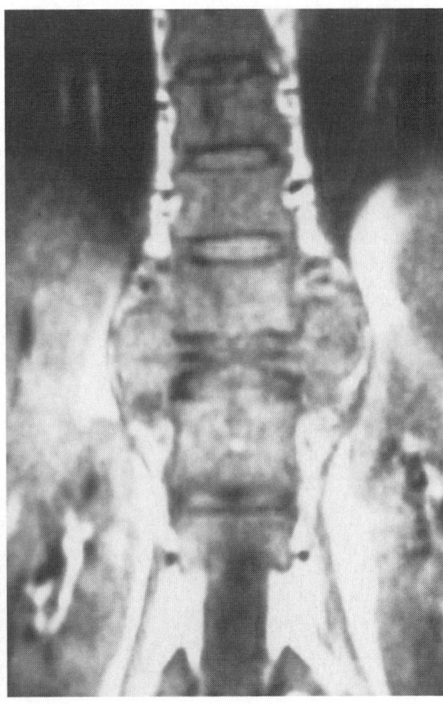

B

Figure 16.75. Tuberculous spondylitis. **A.** T2-weighted image. There is total collapse of the body of T11 and increased intensity of T10, but the intervertebral discs are preserved. There is a long prevertebral abscess extending for several segments. **B.** Coronal T1-weighted image shows the bilateral paraspinal abscess. The collapsed vertebral body is noted. (Courtesy of Dr. Erfan Hospital, Saudi Arabia.)

the low-intensity subarachnoid space. The dorsal epidural fat may disappear in the involved segments. The abscess may be ventral or dorsal, or it may go all around. On T1 following contrast, there is enhancement, which may be a solid, high-intensity band, two lines of enhancement around a nonenhanced portion, or a combination of the two. The epidural abscess may be relatively localized or may extend through various spinal segments (67). There may be solid granuloma, or the abscess may liquefy (Figs. 16.76 and 16.77).

CT alone with contrast usually demonstrates the enhanced abscess wall. It may be combined with myelography to better define the longitudinal extent of the pathologic process, but myelography should be avoided because of the possibility of meningeal contamination.

Incomplete treatment of epidural abscess can occur, and recurrences must be watched for, particularly if only medical antibiotic therapy was used. Surgical treatment combined with medical therapy has been the classic way to handle these abscesses. Contrast enhancement may persist although the patient may have improved clinically, but until the process disappears altogether, recurrence can occur, and follow-up is required.

Subdural Abscess

Subdural abscess in the spine is rare, and the symptoms mimic those of epidural abscess. Most of the reported cases have been iatrogenic (spinal punctures, anesthetics), but about a third have been spontaneous, probably hematogenous, with *Staphylococcus aureus* as the usual pathogen (68). The treatment is surgery and antibiotics. The diagnosis could be made by CT, but MRI is likely to be superior. The surgeon must be forewarned about the need to open the dura. Unfortunately, it may not be possible to differentiate between an epidural and a subdural abscess by imaging methods alone. The history of manipulation preceding the onset, such as a spinal puncture, may favor subdural over epidural abscess.

Spinal Meningitis

Spinal meningitis is usually part of a more generalized inflammation of the meninges, but in some cases it seems to predominate in the spinal meninges. The process can be acute or subacute, and the diagnosis is usually made by spinal puncture rather than by imaging methods, although the latter, namely MRI with contrast enhancement, may be useful, particularly in cases in which no organisms can be grown and when it is necessary to exclude the possibility of an extra-arachnoidal or an extradural infection.

Contrast-enhanced CT may show some circular meningeal enhancement on axial views, but this is the exception. MRI with postenhanced sagittal or coronal T1-weighted images is by far the better procedure (Fig. 16.78).

Arachnoiditis

Arachnoidal adhesions occur most frequently in the thoracic and lower cervical portions of the vertebral canal. Fibrous bands between the pia and arachnoid may be a sequela of acute meningitis or may follow trauma and surgical procedures on the spinal cord. In some instances, adhe-

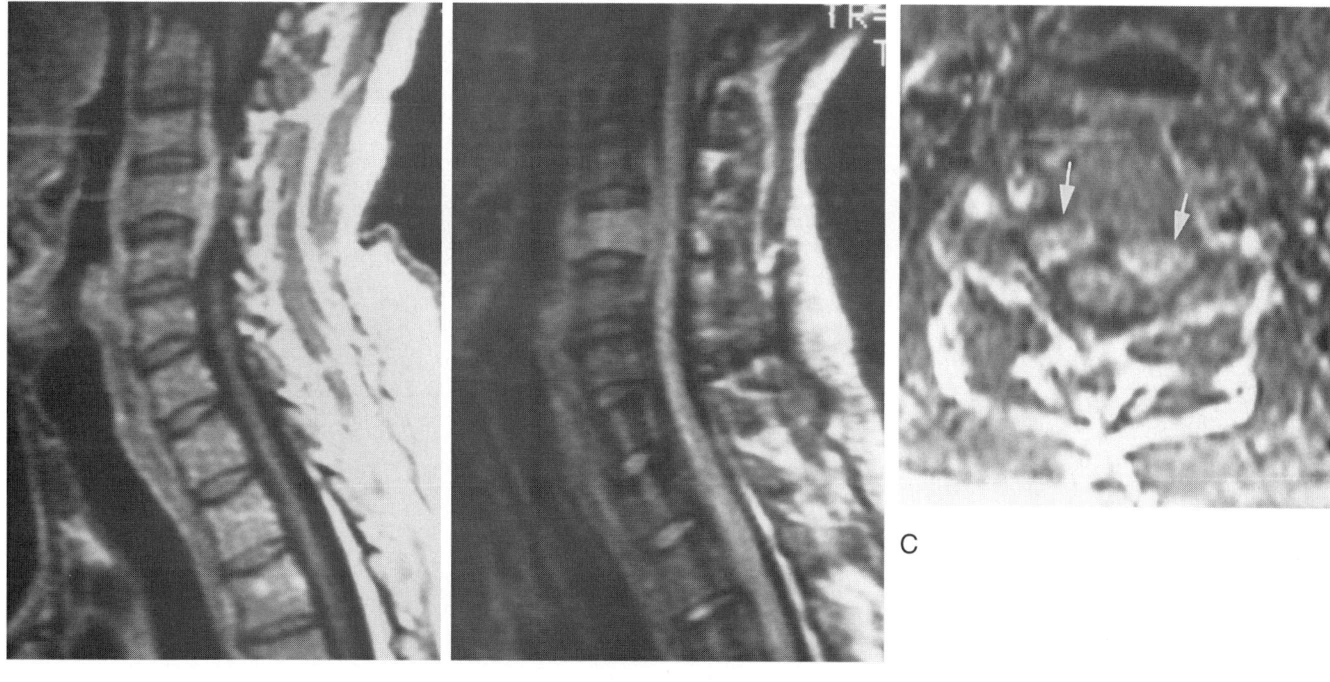

Figure 16.76. Epidural abscess in a 40-year-old patient with AIDS. **A.** A contrast-enhanced T1 sagittal image reveals an enhancing lesion on the ventral side of the spinal canal extending for the length of four cervical vertebral bodies; it is flattening the cord and displacing it dorsally. In addition, there is prevertebral enhancement in the same area, indicating a probable osteomyelitis of the spine. **B.** Proton density weighted sagittal shows hyperintensity of the body of C5; the epidural thickening is much less conspicuous than in A. There is still some CSF space in the area of cord compression. **C.** Axial postcontrast image shows that the abscess is divided at the midline (arrows).

sions occur in association with tumors and degenerative diseases of the spinal cord. The introduction of foreign materials into the spinal subarachnoid space, such as antibiotics, radiopaque substances, and anesthetic agents, may be followed months or years later by the onset of spinal cord symptoms resulting from chronic adhesive arachonoiditis. Important work that establishes beyond reasonable doubt a causal relationship between spinal anesthesia and chronic adhesive arachnoiditis, especially in the use of high, prolonged, or continuous spinal anesthesia, is reported by Kennedy et al. (69). These authors state that high concentrations of anesthetic agents may result in grave spinal cord paralyses. The frequent occurrence of arachnoidal adhesions in the midthoracic region is explained by Williams as resulting from the lowest point of the spine often falling in this area when the patient is supine during anesthesia (70). Adhesive arachnoiditis as a result of the use of a spinal anesthetic has become extremely rare.

Leptomeningeal adhesions develop slowly and gradually and increase in extent. The arachnoid is thickened. The bands that extend between the arachnoid and pia and that also connect the arachnoid and dura may be delicate or dense. Closed cavities containing fluid may be formed; these are leptomeningeal cysts. The fibrous bands and cysts may distort and compress into the spinal cord or spinal nerve roots, or they may interfere with the blood supply.

Myelography serves to establish the correct diagnosis in almost all instances where chronic adhesive arachnoiditis exists. A partial or complete obstruction to the passage of opaque material usually is found at fluoroscopy. Ordinarily there is not one point but numerous points over several vertebral segments at which the radiopaque material will be delayed, deviated from its normal course, or retained in small pockets. If the radiopaque column passes the involved area, residues of contrast material in linear, rounded, irregular forms may remain scattered throughout the abnormal zone. Such multiple reproducible deformities in the myelogram, which extend for a distance and are not accompanied by a filling defect to suggest tumor, usually are indicative of chronic inflammatory disease. It is perhaps worthy of mention that a subdural injection of radiopaque material may cause a somewhat similar appearance at fluoroscopy and in frontal myelograms. A technical error of instillation is usually recognized at the beginning of the fluoroscopic examination, and the subdural position of the radiopaque material can be identified by a lateral film made with the patient prone. The typical configuration of a block produced by arachnoiditis is one in which the special configu-

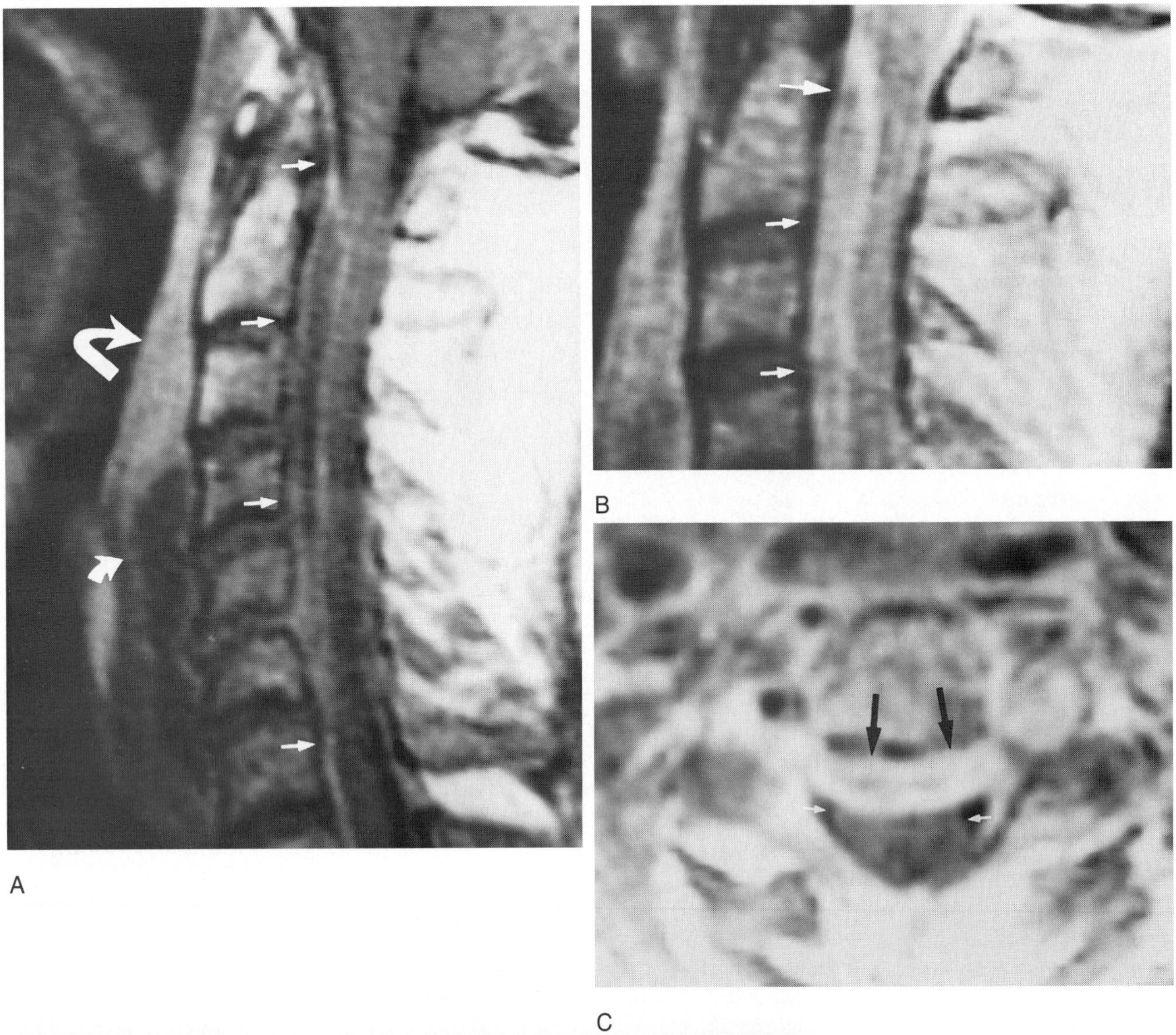

A

B

C

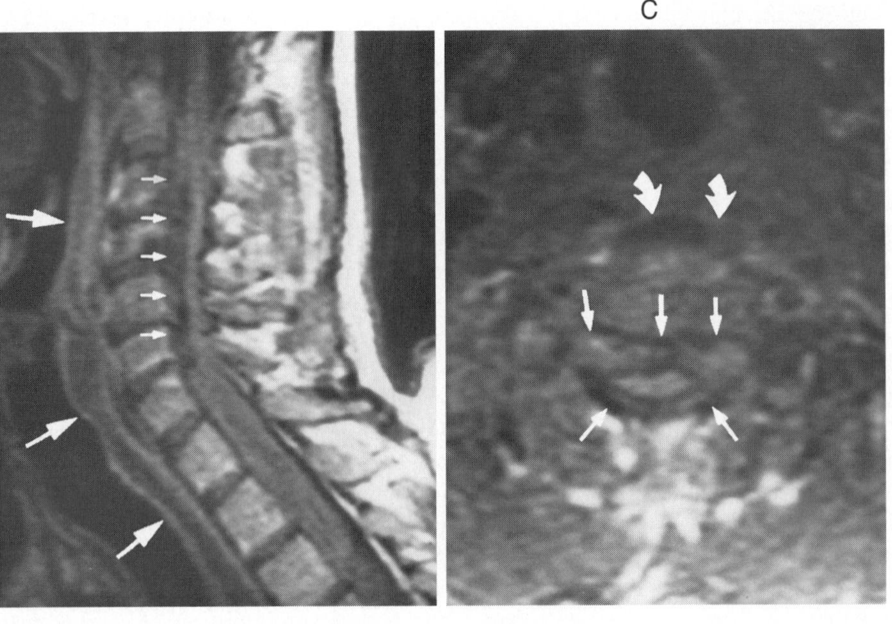

D E

Figure 16.77. Epidural abscess, cervical, two cases. **A.** A patient with a retropharyngeal abscess. The sagittal T1 after contrast shows enhancement of a membrane extending up and down anteriorly to the spinal cord (arrows). There is also enhancement of the prevertebral space, more uniform down to C4 and with cavity formation below that (curved arrow). **B.** In proton density sagittal view both abscesses are hyperintense (arrows). **C.** Postcontrast axial shows the enhanced large epidural abscess (arrows). The spinal cord is flattened (small white arrows). In another case sagittal (**D**) and axial (**E**) views after contrast show no enhancement of the abscess wall; the infection is seen to completely surround the flattened spinal cord (arrows). D shows evidence of a prevertebral abscess with wall enhancement (arrows). In D the epidural abscess extends from C2 through C6 (small white arrows), and the cord is markedly flattened.

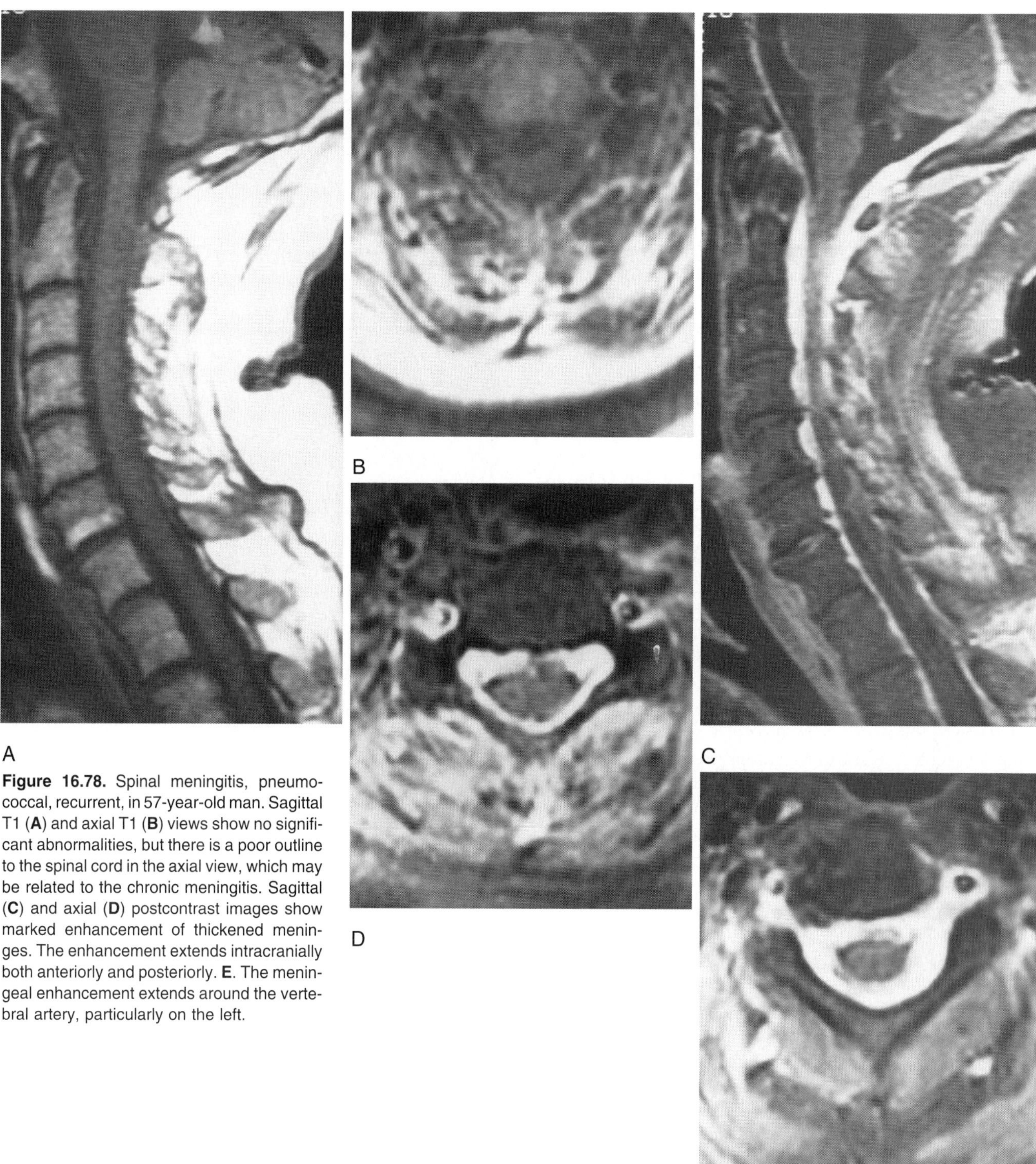

Figure 16.78. Spinal meningitis, pneumococcal, recurrent, in 57-year-old man. Sagittal T1 (**A**) and axial T1 (**B**) views show no significant abnormalities, but there is a poor outline to the spinal cord in the axial view, which may be related to the chronic meningitis. Sagittal (**C**) and axial (**D**) postcontrast images show marked enhancement of thickened meninges. The enhancement extends intracranially both anteriorly and posteriorly. **E**. The meningeal enhancement extends around the vertebral artery, particularly on the left.

ration usually produced by a tumor cannot be seen. The contrast column does not show "cupping" in either the frontal or the lateral roentgenograms, or the column may be split before stopping. The most characteristic appearance of a block produced by adhesions is, therefore, the absence of the usual signs of neoplasms.

Parasitic infestation is a rare cause of chronic leptomeningitis in the United States but is not rare in many countries throughout the world, particularly in Eastern Europe, Asia, and South America. Generally speaking, however, animal parasites are a common cause of nervous system disease. The nervous system is said to be involved in 80 percent of patients with cysticercosis, where humans act as the intermediate host for *Taenia solium*, and neural involvement is frequent with hydatid disease. The larval cysts of *T. solium* and *Taenia echinococcus* are more likely to occur in the brain than in the spinal cord, and in cysticercosis the leptomeninges are more often involved than the parenchyma. Primary hydatid cysts are single and form more frequently in the spinal epidural space than within the dural sac. *Cysticercus cellulosae* may be present in large numbers in the choroid plexus, and it is thought that in this manner they reach the CSF, in which they circulate, and then they gravitate to the lower spinal subarachnoid space.

Thick arachnoidal adhesions are observed most frequently about the base of the brain and the cauda equina.

Spinal arachnoiditis ossificans is a rare form of chronic arachnoiditis. It is probable that it is no more than calcification and ossification in an otherwise nonspecific arachnoidal adhesive process. It has been reported following trauma, subarachnoid hemorrhage, and spinal anesthesia (71). The presence of calcification in arachnoidal adhesions may be a chance finding at autopsy or may be part of a progressive process causing compression of the spinal cord and nerve roots. Except for the presence of calcification, the myelographic appearance is similar to that of other nonspecific arachnoiditis (Fig. 16.79).

The most frequent cause of chronic adhesive arachnoiditis is iatrogenic, due to surgery in the spine, usually lumbar; other causes are myelography, discography and disc chemonucleolysis, spinal anesthesia (intrathecal or epidural), and intrathecal chemotherapeutic agents. Spinal trauma is another frequent cause, and the condition may also result from meningitis.

Although the term *chronic adhesive arachnoiditis* has found its way into the literature, it may not be entirely accurate for many of the instances in which it is found. The term *simple arachnoidal adhesions* is much more appropriate for the great majority of cases where it is found in the lumbar region, for it is not an active chronic inflammatory process. Rather, it is the result of an irritative episode, be it traumatic, chemical, or hemorrhage, that led to the production of inflammation, and finally adhesions where the pia-arachnoid becomes adherent to itself, forming some pockets or loculations, but it does not mean that there exists an active inflammation lasting for the rest of the patient's life.

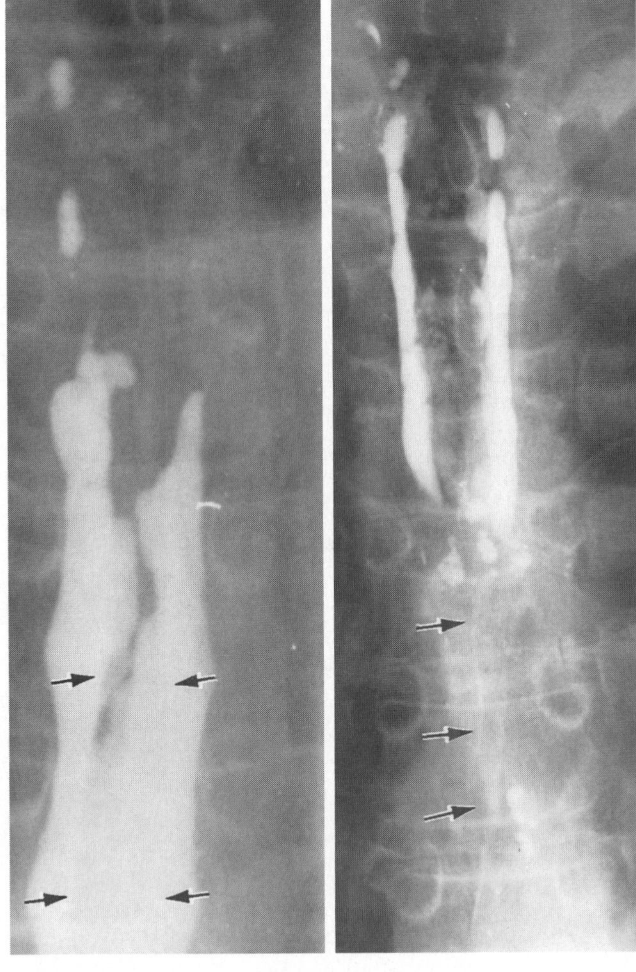

Figure 16.79. Spinal arachnoiditis ossificans, posttraumatic. **A.** Lumbar injection. **B.** Cisternal injection. There is virtually complete block in both directions, and the outline of the contrast column does not reveal any contours suggestive of an intraspinal mass in either the intradural or the extradural space. The cord is atrophic (arrows in A). A thin, elongated shell-like calcification is seen in the area where there is a block to the flow of contrast (arrows in B).

Trauma is a typical example; there may be meningeal disruption and hemorrhage followed by adhesions, and the process may last some weeks or months before it becomes stable, after which no further changes are expected (Fig. 16.79).

The use of Pantopaque myelography was particularly effective in diagnosing arachnoidal adhesions because it does not go through small openings into pockets, whereas the water-soluble contrast does and thus may demonstrate a picture that is less pronounced than that shown by Pantopaque and closer to the true state of the spinal thecal sac (Fig. 16.80*B*). In other words, the picture of arachnoidal adhesions shown by Pantopaque may be an exaggeration of the actual situation. The water-soluble contrast myelogram may show a featureless opaque column without normal root sleeves, leaving the sac without normal-appearing roots

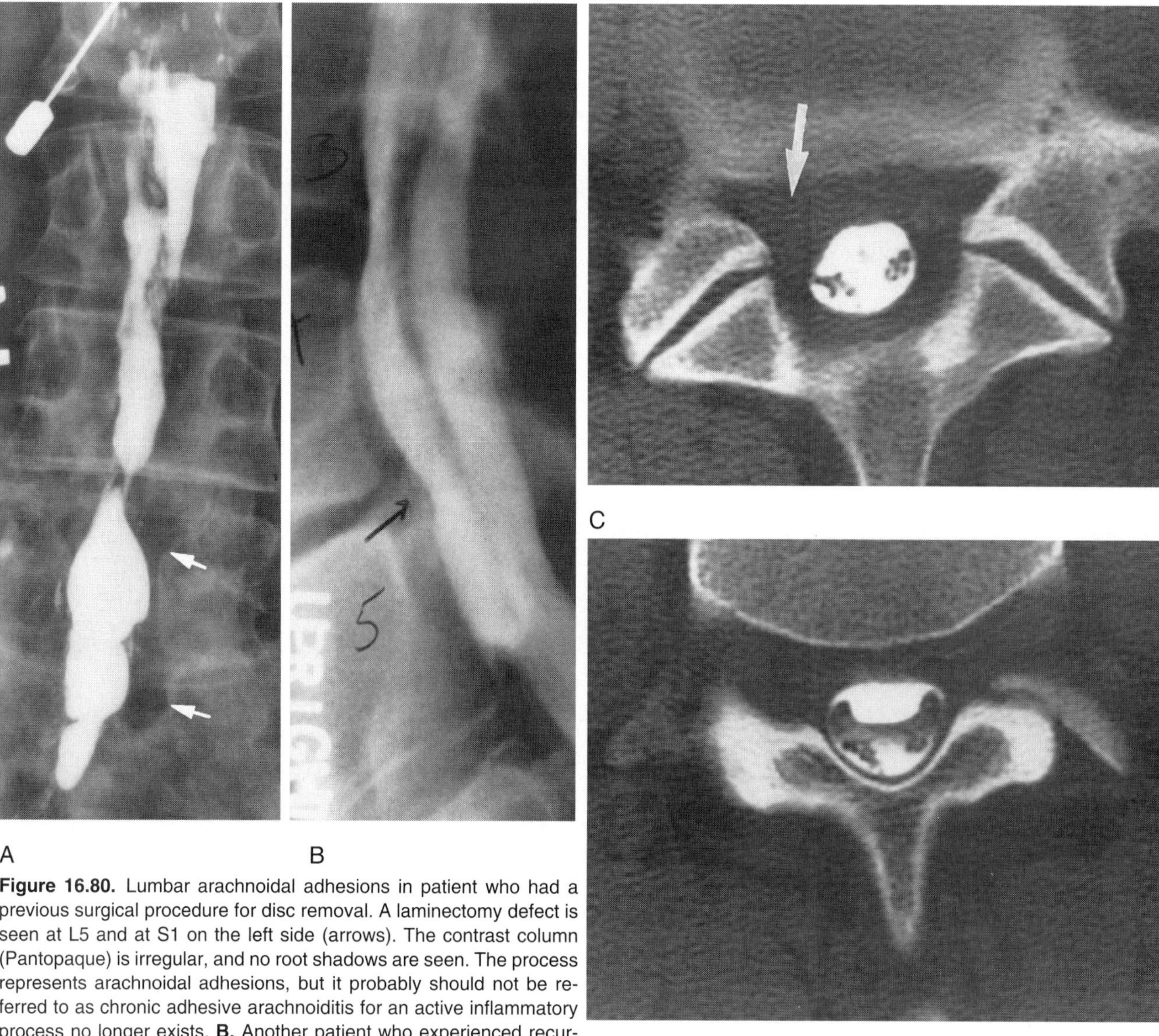

Figure 16.80. Lumbar arachnoidal adhesions in patient who had a previous surgical procedure for disc removal. A laminectomy defect is seen at L5 and at S1 on the left side (arrows). The contrast column (Pantopaque) is irregular, and no root shadows are seen. The process represents arachnoidal adhesions, but it probably should not be referred to as chronic adhesive arachnoiditis for an active inflammatory process no longer exists. **B.** Another patient who experienced recurrence of symptoms some time after surgical removal of a disc. The patient did not have a prior myelogram. The lateral myelogram shows a radiolucent band from L2-L3 down to L5, which on CT axial images was found to be due to adhesion of the roots, which are matted together on both sides (**C** and **D**). In C there is evidence of deformity of the thecal sac on the right side due to a herniated disc (arrow).

running down the sac, or there may be "thickening" of some roots, which may be produced by adhesions between two or more roots. MRI diagnosis of arachnoidal adhesions can be made in the lumbar as well as in the thoracocervical region. Posttraumatic arachnoidal adhesions may lead to the formation of arachnoid pockets around the spinal cord in the thoracic or cervical areas. These pockets or cysts may produce some compression of the spinal cord and sometimes may be associated with syringomyelia. Whether the multiple arachnoidal adhesions lead to the syringomyelia or whether the syrinx is due to central spinal cord hemorrhage and later cavitation cannot be ascertained absolutely; the important point is that if there are signs of cord dysfunction, the treatment, through surgical drainage of the cysts and of the syringomyelic cavity, may improve the patient's symptoms. The diagnosis of posttraumatic arachnoidal adhesions is particularly well seen by MRI. The CSF pockets can be seen to follow the CSF signal on T1- and T2-weighted images, and syringomyelia, if present, is well seen.

In the lumbar region, the most frequent site of occurrence, adhesion between the roots and adhesion of roots to the periphery of the thecal sac, can usually be shown by MRI as well as by CT-myelography (72). Ross et al. have described three types of appearance: (*a*) clumping of a group of roots in the center of the thecal sac, (*b*) adhesion of the roots dorsally against the surface of the sac, giving an appearance suggestive of a thickened dura, and (*c*) diffuse hyperintensity of contents of the thecal sac on T1-weighted images. The myelogram may reveal a complete block to contrast flow in these cases.

INTRASPINAL ARACHNOID CYSTS

These cysts may occur as a complication of epidural anesthesia and may lead to sufficient cord compression to produce paraparesis or paraplegia (73), but the most frequent cause of these cysts produced by arachnoidal adhesions and pocket formation is trauma. It is debatable whether epidural anesthetic agents may be the cause of this complication (74). However, animal experiments can never exclude individual sensitivities to a given anesthetic or other compound. Complications of spinal epidural punctures, on a technical basis, may also be a factor; one of the patients reported by Sklar et al. (73) had only a traumatic spinal lumbar puncture.

Intraspinal meningeal cysts, therefore, constitute a number of different etiologic factors and locations (75). In the congenital variety we may include the intrathoracic meningoceles associated with dural ectasia, the sacral cysts, which may grow with the passage of time, and the epidural cysts in the thoracic region. Neurenteric cysts and epidermoid cysts probably do not belong in this category, for they are not filled with CSF. The encysted dorsal arachnoid diverticula may be added, but they might be considered as acquired by secondary inflammation at their connection with the subarachnoid space.

In the acquired variety, arachnoiditis or arachnoidal inflammation, be it traumatic, infectious (meningitis), inflammatory due to a chemical irritation, or due to the combination of a mild chemical irritation with other factors such as intrathecal hemorrhage, should be considered. The acquired meningeal cysts are usually in the thoracic region. As mentioned earlier, the sacral cysts are acquired in that they grow gradually but existed previously; the same is true of some spontaneous dorsal meningeal cysts in patients with no history of prior surgery or spinal puncture.

Pachymeningitis

Hypertrophic spinal pachymeningitis was first described by Charcot in 1869 and consists of an inflammation of the dura mater leading to thickening of the membrane, which may produce constriction of the spinal canal and interfere with the normal function of the spinal cord. The symptoms consist of local pain, limitation of motion, radicular pain, and, later, diminution of strength in the extremities.

The etiology of a thickened dura varies; syphilis was a frequent occurrence before treatment with modern antibiotics. In addition, nonspecific inflammation and thickening have been reported, also involving the base of the skull (see under "Disease of the Meninges," Chapter 6; see also Fig. 6.52). Thickening due to infiltration of the dura is also seen in mucopolysaccharidoses, particularly the Maroteaux-Lamy variety (Fig. 16.81*B* and *C*). A case has been seen in association with Whipple disease.

The imaging diagnosis of pachymeningitis can be made by MRI because it demonstrates thickening of the membrane outside the subarachnoid space (see Fig. 13.2). It may enhance with contrast. Myelography demonstrates separation between the pedicles and the outer margin of the contrast (Fig. 16.81).

The separation of the subarachnoid space from the bony canal can be shown also by CT-myelography. The meninges can become very thick in chronic cases of meningitis (Fig. 16.78*D* and *E*).

Myelitis

Myelitis is a diagnosis of exclusion. It may be made clinically after other imaging and laboratory tests have failed to demonstrate other possible causes, but in many cases MRI examination may show changes that would assist in the diagnosis. Myelitis may produce an isolated clinical picture of transverse myelitis, or it may be associated with symptoms or signs indicative of involvement of the brain. The latter situation is most common in multiple sclerosis (see Fig. 4.64). Myelitis may be seen in acute disseminated encephalomyelitis (ADEM), usually following a nonspecific viral condition or vaccination; it also may be seen as a manifestation of lupus erythematosus. An important condition to consider in the presence of a chronic picture suggestive of myelitis is arteriovenous malformation of the cord, which may give an image of diffuse enhancement with contrast and hyperintensity on T2.

MRI may show areas of hyperintensity on proton density and T2-weighted images, which may be localized or diffuse. Gadolinium enhancement may or may not show increased uptake (Fig. 16.82). Barakos et al. state that the T2 hyperintensity usually extends for several vertebral segments (76).

Sarcoid can produce a picture of a progressive myelopathy that can be demonstrated by MRI. Multifocal parenchymal enhancement and meningeal enhancement may be seen (77). Acquired immunodeficiency syndrome (AIDS) may be associated with a myelopathic picture owing to cord inflammation (76). MRI may also show enlargement of the cord on T1-weighted images, and this aspect is demonstrable on myelography. Follow-up examination may reveal a return of the spinal cord to normal, or it may show atrophy or diminution in size in the involved segments. In ADEM the changes disappear promptly and the cord returns to normal; in multiple sclerosis the changes may persist for some time.

Hyperintensity on T2-weighted images involving the anterior horns of the gray matter has been reported in poliomyelitis (78). The change may be seen on axial as well as sagittal T2-weighted images.

PARANEOPLASTIC MYELITIS

This is a condition observed in patients with malignant disease elsewhere. In these cases there is also brain involvement, as well as dorsal root ganglia (79).

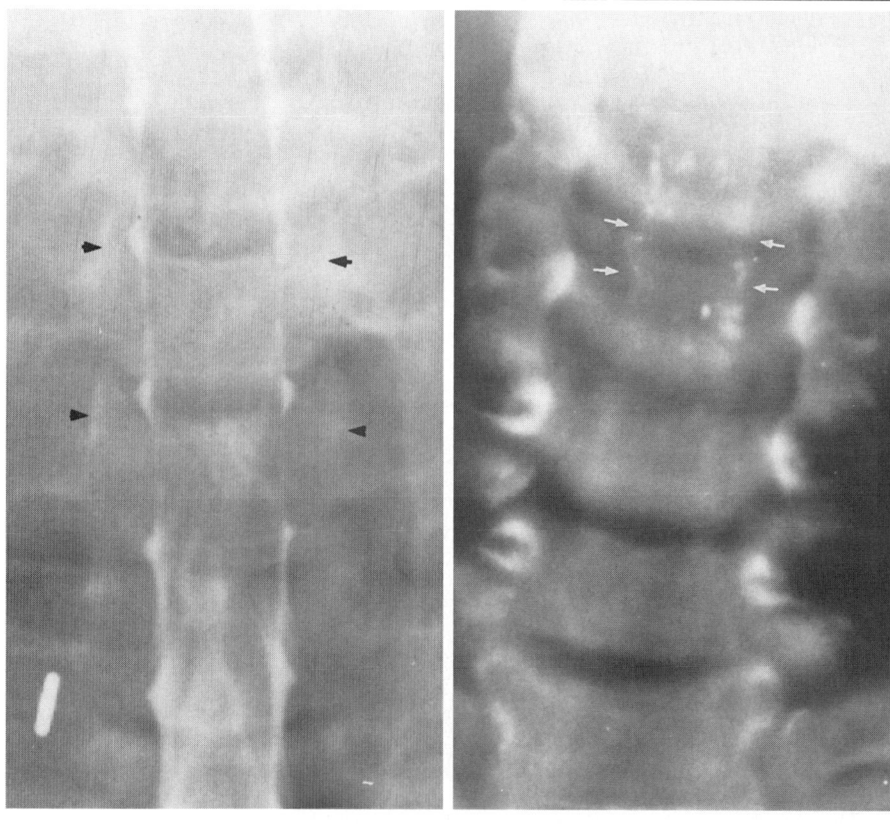

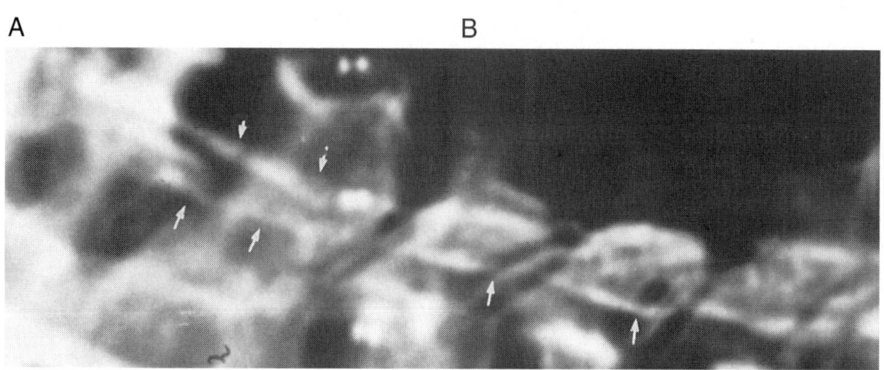

Figure 16.81. Hypertrophic spinal pachymeningitis. **A**. The patient, a 31-year-old man, had complained of neck pain of increasing severity and limitation of motion for 8 months. Myelography demonstrated a partial block to the cephalad flow of contrast, thinning of the contrast outside the cord, and separation of the opaque column from the pedicles (arrowheads). At surgery the dura was greatly thickened (up to 5 mm) and histology revealed marked increase in collagenous material and perivascular round-cell infiltration. The test for syphilis was negative, but the patient had been treated for venereal disease. **B** and **C**. Thickening of dura in patient with mucopolysaccharidosis (Maroteaux-Lamy variety). Frontal (**B**) and lateral (**C**) projections after myelography show the edge of the thecal sac is away from the bony canal margins (arrows).

POSTRADIATION MYELITIS

This is seen in patients treated, most frequently, for head and neck malignancies. In general radiation myelitis is seen between 1 and 2½ years following therapy, but if the radiation dose to the cord has been very high, it may occur earlier. The diagnosis can be made only by MRI, which reveals a segment of T2 hyperintensity, usually in the cervical or the thoracic region. It may enhance with contrast (Fig. 16.83).

MULTIPLE SCLEROSIS

Multiple sclerosis (MS) has been described in Chapter 4. Cord involvement may sometimes be the only manifestation of MS, although in these cases it is fairly common to find typical lesions if an MRI examination of the brain is carried out. For this reason, in any myelopathic syndrome where MS is part of the differential diagnosis the spinal cord as well as the brain should be examined with MRI (see Fig. 4.64). The lesions are T2 bright, they may be single or multiple, and they may or may not contrast enhance.

AMYOTROPHIC LATERAL SCLEROSIS

Amyotrophic lateral sclerosis may show symmetric hyperintensity in the corticospinal tracts beginning at the precentral gyri passing through the brainstem and into the corticospinal tracts in the anterior and lateral cervical spinal cord (80). The distribution is similar to wallerian degeneration, and the bilateral involvement in combination with the clinical findings would be typical of amyotrophic lateral sclerosis.

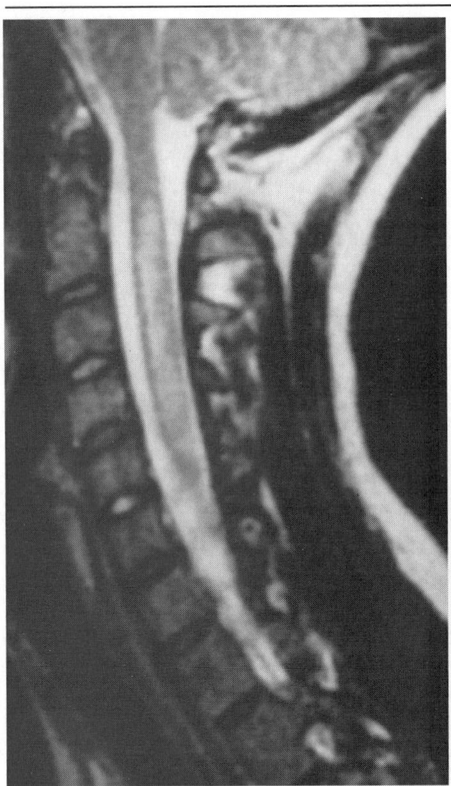

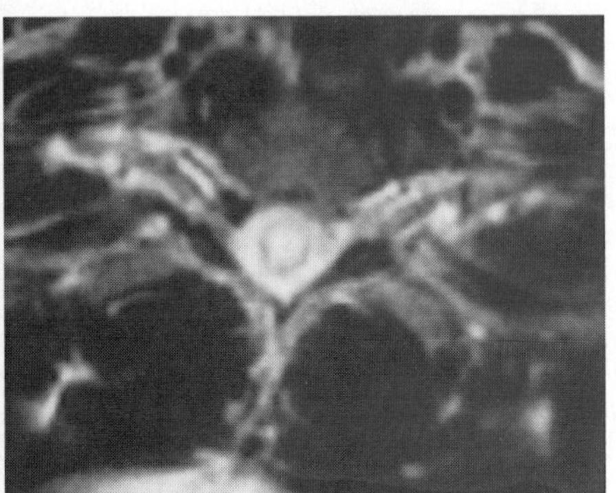

A B

Figure 16.82. Myelitis. **A.** Sagittal T2-weighted MRI shows hyperintensity in the cervical cord; the surrounding CSF is bright. **B.** Axial T2-weighted image shows that the cord is uniformly bright except for a thin normal rim on the periphery. The patient, a 19-year-old boy, was found to have a high Lyme disease titre.

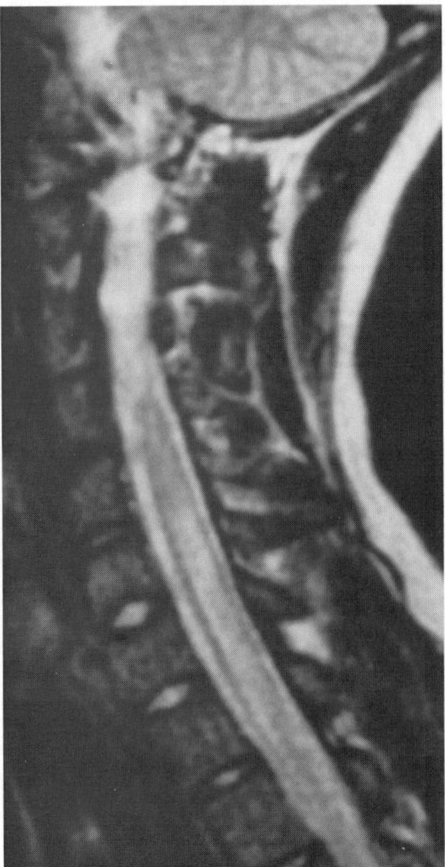

Figure 16.83. Radiation myelitis in a patient who had been treated 20 months previously for a neck malignant lesion. The sagittal T2-weighted image reveals diffuse hyperintensity of the cord extending for three cervical segments.

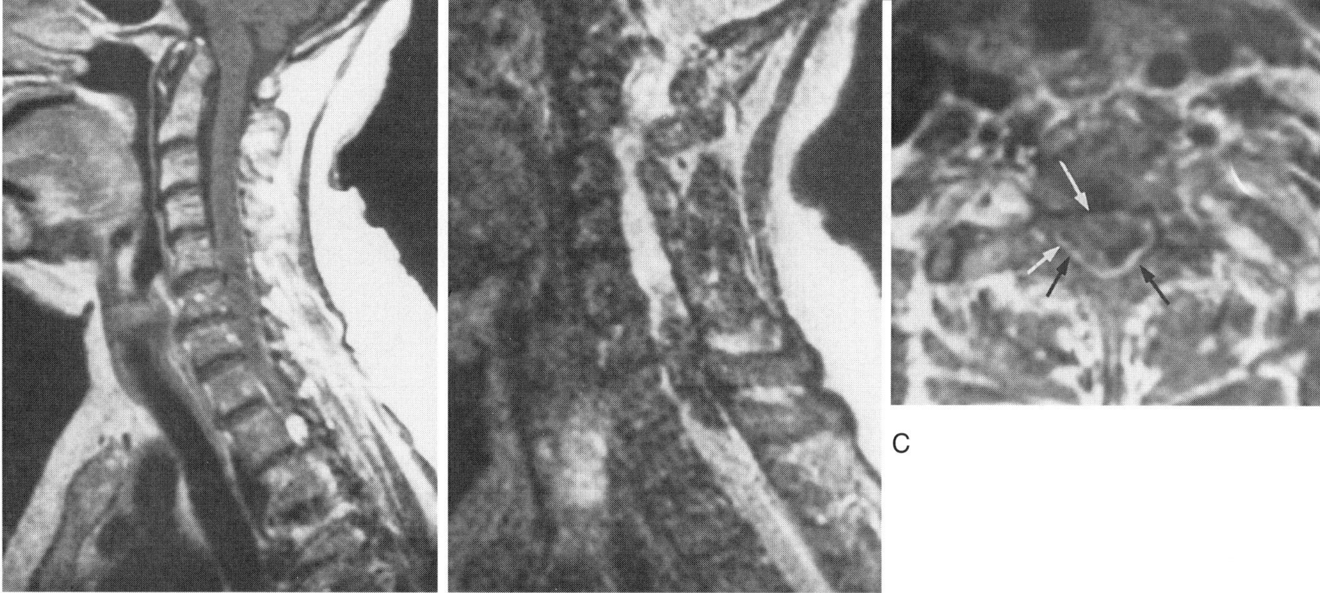

Figure 16.84. Spontaneous spinal epidural hematoma in a 63-year-old woman who complained of onset of severe pain in lower cervical upper thoracic region. **A.** T1-weighted contrast-enhanced sagittal view shows absence of normal dorsal subarachnoid space and considerable thinning of ventral subarachnoid space from C4 down. There is enhancement of the dura on the dorsal side. **B.** T2-weighted image shows a T2-dark dorsal area between C6 and T2, probably related to deoxyhemoglobin. **C.** Axial T1 shows cord compressed and displaced ventrally (white upper arrow) by a slightly hyperintense flat lesion on right side (two arrows, black and white). There is enhancement of the dura (black arrows). Because of the sudden onset, the T2-dark image suggestive of blood in the deoxyhemoglobin stage, and the dural enhancement, a diagnosis of epidural hemorrhage was made and confirmed surgically. The apparent enhancement of the dura on the right side in C does not correlate with the epidural location of the hematoma and suggests that the hematoma may have been subdural. (Courtesy of Stephen Sweriduk, Boston, Mass.)

OTHER CAUSES OF MYELITIS

A cause of myelitis to be considered, particularly in the Caribbean and Japan, is the HTLV II virus. It has been relatively recently recognized and can be diagnosed by appropriate serologic tests. It leads to a paraparesis that usually shows little improvement. In a case seen by the author the patient was thought to have a cervical ridge compressing the cord. This led to a laminectomy. The patient did not improve but progressed slowly to a greater degree of paraparesis, which became stable. MRI revealed atrophy of the cervical spinal cord, and the HTLV II test was performed when it became known (81).

VASCULAR LESIONS OF THE SPINAL CANAL AND SPINAL CORD

Epidural Hemorrhage

This is a condition, usually occurring spontaneously, in which there is a hemorrhage in the epidural space. It is an acute condition, usually requiring emergency treatment, that starts with severe focal back pain, often followed by paraparesis or paraplegia within a relatively short period of time. It presumably arises from rupture of a vascular malformation, an angioma, or a small arteriovenous malformation. Myelography usually reveals an epidural-type block, and CT can demonstrate the hyperdensity of a hemorrhagic lesion in the acute stage (82). MRI may show the hematoma as well as the cord compression. Because of the extradural location of the hematoma, changes in hemoglobin would occur much more rapidly than in the brain (Fig. 16.84).

Circulation of the Spinal Cord

The blood supply of the spinal cord had been described by anatomists, but it took the development of spinal cord angiography for us to be able to understand its distribution as well as its function. Radicular arteries accompany the spinal nerves and supply most of the blood to the spinal cord. However, each one of these radicular arteries does not contribute to the vascular supply of the spinal cord to the same extent. Three vertically arranged territories of supply are recognized (83,84). The majority of the radicular arteries that are present in the embryo regress in the course of development, and in the adult only 6 to 8 functioning arteries that supply the anterior spinal arterial trunk, and between 10 and 23 supplying the posterior spinal arterial trunk remain. The term *radiculomedullary artery* is used to refer to those arteries that actually supply the spinal

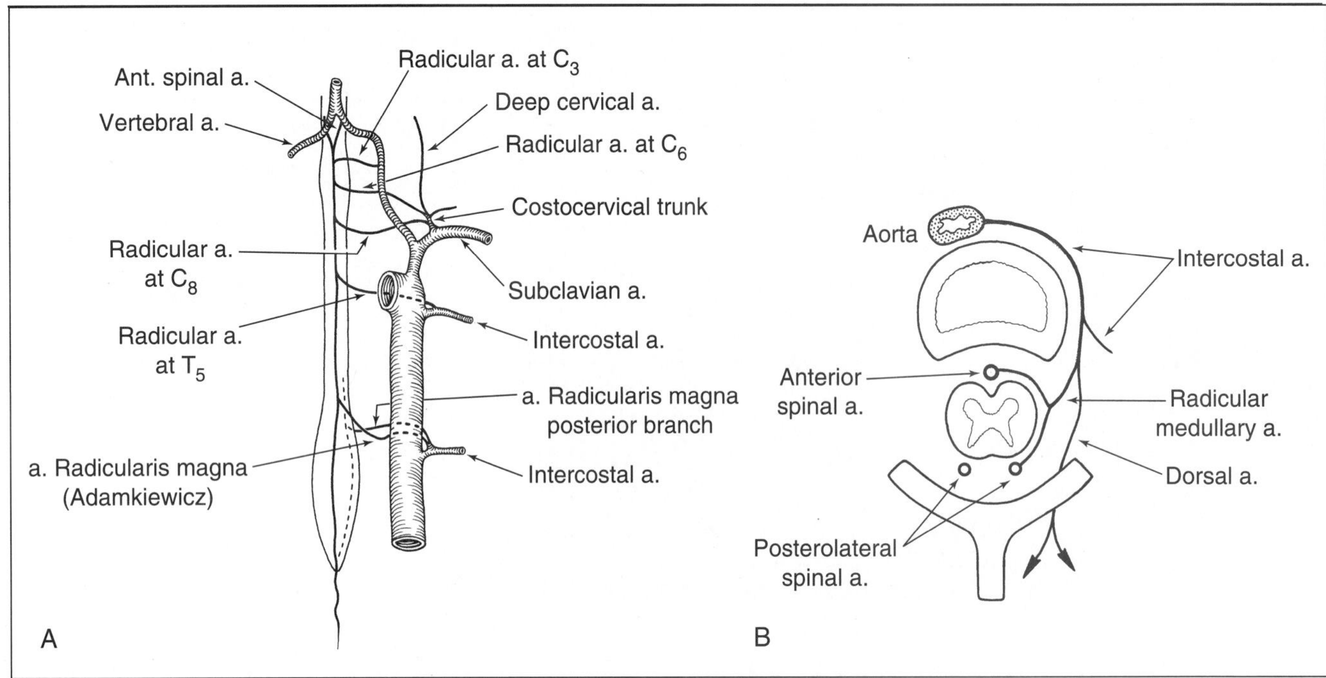

Figure 16.85. Diagram of spinal cord circulation. **A.** Frontal view. **B.** Cross-sectional representation in the horizontal plane.

cord and in the usual case give off two branches, one anterior and one posterior.

The arteries of the spinal cord are arranged along three longitudinal arterial systems: the anterior spinal artery system, the two posterolateral arteries, and the perimedullary plexus, which connects the previous two systems. The anterior spinal artery is formed by the junction of the two arteries arising from the vertebral arteries. The two arteries join to form a single anterior spinal artery. In its upper part this artery could be plexiform (25 percent of cases) and is often double for the first two or three cervical segments (83). (Fig. 16.85). From its cervical portion, the anterior spinal artery is continued down to the lower end of the spinal cord by the anterior radicular branches, which bifurcate as they reach the anterolateral aspect of the spinal cord; one branch is directed cephalad, almost always smaller, and the other branch is directed caudally. Thus the anterior spinal artery is maintained as a single trunk and may be quite small in the midthoracic region; sometimes actual discontinuity exists in the thoracic region. Likewise, the two posterolateral arteries are maintained throughout the length of the spinal cord by the anastomoses of the ascending and descending branches of the posterior radicular arteries and run roughly parallel and medial to the emergence of the posterior roots (Fig. 16.85).

The circulation of the spinal cord can be divided into three major territories:

1. The *superior or cervicodorsal territory* is supplied by the anterior spinal arteries, branches of the vertebral artery, a branch arising from the vertebral artery that accompanies the C3 spinal nerve root, another radicular artery accompanying the C6 nerve root, usually originating from the deep cervical artery, and an artery accompanying the C8 root arising from the costocervical trunk. These levels appear constant, but the side on which they are present varies (Fig. 16.85). Cervical radiculomedullary arteries may also arise from the ascending cervical artery.
2. The *midthoracic region* corresponds to the first seven thoracic spinal segments. The anterior spinal artery receives usually only one radicular artery accompanying the fourth or fifth root on either side arising from the intercostal arteries. As mentioned earlier, the midthoracic region has a relatively poor blood supply.
3. In the *inferior or thoracolumbosacral region*, from the eighth thoracic segment to the conus medullaris, the main arterial supply is the one derived from the *arteria radicularis anterior magna (artery of Adamkiewicz).* This is usually single, arises on the left side in 80 percent of individuals, and reaches the spinal cord accompanying a nerve root between T9 and L2 in 85 percent of the cases (in 75 percent of the cases, it is between T9 and T12). In the remaining 15 percent of the cases, the artery may originate between T5 and T8 (85). In the latter cases a supplemental radicular artery may be encountered farther down. The artery of Adamkiewicz is usually fairly large, giving off a cephalic and a caudal branch, the latter being the larger of the two. Because of this appearance it acquires a hairpin configuration that is characteristic (Fig. 16.85).

The veins of the spinal cord follow essentially the same pattern as the arteries (86). The blood flows out of the spinal cord into the radicular veins to the vertebral venous plexus and the extraspinal network.

Di Chiro et al. were first to demonstrate an intraspinal vascular lesion in the cervical region by means of vertebral angiography (87). These lesions may have been vascular nodules of hemangioblastoma, however, because the patient had retinal angiomatosis and cerebellar vascular nodules as well.

Djindjian et al. were the first to report the diagnosis of an angioma of the spinal cord by angiography (88). For several years Djindjian and coworkers utilized midstream injections into the aorta, after which it was possible via the use of subtraction to visualize the spinal cord circulation. In 1967, Di Chiro and coworkers reported on the use of selective catheterization of individual arteries to demonstrate the circulation of the spinal cord (87). This method was adopted by others very quickly and is now used by all workers in the field. Midstream injections have been reported to produce paraplegia as a complication of the procedure. For further details see Chapters 17 ("Angiography") and 18 ("Endovascular Therapeutic Neuroradiology").

SPINAL CORD INFARCTION

This results from occlusion of one of the feeding arteries of the cord. The circulation of the spinal cord is interesting in that there appears to be circulation moving in the opposite direction in the same artery because of the way that continuity of the anterior spinal artery is obtained by contributions from the radicular arteries. Reversal of circulation can easily be achieved, and it is possibly for this reason that spinal cord ischemic lesions occur less frequently than might be expected (89). The onset is usually abrupt, and men may be more frequently affected than women (10 of 12 cases reported by Yuh et al.).

MRI usually reveals changes, mostly hyperintensity on proton density or on T2-weighted images (Fig. 16.86). The findings may extend for a few to several vertebral segments. Some cases may be associated with aortic occlusion, which may also be visible on the MR examination. The latter cases may also show ischemic changes in the vertebral bodies due to multiple radiculomedullary artery occlusion. Enlargement of the cord due to edema may be demonstrated in the acute stage on T1-weighted images, while later (several months) the cord may be atrophic.

The vascular occlusion is usually arterial and may be due to thrombosis or embolism. Some unusual cases of fibrocartilaginous emboli have been reported in individuals 13 to 77 years of age. A case was reported in which biopsies taken at the time of surgery (the diagnosis had been neoplasm) demonstrated fibrocartilaginous emboli in several of the small arteries included in the specimen (90). Other cases of fibrocartilaginous emboli have been reported (91).

Venous infarction has been reported in association with arteriovenous malformations (92). Causes of spinal cord infarction have been listed as follows: hypertension, aortic surgery, complication from aortography, syphilis, occlusion of vertebral artery, spinal trauma, polycythemia, disc herniation, and thrombophlebitis.

Vascular Malformations

These include arteriovenous communications, cavernous angiomas, and arterial aneurysms.

CAVERNOUS ANGIOMAS

Cavernous angiomas are rare in the spinal cord. They are similar to the ones that occur in the brain, and when they are found in the cord the brain should be carefully examined to rule out similar lesions. The angiomas may produce neurologic signs without rupturing, but they may bleed, leading to the production of a sudden neurologic deficit, usually paraplegia. The diagnosis could be suspected by MRI because the appearance could be somewhat similar to that found in the brain: T1 hypo- or hyperintensity, T2 hyperintensity with area of hypointensity, and little or no alteration of spinal cord contour. Susceptibility images may reveal evidence of old hemorrhage.

ARTERIAL ANEURYSMS

Arterial aneurysms are also quite rare in the spinal cord. They usually occur in the anterior spinal artery, alone or in association with arteriovenous malformations of the cord (93). The aneurysms can be very small or can be large enough to produce cord compression and symptoms related to it (94). They may be associated with conditions other than arteriovenous malformations of the cord, such as coarctation of the aorta. Subarachnoid hemorrhage has been the most frequent presenting symptom. The diagnosis can be made by angiography, and an arteriovenous malformation is usually demonstrated at the same time.

Arteriovenous Malformations and Arteriovenous Fistulas

These are the most important vascular lesions of the spinal cord both because they are more frequent than the others and, particularly, because they are often amenable to surgical and embolization treatment. Thus, an accurate diagnosis, as early as possible, turns out to be most important. Four types have been described: Type I malformations occur in men between 40 and 70 years of age, have a single arterial feeder, and drain into a vein inside the cord. A high percentage (up to half) may be posttraumatic. Type II, occurring mainly in younger patients, have multiple feeders, form a vascular nodule, and are usually found in the upper cervical region (Fig. 16.87). Type III are large and complex, with multiple arterial feeders from more than one vertebral level. Type IV are mostly fed by the anterior spinal artery and are extramedullary. These are true arteriovenous fistulas without a nidus, and the veins are outside the cord. They tend to occur in the thoracolumbar area

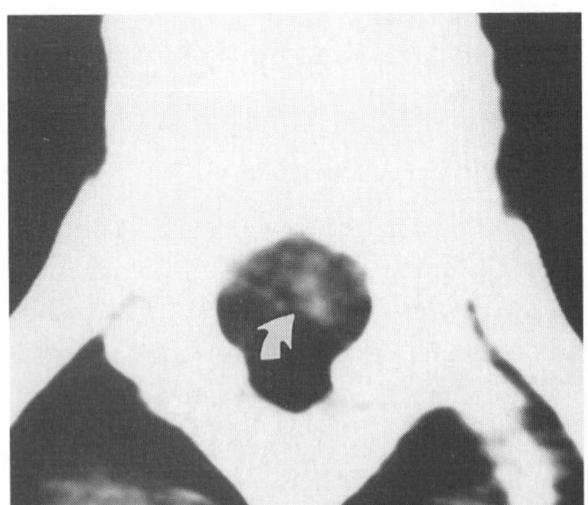

Figure 16.86. Hemorrhagic infarction of lower thoracic spinal cord in a 49-year-old woman with sudden onset of paraplegia and a sensory level. **A.** CT shows increased density compatible with blood (arrow). **B.** Sagittal gradient-echo image, 24 h later, shows marked magnetic susceptibility effect compatible with deoxyhemoglobin. The T1-weighted image was essentially negative at this time. **C.** Myelography was negative except for suggestion of blood vessel shadows, possibly related to an arteriovenous malformation. Spinal angiography (not shown) was negative. **D.** Reexamination by MRI 7 days after onset now showed T1 hyperintensity in appropriate region of cord, consistent with methemoglobin.

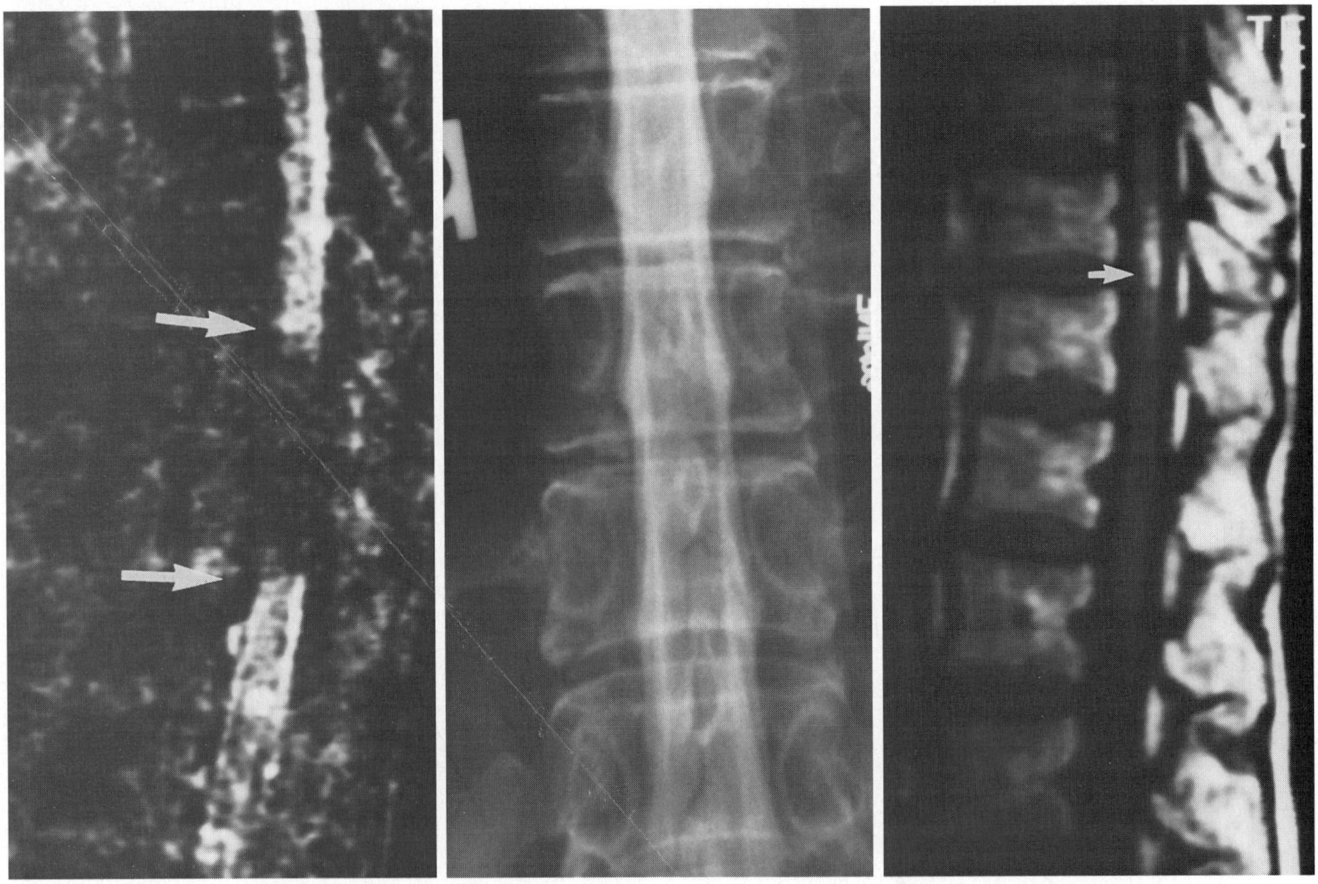

A

B C D

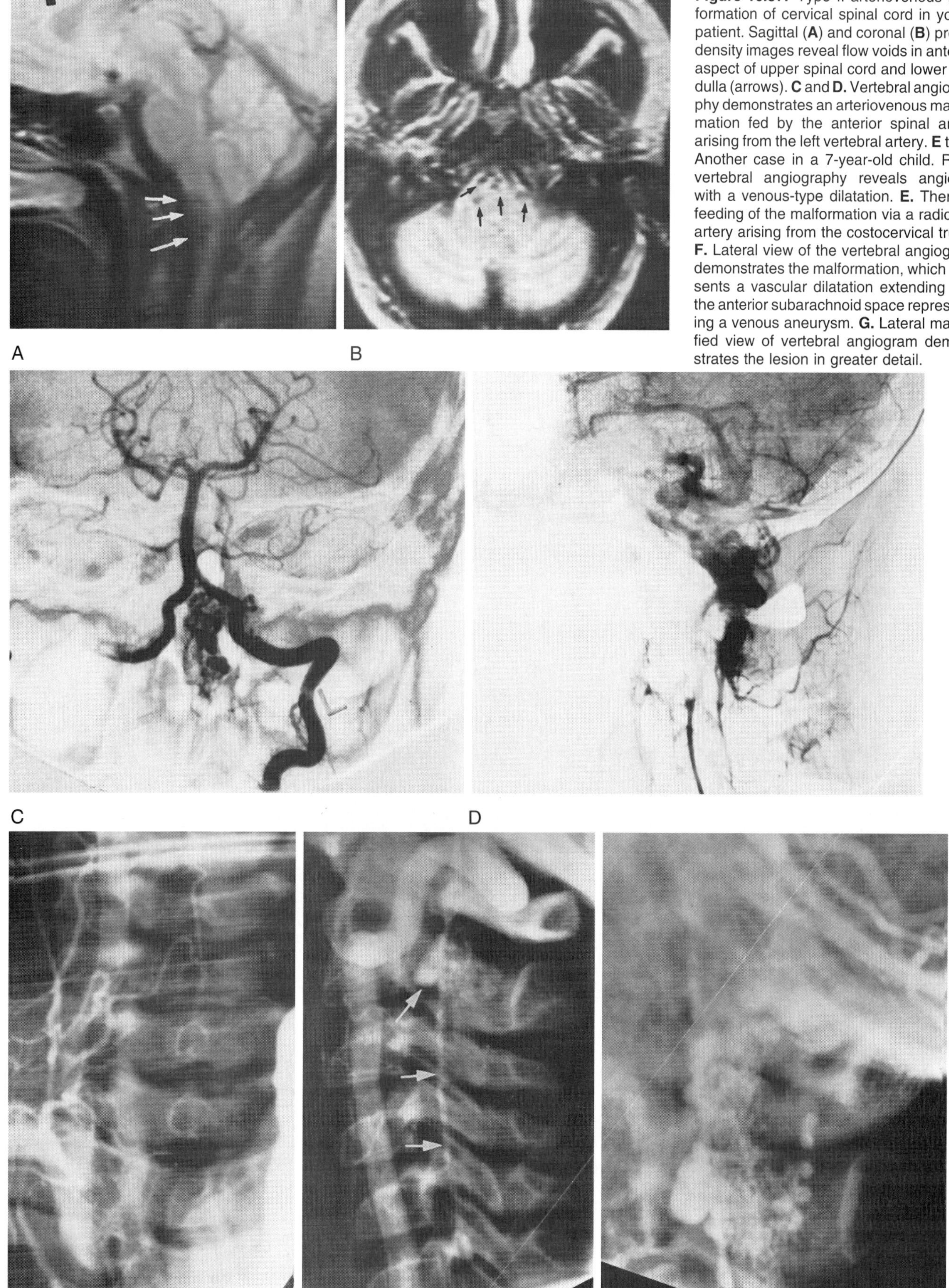

Figure 16.87. Type II arteriovenous malformation of cervical spinal cord in young patient. Sagittal (**A**) and coronal (**B**) proton density images reveal flow voids in anterior aspect of upper spinal cord and lower medulla (arrows). **C** and **D.** Vertebral angiography demonstrates an arteriovenous malformation fed by the anterior spinal artery arising from the left vertebral artery. **E** to **G.** Another case in a 7-year-old child. Right vertebral angiography reveals angioma with a venous-type dilatation. **E.** There is feeding of the malformation via a radicular artery arising from the costocervical trunk. **F.** Lateral view of the vertebral angiogram demonstrates the malformation, which presents a vascular dilatation extending into the anterior subarachnoid space representing a venous aneurysm. **G.** Lateral magnified view of vertebral angiogram demonstrates the lesion in greater detail.

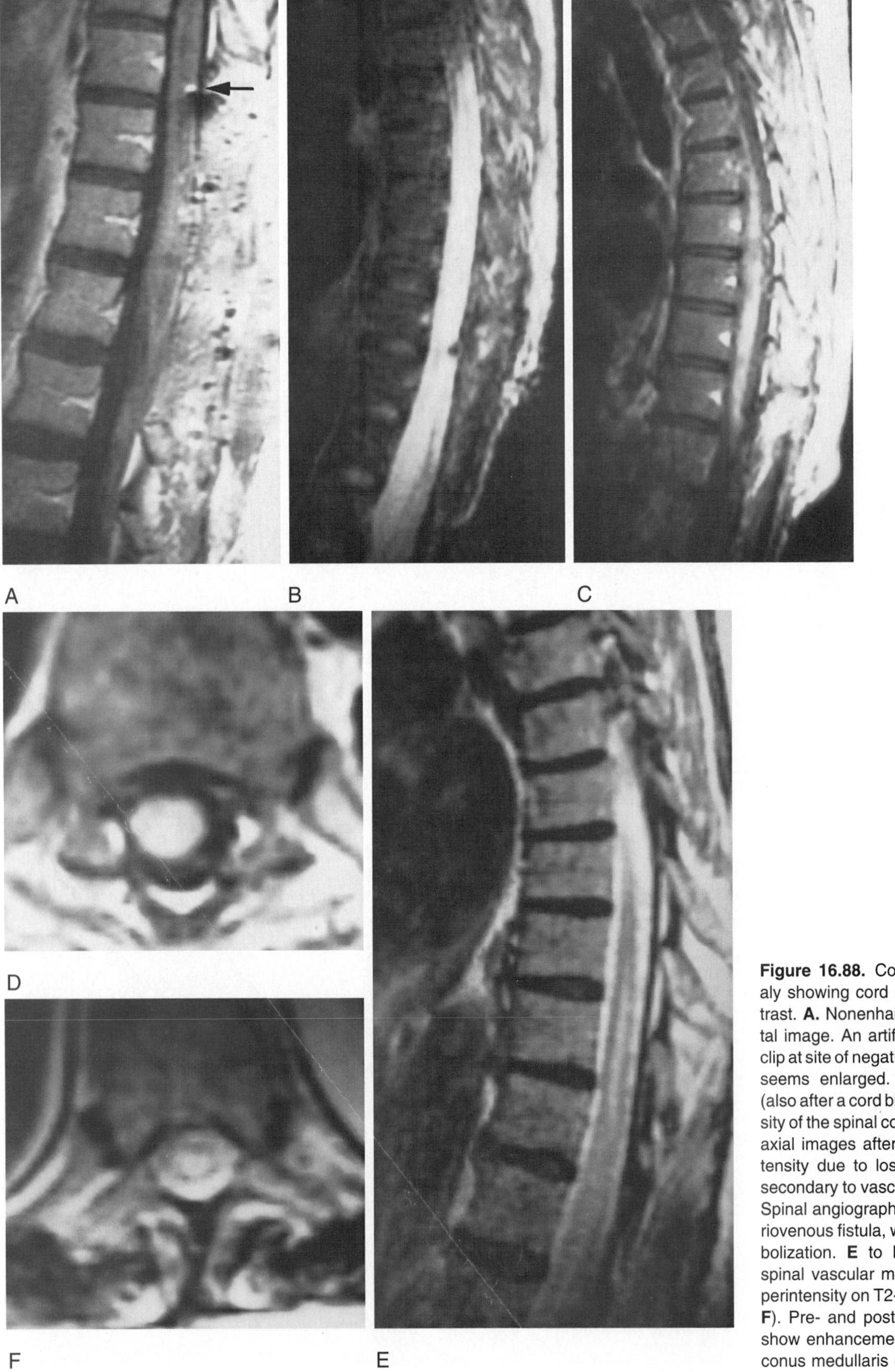

Figure 16.88. Cord arteriovenous anomaly showing cord enhancement after contrast. **A.** Nonenhanced T1-weighted sagittal image. An artifact at arrow is due to a clip at site of negative biopsy (arrow); conus seems enlarged. **B.** T2-weighted image (also after a cord biopsy) shows hyperintensity of the spinal cord. **C** and **D.** Sagittal and axial images after contrast show hyperintensity due to loss of blood-brain barrier secondary to vascular changes in the cord. Spinal angiography demonstrated an arteriovenous fistula, which was treated by embolization. **E** to **H.** Another example of spinal vascular malformation showing hyperintensity on T2-weighted images (**E** and **F**). Pre- and postcontrast sagittal images show enhancement in the lower cord and conus medullaris (**G** and **H**).

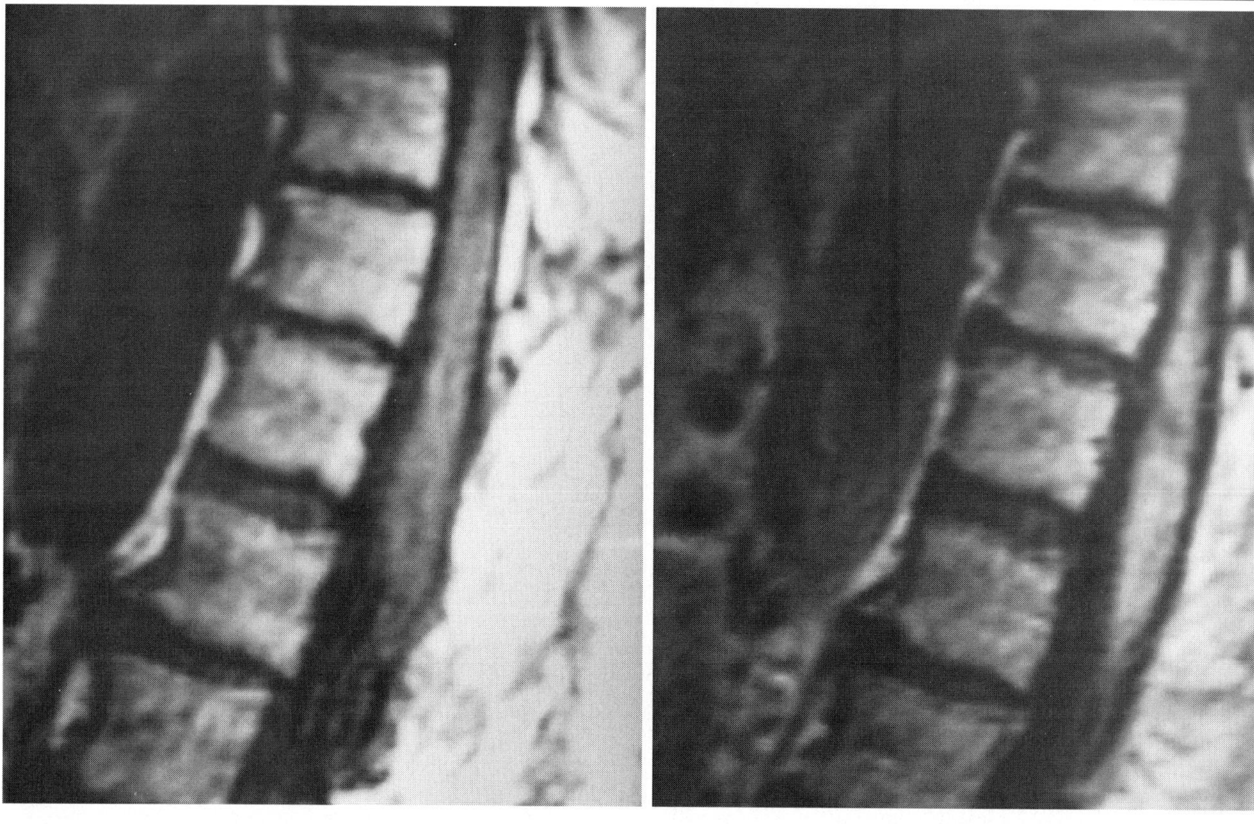

Figure 16.88. *(continued)*

(Fig. 16.90). Further details are found under "Endovascular Therapeutic Neuroradiology," Chapter 18.

The large draining veins of arteriovenous malformations interfere with normal venous drainage, and many of the symptoms associated with these lesions are probably related to venous hypertension in the spinal cord. Paraparesis (progressive or intermittent), impotence, bowel and bladder dysfunction, and sensory disturbances are among the symptoms related to these vascular malformations.

Imaging Findings

The MRI findings are the most important. MRI may reveal hyperintensity of the cord on T2-weighted images, usually in the thoracolumbar area. Most important, contrast enhancement may yield cord enhancement in the involved area (Fig. 16.88). The cord enhancement is indicative of an active process and is of interest because the mechanism is not well understood. The presumptive diagnosis usually is neoplasm because the cord may be slighly increased in size. The cord enhancement may persist for a long time; the author has seen cord enhancement in two examinations separated by several months. A biopsy has been performed in some of our cases and has shown nothing specific (Fig. 16.88).

Myelography with spot films is most important for visualizing the usual serpentine vessels formed by the draining veins (Fig. 16.89). The prominent vessels are most frequently in the dorsal side of the cord, and the patient should be turned to a supine position once prone films are obtained. CT is not helpful, although CT after myelography may demonstrate enlarged peripheral veins. MRI may reveal irregular low-intensity images suggestive of tortuous blood vessels, but sometimes these are inconspicuous and cannot be confidently diagnosed. Gadolinium enhancement may help in deciding whether vessels (usually veins) on the surface of the cord are demonstrable. Spinal angiography is discussed in Chapters 17 and 18.

NEOPLASTIC AND RELATED CONDITIONS OF THE SPINAL CORD, NERVE ROOTS, AND MENINGES

Syringomyelia

This consists of the presence of cavities filled with CSF within the substance of the spinal cord. The cavity may or may not be part of the central canal. When it is, at least part of the wall is covered by ependymal cells, but in most cases the wall of the cavity is not covered by ependyma but by neuroglial hyperplastic tissue in the older cavities and by degenerated neuroglial and neural elements in the younger cavities (95). The cavity is always in the gray matter.

Syringomyelic cavities are often also referred to as *hydromyelia*, and because of the difficulty in deciding between the two pathologic types, both terms are frequently used

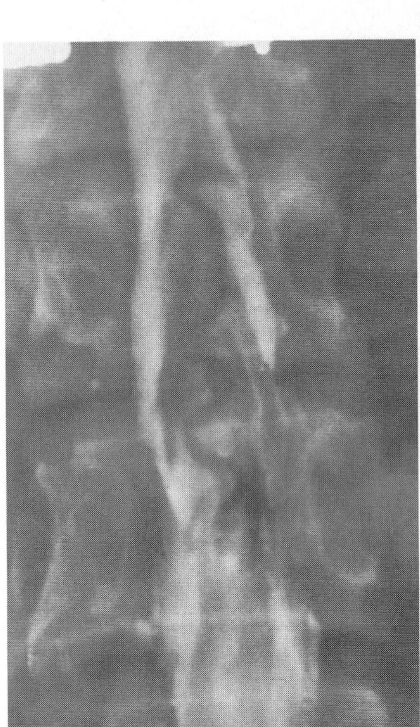

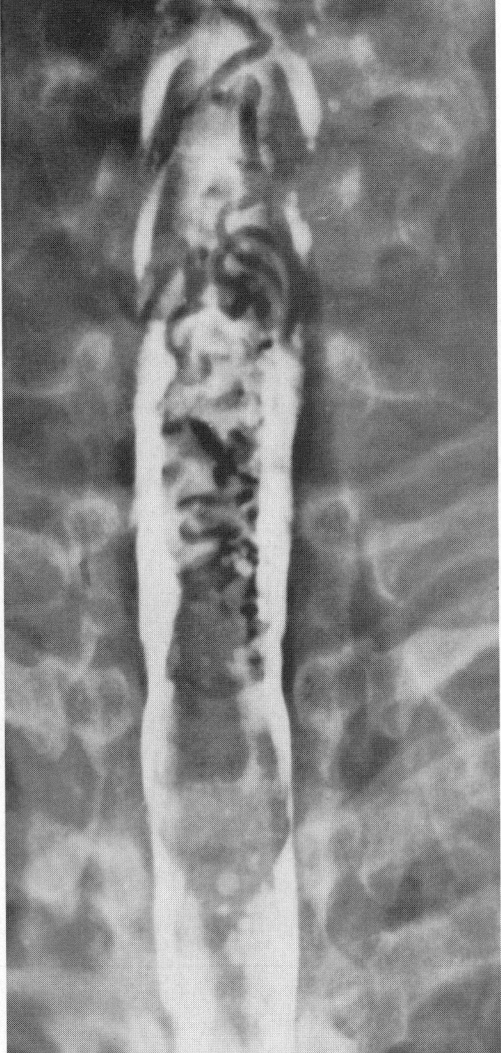

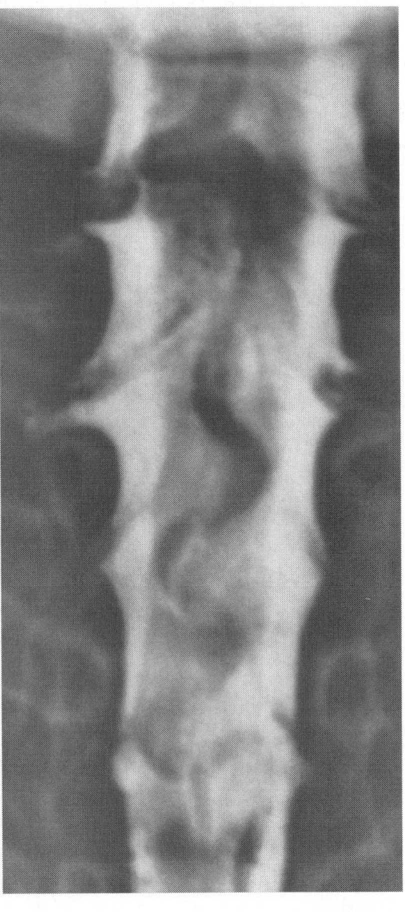

A B C

Figure 16.89. Vascular malformation of spinal cord (three cases). **A.** In the case shown lesion is in the lower thoracic region and is accompanied by a very slight widening of the spinal cord shadow as shown on the myelogram. **B.** The lesion is in the cervical region (in another case) and consists of a large area of involvement with marked dilatation of vessels. Slight cord widening may be present in the upper thoracic region. **C.** Large tortuous vessels in cervical region in 59-year-old woman with coarctation of the aorta. The enlarged channels are arterial and serve as a collateral pathway.

when describing a case. The congenital variety such as the ones associated with Chiari malformations may be referred to as hydromyelia but, here again, the term *syringohydromyelia* may be preferred. The cavity is most conspicuous in the cervical region but often extends for most of the spinal cord down to the lumbar cord enlargement, which is often spared (Fig. 16.91). The cord may be enlarged, and the enlargement is particularly conspicuous in the horizontal position. This is the case when the patient undergoes an MRI examination as well as a CT-myelography examination. It has been shown that a syringohydromyelic cavity may collapse in the erect position, which may indicate that the cavity is not under pressure or that it communicates with the subarachnoid space. The only way that the change in shape of the spinal cord can be shown is by air myelography. It is not necessary to carry out a full-fledged air myelogram, which is rather uncomfortable for the patient; a simple air injection (10 cm^3) in the spinal canal in the sitting position with the head markedly flexed, to hold the air in the cervical spinal canal, is sufficient. The width of the cord can then be compared with an MR sagittal image or with CT myelography or conventional myelography (Fig. 16.92).

Syringomyelia may also be associated with neoplasms, is frequent in posttraumatic myelopathy, may follow a severe inflammatory or vascular focal involvement or hemorrhage, and can be seen in association with severe arachnoiditis. In the cases of hemangioblastoma the syrinx found may well be an intramedullary cyst accompanying the tumor, and the cord may be distended locally.

IMAGING FINDINGS

Syringohydromyelia is easy to diagnose with MRI because the findings are usually very clearly shown on T1- and T2-

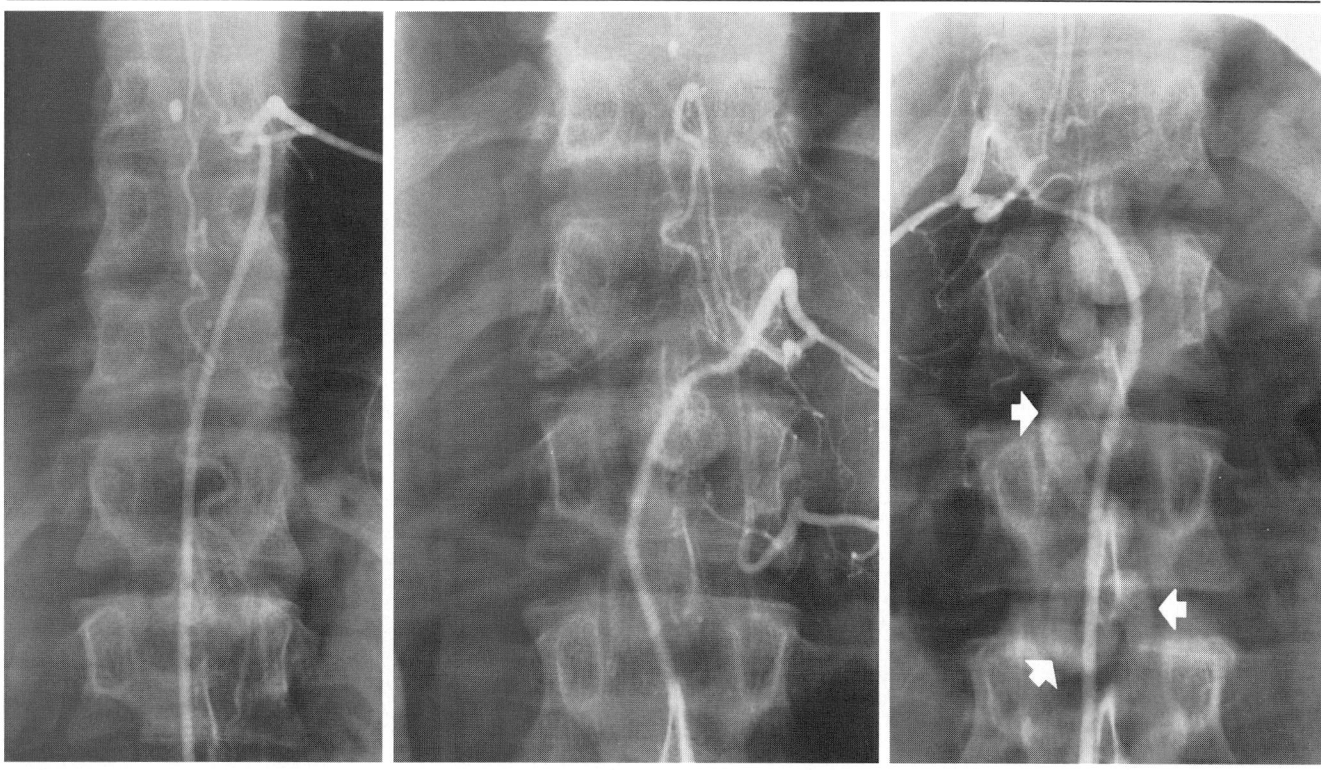

A B C

Figure 16.90. Vascular malformation of spinal cord receiving multiple arterial supply. **A.** The artery of Adamkiewicz arises on the left side at T9. It supplies the arteriovenous malformation. **B.** Supply from the twelfth intercostal artery is also noted. Regurgitation of contrast occurred into the first lumbar artery, indicating supply via this artery as well. **C.** Injection of the right intercostal and lumbar arteries revealed at least one more pedicle arising from the twelfth intercostal artery. A large draining vein is seen (arrows).

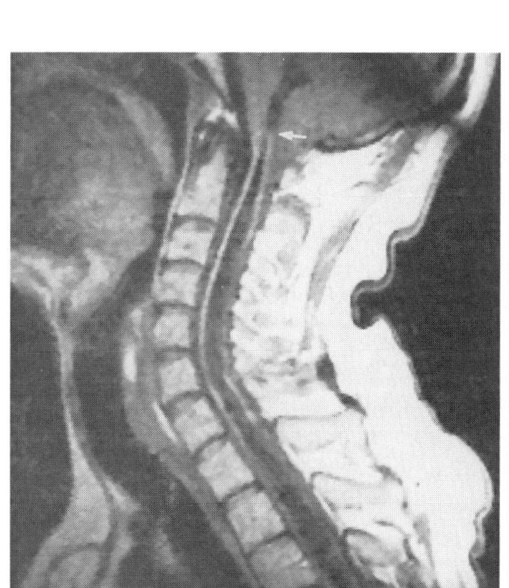

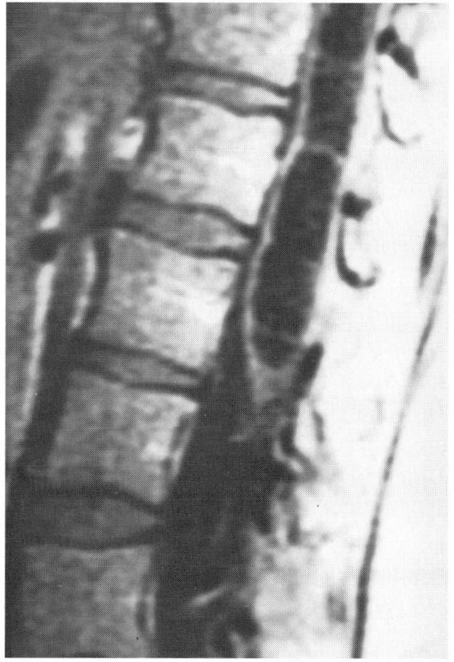

A B

Figure 16.91. Syringomyelia on MRI examination. **A.** The T1-weighted sagittal view shows a large hypointense area running all along the cervical cord, starting at the cervicomedullary junction and extending into the thoracic region. The appearance at the upper end suggests that there is or was a connection with the lower fourth ventricle (arrow). The slightly scalloped margins starting at C6 and continuing caudally are produced by the same bands or incomplete septal demonstrated in Figure 16.93. **B.** Sagittal T1-weighted image in anther patient reveals a large syringomyelic cavity in the thoracic lumbar region, with septation.

Figure 16.92. Syringohydromyelia showing collapse of cavity in erect position. **A.** Prone myelography image shows spinal cord filling entire canal (arrows). There is a small amount of contrast over the dentate ligaments. **B.** Erect lateral view with air in spinal canal shows a small spinal cord and a Chiari-type malformation, a frequent association in patients with syringohydromyelia. The degree of cord collapse is probably increased by the injection of air.

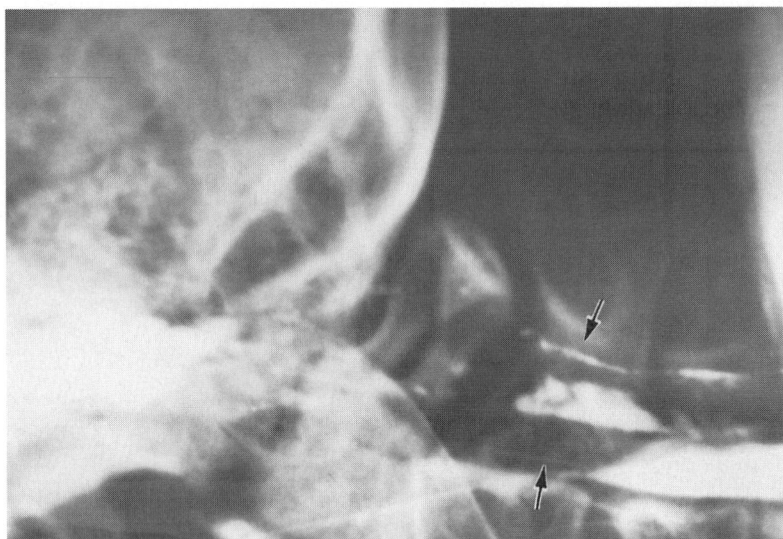

A

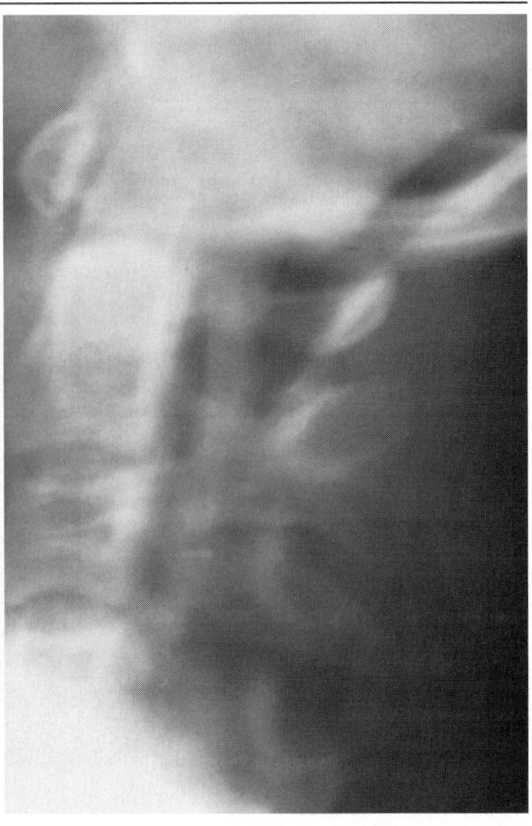

B

weighted images. On T1 images a low-intensity cavity can be seen within the cord on sagittal images, extending for several segments or involving most of the spinal cord (Fig. 16.91). On T2-weighted images the cavity is bright, like CSF. The cavity can be large, showing cord enlargement, or it may not cause significant cord enlargement if there is accompanying cord atrophy, a frequent association in the chronic cases. In order to rule out tumor, it is necessary to perform an examination with contrast. The cavity may be associated with another pathology listed earlier (trauma, arachnoiditis, old myelitis, or arteriovenous malformation).

Myelographic diagnosis and CT-myelography can also be done, but the examination is often laborious unless the contrast enters the spinal cord cavity, as happened occasionally even with Pantopaque (Fig. 16.93). In general, it is necessary to perform a delayed (from 2 to 8 to 10 h) CT examination to detect passage of the contrast material into the spinal cord cavity. This would require maintaining the patient in the horizontal position with the head elevated in order to facilitate the transudation of the contrast across the cord. If the cavity is thin-walled the contrast would pass sooner. Possibly the contrast may enter the canal by way of a direct, very narrow connection between the subarachnoid space and the syrinx cavity, which may occur at the root junctions (Fig. 16.94).

The syrinx cavity may be surgically tapped and shunted into the subarachnoid space. This is particularly effective in cases where upper and lower limits of the cavity are shown by MRI, suggesting a closed cyst. Post et al. have indicated that the presence of demonstrable pulsation on cine-MRI may be a way to determine which cysts should be shunted (96).

Neoplasms

Tumors of the spinal cord and its membranes are similar in type to those found in the cranial cavity. There is, however, considerable difference in the frequency of occurrence of the various types of tumors in the two areas. This is readily understood when the quantity of medullary tissue relative to spinal meninges and spinal nerves is compared with the mass of the brain in relation to its covering. Fifty percent of the neoplasms affecting the spinal cord derive from the meninges or nerves and are about equally divided between meningioma and neurinoma. Gliomas, on the other hand, account for only 10 percent of spinal cord lesions. The mass of the cord is one-seventh that of the brain, where gliomas account for more than half of all primary tumors. Compression of the spinal cord by metastatic tumors from other organs occurs more frequently than cerebral metastases. Two-thirds of all spinal metastases originate in either the lung or the breast.

The difference in behavior of metastatic tumors of the spinal cord compared with those of the brain is also of interest. Intracranial metastases are almost always intrace-

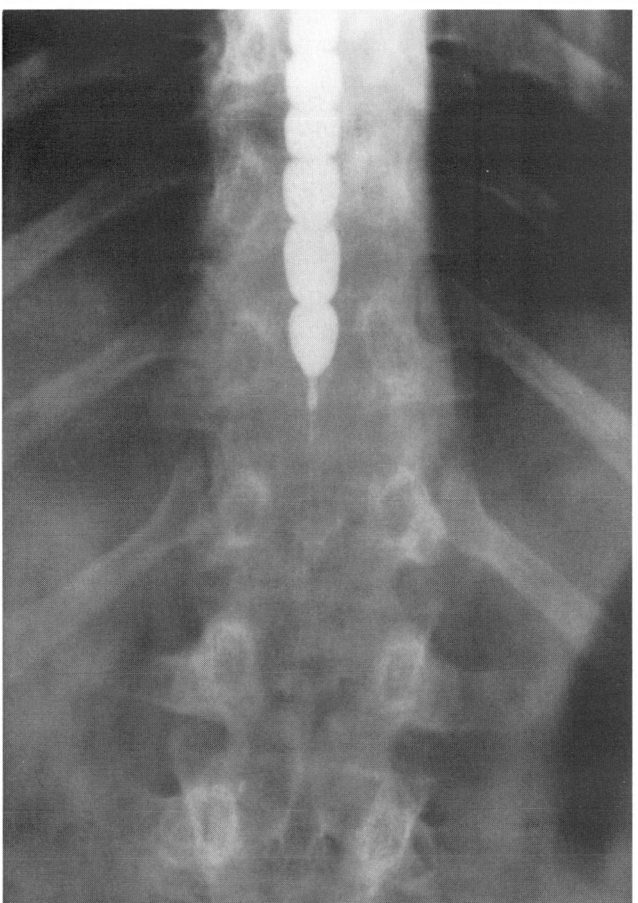

Figure 16.93. Contrast spontaneously entering syringomyelia cavity during myelography. Contrast was found in the canal and entered at the foramen magnum. The segmentation is apparently due to the presence of incomplete septae or strands covered by collagen or blood vessels with hyalinized walls.

rebral, whereas metastases to the spinal cord are usually epidural and rarely extend to the meninges to invade the spinal cord itself. Radiologically, tumors of the spinal cord and its membranes produce changes in the adjacent vertebrae and soft tissues, which indicate their location in approximately 15 percent of cases. In this respect, spinal tumors behave somewhat differently than brain tumors. Localizing changes in adjacent bony structures are observed infrequently with brain tumors, and changes of generalized pressure occur in bony structures at a distance from the lesion. In plain spine radiographs, one or more of three fundamental changes in adjacent portions of the vertebral column may note the presence of tumor:

1. Enlargement of the vertebral canal as manifested by flattening of the cavity of the medial margins of the pedicles with increase in the interpediculate distance, scalloping of the posterior margins of the vertebral body, and thinning of the lamina, all the result of atrophy of the bone by the pulsating pressure of the tumor (Table 16.1, page 790).
2. Enlargement of the intervertebral foramen, which results from an isthmus of tumor in the foramen joining the medial masses of the dumbbell-shaped tumor that lies partially within and partially without the vertebral canal.
3. Calcification within the tumor in the vertebral canal.

Table 16.2.
Relative Incidence of Brain and Spinal Cord Tumors of Various Types in Percentage (Wolf)

Tumor	Brain	Spinal cord
Neurinoma	10	26
Metastatic from other organs	10	25
Meningioma	15	24
Glioma	50	10
Metastatic from brain	—	4
Hemangioblastoma	4	3
Congenital tumors (dermoids, etc.)	5	2
Others	6	6

The relative incidence of intraspinal tumors is shown in Table 16.2.

In addition to the characteristic changes caused by primary spinal cord tumor, metastatic neoplasms may produce abnormalities in plain spine roentgenograms. The spinal cord is frequently affected by an extension of the malignant metastases from the vertebra to the epidural space, and in such instances osteolytic and osteoblastic changes in the adjacent vertebrae may be apparent. An extraneous paraspinal shadow may result from a retropleural tumor, which may extend through one or more intervertebral foramina to invade the epidural tissues. Metastatic epidural tumors usually affect the spinal cord by compression rather than by invasion through the meninges. Tumors arising in the spinal cord do not invade the surrounding bone, although an occasional case of "metastatic" medulloblastoma invading the vertebrae has been reported in the literature. The author has seen at least one case of ependymoma that was diagnosed for the first time upon biopsy of an inguinal lymph node. These are rare occurrences, however. In general, tumors arising from brain or spinal cord tissue do not metastasize outside the central nervous system unless viable cells are accidentally implanted. This could occur sometimes by shunting in a patient who has a neoplasm that invades the ventricles.

INTRAMEDULLARY NEOPLASMS

These make up about 10 percent of primary intraspinal tumors. Ependymoma is more frequent than astrocytoma (Fig. 16.99). Occasionally oligodendroglioma, spongioblastoma, medulloblastoma, and, rarely, gliomas of other histologic types may be encountered. Ependymomas, which constitute 70 percent of the group, originate most frequently in the region of the conus medullaris, where normally, in proportion to the mass of the surrounding neural tissue, there is more ependymal tissue in the walls of the terminal ventricle of the central canal than elsewhere in the nervous system. Ependymoma may extend along the filum terminale for a remarkable distance; in some in-

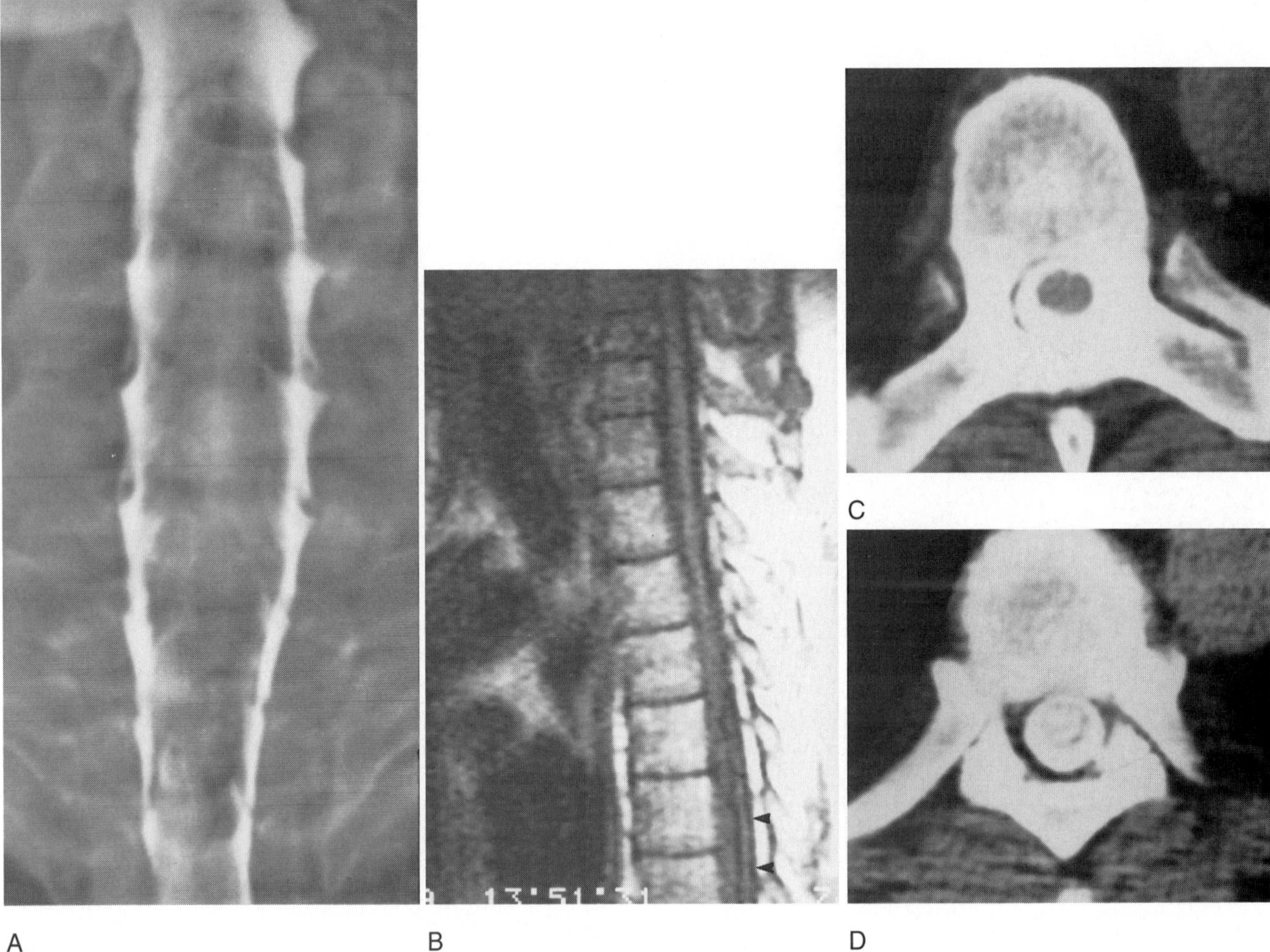

Figure 16.94. Syringohydromyelia with expansion of spinal cord. A. There is marked uniform widening of the spinal cord in the entire cervical area and into the upper thoracic cord. (B to D) Another patient. B. T1-weighted MR image shows syrinx in thoracic region. There is a low-intensity center in the cord (arrowheads). C. CT-myelography shows normal cord appearance surrounded by contrast. D. Axial view 4 h later shows center of cord opacified with a thin rim of normal cord surrounded by subarachnoid contrast.

stances, the lumbosacral portion of the subarachnoid space may fill with tumor throughout its entire length. Because of the great size of some of these tumors, they have been referred to as *giant tumors of the cauda equina*.

Because of the slow growth of the majority of spinal cord gliomas, bone changes in plain spine radiographs may occur. Ependymomas, in particular, may expand the thoracolumbar portion of the vertebral canal for the length of five or six vertebral segments with pressure atrophy of the medial portion of the pedicles and increase in the interpediculate measurements. Scalloping of the posterior margins of the vertebral bodies and thinning of the laminae often are demonstrated in the lateral view (Fig. 16.95).

Spinal cord tumors may start with local pain in the back, approximately at the level of the lesion, and progressive weakness of the extremities. This ordinarily leads to a consultation, and an imaging examination would usually be requested. MRI is by far the most useful examination procedure because the diagnosis can usually be made without the need to carry out any other type of examination. It is necessary to do both noncontrast and contrast-enhanced examinations (Figs. 16.96 to 16.99).

Ependymomas have an isointense or minimally hyperintense appearance with irregularity. They may have a cystic component or may have a syrinx occupying part of the space. They usually enhance with contrast. Astrocytomas tend to have a more heterogeneous appearance, but they may also be partially cystic and they enlarge the spinal cord. In the spinal cord they usually enhance, which is not the case with many of the slowly growing astrocytomas in the cerebral hemispheres. The malignant or glioblastoma-type histologic lesions are uncommon in the spinal cord.

In the study of intramedullary tumors, plain CT or CT with contrast is not very useful because most of the

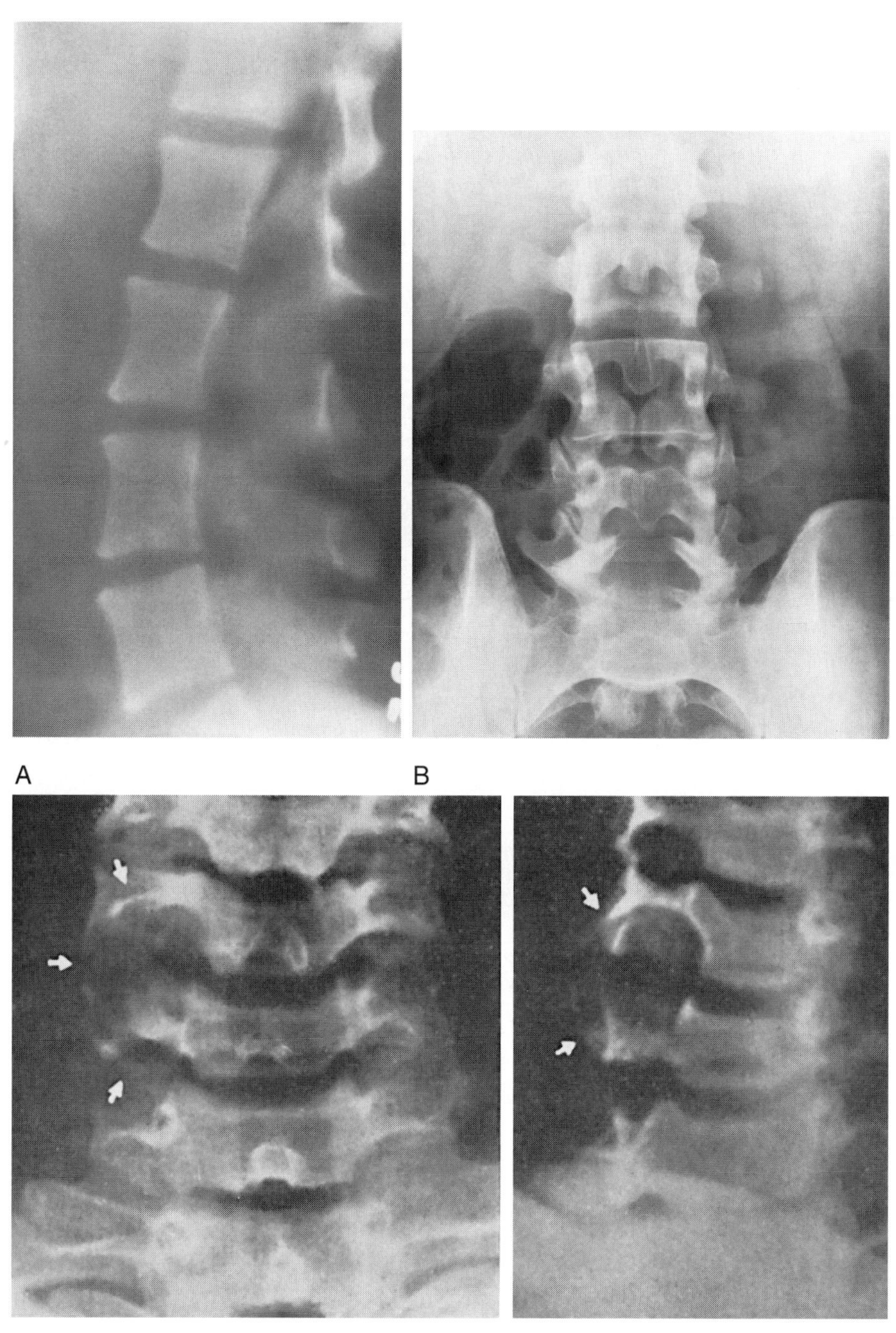

Figure 16.95. Plain-film findings, usually bone remodeling, in slowly growing intraspinal tumors. **A.** Lateral lumbar spine shows marked fusiform widening of spinal canal from L1 through L5. **B.** In the frontal projection there is a spina bifida occulta of L3 and L5 as well as widening of the interpediculate distance owing to pressure erosion and flattening of the pedicles from L2 to L5. The spina bifida would suggest the possibility of a congenital lesion. Patient had a large epidermoid tumor. Frontal (**C**) and left posterior oblique (**D**) cervical spine demonstrate erosion of the C5-C6 intervertebral foramen (arrows) due to a neurofibroma in a patient with neurofibromatosis type I.

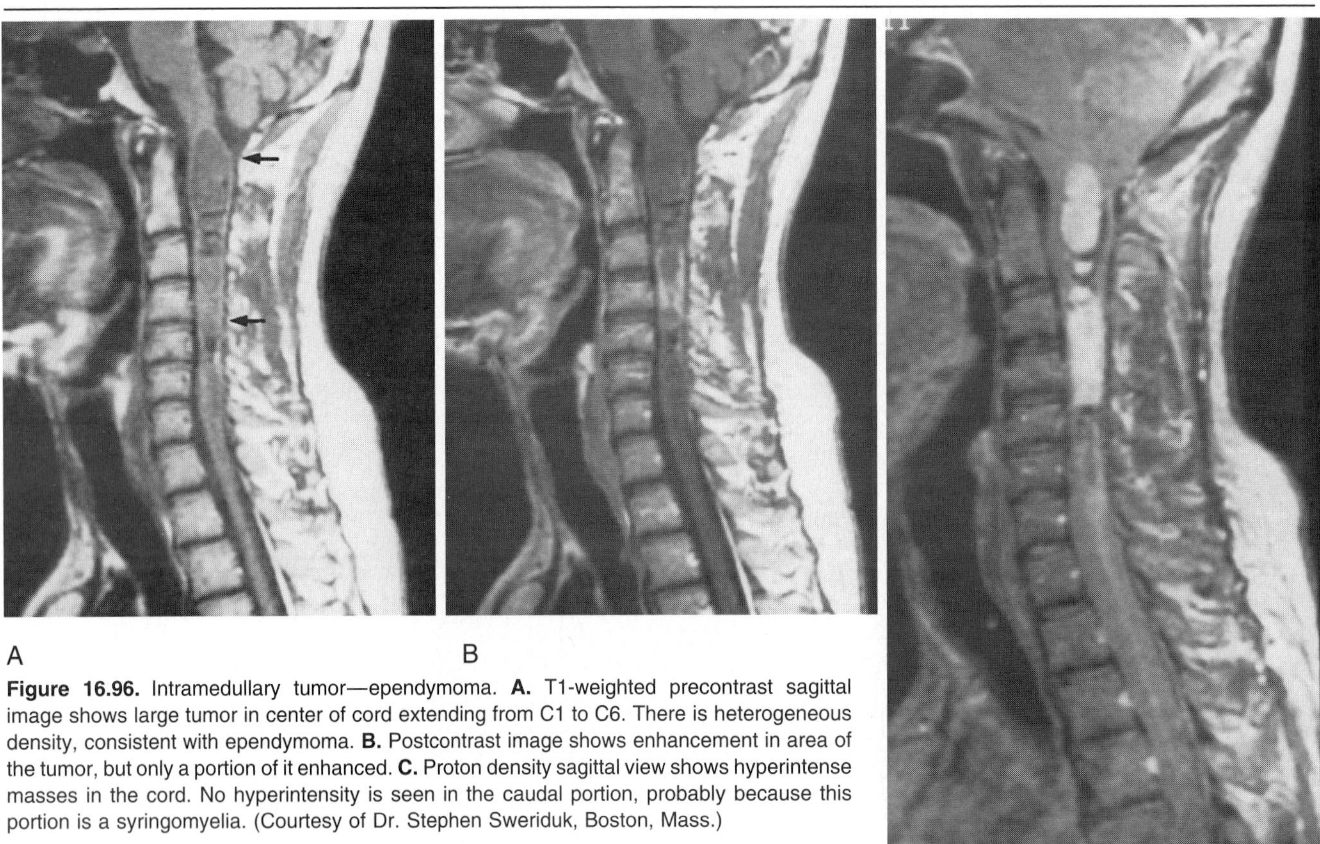

A B

C

Figure 16.96. Intramedullary tumor—ependymoma. **A.** T1-weighted precontrast sagittal image shows large tumor in center of cord extending from C1 to C6. There is heterogeneous density, consistent with ependymoma. **B.** Postcontrast image shows enhancement in area of the tumor, but only a portion of it enhanced. **C.** Proton density sagittal view shows hyperintense masses in the cord. No hyperintensity is seen in the caudal portion, probably because this portion is a syringomyelia. (Courtesy of Dr. Stephen Sweriduk, Boston, Mass.)

A B C

Figure 16.97. Ependymoma in the upper thoracic region. **A.** Precontrast (T1) view shows cord enlargement and inhomogeneous appearance (arrows). **B.** Postcontrast view shows inhomogeneous slight enhancement (arrows). **C.** Axial view shows the enhancement is on the posterolateral aspect of the spinal cord (larger arrow). Small arrows point at unenhanced cord.

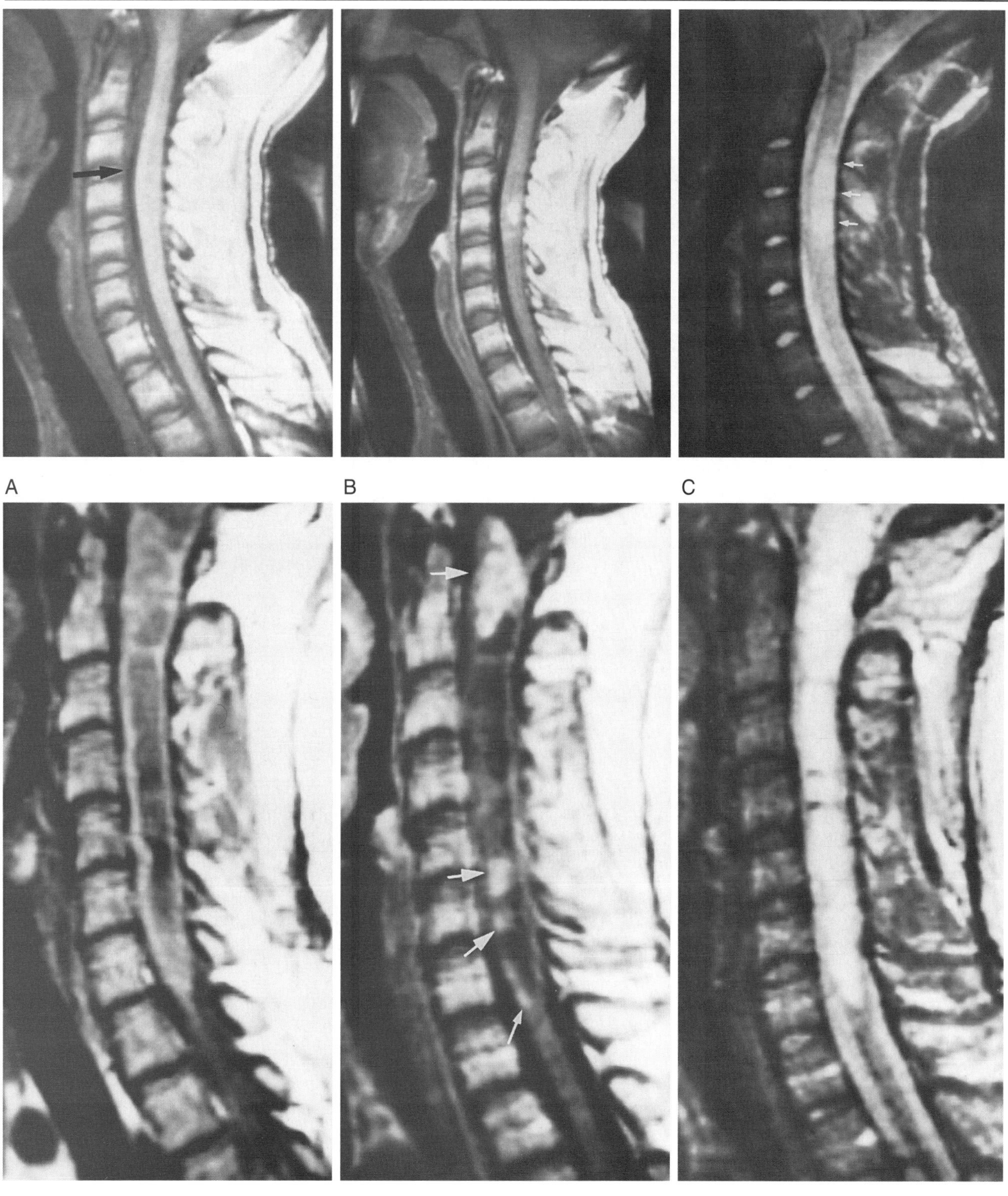

Figure 16.98. Intramedullary tumor—astrocytoma. **A.** Precontrast T1-weighted sagittal view shows focal enlargement of cord (arrow) behind C3-C4. **B.** Postcontrast view shows nodular enhancement. **C.** T2-weighted sagittal reveals a fairly homogeneous area of hyperintensity representing the tumor plus the surrounding edema. **D.** to **F.** Another astrocytoma with a large syrinx and cystic components. **D.** The appearance suggests syringomyelia; however there are nonhomogeneous solid components. **E.** After contrast one large area and some other smaller areas enhance (arrows). Some aspects of the walls of the cyst (syrinx?) are enhancing. **F.** T2-weighted image shows hyperintensity through the tumor and the cysts. The cyst stops caudally at C7.

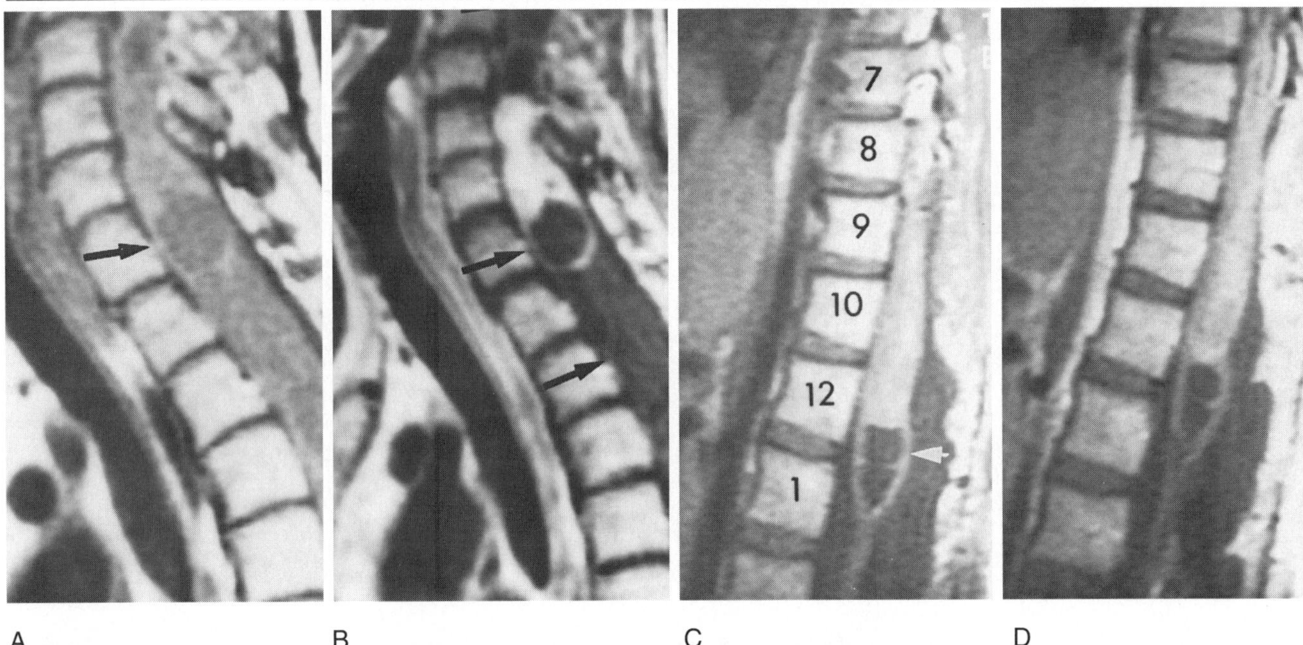

Figure 16.99. Intramedullary tumor—cystic astrocytoma. **A.** Precontrast T1-weighted image shows irregularity in intensity and enlargement up to T7 intraspinal soft tissues over a long area from C2 to T7. A lower-intensity round area is seen (arrow). **B.** Postcontrast sagittal image reveals an area of sharp enhancement surrounding a cystic space, and, below and above the tumor, what appears to be an enlarged cord, probably edema and syringomyelia poorly outlined (arrow). (Courtesy of Dr. Stephen Sweriduk, Boston, Mass.) **C** and **D.** Primary melanoma of spinal cord. **C.** Precontrast T1 shows cord enlargement involving the lower cord and conus. There is a low-intensity area at lower aspect of conus (**C**), which did not enhance in a postcontrast image (**D**). Surgical biopsy demonstrated a melanoma, which was thought to be primary.

time the lesion cannot be visualized. Sometimes slight enhancement can be seen in the area of the tumor. On the other hand, myelography combined with CT is an excellent procedure for examination in institutions where MRI is not available. Myelography is likely to show a widening of the spinal cord; if the mass is large enough, there will be a complete block to the flow of contrast, preceded by an area of widening of the cord. The cord itself would not be displaced to one side or the other, although occasionally an intramedullary tumor can be slightly eccentric so that the cord may appear to be displaced to one side or the tumor may show exophytic growth (Fig. 16.100). CT added to the myelography would assist in eliminating the possibility of an extramedullary tumor with greater assurance.

In the differential diagnosis we should include the possibility of metastatic tumor from the brain or cerebellum to the spinal cord. However, this would be known from the history of the patient, although sometimes a germinoma of the pineal may present first with metastases to the spinal cord (Fig. 16.108). This is rather unusual, however; a CT or MRI examination of the brain would usually reveal the original lesion. Other conditions to consider are vascular malformation of the cord and ischemic lesions of the cord, described previously.

EXTRAMEDULLARY INTRADURAL NEOPLASMS

The majority of these tumors are either meningiomas or neurofibromas. They are located outside the cord but still within the dural membrane. They compress the spinal cord fairly early and usually produce sufficient symptoms so the patient will go to the physician relatively early. An occasional tumor in this location, however, is extremely large, which means the spinal cord would have tolerated the compression, probably indicating that the mass is a soft one.

Meningiomas and Schwannomas (or Neurofibromas)

These two tumors together make up 50 percent of the intraspinal neoplasms, occurring with about equal frequency. Meningiomas tend to occur in the thoracic region in women over 40 years of age, whereas the neurinomas or schwannomas occur in both sexes in about equal frequency and also are distributed equally among the cervical, thoracic, and lumbar regions.

Meningiomas are firmer tumors than the neurinomas and thus are likely to be discovered when they are smaller. Neurinomas can be multiple; in addition, they may extend, with the nerve root from which they originate, through the intervertebral foramen, sometimes producing an enlargement of this foramen, such as is shown in Figure 16.95.

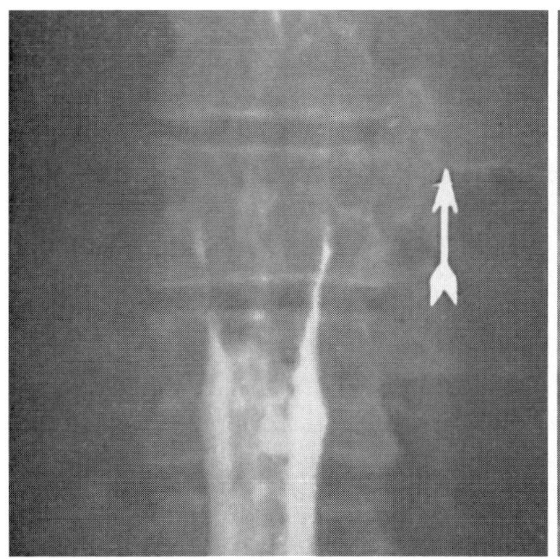
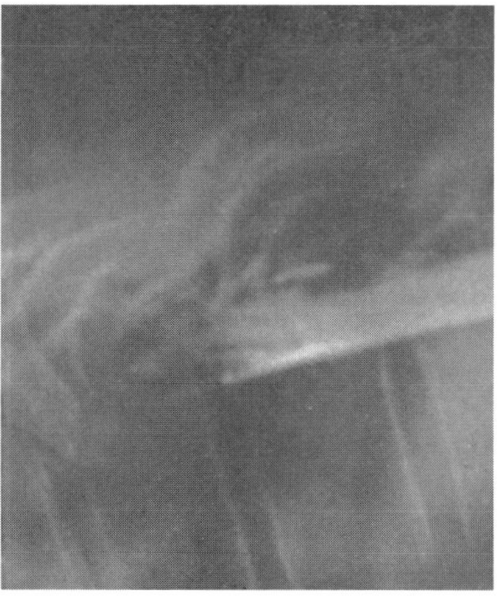

A

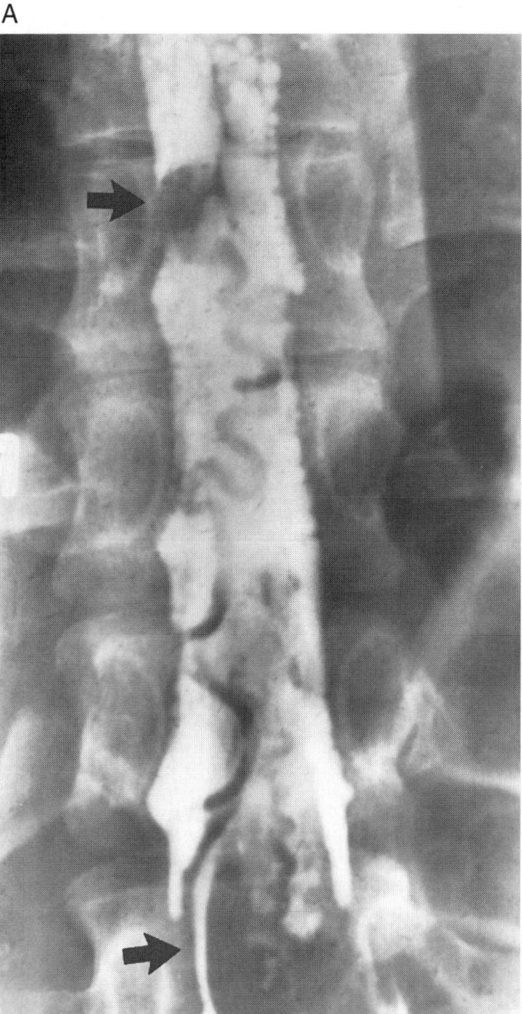

B

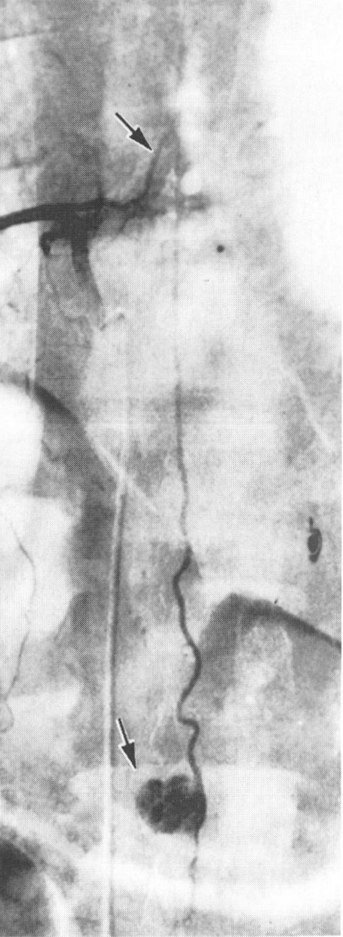

C

Figure 16.100. A. Intramedullary tumor (astrocytoma). The frontal view reveals widening of the cord and finally a complete block to the cephalad flow of contrast. The lateral view, patient prone and tilted head down (right image), shows that the cord widens as it reaches the complete block. **B** and **C.** Hemangioblastoma in another patient. **B.** Myelography reveals an area of cord widening (arrow), and dilated tortuous vascular channels. Another nodule is seen higher up (upper arrow). **C.** Spinal angiography revealed a tumor nodule (arrow). Another nodule was shown on a different injection (not shown here). The patient had von Hippel–Lindau disease.

Plain-film diagnosis can be suspected at times when a meningioma shows sufficient calcification in multiple psammoma bodies to be seen on plain films, but this happens in only about 10 percent of cases, and they may require tomography to be shown. On the other hand, CT scanning can show calcification very clearly, provided that the area where the tumor is located is examined by cross-sectional imaging. Other plain-film findings are erosion of the pedicle, usually only one or two, and enlargement of the intervertebral foramen. When a large neurofibroma is present, the entire spinal canal may be focally enlarged and visible in both frontal and lateral projections. However, plain-film diagnosis of intraspinal tumors is uncommon because only a relatively small percentage of the tumors produce visible changes.

MRI is far superior to the other noninvasive methods of diagnosing extramedullary intradural tumors. Sagittal images can detect the location and the relationship of the tumor mass to the spinal cord as well as the degree of compression of the cord; the exact position of the tumor in relation to the cord can be depicted on axial views of the corresponding area (Figs. 16.101 and 16.106). The tumors usually enhance with contrast, adding further to our ability to diagnose them. Myelography is also quite accurate in diagnosing extramedullary tumors, and a combination of myelography with CT further increases accuracy (Fig. 16.101). If MRI is not available, CT myelography is an excellent diagnostic method.

Some neoplasms can be both intramedullary and extramedullary. This is the case with some congenital tumors

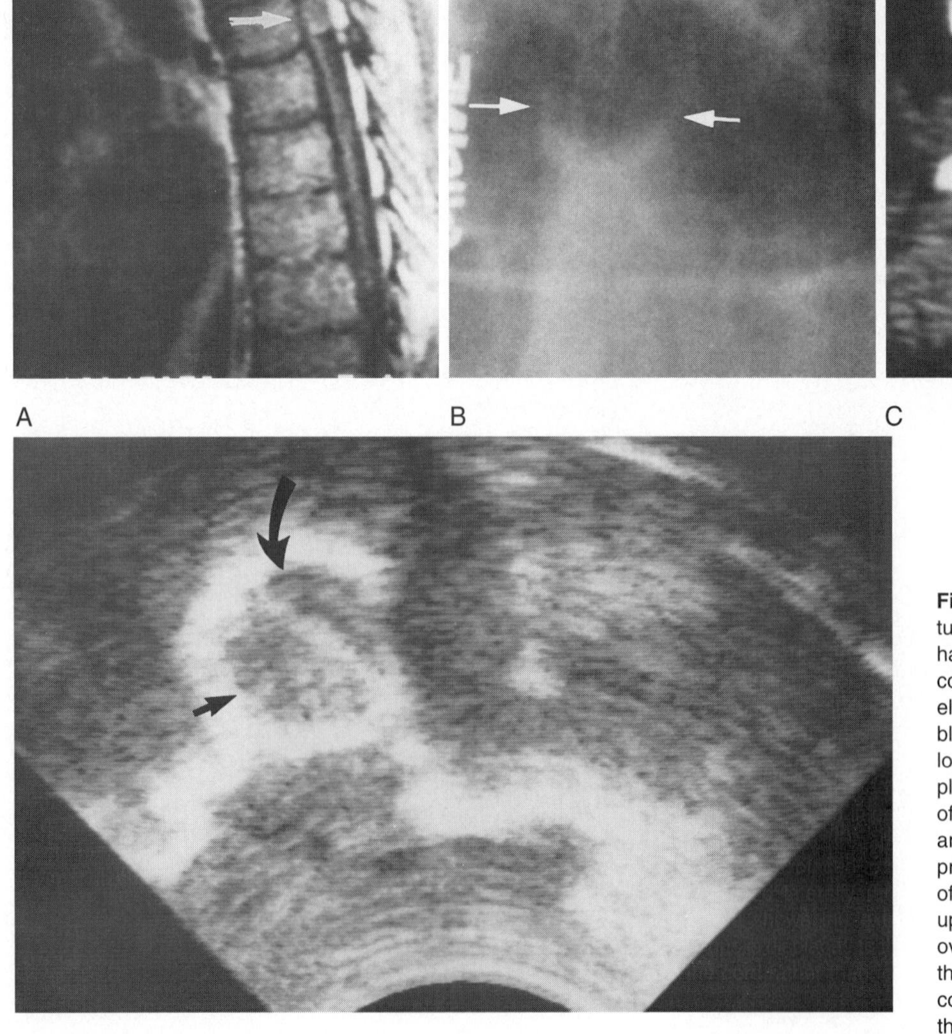

Figure 16.101. Extramedullary intradural tumor—meningioma. **A.** There is an enhancing round tumor flattening the spinal cord in the thoracic region (arrow). **B.** Myelography revealed a typical cup-shaped block of the contrast (arrows). **C.** CT-myelography revealed that the tumor, dorsally placed (arrow), produces a marked degree of flattening of the spinal cord (curved arrow). **D.** Ultrasound in the operating room produced an image almost identical to that of CT-myelography. The image is turned upside down; the ultrasound probe, located over the patient's dorsal skin incision, is at the concave side of the image to facilitate comparison. The arrow points at the tumor; the curved arrow points at the flattened cord.

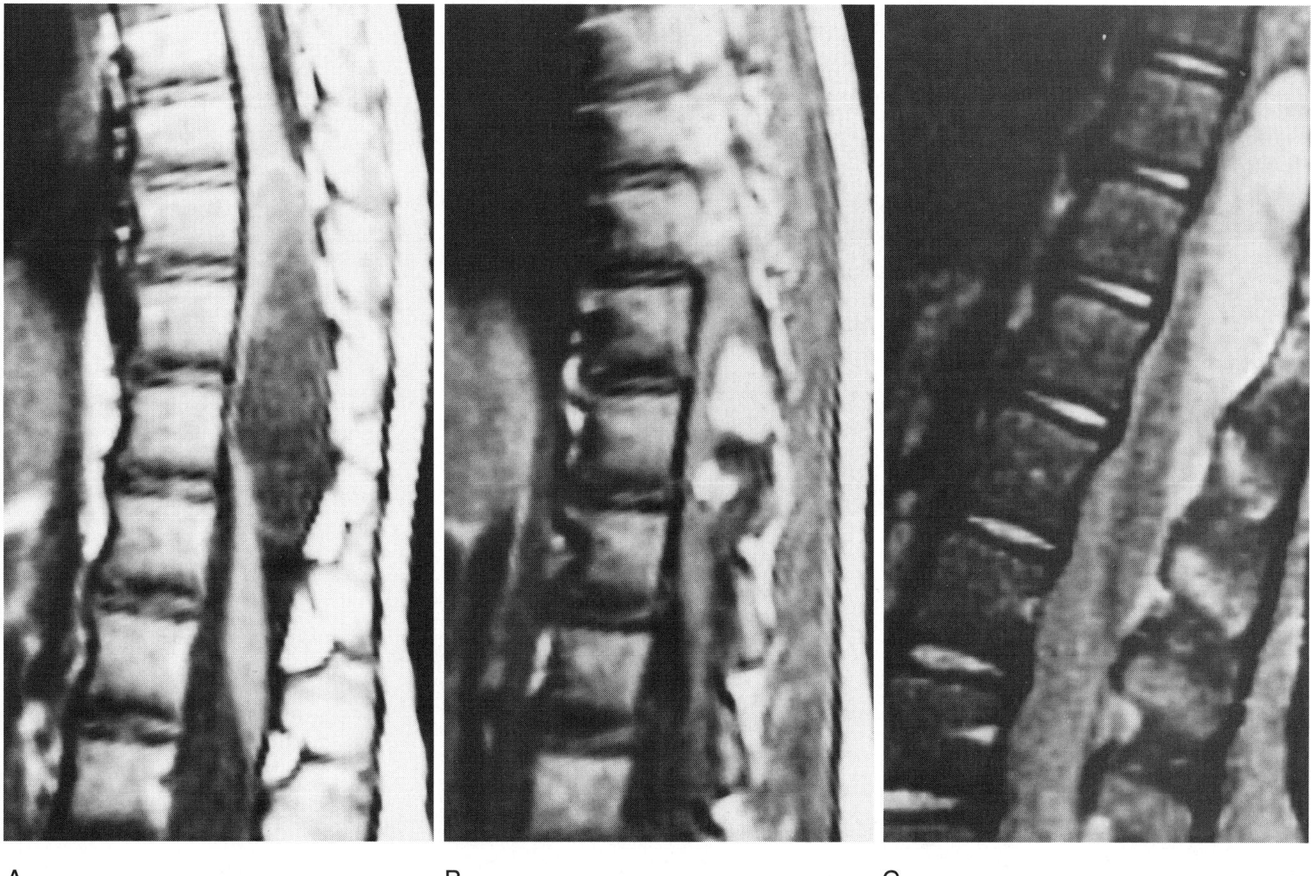

Figure 16.102. Teratoma of spinal canal (in 7-year-old girl). T1-weighted sagittal view shows large mass, which seems to expand the spinal cord. Another section reveals bright areas consistent with fat (no contrast enhancement used). T2-weighted image reveals a tumor, which is partly intramedullary and partly extramedullary. It contains lipomatous tissue as well as other tissue and was classified as a teratoma.

such as lipomas of the spinal cord and teratomas. Epidermoid tumors can also be attached to the cord and may be partly intramedullary (Figs. 16.102 to 16.104). In neurofibromatosis, there may be one or multiple neurofibromas; in addition, there may be an intramedullary tumor, but most of the latter turn out to be astrocytomas (Fig. 16.105). In addition to intramedullary astrocytomas and occasional ependymomas seen in neurofibromatosis, some cases may show an intramedullary schwannoma.

Metastatic Intradural Tumors

The most frequent of these are probably those arising from the tumors of the nervous system, which seed through the CSF. The medulloblastomas are the most frequent, but ependymoblastomas and pineal germinomas and pineoblastomas also occur. Choroidplexus carcinomas may also metastasize (Figs. 16.107 and 16.108; see also Fig. 11.107). Again, MRI with contrast is the best diagnostic method, but myelography can also be used in combination with CT. Intradural metastases from tumors outside the central nervous system may also occur. The majority of these are primary lung and primary breast carcinomas. In addition, melanoma may sometimes produce diffuse meningeal metastases.

The seeding from brain tumors frequently goes to the lumbosacral subarachnoid space. When it is in the spinal cord, the metastatic lesions are most frequently located on the dorsal side of the cord, probably having something to do with the frequent supine position during sleeping. Also, there are more irregularities on the dorsal side of the subarachnoid space, which may cause the cells suspended in the CSF to be caught in these areas. Metastases to the spinal cord via hematogenous spread do occur, but because of the small mass of the spinal cord in comparison to the brain mass, these are rather uncommon. Much more frequently, the metastases from tumors outside the nervous system occur in the epidural space, particularly in the vertebrae.

EXTRADURAL NEOPLASMS

The extradural lesions are by far the most commonly encountered lesions involving the spine and spinal cord. The

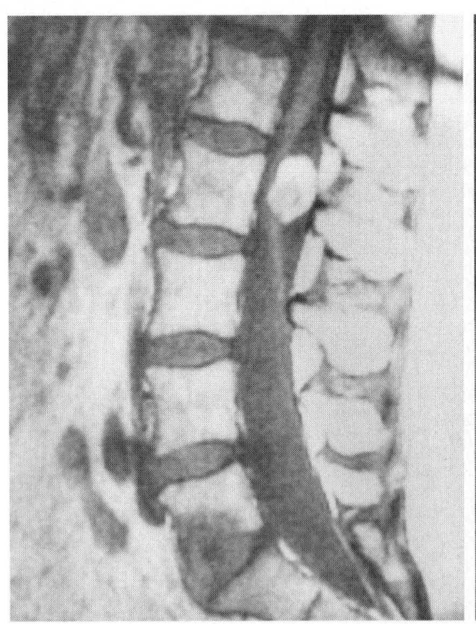

A

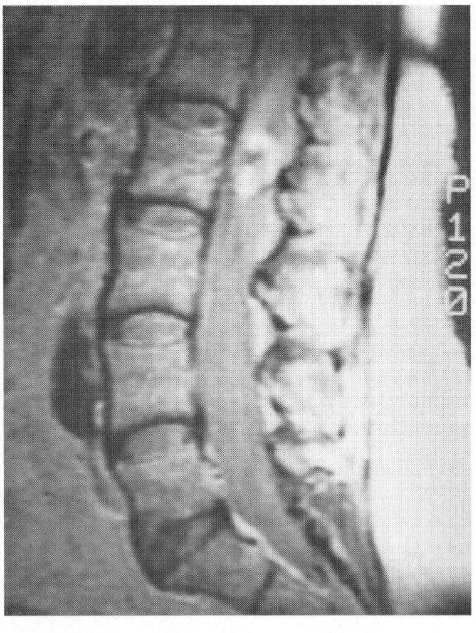

B

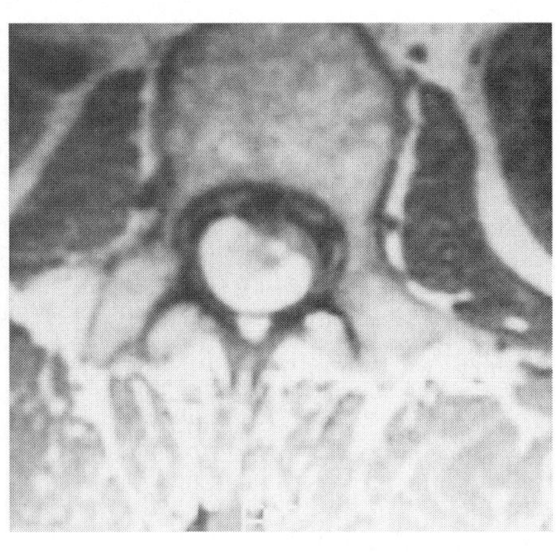

C

Figure 16.103. Dermoid tumor in 61-year-old woman. **A.** T1-weighted sagittal image shows a hyperintense lesion displacing the spinal cord forward. The conus seems to continue below the tumor, and the conus, above the tumor, is also displaced forward. **B.** Proton-density-weighted sagittal shows the mass to be less hyperintense than on T1. The spinal canal below the lesion is enlarged. **C.** T1-weighted noncontrast axial image demonstrates hyperintensity consistent with fat. The lesion was a dermoid tumor.

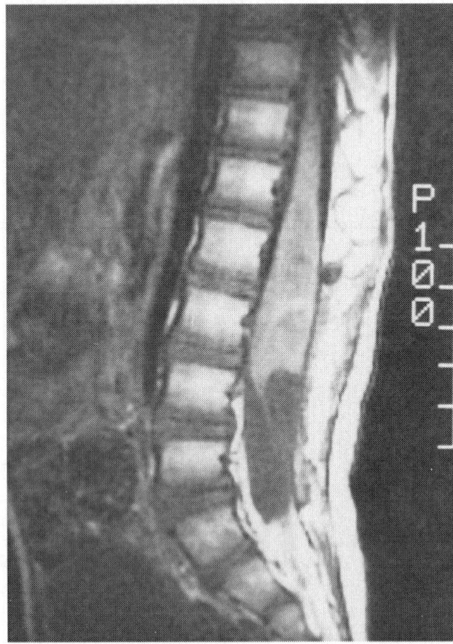

A

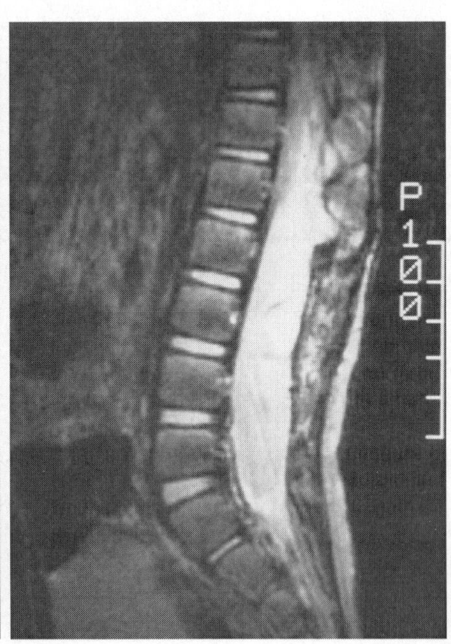

B

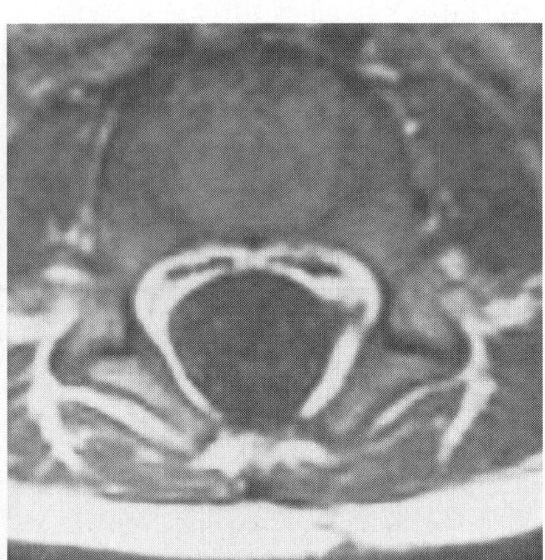

C

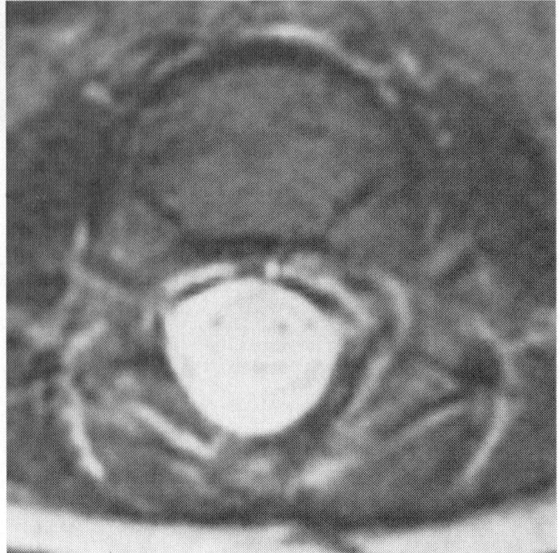

D

Figure 16.104. Congenital tumor, an epidermoid in a 2-year-old girl. **A.** T1-weighted sagittal. The lesion is low-intensity, but there is moderate hyperintensity above it, possibly indicating some fatty component to the lesion. The spinal canal is widened. **B.** T2-weighted sagittal shows that the lower area is now hyperintense. **C** and **D.** T1- and T2-weighted axials show low intensity on T1 (**C**) and high intensity on T2 (**D**) consistent with epidermoid. (Courtesy of Dr. Stephen Sweriduk, Boston, Mass.)

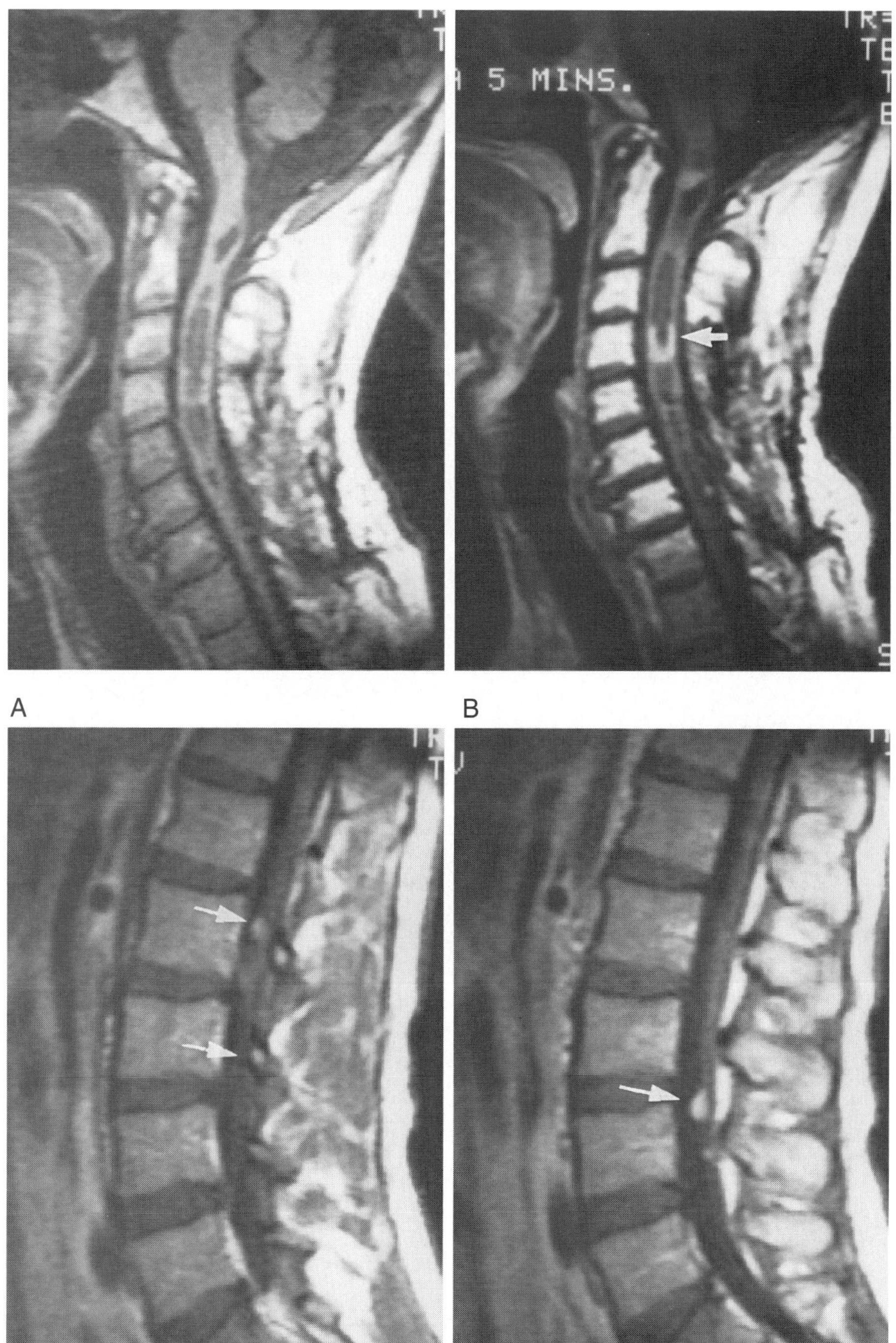

Figure 16.105. Neurofibromatosis type I with an astrocytoma in the cervical region and multiple neurofibromas in lumbar roots. **A.** Precontrast T1 shows syrinx with some solid components. **B.** Postcontrast T1 sagittal 1 year later shows areas of enhancement around part of the cyst (arrow). Note the hyperintensity of all cervical vertebrae due to radiation therapy. **C** and **D.** A number of neurofibromas in lumbar roots are visible after contrast (arrows).

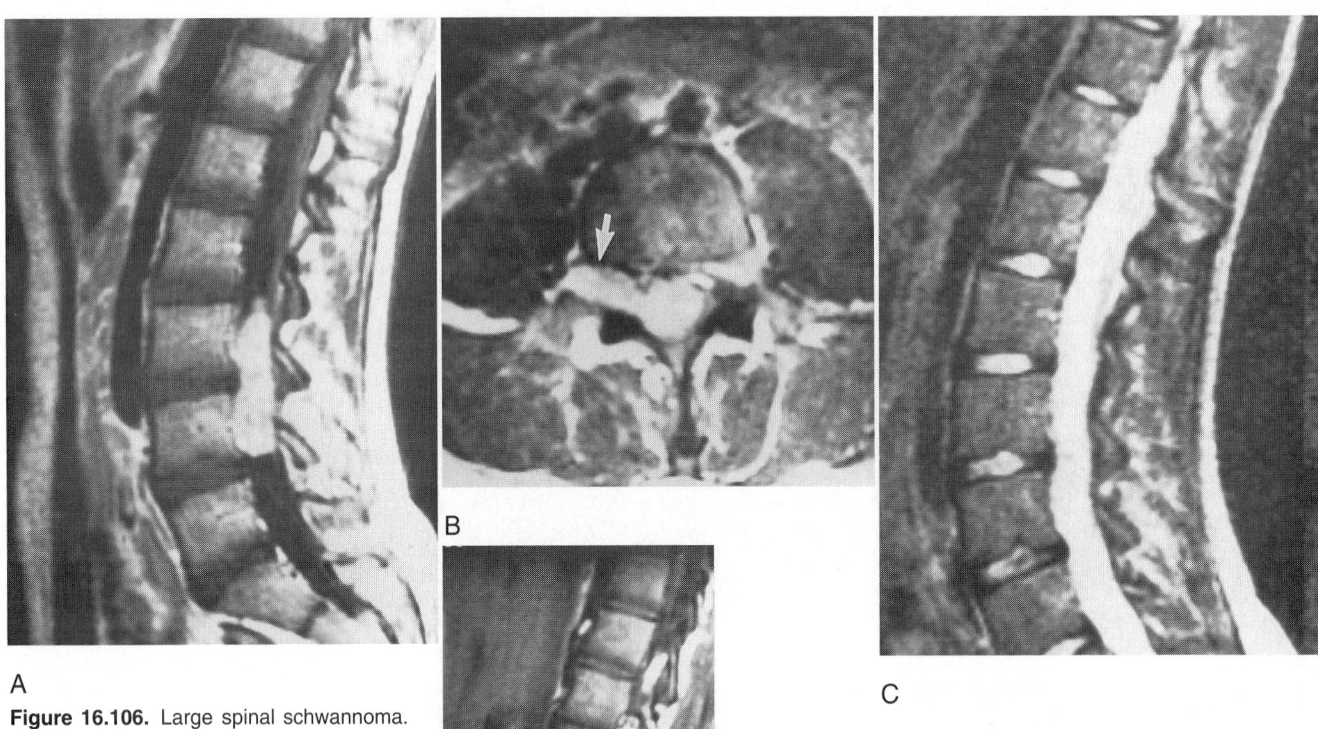

A B C D

Figure 16.106. Large spinal schwannoma. **A.** Large schwannoma seen on enhanced T1 sagittal MRI. These tumors are soft and mold to the shape of the surrounding canal, unlike the meningiomas, which are likely to be firm and maintain their round shape (compare with meningioma in Fig. 16.101). **B.** Postcontrast axial shows that the tumor exits through the neural canal (arrow). **C.** T2-weighted image completely obscures the tumor, which is hyperintense like the surrounding CSF. **D.** Noncontrast sagittal T1 shows the tumor exiting via the intervertebral foramen (arrow). Compare with normal nerves above and below. (Courtesy of Dr. Stephen Sweriduk, Boston, Mass.)

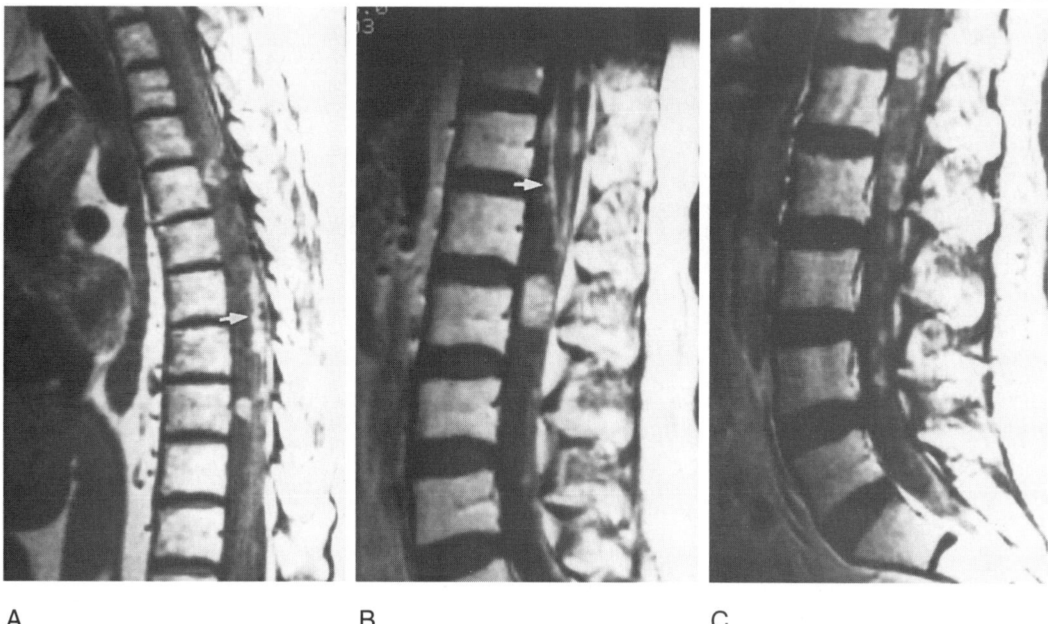

Figure 16.107. Seeding of spinal cord and subarachnoid space from medulloblastoma. **A** to **C.** A number of nodules are demonstrated on sagittal postcontrast T1 images in the thoracic and the lumbar region. The nodules are on the surface of the cord, predominantly in a dorsolateral location. Diffuse meningeal enhancement may also be present (arrows), indicative of meningeal tumor seeding.

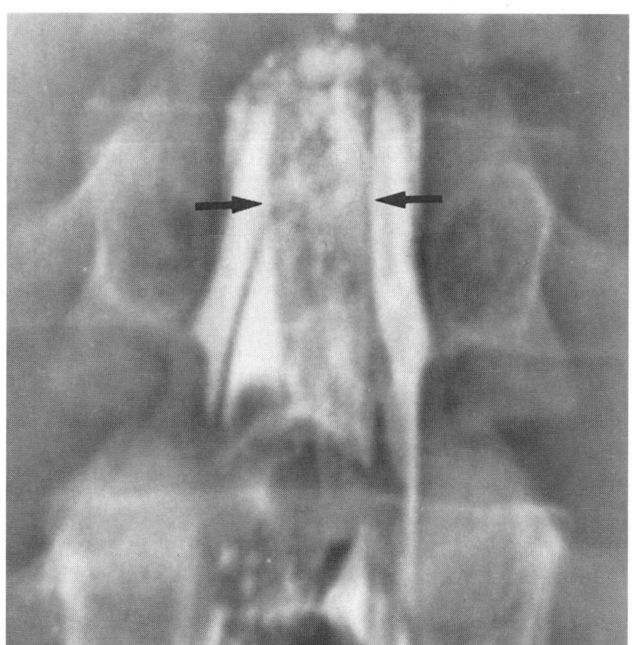

Figure 16.108. Seeding metastases from a pineal germinoma. The myelogram reveals several nodules and a partial block at the level of L2-L3 due to more nodules. The conus (arrows) shows irregularities due to multiple small nodules on its surface. The patient presented with paraparesis before the relatively small pineal tumor was known.

great majority of these, however, are nonneoplastic and include the herniated intervertebral discs, the degenerative osteoarthritic changes described earlier, as well as traumatic conditions and congenital lesions.

In this section we will discuss primarily the extradural neoplasms. These are either benign or malignant in character, although the vast majority are malignant. This situation differs from that of neoplasms occurring in the intradural extramedullary compartment, which are almost all benign. The malignant neoplasms may be primary within the vertebral canal or may represent metastases from elsewhere. Primary extradural tumors, benign and malignant, may arise from the dura, from nerve roots external to the dura, or from connective tissue, fat, blood vessels, lymphatic tissues, and other tissues resident in the epidural space.

Benign extradural tumors include meningiomas, neurinomas, fibromas, lipomas, dermoids or epidermoids, and vascular lesions. Benign tumors are encountered infrequently, in proportion to the occurrence of their intradural counterparts, and usually have an intradural component that can be diagnosed as such by imaging methods, including myelography. Except for the neurinomas, specific changes characteristic of the type of lesion present are not observed on plain films. Erosion, loss of well-defined margins of various portions of the vertebrae found in the vertebral canal, may result from local pressure by the tumor. Extradural neurinomas frequently extend through one or more intervertebral foramina, which may be enlarged; the lesions may be continuous with the large mass in the para-

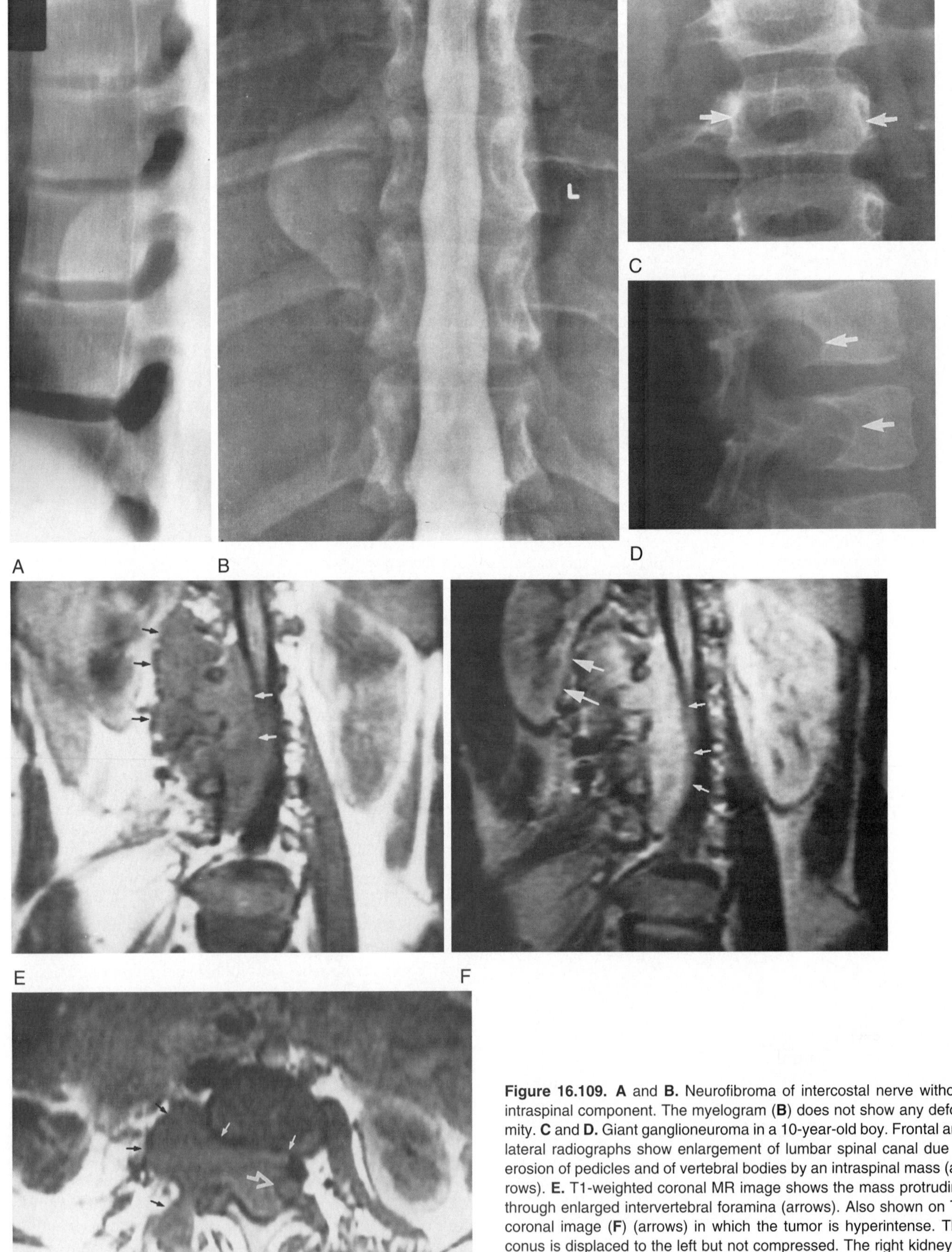

Figure 16.109. **A** and **B.** Neurofibroma of intercostal nerve without intraspinal component. The myelogram (**B**) does not show any deformity. **C** and **D.** Giant ganglioneuroma in a 10-year-old boy. Frontal and lateral radiographs show enlargement of lumbar spinal canal due to erosion of pedicles and of vertebral bodies by an intraspinal mass (arrows). **E.** T1-weighted coronal MR image shows the mass protruding through enlarged intervertebral foramina (arrows). Also shown on T2 coronal image (**F**) (arrows) in which the tumor is hyperintense. The conus is displaced to the left but not compressed. The right kidney is displaced laterally (arrows). **G.** The axial T1-weighted noncontrast image shows the extra- and intraspinal components (arrows). The conus is displaced to the left, but the tumor is soft and partly surrounds the cord rather than flattening it (open arrow).

spinal region (Fig. 16.109). Extradural meningiomas are much less common but may produce local erosion of vertebral pedicles, lamina, or bodies similar to that seen with intrathecal meningiomas. The extradural lipomas are composed of mature fat, which differs little from the areolar tissue of the epidural space. The lesions are frequently associated with spina bifida or some other anomaly of the vertebral column, as explained under "Congenital Anomalies."

CT and MRI usually are sufficient to make a diagnosis of the lesion, which may or may not involve bone. The dura is displaced away from the outer surface of the canal and will produce narrowing of the thecal sac and compression of its contents, be it the spinal cord or, below the first lumbar vertebra, the roots of the cauda equina. MRI may suffice to make a diagnosis, but sometimes myelography followed by CT is also carried out to obtain a more complete picture of the lesion, including the presence and extent of bone destruction.

Myelography usually demonstrates either a broad, long defect on one side or the other of the opaque column or a complete block. A complete block due to an epidural lesion usually has an irregular margin at the point of the block. If the opaque column is looked at from all sides, there will be one side where the opaque column will be narrowed, which is due to the fact that the dura is displaced away from the outer surface of the spinal canal toward the center. The types of lesions encountered include lymphoma, which is the type of epidural lesion that could be primary in the epidural location, or it may be invasion from a retroperitoneal lymphoma (Fig. 16.110). However, the most frequent extradural tumor is metastatic disease to the bones or to the epidural tissues from a tumor elsewhere. Plain-film findings may be diagnostic. Today, however, MRI turns out to be the most useful examination in making an early diagnosis, and, at the same time, in determining whether there is any spinal cord compression, an extremely important question (Figs. 16.111 to 16.113).

In the absence of cross-sectional imaging, if only myelography is available, sometimes it is difficult to differentiate a block produced by an intramedullary tumor and an epidural tumor that is encircling the entire canal. If the head of the opaque column at the block is carefully scrutinized, however, it will be noted that the right and left edges, or the dorsal or ventral edges, whichever is the case, will be displaced toward the center of the canal, that is, toward the center of the cord. This is the opposite of the intramedullary tumors causing a block, which actually produce a slight widening of the column of contrast at the point of the block (Figs. 16.100 and 16.112).

The vast majority of metastatic carcinomas of the epidural space originate in the breast, the lung, or the prostate. Extradural carcinoma most commonly is the secondary extension from an involved vertebra, especially with metastases from the breast. Metastatic carcinoma from the breast may produce osteolytic, osteoblastic, or mixed reactions in the involved vertebrae. Pathologic fracture of one or more vertebrae frequently is demonstrable in spine radiographs. Extension of bronchogenic carcinoma into the epidural space through the intervertebral foramina does occur with or without involvement of the vertebrae themselves. The vertebral change resulting from involvement of the bronchogenic carcinoma is osteolysis. Often there is destruction of half of one or more of the vertebral bodies, the ipsilateral portions of the vertebral arches and posterior portions of the adjacent ridge. A paravertebral soft tissue mass may be visible in the involved area, or the lung carcinoma may be demonstrated in plain spine radiographs.

When the tumor encroaches on the epidural space from one side, the subarachnoid space either at myelography or by MRI is indented and narrowed unilaterally. If there is unilateral collapse of one vertebra, lateral angulation of the subarachnoid space or the spinal column occurs at this level.

Primary tumors of bone that may compress the spinal canal include giant cell tumor, aneurysmal bone cyst, osteoblastoma, osteosarcoma, chordoma, hemangiopericytoma, and myeloma. CT and MRI may help in the differential diagnosis in analyzing the findings seen on plain films. Vertebral hemangiomas are seen fairly frequently on MR images as well as on CT. They are also recognized on plain films of the spine because of the classic vertical striations seen particularly well on lateral views of the spine. On CT axial views the coarse pattern of the bone trabeculae is also fairly typical (Fig. 16.114). Most hemangiomas are small and do not deform the vertebral body. However, some hemangiomas can be large, and may involve the pedicles and lamina; the increase in the size of the bones causes compression of the spinal cord or the roots. Hemangiomas can be multiple. On MRI hemangiomas are usually bright on T1- and T2-weighted images. The brightness on T1 may be associated with blood products. Lipomatous deposits in the vertebral bodies are bright on T1-, but not on T2-weighted images, and are dark on fat-suppressed images.

Extradural sarcoma, either primary or metastatic, does not extend through the dural membrane. Metastatic carcinoma, as a rule, also remains outside the dural sac; an exception is an occasional pulmonary carcinoma, which may invade the dura and present on its internal surface or even invade the spinal cord.

Extradural tumors, usually metastatic, represent the most common lesion producing rapidly developing paraparesis or paraplegia. Under these circumstances it was the usual custom to request emergency myelography. This changed to requesting an emergency MRI examination, which is noninvasive and just as informative or even more so than myelography. If there was a complete block due to compression, it was often difficult to perform a spinal puncture and it was sometimes necessary to perform a C1-C2 puncture. MRI has eliminated all this so that in the last several years we have not performed a single emergency

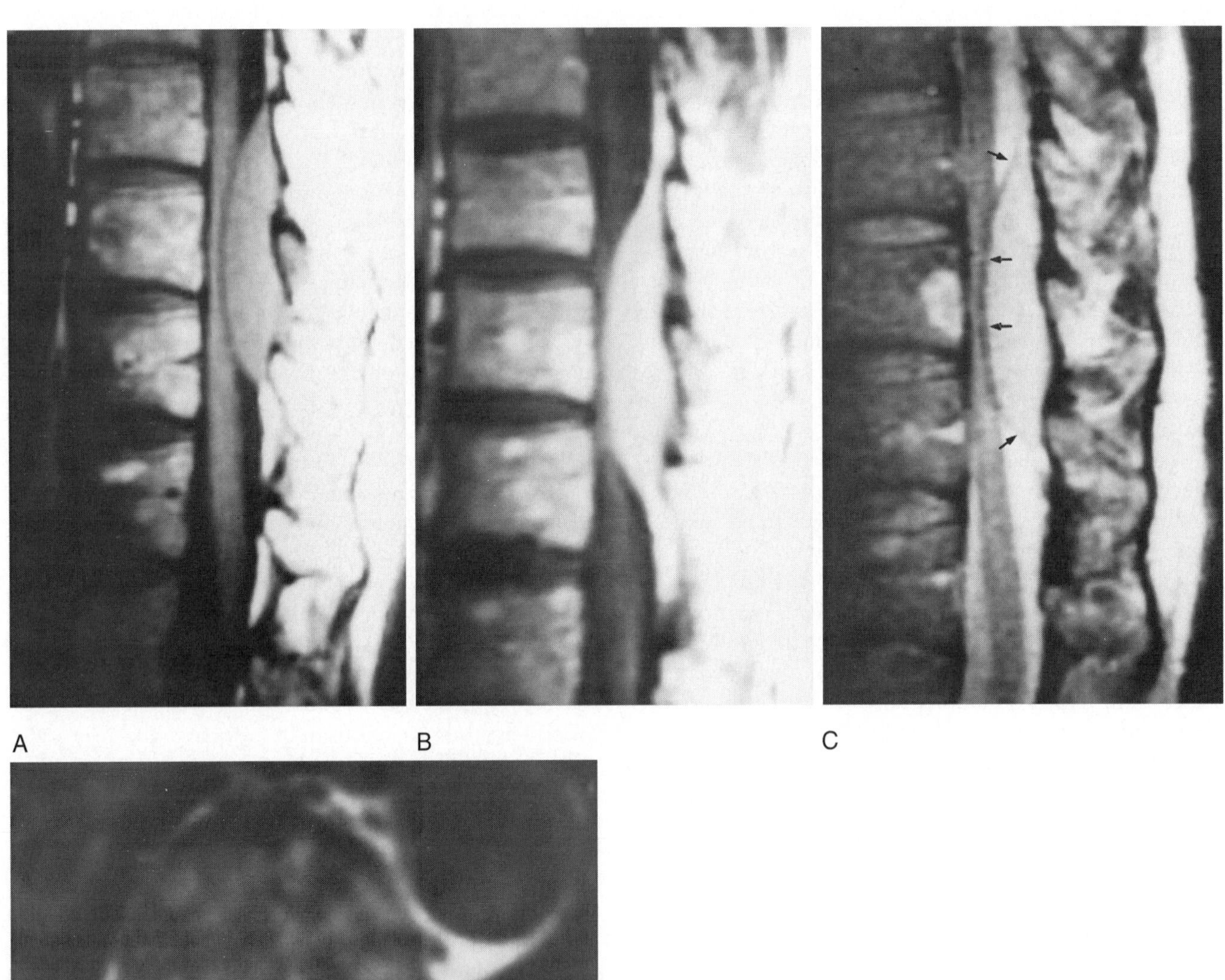

Figure 16.110. Epidural tumor—lymphoma. Precontrast (**A**) and postcontrast (**B**) T1 MRI sagittal view shows a lesion producing a sweeping indentation on the subarachnoid space typical of an epidural location. The lesion enhances brightly. **C.** T2 sagittal view shows that the dura is seen as a low-intensity membrane (arrows). **D.** Axial postcontrast MRI shows that the tumor is in the spinal canal and extends out through the intervertebral foramen on both sides (arrows). No retroperitoneal tumor is seen. (Courtesy of Dr. Stephen Sweriduk, Boston, Mass.)

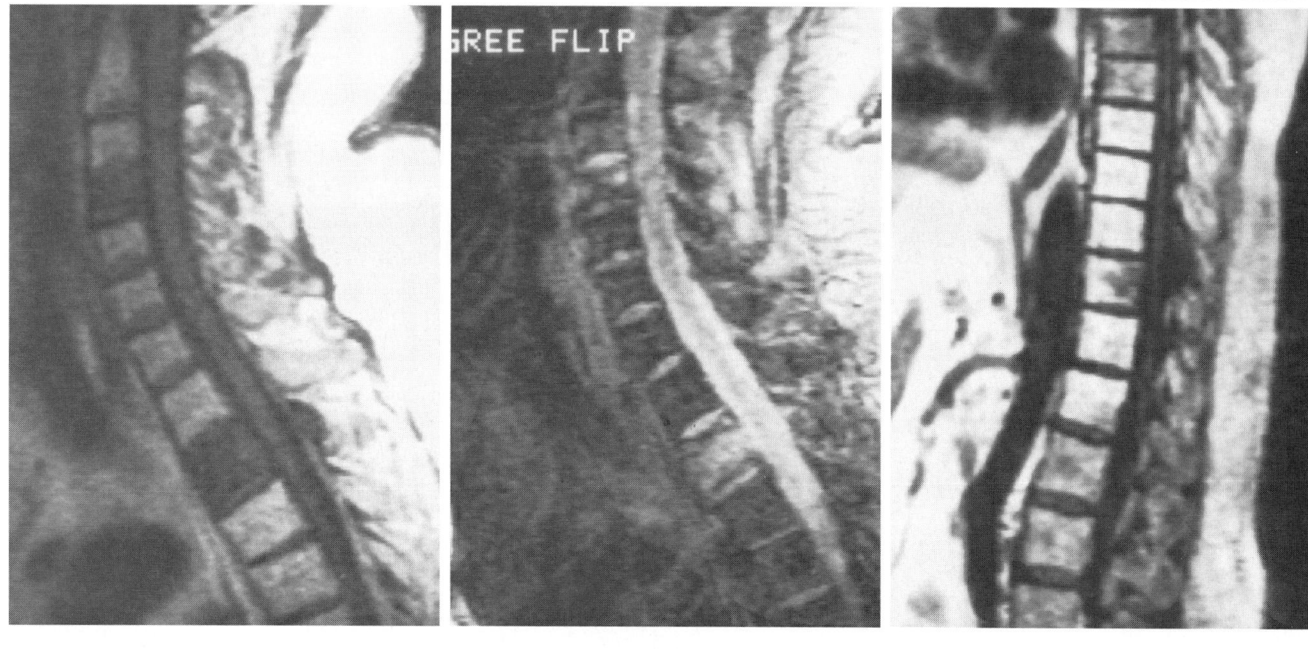

A B C

Figure 16.111. Metastatic prostate carcinoma. **A.** T1-weighted noncontrast view. There are two vertebrae showing bone marrow signal alteration. A frequent cause for this is tumor infiltration. **B.** T2-weighted image shows hyperintensity in the same two vertebral bodies. No evidence of epidural mass or cord compression. **C.** The patient had previously received radiation therapy for involvement of a thoracic vertebra. Typical fatty replacement of bone marrow in T6 to T11 vertebral bodies is seen due to postradiation effect.

myelogram. Compression of the cord can be detected, the degree of compression can be evaluated, and a decision to perform radiation therapy or surgical decompression can be made expeditiously by MRI without contrast (Figs. 16.112 and 16.113).

It is interesting to note that contrast enhancement with MRI is not as helpful as in other tumors in diagnosing malignant epidural tumors (97). Noncontrast MRI is usually sufficient.

Chordoma

In the spine chordomas occur most frequently in the sacral region, but may also be encountered in the cervical region, usually in the first four vertebrae. Occasionally they are found elsewhere in the spine. Their appearance radiographically or on CT is that of bone destruction involving the vertebral bodies and arches, sometimes presenting calcifications within the area of tumor. The calcifications may be residual bone instead of calcium in the tumor. Cord compression is common in the cervical region (Fig. 16.115). Chordomas may involve more than one vertebral body. In the sacrum they may be very destructive and grow very large, also growing into the adjacent soft tissues. Whenever a destructive lesion involving the sacrum is present, particularly if it involves the sacral vertebral body equivalents, chordoma should be included in the differential diagnosis.

TRAUMATIC CONDITIONS OF THE SPINE

A description of all the types of fractures of the vertebrae will not be included here; rather, a discussion of injuries that cause neurologic signs of compression of the roots and the spinal cord will be given. The most common fractures that produce severe neurologic deficit probably involve the cervical spine, at both the upper and lower level near the cervical thoracic junction. In both cases, the injury could be produced by dislocation accompanied by fracture—for instance, of the odontoid process or, in the thoracic region, luxation of the sixth thoracic vertebra on the seventh, which results in compression of the spinal cord between the posterior margin of the body of C-7 and the neural arch of C-6.

Whitley and Fosyth introduced the classification of cervical spine fractures, which was later modified but remains the basic classification (98). They considered flexion injuries, extension injuries, combined flexion and extension injuries, and bursting injuries, which could also be called axial loading or compression injuries. Rotational injuries could be added to these, and combinations are common.

A *flexion injury* usually produces compression of the vertebral bodies as well as of the intervertebral discs. A compression fracture may develop, or, more important, a rupture of the posterior longitudinal ligament which may permit herniation of one of the intervertebral discs, and may also be accompanied by a rupture of the posterior

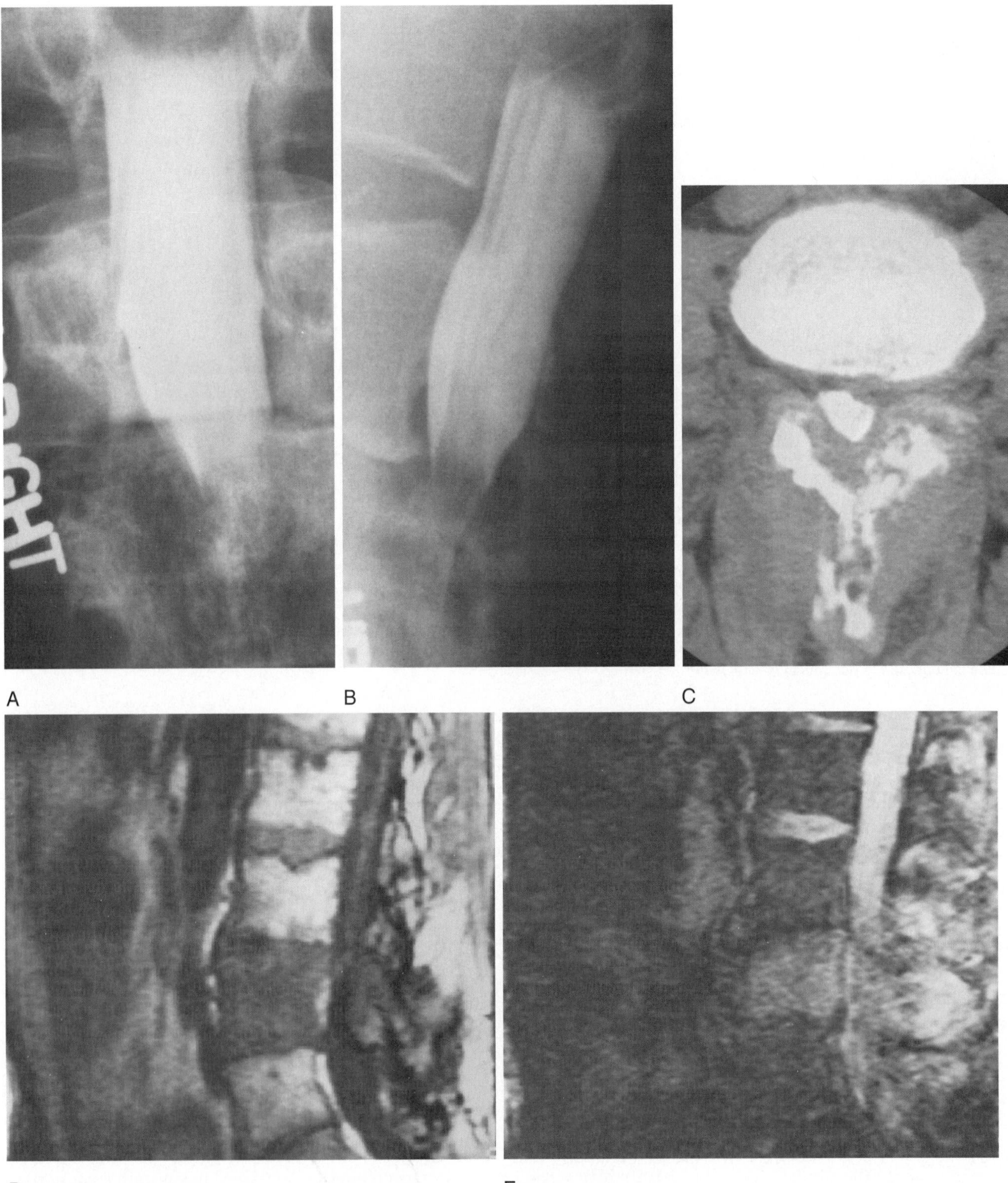

Figure 16.112. Epidural metastases from lung carcinoma. **A** and **B.** Myelography (in erect position) revealed a complete block at the level of L4. There is narrowing of the diameter of the contrast column as it approaches the complete block (contrast injected via a C1-C2 puncture). This is typical of an epidural block. **C.** CT-myelography shows deformity of the thecal sac and in addition demonstrates a soft tissue mass in the canal and bone destruction in the neural arch. **D.** Sagittal T1-weighted MR image shows the loss of marrow of L4. **E.** T2-weighted sagittal reveals hyperintensity of the L4 vertebral body consistent with neoplasm. Today myelography is carried out only rarely because MRI without and with contrast is sufficient to determine the location and the degree of compression of the spinal cord or nerve roots of the cauda equina.

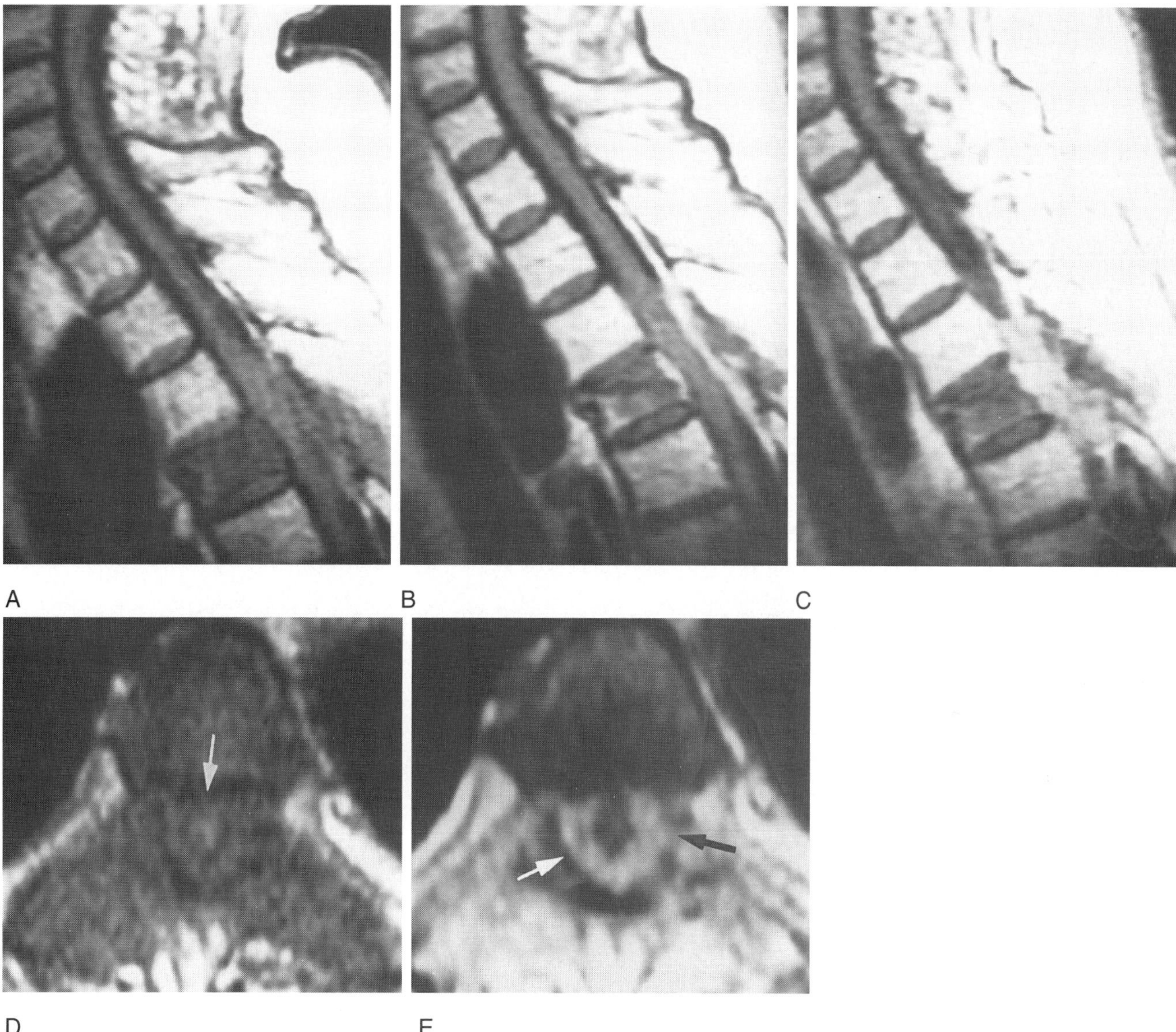

Figure 16.113. Metastatic epidural tumor from a primary lung carcinoma. **A.** There is loss of bone marrow on T1 sagittal views. There is only mild ventral cord compression. Sagittal postcontrast show the tumor in dorsal midline (**B**) and lateral (**C**) surfaces. The involved vertebral body enhances partially. **D.** Axial noncontrast T1-weighted image shows cord surrounded by tumor. The cord is slightly hyperintense (arrow). **E.** Postcontrast view shows enhancement of encircling metastatic tumor (arrows). The cord is circumferentially compressed.

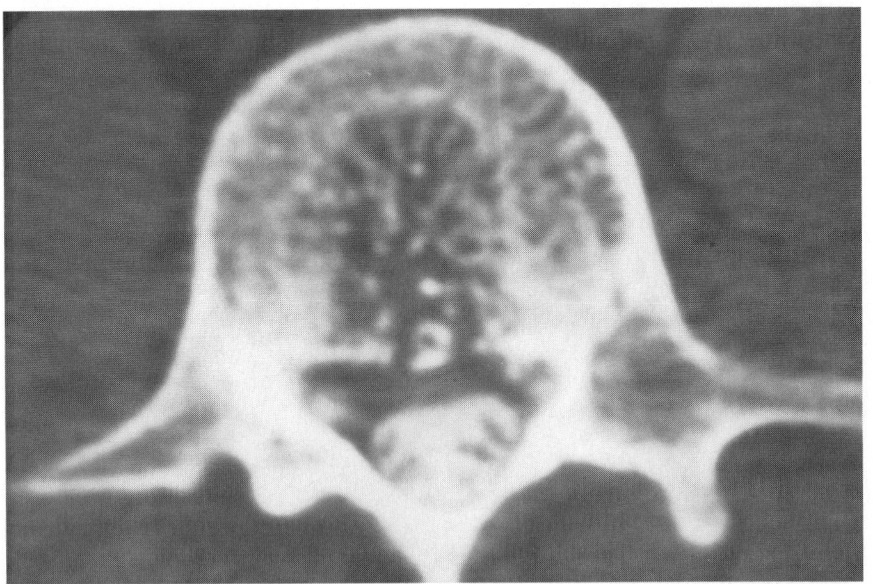

A

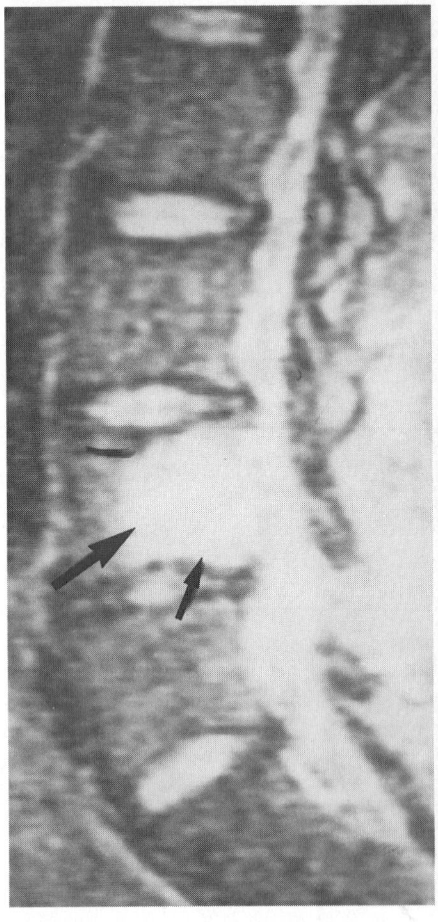

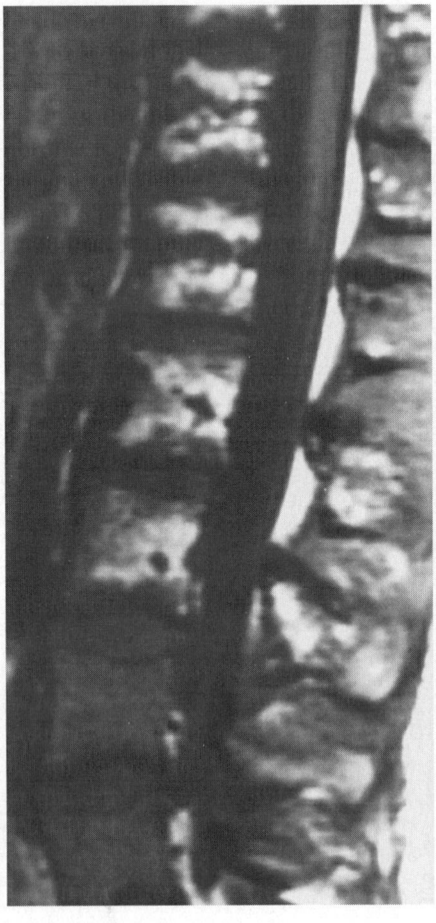

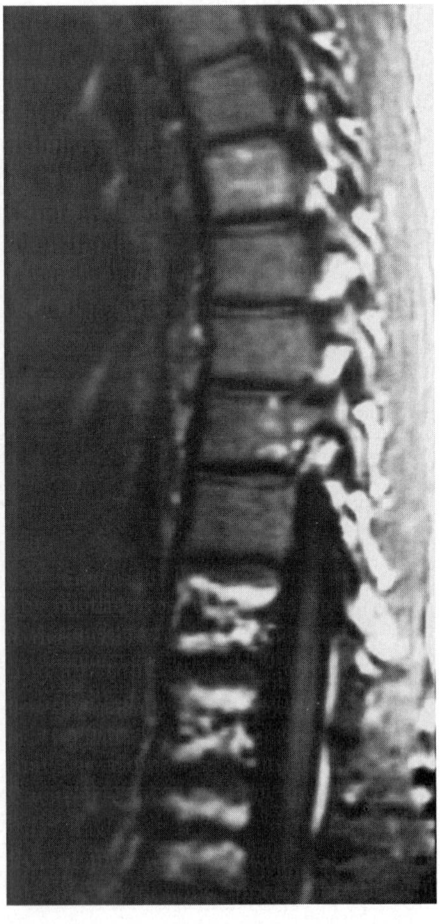

B C D

Figure 16.114. Spinal hemangiomas. **A.** On CT the coarse trabecular pattern is typical. The hemangioma reaches the posterior vertebral margin but does not protrude into the canal. **B.** T2-weighted sagittal MR image shows that the hemangioma is very bright (arrows). This differentiates it from fat deposits in the vertebral bodies, which are fairly common. Hemangiomas are also bright on T1-weighted images, whereas lipomatous deposits are light on T1- but much less bright on T2-weighted images. Also they would be dark on fat-suppressed images. **C** and **D.** Multiple hemangiomas of the vertebral column involving most of the vertebral bodies and many of the arches in a 20-year-old woman. The lesions are all bright on T1-weighted sagittal MR images. The patient did not present any neurologic signs at the time she was seen. There was also one hemangioma in the skull but none in the brain.

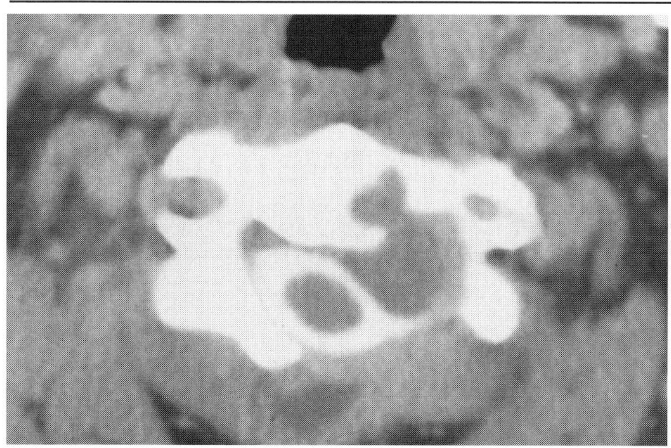
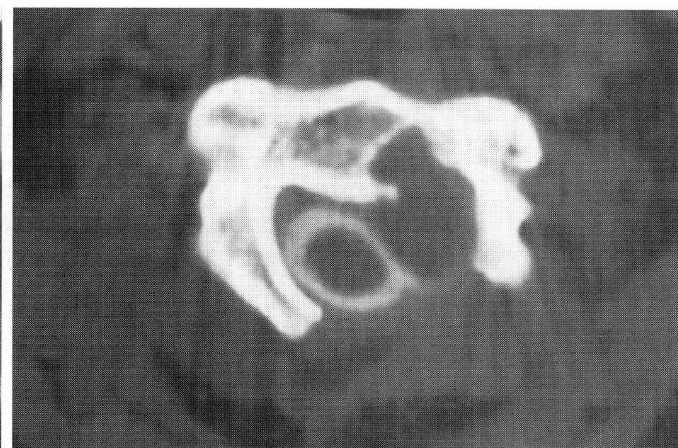

A B

Figure 16.115. Chordoma in cervical region in a 35-year-old man. **A.** The CT-myelogram demonstrates an area of bone destruction involving the body of C3 as well as the adjacent neural arch. The soft-tissue mass is displacing the corresponding nerve root and rotating the spinal cord. **B.** Bone window image to demonstrate the bone destruction, which presents a sharp margin.

interspinous ligaments. The latter can be recognized by the widening of the interspinous space in the lateral view. This can be shown more clearly by flexion lateral views of the cervical spine. The latter cannot be made unless it is determined with certainty that there is no contraindication to taking the films in that position after examining the neutral position lateral views as well as the frontal and transoral views.

The *extension injuries* usually lead to a fracture of the posterior elements. The articular pillars may flatten, and there may be rupture of the anterior common ligament, which, if severe, may lead to subluxation of the vertebra above the disc at the level where the anterior longitudinal ligament ruptured. The posterior longitudinal ligament may also break. Only a fracture of the inferior anterior corner of the vertebral body (teardrop fracture) may be visible; when this is seen, a rupture of the anterior longitudinal ligament should be suspected. Hyperextension injuries may be accompanied by odontoid process fractures.

The bursting injuries are axial-loading injuries where a force is applied to the head in a downward direction. It may be combined with flexion or extension. It may lead to fractures of the vertebral bodies, or it may produce a Jefferson-type fracture, where the atlas bursts at the ring on both sides as the occipital condyles push the atlas down.

Plain film is inadequate to evaluate cervical spine fractures, and CT is usually necessary (Figs. 16.116 and 16.117).

The lateral flexion and rotation injuries produce wedging of the lateral aspect of the vertebral body and its associated lateral mass. One of the effects of flexion injuries is to produce either a bilateral or unilateral subluxation of the articular facets, which become trapped and cannot return to their normal position because the inferoposterior margin of the facets is locked in front of the superior margin of the facet below and thus cannot return to its normal position.

In all of these types of injuries the spinal cord may be involved, and temporary as well as permanent paralysis may result, which, in the cervical region, may involve all four extremities. An important injury to keep in mind is the forward luxation of C-6 on C-7 or C-7 on T1, which will pin the spinal cord and produce a paralysis in most of the cases where it occurs. This area may not be easily radiographed, and it is most important when the patient is examined to always obtain lateral views of the cervical spine where the seventh vertebra is included. MRI is an ideal method for determining the presence of a forward subluxation or dislocation of the lower cervical vertebrae because it can be done rapidly and the spinal cord can be evaluated at the same time. The same is true in the evaluation of any injury in which spinal cord compression is suspected.

In the thoracic region, compression fractures of the vertebral bodies are common, particularly due to osteoporosis or metastatic neoplasm. However, these fractures rarely produce disruption of the spinal canal and cord compression. Severe injuries involving the upper thoracic spine accompanied by dislocation of the thoracic vertebral body usually produce paraplegia (99). Severe spinal injuries involving the lower thoracic-thoracolumbar region produce compression of the conus medullaris. Early CT examination is important in the presence of crush fractures because they may produce fragments that protrude into the spinal canal and compress the spinal cord or spinal nerve roots, depending on whether the fracture occurred in the cervical, thoracic, or lumbar region. Early surgical correction is indicated (Fig. 16.118).

Modern evaluation of spinal injuries that produce neurologic complications, cord contusion, cord compression, radicular compression, or root avulsion includes CT and

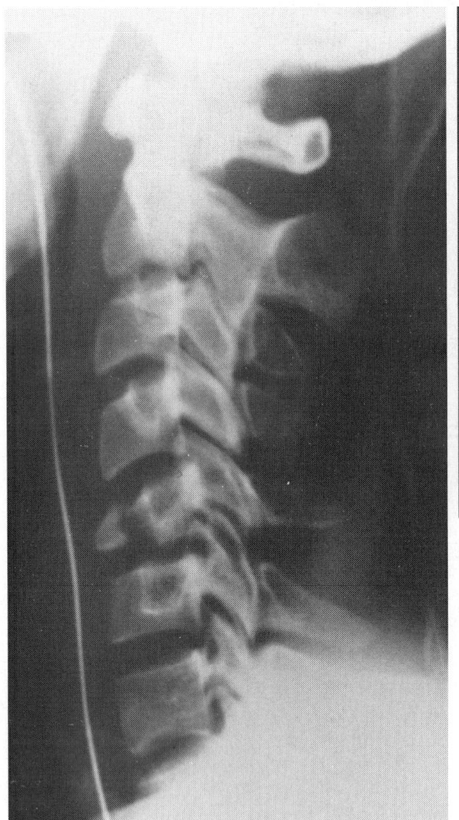

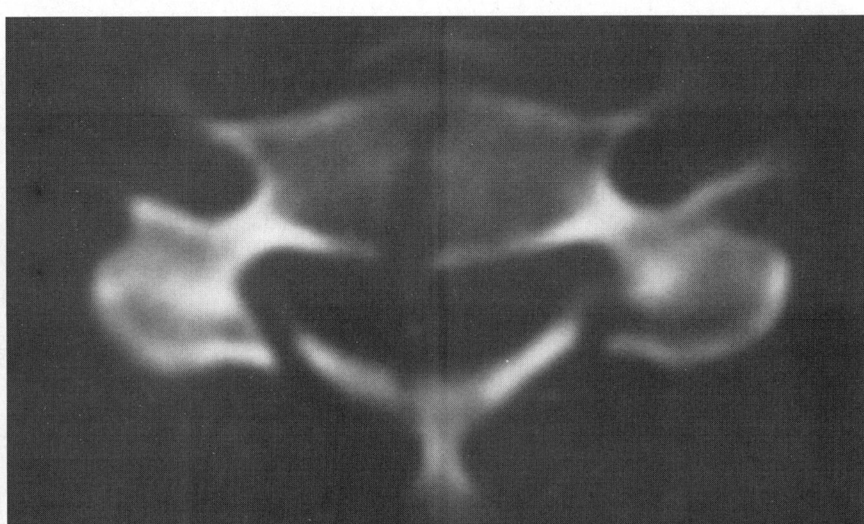

A

B

Figure 16.116. Fracture of fifth cervical vertebra. **A.** Lateral cervical spine shows a compression fracture of C5 and no other abnormalities. The nasogastric tube is not displaced forward, indicating there is no prevertebral hematoma. **B.** Axial CT shows not only the fracture of the vertebral body but also bilateral fractures of the lamina. The neural arch has moved forward, producing flattening of the anteroposterior diameter of the spinal canal and spinal cord compression.

MRI, when possible, is the procedure of choice to allow for an evaluation of the spinal cord in any patient presenting neurologic finding after injury. This is particularly important when there are neurologic findings. Both CT and MRI may be necessary for a more complete evaluation.

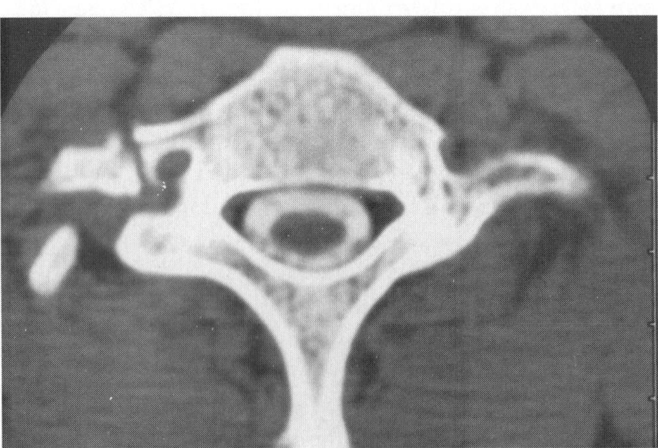

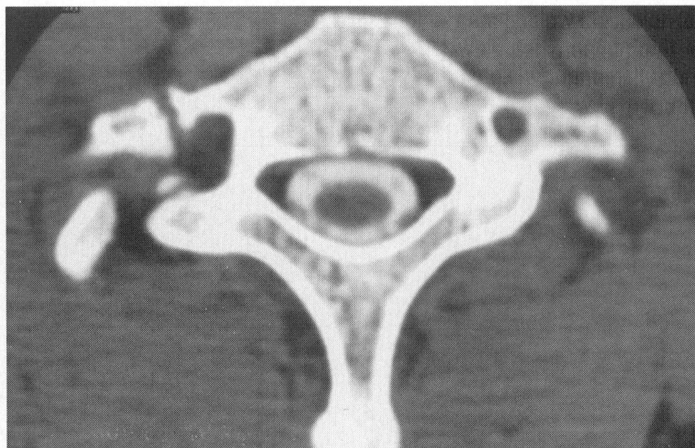

A B

Figure 16.117. Fracture of transverse process of seventh cervical vertebra that produced a radiculopathy thought clinically to be due to a herniated intervertebral disc. The patient sustained an injury involving the right shoulder and neck. The plain-film examination was negative. Several weeks later he was still complaining of radicular-type pain. MRI examination at that time was negative. Because of the persistence of symptoms a herniated disc was suspected. This led to a CT-myelogram, which demonstrated a fracture of the transverse process (**A** and **B**) and no evidence of a disc herniation.

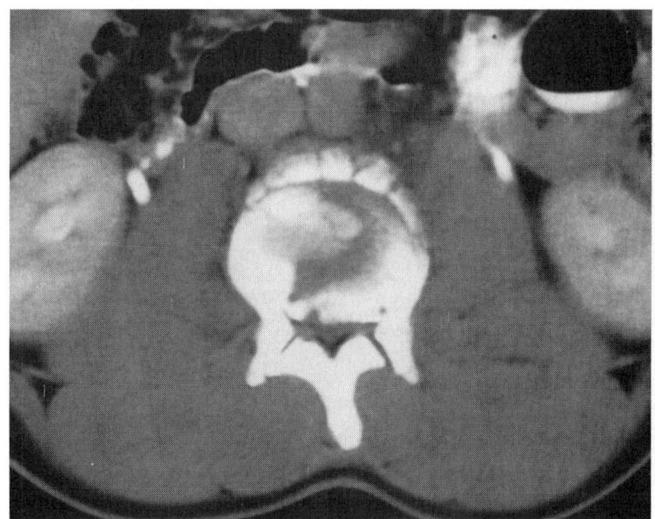

A

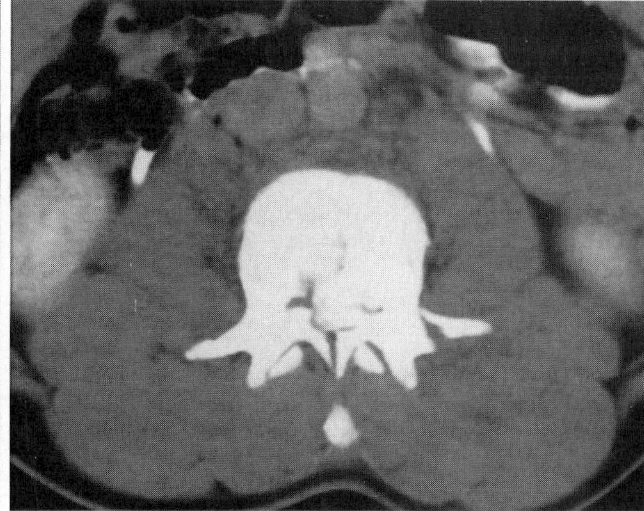

B

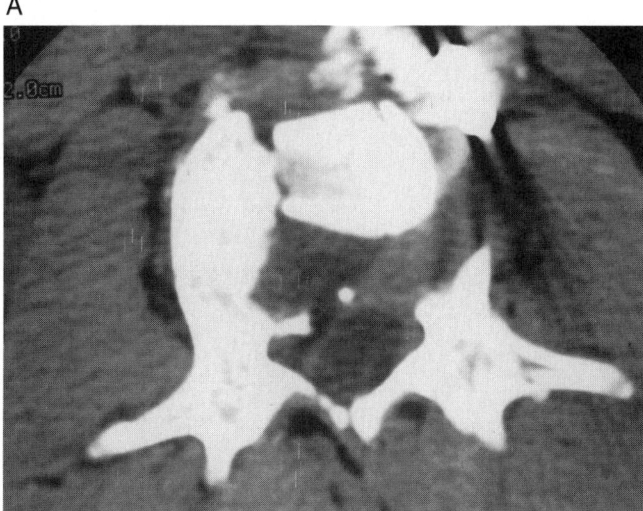

C

Figure 16.118. Crush lumbar vertebral fracture with fragments producing compression of cauda equina roots. **A** and **B.** There is almost total obliteration of the spinal canal. There is paraspinal soft tissue swelling. **C.** Reexamination after surgical intervention reveals a postsurgical decompression and return to a normal canal.

MRI after plain-film examination. Myelography is done if MR is unavailable, is not possible, or is contraindicated. Instruments used to treat fractures are not a contraindication to MR examination if they are aluminum or other diamagnetic metal. The ideal time to perform an MRI examination in a patient who presents with signs of spinal cord damage is early, possibly upon the patient's arrival, after plain-film examination has been obtained and before any specific metallic instrument is applied that could interfere with MRI examination. An open-magnet system instead of the usual tunnel magnet is ideal for examining patients who cannot easily receive life support inside the long tunnel. The traumatized patient with spinal injury and neurologic signs of cord injury should be considered an MRI emergency, because cord evaluation can be accomplished very rapidly and noninvasively. When MRI is unavailable or cannot be performed because the patient is mechanically supported, CT scanning with sagittal and coronal reformatting is excellent for demonstrating deformities of the spinal canal. Unfortunately, it usually does not demonstrate the spinal cord adequately. The latter can be performed after intraspinal injection of a small amount of contrast before the CT examination. The contrast can be allowed to move up by turning the patient on the side and then supine and/or prone. Minimal elevation of the patient's hip area may suffice, which can easily be accomplished in the Stryker frame.

CT examination is essential to study the fracture area, particularly in the cervical region. Fractures are usually underestimated on plain films and one must emphasize the importance of looking for multiple injuries in cervical spine trauma (Fig. 16.116). If the patient shows signs of root avulsion, usually in the cervical area, myelography is ordinarily needed to show the outpouching of the arachnoid associated with tearing of the root, which leaves an opening in the dura through which the arachnoid membrane her-

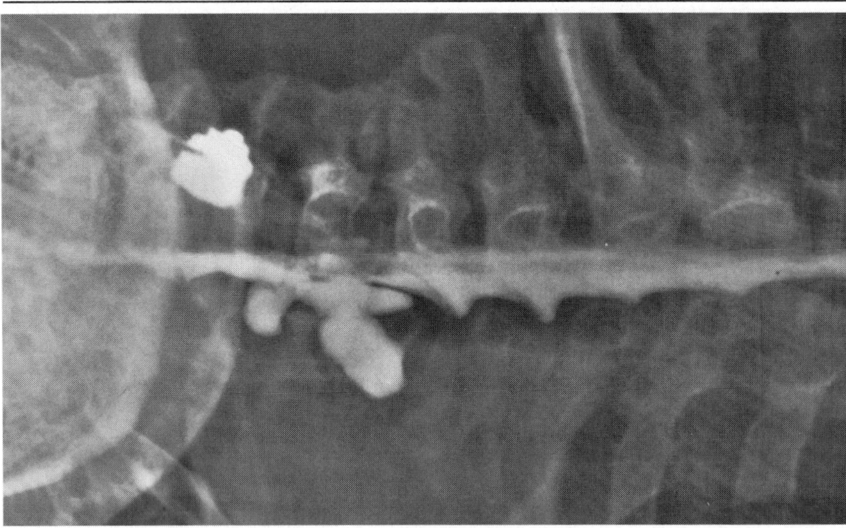

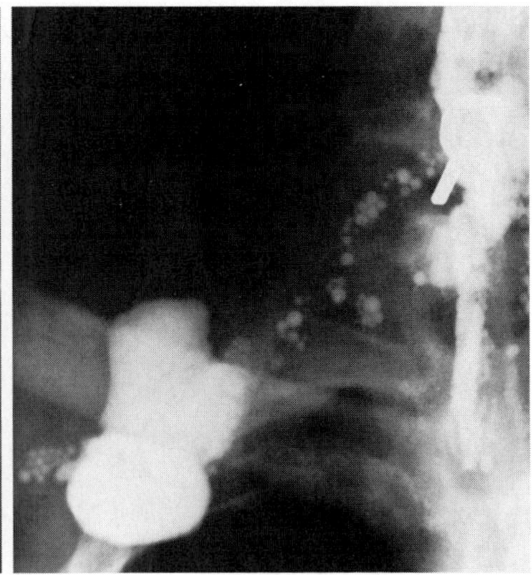

A B

Figure 16.119. Pseudomeningoceles produced by root avulsion in the cervical region. **A.** There is outpouching of contrast out of two of the cervical roots on the right side. To fill these sacs it is necessary to place the patient in the lateral decubitus position on the symptomatic side. **B.** Another case reveals a root avulsion that resulted in considerable extension of the sac to the retroclavicular region along the brachial plexus. The size of the sac will probably continue to grow with time unless it is surgically repaired.

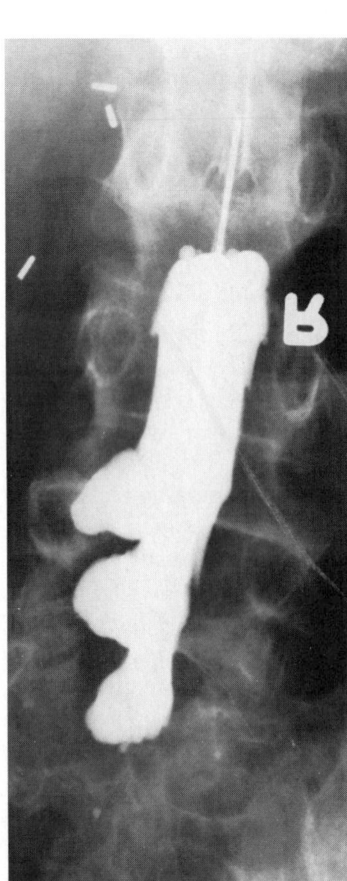

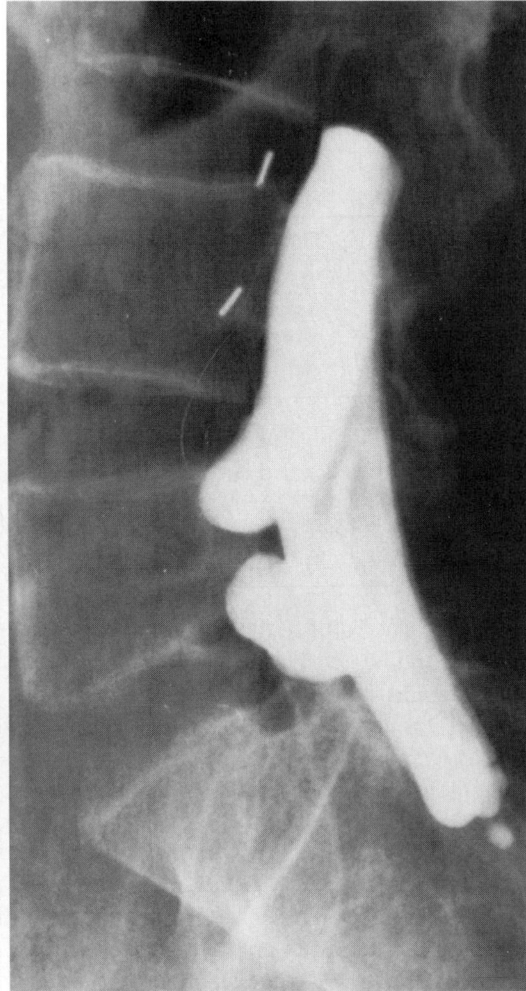

Figure 16.120. Lumbar root avulsion. These are much less common than in the cervical region and result from a type of injury that would pull on the lumbar plexus. The pseudomeningoceles would grow to a large size before becoming stationary.

niates, producing pseudomeningoceles (Fig. 16.119). They are uncommon in the lumbar region (Fig. 16.120).

Brachial plexus injury may be evaluated with CT and, preferably, with MRI. The formation of a pseudomeningocele in association with brachial plexus injury is an indication of root avulsion (100). In the acute stage after injury, CSF may leak out the canal into the brachial plexus area. Later the arachnoid would close, and pseudomeningoceles would form. CT is useful, particularly combined with myelography (101).

REFERENCES

1. Elsberg CA, Dyke CG: The diagnosis and localization of tumors of the spinal cord by means of measurements made on the x-ray films of the vertebrae, and the correlation of clinical and x-ray findings. Bull Neurol Inst New York 1934;3:359.
2. Dandy WE: Roentgenography of the brain after the injection of air into the spinal canal. Ann Surg 1919;70:397–403.
3. Bull JWD: History of neuroradiology. Br J Radiol 1961;34:69–84.
4. Strain WH, Plati JT, Warren SL: Iodinated organic compounds as contrast media for radiographic diagnosis: I-iodinated aracyl esters. J Am Chem Soc 1942;64:1436.
5. Lindblom K: Complications of myelography with abrodil. Acta Radiol 1947;28:69.
6. Castel JC, Dorcier F, Caille JM: Penetration of the brain by nonionic water-soluble tri- and hexoiodinated contrast media. Neuroradiology 1987;29:206–210.
7. Bryan RN, Hershkowitz N: Neuronal effects of water-soluble contrast agents. Invest Radiol 1984;19:329–332.
8. Hershkowitz N, Bryan RN: Neurotoxic effects of water-soluble contrast agents on rat hippocampus. Invest Radiol 1984;19:192–201.
9. Lamb JT: Ioheyol vs. iopamidol for myelography. Invest Radiol 1985;20(suppl 1):537–543.
10. Jinkins JR, Bashir R, Al-Mefty O, et al: Cystic necrosis of the spinal cord in compressive cervical myelopathy: Demonstration by lopamidol CT-myelography. AJR 1986;147:767–775.
11. Dake MD, Dillon WP, Dorwart RH: CT of extraarachnoid metrizamide instillation. AJNR 1986;7:689–692.
12. Lindblom K: Technique and results in myelography and disc punctures. Acta Radiol 1950;34:321.
13. Camp JD: The roentgenologic localization of tumors affecting the spinal cord. Am J Roentgenol 1938;40:540.
14. Camp JD: Contrast myelography past and present. Radiology 1950; 54:477.
15. Horwitz T: The diagnosis of posterior protrusion of the intervertebral disc with special reference to (1) its differentiation from certain degenerative lesions of the disc and its related structures and (2) the interpretation of contrast myelography. Am J Roentgenol 1943; 49:199.
16. Stadnik TW, van Tussebroek FM, Luypaert RR, et al: CT-assisted chemonucleolysis. Eur J Radiol 1988;8:249.
17. Ford LT: Clinical use of chymopapain in lumbar and dorsal disk lesions: An end result study. Clin Orthop 1969;67:81.
18. Lipson SJ, Muir H: Proteoglycans in experimental intervertebral disc degeneration. Spine 1984;6:194–210.
19. Modic MT, Masaryk TJ, Ross JS, et al: Imaging of degenerative disk disease. Radiology 1988;168:177–186.
20. Lindblom K, Hultquist G: Absorption of protruded disc tissue. J Bone Joint Surg Am 1950;32:557–560.
21. Mixter WJ, Barr JS: Rupture of the intervertebral disc and involvement of the spinal canal. N Engl J Med 1934;211:210.
22. Bradford FK, Spurling RG: The Intervertebral Disc. Springfield, IL: Charles C. Thomas, 1945.
23. Jinkins JR, Whittemore AR, Bradley WG: The anatomic basis of vertebrogenic pain and the autonomic syndrome associated with lumbar disk extrusion. AJNR 1989;10:219–231.
24. Sartor K, Richter S: Computed tomography of the spinal canal following intrathecal enhancement: Cervical CT myelography (in German). Abstract in AJNR 1979;1:133.
25. Masaryk TJ, Ross JS, Modic MT, et al: High resolution MR imaging of sequestered lumbar intervertebral disks. AJNR 1988;9: 351–358.
26. Taveras JM: Herniated intervertebral disk: A plea for a more uniform terminology. AJNR 1989;10:1283–1284.
27. Jinkins JR, Gee G, Bazan C: Gadolinium enhanced MRI in the evaluation of the unoperated patient with clinical lumbosacral radiculopathy: Evaluation of 0.1 mmol/kg IV gadopentetate dimeglumine. Paper presented at the Meeting of the American Society of Neuroradiology, Vancouver, Canada, 1993.
28. Lane JI, Koeller KK, Mani RL, et al: Lumbosacral root enhancement: Gadolinium-enhanced MR of the lumbar spine in patients without a history of prior back surgery. Paper presented at the Meeting of the American Society of Neuroradiology, Vancouver, Canada, 1993.
29. Modic MT, Ross JJ, Obuchowski N, et al: Contrast enhancement MR in acute lumbar radiculopathy. Paper presented at the Meeting of the American Society of Neuroradiology, Vancouver, Canada, 1993.
30. Ford LT, Gilvia LA, Murphy WA, et al: Analysis of gas in vacuum lumbar disc. AJR 1977;128:1056–1057.
31. Modic MT, Steinberg PM, Ross JS, et al: Degenerative disk disease: Assessment of changes in vertebral body marrow with MR imaging. Radiology 1988;166:193–199.
32. Rothman SLG, Glenn WV Jr: Multiplanar CT of the Spine. Baltimore: University Park Press, 1985.
33. Wiltse EH Jr, Jackson DW: Fatigue fractures: The basic lesion in isthmic spondylolisthesis. J Bone Joint Surg 1975;57A:17–22.
34. Schlesinger EB, Taveras JM: Factors in the production of "cauda equina" syndromes in lumbar discs. Trans Am Neurol Assoc 1953; 78:263.
35. Roberson GH, Llewellyn HJ, Taveras JM: The narrow lumbar spinal canal syndrome. Radiology 1973;107:89.
36. Cressman MR, Paul RP: Serpentine myelographic defect caused by a redundant nerve root: Case report. J Neurosurg 1968;28:391.
37. Davis RA: Long term outcome analysis of 984 surgically treated herniated lumbar disks. J Neurosurg 1994;80:415–421.
38. Ross JS, Masaryk TJ, Schrader M, et al: MR imaging of the postoperative lumbar spine: Assessment with gadopentetate dimeglumine. AJNR 1990;11:771–776.
39. Hauser OW, Onofrio BM, Miller GM, et al: Cervical neural foraminal canal stenosis: Computerized tomographic myelography diagnosis. J Neurosurg 1993;79:84–88.
40. Pallis C, Jones AM, Spillane JD: Cervical spondylosis: Incidence and implications. Brain 1954;77:24.
41. Brain WR, Wilkinson M: Cervical Spondylosis. Philadelphia: Saunders, 1967.
42. Quaghebeur G, Jeffree M: Synovial cyst of the high cervical spine causing myelopathy. AJNR 1992;13:981–982.
43. Gorey MT, Hyman RA, Black KS, et al: Lumbar synovial cysts eroding bone. AJNR 1992;13:161–163.
44. Patel SC, Sanders WP: Synovial cyst of the cervical spine: Case report and review of the literature. AJNR 1988;9:602–603.
45. Titelbaum DS, Rhodes CH, Brooks JS, et al: Pigmented vilonodular synovitis of a lumbar facet joint. AJNR 1992;13:164–166.
46. Clark LJP, McCormick PW, Domenico DR, et al: Pigmented vilonodular synovitis of the spine. J Neurosurg 1993;79:456–459.
47. Naidich TP, Zimmerman RA, McLone DG, et al: Congenital anomalies of the spine and spinal cord. In Atlas SW (ed), Magnetic Resonance Imaging of the Brain and Spine. New York: Raven Press, 1991.
48. Naidich TP, McLone DG, Mutleur S: A new understanding of dorsal dysraphism with lipoma (lypomyeloschisis): Radiological evaluation and surgical correction. AJNR 1983;4:103–116.

49. Naidich TP, McLone DG: Congenital pathology of the spine and spinal cord. In JM Taveras, J Ferrucci (eds), Radiology: Diagnosis/Imaging/Intervention. Philadelphia: Lippincott, 1995.
50. McLone DG, Naidich TP: Terminal myelocystocele. Neurosurgery 1985;16:36–43.
51. Sigad R, Denys A, Halimi P, et al: Ventriculus terminalis of the conus medullaris: MR imaging in four patients with congenital dilatation. AJNR 1991;12:733–737.
52. Tarlov IM: Sacral Nerve-Root Cysts. Springfield, IL: Charles C. Thomas, 1953.
53. Schievink WI, Reimer R, Folger WN: Surgical treatment of spontaneous intracranial hypotension associated with a spinal arachnoid diverticulum. J Neurosurg 1994;80:736–739.
54. Elsberg CA, Dyke CG, Brewer ED: The symptoms and diagnosis of extradural cysts. Bull Neurol Inst New York 1934;3:395.
55. Hald JK, Bakke SJ, Nakstad PH, et al: Magnetic resonance imaging of an epidural spinal arachnoid cyst. Acta Radiol 1989;30:491–492.
56. Rohrer DC, Burchief KJ, Graber DP: Intraspinal extradural meningeal cyst demonstrating ball-valve mechanism of formation. J Neurosurg 1993;78:122–125.
57. Neuhauser EBD, Witenborg MH, Dehlinger K: Diastematomyelia: Transfixation of the cord or cauda equina with congenital anomalies of the spine. Radiology 1950;54:659.
58. Hilal SK, Martom D, Pollack E: Diastematomyelia in children: Radiographic study of 34 cases. Radiology 1974;112:609.
59. Kennedy PR: New data on diastematomyelia. J Neurosurg 1979; 51:355–361.
60. Jackson FE: Neurenteric cysts: Report of a case of neurenteric cyst with associated chronic meningitis and hydrocephalus. J Neurosurg 1961;18:678.
61. Gerenia GK, Russell EJ, Clasen RA. MR Characteristics of a Neurenteric cyst. AJNR 1988;9:978–980.
62. Kantrowitz LR, Pais MJ, Burnett K, et al. Intraspinal neurenteric cyst containing gastric mucosa: CT and MRI findings. Pediatric Radiol 1986;16:324–327.
63. Matsushima T, Fukui M, Egami H. Epithelial cells in a so-called neurenteric: a light and electron microscopic study. Surg Neurol 1985;24:656–660.
64. Brooks BS, Duvall ER, El Gammal T, et al. Neuroimaging features of neurenteric cysts: analysis of nine cases and review of the literature. AJNR 1993;14:735–746.
65. Thrush A, Enzman D: MR imaging of infectious spondylitis. AJNR 1990;11:1171–1180.
66. Modic MT, Feiglin DH, Piraino DW, et al: Vertebral osteomyelitis: Assessment using MR. Radiology 1985;157:157–166.
67. Numaguchi Y, Rigamonti D, Rothman MI, et al: Spinal epidural abscess: Evaluation with gadolinium-enhanced MR imaging. Radiographics 1993;13:545–554.
68. Bartels RH, de Jong TR, Grotenhuis JA: Spinal subdural abscess: Case report. J Neurosurg 1992;76:307–311.
69. Kennedy R, Effron AS, Perry G: The grave spinal cord paralyses caused by spinal anesthesia. Surg Gynecol Obstet 1950;91:385.
70. Williams JM: Discussion of paper by Kennedy F, Effron AS, Perry G: The grave spinal paralyses caused by spinal anesthesia. Trans Am Neurol Assoc 1950;23.
71. Wise BL, Smith M: Spinal arachnoiditis ossificans. Arch Neurol 1965;13:391.
72. Ross JS, Masaryk TJ, Modic MT, et al: MR imaging of lumbar arachnoiditis. AJNR 1987;8:885–892.
73. Sklar E, Quencer RM, Green BA, et al: Acquired spinal subarachnoid cysts: Evaluation with MR, CT, myelography, and intraoperative sonography. AJNR 1989;10:1097–1104.
74. Nguyen C, Jo K-C, Haughton VM: Effect of lidocaine on the meninges in an experimental animal model. Invest Radiol 1991; 26:745–747.
75. Nabors MW, Pait TG, Byrd EB, et al: Updated assessment and current classification of spinal meningeal cysts. J Neurosurg 1988; 68:366–377.
76. Barakos JA, Mark AS, Dillon WP, et al: MR imaging of acute transverse myelitis and AIDS myelopathy. J Comput Assist Tomogr 1990;14:45–50.
77. Nesbit GM, Miller GM, Baker HL, et al: Spinal cord sarcoidosis: A new finding at MR imaging with Gd-DTPA enhancement. Radiology 1989;173:839–843.
78. Malzberg MS, Rogg JM, Tate CA, et al: Poliomyelitis: Hyperintensity of the anterior horn cells on MR images of the spinal cord. AJR 1993;161:863–865.
79. Henson RA, Urich H: Cancer and the Nervous System. London: Blackwell Scientific Publications, 1982.
80. Friedman DP, Tartaglino LM: Amyotrophic lateral sclerosis: Hyperintensity of the corticospinal tracts on MR images of the spinal cord. AJR 1993;160:604–606.
81. Gajdusek DC: Subacute spongiform encephalopathies: Transmissible cerebral amyloidoses caused by unconventional viruses. In Fields BN, Knipe DM, Chanock RM, et al (eds), Virology, ed 2. New York: Raven Press, 1990.
82. Laissey JP, Milon P, Freger P, et al: Cervical epidural hematomas: CT diagnosis in two cases that resolved spontaneously. AJNR 1990; 11:394–396.
83. Djindjian R: Angiography of the Spinal Cord. Paris: Masson and Cie, 1970.
84. Lasjaunias P, Berenstein AB: Surgical Neuroangiography, ed 3. Berlin: Springer, 1990, pp 40–55.
85. Lazorthes G, Poulhes J, Bastide G, et al: La vascularisation arterielle de la moelle. Neurochirurgie 1958;4:3.
86. Suh TH, Alexander L: Vascular system of the human spinal cord. Arch Neurol Psychiatry 1939;41:659.
87. Di Chiro G, Doppman J, Ommaya AK: Selective arteriography of arteriovenous aneurysms of spinal cord. Radiology 1967;88:1065.
88. Djindjian R, Dumesnil M, Faure C, et al: Etude angiographique d'un angiome intrarachidien. Rev Neurol 1962;106:278.
89. Yuh WTC, Marsh EE III, Wang AK, et al: MR imaging of spinal cord and vertebral body infarction. AJNR 1992;13:145–154.
90. Massachusetts General Hospital—Case Records. Case 5-1991. New Engl J Med 1991;324:322–332.
91. Kestle JRW, Resch L, Tator CH, et al: Intervertebral disc embolization resulting in spinal cord infarction. J Neurosurg 1989;71: 938–941.
92. Larsson EM, Desai P, Hardin CW, et al: Venous infarction of the spinal cord resulting from dural arteriovenous fistula: MR imaging findings. AJNR 1991;12:739–743.
93. Biondi A, Merland JJ, Hodes JE, et al: Aneurysms of spinal arteries associated with intramedullary arteriovenous malformations: Angiographic and clinical aspects. AJNR 1992;13:913–922.
94. Leech PJ, Stokes BAR, Apsimon T, et al: Unruptured aneurysms of the anterior spinal artery presenting as paraparesis. J Neurosurg 1976;45:331–333.
95. Larroche JC: Malformations of the nervous system. In Adams JH, Crosellis JAN, Duchen LW (eds), Greenfield's Neuropathology. New York: Wiley, 1984.
96. Post MJD, Quencer RM, Green BA, et al: Role of sine-MR in evaluation of pulsatile characteristics of post-traumatic spinal and subarachnoid cord cysts. AJNR 1988;9:1001.
97. Sze G, Krol G, Zimmerman RD, et al: Malignant extradural spinal tumors: MR imaging with Gd-DTPA. Radiology 1988;167: 217–223.
98. Whitely JF, Fosyth HF: The classification of cervical spine injuries. AJR 1960;83:633–644.
99. Rogers LF, Thayer C, Weinberg PE, et al: Acute injuries of the upper thoracic spine associated with paraplegia. AJR 1980;134: 67–73.
100. Popovich MJ, Taylor FC, Helmer E: MR imaging of birth-related brachial plexus avulsion. AJNR 1989;10:S98.

101. Armington WG, Harnsberger HR, Osborn AF, et al: Radiolographic evaluation of brachial plexopathy. AJNR 1987;8:361–367.

SELECTED READINGS

Barkovich AJ: Pediatric Neuroradiology. New York: Raven, 1990.

Bobman SA, Atlas SW, Listerud J, et al: Postoperative lumbar spine: Contrast-enhanced chemical shift MR imaging. Radiology 1991;179: 557–562.

Boger DC: Traction device to improve CT imaging of lower cervical spine. AJNR 1968;7:719–721.

Dietemann JL, Romero C, Allal R, et al: CT, myelography and CT-myelography in the evaluation of common cervicobrachial neuralgia. J Neuroradiol 1992;19:167–176.

Djindjian R, Hurth M, Houdart R: Antériographie et ischémie médullaire dorso-lombaire d'origine athéromateuse. (A propos de 5 cas.). Rev Neurol 1970;122:5.

Epstein JE, Epstein BS, Rosenthal AD, et al: Sciatica caused by nerve root entrapment in the lateral recess: The superior facet syndrome. J Neurosurg 1972;36:584–589.

Kerber CW, Sovak M, Ranganathan RS, et al: Iotrol, a new myelographic agent: I. Radiography, CT, CSF clearance, and brain penetration. AJNR 1983;4:317–320.

Naidich TP, Harwood-Nash DC: Diastematomyelia: Hemicord and meningeal sheaths; single and double arachnoid and dural tubes. AJNR 1983;4:633–636.

Nichols DA, Rufenacht DA, Jack CR, et al: Embolization of spinal dural arteriovenous fistula with polyvinyl alcohol particles: Experience in 14 patients. AJNR 1992;13:933–940.

Otake S, Matsuo M, Nishizawa S, et al: Ossification of the posterior longitudinal ligament: MR evaluation. AJNR 1992;13:1059–1067.

Prolo DJ, Oklund SA, Cutcher M: Toward uniformity in evaluating results of lumbar spine operations: A paradigm applied to posterior lumbar interbody fusions. Spine 1986;11:601–606.

Raftopoulos C, Picard GE, Retife C, et al: Endoscopic cure of a giant sacral meningocele associated with Marfan syndrome: Case report. Neurosurgery 1992;30:765–768.

Rothman SLG, Glenn WVG Jr: CT multiplanar reconstruction in 253 cases of lumbar spondylolysis. AJNR 1984;5:81–90.

Teplick JG, Haskin ME: Intravenous contrast-enhanced CT of the postoperative lumbar spine: Improved identification of recurrent disk herniation, scar, arachnoiditis and diskitis. AJNR 1984;5:373–383.

Valk J, van der Knapp MS: Toxic encephalopathy. AJNR 1992;13: 747–760.

Wirth FP, Gado M: Incomplete myelographic block with hypertrophic spinal pachymeningitis. J Neurosurg 1973;38:368–370.

17

Angiography*

* This chapter has been revised with the assistance of John Pile-Spellman, M.D., Associate Professor of Neurosurgery and Radiology, Department of Interventional Neuroradiology, Columbia Presbyterian Medical Center, New York, New York.

CEREBRAL ANGIOGRAPHY

The importance of the cerebral vasculature eluded many of the seers of antiquity, including Aristotle. The Hippocratic physicians, although correcting the errors of the early cardiocentric Hellenic school by placing the brain at the center of control, thought the brain was connected primarily to the spleen and the liver. Herophilus of Alexandria (ca. 300 B.C.) performed some of the first human brain dissections. No human dissections were to be performed for the next 1800 years. Herophilus thought that the base of the brain, the pituitary–rete mirabile, transformed vital spirits to purer animal spirits that were held in the vertebral ventricular system. Galen of Pergamum (A.D. 129–199), without the benefit of human dissection material, concluded that there was a rete mirabile, as his dissections in oxen demonstrated. When, in the Renaissance, Berengario da Carpi in 1522 confirmed that neither rete nor mirabile could be found in over 100 human dissections, the task was left to Vesalius to determine where the vital spirit–animal spirit transformer should be posited. With some artistic license Vesalius placed his critical transformer in the carotid siphon.

Falloppio (1562), Casserio (1627), Vessling (1647), Johannes Welpfer (1658), and Thomas Willis (1664) all described the arterial basal anastomosis that was to bear Willis's name. Arguably, he and his friend Sir Christopher Wren may be considered the earliest endovascular interventionalists—Christopher Wren by injecting material into a horse's vein using a tube made of a quill, Sir Thomas Willis by postulating and then demonstrating collateral cerebral blood flow after carotid occlusion. The study of injected specimens brought increases in the understanding of the cerebral vessels for the next 300 years.

The direct visualization of the cerebral blood vessels in their natural state was first seen by Frans Cornelis Donders, a Dutch ophthalmologist, using a cranial window.

Egas Moniz (1) was not only the originator of carotid angiography, but with his colleagues Almeida Lima and others he laid down the anatomic and pathologic foundations of the method. At a history-making soiree of the Neurological Society of Paris in 1927, he described in detail his successes and also his earlier failures in attempting to opacify the brain and the carotid blood vessels. In the beginning, Moniz used percutaneous puncture for injection of the carotid artery, but his extensive clinical success was with the open method, following exposure of the artery in the neck after a skin incision. The technique of percutaneous carotid angiography, using Thorotrast, was introduced by Loman and Myerson of Boston in 1936 (2). Shimidzu described his experience with the percutaneous method at the imperial University of Tokyo, using water-soluble as well as colloidal contrast media (3); at the same time he recommended techniques of injecting the vertebral and subclavian arteries. The Scandinavian school established the percutaneous carotid puncture, employing water-soluble contrast media (4). Improved contrast agents, coupled with improved fluoroscopy, opened the door for the effective introduction of increased catheter navigation following Seldinger's description. The early 1950s showed a marked increase in activity, with Radner reporting his experience with catheterization of the vertebral arteries and Bierman reporting on the carotid and subclavian arteries. Odman in the 1960s showed a tremendous advancement in anatomic knowledge, led by Salamon and Djinjian as well as Wang and many others.

The Seldinger technique to catheterize individually all of the vessels leading to the brain is employed routinely for all angiographic work.

Technical Considerations

Meticulous technique is most important in obtaining the optimal results in cerebral angiography. Obtaining examinations of consistent and superior quality requires teamwork of a radiologist, technologist, and nurse, who should be well trained and highly practiced in the myriad of skills and knowledge that need to be integrated.

PREPARATION OF PATIENT

The patient should be psychologically and medically prepared to undergo the examination. It is advantageous to see the patient the day before the examination to explain the procedure. The patient should be premedicated lightly for the examination. A variety of medications can be used; we routinely use a combination of an anxiolytic and an analgesic. Medical and logistical considerations dictate the timing and dosing of medication. Early, smaller doses of longer-acting agents are generally safer and have the desired effect.

Patients should be limited to a clear liquid diet, starting at midnight the night before the exam. Intravenous half-normal physiologic saline with 5 percent glucose with fluid maintenance is started early the morning of the procedure. Interventional patients are made NPO at midnight.

Some patients undergoing angiography suffer cognitive impairment, increased intracranial pressure, or incompetent brainstem functions. Close and continuous monitoring and charting during the use of sedation and anesthetic agents is essential. Parameters to be monitored include pulse, blood pressure, cardiac rhythm, pulse oximetry, level of consciousness, motor strength, fluids, medication, and vessels injected. The advent of pulse oximetry has had an extremely beneficial effect on monitoring the effects of narcotics. Respiratory depression leads to the buildup of carbon dioxide and increase in cerebral blood flow with increase in intracranial pressure.

Anesthetics and sedatives can be used during the procedure. In some extremely apprehensive individuals (and children below the age of 12) general anesthesia may be required. Pediatric sedation can be a "cocktail" of secobar-

Table 17.1.
Sedative Dosages for Narcosis in Children

Age (years)	Secobarbital (mg/kg)	Chlorpromazine (mg/kg)	Meperidine (mg/kg)	Atropine
1–4	8–10	1.5	1–1.5	0.02 mg/kg
5–8	5–7	1.0	1–1.5	0.3 mg/pt
9–12	3–4	0.75	1.0	0.4 mg/pt

bital, chlorpromazine, meperidine, and atropine (at dosage levels to be varied according to the age and weight of the child). Dosage levels can be as follows according to Groover et al. (5) (Table 17.1).

More recently, ketamine hydrochloride (2-(20-chlorophenyl)-2-(methylamino)cyclohexanone hydrochloride) has been used for anesthesia in children undergoing neuroradiologic procedures. As yet, it is not possible to indicate whether this is superior to heavy sedation, but the results have been satisfactory. Up to now, an anesthetist has been required during the examination, which complicates the procedures.

When heavy sedation is used, the medication is usually given 1 h before the beginning of the examination. The basic medication has to be varied somewhat depending on the clinical problem; meperidine is used for cerebral angiography. More medication may be added if necessary. Usually, a small additional amount (10 mg) of intravenous (IV) sodium seconal may quiet the child if he or she does not seem to be sufficiently well sedated. Children with brainstem tumors are hypersensitive to chlorpromazine, and in these cases the dose of this drug should be cut to one-half or less.

It has not been our custom to use antihistamine preparations prior to the examination.

Positioning of Patient

The patient is placed in the supine position on a table with an air mattress; a foam pillow or wedge is placed under the knees and the head. A strap is placed across the patient's knees, which are slightly flexed over a pillow. Both wrists are fixed by padded straps to prevent motion of the extremities at an inconvenient time. A blood pressure cuff is put around the arm to make continuous pressure readings, and an IV drip is usually inserted in the left arm so that it does not get in the way of the right-handed operator.

CATHETER FLUSHING DURING ANGIOGRAPHY

It has been customary in our services for many years to flush the needle with saline at least every 2 to 3 min since clots can develop quickly; we use two 5-ml syringes of heparinized saline, aspirating gently 2 to 3 ml of blood with the first, followed by saline injections with the other. Often more than the desired amount of time passes between flushing. If this is the case, it is then necessary to aspirate and fill the tubing completely with blood after disconnecting the syringe filled with saline so that any clots that may have formed may be removed, after which injections can again be made.

INJECTION AND FILMING

Preliminary Filming

After the head has been flexed and a tape placed across the forehead and under the nose, an injection of 2 or 3 ml of contrast material is made. Simultaneous single anteroposterior and lateral films are taken using a 0.5-sec exposure time in order to check that the tip of the needle is in good relationship to the lumen of the artery. The films are rapidly developed; it is desirable to use "rapid-process" film.

The important consideration is that the injection time should be no longer than 1.00 to 1.25 sec. Longer injection times should be avoided because they make the interpretation of physiologic changes more difficult. Simultaneous frontal and lateral serials are usually made.

Compression of Opposite Side during Injection

Single-plane serial filming is used to take the frontal projection while compressing the opposite carotid artery. This is useful to demonstrate an intact circle of Willis. Similarly, compression of the carotid artery during injection of the vertebral and filming in lateral vein can be helpful in demonstrating the intactness of the posterior aspect of the circle of Willis. Compression should be firm in order to stop the flow completely. The technique consists of applying pressure some 2 sec before starting the injection and maintaining it during angiography for not more than 3 to 4 sec (i.e., until the arterial phase is completed). Compression beyond this point is useless. Thus, the total compression time is not more than 6 sec. We use a lead rubber glove or mitten to cover the hand of the operator out of which a hole has been cut at the tip large enough for two fingers. Prolonged compression should be avoided altogether if the patient is considered to have symptomatic extracranial carotid atherosclerosis.

Filming Sequence

It is our custom to expose the first film immediately before the injection of contrast material so that it can be used later for subtraction if required. Immediately thereafter, the injector switch is triggered, and the injection is started as the serialographic series is made. In an uncomplicated case, two films per second are taken during the first 4 sec, and then the sequence is changed to one per second for an additional 6 or 8 sec. If the patient has signs of increased intracranial pressure or is in the older age group, it is advantageous to lengthen the series to cover a span of 10 or even 12 sec since there may be a slow circulation time. In these cases, during the first 4 sec, films might be taken at 2 per second and an additional 6 to 10 films may be made at 1 per second. Generally, simultaneous biplane is preferable to single-plane filming. Where more detail is required and the additional injections will be well tolerated, single-plane filming should be considered.

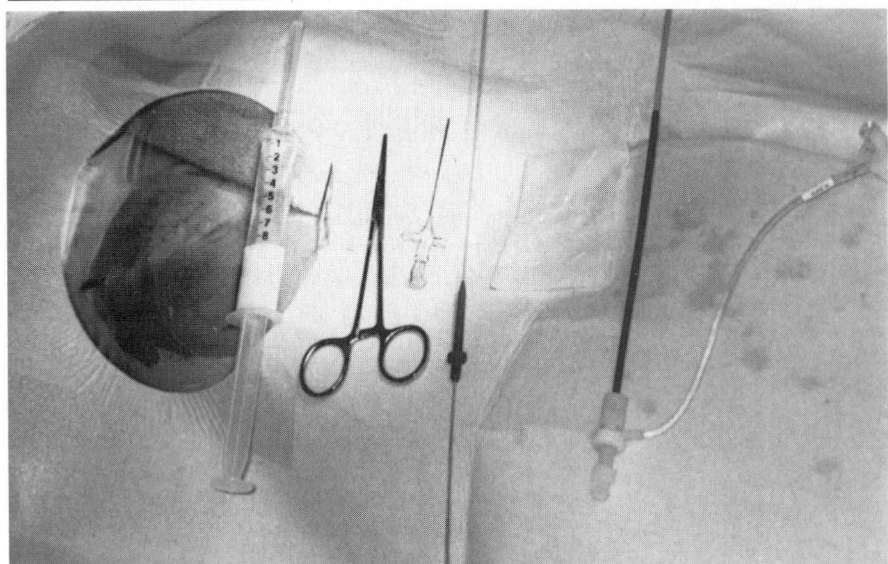

Figure 17.1. Materials needed for puncture. From left to right: syringe full of anesthetic, blade, hemostat, needle, wire, tefla sponge, sheath.

FEMORAL CATHETERIZATION

Catheterization of the femoral artery was originally described by Seldinger and was designed for aortography and angiocardiography (6). By this route it is possible to carry out catheterization of nearly every named artery in the body. The technique is the method of choice for almost all patients. Selective catheterization of the carotid and vertebral arteries requires careful attention to detail. Physicians performing these procedures must undergo a period of training sufficiently long and well supervised to ensure a minimal complication rate. In experienced hands, individual vessel catheterization in the neck is successful in close to 100 percent of cases (Figs. 17.1 to 17.5).

The development of nonthrombogenic catheters has been found to be helpful in preventing clotting and the subsequent injection of such clots into the cerebral vessels. The catheters are impregnated with heparin, and in experiments, both internal and external clot deposition was decreased by the impregnation of the catheters.

Various sizes and shapes of the curves at the ends of the catheters have been suggested to facilitate entering the carotid arteries, but a simple hook appears to be sufficient in most instances. The catheters should have an end hole, and no side holes should be used for selective catheterization. A few of the suggested curves for the tips of the catheters are shown in Figures 18.2 to 18.4. In individuals with tortuous vessels, it is often easier to catheterize the left than the right common carotid artery, although the reverse is usually true in younger patients. Thus, when both sides are to be examined in an atherosclerotic patient, it is advisable to start with the left side. If difficulties are encountered in entering the right common carotid artery, two avenues are available: (*a*) place a larger catheter with side holes into the right innominate artery and inject; or (*b*) remove the catheter and perform a right retrograde brachial angiogram. Further discussion of techniques will be found under "Therapeutic Endovascular Neuroradiology" (Chapter 18).

ARTERIAL PUNCTURE AND CATHETER INTRODUCTION

Table 17.2 lists the tasks involved in prepping and draping the patient and in identifying the artery below the inguinal ligament.

MANIPULATION OF CATHETER

With the advent of the hydrophilic torque control wire, road mapping, and variable stiffness catheters, almost all angiography can be done with a single catheter with a shape similar to a hockey stick. (See Table 17.3.) Complex catheter shapes are needed on occasion.

DIRECT CATHETERIZATION OF BRACHIOCEPHALIC VESSELS

The direct approach to the brachiocephalic arteries is rarely indicated today but occasionally is needed for interventional procedures where proximal occlusions have been performed.

Direct Carotid Artery Puncture

In the classic approach to carotid angiography, with the patient's shoulders elevated by an air bag, the skin is first prepared with local antiseptic, and towels are draped over the lower portion of the neck below the site of the puncture. Local anesthesia is performed by injecting a small amount (less than 1 ml) of 2 percent procaine intradermally at the site of intended puncture; the subcutaneous tissues and the deeper tissues are infiltrated with local anesthetic, making sure that none goes into the bloodstream. A total of 8 to 10 ml of anesthetic is sufficient. The injection of an excessive amount is discouraged because this would be

Table 17.2.
Tasks Involved in Arterial Puncture and Catheter Introduction

Task	Remarks/Variations/Notes
Prep both groins widely.	Iodine preps work by drying. Some patients are sensitive to the preps, which should be washed off after the procedure with peroxide or saline. Care should be taken in the obese or debilitated patient not to allow the soap or iodine prep to flow down the perineum or it will lead to a contact dermatitis.
Identify inguinal ligament.	Between synapsis pubis and superior iliac crest.
Identify femoral artery below inguinal ligament on the inguinal crest.	Positioning is key. The patient must be flat and straight on the table. In large patients with panus, it may be necessary to retract the panus with tape. Lowering the table and standing on a stool so as to work with outstretched and locked elbows often allows one to lean into the vessel using the shoulders, thus keeping the fingers loose so they are more able to feel the pulse. Having to press hard on a deep vessel using the strength of the wrist will, after a short time, tire and numb the hand. In infants, a small towel under the hip to extend the hip is useful. Ultrasound in rare instances is indicated.
Anesthetize over and around artery (Fig. 17.2*A*).	Two to 4 ml 1 percent lidocaine, with addition of 1/2 percent bupivacaine for embolization patients. The pain can be minimized by the following: (*a*) inject the anesthetic slowly over 5 to 10 sec and give it 2 to 3 min to work before the puncture; (*b*) lidocaine jelly under cellophane for 10 min prior to the lidocaine injection will numb skin prior to the lidocaine injection; (*c*) IV analgesics just prior to the injection. Pain and anxiety produce a patient who is moving and hypercoagulable, and who will require higher doses of analgesics.
Make incision (3 mm) over the artery (Fig. 17.2*B*).	Should be as large as the sheath but not larger.
Spread the tissue layers with small forceps (Fig. 17.2*C*).	Allows easy passage of the catheter and avoids entrapment of a hematoma after the catheter is removed if there is bleeding.
Monitor distal femoral pulse by the left index. Steady the proximal artery with the middle and ring finger.	
Holding the needle in the right hand, feel the vessel so the needle is on top of the vessel.	Hold the needle as a *dart* if using a Potts-type needle with an inner hole in needle stylet or as a *piece of bread* for an arterial needle with a flange using the index and middle finger and the thumb.
A double-wall puncture (Fig. 17.3 *A*) is done in a sharp jab, going through both sides. The needle tip should be directed nearly perpendicular over the long axis over the artery and the bevel tip down. Remove the inner needle. Additional lidocaine can be placed in the deep structures. Usually there will be no blood return. At this point, the pulsation of the needle indicates its location. If the needle rocks parallel to the vessel, it is almost certainly in or just above the artery. If the needle rocks perpendicular to the vessel, it is off to the side opposite the initial deflection. If it fails to rock, it is usually not adjacent to the vessel. Retract the needle hub caudad with slight pressure, and slowly withdraw needle until there is brisk, steady blood flow (Fig. 17.4). If the blood flow is slight, pulsate, or the thrill can be felt, the needle tip is not in the middle of a normal femoral artery but can be in a side branch, against the wall, below a stenosis, or in an intimal flap.	A *single-wall puncture* (Fig. 17.3*B*) is done with a short jab, until blood comes back in the inner stylet needle. The puncture should be like a tennis serve, crisp and stereotypic without hesitation. The needle tip should be directed about 45° cephalad with its long axis over the artery and the bevel tip down. Slowly advance the needle until the blood stops. Turn the bevel tip 90°. Usually the blood return begins again. Advance the needle till the blood flow stops. Slowly withdraw needle until brisk, steady blood flow.
While steadying the needle artery with one's left hand, advance the wire through the needle. Advance enough wire so that the amount remaining outside the patient is just longer than the sheath or catheter being inserted.	A gentle curve on the wire directed posteriorly and medially during insertion will help guide it into the femoral artery. Wire advancement should be as smooth as putting a pen in one's pocket. If resistance is felt, stop, look under fluoro, and listen to see if the patient is having any pain. Often the wire has entered a small branch or is having difficulty negotiating a curve and needs to be redirected. If it is subintimal, one must stop. If this is the case, it will usually track along the same course in spite of efforts to redirect it.
Withdraw needle, leaving the wire in place (Fig. 17.5) and compressing the artery, and advance the catheter or sheath over the wire.	The little and ring fingers of the left hand compress the artery, and the index and middle fingers and thumb fix the wire. If the maneuver is done by one person, the wire is delivered back to the left hand. The fingers work in two teams. Assigning the little and ring fingers to the task of compressing the vessel frees up the index finger and thumb. One of the main tricks of gentle and swift angiography is putting the little and the ring fingers to work for every function. It requires practice. Those who have knitted will immediately recognize the maneuvers with the little fingers steadying, delivering, or catching the catheters or wire. Always touch the patient with the palm of little finger. It steadies the hand and gives instant feedback on how the patient is doing.
Remove the wire and confirm blood return.	
Flush the catheter.	Double flushes are used in neuroradiology. Using a small, 5-ml syringe, half filled with saline, gentle aspiration is used to withdraw 2 to 3 ml (three times the dead space of the catheter). Immediately, this syringe is then tightly replaced with a second flush syringe. Again gentle aspiration is performed. Holding the syringe upright and tapping to be sure that all bubbles ascend to the top of the syringe, gently aspirate 0.5 ml and then flush 3 to 4 ml briskly into the catheter. While injecting, turn the stopcock off to be sure that the entire catheter stays filled with heparinized saline between injections.
Connect catheter to a line drip.	Normal saline with 2000 units of heparin per 250 ml with a pressure bag (or pump). Evacuate all unnecessary air from the line, leaving just enough to see the drop in the micro drip chamber. Avoid very high flows to prevent cavitation gas bubbles.

Table 17.3.
Manipulation of the Catheter

Task	Landmarks/Variations
Under fluoroscopic control, advance the guide wire in the aortic arch past the orifice of the target vessel.	In a young patient the guide wire will invariably go into the left vertebral via the proximal subclavian.
While holding the guide wire, advance the catheter. Remove the wire and double flush.	Soft-tip catheters can be advanced without a guide wire in patients without significant atherosclerosis. This practice is not to be recommended in anyone who is over 50 or who has any of the risk factors for arteriosclerotic vascular disease (ASVD).
Gently rotate the catheter tip cephalad.	
Slowly pull the catheter back, catching the tip on an orifice, and confirm with a small injection of contrast.	One can see the catheter tip jump or bob as it catches on the vessel orifice. Injecting small puffs of contrast can also help in identifying the vessel orifice. In difficult arches, or where anatomic variations are suspected, larger injection can be done with road mapping used.
Steady the catheter at this position, inject contrast, and fluoroscopically examine the vessel.	The course of a brachiocephalic vessel should be examined fluoroscopically before a guide wire is advanced. This is particularly true in patients over the age of 45 or with a history of stroke or previous catheterization. With the advent of biplane road-mapping fluoro, this is quick and effective. In those patients meeting the preceding criteria where the catheter cannot be placed at the orifice to obtain this view, one should consider an arch injection.
Under road mapping if available, advance the guide wire into the target vessel.	Do not let the wire go by areas of vessel that may be diseased. Image in the plane that minimizes overlap of vessels: anteroposterior coming off the arch, lateral for going from the common to the internal/external carotid, etc., right anterior oblique for coming off the brachiocephalic into the right vertebral. When selecting the internal carotid, if biplane, or C-arm capabilities are not available, have the patient turn the head away from the side being studied and flex the neck. The steerable guide wires and road mapping not only expedite the angiogram but add significantly to the safety. It will be noticed that, coming off the arch, the right common–internal–middle cerebral artery (and vertebral) axis rotates counterclockwise as it ascends, whereas the left cephalic vessels rotate in a clockwise direction. Rotations of the catheter/wire should be similar to the target vessel.
Advance the catheter over the guide wire, fixing the guide wire so it does not advance.	Movements of the catheter may be swift but must be light and gentle. If there is significant drag of the catheter at the groin site, it is not possible to "feel" the catheter tip; this drag must be avoided and is one of the advantages one quickly notices when routinely using a sheath. It will be noticed that advancing the catheter during systole, when the vessels are slightly larger and straighter, is helpful. By having the electrocardiogram or pulse oximeter beeper on at an audible level and controlling it with flouro, one can quickly identify systole.
Just before the advancing catheter reaches the tip of the guide wire, stop advancing the guide wire and slowly withdraw it.	The catheter can traumatize the blood vessel if the tip of the catheter is advanced past the tip of the wire, particularly if it is up against a tight curve in the blood vessel.
Confirm blood return. Gently double flush.	If there is no blood return, slowly put slight traction on the catheter. Confirm under fluoroscopy that the tip is not against the vessel wall. If it is, slowly turn the catheter tip a half turn. If there is still no blood return, gently aspirate. If there is still no blood return, withdraw the catheter until there is. This usually means that there is spasm or, less commonly, a clot in the distal catheter.
Confirm catheter position with a small amount of contrast.	The catheter tip should not be against the vessel wall, and there should be good flow around the catheter.
Hook up to pump.	Hookups of syringes or injectors tubing to the catheter should always be done making sure that there is free flow of blood and no air bubbles. Connecting flowing fluid columns, meniscus to meniscus, at right angles to each other excludes air. "Palming" the syringe —putting slight pressure on the injector with the thenar eminence as one connects it to the syringe—allows a small amount of fluid to be injected as one is connecting the syringe.
Hook up to the injector.	

equivalent to producing edema of the tissues, which makes palpation of the vessels more difficult. The injection of most of the local anesthetic may be used to help mobilize the vessel in the desired direction. The artery should be more easily palpable after the conclusion of the injection of the anesthetic than before. A small 3-mm skin incision is made at the site of the needle puncture. The artery is then palpated and fixed; an important reference point is the superior margin of the thyroid cartilage. At this level, the bifurcation of the common carotid artery usually takes place. Therefore, if it is decided to inject the common carotid artery, the puncture of the skin should be made as low as possible. If it is decided to puncture the internal carotid artery, this should be done above the bifurcation of the common carotid artery near the origin of the internal carotid artery. It is our custom to go through both the

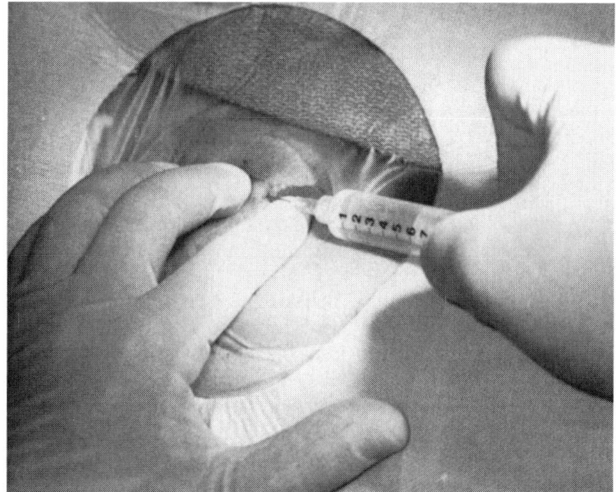

A

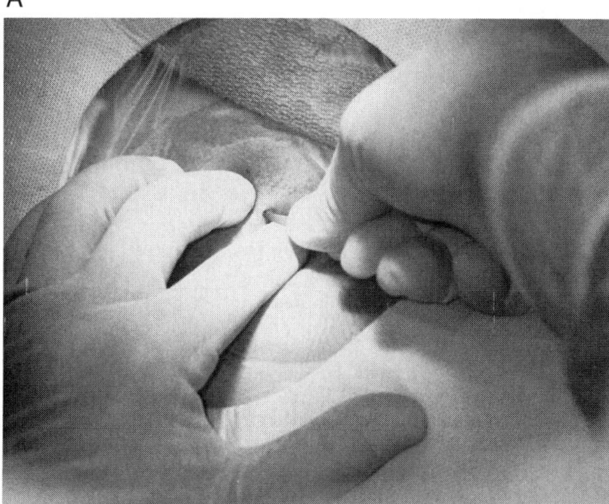

B

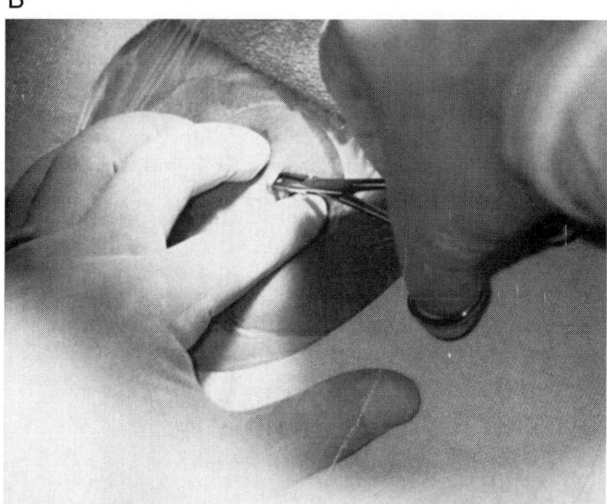

C

Figure 17.2. The skin is covered with translucent sterile plastic, which has a round opening. **A.** Anesthesia is being administered. The anesthetic should be administered around the artery but not necessarily behind it. **B.** A small incision (about 6 mm in length) is made over the artery to facilitate the passage of the catheter. **C.** The incision is spread with a small hemostat, spreading the tissues underneath.

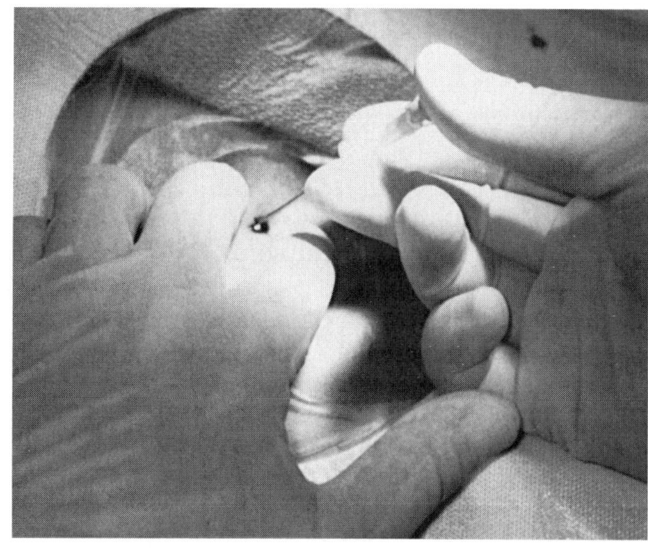

A

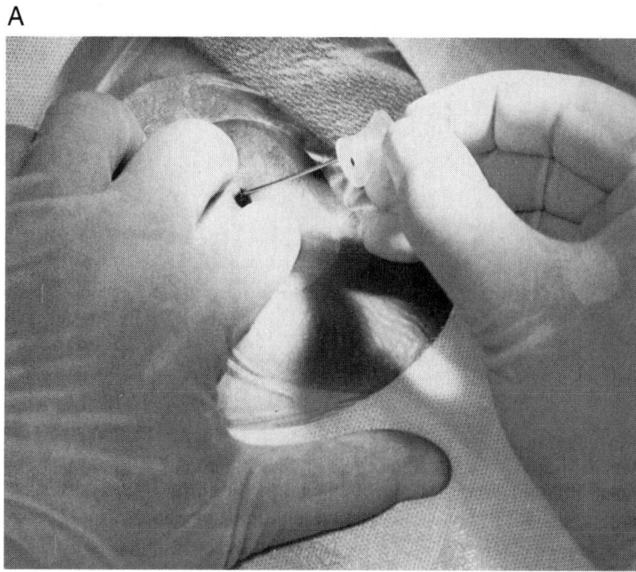

B

Figure 17.3. Technique of needle holding for double-wall puncture (see text) (**A**) and for single-wall puncture (**B**). The latter is preferred, but it increases the chances for dissection.

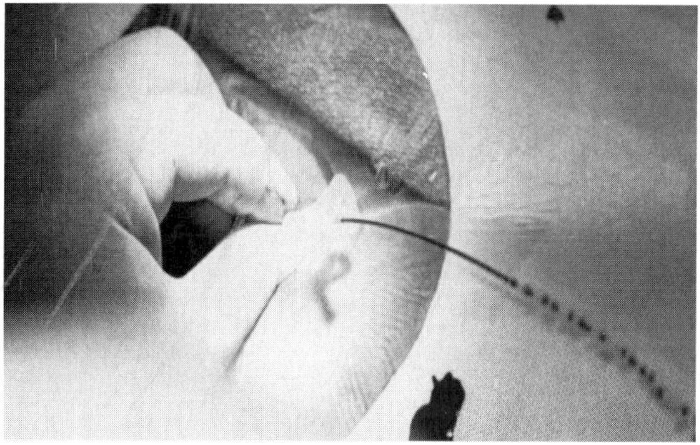

Figure 17.4. Artery has been punctured, and the flow of arterial blood is good.

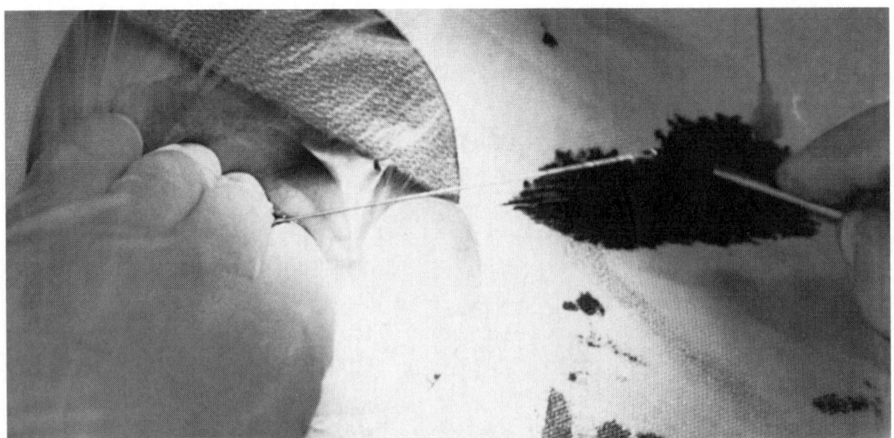

A

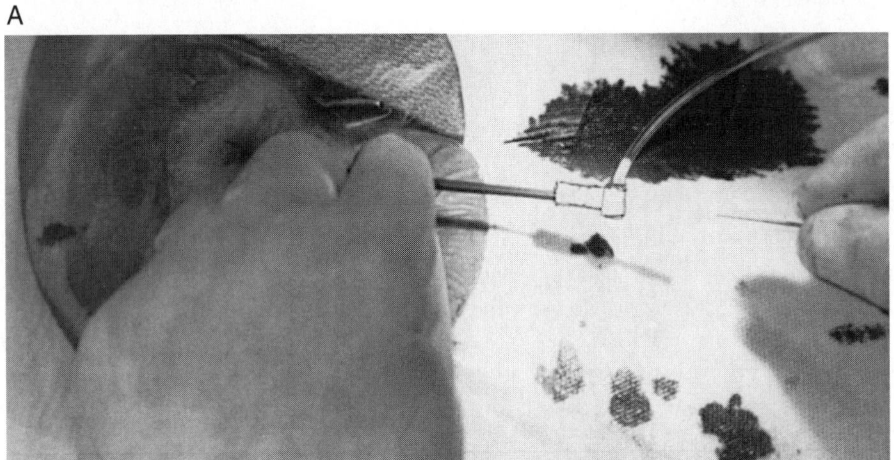

B

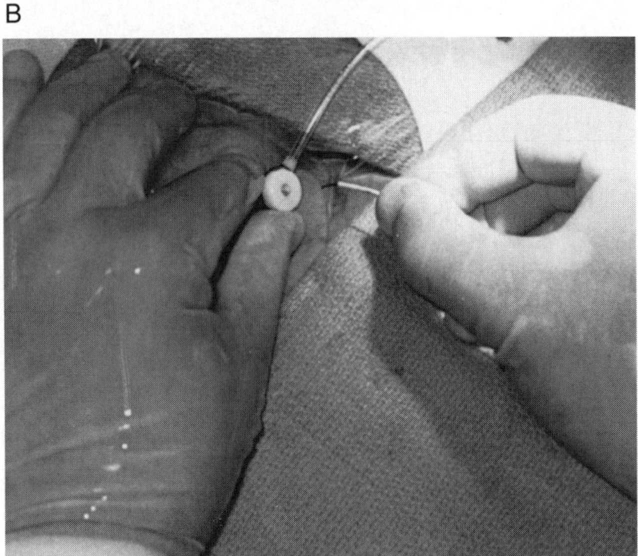

C

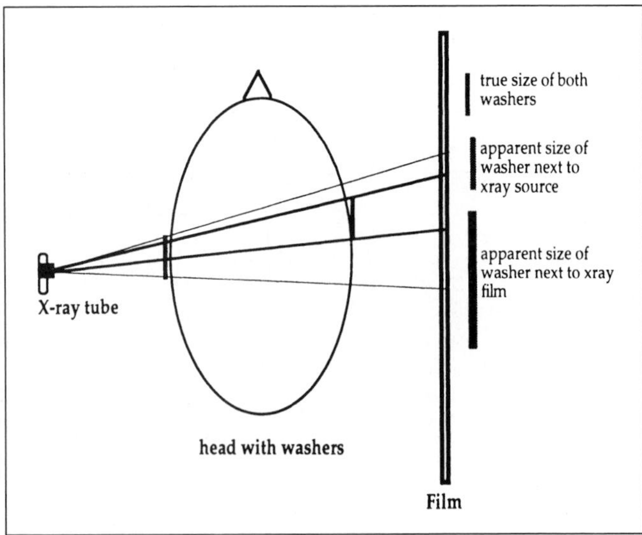

D

Figure 17.5. A. Wire has been inserted through needle and the needle has been removed. Compression is applied on the artery during and after needle removal. **B.** A sheath has been inserted around the wire, after which the wire is removed. **C.** The sheath is ready for the insertion of the catheter. The space between the inner wall of the sheath and the catheter can be irrigated, continuously if desired, to prevent clotting. **D.** Magnification of radiologic images. Markers of equal length appear very different in size. The one close to the x-ray tube appears much larger than the one close to the film or to the image intensifier.

anterior and the posterior arterial walls, then to remove the stylet of the needle and to withdraw slowly. After the needle enters the lumen of the artery upon withdrawal, it can be advanced cephalad in the lumen 1 cm or more.

Puncture at the bifurcation of the common carotid artery should be avoided. This is the worst possible place, for the needle may well pierce three or four arterial walls, thus almost surely resulting in the production of a hematoma. Also, the region of the bifurcation of the common carotid artery is the most frequent place for arteriosclerotic plaques, which may be dislodged by the needle; this increases the incidence of complications.

It is easy to produce injury to the posterior wall of the artery and to lift a flap of intima on injection, which results in the formation of a bleb of contrast material. It is absolutely essential to check needle placement under fluoroscopy in two views; ideally it should be in the center of the lumen.

At the end of the examination the needle is withdrawn and compression of the area of puncture in the neck is maintained for approximately 10 min to prevent the formation of a hematoma. The pressure should be moderately firm and over a long area, made with four fingers rather than with one or two, to prevent direct occlusion of the arterial lumen. In general, compression should not be so vigorous as to stop carotid flow; it is customary to palpate the superficial temporal arterial pulse as compression is being made to make sure that blood is flowing through the carotid system. Approximation of the walls of the carotid artery at the site of a puncture could conceivably cause a clot to form, which would then be dislodged into the bloodstream after pressure is released.

Subclavian Angiography

The first description of percutaneous puncture of the subclavian artery was given by Shimidzu (3). The technique is rather simple; it consists of the insertion of a needle through the triangle formed by the anterior scalene muscle, the omohyoid muscle, and the upper margin of the clavicle. The pulsations of the artery may be felt by flexing the head slightly to relax the neck muscles. The needle is directed downward, backward, and medially, and the artery is entered at or just medial to the anterior extremity of the first rib. A 3-in-long, 17- or 18-gauge needle is necessary. It is advisable to use a needle with a Teflon sleeve; the needle can be withdrawn, and the sleeve will remain in place. The most common complication of subclavian angiography is a pneumothorax, which occurs in approximately 10 percent of patients. A technique for infraclavicular puncture of the subclavian artery has been described (7). This avenue of approach has the advantage of decreasing the incidence of pneumothorax. The occurrence of pneumothorax can also be decreased by connecting a saline-filled plastic tube to the needle. If the needle enters the pleural space, some saline is pulled into the pleural cavity, and this can be seen immediately by the operator. The needle can be withdrawn and its direction changed to avoid reentering the pleural cavity.

Some workers prefer subclavian angiography to the retrograde brachial approach. Since the injection is made closer to the origins of the vessels, it is possible to use smaller amounts of contrast material and filling may well be superior to that obtained by brachial angiography. In addition, the arm pain that occurs with brachial angiography is largely avoided since a blood pressure cuff is applied to the upper arm.

Retrograde Brachial Angiography

Occasionally retrograde brachial angiography can be indicated, where the pathology is clearly related to one vertebral artery and the transfemoral approach is very unattractive. It is necessary to inject large amounts of contrast material of the usual concentration to obtain satisfactory cerebral filling (8). Percutaneous puncture of the brachial artery in the antecubital fossa is carried out without difficulty using a 17-gauge needle in adults. An 18-gauge thin-walled needle is required in small individuals and in older children. The needle may be inserted somewhat higher in the middle of the upper arm. Retrograde brachial angiography is the safest technique of cerebral opacification, as far as intracranial complications are concerned. Injection of 75 ml of contrast material in not more than 2.5 sec at a pressure of 600 lb/in^2 will usually be required, and a blood pressure cuff should be inflated below the injection site. Saline should be used to flush the arteries immediately after administration of the contrast material. It is necessary to thread the needle well into the brachial artery and to fix it to avoid extravasations. If the needle is in a spastic artery, 1 to 2 ml of the local anesthetic, calcium channel blocker, nitroglycerin, or nitroprusside may be injected into the brachial arterial lumen (with the distal blood pressure cuff inflated); this often produces prompt vasal relaxation. A commonly used program during percutaneous brachial angiography, as well as for catheter subclavian angiography via the axillary route, is two films for the first second, four films per second for the next 2 sec, and one film per second for 6 sec.

Axillary Injection Angiography

Although rarely indicated, axillary artery puncture can be performed by the Seldinger method (9). In spite of the fact that the axillary artery is surrounded by the branches of the brachial plexus, it is possible to puncture it by using a gentle technique without any injury to the nerve trunks. The most frequent complication of axillary angiography is a local hematoma.

Direct Vertebral Angiography

Hazardous for the patient and difficult for the angiographer, it is of historical interest that this procedure could be routinely done (10–12). Retrograde catheterization of the vertebral arteries from the femoral route, originally described by Lindgren (13), is now widely employed. Radner (14) recommended the use of the radial artery to introduce a catheter, but this has largely been abandoned since it requires ligation of the artery, and the rate of success is much lower than by the femoral route.

When a catheter is used for vertebral angiography, there is always a danger of obliterating the lumen of the vessel completely, particularly if there is narrowing of the origin of the artery by atherosclerosis. If the patient happens to have a hypoplastic vertebral artery on the opposite side, complications can easily arise. However, by using a small catheter, (0.065-in outside diameter, 0.045-in inside diameter) and by maintaining the tip of the catheter in the vertebral artery only long enough to make the injection (after which the catheter is immediately withdrawn), complications can be minimized.

The great majority of the vertebral angiograms performed in our department are now carried out by direct catheterization via the femoral artery. Less frequently, retrograde brachial injection on the left side is used. The latter can be enhanced by compression of the supraclavicular region on the right side, with pressure directed straight down against the spine. The medial head of the sternocleidomastoid muscle is allowed to roll under the fingers, and pressure is applied medially and downward, toward the spine, between the heads of the muscle. Normally, the right vertebral artery enters the foramen transversarium of the sixth cervical vertebra, and it can be compressed before it enters the bony canal. The degree of filling is almost as satisfactory as that obtained with a good catheter injection, and retrograde flow of contrast material into the opposite vertebral artery is obtained almost routinely, indicating that filling is complete. In older patients for whom catheterization and vascular compression are contraindicated, bilateral retrograde brachial injections are utilized.

Superficial Temporal Catheterization

The technique consists of the introduction of a thin catheter by way of the superficial temporal artery, following surgical exposure of this vessel, in the preauricular region. The catheter can be introduced retrograde into the common carotid artery and even into the aortic arch. It may be kept in mind, however, in dealing with special situations, such as following surgical ligation of the common carotid artery.

Aortic Arch Angiography

The origins of all of the great vessels of the neck are visualized by aortic arch injection. The catheter should be placed in the ascending aorta, for best results, after retrograde passage from the femoral or proximal brachial artery. It is necessary to use an injector capable of delivering 50 to 60 ml of contrast substance within 1.5 sec, and a 76 percent concentration of contrast material is required (meglumine diatrizoate, 66 percent; and sodium diatrizoate, 10 percent). It is recommended that the opacifying medium contain a certain percentage of sodium salt because it has been found that, if the coronary arteries fill, arrhythmia or even ventricular fibrillation may be prevented by using a sodium-containing contrast substance.

Filming in anteroposterior projection with the patient's left shoulder elevated gives a right posterior oblique projection. Simultaneous anteroposterior and lateral serialograms are made, preferably at four films per second for the first 2 to 3 sec and then two films per second for an additional 3 or 4 sec. The technique permits 90° biplane visualization, and the origins of all of the four main vessels are usually visualized with a single injection. If it is necessary to obtain good anatomic detail of the intracranial circulation, catheterization of the individual major arteries may be performed.

Catheterization Materials

An angiogram tray consists of the following items we find useful:

Closed flush system	Kelly clamp
5-ml syringes (3)	Gauze
10-ml syringe (2)	Tefla pad
25-gauge needle	Two-way stopcock
1.5-in needle	Potts-Cournand needle

250 ml normal saline + heparin 4000 units

Nonionic contrast (50 ml)

Morbidity and Complications

CONTRAST MEDIA

The choice of angiographic contrast media has become considerably broader since the introduction of the low-osmolality contrast agents (LOCAs). In the past only the hyperosmolar contrast agents (HOCAs) were available, and these continue to be used for contrast-enhanced computed tomography (CT) scanning unless there is a specific indication for the use of LOCAs. For cerebral angiography the LOCAs, particularly the nonionic, are preferred by most operators at present, but, as explained later, the high-osmolality agents are also satisfactory for many applications.

The new low-osmolality contrast media (LOCM) are somewhat better tolerated by the brain and spinal cord tissue and, in general, should be used for cerebral and spinal angiography, particularly the latter. The higher-osmolality contrast media (HOCM) are safe for cerebral angiography, and a review of complications and morbidity fails to show a significant percentage attributable to the contrast. Thus, the hyperosmolar contrast can be used in all cases, except in the following: where arteritis or arterial spasm associated with subarachnoid hemorrhage is suspected; when the external carotid artery or its branches are being examined to reduce pain; in cases where more than the usual amounts of contrast may be used, such as in neurointerventional procedures; and in cases where a breakdown of the blood-brain barrier may exist, such as in subacute cerebral infarction, for it has been said that hyperosmolar contrast under these circumstances may cause an increase in neurologic deficit (15).

The anticoagulant effect of HOCA, which is considered a safety factor in cerebral angiography, is much lower or is not present with LOCA. There are both ionic and nonionic LOCA; the nonionic are preferred.

HOCA dissociate in solution into an anion and a cation. The anion carries the iodine molecules. The increase in osmolality (from 1200 to 2300 mOsm per kilogram of water) accounts for some of the pharmacologic effects of contrast media hemodilution, vasodilatation, and changes in red cell morphology (16). The electrocardiographic changes and the alterations in myocardial contractility are less demonstrable with LOCA when performing angiocardiography in the experimental animal (17). Nonionic LOCAs do not dissociate in solution.

Most of the reported complications of contrast media usage are with IV use, such as for intravenous urography (IVP), but in the last two decades large amounts of IV contrast have been used for CT—in fact, far more than for IVP. The complication rate seems to be significantly lower in CT than in IVP, possibly because of the lack of any preparation for this examination as compared with IVP, in which the patient takes a physic and enema prior to the examination and is advised not to eat breakfast.

In a prospective study of 100 patients undergoing IV digital subtraction angiography (DSA) for carotid artery disease, Aaron et al. found 55 complications or side effects involving 37 patients (18). Central nervous system (CNS) complications included six major-transient and one major-permanent complication. Systemic complications included 20 major-transient and 2 major-permanent events. The patient's age and the amount of contrast material used did not appear to be significant risk factors. Complications in this series were significantly higher than in previous DSA reports and published data on conventional angiography studies. Many of the patients were in a relatively high-risk group, including 74 patients who had multisystem disease and 30 who had histories of angina.

It appears that complications from intra-arterial injections of contrast are less common (19). The possibility of deleterious effects from the endothelial changes produced by HOCM is difficult to prove in practice. Arterial spasm, encountered in some cases during catheter angiography, appears to be due to mechanical irritation by the catheter rather than to effects of the contrast on the endothelium.

In summary, in cerebral angiography, nonionic LOCA should be used in older subjects, in patients with cardiac or coronary artery disease, when large amounts of contrast are to be used, in neurointerventional procedures, and when the external carotid artery and its branches are being injected because the HOCM produce pain and discomfort. LOCA also should be used when arteritis or cerebral arterial spasm is suspected and in all cases of spinal angiography.

If a patient has a history of severe reaction to contrast media, angiography should be performed after preparing the patient with steroids (20 mg of prednisone 24 and 12 h) for a day prior to angiography. Also an antihistamine preparation such as diphenhydramine hydrochloride is added. This is advisable even if LOCA are to be used.

A certain morbidity always accompanies cerebral angiography (e.g., pain at the puncture). Occasionally, more undesirable reactions occur, such as a local hematoma at the site of puncture, convulsions, and others.

The complications of angiography may be divided into local, embolic, neurologic, general, and miscellaneous. The *local complications* include vessel wall dissection, local hematoma, pseudoaneurysm, fistula formation, thrombosis, and emboli.

The *embolic complications* include plugging of the carotid artery and its branches, which may or may not be symptomatic (20); retinal artery embolism, which may be of thrombotic material or of small fragments of atheromatous plaques; the accidental injection of air; and foreign body emboli due to cotton fibers and talcum powder (21).

The *neurologic complications* are usually the result of interference with the circulation through a vessel and may be due to (*a*) an intramural injection, (*b*) occasionally spasm, (*c*) obstruction of the vessel lumen by a catheter, or, as is most often the case, (*d*) embolism from a clot formed in or on the catheter. We consider technical factors the most important in the production of neurologic complications. Concentration of the examinations in the hands of a small number of individuals who have been specially trained is one way to decrease the complication rate for these procedures.

The most frequent neurologic deficits consist of hemiparesis, dysphasia, unilateral sensory disturbances, and hemianopia. In the various series reported, the incidence of such deficits ranged between 0.2 and 4.5 percent.

Amplatz showed that thrombus formation is minimized by coating catheters and guide wires with benzalkonium chloride–heparin complex (22). Wallace et al. concluded that the patient should be heparinized at the outset of the examination by the intra-arterial injection of 45 units per kilogram of heparin through the inserted catheter (23). The saline solution used during the procedure should contain 1000 units/500 ml, and should be used to irrigate the catheter (3 to 5 ml) every 2 min, each time preceded by aspiration with another syringe as discussed earlier.

In the hands of less experienced operators, nonselective catheterization is the most desirable means of studying the four major cerebral vessels in patients with atherosclerosis. Unfortunately, radiographic contrast is sometimes poor owing to dilution of the contrast medium, and diagnostic studies are not as satisfactory as selective injections.

Although the quality of modern contrast agents is far superior to those used in the past and a wider selection is available, it has been found to be advantageous to restrict the media used for angiography in a given institution to two agents. This simplifies the procedures to a certain extent and has decreased the complication rate even further.

General complications of angiography include disturbances of water metabolism as described by Hudson et al. (24). The retention of water with decreased urine output evidenced on provocative testing was found following cerebral angiography. The state was temporary in the cases reported but lasted as long as 12 to 14 h and was observed in one-half of the patients tested. The disturbance is attributed to an abnormal secretion of antidiuretic hormone (ADH) or to a renal tubular effect. The use of any of the contrast media should be avoided or severely limited in a patient with a serum creatinine value of 2 mg or higher.

The mortality of cerebral angiography is difficult to evaluate because most of the patients who die have a serious illness before the angiogram is performed. Crawford published an interesting study of the pathologic findings in 15 patients coming to autopsy who had cerebral angiography by carotid puncture performed during life (25). In two patients, false aneurysms developed at the site of the puncture, and nine patients had dissecting aneurysms varying from 0.5 to 4.0 cm in length. Five autopsies revealed multiple small cerebral infarcts thought to be due to multiple emboli. In the latter cases, the only possible point of origin found was the site of carotid puncture.

Miscellaneous complications of angiography are numerous, although many are quite rare. They include convulsions; Horner syndrome; aphasia (26,27); hemidysesthesia; apraxia (26); confusion; scotomata; loss of voice and hoarseness due to recurrent laryngeal nerve involvement (26); unilateral focal seizure (28); transient blindness, occurring after insertion of a catheter into the vertebral artery; Brown-Séquard syndrome (29); Wallenberg syndrome (30); brachial nerve palsy following axillary catheterization; homonymous hemianopia (21); transient acute delirium; basilar artery insufficiency (31); unconsciousness with decerebrate rigidity (31); nystagmus (32); transverse myelitis; (33); heart block; ventricular fibrillation; coronary artery spasm (see preceding regarding sodium-containing contrast substances); mediastinal hemorrhage or emphysema (from vasal perforation by a guide wire or catheter); severe hypotension (26); hypertension caused by apprehension (26); severe coughing spasm following injection (28); transient neurogenic shock upon puncture of the artery (28); pain in the arm caused by extravasation of contrast material; general discomfort, chills, and dizziness (27); respiratory arrest and central shock; pneumothorax in subclavian puncture (31,34); retinal hemorrhages; and atelectasis, due to movement of an endotrachial tube from manipulation of the head during a procedure (35).

Transient global amnesia is an unusual neurologic phenomenon that occasionally occurs after angiography, usually of the cerebral vessels. It represents a benign event, and normal function is ultimately restored, but the amnesia may be frightening for both the patient and the physician until its nature is recognized (36). Transient global amnesia has been associated with cerebral angiography performed with the use of ionic agents as well as newer nonionic contrast agents (37).

Involvement of cranial nerves can be seen occasionally after angiography, possibly due to ischemic events involving the blood supply. Lapresle et al. present a review and a personal case of a patient with a regressive paralysis of the IXth, Xth and XIIth as well as the VIIth left cranial nerves (38).

Grzyska et al. reported 1095 patients; 2770 brain supplying arteries have been studied by intra-arterial-DSA (39). Definitive neurologic deficits occurred in 0.09 percent, and transient deficits were observed in 0.45 percent. The reduced complication rate in comparison with former studies seems to be a continued effect of technical progress (DSA) and the use of new nonionic contrast media. In order to reduce the "training hospital effect" (new residents and fellows arriving at midyear) on complication rate, careful supervision of trainees is necessary. Grzyska et al. proposed the average fluoroscopy time per vessel as an objective measure of the investigational skill of a neuroradiologist.

TECHNICAL COMPLICATIONS

Broken guide wires during catheter procedures are not an uncommon complication. The tips of catheters can also break, and for this reason catheters should be carefully inspected and used only once to prevent the possible complications arising from deterioration of the material.

Uchino reviewed the complication rate of cerebral angiography using the transbrachial technique in 333 patients with cerebrovascular disease (40). A total of 342 catheterizations using a sheathless 4-F catheter were attempted, with 337 successes (98.5 percent). There were two major and five minor complications (2.1 percent). A massive hematoma and a pulse deficit were overcome without sequelae. The overall complication incidence was significantly higher in females (5.7 percent) than in males (0.4 percent). This procedure requires extra care in female patients.

Bachman found micro air emboli during cerebral angiography (41). Tiny and not so tiny air emboli may be introduced and can be identified with extreme sensitivity by transcranial Doppler. Their significance is not known but can be identified on each injection. Markus et al. have recently suggested ways of decreasing these emboli (42). First, the media should be allowed to stand before injection. Second, slower injections may lead to fewer cavitation bubbles under pressure.

Ginsberg et al. found no statistically significant difference between glass and plastic syringes for introduction of air emboli (43). Plastic syringes are now routine in most practices.

As noted earlier, injury to the arterial wall is only slight when a clean puncture is performed. If the needle is placed partly in the lumen and partly underneath the endothelium, an intramural injection will take place. A bleb of contrast substance may be introduced into the arterial wall, which may block the flow of contrast substance temporarily and can simulate a thrombosis. The contrast substance may dissect upward for a considerable distance. When a subadventitial injection is made, some of the contrast agent escapes into the surrounding tissues.

In cases where a subintimal bleb is produced at the time of the injection and the distal flow is blocked, the contrast substance will then reflux and be lost via the subclavian artery or aorta. Some of the contrast substance that remains in the common carotid artery after the end of the injection may be pushed upward by the bloodstream, however, and a partial filling of the intracranial vessels is then obtained.

Once a flap of intima has been lifted, it will last for several days. When this is recognized, it is necessary to perform a puncture distal to the lifted flap of intima, or it will not be possible to obtain a satisfactory injection. The occurrence of delayed complications several hours after a poor puncture, and sometimes a day later, may be related to this.

The possibility of intra-arterial clotting above an area of marked stenosis or occlusion should be kept in mind. This may be found in patients with carotid stenosis (44) and also in patients who have undergone carotid ligation. For this reason, puncture of the carotid artery above a common carotid ligation could be hazardous in the first several weeks following ligation. If visualization is needed, the superficial temporal artery approach is recommended. The injection is made retrograde into the superficial temporal artery.

TREATMENT OF COMPLICATIONS

Despite all precautions, complications sometimes occur. The emergency material that should be available in the special procedure room is listed in Table 17.4.

Table 17.4.
Resuscitation in Radiology Department—Emergency Kit

Material in Emergency Cart	
1. *Airway*	3. *Machinery*
Oxygen	Stethoscopes
Oropharyngeal airways	EKG monitor with screen
Nasal airways	Suction (strong)
Endotracheal tubes	Suction catheters
2. *Solutions*	Defibrillator (available)
Lactated Ringers, 1000 ml	4. *Drugs in Emergency Box—All for IV Use*
Dextrose, 10% and 5%	Dextrose, 50%
Sodium Bicarbonate, 5% 500 ml	Amytal
Alcohol sponges	Valium
Tourniquet	Epinephrine
Syringes (plenty)	Isuprel
Intracardiac needles (use disposable spinal needles)	Xylocaine, 2%
Tracheostomy tray	Pressor Amine
	Calcium chloride
	Sodium bicarbonate (ampules)

Radiographic Technique

It is well accepted that at least radiographic projections at right angles (frontal and lateral films) are needed in every cerebral angiogram. In the majority of instances, multiple films in each projection are required for satisfactory diagnosis and localization of abnormalities. In addition to these two views, however, some other films may be required to study special problems.

In order to produce films of good quality, it is essential to immobilize the head; otherwise the patient will move at the time of the injection. The simplest method is to place an adhesive band over the forehead and carry it firmly around the headrest. Another adhesive band is placed under the nose and is also brought around the board. The head should rest on a board that is only as wide as the patient's head to allow the lateral film holder to be placed as close to the side of the head as possible. This method of fixation of the head has been found to be reasonably satisfactory. Other methods of head holding usually interfere with the lateral view because they cast a shadow. It is also possible to place the patient in a plastic (or wooden) box and to add polyurethane foam pads to immobilize the head within the box. This method has the advantage of immobilizing the head more completely for better subtraction radiography. Unfortunately, it interferes with easy positioning of the head; the material of which the box is made also adds a certain amount of tissue-equivalent thickness, increasing the required radiation and producing more scatter.

VIEWS

Lateral View

The lateral view is taken with the patient in the supine position, the film holder being placed along the side of the head—ideally against the side of the head being injected. It is recognized, of course, that not every physical layout will allow such an arrangement, because of restricted space or limitations of the equipment. It has been our custom, for the last several years, to take the lateral view from the same single side regardless of whether the right or left is injected. This simplifies the setup and shortens the technician's preparation time for filming. A biplane simultaneous arrangement is almost mandatory, although it may not be used in every case, as explained previously. In performing biplane simultaneous angiography, the film may have to be farther from the head than is desirable in the lateral projection, particularly when certain types of changers are used. In general, the Franklin-type changer permits the shortest distance from the head to the film during biplane angiography. It must be remembered that the farther away the film is from the head, the more magnification and distortion will be produced. With the use of small focal spots, however, magnification is not such a problem (see text following). A distance of at least 40 in between the target and the film is desirable.

The taking of lateral radiographs with the vertical x-ray beam after turning the head to the side is to be discouraged. It is not possible to obtain straight lateral views when the head has been turned to the side, and the catheter tip may be dislodged from its position in the arterial lumen. On the other hand, it is relatively easy to obtain good, straight, reproducible lateral views when the patient is in the supine position.

Frontal View

The anteroposterior view is made using the vertical x-ray beam. The angulation of the tube varies with the results one wishes to obtain. Our standard frontal angiographic projection includes angling the tube 12° toward the feet from the orbitomeatal line. The aim is to superimpose the upper margins of the petrous pyramids and the upper contours of the orbits. In the majority of patients, this will be accomplished by angling 12° from the orbitomeatal line in the cephalocaudad direction. Because a lateral view is made as a preliminary test, the exact angulation required for each individual patient can be calculated. This is done by tracing the orbitomeatal line from the center of the orbit to the external auditory meatus on the film and by tracing a line following the roofs of the orbit to the upper borders of the petrous pyramids. First, the angle of the orbitomeatal line with the vertical is determined and the calculated angle, usually around 12°, is added to that angle. The central beam enters approximately at the hairline and passes through the center of a line joining points just above the upper margin of the pinna of the ear on each side.

It is important to obtain as close to a standard projection as possible in order to make use of the mental image of the normal angiographic picture in the frontal projection. Usually the view in which the superior orbital margins and the petrous pyramids are superimposed projects "bone-free" the lateral curve of the middle cerebral artery as the horizontal portion turns to become vertical.

Special Views

In certain instances, a greater degree of angulation, as much as 30° or even 35°, is indicated to study special problems. At other times, no angulation of the tube is required, or even a slight degree of angulation cephalad (25° caudocephalad from the orbitomeatal line) is used. The latter angulation projects the orbits squarely through the middle of the cranial cavity; the bifurcation of the internal carotid artery and the proximal portions of the anterior and middle cerebral vessels are seen through the orbit. The projection is usually taken in cases of aneurysms; sometimes it is useful in suprasellar tumors to demonstrate displacement of the horizontal portion of the anterior cerebral artery. Depending on the degree of angulation, the configuration of the middle cerebral vessels, as seen in the frontal projection, will vary (see Fig. 17.56).

Sometimes oblique views are necessary, especially with aneurysms. In order to take an oblique projection, it is best to start by rotating the head between 25 and 30° to the opposite side of that being injected. The angulation of the tube should be decreased by 5° if the standard angiographic angulation (12° caudad) has been used. Occasionally, an oblique view taken with the head rotated to the same side as the injection is necessary to study special problems, particularly aneurysms and sometimes anteriorly placed subdural hematomas. It is usually possible to decide which oblique view to take first by observing the direction of an aneurysm as seen in the preliminary frontal and lateral films. For example, if an aneurysm of the internal carotid artery (at the junction of the posterior communicating artery) is directed posteriorly and medially in relation to the carotid siphon, the head should be rotated to the same side as that being injected, in order to visualize the neck of the aneurysm. On the other hand, if the aneurysm projects posteriorly and laterally, the head should be rotated to the opposite side of that being injected. It is our custom to cone down considerably over the area of interest and to obtain a simultaneous pair of oblique views using the anteroposterior and lateral tubes. If the problem being studied is an aneurysm, it is not necessary to make exposures beyond the arterial phase so that films at two per second for the first 3 sec will suffice. These simultaneous oblique views have been helpful in decreasing the number of injections required to outline accurately the relationship of an aneurysm to the parent vessel and to the surrounding vessels (particularly important with regard to lesions arising in the region of the middle cerebral artery trifurcation). In the case of a large aneurysm, films made more rapidly than two per second may be helpful in studying the filling and emptying pattern of the sac.

When examining the vertebral circulation, it is usually desirable to center the tube for the lateral view more posteriorly than is generally done for carotid angiography. In addition, the routine frontal films should be made in half-axial projection (i.e., film with a 30° angulation caudad in relation to the orbitomeatal line). A reverse (Caldwell) projection is highly useful in vertebral angiography, and base views may be required in certain instances. The value of these views, however, is quite limited without subtraction. Base views are commonly employed in carotid angiography also, and are considered particularly useful in the study of intrasellar masses (45). We have not found the submentovertical projection to be necessary in all cases, since the information is often available on the standard frontal and lateral angiograms (46).

FILMING PROCEDURE

The use of rapid serialographic filming or DSA is essential in both frontal and lateral projections. In this way, all of the phases of the angiogram are recorded as the contrast substance passes through the arteries, the capillaries, and the veins. Simultaneous frontal and lateral filming, as mentioned earlier, makes it possible to get all of the necessary films with a single injection; in addition, if the exposures are properly phased, the same portions of the same vessels are opacified on both views for comparison. There are technical problems, however, and for that reason biplane angiography is not used in every case (see text following).

In some instances, it is desirable to take films more rapidly than two per second during the arterial phase. This is particularly true when lesions such as arteriovenous malformations are being studied. In brachial angiography, it may be desirable to take four films per second for the first 2 to 3 sec in order to ensure that the optimal filling of the arteries, which cannot be controlled when brachial angiography is performed, is recorded on the films. As noted previously, more rapid filming is required in the first 3 or 4 sec (at least two per second), after which one per second for an additional 4 or 5 sec will usually suffice. A late film or two can be made after an interval of 2 sec or longer to record the last portion of the venous phase. The late films usually give very little information except in cases where there are abnormalities of the venous sinuses or the deep veins, or where there is very slow circulation time from increased intracranial pressure. In most of the latter cases, the need for a longer series can be predicted from the clinical findings (e.g., the presence of papilledema). At other times, clinical prediction is not possible, and a second series of films will have to be taken with another injection of contrast material.

From the technical point of view, it is easier to produce radiographs of good quality when only a single serialogram in frontal or in lateral projection is made. When *simultaneous* frontal and lateral views are taken, a certain loss of contrast occurs due to fogging from radiation scatter. This is unavoidable, but it can be minimized to a great extent. The use of crosshatch grids for the lateral projection helps in eliminating lateral film fogging; these are usually of 5:1 ratio. It is even possible to take stereoscopic lateral views with a crosshatch grid because the angulation required is slight, and the low ratio of the grid allows a little angulation without significant cutoff. A 12:1 ratio linear grid is preferable, however, for stereoscopy. In the frontal projection, a crosshatch grid cannot be used because of the beam angulation that is necessary. We have found that by using a high-ratio grid (at least a 12:1, or possibly a 16:1, ratio linear grid) it is possible to obtain almost complete elimination of frontal film fogging. This is further aided by the use of small cones, just large enough to cover the desired field. The best possible coning should be employed, which requires a double diaphragm, one at the window of the x-ray tube and another at the end of the cone. The closer the upper diaphragm opening is to the glass window of the x-ray tube, the more "off-focus" radiation is eliminated. This is important in all radiography but is particularly important when biplane simultaneous angiography is performed. Tubes with a focal spot size of 0.6 mm or less give excellent definition when the beam is properly collimated. In the Puck film changer the exposures alternate, and there is no cross-fogging. The latter is very desirable, and thus the Puck changer has received the widest use, although the pictures are not simultaneous.

Stereoscopic views can be obtained during a serialogram (two or four films per second) by alternate firing of two properly spaced tubes. The alternate firing can be accomplished by having two transformers or by having a high-tension switching device properly synchronized. The latter method works satisfactorily at a considerable saving, since it is carried out with only one transformer.

RADIOGRAPHIC APPARATUS

A minimal radiographic installation for an angiographic room should consist of a 1000- to 1500-milliampere three-phase transformer, a minimum of two radiographic tubes, (one for the anteroposterior and one for the lateral), two adequate film changers capable of taking at least four exposures per second, a table with a movable tabletop suitable for fluoroscopy, a head board that supports the head independent of the film changers, and a fluoroscopic setup for screening in both anteroposterior and lateral projections, with an adequate image intensification and television chain. A mechanical injector capable of delivering 45 to 60 ml of contrast material through a long catheter in 1.5 sec is indispensable for injections into the aortic arch and also for retrograde brachial angiography.

Preferable are biplane high-resolution DSA (1024 line unbroken imaging chain) with or without cut film capabilities with bilateral road mapping on C-arm positioners. Smaller image intensifiers will give higher-resolution pictures at a lower dose. In modern installations DSA has become standard; it yields subtraction images of good quality automatically.

It is recommended that both the anteroposterior and the lateral tubes be equipped with a 0.3-mm focal spot or smaller to permit magnification. Magnification angiography is easily obtainable employing the same target-film distance used in ordinary angiography, but the head is placed midway between the tube and the film, and the grid is removed from the serialographic apparatus. With some adjustment in kilovoltage values, it is possible to obtain serialograms at two exposures per second with considerable increase in small vessel visualization and detail.

Vertebral angiography in the lateral projection with magnification technique should be routine. Whenever exact measurements are needed, such as during the treatment of aneurysms, we place four 10-mm copper washers on both sides of the head as well as anteroposteriorally and laterally.

Tubes equipped with a device for varying the focal spot size are available. The focal spot can be biased down to 0.1 mm and even 0.05 mm, but at these sizes the output of the tube is markedly reduced. When a 0.1-mm focal spot is used, it is possible to obtain 3:1 and even 4:1 direct magnification without appreciable loss of detail (see text following).

We prefer, whenever possible, to use a magnification factor of exactly 2:1 employing the 0.3-mm focal spot. By this means, linear measurements can be divided in half (adding 10 percent), and thus our usual ranges of normal can be easily applied. Otherwise, more complex calculations are required to convert to the actual magnification factor. To obtain a 2:1 magnification, the object is placed midway between the tube target and the film. If the target-film distance is 40 in and the center of the head is 26.3 in from the film, there will be a 3:1 magnification; if the center of the head is 13.6 in from the film, there will be 50 percent (1.5:1) magnification. It is advantageous to use proportions such as these because one can then apply standard measurements without too much difficulty. Ordinary radiographs have approximately 10 percent magnification. Thus, a 2:1 magnification, using the geometry explained earlier, is approximately 10 percent less than twice the size of the radiographic image in the nonmagnified radiograph, but it is actually twice the size of the object itself.

Radiographic magnification requires the use of a small focal-spot x-ray tube, as noted earlier. No grid is needed. The secondary radiation is removed by the air gap present between the object and the film.

Magnification is carried out with a 0.3-mm focal spot or smaller to increase resolution and eliminate some of the loss of detail resulting from the use of intensifying screens because the radiographic images are spread over a larger number of crystals.

With the use of intensifying screens, it is not feasible to obtain all of the film detail because definition is limited by the size of the grains in the screen, as well as by the thickness of the screen. Consequently, if focal spots smaller than 0.3 mm were used, it would be necessary to go to higher magnification ratios (such as 3:1) in order to obtain better definition. In considering these problems, it must be remembered that a 0.3-mm focal spot, when used at higher energies and higher intensities, is actually larger than 0.3 mm. Thus, there probably would be an advantage in having smaller focal spots of the order of 0.1 or 0.05 mm. Although a 0.05-mm focal spot is available, it can be used only at very low intensities (less than 10 milliamperes) as presently designed; smaller focal spots capable of yielding higher-intensity beams are needed. The use of high-definition screens could undoubtedly increase the ability to visualize small vessels, but, unfortunately, such screens require a higher radiation exposure (double that needed for par speed screens).

Venography

ORBITAL VENOGRAPHY

In the rare cases where it is indicated, orbital venography can be quite useful. The frontal veins on the scalp can best be seen by placing the patient in Trendelenburg position or by placing a wide rubber band around the scalp. One of the frontal veins is usually selected for puncture with either a 19- or 21-gauge pediatric scalp vein needle. Alternatively, a 0.0205-inch Seldinger-type guide wire is inserted through the needle and threaded between 1 and 2 cm into the vein. Compression by the patient of the naso-orbital veins will lead to increase opacification of the orbital veins.

An anteroposterior view is essential, with the central beam angled 20° cephalad to the orbitomeatal line; this projects the veins within the orbital margins. Filling of the opposite side is obtained simultaneously and provides comparison. Second, an "off-lateral" series is made, projecting one orbit higher than the other, as superimposition is undesirable. A third projection (the subaxial or submentovertical view) is helpful. The basal projection is particularly valuable for cavernous sinus venography. In selected cases, oblique projections are used.

Serialographic filming is carried out in each projection using either single-plane or biplane apparatus. Films are usually exposed at a rate of one per second for 10 to 12 sec. Magnification techniques may be used from the outset. Subtraction is especially important for the subaxial films.

Measurement of orbital venous pressure is advocated by some as part of orbital venography in order to determine the presence of increased venous pressure owing to compression or obstruction in the region of the cavernous sinus (47). This is accomplished by compressing the opposite orbit and the ipsilateral angular vein in addition to the scalp compression band.

TRANSFEMORAL VEIN APPROACH

This approach can be used to perform venography in the neck or in the head.

DURAL SINUS VENOGRAPHY

Satisfactory opacification of the dural sinuses can be obtained in the venous phase of a carotid angiogram if the opposite carotid artery is compressed and the amount of contrast is increased (12 ml). Vertebral injections usually give excellent opacification of the transverse sinuses, again with an increase in the amount of contrast injected.

JUGULAR VENOGRAPHY

Direct puncture of the internal jugular vein can be performed using the same needle as for carotid puncture. The needle is attached to a syringe filled with saline, and the puncture is made lateral to the carotid pulsation while the patient is asked to perform a Valsalva maneuver. If desired, a narrow plastic compressor may be placed at the base of the neck (48). The needle is then withdrawn slowly while aspirating until a sudden reflux of blood into the syringe is seen. The needle is then replaced by a flexible catheter, using the Seldinger technique, and the tip is advanced into the jugular bulb or the inferior petrosal sinus under fluoroscopic control. Retrograde catheterization after puncturing the antecubital vein or the femoral vein is an alternative method.

If the end of the catheter is in the inferior petrosal sinus, a forceful hand injection of 10 ml of contrast medium will usually fill the cavernous sinuses on both sides. On the other hand, if injection is made into the bulb, 15 to 20 ml may be needed, using an injector with nearly the same pressure as for a carotid arteriogram. If visualization of the cavernous sinuses from a bulb injection is intended, pressure on the jugular vein below the injection site will be necessary. The films are taken with the rapid biplane changers at 0.5-sec intervals. Three series are usually needed: (*a*) lateral; (*b*) transorbital anteroposterior view, with the chin of the patient elevated so that the orbitomeatal line forms a 20° angle with the central beam (central ray should remain perpendicular to the film); and (*c*) submentovertical or subaxial. Normally the cavernous sinuses are symmetrically filled. The carotid artery appears as a filling defect in each cavernous sinus (see Fig. 11.80).

MORBIDITY AND COMPLICATIONS OF VENOGRAPHY

The author has experienced no significant complications from orbital venography or jugular venography. Occasionally, extravasation of contrast material occurs, but this is without significant symptoms or sequelae.

The search for the ideal contrast medium for all angiography and particularly for cerebral angiography continues. In his initial trials, Moniz used strontium bromide but soon changed to sodium iodide, which was employed for several years. In 1931 Moniz and Lima began to use Thorotrast, which is a 25 percent colloidal suspension of thorium dioxide. This is a good medium because it is nonirritating to the endothelium of the vessels. Unfortunately, it is slightly radioactive and, being a colloidal suspension, is picked up by the cells of the reticuloendothelial system, where it is permanently fixed. Hepatoma, bone sarcoma, soft tissue sarcomas, neck fibrosis, and Thorotrast granuloma have been reported many years after the administration of Thorotrast.

Diodrast (35–percent) and later 30 percent Urokon (sodium acetrizoate) were used with equal results. In the 1950s the diatrizoate drugs (Hypaque and Renografin) were found to be preferable. Methylglucamine salts were found by Hilal to have a less convulsant effect and, if nonionics must be used, are preferable for cerebral angiography (49). Broman and Olsson (50), Bassett et al. (51), and Harris (52) found that high-osmotic contrast agents' breakdown of the blood-brain barrier was not ameliorated by steroids. This disruption was proportional to the concentration of the test substance in contact with the capillary endothelium and the time during which the application prevailed. Repeated fractional doses have an enhanced cumulative effect when the interval between the individual injections is short. Latent vascular disease of the brain may be aggravated and may become manifest by the injection of contrast medium. These effects are much more uncommon with contrast media that contain 100 percent methylglucamine salts at 60 percent concentration, and even less so with the low-osmotic agents.

ANTERIOR CIRCULATION ANGIOGRAPHY

The common carotid artery arises on the left side, directly from the aortic arch; on the right side, it is one of the two branches resulting from the bifurcation of the innominate artery (brachiocephalic artery). The common carotid bifurcation is usually situated at the level of the upper portion of the thyroid cartilage (see Figs. 17.6*A* and 17.91), approximately at the upper margin of the body of the fourth cervical vertebra. The level of bifurcation may be higher and sometimes lower than usual. The common carotid artery is rarely absent. When absent, the internal and external carotid arteries usually arise directly from the aorta. On the contrary, anomalous origin of the common carotid artery is fairly frequent. In order to appreciate the relationship of the neck arteries to the various structures, careful study of Figure 17.6 is advised.

Internal Carotid Artery

The internal carotid artery may be divided into four segments: cervical, intrapetrosal, intracavernous, and supraclinoid.

Cervical Portion

From the bifurcation of the common carotid, the internal carotid artery is directed laterally, dorsally, and upward (Fig. 17.6*B*). When the artery is tortuous, the lateral swing is more pronounced. The cervical segment ends as the internal carotid artery enters the carotid canal in the petrous bone; this second segment can be recognized in the frontal projection because of its horizontal direction, which ends in an upward curve (Fig. 17.7). The cervical portion has no branches. Communication between the carotid and vertebral systems may be present (see under "Arterial Variants and Anomalies"). In the distal portion, buckling of the vessel upward and forward may be seen frequently, sometimes appearing as a loop, apparently related to elongation and dilatation with loss of elasticity.

Intrapetrosal Portion

In the lateral projection, the intrapetrosal segment is partly obscured by the heavy density of the petrous bones; the most medial portion of this segment is recognizable as the artery turns upward to emerge from the carotid canal at the petrous tip, thus entering the cranial cavity. The artery is contained for a short distance in a variable space of areolar tissue, extradurally, which permits the vessel to become tortuous. Shortly thereafter the artery enters the lumen of the cavernous sinus (Fig. 17.8). As it enters the cavernous sinus, the artery sometimes presents a circular constriction, which should not be confused with pathologic narrowing (Fig. 17.9).

Intracavernous Portion

Within the cavernous sinus, the internal carotid artery lies near the medial wall of the sinus. As seen in the lateral

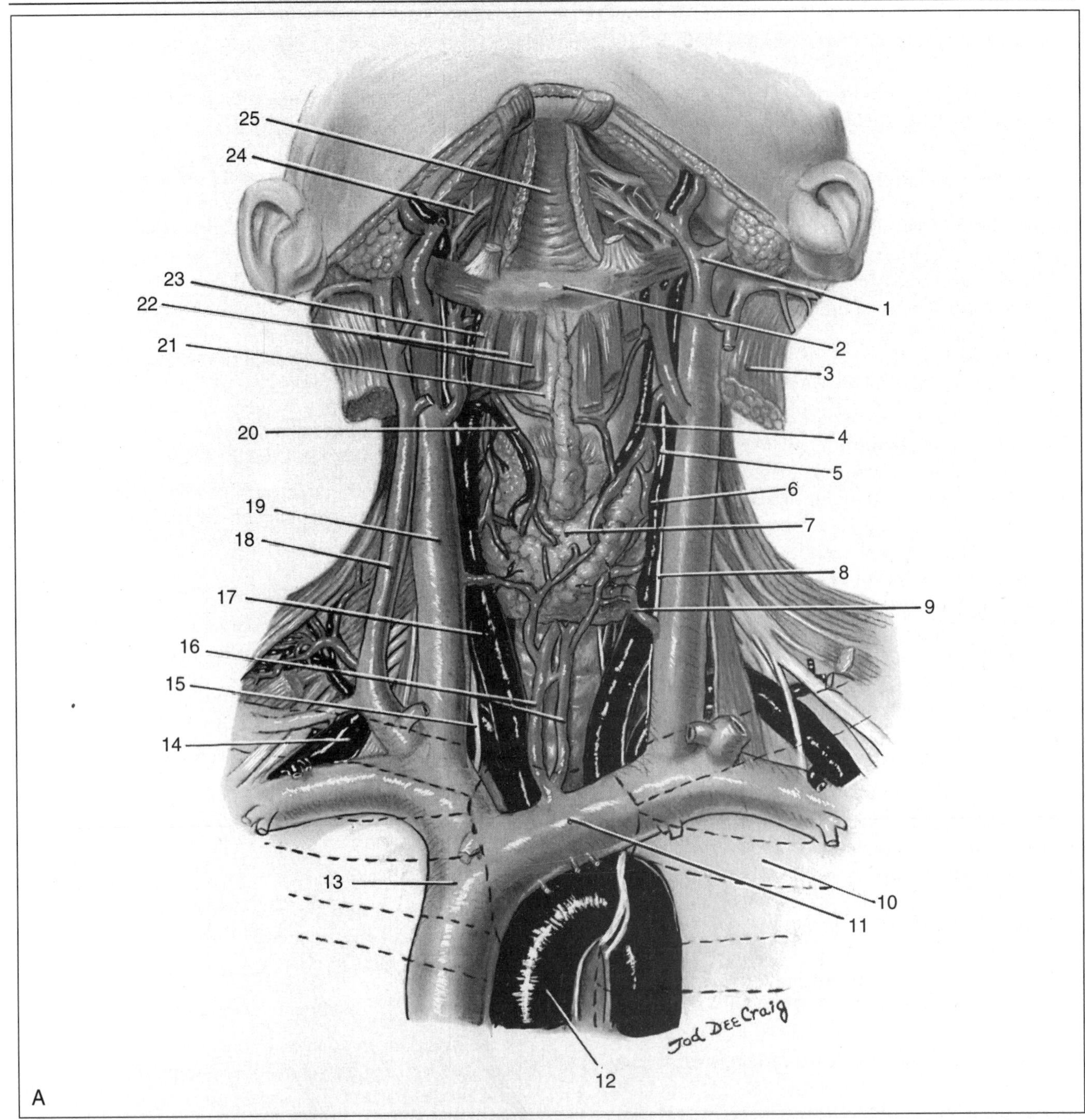

Figure 17.6. A. Diagram to illustrate relationship of carotid arteries with other structures in neck, anterior view. The diagram is intended to indicate the fact that the carotid arteries are surrounded by many structures, which should be kept in mind when doing carotid punctures: (1) facial vein; (2) hyoid bone; (3) sternocleidomastoid muscle; (4) superior thyroid artery; (5) XII nerve (ansa cervicalis); (6) common carotid artery; (7) thyroid gland; (8) X nerve (vagus); (9) middle thyroid vein; (10) first rib; (11) innominate vein; (12) aorta; (13) vena cava; (14) subclavian artery; (15) X nerve (vagus); (16) inferior thyroid vein; (17) common carotid artery; (18) external jugular vein; (19) internal jugular vein; (20) superior thyroid vein; (21) thyroid cartilage; (22) sternohyoid muscle; (23) omohyoid muscle; (24) XII nerve (hypoglossus); (25) milohyoid muscle.

view, the intracavernous segment is roughly horizontal, but a certain degree of tortuosity is common; sometimes marked tortuosity is present even in the absence of arteriosclerosis. The intracavernous segment is usually at or just above the floor of the sella turcica.

In the frontal projection, the intracavernous portion is superimposed on itself, but by following the artery upward it is easy to identify the posterior aspect; by following the intracranial portion of the artery downward, the anterior part of the intracavernous segment can be defined. For our purposes, the intracavernous segment ends at the lower margin of the anterior clinoid process. Usually the poste-

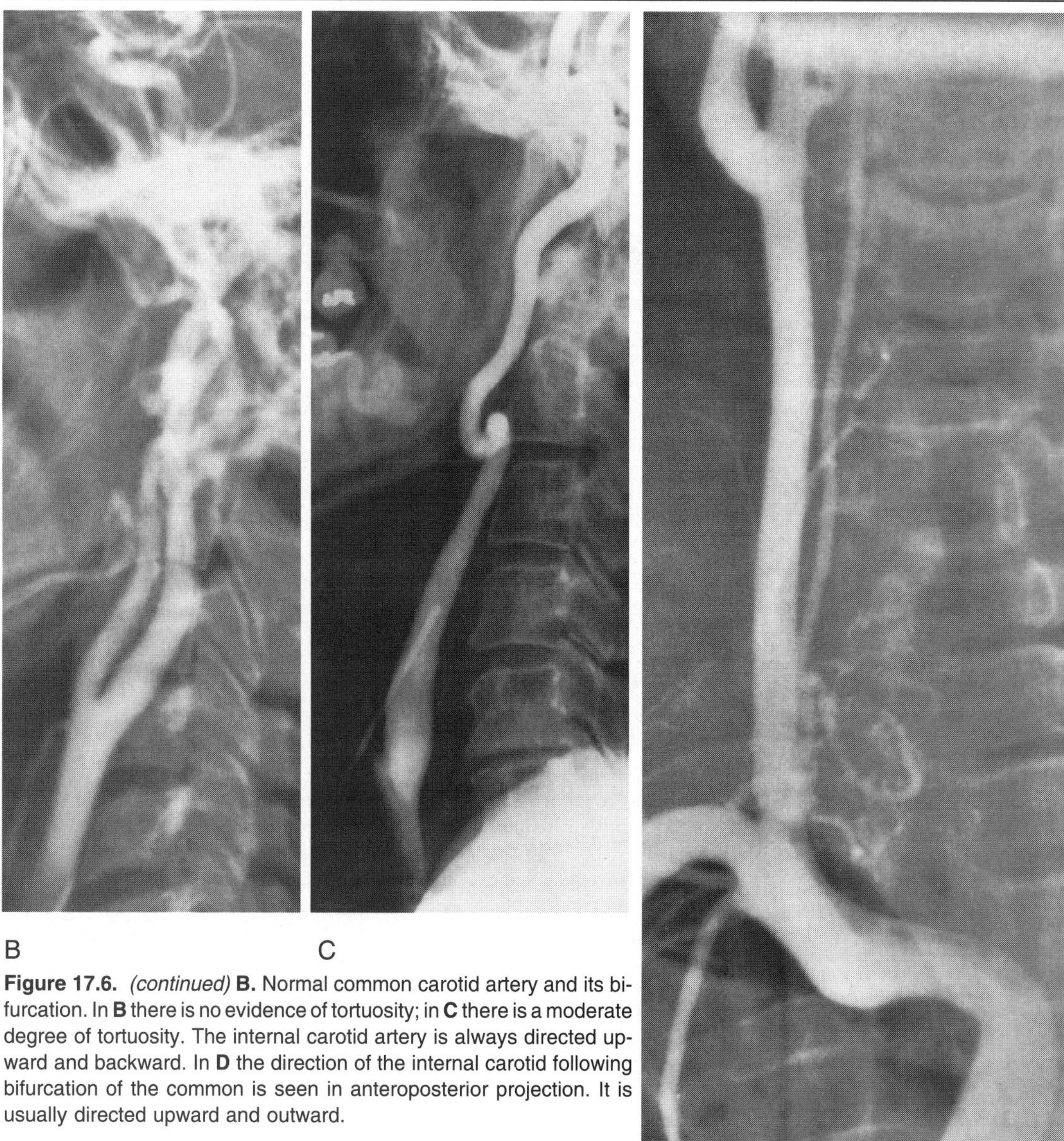

B C D

Figure 17.6. *(continued)* **B.** Normal common carotid artery and its bifurcation. In **B** there is no evidence of tortuosity; in **C** there is a moderate degree of tortuosity. The internal carotid artery is always directed upward and backward. In **D** the direction of the internal carotid following bifurcation of the common is seen in anteroposterior projection. It is usually directed upward and outward.

rior part of the segment is either superimposed upon or slightly medial to the anterior aspect.

Supraclinoid Segment

The fourth portion begins as the artery emerges from the cavernous sinus, after passing under and medial to the anterior clinoid process. At this point the vessel becomes intradural. As the artery emerges, it usually extends upward and backward. It may continue upward and backward to its bifurcation, or it may turn forward and upward, or extend straight upward, before dividing (Fig. 17.10). The point of bifurcation is often difficult to see on lateral films due to superimposition of the anterior and middle cerebral arteries. By following the anterior cerebral artery downward, however, it is usually, although not always, possible to determine the exact point at which bifurcation takes place. It is important to determine this point because in abnormal cases it may be displaced backward, upward, or forward. Unfortunately, variations are common, but usually the point of bifurcation falls on the posterior half of the intracavernous segment if a perpendicular to the plane of the diaphragm a sellae is dropped from the bifurcation. Because of the shape of the intracavernous and supraclinoid segments of the internal carotid artery, Egas Moniz coined the term *carotid siphon* to refer to this portion of the internal carotid artery.

In the frontal projection, the supraclinoid segment of the internal carotid artery is directed upward and laterally to the bifurcation. The apparent lateral inclination of the supraclinoid portion of the internal carotid artery varies with the projection used to take the anteroposterior view.

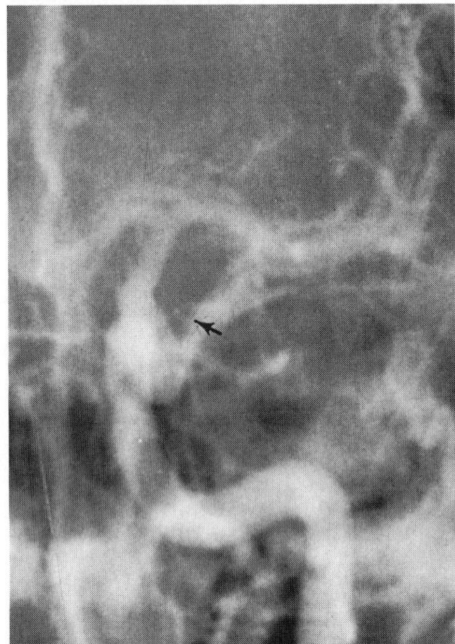

Figure 17.7. Anteroposterior view, normal carotid angiogram. The figure demonstrates the fact that the posterior portion of the intracavernous segment of the internal carotid artery is slightly more medial than the anterior portion. This can be ascertained by following the cervical segment of the internal carotid artery upward, for the posterior portion, and the supraclinoid segment of the artery downward, for the anterior portion. The anterior clinoid process is marked by an arrow.

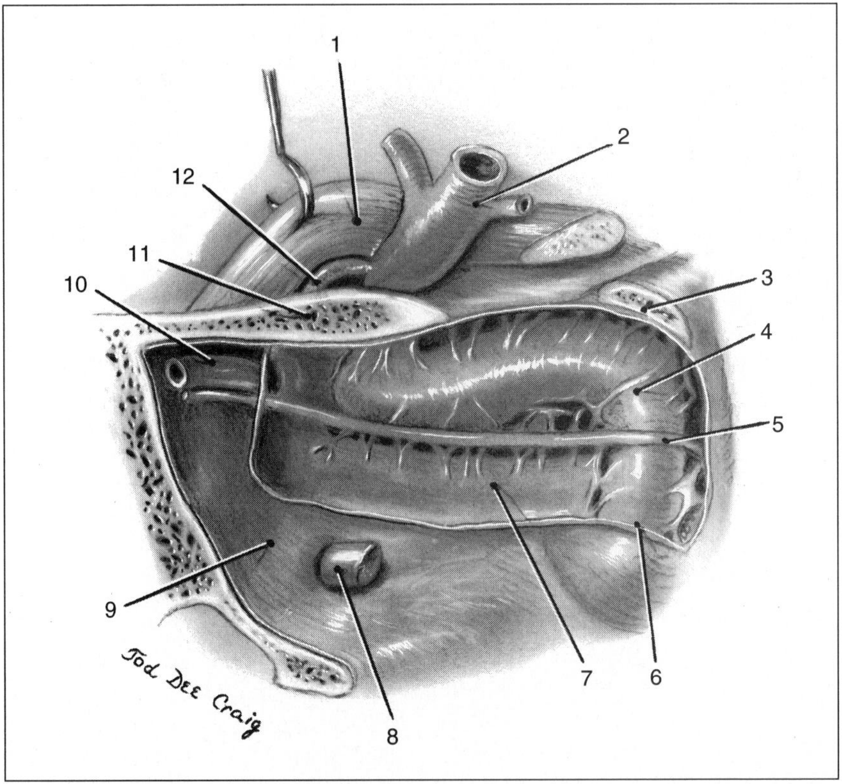

Figure 17.8. Diagram of intracavernous portion of internal carotid artery. (1) Optic nerve; (2) internal carotid artery; (3) posterior clinoid process; (4) internal carotid artery; (5) sixth nerve (abducens); (6) internal orifice of carotid canal; (7) cavernous sinus; (8) superior maxillary nerve; (9) floor of middle fossa; (10) ophthalmic vein; (11) anterior clinoid process; (12) ophthalmic artery.

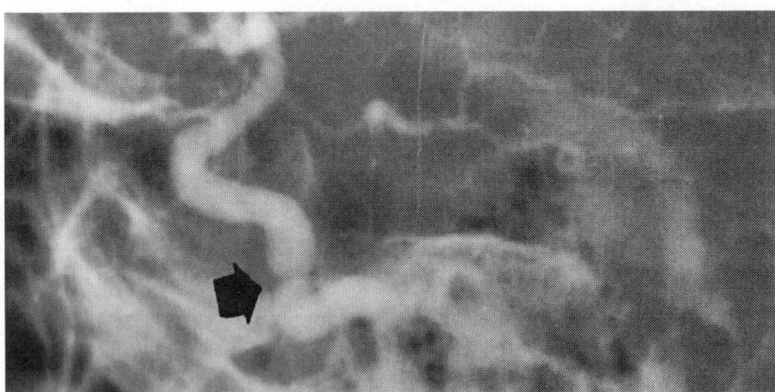

Figure 17.9. Carotid angiogram, lateral view. There is constriction in the precavernous portion of the internal carotid siphon, probably at its entrance into the cavernous sinus. The sylvian triangle is very well outlined in this case.

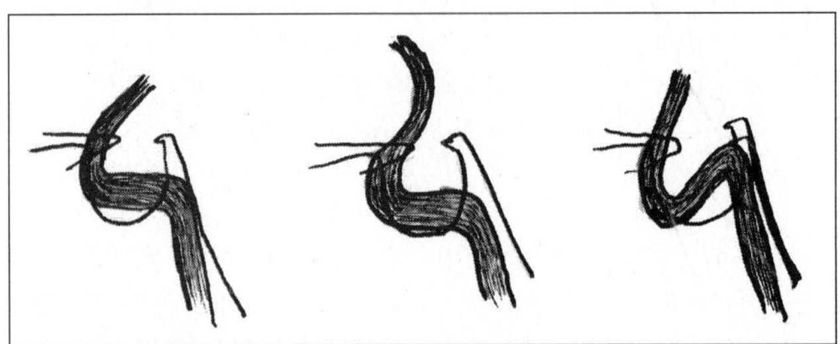

Figure 17.10. Common configurations, relationships of internal carotid siphon with sella turcica in intracavernous and supraclinoid portions.

MINOR BRANCHES OF THE INTERNAL CAROTID ARTERY

All of the major branches of the internal carotid artery arise from the supraclinoid portion of the vessel. However, small branches arise from the intrapetrosal and intracavernous portions. The intrapetrosal branches are not usually visible on the angiogram. These branches are (*a*) the caroticotympanic, which leaves the internal carotid artery in the carotid canal to supply part of the tympanic cavity; and (*b*) the artery of the pterygoid canal (vidian artery), which is inconstant and anastomoses with a branch of the internal maxillary artery.

Intracavernous branches are numerous. McConnell (53) and Parkinson (54, 55) have given excellent anatomic descriptions of these branches. The terminology used by Parkinson is followed here (see Fig. 11.50).

The *meningohypophyseal trunk* was found by Parkinson in all of 200 dissections. It gives off three branches: (*a*) The *artery of the tentorium* is directed backward over the surface of the tentorium and runs at a variable distance from the edge of the tentorial slit. This is the same artery that has been called the artery of Bernasconi and Casinari, which is seen to be enlarged in lesions involving the tentorium, such as meningiomas (56). It may also be visible in normal cases. (*b*) The *dorsal meningeal artery* supplies the dura be-

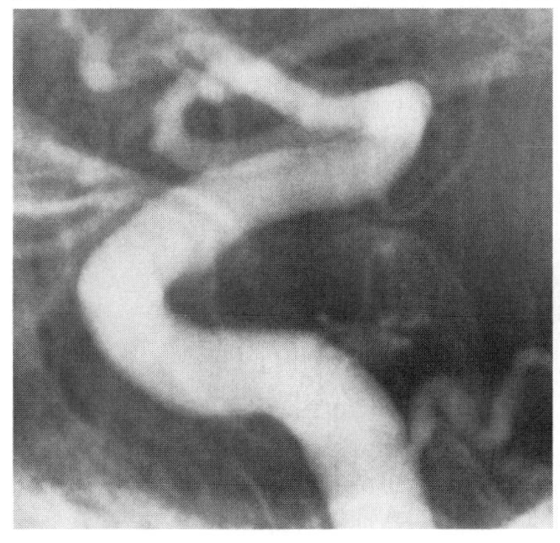

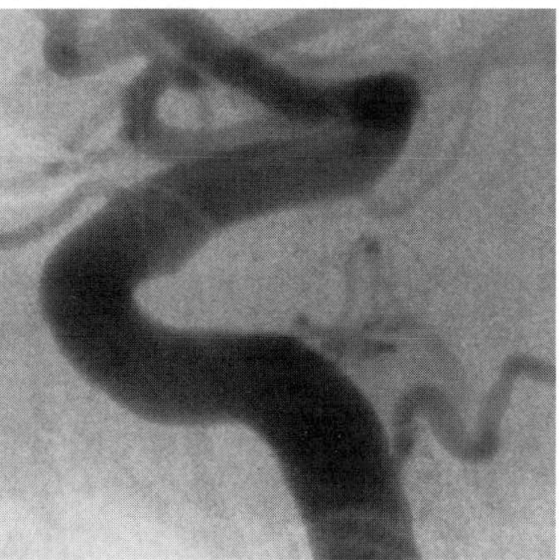

Figure 17.11. Meningohypophyseal artery. There is an enlarged meningohypophyseal artery in this patient, who had a small dural arteriovenous malformation with proptosis. The magnified lateral view (**A**) and the subtraction film (**B**) show the branches, but the subtraction film is much clearer. The larger, inferior artery is probably the artery of the tentorium; the upper branches are twigs of the inferior hypophyseal artery, which is much enlarged, and seems to also supply the back of the clivus.

hind the clivus and cavernous sinus. It anastomoses with the opposite branch behind the dorsum sellae. (*c*) The *inferior hypophyseal artery* supplies the posterior lobe of the pituitary gland. It also anastomoses with the opposite side, and thus an arterial circle is formed around the base of the dorsum sellae.

The *inferior cavernous artery* supplies the wall of the sinus and its contents, and anastomoses with the middle meningeal artery at the foramen spinosum; it was found by Parkinson in 80 percent of specimens. Schnurer and Stattin (57) found the artery of the edge of the tentorium to arise most frequently from what they called the *lateral main stem artery*, which corresponds to the inferior cavernous sinus artery as described by Parkinson, but both the meningohypophyseal and the inferior cavernous trunks give branches to the tentorium. From the same inferior cavernous sinus artery arise branches to the dura of the middle fossa, the gasserian ganglion, and also branches that pass forward and lateral to the lesser wing of the sphenoid and supply the dura of the posterior portion of the anterior cranial fossa. Small branches also pass through the superior orbital fissure or through the bone into the apex of the orbit, where they anastomose with branches of the ophthalmic artery. Thus, there are several anastomotic connections between the internal and external carotid systems at this level (58).

The *capsular artery* arises about 1 cm anterior to the meningohypophyseal trunk and goes under the pituitary gland, following the floor of the sella to anastomose with the opposite side (53). This and the other minor branch arteries can serve as anastomotic pathways between the internal carotid arteries; it has been seen by the author to be markedly enlarged in two cases of "congenital absence" of the cervical portion of the internal carotid artery.

All of the minor branches are visible occasionally on normal angiograms without subtraction. One or more of the branches can be seen almost regularly when subtraction is employed; if subtraction with magnification is used, they can be seen in a high percentage of cases. They may become enlarged in various pathologic states.

Internal carotid injections result in better filling than common carotid injections. The meningohypophyseal and other branches to the pituitary region become enlarged in cases of tumor in this area or in arteriovenous malformations (Fig. 17.11).

Hacker and Alonso (59) and Lehrer (60) described visualization of the posterior lobe of the pituitary gland, which occurs during the arterial phase in normal cases. A homogeneous "stain" can be seen just anterior to the dorsum sellae and partly obscured by bone. Subtraction is necessary to demonstrate this clearly. The pituitary "stain" is obscured by the carotid artery itself if the posterior portion of the siphon is tortuous (Fig. 17.12).

Carotid-cavernous fistulas can lead to marked dilatation of these vessels although they rarely appear to serve as collateral pathways in carotid occlusion.

Minor branches of the supraclinoid segment are also found. The superior hypophyseal arteries, two or more in number on each side, pass above the diaphragm a sellae

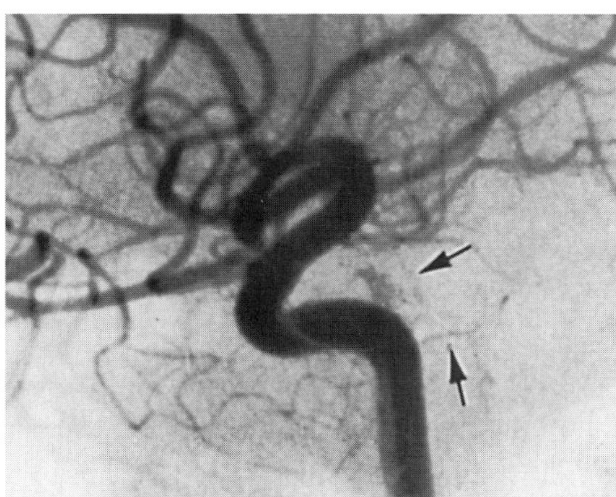

Figure 17.12. Posterior pituitary "blush." The posterior lobe of the pituitary exhibits a faint opacification early in the arterial phase, indicating rapid circulation through this portion of the pituitary gland (arrow). This can be seen well only with subtraction. The meningohypophyseal artery is faintly outlined (lower arrow).

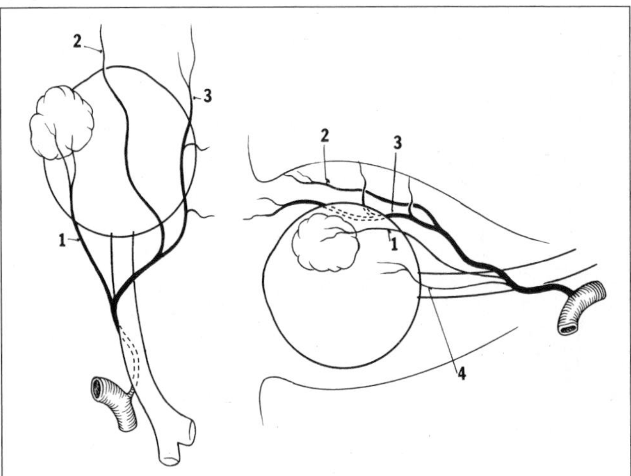

Figure 17.13. Diagram of ophthalmic artery. The artery enters the orbit through the optic foramen under the nerve, then it swings medially and over the nerve: (1) lacrimal artery; (2) supraorbital artery; (3) main trunk with ethmoidal and palpebral branches; (4) central retinal artery.

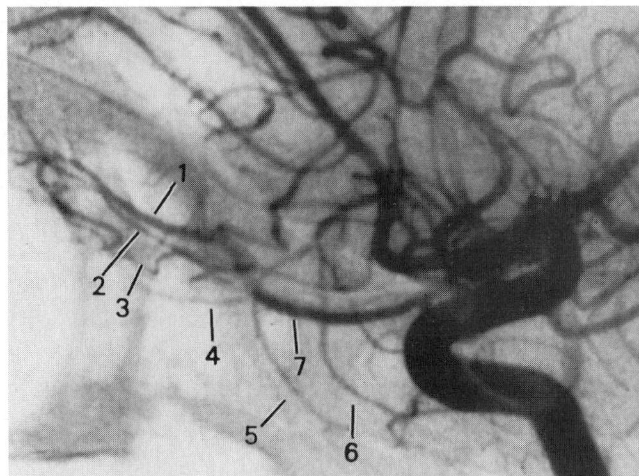

Figure 17.14. Ophthalmic artery, lateral view. (1) ophthalmic artery; (2) supraorbital artery; (3) lacrimal artery; (4) central retinal artery; (5) and (6) anterior temporal branches of middle cerebral artery; (7) trunk of ophthalmic artery.

and branch out over the pituitary stalk, forming a circuminfundibular plexus (see Fig. 11.50). They supply the anterior lobe of the pituitary via this capillary plexus, which forms a portal system of vessels. The arteries are not normally visible on angiograms but may become enlarged with vascular tumors. Baker (61) states that he demonstrated the circuminfundibular plexus in 71 of 75 normal carotid angiograms when magnification and subtraction were employed routinely. Striate branches penetrate the brain via the anterior perforated substance (see under "Anterior Choroidal Artery").

MAJOR BRANCHES OF THE INTERNAL CAROTID ARTERY

The major branches of the internal carotid artery, seen on the cerebral angiogram, follow. The ophthalmic artery arises from the internal carotid artery immediately after it leaves the cavernous sinus, medial to the anterior clinoid process. Although usually subdural in its course, it can be either subarachnoid or intradural. The optic nerve courses first intracranially, then intracanalicularly, and finally intraorbitally. The intraorbital portion of the ophthalmic artery can be divided into three segments: the first, or *straight segment;* the second, or *ring segment;* and the third, or *distal segment.*

The ophthalmic artery enters the orbit through the optic foramen below and lateral to the optic nerve (Fig. 17.13). The artery then turns upward and medially, passing over the nerve to reach the medial wall of the orbit. Its main branches are the lachrymal, which proceeds along the lateral wall, and the supraorbital, which courses approximately in the center of the orbit above the globe. The main trunk of the ophthalmic artery continues along the medial orbital wall, giving off the ethmoidal and the palpebral branches. In the lateral view, the ophthalmic artery trunk can easily be seen, but superimposed bone shadows and superimposition of the branches of the artery make identification difficult without subtraction (Fig. 17.14). In order to visualize the artery and its branches to better advantage in frontal projection, an orbital view is necessary, and a stereoscopic view is preferable in order to separate the ophthalmic from the intracranial arteries. The central retinal artery is not often seen on angiograms, but the arteriolar and capillary blush of the choroid and retina is visible in the late arterial and capillary phases. The blush is identified readily owing to its rostrally concave appearance, corresponding to the posterior aspect of the globe (Fig. 17.15), and this can be used to locate accurately the posterior wall

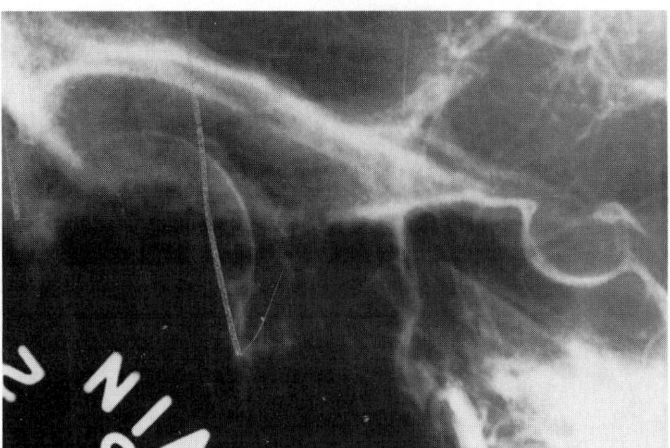

Figure 17.15. Choroid-retinal blush in normal patient. The curvilinear dense shadow marks the posterior margin of the globe, and it is possible to determine the presence of exophthalmus by this means. In addition, it may be possible to follow the results of therapy for conditions causing exophthalmus. This is a graphic means of showing exophthalmus, but CT and MRI are preferred.

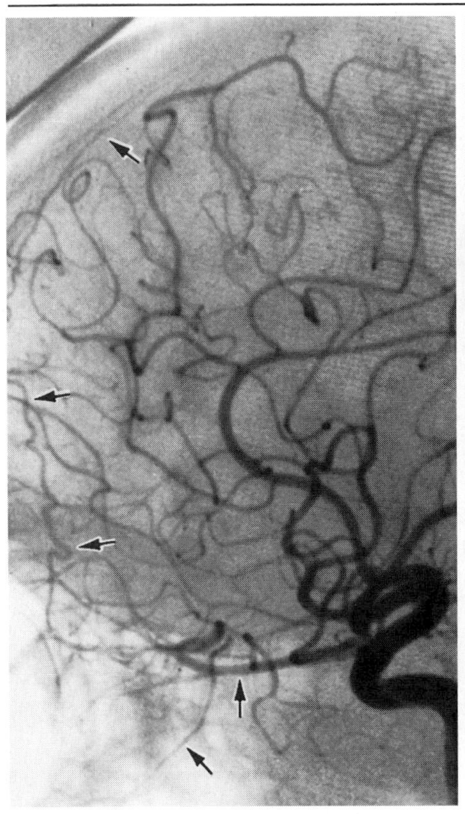
A

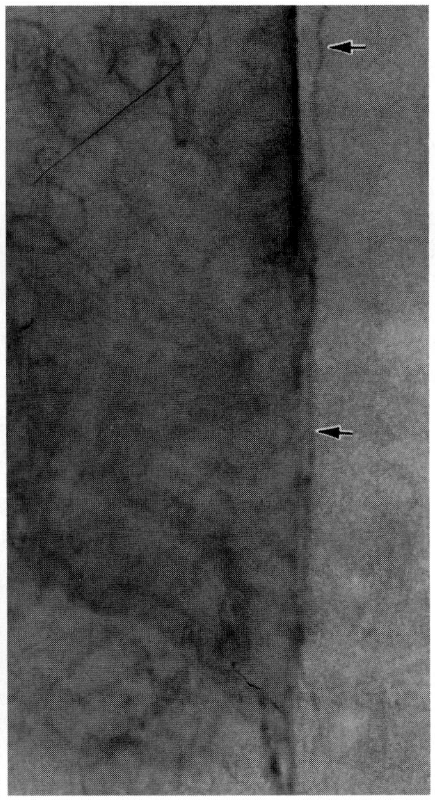
B

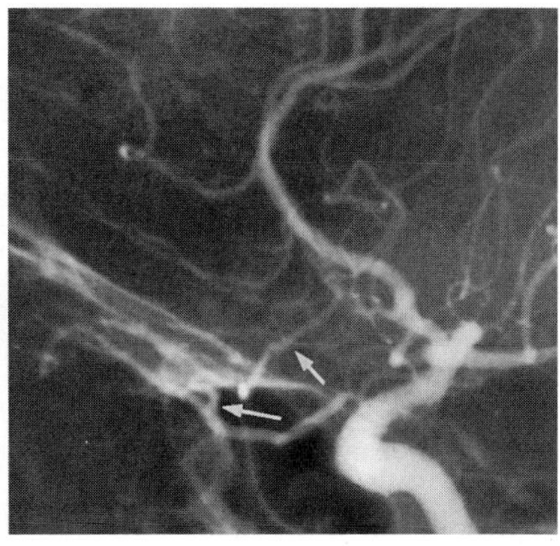
C

Figure 17.16. Normal anterior meningeal artery—artery of the falx. The artery of the falx, a branch of the ophthalmic artery, is seen to ascend a little more posteriorly than usual on the falx (arrows). It can be followed up to the coronal suture. **A.** The ophthalmic artery is large and also gives off an infraorbital branch. **B.** The frontal projection, taken during the capillary phase of the angiogram, demonstrates the anterior meningeal artery (arrows). **C.** Origin of middle meningeal artery from ophthalmic artery (arrows).

of the eyeball. The "retinochoroid blush" is normally 2 to 4 mm posterior to the anterior margin of the frontozygomatic border of the orbit on the corresponding side. If it is anterior to this, exophthalmus may be present. In a straight lateral view, the anterior margin of the lateral orbital border of the side against the film projects dorsal to the one away from the film.

The artery of the falx arises from the anterior ethmoidal branch of the ophthalmic artery. It perforates the cribriform plate and ascends, usually quite close to the attachment of the falx anteriorly to the frontal bone. Sometimes it ascends a little farther away from the anterior falx attachment (Fig. 17.16). The artery may be enlarged in cases of tumors involving the meninges, such as meningiomas, or in arteriovenous malformations supplied by the meningeal circulation. It was seen on arteriograms in 87 percent of normal individuals (62).

The ophthalmic artery may give origin to the middle meningeal artery (Fig. 17.16*C*; see Fig. 11.126). This can most easily be appreciated on lateral film. Sometimes the ophthalmic originates from the meningeal artery (63), in which case the central artery of the retina usually arises directly from the internal carotid artery.

Ducasse et al. studied the arterial vascular system of the orbit in dissections (64). The craniofacial junction is an important location because of possible anastomoses between the internal and external carotid arteries. The anastomoses are situated at the meningeal and palpebral levels and also inside the orbital cavity. There is frequent participation of the external carotid artery to the orbital vascularization by means of three collateral branches. The infraorbital artery, a branch of the maxillary artery, partakes in the arterial supply of the inferior oblique muscle in 85.7 percent of cases. Usually the inferior muscular artery, which is a branch of the ophthalmic artery, also partakes in this supply. In very exceptional cases (2 of 70) the infraorbital artery alone supplies the muscle. The lacrimal artery can come from the external carotid system either from the middle meningeal artery or from the anterior deep temporal artery. This meningolacrimal artery either can be a solo lacrimal artery (14 percent of cases) or can be associated with another classic lacrimal artery, from the ophthalmic artery (43 percent). These lacrimal arteries coming from the external carotid system have the following characteristics: they are thinner than classic arteries, they penetrate the orbit by their own orifice, the Hyrtl canal, and they can participate in the muscular vascularization, especially of the lateral rectus. When these arteries are unique, most often they are encountered when the ophthalmic artery has undercrossed the optic nerve.

The branches of the ophthalmic artery anastomose profusely with those of the external carotid artery (internal maxillary, middle meningeal, superficial temporal, etc.); as a result, the ophthalmic artery is an important anastomotic pathway between internal and external carotid systems.

ARTERIAL VARIANTS AND ANOMALIES OF THE INTERNAL CAROTID ARTERY

The left common carotid artery was found to arise from the right innominate in 9 out of 130 cases examined by Stein et al. (65) (Fig. 17.17). The arrangement is normally encountered in the bovine family. The right subclavian artery originated as the fourth large branch of the aorta and had a retroesophageal course in two instances in the series of Stein et al. In both cases, the right common carotid artery originated directly from the aorta. The site of the bifurcation of the common carotid artery, which usually takes place at the level of the thyroid cartilage, may be higher or lower. Occasionally, the internal carotid artery may be absent (66). The cranial portion of the internal carotid artery can be replaced by branches of the internal maxillary artery entering the skull through the foramen rotundum and foramen ovale, joining intracranially to form a single vessel (67). The opposite internal carotid artery may supply blood by way of transfer collaterals arising from the intracavernous portion of the internal carotid artery. Of 24 such cases reported in the literature, there were 4 with aneurysms of the anterior communicating artery; in 1 case there was cranial nerve involvement due to pressure by an enlarged, tortuous basilar artery (68).

When the internal carotid artery is hypoplastic from birth, the canal of the petrous bone fails to develop normally. This was true in a case report by Prensky and Davis (69). A hypoplastic canal does not necessarily prove that the internal carotid artery was absent in utero; if occlusion of the artery occurs during early infancy, the canal may become narrow as skull growth proceeds. Tomography is required to demonstrate the carotid canals adequately.

Unilateral *internal carotid artery hypoplasia* may be associated with arterial anomalies in the circle of Willis. In a report the middle cerebral artery was supplied via anomalous arteries from the posterior cerebral artery, and the internal carotid artery and ipsilateral common carotid artery also originated from an anomalous brachiocephalic trunk (70).

Two important variants involve the internal carotid artery in its intrapetrosal and its intracavernous portions. When the internal carotid artery enters the carotid canal of the petrous bone, it bends medially and forward. At this point it is very close to the inferior aspect of the tympanic cavity and separated from it only by a thin bit of bone. Sometimes this bony canal wall is incomplete and the internal carotid artery buckles unprotected into the middle ear cavity. It may be indirectly visible behind the hypotympanum, having the appearance of a reddish pulsatile "tumor." The diagnosis of this abnormality should be made by angiography (71). Lapayowker et al. suggest that a vertical line be traced passing through the vestibule approximating the most medial extent of the middle ear (71). Normally the bend of the internal carotid artery is medial to this line (average 5 mm); in a few normal instances the bend of the internal carotid artery touched the vertical vestibular line, but in these cases it was always a good distance below the vestibule. When the carotid artery presents in the middle ear, the lateral margin of the intrapetrosal bend is lateral to the vestibular line in the frontal angiogram (Fig. 17.18 *A*, *B*, *C*). As the vessel buckles laterally, it is usually narrowed and of uneven caliber.

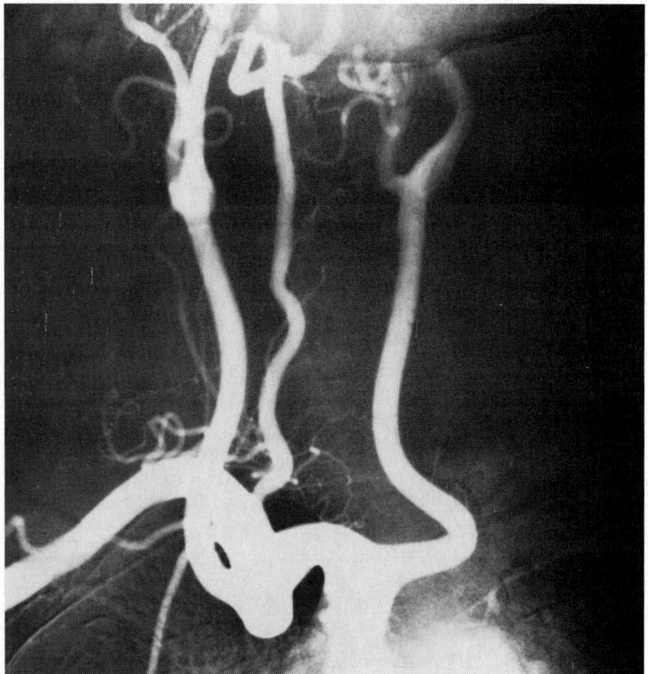

Figure 17.17. Origin of left common carotid from innominate artery (Bovine arch).

A second important variant of the internal carotid artery is encountered in the intracavernous portion. The artery may swing medially more than usual and produce enlargement and deepening of the carotid groove of the sella turcica (Fig. 17.18*D* to *H*). In some cases compression of the optic nerve may result. Numerous other anomalies and variants are described in discussions of the individual vessels.

Carotid-basilar anastomoses may exist at three levels. These anastomotic channels are the result of persistent arteries encountered during embryological development (72). The anastomoses may be seen with greatest frequency just proximal to the intracavernous portion of the internal carotid artery. This is called the *persistent primitive trigeminal artery*, which joins the trunks of the internal carotid and basilar arteries directly. Under certain circumstances the anomaly can be a very important circulatory channel (Fig. 17.19). This persistent artery is sometimes seen in association with other abnormalities such as saccular aneurysms. Saltzman (73) and Lie (74) described three types: type I, in which the rostral parts of the basilar, the posterior cerebral, and superior cerebellar arteries are supplied by the anomalous artery; type II, in which the homolateral

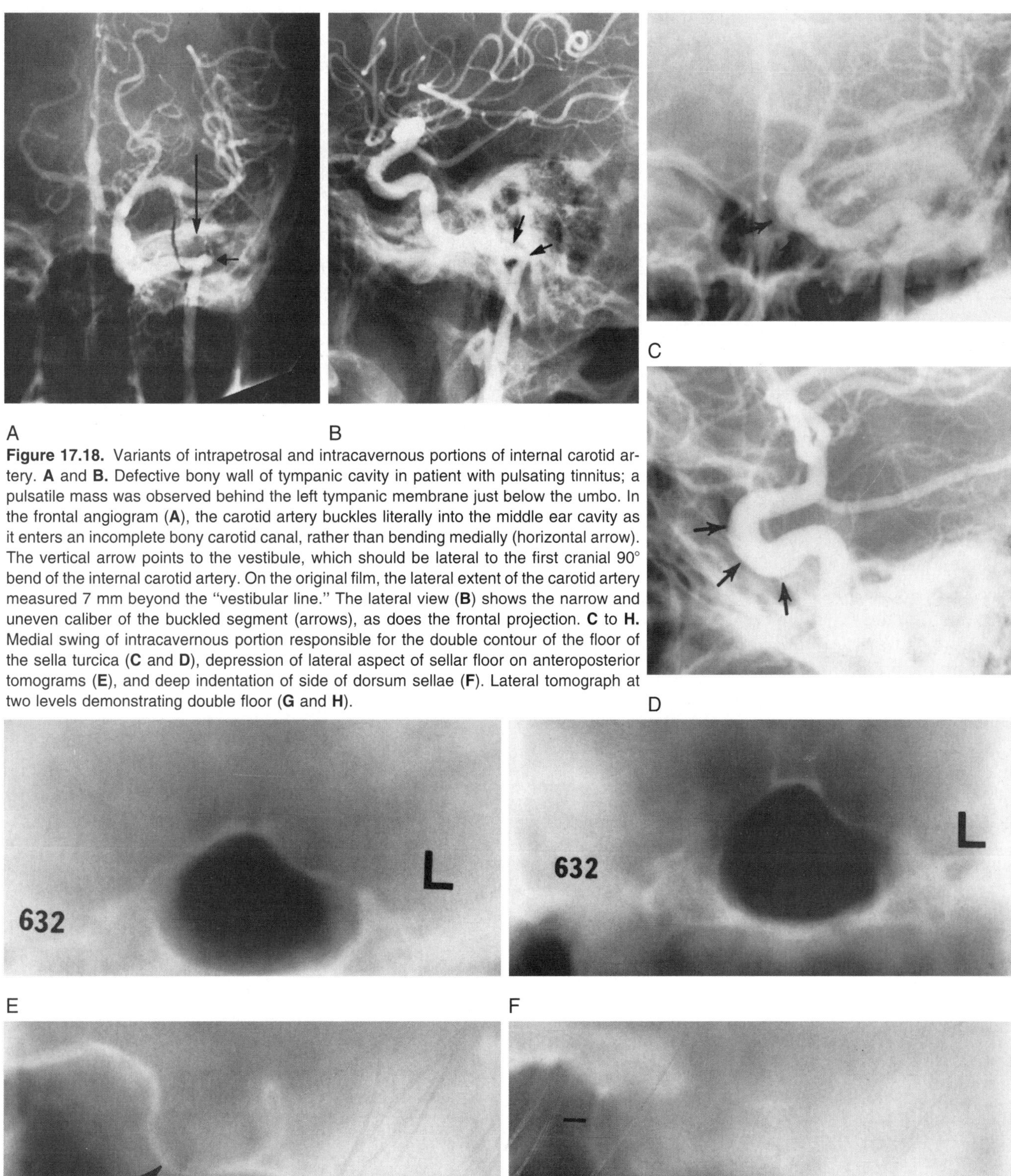

A B

Figure 17.18. Variants of intrapetrosal and intracavernous portions of internal carotid artery. **A** and **B.** Defective bony wall of tympanic cavity in patient with pulsating tinnitus; a pulsatile mass was observed behind the left tympanic membrane just below the umbo. In the frontal angiogram (**A**), the carotid artery buckles literally into the middle ear cavity as it enters an incomplete bony carotid canal, rather than bending medially (horizontal arrow). The vertical arrow points to the vestibule, which should be lateral to the first cranial 90° bend of the internal carotid artery. On the original film, the lateral extent of the carotid artery measured 7 mm beyond the "vestibular line." The lateral view (**B**) shows the narrow and uneven caliber of the buckled segment (arrows), as does the frontal projection. **C** to **H.** Medial swing of intracavernous portion responsible for the double contour of the floor of the sella turcica (**C** and **D**), depression of lateral aspect of sellar floor on anteroposterior tomograms (**E**), and deep indentation of side of dorsum sellae (**F**). Lateral tomograph at two levels demonstrating double floor (**G** and **H**).

C D E F G H

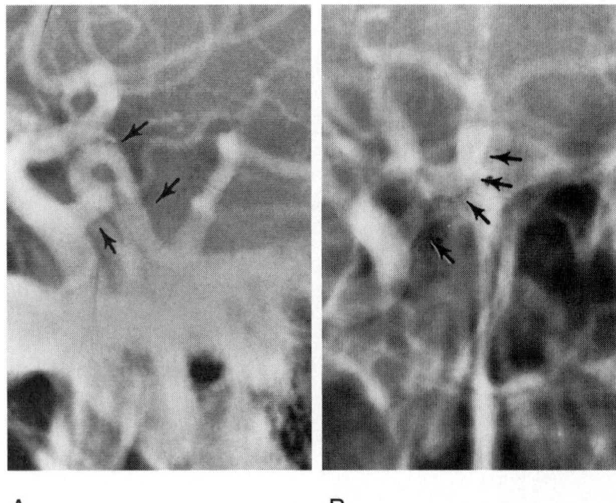

A B

Figure 17.19. Persistent primitive trigeminal artery. **A.** The lateral view demonstrates the origin of the vessel from the posterior portion of the intracavernous segment (sometimes just before the artery enters the cavernous sinus). It has a tortuous course and joins the basilar artery after passing through the anterior and anterolateral aspects of the tentorial incisura. **B.** The frontal projection demonstrates the course of the artery (arrows) and filling of both posterior cerebral and superior cerebellar arteries (see also Fig. 11.53).

posterior cerebral is supplied by the posterior communicating artery and the others by the trigeminal artery; and type III, in which both the posterior cerebral arteries are supplied by posterior communicating arteries. At times, the anomalous artery may communicate directly with a basilar branch (75).

The *persistent primitive acoustic artery* (otic) is in a slightly lower position than the trigeminal artery and arises from the intrapetrosal portion of the internal carotid artery. It joins the basilar artery just caudad to the origins of the anterior inferior cerebellar arteries. It is much less common than the persistent trigeminal artery.

The *persistent primitive hypoglossal artery* also runs with its homologous cranial nerve. This artery arises from the cervical portion of the internal carotid artery and enters the skull via the hypoglossal canal to join the basilar artery. The union is at or near the junction of the vertebrals to form the basilar artery, and the ipsilateral vertebral artery is hypoplastic. The condition is extremely rare (Fig. 17.20*A* and *B*). This persistent artery should not be confused with the *proatlantal intersegmental artery* (PIA), which is also an embryological remnant, connecting the carotid with the vertebral artery (Fig. 17.20*C*). The proatlantal intersegmental artery (PIA) may arise from the external carotid artery and give rise to the occipital artery, supporting the hypothesis that the distal part of the occipital artery is derived from it (76). The anteroposterior view is helpful in differentiating the PIA of external carotid artery origin from the first cervical intersegmental artery.

Sato et al. reported a stroke of the basilar artery territory related to the *persistent primitive first cervical intersegmental artery (proatlantal artery II)* (77).

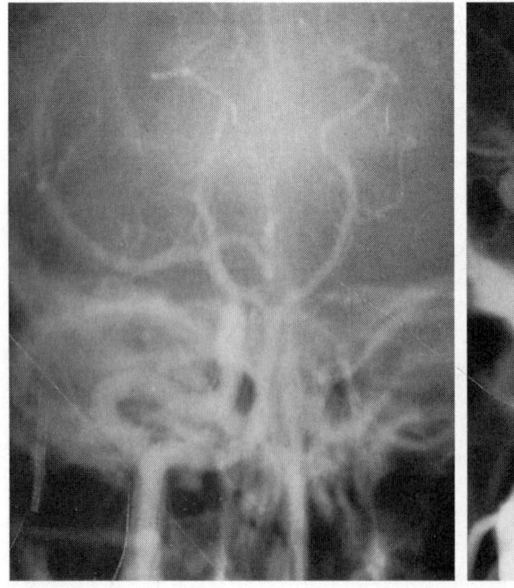

A

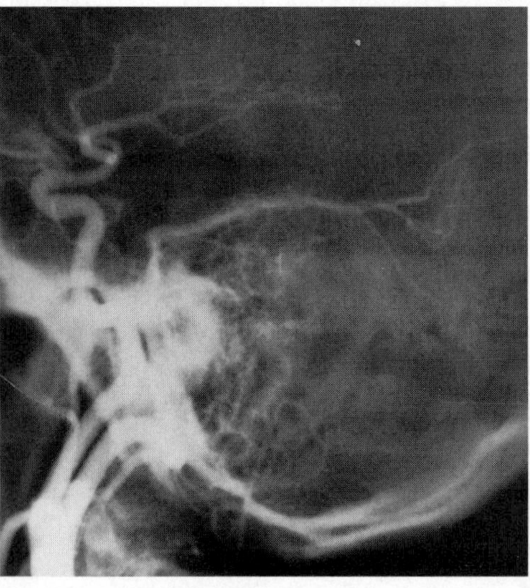

B

C

Figure 17.20. Persistent hypoglossal artery and proatlantal artery. **A.** and **B.** Persistent hypoglossal artery arising from internal carotid at the level of the second cervical vertebra and joining the basilar artery after entering the skull via the hypoglossal foramen. **C.** Example of proatlantal artery. There is occlusion of the internal carotid artery at its origin. A large vessel is seen to join the trunk of the occluded internal carotid artery with the vertebral artery at the level of the atlas (upper arrow).

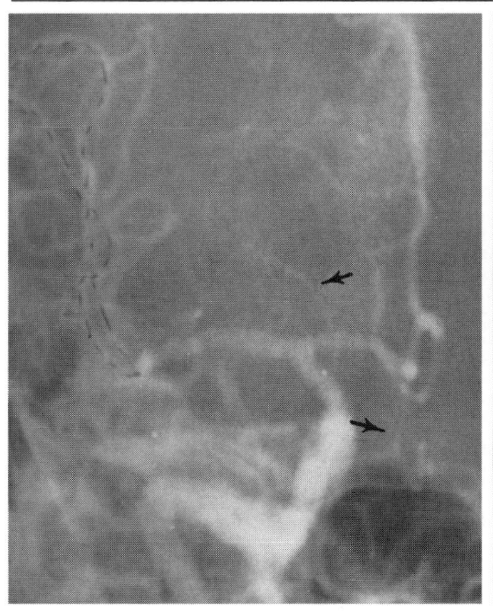

A

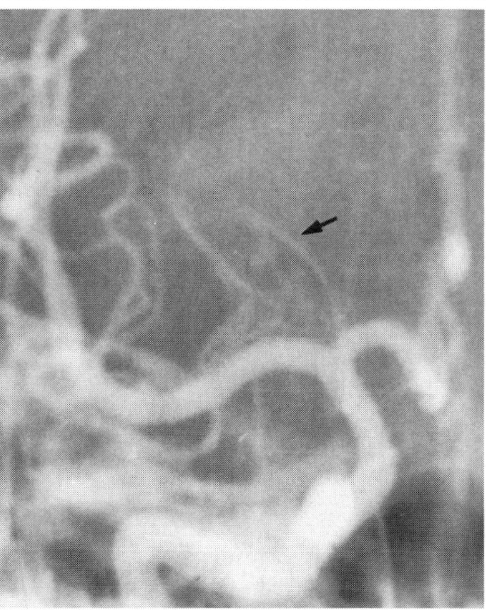

B

Figure 17.21. Normal frontal carotid angiograms to show the anterior choroidal artery. **A.** The frontal view shows the normal curvature of the anterior choroidal in this projection (upper arrow). The lenticulostriate arteries are also shown just lateral to the anterior choroidal artery. The lower arrow in the midline indicates the frontopolar artery, which, because of projection, is thrown downward. The frontal view is not of the same patient as the lateral view. **B.** Another frontal view illustrates the course of the anterior choroidal artery. Its curvature is broader, owing to greater angulation of the tube. The upper portion of the choroidal artery is wider than its lower portion (arrow), indicating the beginning of the plexus (choroidal blush).

Posterior Communicating Artery

This artery, the first intracranial branch of the internal carotid artery, is described together with the posterior cerebral artery (see text following).

Anterior Choroidal Artery

A small and important branch of the internal carotid artery, the anterior choroidal, arises just distal to the origin of the posterior communicating artery in 75 percent of cases. Carpenter and coauthors found that it arose from the middle cerebral artery in 7 of 60 dissections, from the posterior communicating artery in 4, and from the bifurcation of the internal carotid artery at the origins of the anterior and middle cerebral arteries in 2 cases (78). In 1 of the 60 dissections it was absent; it may be double. The relative incidence of these variants has not been confirmed by other authors. Sjogren was able to identify the artery in 93 percent of 100 normal angiograms (79).

Although in 90 percent of the cases the anterior choroidal is the first branch immediately above the posterior communicating artery, one, two, or even three branches may arise from the carotid siphon before the anterior choroidal. These are usually perforating arteries, which enter the anterior perforated substance together with the striate vessels (78). Under certain circumstances the perforating branches arising from the internal carotid artery can become very prominent; they may provide collateral pathways in cases of occlusion at the bifurcation of the internal carotid artery, or in the trunks of the middle and anterior cerebral arteries, as seen in the entity of multiple progressive intracranial arterial occlusion (see under "Moya-Moya," Chapter 10).

After its origin from the posterior aspect of the internal carotid artery, the anterior choroidal is directed posteriorly and slightly medially as it crosses the cisternal space in the parasellar region. This segment has been called the cisternal portion by Sjogren and is about 1 cm in length. The artery, passing laterally, then reaches the medial surface of the tip of the temporal horn, extends around the uncus, and swings laterally and dorsally to enter the temporal horn through the choroidal fissure. Within the temporal horn it supplies the choroid plexus. The latter has been called the plexal portion (Sjogren) and can usually be identified because the shadow of the artery becomes broader at this point (Fig. 17.21). A capillary "blush" is sometimes seen in this region representing the choroid plexus. The anterior choroidal artery supplies, in addition to the choroid plexus, the hippocampus and the basal ganglia.

In the lateral view the anterior choroidal artery is directed backward and slightly downward for a short distance; then it curves upward and backward, describing a gentle arc with a superior convexity (Fig. 17.22), but this is variable. The usual length of the anterior choroidal artery is approximately 3 cm as seen on the films. When longer than 3 cm, the artery may be pathologically elongated and enlarged, although this is not necessarily so. Enlargement of the anterior choroidal artery may indicate the direct blood supply of an intracerebral tumor by this artery, but it may also be enlarged in cases of increased intracranial pressure produced by a tumor in any location. The cause of this is not known but may be a need for greater blood flow in the production of cerebrospinal fluid. The artery may also be enlarged in some cases of cerebral thrombosis. A junctional or infundibular dilatation at the origin of the anterior choroidal from the internal carotid is sometimes seen (Fig. 17.22*A*).

In the frontal projection, the anterior choroidal artery is seen to arise from the internal carotid and to proceed upward and medially for a short distance, after which it turns laterally. After completing its turn around the medial

Figure 17.22. Anterior choroidal artery. **A.** Lateral (arrow). **B.** Frontal projection (arrow). The patient had a small arteriovenous malformation not supplied by the anterior choroidal artery.

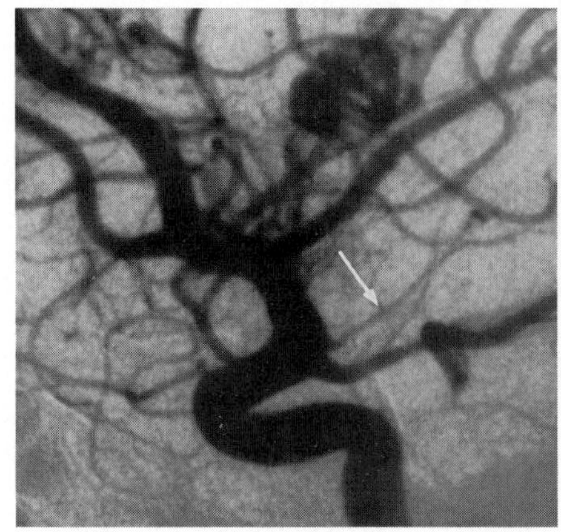

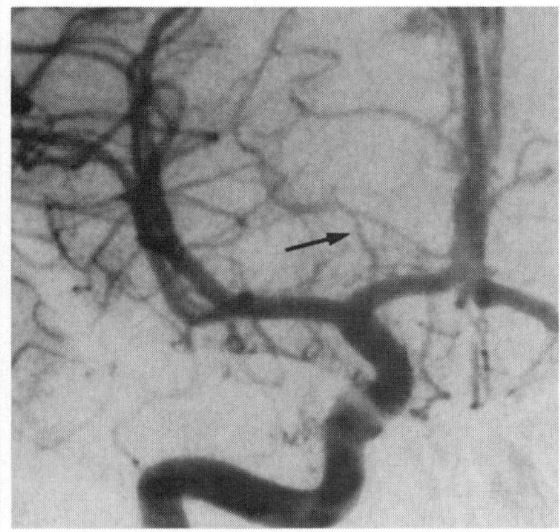

A B

Figure 17.23. Diagram to explain differences in curvature of anterior choroidal artery and in configuration of insular curve of middle cerebral artery with different projections. Left image, steeper craniocaudal angulation; middle, usual angiographic projection (12° above orbitomeatal line); right image, transorbital.

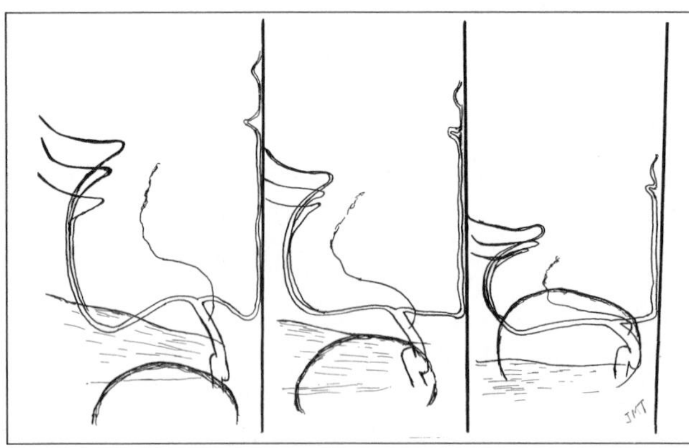

portion of the tip of the temporal lobe, it enters the temporal horn and soon disappears on the angiogram. The curve described by the anterior choroidal artery depends on the projection used. The greater the caudal angulation of the central beam used to make the exposure in relation to the orbitomeatal line, the broader is the curve described by the artery (Fig. 17.23), and vice versa.

The shadow of the artery becomes slightly wider as it forms the choroid plexus, and it is often possible to see the choroid plexus as an area of slightly increased density immediately above the artery (choroid blush). At times the artery can be followed high along its course in the temporal horn. When visible in this manner it may indicate that a pathologic condition is present, as explained previously (Figs. 17.24 and 17.25). Distally, the artery anastomoses with the posterior choroidal artery, which supplies the greater portion of the choroid plexus. The anastomotic pathway is sometimes seen in cases of thrombosis with collateral circulation.

Takahashi investigated the anterior choroidal artery (AChA) angiographically for the origin, size, and course of the stem and for the possible identification of the uncal branch, perforating branches, and plexal segment of the AChA (80). Hypoplastic and hyperplastic types were found (3 and 2.3 percent, respectively). Hypoplasia of the plexal segment of this artery might represent an evolutionary variant in which the artery ceased to acquire choroidal branches, thus remaining in the reptilian stage. The hyperplastic arteries can be classified into subtypes according to the distribution area and course of the vessel. The hyperplastic anomalies are considered to represent a situation in which the AChA has maintained, as a main pathway, an anastomosis with the posterior communicating artery and posterior cerebral artery.

Recent studies reviewed by Helgason of strokes of the anterior choroidal artery have added hemiataxia, acute pseudobulbar mutis, pure motor, pure sensory, and disorders of higher cortical functions to the classic triad of hemisensory, hemimotor, and visual field deficit (81).

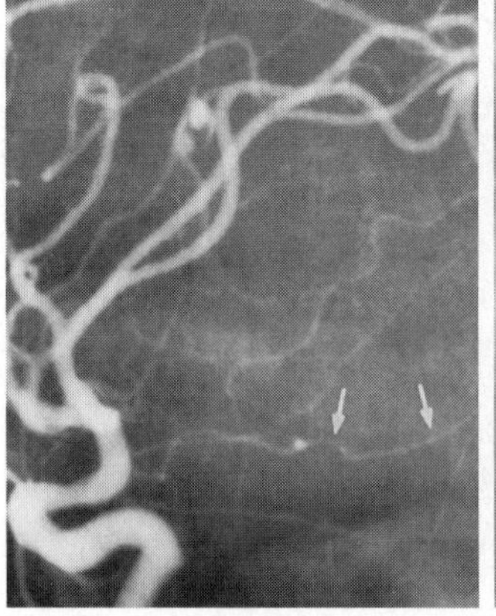

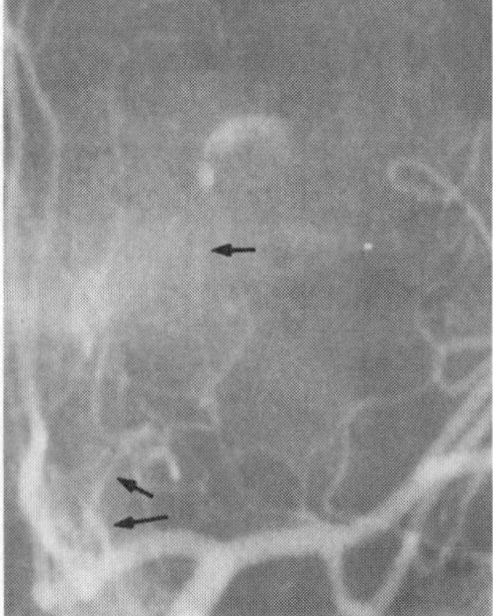

A B

Figure 17.24. Enlarged anterior choroidal artery in patient with basal ganglia hemorrhage. **A.** The lateral projection demonstrates elevation of the middle cerebral group of vessels and an increase in the height of the sylvian triangle. The anterior choroidal artery is enlarged (arrows). **B.** The frontal projection discloses marked lateral displacement of the sylvian vessels toward the inner table of the skull. There is medial displacement of the lenticulostriate arteries; one of them is large (arrow) and leads to an area of increased density representing extravasation of contrast material at the site of hemorrhage. The mass was large, and there is some midline shift of the anterior cerebral artery to the contralateral side. The anterior choroidal is marked by two black arrows.

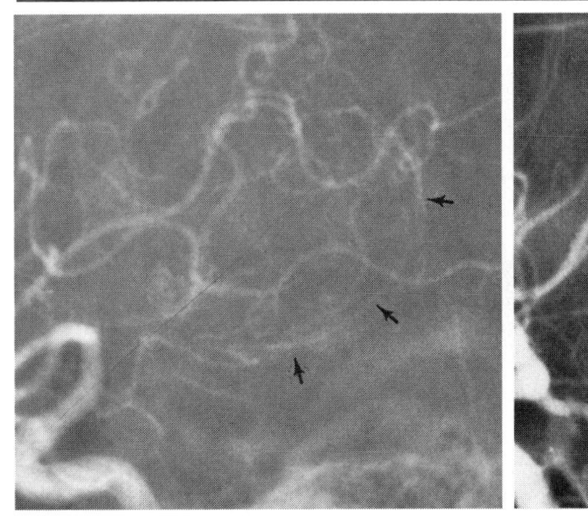

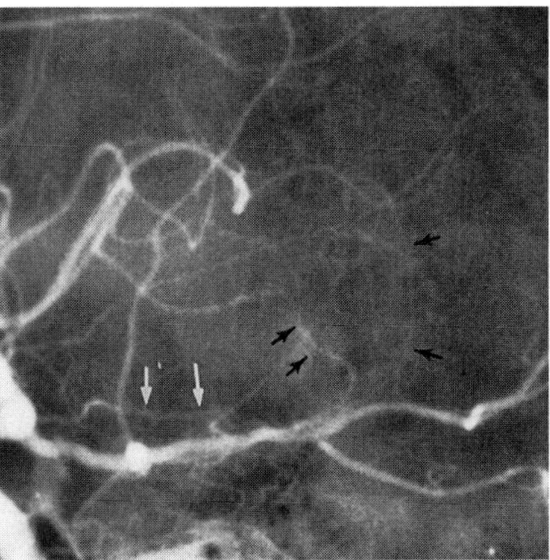

Figure 17.25. Enlarged anterior choroidal artery in patient with thalamic tumor. **A.** The anterior choroidal artery is enlarged, and there is downward displacement of its posterior portion. The curvature shows an increase in its radius due to the thalamic mass (arrows). There is elevation of the middle cerebral branches. **B.** In an angiogram of another case there is downward displacement of the posterior cerebral artery. The lateral posterior choroidal artery is filled (by way of the posterior cerebral artery) and shows widening of its curvature (posterior arrows). The medial posterior choroidal artery is not displaced (double arrows). There is elevation of the middle cerebral branches. The anterior choroidal artery (white arrows) shows elongation and widening of its curvature.

Anterior Cerebral Artery Complex

The anterior cerebral artery (ACA) complex supplies the medial surface of the frontal lobe and parietal lobe as well as the anterior medial limbic structures. Found deep within the hemispheric fissure, it is a good landmark for the midline in anteroposterior view. In lateral view, the anterior cerebral vessel is laid out perpendicular and can be seen in its entirety, the medial terminal branch of the internal carotid.

The ACA complex consists of the ACA, the anterior communicating artery (ACoA), and the perforators.

The ACA has its origin at the bifurcation of the internal carotid artery in the medial part of the sylvian fissure. It has a horizontal and a vertical segment. In its horizontal portion the artery passes medially and forward above the optic nerve until it reaches the ACoA. At this point the artery bends fairly sharply to proceed directly forward and upward along the interhemispheric fissure (Fig. 17.26). It courses beside the anterior aspect of the corpus callosum to the genu, where it turns dorsad. The latter turn may be called the *genu*, or the "knee," of the anterior cerebral artery. The artery continues along the medial surface of the hemisphere directly backward as the pericallosal artery and finally anastomoses with a branch of the posterior cerebral artery.

In the region of the anterior communicating artery, the anterior cerebral artery is usually convex downward initially; then it reverses to describe a slight curve concave downward, followed by another convex forward curve (Fig. 17.27).

In children and in younger individuals these curves are less pronounced than in the older age group, owing to elongation and tortuosity. Throughout their course in the interhemispheric fissure, the anterior cerebral and pericallosal arteries are fairly close to the corpus callosum, but this relationship is variable. The bending of the vessel, which sometimes is quite pronounced in normal individuals, tends to separate the anterior cerebral vessels from the corpus callosum at intervals.

PROXIMAL ACA (A1, PRECOMMUNAL SEGMENT, HORIZONTAL SEGMENT)

The proximal ACA (A1) varies considerably in size. In three-fourths of the cases, the middle cerebral artery is larger than the ACA; in approximately 1 in 20 the ACA is larger; in about 1 in 100 the ACA is angiographically "aplastic." The vessel always runs medially and often anteriorly.

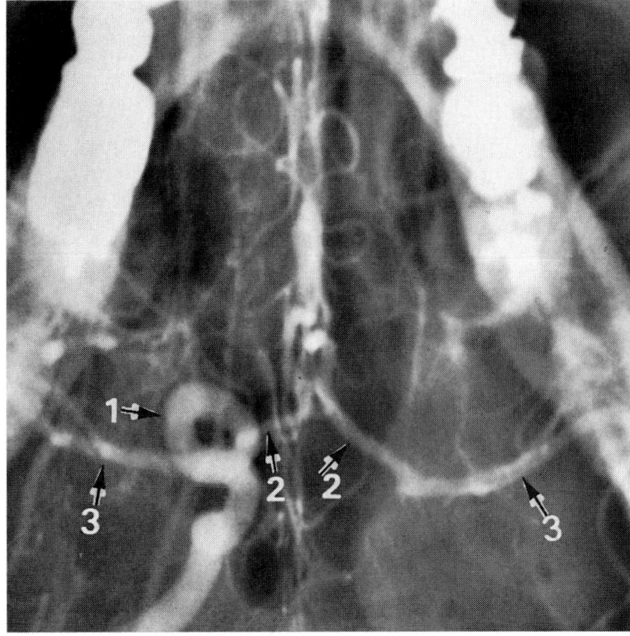

Figure 17.26. Base view of normal carotid artery. The course of the anterior cerebral artery, which is directed medially and forward, is clear. As it reaches the midline it approximates the opposite anterior cerebral and joins it through the anterior communicating artery, which may not be visible as a separate artery owing to its brief course. The two anterior cerebrals then continue their separate courses in the interhemispheric fissure, except in cases where they are united as an azygos vessel for part of their course, usually a short segment distal to the anterior communicating artery. Arrows: (1) intracavernous segment of internal carotid; (2) anterior cerebral arteries; (3) middle cerebral artery.

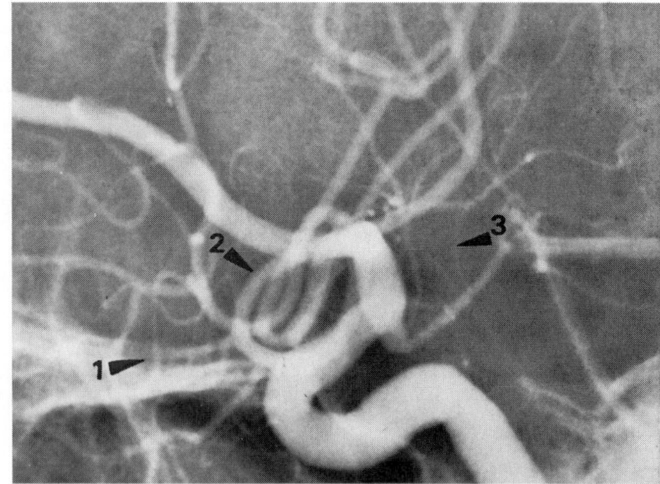

A

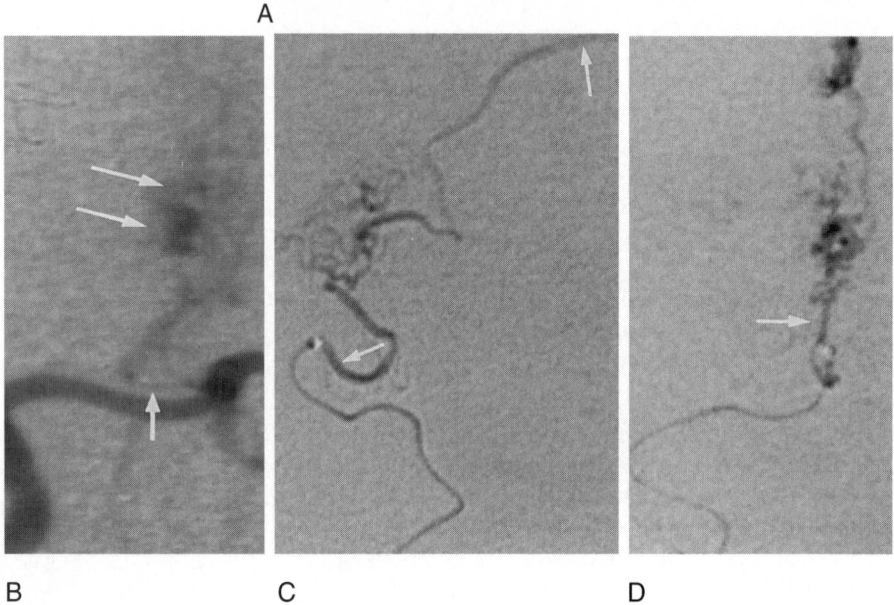

B C D

Figure 17.27. A. Normal anterior cerebral artery; also anterior choroidal artery originating from posterior communicating artery. There is a funnel-shaped junctional dilatation of the posterior communicating artery. The anterior choroidal (arrow 3) is easy to differentiate from the thalamoperforate arteries because of its configuration (compare with Fig. 17.84). The anterior cerebral artery presents a downward convex curve in the region of, and just beyond, the anterior communicating artery, followed by a reverse curve. Arrows: (1) anterior temporal branch of middle cerebral artery; (2) the trunk of the middle cerebral artery is seen to go forward and slightly downward; (3) anterior choroidal artery. **B.** Enlarged perforating branch of anterior cerebral artery just proximal to the anterior communicating artery (arrow) seen in this slightly oblique frontal view. The perforator is supplying a small arteriovenous malformation (upper arrows). Lateral (**C**) and frontal (**D**) superselective injection of the enlarged perforating branch. The malformation is seen. Early draining veins with filling of the internal cerebral vein is seen (arrow).

A method to designate the various segments of the internal carotid artery, the anterior cerebral, the middle cerebral, the vertebral artery, and the basilar artery is shown in Figure 17.28.

In a study, Marinkovic et al. found *hypoplasia of the proximal (A1)* segment of the ACA in 22 percent of the cases (82). Two types of this phenomenon exist: mild and extreme hypoplasia. Mild hypoplasia has been noticed in 14 percent of the specimens. The hypoplastic vessel has ranged from 1.3 to 1.9 mm in diameter (average, 1.6 mm), and it was from 0.6 to 0.9 mm smaller than the opposite A1 portion. An extremely hypoplastic proximal segment has been present in 8 percent of the cases. It has varied from 0.3 to 1.1 mm in size (average, 0.9 mm) and has been more than 1.0 mm smaller than the opposite proximal segment. Both mild and extreme hypoplasia have been associated in 82 percent of the cases with the corresponding variations or malformations of the anterior cerebral, posterior cerebral, posterior communicating, and basilar arteries.

A study by Kitami et al. (83) found that anterior communicating aneurysms are related to changes in the ACA anatomy: (*a*) The aneurysm patients showed significant asymmetry of A1 ($p < .005$) compared with the other patients. (*b*) The left A1 portions were significantly dominant ($p < .05$) to the right in the aneurysm group. (*c*) Angiographic hypoplasias and aplasias of A1 were found in the aneurysm group more frequently than in the other group with statistical significance.

PERFORATORS

One to two dozen small vessels originate from the superior wall of the ACA and the ACoA. The lateral group feed the optic chiasm and anterior perforated substance (84). The medial group enter the supraoptic lamina. They feed the critical structures of the anterior diencephalon, hypothalamus, mesolimbic structures of subcaudate region, anterior commissure, fornix, and septum.

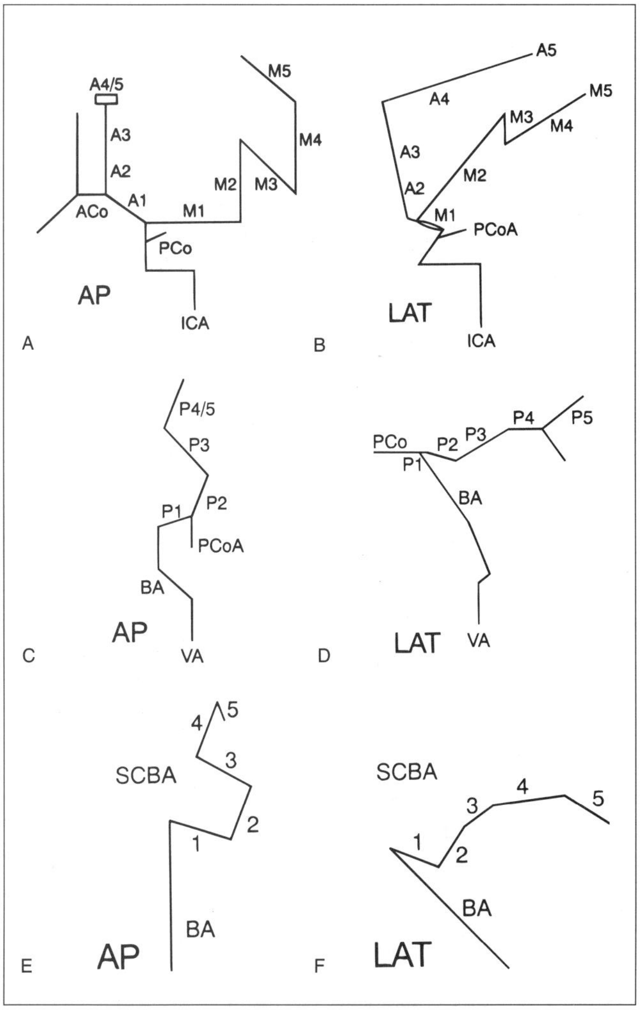

Figure 17.28. Modified Fischer methods to designate the various segments of the long circumferential branches of the internal carotid and vertebrobasilar system. **A.** Frontal carotid system. **B.** Lateral carotid system. **C.** Frontal vertebrobasilar. **D.** Lateral vertebrobasilar showing the vertebrobasilar and posterior cerebral artery. Frontal (**E**) and lateral (**F**) of basilar artery and superior cerebellar artery. ICA = internal carotid; ACO = anterior communicating; A = Anterior cerebral; M = middle cerebral; PCO = posterior communicating; VA = vertebral artery; P = posterior cerebral; BA = basilar artery; SCBA = superior cerebellar artery.

The recurrent artery of Heubner is the largest of the perforators and originates off the ACA in the area of the ACoA (85). It is both a telencephalic and diencephalic vessel. Developmentally the ACA contributed heavily to the striatum. This is a large remnant of that contribution and is in balance with the middle cerebral artery vessels. Coursing back laterally, it supplies the anterior limb of the internal capsule, the anterior inferior portion of the globus pallidus, and the head of the caudate. Additionally, the olfactory trigone and tract, paraterminal gyrus, and medial posterior orbital frontal cortex are the telencephalic portions of this vessel's territory.

In a study by Gomes et al. the recurrent artery of Heubner originated from the A2 segment of the ACA in 57 percent of the cases, from the ACA-ACoA junction in 35 percent, and from the A1 segment in 8 percent (86). The callosal arterial supply from the ACA showed short callosal branches in all brain specimens and long callosal vessels in 10 percent of the specimens.

The artery of Heubner and the perforating branches of the ACA are almost always present (82–88). The recurrent arteries of Heubner varied in number from one to three. They originated from the distal (A2) segment of the ACA in 34 percent of the cases, from the proximal (A1) segment of the ACA in 17 percent, at the level of the ACoA in 21 percent, from the fenestration of the ACA in 8 percent, and in all the other cases (20 percent) from the azygous anterior cerebral artery, accessory middle cerebral artery, frontopolar artery, and, finally, by the common stem with the medial orbitofrontal artery. The artery of Heubner most commonly terminated dorsal and lateral to the carotid bifurcation, at an average distance of 4.8 mm. The mean diameter was 662 μm, that of its extracerebral collateral branches 205 μm, of the terminal branches 462 μm, and of the intracerebral segments 354 μm. Perforating branches varied in number from 1 to 12, with an average of 6.6. The majority of the branches originated from the initial 6.1 mm of the A1 segment. These vessels terminated close to the carotid bifurcation, at an average distance of 3.8 mm. All the perforating branches were divided into small (average, 122 μm in diameter) and large (average, 325 μm). The mean diameter of intracerebral segments was 276 μm, and that of terminal branches 259 μm.

Anastomoses among the perforating arteries were studied in human brains using injection technique with India ink and gelatin, or methylmethacrylate (87). Anastomoses were not found among the perforators of the internal carotid artery and the thalamogeniculate branches. Anastomotic channels involving perforating branches of the AChA, middle cerebral artery, and ACA were noted in 1 percent of the cases. Vascular connections of the premammillary arteries were observed in 30 percent of the brains. They varied from 60 to 280 μm in diameter and from 0.3 to 3.6 (mean, 1.5 mm) in length. Anastomoses among the interpeduncular (thalamoperforate) branches of the posterior cerebral artery were present in 79 percent of the cases. They ranged from 80 to 400 μm (mean, 146 μm) in caliber and from 0.9 to 6.1 mm (mean, 3.3 mm) in length. Since anastomoses among the interpeduncular and the premammillary arteries are much more frequent than those among other perforators, thalamic, subthalamic, and midbrain infarctions seem to be less frequent than capsular and ganglionic ischemic lesions.

ANTERIOR COMMUNICATING ARTERY

A short, small segment invariably connects the ACA and ACoA although it commonly is not demonstrated angiographically. True aplasia of the ACoA artery is rare. The medial perforators off the ACoA are part of the medial group discussed earlier.

The ACoA branches are divided by Marinkovic et al. into the small and the large (88). Small branches were from 1 to 5 in number (mean, 2), and from 70 to 270 μm in diameter (mean, 151 μm). Seventy-six percent of the branches originated directly from the ACoA. They tend to arise closer to the left than to the right ACA. Fourteen percent of them arose from the junctional site of the ACoA with the ACA and 10 percent from the site of origin of the subcallosal artery. Large branches were identified as the *median artery of the corpus callosum* and the *subcallosal artery*, respectively. The former vessel was present in 9 percent of the patients and the latter in 91 percent. The subcallosal artery was from 320 to 640 μm in size (mean, 486 μm). It tended to arise from the middle of the ACoA. Anastomoses involving the ACoA branches are very frequent.

BRANCHES

In studying the branches of the major cerebral arteries, it should be kept in mind that variation is the rule. Regardless of the variation in the course and division of the cortical branches, a fixed area is fed by each vessel (89). A useful nomenclature rests on the vessel's relation to the cistern and distance from its origin (90) (Fig. 17.28). The A1 is the segment between the internal carotid and the ACoA; the A2 segment is distal to the ACoA below the corpus callosum; A3 is the pericallosal portion; A4 is the midsupra callosal portion; and A5 is the terminal portion of the vessel.

Eight named cortical territories are virtually always appreciated regardless of the proximal origin; a single vessel (occasionally two vessels) supplies each territory. They can best be identified in lateral view with the help of a template (91).

Cortical Branches of the ACA	Area
Orbitofrontal artery	Orbital surface of frontal lobe
Frontopolar artery	Anterior aspect frontal lobe
Anterior internal frontal artery Middle internal frontal artery Posterior internal frontal artery	Internal surface of frontal lobe
Paracentral artery	Paracentral lobule
Superior internal parietal	Internal surface of parietal lobe
Pericallosal artery	Branches to corpus callosum Branches to dura

Distally the inferior internal parietal and the posterior pericallosal anastomose with branches of the posterior cerebral artery. The anterior branches anastomose with the homologous branches of the middle cerebral artery. Each vessel has anastomotic branches with its neighbor via gyral anastomoses. If needed, these can be quite robust.

The branches can also be named relative to their trunks. This is analogous to naming the middle cerebral artery by the anterior and posterior division. This clinically useful method of naming allows for the ambiguity inherent in many situations. This system divides the ACA into four branches: the orbitofrontal, frontopolar, callosomarginal, and pericallosal (92). The orbitofrontal and frontopolar are the same for both systems. The callosomarginal is usually the trunk for the internal frontal branches and the paracentral artery. The pericallosal artery usually acts as the trunk for the internal parietal branches and the distal pericallosal artery. The course of each of these is described in the following.

The *orbital branch* or *branches* (sometimes two or three in number) are the first to arise from the ascending portion of the ACA. They extend forward and downward to supply the orbital surface of the frontal lobe. These branches are usually not particularly conspicuous on the angiogram but often can be detected if sought. They may be displaced by subfrontal tumors, thus providing a clue to the extracerebral location of the mass. The orbital branch anastomoses with the orbitofrontal branch of the middle cerebral artery.

The *frontopolar branch* usually arises from the anterior cerebral artery proximal to the maximal bend (knee) of this vessel, but it may arise from the callosomarginal branch of the anterior cerebral artery. From its origin, the artery passes forward and usually upward to reach the region of the anterior pole of the frontal lobe. It ordinarily divides into two or three branches, which surround the anterior border of the frontal lobe and then turn laterally to reach the convexity of the hemisphere.

The origin of the frontopolar artery from the ACA as seen in the anteroposterior view is an important reference point for the remainder of the parent vessel. The relative position of the origin of the vessel depends on the projection used to take the anteroposterior film: if more craniocaudal angulation is used, the point of origin is projected lower; in turn, this can be related to the lateral view to determine corresponding segments in the two projections (Fig. 17.54).

The major branch of the ACA is the *callosomarginal artery*. It usually arises distal to the origin of the frontopolar artery. The callosomarginal artery passes upward, then backward, and gives off the anterior, middle, and posterior internal frontal branches (Fig. 17.29). It may terminate in the paracentral branch around the paracentral lobule. Sometimes the anterior internal frontal branch arises directly from the ACA; at other times the middle and posterior internal frontal branches may arise directly.

The callosomarginal artery is usually contained during part of its course in the callosomarginal sulcus, but as it passes dorsad it may leave this sulcus to traverse the cingulate gyrus, only to enter the cingulate sulcus or another sulcus farther back. This causes the artery or its branches to separate themselves from the midline when entering a

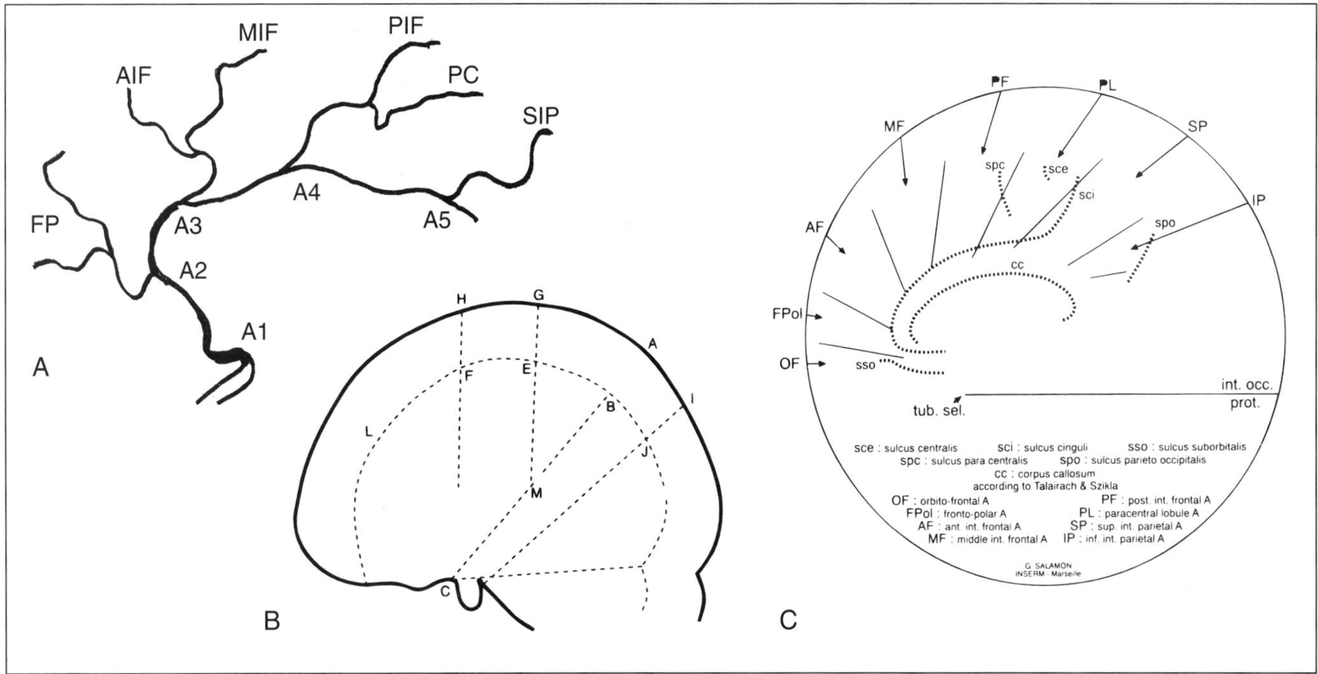

Figure 17.29. A. Diagram of anterior cerebral artery. The denominations A1 to A5 are indicated. FP = frontopolar; AIF = anterior internal frontal; MIF = middle internal frontal; PIF = posterior internal frontal; PC = paracentral; SIP = superior internal parietal. **B.** Procedure of Ring and Waddington (95) for the determination of the vascular territories of the anterior cerebral artery in the lateral projection. (1) A line (L) is constructed, 2.5 cm inside the inner table and parallel to it. (2) The clinoparietal line of Taveras and Wood (92) is drawn from the anterior clinoid process (C) to a point (A), situated 9 cm above the internal occipital protuberance. (3) The intersection of lines (L) and (CA) defines point (B). (4) The midpoint of line (CB) is defined as point (M). (5) From point (M), a vertical line is drawn, parallel to the coronal suture. This line defines point (E), where it crosses line (L), and point (G), where it intersects the inner table. (6) A vertical line (HF) is drawn through the coronal suture parallel to line (GEM). Point (H) is at the inner table and point (F) is on line (L). (7) Point (I) is located at the midpoint of the inner table between point (G) and the internal occipital protuberance. (8) Point (J) is located on line (L) where it intersects a line connecting point (I) with the posterior clinoid process. Space (EFGH) corresponds to the paracentral lobule. Space (EGIJ) corresponds to the precuneus. In front of the plane (HF) is the vascular territory of the internal frontal arteries. The paracentral lobule (EFGH) is supplied by the artery of the paracentral lobule. The precuneus (EGIJ) is vascularized by the internal parietal arteries. **C.** Template suggested by Salamon and Huang (96) to locate territories irrigated by anterior cerebral artery branches.

sulcus and to return to the midline when over a gyrus (Fig. 17.30). When the internal frontal and paracentral branches reach the upper margin of the hemisphere, they go over the top and turn out onto the convexity of the hemisphere, where they anastomose with pre- and postrolandic branches of the middle cerebral artery (Fig. 17.31).

The callosomarginal artery may originate just distal to the ACoA. In such a case, it ascends more or less parallel with the continuing part of the ACA, which then should probably be called the pericallosal artery. It sweeps around parallel to the pericallosal artery but describes a wider arc. With an early origin, the callosomarginal artery gives off not only the anterior, middle, and posterior internal frontal branches but the frontopolar branch as well (Fig. 17.29). In these cases, it will be found, not infrequently, that both pericallosal arteries fill from one side only (Fig. 17.32).

The *pericallosal artery* may be called the terminal branch of the ACA. It is usually fairly close to the outer surface of the corpus callosum except when tortuosity is present. Ordinarily, it gives off the paracentral branch, which may, however, arise from the callosomarginal. The pericallosal artery terminates as the precuneal branch, which supplies the precuneus, or as a posterior callosal branch, which supplies the corpus callosum, and also anastomoses with a branch of the posterior cerebral artery. Sometimes a branch from the right pericallosal artery may supply an area of the left hemisphere after crossing the midline, and vice versa (93) (Fig. 17.33).

The corpus callosum is usually outlined during the intermediate phase of the angiogram owing to the tangential direction of the x-ray beam over the corpus callosum. This causes the capillary network over the surface of the corpus callosum to cast a shadow, sometimes called the "mustache." Asymmetry of this corpus callosum blush may sometimes be useful in diagnosing intracranial masses but should not be relied upon too heavily. Elevation of the corpus callosum on one side may be due to a large ventricle on that side. Sometimes the corpus callosum blush is larger and more prominent on one side than the other. Thus, care should be taken not to "overread" these callosal asymmetries (Fig. 17.34).

The arterial vascularization of the corpus callosum is derived, although in an unequal way, from both of the arterial

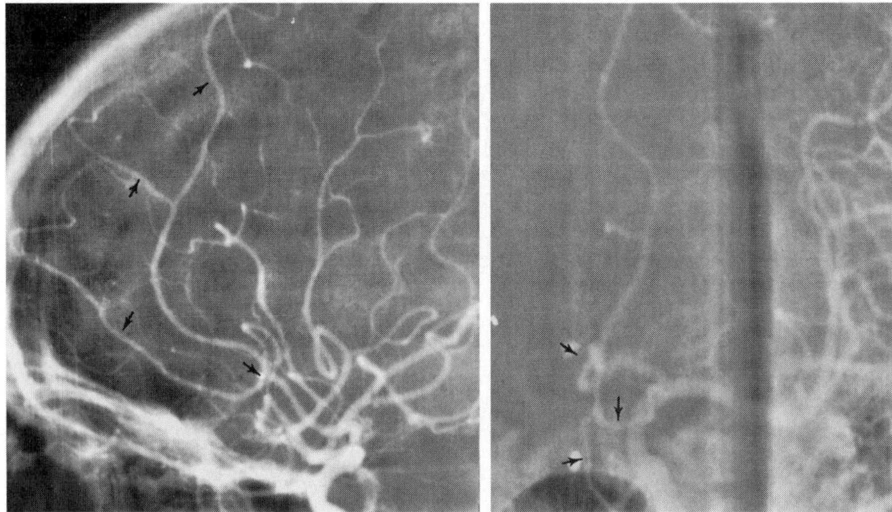

Figure 17.30. Anatomic variant of anterior cerebral artery. **A.** The lateral projection shows a branch of the anterior cerebral artery, the callosomarginal artery from which arise the frontopolar and the anterior and middle internal frontal branches (arrows). The pericallosal artery did not fill from this side but filled from the opposite side when the other carotid was injected. **B.** The frontal projection shows that the callosomarginal separates from the midline, probably because it entered the cingulate sulcus, thus giving the impression of a midline shift. The frontopolar artery and its branches are outlined by the three arrows.

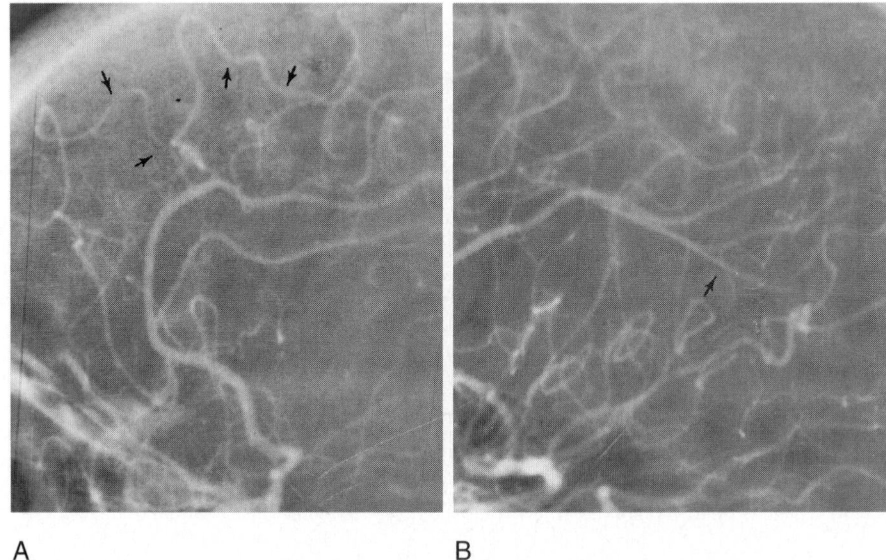

A B

Figure 17.31. **A.** Branches of the anterior cerebral artery going over the upper surface of hemisphere and onto the outer surface of hemisphere (arrows) in a patient with middle cerebral artery occlusion. **B.** Flattening of the posterior portion of the pericallosal artery (arrow). This is a normal variant.

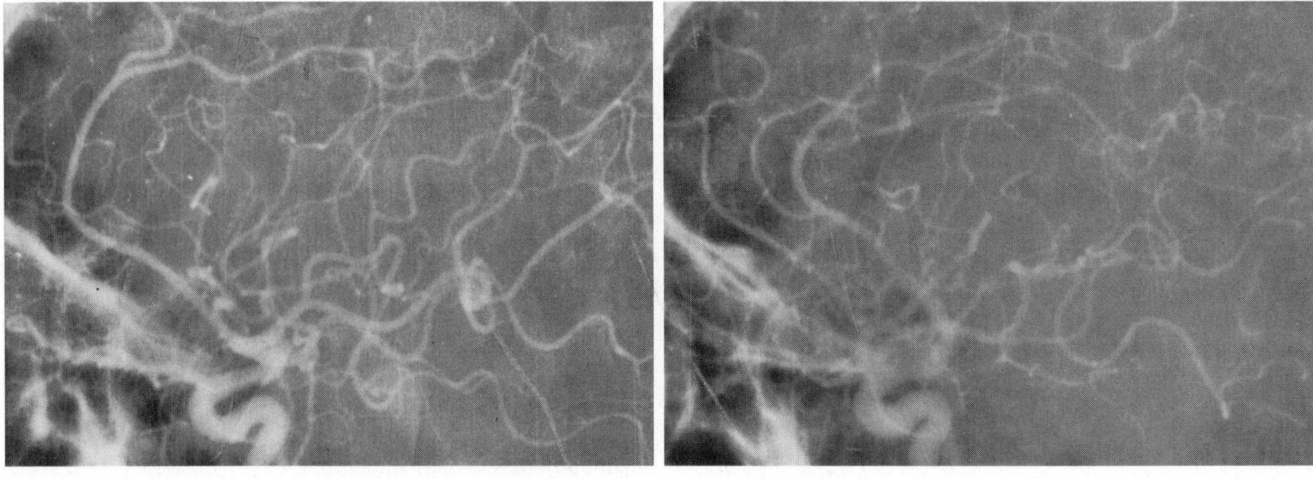

A B

Figure 17.32. Normal carotid angiogram, with both pericallosal arteries arising from one side and simulating ventricular dilatation on opposite side. **A.** When the first side was examined, it showed an apparently wide sweep of the anterior cerebral artery, which suggested ventricular dilatation. **B.** The second side was then injected and showed a normal pericallosal curve; the pericallosal arteries are almost completely superimposed on each other.

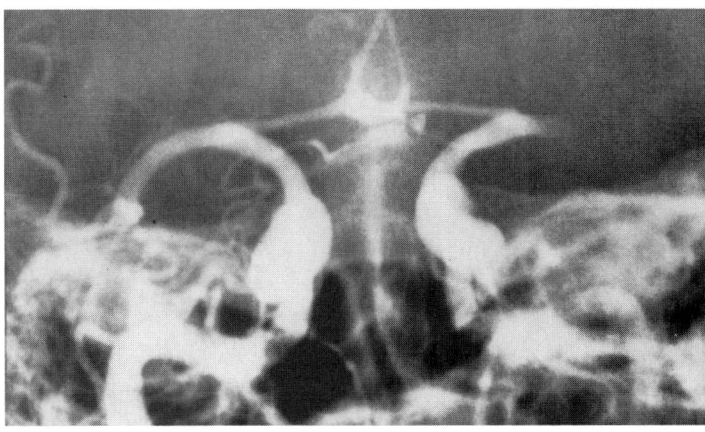
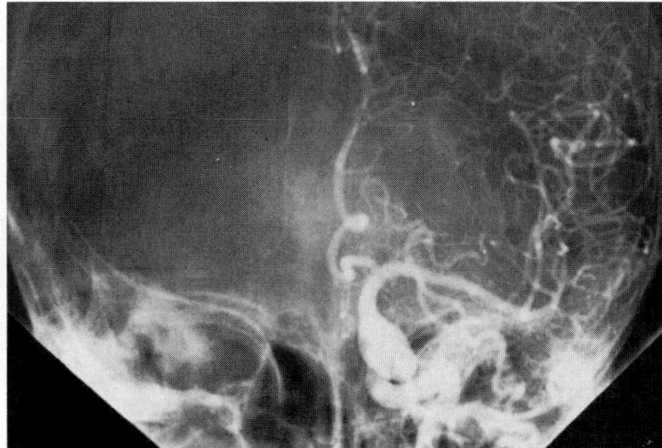

A B

Figure 17.33. Anterior communicating artery and variant of anterior cerebral arteries. **A.** The anterior communicating artery is very clearly visible owing to stretching of the horizontal segment of the anterior cerebral arteries and separation of the anterior cerebral arteries distal to this point. There is enlargement of the right side of the anterior communicating artery, probably due to an aneurysm. Separation of the anterior cerebral arteries in this region is commonly observed with aneurysms of the anterior communicating artery, often due to a hematoma or the mass of the aneurysm. **B.** The pericallosal artery is seen to give branches to both sides. It appears, from the number of branches crossing to the right side, that the major supply is via this route.

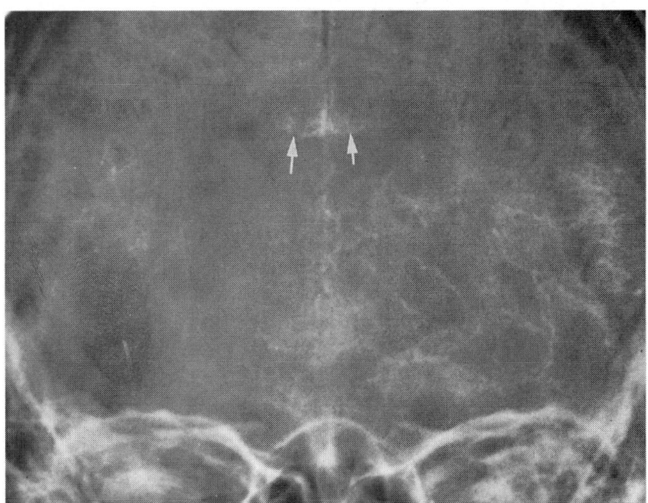

Figure 17.34. Capillary "blush" of corpus callosum in the intermediate phase of an angiogram. The "moustache" produced by the corpus capillary bed is slightly asymmetric, larger on the right, in a normal case (arrows).

systems of the brain: the carotid system and the vertebrobasilar system. According to Wolfram-Gabel et al., the carotid system contributes mainly to this supply by the ACA, which is the main artery of the corpus callosum (94). It accessorily contributes to it by the ACoA, which gives off an inconstant artery called the *median artery of the corpus callosum*. The vertebrobasilar system contributes to the blood supply of the corpus callosum by the terminal branches and by choroidal branches of the posterior cerebral artery. These various arteries give off perforating arteries that are direct or indirect and either short, of medium length, or long. Inside the corpus callosum, these various arteries give off numerous terminal and collateral branches, which run between the nervous fibers. They anastomose with homologous neighboring branches to form a characteristic vascular network. The arrangement of this network is in close connection with the disposition and the orientation of the commisural fibers, which form the different parts of the corpus callosum.

MEASUREMENTS

There is a tremendous range in size of the ACA, but usually the proximal ACA internal diameter is between 1 and 3 mm. The ACA branches can be identified in lateral projection by use of either a template or line tracings, according to the method suggested by Ring and Waddington (95). Salamon and Huang have constructed a template (96) (Fig. 17.29*B* and *C*).

EMBRYOLOGY AND VARIANTS

In the developing embryo the cranial division of the internal carotid artery terminates as the primitive olfactory artery made of two branches, the primary (lateral) one to the nasal fossa and a secondary (medial) one to the olfactory nerve root. The right and left olfactory arteries join, forming the future anterior communicating plexus. The growing of the hemisphere causes enlargement of the medial vessel, which becomes the dominant artery (16- to 18-mm embryo) (97).

In addition to the variants described earlier, others may be encountered. The initial portion of the ACA (A1) is usually horizontal, as seen in frontal films (Fig. 17.33), or it may turn downward. Sometimes, however, it is directed upward, giving a false impression of upward displacement, such as may be produced by a suprasellar or planum sphenoidale mass. The latter configuration is found more

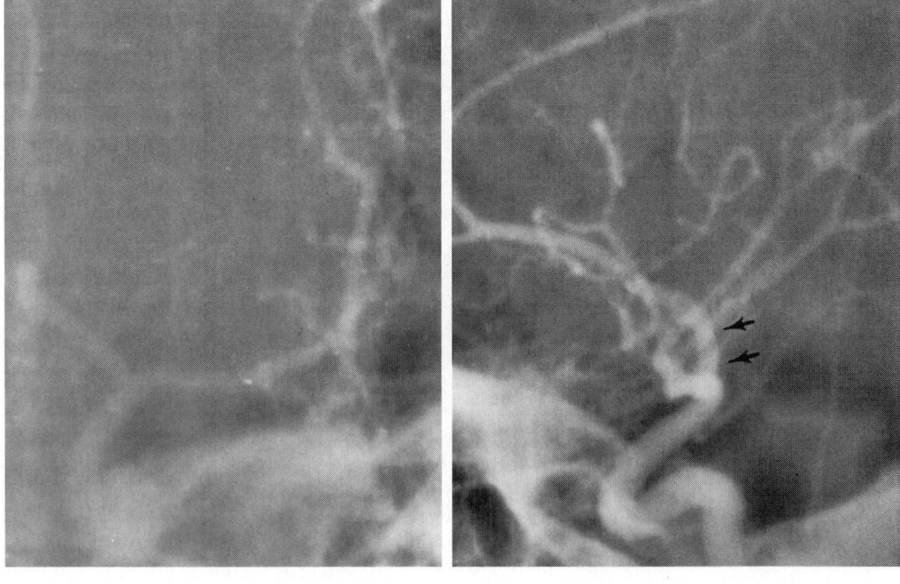

Figure 17.35. Normal carotid angiogram. **A.** The frontal projection shows that the anterior cerebral artery passes upward and medially instead of straight across or slightly downward. **B.** In the lateral projection there is also an upward course of the anterior cerebral artery in its proximal portion (arrows). This appearance is more commonly observed in children than in adults, and it is seen in older individuals where the arteries are atherosclerotic.

frequently in children than in adults (Fig. 17.35). In such cases, the proximal segment of the ACA is often directed more forward than usual, as well as upward.

As seen in the lateral view, the proximal segment of the ascending portion of the ACA (A1) may present a fairly deep curve concave downward, which should not be confused with a suprasellar or subfrontal tumor. More distally, another curve concave upward may be found normally just proximal to the knee (Fig. 17.27). Further dorsad, the pericallosal artery may present a flat segment, which corresponds to the same configuration of the pericallosal sulcus found in some cases (Fig. 17.31*B*). The segment may even present an upward concavity.

PROXIMAL PORTION

The origin of the ACA from the internal carotid artery may take place at the level of the ophthalmic artery. In these cases the artery may pass beneath the optic nerve as it courses medially (98–100).

Frequently one of A1 ACAs feeds both the A2 ACAs. Rarely is the A1 truly absent, although it is not unusual not to demonstrate it angiographically. Therefore, the lack of filling of the trunk of one ACA, even with compression of the opposite side during injection of the contrast substance, indicates that the segment is probably hypoplastic but not absent or thrombosed. Moreover, this hypoplastic segment usually is capable of dilating if partial or complete occlusion of the opposite internal carotid artery occurs. Spasm may also cause the ACA trunk to be thinner on one side. The same can be said for the ACoA. Numerous variations of the ACA have been described and postulated on the basis of embryology. Virtually always, the A1 ACA is cephalad to the optic nerve. In rare cases of duplication, one of the duplicates may lie under the nerve. Rarely, the origin of the ACA can be from the ophthalmic as well as the cavernous carotid.

An *accessory middle cerebral artery* may arise from the horizontal portion of the ACA, proximal to the ACoA, pass laterally, and ascend in the sylvian fissure together with the other branches of the middle cerebral artery (Fig. 17.36). It was found by Jain in 3 percent of cases, but angiographically the authors have recognized it in only a few instances (101). The accessory middle cerebral arteries may represent a variant of the recurrent artery of Heubner (102).

Onishi et al. also reported a patient with an anomalous right ACA originating from the right internal carotid artery immediately distal to the ophthalmic artery and running between the optic nerves associated with congenital skull dysplasia and other systemic bone anomalies, apparently an incomplete form of cleidocranial dysostosis and an aneurysm (103).

The ACoA is usually not clearly visible on the films unless there is some separation of the two anterior arteries (Fig. 17.33). This appearance (i.e., separation of the ACAs at the ACoA) is often seen in association with anterior communicating aneurysms and when observed raises the possibility of an unfilled aneurysm. The ACoA may be single or multiple. Duplications of the ACoA are unusual but appear to be more commonly associated with aneurysms, as are fenestrations.

Ogawa et al. found that 22 percent of patients with aneurysms of the ACoA had vascular anomalies in the vicinity of the ACoA (104). These included a median artery of the corpus callosum (MACC) in 27 cases (13 percent), duplication of the ACoA in 20 (10 percent), and duplication of the A1 segment of the ACA in 1 (0.5 percent). A retrospective study of the angiograms indicated that diagnosis of the A1 or ACoA duplication was not possible; only 11 (41

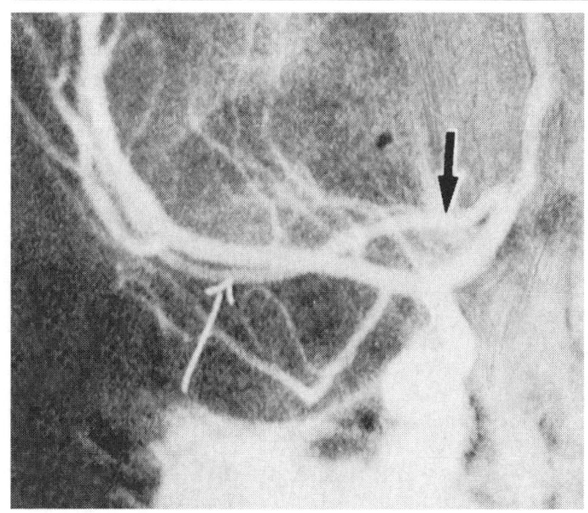

A

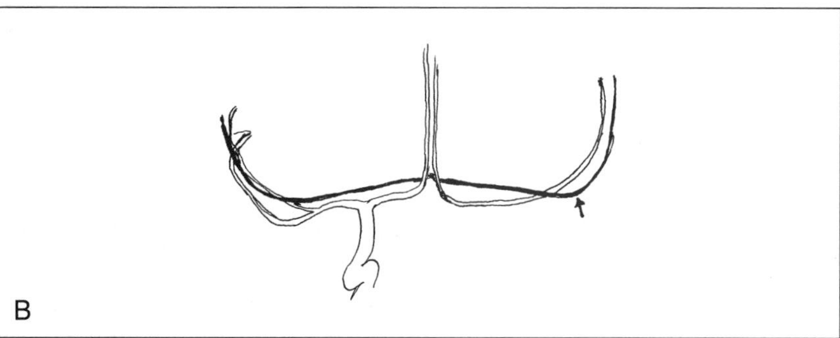

B

Figure 17.36. Branch of middle cerebral artery arising from the anterior cerebral artery in the region of the anterior communicating artery. **A.** The arrows point to the artery. **B.** Drawing from a case in which the middle cerebral branches were seen arising bilaterally from the anterior cerebral arteries (arrow).

percent) of the 27 MACCs were easily identified, while 8 (30 percent) could not be diagnosed. The majority of the cases of ACoA aneurysms with MACC (82 percent) showed trifurcation of the ACoA, A2, and MACC. The operative results in patients with MACC did not differ significantly from the results of the entire ACoA aneurysm series.

DISTAL PORTION

Variations in the distal ACA are sometimes seen. A single unpaired ACA and a segment of fused common proximal trunk are both unusual. In nearly one in six, however, a single ACA vessel supplies bilateral territories. Triplicate ACAs or accessory ACAs can also be seen. There may be a common trunk of the ACAs. In these cases, both horizontal segments join at the midline and thereafter ascend as a common trunk until reaching the falx. At this point they may separate into two groups of branches, one on each side of the falx. Rarely, the pericallosal artery may continue as a single artery giving branches to both sides (Fig. 17.33). The common trunk arrangement is found normally in the horse. There may be an additional ACA, the third vessel arising from the ACoA.

ABNORMALITIES OF THE ANTERIOR CEREBRAL ARTERY

Displacement by Subfalcial Herniations

Because the ACA and its branches are situated more forward, their position may be changed readily by rotation of the head at the time that the frontal film is made. In order to understand the mechanism of shift of the ACA and its branches as seen in the frontal angiogram, it is necessary to recall the relationship of the pericallosal, the frontopolar, and the callosomarginal arteries and their subdivisions with the edge of the falx. A glance at Figure 11.8 suffices to clarify the fact that the falx is narrow in the frontal region and gets progressively wider in its sagittal dimension as it extends backward. It becomes quite thick in the parieto-occipital region, where it joins the tentorium. Brain herniation across the midline occurs easily anteriorly but cannot occur posteriorly because the falx is too wide. The brain can herniate under the falx, but the falx is such a rigid structure that it cannot itself be displaced proportionately to the opposite side by the forces generated. Therefore, the vessels dislocate beneath the falx but return toward the midline as they reach the edge of the falx. Thus, the pericallosal artery, which is situated almost entirely under the edge of the falx, may be displaced throughout its entire extent except for its terminal branch. The frontopolar artery, although passing forward toward the narrow part, is first displaced and then returns to the midline as it reaches the edge of the falx. The callosomarginal artery, depending upon its configuration, is displaced in its more proximal portion, and in its more distal portions it returns to the midline. The same applies to branches of the callosomarginal artery. For this reason, a "step" is often visualized when an artery suddenly changes direction to reach the midline. The presence of a "square step" is almost always an indication of a true shift and is not produced either by rotation of the head at the time that the film was made or by excessive tortuosity of the vessels.

A shift of the anterior cerebral vessels may involve the proximal portion, the central portion, or the distal portion. It may also involve the entire course of the vessels. The way in which the artery is shifted is quite important, and very often it is possible to locate a mass in a general manner, even before looking at the lateral view. Shifts of the anterior cerebral vessels may be divided into several categories.

1. *Round shift.* The ACA and its branches form an arc as they are displaced across the midline. This is typical of frontal tumors. It indicates that the center of the tumor is probably at or near the level of origin of the pericallosal artery along the rostral portion of the anterior cerebral artery (see Fig. 11.8*A* and Fig. 17.37). Such a mass usually displaces the pericallosal artery and also the origins and proximal parts of the frontopolar and callosomarginal arteries.

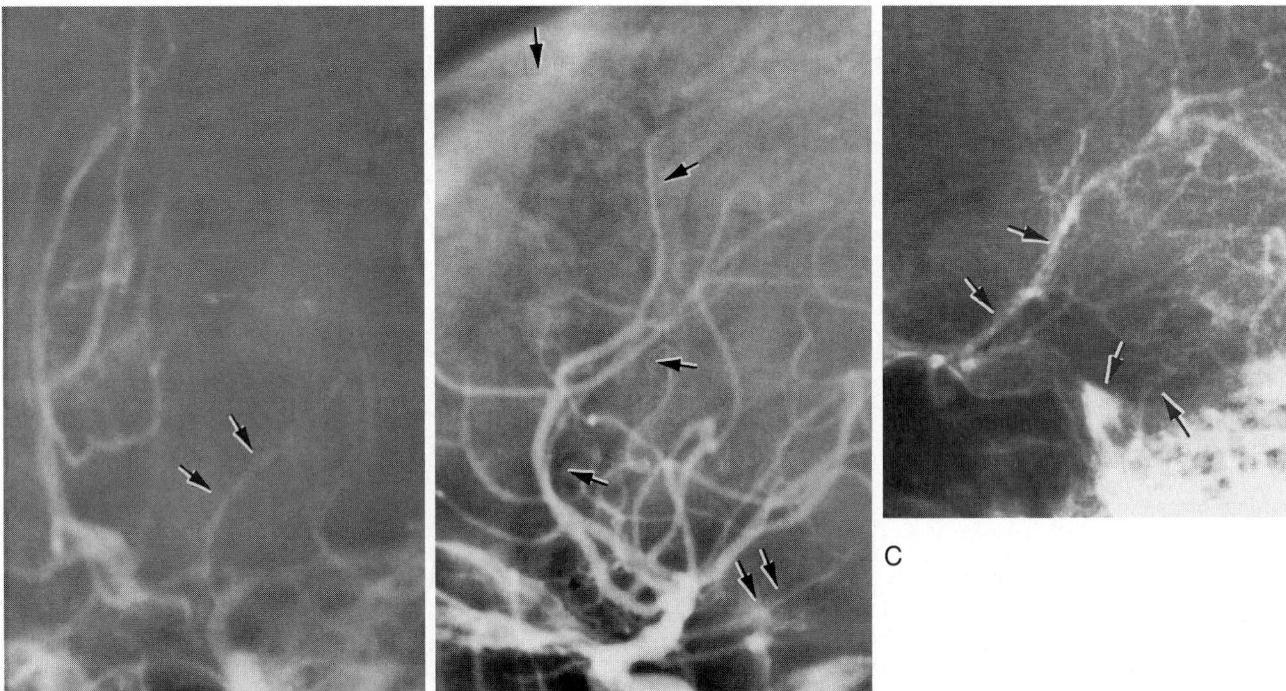

Figure 17.37. Uncal and retroalar herniations in patients with frontal lobe tumors. **A.** The frontal projection shows an increase in the length of the arc described by the anterior choroidal artery, which is at the same time slightly displaced medially (arrows). The tumor was frontal in location, and the increase in the curvature of the anterior choroidal artery cannot be ascribed to infiltration of the medial portion of the temporal lobe by tumor. The typical configuration of the rounded midline shift usually associated with anterior frontal tumors is present. **B.** The lateral projection of the same patient shows disruption of the branches of the anterior cerebral artery, which are stretched, and the curve of the pericaliosal artery, which is blunted (arrows). The anterior choroidal artery is stretched and enlarged (two arrows). The enlargement of the anterior choroidalartery does not necessarily imply that there is blood supply of the tumor by the anterior choroidal artery but is a phenomenon observed in patients with intracranial tumors in any location. **C.** In another patient with a large frontal astrocytoma, the superficial middle cerebral (sylvian) vein (*anterior arrows*) is displaced backward far behind the sphenoid ridge, and its curve is reversed. The uncal herniation is evidenced by compression of the top of the basilar plexus (middle arrow) and backward displacement of the upper part of the anterior pontomesencephalic vein (posterior arrow).

2. *Square shift.* In this type of shift, there is a very well-defined step beneath the falx. As the anterior cerebral artery is followed proximally from the step, it is seen to descend straight downward forming a fairly square angle along the lower portion of the artery. This type of shift indicates that the tumor is situated behind the anterior portion of the artery and the origin of the pericallosal artery (see Fig. 11.8*B*). It is not necessary that the ACA extend straight downward to have a square shift. If the proximal and the distal (immediate subfalcial) portions are *equally displaced,* it is a square shift. The ACA can return toward the midline between the two displaced portions because of its relationship to the falx; if the rostral part of the artery extends more anteriorly than the falx edge, it returns to the midline in that portion only (see Fig. 11.9 and Fig. 17.38).
3. *Proximal shift.* The inferior portion of the anterior cerebral artery is displaced across the midline and the artery, then ascends obliquely toward the midsagittal plane. It is *less shifted* in its upper portion, or it may reach the midline as it ascends, without forming a step under the falx. This usually indicates that the tumor is inferiorly located. The proximal shift is a hallmark of sphenoid ridge meningiomas, but it is often seen with anterior temporal lobe tumors. It is also found with lesions situated subfrontally or in the inferior deep frontal region, but which are not large enough to produce a round shift (see Fig. 11.8*C*).
4. *Distal Shift.* There is a well-defined step under the falx where the vessels are displaced across the midline. The anterior cerebral artery is *less shifted,* or actually is situated in the midline, in its inferior portion. Thus, the vessel is oblique in a direction opposite to that seen with a proximal shift. This is typical of tumors situated posteriorly along the superior convexity of the hemisphere or in the parasagittal region (see Fig. 11.8*D*).

The so-called *frontopolar sign,* as described by Fischer (91), is produced when the ACA is shifted, and the frontopolar artery is also displaced in its proximal portion. As the distal portion of the frontopolar artery reaches the falx anteriorly, it returns to the midline. Upon doing this, it appears to pull the pericallosal artery slightly toward the midline, thus producing a checkrein effect. The frontopo-

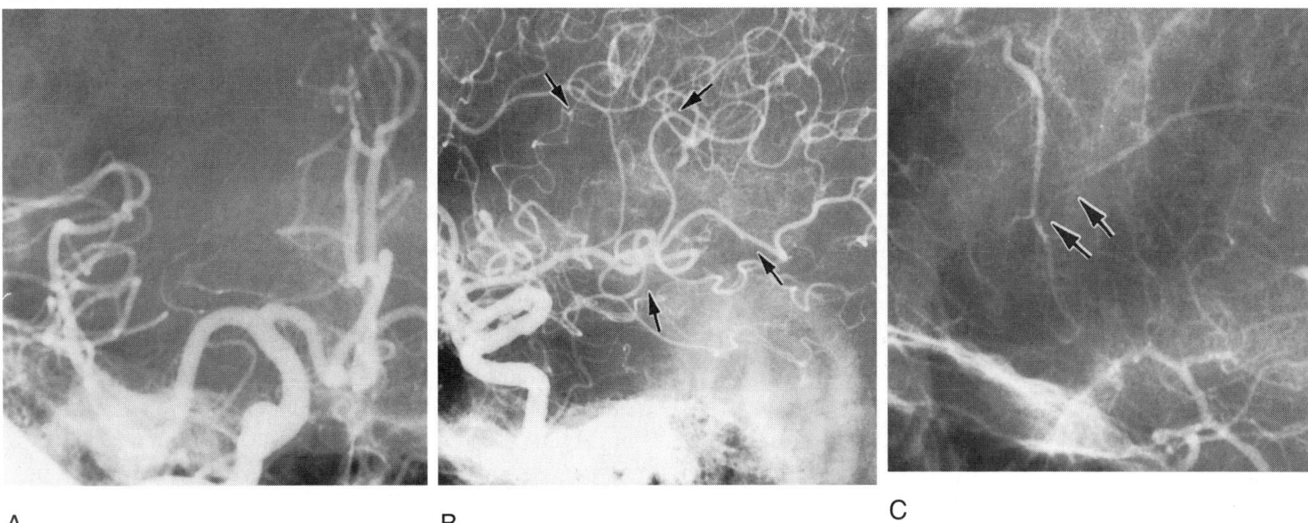

A B C

Figure 17.38. Square shift of anterior cerebral artery. **A.** Proximal and distal shifts of the anterior cerebral artery are demonstrated; the central portion of the anterior cerebral artery returns to the midline. **B.** Lateral view showing the largest portion of the posterior suprasylvian tumor behind the frontal lobe (arrows). **C.** The venous phase shows that the inferior longitudinal sinus, representing the free edge of the falx, indeed crosses the genu of the pericallosal artery, when transferred to B, thus forcing the rostral part of the vessel to return to the midline (arrows).

lar sign indicates that the tumor is behind the coronal plane of the knee of the pericallosal artery. The sign is observed infrequently, and in standard anteroposterior views, the checkrein effect is not produced by the frontopolar but by the callosomarginal artery.

In order to evaluate the significance of arterial shifts, the observer should first glance at the other vessels and try to assess the general tortuosity of the ACA and its branches. The shift of these vessels should be estimated in the proximal and in the distal portions of the artery. The central portion, the general area of the knee of the pericallosal artery, often presents an additional bulge to the opposite side or to the same side, which is normal. In fact, as mentioned above, in some instances where there is a definite shift to the opposite side, the central portion or knee of the pericallosal artery returns to the midline (see Fig. 11.9). There are three possible mechanisms to explain this phenomenon. The knee of the pericallosal artery, as it swings forward, may go past the edge of the falx, as already illustrated in Figure 17.38; the larger frontal horn on the side opposite the tumor may tend to bulge toward the midline; or the artery or arteries may be contained within a sulcus on the side of the tumor during part of their course.

A measured shift of the ACA of 3 mm or more is usually considered significant, but a conclusion should be reached with care because of the normal wavy course or arteriosclerotic tortuosity of the vessels. If the head is rotated toward the side opposite the injection, the ACA and its branches acquire a slightly rounded shape without the formation of a step at the edge of the falx. Rotation to the same side as the injection would produce an ipsilateral curve, the opposite direction to that just described. It is possible to estimate the degree of displacement due to rotation of the head by measuring the distance between the temporal bone (as shown in the anteroposterior film) and the zygomatic process of the frontal bone, and comparing this distance on the two sides. The zygomatic process of the frontal bone is situated in almost the same coronal plane as the knee of the ACA. Since this bony process is almost always visible on the angiogram, it serves as a good landmark for deciding whether the vessel is shifted or rotated.

Herniation of the cingulate gyrus can be suspected on angiograms from the appearance of the callosomarginal branches. The vessels are displaced to the opposite side and, after reaching a certain level, extend downward (i.e., pass caudad, to go under the edge of the falx to reach the midline again) (Fig. 17.39). Complete herniation of the cingulate gyrus is most commonly present with a parasagittal tumor but may be present with any large neoplasm, subdural hematoma, or abscess.

Angiographic findings may be present in connection with nonneoplastic processes that result in vascular displacement. Thus, degenerative changes on one side of the brain may cause a midline shift, which may, on superficial inspection, be thought to be the result of displacement by a mass rather than loss of substance. Such changes are found most frequently in cases of hemiatrophy of the brain resulting from early cerebral damage; this may be caused by trauma or by early vascular occlusion or by an interference with normal growth of any etiology (Fig. 17.40).

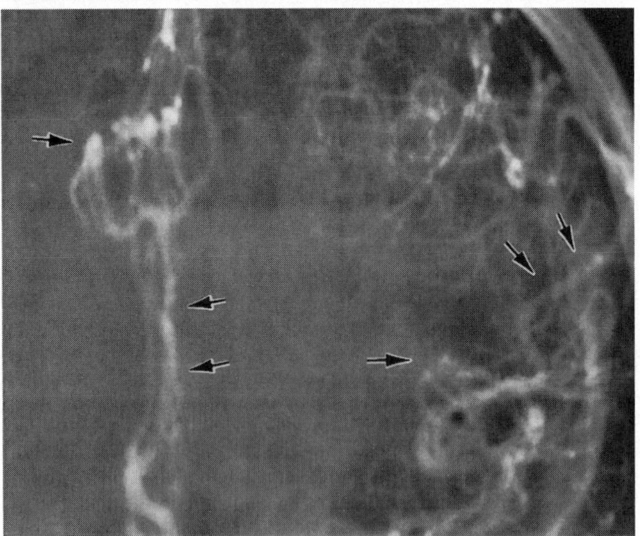

Figure 17.39. High convexity meningioma producing distal shift and herniation of cingulate gyrus. Although the distal portions of the anterior cerebral vessels are markedly displaced across the midline, the central portion of the anterior cerebral artery returns almost to the midline (lower central arrows), but the proximal portion is also shifted. This may be due to greater dilatation of the contralateral frontal horn, or the central segments of the vessels may be within a sulcus instead of on a gyrus so that they are not displaced as far across the midline. There is marked downward displacement of the angiographic sylvian point, with the last emerging vessel extending upward and lateralward (lateral arrows). This is because the center of the neoplasm is high on the convexity, and, although it is a meningioma, the sloping skull surface brings the center of the tumor far medially. The cingulate herniation is denoted by the disposition of the callosomarginal branches, which appear to duplicate their course (upper central arrow). Since the vessels cross the medial aspect of the cingulate gyrus, they are carried contralaterally but must turn back downward to pass under the edge of the falx to reach the midline again before ascending farther.

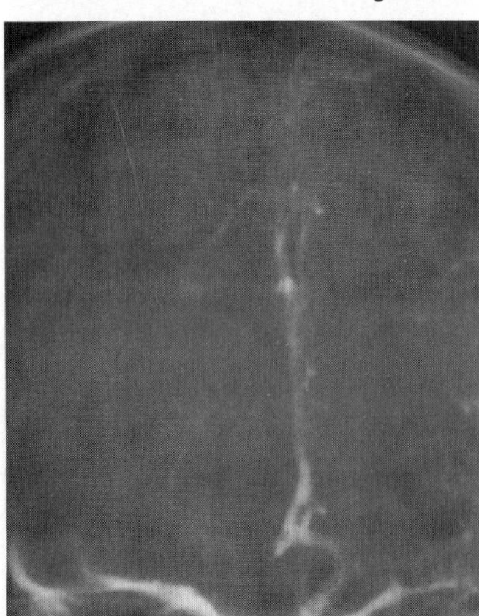

Figure 17.40. Marked off-center position of anterior cerebral vessels in patients with cerebral hemiatrophy. The anterior cerebral artery ascends straight upward and was off center almost 2 cm in the original film. The asymmetry of the skull is plainly visible; the convexity of the skull on the left side, the side of the angiogram, is much less rounded than on the opposite side.

Hydrocephalus and Agenesis of the Corpus Callosum

Severe hydrocephalus will cause stretching of the ACAs around the ventricular system with straightening and elevation of its course. The pial mustache takes on a V shape as the lateral edges of the corpus callosum are bowed upward.

In patients with agenesis of the corpus callosum, the pericallosal artery is either low or absent, with the branches of the ACA having an upward and diagonally radiating pattern toward the convexity.

Middle Cerebral Artery

The middle cerebral artery is the dominant branch of the internal carotid artery and supplies the lateral two-thirds of each of the cerebral hemispheres and the adjacent subcortical regions. This area includes motor, tactile, and auditory areas as well as the associated areas of higher cortical funtion, including language.

The main trunk of the middle cerebral artery (M1) courses above the sphenoid wing in the sylvian vallecula, giving off important lenticulostriate arteries that penetrate the anterior perforated substance. At the anterior portion of the sylvian fissure, at the bottom of the insula, the middle cerebral artery bifurcates or trifurcates and ascends over the insula (M2) before fanning out and passing under the operculum (M3) to reach the lateral surface (M4) and terminate just below the crest of the cerebral hemisphere.

COURSE

The middle cerebral artery is a continuation, or the main branch, of the internal carotid artery. It is never absent in a normal case, for it is more than likely that the corresponding hemisphere would fail to develop normally. When the anterior cerebral artery does not fill, the internal carotid artery extends onward uninterrupted directly laterally to become the middle cerebral artery. Its origin usually is on the medial aspect of the temporal lobe. The proximal portion of the middle cerebral artery is nearly horizontal in its course as it passes laterally and slightly forward. It often extends laterally, forward, and slightly downward (as does

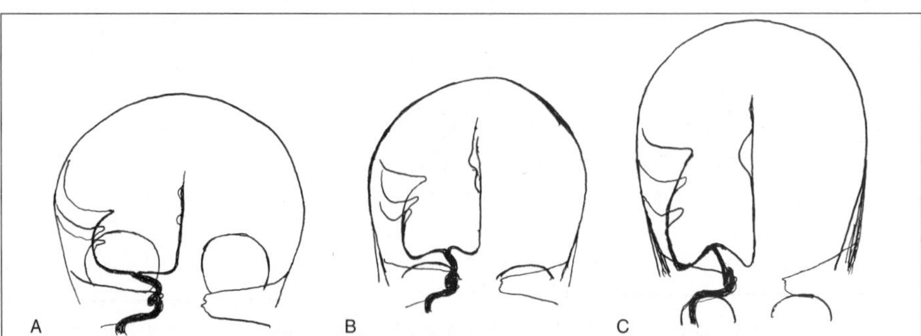

Figure 17.41. Appearance of the internal carotid artery and its branches according to projection. **A.** Orbital view. **B.** Standard angiographic anteroposterior projection. **C.** Half-axial projection.

the anterior cerebral artery); only occasionally does it extend laterally and upward in a normal case when the standard angiographic anteroposterior projection (12° caudad angulation above the orbitomeatal line) is used. It must be realized that because both the anterior and middle cerebral arteries in their "horizontal segments" are directed forward, the standard frontal view tends to project the distal portion of this segment of each artery downward. The slight downward turn of these arteries is therefore exaggerated when a greater degree of caudad angulation is employed. The opposite is true when less caudad angulation is used and when an orbital projection is taken (Fig. 17.41).

As seen in the lateral view, this initial segment is foreshortened by virtue of its lateral direction. Although appearing short, it should be sought since it is usually evident except in children, where it may not be discernible. If the segment is not visible in a straight lateral view, posterior displacement of this portion of the artery may be present (Figs. 17.27 to 17.35). The actual extent of the lateral and forward direction of this segment of the middle cerebral artery may be best shown on a basal view (Figs. 17.42, 17.44 and 17.45).

As the middle cerebral artery extends laterally from the bifurcation, it is situated between the temporal lobe and the lower aspect of the insula or island of Reil (Fig. 17.43). The middle cerebral artery and its branches then turn around the lower part of the island of Reil to continue their course upward and backward in the deepest portion of the sylvian fissure, between the outer surface of the island of Reil and the medial surface of the temporal lobe (Figs. 17.44 and 17.45). By this time the middle cerebral artery has given off several branches, which will be described presently.

Variation in the manner in which the middle cerebral branches originate from the common trunk, as well as in the number of branches formed, is the rule. However, it is best to consider the middle cerebral as bifurcating or trifurcating at, or just before reaching, the end of its horizontal segment. From these branches, other divisions arise that are all contained initially within the sylvian fissure and that leave the fissure at various levels between its anterior and its posterior extent.

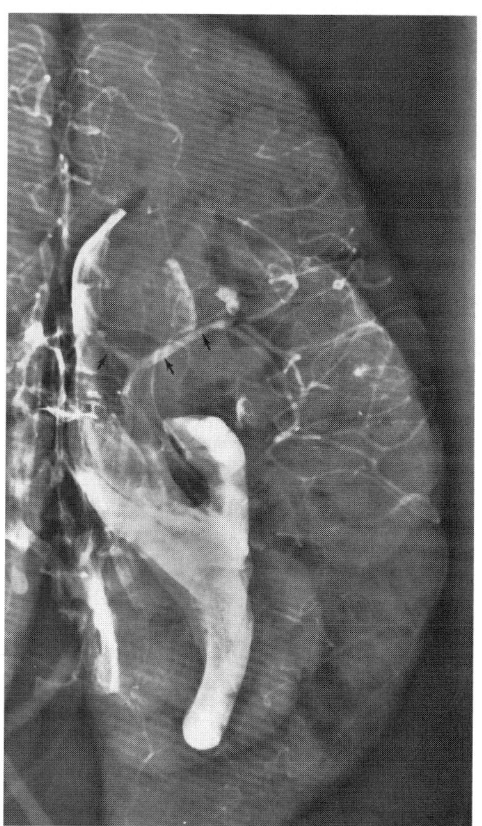

Figure 17.42. Angiogram of specimen in base projection with opacification of the ventricular system. The bifurcation of the internal carotid artery is shown, and its position in relation to the ventricles is seen. The middle cerebral artery describes a curve concave backward (lower arrows). The anterior cerebral artery is directed forward and medially (upper arrow).

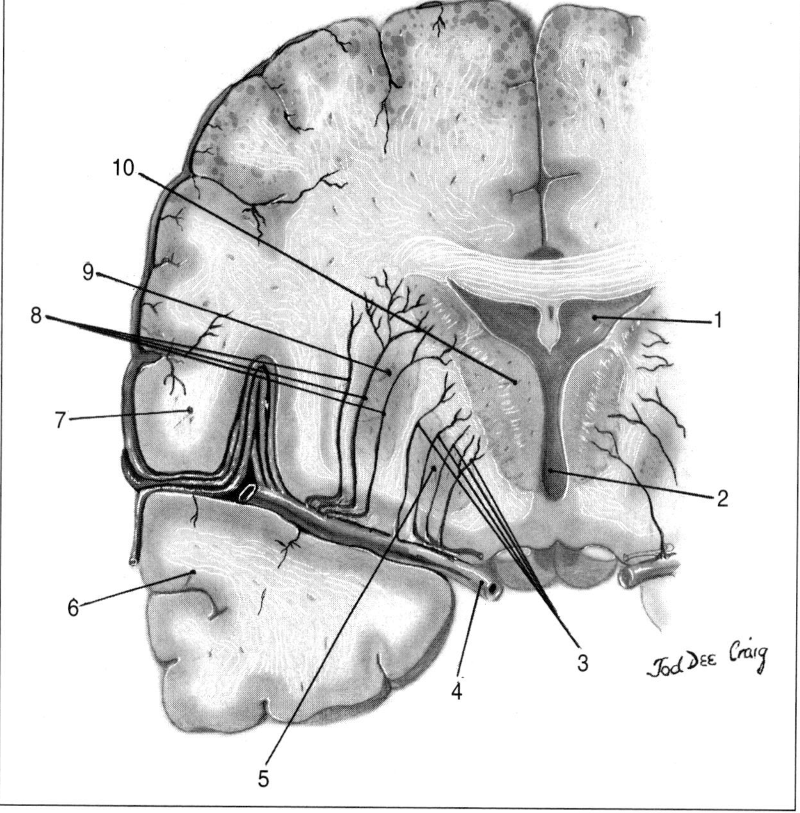

Figure 17.43. Coronal section of the brain through the anterior temporal region—diagrammatic representation. The diagram shows the branches of the middle cerebral artery as they pass upward to the top of the sylvian fissure and then downward before emerging from the fissure: (1) lateral ventricle; (2) third ventricle; (3) medial lenticulostriate arteries mostly arising from artery of Heubner; (4) middle cerebral artery; (5) globus pallidus; (6) temporal lobe; (7) frontoparietal operculum; (8) lateral lenticulostriate arteries; (9) putamen; (10) caudate nucleus.

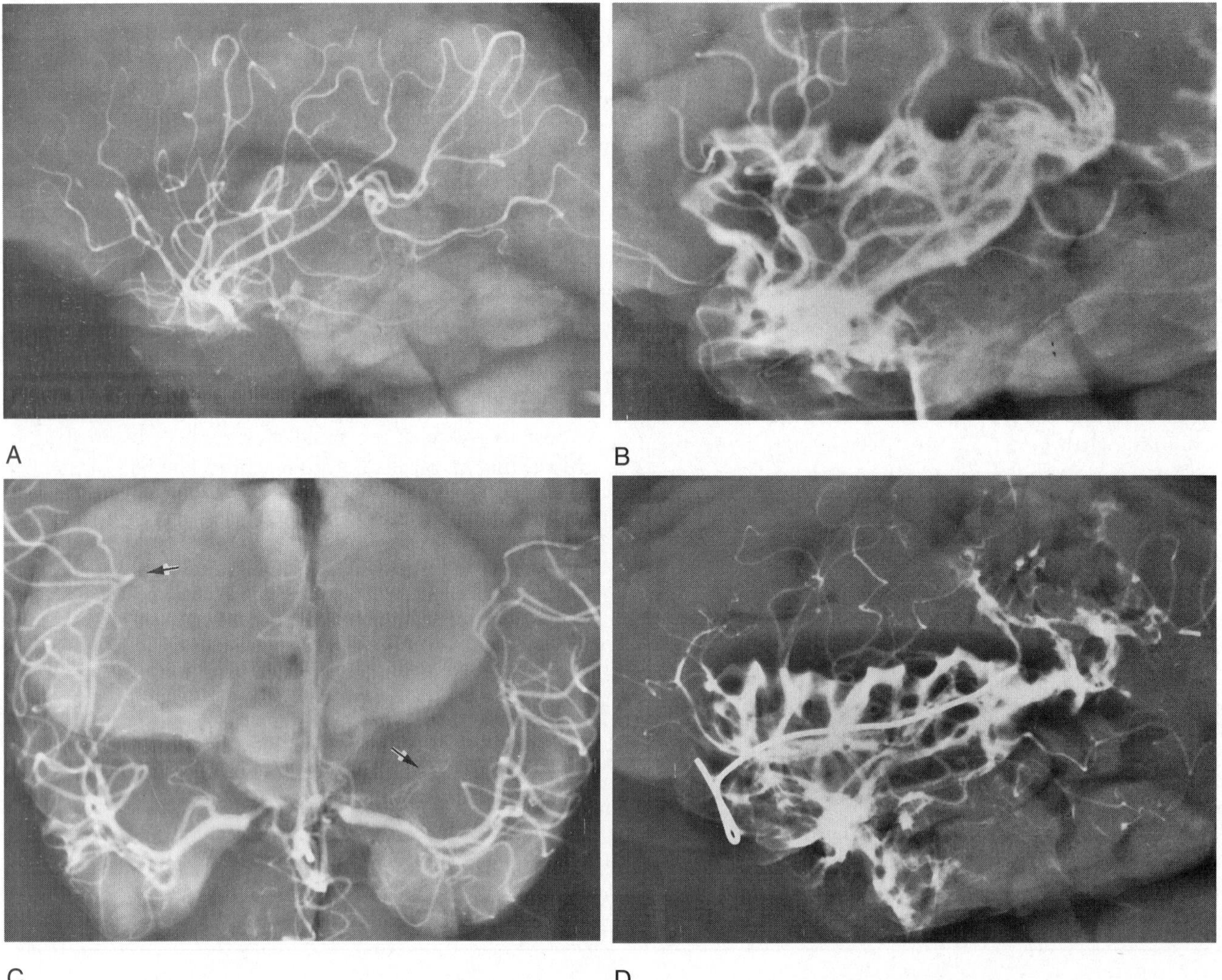

Figure 17.44. Postmortem injection of arteries of brain in normal specimens. **A.** Lateral view, after injection of the middle cerebral artery. **B.** The sylvian triangle can be visualized but becomes much more clearly shown after injecting the sylvian fissure with radiopaque material as shown in a different specimen. **C.** Anteroposterior view of the middle cerebral vessels on both sides demonstrating the configuration of the middle cerebral branches around the insula. The more anterior branches are the lower ones, and the most posterior one forms the angiographic sylvian point (upper arrow). The lenticulostriate arteries are very well shown (lower arrow). **D.** In another specimen wire has been placed over the sylvian fissure to demonstrate its relationship with the sylvian triangle.

BRANCHES

Proximally, a set of striate perforating arteries to the striatum and the surrounding white matter tracts is given off. Distally, the middle cerebral artery bifurcates and gives rise to 13 cortical territories, with their branches feeding the the frontal, parietal, and temporal lobes.

Striate Arteries

These central branches arise from the anterior cerebral and from the middle cerebral arteries; for discussion they will be placed together here since they are also in hemodynamic and developmental balance. The middle cerebral striate arteries supply the lateral portion of the anterior commissure, most of the putamen and lateral segment of the globus pallidus, the superior half of the internal capsule and adjacent corona radiata, and the body and head of the caudate nucleus—except the anterior inferior portion (105).

The striate arteries arising from the horizontal portion of the middle cerebral artery are represented by two groups of three to six small branches, the medial and the lateral striate arteries, which ascend from their origins to penetrate the brain through the anterior perforated substance. The arteries (three to six) of the medial group are usually short, 1.0 to 1.2 cm in length, and small, 0.1 to 0.2 mm in diameter (106). They tend to rise nearly at right angles with the trunk of the middle cerebral artery. They supply the globus pallidus and are not easily seen on carotid angiograms. According to Westberg, the medial lenticulostriate arteries seen in angiograms are usually branches of the artery of Heubner (107, 108) (Figs. 17.43 and 17.46).

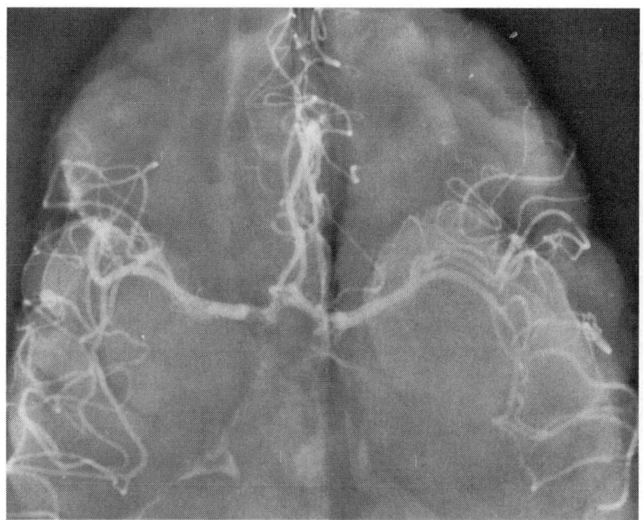

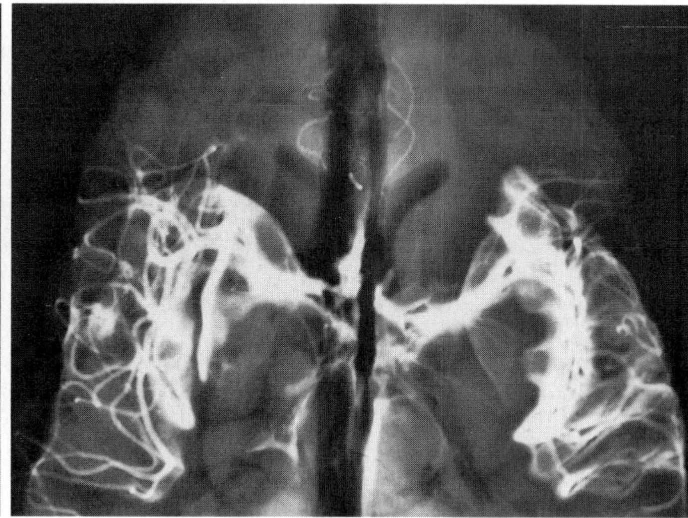

A B

Figure 17.45. Base view, arteriogram of specimen. **A.** The initial picture shows the normal configuration of the middle cerebral artery in the sylvian fissure. **B.** The sylvian fissure was then injected with barium and another film taken.

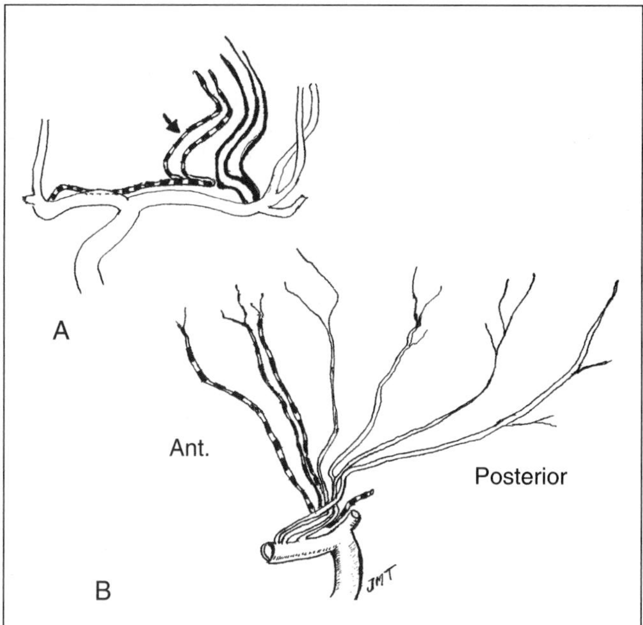

Figure 17.46. Striate arteries according to Westberg (108) and also Stephens and Stillwell (105). The medial striate arteries (arrow) (**A**) are anterior, as seen in the lateral view (**B**). The fan shape of the course of the striate arteries is well shown (B).

The lateral striate group (arteries 0.5 to 0.6 mm in diameter) usually originates from the lateral part of the horizontal segment of the middle cerebral artery but can originate more medially (105). Jain found lateral striate arteries originating from the proximal portion of the trunk of the middle cerebral artery in 54.6 percent of dissections, from the point of the first main bifurcation in 25.6 percent, and from a branch of the middle cerebral in 20.3 percent of cases (101). Thus, it appears that, at least one-half of the time, the origins of the major lateral lenticulostriate arteries are rather medial in position.

Immediately after arising from the middle cerebral artery, the lateral striate arteries are directed medially and posteriorly for a distance of 6 to 10 mm, after which they turn upward and laterally, describing a curve convex medially. As they continue, the curve is reversed, so that an S-shaped curve is formed on the right side and a reversed S on the left (Figs. 17.47 and 17.48) as the observer faces the patient. The configuration is generally similar to that of the AChA.

The medial turn of the lateral striate arteries is rather sharp, and since it is at the same time directed posteriorly, it is best demonstrated in films taken with a standard angiographic projection (12° cephalocaudad angulation from the orbitomeatal line) or in one where a greater degree of caudad angulation is employed.

The striate arteries are usually visible if looked for in radiographs of good quality. Some of these arteries may arise directly from the internal carotid artery. The striate arteries may be enlarged in cases of thrombosis and with neoplasms producing increased intracranial pressure, particularly if the neoplasm is partly supplied by these vessels. It is probable that the prominence of the striate arteries in cases of thrombosis is directly related to the supply of vital areas. The vasodilatation may be associated with metabolic changes, or it may be the result of hypotension in the adjacent capillary beds.

From the horizontal portion of the ACA_1, tiny branches emerge that pierce the brain at the anterior perforated substance and supply the rostrum of the corpus callosum, part of the head of the caudate nucleus, and the septum pellucidum. The artery of Heubner also arises from this segment proximal to the ACoA. From this point the artery of Heubner passes laterally almost parallel with the horizontal portions of the anterior cerebral and of the middle cerebral

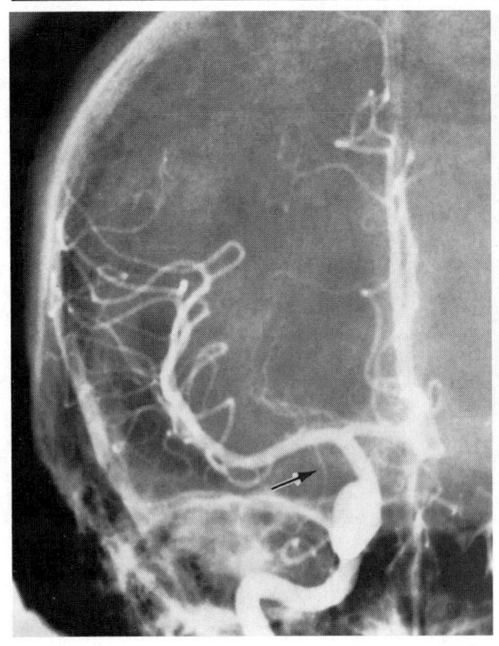

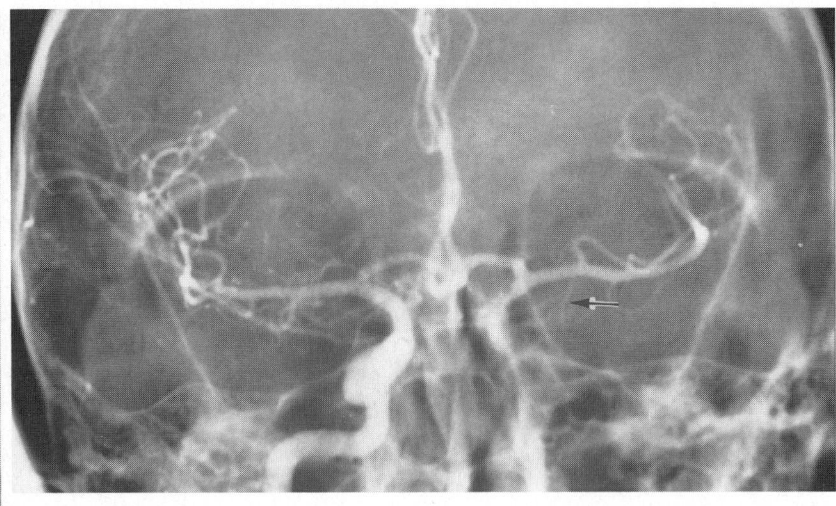

Figure 17.47. Anteroposterior view of carotid angiogram using standard angiographic projection (**A**) and transorbital projection (**B**). The anterior and the middle cerebral arteries appear to extend downward slightly in A but are horizontal or pass upward in B. The arrows in A and B indicate the anterior temporal artery on each side. The lenticulostriate arteries on the right present an S-shaped configuration.

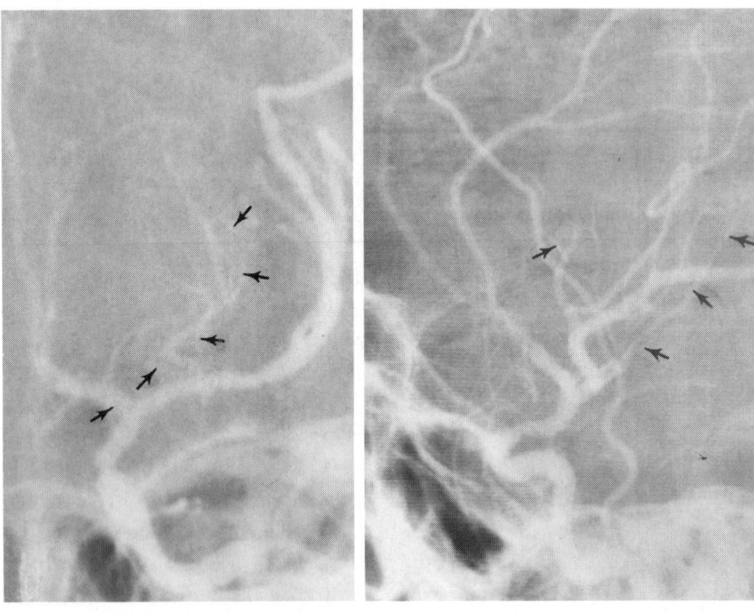

Figure 17.48. Striate arteries in frontal and lateral projection. **A.** The anteroposterior view shows the striate arteries arising from the horizontal portion of the middle cerebral artery (arrows). They describe a reverse S-shaped configuration. In this patient they are well developed, actually enlarged, because this 8-year-old child had an old thrombosis of the middle cerebral vessels and evidently the striate arteries enlarged to provide collateral supply. The anterior choroidal artery (lower arrow) is well shown. There is a slight irregularity of the initial portion of the middle cerebral artery, also extending into the two major branches seen on the films due to the old thrombosis with recanalization. **B.** The lateral view of the same patient shows the proximal part of striate branches unusually well and distributed in a triangular configuration with the apex at the middle cerebral artery (arrows). The irregularity of the arteries of the carotid siphon and the middle cerebral artery is even more conspicuous in the lateral view than in the frontal view, due to the old thrombosis. There are fewer than the usual number of branches present.

arteries until it reaches the origin of the lateral striate branches arising from the middle cerebral artery. At this point the artery swings upward to penetrate the brain through the anterior perforated substance and divides into several branches. The artery of Heubner is slightly tortuous and is usually concealed by the larger middle and anterior cerebral arteries, but it can be demonstrated much more frequently in oblique views. Because of its course, it may also be called the *recurrent striate artery*. Functionally it is considered an important vessel because it supplies the anterior medial aspect of the head of the caudate nucleus and adjoining putamen, part of the septal nucleus, and cells in the rostrolateral area of the olfactory trigone. The artery of Heubner anastomoses with other striate arteries and also with surface branches of the anterior and middle cerebral arteries (109). The latter point is not accepted by some authors who consider the striate arteries as terminal arteries. The recurrent artery of Heubner is infrequently demonstrated on routine angiograms because of the superimposition described earlier but may be seen when angiotomographic techniques are employed. In Jain's study of 300 brains, the artery of Heubner was the most constant of all the branches at the base of the brain and was present bilaterally in all cases (101). Westberg found the artery of Heubner as a single trunk in 32 of 34 specimens; it was absent in a case where the anterior cerebral trunk was also absent, and in another instance it was double (107).

On the lateral projection, the striate arteries are more difficult to visualize because they usually overlie the region of the internal carotid bifurcation and the branches of the middle cerebral artery within the sylvian fissure. Actually they, or the areas they supply, have a fan shape with the apex downward, as seen in the lateral view (Fig. 17.48). In this projection, the branches of the artery of Heubner are the more anteriorly located, and the lateral striate arteries are the posterior ones (Fig. 17.46).

Most reports on small infarcts in the territory of the deep perforators that arise from the internal carotid artery and its branches have focused on the anatomic structures. Recently, it has become possible to map the territories of the deep perforators from the carotid system, based on matching previous anatomic studies with recent data from CT and magnetic resonance imaging (MRI) studies (110). The middle cerebral artery gives origin to two main groups of perforators: the medial and lateral lenticulostriate arteries. Rarely, the thalamotuberal artery may take origin from the middle cerebral artery, but much more commonly it originates from the posterior communicating artery. The ACA gives origin to the anterior lenticulostriate arteries and the recurrent artery of Heubner. The AChA takes its origin from the internal carotid artery and exceptionally from the middle cerebral artery. In addition, a small group of perforators comes directly from the internal carotid artery.

The *anterior perforating arteries*, the group of arteries that enter the brain through the anterior perforated substance (APS), arise from the internal carotid, middle and anterior cerebral, and the anterior choroidal arteries (111). The carotid branches to the APS arise distal to the origin of the AChA. The AChA branches arise from the main or superior branch of the artery. The middle cerebral artery branches to the APS (the lenticulostriate arteries) arise from the M1 and M2 segments and are divided into medial, intermediate, and lateral groups, each of which has a characteristic configuration. The ACA branches arise from the A1 segment and from the recurrent artery. The internal carotid and AChA branches enter the posterior half of the central portion of the APS. The lenticulostriate branches enter the middle and posterior portions of the lateral half of the APS. The A1 segment gives rise to branches that enter the medial half of the APS above the optic nerve and chiasm. The recurrent artery sends branches into the anterior two-thirds of the full mediolateral extent of the APS.

Umansky et al. also studied the perforating branches (PFBs) of the middle cerebral artery (112). Four of five PFBs originated from the main trunk of the middle cerebral artery before its division; the remaining vessels have their origin from branches of the middle cerebral artery as follows: superior trunk vessels 8.5 percent; inferior trunk 6 percent; middle trunk 0.8 percent; early temporal branch 5.3 percent; and early frontal branch 0.4 percent. The number of PFBs in each hemisphere varied from 5 to 29 (mean 14.9 +/− 0.7 vessels). The great majority of PFBs (96 percent) originated along the proximal 17 mm of the middle cerebral artery. The PFBs arising in the first 10 mm had a mean outer diameter of 0.35 +/− 0.01 mm and a mean length of 9.25 +/− 0.19 mm, and those arising from the second 10 mm had a mean outside diameter (OD) of 0.47 +/− 0.02 mm and a mean length of 16.67 +/− 1.4 mm. A clear distinction between a medial and lateral group of PFBs was present in only 14 hemispheres (41 percent). In nine hemispheres (26 percent), perforating vessels from the ACA (A1 segment) and from the recurrent artery of Heubner replaced the medial group of PFBs of the middle cerebral artery. In one case this group originated in an accessory middle cerebral artery. In 9 percent a small anastomosis (OD 0.2 mm) was seen between a PFB of the recurrent artery of Heubner and one of the middle cerebral arteries. Fifty percent of the PFBs originated as single vessels, and 50 percent of the vessels originated as branches of common stems. The OD of the single vessels ranged from 0.1 to 1.1 mm (mean, 0.39 +/− 0.02 mm), and the length ranged from 3 to 20 mm (mean, 10.8 +/− 0.2 mm). The common stems ranged from 0.6 to 1.8 mm (mean, 0.87 +/ − 0.04 mm) in OD and from 1 to 15 mm (mean, 4.1 +/ − 0.4 mm) in length.

Gibo et al. used human brain microdissections to study the middle cerebral artery (113), which was divided into four segments: the *M1 (sphenoidal)* segment coursed posterior and parallel to the sphenoid ridge; the *M2 (insular)* segment lay on the insula; the *M3 (opercular)* segment coursed over the frontoparietal and temporal opercula; and the *M4 (cortical)* segment spread over the cortical surface. The sylvian fissure was divided into a sphenoidal and an operculoinsular compartment. The M1 segment coursed in the sphenoidal compartment, and the M2 and M3 segments coursed in the operculoinsular compartment. The main trunk of the middle cerebral artery divided in one of three ways; bifurcation (78 percent of hemispheres), trifurcation (12 percent), or division into multiple trunks (10 percent). Those that bifurcated were divided into three groups: equal bifurcation (18 percent), inferior trunk dominant (32 percent), or superior trunk dominant (28 percent).

Anterior Branches

After the striate vessels, the first branches to arise from the middle cerebral artery are the anterior temporal branch, which passes downward on the outer surface of the temporal lobe, near the tip, and the orbitofrontal branch (Figs.

17.27 and 17.47). The latter comes out of the sylvian fissure anteriorly and is distributed along the lateral portion and the undersurface of the frontal lobe. The orbitofrontal frequently anastomoses with the orbital branch and the frontopolar branch of the ACA. The anterior temporal (middle cerebral) anastomoses with the anterior temporal branch of the posterior cerebral artery. The orbitofrontal and anterior temporal branches may arise from a common trunk. Vander Eecken found another artery, the temporal polar branch, arising near the anterior temporal artery in 22 of 40 cases (114). When present, it supplies the most anterior portion of the temporal lobe.

After the two or three most anterior branches, which are often not highly conspicuous in the angiogram, comes a series of three or more branches, which we have been in the habit of calling *ascending branches of the middle cerebral artery* (they include one or two prerolandic branches, a rolandic, and an anterior parietal or postrolandic branch). The term *ascending frontoparietal branch* should be avoided because it denotes that only one major branch is found here. This is true in some cases, but the majority will not present this arrangement. The term *candelabra* has also been applied to these from the functional point of view because it is usually possible on clinical grounds to predict which of the main divisions is involved.

Sylvian Segments

It is essential to consider in some detail the middle cerebral artery branches in the sylvian fissure. In order to facilitate the interpretation of cerebral angiograms, one must have a thorough understanding of the relationship of the branches of the middle cerebral artery to the sylvian fissure, with each other, and with the surrounding brain in three dimensions.

The brain is narrower in its transverse diameter anteriorly than it is posteriorly. Therefore, the surface of the anterior portion of the brain is usually projected more medially than the posterior aspect. The discrepancy between the widths of the anterior and the posterior portions is exaggerated in the posteroanterior projection, as opposed to the anteroposterior projection, due to uneven magnification. Frontal angiography is performed with an anteroposterior projection so that the distortion due to magnification is lessened but not eliminated. The insula or island of Reil is closer to the midline along its anterior aspect than it is posteriorly (Fig. 17.49). Actually, in transverse cross section, the insula on its outer surface describes an arc slightly convex outward so that the anterior end and the posterior end are more medially placed than its center (Fig. 17.44 and 17.45).

The outer surface of the insula is hidden by the opercular portions of the frontal, parietal, and temporal lobes (Fig. 17.50). As the branches of the middle cerebral artery enter the sylvian fissure, they are situated against the outer surface of the insula. Some of them (the more anterior ones) are directed straight upward, and most of them are directed upward and backward. As they reach the uppermost portion of the outer surface of the insula, they do not perforate the brain but, rather, reverse their course and are directed downward to the lower margin of the frontoparietal operculum. At this point, they are directed laterally to emerge from the sylvian fissure. Immediately after emerging, the majority of the branches extend upward, or upward and backward, on the outer surface of the hemisphere (Fig. 17.51). If the frontoparietal operculum is removed, it is noted that the superior margin of the insula is transverse and the outer surface of the central lobe is roughly triangular in configuration (Fig. 17.52).

In all there are five to eight branches of the middle cerebral artery on the outer surface of the insula, which, in fanlike fashion, reach the deepest portion of the sulcus formed at the junction of the insula and the frontoparietal operculum. As they reach this area, they must change direction and proceed caudally for a short distance before emerging from the sylvian fissure. For this reason, in the lateral angiogram it is possible to pick the point at which reversal of the course of each artery takes place. If the points are joined, a straight line can be traced from the most anterior to the most posterior portion of the insula. This straight line is the upper side of what will subsequently be called the *sylvian triangle*. It is possible that one of the branches may not reach the highest possible point within the sylvian fissure in its initial course before reversing; conversely, one branch may penetrate deeply into a sulcus so that it actually extends higher than the others. These are normal variations, which are of no pathologic significance unless there is a trend in one direction, involving several branches that appear to be displaced upward or downward.

The last branches to emerge from the sylvian fissure posteriorly are recognized because they produce a dense dot of contrast substance in lateral view. This represents the most posterior point of the sylvian fissure. As can be appreciated, the opercular portion of the brain has a greater vertical dimension anteriorly than it has posteriorly, where it finally disappears at the posterior end of the insula. Therefore, the last branch or branches (they may be two or three in number) do not have an up-and-down course as the more anterior branches do, but they simply come out of the sylvian fissure (toward the lateral film) producing the dot of high density. A glance at Figure 17.53 will clarify this concept.

The inferior side of the sylvian triangle, for our purpose, is formed by a line starting at the posterior point of the sylvian fissure, which we call the *angiographic sylvian point*, and extending along the lower branches of the middle cerebral artery to the anterior extremity of the parent vessel as seen in lateral view. The anterior side of the sylvian triangle can now be traced from this point up to the first opercular branch within the sylvian fissure (i.e., the most anterior one) (Fig. 17.53). The descriptions just given apply to the lateral view, and it is important to relate these to the anteroposterior projection.

In order to understand the anatomy of the middle cerebral vessels as seen in the frontal projection, it must be remembered that the sylvian fissure is inclined backward

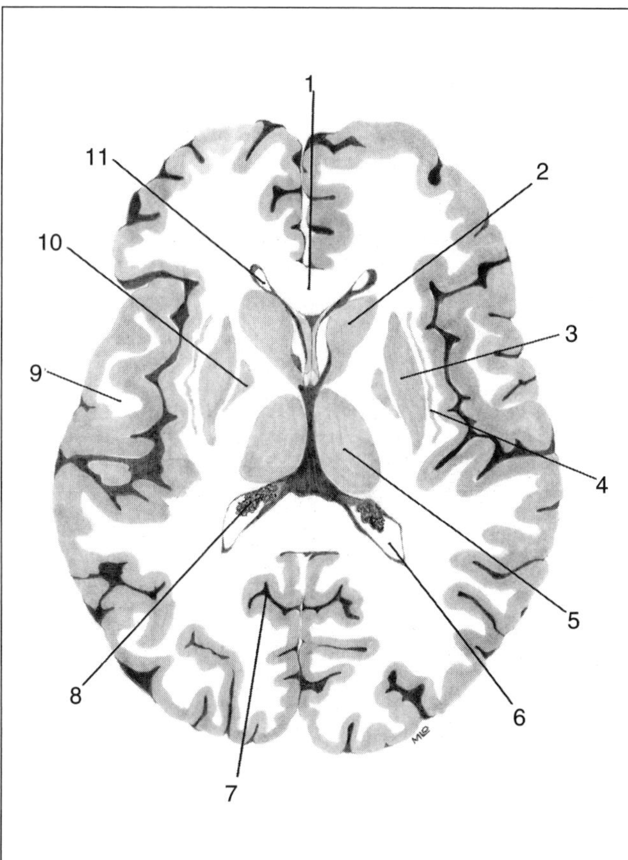

Figure 17.49. Horizontal cross section of the brain. The drawing indicates the configuration of the sylvian fissure and lateral surface of the insula. The anterior aspect of the insular surface is farther medially than the posterior aspect. (1) Genu of corpus callosum; (2) head of caudate nucleus; (3) putamen; (4) claustrum; (5) thalamus; (6) atrium of lateral ventricle; (7) calcarine sulcus; (8) choroid plexus of lateral ventricle; (9) parietal operculum; (10) globus pallidus; (11) anterior horn of lateral ventricle.

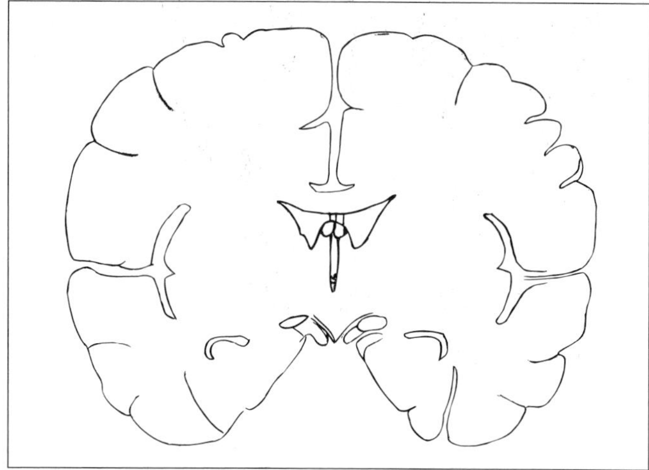

Figure 17.50. Diagram of the coronal section of the brain to show relationships of outer surface of insula to parietal and temporal opercula.

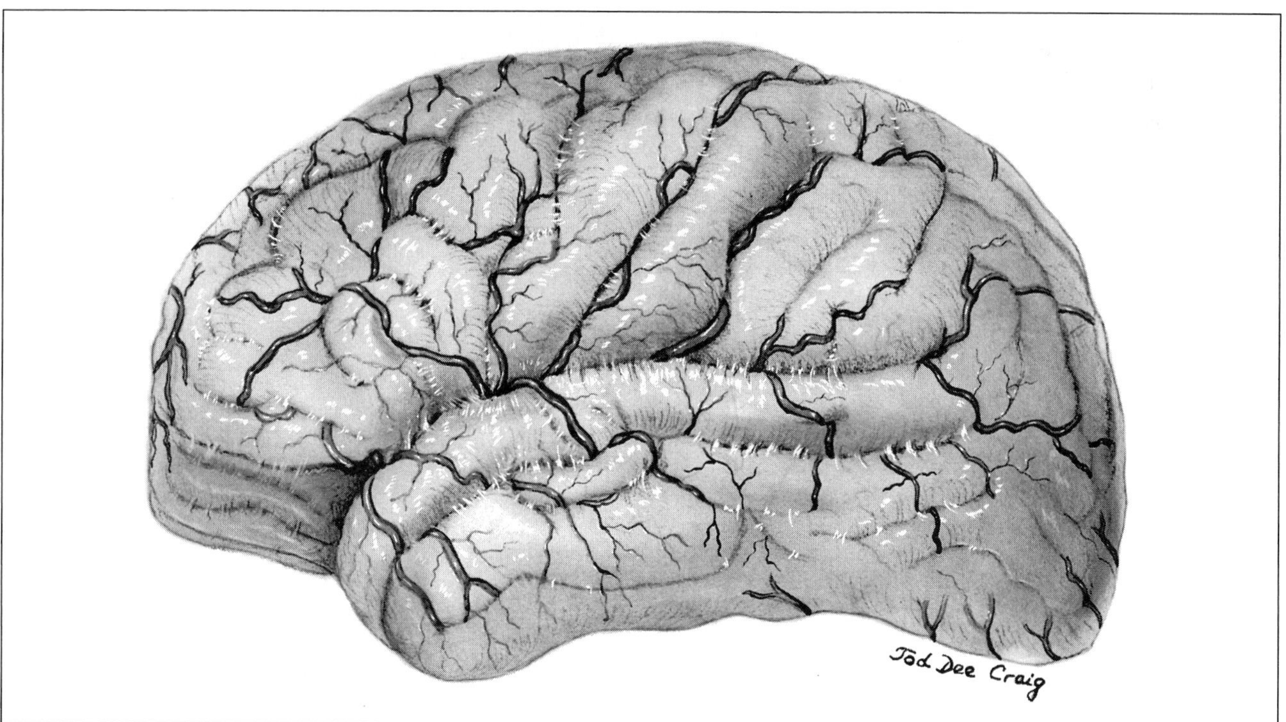

Figure 17.51. Lateral surface of the brain. The cerebral arteries are situated on the surface of the brain, on either the outer surface or the medial surface of the hemisphere. They go in and out of the sulci very frequently. Sometimes they are entirely within a sulcus, and at other times they emerge only to enter the sulcus again.

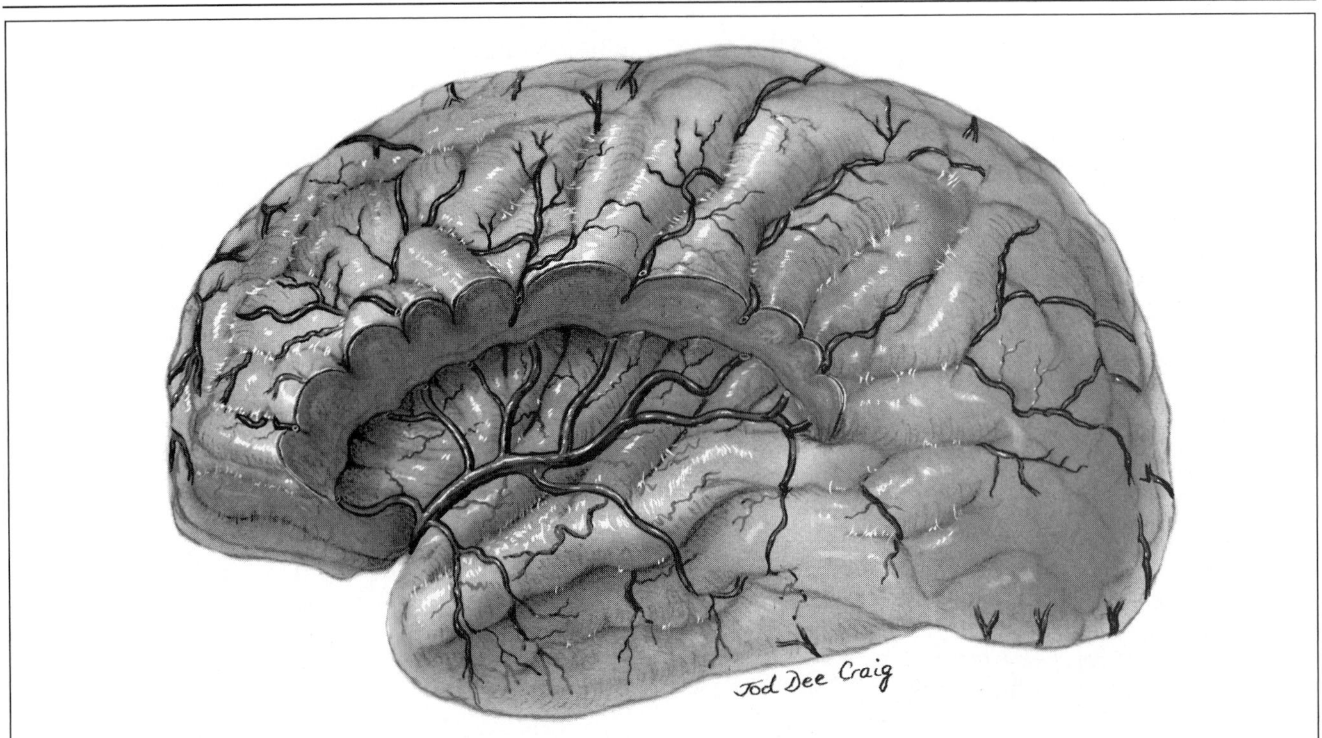

Figure 17.52. Lateral surface of brain with frontoparietal operculum partially removed. The diagram shows the middle cerebral branches over the surface of the insula after the frontoparietal operculum has been cut and the temporal lobe pulled downward. The outer surface of the insula has a triangular configuration, which is not brought out in the sketch because the operculum was sectioned in a curved manner.

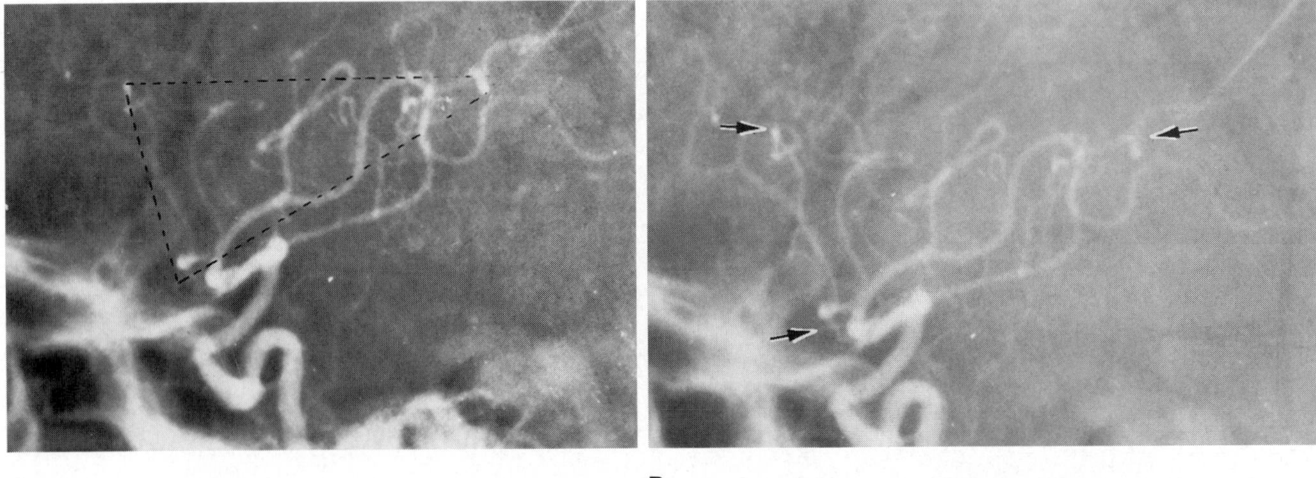

Figure 17.53. Arteriographic demonstration of the sylvian triangle. Normal arteriogram, lateral view. The author's method of determining the sylvian triangle is indicated by dotted lines (**A**). The horizontal arrows (**B**) demonstrate the limits of the triangle. The anterior superior aspect of the sylvian triangle is marked by the top of the first identifiable opercular branch; the anterior inferior aspect of the sylvian triangle is represented by the most anterior portion of the trunk of the middle cerebral artery or the inferior aspect of the first opercular branch, if this is visible, as shown in the figure.

and upward. Therefore, in a film made with the standard frontal angiographic projection (12° cephalocaudad from the orbitomeatal line), the central ray forms an even greater angle with the plane of the sylvian fissure (Fig. 17.54). The anterior branches of the middle cerebral artery are thrown downward and the posterior branches are thrown upward in the frontal film image. One way to remember this point is to keep in mind that anterior moves down and posterior

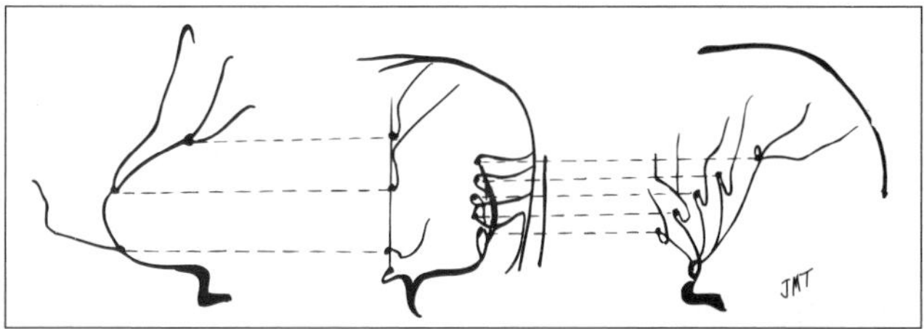

Figure 17.54. Diagrammatic representation of projections of the middle and anterior cerebral arteries and their relative positions according to angulation of the central beam of the x-ray. In both the middle and anterior cerebral diagrams, the head has been tilted with the chin down (see text).

moves up. The same applies to the deep veins of the brain, which will be described later.

Because the branches of the middle cerebral artery first ascend against the outer surface of the insula in the sylvian fissure, descend still within the sylvian fissure, and then are directed laterally to emerge from the fissure, there will be an interlacing of these branches by superimposition in the frontal view. They can still be followed individually, if desired. The more anterior branches may project slightly more medially than the most posterior branches due to the fact that the brain is narrower anteriorly (Fig. 17.49). Even if the anterior branches do not extend farther medially than the posterior branches, they are projected medial to the most lateral aspect of the insula (Fig. 17.55). If the frontal angiographic view were made in posteroanterior projection, the anterior sylvian branches would almost always project medial to the posterior branches.

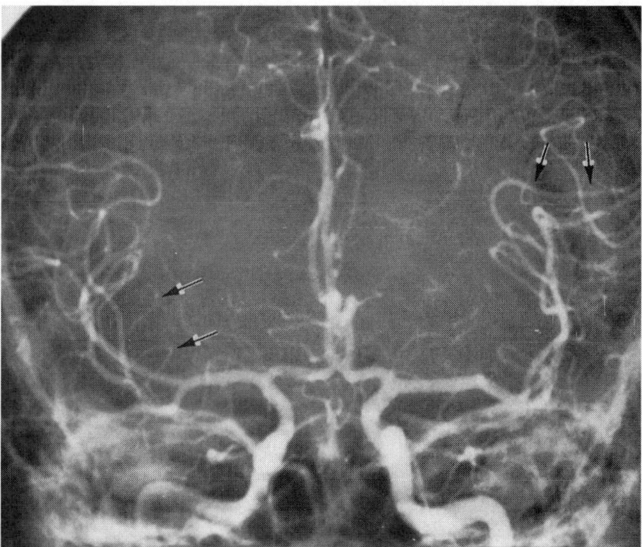

Figure 17.55. Anteroposterior angiogram made with compression of the opposite side during injection. Both angiographic sylvian points are almost exactly equal in height. The distance from each point to the inner table is also almost equal. The left side shows a concave configuration of the last emerging vessels (arrows), which may be related to greater development of the parietal operculum associated with speech. The anterior component loops of the sylvian triangle project slightly more medially than the posterior loops, on the right side (arrows).

The last middle cerebral branch often has a double curve, and as it emerges from the sylvian fissure it is concave upward.

Ascending Branches

After the various branches of the middle cerebral artery emerge from the sylvian fissure, they turn directly upward or, in the case of the more posterior ones, they are directed upward and backward. The most anterior ones may be directed upward and forward. The distribution of the middle cerebral group over the convexity of the hemisphere may be compared with the outstretched hand with the fingers spread apart. The thumb indicates the plane of the sylvian fissure continuing in the direction of the three most posterior branches (posterior parietal, angular, and posterior temporal arteries). The other four fingers represent the ascending branches of the middle cerebral artery (the one or two prerolandic, the rolandic, and the anterior parietal or postrolandic arteries). In some instances the distribution is much more irregular. Sometimes the branches present only a few undulations, whereas at other times they are tortuous. Within their tortuosity, however, they still preserve a certain organization. On glancing at an injected specimen of these branches, one can readily observe that these arteries are sometimes on the convolutions, where they are clearly visible, while at other times they penetrate into the sulci, where they disappear from view (Fig. 17.51), only to emerge again, perhaps a little higher.

In the angiogram, the branches of the middle cerebral artery usually fill well to the superior portion of the convexity of the hemisphere, where they become quite thin and usually disappear after branching and by simply losing their density (i.e., the contrast substance fades away). This is very easy to appreciate in the cases in which the ACA does not fill from one side (see Fig. 10.45). Of course, it is known that many of these branches of the middle cerebral artery anastomose end to end directly with branches of the anterior cerebral artery (see under "Collateral Circulation of the Brain," Chapter 10). However, these anastomoses do not function significantly unless there is a difference in pressure between the anterior and middle cerebral arterial systems, such as may be found in arterial occlusions.

As the posterior branches of the middle cerebral artery ascend and pass backward, they are superimposed upon the branches of the ACA, which are in a different plane, on the medial surface of the hemisphere. The latter include the pericallosal artery and its branches. If these happen to be prominent in their distribution and in their filling with contrast substance (particularly if both pericallosal arteries are filled), an extra density is produced that can suggest increased vascularity and the possible presence of a tumor. Another artifact that is often seen in the middle cerebral distribution is that of a "pseudocloud" in the region of the sylvian triangle; this is produced by the very rich vascularity present in the region and is a normal finding.

In evaluating the relative positions of the ascending branches of the middle cerebral artery, each one can be thought of as following a sulcus or a gyrus (one of the sulci or gyri of the rolandic region). Although this is not the case in most instances (the artery may be on the gyrus at one point and in the sulcus at the next turn), it is helpful to imagine each artery as belonging to a sulcus when the vessels are displaced by a mass.

The middle cerebral branches that supply the anterior and middle thirds of the temporal lobe are often inconspicuous, although they can be seen well through subtraction. They are usually thinner than the other branches and are sometimes superimposed on bone and the regions of the siphon, the anterior choroidal and the posterior communicating vessels, making identification difficult. When there is elevation of the middle cerebral branches by a temporal mass, these branches often become much more conspicuous.

Cortical Branches

There are 13 cortical territories that are virtually always appreciated. Regardless of the proximal origin, a single and occasionally two vessels supply each territory.

Cortical Branches	**Cortical Area Served**
Orbitofrontal artery	Frontal branches
Prefrontal artery	
Precentral artery	
Central artery	
Anterior parietal artery	Parietal branches
Posterior parietal artery	
Angular artery	
Temporo-occipital artery	Temporal branches
Posterior-temporal artery	
Middle-temporal artery	
Inferior temporal artery	
Anterior temporal artery	
Temporal polar artery	

Van der Zwan et al. demonstrated the considerable variation in distribution of the major cerebral arteries in human cadaver studies, particularly in the white matter and distal cortical areas (115). Twenty-six variations in the territory of the ACA, 17 variations in the area of the middle cerebral artery, and 22 variations in the area of the posterior cerebral artery were found in the cortex of 50 hemispheres. Intracerebrally, the anterior, middle, and posterior cerebral arteries contributed in varying degrees to the blood supply of the lobar white matter, the internal capsule, the caudate nucleus, and the lentiform nucleus. The large variation in the area in which the cortical and intracerebral boundaries between these territories were located was demonstrated by illustrating the minimum and maximum extent of each.

Methods of Identification

The branches can be identified in lateral projection by use of either a template or by construction. Ring and Waddington have suggested a relatively simple approach (116). Salamon et al. have constructed a template, helpful to estimate the position of the cortical branches of the middle cerebral artery (Fig. 17.59*C* and *D*) (95). See also Figure 17.29.

Measurements and Landmarks

The normal location of the striates can be determined by measurement. Andersen found that the distance to the most medial artery measured at the apex of the first curve was 26 mm in normal cases; to the most lateral artery, it was 38 mm (117). Salamon et al. observed that the distance from the midline to the most lateral striate artery is about equal to the distance from the inner table to the deepest sylvian vessels, but they did not indicate the range of normal variation (106).

Angiographic Sylvian Point

The most medial extent of the last branch of the middle cerebral artery, before it emerges from the fissure, is called the *angiographic sylvian point* in the frontal view and corresponds to the same point in the lateral projection. On a film with degree of magnification produced by a target film distance of 40 in and with the head approximately 1 in from the film, the deepest portion of the last sylvian vessel is usually not more than 43 mm from the inner table of the skull. The minimal distance encountered in a large group of normal cases was not less than 30 mm. In patients with tortuous vessels from atherosclerosis, an increase of 10 (sometimes more) beyond the 43-mm maximum may be seen. In general, however, the established upper and lower limits of normal (30 to 43 mm) are very useful in confirming medial or lateral displacement of the angiographic sylvian point.

The sylvian point in the frontal angiographic projection is situated close to the center of the distance from the upper margin of the petrous pyramid (or the roof of the orbit, whichever is lower) to a horizontal line drawn tangential to the inner table of the vertex of the skull. If the groove of the superior longitudinal sinus is deep, the internal lateral margin of the bony sinus wall should be used (Fig. 17.56). In a film made in the standard frontal angiographic projection, the angiographic sylvian point can be 9 to 10 mm below the center of the vertex-petrosal distance. If more of the orbits show (i.e., if the petrous pyramids are lower), it tends to be a little lower; in half-axial anteroposterior projections, the point is closer to the center. The sylvian points are usually symmetric, when the right side is compared with the left, in normal cases (Fig. 17.55).

The sylvian point may be localized in the lateral projection, as mentioned earlier, by the one, two, or more vessels seen end-on as they are directed straight out parallel to the x-ray beam to emerge on the surface. Fairly frequently, however, no dense dots can be seen; instead, dense, short loops are present because the x-ray beam did not catch the vessels on end. The exact sylvian point is more difficult to recognize in such cases, but a good approximation is always

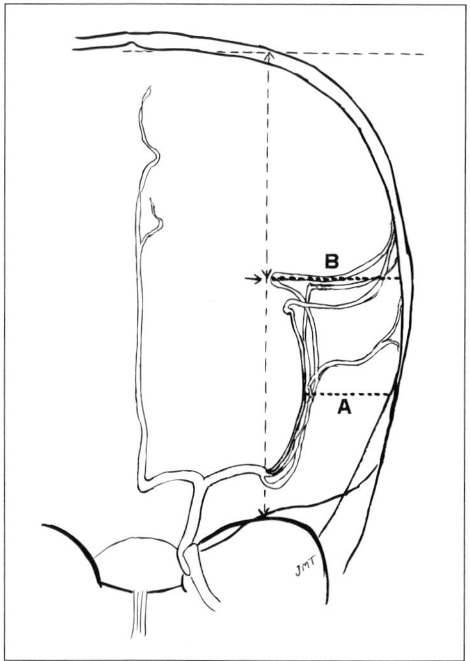

Figure 17.56. Diagram illustrates the method that the author has used to determine the position of the angiographic sylvian point. The arrow in this particular case is almost in the center of the vertical distance from the highest point of the inner table of the skull to the upper margin of the orbit. Distance (**A**) to the medial aspect of the most medial vessel outlining the lateral margin of the insula varies from 20 to 30 mm. Distance (**B**) from the medial margin of the most medial vessel in the region of the sylvian point to the inner table varies from 30 to 43 mm.

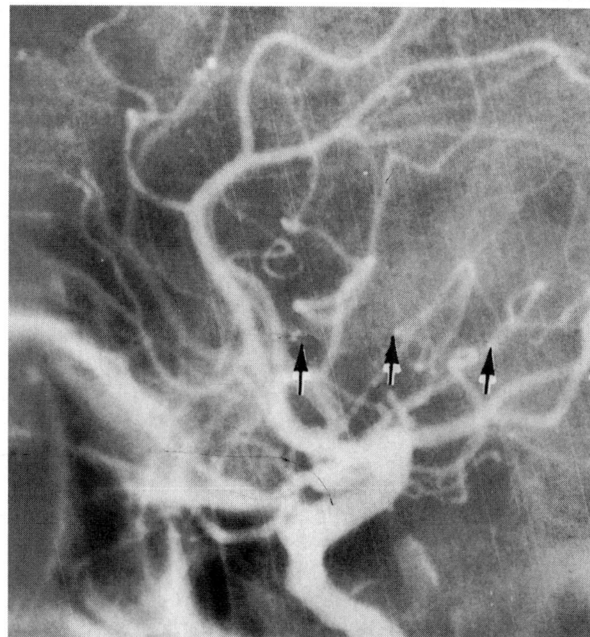

Figure 17.57. Normal lateral carotid angiogram to demonstrate the sylvian triangle and sylvian fissure. The figure illustrates how it is possible to trace the actual position of the sylvian fissure with a fair degree of accuracy by taking the lower portions of the branches of the middle cerebral artery as they return downward and extend laterally to emerge from the sylvian fissure. Absolute accuracy is not possible because the arteries may be either on a gyrus or in a sulcus. The angiographic sylvian point is marked by the most posterior arrow (pointing downward) and is easily determined by following the upper margins of the arterial loops marking the upper contour of the sylvian triangle.

possible. If it is kept in mind that the sylvian point is the apex of the sylvian triangle, the upper side of this triangle can be followed to the point where it meets the last major middle cerebral branches (Fig. 17.57). Stereoscopy can be helpful in identifying the angiographic sylvian point in the lateral view.

The position of the sylvian fissure can be approximated in the lateral view by tracing a line along the points where the opercular vessels turn to leave the fissure after having descended. However, it should be kept in mind that as the opercular branches turn, some may be deep within a sulcus whereas others may be on the surface of a gyrus (Fig. 17.57).

Clinoparietal Line

A line traced in the lateral view from a point 2 cm above the lambda to the anterior clinoid process is usually situated at or just below the lower major branches of the middle cerebral artery. Sometimes the line is just above the lowest major branch in the adult. In children the major middle cerebral branches are always above the clinoparietal line (Fig. 17.58). The actual measurements encountered in a group of normal children varying in age from 5 months to 13 years and in adults are given in Figure 17.59. If the vessels are more than 1 cm above the line in the adult, an infrasylvian mass is suggested.

In the adult, and sometimes in older children, the lambda is not clearly visible on the films. In these cases, a point on the inner table 9 cm above the internal occipital protuberance is taken as the point from which to trace the line (118). It may be noted in Figure 17.59 that in younger children the distance from the clinoparietal line to the lowest major branch of the middle cerebral artery, measured 2 cm behind the carotid artery siphon, is greater than in older children; the distance decreases with advancing age to approach the relationship found in the adult. This is evidently related to brain development (i.e., greater proportional growth of the frontal lobe).

The middle cerebral artery axis can be related to a line drawn from the limbus sphenoidale (point just anterior to the tuberculum sellae) to the midpoint of a chord joining the bregma and internal occipital protuberance (Fig. 17.58*B*). This simple method gives less variation between children and adults than others, partly because the limbus is above the plane of the anterior clinoids in infancy and childhood. In children, the last major branch of the middle cerebral artery is projected, on the average, 5 mm above the line in straight lateral angiograms, with a normal range of 0 to 10 mm (119). In adults, the middle cerebral axis

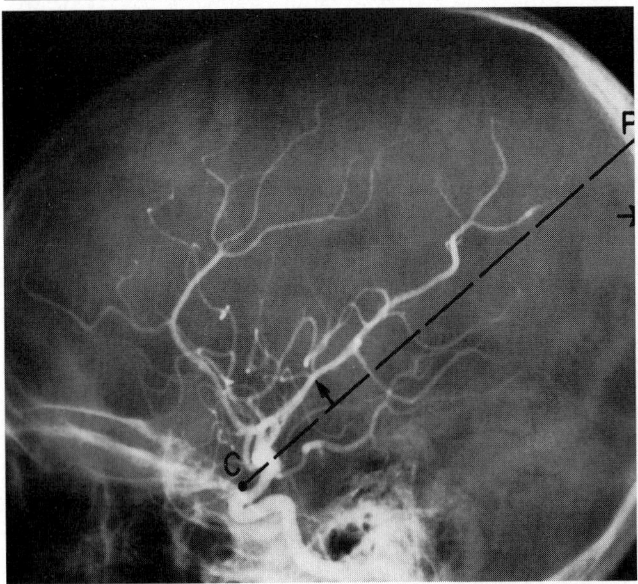

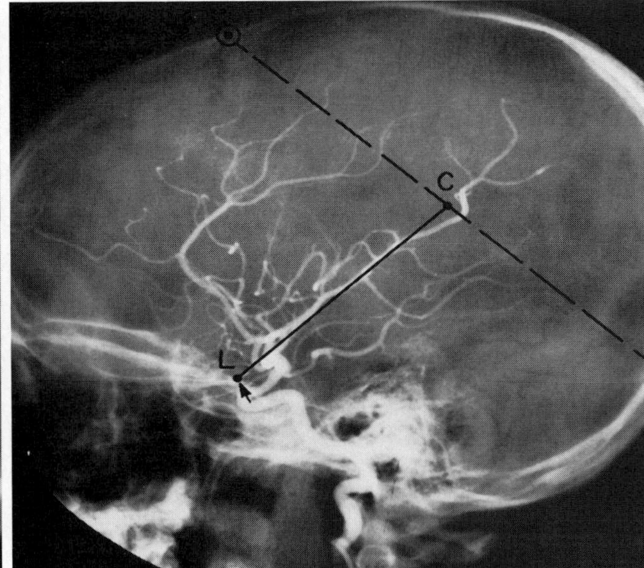

A B

Figure 17.58. Graphic determination of the position of the middle cerebral artery. **A.** The clinoparietal line is plotted on a lateral angiogram made in the early arterial phase. From the lambda (posterior arrow) a line 2 cm long (*a*) is drawn to determine the point *P* along the inner table of the parietal bone. If the lambda cannot be clearly made out, the parietal point can be ascertained by drawing a chord (*b*) 9 cm in length from the torcular to the inner table of the parietal bone. The line *C–P* is then drawn from the anterior clinoid process to the parietal point. On the original radiograph, the distance from the *C–P* line to the lowest major branch of the middle cerebral artery (anterior arrow), as measured 2 cm behind the carotid siphon, was 0.9 cm. **B.** Using the same radiograph illustrated in A, a line is drawn from the limbus sphenoidale (arrow) to the midpoint of a chord joining the bregma and the internal occipital protuberance. The last major branch of the middle cerebral artery, or the middle cerebral artery axis, falls on the limbus-chord line (*L–C*) in this case (see text).

falls on the line in the highest percentage of patients, with a normal range of 6 mm below to 8 mm above the line drawn. In a group of patients with infrasylvian masses, the same authors found the axis more than 10 mm above the limbus-chord line in more than 95 percent of cases.

EMBRYOLOGY AND VARIANTS

Embryology

As Romer pointed out, trivesicular arrangement of the vertebrate brain is organized around sensory organs: nose/prosencephalon, eye/mesencephalon, lateral-line/rhombencephalon (120). A prosencephalic vessel, the middle cerebral artery and its progenitors supply areas involved in olfaction. The internal carotid artery terminates into two olfactory vessels. The lateral olfactory artery homologue with its piriform branch grows tremendously, with the growth of the cortical mantle becoming the middle cerebral artery proper. The middle cerebral artery proper is a late embryologic development. The relay area for olfaction is the striatum, which also grows tremendously. The striatum is fed by a number of striate arteries that collect on the proximal lateral olfactory artery (future middle cerebral artery); initially they go by way of rhinal fissure. Shellshear's principle ("End artery" distributions are constant; conduit vessel distributions vary) allows one to separate the "dancer from the dance" (121); additionally, it appears that "end artery" growth is organized around gray matter, not white matter, course. The end arteries anchor the vessels to the brain. The conduit vessel can shift, grow, and regress in response to global demand and local hemodynamic constraints. Over time, like all branching biological conduit systems, these restraints include "least work" and balance. An excellent and creative synthesis of the variations of the conduit system can be found in Lasjaunias and Berenstein (122).

The course of the conduit portion of the middle cerebral artery is determined by the tremendous growth of the cerebral mantle. The insular (M2) portion of the middle cerebral artery feeds the underlaying cortex and claustrum and holds constant as the remaining cortical areas grow, forcing the frontal, parietal, and temporal lobes to fold and bulge around this restraint (see Fig. 5.1); far from mysterious, similar bulging and folding can be observed when this year's avoirdupois is restrained by last year's vestments.

Variants

An accessory middle cerebral artery originating from the proximal internal carotid, or off the anterior cerebral artery, is rarely seen. Similarly, the unusual middle cerebral takeoff of the anterior choroidal can be appreciated. The striatal arteries vary in number (2 to 20) and origin (M1–M2). The sphenoidal portion (M2) course sags with age, changing from a dorsal-oblique to a basilar-oblique course under the weight of time (123).

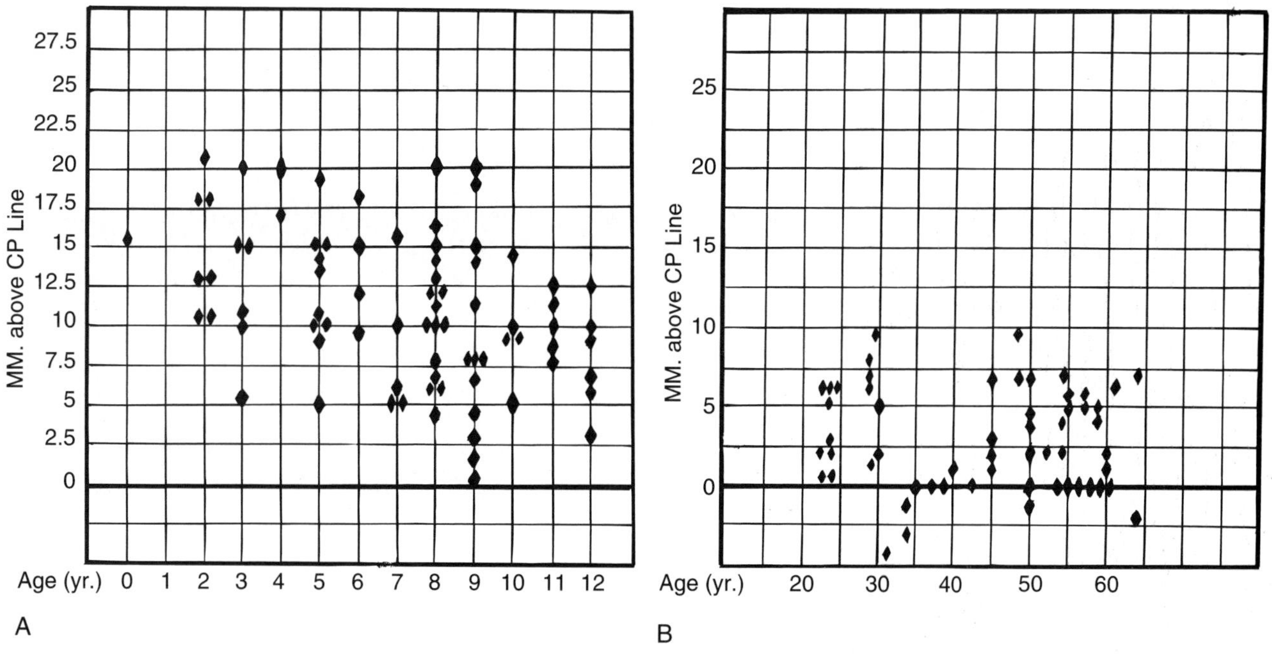

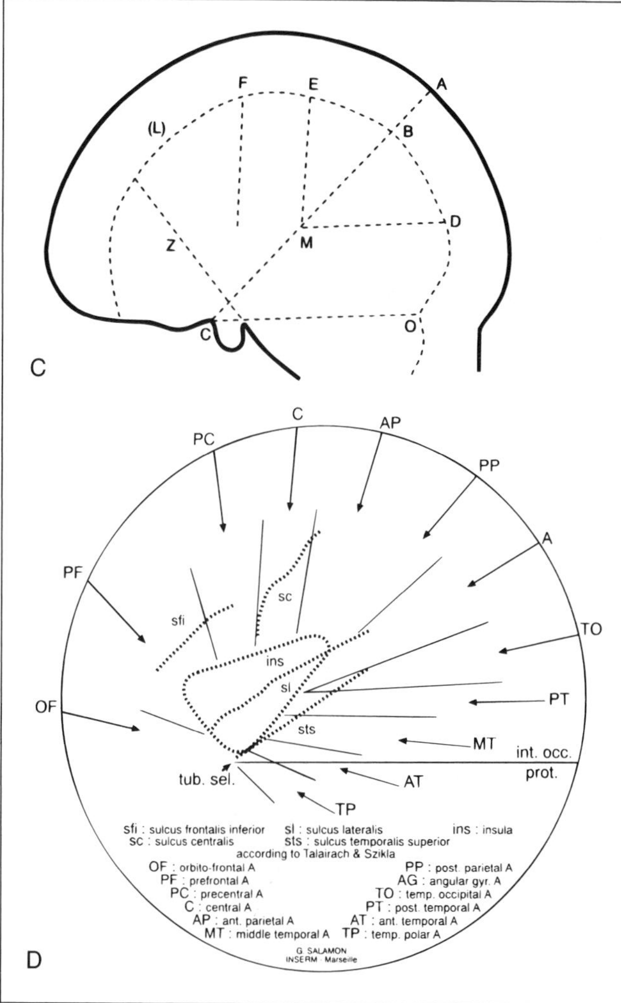

Figure 17.59. Relation of the middle cerebral artery to the clinoparietal line. The graphs indicate the relationship of the lower main branch of the middle cerebral artery to the clinoparietal line in children and in adults. The middle cerebral branches become lower with advancing age (**A**) but remain stationary after growth is completed (**B**). **C.** Schematic representation of the method of Ring and Waddington (116) for determining the vascular territories of the branches of the middle cerebral artery. (1) Construct a line (L), 2.5 cm within the inner table and parallel to it, to a point (O), anterior to the internal occipital protuberance. (2) Construct the clinoparietal line of Taveras and Wood (92) from the anterior clinoid process (C), to a point (A), situated on the inner table 9 cm above the internal occipital protuberance. This line defines point (B) where it crosses line (L). (3) From the midpoint (M) of line (BC), construct a line parallel to line (CO). This defines point (D) where the line crosses line (L). (4) Construct a line parallel to the coronal suture and passing through point (M). This line crosses line (L) at point (E). (5) Construct another vertical line (F), 2.5 cm in front of and parallel to line (ME). (6) Construct a line (Z), connecting the midpoint of the anterior arc of line (L), that is, anterior to point (F), with the dorsum sellae. The clinoparietal line (CA) represents the axis of the middle cerebral artery in adults. Space (OCMD) corresponds to the vascular territory of the posterior temporal artery, and (BME) to that of the posterior parietal artery. The open-ended quadrilateral (EMF) corresponds to the vascular territory of the central artery (or arteries) and permits the identification of the motor area anteriorly and the sensory area posteriorly. In front of and beneath the anterior line (Z) is the vascular territory of the orbitofrontal artery; above and behind is that of the prefrontal or candelabra artery. **D.** Template of Salamon and Huang (96). The template can be placed on the film guided by the tuberculum sellae–internal occipital protuberance line. OF = orbito-frontal artery; PF = prefrontal artery; PC = precentral artery; C = central artery; AP = anterior parietal artery; MT = middle temporal artery; PP = posterior parietal artery; AG = angular gyrus artery; TO = temporal-occipital artery; PT = posttemporal artery; AT = anterior temporal artery; TP = temporopolar artery; SFI = sulcus frontalis inferior; SC = sulcus centralis; sl = sulcus lateralis; sts = sulcus temporalis superior; ins = insula.

Anomalies of the middle cerebral artery have recently been revisited by Umansky et al. (124). They included fenestration (1 percent), located on the first 4 mm of the main trunk of the middle cerebral artery; duplication (1 percent), with vessels arising from the internal carotid artery; accessory middle cerebral artery (2 percent), originating on the A1 segment of the anterior cerebral artery; single-trunk type of middle cerebral artery (4 percent), with no division of its main trunk; and quadrifurcation (four cases, or 4 percent), in which the main trunk of the middle cerebral artery divided into four secondary trunks.

Variable branching patterns of the cortical branches are common. About half of the middle cerebral arteries bifurcate laterally, a quarter trifurcate, a fifth pseudotrifurcate, and 1 in 10 have a proximal branch (pseudobifurcation) or a proximal bifurcation (127). The M1 and M2 portions of the middle cerebral artery can carry important perforators regardless of the branching pattern. A single cortical vascular territory can be served by one or two vessels. The conduit cortical vessels course in the subarachnoid space but may be deep within a sulcus.

Males appear to have larger cerebral vessels (middle cerebral arteries, ACAs) and larger right hemisphere vessels, and females larger left hemisphere vessels (125). Mean diameter was significantly larger by 9.3, 8.8, and 9.7 percent, respectively, in males than in females. There appears to be no correlation of vessel diameter with age.

The cerebral arteries present an optimum blood flow/vessel radius relation. Rositti and Lofgren measured the branch angles and diameters of ACA and its branch segments and found that the bifurcations appear to be optimized to avoid increased hemodynamic stresses both globally and locally in the same manner as extracranial arteries (126).

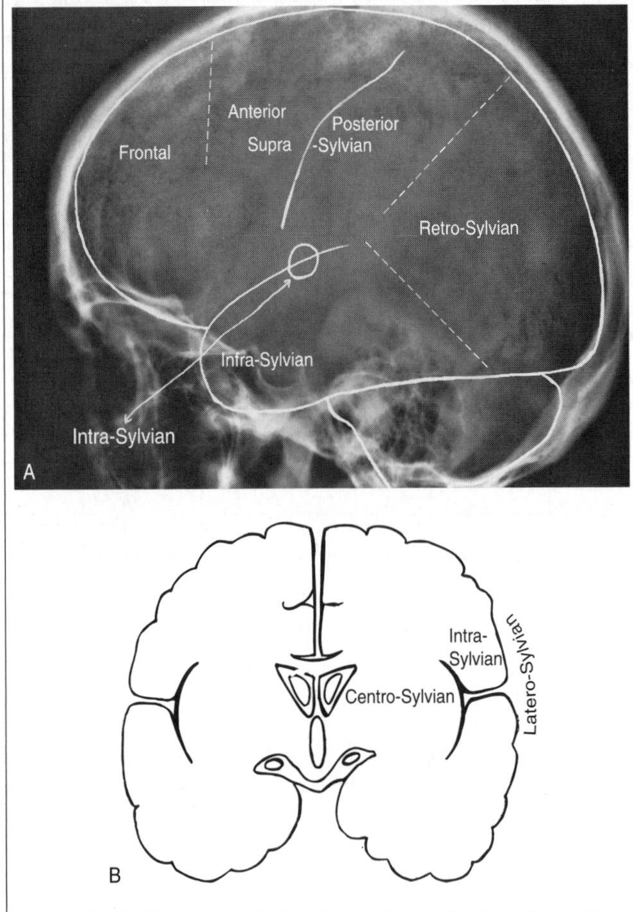

Figure 17.60. Angiographic classification of brain tumors. **A.** Angiographic classification proposed here for brain tumors is, as explained in the text, based on the sylvian fissure, the sylvian triangle, and the angiographic sylvian point. The frontal tumors have to be subdivided into various subgroups, and in addition the suprasylvian, retrosylvian, and infrasylvian masses have to be subdivided, depending on the location of the mass in relation to neighboring parts of the brain. **B.** The masses are classified again according to whether they are lateral or medial to the sylvian fissure.

ABNORMALITIES OF THE VESSELS

A clinically practical classification of mass displacement involving the middle cerebral artery follows and is illustrated in Figure 17.60.

1. Presylvian
2. Suprasylvian
3. Infrasylvian
4. Retrosylvian
5. Intrasylvian
6. Laterosylvian
7. Ventricular dilatation

Frontal Masses (Presylvian)

One of the general signs of frontal (presylvian) masses is that the carotid siphon is downward displaced (Figs. 17.61 and 17.62). The anterior portion of the sylvian triangle may be depressed or deformed. If a mass is inferior frontal, it may deform and elevate the most anterior components of the sylvian triangle (Fig. 17.61); if it is parasagittal in location, it may depress the anterior aspect of the triangle (Fig. 17.62).

Suprasylvian Masses

The lesions of this group include the posterior frontal, frontoparietal, and parietal masses. The supraclinoid portion of the internal carotid artery is displaced downward (closing of the siphon). The ascending branches of the middle cerebral artery often exhibit stretching and bowing with or without loss of undulations. The loss of undulations is often accompanied by spreading of these arteries. Depression of the upper boundary of the sylvian triangle is common.

Parietal convexity tumors characteristically displace the angiographic sylvian point downward. If this point measures more than 1 cm below the center of the distance from

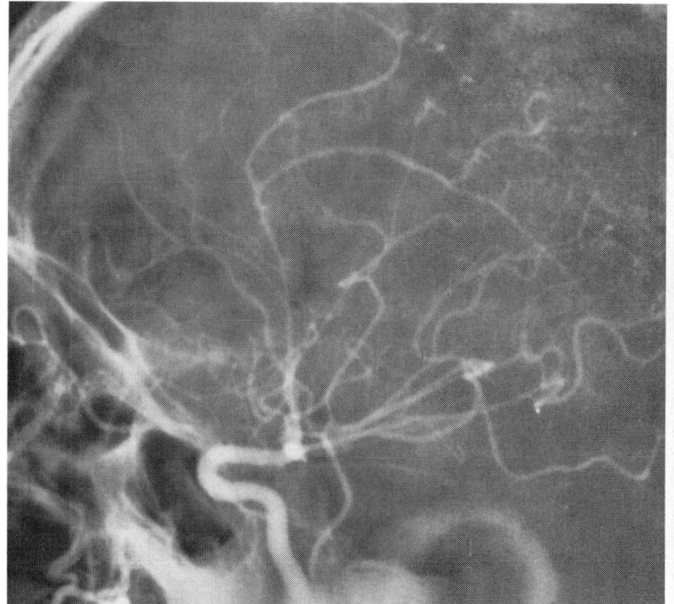

A

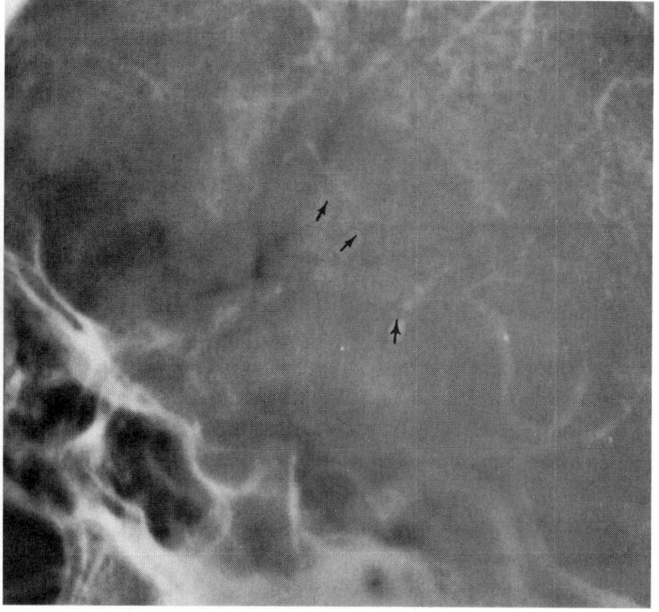

B

Figure 17.61. Inferior frontal (intracerebral) tumor simulating subfrontal mass. **A.** The lateral arterial phase shows elevation of the proximal portion of the pericallosal artery. There is even one branch of the anterior cerebral, the frontopolar artery, that shows perfect bowing very suggestive of a subfrontal mass. In such cases, it is extremely difficult to differentiate intracerebral and extracerebral neoplasms. The configuration is produced by protrusion of the tumor across the midline below the vessels, or exophytic growth, thus elevating some of these branches. It is usually possible with intracerebral tumors to see some fine vessels supplying the undersurface of the frontal lobe, which normally arise from the anterior cerebral artery. However, similar vessels may be seen sometimes in subfrontal tumors as well, and under these circumstances it is not possible to differentiate between the two in the absence of typical abnormal vascularity. **B.** The venous phase shows posterior displacement of the venous angle (arrow) and "humping" of the internal cerebral vein, which is typical of central frontal tumors. There is elevation of the septal vein (double arrow), which confirms the inferior frontal location of the mass.

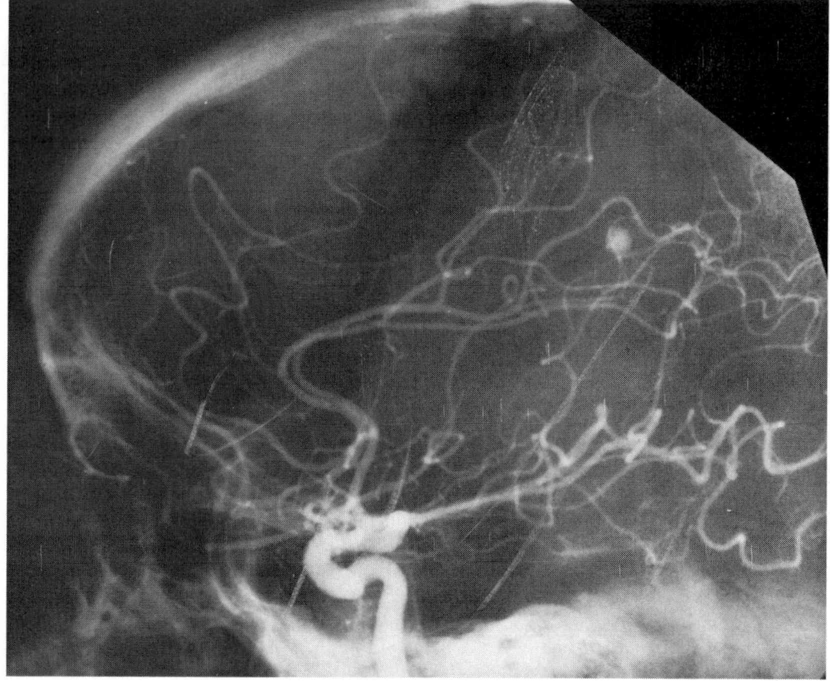

A

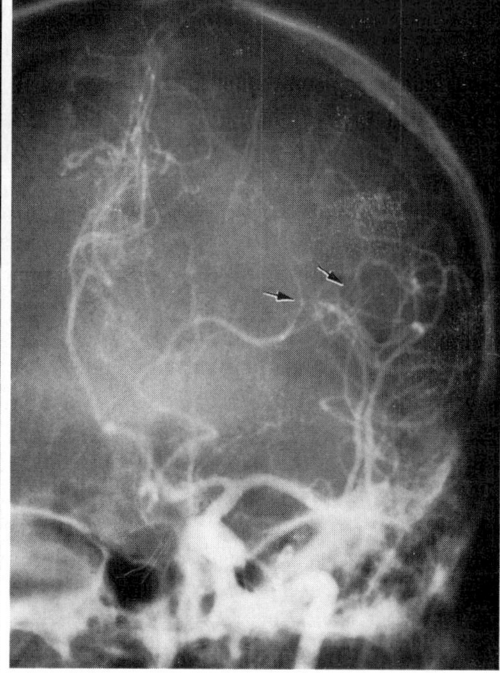

B

Figure 17.62. Frontal parasagittal tumor (meningioma). **A.** In the lateral projection there is downward bowing of a branch of the callosomarginal artery and depression of the pericallosal artery. There is also diffuse depression of the anterior portion of the sylvian triangle. **B.** The frontal view demonstrates a rounded shift. There is lateral displacement of a branch of the anterior cerebral artery (arrows), suggesting that the tumor is either attached to or arising from the falx.

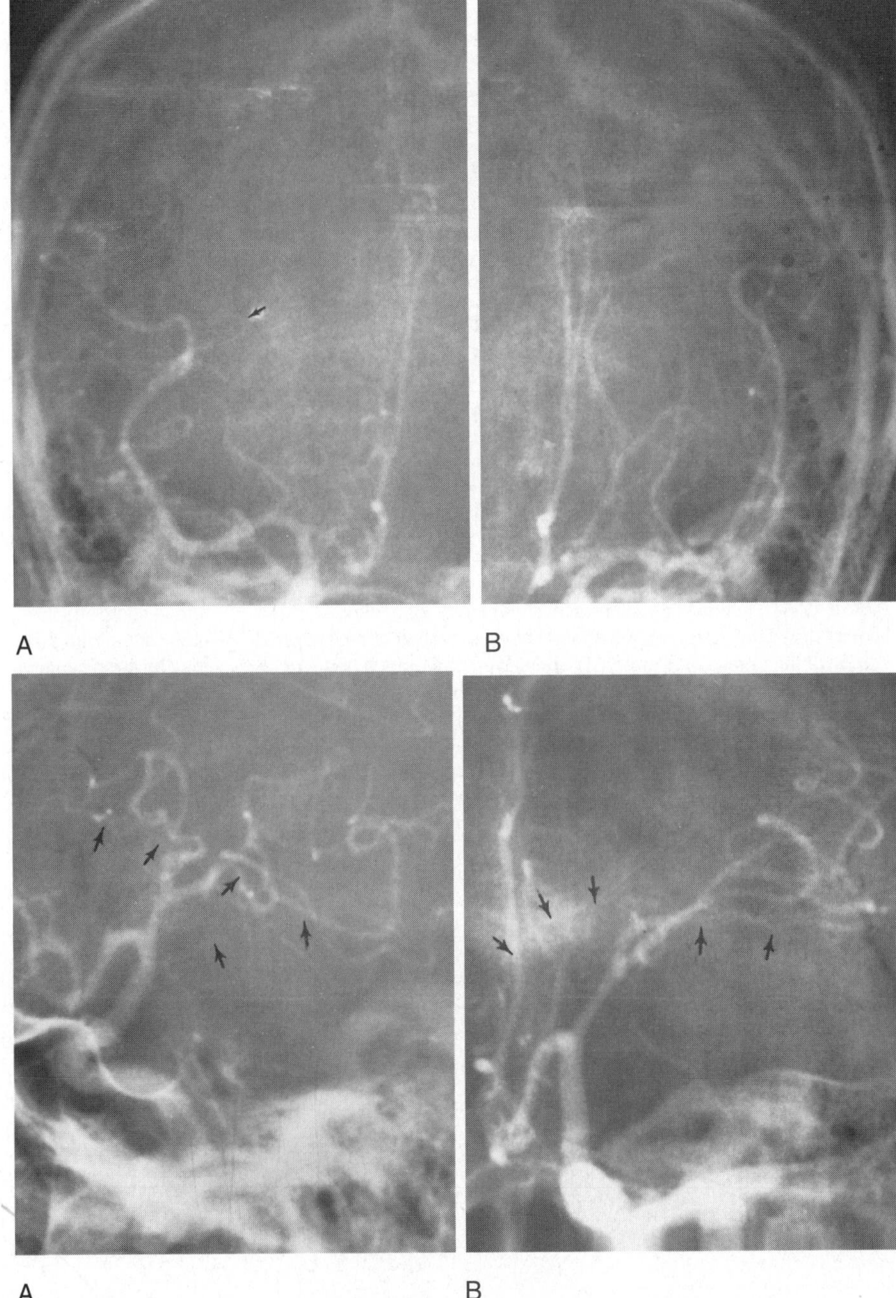

Figure 17.63. Downward displacement of the angiographic sylvian point due to a parietal tumor. On the side of the tumor (**A**) there is downward displacement of the sylvian point (arrow), which is also displaced medially. From this depressed position, the branches emerge from the sylvian fissure obliquely upward and outward; the vessels are directed upward much more than on the opposite (normal) side (**B**). There is only a distal, subfalcial shift. The tumor was situated in the upper part of the hemisphere.

Figure 17.64. Anterior infrasylvian tumor (epidermoidoma). **A.** The lateral view shows upward displacement of the branches of the middle cerebral artery (arrows), which is causing complete disruption of the sylvian triangle. There is marked elevation of the supraclinoid portion of the internal carotid artery with lifting of the bifurcation of this artery. The anterior choroidal artery (lower arrows) is elevated and stretched. **B.** The frontal projection discloses marked elevation of the horizontal portion of the middle cerebral artery, and medial displacement and stretching of the supraclinoid portion of the internal carotid artery with raising of the bifurcation. There is only a slight shift of the anterior cerebral artery across the midline, with the proximal portion displaced to a greater extent. The anterior choroidal artery is seen to describe a wide semicircle, and it is actually beyond the midline (arrows). This artery demarcates the medial extent of the tumor, which was rather large. The midline shift is slight because the tumor was growing very slowly. It might be mentioned that all of the branches of the middle cerebral artery are elevated (lateral arrows) because the entire temporal lobe was lifted upward by the tumor situated under it.

the midline convexity inner table to the upper margin of the orbit or petrous pyramid (whichever is lower), it may be considered as displaced downward (Fig. 17.63).

Infrasylvian Masses

The common features of infrasylvian masses may be listed as follows: (*a*) elevation of the middle cerebral artery and its branches (Figs. 17.64 and 17.65); (*b*) displacement of the middle cerebral artery branches medially, away from the inner table (Fig. 17.66); (*c*) "opening of the siphon," characterized by the displacement of the carotid medially, and its bifurcation often is elevated (Fig. 17.67).

Anterior Temporal Masses

Anterior lesions are characterized by elevation of the horizontal portion of the middle cerebral artery, as seen in frontal view (Fig. 17.68). The anterior portion of the sylvian triangle is elevated.

Posterior Temporal Masses

In these cases, there is frank elevation of the middle cerebral artery branches, as seen in the lateral view. The angiographic sylvian point is elevated, with posterior masses (Fig. 17.69). Such elevation is a characteristic finding of posterior temporal lesions.

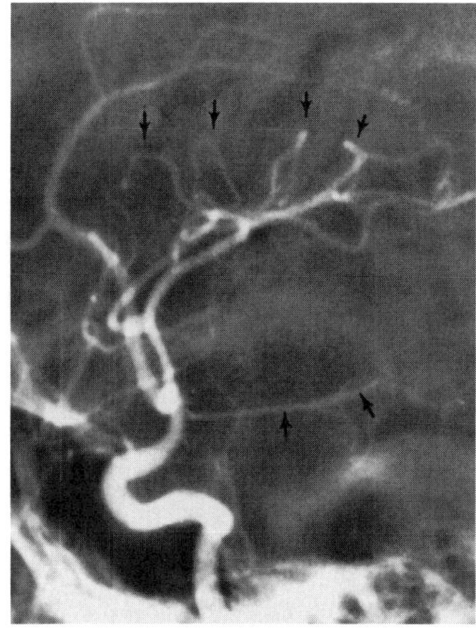

A

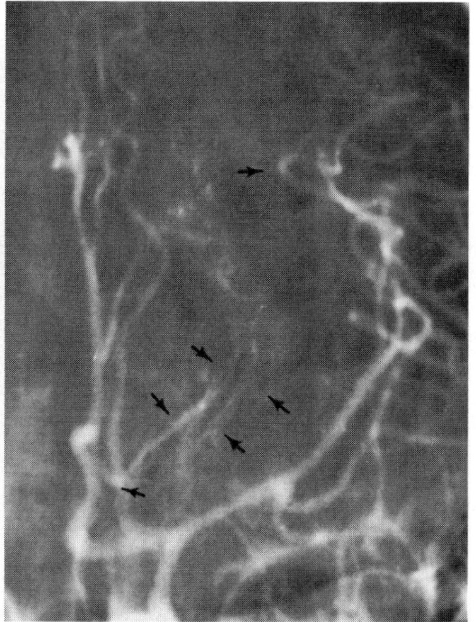

B

Figure 17.65. Temporal tumor occupying the anterior two-thirds of the temporal lobe. **A.** The lateral view shows marked elevation of the middle cerebral artery and its branches. The sylvian triangle is markedly elevated (upper arrows). The supraclinoid portion of the carotid siphon is raised and displaced forward. The anterior choroidal artery is enlarged and straightened (lower arrows). **B.** The frontal projection shows lifting of the horizontal portion of the middle cerebral artery and slight elevation of the angiographic sylvian point (upper arrow). There is medial displacement of the lenticulostriate arteries and of the anterior choroidal artery (lower arrows). There is only a slight degree of midline shift involving the proximal and distal portions of the anterior cerebral artery, with the central portion of the vessel returning to the midline.

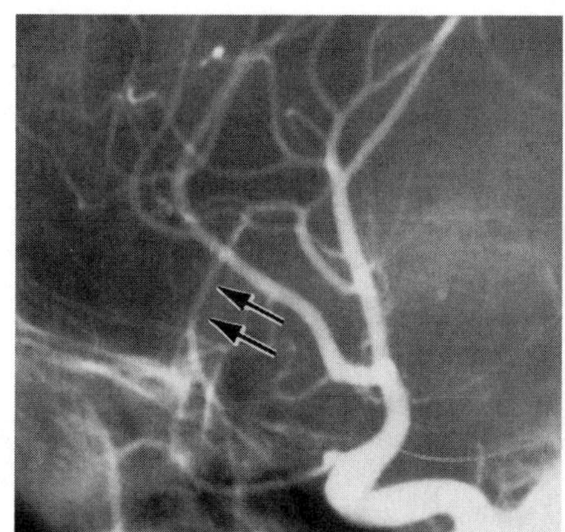

A

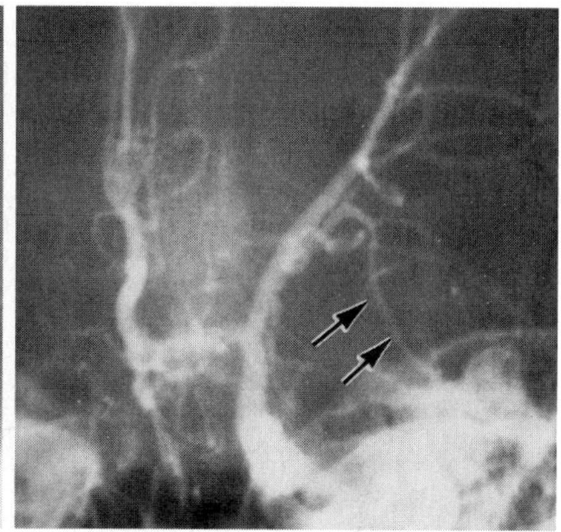

B

Figure 17.66. Large temporal intracerebral tumor showing displacement of the anterior temporal branch of the middle cerebral artery. **A.** There is elevation of the horizontal portion of the middle cerebral artery and upward dislocation of the sylvian triangle. The anterior temporal artery is displaced forward around the mass (arrows). **B.** The deformities are obvious. The anterior temporal branch (arrows) is seen to cross obliquely downward and outward. This appearance is typical of intracerebral tumors.

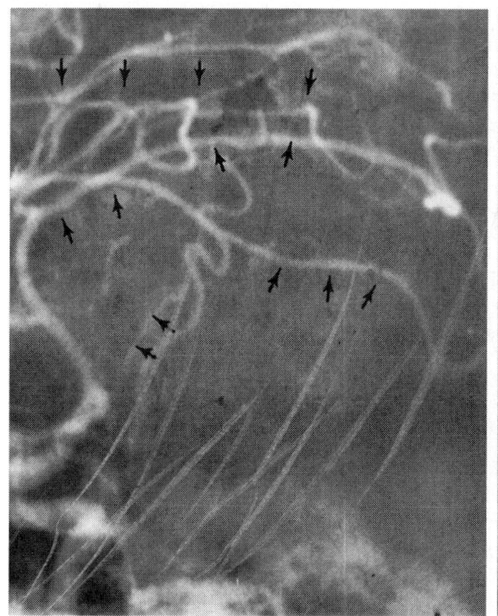

A

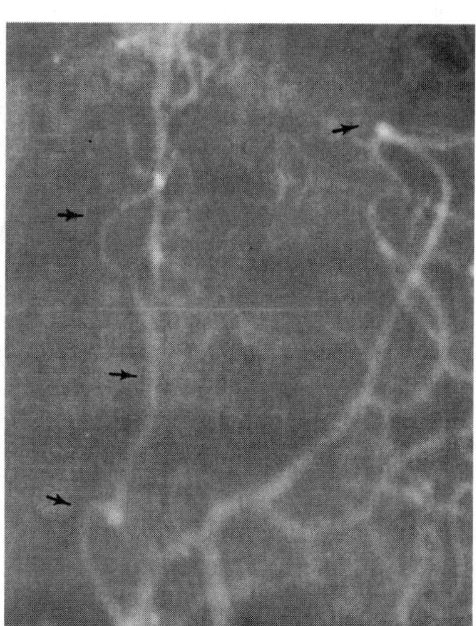

B

Figure 17.67. Middle fossa meningioma. **A.** The lateral view shows a marked degree of elevation of the middle cerebral artery and its branches. The sylvian triangle is extremely high in position (upper arrows) above the level of the pericallosal artery (central arrows). The anterior choroidal artery is markedly elevated, almost vertical in position (two lower arrows). One branch of the middle cerebral artery (posterior three arrows) seems to drape over the tumor, even though it is a meningioma, because the tumor is very deeply placed in the middle fossa. In fact, it could not be removed surgically; thus, some of the lateral aspect of the temporal lobe was not lifted off the floor of the middle fossa. **B.** The frontal projection reveals the marked degree of elevation of the middle cerebral vessels and the extremely high position of the angiographic sylvian point (lateral arrow). The supraclinoid portion of the siphon is displaced medially, and the bifurcation is high. The shift of the anterior cerebral artery is more pronounced in its proximal (inferior) portion and to a lesser degree in its distal segments (upper and lower medial arrows), but the central portion (midline arrow) is practically in the midline.

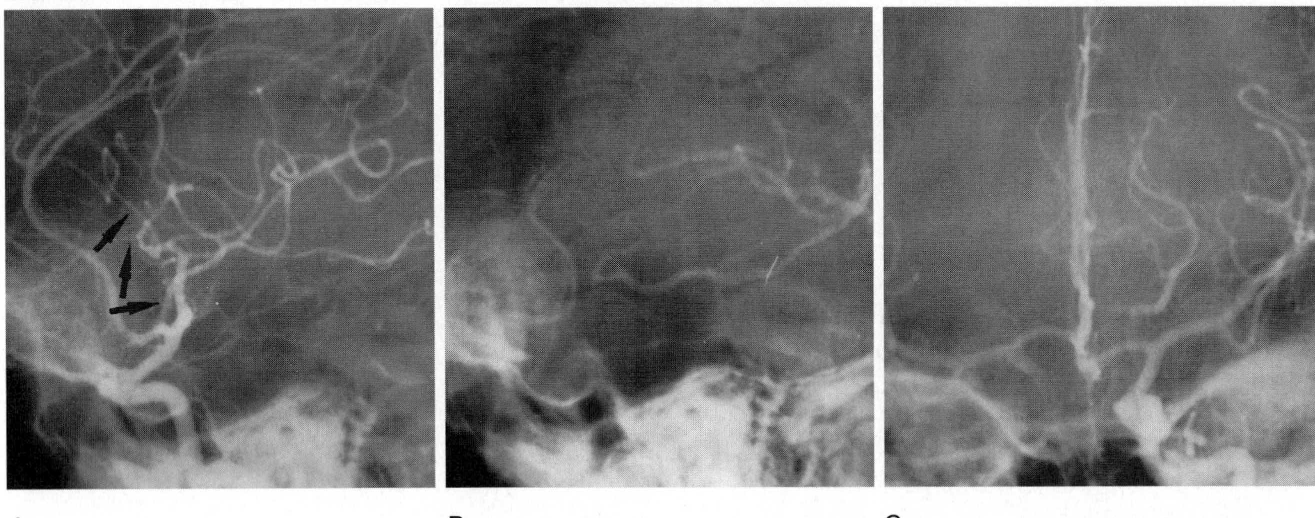

Figure 17.68. Anterior temporal (frontotemporal) extracerebral tumor (sphenoid ridge meningioma). **A.** The lateral arterial phase shows posterior displacement of the horizontal portion of the middle cerebral artery, thus clearing the anterior cerebral artery from any overlying middle cerebral artery branches. The anterior branches of the middle cerebral artery are displaced upward and backward around the tumor (arrows), and the sylvian triangle is disrupted anteriorly. The carotid siphon is closed, which indicates that the tumor mass is wrapped around the sphenoid ridge, growing toward both the frontal and the temporal side. **B.** The venous phase shows posterior displacement of the superficial middle cerebral vein, again emphasizing that the tumor is pushing the tip of the temporal lobe backward. **C.** The frontal film shows elevation of the horizontal portion of the middle cerebral artery. The angiographic sylvian point is only slightly elevated.

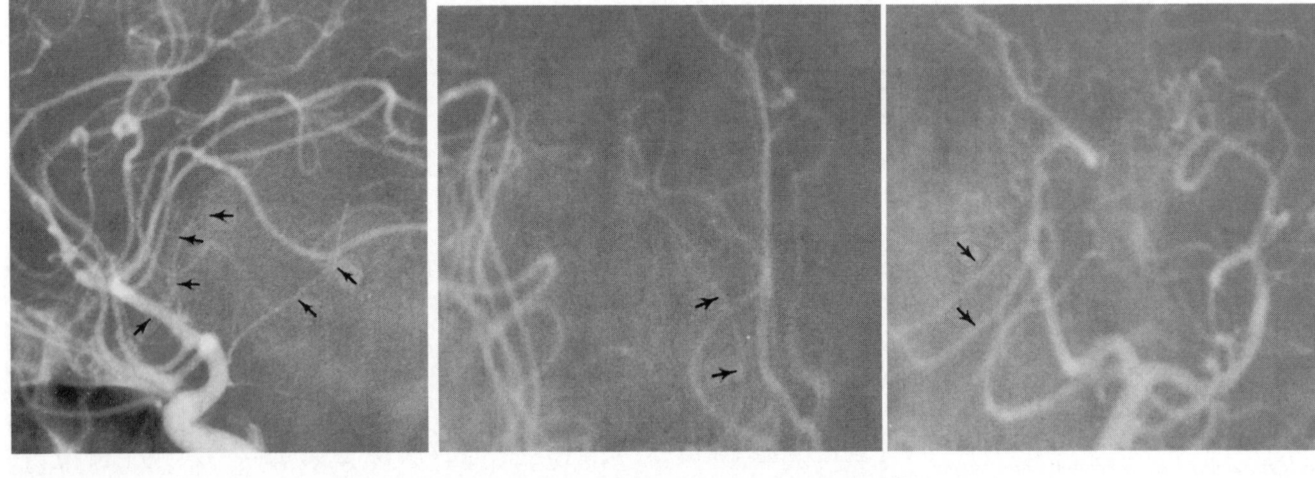

Figure 17.69. Temporal intracerebral tumor occupying entire temporal lobe. **A.** The lateral view shows moderate forward displacement and lifting of the horizontal portion of the middle cerebral artery (anterior arrow), as well as marked elevation of the middle cerebral branches posteriorly. The anterior choroidal artery is elevated, stretched, and enlarged (posterior arrows). The lenticulostriate arteries are also displaced forward (forward arrows). At least two branches of the middle cerebral artery drape over the area occupied by the tumor, indicating the intracerebral position of the mass. **B.** The frontal projection discloses a marked degree of medial displacement and bowing of the anterior choroidal artery (arrows) extending to the most posterior portion of the artery. Because the center of the tumor is more posterior, the supraclinoid portion of the carotid siphon is essentially normal in position. There is medial displacement of the branches of the middle cerebral artery away from the inner table of the skull, which is an indication of involvement of the temporal operculum. **C.** A vertebral angiogram discloses involvement of the posterior temporal branches of the posterior cerebral artery, which are distorted (arrows). There is flattening of the curve of the posterior cerebral artery around the midbrain as compared with the other side. The distortion of the posterior temporal arteries indicates that the tumor has extended far backward, or it is possible that the deformity could be produced by diffuse swelling. The presence of only a small anterior cerebral shift, however, involving chiefly the proximal portion of the artery, would indicate that there is not very much cerebral edema and that the lesion is probably a relatively slowly growing mass. The tumor was an extensive astrocytoma.

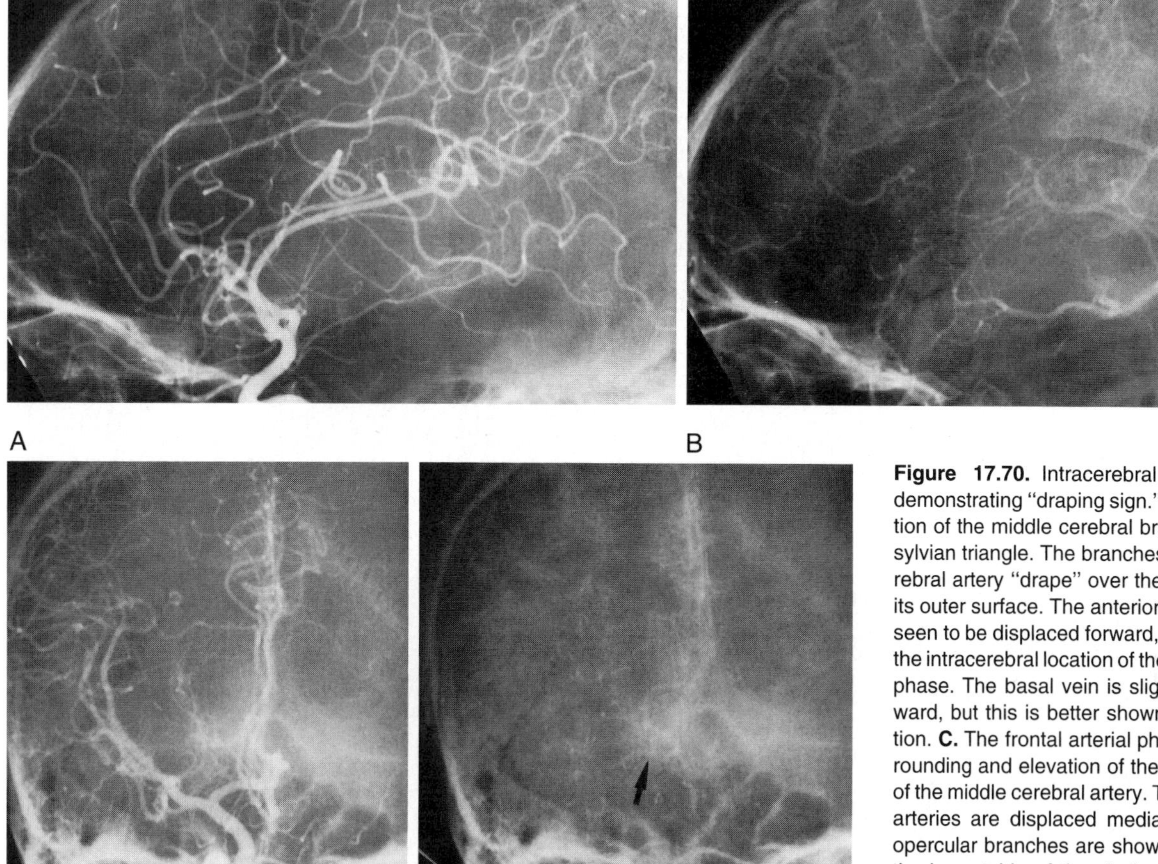

Figure 17.70. Intracerebral temporal tumor demonstrating "draping sign." **A.** There is elevation of the middle cerebral branches and of the sylvian triangle. The branches of the middle cerebral artery "drape" over the temporal lobe on its outer surface. The anterior temporal artery is seen to be displaced forward, further confirming the intracerebral location of the mass. **B.** Venous phase. The basal vein is slightly displaced upward, but this is better shown in frontal projection. **C.** The frontal arterial phase demonstrates rounding and elevation of the horizontal portion of the middle cerebral artery. The lenticulostriate arteries are displaced medially. The temporal opercular branches are shown to stretch out to the inner table of the skull and "drape" downward over the lateral aspect of the temporal lobe. **D.** The frontal venous phase demonstrates well the elevation of the anterior portion of the basal vein (arrow).

Extracerebral Temporal Masses

In general, extracerebral masses produce upward displacement of all of the branches of the middle cerebral artery because they lift the temporal lobe. On the other hand, intracerebral temporal tumors lift the branches within and above the sylvian fissure, while the vessels on the surface of the temporal lobe still descend over and envelop the enlarged lobe. This "draping sign" is seen because the temporal arterial branches drape over the temporal lobe filled with tumor, as seen in the lateral view of the angiogram (Fig. 17.70). Compare with Figure 17.71, a meningioma, in which all anterior branches are elevated.

Retrosylvian Masses

The term *retrosylvian* is applied to all masses that are situated behind the angiographic sylvian point. Angiographically, the most important finding is forward displacement of the angiographic sylvian point. Where the last middle cerebral branches emerge, from the depths of the sylvian fissure onto the surface of the brain, usually indicates the position of the angiographic sylvian point. A forward displacement of the sylvian point results in a telescopic, or closed accordion, deformity of the branches of the middle cerebral artery, which is typical when present (Fig. 17.72).

In frontal projection, the angiographic sylvian point is displaced downward because forward displacement of this point is equivalent to downward displacement in the usual angiographic anteroposterior projection. Therefore, even if the angiographic sylvian point is not displaced downward, as seen in the lateral view, when visualized in the frontal projection, it lies well below the center of the vertex-petrosal reference line described under "Measurements." Use of the sella turcica as a reference point to determine forward displacement is helpful because the angiographic sylvian point is normally well behind and above the dorsum sellae, usually directly above the density of the petrous pyramid. Retrosylvian masses bow the middle cerebral arterial branches.

The inferior retrosylvian tentorial masses produce telescoping of the sylvian triangle and upward displacement of the angiographic sylvian point, as seen in the lateral view.

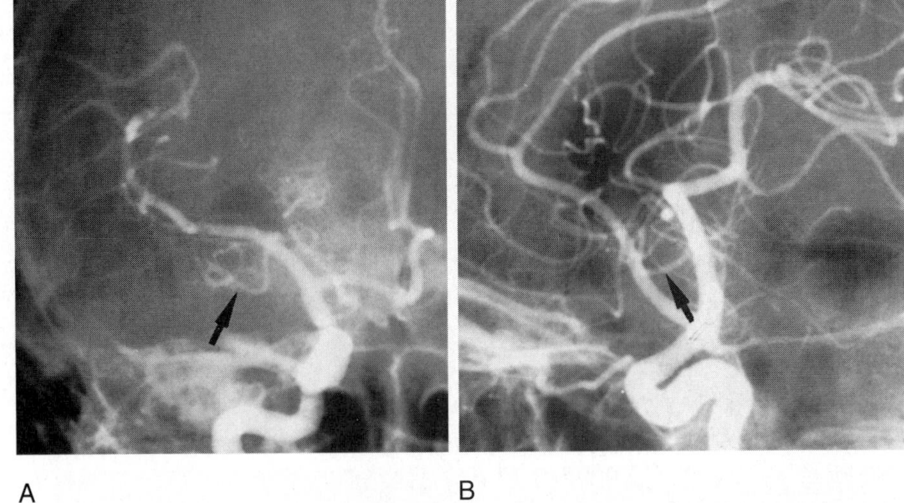

Figure 17.71. Anterior infrasylvian (temporal) tumor, sphenoid ridge meningioma. **A.** The frontal projection demonstrates moderate medial displacement of the supraclinoid portion of the carotid artery and rounded elevation of the middle cerebral artery. There is elevation of the anterior temporal artery (arrow), indicating the extracerebral location of the tumor. A characteristic proximal subfalcial shift is shown. **B.** The lateral view demonstrates the upward dislocation of the middle cerebral artery and the elevation of the anterior temporal branch (arrow).

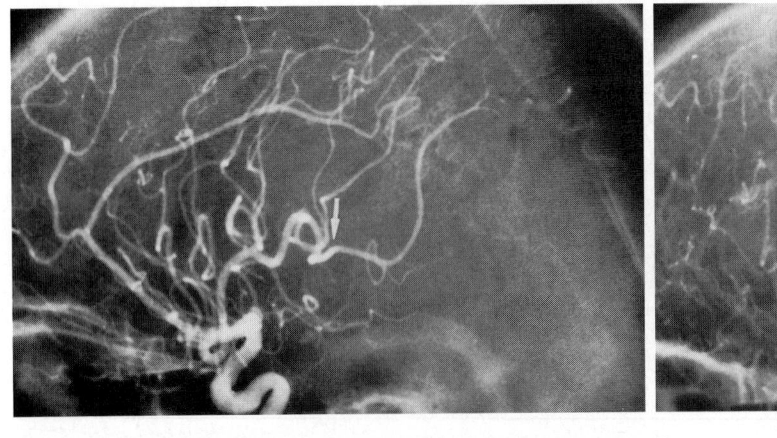

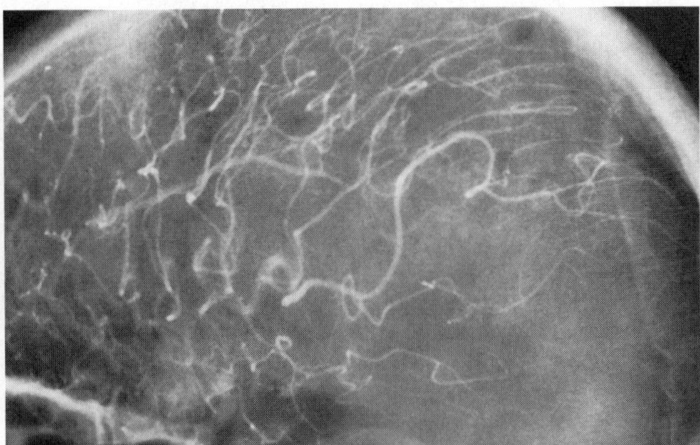

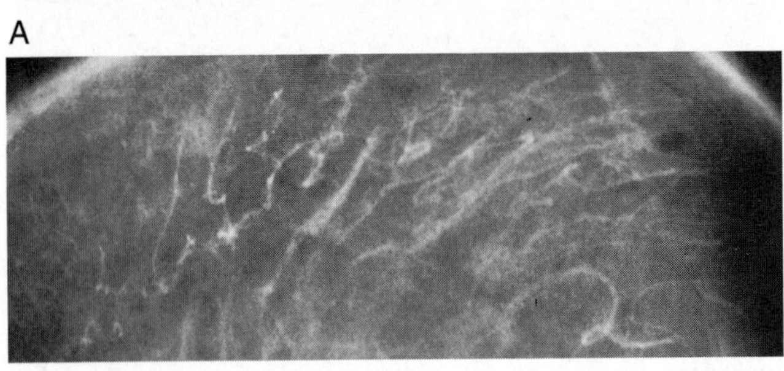

Figure 17.72. Retrosylvian tumor (glioma) producing telescoping of the middle cerebral branches and the "onion peeling" effect. **A** and **B.** The region of the angiographic sylvian point is displaced forward (arrow); it lies almost straight above the dorsum sellae. **C.** The "onion peeling" effect owing to bending of the gyri and sulci of the brain in a concentric manner is evident and is pronounced into the late arterial phase. The "onion peeling" effect extends far beyond the confines of the tumor and is probably associated with edema.

Intrasylvian Masses

As the name indicates, this group comprises masses that occur between the lips of the sylvian fissure. Characteristically, intrasylvian masses cause a very sharp displacement and stretching of the branches of the middle cerebral artery. They produce a rather typical "splitting" of the branches, with some rising above and others situated below the tumor (Fig. 17.73). If the mass bulges out of the sylvian fissure, it may displace the middle cerebral branches away from the inner table of the skull (Fig. 17.74).

Laterosylvian Masses

A typical mass produces medial displacement of the branches of the middle cerebral artery and of the angiographic sylvian point. The displacement is usually easy to evaluate, except in the case of a thin subdural hematoma, where the degree of displacement is only slightly above the normal limit of 43 mm for the sylvian point and 30 mm for the branches over the outer surface of the island of Reil. Because these masses are at the level of the middle cerebral vessels and are extracerebral in location, they simply displace the middle cerebral branches inward and not upward or downward.

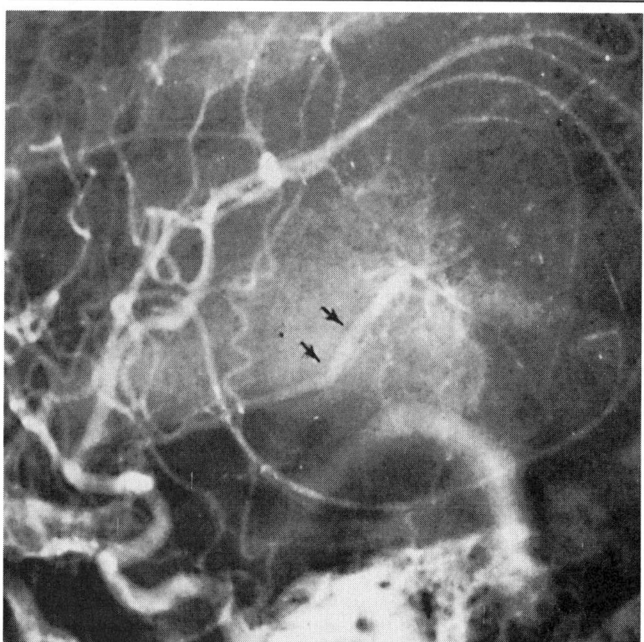

Figure 17.73. Intrasylvian tumor (meningioma). There is "splitting" of the branches of the middle cerebral artery. Such tumors growing in the sylvian fissure displace some branches upward and other branches downward, outlining the mass. A meningeal vessel is supplying the meningioma (arrows).

Ventricular Dilatation

Ventricular dilatation causes diffuse elevation of the vessels that form the sylvian triangle and lateral displacement of the sylvian point.

Posterior Cerebral Artery

As has been pointed out, the posterior cerebral artery is the artery of "seeing and looking," serving almost single-handedly the majority of functions needed for vision (127).

NORMAL GROSS AND ANGIOGRAPHIC ANATOMY

The posterior cerebral artery serves the occipital cortex, thalamus, and mesencephalon. A list of visual ocular areas served by the posterior cerebral artery includes pupillary reflexes, coordination of lateral and horizontal eye movements, and so forth. The proximal segment supplies the midbrain, the mid portion of the thalamus and choroid plexus; the distal branches supply the occipital and temporal cortex.

COURSE

The vessel originates from the distal basilar or the proximal intracranial internal carotid artery. The vessel can be divided into the peduncular (P1–P2), ambient (P2), and quadrigeminal segments (P3). The short (0.5 to 1.0 cm) peduncular segment (P1) courses anteriorly and laterally, with the posterior communicating artery entering at its midportion. The ambient portion extends posteriorly and medially between the midbrain and the parahippocampal gyrus. The quadgrigeminal segment runs in the latter cistern, for which it is named, posteriorly to reach the cortex. The system of Fischer divides it into segments relative to the takeoff of the posterior communicating artery and then similar to the naming of the middle cerebral artery.

As has been pointed out by Lasjaunias and Berenstein, P1 is more like the anterior spinal artery than like a cortical

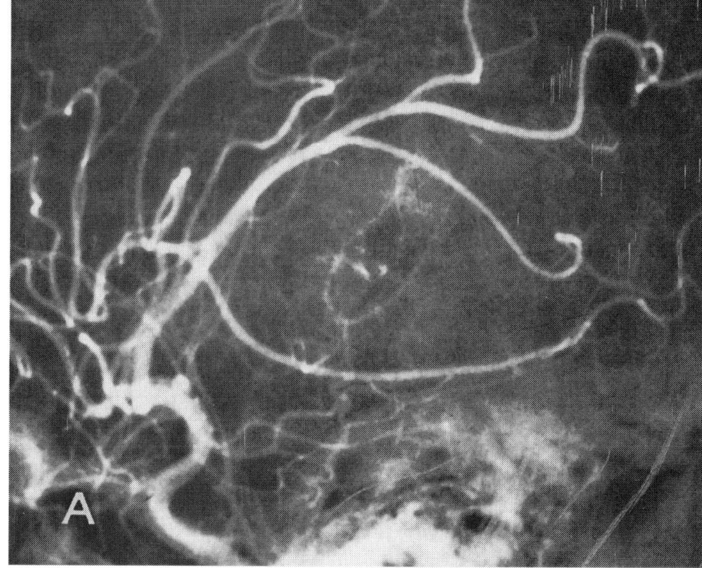

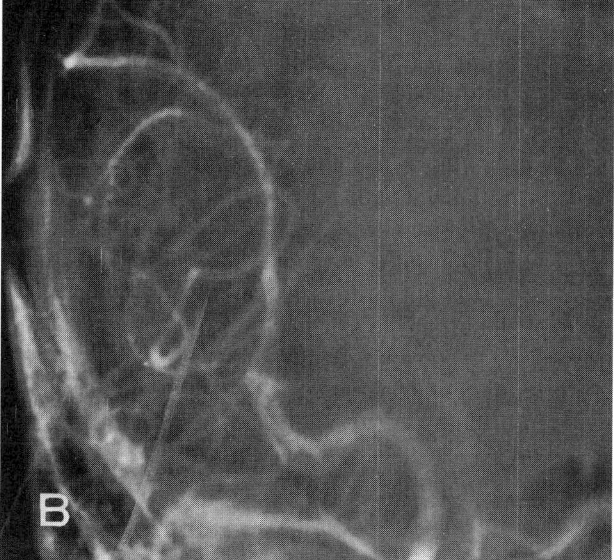

A B

Figure 17.74. Intrasylvian astrocytoma simulating intrasylvian meningioma. **A.** The lateral view shows an appearance quite similar to that noted in the preceding figure. **B.** The frontal projection shows medial displacement of the middle cerebral branches with flattening of the insular curve.

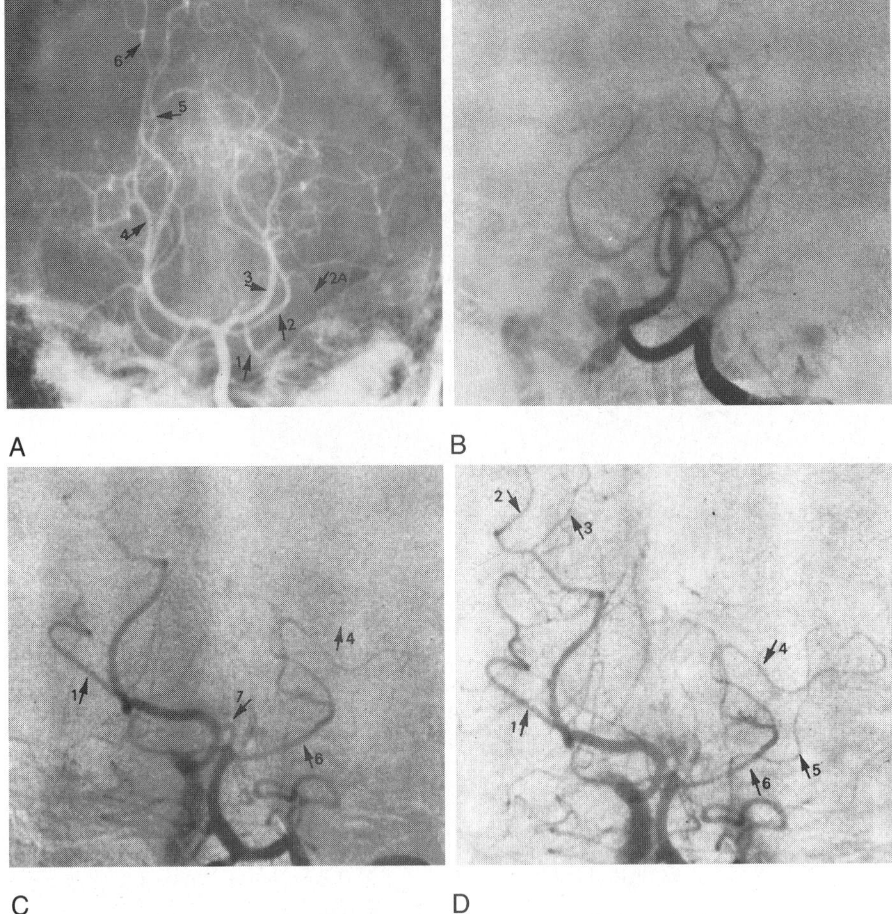

Figure 17.75. Normal vertebral angiograms demonstrating posterior cerebral arteries and posterior communicating arteries. **A.** The arrows refer to (1) posterior communicating artery; (2) superior cerebellar artery; (2A) anterior lateral marginal branch of superior cerebellar artery; (3) posterior cerebral artery; (4) posterior temporal artery; (5) calcarine branch; and (6) parieto-occipital branch of posterior cerebral artery. **B.** Nonfilling of the posterior cerebral artery on the right. **C.** Nonfilling of the posterior cerebral artery on the left. The arrows in C and D refer to (1) posterior temporal branch; (2) parieto-occipital branch; (3) calcarine branch; (4) hemispheric branch of superior cerebellar artery; (5) hemispheric branch of PICA, possibly anastomosing end to end with the hemispheric branch of the superior cerebellar; (6) superior cerebellar artery; and (7) posterior cerebral artery.

branch (122). The interpeduncular perforating arteries (3 to 6) supply the perimedian reticular formation, pretectum and anteromedial roof of the fourth ventricle. Just laterally, the peduncular branches serve the cerebral peduncle, substantia nigra, red nucleus, and part of the tegmentum. The circumflex mesencephalic arteries serve the posterior aspect of the tegmentum (105).

POSTERIOR COMMUNICATING ARTERY

This vessel arises from the dorsal aspect of the carotid siphon and proceeds posteriorly and medially. It is approximately 1.5 cm in length. At its dorsal extremity, it joins the posterior cerebral artery approximately 1.0 cm distal to the bifurcation of the basilar artery (Fig. 17.75). In the lateral view it usually describes a slight curve concave upward (Fig. 17.76). Sometimes it is almost straight, and its junction with the posterior cerebral artery cannot be seen on the films. The latter appearance usually denotes carotid origin of the posterior cerebral artery ("fetal" posterior cerebral) (Fig. 17.77). The posterior communicating and posterior cerebral arteries fill completely or incompletely in a high percentage of carotid angiograms, depending on the location of the injection and other technical factors, including amount of contrast and

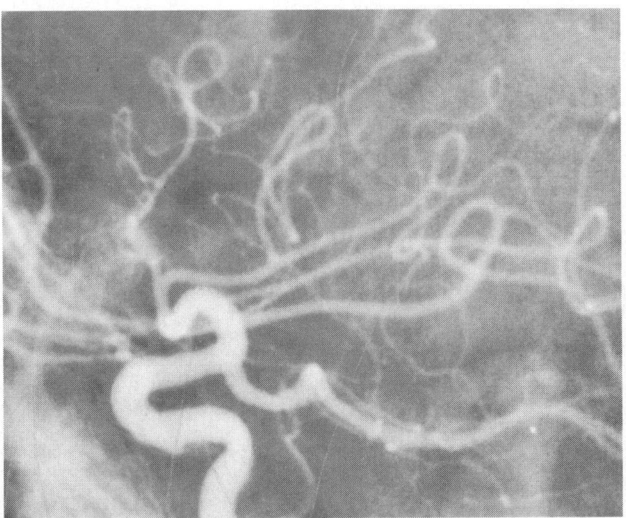

Figure 17.76. Normal carotid angiogram, lateral view. The posterior communicating is well shown and its characteristic upward curvature as it joins the posterior cerebral artery is well demonstrated. Just above the posterior communicating artery is the anterior choroidal. The anterior cerebral artery demonstrates one of its normal variants, namely, the callosomarginal artery is arising from an early bifurcation of the anterior cerebral artery and both pericallosal arteries filled from the opposite side. An appearance such as this may sometimes mislead the observer because it suggests ventricular dilatation.

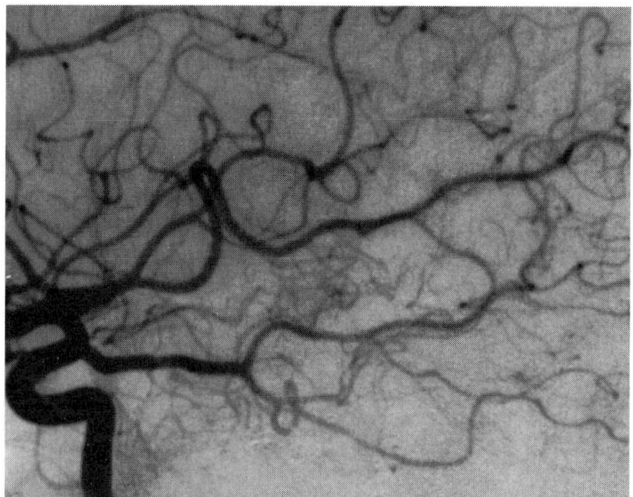

Figure 17.77. Carotid origin of posterior cerebral artery ("fetal" variant). There is no change in the caliber of the posterior communicating artery when it joins the posterior cerebral artery; in fact, the posterior communicating is slightly larger than the posterior cerebral artery, indicating that the blood supply of the posterior cerebral artery is coming from the carotid system.

force of the injection. It fills more frequently in almost one-half of internal carotid injections and in 26 to 30 percent of common carotid injections. One side may fill and not the other, and one side may be larger than the other.

At the junction of the posterior communicating artery with the carotid siphon, there is often a slight dilatation, which we have come to call *junctional dilatation*, and which should not be confused with an aneurysm. The shape of this dilatation may be conical or round (Fig. 17.78), with the posterior communicating artery usually joining the dilatation at its apex. Saltzman has described several cases in which anatomic defects were found in the infundibular or junctional portion of the vessel, similar to those found in aneurysms (128). On the contrary, the work of Fox et al. (129) and Epstein et al. (130) suggests that the dilatation is not "preaneurysmal." One case has been observed in which the entire posterior communicating artery became 3 mm in diameter, the size of a preexisting infundibulum, after carotid ligation. In another case seen by the author, however, a saccular aneurysm was found at the point where only an apparent rounded junctional dilatation had been demonstrated 2 years previously. It is our opinion that the

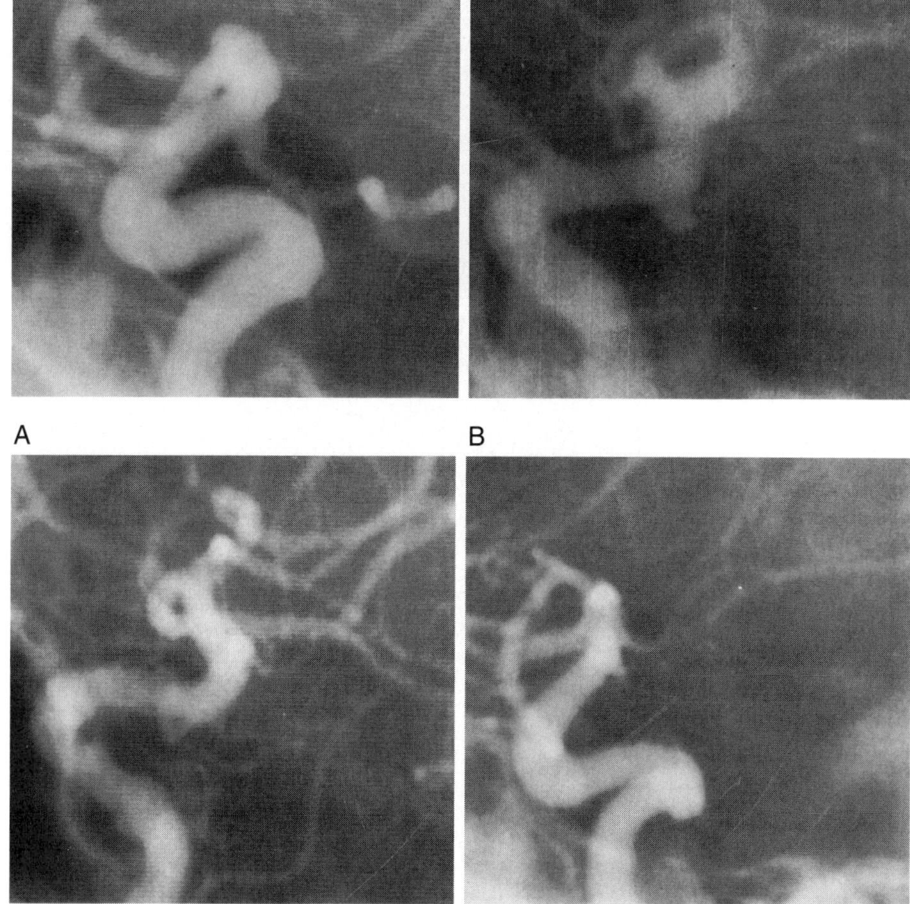

Figure 17.78. Various types of junctional dilatation at origins of the branches of the internal carotid artery. **A.** Funnel shape, with posterior communicating artery arising at apex. **B.** Same shape as above, but posterior communicating artery did not fill. **C.** Dilatation at posterior communicating site and a smaller one at anterior choroidal origin. **D.** Dilatation at anterior choroidal origin (see also "Arterial Aneurysms").

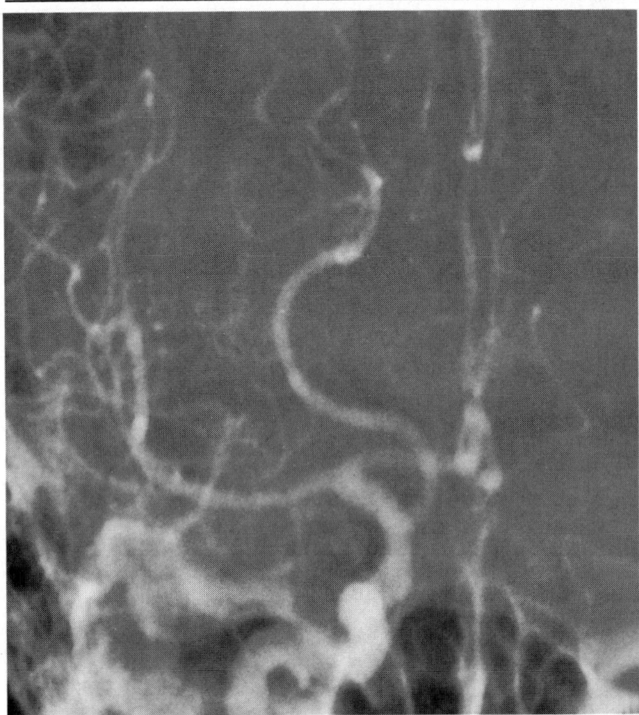

Figure 17.79. Carotid angiogram, normal, showing filling of posterior communicating and posterior cerebral arteries. The posterior communicating artery is directed backward and slightly medially; after joining the posterior cerebral artery, it follows the course of this artery around the brainstem.

dilatation should be considered as a possible aneurysm only when it measures more than 3 mm in diameter or when the posterior communicating artery does not join the dilatation at its apex (see under "Aneurysms," Chapter 10).

In the frontal projection, the posterior communicating artery is partly superimposed on the supraclinoid portion of the internal carotid. The posterior portion usually projects medial to the carotid artery (Fig. 17.79). This is a relatively constant relationship, and deviation should be regarded as probably pathologic.

From the dorsal segment of the posterior communicating artery arise a number of small branches that supply the medial surface of the thalamus and the wall of the third ventricle, but these are demonstrated infrequently on conventional serialograms during carotid angiography. When the posterior communicating artery fills via the basilar artery, the thalamoperforate arteries are usually demonstrated. The branch arising from the posterior communicating artery is the *anterior thalamoperforate artery* (more than one is often present). It supplies the anterior and lateral aspects of the thalamus.

The posterior thalamoperforate arteries arise from the posterior cerebral artery, usually between the bifurcation of the basilar artery and the junction with the posterior communicating artery on each side. They ascend in the interpeduncular fossa and enter the brain behind the mammillary bodies in the posterior perforated substance. They supply the posterior thalamus and adjacent structures and are usually demonstrated on vertebral angiograms of good quality (108, 131) (Figs. 17.80, 17.81, 17.88).

The *tela choroidea of the lateral ventricle* is vascularized by arteries arising from the two systems that form the arterial circle at the base (i.e., the internal carotid system and the vertebral basilar system) (132). This blood supply is given by one anterior choroidal artery and by several posterior choroidal arteries. These arteries anastomose to form multiple indirect and remote links between the carotid and vertebral basilar systems. The capillary networks of the tela choroidea of the lateral ventricle consist of a velar network and a choroidal network. This duality is constantly observed in the choroid formations of the human brain. The venous vascularization of the tela is tributary of the venous circle of the base of the brain through choroidal veins that drain either into the internal cerebral veins or into the basal veins.

PRECOMMUNAL SEGMENT (P1)

The posterior cerebral arteries arise from the bifurcation of the basilar artery just distal to the origins of the superior

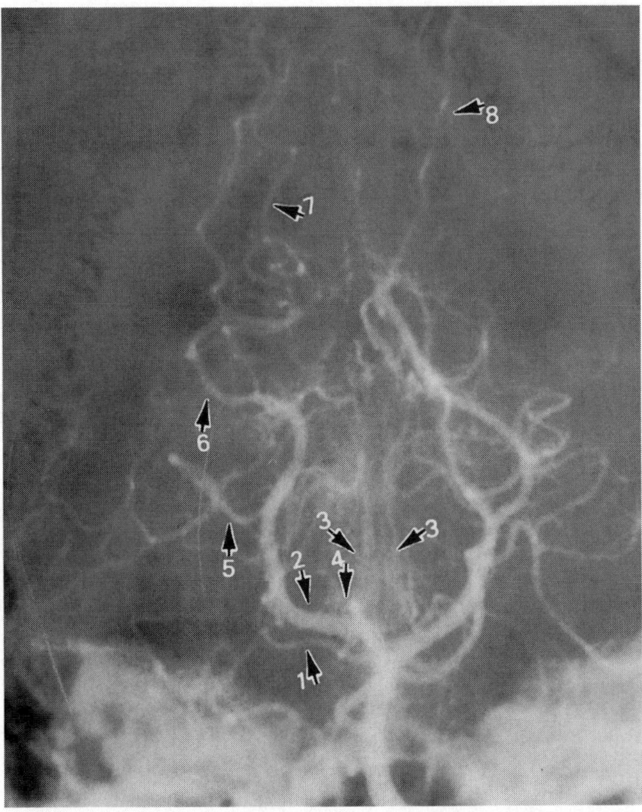

Figure 17.80. Posterior thalamoperforate arteries as seen in the frontal projection. Arrows indicate (1) superior cerebellar artery; (2) posterior cerebral artery; (3) posterior thalamoperforate branches of the posterior cerebral artery; (4) posterior inferior cerebellar artery projecting above the posterior cerebral artery; (5) posterior temporal artery; (6) parieto-occipital branch, which seems to give rise to the calcarine branch (arrow 7) distally; and (8) parieto-occipital branch on left.

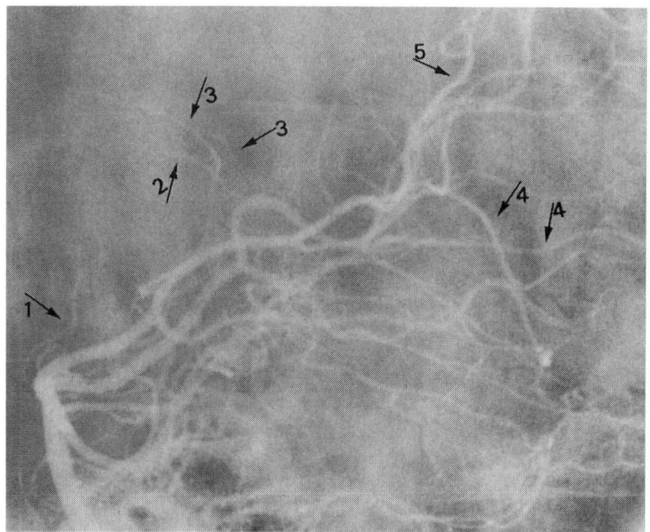

Figure 17.81. Normal vertebral angiogram demonstrating lateral posterior choroidal arteries. Arrows identify (1) posterior thalamoperforate arteries; (2) medial posterior choroidal artery; (3) lateral posterior choroidal arteries; (4) calcarine branches; and (5) parieto-occipital branches.

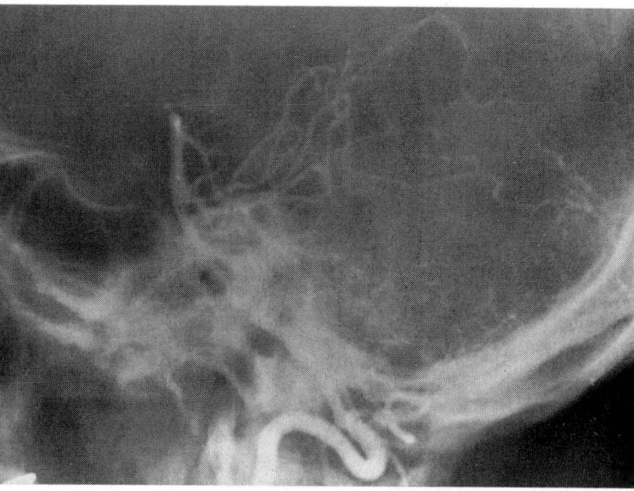

Figure 17.82. Appearance of basilar artery system in lateral projection when posterior cerebral arteries do not fill. Both are filling via the internal carotid artery. Without the numerous overlying branches of the posterior cerebral arteries, it is easier to identify the superior cerebellar artery branches.

cerebellar arteries; the superior cerebellar and posterior cerebral arteries are separated on each side by the third cranial nerve. The artery has a carotid origin on one or both sides in about 15 percent of cases. Actually, in the embryo, the artery is fed by the carotid system, but later the connection with the basilar artery becomes dominant and the posterior communicating artery becomes smaller. In a review of over 200 vertebral angiograms, Saltzman found that both posterior cerebral arteries filled in 88 percent of the cases, only one filled in 10 to 11 percent, and none filled in 2 percent (133) (Fig. 17.82). In the latter group it is presumed that the initial segment of the posterior cerebral artery is either hypoplastic or, rarely, absent. Thus, dual filling of the posterior cerebral artery from both the carotid and basilar systems can occur even in cases that show a dominant carotid origin.

Caruso et al. studied the P1 segment in anatomic dissections (134). Anomalies of the precommunicating segment of the posterior cerebral artery (P1) were found, including a case of duplication of the P1 segment, a large fenestration, and a common orgin with the superior cerebellar artery.

POSTCOMMUNAL SEGMENT (P2–P3)

The posterior cerebral artery first passes laterally and then turns around the cerebral peduncles to the posterolateral aspect of the midbrain (Fig. 17.83). As it turns around the midbrain, the artery often makes a downward swing (concave upward). It may therefore take on an asymmetric and, at times, confusing appearance when the right is compared with the left in frontal projection. The artery is contained within the tentorial incisura and actually follows the medial

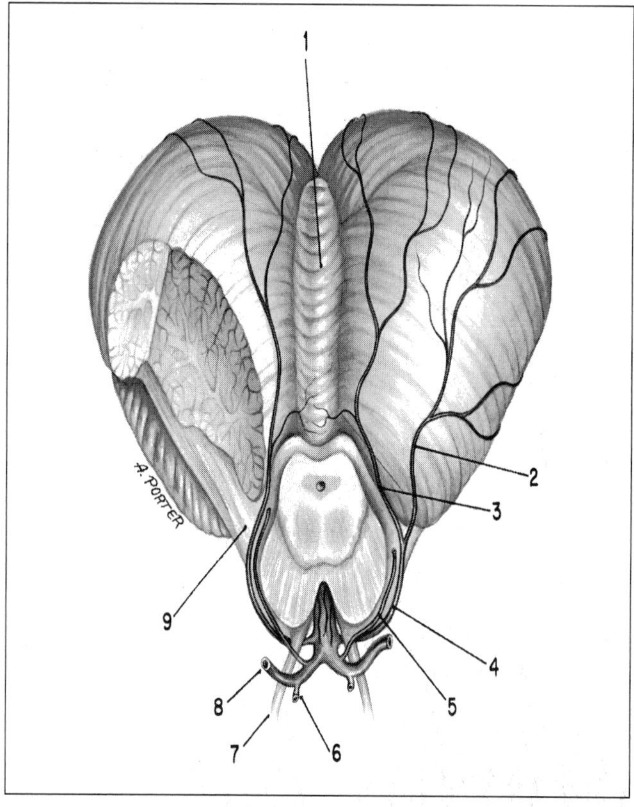

Figure 17.83. Superior view of cerebellum and midbrain that has been cut just above bifurcation of the basilar artery. (1) Superior vermis; (2) hemispheric branch of superior cerebellar artery; (3) vermis branch of superior cerebellar with twigs to supply the precentral area; (4) superior cerebellar artery; (5) medial posterior choroidal artery; (6) posterior communicating artery; (7) third cranial nerve; (8) posterior cerebral artery; and (9) middle cerebellar peduncle.

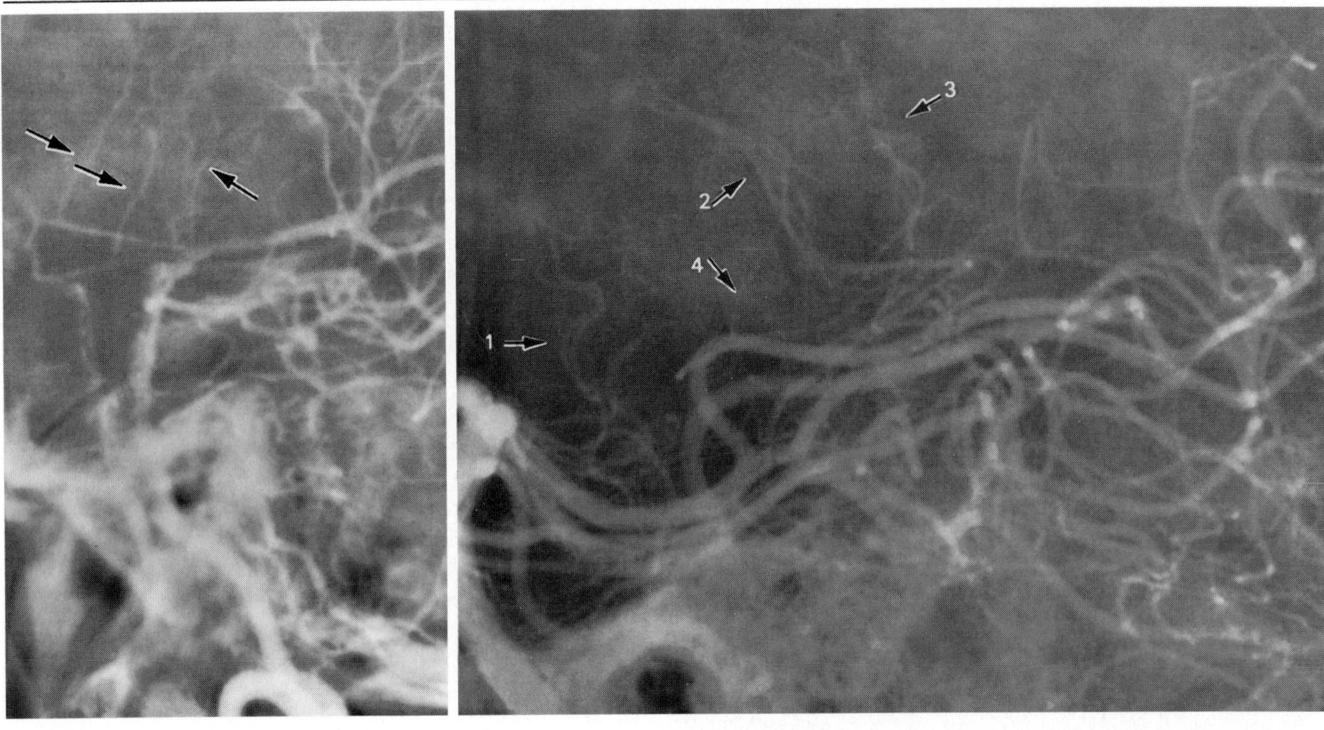

edge of the tentorial slit. As it continues its course dorsad, it rises above the tentorium to run on the medial aspect of the undersurface of the temporal lobe.

POSTERIOR CHOROIDAL ARTERIES

The posterior choroidal arteries originate from the posterior cerebral arteries; there are one medial and two or more lateral arteries on each side (135). The *medial posterior choroidal artery* arises from the posterior cerebral artery just lateral to the bifurcation of the basilar artery (P1). It passes around the midbrain together with, and most frequently obscured by, the parent vessel. As it reaches the posterolateral aspect of the midbrain it ascends, describing a double arch (figure of "3"), and passes just lateral to the pineal body to reach the midline. It then enters the tela choroidea of the third ventricle, following along the roof of this ventricle (Figs. 17.84 and 17.85).

The *lateral posterior choroidal arteries* (at least two in number) arise on each side from the posterior cerebral artery along the lateral and posterolateral aspects of the brain stem. They usually penetrate the choroidal fissure almost immediately and, as they ascend, describe a curve concave forward, corresponding to the posterior aspect of the thalamus (Fig. 17.84). They can be differentiated from the medial posterior choroidal artery in the lateral angiogram because they describe a smooth concave curve, whereas the medial posterior choroidal artery describes a double curve; the medial vessel is usually slightly more anterior in posi-

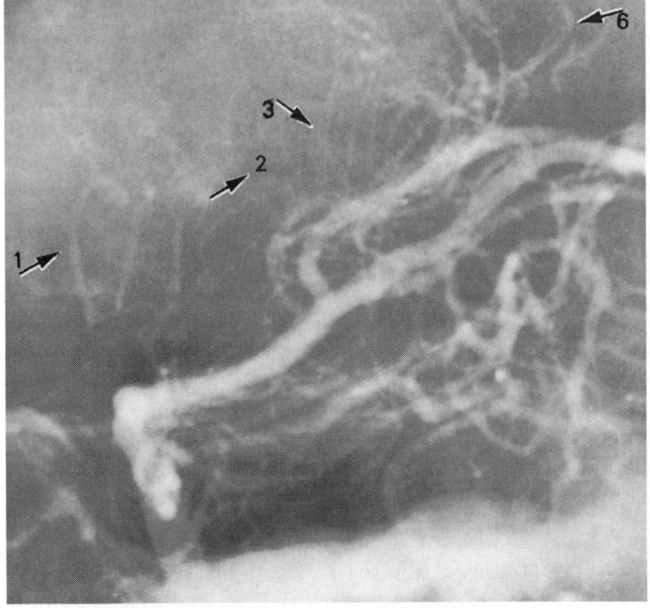

Figure 17.84. Thalamoperforate branches arising from posterior cerebral arteries. **A.** The two anterior arrows mark the anterior thalamoperforate arteries. The posterior arrow marks a posterior thalamoperforate artery arising directly from the posterior cerebral artery. **B.** Arrows indicate (1) posterior thalamoperforate artery; (2) medial posterior choroidal artery; (3) lateral posterior choroidal arteries; and (4) quadrigeminal and geniculate branches. **C.** Arrows indicate (1) anterior thalamoperforate arteries from the posterior communicating artery; (2) posterior thalamoperforate arteries; (3) quadrigeminal and geniculate branches; (4) medial posterior choroidal artery; (5) lateral posterior choroidal arteries; and (6) posterior pericallosal artery.

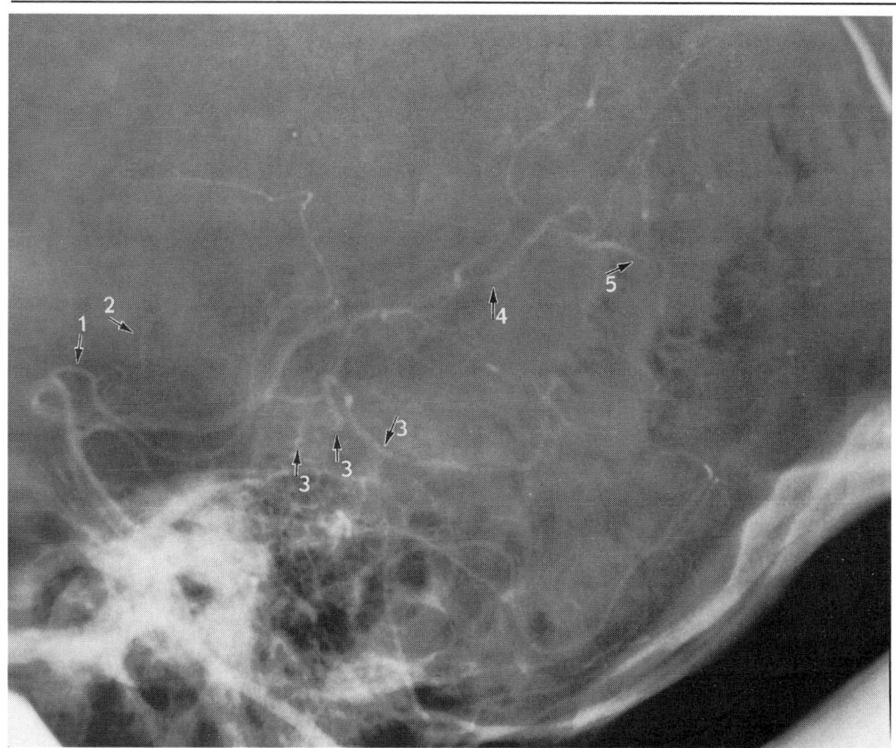

Figure 17.85. Medial posterior choroidal artery demonstrated in lateral projection. The origin of the medial posterior choroidal artery from the initial portion of the posterior cerebral artery is clearly shown in this patient in whom only one posterior cerebral artery filled via the basilar system: (1) medial posterior choroidal artery; (2) posterior thalamoperforate arteries; (3) posterior temporal artery; (4) parieto-occipital branch; and (5) calcarine branch.

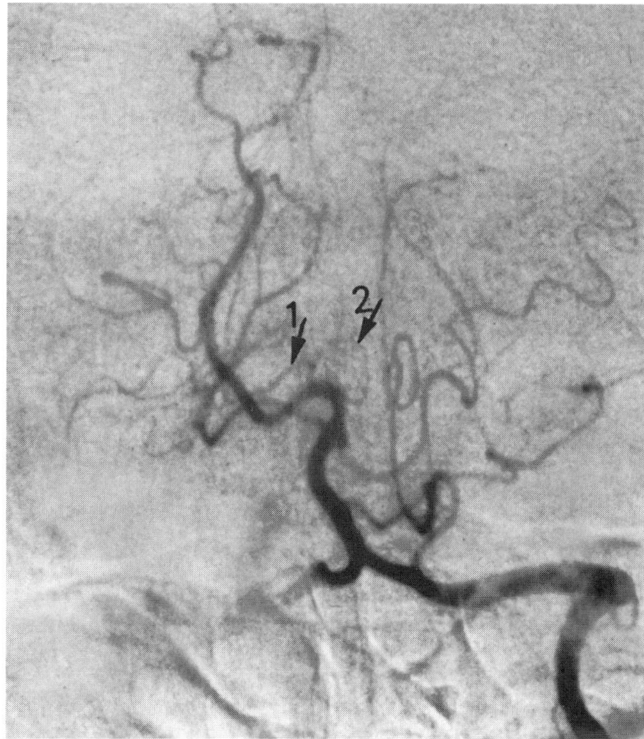

Figure 17.86. Normal vertebral angiogram showing appearance when only one posterior cerebral artery fills, and demonstrating medial posterior choroidal and posterior thalamoperforate arteries: (1) medial posterior choroidal artery as it turns around brainstem; (2) posterior thalamoperforate branches.

tion. On stereoscopic films, the left and right medial posterior choroidal vessels are very near the midline. The posterior choroidal arteries are more difficult to identify on frontal angiographic films, but the thalamoperforate branches can be seen routinely on films of good quality (Figs. 17.80 and 17.86).

CORTICAL BRANCHES (SEE TABLE 17.5)

The posterior cerebral artery gives off an anterior temporal branch, which anastomoses with the corresponding branch

Table 17.5.
Cortical Branches of the Posterior Cerebral Artery

Branches	Area supplied
Parieto-occipital artery	Caudal cuneus, superior occipital gyrus, superior and inferior parietal lobe
Anteroinferior temporal artery(ies)	Medial temporal lobe, hippocampus
Posterior inferior temporal artery(ies)	Medial temporal lobe, hippocampus
Calcarine artery	Visual cortex, inferior cuneus and lingual gyrus
Splenial artery (posterior pericallosal)	Splenium of the corpus callosum
Dural branches	Anterior falx

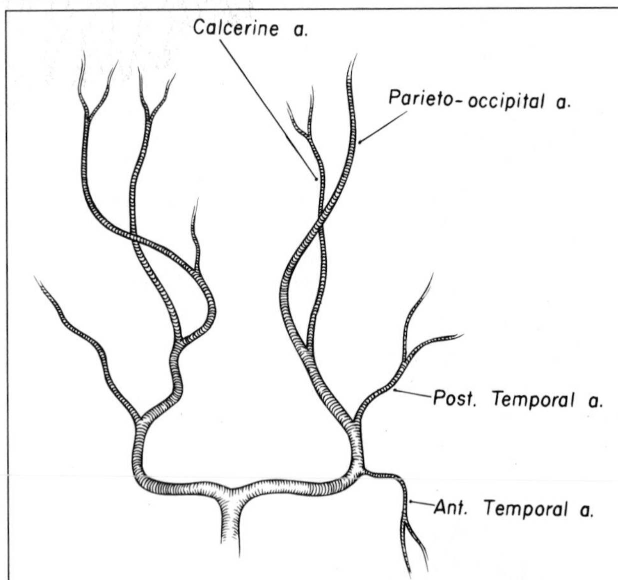

Figure 17.87. Frontal projection of posterior cerebral artery and branches.

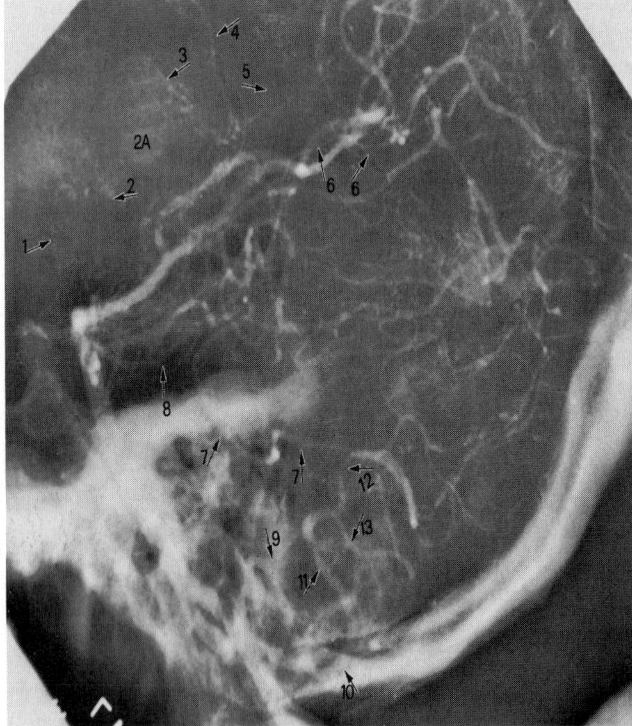

Figure 17.88. Lateral view of vertebral angiogram to demonstrate superior cerebellar arteries. The arrows point to: (1) anterior thalamoperforate arteries arising from the posterior communicating; (2) posterior thalamoperforate arteries; (2A) quadrigeminal and geniculate branches of the posterior cerebral; (3) medial posterior choroidal artery; (4) lateral posterior choroidal arteries; (5) posterior pericallosal branch of posterior cerebral; (6) superior cerebellar arteries passing over the culmen; (7) anterior lateral marginal branch of superior cerebellar artery (in this instance the vessel is larger than usual); (8) anterior aspect of superior cerebellar arteries; (9) lateral medullary portion of posterior inferior cerebellar artery; (10) caudal loop of the posterior inferior cerebellar artery (PICA); (11) posterior medullary segment; (12) supratonsillar and retrotonsillar segments; and (13) tonsillohemispheric branch of PICA.

of the middle cerebral artery along the inferior aspect of the temporal lobe. The vessel is usually inconspicuous on the angiogram.

The posterior temporal artery arises as a single trunk from the midportion of the perimesencephalic segment of the posterior cerebral artery. Sometimes it originates farther distally. The artery supplies the undersurface of the posterior portion of the temporal lobe (fusiform and lingual gyri), and in roughly one-quarter of the cases it supplies part of the visual cortex.

The posterior cerebral artery then bifurcates into two divisions, the calcarine and the parieto-occipital arteries, which supply the medial aspect of the occipital lobe and the precuneus (Fig. 17.87). There is some variation in the arrangement of these branches, as might be expected.

As seen in the lateral projection, it should be remembered that these arterial branches travel first on the undersurface of the temporal lobe, which is slanted downward and laterally to conform to the configuration of the tentorium. Therefore, the posterior temporal branch, which is directed laterally and posteriorly, also passes slightly caudally. For this reason, on the angiogram, that artery and its branches overlie—or project lower than—the superior cerebellar arteries, which are beneath the tentorium (Figs. 17.88 and 17.89).

In the frontal projection the first main branch to leave the posterior cerebral artery is the anterior temporal artery, which may be quite small. The second branch is the posterior temporal artery. In their distal portions, after they cross, the calcarine branch is usually more medial than the parieto-occipital branch (Fig. 17.87). Sometimes the parieto-occipital branch is the first main branch to arise from the stem of the posterior cerebral artery. Identification of the vessels may be difficult without stereoscopic films in the lateral projection because the branches are superimposed when the two posterior cerebral arteries fill.

Functionally, the branches of the posterior cerebral artery can be divided into those feeding the mesencephalon, the diencephalon, the telencephalon, and the choroid.

MEASUREMENTS

The variation of the PCA course and overlap is so great as to make measurements useless. Erdem et al., in an anatomic study of the vascularization of the hippocampus, found that it was supplied by an average of 4.7 arteries per hemisphere (range, 3 to 7 arteries) (136). Based on the origin and caliber of the arteries supplying the hippocampus, the hemispheres were divided into five groups: (*a*) in 57 percent of the hemispheres studied, the origin was mixed and included the anterior choroidal artery

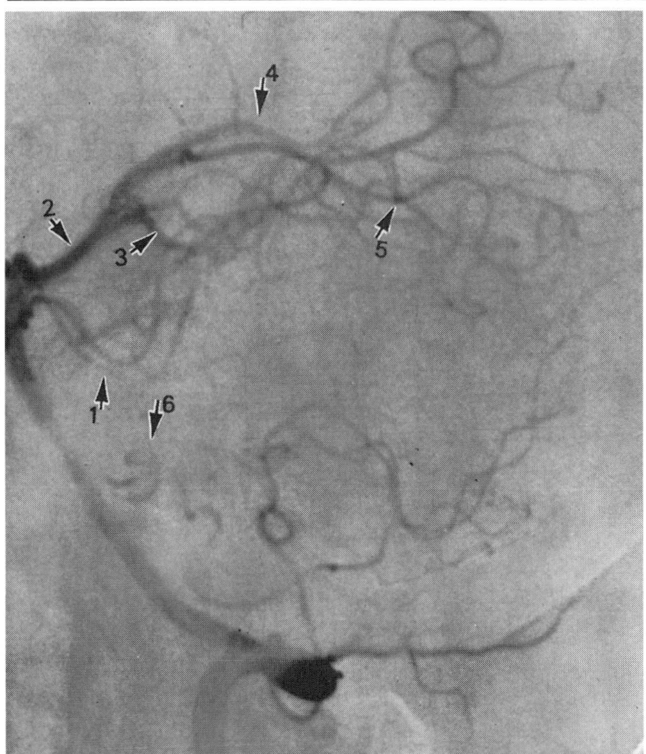

Figure 17.89. Posterior cerebral artery in lateral view. Arrows denote (1) superior cerebellar arteries; (2) posterior cerebral arteries; (3) posterior temporal branch of posterior cerebral artery; (4) parieto-occipital branch of posterior cerebral; (5) calcarine branch of posterior cerebral; and (6) an anterior inferior cerebellar artery, which is giving off a branch following the course of a hemispheric branch. The posterior inferior cerebellar artery has a relatively low origin from the vertebral artery and shows its most common configuration.

(AChA); the main trunk of the posterior cerebral artery (PCA); and the inferior temporal, lateral posterior choroidal, and splenial branches of the PCA; (*b*) in 27 percent, all of the inferior temporal branches of the PCA predominantly supplied the hippocampus; (*c*) in 10 percent, the anterior inferior temporal branch of the PCA was the predominant supplier; (*d*) in 3 percent, the hippocampus was predominantly supplied by arteries originating from the main trunk of the PCA (Uchimura artery); and (*e*) in 3 percent, the AChA gave origin to the hippocampal vessel. It was found as a result of this study that the PCA directly and by its branches contributes much more to the blood supply of the hippocampal formation than the AChA. The uncal sulcus was found to be an important anastomotic site between the hippocampal branches of the AChA and the hippocampal branches of the PCA. In 26.6 percent of hemispheres, one of the hippocampal arteries arose from the lateral posterior choroidal artery. The splenial artery made a loop close to the extraventricular part of the hippocampal tail and gave off multiple vessels to this structure in 36.6 percent of hemispheres. The finding that the AChA passes through the choroid fissure as a trunk and its later division into the lateral plexal and medial perforating branches within the choroid plexus may be of surgical and interventional significance.

The posterior cerebral artery bifurcates in its P2–P3 portion similarly to the middle cerebral artery (137). Three types of divisions were distinguished by location of the division. In the first type (43 percent), the terminal division was located either in the calcarine sulcus or in the quadrigeminal cistern. In the second type (42 percent), the terminal division had the same position, but the distal segment, in addition to its terminal stems, also gave off the common temporal artery. In the third type (16 percent), the terminal division was seen in the ambient cistern. The distal segment of the posterior cerebral artery gave rise to several collateral branches: the collicular artery (3 percent); the anterior (29 percent), middle (30.0 percent), and posterior (29 percent) hippocampal arteries; the proximal (83 percent) and distal (20 percent) lateral posterior choroidal arteries; the proximal (40 percent) and distal (42 percent) medial posterior choroidal arteries; the peduncular, thalamogeniculate, and splenial branches; the lingual gyri artery; and the temporal arteries. Several anatomic variants of the distal segment were observed in this study: fenestration of the distal segment (1 percent), location of the distal segment dorsal to the uncus (3 percent), origin of the collicular (3 percent) and anterior choroidal arteries (1 percent) from the distal segment, and protrusion of the parieto-occipital arterial loop into the lateral ventricle (3 percent).

Milisavljevic et al., in their microdissection study of the *thalamogeniculate (TG) arteries*, showed tremendous variation in number, size, total size, origin and course (138). They varied from 2 to 12 in number (mean, 6), and from 70 to 580 μm in caliber (mean, 350 μm). The average caliber of all the TG vessels per posterior cerebral artery ranged from 700 to 3400 μm (mean, 1970 μm). The TG arteries most often originated as individual vessels; however, in 27 percent of the hemispheres examined, they shared a common site of origin, and in 33 percent of the hemispheres they arose from common stems. The common stems ranged from 320 to 800 μm in diameter (mean, 580 μm). The TG branches arose from the crural or ambient (P2) segment of the posterior cerebral artery in 80 percent of the hemispheres, from the P2 and the quadrigeminal (P3) segment in 20 percent, from both the distal segment of the posterior cerebral artery and the common temporal artery (13 percent), or from the distal segment and either the calcarine (3 percent) or the parieto-occipital artery (3 percent). The TG arteries usually penetrated the medial geniculate body (100 percent), pulvinar thalami (80 percent), brachium of the superior colliculus (53.33 percent), or lateral geniculate body (13.33 percent). The collateral branches of the TG arteries were noted to reach the medial geniculate body (77 percent), pulvinar (70 percent), brachium of the superior colliculus (40 percent), crus cerebri (40 percent), and lateral geniculate body (7 percent). The anastomoses were present in 67 percent, usually between the TG vessels and the medial posterior choroidal artery (33 percent) or the mesencephalothalamic artery (27 percent). They ranged in number from 1 to 3 (mean, 1.2) and in caliber from 90 to 400 μm (mean, 190 μm).

The premammillary artery usally arises from the posterior communicating artery but may come off the posterior cerebral artery (139). The arteries originated from the superior and lateral surfaces of the posterior communicating artery and coursed superiorly, laterally, and posteriorly to enter a triangular perforated space limited by the mammillary body and tuber cinereum medially, the optic tract anterolaterally, and the cerebral peduncle posterolaterally. This space is called the *paramedian perforated substance.* The premammillary artery is small (outside diameter 0.6 +/− 0.2 mm), short (12.0 +/− 2.0 mm), and slightly bigger on the left. Two-thirds of arteries give off branches that supply the cerebral peduncles, optic tract, and paramedian perforated space.

The posterior communicating artery anatomy has been revisited by Pedroza et al. (140). A fetal origin was seen in one in five, and one-third were hypoplastic. Infundibular dilatations were found in 1 in 10 of the arteries. This highly variable vessel is usually larger at its internal carotid artery origin than at the P1 site, and larger and longer on the left (ICA origin outside diameter: 1.5 +/− 0.8 mm on the right and 1.6 +/− 0.6 mm on the left; P1 junction outside diameter: 1.4 +/− 0.7 mm on the right side and 1.6 +/ − 0.6 mm on the left; length: 12.7 +/− 3.2 mm on the right and 12.5 +/− 1.7 mm on the left side). Posterior communicating artery branches originated from the superior (36 percent) or lateral (64 percent) surface of the posterior communicating artery and coursed superiorly, posteriorly, or laterally. These vessels supplied the paramedian perforated substance (21 percent), the tuber cinereum (17 percent), the sulcus between the optic tract and the tuber cinereum (14 percent), the circuminfundibular anastomosis (12 percent), the mammillary bodies (8 percent), the sulcus between the optic tract and the cerebral peduncles (8 percent), and the cerebral peduncles (6 percent). The largest and most constant branch of the posterior communicating artery was the premammillary artery. The number and size of the branches from the posterior communicating artery were independent of the size of the parent artery.

Caplan et al. reviewed occlusions of thalamogeniculate artery and described three clinical syndromes: (*a*) hemisensory loss, hemiataxia, and involuntary movements; (*b*) pure sensory stroke; and (*c*) sensorimotor stroke (141). This is due to involvement of posterolateral and posteromedial portions of the thalamus and of the adjacent internal capsule.

EMBRYOLOGY

The caudal division of the primitive internal carotid artery terminates in the group of vessels that serve (*a*) the mesencephalon, (*b*) posterior choroid, (*c*) diencephalon (dorsomedial part of the forebrain thalamus), and (*d*) optic lobes. These coalesce to form the future posterior cerebral trunk relatively late in development (12-mm embryo). As the occipital lobes enlarge, branches of the posterior cerebral artery become the prominent trunk. The proximal posterior choroidal artery conduit acts as the distal posterior cerebral artery trunk for the developing cortical branches. The posterior choroidal takes over more and more of the distal territory of the anterior choroidal artery. Part of the posterior choroidal territory, in turn, is annexed by the adjacent diencephalic vessel to become the posterior medial choroidal proper. This explains the extensive balance between these three vessels.

There is a posterior shift of the posterior cerebral artery origin from the internal carotid to the basilar system. In the prechoroidal stage, the trigeminal carotid off the proximal internal carotid homologue feeds the basilar artery just caudad to the anterior superior cerebellar artery. This vessel regresses during the choroidal stage, with flow coming for this territory from the caudal division of the internal carotid artery.

VARIANTS

The origin of the posterior cerebral artery is usually off the basilar, but it is not uncommon for the takeoff to retain its origin off the internal carotid and thus "fetal origin" posterior cerebral artery. The posterior communicating artery may be continuous with the parieto-occipital branch of the posterior cerebral artery and another branch may arise from the carotid siphon, which is continuous with the posterior temporal branch. This is not a rare anomaly (Fig. 17.90).

Although unusual, the posterior laterial choroidal artery may be absent, with its territory being taken over by the anterior choroidal artery. Accessory blood supply to the visual cortex is sometimes supplied by other cortical branches, such as the parieto-occipital branches.

ABNORMALITIES OF POSTERIOR CEREBRAL VESSELS

Displacement

Transtentorial herniations, most commonly consisting of a hernia of the hippocampal gyrus through the incisura of the tentorium, are frequently found at autopsy; they are often a prime cause of death owing to compression of, and hemorrhage into, the mesencephalon. The hemorrhage may be venous or arterial or both. According to Johnson and Yates, arterial bleeding may be seen in the more acute cases; it is due to sudden elongation of the arteries with rupture of the vessels as a result of lateral flattening of the midbrain with consequent increase in anteroposterior diameter (142).

The hernia may be anterior, involving only the uncus

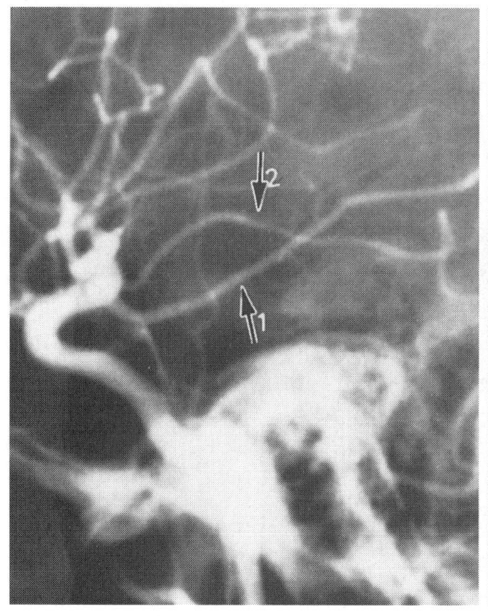

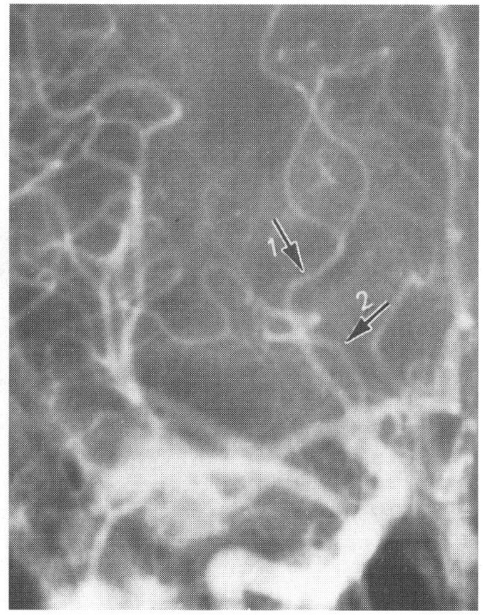

A B

Figure 17.90. Carotid angiogram demonstrating dual direct origin of posterior cerebral artery. **A.** The lower vessel arising from the carotid siphon (arrow 1) gives origin to the parieto-occipital and calcarine branches. The vessel immediately above (arrow 2) is the posterior temporal branch of the posterior cerebral artery. **B.** Simultaneous frontal projection.

and the anterior portion of the hippocampus, or it may be posterior (see Figs. 4.31 to 4.34). Anterior and posterior herniations may combine to form a complete downward herniation. The herniation may sometimes be bilateral but usually is on only the side of the mass lesion.

The presence of transtentorial herniations does not necessarily indicate a fatal outcome. On the contrary, the majority of patients recover, following simple surgical removal of the causative factor or simple decompression. Sometimes removal of the herniated portion of brain or sectioning of the tentorial edge may have to be performed.

Lateral displacement of the upper brainstem (midbrain) is often present in association with a midline cerebral dislocation, especially in connection with masses involving the lower portions of the hemisphere, the deep masses, temporal lobe masses, and subdural hematomas. When a marked lateral displacement of the midbrain exists, the structure may be compressed against the side of the tentorium opposite the mass, thus producing ipsilateral neurologic signs. Any case in which a marked midline shift is present is a candidate for transtentorial herniation of the hippocampus. These cases should therefore be handled with great care to prevent a potential or a small hernia from becoming a large one.

Central incisural herniations, both upward and downward, can be seen. Upward herniations of the contents of the posterior fossa, usually the cerebellum, through the tentorial incisura may occur in connection with masses involving the posterior fossa. They usually occur behind the quadrigeminal plate, in which case the brainstem is displaced forward against the clivus. Herniation may be posterolateral in location, on one or both sides.

Although the proximal posterior cerebral artery is variable in its course, making confident interpretation of displacement difficult, its close proximity to the midbrain, thalamus, and choroidal fissure will usually lead to displacement in cases with masses in this area.

The peduncular segment (P1) is displaced medially and posteriorly by uncal herniations. Midbrain masses may displace the segment laterally. The redundant ambient (P2) segment may be straightened and displaced medially and inferiorly by posterior transtentorial (posterior hippocampus) herniations. Similarly, large masses of the ambient cistern may straighten and laterally displace the ambient portion.

The quadrigeminal segment of the posterior cerebral artery (P3) is extremely variable. Dandy-Walker cysts may displace this segment laterally, superiorly, and posteriorly, while posterior hippocampal lesions may displace the segment medially and inferiorly.

POSTERIOR CIRCULATION ANGIOGRAPHY

The usefulness of diagnostic posterior circulation angiography is limited to determining the fine vascular status prior to therapy. The indications for angiography in the diagnosis of infratentorial masses have been replaced by CT and MRI. Some of the definite indications for vertebral angiography are (*a*) to diagnose or access a posterior fossa aneurysm; (*b*) to demonstrate abnormal circulation patterns whenever a posterior fossa lesion is suspected clinically of being either a hemangioblastoma or an arteriovenous malformation; and (*c*) to show tumor circulation when it is suspected that a lesion may be a meningioma, particularly in the case of a mass that may require embolization. Knowledge of the vascular anatomy gleaned from angiography, however, is extremely useful since it can increasingly be appreciated on magnetic resonance angiography (MRA).

Vertebral Angiography

VERTEBRAL ARTERY

The vertebral artery originates in the neck and is the first branch of the subclavian artery on each side. From its origin, the artery is directed upward and medially to enter the foramen transversarium of the sixth cervical vertebra. Here, it ascends on each side of the neck, contained within the foramina transversaria, until it reaches the second cervical vertebra. It emerges from the foramen transversarium of the second cervical vertebra and proceeds laterally to enter the foramen transversarium of the atlas. It then travels posteriorly to wind itself behind the superior articular process of the atlas. At this point it may be surrounded by a complete ring of bone, forming a foramen, which is visible on plain films in the lateral projection. Most often, however, only a ligament is present behind the artery. Sometimes an incomplete ring of bone is present. The artery then proceeds forward, upward, and medially, piercing the dura as it enters the foramen magnum (Fig. 17.91), and finally reaching the posterior surface of the clivus. There, both left and right vertebral arteries unite to form the basilar artery at the lower border of the pons.

Anatomic Variations

The vertebral artery may sometimes arise from the common carotid artery, from the inferior thyroid artery, from the innominate artery, or directly from the aorta. Either side may originate from an anomalous site. The left vertebral artery arises directly from the aorta in 6 percent of cases (14, 143). The vertebral artery may present variations in its course within the foramina transversaria: it may not penetrate at the sixth cervical vertebra but enter instead at the fifth cervical vertebra, or higher (Fig. 17.92). Occasionally, it has been seen to emerge from its bony canal between the third and the second cervical vertebrae, only to go back into the foramen transversarium at the atlas. In the rare cases in which the right vertebral artery comes off the aorta, behind the left subclavian artery, the vertebral artery passes behind the esophagus as it goes laterally to enter the foramen transversarium of the sixth cervical vertebra. Duplication or "fenestration" of the vertebral artery is sometimes seen (144). The anomaly consists of a splitting of the artery into two components—not necessarily of equal size—that join together a short distance above (Fig. 17.93). Double

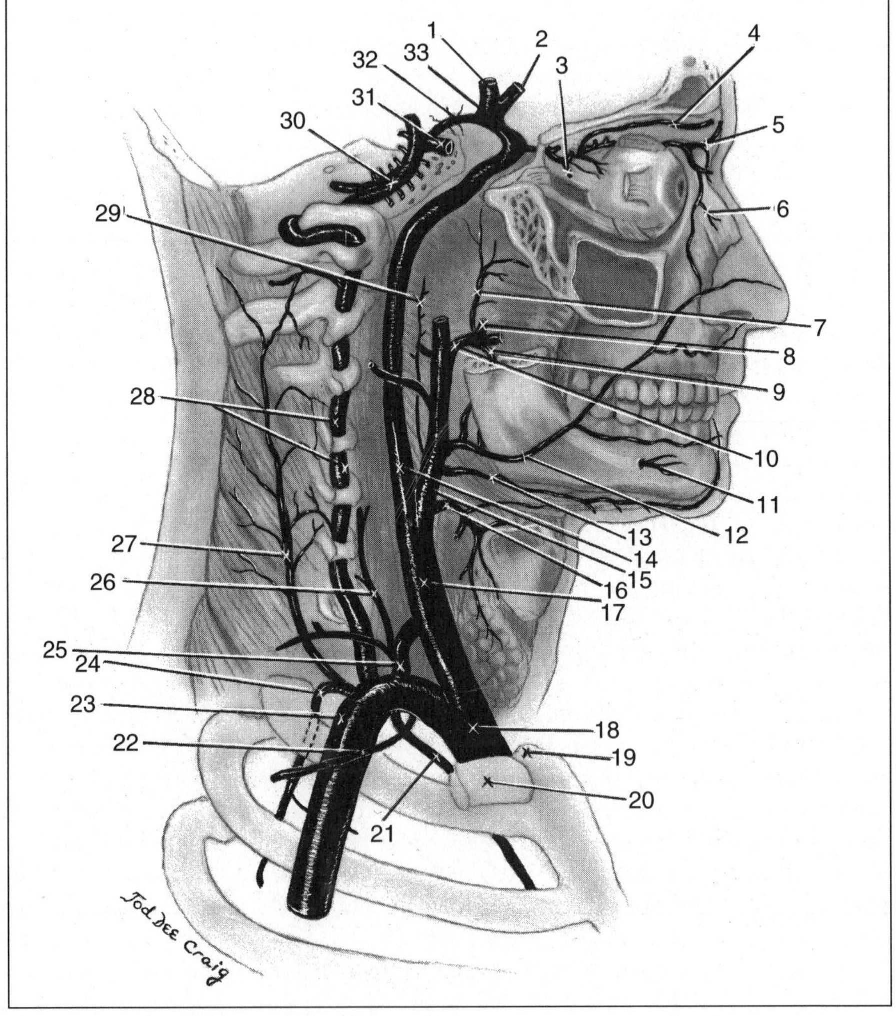

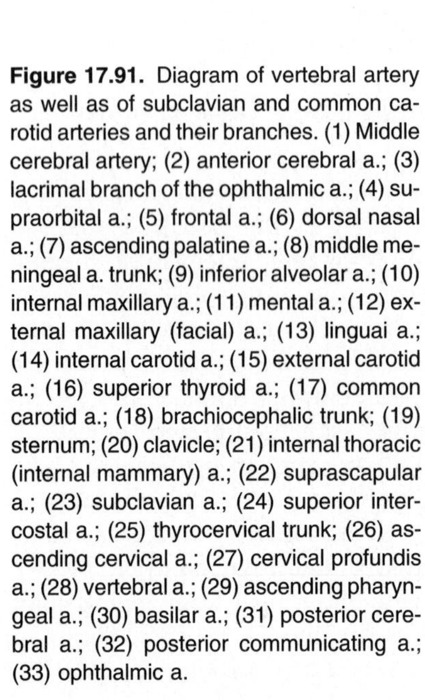
Figure 17.91. Diagram of vertebral artery as well as of subclavian and common carotid arteries and their branches. (1) Middle cerebral artery; (2) anterior cerebral a.; (3) lacrimal branch of the ophthalmic a.; (4) supraorbital a.; (5) frontal a.; (6) dorsal nasal a.; (7) ascending palatine a.; (8) middle meningeal a. trunk; (9) inferior alveolar a.; (10) internal maxillary a.; (11) mental a.; (12) external maxillary (facial) a.; (13) linguai a.; (14) internal carotid a.; (15) external carotid a.; (16) superior thyroid a.; (17) common carotid a.; (18) brachiocephalic trunk; (19) sternum; (20) clavicle; (21) internal thoracic (internal mammary) a.; (22) suprascapular a.; (23) subclavian a.; (24) superior intercostal a.; (25) thyrocervical trunk; (26) ascending cervical a.; (27) cervical profundis a.; (28) vertebral a.; (29) ascending pharyngeal a.; (30) basilar a.; (31) posterior cerebral a.; (32) posterior communicating a.; (33) ophthalmic a.

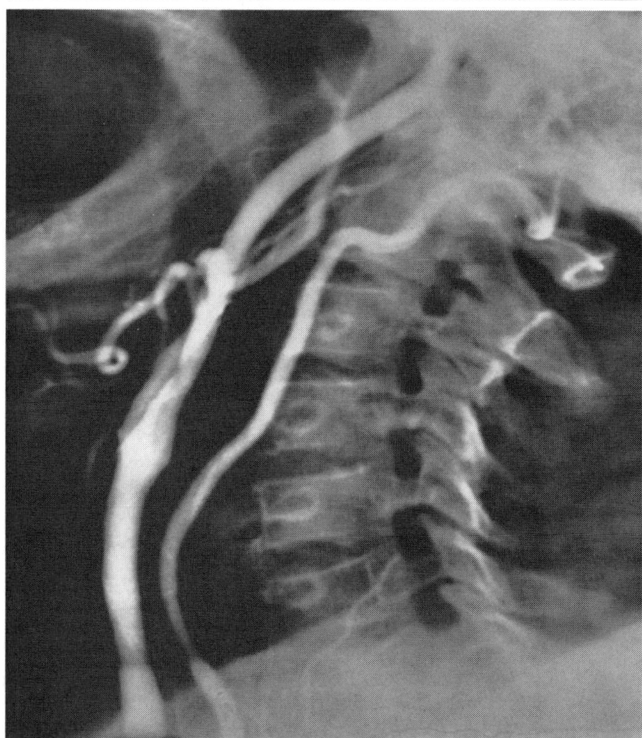

Figure 17.92. Anomaly of the vertebral artery. The artery enters the foramen transversarium of the fourth cervical vertebra instead of at C6, which is usually the case. The appearance gives the impression of forward displacement.

origin of the vertebral artery joining to form a common trunk occurs rarely. Cavdar and Arisen gives an excellent review of the variations and presents a case with a left vertebral artery arising directly from the arch of the aorta, and a double-originating vertebral artery on the right (145).

The left vertebral artery is larger than the right in a higher percentage of cases (42 percent); the right and left vertebral arteries are approximately of the same caliber in 26 percent; and the right side is larger than the left in 32 percent (146). One vertebral artery, usually the right, may be hypoplastic. The vertebral artery may also be hypoplastic in its intracranial segment. It may end at the posterior inferior cerebellar artery (Fig. 17.104*B*) or it may continue as a very thin vessel to merge with the opposite artery. The anatomic relationships of the cervical portion of the vertebral artery are illustrated in Figure 17.91.

Within the foramina transversaria of the cervical vertebrae, after it ascends to the skull, the vertebral artery is surrounded by a plexus of veins that come together in their lower portion and form the vertebral vein. The vein emerges from the foramen transversarium of the sixth cervical vertebra and accompanies the vertebral artery for a short segment. Arteriovenous fistulas between the vertebral artery and surrounding venous plexus occur as a result of trauma or surgical intervention.

Chopard et al. studied the connective muscular components of the walls of the terminal segments of the vertebral arteries as well as the basilar artery utilizing light micros-

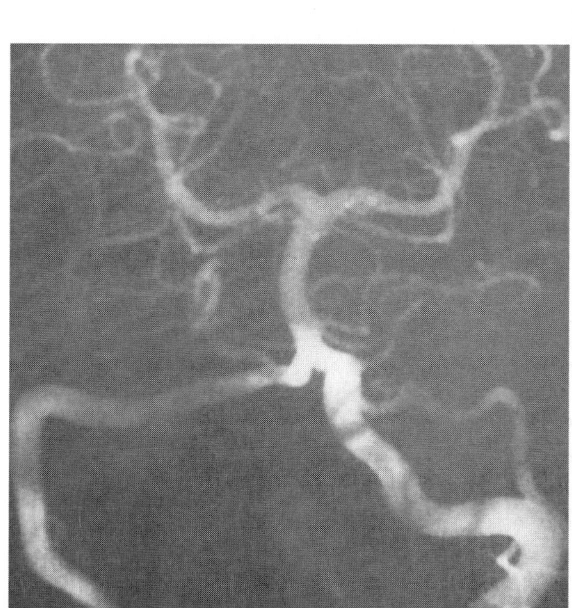

A

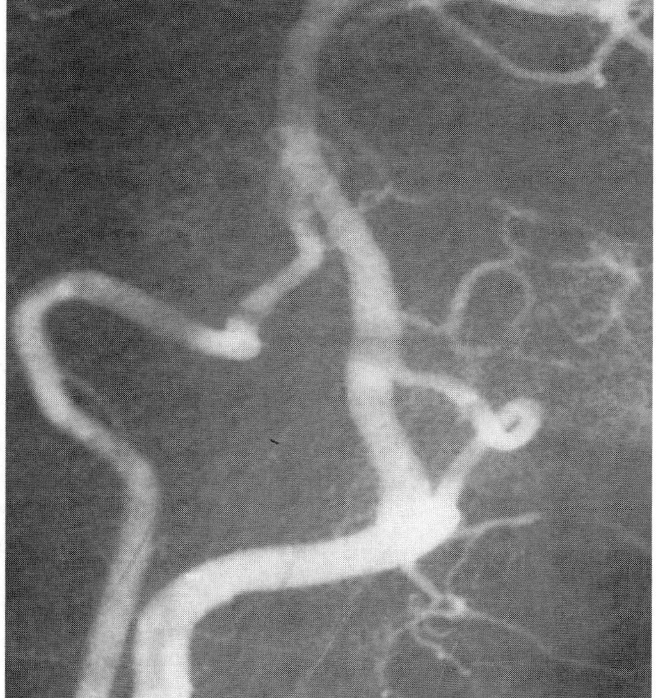

B

Figure 17.93. Fenestration of the vertebral artery (left). **A.** Frontal view. The larger of the two components follows an anomalous course and does not ascend to go through the foramen transversarium of the atlas. **B.** Oblique view demonstrates the fenestration more completely.

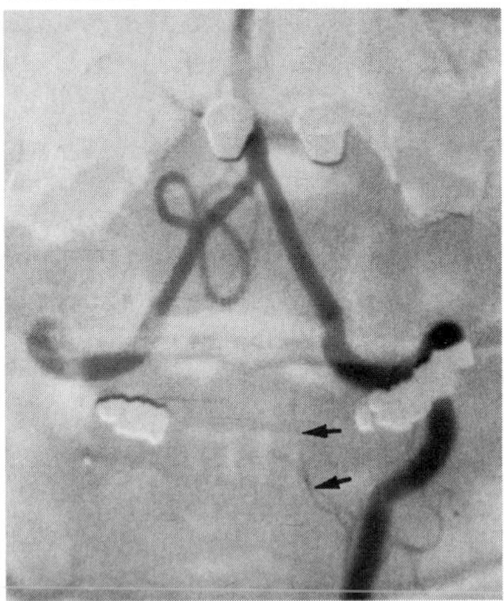

Figure 17.94. Anterior meningeal artery. Two small branches are seen arising from the cervical portion of the vertebral artery at the level of the body of C2 (arrows).

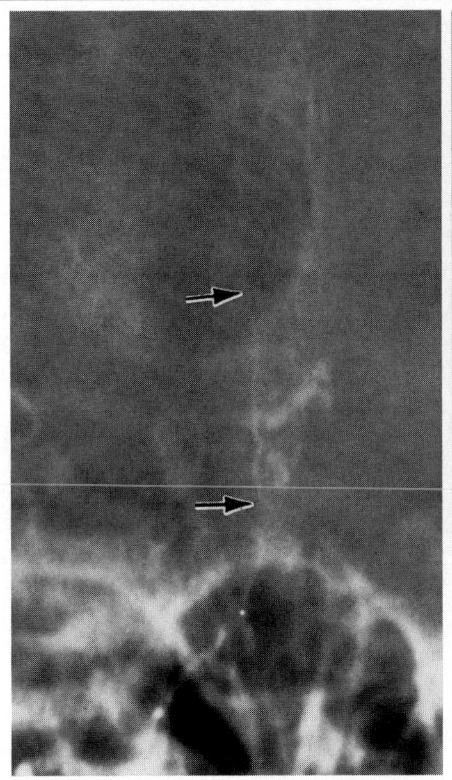

A

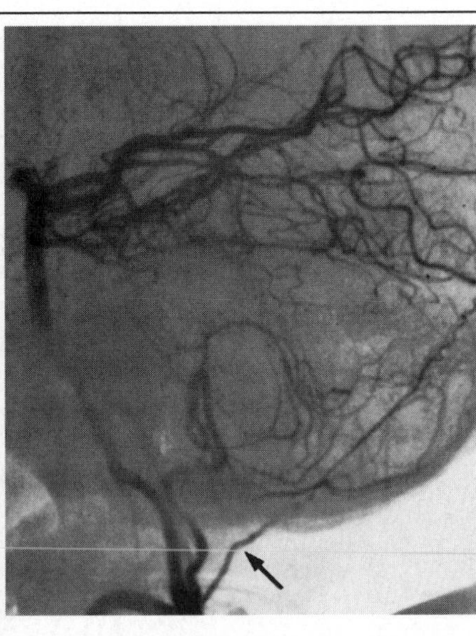

B

Figure 17.95. Posterior meningeal artery. The frontal and lateral projections (**A** and **B**) demonstrate the posterior meningeal artery ascending near the midline in the falx cerebelli. Because the head is slightly rotated to the left side, the vessel in the frontal projection appears to be off center to the right (arrows).

copy (147). The vertebral arteries had elastic lamina and external layer of tunica media in contrast to the basilar artery, where the elastic tissue is localized mainly in the tunica media and is distributed heterogeneously.

Chopard et al. showed that the vertebral artery is fixed to adjacent structures in the fibrous osteomuscular tunnel by means of a continuous lamina of collagen along its entire course and that there is considerable independence between the artery and the branches of the spinal nerves (148).

Cervical Branches

In its *cervical portion*, the vertebral artery gives rise to spinal and muscular branches. The spinal branches enter the vertebral canal through the intervertebral foramina. They supply the spinal cord and the meninges; some anastomose with the anterior and posterior spinal arteries of the cord. There are ascending and descending branches inside the intervertebral foramina that anastomose with each other, thus forming an anastomotic chain on each side, behind the vertebral bodies, near the pedicles. The muscular branches supply the paraspinal muscles; they anastomose with branches of the external occipital and the ascending pharyngeal arteries, which also supply the muscles.

Greitz and Lauren described an *anterior meningeal artery*, which arises at the level of the body of the axis (149). This artery ascends over the dura after entering the spinal canal through the intervertebral foramen. It ends by dividing into two or more small branches supplying the dura along the anterior aspect of the foramen magnum (Fig. 17.94). In one of Greitz's cases, it supplied a glomus jugulare tumor. In other cases seen by the author the anterior meningeal arteries were enlarged, and they supplied, in turn, a metastatic tumor of the clivus, a meningioma of the clivus, a dural arteriovenous malformation, an acoustic neurinoma, a chordoma, and a primary nasopharyngeal carcinoma. The anterior meningeal branch of the vertebral artery is seen infrequently in normal vertebral angiograms (probably less than 10 percent of cases).

The *posterior meningeal branch* springs from the vertebral artery before piercing the dura mater just below the level of the foramen magnum. It gives off small branches between the bone and the dura mater, and its main branch supplies the falx cerebelli (150). It is often seen on vertebral angiograms—13 percent in the cases reported by Hawkins and Melcher (151). However, in the specimens of the falx cerebelli examined microscopically by the same authors (13 cadavers), the artery was present in all. The falx cerebelli is a small band of dura mater, crescentic in shape, extending from the posterior aspect of the tentorium, at the straight sinus, to the posterior aspect of the foramen magnum. It seldom measures more than 1 cm in depth and becomes narrower as it reaches the foramen magnum. It often divides here into two ridges before merging with the other reflections of the dura mater. Because the artery runs on the edge of the shallow falx, it is separated from the inner

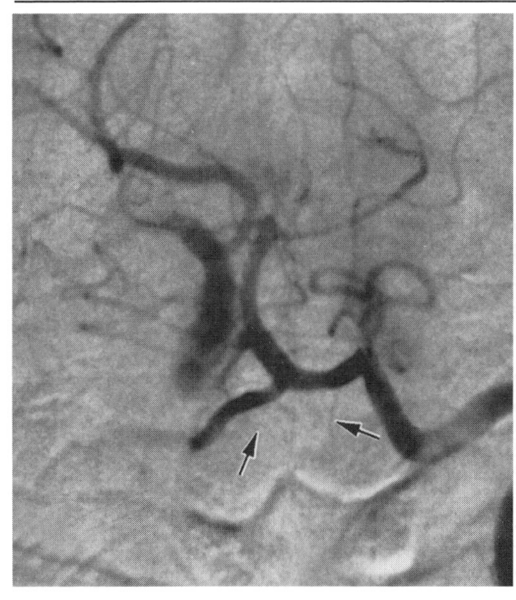

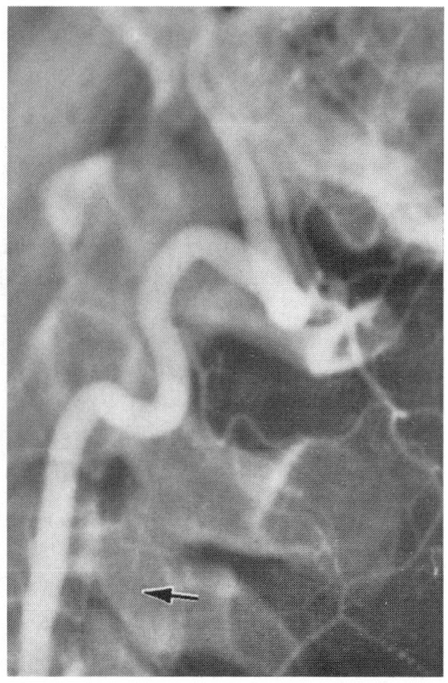

A B

Figure 17.96. Anterior spinal artery. **A.** The frontal projection demonstrates the artery very faintly (arrows) unless the vessel is enlarged such as may be the case in arteriovenous malformations. **B.** In the lateral projection, the artery is much more clearly outlined. The artery, which marks the anterior aspect of the spinal cord, is situated 6 mm behind the posterior margins of the vertebral bodies in this instance. The distance here is due to the fact that the patient is lying in the supine position during the angiographic procedure and the cord drops to the dorsal side of the canal.

table of the occipital bone by a distance of about 1 cm (Fig. 17.95). The separation is also due to the fact that the falx cerebelli rests on a ridge, which is the lower component of the occipital cruciate eminence. The configuration of the posterior meningeal branch is such that it is not easily confused with a hemispheric or vermian branch of the posterior inferior cerebellar artery.

Intracranial Branches

The *intracranial portion* gives rise to three principal circulations: the spinal arteries, the posterior inferior cerebellar artery, and the medullary branches.

Spinal Arteries According to Schechter and Zingesser, the anterior spinal vessels can be identified in vertebral angiography in as many as 50 percent of the cases where, following injection of one vertebral artery, satisfactory filling of the opposite artery is obtained by regurgitation (152). To be sure, the arteries can be visualized only very faintly and perhaps solely in the lateral projection, but if looked for they can usually be identified. It is somewhat more difficult to see them in such a high percentage of cases in the frontal projection, but, with subtraction, identification may be accomplished more readily (Fig. 17.96). A more complete discussion of the anterior spinal arteries and other branches of the vertebral arteries to the spinal cord is given under "Spinal Angiography."

There are always one or two anterior spinal arteries (right or left), which proceed from the intracranial segment of the vertebral arteries (153). These arteries have a descending course, with distribution into the ventral face of the medulla oblongata and the first cervical segments of the medulla spinalis. In cases where there are two anterior spinal arteries, they anastomose with each other to form the common, unpaired, and median anterior spinal artery. The different observed locations of the origins of anterior spinal arteries may be systematized into three types: bilateral origin (type I; 78 percent); unilateral origin (type II; 10 percent); and origin in an intervertebral transversal anastomosis (type III; 13 percent). The bilateral type can subdivide, according to the caliber of the arteries, into the subtypes *balanced* (type Ia; 23 percent), *right dominated* (type Ib; 32 percent), and *left dominated* (type Ic; 23 percent). The collaterals of the anterior spinal arteries also supply the ventral face of the medulla oblongata.

The posterior spinal plexus of arteries is seen in a much lower proportion of cases. Krayenbuhl and Yasargil refer to identification of all of the spinal arteries in only a few of their cases (146). This is probably due to poor filling or to failure to use subtraction techniques. The use of subtraction greatly increases the percentage of cases in which the anterior spinal vessels as well as the posterior spinal plexus of arteries can be visualized on radiographs.

Posterior Inferior Cerebellar Artery The artery is present bilaterally and is of the same caliber on both sides in approximately 25 percent of cases (146). In the remaining 75 percent of cases, it is asymmetric. Sometimes both arteries are very small; one or both may be absent; or they may arise from the anterior inferior cerebellar or from the basilar artery.

The posterior inferior cerebellar artery (PICA) is the largest branch of the vertebral artery and supplies the inferior and posterior aspects of the ipsilateral cerebellar hemisphere, the tonsil, and the choroid plexus of the fourth ventricle. It arises on each anterolateral aspect of the medulla oblongata. It passes laterally between the origins of the vagus and accessory nerves around the medulla and reaches the posterior lateral aspect of the medulla. This

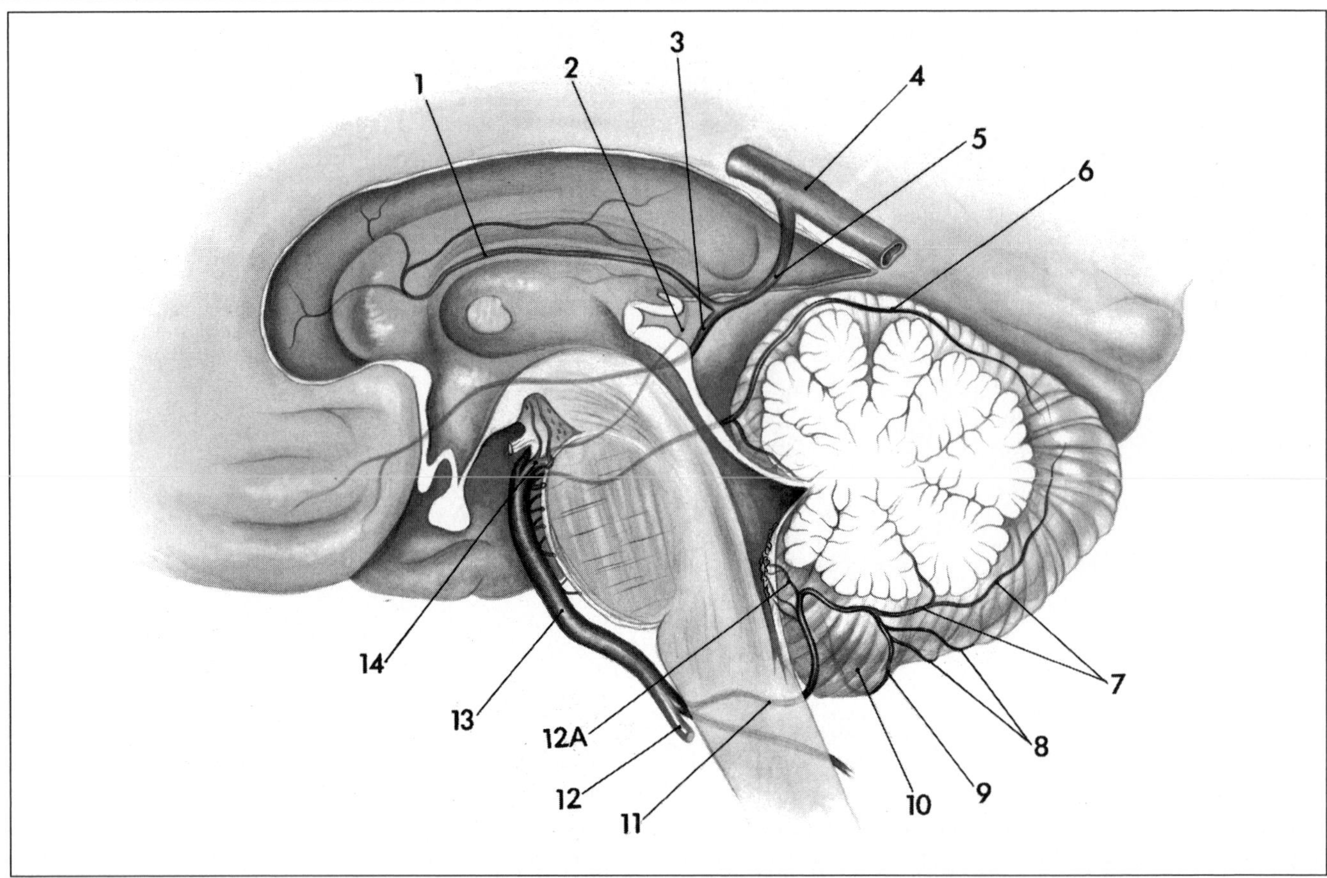

Figure 17.97. Diagrammatic configuration of the basilar artery, posterior inferior cerebellar artery, and cerebral structures. (1) Internal cerebral vein; (2) medial posterior choroidal artery; (3) basal vein of Rosenthal; (4) straight sinus; (5) vein of Galen; (6) superior cerebellar artery, vermian branch; (7) vermian branch of posterior inferior cerebellar artery (PICA); (8) hemispheric branches arising from tonsillohemispheric division of PICA; (9) retrotonsillar segment of PICA continuing on the lateral surface of the hemisphere; (10) cerebellar tonsil; (11) perimedullary segment of the PICA; (12) vertebral artery; (12A) choroidal branches; (13) basilar artery; (14) posterior cerebral artery.

segment is called the *perimedullary segment* of the posterior inferior cerebellar artery. The artery then turns upward fairly sharply, describing a curve convex downward referred to as the *caudal curve* or caudal loop. The artery continues upward and medially in its retromedullary segment, describing a second curve concave downward termed the *cranial curve* or loop of the PICA. At that point it approximates the inferior aspect of the fourth ventricle (Figs. 17.97 and 17.98). As it bends, it goes over the upper aspect of the tonsil on its medial side. For this reason Huang and Wolf prefer to call this the *supratonsillar segment* of the PICA, which is a more descriptive term than cranial curve or cranial loop (154). In this segment the PICA may course over the top of the tonsil, somewhat more medially, or it may have a transverse course. The artery here turns downward and backward in the retrotonsillar fissure (superior retrotonsillar segment).

The posterior inferior cerebellar artery divides into two main branches, the *vermian branch*, which is near the midline and ascends along the cerebellar vermis, and the *tonsillohemispheric branch*. The tonsillohemispheric branch originates from the trunk of the PICA in the upper retromedullary portion. It enters the retrotonsillar fissure, curving downward around the tonsil to reach the lower aspect of this fissure. It then continues on the inferior surface of the cerebellar hemisphere, giving several branches (Fig. 17.99). This is the most common configuration—12 of 30 according to Greitz and Sjogren (155).

In the next most common arrangement, the tonsillohemispheric branch swings forward around the anterior aspect of the tonsil (Fig. 17.100). A number of other variants of the posterior inferior cerebellar artery and its branches, according to Huang and Wolf, are illustrated in Figure 17.101 (154). The hemispheric branches pass downward and under the inferior aspect of the cerebellar hemisphere and ascend on the lateral side (Fig. 17.98).

The caudal curve of the PICA is usually above the level of the foramen magnum, but, in certain normal instances, it can extend a fair distance below the level of the foramen magnum (Fig. 17.102). However, the tonsillar branches of

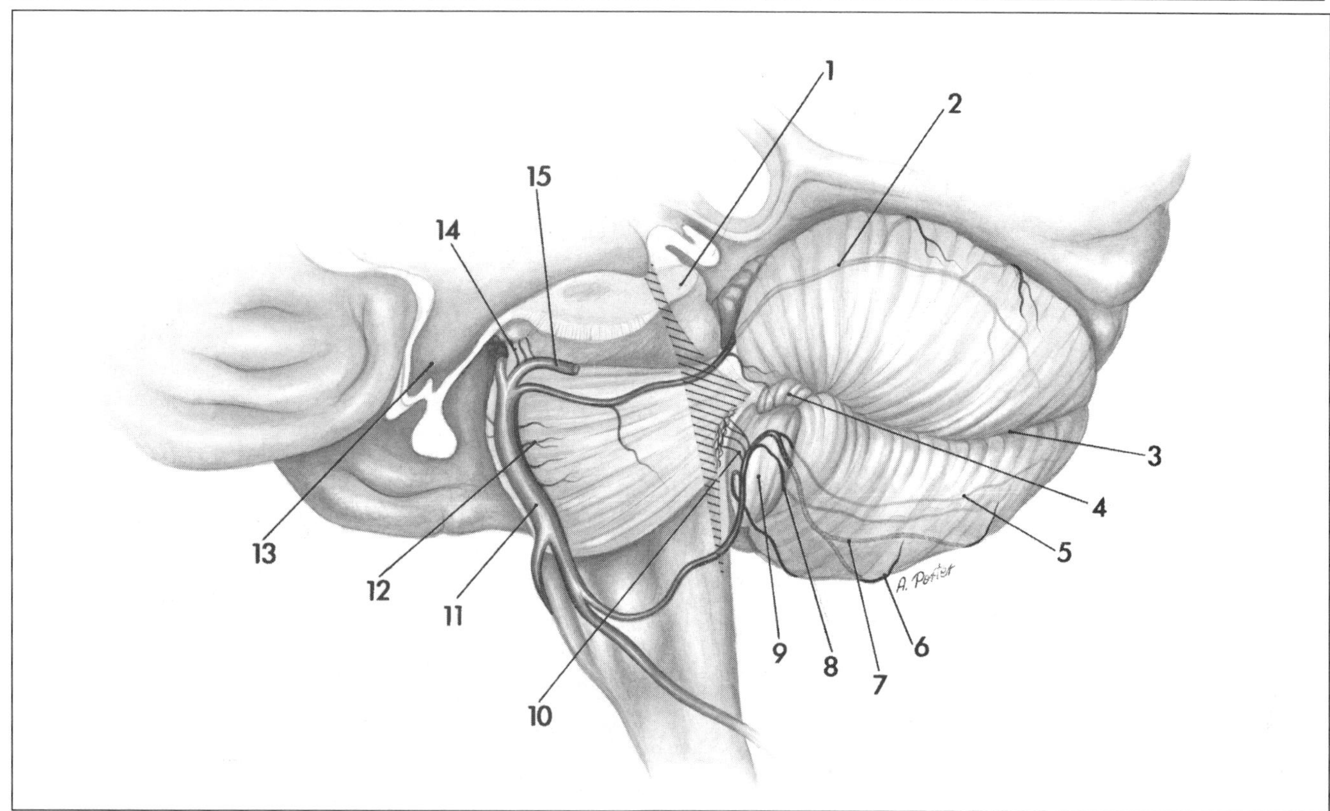

Figure 17.98. Diagrammatic configuration of the basilar artery, posterior inferior cerebellar artery (PICA), and cerebral structures. (1) Quadrigeminal plate; (2) vermian branch of superior cerebellar artery; (3) great horizontal fissure of the cerebellum; (4) flocculus; (5) vermian branches of the posterior inferior cerebellar artery; (6, 7, and 8) hemispheric branches from the tonsillohemispheric division and directly from the PICA; (9) tonsil; (10) choroidal branches of the PICA; (11) basilar artery; (12) pontine branches of basilar artery; (13) third ventricle. The fourth ventricle is outlined as a point of reference. The cerebellar tonsil on the side shown has been removed to expose the PICA.

the tonsillohemispheric division are always above the foramen magnum and do not project downward unless there is tonsillar herniation (Figs. 17.99*A* and 17.102). Thus, in order to diagnose tonsillar herniation it is necessary to identify the tonsillar branches.

Out of the cephalic curve of the posterior inferior cerebellar artery, there are minute branches that supply the choroid plexus of the fourth ventricle. The anterior aspect of the uppermost portion of this curve has been termed (by Huang and Wolf) the *choroidal point.* The estimation of this point can be important in determining displacement of the inferior aspect of the fourth ventricle and is shown in the diagram illustrated in Figure 17.103. The choroid plexus of the fourth ventricle is usually not identified in vertebral angiograms even when there is good filling. However, with subtraction or with the addition of angiotomography it will be possible to identify the choroid plexus in a higher proportion of cases. This should be a useful landmark in vertebral angiography for, unfortunately, the relationship of the cephalic curve to the lower portion of the fourth ventricle is not constant due to the variability of the origin and the different configurations of the PICA.

The vermian branch of the posterior inferior cerebellar artery is important in that it occupies an almost midline position. In that respect it is equivalent to the pericallosal artery of the carotid system. Unfortunately, it is situated very far posteriorly so that any degree of rotation of the head tends to project the artery off the midline. It is usually easy to identify the vermian branch in the lateral view because it is almost always separated from the cranium by a distance of 1 to 2 cm. The hemispheric branches, in contrast, are seen to curve downward and approximate the inner table of the skull (Figs. 17.97 and 17.98). The vermian branch can also be recognized because it almost always makes a curve concave upward at the anterior inferior aspect of the pyramid of the vermis (Figs. 17.97; 17.103). The term *copula pyramidis* has been coined to refer to the band of tissue connecting the pyramid of the vermis with the biventral lobules of the cerebellum on each side (156). This curve is almost always recognizable and lies above and a little behind the posterior margin of the foramen magnum. It is an important anatomic reference point (Figs. 17.99, 17.100, 17.102). The vermian branch may give off a variable number of twigs that curve around the periphery of the cerebellar lobes. As mentioned elsewhere, stereoscopy is helpful in identifying these branches.

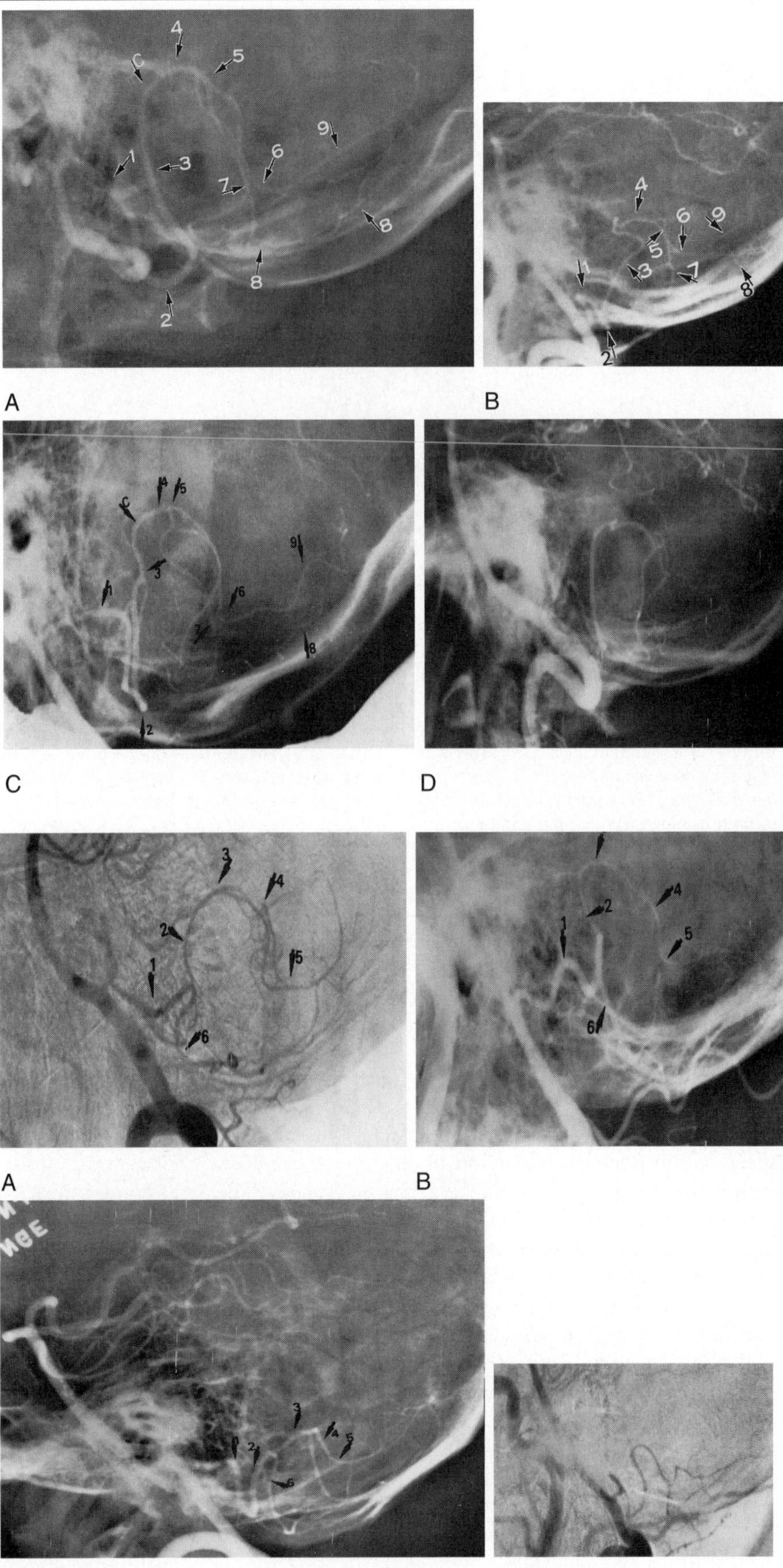

Figure 17.99. Common configuration of posterior inferior cerebellar artery (PICA) in lateral projection. **A** and **B.** The vertebral artery (**A**) ends in the PICA. It has either a very tiny or no connection with the other vertebral artery to form the basilar. The caudal loop in A and B goes below the foramen magnum. The perimedullary segments are composed of the (1) lateral medullary segment; (2) caudal loop; (3) posterior medullary segment; (4) supratonsillar segment; (5) superior retrotonsillar portion and origin of tonsillohemispheric branch; (6) copular area (retrotonsillar curve of vermian branch); (7) inferior retrotonsillar portion of tonsillohemispheric branch; (8) hemispheric branches; (9) vermian branch; (c) choroidal point. **C.** Another typical configuration of the PICA of the same general type. The numbers correspond to those in A. **D.** Another example. The tonsillar curve is so pronounced in some cases that it may suggest a tumor.

Figure 17.100. Second most common configuration of posterior inferior cerebellar artery. **A** and **B.** (1) Perimedullary segment; (2) retromedullary segment; (3) supratonsillar segment; (4) superior retrotonsillar segment; (5) retrotonsillar curve of vermian branch (copular point); (6) tonsillohemispheric branch. **C.** This appearance is actually of the same type as A and B, and the numbers correspond to the same segments. **D.** In this instance there is no vermian branch identifiable on the films.

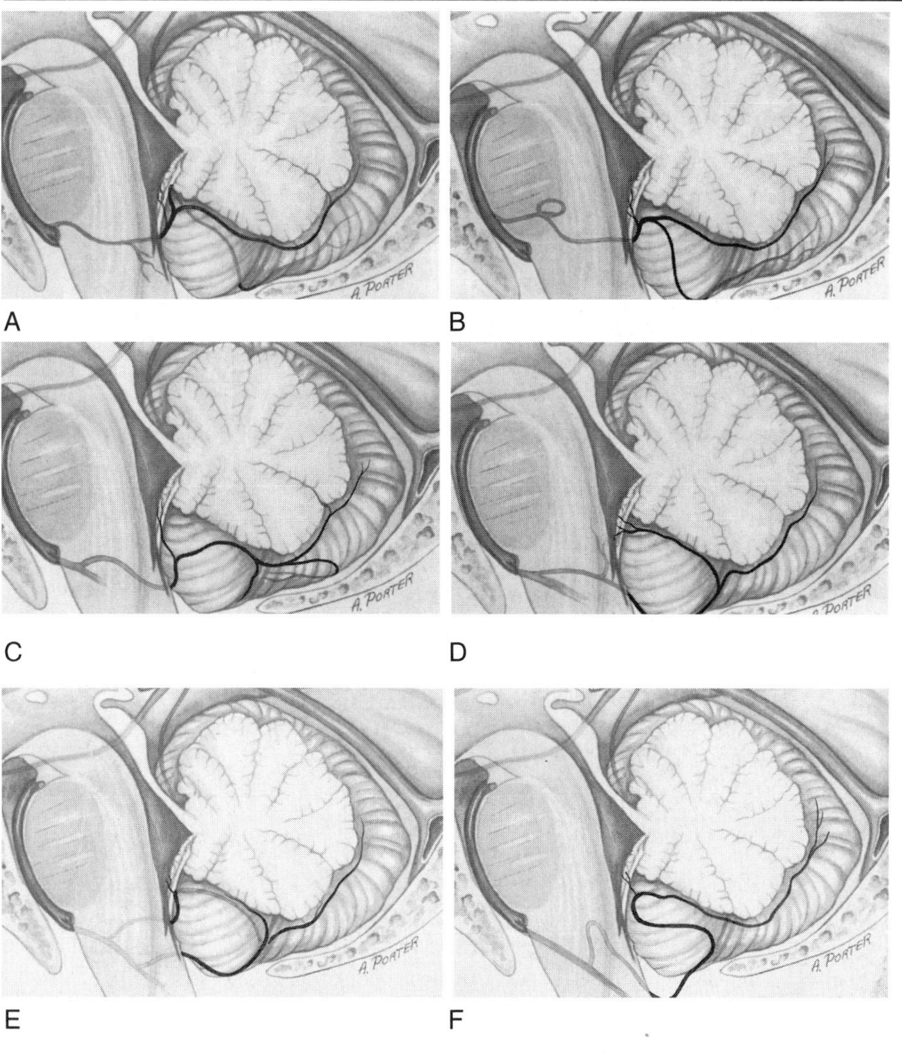

Figure 17.101. Additional variants of posterior inferior cerebellar artery (PICA) according to Huang and Wolf (154). **A.** The anterior and lateral medullary segments are located high, and there is no real caudal curve. A branch to the medulla is prominent in this instance. **B.** The PICA is originating from the basilar artery, and in this instance no caudal curve is present. **C.** There is no supratonsillar segment of the PICA, which runs on the medial side of the tonsil. **D.** The PICA trunk makes a curve below the tonsil. **E.** The PICA is divided into two separate trunks arising from the vertebral artery. **F.** Tortuous PICA extending below the foramen magnum.

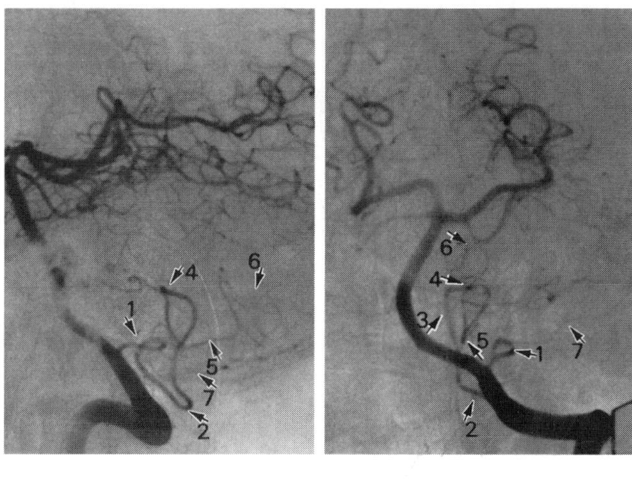

Figure 17.102. Posterior inferior cerebellar artery (PICA) extending below the foramen magnum in the normal case. The numbered arrows 1 through 5 are the same in both the lateral (**A**) and the frontal (**B**) views. (1) Perimedullary segment; (2) caudal loop; (3) posterior medullary segment; (4) supratonsillar segment; (5) segment running on the medial surface of the tonsil; (6) vermian branch of PICA in frontal view; in the lateral view, 6, represents the retrotonsillar curve of the vermian branch (copular point); (7) hemispheric branch.

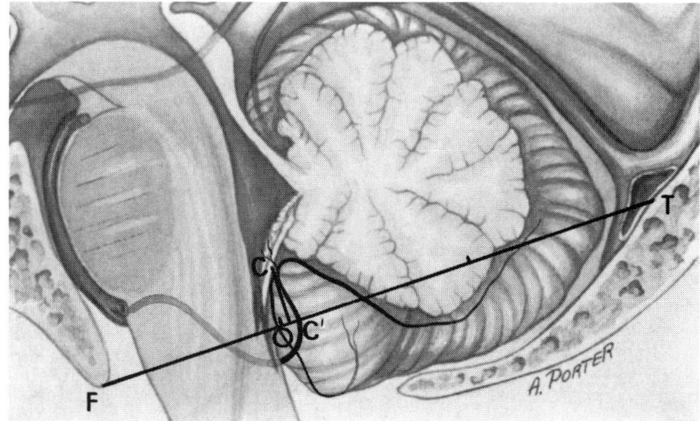

Figure 17.103. Normal measurements of choroidal point. The choroidal point as defined by Huang and Wolf (157) is the point at which the posterior medullary segment joins the supratonsillar segment. A perpendicular line from the choroidal point C to the foramen magnum (at the basion-torcular) line falls at C′. C′ in 90 percent of the cases was located from 1 mm anterior, to 3 mm posterior, to the junction of the anterior and middle thirds of the F–T line (O).

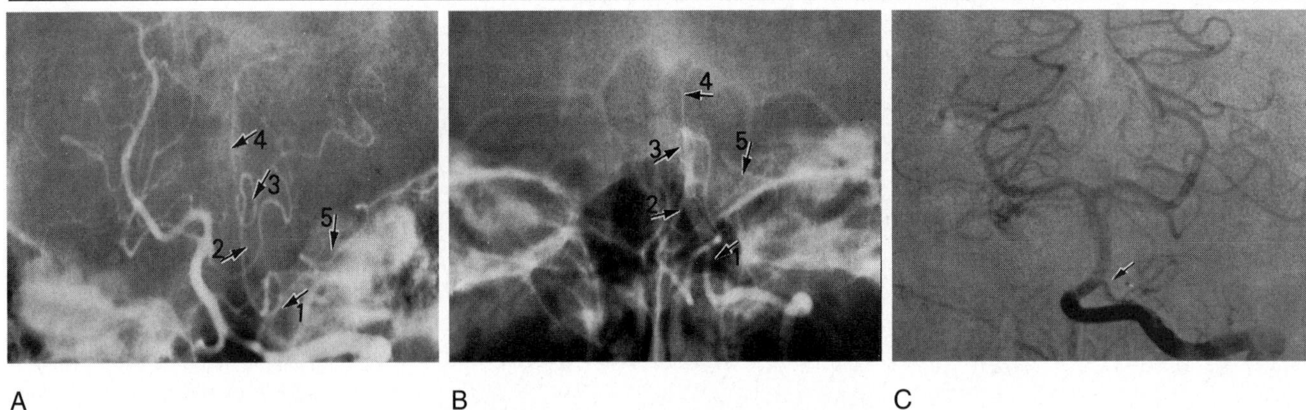

Figure 17.104. Anteroposterior projections of vertebral angiograms to demonstrate posterior inferior cerebellar artery (PICA). **A.** The perimedullary segment (arrow 1), the retromedullary segment (arrow 2), the supra- and superior retrotonsillar segments (arrow 3), and the vermian branch (arrow 4) are well demonstrated in this patient who does not have filling of the posterior cerebral artery on the left side. The anterior inferior cerebellar artery (arrow 5) crosses the proximal segments of the PICA. **B.** The PICA originates from the basilar artery (arrow). Arrows 1, 2, 3, and 4 represent the perimedullary, retromedullary, supra- and retrotonsillar, and vermian segments. Arrow 5 points to a hemispheric branch. **C.** Frontal projection showing the vertebral artery ending in the PICA.

In the *frontal projection*, the cranial curve of the PICA is very close to the midline, and lateral displacements of this portion of the vessel are usually meaningful (Fig. 17.104). The same applies to forward and backward displacement of the choroidal point area. Elongation of the top of the cranial curve (supratonsillar segment) can also be significant. It is seen with enlargement of the fourth ventricle as a result of tumor or from other causes (154, 157).

As in other areas, it is necessary to look at vertebral angiograms with understanding of the relationships of the vessels with various neural structures. Some of these are illustrated by diagrams in Figures 17.97, 17.98, 17.101, 17.105, and 17.110. The student of the posterior fossa is advised to take stereoscopic lateral and anteroposterior views either by making two consecutive injections (having the patient immobilized between the injections) or by taking a single-injection serial that is so arranged that every alternate picture is a stereoscopic mate of the preceding and following film. Subtraction is necessary because it eliminates some of the obscuring bone structures. The frequent anatomic variations of these arteries further increase the difficulty of accurately identifying the various branches of the PICA without stereoscopic films.

The use of routine magnification for the lateral serialogram has been very helpful. This can also be done in the frontal view. Another helpful technical refinement is to obtain two frontal serialograms, one in half-axial and the other in an exaggerated transorbital projection (Fig. 17.106). This can be combined with subtraction to further improve visualization (Fig. 17.106*C*). Superselective injection of the PICA can be accomplished (Fig. 17.107). A base view is often helpful in delineating the anatomy but also requires subtraction for clearest visualization of the vessels (Fig. 17.108). Digital angiography equipment has been a helpful addition to angiography in providing easy routine subtraction.

The vermian branch is sometimes seen to anastomose directly with the corresponding branch of the superior cerebellar artery (Fig. 17.99*C*). This is particularly conspicuous in cases where there is partial or complete occlusion

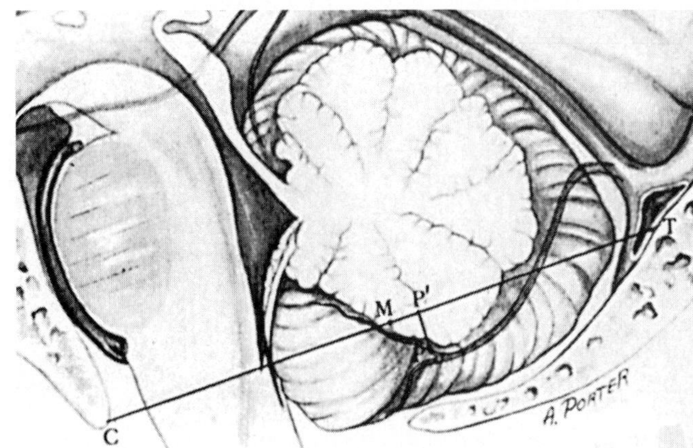

Figure 17.105. Relationship of the copular point to the clivus-torcular line. Huang and Wolf (157) found that the copular point (P) usually falls within a circle of 6 or 6.0 mm radius centered at a point 4 mm behind the midpoint (M) of the C-T line and 4 mm below this line. (More specifically, the line is actually drawn from the basion to the internal occipital protuberance.) By tracing the inferior vermian vein back to its origin, the copular point is usually found to be situated approximately 1 cm above and behind the posterior edge of the foramen magnum.

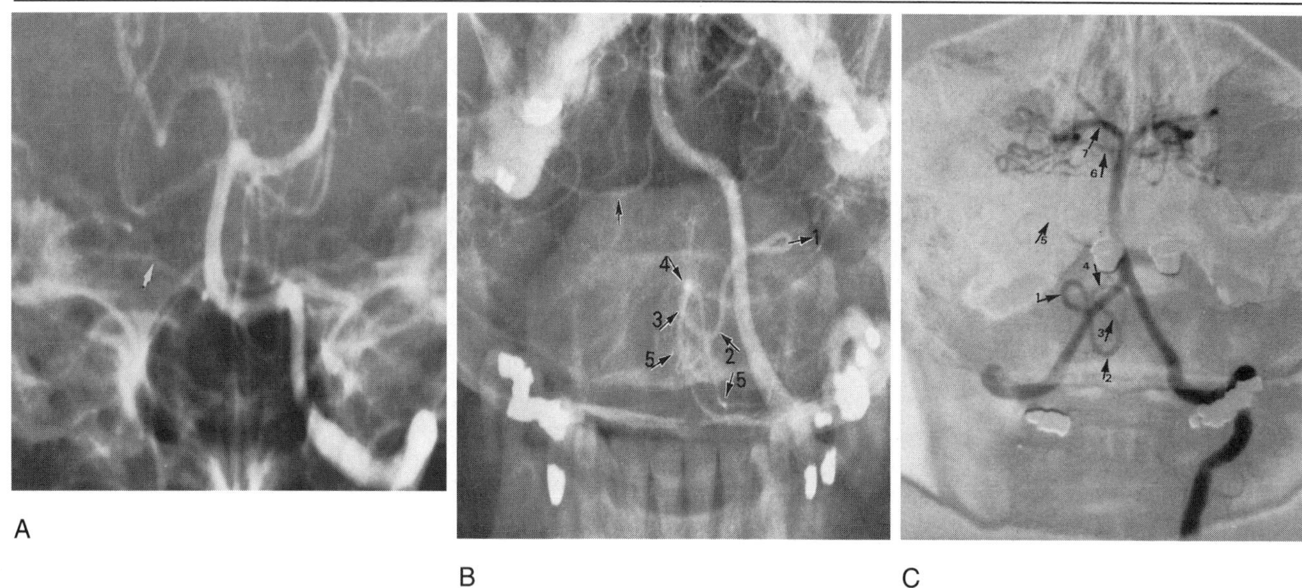

Figure 17.106. Standard frontal and transfacial projections of vertebral-basilar arteries. The posterior inferior cerebellar artery is much more clearly visualized in the film taken without angulation through the open mouth (**B**). The arrows represent (1) perimedullary segment; (2) caudal curve; (3) retromedullary segment; (4) supratonsillar segment seen on end; (5) retrotonsillar and tonsillohemispheric branches. The upper arrow points to the anterior inferior cerebellar artery, which is poorly demonstrated in the routine angle view (**A**) because it overlies bone. **C.** Subtraction to demonstrate vessels through bony structures. The superior cerebellar (6) and posterior cerebral (7) arterial branches overlie each other, but displacement of the trunks of these arteries in the plane of the projection can be easily ascertained. Arrows 1 through 4 correspond to those in B, whereas 5 points to the anterior inferior cerebellar artery.

of the basilar artery (see Fig. 10.68). Anastomosis may also take place between the hemispheric branches of the posterior inferior cerebellar and the superior cerebellar arteries. The vermian branch of the PICA can be absent.

Medullary Branches These are several small branches that arise from the vertebral artery or its branches that are distributed to the medulla oblongata. The branches are usually not apparent on normal vertebral angiograms but may be visible if they become enlarged.

BASILAR ARTERY

The basilar artery results from the fusion of the two vertebral arteries. The junction usually takes place along the lower aspect of the pons, in front of which the vessel ascends to its bifurcation, generally behind or just above the top of the dorsum sellae. It tends to lie in a very shallow groove in front of the pons (Fig. 17.109). In older individuals the artery is naturally tortuous and the junction of the two vertebral arteries is usually displaced toward the side of the smaller vessel, thus placing the proximal part of the basilar artery off the midline. The off-center position of this portion of the artery indicates which of the two vertebral arteries is dominant. The basilar artery may be divided or fenestrated, just distal to the junction of the two vertebral arteries (see Fig. 10.95).

The basilar artery is separated from the clivus by a distance of only 2 to 3 mm, but the relationship of the anterior margin of the basilar artery with the clivus is somewhat variable. The distance to the clivus is slightly greater in children and may increase along the upper portion of the basilar artery as compared with the lower part. In addition, when the artery is tortuous it may be displaced backward as it moves away from the midline because the clivus is concave. Although the bifurcation of the basilar artery is usually at the level of, or slightly above, the tip of the dorsum sellae, sometimes it is just below the level of the top of the dorsum.

When the artery is arteriosclerotic, the point of bifurcation may be considerably higher than normal and may produce an indentation of the floor of the third ventricle, which is clearly visible on air studies (see Fig. 10.70). The higher or lower position of the bifurcation of the basilar artery produces different configurations of the posterior cerebral and superior cerebellar arteries, especially as seen in frontal projection.

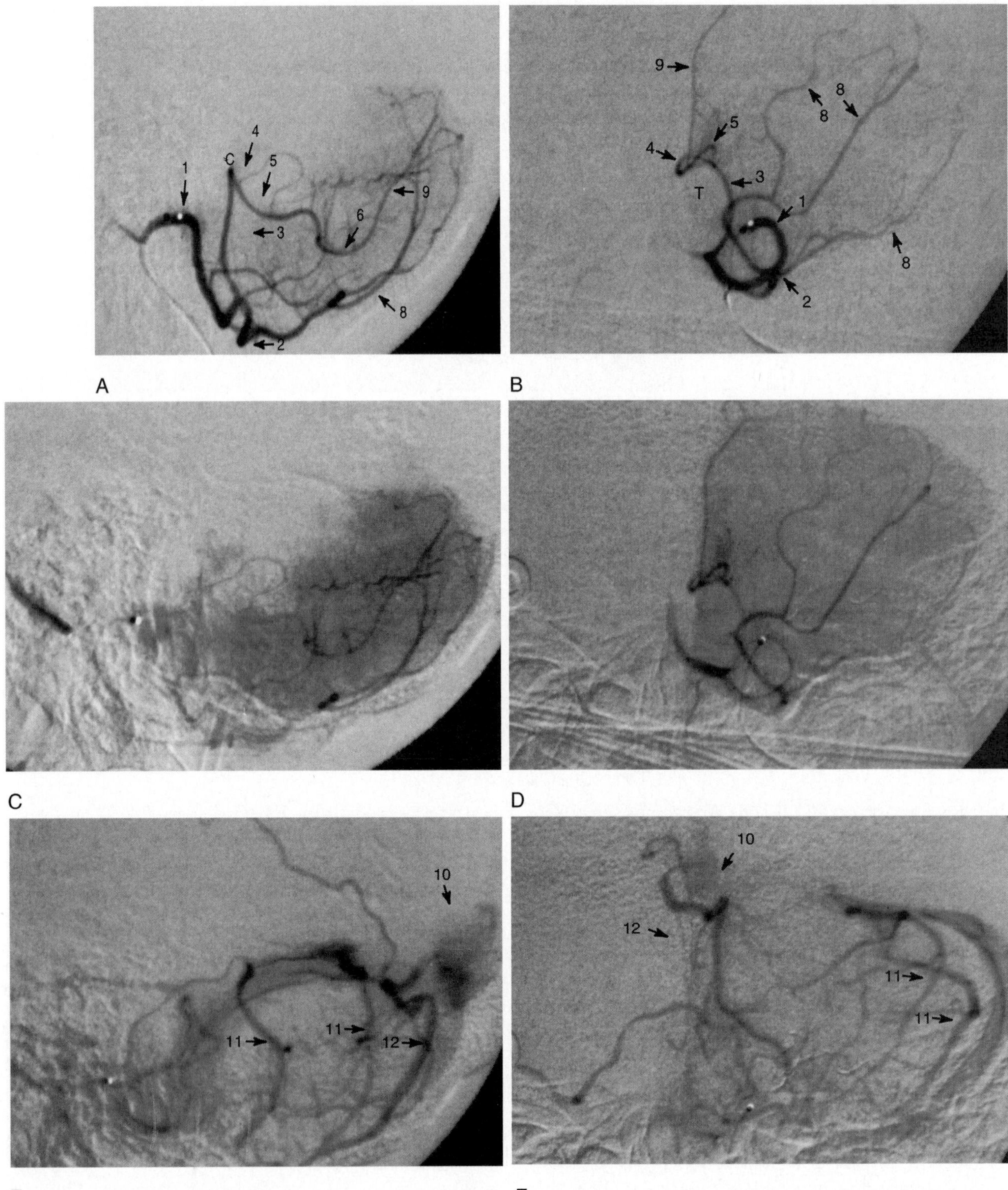

Figure 17.107. Superselective injection of PICA. The numbers indicate (1) lateral medullary segment; (2) caudal loop; (3) posterior medullary segment; (4) supratonsillar segment; (5) superior retrotonsillar portion; (6) copular area (retrotonsillar curve of vermian branch); (7) inferior retrotonsillar portion of tonsillohemispheric branch; (8) hemispheric branches; (9) vermian branch; choroidal point is at C. **A.** Lateral. **B.** Frontal view. **C.** Lateral intermediate phase. **D.** Frontal intermediate phase. **E** and **F.** Lateral and frontal views, venous phase. (10) lower aspect of torcula; (11) hemispheric veins; (12) vermian vein. The vermian vein in the lateral view appears to be farther back than usual. This may be due to some rotation of the head because the vermian vein in normal cases is situated about 1 cm away from the inner table.

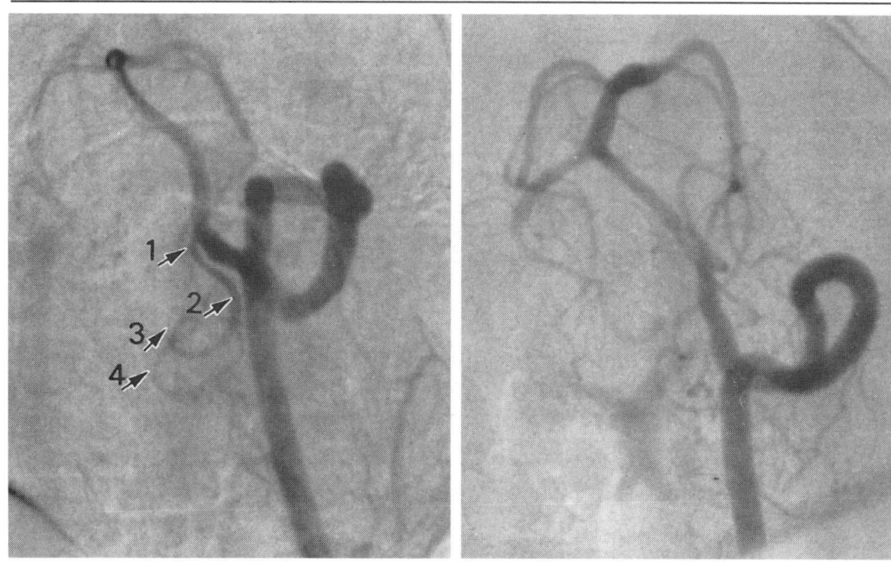

Figure 17.108. Basal projection of vertebral-basilar system. **A.** The mentovertical view and modified base view (**B**) are often useful to visualize vascular displacements and sometimes to demonstrate saccular aneurysms. The posterior inferior cerebellar artery is labeled with numbered arrows (A): (1) premedullary segment; (2) lateral medullary segment; (3) posterior medullary segment; (4) supra- and retrotonsillar segments.

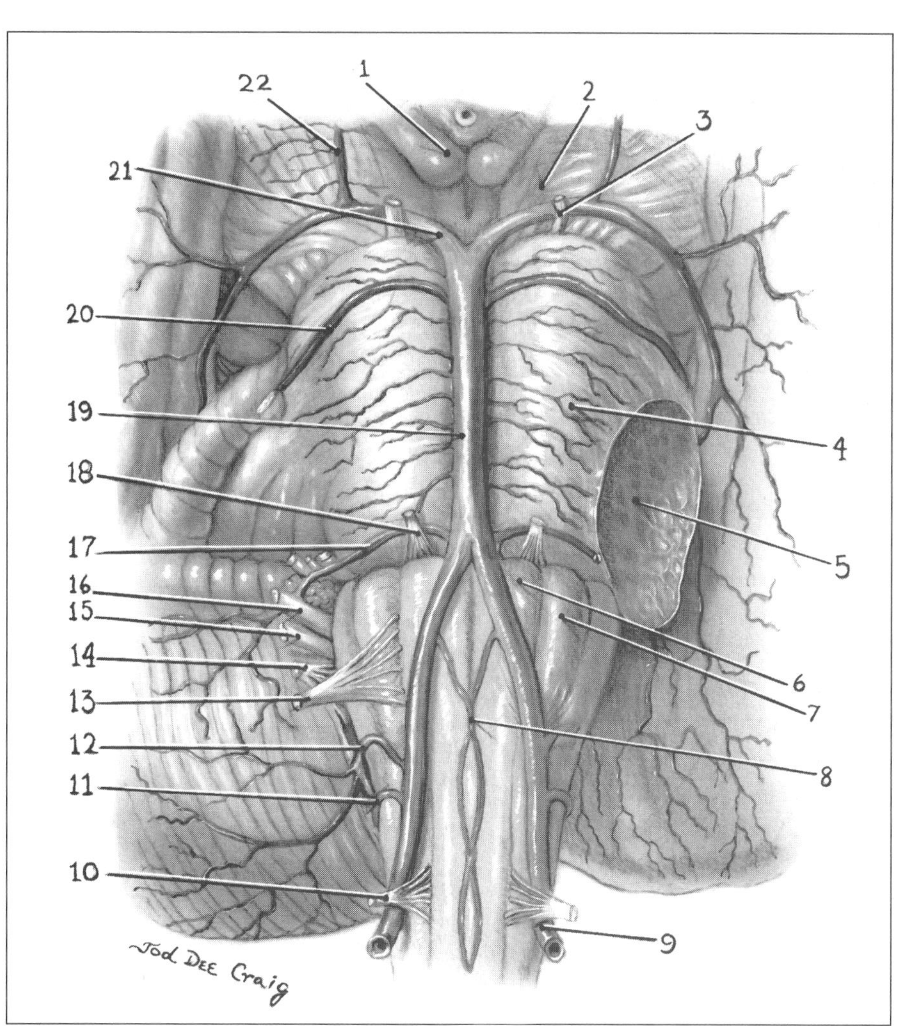

Figure 17.109. Diagram of vertebral and basilar arteries and their branches. A frontal view of the pons and medulla shows the branches of the vertebral and basilar arteries and related structures: (1) mammillary body; (2) cerebral peduncle; (3) III cranial nerve (oculomotor); (4) pons; (5) cross section of brachium pontis (middle cerebellar peduncle); (6) pyramid of medulla; (7) olive; (8) anterior spinal artery; (9) vertebral artery; (10) first cervical nerve root; (11) posterior spinal artery; (12) posterior inferior cerebellar artery; (13) XII cranial nerve (hypoglossus); (14) XI cranial nerve (spinal accessory); (15) X cranial nerve (vagus); (16) IX cranial nerve (glossopharyngeal); (17) anterior inferior cerebellar artery; (18) VI cranial nerve (abducens); (19) basilar artery; (20) superior cerebellar artery; (21) posterior cerebral artery; (22) posterior communicating artery (after Testut).

Minor Branches

The basilar artery gives off many branches, most of which are small and supply the pons (Fig. 17.109). These branches are not usually perceived on vertebral angiograms even with the use of tomography. With subtraction it is possible to demonstrate, during the intermediate phase, a general staining of the pons and cerebellum (cerebrogram phase), which sometimes allows visualization of the total structures and the cavity of the fourth ventricle. This technique, however, necessitates the injection of larger amounts of contrast material (158). Caruso et al. studied the perforating branches of the upper basilar artery and of the first (P1) segment of the posterior cerebral artery in 50 human brain cadavers (159). No vertical branches arose from the basilar bifurcation. The upper basilar artery gave rise to horizontal branches, which were studied with reference to their angle of origin. Perforating arteries arising from P1 segments were found in all specimens. Rare branches were found to come from the inferior and anterior surfaces of P1 segments.

The midbrain and posterior diencephalon (interpeduncular fossa) microvascular anatomy is primarily from that of perforating arteries originating from the last 5 mm of the basilar artery, from the initial 7 mm of both superior cerebellar arteries, and from the initial segment (P1 segment) of the posterior cerebral artery (160). The perforating branches penetrated a small space in the upper part of the interpeduncular fossa. The anterior two-thirds of this space was occupied by the posterior perforated substance, and the posterior one-third was the site of penetration of the branches that supply the inferior mesencephalon. The posterior perforated substance was divided into anterior and posterior halves. The anterior half was perforated by the paramedian thalamic arteries (diameter 0.6 +/− 0.1 mm), while the superior paramedian mesencephalic arteries (diameter 0.2 +/− 0.06 mm) perforated the posterior half. The perforating arteries originated from a trunk exclusive to the anterior half in 30 percent, from a trunk supplying both halves in 60 percent, and from a trunk exclusive to the posterior half in 13 percent of specimens. There were many naturally occurring anastomoses between the perforating branches. The paramedian inferior mesencephalic arteries penetrating the posterior one-third of the upper part of the interpeduncular fossa arose from the P1 segment in 32 percent, from the proximal 7 mm of the SCA in 45 percent, and from the last 5 mm of the basilar artery in 23 percent.

Torche et al. recently studied the microvascular anatomy of the basilar artery between the superior cerebellar artery and the vertebrobasilar junction (i.e., the *lower basilar artery*) in injected cadaver brains (161). The length of this segment of the basilar artery was 28 +/− 1.35 mm and its course was straight in 45 percent of brains, curved in 35 percent, and tortuous in 20 percent. The average number of perforators was 17 per brain. Of these, 35 percent were median and 65 percent were lateral. Median branches were about half the size (a mean length of 5.8 +/− 1.25 mm), whereas left and right lateral branches had a mean length of 16 +/− 1.25 mm and 16 +/− 1.58 mm, respectively.

Anterior Inferior Cerebellar Artery

The *anterior inferior cerebellar artery* (AICA or *middle* cerebellar artery of the French anatomists) normally arises from the basilar artery above the junction of the two vertebral arteries and is usually present on both sides. The size and course of this artery are variable and are dependent, in part, upon the size and distribution of the PICA. The variation in size of the AICA is in inverse proportion to the PICA. After its origin from the basilar artery, the AICA extends laterally and downward across the lower pons (Fig. 17.110). As it reaches the seventh and eighth nerves it continues horizontally with these nerves, passing behind the internal auditory canal, into which it frequently makes a tight loop. It then reverses its course and enters the cerebellum (Fig. 17.111). The AICA gives origin to the *internal auditory artery;* in one-third of cases, however, the internal auditory arises directly from the basilar artery. According to Smaltino et al., direct origin of the internal auditory artery from the basilar artery is uncommon (3 percent) (162). These authors refer to the *cerebellolabyrinthine artery*, which gives origin to the auditory artery. The cerebellolabyrinthine artery may originate from the basilar artery as a common trunk with the anterior inferior cerebellar artery, or it may originate separately just above the AICA. In 85 percent of the cases the AICA arose at the same level on both sides. The two sides are equal in size in 15 percent, the right larger in 48 percent, and the left larger in 37 percent of patients (163). The AICA can be injected alone via superselective catheterization (Fig. 17.111*C* to *G*).

Kim et al. studied the variability of the anatomic relationship of the AICA to the facial (seventh) and vestibulocochlear (eighth) nerves in 52 cerebellopontine angles (CPAs) (164). The AICA originated from the basilar artery (98.1 percent) or from the vertebral artery (1.9 percent) as a single (92.3 percent of CPAs) or duplicate (7.7 percent) artery. Each of the 52 CPAs had one or more arterial trunks that coursed in close proximity to the seventh and eighth cranial nerves and thus were said to be nerve related. The nerve-related arterial trunks were divided into three segments based on their relationship to the nerves and meatus: the premeatal, meatal, and postmeatal segments. The nerve-related branches of the AICA gave rise to the internal auditory artery in 92.3 percent of the CPAs, the recurrent perforating artery in 78.8 percent, and the subarcuate artery in 30.8 percent.

Woischneck and Hussein (165) found the following in their study of the *anterior inferior cerebellar artery* (AICA) at microdissection: (*a*) there is a reciprocal relationship between the development of the AICA and the PICA; (*b*) we

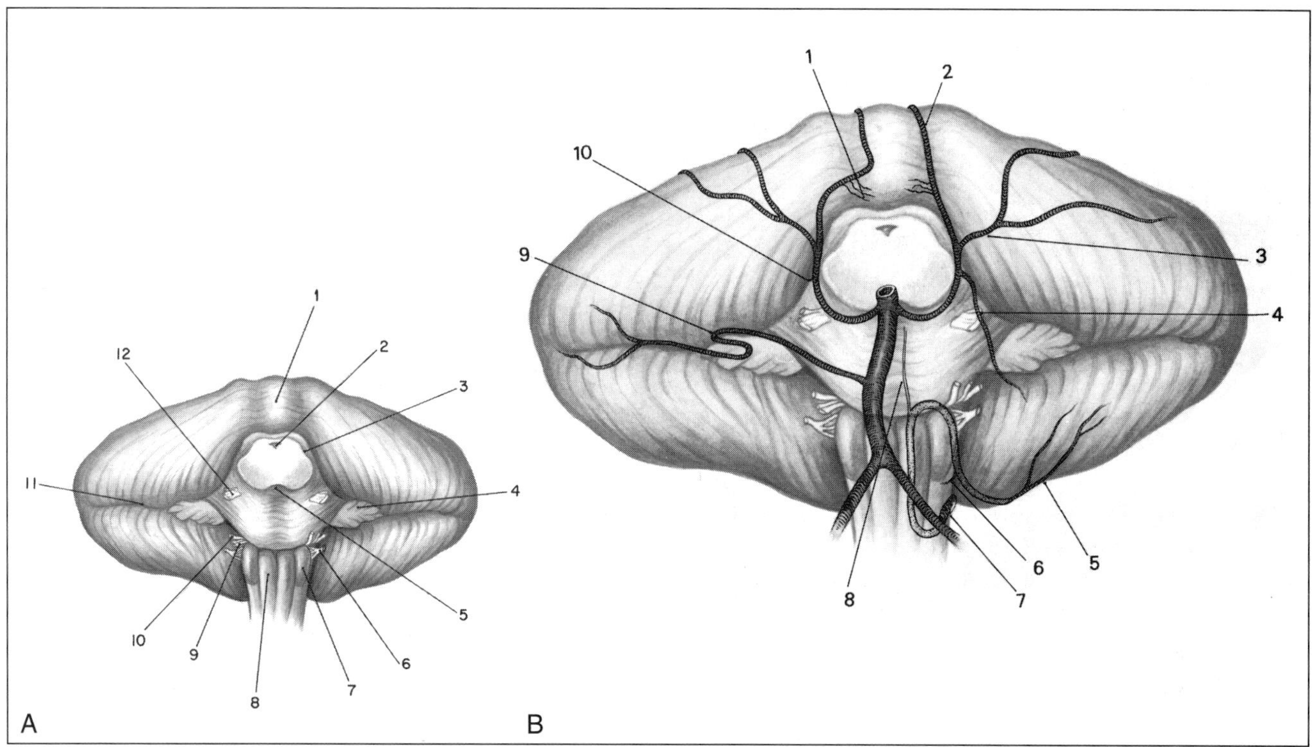

Figure 17.110. Diagram to illustrate the anatomy of the brainstem and cerebellum as seen in angled anteroposterior projection similar to that used in cerebral angiography. **A.** (1) Superior vermis; (2) aqueduct of Sylvius; (3) lateral mesencephalic sulcus; (4) flocculus; (5) interpeduncular fossa; (6) vagus (X) nerve; (7) olive; (8) pyramid; (9) facial (VII) nerve; (10) acoustic (VIII) nerve; (11) great horizontal fissure of cerebellum; and (12) trigeminal (V) nerve. **B.** (1) Precentral arterial branches of the superior cerebellar artery; (2) superior vermian branch of superior cerebellar artery; (3) hemispheric branch; (4) anterior lateral marginal branch; (5) hemispheric branch of the tonsillohemispheric division of the posterior inferior cerebellar artery (PICA); (6) tonsillar branch; (7) perimedullary segment of PICA; (8) vermian branch of PICA; (9) anterior inferior cerebellar artery; and (10) superior cerebellar artery. (The right side in this drawing is slightly different from the left.)

can draw no conclusions concerning the pattern of the AICA on one side to the pattern on the other side; (*c*) the size of the AICA at the level of the basilar artery gives an indirect indication of the peripheral course; and (*d*) the AICA and the cranial nerves are in a constant relationship to each other.

Superior Cerebellar Artery

The artery is paired and arises at or near the bifurcation of the basilar artery. Sometimes it almost appears to have a common origin with the posterior cerebral artery. As it leaves the basilar artery it turns somewhat downward to a variable degree to go around the anterolateral aspect of the upper pons. The downward swing may be lower on one side than on the other, thus producing a slight asymmetry in normal cases; in frontal view the curve is then wider on one side than on the other. In general, however, the curves, convex downward, are reasonably symmetric on the two sides (Fig. 17.112). After passing one-half the distance around the pons, the superior cerebellar artery turns dorsad and gives off a branch called the *lateral branch* or *anterior lateral marginal artery* (166) (Fig. 17.113*A*). This branch passes in front of the brachium pontis and anterior aspect of the cerebellar hemisphere and may give off twigs to the lateral aspect of the precentral cerebellar fissure. Sometimes the lateral branch is very large in relation to the others (Figs. 17.88 and 17.113*A*).

As it continues its course around the brainstem, the superior cerebellar artery gives off one or two *hemispheric branches*, which ramify over the superior surface of the cerebellar hemisphere (Fig. 17.83). The main stem continues as the *superior vermian branch*, which ascends to reach the culmen and then descends posteriorly, maintaining its close relationship to the vermis. There it may anastomose end to end with the vermian branch of the posterior inferior cerebellar artery. At its highest point (the culmen), in lateral view, the artery is usually not projected higher than either of the posterior cerebral arteries (Figs. 17.100, 17.112, 17.113, and 17.114). The latter are supratentorial but more lateral in position. It is not uncommon, however, to find a normal case in which the highest curve of a superior cerebellar artery projects slightly above one or both posterior cerebral arteries. In general, however, this relationship should be regarded with suspicion for it may be a sign of either upward transtentorial bulging of the cerebellum or downward pressure exerted upon the posterior

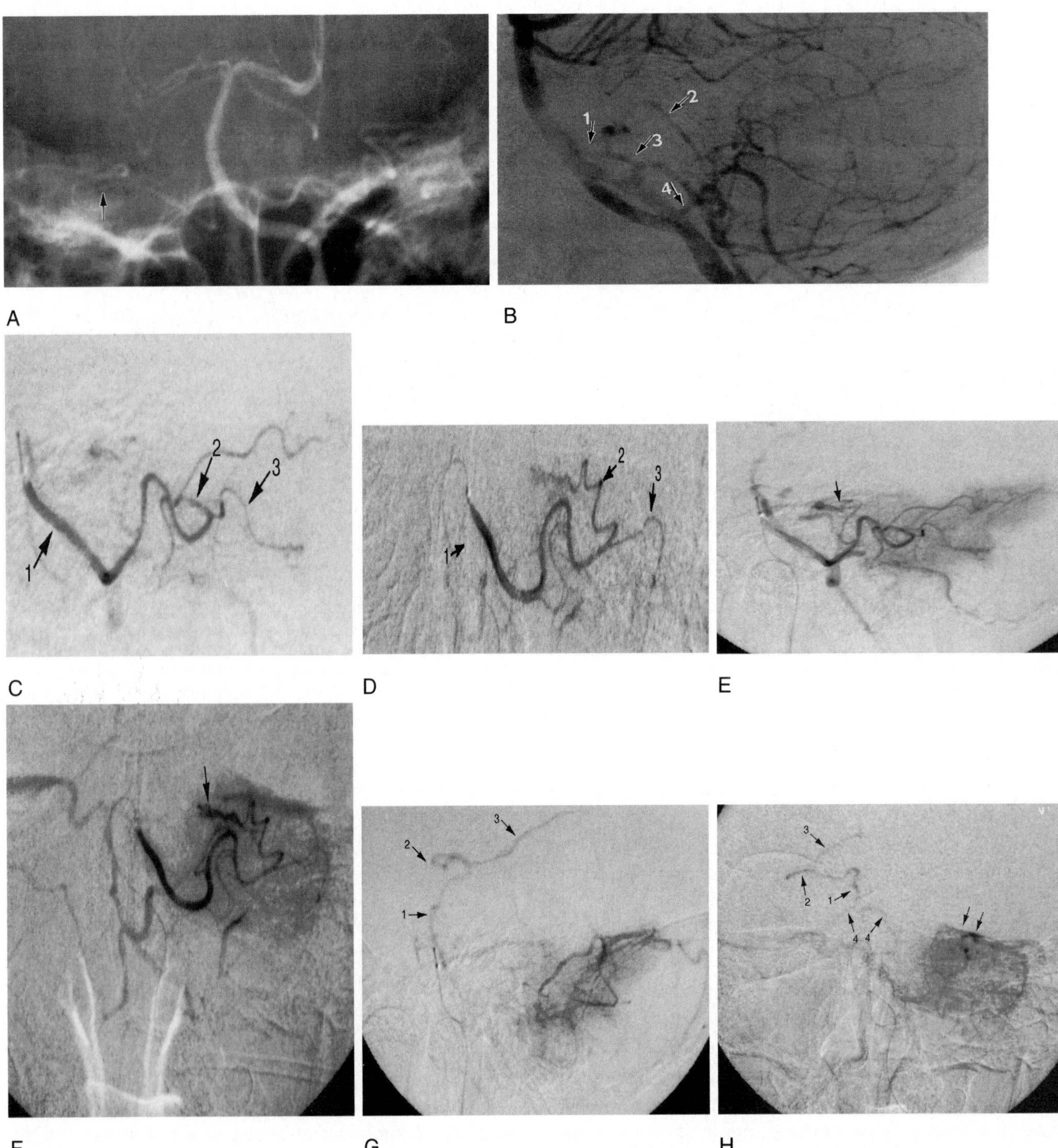

Figure 17.111. Examples of normal vertebral angiograms to demonstrate anterior inferior cerebellar artery (AICA). **A.** Both AICAs fill well. The right is disposed according to the classic description and makes a tight curve into the internal auditory canal. The left is somewhat larger and less typical. It appears to give origin to branches that normally arise from the posterior inferior cerebellar artery (PICA), which does not fill on this side. **B.** The numbered arrows are (1) common trunk of AICA and PICA on right; (2) AICA; (3) PICA; and (4) PICA on the opposite side. **C** to **H.** Superselective injection of AICA. **C** and **D.** Lateral and frontal views, arterial phase: (1) trunk of AICA; (2) branch supplying a small arteriovenous malformation; (3) hemispheric branch. **E** and **F.** Lateral and frontal intermediate phase. The arrow indicates an early filling vein associated with the small arteriovenous malformation. The capillary blush indicates the area normally supplied by the artery. **G** and **H.** Lateral and frontal views, venous phase. The arteriovenous malformation drains into the superior group: (1) anterior pontomesencephalic vein; (2) peripeduncular vein tributary to the basal vein (3); (4) transverse pontine veins. The double arrows are over the lateral sinus.

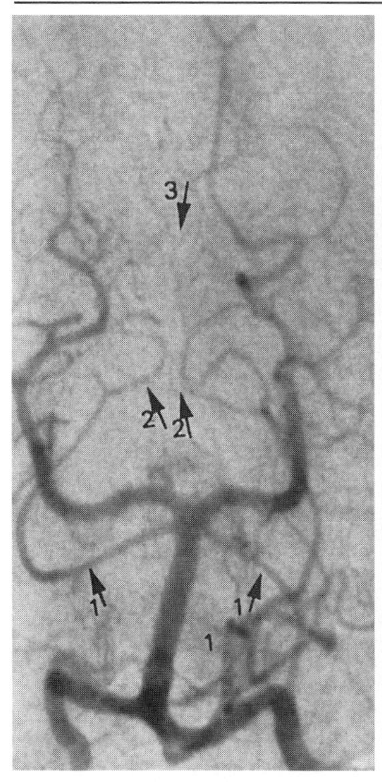

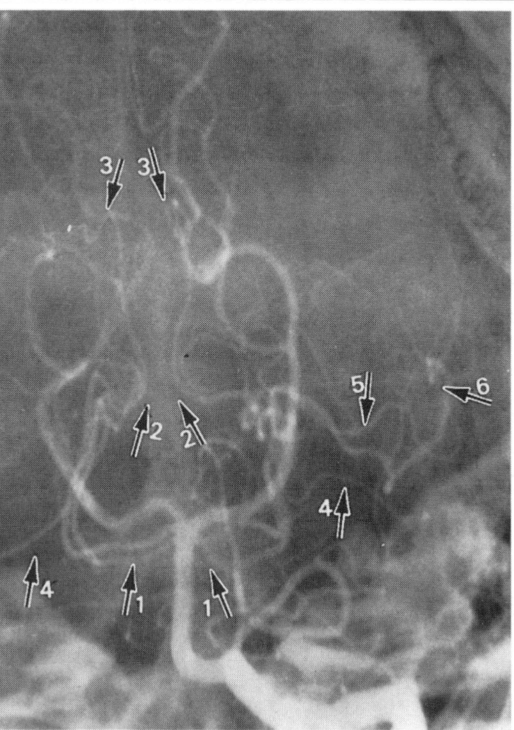

Figure 17.112. Frontal views of superior cerebellar arteries. **A.** A typical example of superior cerebellar arteries (1) arising just caudal to the origins of the posterior cerebral arteries is shown by left vertebral angiography. The arteries then pass around the brainstem and come fairly close together near the midline (2) behind the midbrain. They usually continue as superior vermian branches after giving off hemispheric branches. As described in the text, the vermian branches turn downward over the upper vermis and in the frontal projection they end approximately where arrow 3 is located. Any vessels beyond that point are posterior cerebral branches and are supratentorial in location. **B.** An example of double superior cerebellar arteries on both sides is shown. (Unilateral duplication is more common.) Arrows: (1) split trunk of superior cerebellar artery bilaterally; (2) superior vermian branches; (3) superior vermian branches seen end-on as they turn downward over the vermis; (4) anterior marginal branch; (5) hemispheric branch of the superior cerebellar artery; and (6) posterior temporal branch of posterior cerebral artery.

cerebral arteries, flattening them against the tentorial surface. The configuration of the superior cerebellar arteries is best demonstrated by vertebral angiography when there is bilateral carotid origin of the posterior cerebral arteries.

There are inconstant small branches arising from the preculminate segment, which outline the precentral cerebellar fissure and can be seen in the lateral view in some cases. Huang et al. have designated these the *precentral cerebellar arteries* (166). They are important because of their location at the anterior medullary velum, thus indicating the position of the upper aspect of the fourth ventricle, in a manner similar to the precentral cerebellar vein (see text following).

The superior cerebellar artery may be double, or even triple, on one or both sides (Fig. 17.112*B*); it is rarely absent. The configuration of the superior cerebellar artery is best seen in lateral projection when the posterior cerebral artery does not fill (Fig. 17.82). Hardy et al. studied the superior cerebellar artery in 50 cerebellar hemispheres (167). Forty-three superior cerebellar arteries arose as a single trunk, and 7 arose as duplicate trunks. One solitary trunk and the rostral trunk of one duplicate vessel arose from the posterior cerebral artery. The remainder arose from the basilar artery. The superior cerebellar artery was divided into four segments: the anterior pontomesencephalic segment lay below the oculomotor nerve; the lateral pontomesencephalic segment coursed below the trochlear and above the trigeminal nerve; the cerebellomesencephalic segment coursed in the groove between the cerebellum and the upper brainstem; and the cortical segment was distributed to the cerebellar surface. The superior cerebellar arteries arising as a single trunk bifurcated into a rostral and a caudal trunk, corresponding to the trunks formed by a duplicate origin. The rostral trunk supplied the medial and the caudal trunk supplied the lateral parts of the cerebellar cortex. The superior cerebellar artery gave off perforating, precerebellar, and cortical arteries. The perforating arteries penetrated the interpeduncular fossa, the cerebral peduncles, the junctions of the superior and middle cerebellar peduncles, and the colliculi. The precerebellar branches arose within the cerebellomesencephalic groove and supplied the adjoining parts of the cerebellum and brainstem. The cortical branches were divided into vermian, hemispheric, and marginal arteries. The 50 superior cerebellar arteries had points of contact with 32 oculomotor, 46 trochlear, and 26 trigeminal nerves.

Surgical revascularization for vertebrobasilar system requires that we identify the best sites at which to perform bypass procedures (168). The ideal sites for an anastomosis were identified as the pretonsillar segment of the PICA, the second portion of the AICA, the perimesencephalic segment of the superior cerebellar artery, and the perimesencephalic part of the posterior cerebral artery. These were the best sites because of their outer diameter, degree of mobility, least number of branches, and frequency of occurrence.

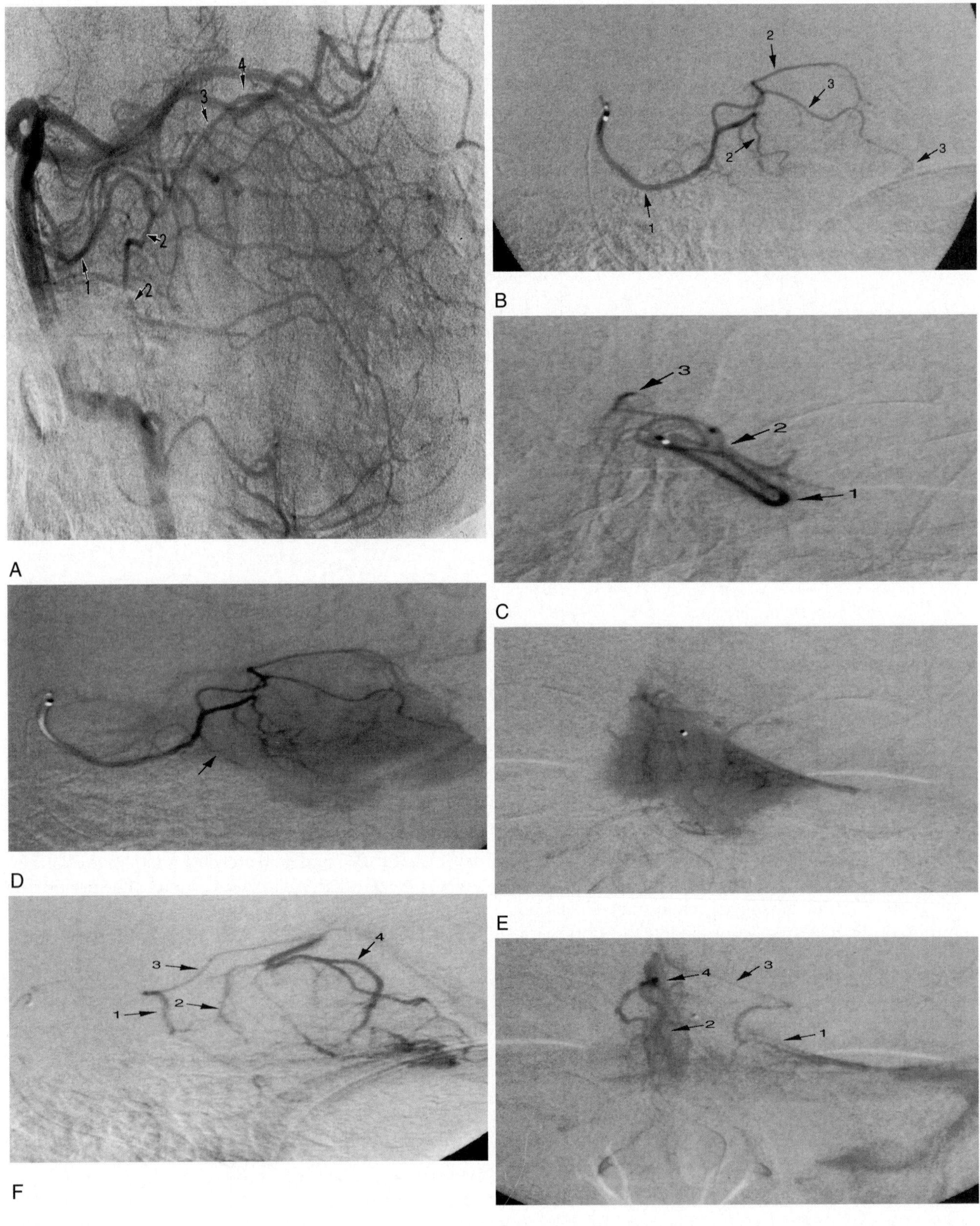

Figure 17.113. Superior cerebellar artery. **A.** The arrows point to (1) proximal superior cerebellar arteries; (2) anterior lateral marginal branch; and (3) and (4) vermian branches. **B** to **F.** Superselective angiography of superior cerebellar artery. Lateral (**B**) and frontal (**C**) views, arterial phase: (1) perimesencephalic portion; (2) hemispheric branch; (3) vermian branch. Lateral (**D**) and frontal (**E**) view, intermediate phase. The cerebrogram, intermediate phase, indicates the areas supplied by this artery. Lateral (**F**) and frontal (**G**) view, venous phase: (1) anterior pontomesencephalic veins; (3) basal vein; (4) superior vermian vein.

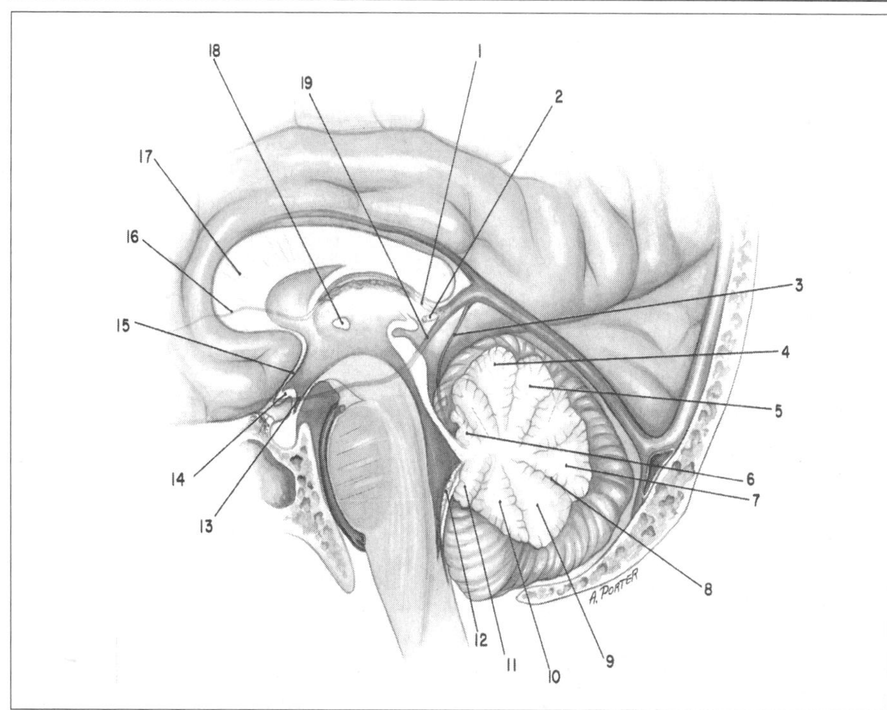

Figure 17.114. Diagrammatic cross section of the posterior fossa structures and the third ventricle. (1) Internal cerebral vein; (2) cut contralateral basal vein; (3) precentral cerebellar vein; (4 and 5) culmen of vermis; (6) central lobule of cerebellum; (7) tuber of vermis (just above it are the folium and the declive); (8) prepyramidal sulcus; (9) pyramis; (10) uvula; (11) nodule; (12) choroid plexus of fourth ventricle; (13) infundibular recess of third ventricle; (14) optic chiasm; (15) lamina terminalis; (16) septal vein; (17) corpus callosum; (18) massa intermedia; (19) posterior aspect of basal vein.

Cerebral Veins

SUPERFICIAL CEREBRAL VEINS

The superficial cerebral veins are extremely variable in their configuration. Most of these veins run upward to end in the superior longitudinal sinus *(superior cerebral veins).* The great majority ascend upward and backward, but as they reach the superior convexity of the brain, they turn rostrad and enter the superior longitudinal sinus against the flow of the bloodstream. Only one or two of the anterior frontal veins join the longitudinal sinus in the direction of the bloodstream. Blood flow in the superior cerebral veins is toward the sinus. The largest of these veins is the *vein of Trolard,* the position (as well as the size) of which is variable. The vein of Trolard anastomoses with the *vein of Labbé,* which is directed downward and backward to end in the lateral sinus. Together they form an important venous anastomotic pathway. Like the vein of Trolard, the vein of Labbé is quite variable in position, size, and configuration (Figs. 17.115 and 17.129).

Another of the descending veins is the superficial *middle cerebral vein* or veins; they may be two in number. These veins run in the sylvian fissure downward and forward and then medially along the sphenoid ridge to end in the sphenoparietal sinus or enter directly the cavernous sinus (Figs. 17.116 and 17.137).

The *inferior cerebral veins* drain the undersurface of the hemisphere. The veins under the temporal lobe join the middle cerebral and basal veins; those on the orbital surface of the frontal lobe join the superficial frontal veins and empty into the superior sagittal sinus.

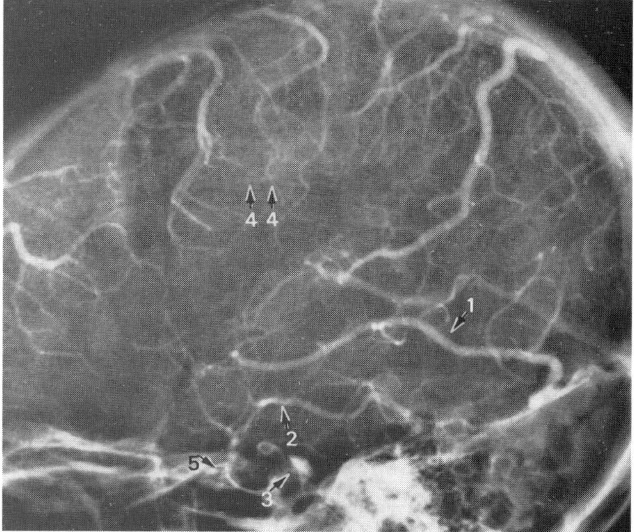

Figure 17.115. Normal venogram. A lateral view shows the superficial superior cerebral veins curving rostrad to join the superior sagittal sinus. The inferior veins usually drain toward the middle cerebral or sylvian vein and by way of the vein of Labbé (arrow 1). The basal vein is outlined and is seen to receive tributaries from the basal ganglia arranged in a fan shape. It runs horizontally, not joining the internal cerebral vein but ending in the superior petrosal sinus (arrow 2). The density behind the clivus is produced by the basilar plexus (arrow 3). The inferior sagittal sinus is faintly outlined with contrast (arrow 4). An uncal vein is also seen (arrow 5).

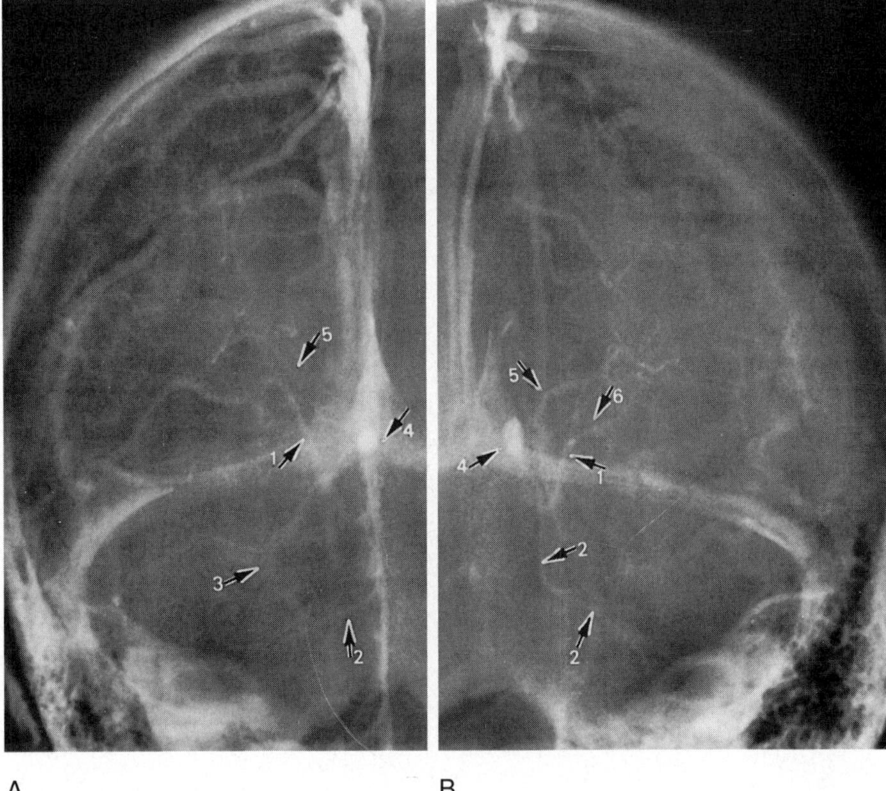

Figure 17.116. Normal frontal venography. **A** and **B**. Right and left venograms demonstrate the thalamostriate vein (arrow 1) outlining the ventricle on each side (the head is slightly rotated on the left angiogram). The septal vein is seen on both sides (arrow 2). Arrows: (3) basal vein; (4) internal cerebral vein seen end-on; (5) medial atrial vein; (6) anterior caudate vein. The superficial veins are seen to drain upward on the surface of the hemisphere to join the superior sagittal sinus; some are on the medial surface of the hemisphere.

On the angiogram the frontal veins fill slightly before the posterior frontal and parietal veins. Actually, if a serial study is made, it is observed how, in very rapid succession, the frontal veins appear first very faintly, and shortly thereafter the parietal veins fill. The deep veins are usually the last ones to fill, but the pattern is variable; they frequently remain filled longer than the superficial veins (at least with sufficient concentration of contrast substance to be well visualized) (see under "Physiology," Chapter 10).

DEEP CEREBRAL VEINS

The deep cerebral veins are more important than the superficial veins from the angiographic point of view. The principal vessels are the insular and striate veins, the subependymal veins, the basal vein, and the vein of Galen.

There are a variable number of veins over the surface of the insula that have a configuration similar to the branches of the middle cerebral artery in the same location (i.e., they assume a triangular configuration so that a "venous sylvian triangle" is visible in many instances). If it is not clearly seen frequently, it is because of superimposition of other veins. These veins usually drain into the deep middle cerebral vein, which in turn empties into the basal cerebral vein. When the deep middle cerebral vein does not empty into the basal vein, it is seen to descend and to empty into the sphenoparietal sinus. In addition to the insular veins, the deep middle cerebral vein receives the striate veins and veins from the inferior aspect of the frontal lobe. Wolf et al. have also identified the *uncal vein*, which runs on the medial aspect of the temporal lobe in front of the uncus (169). It drains into the sphenoparietal venous sinus (sinus of the lesser wing) or directly into the cavernous sinus (Fig. 17.137). *Stereoscopic serial examinations* are extremely useful in detecting the relationship of the various venous systems. The use of serial angiography is required to ascertain the direction of drainage of the channels and to observe the emptying patterns.

SUBEPENDYMAL VEINS

Internal Cerebral Vein

The vessel is paired, and the two veins are situated just off the midline so that they are, for their greater extent, placed one against the other, at the roof of the third ventricle in the tela choroidea (Fig. 17.117). Their configuration is that of the roof of the third ventricle as seen in the lateral projection. The veins begin at the foramen of Monro and extend slightly upward and backward, and after reaching their highest point gradually descend downward and backward, forming a fairly regular, semicircular, or somewhat elliptic curve. *The anterior slope of the curve is approximately equal in length and arc to the posterior slope*, but variations are fairly common. The internal cerebral veins leave the roof of the third ventricle just above the suprapineal recess and enter the upper portion of the quadrigeminal cistern where they join to form the great vein of Galen. The vein of Galen

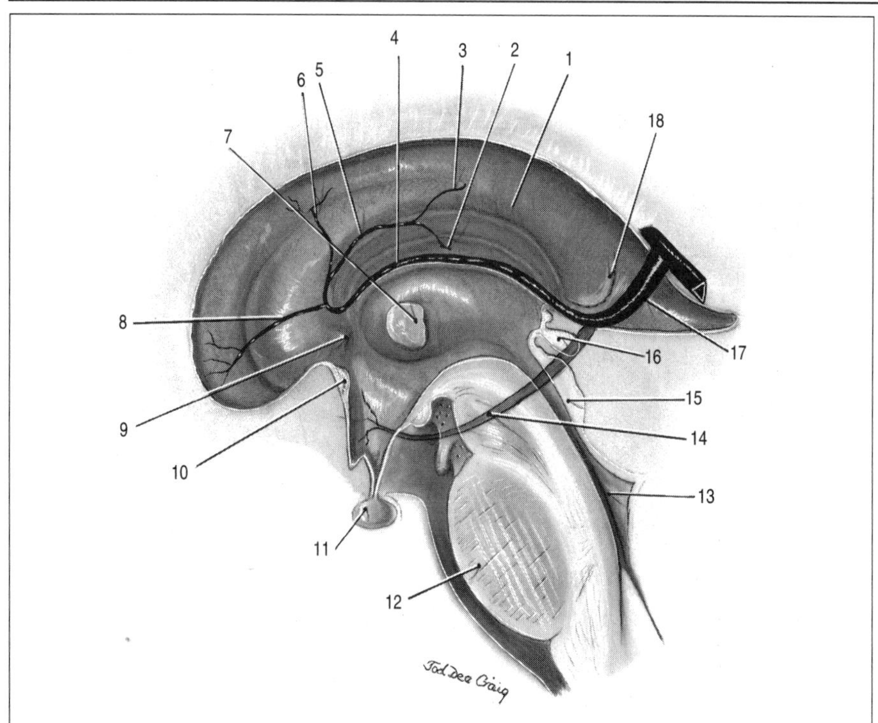

Figure 17.117. Diagrammatic representation of deep cerebral veins and their relation with adjacent brain structures in lateral projection. (1) Lateral ventricle; (2) terminal branch of thalamostriate vein; (3) posterior caudate veins; (4) internal cerebral vein; (5) thalamostriate vein; (6) anterior caudate vein; (7) massa intermedia; (8) septal vein; (9) foramen of Monro; (10) anterior commissure; (11) hypophysis; (12) pons; (13) fourth ventricle; (14) basal vein passing schematically behind the midbrain; (15) quadrigeminal plate; (16) pineal; (17) vein of Galen; (18) splenium of corpus callosum.

describes a curve concave upward and ends as it joins the straight sinus (Fig. 17.117).

The main tributary of the internal cerebral vein on each side is the *thalamostriate vein* or *terminal vein.* This vein is itself formed by tributaries running on the wall of the lateral ventricle, and it also receives the *choroid vein,* which runs along the choroid plexus of the lateral ventricle. From its junction with the internal cerebral vein, the thalamostriate vein can be followed backward and slightly upward in the groove formed by the caudate nucleus and the thalamus (Fig. 17.118). The vein is therefore situated on the inferior and lateral aspect of the ventricular wall and actually outlines the approximate size of the lateral ventricle (Fig. 17.116). If the ventricle has become enlarged, the arc, concave upward and described by the thalamostriate vein, becomes much wider (Fig. 17.119). If the ventricle is narrowed, such as may occur when there is medial displacement by a mass, the arc will be reduced or flattened.

The *venous angle* is the point of junction of the thalamostriate vein with the internal cerebral vein. At this point the *septal vein,* extending backward from the frontal horn of the lateral ventricle on each side, usually joins the internal cerebral vein. In most cases the junction is situated at the foramen of Monro (Fig. 17.120). At times, however, the thalamostriate vein does not join the internal cerebral vein at the foramen of Monro, but behind the foramen (Figs. 17.121 and 17.122). This anatomic variant is fairly common and has been referred to as a *false venous angle.* In some patients with a false angle, the usual arc of the internal cerebral vein is completed by the septal vein (Fig. 17.121); in others, the septal vein joins the thalamostriate vein and the usual arc of the internal cerebral vein is not completed. In the latter cases, the appearance is often suggestive of upward displacement of the internal cerebral and septal veins (Figs. 17.121 and 17.122). It can usually be appreciated that an anomaly is present and not a displacement because the foramen of Monro is situated directly above (or a little behind) the dorsum sella; in the case of a false venous angle, the junction takes place considerably behind the sella turcica, too far back to represent the foramen of Monro. Additionally, if the foramen of Monro were displaced backward (as by a frontal pole tumor), the arc of the internal cerebral vein would be high (i.e., the vein is "humped"). With a normal but false venous angle, the arc is flatter, or no arc is present (Fig. 17.122).

There are numerous veins in the depths of the cerebral hemispheres distributed in radial fashion *(medullary veins).* The deeper ones drain into the deep cerebral veins, and the more superficial ones drain into the superficial cerebral veins. There are anastomoses between the two groups, allowing blood to flow from the superficial to the deep system in case of occlusion of superficial veins and contrariwise in the case of obstruction of the deep veins, such as is encountered in certain types of venous sinus thrombosis. The arrangement of the medullary veins is schematically shown in Figure 17.123. The medullary veins may become enlarged with arteriovenous malformations and with malignant tumors (Fig. 17.124). *These veins, however, are not visible* on the average angiogram except when they are pathologic. Magnification will sometimes show very fine,

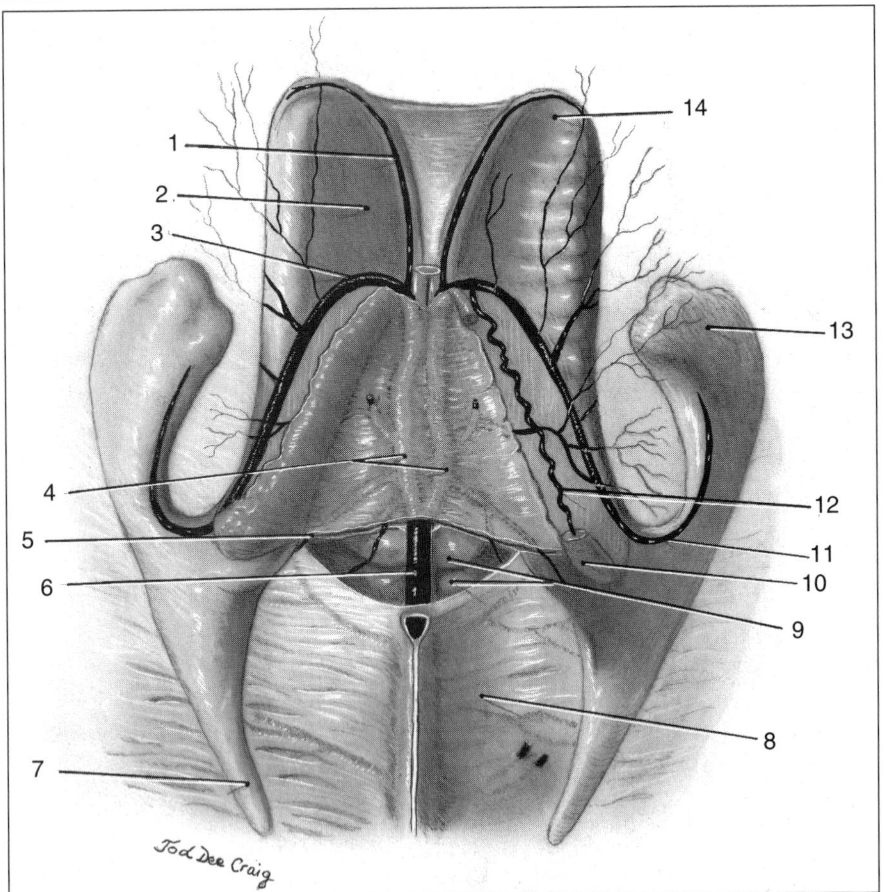

Figure 17.118. Diagrammatic representation of deep cerebral veins seen from above. The two thalamostriate veins are seen to join a septal vein to form the internal cerebral vein on each side. The internal cerebral veins are contained within the velum interpositum and join posteriorly to form the vein of Galen. The choroid plexus was removed on the right side to show the choroid vein. The thalamostriate vein is drawn to the temporal horn. This is seen sometimes but is by no means a constant feature. Variation in the configuration of the veins is, of course, the rule. (1) Septal vein; (2) anterior horn at the junction with the body of the lateral ventricle; (3) thalamostriate vein; (4) internal cerebral veins; (5) the two leaves of the velum interpositum; (6) vein of Galen; (7) occipital horn; (8) tentorium; (9) quadrigeminal tubercles; (10) choroid plexus; (11) initial segment of the thalamostriate vein or terminal vein; (12) choroid vein; (13) temporal horn; (14) frontal horn of the lateral ventricle. (See also Fig. 17-117.) Medial to the thalamostriate vein is the thalamus and anterolaterally is the caudate nucleus.

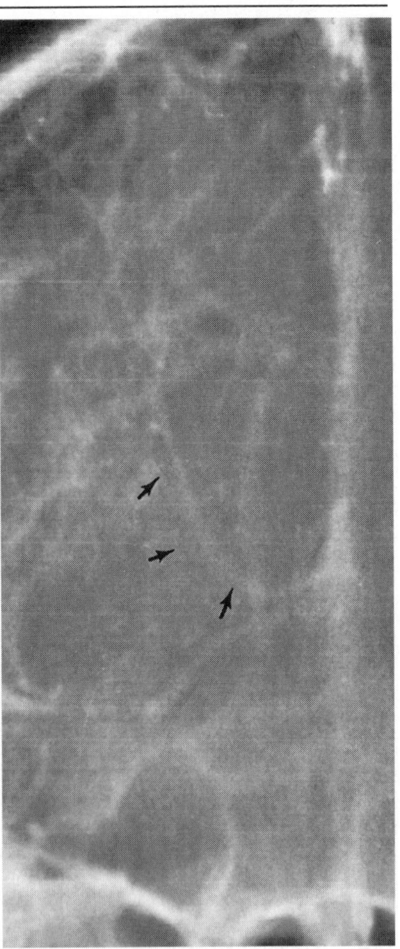

Figure 17.119. Ventricular dilatation, moderate, demonstrated by the wide curve of the thalamostriate vein (arrows).

normal, medullary veins; to be considered normal, however, the veins must be very thin. If seen, they should always be regarded with suspicion for it may be an indication of a pathologic process.

The deeper veins *become visible only as they reach the ventricular wall* and from that point to their junction with the internal cerebral vein, or thalamostriate vein, they are well shown (Figs. 17.121 and 17.125). These small subependymal veins make it possible to outline the ventricular surface on the lateral angiogram fairly accurately, and enlargement of the ventricle can be seen readily in this way.

A small vein is often seen that joins the anterior portion of the vein of Galen just behind the junction of the two internal cerebral veins. This small vein is the *posterior callosal vein;* it extends around the splenium of the corpus callosum before it joins the vein of Galen. Actually, the vein of Galen approximates the position and shape of the splenium of the corpus callosum, but its relationship with this structure is variable. The posterior callosal vein (vein of the corpus callosum or splenial vein) is seen in a fairly high percentage of cases if looked for carefully. Ring found it in over 95 percent of 100 normal angiograms (170). Occasionally, however, the vein is absent. Presumably, the junction of this vein with the posterior aspect of the internal cerebral vein or the vein of Galen indicates fairly accurately the position of the inferior margin of the splenium of the corpus callosum. The author has not found this structure very helpful except as evidence of involvement of the corpus callosum by a tumor if the arc of the vein is widened.

Attempts have been made to determine if the position

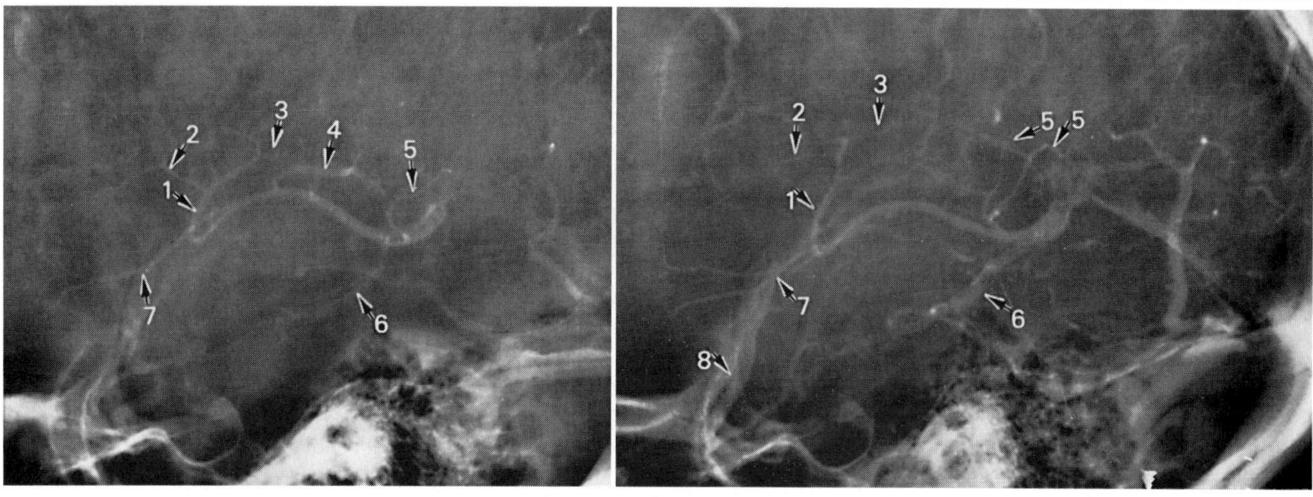

A B

Figure 17.120. Normal venogram—subependymal veins. The films represent the right (**A**) and left (**B**) sides of the same patient. The configuration of the two internal cerebral veins is similar. The inferior sagittal sinus is seen on the left but not on the right. Arrows: (1) thalamostriate vein; (2) anterior caudate vein; (3) posterior caudate vein; (4) medial subependymal vein perforating roof of third ventricle to join internal cerebral vein; (5) medial atrial vein; (6) basal vein; (7) septal vein joining internal cerebral behind the foramen of Monro in A and at the foramen in B; (8) superficial middle cerebral vein draining into sphenoparietal sinus (sinus of the lesser sphenoid wing).

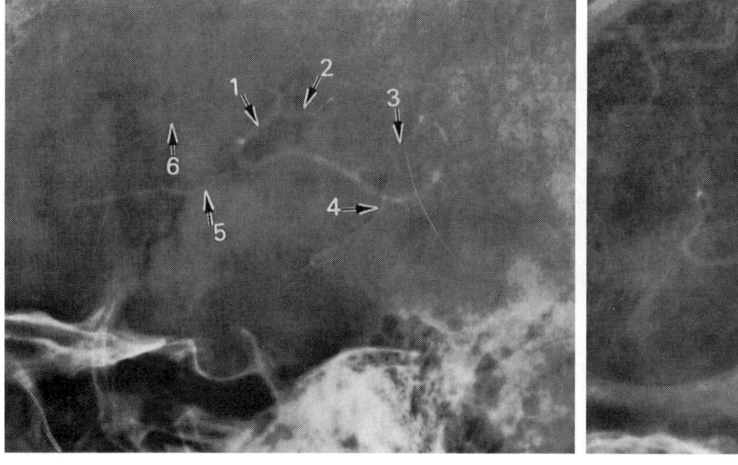

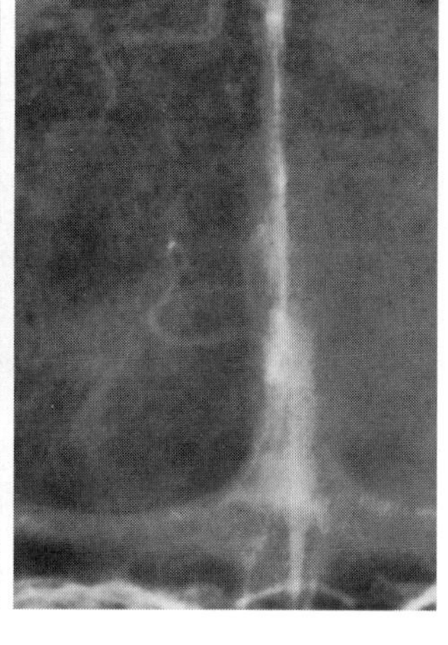

A B

Figure 17.121. Normal venogram—false venous angle. **A.** The appearance suggests a normal configuration of the internal cerebral vein, but the septal vein makes a slight curve, convex downward, before joining the thalamostriate vein, which is usually at the foramen of Monro. The junction with the thalamostriate vein is about 1 cm behind the foramen of Monro. Arrows: (1) thalamostriate vein; (2) posterior caudate vein; (3) medial atrial vein; (4) inferior ventricular (atriotemporal) vein; (5) septal vein—the arrow is in the expected position of the foramen of Monro; (6) anterior caudate veins. **B.** In the frontal projection, the thalamostriate vein is seen to travel on the floor of the lateral ventricle transversely to join the internal cerebral vein, further confirming that the junction of these veins is behind the foramen of Monro.

of the internal cerebral vein is normal by measurement in the lateral view. At least three different methods have been proposed to determine if the position of the foramen of Monro is normal or abnormal, based on the venous angle. Because of the variations in the point at which the internal cerebral and thalamostriate veins join, this determination by angiography is not too accurate. The simplest methods are those proposed by Wolf et al. (171), by Laine and coauthors (172), and by Ring (170). In a comparative study of the methods proposed by Wolf and by Laine, Ring found that the method of Laine is slightly more accurate. The method proposed by Wolf et al. is also of help in determining the presence of upward or downward displacement of the middle and posterior portions of the internal cerebral vein.

Like all biologic measurements, only gross separations from the normal fall outside of the usual limits in all cases. Minor displacements may fall within accepted limits and, vice versa, normal veins may sometimes measure beyond the usual limits. Ring found that 19 percent of patients present a false venous angle (170). In the majority of these cases, it is easy to determine that a false venous angle is present, as noted previously. At times, however, it is not realized that this anatomic variation is present and, therefore, a false conclusion could be reached. With experience, it may be possible to largely eliminate this source of error,

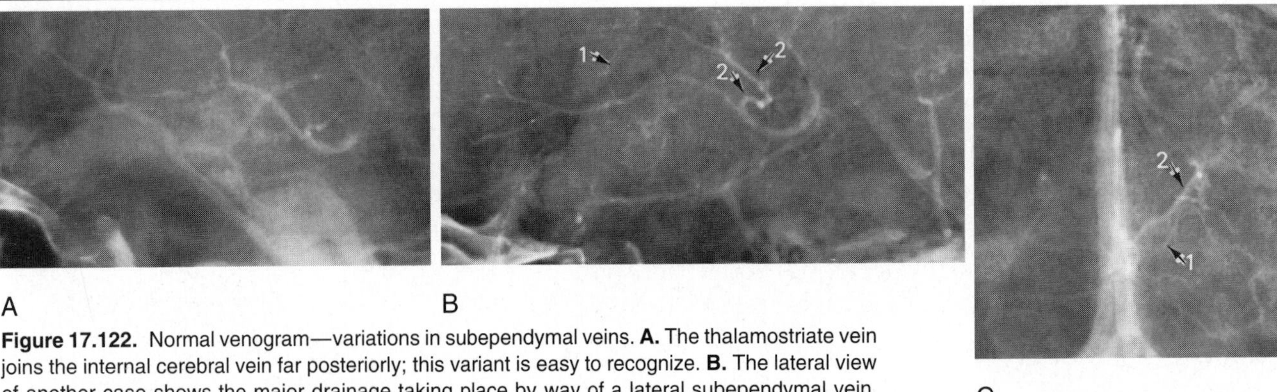

Figure 17.122. Normal venogram—variations in subependymal veins. **A.** The thalamostriate vein joins the internal cerebral vein far posteriorly; this variant is easy to recognize. **B.** The lateral view of another case shows the major drainage taking place by way of a lateral subependymal vein. There is a small vein in the normal location of the thalamostriate vein at the foramen of Monro, which can be recognized in the frontal projection (C). Arrows: (1) small vein in the place of the thalamostriate vein; (2) lateral subependymal veins. **C.** In the anteroposterior view of B, the arrow numbers correspond to those in B. It is noteworthy that, in spite of the venous variants, the size of the ventricle can be estimated accurately. The fine-speckled appearance paralleling the large subependymal vein in B represents fine subependymal veins along the roof of the ventricle.

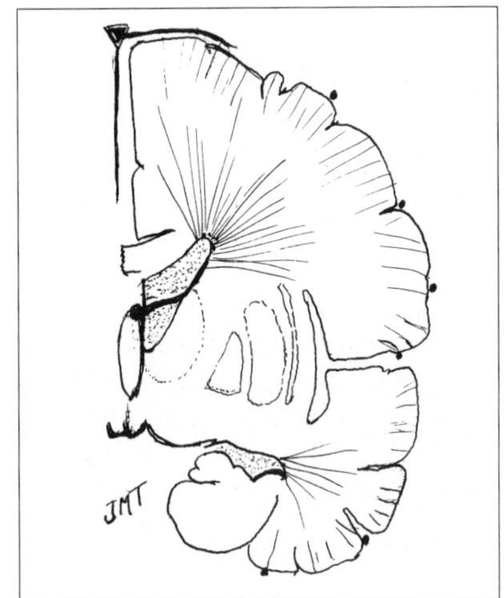

Figure 17.123. Diagrammatic representation of medullary veins of brain. The drawing represents a coronal section depicting the fan-shaped distribution of the medullary veins. They extend radially toward the ventricular wall and outward toward the surface of the hemisphere.

but this anatomic variant tends to decrease the accuracy of any method of locating the posterior aspect of the foramen of Monro based on angiograms.

The arc of the internal cerebral vein differs with the shape of the head. In a patient with a dolichocephalic head, the arc of the internal cerebral vein is flatter than in a patient with brachycephaly. In the latter instance, the vein describes a high arching curve. The arc is often higher in children than in adults.

Wolf and Huang have proposed that the subependymal veins of the lateral ventricle (all of the veins referred to previously, except the medullary veins, are subependymal) be divided into medial and lateral groups (173). The *medial group* is on the medial wall of the ventricle and comprises the septal vein, the medial atrial veins, small veins arising from the corpus callosum and septum, the vein of the posterior horn (which joins the atrial veins), and the vein of the hippocampus (on the medial side of the temporal horn), which empties into the basal vein (Figs. 17.120 and 17.121). The *lateral subependymal venous group* includes the thalamostriate vein, which receives the anterior caudate and the posterior caudate (posterior terminal) veins. It also includes the *inferior ventricular vein* (or atriotemporal vein), which is sometimes large; it is laterally situated and usually conforms to the shape of the atrium or of the caudate nucleus. It originates in the posterior portion of the body of the lateral ventricle, swings around the anterior wall of the atrium, and ends in the basal vein after passing through the choroidal fissure (Fig. 17.126). Sometimes, prominent *lateral atrial veins* are seen to drain into the basal vein.

Basal Vein (Basal Cerebral Vein)

The basal vein (*vein of Rosenthal*) originates on the medial aspect of the anterior portion of the temporal lobe by tributaries arising from the medial surface and the temporal horn. It also receives veins coming from the hippocampal gyrus, the interpeduncular fossa, and the midbrain. The basal vein receives a small *anterior cerebral vein*, which passes laterally with the anterior cerebral artery, and the *deep middle cerebral vein* (Fig. 17.127). It also receives many fine branches, the *inferior striate veins*, which leave the corpus striatum at the anterior perforated substance. From these origins the basal vein passes backward and goes around the brainstem as it extends upward to join the two internal cerebral veins immediately before they fuse to form the vein of Galen. Variations from this usual confluence are

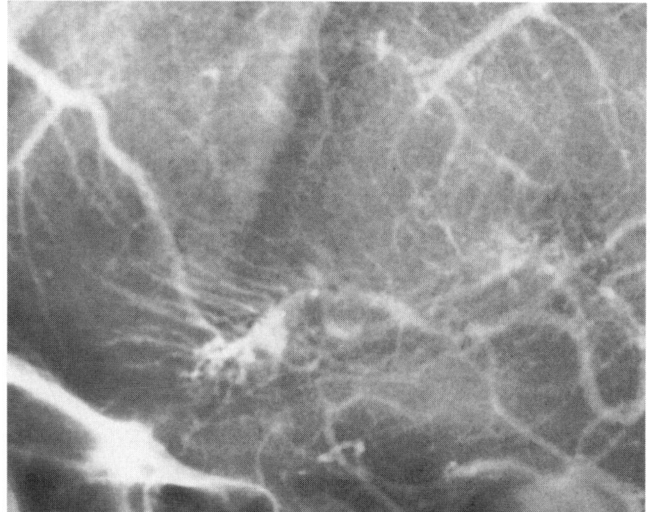

A

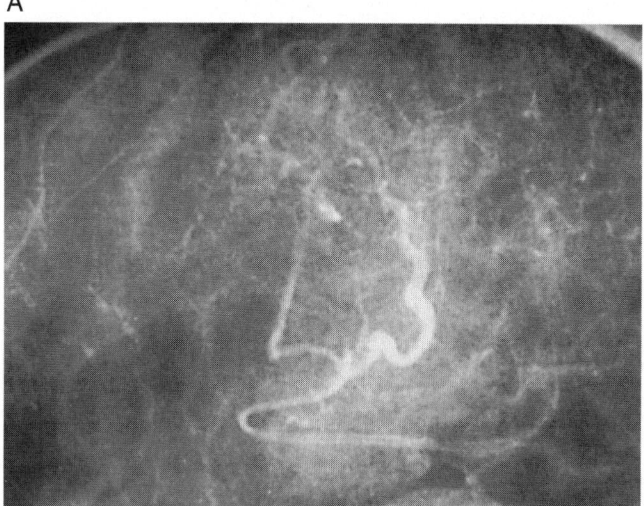

B

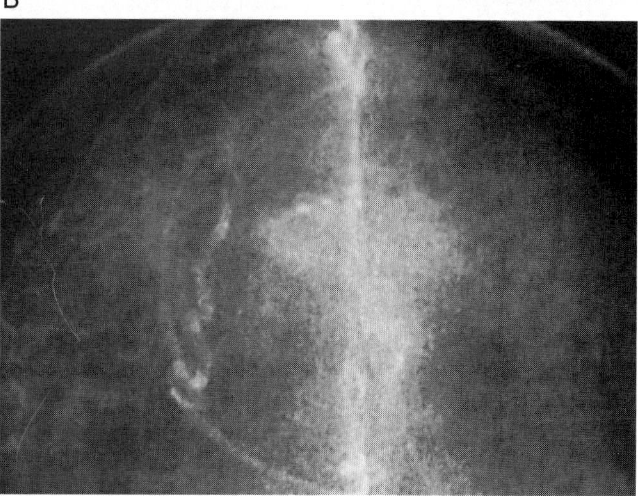

C

Figure 17.124. Enlarged medullary veins in two patients with glioblastoma multiforme. **A.** The enlargement of the medullary veins in radial fashion is evident. **B** and **C.** In another patient the drainage of veins into the deep veins as well as into the superior superficial cerebral veins can be seen.

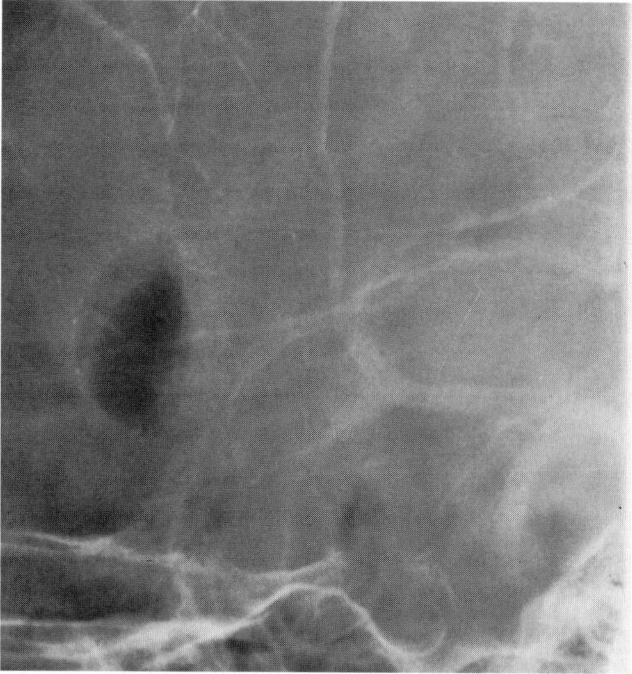

Figure 17.125. Normal venogram. The veins of the frontal horn draining into the septal vein become visible at the wall of the ventricle and thus faithfully outline the ventricular contour in normal cases.

very common. The basal vein may not join the internal cerebral vein at the vein of Galen but may end directly in the straight sinus. It may join the vein of Galen just before this vein enters the straight sinus.

The basal veins are somewhat similar in their configuration to the posterior cerebral arteries but are situated slightly higher. These relationships are explained in Figure 17.128. Because the basal vein is higher in position than the posterior cerebral artery, it does not behave in a manner identical with the artery when displaced by various pathologic processes. When seen in the lateral projection, the basal vein originates above the sella turcica, and from its origin it first passes slightly downward before going upward and continuing backward (Fig. 17.129). The degree of downward curve from its origin is somewhat variable, and care should be taken not to consider the anterior portion of this vein to be displaced upward unless it is a definite change. The anterior portion is usually considered elevated if the change in curve takes place posteriorly, instead of approximately 1.5 cm above and behind the sella turcica, the point where the curve usually changes.

The anterior portion of the basal vein fills earliest and is often empty in the later phases of the angiogram. Thus, the branches that form the basal vein fill at a time when superimposition of the other veins tends to obscure them. Nevertheless, by concentrating on the proper region, it is possible to visualize these branches (anterior cerebral veins, inferior striate veins, deep middle cerebral veins) (Figs. 17.130 and 17.131).

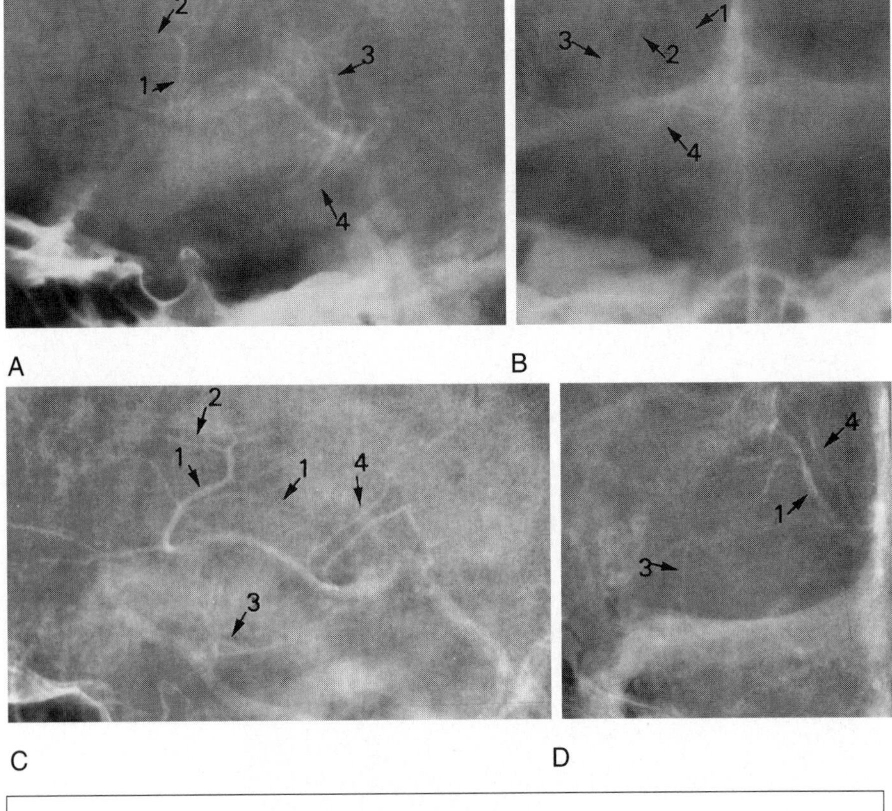

Figure 17.126. Normal venogram. **A.** Lateral projection. The internal cerebral vein has a "humped" configuration in a patient who has a slightly brachycephalic head. The inferior ventricular vein is seen to originate in the body of the lateral ventricle and to swing around the atrium to join the basal vein. **B.** Frontal projection. Arrows: (1) thalamostriate vein; (2) anterior caudate vein; (3) inferior ventricular vein (retrothalamic); (4) basal vein. **C** and **D.** The lateral and anteroposterior venograms of another patient show (1) thalamostriate (terminal) vein; (2) anterior caudate vein; (4) medial atrial veins. An inferior ventricular vein (3) is also present but is superimposed on the basal vein in the lateral view. The numbered arrows apply to all figures.

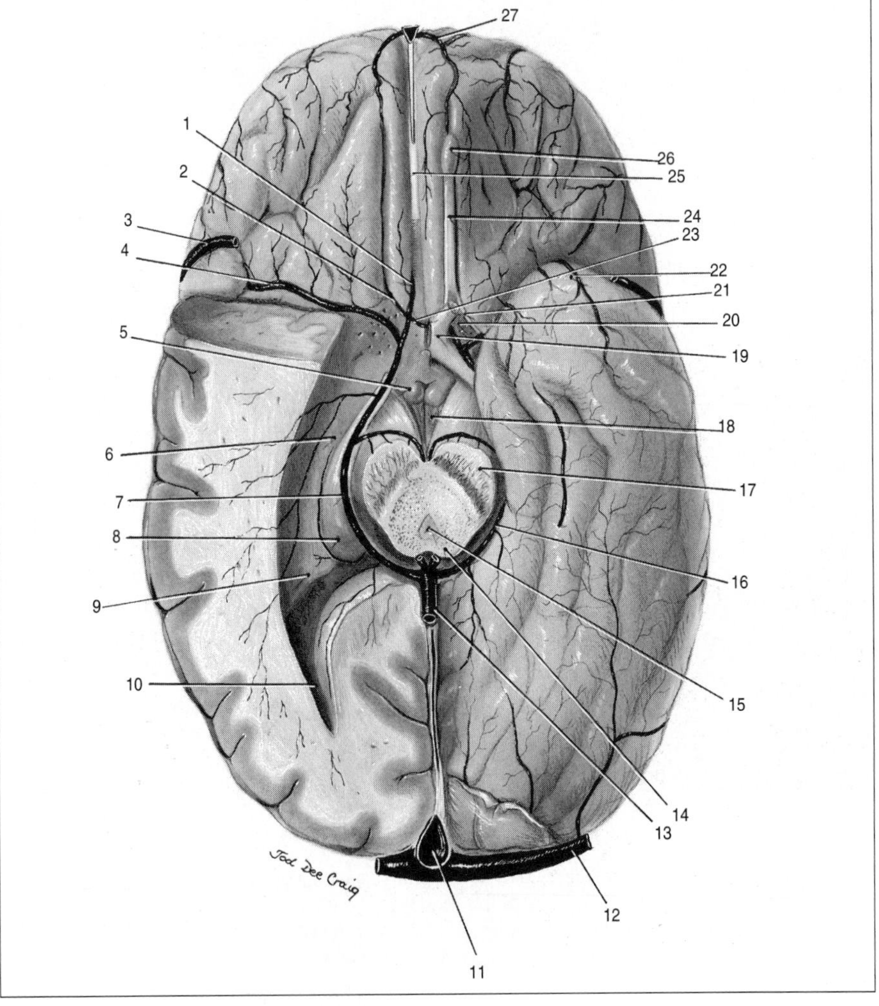

Figure 17.127. Diagram depicting basal vein, its origins and relations with midbrain. The tip of the temporal lobe on the right side has been removed and a horizontal cross section of the temporal and occipital lobes has been done to open the temporal horn, occipital horn, and atrium of the ventricle. (1) Anterior cerebral vein; (2) olfactory vein; (3) superficial middle cerebral vein; (4) deep middle cerebral vein; (5) mammillary body; (6) temporal horn of the lateral ventricle; (7) basal vein; (8) hippocampus major; (9) collateral eminence; (10) posterior horn of the lateral ventricle; (11) superior sagittal sinus joining; (12) transverse sinus; (13) vein of Galen; (14) quadrigeminal plate; (15) aqueduct of Sylvius; (16) basal vein; (17) cerebral peduncle and peripeduncular vein; (18) posterior perforated substance; (19) optic chiasm; (20) anterior perforated substance; (21) lateral olfactory striae; (22) anterior tip of the temporal lobe; (23) anterior communicating vein; (24) olfactory tract; (25) longitudinal (interhemispheric) fissure; (26) olfactory bulb; (27) superficial cerebral vein.

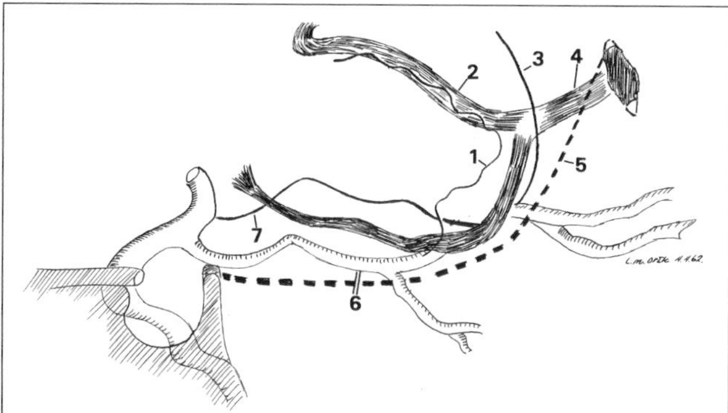

Figure 17.128. Diagram representing the relationship of the posterior cerebral artery and basal vein with tentorial incisura, posterior choroidal arteries, and anterior choroidal artery. (1) Medial posterior choroidal artery; (2) internal cerebral vein; (3) lateral posterior choroidal artery; (4) vein of Galen; (5) tentorial edge; (6) posterior cerebral artery; (7) anterior choroidal artery.

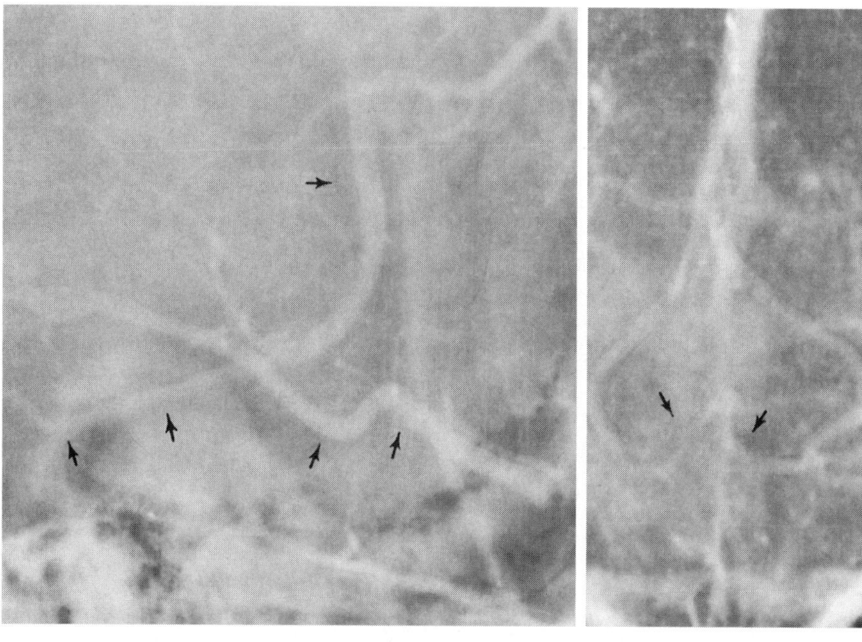

Figure 17.129. Normal venogram lateral view. **A.** The basal vein (lower anterior arrows) shows its typical configuration, with its downward and backward course and then formation of an angle just behind the dorsum sellae. In most instances, the angle is less well marked than the one shown in this case. The figure also illustrates an anomaly of the vein of Galen, which joins the inferior longitudinal sinus very high (upper arrow), flowing into a steep, straight sinus. The vein of Labbé (lower posterior arrows) does not join the lateral sinus, as is the case usually, but extends through a connecting vein to join an eccentrically placed superior longitudinal sinus. **B.** The anteroposterior film demonstrates bilateral filling of the basal veins because cross-compression was done during injection and a slightly greater amount of contrast material was used. The configuration of the basal veins in their anterior portions demonstrates their position around the midbrain. The branches coming from the interpeduncular fossa are clearly demonstrated (arrows). (Compare with appearance shown on diagram in Figure 17.127.)

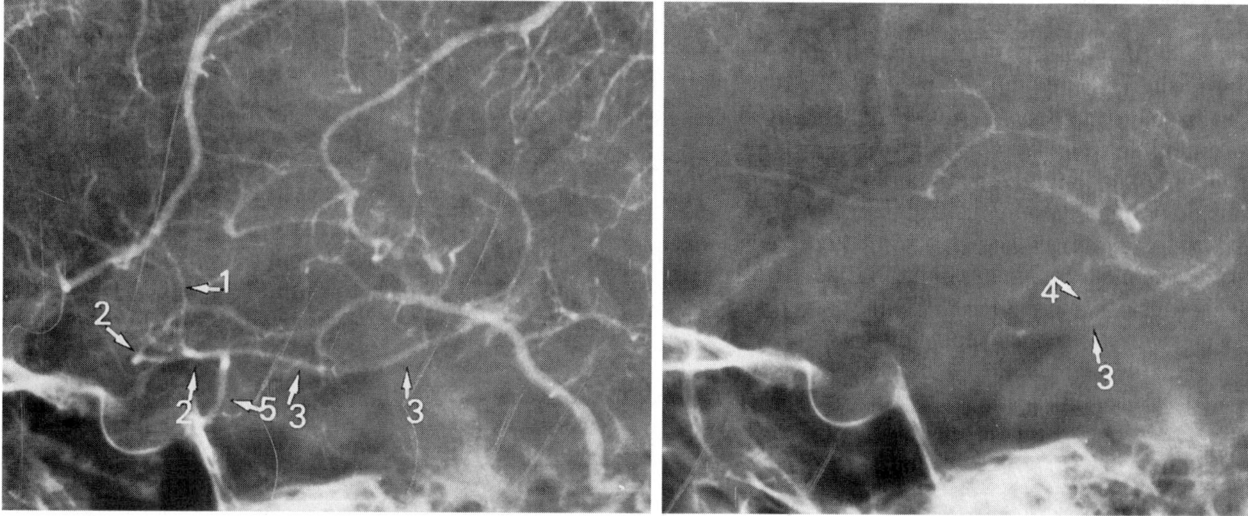

Figure 17.130. Normal venogram to demonstrate sequential filling of the basal vein. The lateral view shows inferior striate veins and the deep middle cerebral vein opacified (**A**), which, in a later phase, emptied, leaving only the posterior part of the basal vein filled (**B**). Arrows: (1) inferior striate veins; (2) deep middle cerebral vein; (3) basal vein; (4) inferior ventricular vein; (5) medial temporal (uncal) vein ending in the cavernous sinus.

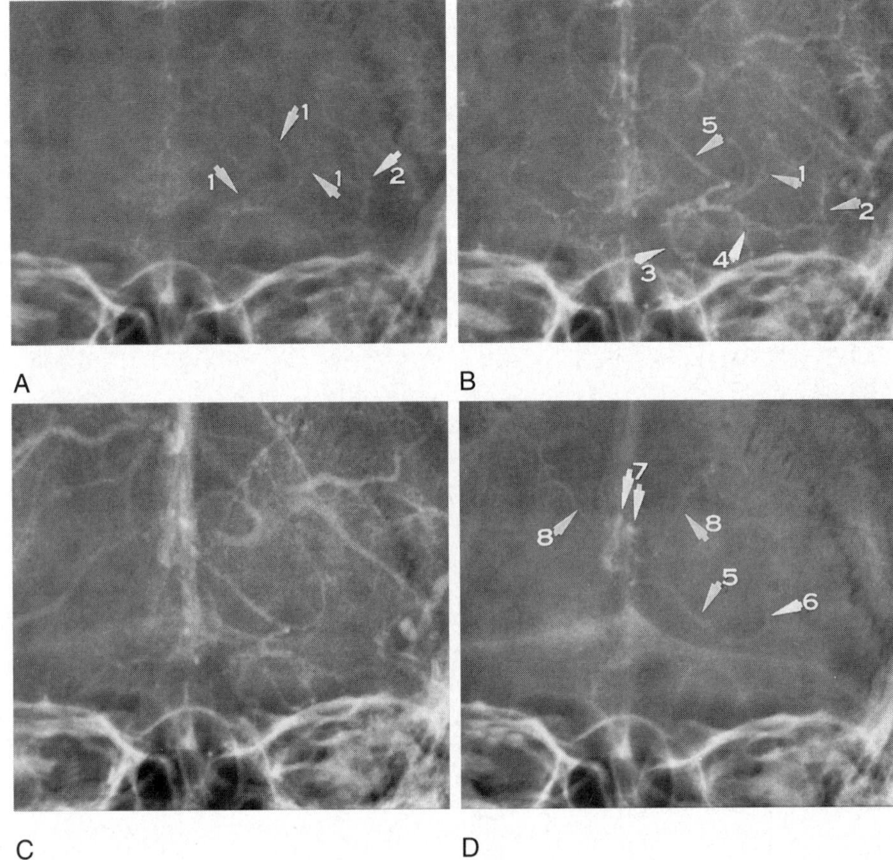

Figure 17.131. Anteroposterior venogram to demonstrate sequence of filling of tributaries of basal vein. **A.** The first film taken in the early venous phase demonstrates inferior striate veins (1) and insular veins (2). **B.** A film taken slightly later demonstrates filling of a medial temporal (uncal) vein (3), the deep middle cerebral vein (4) which receives striate (1) and insular veins (2). The anterior two-thirds of the basal vein is visible (5). The opposite side is now beginning to fill (the injection being made with cross compression). **C.** One second later, the basal vein is well filled; the striate and insular veins are empty, and the deep middle cerebral and medial temporal veins are almost empty. **D.** Two seconds later, the subependymal veins remain filled; only the posterior portion of the basal vein is seen: (5) basal vein; (6) inferior ventricular vein (visible in C also); (7) internal cerebral veins; (8) thalamostriate veins.

The appearance of the internal cerebral vein as seen in the *frontal projection* is that of a short band of increased density near the midline. The length of the vertical band of increased density in the midline produced by the internal cerebral vein varies, depending on the degree of angulation of the x-ray tube used to make the radiograph. The greater the degree of angulation, the longer the internal cerebral vein will appear to be in the frontal projection. The inferior portion of the shadow represents the anterior portion of the vein if there is considerable angulation. If the projection is such that the orbits are high on the film, the vein is either seen endwise or the posterior portion may be lower than the anterior portion. The curves described by the thalamostriate and the basal veins are best shown on a very good angiogram or on a diagram (Figs. 17.116, 17.117, and 17.129). The distance of the upper end of the thalamostriate vein from the midline can be used to estimate ventricular size. Twenty millimeters is considered the upper limit of normal, and the presence of anatomic variants does not vitiate the results (Fig. 17.132). It is also possible to esti-

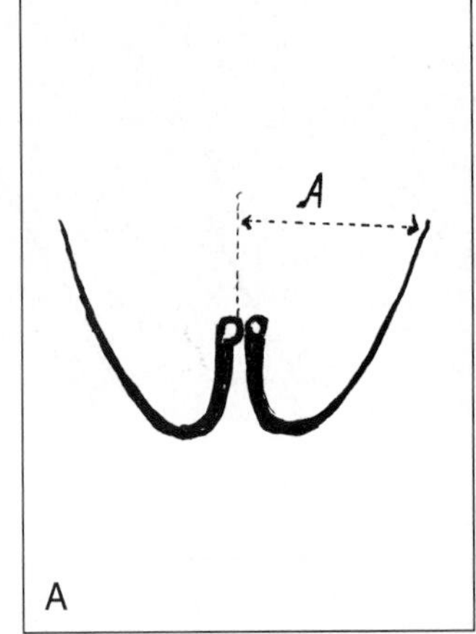

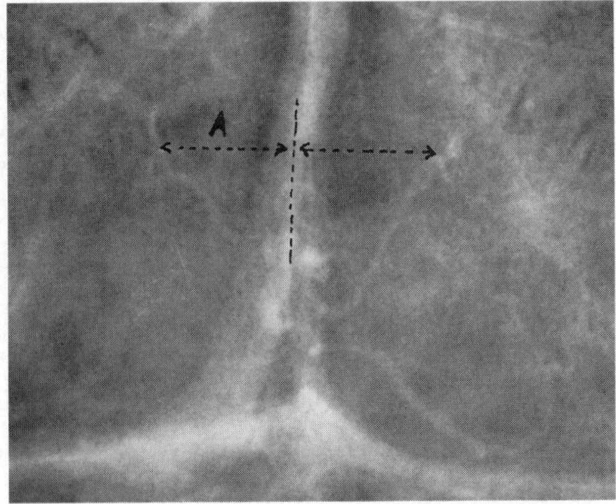

Figure 17.132. Method of estimating ventricular size from the frontal venogram. **A.** The measurement is taken from the midline to the uppermost portion of the veins connected with the thalamostriate veins (lateral subependymal veins). Normal measurements are less than 20 mm. **B.** When there is an anomalous venous angle, the same method can be followed. On the right, the thalamostriate vein follows the floor of the lateral ventricle to join the internal cerebral vein, but measurement A can be obtained as easily on the right as on the left side.

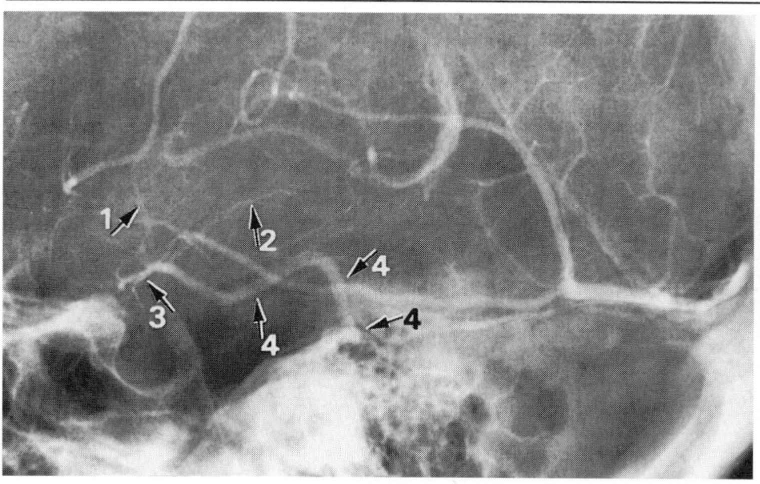

A

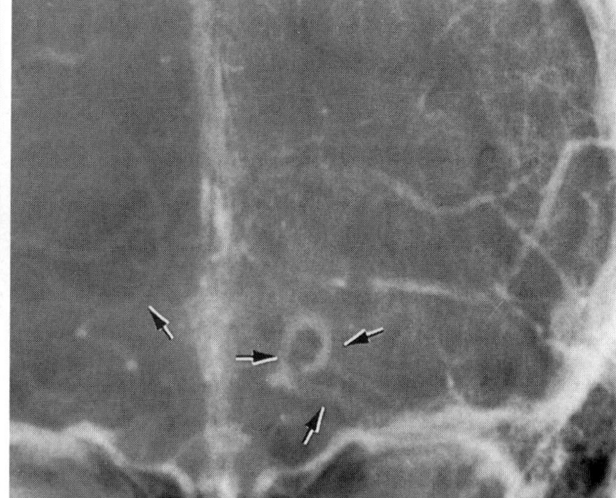

B

Figure 17.133. Variation of basal vein—lateral mesencephalic vein. **A.** The posterior portion of the basal vein does not fill. Its anterior portion receives the usual tributaries: striate (1), insular (2), deep middle cerebral (3). As the vein turns around the midbrain, however, it curves downward and joins the superior petrosal sinus (4). **B.** The appearance is shown in the same patient in a frontal view taken with cross compression. It demonstrates a normal basal vein on the right (arrow) and the lateral mesencephalic variant on the left (arrows).

mate ventricular size in the lateral view. A measurement of 20 mm from the upper margin of the internal cerebral vein to the tips of the visible subependymal veins is close to the upper limits of normal in lateral view, taken without magnification. The curve of the basal veins is again related to the angulation of the tube; the greater the angulation, the longer the sweep. The septal vein is difficult to visualize on most frontal angiograms. In half-axial projection, however, the septal veins are often well shown (Fig. 17.116).

The basal cerebral vein in humans is formed by the fusion of several secondary anastomotic channels derived from primitive veins (174, 175). As a result of this, variations in the filling and configuration of the vessels are common. The variations are due to failure of fusion of the different components of the vein and have been well documented angiographically by Wolf et al. (176). The most frequent variant is drainage of the vein via the lateral mesencephalic vein into the superior petrosal sinus. In these cases the anterior aspect of the basal cerebral vein has its usual configuration, but as the vein turns around the midbrain, it descends in the lateral mesencephalic sulcus via the lateral mesencephalic vein and does not continue backward and upward to join the vein of Galen. In some cases, however, the posterior segment of the basal vein may also be present. The basal vein occasionally may drain into the pontine plexus of veins or into the transverse (lateral) sinus (180). Some variants are illustrated in Figures 17.133 and 17.134.

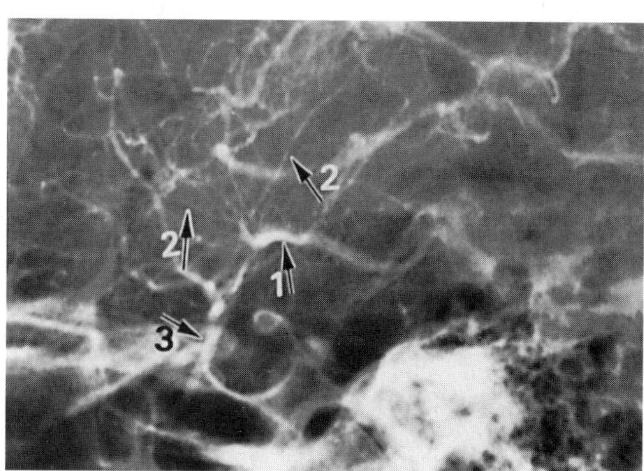

A

B

Figure 17.134. Normal venogram to demonstrate lateral mesencephalic and uncal veins. **A.** The posterior portion of the basal vein is not seen. The tributaries of the basal vein are well shown (arrows 1 and 2). A vein descends toward the sphenoparietal sinus, which is an uncal vein (arrow 3). **B.** In the frontal projection, a lateral mesencephalic vein is shown on both sides. The arrow points to the uncal vein.

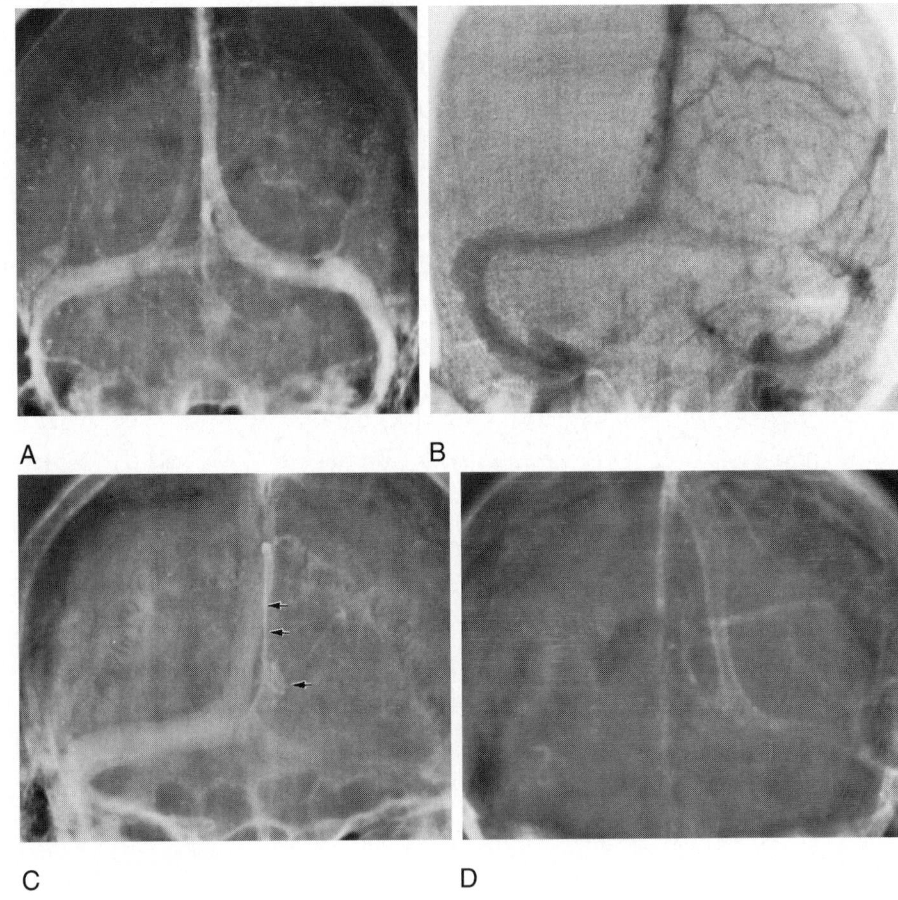

Figure 17.135. Variations of sinuses in region of torcular Herophili. **A.** The superior longitudinal sinus divides into two branches, which are then connected by a transverse component. **B.** The right sinus drains the left hemisphere, which is common, but some drainage occurs also via the left side. **C.** The posterior portion of the superior longitudinal sinus is slightly deviated to the right. There is little filling of the left transverse sinus. The thalamostriate vein is shown joining the internal cerebral vein (lower arrow). The inferior longitudinal sinus outlines the position of the free edge of the falx (two arrows). **D.** An anomaly of the superior longitudinal sinus is demonstrated, which, in its posterior portion, is markedly off center in position. Most often the deviation is to the right, rarely to the left.

DURAL SINUSES

The *superior longitudinal sinus* is seen in a discontinuous manner because only part of the blood draining into the sinus is opacified with contrast substance in unilateral angiography. If it is desired to outline the superior longitudinal sinus more fully, compression of the opposite carotid artery during the injection of a larger amount of contrast substance (12 ml) is usually satisfactory. To examine the superior longitudinal sinus, the lateral projection is essential; also, a half-axial projection (taken with slight rotation of the head toward one side to prevent superimposition of the anterior on the posterior aspects of the sinus) is important.

The *lateral sinuses* are often quite well shown on the anteroposterior projection. One sinus (the right) is usually larger than the other, and sometimes practically all the contrast substance drains through one side. It should be kept in mind that "streaming" or "laminar flow" is the rule in the superior longitudinal and lateral sinuses so that it is possible, if only one side is injected, that the contrast substance would turn toward the lateral sinus on the same side, unless this sinus is much smaller than the opposite one. Drainage of contrast substance through the lateral sinus on the side of the injection, therefore, does not mean that the opposite side is hypoplastic or obstructed.

The posterior portion of the superior longitudinal sinus is often situated off center, even in perfectly aligned anteroposterior films, almost always to the right (Fig. 17.135). This is a normal variant. Sometimes it is placed far laterally; instances are known in which it was so laterally situated that upon placing a burr hole for ventriculography that the outer sinus wall was pierced, with resultant fatal bleeding. In these extreme cases, the sinus is lateral to the attachment of the falx.

The *inferior longitudinal sinus* is not always shown in angiograms (Figs. 17.120 and 17.121). On the other hand, the *straight sinus* (which receives the vein of Galen) is shown in almost all cases, although opacification may be very faint. The vein of Galen usually joins the straight sinus at the junction of the falx and tentorium, but sometimes they may join higher along the posterior part of the falx, or at least it would so appear in some angiograms (Fig. 17.129). The height of the tentorium also is variable; at times, the straight sinus is bifid, extending around a defect in the tentorium.

The *sphenoparietal* sinus, which runs on the inferior aspect of the sphenoid ridge (Fig. 17.136), is often shown on the angiogram. Sometimes a slight area of increased density can be seen adjacent to the sella turcica; this is produced by the *cavernous sinus.* The *petrosal sinuses* (*superior* and *inferior*) are shown fairly frequently. The inferior petrosal si-

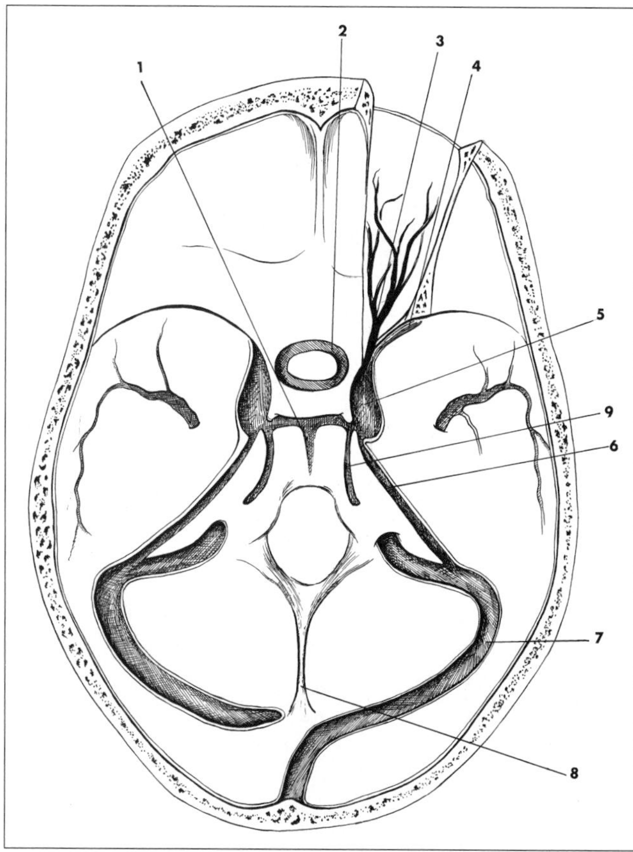

nuses are seen just behind the dorsum sella and cannot be distinguished from portions of the basilar plexus (Fig. 17.137). The torcular Herophili is usually seen at the inferior portion of the superior longitudinal sinus where this joins the straight sinus. Its anterior aspect often presents a rounded configuration (Fig. 17.137). Variations of the confluence of the sinuses are frequent (Fig. 17.135). From this point the lateral sinuses arise and are often seen in the lateral projection as a band of increased density (Fig. 17.137). The lateral sinus may be equal on both sides, but in the majority of cases the right sinus is larger; occasionally the left lateral sinus is absent (Fig. 17.135). The various sinuses join and form the internal jugular veins, which are often visualized on the films in the later phases of the serialogram. The jugular vein is usually wider than the internal carotid artery.

Excellent visualization of the internal jugular vein and its tributaries may be obtained by means of jugular venography. The petrosal sinuses can be injected by advancing a catheter cephalad in the jugular vein. Reflux into the cavernous sinuses and ophthalmic veins, as well as into the lateral sinuses, is usually obtained (Fig. 17.138).

Figure 17.136. Diagram of dural sinuses. (1) Basilar plexus; (2) circular sinus; (3) superior ophthalmic vein; (4) sphenoparietal sinus; (5) cavernous sinus; (6) superior petrosal sinus; (7) transverse sinus; (8) occipital sinus; (9) inferior petrosal sinus.

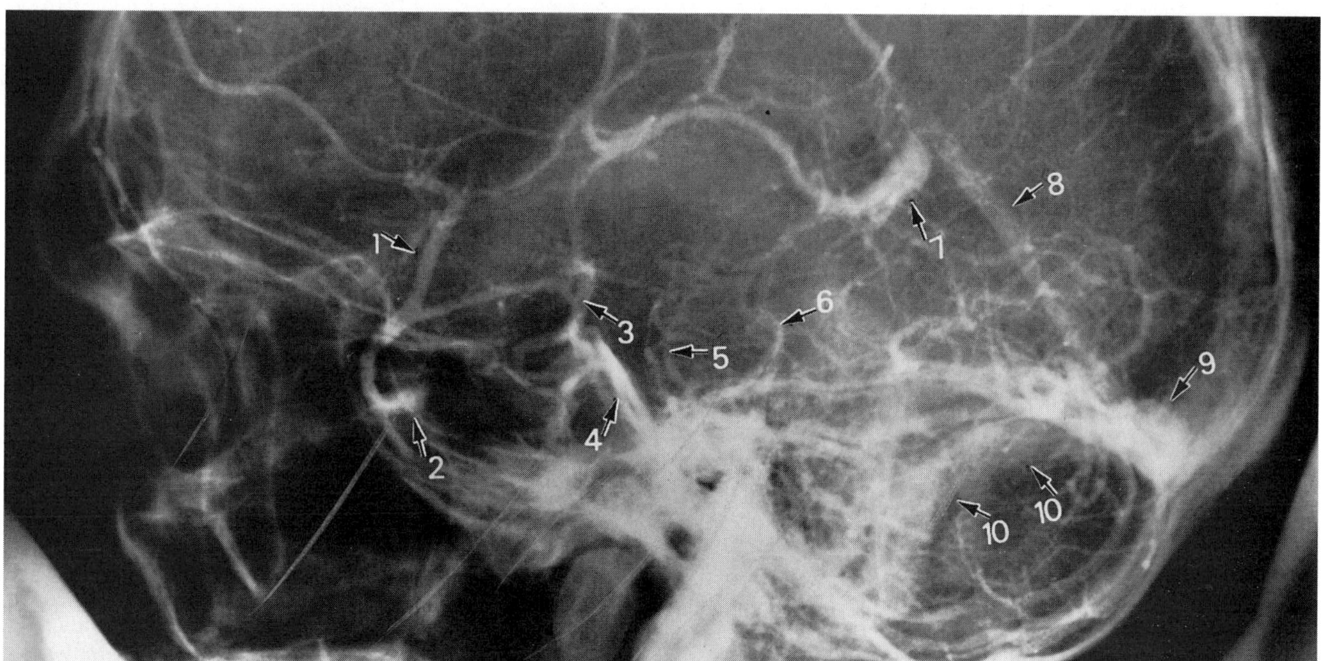

Figure 17.137. Normal venous phase of the right brachial angiogram. (1) Superficial middle cerebral vein draining into (2) sphenoparietal sinus; (3) uncal (medial temporal) vein draining into cavernous sinus; (4) inferior petrosal sinus; (5) anterior pontomesencephalic veins; (6) lateral anastomotic mesencephalic vein; (7) vein of Galen; (8) straight sinus; (9) torcular Herophili; (10) lateral sinus. The superior longitudinal sinus is seen throughout its course.

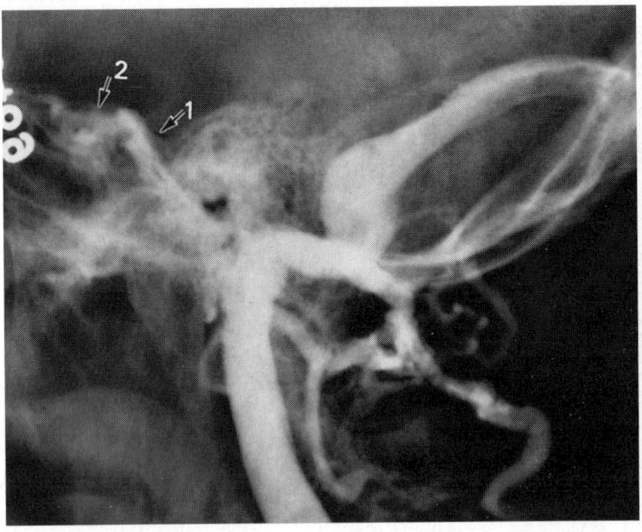

A

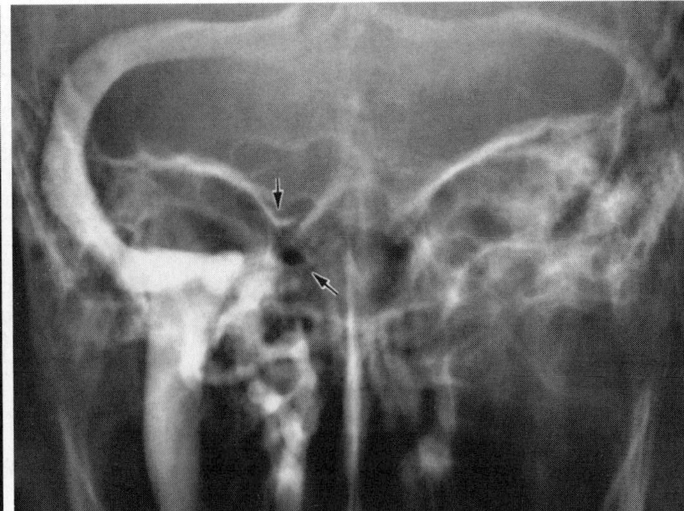

B

Figure 17.138. Normal jugular venogram with filling of intracranial sinuses. **A.** The lateral view demonstrates filling of the jugular vein and lateral sinus with regurgitation through emissary channels into the deep cervical veins. The inferior petrosal sinus (1) and cavernous sinus (2) are filled. **B.** In the anteroposterior view, the filling of the cavernous sinus is not well shown. The radiolucency caused by the internal carotid artery is demonstrated (arrows). **C.** The base view shows the inferior petrosal sinus (1) and cavernous sinus (2) clearly with the internal carotid artery contained within the latter. The posterior aspect of the cavernous sinus is normally more medial than the anterior part, but the appearance is exaggerated in this case. There is some lateral displacement of the anterior portion of the cavernous sinus owing to a pituitary adenoma.

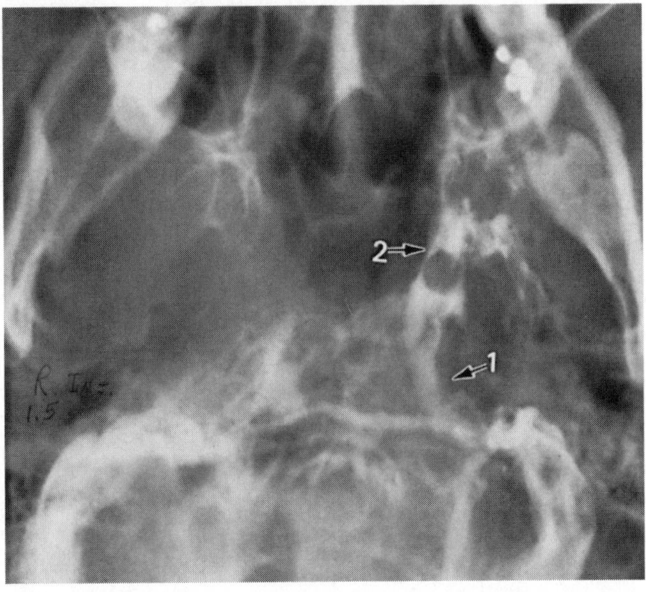

C

VEINS OF POSTERIOR FOSSA

Huang and Wolf (177) have divided these veins into three groups based partly on location and partly on direction of drainage:

1. A *superior group* that drains upward or deeply into the galenic system.
2. An *anterior group* that drains forward into the petrosal sinuses.
3. A *posterior group* that drains backward or laterally into the torcular Herophili or the neighboring straight and lateral sinuses.

Superiorly Draining Group

The first division includes the following vessels:

1. The *posterior mesencephalic vein* may be identical to the posterior part of the basal vein of Rosenthal or may run parallel to it in the perimesencephalic space. The two veins are usually indistinguishable unless they have a different configuration in vertebral as compared with carotid angiography or unless they are multiple (Fig. 17.139). The word *posterior* denotes only that venous drainage is in that direction.
2. The *precentral cerebellar vein* is a most important structure from the angiographic point of view (178). It first runs between the central lobule and the lingula of the cerebellum and roughly parallels the anterior medullary velum of the fourth ventricle. The vein arises deep within the precentral fissure, often from two "brachial" veins, and courses upward and slightly forward until it reaches the lower portion of the quadrigeminal or collicular plate. At this point it bends backward and continues upward to join the vein of Galen (Fig. 17.114). The bend has been termed by Huang and Wolf the *colliculocentral point.* The most rostral extension of the curve is an important landmark both for identification of the vein and for measurement to determine if it lies in normal position (Figs. 17.139 and 17.140). The precentral vein is a single midline vessel, but its two chief tributaries may not unite until they almost reach the level of the vein of Galen.

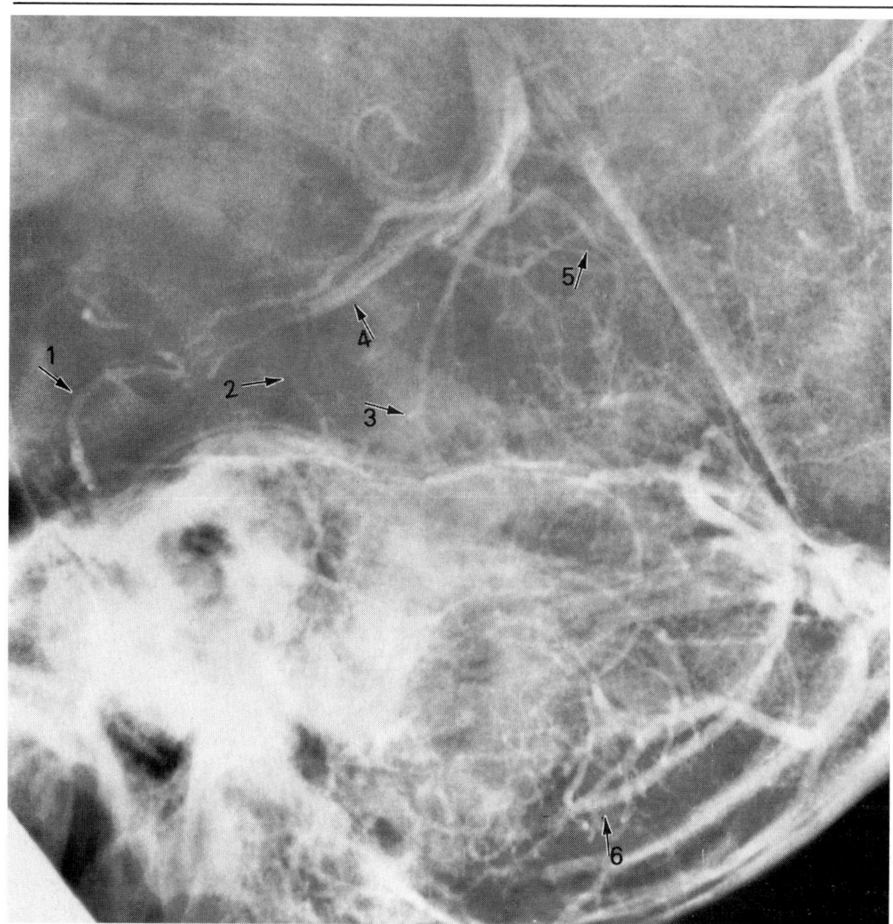

Figure 17.139. Posterior mesencephalic vein and other veins of vertebral system as seen in the lateral view. The arrows are numbered as follows: (1) anterior pontomesencephalic vein; (2) lateral mesencephalic vein; (3) precentral cerebellar vein; (4) posterior mesencephalic vein (actually three veins are seen in this particular angiogram, and it is probable that some of these represent portions of the basal vein—see text); (5) superior vermian vein; and (6) inferior vermian vein. The anterior pontomesencephalic venous system is well shown anteriorly.

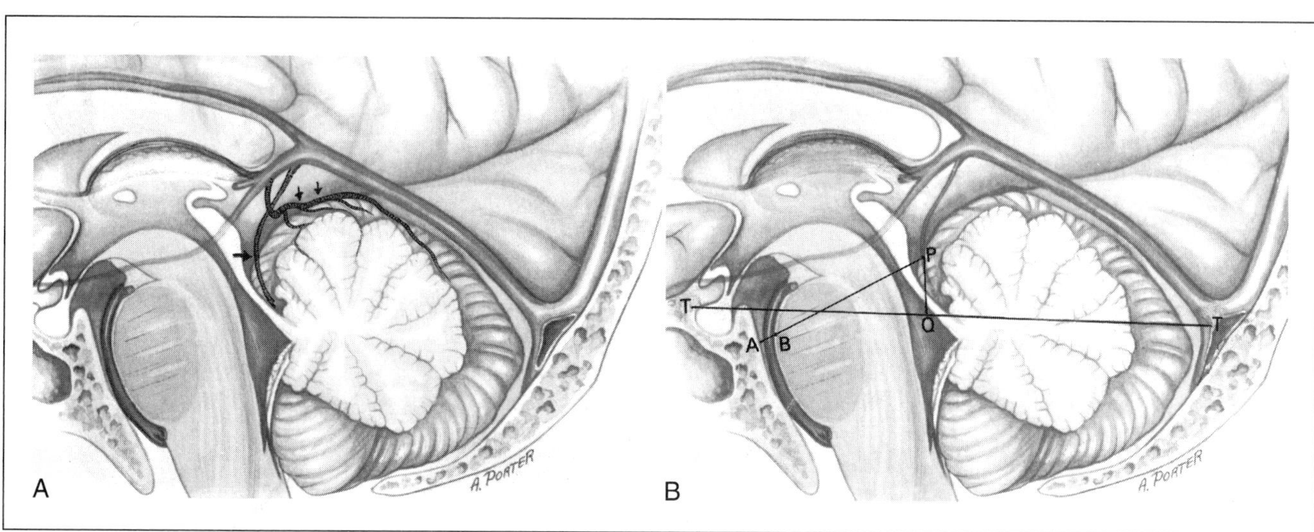

Figure 17.140. Precentral cerebellar vein. **A.** The diagram shows the normal position of the precentral cerebellar vein (arrow) and points of reference. It also demonstrates the relationship of the precentral cerebellar vein to the superior vermian vein (double arrow). **B.** Measurements of the colliculocentral point of the precentral cerebellar vein (according to Huang and Wolf [177].

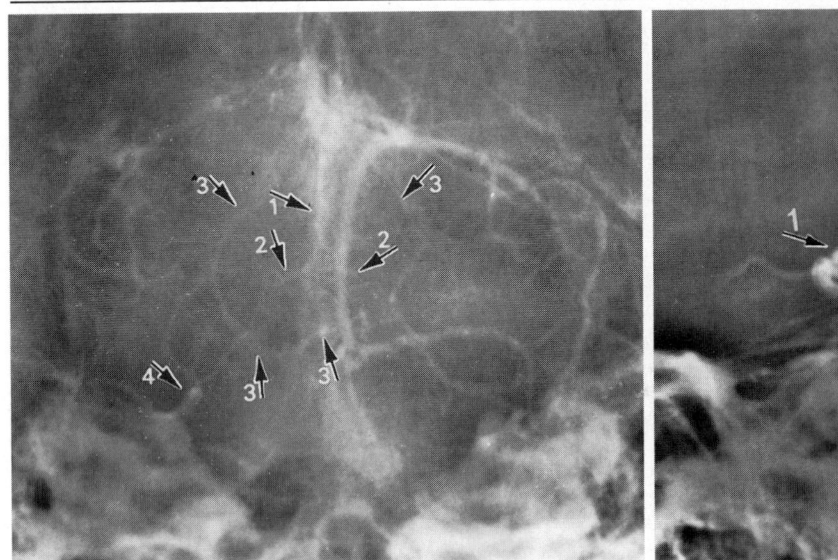

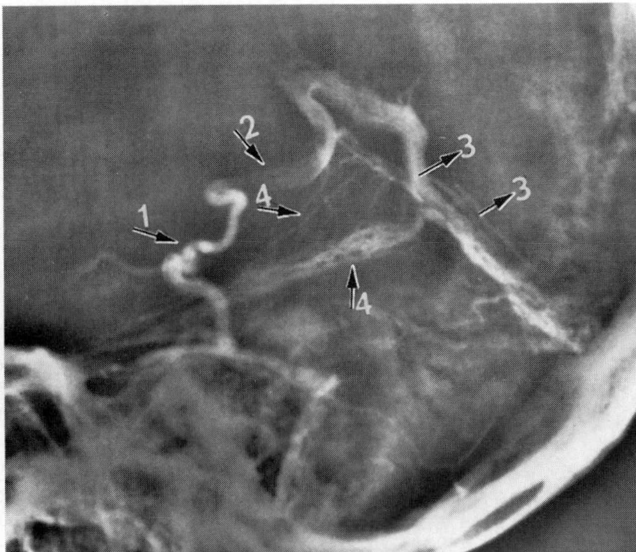

A B

Figure 17.141. A. Normal vertebral angiogram, venous phase, frontal projection. Arrows denote (1) precentral cerebellar vein; (2) brachial tributaries of the precentral cerebellar vein (both the precentral vein and its tributaries are quite faint in most instances, certainly much smaller than the inferior vermian vein); (3) posterior mesencephalic veins or basal veins on both sides outlining the peduncles and the interpeduncular fossa; and (4) petrosal vein. **B.** Enlarged lateral anastomotic mesencephalic vein in a patient with dural venous sinus thrombosis. Arrows identify (1) enlarged lateral anastomotic mesencephalic vein, ending in superior petrosal sinus; (2) posterior mesencephalic (or basal) vein; (3) partially recannalized straight sinus; (4) enlarged venous channels running on the surface of the tentorium. The filling was obtained by injection of the jugular vein in a retrograde fashion.

Sometimes the vein may end in the posterior part of the internal cerebral vein on one or both sides. Because the precentral cerebellar vein is thin, it is not easily demonstrated in the frontal projection. This is particularly true when the inferior vermian veins are prominent. The precentral cerebellar vein may be confused with a paracentral vein, which has a rather similar position, but it is not in the midline. The latter can be recognized in the lateral view because it is straight and lacks the bend at the colliculocentral point; in the frontal projection it does not reach the midline until it joins the vein of Galen (Fig. 17.141). The precentral cerebellar vein is not always identifiable on vertebral angiograms; however, it can be seen in approximately 75 percent of the cases. The normal position of the precentral vein is shown in the diagram in Figure 17.140, together with the method suggested by Huang et al. to determine its position (166). The measurements have been found very useful by the present author.

3. The third vein of the group is the *superior vermian vein*, which drains the upper vermis and other adjacent parts of the cerebellum and ends superiorly in the vein of Galen (Figs. 17.139 and 17.140). It may join the precentral vein before reaching its usual termination and it may be more conspicuous than the precentral vein. It usually has a double curve (convex upward, then downward, as it extends forward) and enters the vein of Galen rostral to the precentral vein, so that it can be differentiated from the latter without difficulty, in the average case.
4. Another important vein in this group is the *lateral mesencephalic vein*, which runs in the sulcus between the peduncle and the tegmentum of the midbrain and ends either in the basal vein or in the posterior mesencephalic vein. It is of variable size and may become a prominent anastomotic pathway between the basal vein and the petrosal vein (Figs. 17.139 and 141). In some instances the posterior portion of the basal vein is absent and its anterior tributaries drain via this *lateral anastomotic mesencephalic vein* into the petrosal vein (176) (Fig. 17.141B). In other cases, it is obvious from the relative sizes of the posterior portion of the basal vein compared with the lateral anastomotic mesencephalic vein that the main direction of blood flow is via the lateral mesencephalic vein even though the posterior portion of the basal vein is patent.

It should be reemphasized that the posterior mesencephalic vein that is seen almost constantly on vertebral angiograms may well be the same structure as the posterior portion of the basal vein of Rosenthal, for they are indistinguishable. However, in some instances there appear to be two or more veins in the same area (Fig. 17.139). Many times this phenomenon may be due to superimposition of

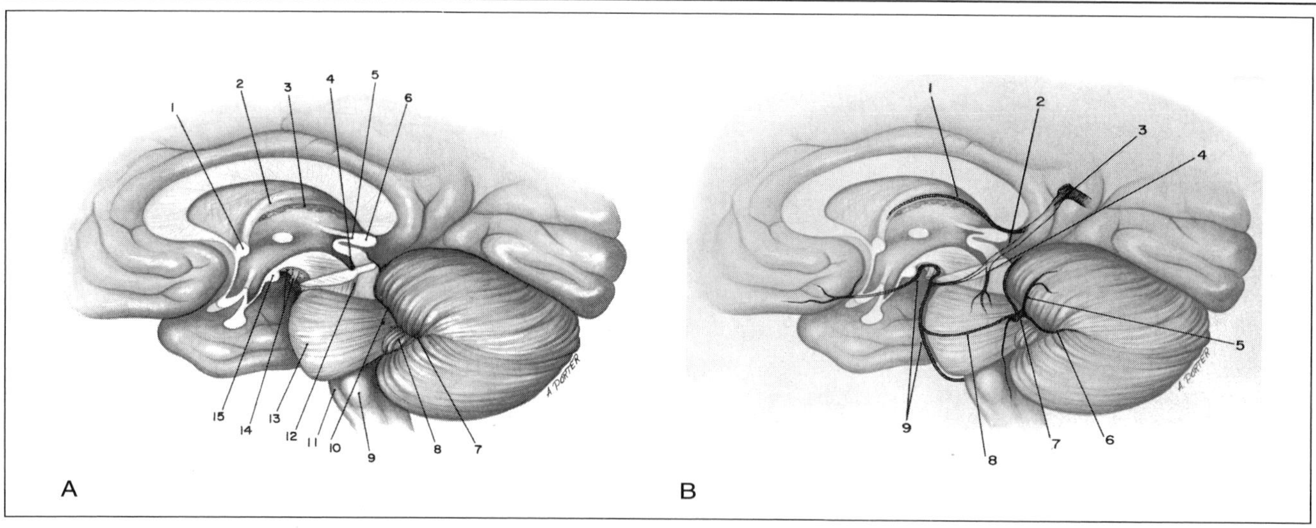

Figure 17.142. A. Posterior fossa structures in the midbrain region. Numbers indicate (1) anterior commissure; (2) fornix; (3) choroid plexus; (4) aqueduct of Sylvius; (5) pineal recess; (6) pineal body; (7) great horizontal fissure of the cerebellum; (8) flocculus; (9) olive of medulla; (10) middle cerebellar peduncle (brachium pontis); (11) pyramid; (12) lateral mesencephalic sulcus; (13) pons; (14) third cranial nerve, interpeduncular fossa, and posterior perforated substance; and (15) mammillary tubercule. **B.** Veins of lateral and anterior aspects of posterior fossa. Numbers identify (1) internal cerebral vein; (2) basal vein; (3) vein of Galen; (4) lateral mesencephalic vein; (5) cerebellar tributary of petrosal vein; (6) vein running in the great horizontal fissure of the cerebellum; (7) petrosal vein; (8) transverse pontine vein; and (9) anterior pontomesencephalic venous system demonstrating its three segments: the anterior, the interpeduncular, and the prepontine segment.

the two sides, and without stereoscopic films it is not possible to be certain of the anatomy. In cases of venous sinus thrombosis the anastomotic venous channels can become very prominent (Fig. 17.141).

Anteriorly Draining Group

The second division of veins is the *anterior* or *petrosal group* (178). The *petrosal vein* is one of the major collecting venous trunks in the posterior fossa. Several tributaries converge to the petrosal vein from the anterior surface of the medulla and pons, and from the upper and lower anterior cerebellum. The vein runs a short course in the cerebellopontine angle cistern and empties into the superior petrosal sinus. It is often displaced by tumor of the area, especially acoustic neurinomas, and compressed by these and other tumors.

The most important group of tributaries of the petrosal vein is the *anterior pontomesencephalic "vein,"* which most commonly is a group of veins or network of veinlets in front of the upper brainstem; occasionally, it is found as a single vein. When viewed from the lateral aspect, the network outlines the interpeduncular fossa and pons. Huang et al. divided the vein into three parts (178). The "first segment" arises in the region of the anterior perforated substance, in the same area where some of the tributaries of the basal vein of Rosenthal originate. It then runs backward below the optic tract to reach the interpeduncular fossa. The "second segment" is in the interpeduncular fossa, the deepest aspect of which is rather well demarcated by the veins. The "third segment" outlines the anterior aspect of the pons, assuming the shape of the belly of the pons (Figs. 17.139 and 17.142). The most important parts are "segments 2 and 3," for they outline with fairly consistent accuracy the interpeduncular fossa and the anterior border of the pons. The basilar artery is not an accurate marker for the ventral margin of the pons because it is not always midline and is not closely attached to the pons except by the short pontine branches that arise from it. In vertebral angiography only "segments 2 and 3" ordinarily fill (Fig. 17.143). The pontomesencephalic vein may drain directly into the inferior petrosal sinus; sometimes, there is a direct connection between the pontine veins and the basilar plexus situated behind the clivus.

In addition to the anterior pontomesencephalic vein there are the other tributaries of the petrosal vein mentioned earlier, but these are rarely useful in diagnosis. Some are difficult to identify with certainty. This is true for the brachial veins stemming from the lateral aspects of the precentral cerebellar fissure and for the vein of the lateral recess of the fourth ventricle, as well as several others, as described by Huang et al. (166). Undoubtedly, with stereoscopic subtraction views it is possible to determine the relationship of these veins to the various neural structures. This can be done successfully if one keeps in mind that, with few exceptions, all of these veins are on the surface of either the pons, the medulla, or the cerebellum (or in anatomically

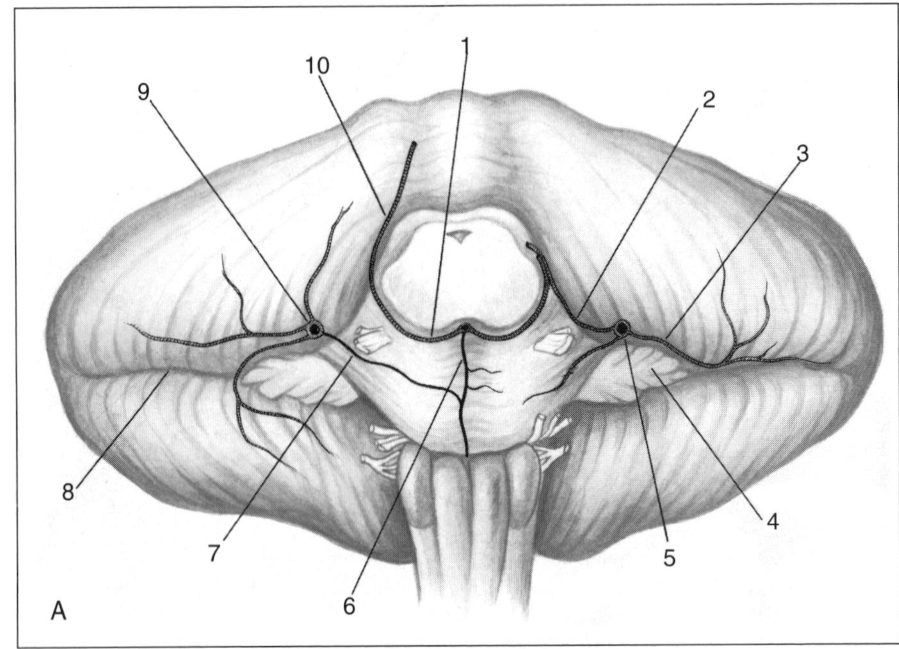

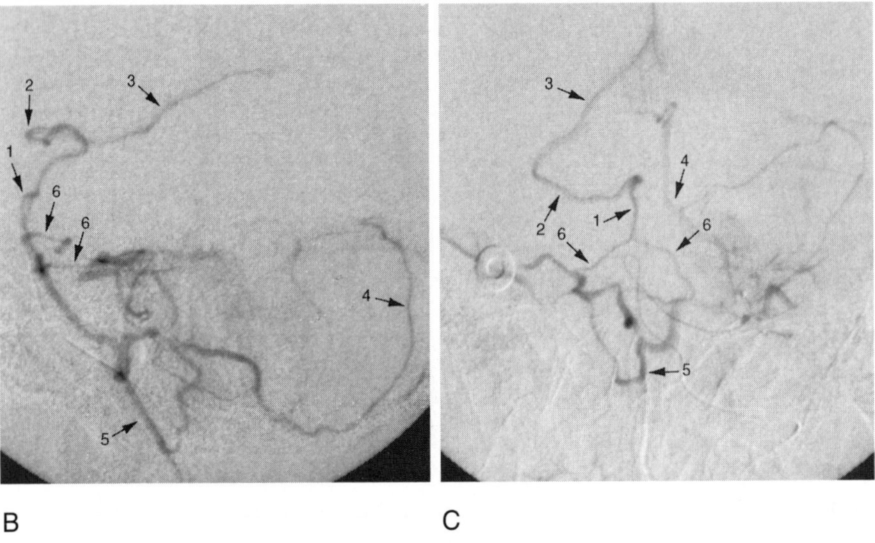

Figure 17.143. A. Anterior and lateral veins of posterior fossa. Numbers indicate (1) peripeduncular portion of basal vein (or posterior mesencephalic vein); (2) lateral mesencephalic vein; (3) lateral tributary of the petrosal vein, receiving vein from the cerebellar hemisphere, and a vein running along the great horizontal fissure; (4) flocculus; (5) petrosal vein; (6) pontine segment of anterior pontomesencephalic vein; (7) transverse pontine vein; (8) great horizontal fissure; (9) petrosal vein receiving various tributaries; and (10) posterior mesencephalic or basal vein. **B** and **C.** Venous phase after superselective injection of the anterior inferior cerebellar artery in a patient who had a small arteriovenous malformation in the left side of the cerebellum. **B.** Lateral view. The arrows show (1) anterior pontomesencephalic vein; (2) peripeduncular portion of the basal vein; (3) basal vein; (4) inferior vermian vein; (5) anterior medullary veins; (6) transverse pontine veins. **C.** Frontal view. The numbered arrows are the same as B.

defined fissures) rather than in the depths or parenchyma of these structures (Figs. 17.142 and 17.143).

Posteriorly Draining Group

The third group comprises those veins that empty posteriorly or laterally into the torcular Herophili or neighboring straight sinus or into the lateral sinuses. These include the *inferior vermian* veins, which are usually paired and run on each side of the vermis. In the frontal (half-axial) projection they are very prominent in many instances, and they tend to obscure the precentral cerebellar vein (Figs. 17.141 and 17.145). In general, the inferior vermian veins serve as markers for the midline of the cerebellum, although they are actually paramedian in location. In this role they are useful in diagnosing posterior fossa tumors because they are dislocated along with any displacement of the vermis. The inferior vermian vein receives on each side tributaries from the posterior inferior aspect of the cerebellar hemisphere. It ends superiorly in the posterior portion of the straight sinus or in the proximal segment of the lateral sinus. Before emptying into the sinus, the inferior vermian vein may receive tributaries from the superior one-half of the vermis, especially the declival portion (Fig. 17.144).

The point where the tonsillar tributaries—superior and inferior—join to form the inferior vermian vein has been called the *copular point* (conjunction). This point can be recognized with ease in some cases but not in all. It is helpful when the superior retrotonsillar vein makes a distinct curve concave upward at the lower portion of the pyramid. In establishing the normal position of the point, Huang et al. traced a line from the basion to the torcular. The copular point usually falls within a circle of 6-mm radius centered

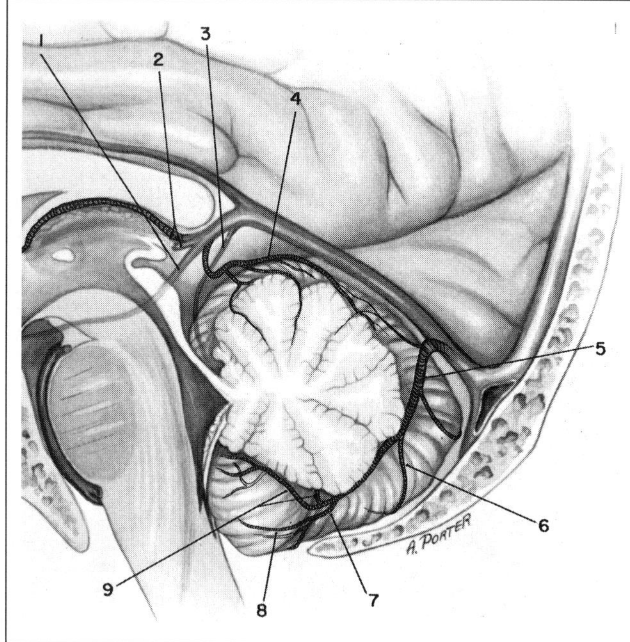

A

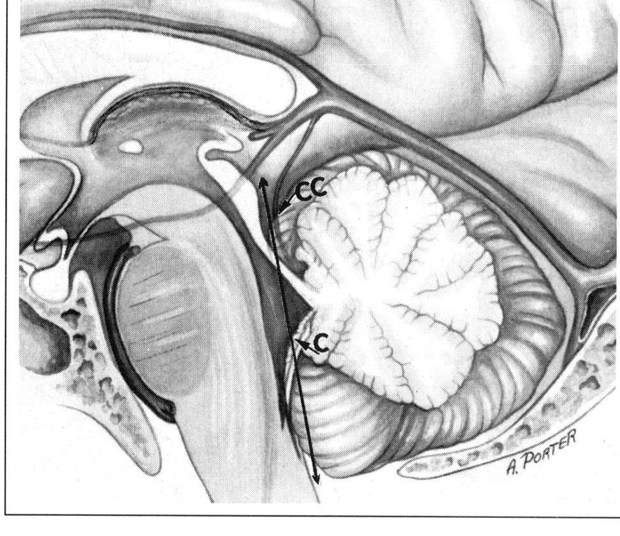

B

Figure 17.144. A. Superior and inferior vermian veins and their relation to cerebellum and sinuses. The veins numbered are (1) basal vein; (2) internal cerebral veins; (3) precentral cerebellar vein; (4) superior vermian vein and tributaries; (5) inferior vermian vein receiving a tributary from the upper vermis; (6) hemispheric tributaries of inferior vermian vein; (7) region of the copular point; (8) inferior retrotonsillar veins; and (9) superior retrotonsillar and medial tonsillar veins. **B.** Division of posterior fossa into anterior and posterior compartments by a plane represented by line C–C–C (double-headed arrow) passing through fourth ventricle. The term *C–C–C line* is derived from the choroid point of the posterior inferior cerebellar artery and the colliculocentral point of the precentral cerebellar vein.

at a point 4 mm below the basion-torcular or clivus-torcular line and 4 mm behind the midpoint of the line (Fig. 17.144). In only 3 cases out of the 50 studied did the copular point fall outside this circle. It appears, then, that with knowledge of the anatomy of this area it is possible to have another parameter for evaluation of the position of the retrotonsillar area and the inferior part of the fourth ventricle. This is particularly true if stereoscopic pairs are used to identify the origin of the inferior vermian vein in the lateral view.

In the frontal projection the inferior vermian veins can be seen to receive tonsillar tributaries that are usually more lateral than the vermian veins. They may be recognized as they curve inward to join the inferior vermian vein or, often, the inferior retrotonsillar vein. Corresponding medial tonsillar veins extend laterally. Unfortunately the relationships are not constant; the tonsillar branches may pass straight downward or upward to join the vermian vein or one of its tributaries (Fig. 17.145). Inferior hemispheric veins, the suprapyramidal vessels, and other tributaries join the inferior vermian vein more distally.

Other veins in the posteriorly draining group include the superior hemispheric veins and declival veins. If the correct position of these veins is identified, they can be useful in a given case in evaluating a mass in the posterior compartment of the posterior fossa. The inferior vermian vein is always approximately 1 cm away from the inner table of the occipital bone, whereas the hemispheric cerebellar veins extend to the inner table.

Physiology of Posterior Fossa Circulation

Greitz studied the circulation times in vertebral angiograms and found them to be comparable to those encountered in the carotid system (179). The *circulation time* (or arteriovenous circulation time) was measured from the time of maximal filling of the basilar artery to maximal filling of the local veins, as seen in half-axial projection. The veins used in the study were the cerebellar hemispheric veins and the petrosal veins. The circulation in the territory of the posterior cerebral arteries (supratentorial) was also evaluated. In the intermediate (capillary) phase there is uniform "staining" of the posterior fossa.

Greitz found that the mean value for the circulation time was between 3.5 and 3.7 sec. On the average it was slightly longer on the injected side than on the noninjected side—which is difficult to explain. The occipital circulation time was essentially the same as that in the infratentorial region. He found good correlation between the circulation times and regional blood flow measurements of the posterior fossa using the xenon washout technique, in a manner similar to that employed in carotid angiography (180).

With infratentorial tumors, the circulation was slower on the side of the tumor than on the other side in some

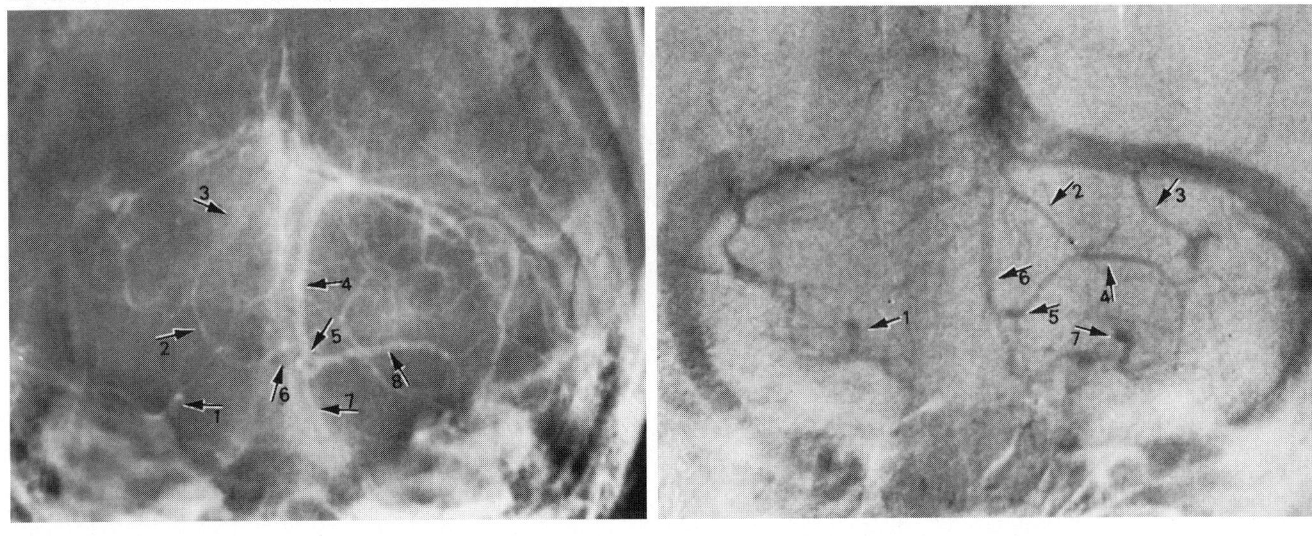

A B

Figure 17.145. Normal vertebral angiogram, venous phase, frontal projection. **A.** The veins are numbered as follows: (1) petrosal vein; (2) peripeduncular portion of the basal vein; (3) basal vein (or posterior mesencephalic vein); (4) inferior vermian vein; (5) copular point of inferior vermian vein; (6) interpeduncular portion of anterior pontomesencephalic vein; (7) inferior retrotonsillar vein; and (8) inferior hemispheric vein coming from the region of the biventral lobule of the cerebellum. **B.** The numbered arrows are (1) petrosal veins on both sides; (2) superior hemispheric vein; (3) hemispheric vein ending in the lateral sinus; (4) inferior hemispheric vein in the region of the biventral lobule; (5) copular point; and (6) inferior vermian vein.

cases. Lengthening of the overall circulation time (more than 1 sec over the mean) was more common. Greitz observed an obvious trend for the circulation to be faster in the occipital region supplied by the vertebral artery than in the infratentorial region, in cases of infratentorial tumors; this gave the posterior fossa an "empty" appearance in the early venous phase when only the occipital veins were filled (12 of 35 cases). See Chapter 10 for further details on cerebral circulation physiology.

NONCEREBRAL CRANIOFACIAL ANGIOGRAPHY

The face, skull, and neck are supplied primarily by the external carotid artery, with contributions from the vertebral artery and cervical branches of the subclavian. The indications for external carotid angiography include (*a*) presumed or suspected hypervascular cranial-vault-facial or base of the skull lesions (meningiomas, glomus jugulare, nasopharyngeal angiofibromas, metastatic tumors, arteriovenous malformations, and carotid-cavernous fistulas); (*b*) suspected arteritic process involving the branches of the external carotid artery; (*c*) prior to revascularization procedures such as mca-eca bypass; and (*d*) extensive head and neck tumors before surgical intervention. External carotid angiography is also indicated in the study of arteriovenous malformations of the head, particularly dural arteriovenous malformations, usually supplied primarily by branches of the external carotid artery.

Along with the cervical branches off the subclavian and vertebral arteries, the external carotid artery feeds the face and neck. These branches have extensive anastomoses with each other as well as with the intracranial and intraspinal blood supply. Intimate and facile knowledge of the external carotid circulation is essential for those involved in the practice of intervention in this area. Students of the external carotid artery are advised to study Lasjounias and Berenstein (122).

Organizing Principles of the Extended Carotid Artery

The lack of an exegesis on blood vessel organizational principles has not deterred the author from offering some principles that he finds helpful. What we see angiographically is the dynamic balance of present needs and possibilities working with past solutions. Six principles are offered: (*a*) minimal work; (*b*) functional grouping; (*c*) anatomy chases physiology; (*d*) everything is connected to everything; (*e*) historical dominion; and (*f*) phenotypic variation. If these principles are present, they emerge from cellular mechanisms.

The concept of *minimal work* is overriding in life. Arteries minimize the work associated with carrying blood. Since the work of perfusion is related to an inverse of the radius to the fourth power, a single, ever-so-slightly larger conduit vessel is favored over two slightly smaller vessels. This factor favors the growth of one territory at the expense of its neighbors. Growth, regression, and annexation are in balance. In a situation where one vessel has grown to take over a territory from its neighbor, it will do so at the cost of the neighbor's size. The least work factor also explains why a bifurcation of a large blood vessel at equal angles bifurcates at a small angle (ca. 25°) and a small vessel comes off at a steeper angle (90°).

As in the brain, a Shellshear rule of sorts also holds: "end artery" distributions are constant, while conduit vessel distributions vary; and a single vessel supplies a single functional group (121). Conduit vessels collect a number these functional groups. The functional groups consist of tissues of the same type that perform one task, such as muscle, nerve, bone, gland, or subcutaneous tissue. *Supplies to these functional groups are quite constant.* The course of the arteries is usually associated with the nerves and enters the muscles with them at the motor point. There is tremendous variation in the conduit vessels.

As John Hunter has pointed out, blood vessels grow to living tissue: *anatomy chases physiology*, form follows function. Tissue resilience is the reason all ablative methods of treatment such as embolization, surgery, and radiosurgery can work. The pathologic tissue is hurt more than the normal tissue. Understanding the range of physiologic stress that a given tissue can take and still remain viable is at the center of successful results. The external carotid embolizations offer a window to this very dynamic process and constant observation of the tissues that have been embolized over the hours. This is a dynamic process, and the postoperative care is critical. Ambrose Paré, the barber-surgeon, understood this gift when he stated, "We dress the wounds. God heals the patient."

Everything is connected to everything else, at almost every level. Given enough time and enough need in a young enough tissue, these connections can become massive. These collateral anastomsoses can often be counted on to avoid ischemia from vessel occlusion—but often not. They can be helpful in controlling embolization, but blood vessels are derived from a network, then an arcade, and finally are conduit systems. A tremendous amount of congenital variation is present.

The *historical dominion* of blood vessel organization is clear. The variations that are seen can be seen in "caricature" in other animals and during different stages of development.

The tissues of the head and neck are organized into layers (Fig. 17.146). The named blood vessels of the extracranial circulation (occipital, facial, etc.) can be thought of as primary conduits to a territory of one of the layers. It is from this primary function that the name is often given.

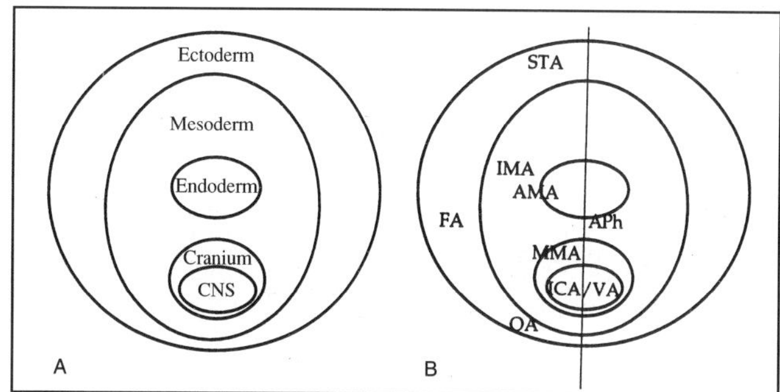

Figure 17.146. A. A useful but violent simplification is that the blood vessels feed a dominant tissue type. Vessels that are in the cutaneous ectoderm, the superficial temporal artery (STA), the facial artery (FA), the transverse facial (TFA) and the occipital artery (OA) have in their subcutaneous course a very tortuous appearance. **B.** The mesoderm is fed by branches of the internal maxillary artery (IMA); the endoderm by the ascending pharyngeal (APh) and accessory meningeal (AmA); the pericranium by the middle meningeal (stapedial system); the neuroectoderm by the internal carotid and the vertebral system.

ANASTOMOSIS

Anastomoses exist at boundaries. A grouping of the anastomotic types used by the author includes four categories: (*a*) those within functional groups; (*b*) those between somatic levels; (*c*) those between end arteries; and (*d*) those between tissue layers. Those within functional groups are always present and easy to identify. Injection of one pedicle of the middle meningeal will fill the neighboring branches. The anterior deep temporal can be counted on to fill the middle deep temporal, feeding the temporalis, and so on. The second type of anastomosis is seen at the boundary between somatic levels. This intermetameric connection is easily demonstrated in the spinal region but is present in the other areas. The connections are so numerous that a "grid" of vessels is formed. These connections will be repeated at every level. The third class of anastomosis is at the end of the vascular territory; there are no end arteries, only loops. Each vessel at the end of its territory will bifurcate and anastomoses its neighbor's bifurcated end artery. This pattern is also constant. The last group, the least numerous, can be the most surprising—that of anastomosis between layers such as the connections of the internal maxillary artery to the internal carotid artery; of the occipital or superficial temporal to the meningeal arteries. Attention to the location and type of anastomosis is critical during intervention.

Angiographic Protocols

Angiographic studies must include the target vessels and the vessel field across the target. The latter can include many anastomoses. One view of these anastomotic vessels' involvement is usually adequate. Images should be obtained perpendicular to the greatest change in anatomy. In the neck this is usually in the lateral view. The distal internal maxillary artery and assessment of midline collateral paths are best seen in an anteroposterior view.

Any blood vessels that are seen to cross are in different planes. Global injections are useful for global assessments;

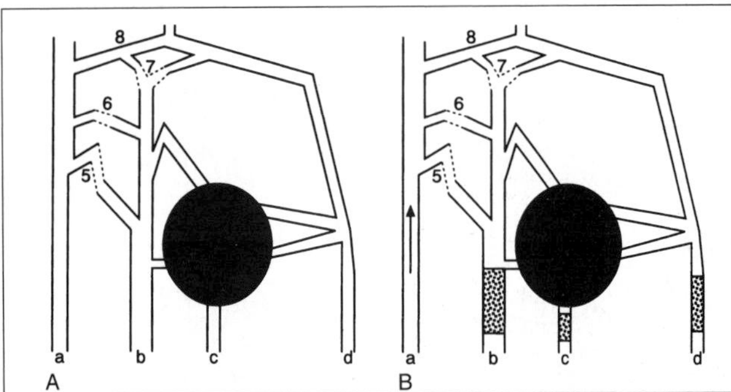

Figure 17.147. A. Three vascular pedicles (b, c, d) can be seen to feed the tumor; (c) is "dedicated"; (d) is dedicated with distal anastomosis; (b) gives off feeders with large vessels of passage, some of which feed it by recurrent vessels; and a vessel (a) is collateral to the vessels. If the flow to the tumor/arteriovenous malformation is low and an adequate injection is done, an angiogram that involves b,c,d would be adequate. If the flow is very high, reversal in flow in the distal portion of (b) will take place so that (a) will fill the distal tumor via 6. In this situation, a control angiogram must include a, b, c, and d. **B.** Proximal embolization of b, c, and d will lead to the incorrect view that the tumor has been embolized totally where in fact none of the tumor per se has been occluded. Injecting vessel (a) will lead to the proper assessment and avoid an unpleasant surprise.

subselective injections are useful for selective treatment. Blood vessels running in a bone groove (middle meningeal) or in a muscle (middle deep temporal) are relatively straight in their course since they are contained in their position. Along the course of a blood vessel there are spots where the vessel is constrained. At these points the vessel location can always be identified, and the vessel can be hurt by trauma. The infraorbital foramina, foramen spinosum, optic, jugular, and jugular canal are such examples. The blood vessels in fat or in the subarachnoid space are free to move around, and their course is quite variable.

The dictum to explore a lesion from normal tissue through to normal tissue, as in surgery, also holds in imaging. Vascular anatomy is topological, not orthogonal. Blood vessels feeding a vascular axis, or its anastomoses, can originate at some distance from the site of its neighbor. Just as the lesion should always be imaged on the middle of the film, not the edge, the vessel should be imaged in the middle of the "vascular field," not on the edge. Knowledge of the primary and collateral pathways is needed to study a lesion adequately. A schematic tumor is shown in Figure 17.147.

BALANCE POINTS

The abundance of collateral anastomoses has led to a dynamic balance. These watershed anastomoses have been described as *balance points* and are important to realize because inadvertent disconnection of these points can have lasting effects.

Normal Gross and Radiographic Anatomy

The external carotid artery is the smaller of the two branches resulting from the bifurcation of the common carotid artery. It supplies all of the head and neck structures. The appearance in frontal and lateral projections is shown diagrammatically and on radiographs in Figures 17.148 to 17.150.

There are 12 branches of the external carotid artery (see Table 17.6).

The branches of the external carotid artery anastomose with those of the opposite side, but, in addition, anastomoses exist between the external and internal carotid branches and between the vertebral and external carotid circulations as follows: (*a*) the ophthalmic artery and its branches anastomose with branches of the internal maxillary and the middle meningeal at several points (Fig. 17.151; 17.14; see also Fig. 10.5); (*b*) the transdural external-internal carotid anastomoses, where meningeal artery branches cross the subdural space and anastomose with branches of the middle cerebral and the posterior cerebral arteries on the outer surface of the hemisphere, and with branches of the anterior cerebral artery on the anterior surface, and on the inner surface (at the falx cerebri) (see Figs. 10.53 and 10.54); (*c*) between the branches of the internal carotid artery arising from the intracavernous portion and the branches of the external carotid artery at the base of the skull; and (*d*) between the external carotid and the vertebral artery branches, usually via the muscular branches of the vertebral artery, but transdural anastomoses exist also in the posterior fossa.

Embryology and Variants

The stapedial artery, which (embryologically) fed the dura and the orbit, was in large part annexed by the external carotid artery. The remaining was annexed by the internal carotid artery. The largest remaining pedicle of the stapedial artery is the middle meningeal. This takeover by the external carotid artery in large part accounts for the tremendous number of anastomoses between the two groups.

ABNORMAL VESSELS

A variety of vascular lesions can be seen in the head and neck and demonstrated on angiography. They will be discussed briefly in the following and additionally in the section on "Endovascular Therapeutic Neuroradiology" (Chapter 18).

Vascular Lesions

Arterial aneurysms arising from the external carotid artery are usually posttraumatic, associated with skull fractures or with puncture wounds. These may involve the meningeal vessels most frequently and are common in association with linear fractures of the skull (see Fig. 7.15). Their rupture may be responsible for some cases of delayed epidural he-

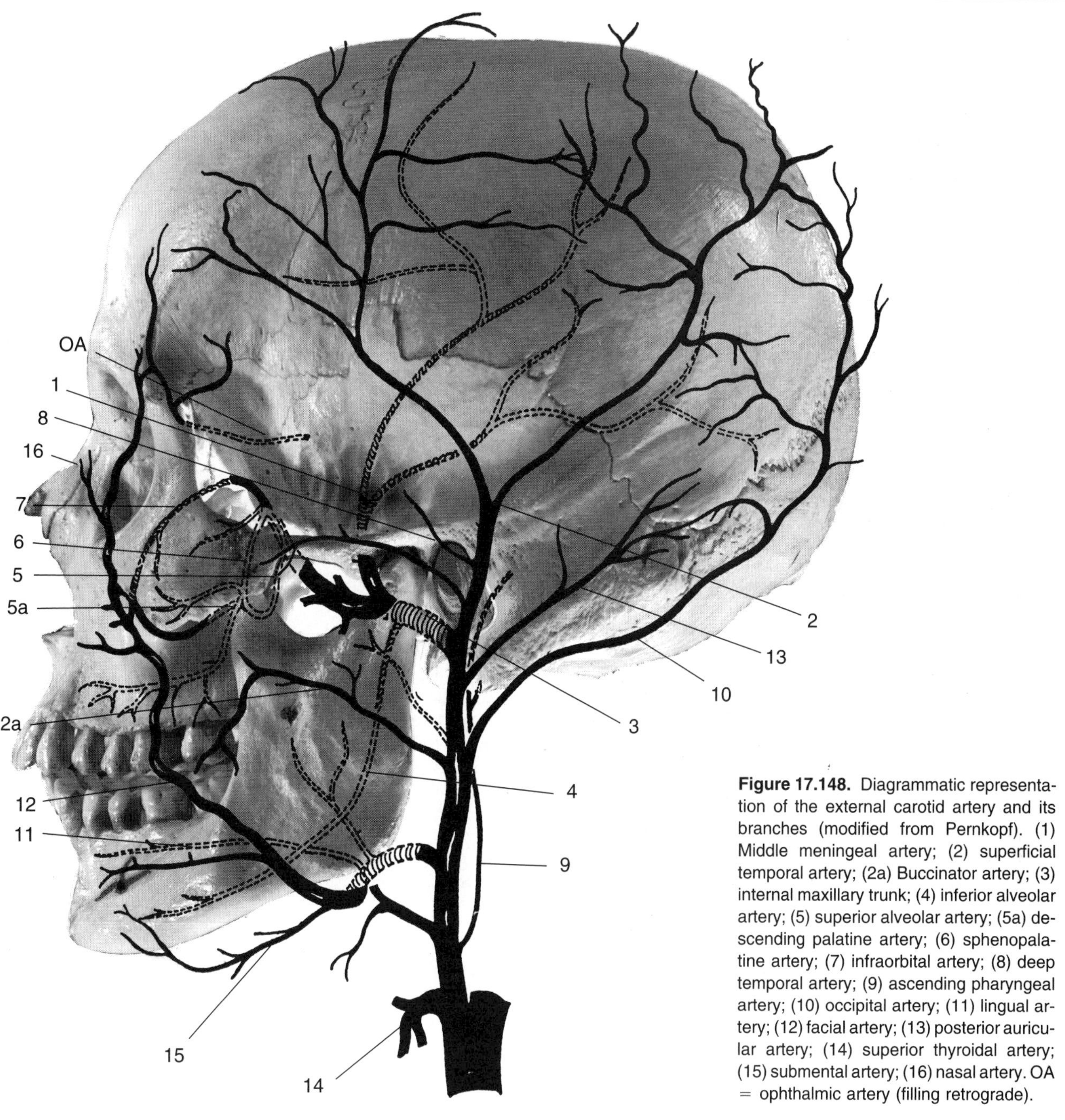

Figure 17.148. Diagrammatic representation of the external carotid artery and its branches (modified from Pernkopf). (1) Middle meningeal artery; (2) superficial temporal artery; (2a) Buccinator artery; (3) internal maxillary trunk; (4) inferior alveolar artery; (5) superior alveolar artery; (5a) descending palatine artery; (6) sphenopalatine artery; (7) infraorbital artery; (8) deep temporal artery; (9) ascending pharyngeal artery; (10) occipital artery; (11) lingual artery; (12) facial artery; (13) posterior auricular artery; (14) superior thyroidal artery; (15) submental artery; (16) nasal artery. OA = ophthalmic artery (filling retrograde).

matomas. Aneurysms associated with inflammatory conditions such as pharyngeal abscess and other severe infections may be seen at times (see Figs. 10.86 and 6.3). Congenital aneurysms of branches of the external carotid artery are exceedingly rare.

Arteriovenous Lesions

These may be congenital or acquired. The congenital arteriovenous malformations may be encountered in several locations.

Dural Arteriovenous Malformations

The arteriovenous communication may be at various levels, but frequently it involves the walls of the dural sinuses. This results in enlargement of these sinuses and interference with venous flow in the brain (Fig. 17.152). The important feature of these dural arteriovenous malformations, which are usually almost totally supplied by the external carotid artery, is the increased pressure in the dural venous sinuses, which in turn leads to chronic increased intracranial pressure (181). The lesions are more common in the

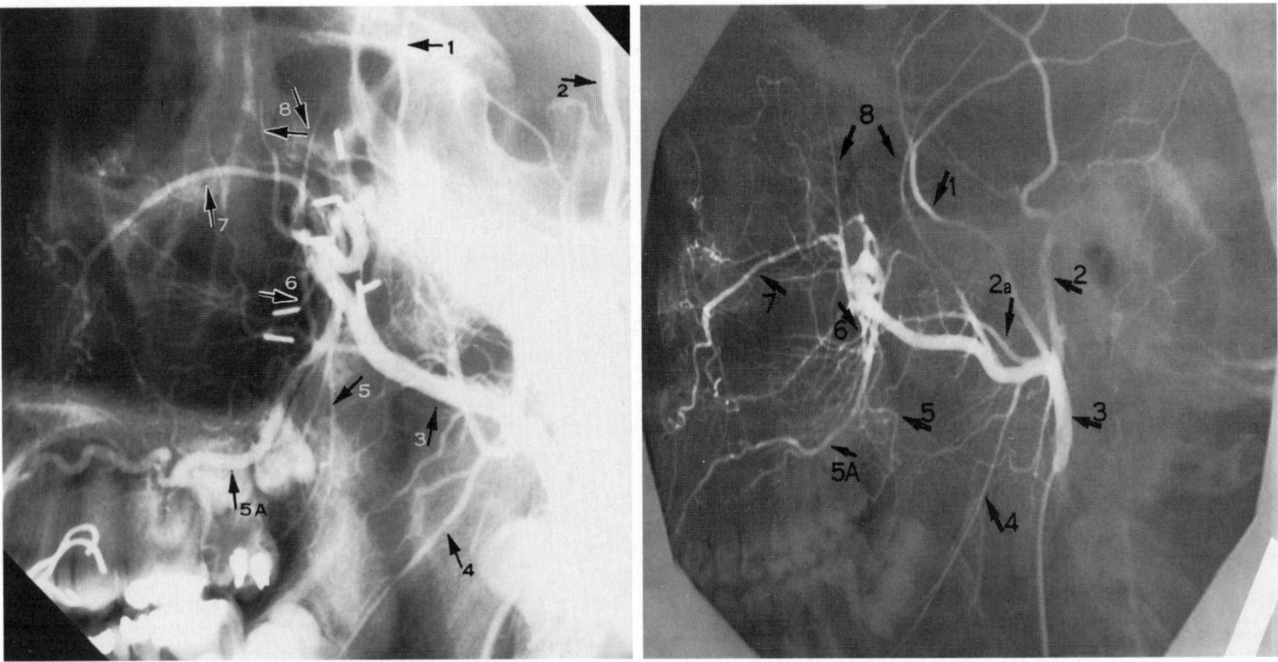

A B

Figure 17.149. Lateral (**A**), and anteroposterior (**B**) angiogram of the distal external carotid artery. The following numbering system is used for all external carotid injections: (1) middle meningeal; (1a) accessory meningeal artery; (2) superficial temporal artery; (2a) transverse facial artery; (3) internal maxillary artery; (4) inferior alveolar artery; (5) superior alveolar artery; (5a) descending palatine; (6) sphenopalatine; (7) infraorbital artery; (8) deep temporal arteries; (9) ascending pharyngeal artery; (10) occipital artery; (11) lingual artery; (12) facial artery; (13) posterior auricular; (14) superior thyroidal; ICA = internal carotid artery; OA = ophthalmic artery; TA = tentorial artery. The hypervascular nasal mucosa in this patient with nosebleeds. Note that over the skull there are three layers fed by the superficial temporal, the deep temporal, and the middle meningeal. The dilated vessels are due to a tumor of the calvarium. The numbered arrows correspond in A and B. The same numbers are used in subsequent figures to indicate the vessels.

posterior fossa or in the region of the torcular Herophili than elsewhere. Diagnosis is easy if selective internal and external carotid angiography is carried out. Thrombosis of the draining dural sinuses may occur spontaneously, which leads to further increase in intracranial venous pressure. In fact, it appears that in a large proportion of the cases thrombosis of the sinuses preceded the development of the arteriovenous communication (see Chapter 10 for further details).

Cavernous Sinus Lesions

In the case of cavernous sinus malformations, the chief manifestation is pulsating exophthalmos similar to a carotid cavernous fistula, but the exophthalmos may be minimal (182). Other manifestations such as dilated conjunctival veins and diplopia may be seen; a bruit may be heard, and increased intraocular pressure is often found on examination. Angiography may demonstrate a supply via meningeal branches of the internal carotid artery (Fig. 17.11), or it may stem exclusively from branches of the external carotid artery (Fig. 17.153).

Arteriovenous Communications

Arteriovenous communications may be found in the external carotid as an isolated phenomenon or in association with the Rendu-Osler-Weber syndrome and in the Wyburn-Mason (Bonnet-Dechaume-Blanc) syndrome. These entities are characterized by the presence of angiomas and arteriovenous communications in various locations, including the retina, the intracranial vessels, the external carotid branches, arteries of the extremities, and others.

In addition, a certain percentage of arteriovenous malformations normally supplied by the internal carotid or vertebral and basilar systems receive some blood supply from the external carotid artery via the external-internal carotid transdural anastomoses referred to earlier. The external carotid supply of these arteriovenous lesions may increase following surgical intervention or ligation of main feeding arteries. Supply to cerebral arteriovenous malformations through meningeal branches of the internal carotid and vertebral arteries is also observed (Fig. 17.153). The mechanism involved in the supply of cerebral and cerebellar arteriovenous malformations via transdural

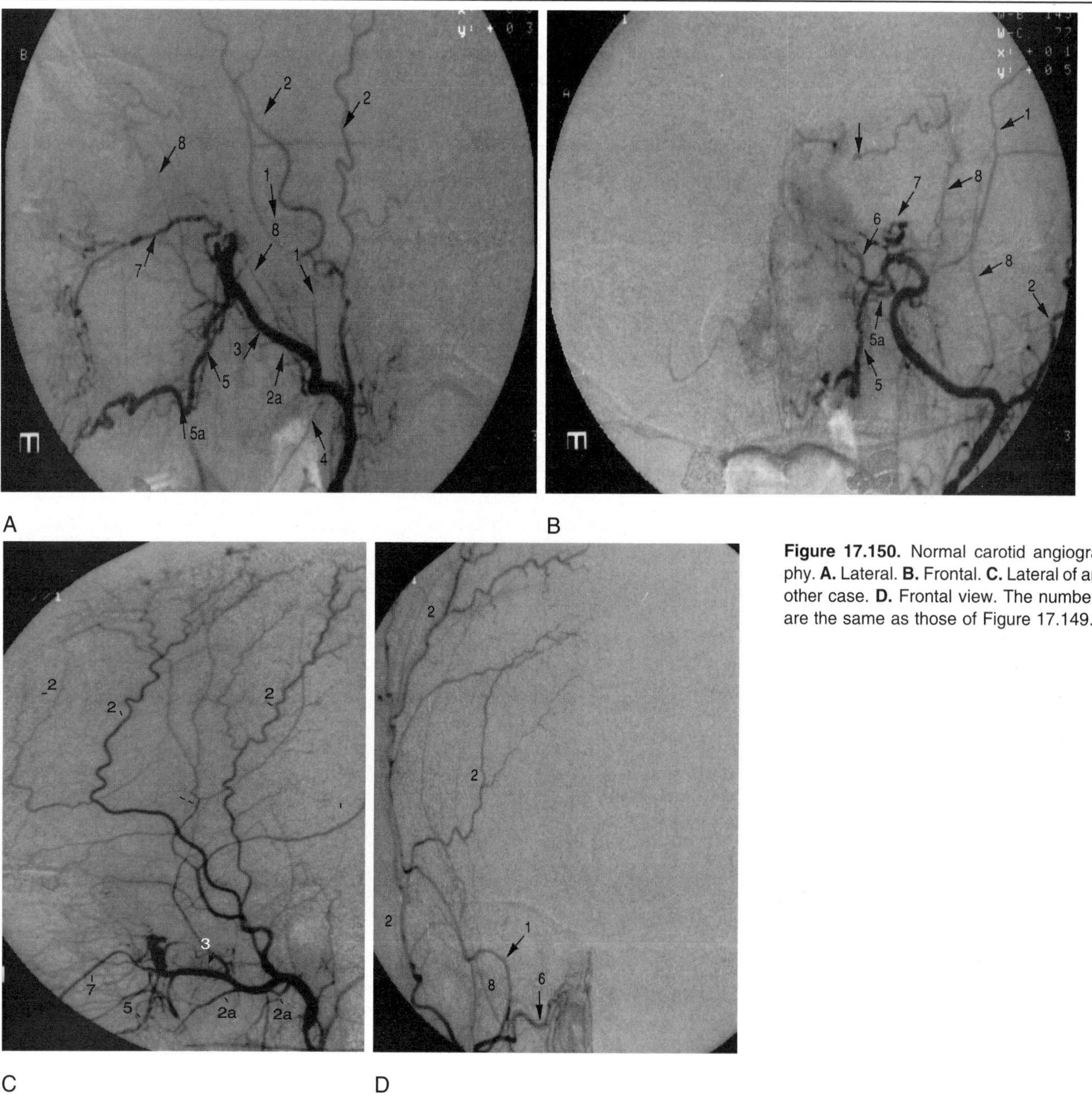

Figure 17.150. Normal carotid angiography. **A.** Lateral. **B.** Frontal. **C.** Lateral of another case. **D.** Frontal view. The numbers are the same as those of Figure 17.149.

communications of the cerebral with the meningeal arteries is as follows: the arteriovenous malformation creates a low-pressure area into which flow from adjacent arterial territories takes place. This leads to enlargement of preexisting transdural anastomoses. The same mechanism is operative in cases of intracranial arterial occlusions described earlier (see Chapter 10). In other cases, the blood supply to the malformation is about equal from both systems, and it is probable that in these cases embryologic factors must be responsible. Newton and Cronqvist refer to these as mixed pial-dural malformations (183).

Venous Malformations

Venous malformations in the external carotid territory are fairly common. There is a normal arterial supply with partial filling of the dependent portion of the dilated veins on late views. In the past they have often been labeled hemangiomas.

Arteriovenous Malformations of Scalp (Cirsoid Aneurysms)

These lesions are usually congenital and may behave like an arteriovenous fistula, which can be dealt with by simple

Table 17.6.
Branches of the External Carotid Artery

Name	Origin	Course	Branches	Tissues fed	Anastomosis
Superior Thyroidal	ECA, CCA	anterior inferior		larynx, superior thyroid, Sternocleidomastoid	Inferior thyroidal
Ascending Pharyngeal	ECA, OA	superiorly, medial	Pharyngeal A. Inferior Tympanic A. Neuromeningeal A. (C3)X–XI Musculo-spinal A	superior ¶ middle pharynx, petrous pyramid, posterior fossa meninges	VA ICA IMA
Lingual	ECA, L-Ft	superior, medial	Lingual Submental	tongue, submental gland	Ophthal
Facial	ECA, LF	anterior lateral cephalad	Ascending Palatine A., Glandular A. Submental A. Labial A. Nasal A.	face, lips, nose submental gland	Ophthal IMA, STA Sup Thyroid
Occipital	ECA	cephalad posterolateral	posterior neck muscles posterior meningeal Mastoid branches	occipital muscular cutaneous, posterior meninges	VA STA, VA, AscCer
Posterior auricular	ECA,	cephalad posterior	auricular, mastoid	ear, mastoid, facial canal	MMA, OcA,
Internal maxillary	ECA	anterior anterior medial	Mandibular portion Pterygoid portion Pterygopalatine portion	Maxilla Mandible lateral Dura Muscles of Mastication	ICA, OphA, OcA, P FA, IMA ICA, AscPhryg, FA
Superficial temporal	ECA	superior	scalp	zygomatic-orbital frontal parietal	FA, PAurA., TFA
Inferior thyroidal	SC, CCA			thyroid	
Ascending cervical	SC thycrv	superior		anterior prevertebral	AscPhy, VA
Deep cervical	SC cstcrv	superior	posterior	posterior paravertebral	OA, VA
Mandibular portion	ECA	anterior	Anterior Tympanic A. Deep Auricular A. Middle Meningeal A. Accessory Meningeal A. Inferior Tympanic A. Inferior Alveolar A.	Ear Dura Mandible	ICA, OphA
Pterygoid portion	ECA	anterior	Mid Deep Temporal A. Pterygoid A. Masseteric A. Buccal A.	Cheek Muscles of Mastication	OphA Asc Phryg
Pterygopalatine portion	ECA	medial	Posterior Superior Alveolar Infraorbital A. Greater Descending Palatine A. Artery of Foramen Rotundum Artery of pterygoid canal Sphenopalatine A.	Maxilla Medial mastication muscles	FA ICA OphA

ligation or excision, or they may involve a broader group of vessels presenting many arterialized veins, which is difficult to treat surgically. Treatment by percutaneous embolization may be useful in these cases.

Arteriovenous Malformations of Orbit

These malformations may be supplied by branches of the ophthalmic artery as well as by branches of the external carotid artery. It is important to delineate the complete supply of these lesions prior to surgical intervention in order to prevent recurrence (Fig. 17.154).

Acquired Arteriovenous Communications

These include the posttraumatic carotid cavernous fistulas supplied by the external carotid artery, which are uncommon, and the arteriovenous communications found follow-

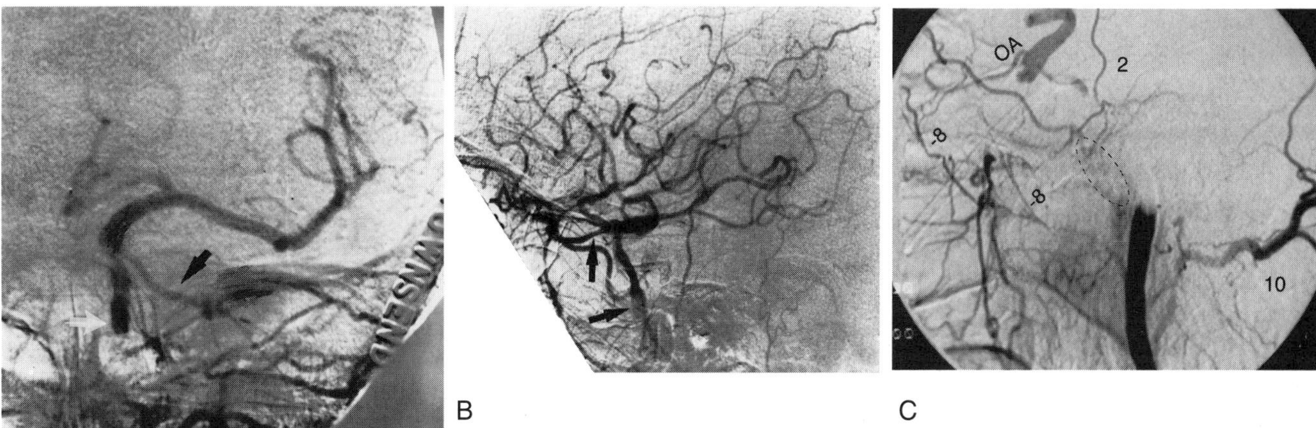

Figure 17.151. Collateral circulation through the ophthalmic artery supplying the occluded internal carotid circulation rather adequately. **A.** Frontal view. Large ophthalmic artery (upper arrow). Proximal retrograde filling in internal carotid artery down to point of complete occlusion (white arrow). **B.** Lateral view. Proximal regurgitation into internal carotid (lower arrow). Ophthalmic artery (upper arrow). **C.** In another example, following balloon occlusion of the internal carotid artery below the intrapetrosal portion. The intracranial carotid is filled via collateral through the opthalmic artery: (2) superficial temporal artery; (8) deep temporal artery; (10) occipital artery; (OA) ophthalmic a.

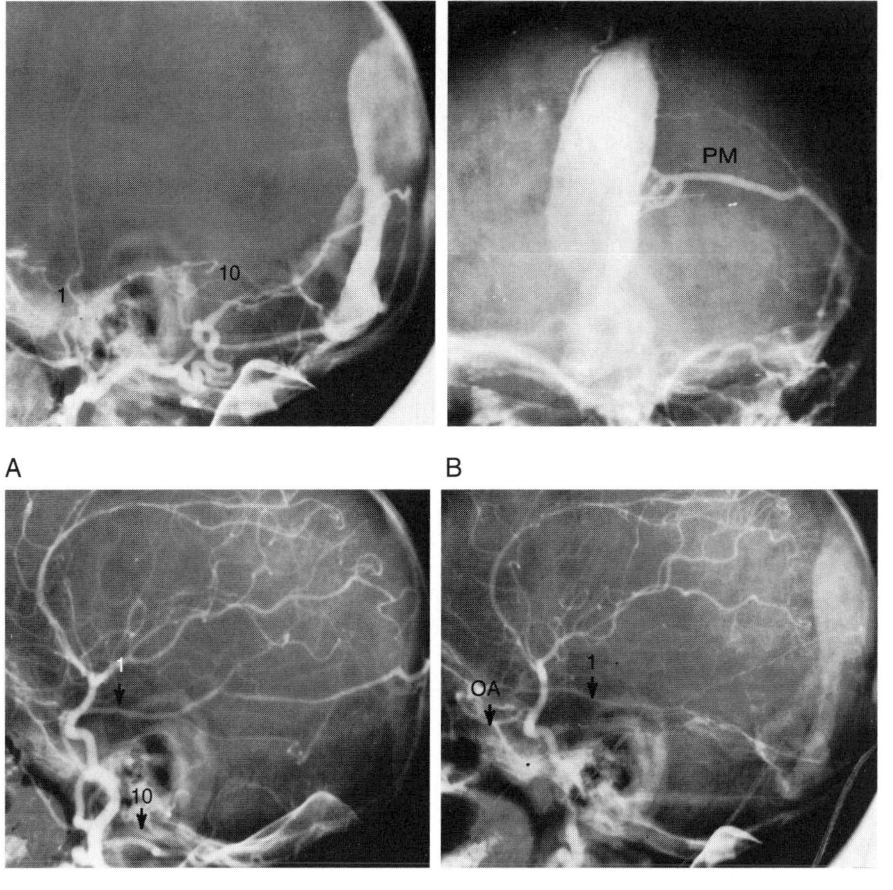

Figure 17.152. Posterior sagittal sinus dural arteriovenous malformation. **A.** Lateral left external carotid artery with filling of the arteriovenous malformation via transmastoid branches of the occipital artery (10) to reach the dural location, where they run straight in the periosteum/dura. The middle meningeal artery (1) gives off dural branches that pass posteriorly over the tentorium. The major territory of the middle meningeal feeds via the middle meningeal that comes off the ophthalmic artery seen on the left lateral internal carotid artery injection (**D**). **C.** Lateral right common carotid artery injection showing the dilated middle meningeal branch (1) with filling of the arteriovenous malformation; note that the vessel enlarges as it gets closer to the fistulous site. The posterior meningeal (PM) is well seen in **B**.

Figure 17.153. Nonmiddle meningeal dural branches. **A.** Lateral internal carotid artery angiogram in a patient with a medial frontal arteriovenous malformation fed primarily by the dilated branches of the anterior cerebral artery and the middle cerebral artery. The tentorial branch (arrow) is seen coming off the posterior petrous internal carotid artery. The anterior choroidal is also well demonstrated (arrowhead). **B** to **E.** Right cavernous sinus dural arteriovenous malformation fed by the distal branches of the internal maxillary artery. **B.** Lateral right external carotid shows filling of the cavernous sinus (arrow) with filling of the superior ophthalmic vein (OV) in C as well as some reflux into the intracranial venous system. **C.** The internal maxillary artery fills the cavernous dural arteriovenous malformation via the artery of the foramen rotundum and the artery of the foramen ovale (accessory meningeal) as well as the middle meningeal. (OV) and (arrows) show ophthalmic vein. **D** and **E.** The course of the vessels up the lateral wall of the cavernous sinus can be seen on the left internal maxillary and ascending pharyngeal injection with filling of the arteriovenous malformation across small anastomotic branches. **E.** Anteroposterior view shows the filling across the cavernous sinus. In Figure E, IPS refers to the inferior petrosalsinus. (1) middle meningeal a; (2) superficial temperal a.

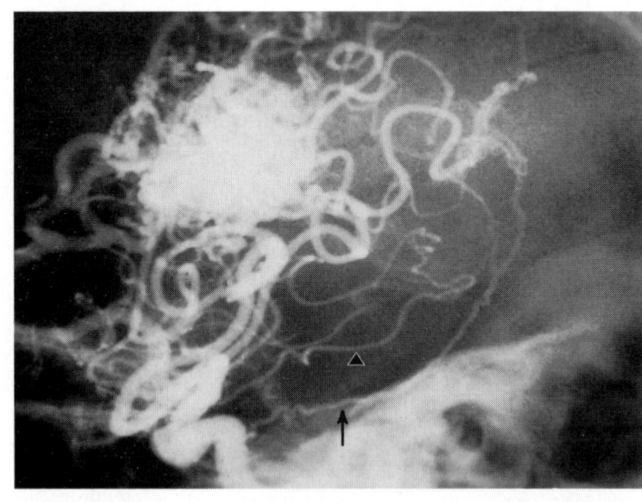

A

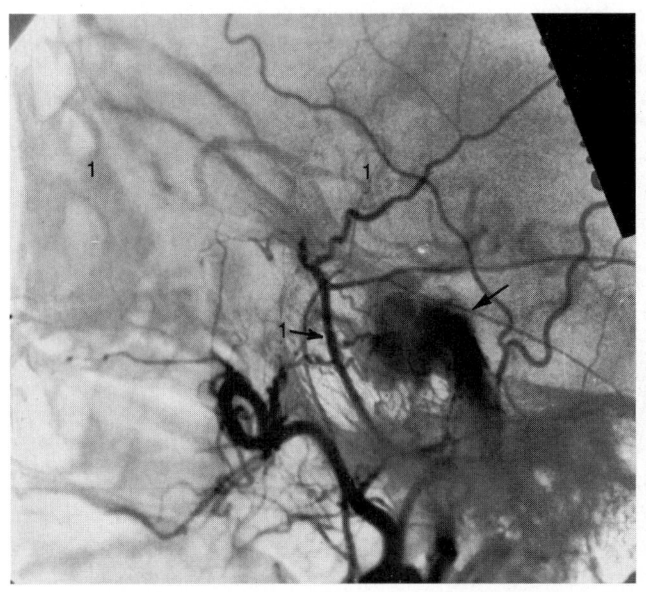

B

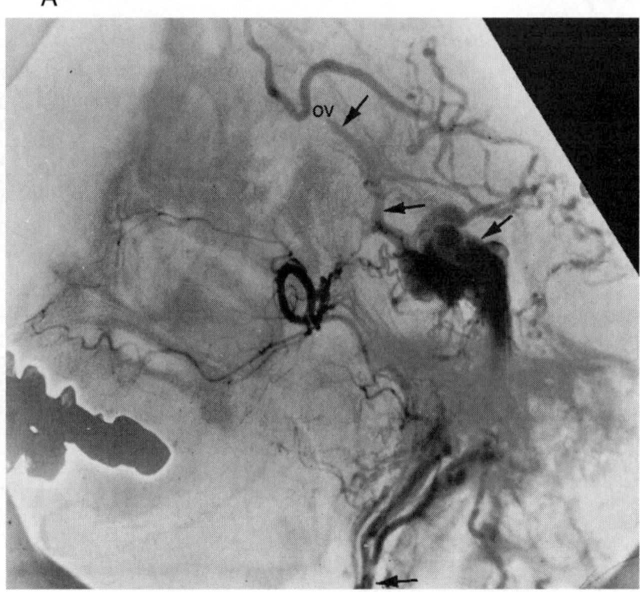

C

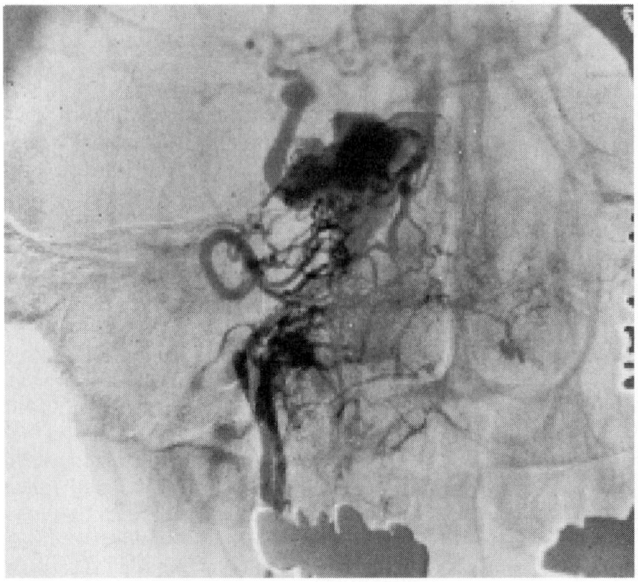

D

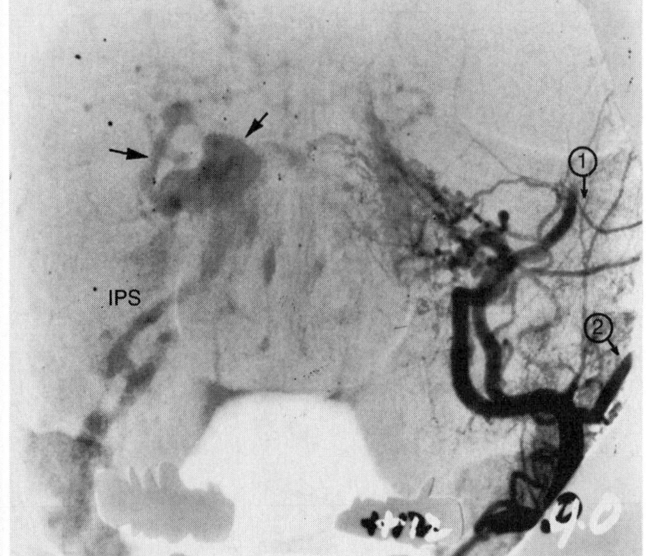

E

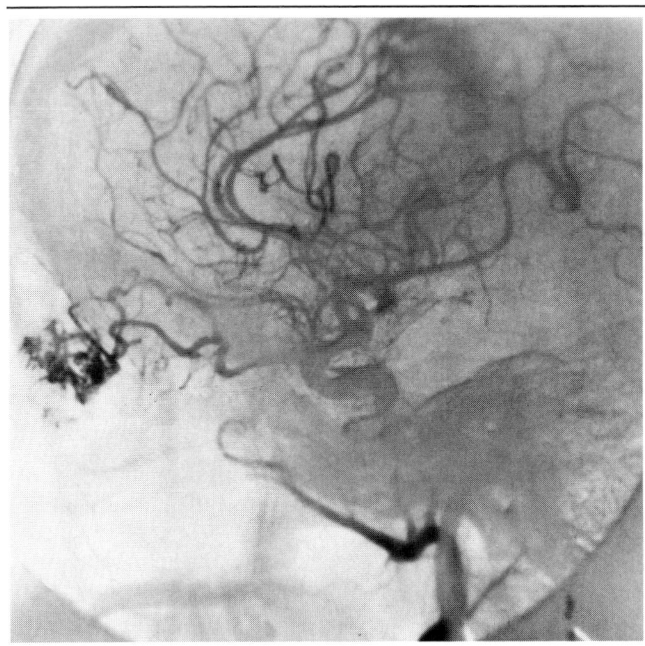

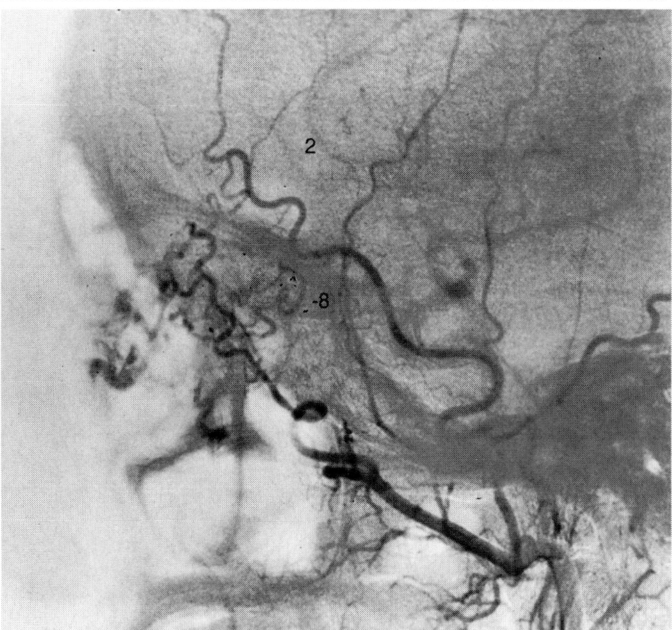

A B

Figure 17.154. Orbital arteriovenous malformation supplied by the ophthalmic and internal carotid arteries. **A.** Common carotid artery injection with filling of the arteriovenous malformation by the distal portion of the ophthalmic artery. Note that the three portions of the intraconal vessel are well seen. Anastomosis between the medial and lateral distal ophthalmic branches across the top of the orbit is identified. **B.** Lateral external carotid artery angiogram with filling of the orbital arteriovenous malformation via the transmalar branches of the dilated (8) anterior deep temporal artery and superficial temporal artery (2) branches in the region of the lateral orbital rim.

ing skull fractures. These involve the middle meningeal vessels and are demonstrated on angiograms performed soon after trauma. The ruptured meningeal vessels are seen to empty into the surrounding veins, thus avoiding the formation of an epidural hematoma (184).

Arterial Occlusions

These are usually not clinically significant because of the abundant anastomoses that exist. They may be spontaneous, usually related to atherosclerosis, or associated with certain inflammatory conditions such as mucormycosis and other severe infections. Simultaneous occlusion of the external and internal carotid may interfere with the development of adequate collateral circulation, particularly via the ophthalmic artery. As mentioned earlier, extensive collateral anastomoses exist between the external and internal carotid systems (see under "Collateral Circulation of the Brain," Chapter 10). At times the external carotid may "steal" from the internal carotid system, and this may be a cause of transient ischemic attacks.

NEOPLASMS

A few conditions that may involve the external carotid arteries and grow intracranially deserve special mention.

Glomus Jugulare Tumors

These are usually supplied by the external carotid via the ascending pharyngeal and other branches of the external carotid artery. As mentioned earlier, they may produce an intracranial mass in the lower cerebellopontine angle region, which is extradural in location. The blood supply is fairly characteristic (Figs. 17.155 and 17.156). The vascularity of these tumors can be reduced by percutaneous embolization prior to surgical intervention, thereby making surgical intervention much easier. Occlusion of the jugular vein is common owing to invasion by tumor. In these cases diagnosis of occlusion may be made by observing retrograde venous flow or by jugular venography (see Fig. 11.113).

Nasopharyngeal Angiofibromas

These occur in children or adolescents and characteristically produce a concave deformity of the posterior wall of the maxillary antrum and posterior displacement and pressure erosion of the pterygoid process. The blood supply is rich, and surgical intervention is very bloody (Fig. 17.157). Recurrence is common following surgical excision because of failure to achieve complete removal. The recurrences are more likely to receive blood supply from the intracavernous branches of the internal carotid artery, par-

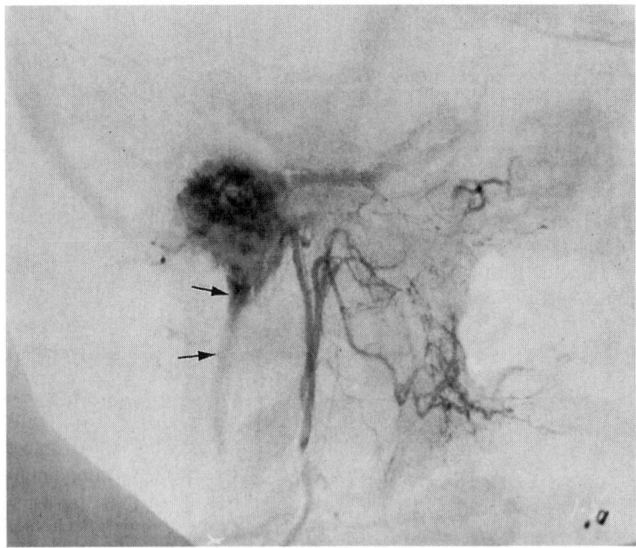

A

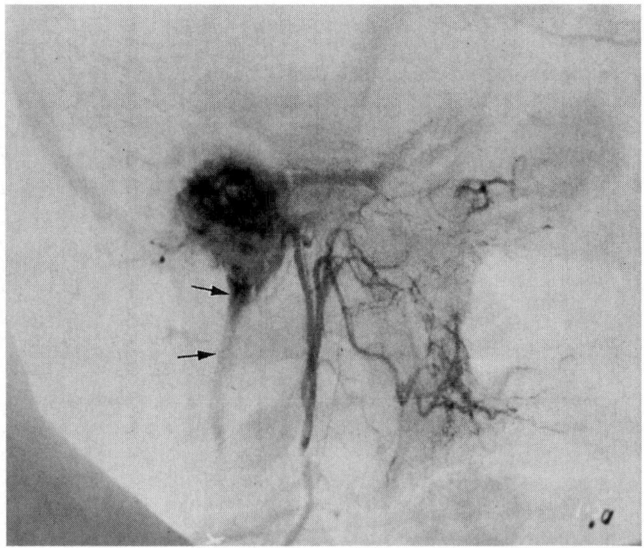

B

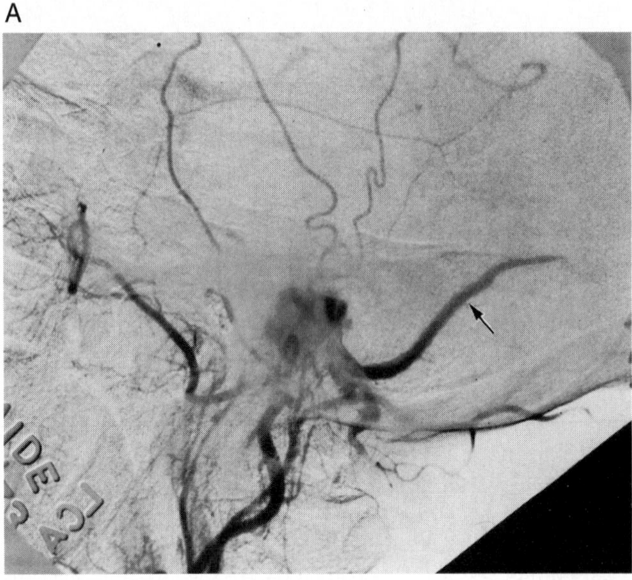

C

Figure 17.155. Glomus jugulare tumor shown by selective catheterization of the ascending pharyngeal artery with occlusion of the jugular vein and retrograde filling of the sigmoid sinus. **A.** Frontal oblique view of the ascending pharyngeal artery showing the hypervascular blush of the glomus jugulare tumor in the jugular canal. The dominant feeder is the neuromeningeal branch of the ascending pharyngeal. The jugular vein fills poorly (arrows) and there is reflux up the inferior petrosal sinus in this view. The superior pharyngeal branches and the inferior tympanic branches are seen. **B** and **C.** Lateral view of the external carotid artery is seen; the dominant feeders are the ascending pharyngeal. Note the close approximation of the ascending pharyngeal and the internal carotid seen behind it partially opacified. The posterior auricular also feeds the tumor. Reflux up the sigmoid sinus is seen.

ticularly after ligation of the internal maxillary artery. The tumors tend to grow through normal openings such as the ostium of the sphenoid sinus, and the inferior and superior orbital fissures. In order to decrease the need for blood transfusions during surgical removal, embolization of the internal maxillary artery under fluoroscopic control prior to surgery has been found beneficial.

Carotid Body Tumors

Carotid body tumors derive their blood supply primarily from the external carotid artery but may receive branches from the internal carotid bulb. Usually they displace the internal carotid artery but do not cause obstruction of this vessel. The angiographic appearance suggests a malignant tumor because of the irregular vessels and the multiple irregular draining veins found in them. At other times the "stain" is more homogeneous. (Fig. 17.158*A* and *B*). The glomus intravagale tumors occur in the same area (Fig. 17.158*C* and *D*).

Other Tumors

Malignant nasopharyngeal tumors may grow extradurally and may receive a blood supply from the external carotid artery or from intracavernous branches of the internal carotid artery. The great majority of meningiomas receive at least partial blood supply from branches of the middle meningeal artery; from meningeal arterial branches arising from the ophthalmic, the vertebral, and the external carotid arteries; or from meningeal branches of the internal carotid artery. The case shown in Figure 17.157*B* is a parasellar meningioma receiving its blood supply exclusively from the intracavernous branches of the internal carotid artery and no demonstrable supply from the external carotid vessels on selective external carotid angiography.

Acoustic neurinomas may receive their blood supply from branches of the external carotid artery instead of the vertebral system. Any tumor involving the bones of the vault may be expected to receive its blood supply from the

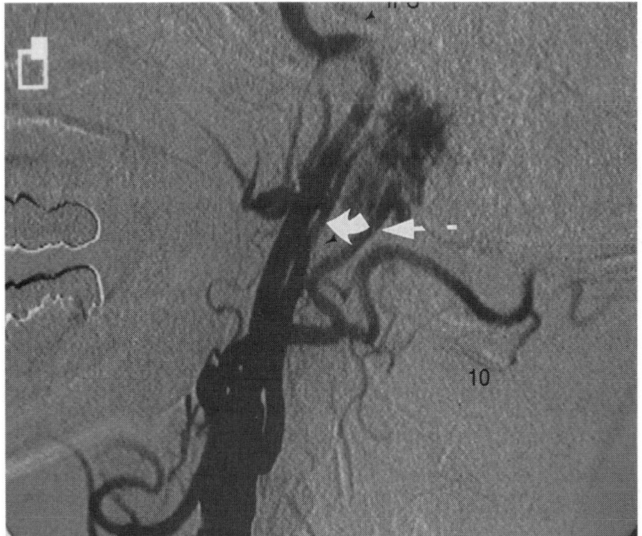

Figure 17.156. Lateral common carotid injection of a patient with a glomus jugulare tumor. The filling, as in the previous case (Fig. 17.155), is by the posterior auricular (arrow) and the ascending pharyngeal (curved arrow). There is reflux up the inferior petrosal sinus (IPS). The internal carotid artery (ICA) is seen just anterior to the mass; (10) occipital artery.

external carotid artery via the superficial temporal and occipital arteries as well as via the meningeal arteries. Increased size of the external carotid branches supplying the skull is observed in Paget disease, and sarcomatous degeneration in this condition is accompanied by further increase in the size of the arteries and by pooling within venous lakes in the region of the tumor.

Technique

External carotid artery catheterization is made via the femoral route, although in rare occasions other older approaches may be needed for treatment. Selection of each of the vessels of the external carotid can be performed. For further details see under "Therapeutic Endovascular Neuroradiology" (Chapter 18).

COMPLETE LISTING OF ARTERIAL AND VENOUS SYSTEM

Following is a complete listing of the arteries of the carotid system (internal and external), the vertebral system, and the basilar system. Also included is a listing of the cerebral veins and the dural sinuses.

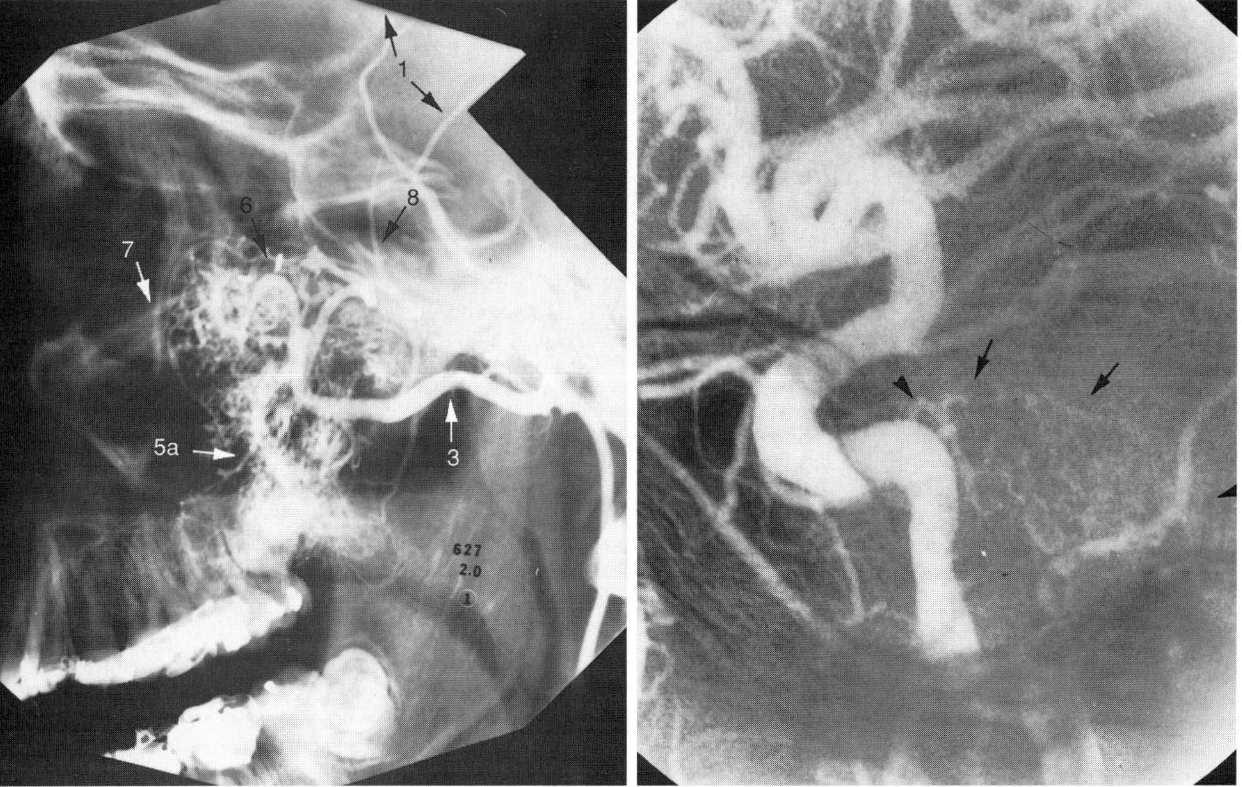

Figure 17.157. A. Nasopharyngeal angiofibroma. A lateral external carotid injection showing an enlarged internal maxillary artery (3) with hypervascular mass in the nasopharynx. The blood vessels feeding it include the sphenopalatine (6) and the descending palatine (5a). The middle meningeal (1), masseteric artery and middle deep temporal artery (8), and the infraorbital artery (7), although not feeding the tumor, are well seen. **B.** Lateral common carotid injection in a patient with a parasellar meningioma (arrows) showing a dilated meningohypophyseal branch of the internal carotid artery (arrowhead).

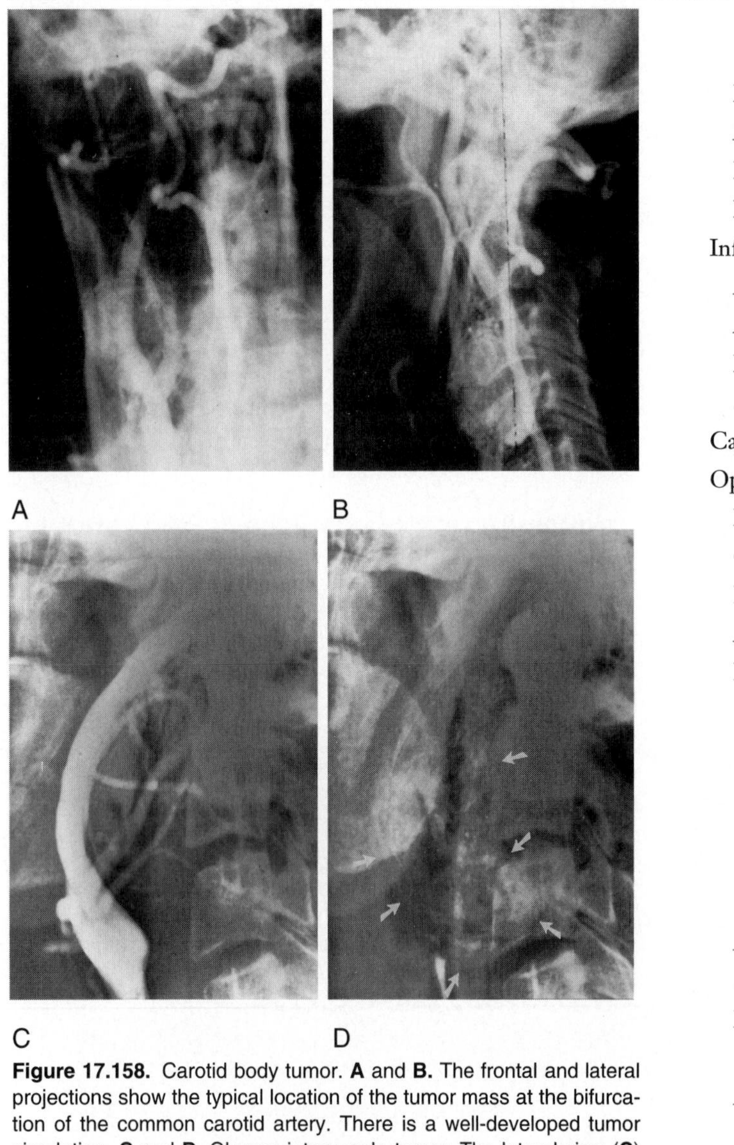

Figure 17.158. Carotid body tumor. **A** and **B.** The frontal and lateral projections show the typical location of the tumor mass at the bifurcation of the common carotid artery. There is a well-developed tumor circulation. **C** and **D.** Glomus intravagale tumor. The lateral view (**C**) shows that both the internal and external carotid arteries are displaced forward. This is different from the carotid body tumor, where these arteries are usually splayed. The delayed film (**D**) shows a somewhat homogeneous blush where numerous fine vessels are visible (arrows).

CEREBRAL AND CRANIOFACIAL ARTERIES

Internal carotid artery

- Caroticotympanic artery
- Mandibular artery
- Vidian artery
  - Sphenoidal branch
- Meningohypophyseal trunk
  - Marginal tentorial artery
  - Lateral clival artery
    - Medial branch
    - Lateral branch
  - Posteroinferior hypophyseal artery
  - Medial clival artery
  - Recurrent artery of foramen lacerum
  - Lateral artery of trigeminal ganglion
- Inferolateral trunk
  - Anteromedial branch
  - Anterolateral branch
  - Posterior branch
  - Superior branch
- Capsular artery
- Ophthalmic artery
  - Lateral ciliary artery
  - Central retinal artery
  - Deep recurrent ophthalmic artery
  - Medial ciliary artery
  - Lacrymal artery
    - Recurrent meningeal artery
      - Recurrent tentorial artery
      - Meningeal branch for sphenoidal ridge
      - Anterior frontal meningeal branch
    - Lateral muscular artery
    - Meningo-ophthalmic artery
  - Muscular arteries
  - Supraorbital artery
  - Posterior ethmoidal artery
    - Jugum sphenoidale branch
  - Anterior ethmoidal artery
    - Anterior falcine artery
- Superior hypophyseal arteries
- Anterior choroidal artery
  - Cisternal segment
    - Temporal branches
    - Perforating branches
  - Choroidal segment

Anterior Cerebral Artery

- Medial striate arteries
- Heubner artery
- Anterior communicating artery
  - Perforating arteries
- Orbitofrontal artery
- Frontopolar artery
- Callosomarginal artery
  - Anterior internal frontal artery

- Middle internal frontal artery
- Posterior internal frontal artery

Pericallosal artery
- Paracentral artery
- Superior internal parietal artery
- Inferior internal parietal artery

Middle Cerebral Artery

Medial striate arteries
Lateral striate arteries (lenticulostriate arteries)
Orbitofrontal artery
Operculofrontal artery (candelabra artery)
Central sulcus artery
Posterior parietal artery
Angular artery
Posterior temporal artery
Middle temporal artery
Anterior temporal artery
Temporopolar artery

Vertebral Artery

Muscular branches
Radicular branches
- Anterior anastomotic arteries *(transverse foramen; C3, C4)*
- Posterior anastomotic arteries *(transverse foramen; C2)*

Meningeal branches
- Odontoid arch system
- Artery of falx cerebelli
- Posterior meningeal artery
  - Cerebellar fossa branch

Medullary branches
Posterior inferior cerebellar artery
- Lateral branch (tonsillohemispheric branch)
- Medial branch (vermian branch)
- Meningeal branches

Anterior spinal artery

Basilar Artery

Pontine branches (pontine arteries)
- Medial arteries
- Transverse arteries

Anterior inferior cerebellar artery
- Internal auditory artery
  - Vestibular branch to seventh nerve
  - Cochlear branches
  - Vestibulocochlear branches
- Rostrolateral branch
  - Ascending branch
  - Descending branch
- Caudomedial artery
  - Branches to choroid plexus
  - Medial branch
  - Lateral branch
- Meningeal branches

Superior cerebellar artery
- Perforating branches to pontomesencephalic junction
- Lateral (marginal) branch
- Medial (hemispheric) branch
- Meningeal branches

Posterior Cerebral Artery

Paramedian arteries
Posterior communicating artery
- Anterior thalamoperforate arteries

Short circumferential arteries
Long circumferential arteries
- Quadrigeminal artery

Posterior thalamoperforate arteries
Thalamogeniculate arteries
Posterior choroidal artery
- Medial posterior choroidal artery
- Lateral posterior choroidal artery

Hippocampal artery
Anterior temporal artery
Middle temporal artery
Posterior temporal artery
Temporo-occipital artery
Parieto-occipital arteries
Calcarine artery
Posterior pericallosal artery
Meningeal branches

External Carotid Artery

Superior thyroid artery
- Hyoid branch
  - Submental branch
  - Anterior anastomotic branch
- Superior laryngeal artery (foramen of thyrohyoidian membrane)
  - Ventral trunk
    - Epiglottic branch
  - Dorsal trunk

Lateral longitudinal arterial arcade of laryngeal arteries
Glandular trunk (posterior branch)
Cricothyroid artery
Medial longitudinal arterial arcade of laryngeal arteries
Superior marginal glandular arcade
Posterior glandular arcade
Lateral grandular arcade
Sternomastoid artery
Lingual artery
Suprahyoid branch
Deep lingual artery
Sublingual artery
Sublingual anastomosis
Periglandular ring
Medial mandibular branch
Facial artery
Ascending palatine artery
Submandibular artery
Submental artery
Sublingual anastomosis
Periglandular ring
Anterior hyoid branch
Posterior hyoid branch
Inferior masseteric artery
Jugal trunk
Buccomasseteric trunk
Posterior jugal artery
Middle mental artery
Inferior labial artery
Middle jugal artery
Superior labial artery
Anterior jugal artery
Alar artery
Nasal arcade
Angular artery
Occipital artery
Stylomastoid artery (stylomastoid foramen)
C1 posterior anastomotic branch
C2 posterior anastomotic branch
Meningeal branch
Artery of falx cerebelli
Mastoid branch
Cerebellar fossa branch
Cerebellopontine angle branch
Osteocutaneous branch
Cutaneous branch
Torcular branch
Ascending pharyngeal artery
Inferior pharyngeal artery
Middle pharyngeal artery
Superior pharyngeal branch
Inferior eustachian tube artery
Mandibular anastomosis (foramen lacerum)
Carotid branch (foramen lacerum)
Inferior tympanic artery (jacobson canal)
Musculospinal artery
Prevertebral branch
Neuromeningeal trunk
Hypoglossal branch (hypoglossal canal)
Cerebellar fossa branch
Foramen magnum branch
Clival branch
Odontoid arterial arch
Jugular branch (jugular foramen)
Cerebellar fossa branch
Cerebellopontine angle branch
Inferior petrosal branch
Posterior auricular artery
Stylomastoid artery (stylomastoid foramen)
Muscular branch
Stylomuscular artery
Auricular branch
Cutaneous branch
Retroauricular arterial arch
Superficial temporal artery
Zygomatico-orbital branch
Posterior deep temporal artery
Frontoparietal branch
Parieto-occipital branch
Anterior auricular branch
Retroauricular arterial arch
Transverse facial artery
Jugal branch
Superior masseteric artery
Internal maxillary artery
Anterior tympanic artery (anterior tympanic canal)
Middle masseteric artery
Inferior alveolar artery
Middle meningeal artery (foramen spinosum)
Cavernous branch
Petrous branch
Superior tympanic artery
Petrosquamosal branch

Basal tentorial branch
Posterior fossa branch
Parieto-occipital branch
Middle cranial fossa branch
Frontal branch
Sphenoidal branch
Tentorial branch
Meningolacrimal artery
Accessory meningeal artery
Cavernous branch (foramen ovale)
Eustachian tube branch
Palatine branch
Middle deep temporal artery
Deep masseteric artery
Buccal artery
Greater palatine artery (posterior palatine canal)
Pterygoid branch
Pterygoid artery
Antral artery
Anterior deep temporal artery
Orbital branch (malar bone foramen)
Musculocutaneous branch
Infraorbital artery
Orbital branch
Jugal branch (infraorbital canal)
Superior alveolar artery
Antral branch (antral foramen)
Jugal branch
Alveolar branch (superior alveolar canal)
Sphenopalatine artery
Septal branch
Turbinate branch
Pterygovaginal artery
Vidian artery (vidian canal)
Artery of foramen rotundum (foramen rotundum)

Subclavian Artery

Ascending cervical artery
Muscular branches
Radicular branches
Anterior anastomotic arteries (*transverse foramen; C3, C4*)
Deep cervical artery
Muscular branches
Radicular branches
Posterior anastomotic arteries (*transverse foramen; C2, C3*)

DURAL SINUSES AND VEINS

Dural sinuses

(Superior sinus group)
Superior sagittal sinus
Inferior sagittal sinus
Straight sinus
Tentorial sinus
Confluence of sinuses (torcular Herophili)
Transverse sinus
Sigmoid sinus
Occipital sinus
Marginal sinus
(Basal sinus group)
Cavernous sinus
Anterior intercavernous sinus
Posterior intercavernous sinus
Basilar plexus
Foramen ovale plexus
Pterygoid plexus
Sphenoparietal sinus
Superior petrosal sinus
Inferior petrosal sinus

Supratentorial Cerebral Veins

(Superficial veins)
(Ascending cerebral veins)
Frontal ascending veins
Frontoparietal vein (Trolard)
Central vein (Rolando)
Parietal ascending veins
Occipital ascending veins
(Descending cerebral veins)
Superficial middle cerebral vein (sylvian)
Temporo-occipital vein (Labbé)
(Deep veins)
Vein of Galen
(Tributaries of vein of Galen)
Dorsal callosal vein
Internal occipital vein
Internal cerebral vein
Medial atrial vein
Anterior thalamic vein
Superior thalamic vein
Direct lateral vein
Septal vein

Posterior septal vein
Thalamostriate vein
Anterior caudate vein
Longitudinal caudate vein
Transverse caudate vein
Upper choroidal vein
Basal vein of Rosenthal
Inferior temporo-occipital vein
Calcarine vein
Inferior thalamic vein
Posterior thalamic vein
Inferior striatum veins
Peduncular vein
Lateral atrial vein
Inferior ventricular vein
Inferior choroidal vein
Hippocampal veins
Anterior cerebral vein
Olfactory vein
Anterior pericallosal vein
Anterior communicating
Deep middle cerebral vein
Fronto-orbital vein
Anterior insular vein
Middle insular vein
Posterior insular vein

Posterior Fossa Veins

(Superior group)
Vein of Galen
(Cerebellar veins)
Precentral cerebellar vein
Superior cerebellar vein
Superior vermian vein
Superior hemispheric vein
(Mesencephalic veins)
Posterior mesencephalic vein
Lateral mesencephalic vein
Anterior pontomesencephalic vein
(Anterior group)
Petrosal vein
(Veins on the anterior surface of brainstem)
(Longitudinal veins)
Lateral pontomesencephalic vein
Anterior medullary vein
(Transverse veins)
Transverse pontine vein
Peduncular vein
(Veins of wings of precentral cerebellar fissure)
Brachial vein
(Veins of cerebellar hemisphere)
Anterior lateral marginal vein
Superior hemispheric vein
Inferior hemispheric vein
Vein of great horizontal fissure
(Veins of cerebellomedullary fissure [retro-olivary veins])
Lateral pontine vein
Vein of lateral recess of fourth ventricle
(Posterior group)
Straight sinus
Inferior vermian vein
Superior retrotonsillar vein
Inferior retrotonsillar vein
Transverse sinus
Inferior hemispheric vein

Extracerebral Veins

(Intracranial extracerebral veins)
Anterior meningeal vein
Middle meningeal vein
Diploic veins
(Extracranial extracerebral veins)
Superficial temporal veins
Medial temporal veins
Occipital veins
External jugular vein
Supratrochlear vein
Supraorbital vein
Angular vein
Facial vein
Submental vein
Retromandibular vein
(Deep head veins)
External palatine vein
Pterygoid plexus
Medial meningeal vein
Pterygoid canal vein
Deep temporal vein
Sternocleidomastoid veins

Orbital Veins

Superior ophthalmic vein
  Anterior anastomotic vein
  Middle anastomotic vein
  Posterior anastomotic vein
  Lacrimal vein
Middle ophthalmic vein
Inferior ophthalmic vein

SPINAL ANGIOGRAPHY

Background and Indications

Indications for spinal angiography include suspected arteriovenous malformations and suspected hypervascular tumors. Often the dural spinal arteriovenous malformations are missed until too late in their course. Spinal angiography should always be strongly considered in patients with unexplained progressive spinal-related neurologic deficits. In relentlessly progressive situations, repeat spinal angiography should be considered. MRI/magnetic resonance angiography (MRA) can rule in spinal angiography but cannot rule it out.

Technique

Spinal angiography is a long, tedious, and demanding technique. The individual parts are straightforward, and they must be repeated over and over again, in spite of patient, team, and operator fatigue.

Incomplete or inadequate spinal angiograms can do more harm than good. What constitutes a complete spinal angiogram? A complete study is one where the pathologic, normal, and collateral vasculature to the targets has been demonstrated (Fig. 17.159) Specifically, it depends on the disease being studied. What constitutes adequate opacification of a vessel? Occasionally more than one level and/or side will be visualized during angiography. This can happen because of a common origin, reflux, or filling through collaterals. If there is no disease seen, *and* there is staining of the vertebral body segment at the site of additional filling, selective angiography at this point does not need to be performed (Table 17.7).

PATIENT PREPARATION

Although spinal angiography can be done under IV sedation, often general anesthesia is safer, easier, and more effective. A variety of considerations go into the decision that have been outlined in the following. We tend to favor general anesthesia since movement causes a marked deterioration of the images, increased use of contrast, and significant patient discomfort. In patients with pathology such as paraspinal tumors, where the spinal angiogram is going to

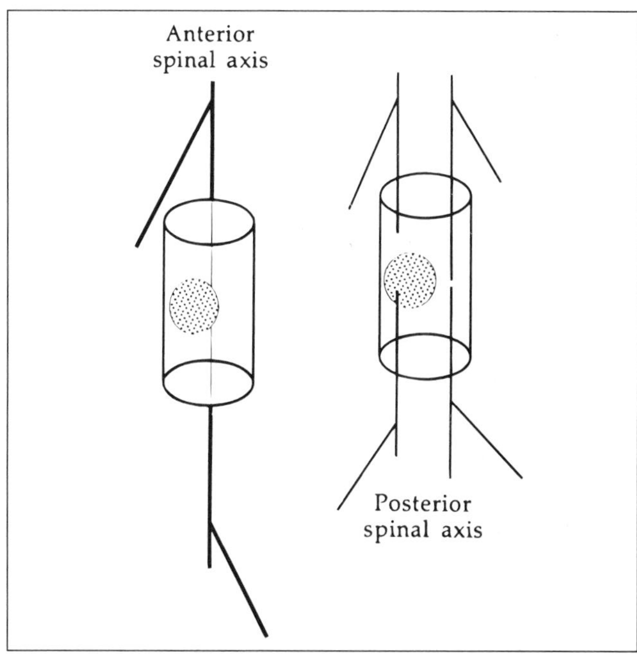

Figure 17.159. "Complete" angiogram of the spinal cord requires that the anterior and the posterior spinal axes be injected on both sides of the suspected lesion.

Table 17.7.
Indications for Spinal Angiography

	Spine tumor	Spinal cord tumor/AVM	Spinal dural AVM
Complete angiogram?	• Two levels above • Two levels below pathology	• Anterior spinal axis • Posterior spinal axis *both* sides of the intrinsic lesion (spinal cord mass)	• Feeders to all dural shunts • Anterior spinal artery circulation on late films
Where to start?	• Level of the vertebral body involvement • Flush aortography can be helpful	• Below the area of the abnormality (see Chipault Rule)	• Thoracolumbar junction • Bilateral femoral simultaneous can be used in difficult cases
What to identify?	• Feeders to tumor	• Both ends and both sides of the anterior and posterior spinal axes wherever they originate	• Stasis in anterior spinal artery • Arteriovenous shunt site(s) • Draining veins

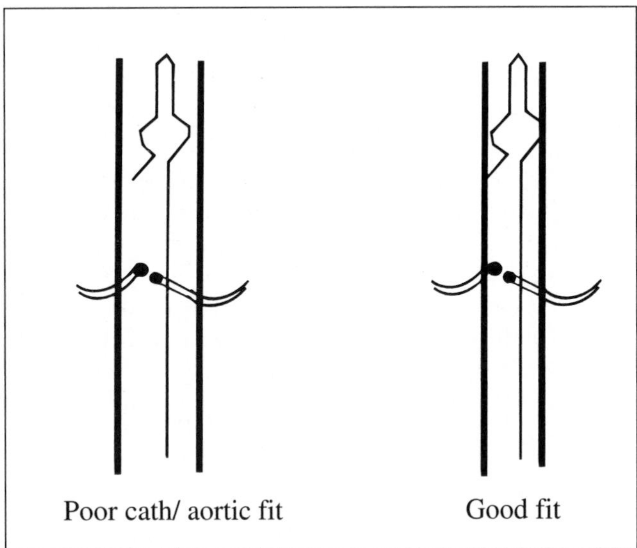

Figure 17.160. The aorta (heavy line) gives off two small arcing vessels, the intercostals or the lumbars. These paired vessels angle acutely from the aorta. The catheter, the thin shepherd's hook, must be wide enough so that it touches the opposite wall.

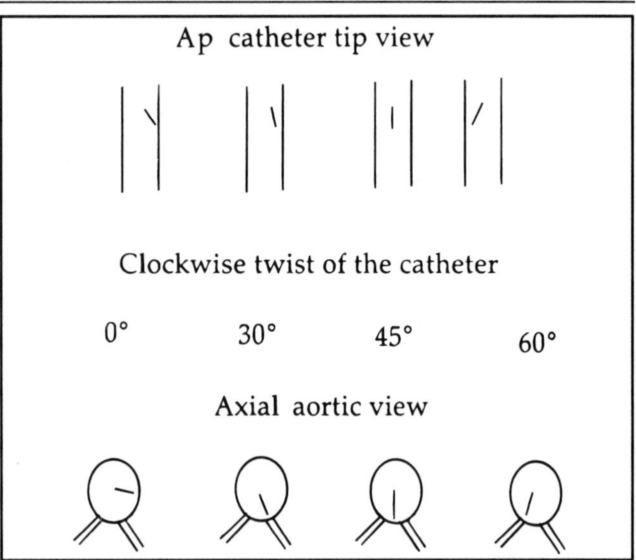

Figure 17.161. The top row shows how the catheter tip looks as seen on anteroposterior fluoroscopy, as the catheter is rotated around in a clockwise position (middle row). The bottom row shows an axial view as the catheter is rotated clockwise around the vessel, with the tip of the catheter in the desirable position (tip pointing dorsally).

be limited, we tend to favor monitored awake sedation unless the pain would not allow the patient to cooperate. Patients under 10 years of age usually require general anesthesia. If embolization is being done at the same time and general anesthesia is being used, sensory and motor-evoked responses should be performed. These methods are sensitive to spinal cord stress. If the baseline is severely abnormal or interactions with anesthetic agents are profound, a wake-up call is needed. The patients are allowed to wake up with the cuffed endotracheal tube in place. This option should be thoroughly discussed with the patient. During the transition from awake to asleep, the patient will pass through stage 2 anesthesia. At least seven staff are needed for this. One person holds both legs, two are assigned to hold an arm and the ipsilateral chest, and one holds the head and talks to the patient. The anesthesiologist and the neurointerventionalist remain at their stations to perform and do not participate in restraining the patient.

CATHETERS

The spinal arteries come off at a downward angle off the aorta, vertebral, and iliacs. Catheterization of all of these vessels can be performed superselectively. A reverse curve is quite useful in expediting catheterization. The shepherd's hook catheter is quite useful. Pick a size so that the catheter tip is held against the aorta (Fig. 17.160). The catheter tip should be very soft.

The shepherd's hook or Michaelson catheter is reformed in either the subclavian or the iliac. The catheter tip is positioned on the left lateral wall of the aorta. When the catheter is turned clockwise, the catheter tip will move from the patient's left to right in anteroposterior view when it is facing the posterior wall (Fig. 17.161). The orifice of the lumbar and thoracic vessels is off the posterior wall. When the catheter tip catches the orifice it bobs, and gentle injection will confirm its location. The catheter tip is then advanced by retracting on the catheter hub while injecting a small amount of contrast as one seats the catheter tip. After the run, the catheter is then backed out of the orifice by advancing the catheter at the groin. If the catheter tip is seated in the left vessel, a slight clockwise twist will place the catheter tip in the right-sided vessel and vice versa, since the orifices are usually right next to each other. Also, identifying where the orifice is, relative to one pedicle and level, gives an indication of the location at the level above and below. The catheter should be kept full of contrast since it can be difficult to see the catheter in heavy patients.

The injection rate is low, at 1 to 2 ml per second. The filming is two films per second for 3 sec, one film per second for 10 sec, and one film every other second for the next 10 sec.

Normal Vascular Anatomy

ARTERIES

The excellent text by Thron, with its beautiful microradiographs, is recommended to the student of spinal cord anatomy (185). The blood supply to the spinal cord is initially metameric to each of the 31 somites, with feeding vessels to both the posterior aspect and the anterior part. Fusion of the anterior contribution into a single anterior spinal artery axis occurs with contribution from four to eight of the original levels.

The vertebral body feeder vessel is used as a marker as to the level from which the cord vessel originates. As the

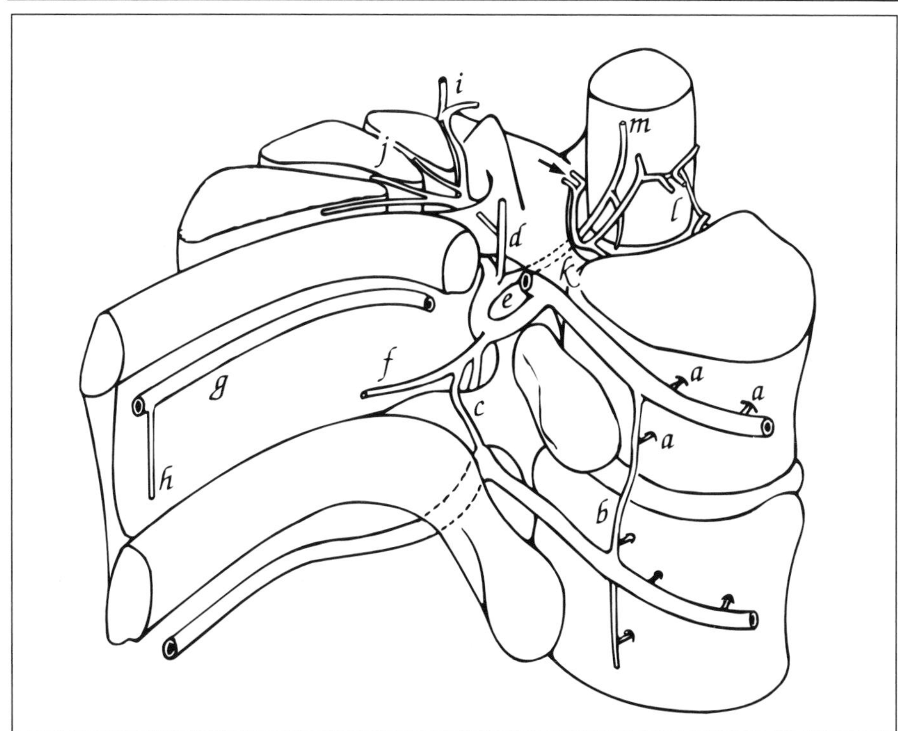

Figure 17.162. Extradural and extraspinal branches of the intercostal system. (a) Vertebral body arteries; (b) anterolateral anastomotic artery; (c and d) pretransverse anastomoses; (e) dorsospinal artery; (f) first perforating muscular branch; (g) lateral muscular branch; (h) second perforating muscular branch; (i) dorsal muscular branch (medial division and longitudinal anastomosis); (j) medial and lateral muscular branches of the dorsal muscular group; (k) meningoradicular artery; (l) retrocorporeal anastomosis; (m) dural branch; (arrow) prelaminar artery or dorsal epidural branch. (Modified from Lasjaunias and Berenstein, Surgical Neuroangiography [Berlin: Springer, 1990].)

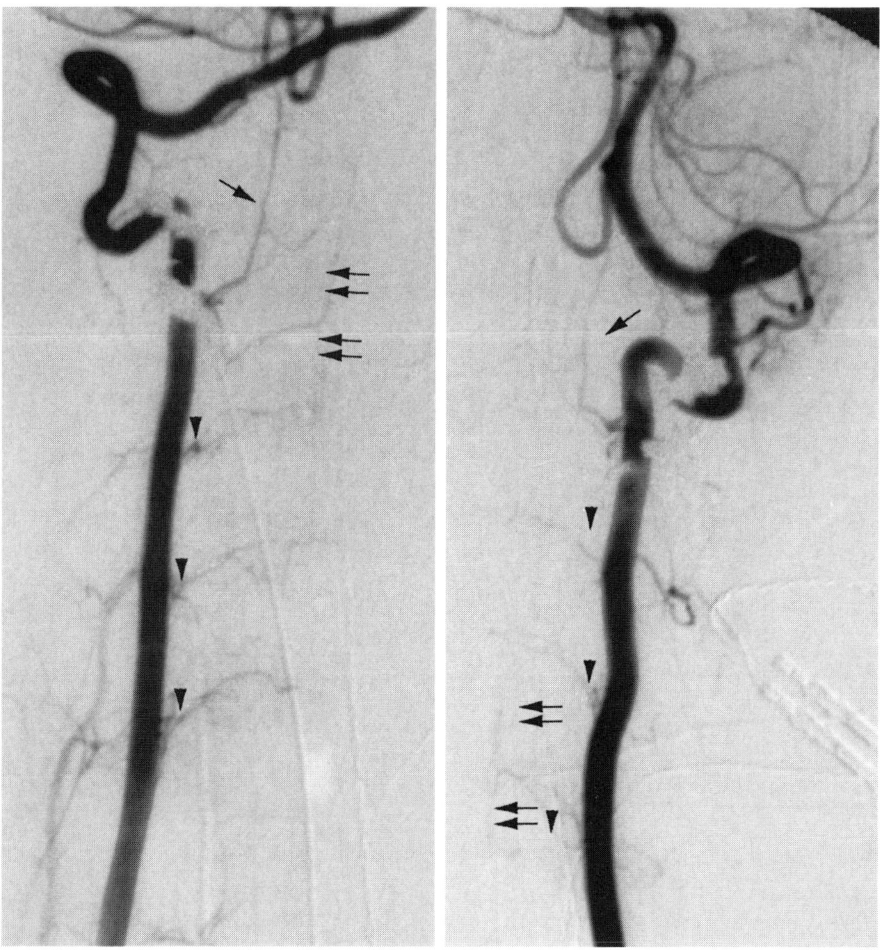

Figure 17.163. A and **B.** Anteroposterior vertebral right and left. The vertebral artery gives off a meningoradicular artery (arrowheads) at each level and on each side. The vertebral gives off the artery of C3 (one arrow), which communicates with the ascending pharyngeal, as well as the metameric reflux into the deep cervical anastomoses. The artery of the cervical enlargement, coming off both the right C3 and left C6 (double arrows) meningoradicular artery, is identified. Note that when duplicated it forms a diamond. (This should not be confused with the hexagon-square-hexagon seen in retrocorporeal dural anastomoses.)

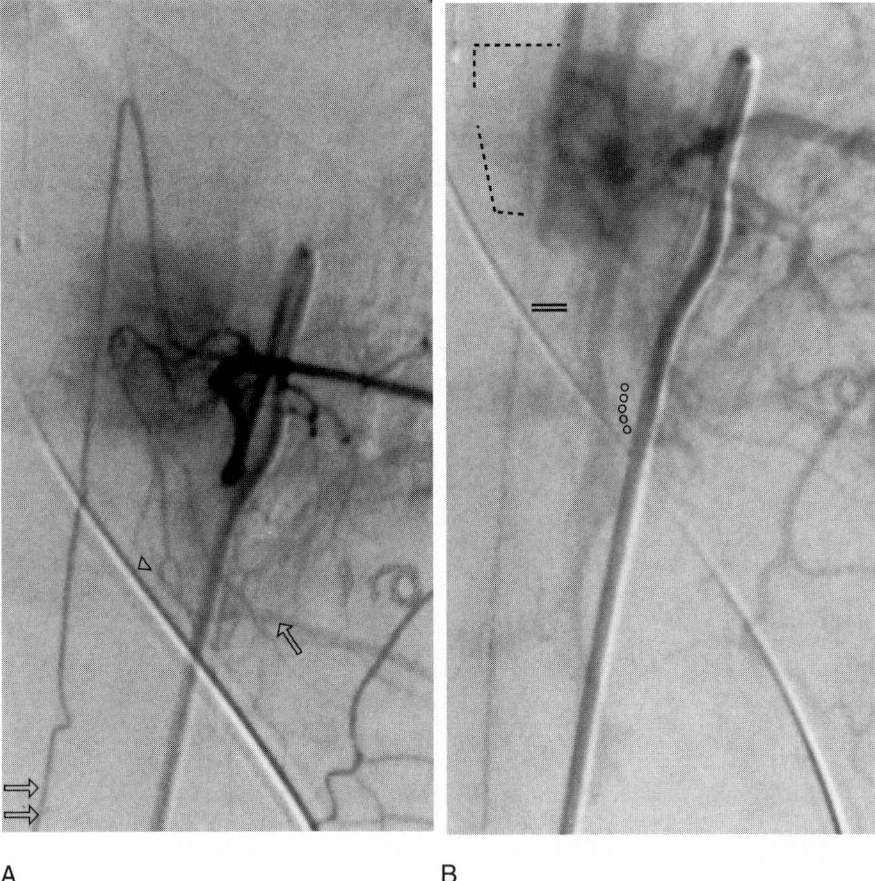

Figure 17.164. A and **B.** Anteroposterior left intercostal T9 early and late. The intercostal gives off a meningoradicular artery (arrowhead) that feeds the artery of the thoracolumbar enlargement (double arrow) (artery of Adamkiewicz). The characteristic hairpin turn is seen where the radicular artery reaches the anterior spinal axis. Note that it feeds both the ascending and descending limb. The overlaying dorsal spinal (double cross) and dorsal muscular (circle and stick) arteries can obscure the exact takeoff. The intercostal (open arrow) is well seen. Note the dense hemiblush (dotted line in B) of the vertebral body and pedicle opacified by the multiple vertebral body arteries arising from the intercostal trunk and the retrocorporeal vessels. The late phase shows a midline longitudinal vein (double sticks), presumably dorsal, and a very faint spinal cord blush. The characteristic scalloped appearance of the epidural venous plexus (row of circles) is opacified by the drainage from the basivertebral plexus and is seen to drain into the intercostal vein.

vertebral bodies grow in length faster than the spinal cord, the contribution to the spinal cord takes on an upward oblique course, which is greatest for the conus and decreases at ascending levels. This observation has been synthesized into *Chipault law.* The cord level at a given spinous process is related by this law:

1 for the cervical region

2 for the top six thoracic bodies

3 for the T6–11

Lumbar levels for last two thoracic spinous processes

Sacral levels for the thoracic level

The blood vessels supplying the spinal cord come off the vertebral arteries, aorta, hypogastrics, or their neighbors, the ascending cervicals, deep cervicals, and the bronchiolar or lateral sacral vessels. The vessels can be appreciated from Figures 17.162 through 17.164.

There are numerous anastomoses and thus variations in the blood supply of the spine, giving the vascular supply almost a network appearance. The cervical region, thoracolumbar region, and sacrococcygeal region have similar components but are packaged slightly differently. The cervical region has four longitudinal axes, and the components can originate from the external carotid artery (ascending pharyngeal, occipital), the ascending cervical artery, the deep cervical artery, or the vertebral arteries. The thoracolumbar region originates off the aorta, and the sacrococcygeal area comes off the internal iliacs or middle sacral arteries (Table 17.8).

The blood supply to the spinal cord is via *radicular arteries* that course along a nerve root, ascending from the bony foramina of origin to the somite. When they reach the cord, they split into a cephalic and a caudal division. This course gives the characteristic hairpin appearance. This can be seen on both the radicular vessel that feeds the anterior spinal axis and the vessel that feeds the posterior lateral axis (Table 17.9) (Figs. 17.164 to 17.167).

The anteriorly coursing radicular vessels reach the midline and join a longitudinal axis with the anterior spinal artery, which then gives off a sulcal artery at each level and for each side. In common parlance, the entire radicular-anterior spinal-sulcal artery complex is termed the *anterior spinal artery* (see Fig. 16.85). This vessel supplies the anterior two-thirds of the spinal cord, including the motor nuclei. Ischemia to this area gives an eerie and devastating anterior cord syndrome with loss of motor strength, pain and temperature, and sparing of the dorsal columns with intact position sense. The patient cannot move his or her extremities or feel pain but can tell the position of the extremities. The anterior spinal artery supplying the gray

Table 17.8.
Origin and Distribution of Spinal Arteries

Name	Origin	Course	Branches	Tissues fed
A. Ascending pharyngeal artery, occipital artery, ascending cervical artery, deep cervical artery, vertebral artery	ECA, Subclavian A	See discussion of each		Spine, surrounding muscles, spinal cord
B. Lumbar or intercostal artery	Aorta, IIA	Posterior lateral	Vertebral body artery (3) vertebral longitudinal artery	Spine, surrounding muscles, spinal cord
C. Middle sacral artery, hypogastric artery	Aorta, IIA			Spine, surrounding muscles, spinal cord
Vertebral body artery	Lumbar/intercostal arteries	Media	Ipsilateral and contralateral vertebral body arteries	Vertebral bodies
Lateral muscular (ventral division) artery	Lumbar/intercostal artery	Lateral	Muscular and cutaneous	Muscles and skin
Dorsal spinal artery	Lumbar/intercostal arteries	Lateral → posterior → medial	Muscular (first perforating)	
Dorsal muscular artery	Dorsal spinal artery	Posterior	Medial and lateral	Extensor muscles of the BA
Meningoradicular artery	Dorsal spinal artery	Medial	Radicular artery, retrocorporeal anastomotic artery, dural artery, prelaminar artery	Spinal and dura
(Radiculomedullary) anterior spinal artery	Radicular artery		Rostral and caudal divisions of anterior spinal artery axis, cord	Anterior portion of cord, and nerves
(Radicular-pial) → posterior spinal artery				Posterior portion of cord, and nerves

matter of the cord compensates by being larger, having an intact longitudinal axis, and having large vessels that feed the areas of highest demand, the cervical and thoracolumbar enlargements. The radicular artery that contributes to the anterior spinal artery of the cervical region is called the *artery of the cervical enlargement.* Similarly, in the thoracolumbar region it is known as the *artery of the thoracolumbar enlargement,* or the *artery of Adamkiewicz.* Four to eight radicular arteries, from 200 to 800 μm in size, contribute to the anterior spinal artery axis. The origin is highly variable and can come off almost any level.

The posteriorly coursing radicular arteries reach the posterior lateral aspect of the cord, where they then anastomose with a pial network that, when intact longitudinally, is called the *posterior lateral spinal artery.* These are about twice as numerous and half the size of the anterior spinal artery.

Anastomotic connections in the cord are many, are difficult to identify, and often are not adequate for collateral supply. They include anastomosis around the outside of the cord, the most constant one being a loop or basket around the conus medullaris, often referred to as the *arterial basket of Lazorthes.* Around the cord a pial network is present, in which descending and ascending anastomoses have been identified on microradiographs. Duplication of the anterior spinal artery is common in the cervical region, yet is rare below.

VEINS

The veins drain longitudinally. There is an extradural and intradural venous system. The cord is drained by intrinsic veins originating in the deep cord gray matter and passing radially out to the edge of the cord to be collected in extrinsic veins on the limbus of the cord. Two major veins, the duplicated *ventral spinal vein* and the *dorsal spinal vein,* are both relatively larger caudally than cephalically (1000 to 100 μm) and anastomose with each other as well as with the venous plexus on the surface of the cord. These then drain into a *radicular vein.* The latter courses along the

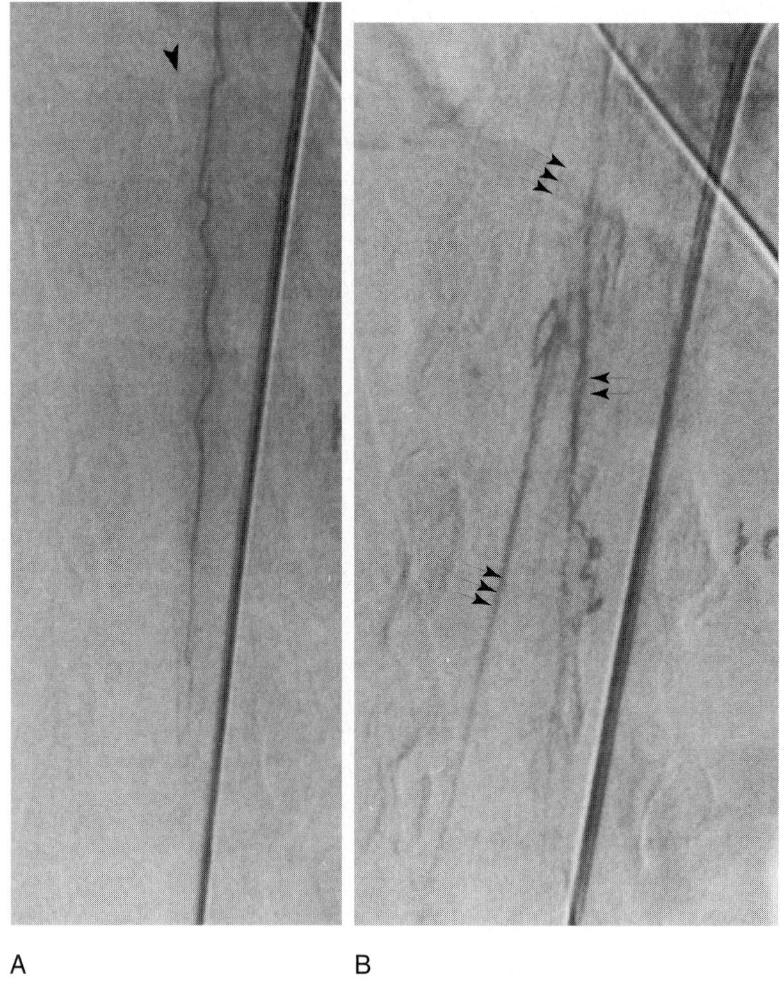

Figure 17.165. Anteroposterior left intercostal T9 injection centered at T12 arterial and venous. **A.** The anterior spinal axis is well filled. Note the faint filling of the arterial basket of Lazorthes (arrowhead) at the end of the conus. **B.** The venous phase shows well the midline longitudinal veins (double arrow) as well as an anastomotic connection to the other longitudinal vein that then drains out radicular veins (triple arrows) on the right at both T11 and T2.

Table 17.9.
Identification of Spinal Arteries

	Anterior spinal	Posteriolateral	Comment
Size	200–800 μm	100–400 μm	Variation and disease dependent
Length	Often over many segments particularly in the cervical or thoracolumbar region; both arms usually seen	Usually over a couple of segments	
Location	Midline Anterior spinal canal	Slightly off midline Posterior spinal canal	*Beware:* slight rotation of the cord or patient can distort the location
Shape	Hairpin, diamond, T	Hairpin, T	The characteristic hairpin is due to the long oblique ascending course of the radicular artery and the descending straighter anterior spinal or posterior spinal proper segment.

nerve root, reaching the epidural venous plexus after "tunneling" through the dura for some distance. There are no valves per se, but the tunneling and the angle of the drainage pathways may functionally act that way.

In Figure 17.168 the epidural system consists of two longitudinal axes. The paired basivertebral *veins* (1) are the headwaters of the epidural plexus beginning at the back of the vertebral body. They send venous blood laterally across the *retrocorporal venous plexus (anterior internal plexus)* (2) to the paired *anterior internal vertebral veins* (3), which lie inside the spinal canal. The *suprapedicular communicating vein* (4) and the *infrapedicular communicating veins* (5) connect

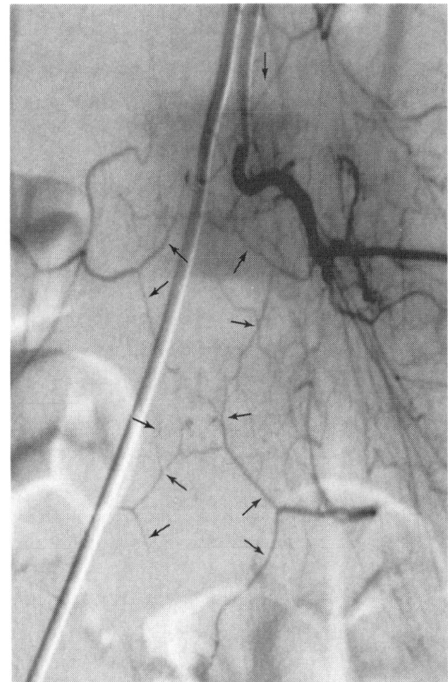

Figure 17.166. Anteroposterior left L3 lumbar artery. Filling of the retrocorporeal dural anastomoses has a characteristic pattern of repeated hexagon-square-hexagon. The small square is centered around the midportion of the vertebral body. This pattern is highly recognizable.

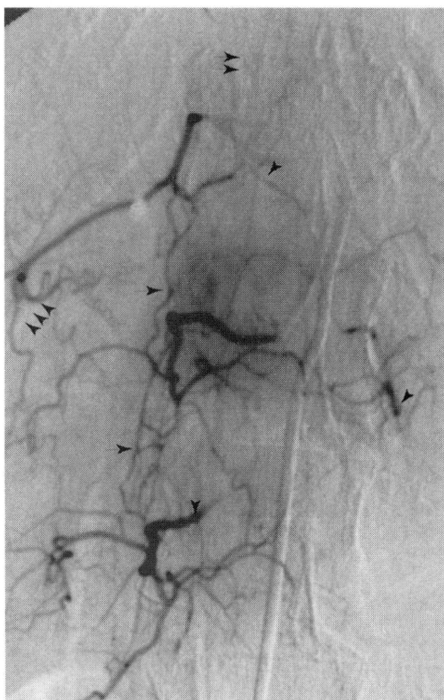

Figure 17.167. Anteroposterior right L1 lumbar artery. Injection of the right L1 opacifies the T12 and L2 (arrowheads) levels primarily via the well-developed prelongitudinal anastomotic arteries (two single arrows), as well as via muscular anastomoses (three arrows). Note filling of the radiculomedullary vessel that fills a posterior lateral axis (double arrow).

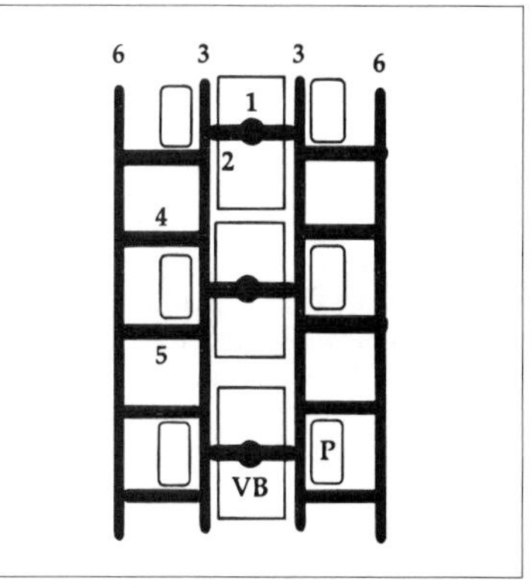

Figure 17.168. The epidural venous plexus can appear like a Jacob's ladder: (1) basivertebral veins; (2) retrocorporeal venous plexus (anterior internal plexus); (3) anterior internal vertebral veins (vertical) (AIVV); (4) suprapedicular communicating vein (SPCV); (5) infrapedicular communicating veins (IPCV); (6) external venous plexus. VB = vertebral body.

the intraspinal canal drainage to the longitudinal axis. In the cervical region this is called the *vertebral vein;* in the thoracic region, the *azygous vein;* and in the lumbosacral region, the *ascending lumbosacral veins.* These drain into the innominate veins, superior vena cava, left renal vein, and iliac veins.

REFERENCES

1. Moniz E: Arterial encephalography: Its importance in the location of cerebral tumors. Rev Neurol 1927;1:48–72.
2. Loman J, Myerson A: Visualization of cerebral vessels by direct intracarotid injection of thorium dioxide (Thoratrast). Am J Roentgenol 1936;35:188–193.
3. Shimidzu K: Beiträge zur Arteriographie des Gehirnseintache percutane Methode. Arch Klin Chir 1937;188:295.
4. Engeset A: Cerebral angiography with perabrodil (carotis angiography). Acta Radiol Suppl 56, 1944.
5. Groover RV, Chutorian AM, Nellhaus G: Neuroradiologic procedures in children: Comparison of heavy sedation and general anesthesia. Acta Radiol 1966;5:180.
6. Seldinger S: Catheter replacement of the needle in percutaneous arteriography: A new technique. Acta Radiol 1953;39:368–376.
7. Amplatz K: A new subclavian artery catheterization technique: Preliminary report. Radiology 1962;78:963–966.
8. Pygott F, Hutton CF: Vertebral arteriography by percutaneous brachial artery catheterization. Br J Radiol 1959;32:114.
9. Newton TH: The axillary approach to arteriography of the aorta and its branches. Am J Roentgenol 1963;89:275.
10. Sugar O, Holden LB, Powell CB: Vertebral angiography. Am J Roentgenol 1949;61:166.
11. Lindgren E: Percutaneous angiography of the vertebral artery. Acta Radiol 1950;33:389–404.
12. Lindgren E: Technique of direct (percutaneous) cerebral angiography. Br J Radiol 1947;20:326–331.
13. Lindgren E: Another method of vertebral angiography. Acta Radiol 1956;46:257–261.
14. Radner S: Vertebral angiography by catheterization: A new method employed in 221 cases. Acta Radiol 1951; Suppl 87.
15. Pullicino P, Kendall BE: Contrast enhancement in ischemic lesions: I. Relationship to progress. Neuroradiology 1980;19: 235–240.
16. McClennan BL: Low osmolality contrast media: Premises and promises. Radiology 1987;162:1–8.
17. Wisneski JA, Gertz EW, Neese RA, et al: Absence of myocardial biochemical toxicity with a non-ionic contrast agent (iopamidol). Am Heart J 1985;110:609–617.
18. Aaron JO, Hesselink JR, Oot R, et al: Complications of intravenous DSA performed for carotid artery disease: A prospective study. Radiology 1984;153:675–678.
19. Lasser EC: Adverse systemic reactions to contrast media. In M Sovak (ed), Radiocontrast Agents. New York: Springer, 1984, pp 525–532.
20. Rumbaugh CL, Davis DO, Gilson M: Experimental cerebral emboli: Angiographic evaluation of autologous emboli in the dog. Invest Radiol 1968;3:330–336.
21. Mishkin MM: Petechial reactions to angiography. Acta Radiol Diag 1966;5:413.
22. Amplatz K: A simple non-thrombogenic coating. Invest Radiol 1971;6:280.
23. Wallace S, Medellin H, DeJong D, et al: Systemic heparinization for angiography. Am J Roentgenol 1972;116:204.

24. Hudson JD, Joynt RJ, Pribram HFW: Water retention following neuroradiologic procedures. Arch Neurol 1967;16:624.
25. Crawford T: The pathological effects of cerebral arteriography. J Neurol Neurosurg Psychiatry 1956;19:217.
26. Allen JH, Parera C, Potts DG: The relation of arterial trauma to complications of cerebral angiography. Am J Roentgenol Radium Ther Nucl Med 1965;95:845.
27. Chase NE, Kricheff II: The comparison of the complication rates of meglumine iothalamate and sodium diatrizoate in cerebral angiography. Am J Roentgenol Radium Ther Nucl Med 1965;95:852.
28. Baird RM, Lapayowker MS, Murtagh F, et al: Percutaneous retrograde brachial arteriography. Am J Roetgenol Radium Ther Nucl Med 1965;94:19.
29. Sugar O, Bucy PC: Some complications of vertebral angiography. J Neurosurg 1954;11:607.
30. Hauge R: Catheter vertebral angiography. Acta Radiol Suppl 1954; 109.
31. Pribram HFW: Complications of angiography in cerebrovascular disease. Radiology 1965;85:33.
32. Takahashi M, Wilson G, Hanafee W: Catheter vertebral angiography: A review of 30 examinations. J Neurosurg 1969;30:722.
33. Wilson GH, Hanafee WN: Angiographic findings in 16 patients with juvenile nasopharyngeal angiofibroma. Radiology 1969;92: 279.
34. Hass WR, Fields WS, North RR, et al: Joint study of extracranial arterial occlusion: II. Arteriography, techniques, sites, and complications. JAMA 1968;203:961.
35. Alberti J, Hanafee W, Wilson G, et al: Unsuspected pulmonary collapse during neurologic procedures. Radiology 1967;89:316.
36. Brady AP, Hough DM, Lo R, et al: Transient global amnesia after cerebral angiography with iohexol. Can Assoc Radiol J 1993;44: 450–452.
37. Giang DW, Kido DK: Transient global amnesia associated with cerebral angiography performed with use of iopamidol. Radiology 1989;172:195–196.
38. Lapresle J, Lasjaunias P, Thevenier D: Transitory paralysis of cranial nerves IX, X and XII as well as the left VII after angiography: Contribution to the ischemic pathology of the cranial nerves. Rev Neurol 1980;136:787–791.
39. Grzyska U, Freitag J, Zeumer H: Selective cerebral intraarterial DSA: Complication rate and control of risk factors. Neuroradiology 1990;32:296–299.
40. Uchino A. Local complications in transbrachial cerebral angiography using the 4-F catheter. Neurologia Medic Chirurgica 1991; 31:647–649.
41. Bachman DM: Microscopic air embolism during cerebral angiography, letter; comment. Lancet 1993;341:1537–1538.
42. Markus H, Loh A, Israel D, et al: Microscopic air embolism during cerebral angiography and strategies of its avoidance. Lancet 1993; 341:784–787.
43. Ginsberg LE, Stump DA, King JC, et al: Air embolus risk with glass versus plastic syringes: In vitro study and implications for neuroangiography. Radiology 1994;191:813–816.
44. Roberson GH, Scott WR: Thrombi at the site of carotid stenosis. Radiology 1973;109:353.
45. Ecker AD: The Normal Cerebral Angiogram. Springfield, IL: Charles C Thomas, 1951.
46. Chase NE, Taveras JM: Carotid angiography in the diagnosis of extradural parasellar tumor. Acta Radiol 1963;1:214.
47. Vignaud J, Clay C, Bilaniuk LT. Venography of the orbit; an analytical report of 413 cases. Radiology 1974;110:373–382.
48. Tenner MS, Trokel SL: A simple device for jugular-vein compression: A technical note. Radiology 1970;96:60.
49. Hilal SK: Hemodynamic response in the cerebral vessels to angiographic contrast media. Acta Radiol 1966;5:211.
50. Broman T, Olsson O: Experimental study of contrast media for cerebral angiography with reference to possible injurious effects on the cerebral blood vessels. Acta Radiol 1949;31:321.
51. Bassett RC, Rogers JS, Cherry GR, et al: The effect of contrast media on the blood-brain barrier. J Neurosurg 1953;10:38.
52. Harris AB: Steroids and blood-brain barrier alterations in sodium acetrizoate injury. Arch Neurol 1967;17:282.
53. McConnell EM: The arterial blood supply of the human hypophysis cerebri. Anat Rec 1953;115:175.
54. Parkinson D: Collateral circulation of cavernous carotid artery: Anatomy. Can J Surg 1964;7:251.
55. Parkinson D: A surgical approach to the cavernous portion of the carotid artery: Anatomical studies and case report. J Neurosurg 1965;23:474.
56. Bernasconi V, Casinari V: Caratteritische angiografiche die meningiomi del tentorio. Radiol Med 1957;43:1015.
57. Schnurer LB, Stattin S: Vascular supply of intracranial dura from internal carotid artery with special reference to its angiographic significance. Acta Radiol Diagn 1963;1:441.
58. Margolis MT, Newton TH: Collateral pathways between the cavernous portion of the internal carotid and external carotid arteries. Radiology 1969;93:834.
59. Hacker H, Alonso A: Uberdie angiographische Dartstellung eines kappillaren Gefassnetzes am dorsum sellae and seine Deutung als neurohypophyse. Fortschr Rontgenstr 1968;108:141.
60. Lehrer HZ: Angiographic visualization of the posterior pituitary and clinical stress. Radiology 1970;94:7.
61. Baker HL Jr: The angiographic delineation of sellar and parasellar masses. Radiology 1972;104:67.
62. Pollock JA, Newton TH: The anterior falx artery: Normal and pathologic anatomy. Radiology 1968;91:1089.
63. Brucher J: Origin of ophthalmic artery from the middle meningeal artery. Radiology 1969;93:51.
64. Ducasse A, Segal A, Delatre JF, et al: Participation of the external carotid artery in orbital vascularization. (French). J Fr Ophtalmol 1985;8:333–339.
65. Stein BM, McCormick W, Rodriquez JN, et al: Incidence and significance of occlusive vascular disease of the extracranial arteries as demonstrated by postmortem angiography. Trans Am Neurol Assoc 1961;86:60.
66. Teal JS, Rumbaugh CL, Bergeron RT, et al: Congenital absence of the internal carotid artery associated with cerebral hemiatrophy, absence of the external carotid artery, and persistence of the stapedial artery. Am J Roentgenol Radium Ther Nucl Med 1973;118: 534.
67. Gray H: Anatomy of the Human Body, Charles Mayo Goss (ed). ed 23. Philadelphia: Lea and Febiger, 1959.
68. Turnbull I: Agenesis of the internal carotid artery. Neurology 1962;12:588.
69. Prensky AL, Davis DO: Obstruction of major cerebral vessels in early childhood without neurological signs. Neurology 1970;20: 945.
70. Tanaka K, Yonekawa Y, Matsuba K: Hypoplasia of the internal carotid artery: Report of an unusual case. Neurol Med Chir 1991; 31:290–291.
71. Lapayowker MS, Liebman EP, Ronis ML, Safer JN: Presentation of the internal carotid artery as a tumor of the middle ear. Radiology 1971;98:293.
72. Padget DH: The circle of Willis, its embryology and anatomy. In WE Dandy (ed), Intracranial Aneurysms. Ithaca, NY: Comstock, 1944, p 67.
73. Saltzman GF: Patent primitive trigeminal artery studied by cerebral angiography. Acta Radiol 1959;51:329.
74. Lie TA: Congenital Anomalies of the Carotid Arteries. Amsterdam: Excerpta Medica Foundation, 1968.
75. Teal JS, Rumbaugh CL, Bergeron RT, et al: Persistent carotid-superior cerebellar artery anastomosis: A variant of persistent trigeminal artery. Radiology 1972;103:335.

76. Obayashi T, Furuse M: The proatlantal intersegmental artery: A case report and review of the literature. Arch Neurol 1980;37: 387–389.
77. Sato H, Ogawa A, Kitahara M, et al: Persistent primitive first cervical intersegmental artery (proatlantal artery II) with occlusion of the basilar artery: A case report, review (Japanese). Brain & Nerve 1988;40:219–224.
78. Carpenter MB, Noback CR, Moss ML: The anterior choroidal artery: Its origins, course, distribution, and variations. Arch Neurol Psychiatry 1954;71:714.
79. Sjogren SE: The anterior choroidal artery. Acta Radiol 1956;46: 143–157.
80. Takahashi S, Suga T, Kawata Y, et al: Anterior choroidal artery: Angiographic analysis of variation and anomalies. AJNR 1990;11: 719–729.
81. Helgason CM: A new view of anterior choroidal artery territory infarction. J Neurol 1988;235:387–391.
82. Marinkovic S, Kovacevic M, Milisavljevic M: Hypoplasia of the proximal segment of the anterior cerebral artery. Anat Anz 1989; 168:145–154.
83. Kitami K, Kamiyana H, Yasui N: Angiographic analysis of the anterior cerebral arteries with cerebral aneurysms—with special interest in the morphological aspect including so-called vascular anomalies (Japanese). No Shinkei Geka 1985;13:1161–1167.
84. Lazorthes G: Vascularisation et circulation cérébrales. Paris: Masson, 1961.
85. Heubner A.—Zur Topographie der Ennahrungsgebiete der eincelen Hirnarterien. Zentalbl Med Wiss 1872;52:817–826.
86. Gomes FB, Dujoyny M, Umansky F, et al: Microanatomy of the anterior cerebral artery. Surg Neurol 1986;26:129–141.
87. Marinkovic S, Milisavljevic M, Marinkovic Z: Anastomoses among the perforating arteries of the brain: Microanatomy and clinical significance. Neurologija 1990;39:107–114.
88. Marinkovic S, Milisavljevic M, Marinkovic Z: Branches of the anterior communicating artery. Microsurgical anatomy. Acta Neurochir 1990;106:78–85.
89. Foix Ch, Hillemand P: Les arteres cerebrales. C R Seances Soc Biol 1925;92:31–33.
90. Fischer E: Die Lageabweichungen der vorderen Hirnarterie im Gefasbild. Zentralbl Neurochir 1938;3:300–313.
91. Salamon G: Atlas de la vacularisation arterielle du cerveau chez l'homme. Paris: Sandoz, 1973.
92. Taveras JM, Wood EW: Diagnostic Neuroradiology. Baltimore, MD: Williams and Wilkins, 1964, p 501.
93. Vander Eecken HM: Discussion of "Collateral Circulation of the Brain." Proceedings of International Conference on Vascular Diseases of the Brain. Neurology 1961;11:16.
94. Wolfram-Gabel R, Maillot C, Koritke JG: Arterial vascularization of the corpus callosum in man (French). Arch Anat Histol Embryol 1989;72:43–55.
95. Ring BA, Waddington MM: Roentgenographic anatomy of the pericallosal arteries. AJR 1968;104:109–118.
96. Salamon G, Huang YP: Radiologic Anatomy of the Brain. Berlin: Springer, 1976.
97. Padget DH: The development of the cranial arteries in the human embryo. Contrib Embryol Carnegie Inst 1948;32:205.
98. Teal JS, Rumbaugh CL, Segall HD, et al: Anomalous branches of the internal carotid artery. Radiology 1973;106:123.
99. Mercier P, Velut S, Fournier D, et al: A rare embryologic variation: Carotid-anterior cerebral artery anastomosis or infraoptic course of the anterior cerebral artery (Review). Surg Radiol Anat 1989; 11:73–77.
100. Mäurer J, Mäurer E, Perneczky A: Surgically verified variations in the A1 segment of the anterior cerebral artery. J Neurosurg 1991; 75:950–953.
101. Jain KK: Some observations on the anatomy of the middle cerebral artery. Can J Surg 1964;7:134.
102. Tran-Dinh H: The accessory middle cerebral artery: A variant of the recurrent artery of Heubner (A centralis longa)? Acta Anat 1986;126:167–171.
103. Onishi H, Yamashita J, Enkaku F, Fujisawa H: Anomalous origin of the anterior cerebral artery and congenital skull dysplasia: Case report. Neurol Med Chir 1992;32:296–299.
104. Ogawa A, Suzuki M, Sakurai Y, et al: Vascular anomalies associated with aneurysms of the anterior communicating artery: Microsurgical observations. J Neurosurg 1990;72:706–709.
105. Stephens RB, Stillwell DL: Arteries and Veins of the Brain. Springfield, IL: Charles C Thomas, 1969.
106. Salamon G, Boudouresques J, Combalbert A, et al: Les arteres lenticulostriées. Etude arteriographique. Leur interet dans le diagnostic des hematomes intracerebraux. Rev Neurol 1966;114:361.
107. Westberg G: The recurrent artery of Heubner and the arteries of the central ganglia. Acta Radiol Diagn 1963;1:949.
108. Westberg G: Arteries of the basal ganglia. Acta Radiol 1966;5:581.
109. Kaplan HA: Vascular supply of the base of the brain. In WS Fields (ed), Pathogenesis and Treatment of Parkinsonism. Springfield, IL: Charles C Thomas, 1958.
110. Ghika JA, Bogousslavsky J, Regli F: Deep perforators from the carotid system: Template of the vascular territories (Review). Arch Neurol 1990;47:1097–1100.
111. Rosner SS, Rhoton A Jr, Ono M, et al: Microsurgical anatomy of the anterior perforating arteries. J Neurosurg 1984;61:468–485.
112. Umansky F, Gomes FB, Dujovny M, et al: The perforating branches of the middle cerebral artery: A microanatomical study. J Neurosurg 1985;62:261–268.
113. Gibo H, Carver CC, Rhoton A Jr., et al: Microsurgical anatomy of the middle cerebral artery. J Neurosurg 1981;54:151–169.
114. Vander Eecken HM: The Anastomoses between the Leptomeningeal Arteries of the Brain: Their Morphological, Pathological and Clinical Significance. Springfield, IL: Charles C Thomas, 1959.
115. Van der Zwan A, Hillen B, Tulleken CA: Variability of the territories of the major cerebral arteries. J Neurosurg 1992;77:927–940.
116. Ring BA, Waddington MM: Angiographic identification of the motor strip. J Neurosurg 1967;26:249–254.
117. Andersen PE: The lenticulo-striate arteries and their diagnostic value: A preliminary report. Acta Radiol 1958;50:84.
118. Taveras JM, Poser CM: Roentgenologic aspects of cerebral angiography in children. Am J Roentgenol Radium Ther Nucl Med 1959; 82:371.
119. Jimenez JP, Goree JA: The normal middle cerebral artery axis. Am J Roentgenol Radium Ther Nucl Med 1967;101:88.
120. Romer AS: The Vertebrate Body, ed 4. London: Saunders, 1970.
121. Shellshear JL. A contribution to the knowledge of the arterial supply of the cerebral cortex in man. Brain 1927;50:236–253.
122. Lasjaunias P, Berenstein A: Surgical Neuroangiography. Berlin: Springer, 1990.
123. Krayenbuhl Y, Yasargil MG: Cerebral Angiography. Philadelphia: Lippincott, 1968.
124. Umansky F, Juarez SM, Dujovny M, et al: Microsurgical anatomy of the proximal segments of the middle cerebral artery. J Neurosurg 1984;61:458–467.
125. Muller HR, Brunholzl C, Radu EW, Buser M: Sex and size differences of cerebral arterial caliber. Neuroradiology 1991;33: 212–216.
126. Rositti S, Lofgren J: Optimality principles and flow orderliness at the branching points of cerebral arteries. Stroke 1993;24: 1029–1032.
127. Hoyt WF, Newton TH, Margolis MT: The posterior cerebral artery: Embryology and developmental anomalies. In TH Newton, GD Potts (eds), Radiology of the Skull and Brain. St. Louis, MO: Mosby, 1974, p 1540.
128. Saltzman GF: Angiographic demonstration of the posterior communicating and posterior cerebral arteries: I. Normal angiography. Acta Radiol 1959;51:1.

129. Fox JL, Boez TC, Jakoby RH: Differentiation of aneurysm from infundibulum of the posterior communicating artery. J Neurosurg 1964;21:135–138.
130. Epstein BS, Ransohoff J, Budzilovich GN: The clinical significance of junctional dilatation of the posterior communicating artery. J Neurosurg 1970;33:529.
131. Hara K, Fujino Y: The thalamoperforate artery. Acta Radiol 1965; 5:192.
132. Wolfram-Gabel R, Maillot C, Koritke JG, et al: The vascularization of the human tela choroidea of the lateral ventricle (French). Acta Anat 1987;128:301–321.
133. Saltzman, GF: Angiographic demonstration of the posterior communicating and posterior cerebral arteries: I. Normal angiography. Acta Radiol 1959;51: 1; II. Pathologic angiography. Acta Radiol 1959;52:114.
134. Caruso G, Vincentelli F, Rabehanta P, et al: Anomalies of the P1 segment of the posterior cerebral artery: Early bifurcation or duplication, fenestration, common trunk with the superior cerebellar artery. Acta Neurochir 1991;109:66–71.
135. Galloway JR, Greitz T: The medial and lateral choroid arteries: An anatomic and roentgenographic study. Acta Radiol 1960;53: 353.
136. Erdem A, Yasargil G, Roth P: Microsurgical anatomy of the hippocampal arteries. J Neurosurg 1993;79:256–265.
137. Marinkovic S, Milisavljevic M, Kovacevic M. Interpeduncular perforating branches of the posterior cerebral artery. Microsurgical anatomy of their extracerebral and intracerebral segments. Surg Neurol 1986;26:349–359.
138. Milisavljevic MM, Marinkovic S, Gibo H, et al: The thalamogeniculate perforators of the posterior cerebral artery: The microsurgical anatomy. Neurosurgery 1991;28:523–529.
139. Pedroza A, Dujovny M, Cabezudo-Artero JC, et al: Microanatomy of the premamillary artery. Acta Neurochir 1987;86:50–55.
140. Pedroza A, Dujovny M, Artero JC, et al: Microanatomy of the posterior communicating artery. Neurosurgery 1987;20:228–235.
141. Caplan LR, De Witt LD, Pessin MS, et al: Lateral thalamic infarcts (Review). Arch Neurol 1988;45:959–964.
142. Johnson RT, Yates PO: Clinico-pathological aspects of pressure changes at the tentorium. Acta Radiol 1956;46:242.
143. Stein BM, McCormick W, Rodriquez JN, et al: Postmortem angiography of cerebral vascular system. Arch Neurol 1962;7:545.
144. Teal JS, Rumbaugh CL, Bergeron RT, et al: Angiographic demonstration of fenestration of the intradural arteries. Radiology 1973; 106:123.
145. Cavdar S, Arisen E: Variations in the extracranial origin of the human vertebral artery. Acta Anat 1989;135:236–238.
146. Krayenbuhl Y, Yasargil MG: Die vaskularen Erkrankungen im Gebiet der Arteria Vertebralis und Arteria Basialis. Stuttgart: Thieme, 1957.
147. Chopard RP, Lucas GA, Laudana A: Microscopic anatomy of the human vertebro-basilar system. Arq Neuropsiquiatr 1991;49: 430–433.
148. Chopard RP, de Miranda Neto MH, Lucas GA, et al: The vertebral artery: Its relationship with adjoining tissues in its course intra and inter transverse processes in man. Rev Paul Med 1992;110: 245–250.
149. Greitz T, Lauren T: Anterior meningeal branch of the vertebral artery. Acta Radiol Diag 1968;7:219.
150. Dilenge D, David M: La Branche meningie de l'artere vertebrale. Neurochirurgie 1967;13:121.
151. Hawkins TD, Melcher DH: A meningeal artery in the falx cerebelli. Clin Radiol 1966;17:377.
152. Schechter MM, Zingesser LH: The spinal arteries. Acta Radiol 1966;5:1124–1131.
153. Rodriguez-Baeza A, Muset-Lara A, Rodriguez-Pazos M, et al: Anterior spinal arteries: Origin and distribution in man. Acta Anat 1989;136:217–221.
154. Huang YP, Wolf BS: Angiographic features of fourth ventricle tumors with special reference to the posterior inferior cerebellar artery. Am J Roentgenol Radium Ther Nucl Med 1969;107:543.
155. Greitz T, Sjogren S: The posterior inferior cerebellar artery. Acta Radiol 1963;1:284.
156. Angevine JB Jr, Mancall EL, Yakovlev PI: The Human Cerebellum: An Atlas of Gross Topography in Spinal Sections. Boston: Little, Brown, 1961.
157. Huang YP, Wolf BS: Angiographic features of brain stem tumors and differential diagnosis from fourth ventricle tumors. Am J Roentgenol Radium Ther Nucl Med 1970;110:1.
158. Aubin M, Metzger J, Kobayashi N, et al: Visibilité et contours des structures de la fosse posterieure sur les temps capillaires et veineuz de l'angiographie vertebrale. Paper presented at the Ninth Symposium Neuroradiologicum, Gothenberg, Sweden, 24–29 August 1970.
159. Caruso G, Vincenelli F, Giudicelli G, et al: Perforating branches of the basilar bifurcation. J Neurosurg 1990;73:259–265.
160. Pedroza A, Dujovny M, Ausman JI, et al: Microvascular anatomy of the interpeduncular fossa. J Neurosurg 1986;64:484–493.
161. Torche M, Mahmood A, Araujo R, et al: Microsurgical anatomy of the lower basilar artery. Neurol Res 1992;14:259–262.
162. Smaltino F, Bernini FP, Elefante R: Normal and pathological findings of the angiographic examination of the internal auditory artery. Neuroradiology 1971;2:216.
163. Bebin J: The cerebellopontine angle, the blood supply of the brain stem and the reticular formation. Part 1. Henry Ford Hosp Med J 1968;16:61.
164. Kim HN, Kim YH, Park IY, et al: Variability of the surgical anatomy of the neurovascular complex of the cerebellopontine angle. Ann Otol Rhinol Laryngol 1990;99:288–296.
165. Woischneck D, Hussein S: The anterior inferior cerebellar artery (AICA): Clinical and radiological significance. Neurosurg Rev 1991;14:293–295.
166. Huang YP, Wolf BS, Antin SP, et al: Angiographic features of aqueductal stenosis. Am J Roentgenol Radium Ther Nucl Med 1968;104:90.
167. Hardy DG, Peace DA, Rhoton A Jr: Microsurgical anatomy of the superior cerebellar artery. Neurosurgery 1980;6:10–28.
168. Shrontz C, Jujovny M, Ausman JI, et al: Surgical anatomy of the arteries of the posterior fossa. J Neurosurg 1986;65:540–544.
169. Wolf BS, Huang YP, Newman CM: The superficial sylvian venous drainage system. Am J Roentgenol Radium Ther Nucl Med 1963; 89:398.
170. Ring BA: Variations of the striate and other cerebral veins affecting measurements of the "venous angle." Acta Radiol 1959;52:433.
171. Wolf BS, Newman CM, Schlesinger B: The diagnostic value of the deep cerebral veins in cerebral angiography. Radiology 1955; 64:161.
172. Laine E, Delandtsheer JM, Galibert P, et al: Phlebography in tumors of hemispheres and central grey matter. Acta Radiol 1956; 46:203.
173. Wolf BS, Huang YP: The subependymal veins of the lateral ventricles. Am J Roentgenol Radium Ther Nucl Med 1964;91:406.
174. Padget DH: The cranial venous system in man in reference to development, adult configuration, and relation to the arteries. Am J Anat 1956;98:307.
175. Padget DH: The development of the cranial venous system in man, from the viewpoint of comparative anatomy. Contrib Embryol 1957;36:79.
176. Wolf BS, Huang YP, Newman CM: The lateral anastomotic mesencephalic vein and other variations in drainage of the basal cerebral vein. Am J Roentgenol 1963;89:411.
177. Huang YP, Wolf BS: The veins of the posterior fossa–superior or galenic draining group. Am J Roentgenol 1965;95:808.
178. Huang YP, Wolf BS, Antin SP, et al: The veins of the posterior fossa–anterior or petrosal draining group. Am J Roentgenol 1968; 104:36.
179. Greitz T: A radiologic study of the brain circulation by rapid serial angiography of the carotid artery. Acta Radiol Suppl 1956;140.

180. Greitz T, Cronqvist S: Cerebral circulation studied with angiography and isotope technique: A comparative study. In J Taveras, H Fischgold, D Dilenge (eds), Recent Advances in the Studies of Cerebral Circulation. Springfield, IL: Charles C Thomas, 1970.

181. Newton TH, Weidner W, Greitz T: Dural arteriovenous malformation in the posterior fossa. Radiology 1968;90:27.

182. Newton TH, Hoyt WF: Dural arteriovenous shunts in the region of the cavernous sinus. Neuroradiology 1970;1:71.

183. Newton TH, Cronqvist S: Involvement of dural arteries in intracranial arteriovenous malformations. Radiology 1969;93:1071.

184. Schechter MM, Zingesser LH, Rayport M: Torn meningeal vessels: An evaluation of a clinical spectrum through the use of angiography. Radiology 1966;86:686.

185. Thron AK: Vascular anatomy of the spinal cord: Neuroradiological investigations and clinical syndromes. Berlin: Springer, 1988.

SELECTED READINGS

Baker HL Jr: Cerebellopontine angle myelography. J Neurosurg 1972; 104:67.

Cohen AM, Doershuk CF, Stern RC: Bronchial artery embolization to control hemoptysis in cystic fibrosis. Radiology 1990;175:401–405.

Crowell RM, Morawetz RB: The anterior communicating artery has significant branches. Stroke 1977;8:272–273.

Dawson P: New contrast agents: Chemistry and pharmacology. Invest Radiol 1984;19:S293–S300.

Fisher CM: The posterior cerebral artery syndrome. Can J Neurol Sci 1986;13:232–239.

Gibo H, Lenkey C, Rhoton A Jr: Microsurgical anatomy of the supraclinoid portion of the internal carotid artery. J Neurosurg 1981;55: 560–574.

Gorczyca W, Mohr G: Microvascular anatomy of Heubner's recurrent artery. Neurol Res 1987;9:259–264.

Hankey GJ, Warlow CP, Sellar RJ: Cerebral angiographic risk in mild cerebrovascular disease (Review). Stroke 1990;21:209–222.

Hassler O, Saltzman GF: Angiographic and histologic changes in infundibular widening of the posterior communicating artery. Acta Radiol 1963;1:321.

Hilal SK, Tookoian H, Wood EH: Displacement of the aqueduct of Sylvius by posterior fossa tumors. Acta Radiol 1969;9:167.

Hunt WE, Hess RM: Surgical risk as related to time of intervention in the repair of intracranial aneurysms. J Neurosurg 1968;28:14.

Krayenbuhl H, Richter HR: Die Zerebrale Angiographie. Stuttgart: Thieme, 1952.

Lazorthes G, Poulhes J, Bastide G, et al: La vascularisation arterielle de la moelle. Neurochirurgie 1958;4:3.

Lemos VP, Medeiros MM, De Carvalho RC: Neuroanatomical study of the orbitofrontal branch of the anterior cerebral artery in human brains (Portuguese). Arq Neuropsiquiatr 1984;42:9–13.

Lussenhop AJ: Artificial embolization for cerebral arteriovenous malformations. Progr Neurol Surg 1969;3:320.

Madden JA: The effect of carbon dioxide on cerebral arteries (Review). Pharmacol Ther 1993;59:229–250.

Mahmood A, Dujovny M, Torche M, et al: Microvascular anatomy of foramen caecum medullae oblongatae. J Neurosurg 1991;75:299–304.

Marinkovic SV, Milisavljevic MM, Vuckovic VD: Microvascular anatomy of the uncus and the parahippocampal gyrus. Neurosurgery 1991;29: 805–814.

Pascual-Castroviejo I: Persistence of the stapedial artery in a first arch anomaly: A case report. Cleft Palate J 1988;20:146–150.

Saeki N, Rhoton A Jr: Microsurgical anatomy of the upper basilar artery and the posterior circle of Willis. J Neurosurg 1984;61:468–485.

Saunders WP, Sorek PA, Mehta BA: Fenestration of intracranial arteries with special attention to associated aneurysms and other anomalies. AJNR 1993;14:675–680.

Serbinenko FA: Balloon catheterization and occlusion of major cerebral vessels. J Neurosurg 1974;41:125.

Sheffield Ea, Weller RO: Age changes at cerebral artery bifurcations and the pathogenesis of berry aneurysms. J Neurol Sci 1980;46;341–352.

Sjogren SE: Percutaneous vertebral angiography. Acta Radiol 1953;40: 113.

Sliwa JA, Maclean IC: Ischemic myelopathy: A review of spinal vasculature and related clinical syndromes. Arch Phys Med Rehabil 1992;73: 365–372.

Stehbens WE: Etiology of intracranial berry aneurysms. J Neurosurg 1989;70:823–831.

Stern J, Correll JW, Bryan N: Persistent hypoglossal artery and persistent trigeminal artery presenting with posterior fossa transient ischemic attacks: Report of two cases. J Neurosurg 1978;49:614–619.

Takahashi S, Hoshino F, Uemura K, et al: Accessory middle cerebral artery: Is it a variant form of the recurrent artery of Heubner? AJNR 1989;10:563–568.

Teal JS, Bergeron RT, Rumbaugh CL, et al: Aneurysms of the petrous or cavernous portion of the internal carotid artery associated with nonpenetrating head trauma. J Neurosurg 1973;38:568.

Vitte E, Feron JM, Guerin-Surville H, et al: Anatomical study of digital compression of the vertebral artery at its origin and at the suboccipital triangle. Anat Clin 1985;7:77–82.

Yamamoto I, Rhoton A Jr, Peace DA: Microsurgery of the third ventricle: Part I. Microsurgical anatomy. Neurosurgery 1981;8:334–356.

18

Endovascular Therapeutic Neuroradiology

John Pile-Spellman

18.1 Introduction

Interventional neuroradiology grows along out of both surgical and radiologic tradition. It is a clinical practice that requires the integration of radiologic and clinical skills, with the advent of new materials and greater understanding of the disease. Endovascular procedures will continue to have an ever-increasing impact on clinical care.

This chapter represents the interventional neuroradiology portion of this work. We have chosen the title "Endovascular Therapeutic Neuroradiology" because all of the items discussed take an endovascular approach. There are three other areas that could be included in a chapter on interventional neuroradiology: stereotactic biopsies of cerebral lesions; percutaneous discectomy; and percutaneous injection of plastic material into collapsed vertebral bodies, particularly in the thoracic region. However, it is likely that these would be handled by either neurosurgeons or orthopedic surgeons, as is the case at the Massachusetts

General Hospital and the Neurological Institute of Columbia Presbyterian Medical Center.

The chapter is divided into twelve sections including this introduction. Each section is separated as a subchapter with its own bibliographic references for the convenience of the reader. The sections are as follows:

18.1. Introduction
18.2. Materials and Methods (by John Pile-Spellman and William L. Young)
18.3. Arteriovenous fistulas
18.4. Cerebral Arteriovenous Malformations
18.5. Dural Arteriovenous Malformations
18.6. Spinal Arteriovenous Malformations
18.7. Aneurysms
18.8. Vasospasm
18.9. Hyperacute Intra-arterial Thrombolytic Therapy for Thromboembolic Stroke (by John Pile-Spellman and Ichiro Nakara)
18.10. Brachiocephalic Angioplasty
18.11. Craniofacial Pathology (by Lotfi Hacein-Bey and John Pile-Spellman)
18.12. Endovascular Management of Injuries to the Extracranial Carotid and Vertebral Arteries (by E. Sander Connolly, Jr., and John Pile-Spellman)

Although the references are numbered separately for each section, the tables and illustrations are numbered in sequence throughout the entire chapter.

18.2 Materials and Methods for Interventional Neuroradiology (INR)

John Pile-Spellman and William L. Young*

Key Points

1. Transfemoral arterial access with a triaxial system under full heparinization is the most common approach, although many approaches are needed.
2. An embolic agent should be controllable, radiodense, as permanent as needed, and have Food and Drug Administration (FDA) approval.
3. Treat the abnormal vessels, and spare the normal vessels.
4. Tailored anesthetic care adds profoundly to the success and safety of endovascular treatment.
5. Postoperative monitoring and management are critical.
6. Interventional materials and methods can be considered extensions of our hands and minds. Sympathetic understanding of materials and methods is needed to use them effectively.

Access

It is now possible to access a target region safely using various devices and materials. The routine approach is the transfemoral arterial approach, but a variety of approaches can be used, including direct cutaneous, transfemoral venous, transcarotid, and transjugular. A triaxial system consists of a sheath, a guiding catheter, and a microcatheter. Figure 18.1 illustrates the most commonly used system. The system must work together as a unit (1–4).

PUMPS, TUBING, AND PRESSURE TRANSDUCERS

The space between the catheters must be perfused with heparinized saline (2000 units heparin/500 ml normal saline) to avoid clot formation and subsequent embolization. Air must be excluded. High-pressure tubing can be used with either pressure packs or pumps. Pressure transducers within the circuit give a great deal of useful information. The femoral line is used to monitor the patient's systemic blood pressure and can be used to draw blood activated coagulated time (ACT) and arterial blood gas (ABG) tests as required. The microcatheter or distal catheter can give information regarding the pathophysiology of the brain vessels (5,6,7). In arteriovenous malformations (AVMs) there is usually a 30 to 60 percent drop in the mean pressure, and across a significant stenosis there is also such a drop (8,9). If the catheters become occluded, there is a loss of the waveform and a rise in the pressure. Catheters that are wedged should not be perfused with a pressure pack. If it is necessary to infuse a wedged catheter, perfusion by hand under fluoroscopic control is preferred. Alternatively, a pressure-regulated pump that is equipped to have both pressure and volume limits can be used. Inadvertent perfusion of a wedged catheter can lead to overperfusion and rupture.

SHEATHS AND SIZES

There is a confusing array of size units. French, gauge, mils(1/1000 inch), millimeters, microns, and United States Pharmacopeia (USP) are used sometimes in reference to the inner diameter and sometimes to the outer diameter. See Tables 18.1 and 18.2. In addition, critical tolerances are not given. Hydrophilic catheters swell slightly when placed in the body, and slight kinking in storage or in the body, tapering of the tip, or irregularity of the inner surface all decrease tolerances. If not allowed for, these lowered tolerances can add dangerously to the difficulty of the procedure. For this reason, a family of sheaths, guiding cathe-

* Associate Professor of Anesthesiology (in Neurological Surgery and in Radiology), Department of Anesthesiology, Columbia University College of Physicians & Surgeons, New York, New York.

Table 18.1.
Device Measurements

French (F)	Gauge (Gg)	Mils	Millimeters	Microns	USP*
Outer catheter: inner sheath's diameter in millimeters.	Needles: higher number = smaller needle size, †OD.	Guide wire: thousandth of an inch called "038" or just "38," written as .038.	Inner catheter: most important, most variable, and most often not given.	Emboli: 1 millimeter = 1000 microns.	Suture: smallest called "4-0," largest called "4," with 0 being in the middle (i.e., 4, 3, 2, 1, 0,000,000).

* United States Pharmacopeia.
† OD = outer diameter

ters, and microcatheters should be on hand. Any alteration should be checked in vitro prior to use.

The sheath consists of a short piece of tubing, a side-in, and a check flow valve. The size of the sheath is the inner diameter or the size of the guiding catheter that it will accept. A half-size-larger sheath than the guiding catheter is used to allow pressure monitoring and blood samples to be removed. A thin wall and a nonkinkable shaft are characteristics to evaluate in the selection of sheaths. The check valve consists of a flap, or O-ring. A good check valve should allow a wide range of catheters to advance without leaking. We prefer using a sheath in almost all angiographic procedures. Advantages include (a) greater ease of manipulation of the catheter, (b) less trauma to the femoral vessels caused by the repeated manipulation, (c) ease of exchange for a different catheter, (d) a more horizonal and thus a lower puncture site with less bending of the catheter at that spot, (e) an independent arterial port for monitoring, (f) fewer hematomas or spasm, and (g) perfusion of the leg below the puncture site. These more than compensate for the slightly larger size required and the additional effort.

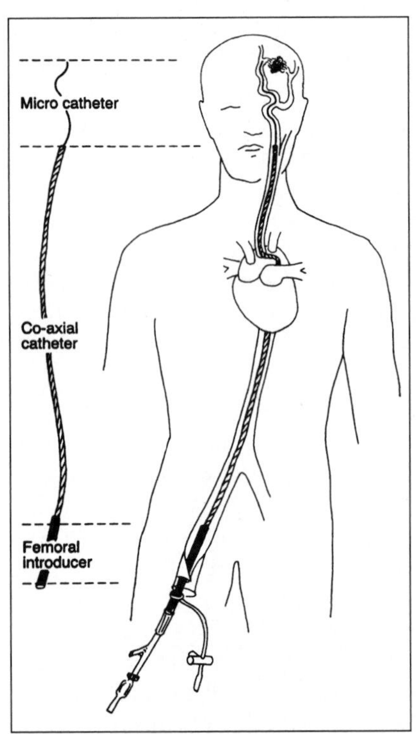

Figure 18.1. Triaxial catheter system.

GUIDING CATHETERS

Large French (5F to 8F) catheters are usually used to deliver materials and to deliver adequate contrast simultaneously. Thin-walled, nonthrombogenic, nonkinkable, low-friction, trackable, shapable, atraumatic, highly flexible, high-tensile-strength catheters are needed, particularly in catheterizing tortuous vessels. No one material or design meets all requirements. Compromises have been made in the past. The characteristics of a polymer are determined more by the exact nature of the building blocks and links than by the class to which the polymer belongs. Catheters made of Teflon, polyethylene, polyurethane, polypropylene, silicone, polyvinylchloride, and pursil are all available in a range of characteristics, and the exact operating characteristics cannot be determined by the class of material. Recent advances have been made in the fabrication of these materials. Future development will most likely be in the "designer polymers" for specific endovascular applications.

There must be a close fit between the catheter and the wire to avoid inadvertent direction or clot formation between the guiding catheter and the inner aspect of the catheter. All attempts must be made to avoid clot formation. These include (a) full heparinization after the sheath is placed but prior to catheter placement, (b) care in avoiding

Table 18.2.
Approximate Size Equivalents

French	Millimeters	Mils	Gauge
1.0	0.33	13	29
1.5	0.50	20	25
2.0	0.66	26	
2.7	0.90	35	
2.9	0.96	38	
3.0	1.00	40	19.5
3.7	1.25	49	18
4.0	1.35	52	
5.0	1.67	66	16
6.0	2.00	78	14.5
7.0	2.30	92	—

* OD = outer diameter

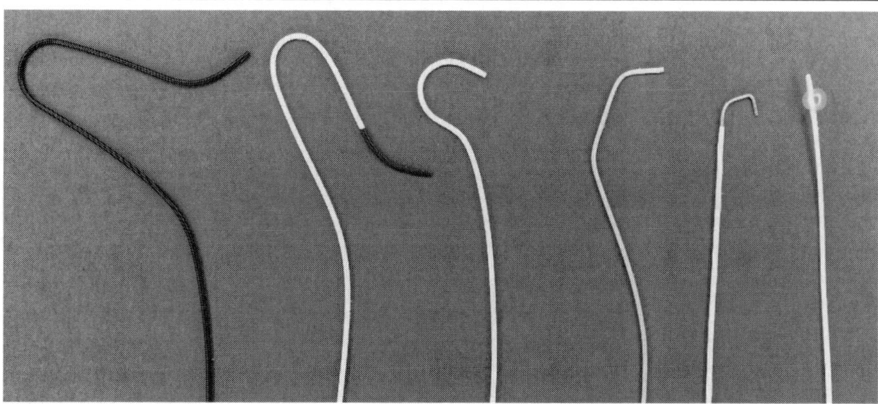

Figure 18.2. Catheter shapes: the hockey stick, the C shape, and the "reformed" (Simmons) catheter. **A.** Simmons hydrophilic coating. **B.** Simmons shape with a soft tip and very radiodense tip. **C.** C shape. **D.** H_1-H_2. (Hockey stick) **E.** Coaxial catheter. **F.** Balloon occlusion catheter.

any unflushed dead space, (c) withdrawing and flushing guiding and inner catheters if catheterization is unsuccessful after a short time, and (d) limiting the total surface area in all ways practical if the catheter is exposed to blood. A smaller inner catheter is temporarily used during placement for guiding catheters greater than 6F. The usual combinations are a 5F to 7F catheter and a 4F to 6F catheter. The guiding catheter can be given a gentle distal curve to allow it to sit gently in the vessel.

CATHETER SHAPES

Prior to the introduction of the torquable guide and road mapping, a complex array of catheter shapes was needed to routinely catheterize the vessels of the ectatic arch. The exact detail of each catheter manipulation was developed by the early workers. These catheters acquired an even more confusing array of names as "designer catheters" with individual modifications appeared. Catheters have three basic shapes (Fig. 18.2): the hockey stick, the C shape, and the "reformed" catheter. These have undergone a vast array of modifications. Figure 18.3 shows some of the modifications that the basic hockey stick shape can undergo.

The reformed catheter is formed in the subclavian, iliacs, or off the aortic valve. This catheter is highly useful when catheterizing smaller vessels originating at very acute angles from larger tortuous vessels such as a left common carotid artery in an elderly hypertensive individual. The tip is generally very soft and has a stiff proximal portion. It can be used

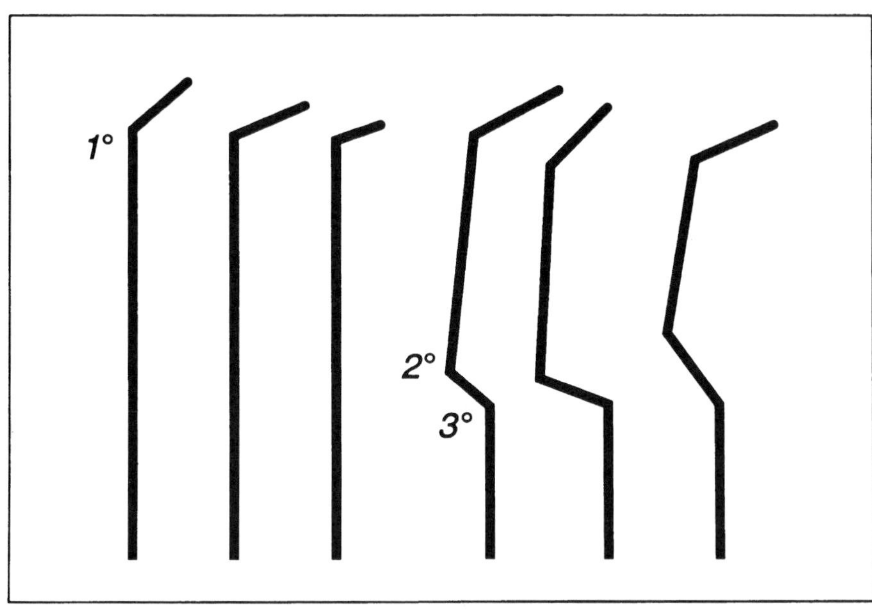

Figure 18.3. Catheter shape modifications: (1) the length of the components, (2) the primary curve angle, (3) secondary and tertiary curves proximally on the shaft, and (4) tapering distally or stiffening proximally.

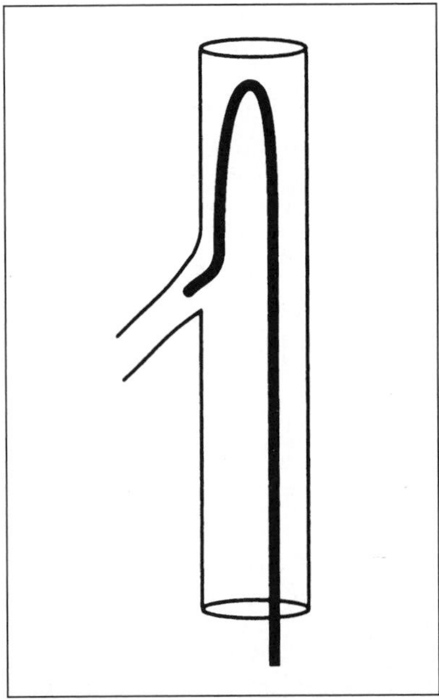

Figure 18.4. Reformed, or Simmons, catheter. The reformed catheter is reshaped in the subclavian, iliacs, or off the aortic valve. This catheter is highly useful when catheterizing vessels coming at a very acute angle off a large tortuous vessel such as a left common carotid in an elderly hypertensive individual. The tip is generally very soft and has a stiff proximal portion. It can be used with or without a guide wire. Note that when the proximal end of the catheter is withdrawn, the distal tip of the catheter advances. More distal subselective catheterization is usually not possible.

with or without a guidewire. Usually more distal subselective catheterization is not possible (Fig. 18.4).

MICROCATHETERS

Catheters with distal tips of from 1F to 3F are called microcatheters (10,11). They can be used to reach almost any distal field vessel in the body. They are introduced through a guiding catheter. Since torquability is absent in these catheters, the different shapes are even more important. Generally the catheter shape that slightly exaggerates the curve around the vessel one is negotiating works best. Once the catheter has negotiated the curve, a straight catheter offers the least resistance. A straight catheter will tend to stay on the outside of a curve, and a curved catheter tip will tend to cross back to the inside wall sooner after rounding the curve. Small, branching, low-flow vessels with tight curves (>90°) and many proximal curves can be challenging to navigate through. Since most of the materials are thermoplastic at temperatures close to body temperature, over time they will take on the shape of the vessels they are in. This can be used to advantage and explains why the microcatheter appears to get "stuck" if left in the same place over time, since its shape conforms to the entire length of the vessel. The authors routinely shape the distal end of the catheter and find a 4-mm hockey stick shape to be the most universally useful. An array of microcatheters is made.* Double-lumen catheters have also been used for embolization (12,13).

Wire-Directed Catheters

The wire or geometry-directed catheters are of variable stiffness but stiff enough to be advanced without a wire in a straight vessel. They are preferred catheters in the external circulation, when navigating without the aid of flow, and when nonliquid emboli are used. A significant amount of force is usually needed to get wire-directed catheters around more than four or five right angles; thus it is usually difficult to get past the M2–3 or similar areas. The tiny microwire, although extremely soft, can, if forcibly advanced with the catheter, wedge and perforate a thin-walled vessel. In addition, care must be taken to avoid pushing too hard in the neck lest small dissections develop (14,15).

Flow-Directed Catheters

Flow-directed microcatheters have a very soft, floppy, distal segment that is carried by the blood flow (16). The stiff proximal portion allows the distal segment to be advanced through the catheter. These devices allow very gentle catheterization of the vessels that have significant antegrade flow. Easily plugged, these tiny-lumen catheters are usually reserved for liquid agents such as acrylate adhesives, ethanol, or very dilute and small embolic agents (polyvinyl alcohol 150 μ, 6-0 silk). With these catheters it is usually possible to reach almost any vessel, even those with very small flows, by using the appropriate curve and manipulation. If they become wedged in a tiny vessel, overinflation can lead to rupture. To avoid this occurrence, the authors keep them filled with contrast at all times and only flush them under fluoroscopy. Calibrated leak balloons (17–19) and double-lumen balloons (12,13) have been supplanted by these newer designs (20).

WIRES

Guide wires are essential. One can use the heparin-coated wound spring catheters or the newer smooth, hydrophilic, soft-metal-core torquable. The guide wire is advanced into the vessel and the catheter advanced over it. The newer torquable wires offer such excellent control that it is uncommon to need the complex array of catheter shapes previously used. The wire should fit closely but glide freely.

Exchange wires that are at least twice the length of the catheter are useful when various catheters and wires are needed to negotiate difficult proximal curves. Two-piece micro exchange extension wires can be very useful. Exchange wires are essential for angioplasty because the stenotic lesion should be crossed as few times as possible before, during, and after angioplasty. A group of torque-

* For example, by Target, Temecula, Calif.; Microvena, Vadnais Heights, Calif.; ITC, San Francisco, Calif.; Nycomed-Ingenor, Paris, France; Balt, Montmorency, France; and Cook, Cook, Inc., Bloomington, Ill.

Table 18.3.
Provocative Agents

Agent	Dose	Use	Comment
Lidocaine (Xylocaine)	20 mg/ml	Peripheral nerves, white matter tracts, cerebellar gray matter	Opacified with powder metrizamide. May be used for cerebral gray matter if pretreated with amobarbital. Also useful for treating spasm.
Amobarbital (Amytal)	20 mg/ml	Gray matter	Opacified with nonionic contrast.
Saline	NS*	Flow arrest	Rarely used.

* NS = normal saline

controlled, hydrophilic, tapered wires in exchange lengths are highly effective for this purpose.

Agents

Materials that are delivered through catheters include agents for opacification, functional blockade, thrombolysis, angioplasty, spasmolytics, and cytotoxic agents, chemotherapy, or occlusion.

OPACIFICATION

Contrast agents are the routine opacification agents used during embolization. Liquid nonionics are favored whenever possible. Lyophilized nonionic metrizamide* is used to opacify liquid agents such as Xylocaine or ethanol. Ionic contrast agents† are used when the lowest viscosity is needed, such as with microcatheters, microballoons, or microemboli in tiny flow-directed catheters. Metals such as gold, platinum, tantalum, and bismuth have all been used and can be seen quite well. Gold and platinum markers can be seen quite well and have been incorporated into devices. Tantalum (atomic number 73) is a heavy, hard, extremely noncorrosive material that can be ground into a fine powder in the micrometer range. It is used to opacify acrylates.

FUNCTIONAL BLOCKADE

Temporary neurologic blockade combined with focused monitoring is useful prior to permanent occlusion of a vessel. The exact nature of the test blockade must be replicated by the permanent blockade. An extremely robust approach, it cannot replace detailed knowledge of the anatomy or the appreciation that "the same man never crosses the same river twice" (Xeno). In its simplest form, saline is injected into a cutaneous vessel, and the cutaneous distribution is observed for the characteristic transient pallor. In its more complex forms, anesthetics opacified with contrast are injected under fluoroscopic control while complex serial neurologic monitoring is performed, including monitoring of sensory, motor-evoked electroencephalographic responses and highly tailored serial neuropsychiatric and neurologic exams. The latter examinations are always included in the treatment of patients (Table 18.3).

* Amipaque (Metrizamide), Winthrop, New York.

† Conray (iothalamatoameglumine), Mallinckrodt Medical, St. Louis, Mo.

THROMBOLYSIS

Dissolution of a thrombus is mediated by fibrinolysis within the thrombus (thrombolysis). Degradation of fibrin is catalyzed by plasmin activated from plasminogen. Normally, a fibrinolytic system exists in circulating blood as plasminogen, which is the precursor of plasmin and has no enzyme activity. Formation of plasmin is promoted by the appearance of the plasminogen activator. Exogenous plasminogen activators, such as urokinase (UK), streptokinase (SK), or acylated plasminogen-streptokinase activator complex (APSAC), have been used in thrombolytic therapy. Urokinase, which is a serine protease produced from human urine or fetal renal cell culture, directly activates plasminogen. In contrast, SK, derived from culture of beta-hemolytic streptococcus, has no direct effect on plasminogen. SK combines with plasminogen to form a plasminogen-streptokinase complex, which activates circulating plasminogen to form plasmin. Free plasmin in the circulating blood activated by these agents degrades fibrin and fibrinogen, causing fibrinolysis. These exogenous agents also inactivate prothrombin (II) factors V and VIII, thereby inhibiting systemic coagulation. Also, fibrin degradation products (FDPs) act as potent anticoagulants. Thus, a large dose of these agents could cause a prolonged systemic anticoagulant state. SK is less expensive than UK, and mass production is easy. However, the half-life of SK is longer (18 to 83 min) than that of UK (11 to 18 min), and SK has more side effects, such as fever or allergy, compared with UK, because of its immunogenetic property. Activity may be unstable in patients with a previous streptococcus infection. APSAC has been considered to be more fibrin specific in ongoing studies.

In contrast to these exogenous plasminogen activators, which act nonspecifically on circulating plasminogen, tissue plasminogen activator (tPA) and single-chain urokinase plasminogen activator (scuPA) are endogenous plasminogen activators with high fibrin specificity. tPA is a serine protease with a short half-life (5 to 8 min). It was produced initially from melanoma cell culture, and recently by recombinant DNA technique. Although associated with fibrin, tPA is activated in the thrombus and converts plasminogen to plasmin, which is protected from the neutralizing effect of alpha$_2$-antiplasmin by fibrin, as already described. The agent scuPA has no direct activity to

Table 18.4.
Thrombolytic Agents

	Streptokinase	Urokinase (UK)	tPA*	proUK†
Half-life	30 min	15 min	6 min	
Activity	High	High	Higher	Higher
Specificity	Low	Low	High	High

* tPA = tissue plasminogen activator.
† proUK = prourokinase.

plasminogen but is activated and converted to UK by plasmin in the thrombus, which causes the localized fibrinolysis. Endogenous plasminogen activators have been considered to have few anticoagulant effects. However, high doses of tPA may produce systemic fibrinogenolysis and plasminogen destruction through inactivation of clotting factors (Table 18.4). The indications, contraindications, and optimal doses are unknown for thrombolysis.

ANGIOPLASTY

Angioplasty for stenotic brachiocephalic lesions is practical for patients when indicated. The exact indications, contraindications, and preferred methods are not known. Three methods have been used, each requiring equipment modifications. The first is to perform angioplasty without cerebral protection. The second is to use distal cerebral protection. The third uses proximal occlusion with aspiration.

No Embolic Cerebral Protection

The lesion is crossed with soft tapered wire and then by a small, low-profile catheter. The wire is exchanged for stiff exchange wire such as a Rosen. The angioplasty catheter is then exchanged, and the exchange wire is removed. One inflates the angioplasty balloon while perfusing distally with oxygenated blood. Blood from the distal catheter is then aspirated while the balloon is being deflated. The wire is replaced and exchanged for a diagnostic catheter. The process is repeated if needed. Routine angioplasty catheters can be used for this procedure. A side hole on the angioplasty catheter allows for the perfusion during angioplasty.

Distal Embolic Cerebral Protection

A large guiding catheter is placed proximal to the lesion (21). A microballoon catheter wire that acts as the angioplasty catheter's guide wire is placed above the stenosis and inflated. The angioplasty catheter is placed across the lesion and inflated and aspirated. The angioplasty balloon is removed and the debris is aspirated from the guiding catheter. The micro-occlusion balloon is then deflated and an angiogram obtained. Materials for this method must be fabricated from available materials.

Proximal Embolic Cerebral Protection

A guiding occlusion balloon catheter is placed and inflated in the parent vessel proximal to the intracranial and extracranial feeder. The lesion is then crossed with a wire, followed by the angioplasty catheter at the level of the stenosis; the catheter is inflated and removed. The guiding catheter is then aspirated for debris and deflated, and an angiogram is obtained.

Angioplasty for the large brachiocephalic vessels with atherosclerotic vascular disease requires strong balloons (10 to 15 atm) with a low profile (4F to 5F) and excellent trackability. The Stealth catheter has a significantly weaker balloon but can be used to navigate intracranially. The balloon should be sized to approximate the native vessel and should cover well the area of narrowing. Antispasmotics, anticoagulants, antiplatelets, and usually thrombolytics should be given prior to angioplasty.

Angioplasty for Vasospasm

The nondetachable silicone balloon,* the latex balloon,† or the Stealth catheter can be used (22–25). The authors favor the latex balloon mounted nondetachably on a wire-guided microcatheter, as others have reported (26,27). The acute angle of the anterior cerebral artery is difficult to navigate. See Table 18.5.

There are no stents currently available. Stents designed for other purposes have been used, and early results are promising. Covered stents would appear to address the problem of emboli.

SPASMOLYSIS

Occasionally, spasm can develop during a catheter manipulation or angioplasty. Pretreatment with nimodipine is helpful. Intra-arterial nitrogylcerin, verapamil, nitroprusside, or papaverine can be used. Sublingual nimodipine or nitroglycerine paste can also be used.

There is some indication that intra-arterial papaverine can be of benefit for cerebral vasospasm from subarachnoid hemorrhage. Papaverine can dilate vasospastic cerebral blood vessels and is associated with increased intracranial pressure. See Table 18.6.

CHEMOTHERAPY

Intra-arterial chemotherapy has been used for intra- and extracranial tumors to help limit the systemic toxicity. The dose to the target appears to be substantially increased. Advances in this field have been limited by the difficulty of confidently assessing beneficial effects and by the continued local toxicity in the perfused territory. The indications, contraindications, and dosages for intra-arterial chemotherapy are not known. See Table 18.7.

* ITC, San Francisco, Calif.

† Nycomed-Ingenor, Paris, France.

Table 18.5.
Angioplasty Balloons

Balloon	Profile/Atmospheres (atm)	Use
Angioplasty balloon, routine	4–7F/10–15 atm	Brachiocephalic atherosclerotic vascular disease
Stealth balloon	3F/6 atm	Intracranial atherosclerotic vascular disease/vasospasm
Latex balloon	2F/2–3 atm	Vasospasm
Latex occlusion balloon	6–7F/2–3 atm	Test occlusion
Silicone balloon	1–2F/0.5 atm	Vasospasm

Table 18.6.
Spasmolytic Agents

Agent	Dose	Comment
Lidocaine	20 mg/ml	Opacified with dry metrizamide
Verapamil	1 mg	
Nitroglycerin	50–100 μg	
Papaverine	10 mg	Monitor intracranial pressure
Nitropaste	1–2″	
Nimodipine	30 mg sl/po q10°	

OCCLUSION

A variety of agents can be used to occlude vessels (28,29,30). The choice is determined by a variety of considerations. Agents can be liquid, particulate, cocktails, or implantable devices.

Liquid Occlusive Agents

The liquid agents allow for the greatest variety of injection techniques. There are a great variety of agents, and complete understanding and facility with a small group of them is surely advisable (Table 18.8).

The cyanoacrylates are extremely useful for AVMs (31–37). See Table 18.9. A relatively small amount (0.2 to 1.0 ml) of a very-low-viscosity acrylate can produce a tremendous amount of permanent occlusion in a highly controllable fashion. This agent is unforgiving, and one needs a significant amount of experience to avoid catastrophic misadventures. The ability to change the polymerization times is a very important attribute that allows for a wide range of AVM flow types to be treated (38). Polymerization occurs when the glue comes into contact with ions in the blood or on the vascular endothelium. Mixing iophendylate with cyanoacrylate causes slowing of the polymerization, allowing flow-directed embolization into the nidus of an AVM or into the central neovascularity of a tumor or hemangioma. Brothers et al. (31) performed in vivo and in vitro comparisons of isobutyl-2-cyanoacrylate (IBCA) with NBCA (*N*-butyl-2-cyanoacrylate, Histoacryl), a tissue adhesive approved for surgical use in Europe. Polymerization times in static plasma were compared, and the effect of the addition of iophendylate oil or glacial acetic acid on polymerization was assessed. Polymerization times in vivo were compared after intra-arterial injection into the internal carotid artery in pigs using a standardized technique. Their results showed that although NBCA polymerization is demonstrably faster than IBCA in vitro, intra-arterial injections of each glue show no significant difference in polymerization times. Like IBCA, NBCA polymerization can be predictably prolonged by the addition of oil or glacial acetic acid, though the effect is less for NBCA. Brothers et al. concluded that NBCA has clinical and biological behaviors similar to IBCA and therefore was an acceptable alternative to IBCA for intravascular use. More recently, Widlus et al. (39) also showed that the in vitro cyanoacrylate glue polymerization time can be changed. The authors attempted to define the relationship between the iophendylate-glue ratio and polymerization time with an in vivo swine model. In this model, glue setup occurred much more rapidly than predicted on the basis of in vitro studies. This appeared to be due to glue polymerizing on the endothelium at vessel bifurcations and at areas of acute angulation or marked vessel narrowing. On the basis of these data, the authors substantially increased the iophendylate-glue ratio in their most recent AVM embolization procedures and achieved nidus occlusion in each case. Using the authors' guidelines, it is possible to achieve optimal distal flow–directed embolization with cyanoacrylate. The hard, strong acrylates such as the isobutyl cyanoacrylates can increase the difficulty of surgical removal.

The long-term histopathologic effects of cyanoacrylates on tissues appear to be relatively benign. Brothers et al. (31) found that the histopathologic reactions were similar for both IBCA and NBCA. Acute vasculitis was observed, which became chronic and granulomatous after about 1 month. Both glues showed frequent foci of extravascular extrusion through the embolized pig rete and recanaliza-

Table 18.7.
Chemotherapeutic Agents

Agent	Dose: interval	Comment/Toxicity
BCNU*	80–240 mg/m^2: 6 wk	Glioblastoma/myelosuppression
Cisplatin	75 mg/m^2: 4 wk	Glioblastoma/head and neck tumor, myelosuppression, renal failure

* BCNU = 1,3 bis 2 chloroethyl-1-nitrosourrea

Table 18.8.
Liquid Occlusive Agents

	Cyanoacrylates	Ethanol	Thrombin Admixtures	Estrogen	Socadecol™
Purpose	AVMs*	VMs,† tumors	preop AVMs*	Tumors	VMs†
Size/viscosity	Low viscosity	Low viscosity		Low viscosity	
Delivery system	1F	1F	3F	1F	2F
Permanence	4+	2+	2+	2+	3+
Penetration	Small arteries	Capillaries	Small arteries	Capillaries	Small arteries
Ease of use	1+	3+	2+	4+	4+
Regulator status	Not FDA-approved	NA‡	NA	Off label use§	Approved
Opacification	Tantalum	Metrizamide	Metrizamide	Contrast	Metrizamide
Comment	Preferred agent for AVMs, control polymerization time with iophendylate (Pantopaque) or glacial acetic acid	Artery or vein, cytotoxic	Control of polymerization time, thrombin excess needed		Venous or artery
Considerations	Highly operator-dependent	Painful, vasospastic, pulmonary reactions			Painless

* AVM = arteriovenous malformation.
† VM = venous malformation.
‡ NA = not available.
§ Not FDA-approved for this use.

tion of previously occluded embolized vessels. An initial giant cell reaction subsided after a few years. If the reaction does persist, it appears to be effectively treated with steroids (40). Histoacryl (*N*-butyl-2-cyanoacrylate) is one of the least histotoxic cyanoacrylate derivatives and is used as a tissue adhesive for skin closure (as for blepharoplasty incisions). Acute inflammation and prolonged foreign-body giant cell response can occasionally be seen. Acrylates produce some cell inhibitions. This cell inhibition is in a linear proportion with the amount of formaldehyde released upon polymer degradation (41,42). Allergic reactions to cyanoacrylate adhesives are extremely rare, but should not be considered impossible (43).

We find *ethanol* useful for venous malformations (VMs), tumors, and occasionally AVMs. Dehydrated ethanol is opacified with metrizamide and injected under fluoroscopy; general anesthesia is usually required. Ethanol produces a chemical burn, with denaturing of protein leading to cytotoxic and vascular destruction. It is related to the dosage, concentration, and length of exposure (44–48). Proximal arterial spasm can develop. As with all other embolic agents, any significant amount returning to the systemic circulation should be avoided. Profound drops in the PO_2 are seen when this agent enters the pulmonary circulation. Close monitoring and various strategies are needed to limit this potentially dangerous problem.

Socadecol* is a painless sclerosing agent that can be opacified with metrizamide. There is little in the way of cytotoxic effect. It is essentially a soap, and relatively long exposure of the vessel is necessary for it to be effective (49,50). Ethibloc† (ethanol and corn protein) precipitates and causes an inflammatory reaction (51–53). Some operators achieve excellent results, but this author has little experience. Silicone is no longer used (54). Newer agents are under development (55–58).

Table 18.9.
Advantages of Acrylate as Embolic Material

Essentially permanent
Very liquid, flows through very small, soft tubes
Highly controllable solidification time
Malleable at time of surgery
Can be made radiopaque
Can be delivered without pressure or flushing
No demonstrated short-term toxicity

Nonliquid Occlusive Agents

The most commonly used materials for the treatment of tumors are the particulate agents (Table 18.10). PVA‡ has been used for many years and is available in a variety of approximate ranges (150 to 300 μ, 300 to 500 μ, 500 to 1000 μ) (59–64). It is highly effective for preoperative tumor embolization and is available in different sizes. The different sizes can be used in the same vessel as the flow changes, starting with large particles to occlude the larger AV shunts within a tumor, followed by smaller sizes to occlude the tumor bed proper, and switching back to the larger materials for proximal occlusion of the feeder. Tiny potentially dangerous collaterals can be avoided by using larger-sized particles with dynamic flow

* Sodium tetradecyl sulfate, Elkins-Sinn, Cherry Hill, N.J.

† Ethica, Hamburg, Germany.

‡ Polyvinyl alcohol foam (PVA), available as Ivalon, !VALON®, Inc., San Diego, Calif., or Contour®, Intervention Therapeutics Corp., So. San Francisco, Calif.

Table 18.10.
Particulate Occlusive Agents

	PVA*	Avatine	Gelfoam	Suture	Beads
Purpose	Tumors, AVMs	Tumors, AVMs	Tumors	Tumors	AVMs
Size	100–1000 μ	75–150 μ	Cut to size	.0035–.023″	1–7 mm
Delivery system	>.018″	>.018″	>.018″	>.010″	>6F
Permanence	2+	2+	1+	2+	4+
Penetration	Small arteries	Small arteries	Small arteries	Small arteries	Small arteries
Ease of use	1+	1+	2+	3+	2+
Regulator status	NA†	NA	NA	Not approved for this use	Approved
Opacification	Contrast	Contrast	Contrast	Contrast	Contrast
Comments	Irregular shape, available in size ranges	Giant cell reaction	Allows proximal occlusion of small vessels	Like Gelfoam but smaller, and many required	Giant cell reaction, high flow
Considerations	Requires "flush"	Requires "flush"	Requires "flush"	Requires repeated "flushes"	Requires "flush" and luck, no control

* PVA = polyvinyl alcohol.
† NA = not available.

control. It is important to recognize that the particle size is approximate. If the mixture has a cloudy appearance, it has a great number of small particles. The PVA should always be "washed" in saline and decanted to get rid of any small particles that are suspended in the supernatant if these particles are not wanted. PVA creates a moderate inflammatory reaction and is prone to revascularize (65). Gelfoam powder is no longer available. Gelfoam plugs are cut to size, loaded in a syringe, and injected. They are useful for temporary occlusion (days). Suture material is highly effective and can be cut in 5- to 10-mm lengths. Often hundreds of pieces are needed to occlude a vessel. Avatine† (microfibrillar collagen), a processed collagen powder, causes a significant giant cell reaction and appears to be more permanent than Gelfoam. Beads are no longer used.

A variety of balloons, coils, and other devices have been used to occlude vessels or vessel segments. The choice depends on (a) the vessel size, (b) the nature of the vessel or segment to be occluded, (c) access, (d) the location of occlusion tolerance, (e) traction and manipulation tolerance, (f) flow force, and (g) availability. For discrete occlusion of a large vessel such as an internal carotid artery, where the vessel is tolerant to traction and manipulation and tolerance to the exact occlusion location and a high flow force must be resisted, balloons are preferred. For medium-sized vessels with similar characteristics, spring coils have many advantages. For sensitive segments that will not tolerate manipulation or traction, such as acute aneurysms, the Guglielmi electrolytic detachable coils (GDC™) clearly is the preferred method. Silastic spheres are of historical interest (66,67).

Balloons represent an important group of occluding agents that have special applications (69–77,79). They can be either nondetachable or detachable. The latter constitute the most important group and were responsible early-on for the launching of what might be called the second phase of progress in endovascular therapy by Serbinenko (75) and others (68) (Fig. 18.5).

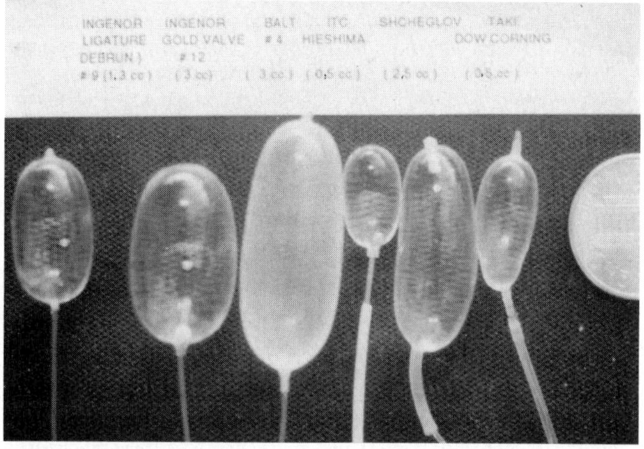

Figure 18.5. Detachable balloon. There have been a variety of detachable balloons, including the (1) Ingenor-Ligature (68), (2) Ingenor-Gold valve (69), (3) DBS ITC, (70,71,72,73), (4) Taki-Dow Corning (74), (5) Shcheglov (75, 76), and (6) Balt. The latex balloons have the highest deflated/inflated size ratios, are relatively thrombogenic and mitogenic, and degrade over time. The silicone balloons are biologically inert. Permanence of either type requires the presence of a solidifing agent such as isomolar (HEMA) 2-hydroxyethl-methaacrylate (not available) or low-viscosity silicone, or the use of tandem occlusion (77–79).

Recently coils have been replacing detachable balloons for many uses, particularly in the obliteration of saccular aneurysms (Figs. 18.6 and 18.38; Table 18.11). Coils are also highly effective for vessel occlusion (80–88).

Balloons and coils do migrate and can usually be retrieved. Retrieval systems for the microwires and balloons* and for the regular-size coils and catheters† should

* Avatine, Medchem Products, Woburn, Mass.

* Target, Temecula, Calif.; Microvena, Vadnais Heights, Calif.
† Cook, Cook, Inc., Bloomington, Ill.

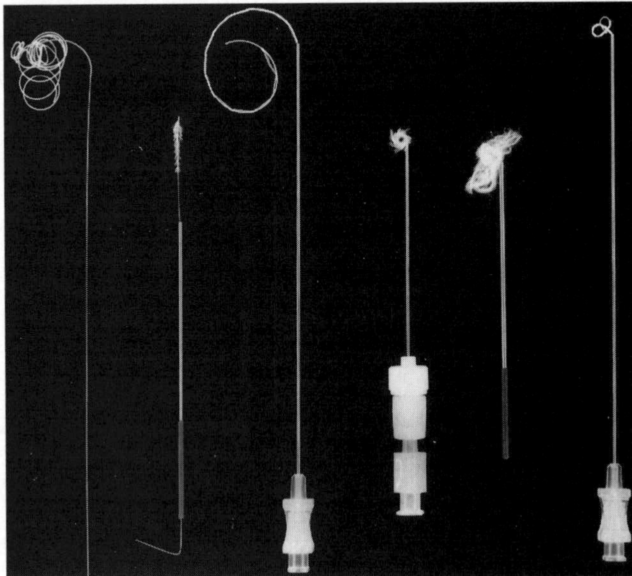

Figure 18.6. There are three types of coils. The first, steel spring emboli, are essentially short pieces of guide wire (with steel wire mandrils) that have been curved and fitted with dacron fibers to make them highly thrombogenic (80–82). The second type is platinum microcoils (with steel wire mandrils), which are essentially short pieces of microwires with or without the dacron fibers (83–86). The third type are platinum coils, without the mandril, soldered on a Teflon-insulated stainless steel wire that allows electrolytic detachment (87, 88). Each class has very different operating characteristics. From left to right: **A.** 8 mm/20mm Guglielmi detachable coil (GDC). Use: The stainless steel Teflon covered mandrill is connected to the floppy platinum coil. These are extremely useful for treating aneurysms. The coil is electrolitically detached. Vendor: Target Therapeutics. **B.** Hilal embolization microcoils 018-1.5-2 Cook. Use: These small platinum micro-coils can be injected or pushed through a #18 microcatheter and are useful for occluding external carotid artery segments. Vendor: Cook. **C.** Vein of galen fibered platinum coils 016/20mm/100mm. Use: These coils are useful for either transvenous or transvascular occlusion of large venous sacks, including the vein of Galen or sinuses. Vendor: Target Therapeutics. **D.** 18S-2/3 Tornado coils. Use: These cook coils are extremely useful for obliterating vessels in both the external and internal cranial vessels. They are also easily delivered. Vendor: Cook. **E.** Steel spring emboli 38-5cm–4mm. Use: These heavy-duty fiber-covered coils are useful for obliterating external carotid artery vessels. They are pushed with a #18 wire through a #5 French catheter. **F.** Complex helical fiber platinum coil 016 4–7/40. Use: These coils are similar in use to **B** and **D**.

be kept handy. They are not easy to use, but one is very grateful to have any tool at all in some situations.

Gels and Cocktails

A variety of "cocktails" consisting of mixtures of some of the agents discussed in text preceding have been tried in the hope of deriving benefits from each. Ethanol (30 percent), PVA Gelfoam powder, and contrast have been used with some success for AVMs. Chemotherapeutic agents, PVA, and contrast have been used to treat tumors.

A variety of specifically fabricated polymers are just now becoming available. Hylan* and EVAL† are among the first of this new "designer" group that will no doubt offer many advantages.

INR Considerations Pertinent to Anesthetic Care

GENERAL COMMENTS AND SCOPE OF INR PROCEDURES

The procedures performed in INR practice are inherently dangerous. Despite tremendous advances in neuroradiology (cerebral angiography was a *surgical* procedure in the 1950s [89]), standard *diagnostic* cerebral angiography has a low but significant morbidity associated with it. In 1984, Earnest et al. reported an overall incidence of complications of 8.5 percent, neurologic complications of 2.6 percent, and permanent neurologic deficit of 0.33 percent in a prospective study of 1517 patients (90). In 1987, Dion et al. reported a 1.3 percent neurologic complication rate in the first 24 h (0.1 percent permanent) in 1002 procedures and a 1.8 percent rate (0.3 percent permanent) for late cerebral ischemic events between 24 and 72 h after angiography (91).

Even in experienced hands, the complication rate may be considerably higher for many reasons (e.g., patient selection). Purdy et al. reported an incidence of intracranial hemorrhage (ICH) during AVM embolization of 11 percent (7 out of 63), with a poor outcome in 5 percent (3 out of 63) (92). A primary goal of anesthesia coverage is immediate intervention in the event of a catastrophe such as ICH.

In the authors' practice, anesthetics are given by anesthesiologists. The contribution of their specialized skill and knowledge to the care of these patients is essential, since there are many anesthetic considerations (Tables 18.12 and 18.13).

INR TREATMENT GOALS

Many of the considerations described in text following are also applicable to certain complex neuroradiologic diagnostic procedures (1,28,93–95,96–98,99–104). *Superselective angiography* can define complex angioarchitecture not visualized on routine angiography. Proximal carotid or vertebral artery *test occlusion* may be used. Finally, *provocative testing* with deliberate hypotension during test occlusions and superselective anesthesia functional examination (SAFE), such as intra-arterial amobarbital administration into vascular territories at risk, fall into this category.

PREPROCEDURE ANESTHETIC CONSIDERATIONS

In adults, the basic anesthetic approach is conscious sedation. This allows for intermittent assessment of neuro-

* Hylan, Biomatrix, Ridgefield, NJ.

† Taki.

Table 18.11.
Devices and Occlusive Agents

	Latex Balloons	Silicone Balloons	Spring Coils	Micro Coils	GDC*
Purpose	Fistulas, discrete large vessel occlusions, aneurysms	Fistulas, discrete large vessel occlusions	Medium vessel occlusions	Small vessel occlusions	Aneurysms
Size	4–15 mm diameter 5–20 mm length		.025–.052″ spring, 3–10 mm helix or cloverleaf, 10–50 mm length		1–7 mm
Delivery system	7–8F	7–8F	3–7F	>.010	2–3F
Permanence	2+ (deflate)	2+ (deflate)	4+	4+	4+
Penetration	Large arteries, fistulas	Large arteries, fistulas	Medium to large arteries	Small to medium arteries	4–25 mm aneurysms
Ease of use	1+	1+	2+	3+	2+
Regulator status	IDE†-approved	Withdrawn	Approved	Approved for this use	Approved
Company	Nycomed-Ingenor, Paris, France Balt, Montmorency, France	ITC	Cook, Cook, Inc., Bloomington, Ill.	Cook, Cook, Inc., Bloomington, Ill. Target, Temecula, Calif.	Target, Temecula, Calif.
Opacification	Contrast, silicone	Contrast HEMA‡	NA§	NA§	NA§
Comment	Valve; latex ligature, rubber plug, miter valve	Valve; miter valve	Cannot be remanipulated; emboli possible	Cannot be remanipulated; emboli possible	Can be remanipulated prior to detachment
Considerations	Traction detachment (50–200 grams of traction)	Traction detachment (20–70 grams of traction)	Advanced through the catheter by pushing with a guide wire	Advanced through the catheter by pushing with a guide wire	Protects from acute rebleed; promising continued advances

* GDC = Guglielmi detachable coils.
† IDE = investigational device exemption.
‡ HEMA = Hydroxy-ethylmeth-acrylate.
§ NA = not available.

Table 18.12.
Interventional Neuroradiologic Procedures and Primary Anesthetic Considerations

Procedure	Anesthetic Considerations
Therapeutic embolization of vascular malformations	
Intracranial arteriovenous malformations (AVMs)	Deliberate hypotension, postprocedure normal pressure perfusion breakthrough (NPPB)
Dural AVMs	Deliberate hypercapnia
Extracranial AVMs	Deliberate hypercapnia
Carotid-cavernous fistulas	Deliberate hypercapnia, postprocedure NPPB
Cerebral aneurysms	Aneurysmal rupture, blood pressure control*
Sclerotherapy of venous angiomas	Airway swelling, hypoxia, hypoglycemia, intoxication from ethanol
Balloon angioplasty of occlusive cerebrovascular disease	Cerebral ischemia, deliberate hypertension, concomitant coronary artery disease
Balloon angioplasty of cerebral vasospasm secondary to aneurysmal subarachnoid hemorrhage	Cerebral ischemia, blood pressure control*
Therapeutic carotid occlusion for giant aneurysms and skull base tumors	Cerebral ischemia, blood pressure control*
Thrombolysis of acute thromboembolic stroke	Postprocedure intracranial hemorrhage, concomitant coronary artery disease, blood pressure control*
Intra-arterial chemotherapy of head and neck tumors	Airway swelling, intracranial hypertension
Embolization for epistaxis	Airway control

* Blood pressure control = deliberate hypo- and/or hypertension.

Table 18.13.
Anesthesia Setup: Drugs and Equipment Recommended for Typical Conscious Sedation INR Cases

Equipment
Portable monitor for transport
O_2 tank for transport
Laryngoscopy and airway supplies
Source of suction
Anesthesia machine with ventilator
Routine drugs
Midazolam
Fentanyl
Droperidol
Propofol for bolus and infusion
Heparin
Phenylephrine for bolus and infusion
Esmolol for infusion
Labetalol
Emergency drugs
Protamine
Thiopental
Succinylcholine
Nondepolarizing muscle relaxant
Atropine
Lidocaine
Ephedrine
Mannitol

logic function during manipulation of the vasculature. Small children and uncooperative adult patients will generally require general anesthesia with endotracheal intubation; general anesthesia is also used for certain procedures. Preprocedure considerations include the following.

History

In addition to the usual disease-specific and preanesthetic evaluation of the neurosurgical patient, previous experience with angiography, history of prior anticoagulation or coagulation disorders, protamine allergy (including insulin use, fish allergy, and prior vasectomy), recent steroid use, and contrast reactions (including general atopy and iodine or shellfish allergies) should be noted. Neck, back, or joint problems may influence the ability to secure the airway or for the patient to tolerate lying supine for several hours. In the population with occlusive cerebrovascular disease, control of preprocedure essential hypertension is critical for perioperative hemodynamic stability, as lucidly reviewed by Gelb and Herrick (105). The possibility of pregnancy in female patients should be determined.

Physical Examination

Conscious sedation may predispose certain patients to airway obstruction; checking the patency of the nares will let the anesthetist know which side is less likely to present a problem if the need arises to place a nasal cannula intraoperatively. Of special concern is the patient with a tumor or venous malformation that involves the upper airway (see section on "Craniofacial Embolization" this chapter). The potential for postprocedure swelling that might impinge upon the airway should be carefully discussed with the INR team.

Laboratory Testing

In addition to general preanesthetic considerations, evaluation of hemostatic function should be considered.

Premedication

An anxiolytic may be given, if appropriate to the patient's sensorium. In cases where deliberate hypotension is to be used, a preoperative regime of a beta blocker or angiotensin-converting enzyme inhibitor such as captopril may be considered, although intraoperative therapy with an intravenous hypotensive agent without pretreatment is probably adequate in most cases. In patients in whom oral secretions are foreseen to be or have previously been a problem, atropine or glycopyrrolate can be administered intravenously in the angiography suite.

Prophylaxis for cerebral ischemia is in a state of development. The authors have routinely placed patients on oral nimodipine in those cases that entail an appreciable risk of cerebral ischemia. Because of the data supporting nimodipine for treatment of cerebral ischemia in the setting of ischemic stroke (106) and subarachnoid hemorrhage (SAH) (107–109), coupled with the lack of impressive side effects (110,111), the authors' personal bias is to expectantly treat with nimodipine. Nimodipine is also felt to lessen the incidence of traumatic vessel spasm during catheter passage; nifedipine is used by some for this purpose (112). The preceding notwithstanding, use of nimodipine for such prophylactic purposes has not been documented to be effective by randomized, controlled studies.

Other authors have described additional considerations for premedication, including corticosteroids, anticonvulsants, aspirin, and antibiotics (28).

Room Preparation

Ideally, the INR suite should be equipped for anesthetic care exactly as a standard operating room. Suction, gas evacuation, oxygen, and nitrous oxide should be available from wall outlets. Dedicated 20-A power lines, including emergency circuits, should be available. A dedicated phone line for the anesthesia team for laboratory communication and management of neurologic catastrophes is essential. A refrigerator for drugs should be in the room. Emergency equipment for cardiopulmonary resuscitation, including a defibrillator and materials for surgical airway access, should be immediately available. The anesthesia machine should ideally have the ability to provide CO_2 gas. Adequate spotlighting should be available to maintain the anesthesia record and to observe monitors, since the room lights are often dimmed for viewing of the fluoroscopy screens.

Many angiography suites have doors that automatically switch off fluoroscopy when they are opened. This can be detrimental in emergencies (e.g., if someone enters the room during a critical manipulation of the intracerebral catheters). An entry "maze" is preferable that allows room access at all times but still provides radiation protection to those outside the room.

Because the risk of intracranial hemorrhage or vascular occlusion is ever present, airway, intubation, and induction materials must be prepared for immediate use and be kept near the head of the table. Long or extension tubing from the anesthesia circuit is desirable.

CONDUCT OF ANESTHESIA

Patient Positioning

Since the procedures may take many hours, having the patient as comfortable as possible before beginning sedation is essential. A comfortable air or foam mattress and some type of device for good head and neck positioning are needed. After the femoral introducer sheath has been placed, a pillow placed under the knees to obtain a modest amount of flexion may improve patient tolerance to prolonged periods of lying supine. No amount of conscious sedation can substitute for careful patient positioning. Because patients may return for multiple treatments, continued patient acceptance is important. Since head position needs to be maintained constant, a headrest that discourages movement or paper tape across the patient's forehead is used as a "reminder." Use of rigid fixation should be avoided because it might increase the likelihood of aspiration if emesis occurs.

Intravenous Vascular Access

For major cases, two intravenous lines should be available, one at least 18 gauge or greater (in adults). To maximize the distance between the fluoroscopy unit and the anesthetist, IV lines are prepared with two anesthesia extension tubings. In one line, a stopcock or infusion port near the patient can be used for continuous drug infusions. The other line may be used for bolus injections through a port farthest from the image intensifier during fluoroscopy to minimize radiation exposure. When the patient is draped with arms restrained and advanced toward the image intensifier, access to IV sites is difficult. Therefore, anesthetics and vasoactive drugs should be in-line and ready to infuse before the patient is moved into final position, and all lines should be clearly labeled.

Arterial Pressure Monitoring

The authors use direct transduction of arterial pressure in any intracranial or spinal cord procedure; it is certainly indicated whenever the likelihood exists for manipulation of systemic pressure with vasoactive agents, in procedures involving the posterior fossa or upper cervical cord, or when there are mitigating medical considerations. There is little, if any, additional risk to the patient, since the arterial system is cannulated as part of the treatment. For the typical intracranial procedure, three arterial pressures are easily monitored and a pressure measurement is set up. Pressure transducers and access stopcocks for blood withdrawal and zeroing are mounted on either the sterile field or toward the anesthesia team, depending on local preferences. The advantage of having the stopcocks and transducers on the field is that the radiology team assumes the care of the various connections as part of their setup, and the likelihood of inadvertently flushing or injecting the wrong catheter is greatly reduced.

The first pressure is femoral artery pressure. Although some institutions also perform radial artery catheterizations, the femoral artery introducer sheath is easily used as the real-time monitor of arterial pressure. This spares the patient radial artery cannulation. A disadvantage is that it consistently underestimates the systolic pressure and overestimates the diastolic pressure because of the coaxial catheter passing through it. This effect can be minimized by using a femoral sheath 1/2F larger than will accommodate the coaxial catheter. However, the mean pressures are reliable and may be used safely to monitor the induction of either hyper- or hypotension. In addition, the disparity between femoral artery values can be compared with the blood pressure cuff. The femoral catheter is continually flushed with an intraflow device at 3 ml/h of heparinized saline, which does not appreciably influence the mean pressure recording.

The second pressure is derived from the coaxial catheter in the carotid or the vertebral artery. The reasons for monitoring this pressure are several. Thrombus formation and vascular spasm at the catheter tip or migration of the catheter may be diagnosed by damping of the waveform. Also, leaks in the introducer collar for the superselective catheter will appear as a loss of pressure in the coaxial tracing. A high-volume (100 ml/h) continuous heparinized flush is passed through the coaxial tip to discourage thrombus formation (this infusion characteristically results in a 20-mm Hg increase in the coaxial pressure and should be turned off for quantitative readings). A flush system malfunction may be readily detected by a change in or loss of the waveform.

Finally, the pressure at the tip of the superselective or balloon catheter may be monitored. This is useful during intracranial AVM embolization and for measuring "stump" pressures during balloon occlusions. The use of microcatheters for mean pressure measurements has been validated by Duckwiler et al. (6).

Other Systemic Monitoring

Other monitors should include a five-lead electrocardiogram (ECG) (ideally with automated segment trending) and automatic blood pressure cuff. In patients at risk for myocardial ischemia, a baseline recording of the ECG may be helpful for later comparisons during hemodynamic manipulation. A pulse oximeter probe is placed on the great toe of the leg that will receive the femoral catheters. This can give an early warning of femoral artery obstruction or

Table 18.14.
Management of Neurologic Catastrophes*

Initial resuscitation
- Communicate with radiologists
- Call for assistance
- Secure the airway and hyperventilate with 100% O_2
- Determine if problem is hemorrhagic or occlusive
  - Hemorrhagic: immediate heparin reversal (1 mg protamine for each 100 units of heparin given) and low normal pressure
  - Occlusive: deliberate hypertension, titrated to neurologic exam, angiography, or physiologic imaging studies (transcranial Doppler, cerebral blood flow, etc.)

Further resuscitation
- Head up 15° in neutral position
- Titrate of ventilation to a Pa_{CO_2} of 26–28 mmHg
- Mannitol 0.5 g/kg, rapid IV infusion
- Anticonvulsants: phenytoin (give slowly: 50 mg/min) and phenobarbital
- Titrate thiopental infusion to EEG burst suppression
- Allow body temperature to fall as quickly as possible to 33–34°C
- Consider dexamethasone 10 mg†

* These are only general recommendations, and drug doses must be adapted to specific clinical situations and in accordance with a patient's preexisting medical condition. In some cases of asymptomatic or minor vessel puncture or occlusion, less aggressive management may be appropriate.

† Steroids are of dubious value in the treatment of focal cerebral ischemia (172) but may have a place for reducing mass effect from a hemorrhage, if clinically appropriate.

distal thromboembolism. It is also useful when the femoral sheath must be removed and the site compressed for hemostasis, particularly in smaller children, where overvigorous compression can lead to permanent occlusion of the vessel.

Oxygen (2 to 4 l/min) is given by nasal cannula with a plastic catheter in place to monitor Pet_{CO_2}. In the authors' practice this is accomplished using a "suction" type of end-tidal monitor* and a truncated 14-gauge catheter placed in one of the prongs of the nasal cannula. For the spontaneously breathing patient, an indicator of respiratory rate is recommended if Pet_{CO_2} is not available and may be useful for detecting abnormal respiratory patterns during procedures involving the posterior fossa. Peripheral temperature may be monitored in a number of ways, such as through skin sensors or an axillary probe. In the authors' experience, tympanic temperatures correlate best with brain temperatures (113). Shivering is a troublesome problem because it results in patient motion and imaging degradation, and every effort should be made to keep the patient's temperature near normal (except in the case of a neurologic catastrophe; see Table 18.14).

All patients undergoing transfemoral procedures receive bladder catheters to assist in fluid management as well as to provide comfort. A large volume of heparinized flush solution may be necessary over the course of the procedure. Radiographic contrast is an osmotic diuretic; the administration of diuretics such as mannitol or furosemide may be required.

After placement of monitors, sufficient slack is needed on all monitoring lines, intravenous lines, and airway connections to advance the patient toward the image intensifier. The timing and amount of contrast material administered should be noted by the anesthesia team.

When the patient's condition warrants placement of a central venous or pulmonary artery catheter, central catheters may be positioned by taking advantage of fluoroscopy. Similarly, the endotracheal tube position for general anesthesia cases is easily verified by fluoroscopy of the chest during passage of the coaxial catheters.

CNS Monitoring

During many procedures the neurologic exam provides adequate monitoring of central nervous system integrity as an index of distal ischemia. The authors routinely perform repeated focused neurologic and neuropsychiatric testing on the awake patient. Adjuncts, especially useful during general anesthesia or planned proximal occlusions, include an EEG (114, 115), evaluation of somatosensory (116) and motor-evoked potentials,† transcranial Doppler ultrasound (TCD) examination (117), and xenon 133 cerebral blood flow (CBF) monitoring (93).

Other methods of determining the cerebral hemodynamic effect of proximal carotid or vertebral occlusion that may be used during the period of anesthesia care include CBF measurement with stable xenon CT scanning or single photon emission computerized tomography (SPECT) (118–121). There is still debate as to which of the physiologic imaging procedures yields the most appropriate information for a given clinical setting (122).

Anesthetic Techniques

Conscious Sedation The primary goals of conscious sedation are to alleviate pain or discomfort, prevent anxiety, and produce patient immobility, but at the same time to allow for a rapid decrease in the level of sedation when neurologic testing is required.

The procedures, in general, are not painful, with the exception of sclerotherapy and chemotherapy. There is an element of pain (frequently described as burning) associated with injection of contrast into the cerebral arteries and with distention or traction on them. However, discomfort from long periods of lying still is the main complaint. Insertion of the bladder catheter and to a lesser extent the initial groin puncture for the femoral cannulation are two notable points of discomfort.

The procedure is also psychologically stressful. There is a risk of serious stroke or death. This may be particularly important in a patient who has already suffered a preoperative hemorrhage or stroke. Movement by the patient will decrease the usefulness of the road-mapping techniques and could potentially result in a complication.

Anesthetic agents are selected to meet the above goals. The authors' primary approach to conscious sedation is to

* Ohmeda RGM.

† Roger Emmerson, M.D., personal material.

establish a base of neuroleptic anesthesia by titration of 2 to 4 μg/kg of fentanyl, 2.5 to 5 mg of droperidol, and 3 to 5 mg of midazolam after intravenous access and oxygen administration have been started. The goal of this initial drug titration is to render the patient immobile and generally unaware of the surroundings, but still arousable with adequate spontaneous ventilation. A small bolus of propofol may be useful just as a (well-lubricated) bladder catheter is passed in males.

When the patient is in final position and draping begins, a propofol infusion is started at very low levels (10 to 20 μg/kg/min) and then titrated slowly to result in an unconscious patient with a patent airway. The use of propofol gives the anesthetist some degree of control when a rapid return to consciousness is needed for neurologic assessment.

All patients should receive supplemental oxygen during conscious sedation techniques. Placement of nasopharyngeal airways may cause troublesome bleeding in anticoagulated patients and is generally avoided. If the need for a nasopharyngeal airway is expected, it is prudent to place it before anticoagulation and observe meticulous hemostasis.

The authors feel that droperidol is an excellent addition to the neuroleptic technique because of its antiemetic effect, its alpha-adrenergic blockade, and the impression that it renders a calmer, more motionless patient than do benzodiazepines alone. Postprocedure dysphoria is a theoretical concern, and dopa-adrenergic blockade can result in extrapyramidal symptoms in normal patients as well as in those with Parkinson disease (123). The authors had one patient with a basal ganglia AVM who developed mild dyskinetic movements after droperidol administration that resolved within several hours after the procedure was finished.

A variety of other sedation regimens and variations are certainly possible (1,112,124–126) and must be based on the experience of the practitioner and the goals of anesthetic management for a particular procedure. In the authors' experience and in that of others, chloral hydrate- and ketamine-based techniques have little to offer (125). A predominantly propofol-based technique is possible and intuitively appealing. Enthusiasm for this method, however, quickly waned at the author's institution because of an unacceptably high incidence of upper airway obstruction, which led to nasopharyngeal airway placement in an anticoagulated patient and enough epistaxis to complicate airway control. In addition, troublesome behavioral disinhibition seemed to occur frequently.

General Anesthesia with Endotracheal Intubation Small children and uncooperative adult patients require general anesthesia with endotracheal intubation. Although deep intravenous anesthesia without endotracheal intubation has been proposed in these patients (126), prolonged periods on the procedure table may result in patient motion. General anesthesia is also used for certain specific procedures such as aneurysm ablation, sclerotherapy, and certain cases of chemotherapy. There is no evidence or suggestion that general anesthesia with endotracheal intubation should differ in the INR suite from its usual intraoperative application, be it for adult or pediatric cases. Anesthetic choice and cerebral protection during neurosurgical procedures are extensively reviewed elsewhere (127).

When general anesthesia is used, it is frequently to obtain a motionless patient to improve the quality of the images. This is especially pertinent to INR treatment of spinal pathology, where sometimes exhaustive multilevel angiography must be performed. Because chest excursion during positive pressure ventilation may interfere with "road mapping," radiologists frequently request apnea for digital subtraction angiogram (DSA) in spinal procedures. An effective alternative to apnea is to adjust the ventilator to a relatively rapid rate and small tidal volume. Adequate gas exchange can be maintained during brief periods without degrading the image quality by excessive chest excursion.

Anticoagulation

Careful management of coagulation is required to prevent thromboembolic complications during and after the procedures, although algorithms for anticoagulation remain controversial (1,92,104). Anticoagulation is certainly indicated whenever permanent or test occlusion is performed. Distal thromboembolism or clot propagation can be major sources of complications after major vascular occlusion.

Whether heparinization should be used for *every* case of intracranial catheterization is not clear. Some would argue that anticoagulation increases the risk of intracranial hemorrhage. The authors feel strongly that heparinization should be routinely performed during *any* superselective catheterization. In addition to thrombus formation from foreign bodies in the circulation, a considerable amount of thrombogenic endothelial damage may be done by the passage of the superselective catheter. We routinely heparinize the patient from just after the placement of the sheath until the next morning.

After placement of the femoral introducer catheter, a baseline activated clotting time (ACT) is obtained. Heparin, 5000 units/70 kg, is given and another ACT is checked. The target is at least two to three times baseline. ACT is monitored at least every hour. If an ACT is not drawn on schedule due to some extenuating circumstance, heparin, 2000 units, is given empirically every hour. The risk of overdosing the patient on heparin in this fashion is minimal compared to the risk of inadvertent thrombus formation. Heparin dose and ACT may be entered in a graphic manner on the anesthesia record so that it is easier to follow trends at a glance.

In the authors' practice, heparin is continued through the first postprocedure night. The rationale for postprocedure anticoagulation is to protect against both the thrombogenic effects of endothelial trauma and the inherently thrombogenic nature of the materials instilled, such as glue or coils, which can cause retrograde thrombosis in embolized vessels. A period of 24 h is felt to be sufficient for a "pseudoendothelial" layer to form and prevent either retrograde or antegrade thrombus formation that may propagate along the arterial tree (and the venous system in AVMs) with potentially disastrous results. The heparin effect is then allowed to wane on the first postprocedure day. Because the patient is heparinized, the large introducer sheath in the groin is left in place the first postprocedure night and removed before discharge to the floor on the following morning.

Sometimes the procedure may be aborted before any foreign material is deposited or significant endothelial trauma has taken place. For example, superselective angiography or provocative testing may reveal that a lesion is not amenable to treatment. In this event, heparin is electively reversed with protamine at the conclusion of the procedure and the femoral catheter is removed in the angiography suite.

An occasional patient may be refractory to attempts to obtain adequate anticoagulation. Switching from bovine to porcine heparin or vice versa may be of use. If antithrombin III deficiency is suspected, administration of fresh-frozen plasma may be necessary.

Other Laboratory Tests to Monitor

A baseline arterial blood gas at the time of the first ACT is useful to determine a baseline PaO_2-to-SaO_2 gradient as well as the $PaCO_2$-to-$PetCO_2$ gradient. Although the correlation between $PaCO_2$ and $PetCO_2$ is usually good during general anesthesia (128), monitoring $PetCO_2$ through the nasal cannula is less precise and the discrepancy between end-tidal and arterial values is greater.

The patients receive large quantities of fluid and contrast and may diurese considerably, and a baseline hematocrit determination is helpful. The issue of optimal hematocrit in the brain-injured patient is controversial (129,130), especially in the setting of aneurysmal SAH, and beyond the scope of this review. Based on available evidence, both extremes of hemodilution and hemoconcentration should be avoided. Because intravenous ethanol administration may result in hypoglycemia (131), monitoring blood glucose may be useful during sclerotherapy.

Superselective Anesthesia Functional Examination (SAFE)

SAFE is carried out to determine, prior to therapeutic embolization, if the tip of the catheter has been inadvertently placed proximal to the origin of nutritive vessels to eloquent regions, either in the brain or spinal cord (115,132,133). Such testing is really a variation and extension of the Wada and Rasmussen test (134), in which amobarbital is injected into the internal carotid artery to determine hemispheric dominance and language function.

Before testing, the level of sedation should be decreased by stopping the propofol infusion. In rare instances (to be avoided) it may be necessary to use naloxone or flumazenil to antagonize other intravenous agents. A baseline, focused neurologic exam under residual light sedation is performed. Sodium amobarbital (30 mg) or lidocaine (30 mg), mixed with contrast, is then given via the superselective catheter and an angiogram obtained of the distribution of the drug/contrast mixture. The doses and volume (0.5 to 3 ml) of agent may be altered to fit the clinical situation. Sodium amobarbital is used for investigating gray matter areas. Lidocaine may be used for evaluating the integrity of white matter tracts, especially in the spinal cord (135,136). Injection of lidocaine may result in seizures when used in the brain, particularly in areas such as the motor strip. Besides being disquieting to the patient and increasing the risk of aspiration, seizure activity can result in a transient focal neurologic deficit. A postictal paralysis, for example, can confuse interpretation of the test. For this reason, the barbiturate is usually given first, followed by lidocaine. If the amobarbital is negative, it may protect against cortical seizure but not significantly interfere with assessment of lidocaine's effect on white matter tracts. Not all authors agree on the use of lidocaine for intracerebral testing (137).

After drug injection, the neurologic examination is repeated. Attention is directed to areas at risk as well as "quiet areas" where a deficit might be missed if only a motor or sensory exam is performed, such as a dominant parietal lobe.

SAFE is generally reliable, but false-positive tests can occur with overinjection and reflux into normal vessels. Underinjection, or a "sump" effect from an AVM, may lead to false-negative results (95). Systemic recirculation of the anesthetic may, in some cases, result in generalized sedation. Rauch et al. described the use of EEG monitoring, coupled with a clinical exam, to enhance the sensitivity of SAFE (137).

Deliberate Hypotension

The two primary indications for elective deliberate hypotension are (a) to slow flow in an AVM feeding artery before injection of glue and (b) to test cerebrovascular reserve in patients undergoing carotid occlusion. In most cases, the level of sedation is decreased so that neurologic exams can be followed during the period of deliberate hypotension. In awake patients, nausea and vomiting can be a major problem. It is for this reason that droperidol is an attractive choice as part of the sedative regime. An additional dose of droperidol (1.25 mg) may be given for antiemesis just before starting hypotension (which usually begins at least 2 h after the initial dose). Before beginning hypotension, one should confirm that the patient is fully oxygenated and the airway unobstructed.

The authors' first-line agent is usually esmolol, given as a 1 mg/kg bolus and titrated to target systemic blood pressure at an infusion rate beginning at 0.5 mg/kg/min. High levels of infusion are often needed, and boluses of labetalol (in the range of 50 to 100 mg) are useful as an adjunct. Adrenergic blockers have the advantage of not directly affecting cerebral blood flow (138) and have the theoretical advantage of shifting the autoregulatory curve to the right (139). Trimethaphan probably also shares such an effect (140). A disadvantage is that the large doses needed for awake patients frequently cause pupillary dilatation, and this may confound the neurologic exam.

Sodium nitroprusside (SNP) and nitroglycerin have been described for use during INR procedures (112). The authors tend to avoid these cerebral vasodilators, including dihydralazine, because of the theoretical potential for cerebral steal, unless there is some specific indication (e.g., coronary artery disease for nitroglycerin). The greatest disadvantage of nitroglycerin and SNP is that it is easy to overshoot and render the patient momentarily severely hypotensive. Although this can be treated without incident in the patient under general anesthesia with endotracheal intubation, the onset of hypotension-induced emesis and nausea in an awake patient can be disastrous in the INR setting from several standpoints. It can decrease the total amount of time available to the team for the procedure because of continued discomfort and can interfere with angiographic visualization because of motion artifact. The nausea may be confused with acute intracranial hypertension from vascular perforation. Retching can cause migration of the intracranial catheters from their desired location, cause further endothelial damage, or produce vessel perforation.

Blood Pressure Augmentation (Deliberate Hypertension)

Not infrequently the patient will experience cerebral ischemia from either a planned or inadvertent vascular occlusion. As reviewed recently by Young and Cole, the systemic blood pressure should be increased to drive adequate flow via collaterals to the area of ischemia as a temporizing measure (141). The primary routes of collateral circulation are the Willisian channels (anterior communicating artery [ACA] and posterior communicating artery [PCoA] and the ophthalmic via the external carotid artery). The second main recourse for collateral flow in the hemispheres is the surface connections between pial arteries that bridge major arterial territories (ACA-PCA, ACA-MCA [middle cerebral artery], MCA-PCA). These connections are called by various names. *Pial-to-pial anastomoses* or *collaterals* seem to be the most logical, but they are also called *leptomeningeal pathways* (142). These pathways may protect the so-called *border zones* or *watershed areas* between vascular territories. There is a considerable amount of confusion in terminology in this domain (143). Physiologically, a more precise term might be *equal pressure boundary* (144), where, under normal circumstances, pial flow does not cross collateral pathways into an adjacent territory because the pressure on either side of this distal territorial boundary is equal. There is considerable variation in the anatomic location of these boundaries, and they may change during the course of treatment if the vascular architecture is altered, such as after multiple AVM embolizations. Collateral pathways are most efficacious during chronic ischemia, when they may gradually enlarge over time. Acutely, it is frequently necessary to augment blood pressure to drive flow across them effectively. Absence of adequate collateral pathways, especially in the circle of Willis, is a normal anatomic variant, so deliberate hypertension is not guaranteed to succeed. Deliberate hypertension to treat acute cerebral ischemia by improving pial-to-pial collateral flow across a "watershed" is useful.

The authors' first-line agent is phenylephrine (about 1 μg/kg) in a bolus followed by titrated infusion to increase the pressure up to levels that reverse the neurologic deficit, empirically, 30 to 40 percent above baseline. The ECG and ST-segment monitor should be carefully inspected for signs of myocardial ischemia. Blood pressure goals must be tempered by the patient's preexisting medical status. Based on the best available evidence, deliberate hypertension in the face of symptomatic cerebral ischemia from vascular occlusion during AVM embolization should not be avoided because of fear of rupturing the malformation (145).

If the heart rate is very low to start, for example, because of preoperative beta blockade or sinus node disease, an alternate choice would be dopamine, with or without phenylephrine. In the authors' experience, the use of dopamine alone to induce hypertension frequently results in unacceptable tachycardia.

Deliberate Hypercapnia

Venous malformations of the face or dural fistulas have the potential to drain into intracerebral veins or sinuses. During general anesthesia, hypercapnia is desirable when agents are injected into the venous circulation. By increasing the $Pa{CO_2}$ to 50 to 60 mm Hg, cerebral venous outflow will greatly exceed extracranial venous outflow and the pressure gradient will favor movement of a sclerosing agent, chemotherapeutic agent, or glue away from vital intracranial drainage pathways. Although actual pressure gradients have never been studied, increased intracranial outflow is readily demonstrable in clinical practice with angiography. Addition of CO_2 gas to the inspired gas mixture is the easiest and safest way to achieve hypercapnia. Airway collapse and atelectasis are prevented by maintaining adequate tidal volume. However, hypoventilation may be employed if CO_2 gas is not available; in this case, addition of positive end-expiratory pressure may be useful to maintain oxygenation.

Transport and Postprocedure Considerations

After intracranial or intraspinal procedures, patients spend the first postprocedure night in the intensive care unit

(ICU). Complicated cases may go first to a CT or SPECT scan; only rarely is an emergent craniotomy indicated. Patients should receive oxygen during transport. Arterial blood pressure and, if the situation dictates, oxygen saturation should be monitored en route. Blood pressure control, either modest hypotension in the case of AVM embolization or deliberate hypertension in the patient with occlusive or vasospastic cerebrovascular disease, should be continued during transport.

Postprocedure nausea and vomiting can be due to anesthetic agents or the large volumes of contrast agent. This general topic is reviewed elsewhere (146). For procedures in the posterior fossa, small degrees of ischemia and swelling from contrast not infrequently result in symptomatic local brain swelling in the postprocedure period. In the more capacious supratentorial compartment, such minor swelling is rarely symptomatic. In the posterior fossa, this may present as delayed deficits or decreased sensorium during the course of the first evening after the procedure, particularly if CSF pathways become obstructed. This eventuality should be factored into decisions regarding airway management.

COMPLICATIONS AND SPECIAL CONSIDERATIONS

Management of Neurologic Catastrophes

Complications during instrumentation of the cerebral vasculature can be rapid and dramatic and require a multidisciplinary collaboration (92). Having a well-thought-out plan for dealing with intracranial catastrophe may make the difference between an uneventful outcome and death. A catastrophe plan outline is shown in Table 18.14, based on currently recommended approaches to the treatment of acute cerebral injury (127,147).

If a neurologic catastrophe occurs, rapid and effective communication between the anesthesia and radiology teams is vital. The appropriate neurology and neurosurgical consultants should be contacted as soon as possible. The anesthetist should know enough about the nature and extent of the problem to treat it effectively. The primary responsibility of the anesthesia team is to secure the airway and preserve gas exchange. If endotracheal intubation is necessary, a thiopental and relaxant induction should not be avoided because of the possibility of a transient decrease in perfusion pressure.

Simultaneous with airway maintenance, the first branch in the decision-making algorithm is for the anesthesiologist to communicate with the INR team and determine whether the problem is hemorrhagic or occlusive.

In the setting of vascular occlusion, a method to increase distal perfusion by blood pressure augmentation either with or without direct thrombolysis is the primary strategy. Note that thiopental will probably provide some degree of protection even after an occlusion (148). An example of using deliberate hypertension in the setting of acute hemispheric ischemia from middle cerebral artery (MCA) occlusion is shown in Figure 18.7.

If the problem is hemorrhagic, *immediate* reversal of heparin is indicated. Protamine is given as rapidly as possible to reverse heparin without undue regard for the systemic blood pressure. The cardiac output need only be as high as is necessary to achieve reversal of heparin.* The dispatch with which heparin is reversed may very well be the critical step between a good and a poor outcome from the bleed.

As an emergency reversal dose, 1 mg protamine can be given for each 100 units heparin total dosage during the case. The ACT can then be used to fine-tune the final protamine dose. Blood pressure control requires second-to-second communication with the radiologist. While bleeding is in process and during reversal of heparin, the blood pressure should be kept as low as possible.† In concert with securing the airway, thiopental should be considered as a first-line method of lowering blood pressure; it will also prevent seizure activity from acute SAH. Once the bleeding has been controlled, especially if by temporary vascular occlusion, blood pressure should be kept as high as clinically appropriate after consulting with the INR team.

Bleeding catastrophes are usually heralded by headache, nausea, vomiting, and vascular pain related to the area of perforation. The radiologist can often see the contrast extravasating seconds before the patient becomes symptomatic. In cases of vessel puncture, heparin reversal *before* withdrawing the offending wire or catheter back into the lumen of the vessel will keep the perforation partially blocked until hemostatic function is restored. Rupture or perforation of vessels is often treatable with glue, coils, or balloons. An example of vessel perforation and resultant symptomatic intracerebral hemorrhage (ICH) is shown in Figure 18.8.

If an episode of suspected contrast extravasation or vessel puncture turns out not to be a bleed, the patient can be reheparinized. If significant mass effect is present, the decision to intervene operatively can be undertaken after consultation with the other specialists involved.

Pronounced tissue swelling can follow treatment with sclerosing agents (Fig 18.9).

Contrast Reactions

Despite a controversy over the general utilization of nonionic agents and the cost-effectiveness for radiologic imaging, for INR purposes the lower osmotic activity allows for relatively generous use in single cerebral vessels. A single vascular pedicle may receive in the vicinity of 100 to 200 ml of contrast during the course of a procedure. This could not be accomplished with older ionic agents.

---

* Because of experience with cardiopulmonary bypass and postbypass left ventricular dysfunction, most anesthesiologists are reluctant to administer protamine rapidly enough.

† These are recommendations based on clinical experience and intuition. Ideally, some index of cerebral perfusion would be used to optimize both cerebral perfusion pressure (CPP) and cerebral blood flow (CBF). See Eng et al. (149).

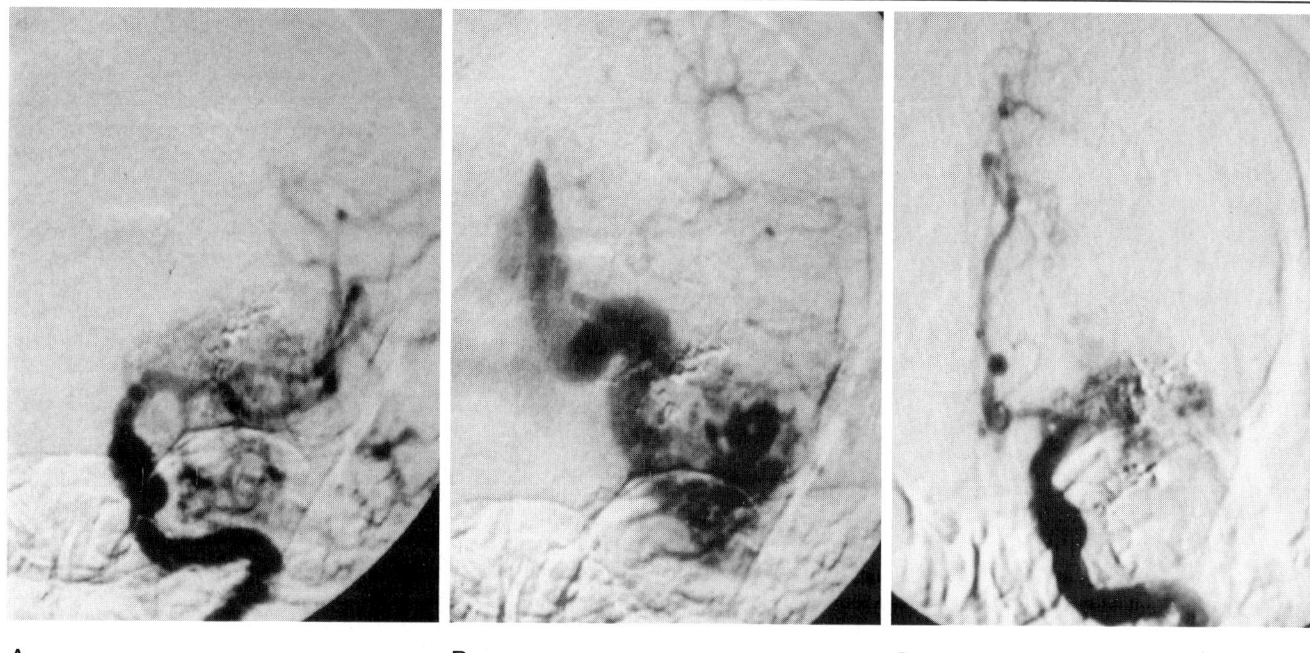

Figure 18.7. Acute middle cerebral occlusion occurring during an interventional procedure. The patient was a 54-year-old woman undergoing a glue embolization of an arteriovenous malformation. **A.** Left carotid angiography demonstrates an AVM supplied by branches of the middle cerebral artery and draining mostly by way of the basal vein into the vein of Galen **B.** During the embolization procedure the catheter became trapped by the glue in the middle cerebral artery. This caused occlusion of the cerebral artery, leading to profound hemiplegia and aphasia. **C.** A repeat injection of contrast shows the middle cerebral artery occlusion, but the anterior cerebral artery is now filling. The patient was immediately treated with induced hypertension (following reversal of the heparin effect with protamine), in order to contribute to the opening of the anastomoses between the anterior and middle cerebral arteries on the surface of the brain. Within an hour, the patient improved and had only minor residual neurologic deficit, which persisted. A CT examination revealed a small temporal infarct. Reprinted with permission from Young WL, Pile-Spellman J, Anesthesia for Interventional Neuroradiology. Anesthesiology, Vol. 80, No. 2, February 1994, p. 441.

For patients having a history of reactions, pretreatment with steroids and antihistamines is recommended (150). Prednisone, 50 mg the evening before and the morning of the procedure, and diphenhydramine, 50 mg IV before starting the procedure, is the current regimen at the authors' institution.

To prevent renal complications, intraoperative fluid management should be aimed at maintaining euvolemia to offset the diuretic effect of the injected contrast. Maintaining an isotonic or slightly hypertonic state for neurosurgical patients (151) is generally not a problem because contrast-induced diuresis usually encourages a hypertonic state. However, patients who have undergone diagnostic procedures in the previous week before an INR procedure are frequently quite volume depleted and can be hemodynamically unstable.

Synthesis and Comment

A major consideration for anesthetic management during INR is that although the patients receive IV sedative drugs, the routine and potential emergency management of these cases is much more interactive than a typical "monitored anesthesia care" (MAC) case because of frequent changes in level of consciousness and manipulation of systemic arterial blood pressure. In addition, the nature of many of the potential complications requires immediate intervention by the anesthesiologist. Although MAC is appropriate for a diagnostic procedure or a minor surgical procedure that is performed primarily with local anesthesia supplemented by minimal sedation, active manipulation of hemodynamics and sensorium renders a description more akin to dynamic akinetic sedation/controlled hemodynamics (DASCH). *Dynamic* refers to repeated lightening and deepening of sedation, *akinetic* stresses the importance of an immobile patient, and *controlled hemodynamics* refers to the physiologic trespass by manipulation of blood pressure. The goals of the anesthetic technique produce a high level of expectations and degree of interaction of the INR and anesthesia teams. New staff to the INR environment must be aware that the anesthetic care of these patients may be potentially much more involved than in other, superficially similar, settings.

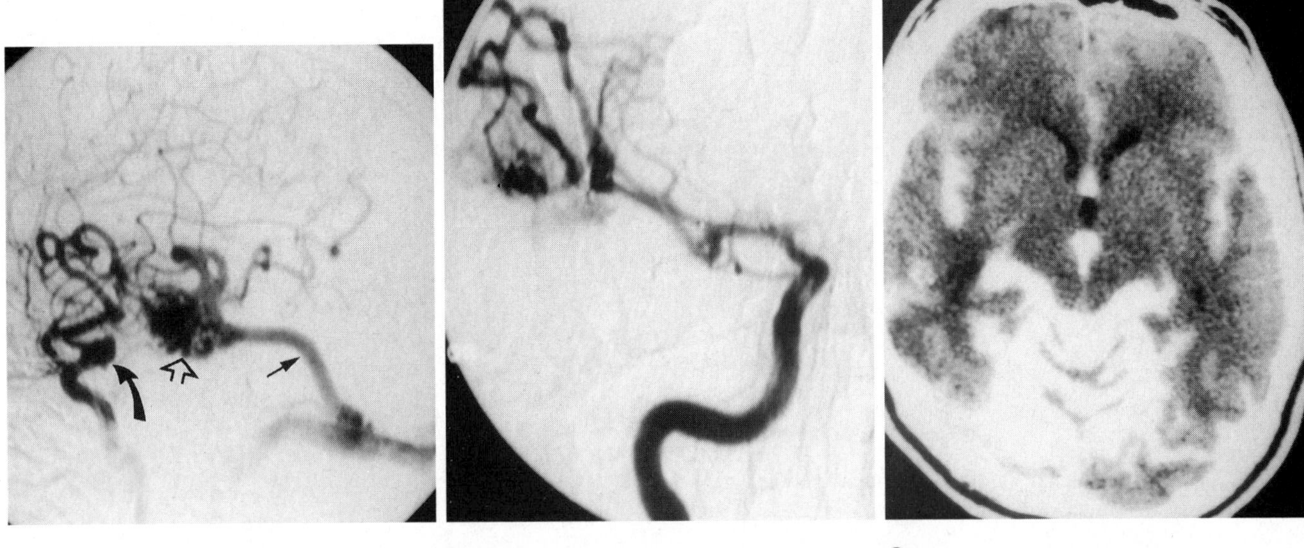

A B C

Figure 18.8. Example of vessel perforation during interventional procedure. The patient was a 50-year-old man who originally presented with spontaneous intracranial hemorrhage. **A.** Lateral carotid angiogram of a right posterior temporal arteriovenous malformation (open arrow) supplied by two middle cerebral artery (MCA) branches with superficial drainage into the vein of Labbe (arrow). An aneurysm is shown at the bifurcation of the middle cerebral artery (curved arrow). During the manipulation of the microcatheter toward the AVM, the microcatheter entered the aneurysmal sac, perforating it. The patient became acutely bradycardic (65 decreased to 35 beats per minute), hypertensive (MAP 90 rose to 140 mm of mercury), and comatose. An injection of contrast showed a small hematoma in the brain (not shown). A repeat angiogram following the perforation before the removal of catheters showed considerable spasm and the aneurysmal sac was no longer visible **(B).** Anesthesia was induced immediately with thiopental and succinylcholine, the trachea was intubated, and modest hyperventilation was started. Protamine was given simultaneously with the induction sequence. The blood pressure target was 20–30% below the patient's baseline mean arterial pressure. When the thiopental effect waned after 10 min the patient began to spontaneously move all four extremities. At this time, it was elected to place the patient in burst-suppression with thiopental and to obtain a CT scan **(C)**, which demonstrated a fairly large amount of subarachnoid blood. Some of the hyperdensity may be due to additional contrast medium mixed with blood. The patient was brought to the intensive care unit, allowed to emerge from the thiopental, and extubated neurologically intact. He made an uneventful recovery and underwent surgical resection without complications. Reprinted with permission from Young WL, Pile-Spellman J, Anesthesia for Interventional Neuroradiology, Anesthesiology, Vol. 80, No. 2, February 1994, p. 444.

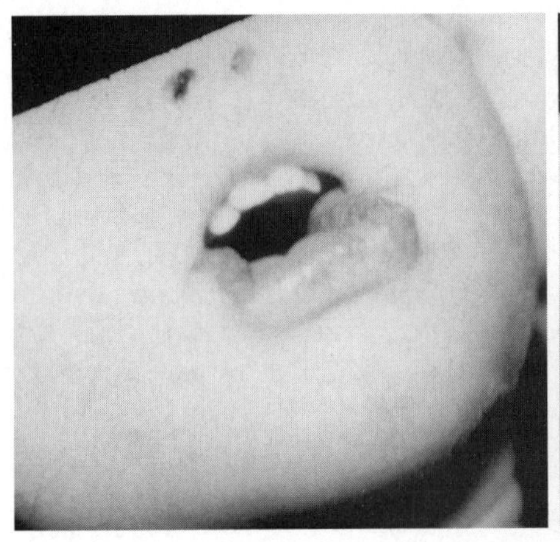

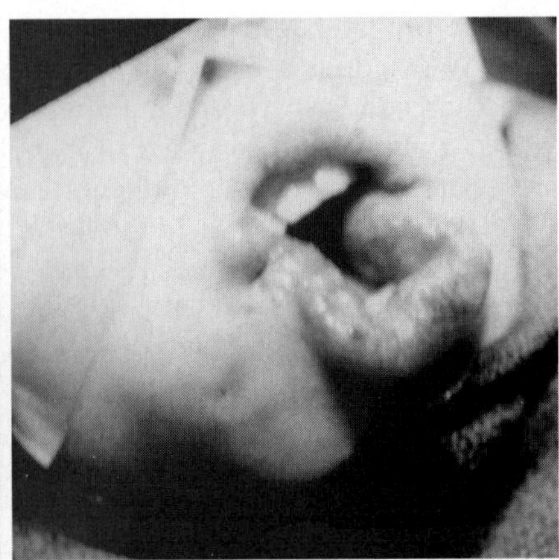

A B

Figure 18.9. Example of marked soft tissue swelling after 95% ethanol sclerotherapy, in a 5-year-old girl with a venous malformation of the lower lip. **(A)** Prior to the injections; **(B)** following the ethanol injections demonstrating the dramatic degree of swelling of the lower lip. Reprinted with permission from Young WL, Pile-Spellman J, Anesthesia for interventional neuroradiology. Anesthesiology, Vol. 80, No. 2, February 1994, p. 448.

Radiation Safety

As a potential risk to anesthesia personnel (152), there are three sources of radiation exposure typically encountered from the imaging equipment: *direct* (from the x-ray tube), *leakage* (through the collimators' protective shielding), and *scattered* (reflected from the patient and the area surrounding the body part being imaged). The annual recommended limit for occupational whole-body exposure is 5000 mRems (153). With proper precautions the anesthesia team should be exposed to less than 0.1 mRem/h.

Specific Procedures

THERAPEUTIC EMBOLIZATION OF INTRACRANIAL AVMs

The main anesthetic goal is to render the patient comfortable and, if possible, unconscious during periods when it is not necessary to be awake. During SAFE and neurologic exams, the patient should be awake and responsive. Despite best efforts, patients usually will not tolerate more than 4 to 5 hours of conscious sedation and will not remain still enough to allow satisfactory performance of the neuroimaging procedures. As the superselective catheter is passed distally, pressure measurements may be made at the tip of the catheter. The pressure will typically decrease in a stepwise fashion as it is advanced distally (6,154). When the catheter has been placed in position for potential glue injection, the level of sedation is decreased and a baseline neurologic exam is performed. SAFE is then performed. If this test is positive, that is, a focal neurologic deficit is encountered, then the catheter is repositioned or embolization of that pedicle may be aborted. If negative, the glue or embolic material can be injected.

Once the superselective catheter is in optimal position, profound but tolerable systemic hypotension is induced while the radiologists prepare the glue for injection. Hypotension slows the flow through the fistula and provides for a more controlled deposition of embolic material, particularly of the glues. Deliberate hypotension is used to achieve *flow arrest.* Ideally, there would be zero flow through the AVM, so that the distribution of glue would be totally controlled by the radiologist who is injecting the glue. Adequate flow arrest appears to occur at a different systemic pressure for each patient. In fact, it seems that flow through the fistula remains relatively constant until a certain pressure is reached, when it drops off sharply. Typically, the authors' institution will reduce systemic mean arterial pressure (MAP) to about 50 mm Hg, but greater or lesser degrees depend on the speed of the contrast transit through the fistula.

Since AVM feeding arteries supply variable degrees of normal brain, abrupt restoration of normal systemic pressure to a chronically hypotensive vascular bed may overwhelm autoregulatory capacity and result in hemorrhage or swelling (normal perfusion pressure breakthrough, NPPB). It is for this reason that the target range for post-treatment blood pressure is strict maintenance of 10 to 20 percent below the patient's normal ward blood pressure. An alternative approach to explain hemorrhage and swelling after AVM treatment has been termed *venous overload* (155) or *occlusive hyperemia* (156), emphasizing that venous outflow obstruction can also result in complications. The exact pathophysiology of hemodynamic complications after treatment of AVMs remains controversial (157).

Although any injected embolic material can occlude normal vessels, injection of the glue is fraught with particular hazards. Injection of glue is a critical moment (not unlike the moment when a surgeon closes the clip on the neck of an aneurysm). The catheter may become glued to the vessel. If the catheter cannot be removed by intermittent firm, gentle traction, it may be necessary to leave it intravascularly, where it will eventually endothelialize. Similarly, the catheter, as it is withdrawn, may drag a piece of glue into the proximal part of the artery and occlude it. In this event, territories fed by nutrient vessels distal to the occlusion may become ischemic. As mentioned, venous outflow obstruction can result in intracranial hypertension (ICH). Glue may also pass into the pulmonary circulation. Small amounts (less than 0.5 ml) may not be clinically significant. Larger amounts, however, may result in a syndrome akin to acute idiopathic pulmonary embolism. Since the glue is extremely thrombogenic, it may pick up thrombus en route and form more clot once lodged in the pulmonary vasculature. This is of particular concern in small children with large AVMs. At the time of gluing, the anesthetist must be ready to intervene immediately in the event of catastrophe.

TREATMENT OF SPINAL CORD LESIONS

For cases done with general anesthesia with endotracheal intubation, an intraoperative wake-up test may be requested. The authors find it useful to review the wake-up procedure with the patient the night before and again the morning of the procedure. Several practice neurologic exams are performed with the patient, both awake and after initial sedation has been given. Our preferred regimen for patients requiring general anesthesia who are scheduled for intraoperative wake-up is a N_2O/narcotic/propofol. Neuromuscular blockade, if used, should be readily reversible for the wake-up test.

Somatosensory and motor-evoked responses may be helpful in most anesthetized and sedated patients. When using motor-evoked potential monitoring with transcranial magnet stimulation during general anesthesia, we titrate neuromuscular blockade to a reduction of single twitch height (T1) to about 40 to 50 of baseline.* Optimal anesthetic regimens for the use of intraoperative motor-evoked potentials have yet to be formulated and are discussed elsewhere (158,159). Pressure measurements from balloon catheters placed in the rectum may be of occasional use in

* David C. Adams, M.D., personal communication.

assessing sacral root function. Triple-lumen bladder catheters can also be used to do intraprocedural cystometrics.

CAROTID TEST OCCLUSION AND THERAPEUTIC CAROTID OCCLUSION

First, after routine carotid and vertebral angiograms, the anatomic integrity of the circle of Willis is assessed. A double-lumen balloon catheter is placed in the carotid artery. The balloon is long enough so that distal ICA branches that may serve as a source of collateral circulation are blocked. A baseline neurologic examination is performed, transcranial Doppler (TCD) velocity of the MCA is recorded, and cerebral blood flow (CBF) is measured by intracarotid xenon 133 injection. Baseline femoral and carotid pressures are noted.

The balloon is then inflated; the stump pressure in the carotid distal to the balloon is recorded.* When the balloon is inflated, focal headache may occur (163). It is the authors' clinical impression that the blood pressure often increases 10 to 15 percent with inflation of the balloon. Although it is probably wisest not to treat modest increases in blood pressure aggressively, treatment of hemodynamically significant bradycardia with atropine is indicated.

The neurologic examination is repeated. As in the case with SAFE, attention is directed to areas at risk, such as watershed regions, as well as "quiet areas." After a few minutes of equilibration, xenon 133 CBF and TCD values are measured. Immediately thereafter, a SPECT tracer can be given. At the present time, Ceretec (^{99m}technetium-labeled HMPAO†) is used. Ceretec is a tracer that rapidly crosses the blood-brain barrier, binds to cerebral tissues, and takes a "snapshot" of the blood flow distribution (not quantitative CBF levels) to the brain at that instant; the relatively long half-life of Ceretec (about 6 h) allows the patient to go to the nuclear medicine department after the procedure to have the "snapshot" developed by placement in the SPECT scanner.

To assess the extent of cerebrovascular reserve more completely, deliberate hypotension is begun after 15 min of observation of the patient at spontaneous postocclusion MAP. The *lack* of cerebral ischemic symptoms at relative normotension does not yield information on the status of cerebrovascular reserve. The blood pressure is lowered gradually to determine at what point the patient begins to show evidence of cerebral ischemia (93). We usually begin with esmolol (and consider adding nitroglycerin in a patient with coronary artery disease) and slowly bring the pressure down as the radiologist continually assesses neurologic function. One must proceed cautiously with blood pressure reduction to interpret the neurologic exam rationally. Frequently, the first sign of impending cerebral ischemia is yawning. If the radiologist feels that the patient is becoming symptomatic, the balloon is deflated and the hypotensive agent(s) are discontinued. Depending on the clinical circumstances, phenylephrine (or another clinically appropriate agent) can be used to bring the blood pressure back toward normal levels.

The patient's hematocrit, Pa_{CO_2}, and blood pressure at the time when the test occlusion is considered "passed" or "failed" should be carefully noted. The lowest systemic pressure obtained before symptoms, if any, and the results of the other imaging modalities are considered in formulating a treatment plan regarding INR occlusion or the advisability of vascular sacrifice during surgical resection.

* Although normal stump pressure does not guarantee normal CBF, very low stump pressure certainly implies low CBF (160), and there appears to be a good correlation between stump pressures and other indices of CBF (160–162).

† Hexamethylpropylamineoxime.

INTRACRANIAL ANEURYSM PROCEDURES

Coil Aneurysm Ablation

Because these procedures can be quite long (especially for large lesions requiring multiple GDC coils) and there is a lesser need to follow the neurologic exam, these cases are most often done under general anesthesia with endotracheal intubation for placement of coils.

The anesthetist should be prepared for aneurysmal rupture and acute subarachnoid hemorrhage (SAH) at all times, either from spontaneous rupture of a leaky sac or from direct violation of the aneurysm wall by the vascular manipulation.

Balloon Angioplasty of Cerebral Vasospasm from Aneurysmal SAH

Angioplasty is usually reserved for patients who have already had the symptomatic lesion surgically clipped (for fear of rerupture) and is done early in the course of symptomatic ischemia to prevent transformation of a bland infarct into a hemorrhagic one. These procedures are commonly performed in patients who are in extremis and are therefore frequently intubated, on vasopressor agents, and have either ventricular drainage or other ICP monitoring equipment in place. Blood pressure management after angioplasty must take into consideration the presence and age of any existing cerebral ischemia or cerebral infarction. If deliberate hypertension was being used to ameliorate a focal neurologic deficit before angioplasty, after angiographic demonstration of the significantly widened spastic segment, blood pressure should probably be managed in the normal range.

OTHER CNS VASCULAR MALFORMATIONS

Dural AVMs

Dural AVM, initially thought to be a congenital disorder, is currently considered an acquired lesion resulting from venous dural sinus stenosis or occlusion, opening of potential arteriovenous shunts, and subsequent recanalization. Dural AVMs may be fed by multiple intra- and extracranial arteries, and multistaged embolization is usually performed (164). SAFE is performed as in cases of intracranial AVMs. NBCA is usually used as an embolic agent. Both transarterial and transvenous approaches can be utilized to access the dural sinuses.

Carotid-Cavernous and Vertebral Fistulas

Both carotid-cavernous fistulas and vertebral fistulas may induce arterial hypotension and venous hypertension in neighboring circulatory regions, analogous to true cerebral AVMs. NPPB has rarely been described after fistula interruption (165), so attention to postprocedure blood pressure control may be warranted.

Vein of Galen Malformations

Patients with vein of Galen malformations may have intractable congestive heart failure, intractable seizures, hydrocephalus, and mental retardation (102). Several approaches have been attempted, including transarterial and transvenous (166). Anesthetic considerations for INR therapy are the same as for surgical treatment (167). In infants with high-output failure, preexisting right-to-left shunts, and pulmonary hypertension, a relatively small pulmonary glue embolism can be fatal.

SCLEROTHERAPY OF VENOUS ANGIOMAS

Venous angiomas may occur anywhere in the body and are usually treated at multiple sessions. The procedures are short (30 to 60 min) but painful, and general anesthesia with endotracheal intubation is used. Complex airway involvement may require endotracheal intubation with fiberoptic techniques (168) or elective preprocedure tracheostomy (169). Since *marked* swelling occurs immediately after ethanol injection, the ability of the patient to maintain a patent airway must be carefully considered in the discussion with the radiologist. An example of acute swelling is shown in Figure 18.9. More graphic examples of venous malformations impinging on the airway are shown elsewhere (169,170).

Ethanol has several noteworthy side effects. First, upon injection it can cause changes in the pulmonary vasculature and create a short-lived shunt or a ventilation-perfusion mismatch. Desaturation on the pulse oximeter is frequently noted after injection; in the authors' experience at least a 2 to 3 percent drop in oxygen saturation is noted in about 25 percent of cases and, rarely, more significant decreases. There have been unpublished anecdotal reports of cardiac arrest during ethanol sclerotherapy, as well as of hypoglycemia. The systemic effects of ethanol in this setting need further study.

Placing the patient on 100 percent oxygen during ethanol injection is a possible consideration. The authors favor placing the patient on 30 percent oxygen and assiduously avoiding any drainage back to the lungs. If any is seen, one must stop injecting, or try to stop its drainage by reflux, increase to 100 percent oxygen and increase the ventilation rate. Usually the drop in PO_2 is only transient. Hypercapnia is also used (see text preceding). The predictable intoxication and other side effects of ethanol may be evident after emergence from anesthesia; postemergence agitation is seen in children.

INTRA-ARTERIAL CHEMOTHERAPY AND EMBOLIZATION OF TUMORS

Hypervascular tumors can swell if there is venous occlusion, hemorrhage into the tumor bed, or significant tissue necrosis. These conditions are most likely to be seen when there is incomplete embolization of feeding arteries. Patients may present with an already compromised airway, and treatment may result in further compromise. Systemic effects of chemotherapeutic agents are minimal because, although standard IV doses are used, the drugs appear to become trapped in the tissue being embolized.

Paragangliomas present the possibility for catecholamine release from the tumor during the course of embolization (171), and the means to treat a hypertensive crisis should be at hand. In addition, swelling after embolization of carotid body tumors may result in symptomatic bradycardia.

MANAGEMENT OF OCCLUSIVE CEREBROVASCULAR DISEASE

Angioplasty

Anesthetic considerations for this procedure include those discussed for deliberate hypertension and the general considerations pertinent to the care of the carotid endarterectomy patient.

Thrombolysis of Acute Thromboembolic Stroke

Anesthetic considerations for these patients include the usual concerns for elderly patients with symptomatic and most probably widespread atherosclerotic disease. Blood pressure management is a particularly important consideration. Patients with acute thromboembolic stroke are commonly spontaneously hypertensive and, in the face of a nonhemorrhagic focal neurologic deficit, should not have their blood pressure aggressively treated (172). After clot lysis, blood pressure should probably be maintained in the normal range and ideally titrated to some index of CBF to prevent hyperperfusion injury. The pathogenesis of hemorrhagic transformation may be related to collateral blood flow to ischemic regions, acting in concert with systemic hypertension (173), but studies in this specific clinical setting are lacking, concerning both blood pressure management and the use of other cerebral protective techniques.

As INR methods develop, this area could evolve into one of the most interactive areas with anesthesia care because of the high incidence of systemic disease present in these patients, coupled with the high morbidity associated with acute thromboembolic stroke.

TREATMENT OF EPISTAXIS

Maintenance of an unobstructed airway and adequate gas exchange with minimal sedation are the primary goals of anesthetic management in these cases.

REFERENCES

1. Eskridge JM: Interventional neuroradiology. Radiology 1989;172: 991–1006.
2. Vinuela F, Fox AJ: Interventional neuroradiology and the management of arteriovenous fistulas. Neurol Clin 1983;1:131–154.
3. Gerlock AJ, Mirfakhraee M: Materials and techniques for peripheral visceral embolization. In Essentials of Diagnostic and Interventional Angiographic Techniques. Philadelphia: Saunders, 1985, 131–173.
4. Halbach VV, Higashida RT, Hieshima GB: Interventional neuroradiology (review). Am J Roentgenol 1989;153:467–476.
5. Duckwiler GR, Dion JE, Vinuela F, Martin N, Jabour B, Bentson J. Intravascular microcatheter pressure monitoring: Experimental work and early clinical evaluation (abstract). AJNR 1989;10:876.
6. Duckwiler G, Dion J, Vinuela F, Jabour B, Martin N, Bentson J: Intravascular microcatheter pressure monitoring: Experimental results and early clinical evaluation. Am J Neuroradiol 1990;11: 169–175.
7. Jungreis CA, Horton JA, Hecht ST: Blood pressure changes in feeders to cerebral arteriovenous malformations during therapeutic embolization. Am J Neuroradiol 1989;10:575–578.
8. Fleischer LH, Young WL, Pile-Spellman J, et al: The relationship of transcranial Doppler flow velocities and arteriovenous malformation feeding artery pressures (abstract). Poster presentation at the 1994 Annual Meeting of the American Association of Neurological Surgeons, San Diego, April 9–14, 1994.
9. Ornstein E, Blesser WB, Young WL, Pile-Spellman J: A computer simulation of the haemodynamic effects of intracranial arteriovenous malformation occlusion. Neurol Res 1994;16:345–352.
10. Jungreis CA, Berenstein A, Choi IS: Use of an open-ended guidewire: Steerable microguidewire assembly system in surgical neuroangiographic procedures. AJNR 1987;8:237–241.
11. Partington CR, Graves VB, Rufenacht DA, et al: Biocompatibility of 1-French polyethylene catheters used in interventional neuroradiology procedures: A study with rats and dogs. AJNR 1990;11: 881–885.
12. ApSimon HT, Hartley DE: Embolization of small vessels with a double-lumen microballoon catheter: I. Design and construction. Radiology 1984;151:55–57.
13. ApSimon HT, Hartley DE, Maddren L, Harper C: Embolization of small vessels with a double-lumen microballoon catheter: II. Laboratory, animal, and histological studies. Work in progress. Radiology 1984;151:59–64.
14. Kikuchi Y, Strother CM, Boyer M: New catheter for endovascular interventional procedures. Radiology 1987;165:870–871.
15. Wolpert SM, Kwan ES, Heros D, Kasdon DL, Hedges T III: Selective delivery of chemotherapeutic agents with a new catheter system. Radiology 1988;166:547–549.
16. Dion JE, Duckwiler GR, Lylyk P, Vinuela F, Bentson J: Progressive Suppleness Pursil Catheter: A new tool for superselective angiography and embolization. AJNR 1989;10:1068–1070.
17. Debrun CM, Vinuela FV, Fox AJ, Kan S: Two different calibrated leak balloons: Experimental work and application in humans. AJNR 1982;3:407–414.
18. Kerber C: Balloon catheter with a calibrated leak: A new system for superselective angiography and occlusive catheter therapy. Radiology 1976;120:547–550.
19. O'Reilly GV, Kleefield J, Forrest MD, Wang AM: Calibrated-leak balloon: Accurate placement of the leak. AJNR 1985;6:90–91.
20. Bank WO, Trainer FG, Edwards MS, Newton TH: Arterial injury during intracerebral manipulation of intracerebral microcatheters. Neuroradiology 1982;22:274.
21. Theron J, Courtheoux P, Alachkar F, Bouvard G, Maiza D: New triple coaxial catheter system for carotid angioplasty with cerebral protection (followed with Commentary by Ferguson R: Getting it right the first time, pp 875–877). Am J Neuroradiol 1990;11: 869–874.
22. Higashida RT, Halbach VV, Cahan LD, et al: Transluminal angioplasty for treatment of intracranial arterial vasospasm. J Neurosurg 1989;71:648–653.
23. Higashida RT, Halbach VV, Dormandy B, Bell J, Brant-Zawadzki M, Hieshima GB: New microballoon device for transluminal angioplasty of intracranial arterial vasospasm. AJNR 1990;11: 233–238.
24. Newell DW, Eskridge JM, Mayberg MR, Grady MS, Winn HR: Angioplasty for the treatment of symptomatic vasospasm following subarachnoid hemorrhage. J Neurosurg 1989;71:654–660.
25. Zubkov YN, Nikiforov BM, Shustin VA: Balloon catheter technique for dilatation of constricted cerebral arteries after aneurysmal SAH. Acta Neurochir 1984;70:65–79.
26. Brothers MF, Holgate R: Intracranial angioplasty for treatment of vasospasm after subarachnoid hemorrhage: Technique and modifications to improve branch access. AJNR 1990;11:239–248.
27. Nelson M: A versatile, steerable, flow-guided catheter for delivery of detachable balloons. AJNR 1990;11:657–658.
28. Berenstein A, Kricheff II: Catheter and material selection for transarterial embolization: Technical considerations. Radiology 1979; 132:619–631.
29. Berenstein A, Kricheff II: Microembolization techniques of vascular occlusion: Radiologic, pathologic, and clinical correlation. AJNR 1981;2:261–267.
30. Kunstlinger F, Brunelle F, Chaumont P, Doyon D: Vascular occlusive agents (review). Am J Roentgenol 1981;136:151–156.
31. Brothers MF, Kaufmann JC, Fox AJ, Deveikis JP: n-Butyl 2-cyanoacrylate—substitute for IBCA in interventional neuroradiology: Histopathologic and polymerization time studies. AJNR 1989;10: 777–786.
32. Cromwell LD, Freeny PC, Kerber CW, Kunz LL, Harris AB, Shaw CM: Histologic analysis of tissue response to bucrylate-pantopaque mixture. Am J Roentgenol 1986;147:627–631.
33. Cromwell LD, Kerber CW: Modification of cyanoacrylate for therapeutic embolization: Preliminary experience. Am J Roentgenol 1979;132:799–801.
34. Goldman ML, Philip PK, Sarrafizadeh MS, Marar HG, Singh N: Transcatheter embolization with bucrylate (in 100 patients). Radiographics 1982;2:340–375.
35. Kish KK, Rapp SM, Wilner HI, Wolfe D, Thomas LM, Barr J: Histopathologic effects of transarterial bucrylate occlusion of intracerebral arteries in mongrel dogs. AJNR 1983;4:385–387.
36. Klara PM, George ED, McDonnell DE, Pevsner PH: Morphological studies of human arteriovenous malformations: Effects of isobutyl 2-cyanoacrylate embolization. J Neurosurg 1985;63:421–425.
37. Marck P, Cummings JE, Galil K: Weak mutagenicity of isobutyl-2-cyanoacrylate tissue adhesive. J Dent Res 1982;61:288–292.
38. Spiegel SM, Vinuela F, Goldwasser MJ, Fox AJ, Pelz DM: Adjusting polymerization time of isobutyl-2-cyanoacrylate. AJNR 1986; 7:109–112.
39. Widlus DM, Lammert GK, Brant A, et al: In vivo evaluation of iophendylate-cyanoacrylate mixtures. Radiology 1992;185: 269–273.
40. Ueki T, Takeo G, Kinoshita J, Tsujihata M, Nagataki S: A case of foreign-body granuloma treated with steroid hormone. Rinsho Shinkeigaku 1992;32:1028–1031.
41. Morikawa K: Biochemical study on the application of alpha-cyanoacrylate instant adhesives in dentistry. Shikwa Gakuho 1990;90: 201–224.
42. Zhou D: Long-term pathological findings of cerebral arteriovenous malformation after embolization. Chung Hua Wai Ko Tsa Chih 1991;29:377–378.

43. Tomb RR, Lepoittevin JP, Durepaire F, Grosshans E: Ectopic contact dermatitis from ethyl cyanoacrylate instant adhesives. Contact Dermatitis 1993;28:206–208.
44. Berenstein A, Choi IS: Treatment of venous angiomas by direct alcohol injection (abstract). AJNR 1983;4:1144.
45. Choi IS, Berenstein A, Scott J: Use of ethyl alcohol in the treatment of malignant tumors. AJNR 1985;6:462.
46. Ellman BA, Parkhill BJ, Marcus PB, Curry TS, Peters PC: Renal ablation with absolute ethanol: Mechanism of action. Invest Radiol 1984;19:416–423.
47. Pevsner PH, Klara P, Doppman J, George E, Girton M: Ethyl alcohol: Experimental agent for interventional therapy of neurovascular lesions. AJNR 1983;4:388–390.
48. Yakes WF, Haas DK, Parker SH, et al: Symptomatic vascular malformations: Ethanol embolotherapy. Radiology 1989;170: 1059–1066.
49. Cho KJ, Williams DM, Brady TM, et al: Transcatheter embolization with sodium tetradecyl sulfate: Experimental and clinical results. Radiology 1984;153:95–99.
50. Dion JE: Abstracts of the annual meeting of the ASNR. ASNR 1991;138.
51. Dubois JM, Sebag GH, De Prost Y, Teillac D, Chretien B, Brunelle FO: Soft-tissue venous malformations in children: Percutaneous sclerotherapy with Ethibloc. Radiology 1991;180:195–198.
52. Kauffmann GW, Rassweiler J, Richter G, Hauenstein KH, Rohrbach R, Friedburg H: Capillary embolization with Ethibloc: New embolization concept tested in dog kidneys. Am J Roentgenol 1981; 137:1163–1168.
53. Wright KC, Bowers T, Chuang VP, Tsai CC: Experimental evaluation of Ethibloc for nonsurgical nephrectomy. Radiology 1982; 145:339–342.
54. Berenstein A: Flow-controlled silicone fluid embolization. Am J Roentgenol 1980;134:1213–1218.
55. Leudke MD, Pile-Spellman JM, Ecker HM: Percutaneous treatment of facial arteriovenous malformations with cryoprecipitate: Adjunct to surgery. AJNR 1989;10:882.
56. Leudke MD, Pile-Spellman JM, Huggins CE, Davis KR, Chin JK: Cryoprecipitate admixtures: In vitro testing as embolic agent (abstract). AJNR 1988;9:1030.
57. Shimizu Y, Nagamine Y, Fujiwara S, Suzuki J, Yamamoto T, Iwasaki Y: An experimental study of vascular damage in estrogen-induced embolization. Surg Neurol 1987;28:23–30.
58. Taki W, Yonekawa Y, Iwata H, Uno A, Yamashita K, Amemiya H: A new liquid material for embolization of arteriovenous malformations. AJNR 1990;11:163–168.
59. Berenstein A, Graeb DA: Convenient preparation of ready-to-use particles in polyvinyl alcohol foam suspension for embolization. Radiology 1982;145:846.
60. Chuang VP, Tsai CC, Soo CS, Wright K, Wallace S, Charnsangavej C: Experimental canine hepatic artery embolization with polyvinyl alcohol foam particles. Radiology 1982;145:21–25.
61. Wright KC, Anderson JH, Gianturco C, Wallace S, Chuang VP: Partial splenic embolization using polyvinyl alcohol foam, dextran, polystyrene, or silicone: An experimental study in dogs. Radiology 1982;142:351–354.
62. Herrera M, Rysavy J, Kotula S, Rusnak B, Castaneda-Zuniga WR, Amplatz K: Ivalon shavings: Technical considerations of a new embolic agent. Radiology 1982;144:638–640.
63. Kerber CW, Bank WP, Horton JA: Polyvinyl alcohol foam: Prepacking emboli for therapeutic embolization. Radiology 1988;130: 1193–1194.
64. Szwarc IA, Carrasco CH, Wallace S, Richli W: Radiopaque suspension of polyvinyl alcohol foam for embolization. Am J Roentgenol 1986;146:591–592.
65. Repa I, Moradian GP, Dehner LP, et al: Mortalities associated with use of a commercial suspension of polyvinyl alcohol. Radiology 1989;170:395–399.
66. Lussenhop AJ, Spence WT: Artificial embolization of cerebral arteries. Report of use in a case of arteriovenous malformation. JAMA 1960;172:1153–1155.
67. Russell EJ, Levy JM: Direct catheter redirection of a symptomatic errant intracranial silastic sphere embolus. Radiology 1987;165: 631–633.
68. Debrun G, Lacour P, Caron J-P, Hurth M, Comoy J, Keravel Y: Detachable balloon and calibrated-leak balloon techniques in the treatment of cerebral vascular lesions. J Neurosurg 1978;49: 635–649.
69. O'Reilly GV, Kleefield J, Forrest MD, Svendsen PA, Serur JR: Fabrication of microballoons for interventional neuroradiology: Preliminary report. AJNR 1984;5:625–628.
70. Higashida RT, Halbach VV, Dowd CF, Barnwell SL, Hieshima GB: Intracranial aneurysms: Interventional neurovascular treatment with detachable balloons—results in 215 cases. Radiology 1991;178:663–670.
71. Higashida RT, Halback VV, Dormandy B, Bell JD, Hieshima GB: Endovascular treatment of intracranial aneurysms with a new silicone microballoon device: Technical considerations and indications for therapy. Radiology 1990;174:687–691.
72. Kaufman SL, Strandberg JD, Barth KH, Gross GS, White R Jr: Therapeutic embolization with detachable silicone balloons: Long-term effects in swine. Invest Radiol 1979;14:156–161.
73. White R Jr, Kaufman SL, Barth KH, DeCaprio V, Strandberg JD: Therapeutic embolization with detachable silicone balloons: Early clinical experience. JAMA 1979;241:1257–1260.
74. Taki W, Handa H, Miyake H, et al: New detachable balloon technique for traumatic carotid-cavernous sinus fistulae. AJNR 1985; 6:961–694.
75. Serbinenko FA: Balloon catheterization and occlusion of major cerebral vessels. J Neurosurg 1974;41:125–145.
76. Romodanov AP, Scheglov VI: Intravascular occlusion of saccular aneurysms of the cerebral arteries by means of a detachable balloon. In H. Krayenbuhl (ed), Advances in Technical Standards in Neurosurgery. Vienna: Springer-Verlag, 1982:25–49.
77. Goto K, Halbach VV, Hardin CW, Higashida RT, Hieshima GB: Permanent inflation of detachable balloons with a low-viscosity, hydrophilic polymerizing system. Radiology 1988;169:787–790.
78. Monsein LH, Debrun GM, Chazaly JR: Hydroxyethyl methylacrylate and latex balloons. AJNR 1990;11:663–664.
79. Taki W, Handa H, Yamagata S, Ishikawa M, Iwata H, Ikada Y: Radiopaque solidifying liquids for releasable balloon technique: A technical note. Surg Neurol 1980;13:140–142.
80. Braun IF, Hoffman J Jr, Casarella WJ, Davis PC: Use of coils for transcatheter carotid occlusion. AJNR 1985;6:953–956.
81. Chuang VP, Wallace S, Gianturco C, Soo CS: Complications of coil embolization: Prevention and management. Am J Roentgenol 1981;137:809–813.
82. Rao VR, Mandalam RK, Joseph S, et al: Embolization of large saccular aneurysms with Gianturco coils. Radiology 1990;175: 407–410.
83. Graves VB, Partington CR, Rufenacht DA, Rappe AH, Strother CM: Treatment of carotid artery aneurysms with platinum coils: An experimental study in dogs. AJNR 1990;11:249–252.
84. Hilal SK, Khandji AG, Chi TL, Stein BM, Bello JM, Silver AJ: Synthetic fiber-coated platinum coils successfully used for endovascular treatment of arteriovenous malformations, aneurysm and direct arteriovenous fistulas of CNS (abstract). AJNR 1988;9:1030.
85. Morse SS, Clark RA, Puffenbarger A: Platinum microcoils for therapeutic embolization: Nonneuroradiologic applications. Am J Roentgenol 1990;155:401–403.
86. Yang PJ, Halbach VV, Higashida RT, Hieshima GB: Platinum wire: A new transvascular embolic agent. AJNR 1988;9:547–550.
87. Guglielmi G, Vinuela F, Sepetka I, Macellari V: Electrothrombosis of saccular aneurysms via endovascular approach: 1. Electrochemical basis, technique, and experimental results. J Neurosurg 1991; 75:1–7.

88. Guglielmi G, Vinuela F, Dion J, Duckwiler G: Electrothrombosis of saccular aneurysms via endovascular approach: 2. Preliminary clinical experience (see comments). J Neurosurg 1991;75:8–14.
89. Dyken ML: Controversies in stroke: Past and present (The Willis Lecture). Stroke 1993;24:1251–1258.
90. Earnest F IV, Forbes G, Sandok BA, et al: Complications of cerebral angiography: Prospective assessment of risk. AJR 1984;142: 247–253.
91. Dion JE, Gates PC, Fox AJ, Barnett HJM, RitaJ B: Clinical events following neuroangiography: A prospective study. Stroke 1987;18: 997–1004.
92. Purdy PD, Batjer HH, Samson D: Management of hemorrhagic complications from preoperative embolization of arteriovenous malformations. J Neurosurg 1991;74:205–211.
93. Anon VV, Aymard A, Gobin YP, et al: Balloon occlusion of the internal carotid artery in 40 cases of giant intracavernous aneurysm: Technical aspects, cerebral monitoring, and results. Neuroradiology 1992;34:245–251.
94. Anson JA, Spetzler RF: Interventional neuroradiology for spinal pathology. Clin Neurosurg 1992;39:388–417.
95. Barnwell SL: Interventional neuroradiology (review). West J Med 1993;158:162–170.
96. Brown MM: Surgery, angioplasty, and interventional neuroradiology. Curr Opin Neurol Neurosurg 1993;6:66–73.
97. Bryan RN: Remarks on interventional neuroradiology. Am J Neuroradiol 1990;11:630–632.
98. Duckwiler GR, Dion JE, Vinuela F, Bentson J: A survey of vascular interventional procedures in neuroradiology. Am J Neuroradiol 1990;11:621–623.
99. Halbach VV, Higashida RT, Hieshima GB: Interventional neuroradiology (review). Am J Roentgenol 1989;153:467–476.
100. Luessenhop AJ: Interventional neuroradiology: A neurosurgeon's perspective. Am J Neuroradiol 1990;11:625–629.
101. Purdy PD, Batjer HH, Risser RC, Samson D: Arteriovenous malformations of the brain: Choosing embolic materials to enhance safety and ease of excision. J Neurosurg 1992;77:217–222.
102. Setton A, Berenstein A: Interventional neuroradiology. Curr Opin Neurol Neurosurg 1992;5:870–880.
103. Vinuela F, Dion J, Duckwiler G, Guest Editors: Interventional Neuroradiology. Neuroimag Clin North Am 1992;2:1–388.
104. Vinuela F, Halbach VV, Dion JE: Interventional Neuroradiology: Endovascular Therapy of the Central Nervous System. New York: Raven, 1992:209.
105. Gelb AW, Herrick IA: Preoperative hypertension does predict post-carotid endarterectomy hypertension (letter to the editor). [comment (with response) on Shuaib A, Hunter M, Anderson MA: Multiple intracranial hemorrhages after carotid endarterectomy, Can J Neurol Sci 16:345–347, 1989]. Can J Neurolog Sci 1990; 17:95–97.
106. Gelmers HJ, Gorter K, De Weerdt CJ, Wiezer MJ: A controlled trial of nimodipine in acute ischemic stroke. New Engl J Med 1988; 318:203–207.
107. Mee E, Dorrance D, Lowe D, Neil-Dwyer G: Controlled study of nimodipine in aneurysm patients treated early after subarachnoid hemorrhage. Neurosurgery 1988;22:484–491.
108. Ohman J, Heiskanen O: Effect of nimodipine on the outcome of patients after aneurysmal subarachnoid hemorrhage and surgery. J Neurosurg 1988;69:683–686.
109. Pickard JD, Murray GD, Illingworth R, et al: Effect of oral nimodipine on cerebral infarction and outcome after subarachnoid haemorrhage: British aneurysm nimodipine trial. Br Med J 1989;298: 636–642.
110. Stullken EH, Johnston WE, Prough DS, Balestrieri EF, McWhorter JM: Implications of nimodipine prophylaxis of cerebral vasospasm on anesthetic management during intracranial aneurysm clipping. J Neurosurg 1985;62:200–205.
111. Warner DS, Sokoll MD, Maktabi M, Godersky JC, Adams HP: Nicardipine HCI: Clinical experience in patients undergoing anaesthesia for intracranial aneurysm clipping. Can J Anaesth 1989; 36:219–223.
112. O'Mahony BJ, Bolsin SNC: Anaesthesia for closed embolisation of cerebral arteriovenous malformations. Anaesth Intensive Care 1988;16:318–323.
113. Stone JG, Young WL, Smith CR, Solomon RA, Ostapkovich N, Wang A: Do temperatures recorded at standard monitoring sites reflect actual brain temperature during deep hypothermia? (abstract). Anesthesiology 1991;75:A483.
114. Berenstein A, Ransohoff J, Kupersmith M, Flamm E, Graeb D: Transvascular treatment of giant aneurysms of the cavernous carotid and vertebral arteries. Surg Neurol 1984;21:3–12.
115. Rauch RA, Vinuela F, Dion J, et al: Preembolization functional evaluation in brain arteriovenous malformations: The superselective amytal test. AJNR 1992;13:303–308.
116. Berenstein A, Young W, Ransohoff J, Benjamin V, Merkan H: Somatosensory evoked potentials during spinal angiography and therapeutic transvascular embolization. J Neurosurg 1984;60: 777–785.
117. Giller CA, Mathews D, Walker B, Purdy PD, Roseland A: Prediction of tolerance to carotid artery occlusion using transcranial Doppler ultrasound (abstract). J Neurosurg 1993;78:366A.
118. Eckard DA, Purdy PD, Bonte FJ: Temporary balloon occlusion of the carotid artery combined with brain blood flow imaging as a test to predict tolerance prior to permanent carotid sacrifice. Am J Neuroradiol 1992;13:1565–1569.
119. Moody EB, Dawson RC III, Sandler MP: ^{99m}Tc-HMPAO SPECT imaging in interventional neuroradiology: Validation of balloon test occlusion. Am J Neuroradiol 1991;12:1043–1044.
120. Nakano S, Kinoshita K, Jinnouchi S, Hoshi H, Watanabe K: Critical cerebral blood flow thresholds studied by SPECT using Xenon-133 and Iodine-123 Iodoamphetamine. J Nucl Med 1989;30: 337–342.
121. Yudd AP, Van Heertum RL, Masdeu JC: Interventions and functional brain imaging. Sem Nucl Med 1991;21:153–158.
122. Purdy PD: Imaging cerebral blood flow in interventional neuroradiology: Choice of technique and indications (commentary). Am J Neuroradiol 1991;12:424–427.
123. Patton CM Jr: Rapid induction of acute dyskinesia by droperidol. Anesthesiology 1975;43:126–127.
124. Brann CA, Janik DJ: Anesthesia in the radiology suite. Probl Anesth 1992;6:413–429.
125. Ferrer-Brechner T, Winter J: Anesthetic considerations for cerebral computer tomography. Anesth Analg 1977;56:344–347.
126. Glauber DT, Audenaert SM: Anesthesia for children undergoing craniospinal radiotherapy. Anesthesiology 1987;67:801–803.
127. Drummond JC: Cerebral ischemia: State of the art management. Anesth Analg 1992 (suppl to vol 74):1992 Review Course Lectures: 120–128.
128. Young WL, Prohovnik I, Ornstein E, Ostapkovich N, Matteo RS: Cerebral blood flow reactivity to changes in carbon dioxide calculated using end-tidal *versus* arterial tensions. J Cereb Blood Flow Metab 1991;11:1031–1035.
129. Korosue K, Heros RC: Mechanism of cerebral blood flow augmentation by hemodilution in rabbits. Stroke 1992;23:1487–1493.
130. Todd MM, Weeks JB, Warner DS: Cerebral blood flow, blood volume, and brain tissue hematocrit during isovolemic hemodilution with hetastarch in rats. Am J Physiol 1992;263:H75–H82.
131. Service FJ: Hypoglycemic disorders. In JB Wyngaarden, LH Smith Jr (eds), Cecil Textbook of Medicine. Philadelphia: Saunders, 1985: 1341–1349.
132. Peters KR, Quisling RG, Gilmore R, Mickle P, Kuperus JH: Intraarterial use of sodium methohexital for provocative testing during brain embolotherapy. Am J Neuroradiol 1993;14:171–174.

133. Purdy PD, Batjer HH, Samson D, Risser RC, Bowman GW: Intra-arterial sodium amytal administration to guide preoperative embolization of cerebral arteriovenous malformations. J Neurosurg Anesth 1991;3:103–106.
134. Wada J, Rassmussen T: Intracarotid injection of sodium amytal for the lateralization of cerebral speech dominance: Experimental and clinical observations. J Neurosurg 1960;17:266–282.
135. Doppman JL, Girton M, Oldfield EH: Spinal Wada test. Radiology 1986;161:319–321.
136. Horton JA, Latchaw RE, Gold LHA, Pang D: Embolization of intramedullary arteriovenous malformations of the spinal cord. Am J Neuroradiol 1986;7:113–118.
137. Rauch RA, Vinuela F, Dion J, et al: Preembolization functional evaluation in brain arteriovenous malformations: The ability of superselective amytal test to predict neurologic dysfunction before embolization. AJNR 1992;13:309–314.
138. Schroeder T, Schierbeck J, Howardy P, Knudsen L, Skafte-Holm P, Gefke K: Effect of labetalol on cerebral blood flow and middle cerebral arterial flow velocity in healthy volunteers. Neurol Res 1991;13:10–12.
139. Fitch W, Ferguson GG, Sengupta D, Garibi J, Harper AM: Autoregulation of cerebral blood flow during controlled hypotension in baboons. J Neurol Neurosurg Psychiatry 1976;39:1014–1022.
140. Werner C, Hoffman WE, Thomas C, Miletich DJ, Albrecht RF: Ganglionic blockade improves neurologic outcome from incomplete ischemia in rats: Partial reversal by exogenous catecholamines. Anesthesiology 1990;73:923–929.
141. Young WL, Cole DJ: Deliberate hypertension: Rationale and application for augmenting cerebral blood flow. Probl Anesth 1993; 7:140–153.
142. Day AL: Arterial distributions and variants. In JH Wood (ed), Cerebral Blood Flow: Physiologic and Clinical Aspects. New York: McGraw-Hill, 1987:19–36.
143. Bladin CF, Chambers BR, Donnan GA: Confusing stroke terminology: Watershed or borderzone infarction (letter to the editor) [Comment on (with response by) van der Zwan A, Hillen B: Review of the variability of the territories of the major cerebral arteries. Stroke 22:1078–1084, 1991]. Stroke 1993;24:477–478.
144. Van der Zwan A, Hillen B, Tulleken CAF, Dujovny M, Dragovic L: Variability of the territories of the major cerebral arteries. J Neurosurg 1992;77:927–940.
145. Szabo MD, Crosby G, Sundaram P, Dodson BA, Kjellberg RN: Hypertension does not cause spontaneous hemorrhage of intracranial arteriovenous malformations. Anesthesiology 1989;70: 761–763.
146. Watcha MF, White PF: Postoperative nausea and vomiting: Its etiology, treatment, and prevention. Anesthesiology 1992;77: 162–184.
147. Young WL, McCormick PC: Perioperative management of intracranial catastrophes. Crit Care Clinic 1989;5:821–844.
148. Selman WR, Spetzler RF, Roessmann UR, Rosenblatt JI, Crumrine RC: Barbiturate-induced coma therapy for focal cerebral ischemia: Effect after temporary and permanent MCA occlusion. J Neurosurg 1981;55:220–226.
149. Eng CC, Lam AM, Byrd S, Newell DW: The diagnosis and management of a perianesthetic cerebral aneurysmal rupture aided with transcranial Doppler ultrasonography. Anesthesiology 1993;78: 191–194.
150. Goldberg M: Systemic reactions to intravascular contrast media: A guide for the anesthesiologist (review). Anesthesiology 1984;60: 46–56.
151. Todd MM, Warner DS: Perioperative fluid management in neurosurgery. Curr Opin Anaesth 1989;2:599–563.
152. Aidinis SJ, Zimmerman RA, Shapiro HM, Bilanuick LT, Broennie AM: Anesthesia for brain computer tomography. Anesthesiology 1976;44:420–425.
153. Sorenson JA, Phelps ME: Physics in Nuclear Medicine, ed 2. Philadelphia: Saunders/Harcourt Brace Jovanovich, 1987:590.
154. Fleischer LH, Young WL, Pile-Spellman J, et al: Relationship of transcranial Doppler flow velocities and arteriovenous malformation feeding artery pressures. Stroke 1993;24:1897–1902.
155. Wilson CB, Hieshima G: Occlusive hyperemia: A new way to think about an old problem (editorial). J Neurosurg 1993;78:165–166.
156. Al-Rodhan NRF, Sundt TM Jr, Piepgras DG, Nichols DA, Rufenacht D, Stevens LN: Occlusive hyperemia: A theory for the hemodynamic complications following resection of intracerebral arteriovenous malformations. J Neurosurg 1993;78:167–175.
157. Young WL, Kader A, Prohovnik I, et al: Pressure autoregulation is intact after arteriovenous malformation resection. Neurosurgery 1993;32:491–497.
158. Kalkman CJ, Drummond JC, Ribberink AA, Patel PM, Sano T, Bickford RG: Effects of propofol, etomidate, midazolam, and fentanyl on motor evoked responses to transcranial electrical or magnetic stimulation in humans. Anesthesiology 1992;76:502–509.
159. Losasso TJ, Boudreaux JK, Muzzi DA, Cucchiara RF, Daube JR: The effect of anesthetic agents on transcranial magnetic motor evoked potentials (TMEP) in neurosurgical patients (abstract). J Neurosurg Anesth 1991;3:200.
160. McKay RD, Sundt TM, Michenfelder JD, et al: Internal carotid artery stump pressure and cerebral blood flow during carotid endarterectomy: Modification by halothane, enflurane, and innovar. Anesthesiology 1976;45:390–399.
161. Jorgensen LG, Schroeder TV: Transcranial Doppler for detection of cerebral ischaemia during carotid endarterectomy. Eur J Vasc Surg 1992;6:142–147.
162. Kofke WA, Barker D, Brauer P, et al: Comparison of 3-D Xe CBF, transcranial Doppler, and carotid stump pressure during carotid balloon test occlusion in humans (abstract). J Neurosurg Anesth 1991;3:207.
163. Nichols FT III, Mawad M, Mohr JP, Stein B, Hilal S, Michelsen WJ: Focal headache during balloon inflation in the internal carotid and middle cerebral arteries. Stroke 1990;21:555–559.
164. Halbach VV, Higashida RT, Hieshima GB, Goto K, Norman D, Newton TH: Dural fistulas involving the transverse and sigmoid sinuses: Results of treatment in 28 patients. Radiology 1987;163: 443–447.
165. Halbach V, Higashida RT, Hieshima G, Norman D: Normal perfusion pressure breakthrough occurring during treatment of carotid and vertebral fistulas. Am J Neuroradiol 1987;8:751–756.
166. Lylyk P, Vinuela F, Dion JE, et al: Therapeutic alternatives for vein of Galen vascular malformations. J Neurosurg 1993;78:438–445.
167. McLeod ME, Creighton RE, Humphreys RP: Anaesthetic management of arteriovenous malformations of the vein of Galen. Can Anaesth Soc J 1982;29:307–312.
168. Roberts JT, Pile-Spellman J, Joseph M, Glinski E, Chin J, Hacein-Bey L: A patient with massive oral-facial venous malformation. J Clin Anesth 1991;3:76–79.
169. Szlavy L, Taveras JM: Noncoronary Angioplasty and Interventional Radiologic Treatment of Vascular Malformations. Baltimore: Williams and Williams, 1995.
170. Lasjaunias P, Berenstein A: Endovascular treatment of the craniofacial lesions. In Surgical Neuroangiography, vol 2. Heidelberg: Springer-Verlag, 1987:389–397.
171. LaMuraglia GM, Fabian RL, Brewster DC, et al: The current surgical management of carotid body paragangliomas. J Vasc Surg 1992;15:1038–1045.
172. Schell RM, Cole DJ: Cerebral protection and neuroanesthesia. Anesth Clin North Am 1992;10:453–469.
173. Lyden PD, Zivin JA: Hemorrhagic transformation after cerebral ischemia: Mechanisms and incidence. Cerebrovasc Brain Metab Rev 1993;5:1–16.

18.3 Arteriovenous Fistulas

Key Points

1. An arteriovenous fistula (AVF) is a single hole in an artery connected to a vein.
2. AVFs are excellent models for the pathophysiology and treatment of many conditions, including arteriovenous malformations (AVMs), venous thrombosis, and ischemia.
3. AVFs usually are:
   - posttraumatic.
   - symptomatic.
   - in need of treatment.
4. Urgent treatment is indicated for:
   - cortical drainage.
   - bleeding.
   - symptomatic venous hypertension.
5. Assess prior to treatment:
   - systemic or associated disease.
   - adequate collateral arteries and veins.
   - anatomic and pathophysiologic details of specific patient.
6. Occlude the fistula site; spare the parent vessel. Approach the arterial side first.

Etiology, Importance, and Classification

An arteriovenous fistula (AVF) is a single hole between an artery and a vein. Fistulas can be classified as to (a) etiology, (b) location, (c) angioarchitecture, (d) flow, or (e) clinical presentation. AVFs can be developmental, traumatic, iatrogenic, degenerative, aneurysm rupture, infectious, and even tumoral in *etiology* (1–18) (Table 18.15). Fistulas tend to be acquired, where as arteriovenous malformations (AVMs) tend to be congenital. The most common cause of a fistula is trauma.

The *location* classification of AVFs rests on identifying either (a) the artery and vein involved in the fistula or, less commonly, (b) the space in which the fistula site exists.

Table 18.15.
Etiologies of Fistulas

Traumatic
Direct or indirect
Iatrogenic
Spontaneous
Congenital/Acquired
Ruptured aneurysm
Tumor necrosis
Thrombosis and recanalization
Idiopathic
Systemic/Predisposition
Ehlers-Danlos syndrome
Fibromuscular dysplasia
Neurofibromatosis

This classification rests on angiographic information and is the most useful. There are various kinds of fistulas: carotid-cavernous fistula (CCF), vertebral-jugular fistula, middle cerebral artery–middle cerebral vein fistula, and others. *Fistula sites* can be extracranial, peridural artery-sinus, intradural artery-sinus, intracranial, peridural artery-sinus/vein, pial artery-vein, or medullary artery-vein.

The angioarchitecture classification can also be confusing, since fistulas are classified as a subset of AVMs (19). It is probably more helpful to think of AVMs as a collection of AVFs than of an AVF as a piece of an AVM.

Flow classification rests on the angiographic picture, or auscultation. Flows are classified as *high flow* or *low flow*. This classification is a rule of thumb that often separates those AVFs (AVMs) that do not have associated venous thrombosis from those that do. Prior to selective angiography this classification also was used to separate the low-flow dural AVFs from the high-flow spinal AVFs.

The *clinical classification* rests on how the patient presents. Since the clinical presentation is often startling and often points in the direction of the diagnostic and therapeutic options, it is useful as a first approximation. Clinical presentation also gives some indication as to the pathophysiology involved. The details can only be given by angiography. Published series are often grouped by this classification.

Pathology and Pathophysiology

Arteriovenous fistulas have had a unique role in the development of interventional neuroradiology and endovascular surgery (20). Together with other forms of arteriovenous shunting, they have helped highlight therapeutic and pathophysiologic considerations. The details of each type need to be appreciated before treatment can be undertaken. The changes associated with fistulas can be divided into anatomic or physiologic.

The physiologic changes are related to the progressive neurologic dysfunction. They include venous hypertension and congestion of the surrounding tissue, as well as an increase in velocity and flow in the feeding arteries and draining veins (Table 18.16).

The anatomic (morphologic) changes are thought to cause the catastrophic bleeds. They include the high-flow angiopathy seen on both the venous and the arterial side. These changes are all compensatory to the high flow and low pressure, but can become either ineffective or overeffective. At a macroscopic level there is *primarily segmental dilatation* of the blood vessel leading to ectasia. If the dilatation is nonsegmental or involves a weakened segment, *aneurysm* formation is also seen. If the responses are hyperactive, *stenosis* and even *thrombosis* can ensue. At the microscopic level, changes occur in the structural makeup

Table 18.16.
Physiologic Effect of an AV Shunt on Tissues (See Fig. 18.10*B*)

Vessel Δ fistula	Velocity	Pressure	Diameter	Resistance	Po_2	Comments
Feeding artery (1)	+++	−−−	++	−−−	=	
Vessel of passage (2)	+	−−	=	−	=	
Adjacent territory artery (3)	−	−−	=	=	=	
Collateral arteries (4)	++	−−	+++		=	Normally not seen.
Dedicated feeder (5)	++++	−−−	++++	−−−	=	Physiologically dedicated but can be in contact with large areas of tissue if retrograde filling via arterial collateral happens.
Fistula (6)	++++	−−−−−	Prime event	−−−−−−−	=	Due to Poiseuille's law, very sensitive to the size of the fistula.
Capillary (7)	?(−)	?(+)	?(+)	?(−)	?(=)	Using the eye as an example, there is tremendous increase in the hyperemia.
Adjacent territory vein (8)	−	+	+	=	=	
Vein of passage (9)	−	+	?	=	+	Name does not fit, but it is symmetrical with the artery.
Veins collateral (10)	+++	+++	+++	−−−	++	Veins may begin to play a role in the development of resistance, a role they are not prepared to assume.
Dedicated draining veins	++++	++++	++++	−−−−	+++	
Draining veins	++	−−	+++	−−	++	
Interstitial fluid	?	++	++	?	?	Using the eye as an example.
Extracellular fluid (CSF)	+	+	+	?	?	Noncommunicating and communicating hydrocephalus can occur as a result of AVFs.

of the vessel (21). The endothelium is denuded, and the internal elastic membrane is thickened and then frayed and broken. The muscle layer is thinned and replaced with primitive myointimal cells. Vasa vasorum develop. These changes are seen on both the arterial and venous side. It is the impression that symptomatic thrombus and stenosis is more common on the venous side and aneurysm formation is more common on the arterial side.

CLINICAL-PATHOLOGIC CORRELATES

A fistula within the subarachnoid space or draining into the intracranial or intraspinal veins presents a serious risk of bleeding (Table 18.15). The larger the fistula and the more the associated venous stenosis and thrombosis, the greater the chance of venous hypertension and mass effect. The larger the fistula and the younger the patient, the greater the chance of congestive heart failure (Table 18.17).

The progressive effects of the fistula on the cerebral vascular physiology are related to both the arterial and the venous state, but appear to be more sensitive to venous occlusion both clinically and experimentally (22).

A model of a rat arteriovenous fistula was created anastomosing a proximal common carotid artery to distal external jugular vein, the primary vessel draining intracranial venous blood (22). In rats with an AVF, occlusion of venous outflow increased torcular pressure and created severe ischemic changes. Torcular pressure and systemic arterial pressure had a positive linear relationship. Histologic examination revealed venous infarction, subarachnoid hemorrhage, and severe brain edema. This model of cerebrovascular "steal" with venous hypertension reproduces both hemodynamic and hemorrhagic complications of human AVFs and emphasizes the importance of venous outflow obstruction and venous hypertension in the pathophysiology of these lesions.

In 44 cats, a fistula between the left distal common carotid artery and the jugular vein was created and the left vertebral artery was simultaneously occluded, producing a chronic cerebral venous ischemic state. Six weeks later, pial arterial behavior, disruption of the blood-brain barrier (BBB), and cerebral histologic changes were investigated using three experimental methods. The results indicate that the perfusion pressure breakthrough threshold in the chronically ischemic brain may not be reduced by the restoration of normal blood flow, but may be decreased by the addition of new ischemic insults or hypertension (22).

Table 18.17.
Fistula Location

Fistula Site	Usual Etiology	Usual Venous Drainage	Usual Symptom	Comments
Extracranial brachiocephalic artery	Trauma, FMD*, iatrogenic	Extracranial	Swelling, pain	(FA-FV F)† Thick-walled artery and veins
Extracranial peridural artery and sinus	FMD*, aneurysm	Sinus +/− cerebral veins	Discomfort, bruit, pressure, neuropathy	Vertebral AVF, only rarely has neurologic consequences
Interdural artery and sinus	Trauma, FMD*, iatrogenic	Cerebral veins +/− sinus	Bruit, discomfort, pressure, neuropathy, venous hypertension	Carotid-cavernous fistula
Intracranial peridural artery, sinus, and vein	FMD*, aneurysm	Sinus +/− cerebral veins	Discomfort, bruit, pressure, neuropathy	VGAM‡
Pial artery and vein	Congenital, trauma	Cerebral veins	Seizures, headache, hemorrhage, venous hypertension	Spinal type IV
Medullary artery and vein	Congenital	Cerebral veins	Hemorrhage	As an isolated finding, extremely rare

* FMD = fibromuscular dysplasia.
† FA-FV F = facial artery-facial vein fistula.
‡ VGAM = vein of Galen arterial malformation.

The location of the fistula determines the nature of the blood vessel, the possible source of collaterals, and the probable venous drainage. As one progresses from extracranial to medullary, the arteries become smaller, thinner, and stiffer (from less elastic tissue) and have tighter turns, more branches, fewer collaterals, and more intracranial venous drainage. All these factors increase the difficulty as well as the risk of treatment. Over time fistulas tend to get larger, recruiting more arterial collaterals as the fistula hole enlarges. Rarely, true fistulas can obliterate spontaneously, but the natural history is one of increasing problems (23,24).

Work-up and Management

The clinical presentation most commonly includes some discomfort, pain, or headache presumably related to vessel or tissue distention. In posttraumatic fistulas this develops days to weeks after the trauma. Some dysfunction of the surrounding tissues is also present. This can be due to mass effect from the veins or venous hypertension. Symptoms from mass effect are usually relatively mild but in the globe, thalamus, or spinal cord can be significant. Venous hypertension leads to a loss of an effective arteriovenous (AV) gradient, impaired venous, and cerebrospinal fluid (CSF) drainage in the tissues. In some cases this can lead to local ischemia, tissue edema, and hydrocephalus. This constellation is more common when there is associated venous outlet obstructions and a large fistula.

The clinical findings of a carotid-cavernous fistula offer insight into the general condition of venous and tissue hypertension, since one can see the tissues affected. Proptosis, chemosis, impaired optic mobility, ophthalmoplegia, glaucoma, ischemic neovascularity of the retina, and mass effect can be seen (25–29). These changes in the spinal cord or brain can be inferred (30–34). Seizure may be related to any of these etiologies. Hemorrhage is related either to the initial disruption of the vessel and tissues or failure of the vessels to adapt to the increased flow and pressure in the veins (25). Hemorrhages in these patients are extremely dangerous, with a high chance of fatal recurrence. High-output cardiac failure is distinctly uncommon except in the very young before the sutures close.

The development and resolution of reversible retinal superficial cotton-wool spots and *deep gray intraretinal lesions* paralleling visual deterioration and improvement in carotid-cavernous fistulas have been reported. It has been postulated that the deep intraretinal lesions are clinical manifestations of a zone of retinal microvascular watershed ischemia, and that their presence may be an important diagnostic guide to the presence of reversible ocular ischemia (35). *Globe tenting* is a change in the posterior globe configuration that results in a tented or conical appearance and is objectively defined as a posterior globe angle of less than 130°. It is caused by an acute or subacute intraorbital mass effect producing significant proptosis with tethering of the globe by the stretched optic nerve that can be seen in traumatic carotid-cavernous fistula (CCF). Progressive narrowing of the posterior globe angle has correlated with an increase in proptosis and in optic nerve length, as well as with more severe visual impairment. Tenting with a posterior globe angle of 120 to 130° has correlated with mild visual symptoms and a good recovery. A posterior globe angle of less than 120° with acute proptosis constitutes a surgical emergency; a delay in surgical decompression in these patients may prevent complete recovery of visual function (36).

In acute traumatic fistulas, the arteries are severely disrupted, with associated dissections, pseudoaneurysms, and perivascular hematomas and thrombi, as well as with significant surrounding tissue trauma (37). If treatment can be delayed until the fistula matures, it should be. If not, extreme care must be taken not to disrupt the vessel further by manipulations. Assessment of these associated findings prior to treatment is essential, since they can severely limit the approach to treatment and prejudice the outcome (38–40).

DIAGNOSIS

Cross-sectional imaging is most helpful in determining the extent of involvement of the fistula (41), venous hypertension (42), and the condition of the surrounding tissue (43). For traumatic fistulas with associated bone fractures (44), computed tomography (CT) is indicated. Magnetic resonance imaging (MRI) or magnetic resonance angiography (MRA) demonstrates the arteriovenous anatomy, venous hypertension, and surrounding tissue changes. Color-flow Doppler and TCD are relatively sensitive (95 percent) and specific (90 percent) for high-flow conditions such as AVMs and fistulas (45–48). In patients with large shunts and venous hypertension, SPECT can indicate the scope of hemodynamic derangement (49).

Treatment planning rests on complete angiography. The high flow associated with the lesion requires high-speed angiography (4/sec) to identify the exact fistula site. Filling the fistula via collateral injections or distal-to-flow arrest can also help identify the exact location of the fistula. The nature and adequacy of distal collateral flow can be suggested by angiographic studies and determined by test occlusions. This should be done whenever there may be advertent or inadvertent parent vessel occlusion with fistula (50).

MANAGEMENT

The goals are usually to obliterate the fistulous connection between the artery and vein and to spare the parent artery. Obliteration of the parent vessel across the fistula site is necessary when the parent vessel is dysplastic and adequate collateral circulation has been demonstrated.

Treatment is indicated for nearly all AVFs of the cranial cephalic region. The decisions regarding treatment require angiography. Indications for treatment include (a) the presence of subarachnoid veins, (b) intractable headache or bruit with disruption of sleeping, work, or social performance, and (c) neurologic or functional deficit related to tissue edema or mass effect. Indications for urgent and emergent treatment include (a) recurrent bleeding, particularly in patients with trauma, (b) progressive loss of neurologic function of the areas involved, and (c) pseudoaneurysm or aneurysm (51–53).

Spontaneous clinical cures should always be confirmed by angiography because they may represent obliteration of the superficial drainage with increased cerebral cortical venous drainage and risk of bleeding (54).

ENDOVASCULAR CARE

Endovascular Strategy

The first step is to identify the exact site of the fistula clearly. This can usually only be done during superselective studies. Occasionally use of high-speed angiography, cross filling, or controlled hypotension can help identify a fistula. The typical transition site from artery–fistula–vein must be seen. The artery shows a slight increase in size as it reaches the fistula. At the fistula, a narrowing can usually be identified. There is almost always a poststenotic venous dilatation. Tremendous turbulence can be identified at the fistula site by vigorous movement of the catheter tip. The catheter stops moving as soon as it passes into the venous pouch. Movement of contrast tends to be much more rapid on the arterial side than on the venous side. Knowledge of the course of the normal vessels is critical to avoid inadvertent proximal or distal occlusion. The target of the treatment is the fistula, and it must be clearly in the therapeutic sites (Fig. 18.10).

Associated disease and conditions such as associated trauma, planned surgery, or cardiac disease can limit the therapeutic options and add to the technical difficulty. Assessment of collateral circulation and cerebral vascular reserve is helpful in the event of inadvertent proximal occlusion.

Care must be taken in placing the therapeutic occlusion device (Fig. 18.11). Generally, the arterial side should be approached first. The arterial approach tends to give the best view and control, is the most forgiving to misadventure, and thus offers the greatest chance of success. Partial arterial treatment can also be an adjuvant prior to the surgical or the transvenous approach. The transvenous approach is highly effective if the venous structure can tolerate the increased pressure associated with occlusion, and if the occluded segment is not the drainage for some unrecognized normal venous drainage. A combined interventional and surgical approach is occasionally needed. Rarely, radiation is indicated.

Based on many years' experience, one author believes that arterial side occlusion leads to recurrence, whereas venous side occlusion leads to permanent cure. Sinus thrombosis precedes the development of dural AVMs, and arterialized venous pressure within the cranium or the orbit is thought to be the source of morbidity. Vein of Galen aneurysms embrace some features of cerebral AVMs, such as a reticulum, and some features of dural fistulas, namely, evidence of previous sinus anomaly and direct drainage into a sinus. These aneurysms are also permanently cured by venous side thrombosis, although the dangers inherent in their reticulum demand that this be done in stages or preceded by arterial side embolization. A very limited experience with venous end occlusion of cerebral (and spinal) AVMs suggests that they, too, can be permanently cured by venous side occlusion without excision. Their reticulum demands maximum, multistage, preliminary arterial side embolization together with intraoperative hypotension during the venous occlusion stage in order to minimize intracerebral hemorrhage or swelling. The theory is advanced that dural fistulas, vein of Galen aneurysms, and AVMs are venous- rather than arterial-based lesions, which

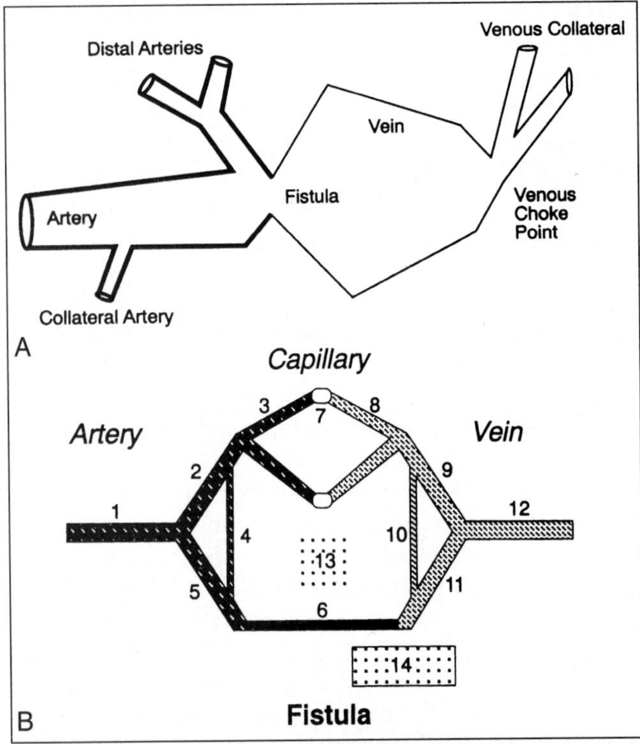

Figure 18.10. A. Diagram of a fistula, artery, and vein. **B.** A simple schematic of an arteriovenous fistula (AVF) and the surrounding brain tissue: feeding artery (1), vessel of passage (2), adjacent territory artery (3), arterial collateral (4), dedicated feeder (5), fistula (6), capillary (7), adjacent territory vein (8), vein of passage (9), collateral veins (10), dedicated draining veins (11, 12), interstitial fluid (13), and extracellular fluid (CSF) (14). (See Table 18.16.)

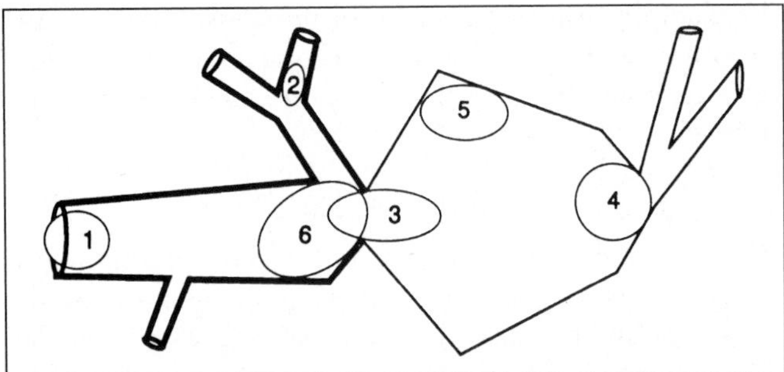

Figure 18.11. Occlusion of a fistula with sparing of the parent vessel (3) without distal arterial (2) or venous migration (4) is required to cure the condition without causing a complication. Parent vessel obliteration is also usually effective if it does not cause distal ischemia and effectively traps both the proximal and distal arterial supply (6). Migration of the embolus is tolerated as long as the embolus does not migrate into a venous choke point.

is consistent with the experience that permanent cure has been effected by venous side occlusion without excision in all three anomalies. It is speculated that there may be a developmental link between AVMs and the venous malformations, the AVM being essentially a fistulized venous malformation (55).

Endovascular Tactics

The endovascular tactic depends on the location, size, and strength of the parent vessel (see Table 18.18).

Endovascular therapy for the treatment of fistulas of the proximal vertebral and internal carotid is initially through the arterial route with detachable balloons (Fig. 18.12).

Table 18.18.
Types of Treatment for Fistulas

Treatment	Advantages	Disadvantages	Fistula Location	Materials	Technical Points
Transarterial with parent artery sparing	No ischemia	Inadvertent parent vessel occlusion	Off important vessel of passage	Balloons, coils, NBCA*	Must avoid proximal occlusion
Transarterial with parent artery occlusion	Severely damaged vessel	Decreased cerebral vascular reserve	Off nonessential or redundant vessel	Balloon, coils, NBCA*	Must effectively "trap" fistula
Transvenous occlusion with parent vessel sparing	Only access after parent vessel occlusion	Inadvertent vein occlusion	Nonsubarchnoid veins	Coils, silk, balloons, NBCA*	
Transcutaneous (surgery plus embolization)	Isolated vascular segments	Logistically difficult	Trapped venous segment with collateral flow feeding the fistula	Coils, NBCA*	
Surgery	Excellent when feeder is superficial and draining vein is deep	Tremendous bleeding, confusion as to site of fistula			
Radiosurgery	Noninvasive	Generally ineffective, radiation to surrounding structures	Cavernous	Linac, gamma knife, proton-beam	

* NBCA = *N*-butyl-2-cyanoacrylate.

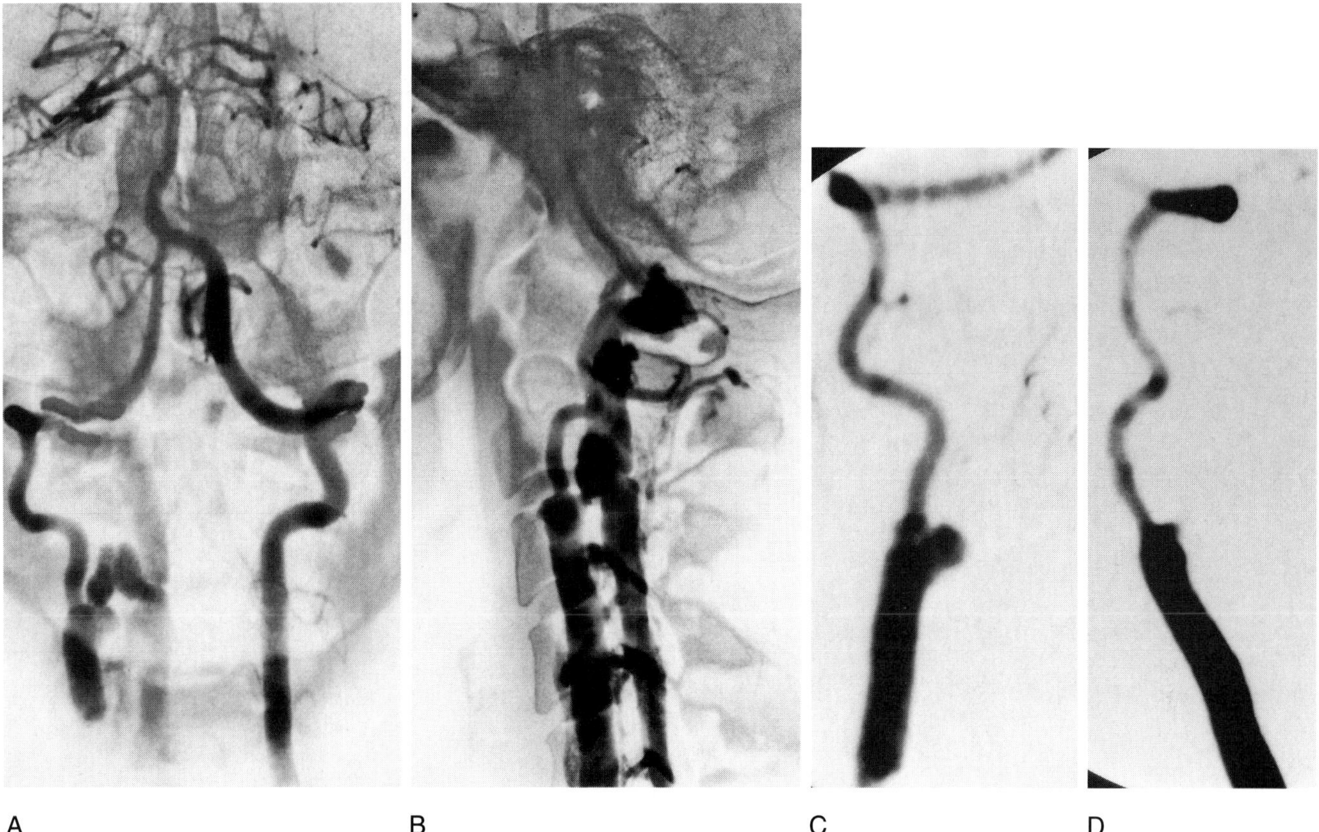

Figure 18.12. Vertebral artery fistula in a 38-year-old female with right neck bruit. Anteroposterior (**A**) and lateral (**B**) left vertebral angiogram. The right-side fistula is seen from the angiogram injection. There is engorgement of the perivertebral venous plexus. **C** and **D.** Right vertebral posttreatment angiogram showing successful balloon occlusion of the fistula; note the discrepancy in vessel size below and above the level of the fistula (C, anteroposterior view; D, lateral view).

Coils and tissue adhesives are the treatment of choice for distal vessels (Fig. 18.13).

Debrun outlined three strategies of *balloon therapy* for traumatic CCFs with occlusion of the fistula while maintaining the carotid blood flow (56). The most common technique uses the end-arterial route: introducing the balloon catheter in the neck or the groin. If the balloon is detached in the cavernous sinus, the carotid blood flow will be preserved (Fig. 18.14). A second approach uses the venous retrograde route through the jugular vein, inferior petrosal sinus, and cavernous sinus. Elegant and safe, this method is appropriate when the fistula drains posteriorly. A third approach involves surgical exposure of the cavernous sinus and direct introduction of the balloon. This is sometimes the only recourse when the fistula has been previously treated with internal carotid ligation.

CCFs can be successfully treated by the endovascular approach *through the vertebrobasilar system*, after the internal carotid artery has been occluded during initial treatment, by navigating through the dilated posterior communicating artery (57).

The use of a PVA embolus captive on a nylon suture has also been used for emboli (58).

Placement of platinum spring microcoils in the cavernous sinus from a transarterial route with the guide wire has some success in spite of the problems of protrusion into the parent vessel and migration into the outflow vein (59). CCFs caused by a ruptured intracavernous aneurysm have been successfully treated with GDC coils via an endovascular transvenous approach (60).

Endovascular therapy is the treatment of choice for vertebral AVFs. Beaujeux et al. summarized the Salstpier 12-year experience with 46 vertebral AVFs (61). Thirty percent were asymptomatic, tinnitus occurred in 45 percent, vertigo in 13 percent, neurologic deficit in 7 percent, and pain in 5 percent. Of the 46 AVFs, 41 percent were caused by trauma and 59 percent were spontaneous. The fistula was found at C1 to C2 in 46 percent of cases, at C2 to C5 in 11 percent, and below C5 in 44 percent. Thirty-four patients (35 vertebral AVFs) were treated with the endovascular technique. Embolization was performed with latex balloons filled with contrast medium in most cases. Endovascular therapy resulted in complete occlusion in 32 cases

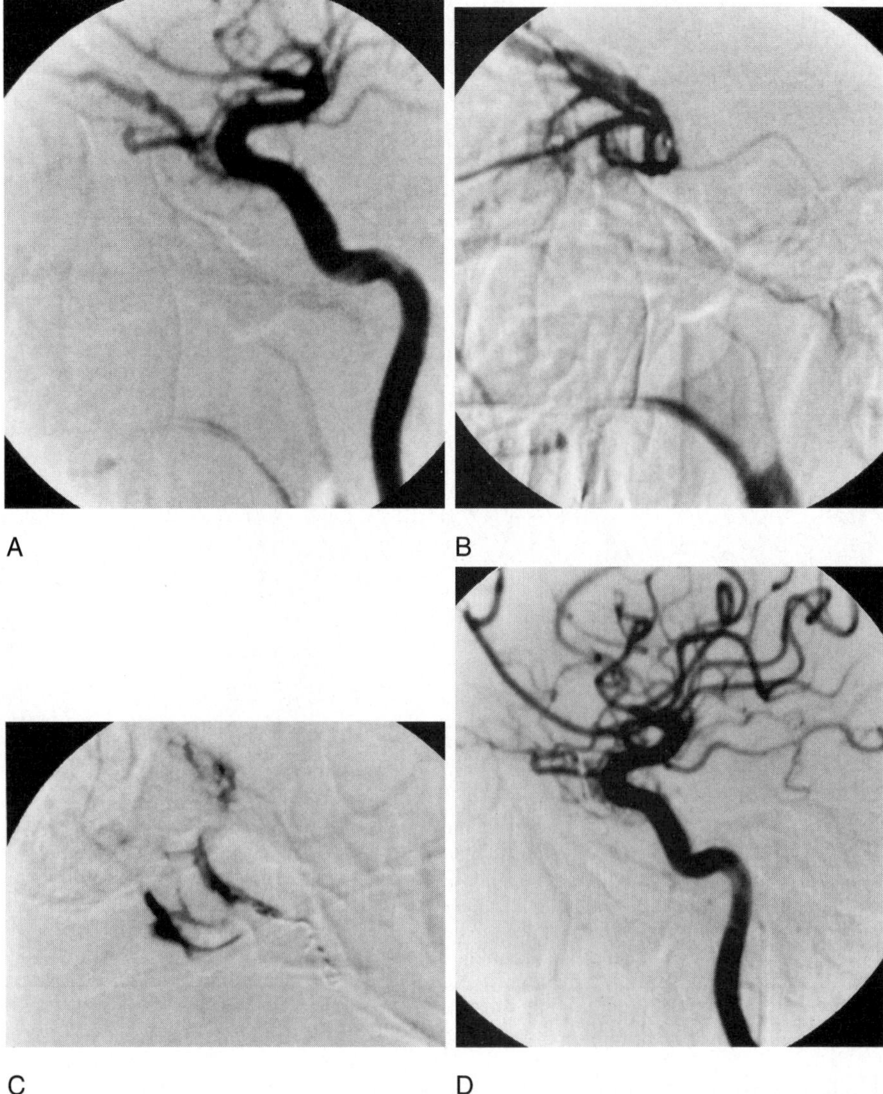

Figure 18.13. Right cavernous sinus AVF in a 26-year-old male with right eye proptosis, chemosis, and glaucoma. **A.** Right internal carotid artery (ICA) angiogram. The AVF is between the cavernous ICA branches and the anterior cavernous sinus draining the ophthalmic veins. **B.** Transvenous approach. The catheter tip is in the superior petrosal sinus–cavernous sinus. **C.** Deposition of coils through a microcatheter in the anterior cavernous sinus. **D.** Right ICA angiogram postembolization. The fistula is not seen.

(91 percent) and partial occlusion in 3 (9 percent). The vertebral artery could not be preserved in 3 patients. Endovascular balloon treatment of vertebral AVFs is effective in occluding the shunt, avoids general anesthesia and surgical intervention, and results in minimal morbidity. Endovascular therapy is the treatment of choice for vertebral AVFs (60). Transcatheter platinum coil obliteration of a cerebellar arteriovenous fistula is highly effective (62).

Transvenous embolization of fistulas is highly effective but is usually used only when the arterial route has been unsuccessful, when arterial access has been hampered by earlier ligations, or in types I and III vein of Galen AVMs or AVFs. The transvenous approach to the CCF through the inferior petrosal sinus or the superior ophthalmic vein with mini coils, liquid adhesives, balloons, and combinations has been used in patients that have failed the transarterial approach (63). In this difficult patient population, almost four-fifths were cured. Fatal complications may occur.

Vein of Galen aneurysms (types I and II) have been treated by percutaneous transvenous endovascular occlusion of the aneurysmal vein via the femoral vein or the jugular vein. In spite of multipedicular feeders and intervening arterial network, treatment was possible. Measurement of intra-aneurysmal pressure during the course of treatment allowed better understanding of the hemodynamics of the lesions, guided the amount of occlusion to be accomplished during each treatment session, and thus may have prevented the phenomenon of normal perfusion pressure breakthrough. The percutaneous transvenous approach offers all the advantages of the transtorcular approach but avoids surgery. Because of excellent angiographic and clinical results—five complete and two partial occlusions, with favorable outcomes and no major complications—some authors believe that this technique is better for the treatment of multipedicular vein of Galen aneurysms than transarterial embolization or surgery (64).

Galenic AV fistulas embolized via a transtorcular venous approach show significant symptomatic improvement in 80 percent of cases and a 20 percent failure rate with disease related mortality (65).

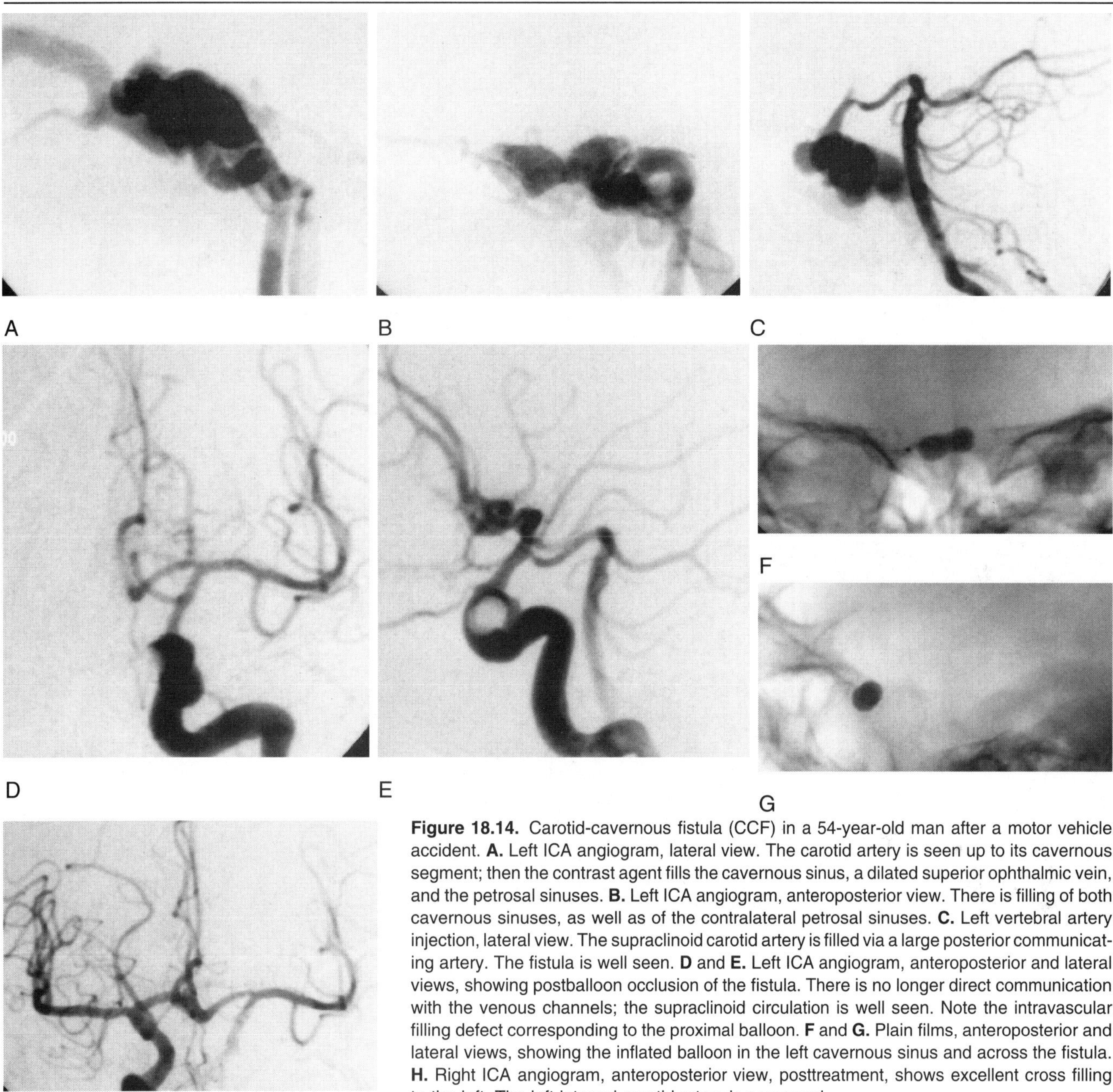

Figure 18.14. Carotid-cavernous fistula (CCF) in a 54-year-old man after a motor vehicle accident. **A.** Left ICA angiogram, lateral view. The carotid artery is seen up to its cavernous segment; then the contrast agent fills the cavernous sinus, a dilated superior ophthalmic vein, and the petrosal sinuses. **B.** Left ICA angiogram, anteroposterior view. There is filling of both cavernous sinuses, as well as of the contralateral petrosal sinuses. **C.** Left vertebral artery injection, lateral view. The supraclinoid carotid artery is filled via a large posterior communicating artery. The fistula is well seen. **D** and **E.** Left ICA angiogram, anteroposterior and lateral views, showing postballoon occlusion of the fistula. There is no longer direct communication with the venous channels; the supraclinoid circulation is well seen. Note the intravascular filling defect corresponding to the proximal balloon. **F** and **G.** Plain films, anteroposterior and lateral views, showing the inflated balloon in the left cavernous sinus and across the fistula. **H.** Right ICA angiogram, anteroposterior view, posttreatment, shows excellent cross filling to the left. The left internal carotid artery is preserved.

Transarterial balloon embolization is the preferred treatment for fistulas with large (1- to 3-mm) holes in strong, thick-walled vessels (carotid-cavernous, vertebral, external carotid–jugular vein fistulas) (Figs. 18.14 and 18.15).

Intravascular detachable balloon techniques, with preserving of the parent vessel, were reported in 12 out of 17 posttraumatic carotid-cavernous sinus fistulas (66).

Occlusion of the carotid artery or a unilateral double CCF makes the transarterial approach hazardous or impossible and requires complex methods. In such cases transvenous embolization can be an alternative treatment, although it is sometimes difficult or impossible to perform. Three cases of direct traumatic CCF and their treatments are described. Unilateral double CCFs have been treated with detachable balloons. If previous trapping has been performed, percutaneous angioplasty with subsequent plastic embolization of the fistula can be curative. When transarterial and transvenous approaches are impossible, combining a surgical procedure and an interventional technique may be needed (67,68).

Direct transcutaneous puncture of the cavernous sinus through an intact orbit for embolization of a recurrent CCF after 10 prior operations has been successful for obliteration (69).

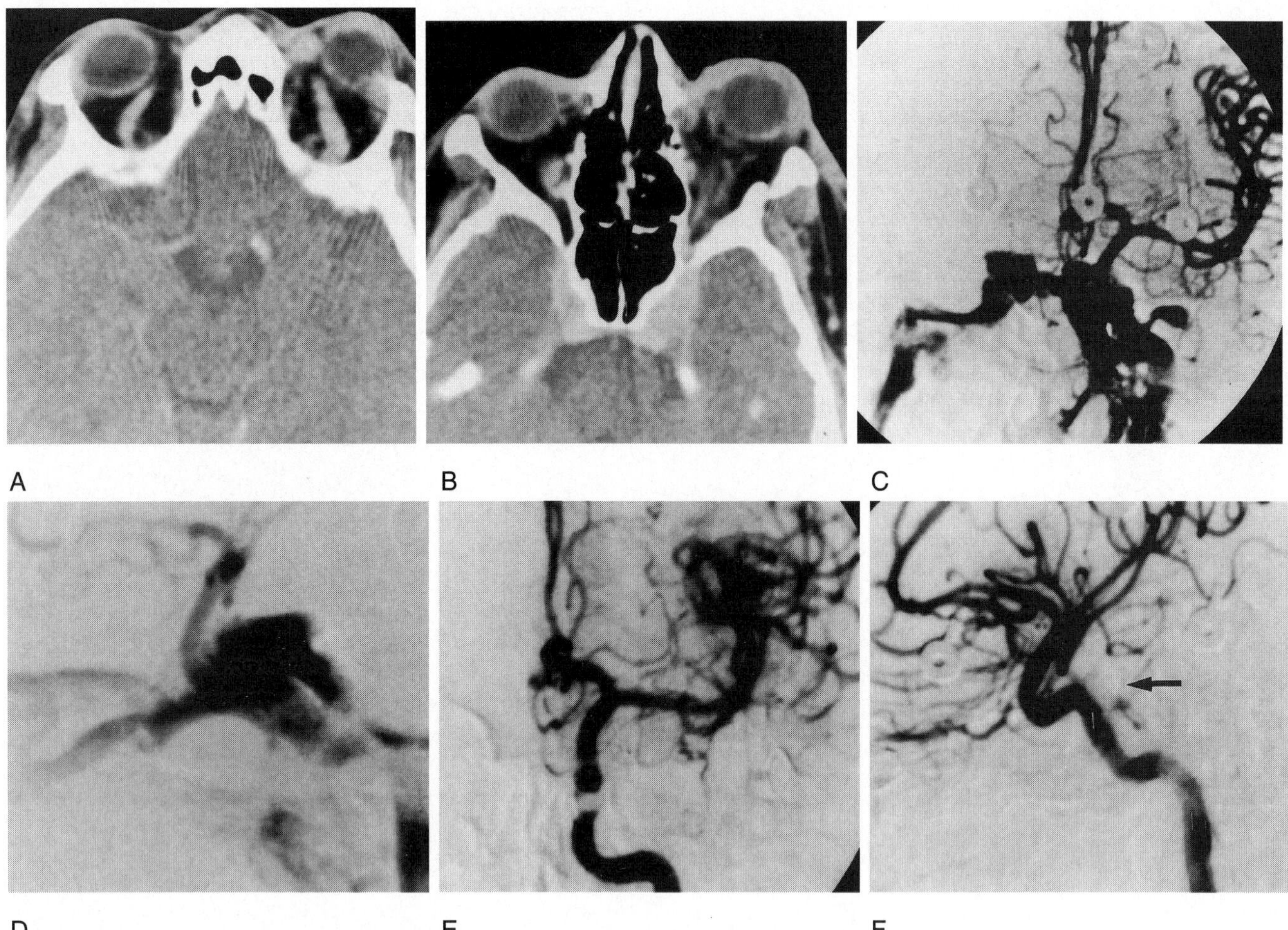

A B C

D E F

Figure 18.15. Traumatic left carotid-cavernous fistula in a 27-year-old female. **A** and **B.** CT examination with contrast. **A.** CT scan shows a prominent left superior ophthalmic vein and left proptosis. **B.** CT scan shows prominent cavernous sinuses, left greater than right, as well as thickened left episcleral tissue. **C** and **D.** Pretreatment angiograms. **C.** Left angiogram, anteroposterior view, shows early filling of the left superior ophthalmic vein from the left ICA, bilateral cavernous sinus filling, and filling of the right superior ophthalmic vein. **D.** Left ICA angiogram, lateral view, ICA shows AV shunting; the rent is most likely in the C4 segment of the left ICA. **E** and **F.** Posttreatment angiograms. **E.** Left ICA angiogram, anteroposterior view. **F.** Left ICA angiogram, lateral view, shows the fistula occluded with one balloon (arrow) with preservation of the left ICA.

In dural CCFs not requiring emergent treatment, combined carotid artery and jugular vein compression was preferred and resulted in complete cure or sufficient improvement in all but one patient. This method is recommended as the first stage of treatment in a dural CCF with an uncomplicated course (70).

Results and Complications

The results from embolization for fistulas are usually excellent, with a high cure rate and relatively low morbidity.

In a University of California–Los Angeles study from 1974 to 1986, 148 patients with CCF were evaluated for intravascular therapy (71). Four patients died from hemorrhage before treatment could be instituted, and the CCF closed spontaneously in 5. Therapeutic approaches that resulted in complete occlusion in the remaining 139 cases were transarterial in 118, were transvenous in 15, and involved external compression of the carotid artery and jugular vein in 6. The current treatment of choice of the direct CCF is intravascular embolization using detachable balloons, particulate emboli, or liquid adhesive agents to occlude the CCF while attempting to preserve the carotid artery. In 15 patients it was technically too difficult to use the transarterial approach. The patients were therefore treated from a transvenous approach, including access via the femoral vein superior ophthalmic vein, intraoperatively from the inferior petrosal sinus, or by direct puncture of the cavernous sinus. Embolic agents used included detachable silicone balloons, steel minicoils, particulate emboli, and isobutyl-2-cyanoacrylate (IBCA). In 14 of these 15 patients total obliteration was achieved with marked improvement in symptoms. Complications occurred in 3 patients, including perforation of the cavernous sinus resulting in subarachnoid hemorrhage, delayed pontine hemorrhage from subtotal occlusion of the fistula, and transient increased proptosis.

Out of 65 CCFs studied at University Hospital, London, Canada, from 1978 to 1982, 20 were spontaneous CCFs. Of these 20 fistulas, 17 were unilateral and 3 were bilateral. In 18 cases the angiographic findings were typical of an AVM, and in 2 a ruptured giant intracavernous aneurysm was found. These patients were treated according to whether they had a nonresolving or progressive cavernous sinus syndrome or deterioration of vision. The cavernous dural AVMs were treated with polyvinyl alcohol and/or IBCA embolization of the external carotid artery blood supply. Two patients underwent postembolization surgical procedures. The detachable balloon technique was used to occlude the fistulas associated with the two giant ruptured intracavernous aneurysms and a small dural intracavernous AVM. Eight patients received no therapy; in 2, spontaneous obliteration of the fistula occurred. Of the 9 cavernous AVMs embolized with particles and/or IBCA, successful transvascular embolization was achieved in 7 cases, and partial embolization followed by surgery in 2 cases. Successful balloon obliteration of the giant intracavernous ruptured aneurysm was obtained in 2 cases. In 1 patient, right hemiplegia with aphasia resulted from reflux of IBCA emboli through the artery of the foramen rotundum into the left middle cerebral artery (72).

Treatment of non-Galenic cerebral vascular fistulas is also excellent (73). The younger the patients, the more likely they are to have feeding from more than one long circumferential source and to have cardiac failure. These fistulas usually have one primary venous source and can be effectively treated by either the surgical or endovascular approach. Control of the embolic agent can be difficult, and tandem balloon methods are useful.

The complications from endovascular therapy for fistulas are uncommon but include distal emboli, vessel rupture, augmentation of venous hypertension, and, rarely, normal pressure perfusion breakthrough. Venous occlusion appears to be the cause of significant morbidity.

Attempts at balloon occlusion of a patient with Ehlers-Danlos syndrome and CCF were unsuccessful and caused multiple arterial dissections and lacerations eventually leading to massive retroperitoneal hemorrhage and death (74). Neurologic deficits after abrupt closure of carotid and vertebral fistulas have been reported in less than 3 percent of cases. Immediate massive cerebral edema, brain herniation, and even death can ensue.

Normal perfusion pressure breakthrough occurred in some patients. Large fistulas that had been present for decades were thought to be the cause, and slow occlusion under hypotension is indicated in these patients (75).

Balloon embolization of CCF has been complicated by fatal cavernous sinus and brainstem venous thrombosis related to balloon migration into the venous outflow, and this uncommon complication has been as high as 4 percent in some series (76,77).

THERAPEUTIC OPTIONS

Surgery

Surgery is indicated today when endovascular methods fail, as well as in cerebral pial fistulas that are anatomically favorable. In these cases, which can be the most difficult, a combined approach with intraoperative angiography and temporary occlusion can be helpful.

In 74 patients with CCF, two-thirds underwent carotid artery surgery because of the fistula, with 28 percent having further visual loss and 5 (10 percent) having cerebral ischemia (78).

Surgical identification of the fistula and confirmation of its obliteration achieved with intraoperative angiography have been found useful. Dissection, control of bleeding, and carotid blood flow were facilitated by temporary balloon occlusion of the cavernous carotid artery (79).

Radiation

Stereotactic radiation can be considered for those patients for whom embolization and surgery cannot be considered or for whom embolization or surgery has been ineffective. Bitoh et al. reported that two patients with spontaneous CCFs were successfully treated with cobalt 60 irradiation to the sellar region. The total radiation doses were 3200 rad and 3024 rad. The patients responded satisfactorily to the treatment, showing disappearance of the fistulas on angiograms and patency of the internal and external carotid arteries (80). Focal radiation after embolization can be useful to obliterate fistulas completely after partial embolization. Four cases of mixed internal and external CCFs were successfully treated with embolization of feeders from the external carotid artery (branches of the internal maxillary artery (IMA)) using Ivalon. Focal irradiation to the cavernous sinus was done with total doses of approximately 30 Gy (81,82).

Summary

An AVF is a single hole in an artery connected to a vein. The AVF is an excellent model for the pathophysiology and treatment of many conditions, including AVMs, venous thrombosis, and ischemia. AVFs usually are posttraumatic, symptomatic, and in need of treatment. Urgent treatment is indicated for cortical drainage, bleeding, and symptomatic venous hypertension. Assess, prior to treatment, systemic or associated disease, adequate collateral arteries and veins, as well as the anatomical pathophysiologic details of specific patients. Occlude the fistula site; spare the parent vessel. Approach the arterial side first.

REFERENCES

1. Eggers F, Lukin R, Chambers AA, Tomsick TA, Sawaya R: Iatrogenic carotid-cavernous fistula following Fogarty catheter thromboendarterectomy: Case report. J Neurosurg 1979;51:543–545.
2. Kushner FH: Carotid-cavernous fistula as a complication of carotid endarterectomy. Ann Ophthalmol 1981;13:979–982.
3. Fuentes JM, Benezech J, Joyeux A, Vlahovitch B, Thevenet A, Vavdin F: Iatrogenic carotid-cavernous fistulas, complications of carotid thrombectomy. Neurochirurgie 1985;31:265–270.

4. Feuerman TF, Hieshima GB, Bentson JR, Batzdorf U: Carotid-cavernous fistula following nasopharyngeal biopsy. Arch Otolaryngol 1984;110:412–414.
5. Lister JR, Sypert GW: Traumatic false aneurysm and carotid-cavernous fistula: A complication of sphenoidotomy. Neurosurgery 1979;5:473–475.
6. Freitas MA, Filho CA, Lima R, Marchiori E: Traumatic ophthalmic fistula simulating carotid-cavernous fistula. Neurosurgery 1983;12: 102–104.
7. Habal MB: A carotid cavernous sinus fistula after maxillary osteotomy. Plast Reconstr Surg 1986;77:981–987.
8. Gokalp HZ, Kanpolat Y, Tumer B: Carotid-cavernous fistula following percutaneous trigeminal ganglion approach. Clin Neurol Neurosurg 1980;82:269–272.
9. Kupersmith MJ, Hurst R, Berenstein A, Choi IS, Jafar J, Ransohoff J: The benign course of cavernous carotid artery aneurysms. J Neurosurg 1992;77:690–693.
10. Bellot J, Gherardi R, Poirier J, Lacour P, Debrun G, Barbizet J: Fibromuscular dysplasia of cervico-cephalic arteries with multiple dissections and a carotid-cavernous fistula: A pathological study. Stroke 1985;16:255–261.
11. Canova A, Esposito S, Patricolo A, Volpini A, Baciocco A: Spontaneous obliteration of a carotid-cavernous fistula associated with fibromuscular dysplasia of the internal carotid artery. J Neurosurg Sci 1987;31:37–40.
12. Dany F, Fraysse A, Priollet P, et al: Dysmorphic syndrome and vascular dysplasia: An atypical form of type IV Ehlers-Danlos syndrome. J Mal Vasc 1986;11:263–269.
13. de Campos JM, Ferro MO, Burzaco JA, et al.: Spontaneous carotid cavernous fistula in osteogenesis imperfecta. J Neurosurg 1982;56: 590–593.
14. Singman R, Asaikar S, Hotson G, Prose NS: Aplasia cutis congenita and arteriovenous fistula: Case report and review. Arch Neurol 1990; 47:1255–1258.
15. Chen MN, Nakazawa S, Hori M. A case of primary intracranial choriocarcinoma with a carotid-cavernous fistula. No Shinkei Geka 1993;21:1031–1034.
16. Weir B, MacDonald N, Mielke B: Intracranial vascular complications of choriocarcinoma. Neurosurgery 1978;2:138–142.
17. Saff G, Frau M, Murtagh FR, Silbiger ML: Mucormycosis associated with carotid cavernous fistula and cavernous carotid mycotic aneurysm. J Fla Med Assoc 1989;76:863–865.
18. Toya S, Shiobara R, Izumi J, Shinomiya Y, Shiga H, Kimura C: Spontaneous carotid-cavernous fistula during pregnancy or in the postpartum stage: Report of two cases. J Neurosurg 1981;54: 252–256.
19. Seidenwurm D, Berenstein A, Hyman A, Kowalski H: Vein of Galen malformation: Correlation of clinical presentation, arteriography, and MR imaging. AJNR 1991;12:347–354.
20. Pool JL: The development of modern intracranial aneurysm surgery. Neurosurgery 1977;1:233–237.
21. Pile-Spellman J, Baker KF, Liszezak TM, et al: High flow angiopathy: Cerebral blood vessel changes in experimental chronic arteriovenous fistula. Am J Neuroradiology 1986;7:811–815.
22. Bederson JB, Wiestler OD, Brustle O, Roth P, Frick R, Yasargil MG: Intracranial venous hypertension and the effects of venous outflow obstruction in a rat model of arteriovenous fistula. Neurosurgery 1991;29:341–350.
23. Konig A, Herrmann HD: Spontaneous healing of a cavernous carotid sinus fistula caused by a gun shot injury. Neurochirurgia 1985; 28:22–24.
24. Santosh C, Teasdale E, Molyneux A: Spontaneous closure of an intracranial middle cerebral arteriovenous fistula. Neuroradiology 1991;33:65–66.
25. Cahill DW, Rao KC, Ducker TB: Delayed carotid-cavernous fistula and multiple cranial neuropathy following basal skull fracture. Surg Neurol 1981;16:17–22.
26. Barke RM, Yoshizumi MO, Hepler RS, Krauss HR, Jabour BA: Spontaneous dural carotid-cavernous fistula with central retinal vein occlusion and iris neovascularization. Ann Ophthalmol 1991;23: 11–17.
27. Brunette I, Boghen D: Central retinal vein occlusion complicating spontaneous carotid-cavernous fistula: Case report. Arch Ophthalmol 1987;105:464–465.
28. Suzuki Y, Kase M, Yokoi M, Arikado T, Miyasaka K: Development of central retinal vein occlusion in dural carotid-cavernous fistula. Ophthalmologica 1989;199:28–33.
29. Buus DR, Tse DT, Parrish R II: Spontaneous carotid cavernous fistula presenting with acute angle closure glaucoma. Arch Ophthalmol 1989;107:596–597.
30. Barnes BD, Rosenblum ML, Pitts LH, Winestock DP, Parker H, Nohr ML: Carotid-cavernous fistula: Demonstration of asymptomatic vascular "steal." J Neurosurg 1978;49:49–55.
31. Chung TS, Lee JD, Suh JH, Kim DI, Park CY: Increased cerebral perfusion after detachable balloon embolization of carotid cavernous fistula on technetium-99m-HMPAO brain SPECT. J Nucl Med 1993;34:1987–1989.
32. Teng MM, Chang T, Pan DH, et al: Brainstem edema: An unusual complication of carotid cavernous fistula. AJNR 1991;12:139–142.
33. Dohrmann PJ, Batjer HH, Samson D, Suss RA: Recurrent subarachnoid hemorrhage complicating a traumatic carotid-cavernous fistula. Neurosurgery 1985;17:480–483.
34. Olteanu-Nerbe V, Bauer M, Vogl T, Marguth F: Endovascular treatment of traumatic arteriovenous fistulas of the vertebral artery. Neurosurg Rev 1993;16:267–273.
35. Cherny M, O'Day J, Currie J: Intraretinal gray lesions as a sign of reversible visual loss following prolonged ophthalmic artery hypoperfusion. J Clin Neuro Ophthalmol 1991;11:228–232.
36. Dalley RW, Robertson WD, Rootman J: Globe tenting: A sign of increased orbital tension. AJNR 1989;10:181–186.
37. Corradino G, Wolf AL, Mirvis S, Joslyn J: Fractures of the clivus: Classification and clinical features. Neurosurgery 1990;27:592–596.
38. Ahuja A, Guterman LR, Hopkins LN: Carotid cavernous fistula and false aneurysm of the cavernous carotid artery: Complications of transsphenoidal surgery. Neurosurgery 1992;31:774–778.
39. Chaloupka JC, Kibble MB, Hoffman JC: Ascending pharyngeal artery–internal jugular vein fistula complicating radical neck dissection. Neuroradiology 1992;34:524–525.
40. Bullock R, van Dellen JR: Acute carotid-cavernous fistula with retained knife blade after transorbital stab wound. Surg Neurol 1985; 24:555–558.
41. Lanzieri CF, Duchesneau PM, Rosenbloom SA, Smith AS, Rosenbaum AE: The significance of asymmetry of the foramen of Vesalius. AJNR 1988;9:1201–1204.
42. Ahmadi J, Teal JS, Segall HD, Zee CS, Han JS, Becker TS: Computed tomography of carotid-cavernous fistula. AJNR 1983;4: 131–136.
43. Chung JW, Chang KH, Han MH, Kim BH, Song CS: Computed tomography of cavernous sinus diseases. Neuroradiology 1988;30: 319–328.
44. Claeys MH, Achten E, De Laey JJ: Non-invasive diagnosis of the localisation of the fistula in dural carotid shunt: A case presentation. Bull Soc Belge Ophthalmol 1992;245:39–43.
45. Erickson SJ, Hendrix LE, Massaro BM, et al: Color Doppler flow imaging of the normal and abnormal orbit. Radiology 1989;173: 511–516.
46. Munk P, Downey D, Nicolle D, Vellet AD, Rankin R, Lin DT: The role of colour flow Doppler ultrasonography in the investigation of disease in the eye and orbit. Can J Ophthalmol 1993;28:171–176.
47. Sommer C, Mullges W, Ringelstein EB: Noninvasive assessment of intracranial fistulas and other small arteriovenous malformations. Neurosurgery 1992;30:522–528.
48. Manchola IF, De Salles AA, Foo TK, Ackerman RH, Candia GT, Kjellberg RN: Arteriovenous malformation hemodynamics: A transcranial Doppler study. Neurosurgery 1993;33:556–562.
49. Watanabe A, Ishii R, Suzuki Y, et al: The cerebral circulation in cases of carotid cavernous fistula: Findings of single photon emission computed tomography. Neuroradiology 1990;32:108–113.

50. Cares HL, Roberson GH, Grand W, Hopkins LN: A safe technique for the precise localization of carotid-cavernous fistula during balloon obliteration: Technical note. J Neurosurg 1978;49:146–149.
51. Halbach VV, Hieshima GB, Higashida RT, Reicher M: Carotid cavernous fistulae: Indications for urgent treatment. Am J Roentgenol 1987;149:587–593.
52. Wilson CB, Markesbery W: Traumatic carotid-cavernous fistula with fatal epistaxis: Report of a case. J Neurosurg 1966;24:111–113.
53. Kurata A, Takano M, Tokiwa K, Miyasaka Y, Yada K, Kan S: Spontaneous carotid cavernous fistula presenting only with cranial nerve palsies. AJNR 1993;14:1097–1101.
54. Lin TK, Chang CN, Wai YY: Spontaneous intracerebral hematoma from occult carotid-cavernous fistula during pregnancy and puerperium: Case report. J Neurosurg 1992;76:714–717.
55. Mullan S: Reflections upon the nature and management of intracranial and intraspinal vascular malformations and fistulae. J Neurosurg 1994;80:606–616.
56. Debrun GM: Treatment of traumatic carotid-cavernous fistula using detachable balloon catheters. AJNR 1983;4:355–356.
57. Garcia-Cervigon E, Bien S, Laurent A, Weitzner I Jr, Biondi A, Merland JJ: Treatment of a recurrent traumatic carotid-cavernous fistula: Vertebro-basilar approach after surgical occlusion of the internal carotid artery. Neuroradiology 1988;30:355–357.
58. Ebina K, Iwabuchi T: Closure of traumatic internal carotid-cavernous fistula with an improved type of captive embolus. No Shinkei Geka 1978;6:59–66.
59. Halbach VV, Higashida RT, Barnwell SL, Dowd CF, Hieshima GB: Transarterial platinum coil embolization of carotid-cavernous fistulas. AJNR 1991;12:429–433.
60. Guglielmi G, Vinuela F, Briganti F, Duckwiler G: Carotid-cavernous fistula caused by a ruptured intracavernous aneurysm: Endovascular treatment by electrothrombosis with detachable coils. Neurosurgery 1992;31:591–596.
61. Beaujeux RL, Reizine DC, Casasco A, et al: Endovascular treatment of vertebral arteriovenous fistula. Radiology 1992;183:361–367.
62. Smith MD, Russell EJ, Levy R, Crowell RM: Transcatheter obliteration of a cerebellar arteriovenous fistula with platinum coils. AJNR 1990;11:1199–1202.
63. Halbach VV, Higashida RT, Hieshima GB, Hardin GW, Yang PJ: Transvenous embolization of direct carotid cavernous fistulas. AJNR 1988;9:741–747.
64. Casasco A, Lylyk P, Hodes JE, Kohan G, Aymard A, Merland JJ: Percutaneous transvenous catheterization and embolization of vein of Galen aneurysms. Neurosurgery 1991;28:260–266.
65. Hanner JS, Quisling RG, Mickle JP, Hawkins JS: Gianturco coil embolization of vein of Galen aneurysms: Technical aspects. Radiographics 1988;8:935–946.
66. Debrun G, Lacour P, Caron JP, Hurth M, Comoy J, Keravel Y: Detachable balloon and calibrated-leak balloon techniques in the treatment of cerebral vascular lesions. J Neurosurg 1978;49: 635–649.
67. Pierot L, Moret J, Boulin A, Castaings L: Endovascular treatment of post-traumatic complex carotid-cavernous fistulas, using the arterial approach. J Neuroradiol 1992;19:79–87.
68. Pilla TJ, Tantana S, Smith KR: Percutaneous transluminal angioplasty prior to carotid cavernous fistula embolization. AJNR 1988; 9:789–790.
69. Teng MM, Guo WY, Lee LS, Chang T: Direct puncture of the cavernous sinus for obliteration of a recurrent carotid-cavernous fistula. Neurosurgery 1988;23:104–107.
70. Mobius E, Berg-Dammer E, Kuhne D, de Silva RD: Clinical aspects and treatment of spontaneous carotid artery-cavernous sinus fistula. Fortschr Neurol Psychiatr 1989;57:518–526.
71. Goto K, Hieshima GB, Higashida RT, et al: Treatment of direct carotid cavernous sinus fistulae: Various therapeutic approaches and results in 148 cases. Acta Radiol Suppl 1986;369:576–579.
72. Vinuela F, Fox AJ, Debrun GM, Peerless SJ, Drake CG: Spontaneous carotid-cavernous fistulas: Clinical, radiological, and therapeutic considerations. Experience with 20 cases. J Neurosurg 1984; 60:976–684.
73. Lownie SP, Duckwiler GR, Fox AJ, Drake CD: Therapeutic management of non–vein of Galen arteriovenous malformation. Interventional Neuroradiology 1992;1:87–113.
74. Lach B, Nair SG, Russell NA, Benoit BG: Spontaneous carotid-cavernous fistula and multiple arterial dissections in type IV Ehlers-Danlos syndrome: Case report. J Neurosurg 1987;66:462–467.
75. Halbach VV, Higashida RT, Hieshima GB, Norman D: Normal perfusion pressure breakthrough occurring during treatment of carotid and vertebral fistulas. AJNR 1987;8:751–756.
76. Santhosh J, Rao VR, Ravimandalam K, Gupta AK, Unni NM, Rao AS: Endovascular management of carotid cavernous fistulae: Observation on angiographic and clinical results. Acta Neurol Scand 1993; 88:320–326.
77. Wilms G, Peene P, Herpels V, van Laer L, Baert AL: Balloon embolisation of carotid-cavernous fistula: Fatal cavernous sinus and brain stem venous thrombosis by balloon migration. Rofo Fortschr Geb Rontgenstr Neuen Bildgeb Verfahr 1992;156:393–395.
78. Palestine AG, Younge BR, Piepgras DG: Visual prognosis in carotid-cavernous fistula. Arch Ophthalmol 1981;99:1600–1603.
79. LeRoux PD, Elliott JP, Eskridge JM, Mayberg M: Intraoperative angiography and temporary balloon occlusion facilitating surgical obliteration of a traumatic carotid cavernous fistula: A case report. Surg Neurol 1990;34:260–265.
80. Bitoh S, Hasegawa H, Fujiwara M, Nakao K: Irradiation of spontaneous carotid-cavernous fistulas. Surg Neurol 1982;17:282–286.
81. Mizobuchi M, Mino S, Nagao S, Ohmoto T, Ohkawa M: Carotid-cavernous fistula successfully treated with embolization and radiation therapy: Report of three cases. No Shinkei Geka 1991;19: 83–87.
82. Pierot L, Poisson M, Jason M, Pontvert D, Chiras J: Treatment of type D dural carotid-cavernous fistula by embolization followed by irradiation. Neuroradiology 1992;34:77–80.

18.4 Cerebral Arteriovenous Malformations

Key Points

1. The goal is to decrease the risk of bleeding.
2. The risk of bleeding from an arteriovenous malformation (AVM) is in the range of 3 percent per year. Approximately one-third of these patients will die from the bleed, one-third will have a significant stroke, and one-third will be unscathed.
3. The risk of bleeding is higher in the smaller, higher-pressure AVMs with aneurysms or venous occlusive disease.
4. The first goal of treatment is total obliteration.

5. Superselective Wada testing prior to embolization helps determine functional neurologic localization and decreases the risk of embolization.
6. Permanent obliteration of the feeding artery-nidus-vein complex is highly effective in reducing the size of the AVM.
7. Partial treatment is indicated for adjuvant treatment of intranidal aneurysms and for progressive "steal." Partial obliteration per se by any method is not known to decrease the risk of bleeding.

Background

Arteriovenous malformations (AVMs) are the most common of the vascular malformations and carry the greatest morbidity. After a brief discussion of the other vascular malformations, the rest of this section will discuss solely AVMs. Vascular malformations are relatively uncommon. They can be divided by location, etiology, pathophysiology, clinical presentation, and type of treatment (Table 18.19).

TYPES OF VASCULAR ANOMALIES

The classification of vascular anomalies by McCormick includes cavernous angiomas, telangiectasia, venous angiomas, varix, AVMs, and cryptic AVMs (1,2). Most types have a characteristic signature. Endovascular therapy is *not* helpful in the treatment of cavernous angiomas, telangiectasia, venous angiomas, or venous varix.

CEREBRAL AVMs

AVMs can be found throughout the central nervous system and its coverings. The center of these AVMs, the *nidus*, is the collection of blood vessels where the AV shunting takes place. AVMs appear to be organized around neural or vascular structures, being wedge, round, or discoid in shape. Assessment of the size, location, and angioarchitecture of the nidus determines the treatment strategy. Cerebral AVMs are found equally throughout the substance of the brain. Varying in size, they are believed to be congenital. The pathologic characteristic feature is an absence of capillaries. The angiographic signature is a profound AV shunting. Superselective injections into the feeding pedicle will almost always reveal multiple but angiographically discrete fistulas. These direct holes between the artery and vein can be tiny but usually are in the range of 0.5 to 2.0 mm, as seen angiographically and by the size of the spherical emboli that pass through them.

Cerebral AVFs are where large, named vessels anastomose directly with the surrounding veins. They can be congenital or aquired (see section on AVFs in text preceding).

Table 18.19.
Location, Etiology, Pathophysiology, Clinical Presentation, Signature, and Treatment of Vascular Malformations

Malformations	Pathology	Etiology	Clinical Presentation	Pathophysiology	Signature	Treatment
Cavernous angiomas	Compact, sinusoidal vessels, separate from neural tissue, no arteries, much Ca++	Congenital	Incidental or bleeding	? Recurrent small bleedings	"Cat's eye" on MRI	Wait and watch, surgery if repeated bleeding
Telangiectasis	Small, capillarylike	Congenital	Incidental			No treatment indicated
Venous malformations	Only venous, single draining vein, normal brain	Congenital	Incidental	Normal unless associated with cavernous malformation	Venous "hydra" without shunts	Contraindicated
Dural AVMs	Shunt in dura, dilated cerebral veins	Acquired, traumatic for single hole, postsinus venous thrombosis	Bruit, seizure, proptosis, chemosis, bleeding	Venous hypertension due to AV shunting and venous occlusion	External carotid artery feeders, thrombosis of a sinus	Embolization surgery
Cerebral AVMs	Arteries and veins only, cliotic plane, focal Ca++	Congenital	Seizure, bleeding, headache	High-flow angiopathy and venous occlusive disease, leading to bleeding	Dilated arteries and veins with early AV shunting, little mass effect relative to mass size	Surgery, radiosurgery, embolization
AVFs	Single arteries and veins	Congenital or acquired	Mass effect, congestive heart failure, seizures	Large mass effect, low arterial feeder pressure	Massively dilated AV unit	Surgery
Cryptic AVMs	Like AVMs but very small	Congenital	Bleeding	?	Small angiographically occult AVM	

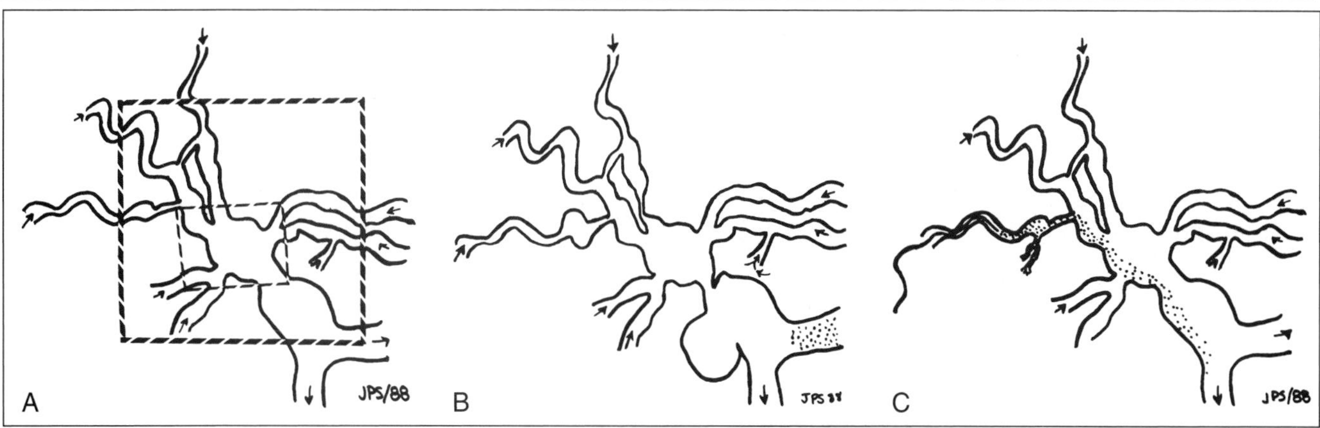

Figure 18.16. A. Diagram of an AVM with the arteriovenous connections outlined by the inner box. This may be thought of as the true nidus. The outer box represents the abnormally dilated arteries and veins. **B.** Over time, high-flow venopathy and arteriopathy create stenosis, aneurysms, and thrombosis. **C.** Embolization of a pedicle can lead to partial obliteration of the artery feeders and venous drainage.

INCIDENCE AND PREVALENCE

The Cooperative Study of Intracranial Aneurysms and Subarachnoid Hemorrhage found that cerebral AVMs accounted for 8.6 percent of bleeds and 1 percent of all strokes (3). The prevalence may be as high as 4.3 percent in the important autopsy series by McCormick (1,2). Of these patients found at autopsy, only one in eight had been symptomatic. AVMs appear to be congenital without a hereditory basis. There is a male predominance.

PATHOPHYSIOLOGY

Cerebral AVMs cause hemorrhage, seizures, mass effect, progressive neurologic headache, and bruits. The pathophysiology is similar to that of AVFs and is covered in great detail in that section. AVMs have AV shunting; the increased flow can place profound stress on the cerebral vasculature, causing an aquired high-flow angiopathy (Fig. 18.16). The feeding arteries and draining veins undergo changes including stenosis, thrombosis, aneurysm formation, and total loss of the blood-brain barrier and with it, presumably, of autoregulation. Much of the pathophysiologic changes are related to these factors. Histologically, the vessel tries to cope with the stress, but over the long run these mechanisms may fail. The endothelium first becomes plump and thickened, and there is thickening of the internal elastic membrane. As the flow increases, the endothelium is stripped off and replaced by a carpet of degranulated cells, presumably platelets. The internal elastic membrane becomes frayed and eventually thinned. The muscularis undergoes a dedifferentiation into myointimal cells, and there is development of vasavasorum (1,4).

Exactly why cerebral AVMs bleed is unclear, but certain aspects are known to be related to hemorrhage (Table 18.20) (5). It should be noted that pregnancy has been removed from the list. The risk of bleeding or rebleeding in AVMs is in the range of 3 percent per year. Approximately one-third of these patients will die from the bleed, one-third will have a significant stroke, and one-third will be unscathed. The risk of a rebleed in the first year is in the range of 6 to 10 percent (7,8).

Table 18.20.
Hemorrhage Risk Factors for AVMs

Small size	Paucity of venous drainage
Feeding artery pseudoaneurysms	Venous stenosis
Intranidal aneurysms	Deep venous drainage
High-pressure arterial feeders	Temporal lobe location

Classification, Clinical Features, and Prognosis

Cerebral AVMs can be divided by a number of classifications. The classification of Parkinson and Pachers (Table 18.21) is an angioarchitecture classification that may be useful in understanding the AVM structure (9). The Spetzler classification is directed at accessing the difficulty of treatment by direct surgical approach. The Spetzler-Martin classification (Table 18.22) is useful in understanding the expected surgical outcome for a given size of AVM, its eloquence, and the presence or absence of deep drainage (10,11). Clearly, the larger the size of AVM, the more difficult the surgery. However, it is not until AVMs are larger than 5 cm that size is a truly limiting factor. The eloquence of the location is critical even for small AVMs. The third characteristic, deep venous drainage, may be a marker for several things, including venous hypertension and thrombosis, both of which may add to the difficulty of surgery.

If there were a classification to stratify outcomes for ra-

Table 18.21.
Parkinson and Pachers Classification

Parkinson Classification according to the morphology, 1980

Type I: **Multiple unit AVM** consists of multiple arteries and multiple draining veins.
"Multi-clustered units consist of a pair of single artery and single vein." ???
Type II: **Single unit AVM** including a single artery, single fistula, and single draining vein.
Type III: **Straight line AVM** is a direct arteriovenous shunt, in which one or major arteries proceed without subdivision or diminution of caliber directly into a venous sinus.
(corresponding to so-called single AVF)
Type IV: **Combined AVM** is fed by cerebral and extracerebral vessels.
(corresponding to so-called mixed AVM)
Type V: **Venous wall AVM** consists of purely extracerebral arteries draining into a dural sinus.
(corresponding to so-called dural AVF)
Intracerebral AVM seems to include Type I, II, III, IV.

Source: Parkinson D, et al: Arteriovenous malformations. Summary of 100 consecutive supratentorial cases. J Neurosurg 53: 285–29, 1980.

diosurgery, it would weigh size more critically into the grade. Radiosurgery has become an increasingly popular approach to AVM treatment with the introduction of the Linac (12). The outcome from radiosurgery is primarily a function of dose, which in turn is a function of the size of the AVM. The type of ionizing radiation appears to be less important than the dose to the AVM versus that to the normal brain. To obliterate an AVM, it is necessary to get 20 Gy to the AVM in a single treatment. To avoid hurting normal brain, the dose must be kept to less than 60 Gy, and to avoid causing necrosis of the center of the AVM,

Table 18.22.
Spetzler-Martin Classification

Feature	Point
size*	
small (<3 cm)	1
medium (3–6 cm)	2
large (>6 cm)	3
eloquence of adjacent brain†	
noneloquent	0
eloquent	1
pattern of venous drainage‡	
superficial only	0
deep	1

Source: Spetzler RF, et al: A proposal grading system for arteriovenous malformations. J Neurosurg 65: 476–483, 1986.
* the largest diameter of the nidus of the angiograms
† superficial: through the cortical venous system
deep: any/all drainage thru deep veins such as internal cerebral vein, basal vein, precentral cerebellar vein
post. fossa: only cerebellar hemispheric veins draining directly into the straight sinus or transverse sinus are considered "superficial"
‡ regions, if injured, resulting in a disabling neurological deficit: sensorimotor, language, visual cortex, hypothalamus, thalamus, internal capsule, brain stem, cerebellar peduncles, deep cerebellar nuclei

Table 18.23.
Factors Influencing Results in Embolization of AVMs

Extent:	number of named pedicles eloquence of area
Angioarchitecture:	direct dedicated feeders, vessels of passage, or collateral vessels

the dose must be below 80 Gy. These items must all be calculated and considered in radiosurgery planning. Partial permanent embolization prior to radiosurgery in AVMs larger than 2.5 cm is a conceptually attractive option. The expected benefit from such an approach may be difficult to appreciate, since the partial embolization may not be in a location that can decrease the targeted size.

Factors that have entered into a embolization outcome are under development at the author's institution (Table 18.23). The factors depend on the angioarchitecture, the extent of the lesion, and the eloquence of the tissue. The angioarchitecture is the most important factor in terms of safe embolization (Fig. 18.17). The AVM can be fed by direct feeders, vessels of passage, or collateral vessels. The direct dedicated feeders are safe to embolize, whereas collateral flow to the AVM will almost always exact a toll on normal tissue embolization. The AVM can be fed by long or short circumferentials or by perforators. The long circumferentials have many anastomotic collaterals and serve tissue that tends to have the greatest neuronal redundancy. The short circumferentials (in which we include the choroidal anterior) are more dangerous because they serve deep white matter tracts and important nuclei. The perforators are also dangerous because they serve the deep white matter and basal ganglia. If vessels and areas serve neurologically quiet areas, damage to the tissue will not have a measurable effect on outcome (see Figure 18.10).

Work-up

CLINICAL

When cerebral AVMs become symptomatic, patients present with hemorrhage, seizures, headache, or bruit. The work-up of a patient with an AVM (Table 18.24) is aimed at identifying any neurologic deficit that the AVM may have caused, as well as the general health of the patient. Subtle neurologic findings and cognitive changes can often be identified even in the asymptomatic patient. These changes, if not appreciated, can cause confusion and concern in the later management of the patient. Conditions that could shorten a person's expected life span weigh heavily into the decision to stay treatment and must be assessed in this actuarial light.

Other causes for the presenting symptoms should be explored, although in the young and healthy patient they are unlikely to be found. In patients presenting with hemorrhage, the course can be quite stormy, particularly if there is significant blood.

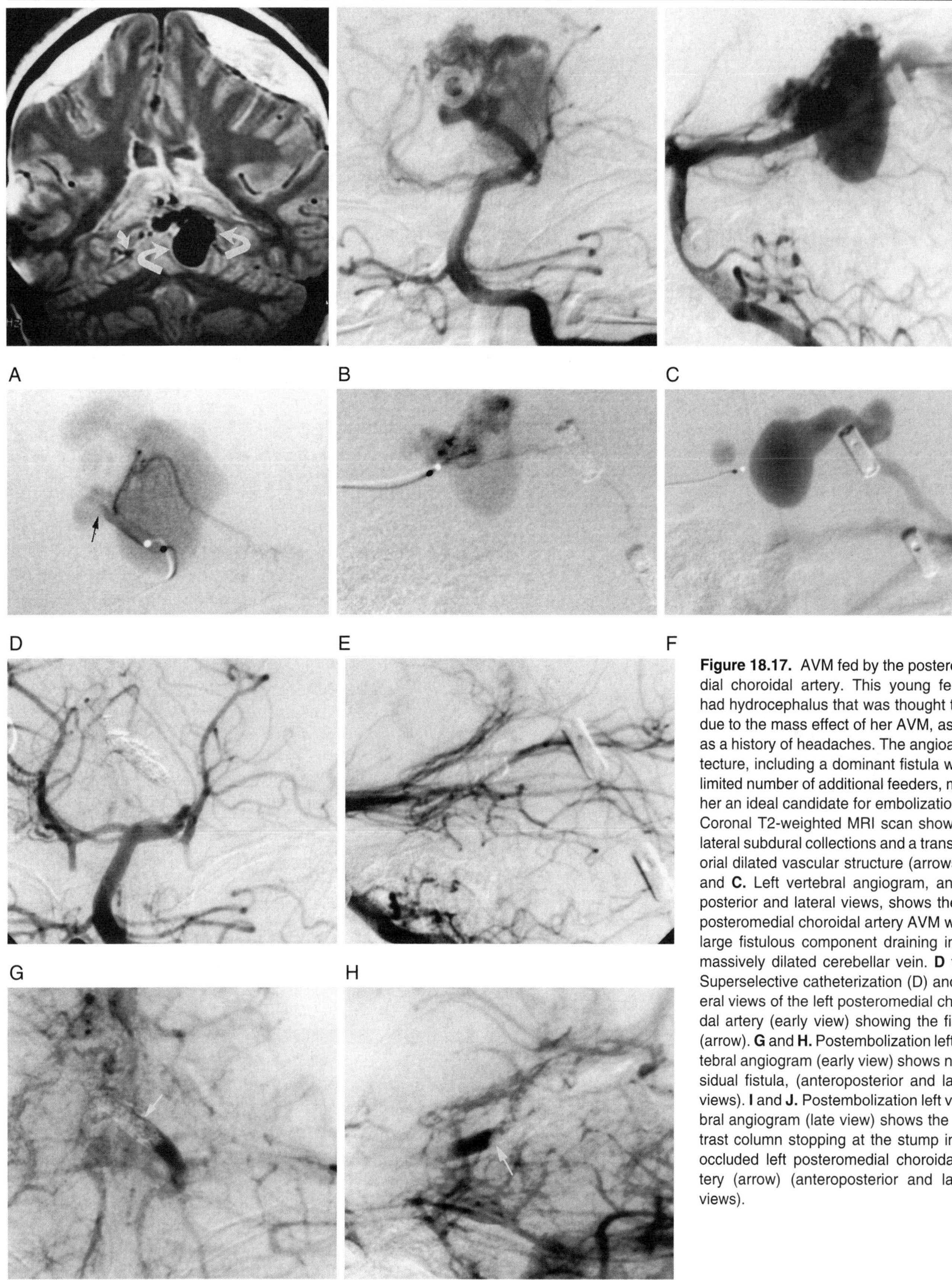

Figure 18.17. AVM fed by the posteromedial choroidal artery. This young female had hydrocephalus that was thought to be due to the mass effect of her AVM, as well as a history of headaches. The angioarchitecture, including a dominant fistula with a limited number of additional feeders, made her an ideal candidate for embolization. **A.** Coronal T2-weighted MRI scan shows bilateral subdural collections and a transtentorial dilated vascular structure (arrows). **B** and **C.** Left vertebral angiogram, anteroposterior and lateral views, shows the left posteromedial choroidal artery AVM with a large fistulous component draining into a massively dilated cerebellar vein. **D** to **F.** Superselective catheterization (D) and lateral views of the left posteromedial choroidal artery (early view) showing the fistula (arrow). **G** and **H.** Postembolization left vertebral angiogram (early view) shows no residual fistula, (anteroposterior and lateral views). **I** and **J.** Postembolization left vertebral angiogram (late view) shows the contrast column stopping at the stump in the occluded left posteromedial choroidal artery (arrow) (anteroposterior and lateral views).

Table 18.24.
Work-up of a Patient with an AVM

Item	Studies	Criteria/Comments
Volume, location, extent	MRI, CT	
Angioarchitecture	Superselective angiogram	Flow rate, nidal aneurysm
Functional involvement	Functional MRI/SPECT, superselective Wada testing	Clearest for superselective Wada testing
Baseline deficits	Complete and formal neurologic and psychological testing	Useful in assuring patient of present state

RADIOLOGICAL

The radiological examination of a patient with an AVM usually includes a CT, MRI, and selective angiogram. In patients with acute bleeds, CT is often the initial study. SPECT scans can be particularly helpful in those rare cases when associated ischemia is suspected to be the cause of progressive neurologic deterioration or when normal pressure perfusion breakthrough may develop. Robust adaptive changes of the brain to chronic regional hyptotension can usually be demonstrated (13).

MRI is extremely useful in determining the exact size and location of the AVM. The exact relationship between the AVM and the deep gray matter or primary motor and sensory cortical areas can be identified. Previous bleeds, infarctions, edema, venous or sinus thrombosis, mass effect, and the feeding arteries and veins coursing through the white matter can all be clearly identified. Gadolinium complex of diethylene Pentaacetic acid first-pass studies appear to be more sensitive than T2-weighted images or MR angiography because of their high intrinsic sensitivity to regional blood flow and volume.

The high-speed selective angiogram is the road map used to guide all treatments. Superselective angiograms of feeding pedicles can be helpful. The angioarchitecture, feeding arteries and draining veins, relative flow rates, associated aneurysms, stenosis, occlusions, shift in watershed, apparent compartments, and degree of ectasia should all be identified prior to formulating an endovascular approach. Stereo views may show the exact configuration of the arteries and veins with the nidus, and can be quite helpful prior to surgery, particularly in the effort to spare normal brain.

LABORATORY

Transcranial Doppler can usually identify the presence of high-velocity blood flow in the cisternal vessels feeding an AVM and can be used to follow treatment (14). Baseline and intraoperative neuropsychological testing, sensory- or motor-evoked responces (15), and formal visual fields are indicated if the lesion or location suggests that these functions could be involved.

Management

Communication in the development and execution of the goals, strategies, and tactics of the treatment is essential if the best result is to be achieved. Going over the plan in detail with the patient allows the patient to participate fully and actively in the healing process and helps avoid confusion and unnecessary suffering. Endovascular treatment of AVMs requires the coordination of a large team to address complex, difficult, and overlapping problems. Active participation from stroke neurologists, cerebral vascular neurosurgeons, radiosurgeons, and interventional neuroradiologists helps immeasurably in addressing complex AVMs (16,17). Input from anesthesiologists, nurses, and radiographic technologists is essential for developing tactics and executing a plan (18–20).

GOALS

The goals of embolization treatment can be definitive, adjuvant, or palliative. Reaching one goal can allow one to reassess to reach a more ambitious goal. Often it is difficult before superselective pedicle angiography and provocative testing to tell exactly what can be treated safely and effectively.

APPROACH TO CEREBRAL AVMs

Indications

In otherwise healthy patients under 55 with an AVM that can be treated with a high efficacy and low accepted morbidity, treatment should be strongly considered. The younger the patient and the greater the likelihood of an effective and safe treatment, the more strongly should the treatment be advised. Partial, incomplete treatment by any means is unlikely to benefit the patient unless it is aimed at a high-risk portion of the AVM.

Definitive embolization of cerebral AVMs can be considered likely to succeed in patients with Parkinson and Pachers types 2, 3, and 5; in Spetzler-Martin grades 1 and 2; and in those with favorable endovascular characteristics (Fig. 18.18; see Tables 18.21 and 18.22). The wisdom of such an approach depends on the risk and benefits of other therapeutic options for the patient.

Adjuvant embolization of cerebral AVMs can be considered in those patients with Parkinson and Pachers types 1 and 4, in Spetzler-Martin grade 2 and above, in AVMs larger than 2.5 cm in diameter, and when endovascular characteristics are thought to make the additional risk of the procedure less than the benefit it will offer (Fig. 18.19) (21). Adjuvant embolization may be particularly helpful for (a) deep feeders, (b) AVMs in eloquent areas, (c) AVMs with perforators or choroidals (22), (d) AVMs with very high flow states, (e) massive AVMs, or (f) AVMs with symp-

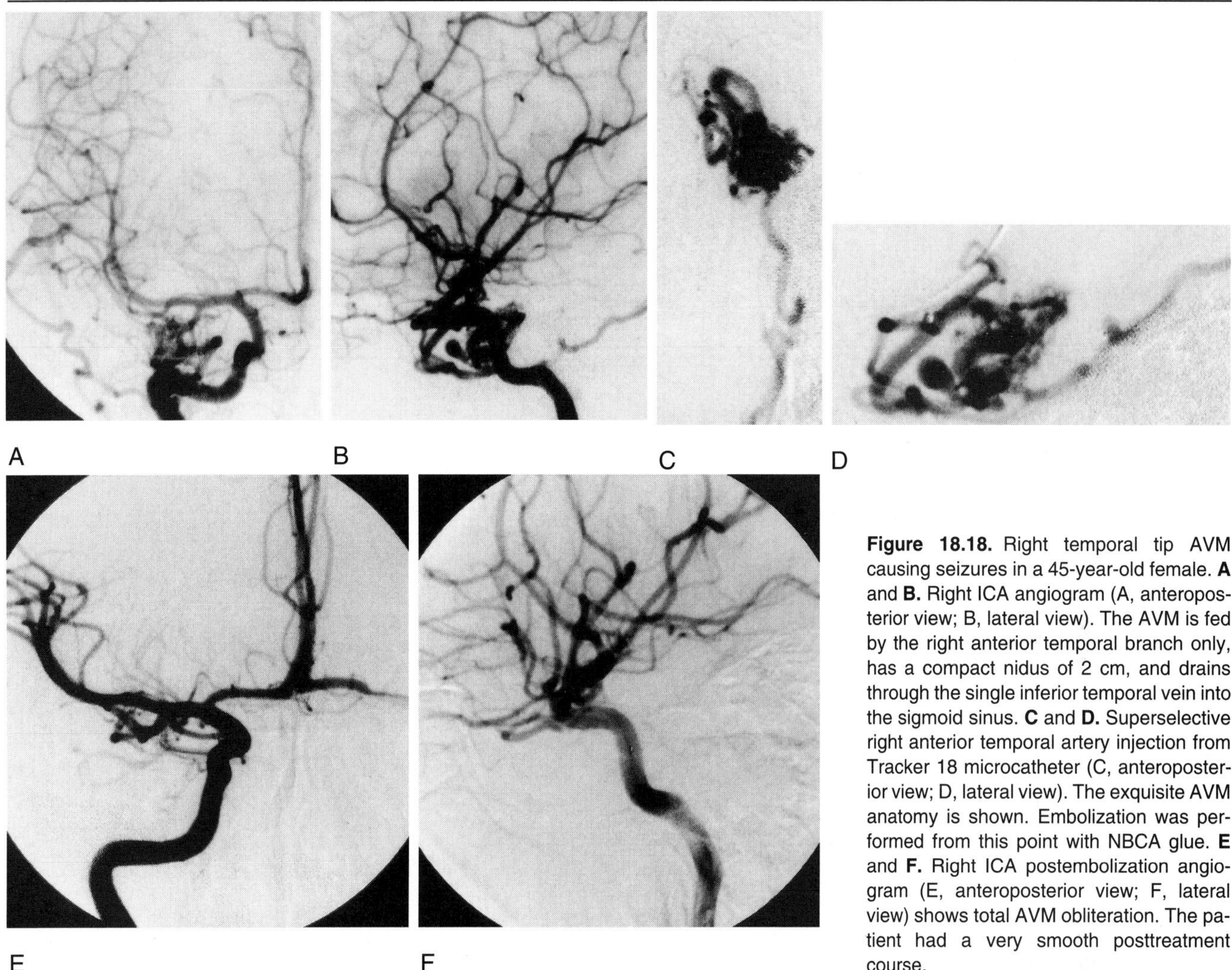

Figure 18.18. Right temporal tip AVM causing seizures in a 45-year-old female. **A** and **B.** Right ICA angiogram (A, anteroposterior view; B, lateral view). The AVM is fed by the right anterior temporal branch only, has a compact nidus of 2 cm, and drains through the single inferior temporal vein into the sigmoid sinus. **C** and **D.** Superselective right anterior temporal artery injection from Tracker 18 microcatheter (C, anteroposterior view; D, lateral view). The exquisite AVM anatomy is shown. Embolization was performed from this point with NBCA glue. **E** and **F.** Right ICA postembolization angiogram (E, anteroposterior view; F, lateral view) shows total AVM obliteration. The patient had a very smooth posttreatment course.

tomatic venous hypertension (23). Embolization usually decreases the size of the AVM and thus the grade (24). Permanent agents such as NBCA have many advantages over less lasting agents and allow a much wider range of therapeutic options. They give more freedom in the staging of the embolization, allow definitive embolization treatment to be appreciated, and allow radiosurgery to be used on the remaining AVM (Fig. 18.20). The combination of radiosurgery and embolization has been encouraging by some reports (25). However, the acrylates can recannalize. Rarely, unplanned acute surgery may be needed to evacuate blood and to relieve mass effect from an intracranial bleed associated with embolization and can be quite effective if done emergently (26).

Palliative embolization of cerebral AVMs is occasionally indicated and can be quite effective. The indications include (a) progressive neurologic deterioration (Fig. 18.21) (27), (b) medically intractable seizures, (c) dangerous pseudoaneurysms associated with bleeds (Fig. 18.22), (d) intractable headaches, and (e) cardiac failure (28). The headache can be associated with a dural component or large venous aneurysm, particularly in the area of the thalamus or incisura. Neurologic changes can occasionally be reversed with embolization (29), though this is not an indication for treatment.

Endovascular Strategy

Staging the embolization allows large hemodynamic changes to be made slowly and compensatory mechanisms to be implemented before additional stress is placed on the critical tissue. These factors can be particularly important in highly eloquent areas such as the motor strip and deep white matter tracts. In large AVMs it is possible to do noncontiguous, noncomplementary areas at the same sitting.

It is important to realize that one area can compensate quite adequately for another, but if the second area is also damaged, profound dysfunction can occur. The primary sensory and motor areas of the cortex offer such an arrangement for the hand, and the primary motor and accessory motor areas for the foot are another.

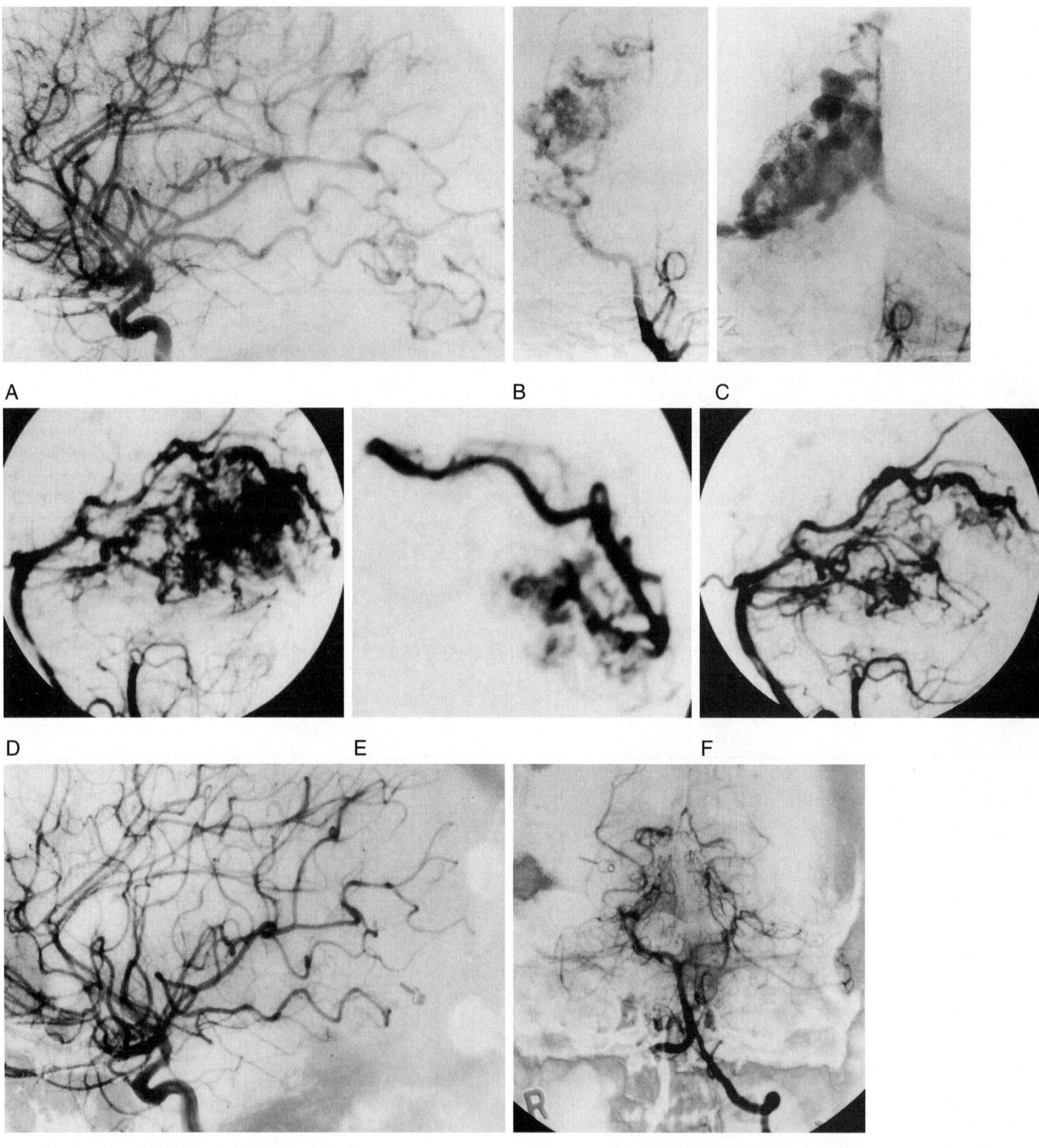

Figure 18.19. A 37-year-old female with seizures and migraine headaches from a right occipital cortical AVM. The patient had adjuvant embolization of deep feeders prior to definitive surgery. **A.** Right ICA lateral view of the parieto-occipital gyral feeders. **B.** Left vertebral angiogram (early), anteroposterior view. **C.** Left vertebral angiogram (late), anteroposterior view, shows the important right posterior cerebral artery (PCA) contribution to the AVM, the large nidus, and drainage to the sagittal sinus. **D.** Left vertebral artery angiogram, lateral view, shows the massive right parieto-occipital branch to the AVM. **E.** Superselective right PCA angiogram shows the diffuse nidus. **F.** Left vertebral artery injection, postembolization, shows marked reduction in the AVM nidus size. **G** and **H.** Postsurgery angiogram shows total AVM excision (G, lateral view; H, anteroposterior view).

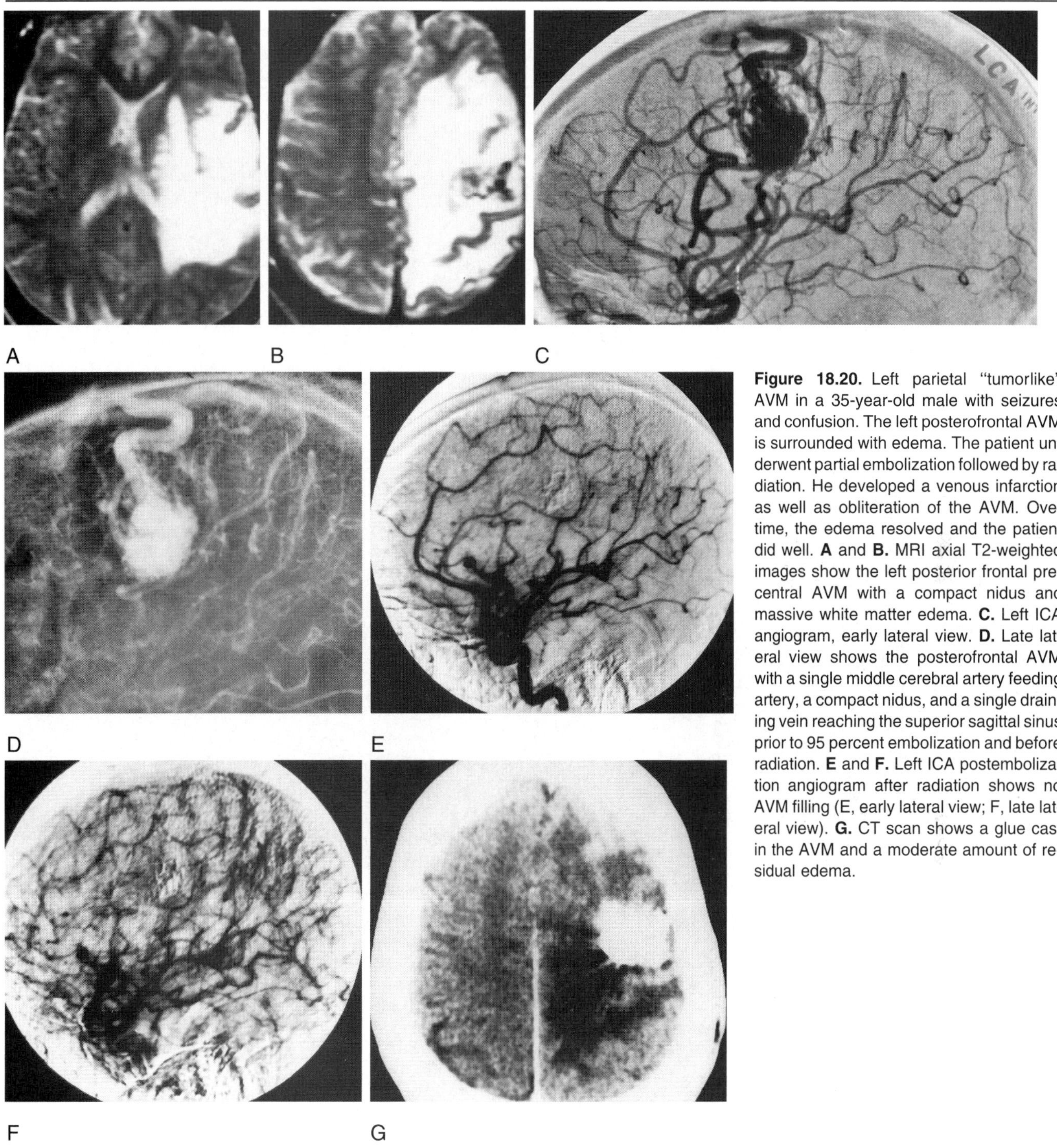

Figure 18.20. Left parietal "tumorlike" AVM in a 35-year-old male with seizures and confusion. The left posterofrontal AVM is surrounded with edema. The patient underwent partial embolization followed by radiation. He developed a venous infarction as well as obliteration of the AVM. Over time, the edema resolved and the patient did well. **A** and **B.** MRI axial T2-weighted images show the left posterior frontal precentral AVM with a compact nidus and massive white matter edema. **C.** Left ICA angiogram, early lateral view. **D.** Late lateral view shows the posterofrontal AVM with a single middle cerebral artery feeding artery, a compact nidus, and a single draining vein reaching the superior sagittal sinus prior to 95 percent embolization and before radiation. **E** and **F.** Left ICA postembolization angiogram after radiation shows no AVM filling (E, early lateral view; F, late lateral view). **G.** CT scan shows a glue cast in the AVM and a moderate amount of residual edema.

What can be done depends largely on the size of the AVM and whether there is involvement of the deep gray matter (particularly the thalamus) or the primary efferent or afferent white matter tracts (Fig. 18.23). The magnitude of risk for an untreated AVM depends on whether there are aneurysms or deep venous drainage. An algorithm that the author tends to follow is based on size, eloquence, and angiographic risk factors for bleeding if untreated (see Table 18.23).

Endovascular Tactics

Endovascular tactics depend on the strategy and the goals. The vascular anatomy, including the size of the vessels, number of loops, collateral flow, watershed anastomosis, anomalies, venous outflow, and functional anatomy, all need to be considered.

Usually it is best to go after the largest macrofistula component of the AVM first to slow the flow down. This permits greater understanding of the remaining AVM and de-

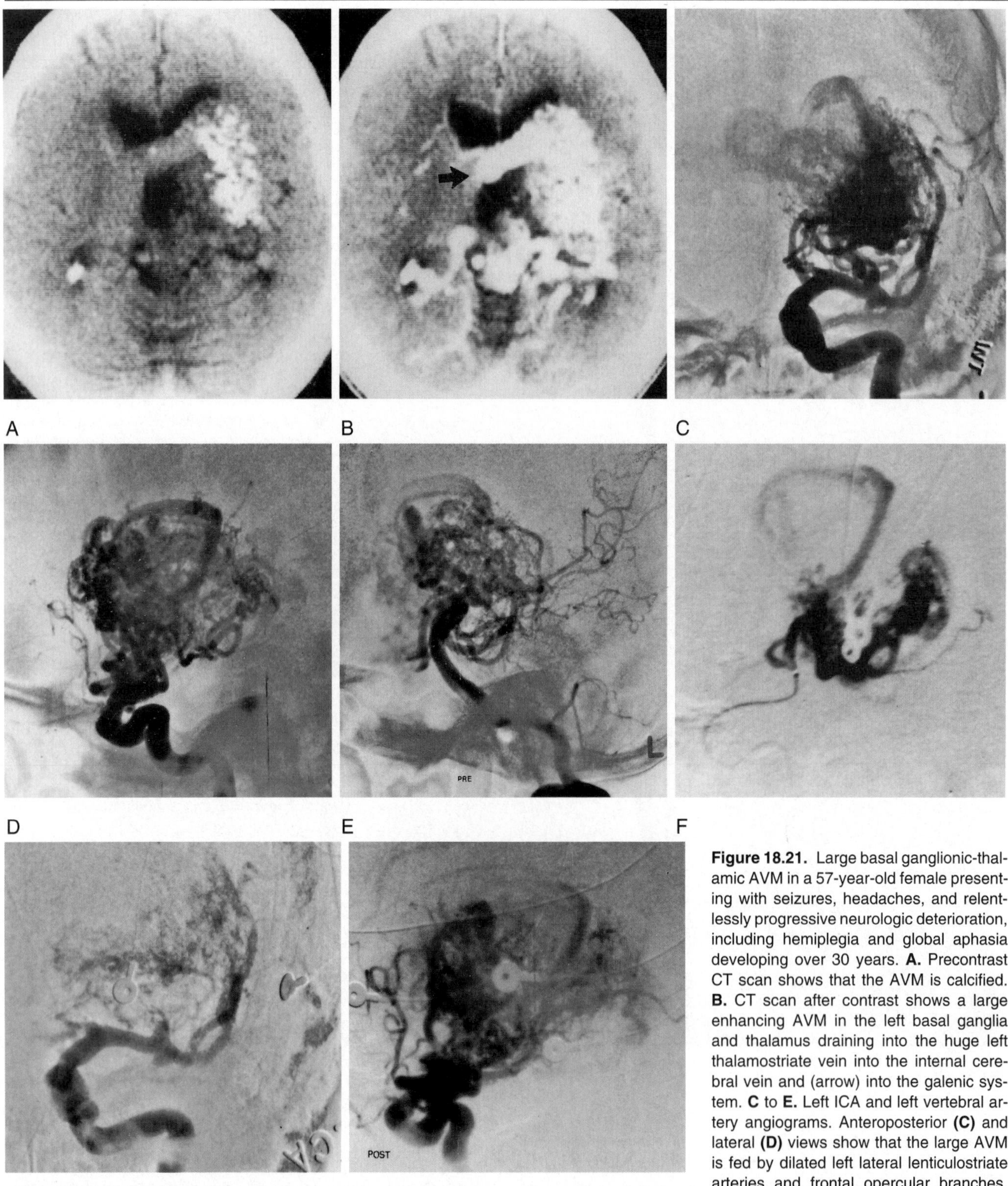

Figure 18.21. Large basal ganglionic-thalamic AVM in a 57-year-old female presenting with seizures, headaches, and relentlessly progressive neurologic deterioration, including hemiplegia and global aphasia developing over 30 years. **A.** Precontrast CT scan shows that the AVM is calcified. **B.** CT scan after contrast shows a large enhancing AVM in the left basal ganglia and thalamus draining into the huge left thalamostriate vein into the internal cerebral vein and (arrow) into the galenic system. **C** to **E.** Left ICA and left vertebral artery angiograms. Anteroposterior **(C)** and lateral **(D)** views show that the large AVM is fed by dilated left lateral lenticulostriate arteries and frontal opercular branches. The ACA is not seen from this injection. **E.** Left angiogram showing PCA and PCoA feeders to the thalamus and basal ganglia. **F.** Superselective left lenticulostriate injection. Sodium amobarbital testing was carried out at this point, which was negative. NBCA glue embolization was performed into perforating branches and other lenticulostriate arteries. **G** and **H.** Left ICA angiogram postembolization shows that the nidus is smaller; the ACA is seen (G, anteroposterior view; H, lateral view). With repeated embolizations the patient gradually recovered significant speech, progressing from a severely global aphasia to a moderately severe motor aphasia. Anteroposterior and lateral views, postembolization, compare with C and D.

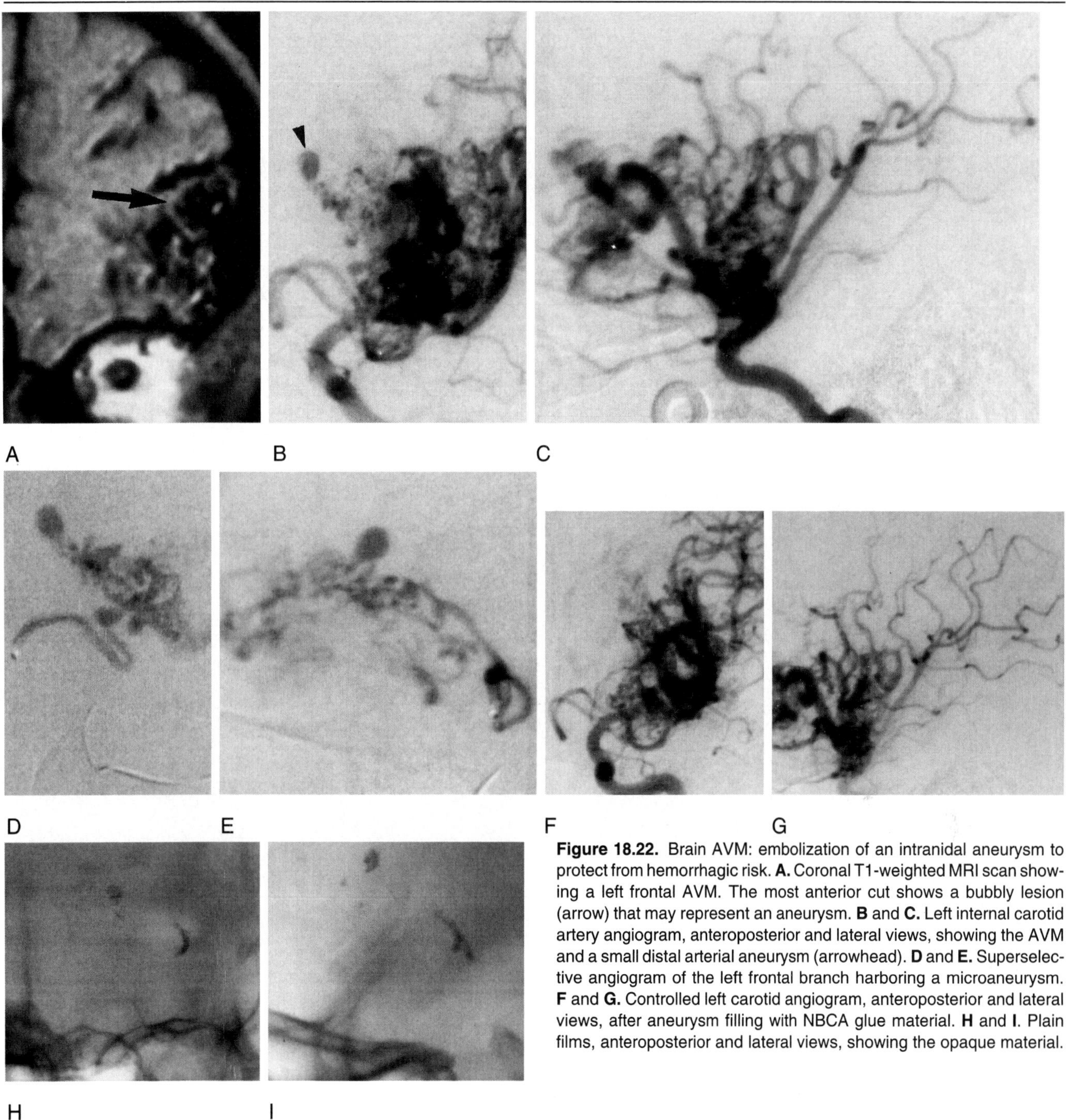

Figure 18.22. Brain AVM: embolization of an intranidal aneurysm to protect from hemorrhagic risk. **A.** Coronal T1-weighted MRI scan showing a left frontal AVM. The most anterior cut shows a bubbly lesion (arrow) that may represent an aneurysm. **B** and **C.** Left internal carotid artery angiogram, anteroposterior and lateral views, showing the AVM and a small distal arterial aneurysm (arrowhead). **D** and **E.** Superselective angiogram of the left frontal branch harboring a microaneurysm. **F** and **G.** Controlled left carotid angiogram, anteroposterior and lateral views, after aneurysm filling with NBCA glue material. **H** and **I**. Plain films, anteroposterior and lateral views, showing the opaque material.

creases some of the venous hypertension. However, it is usually the deep periventricular feeders that are the most challenging surgically and that are the source of bleeds. Hypotension is often useful to allow more control during embolization and to keep the embolization material from passing into the cranial or systemic venous system. Total flow arrest can also be helpful and can be done by a second catheter with a balloon introduced into the system. Staged embolization should be considered when there are a number of feeders involving eloquent areas or when normal pressure perfusion breakthrough is a possibility (30). Surgical exposure of the AVM feeders in those rare cases in which it is needed can be helpful. The technique for the pediatric patient is similar, though it requires miniaturization of the materials and additional attention to details (31).

METHODS

The technical methods can be broken down in a step-by-step way to include preoperative, operative, and postoperative considerations (Table 18.25). As with all crafts, the

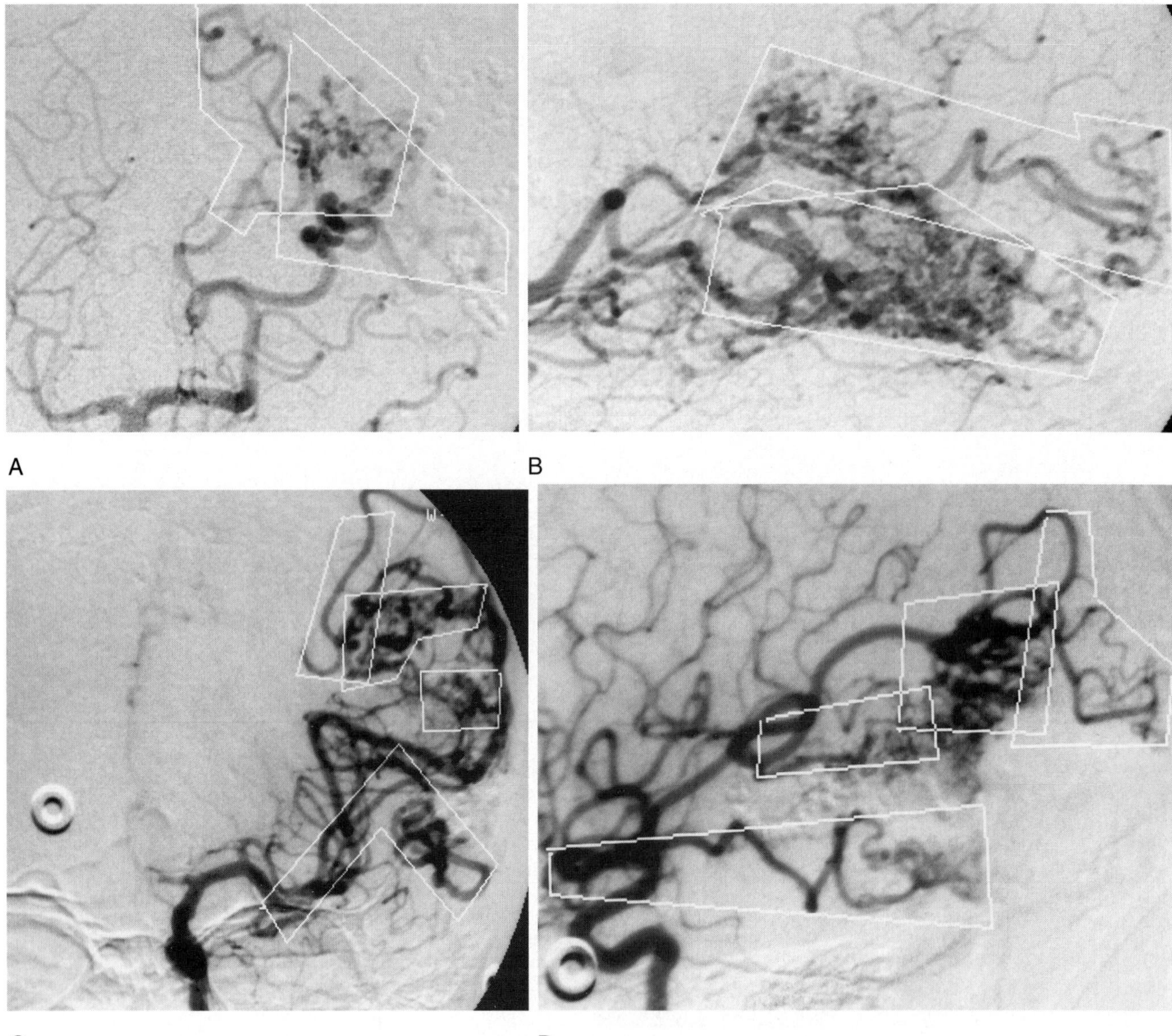

Figure 18.23. Brain AVM superselective exploration in a 40-year-old female with seizures from a large temporo-occipital AVM. The patient was treated 10 years previously with silastic sphere embolization. Because of the eloquent nature of the brain surrounding the AVM, superselective angiographic exploration was carried out, with superselective intra-arterial sodium amobarbital injections and neurologic functional mapping. There had been displacement of the sensory language function in this patient, from the expected location. **A** and **B.** Left vertebral artery angiogram, anteroposterior and lateral views. Arterial territories contributing to the AVM. **C** and **D.** Left ICA angiogram, anteroposterior and lateral views. The boxes designate the vascular territories associated with a given artery feeding the AVM. It can be demonstrated by superselective angiography.

Table 18.25.
Treatment Guidelines for AVMs

Preoperative
1. Evaluate goal of embolization and timing of treatment.
2. Calcium channel blockers 12 h prior, anxiolytics on call.
3. Anticonvulsant levels, complete blood count, coagulation profile.

Operative
1. Monitoring, ECG, O_2 saturation, baseline neurologic exam, blood pressure.
2. Mild anesthetic (see section on anesthetics this chapter).
3. Foley catheter, intravenous access (patient needs 2 intravenous lines).
4. 7.5F sheath.
5. Heparinization (ACT 2.5 × normal).
6. 7F guiding catheter in parent vessel.
7. Biplane angiogram.
8. Road map.
9. Navigate microcatheter into fistula position.
10. Superselective angiogram through microcatheter.
11. Tailored neurologic examination.
12. Amytal 30 mg/Xylocaine 40 mg superselective angiograms.
13. Repeat neurologic examination.
14. Relative hypotension.
15. Embolization: acrylate embolization (NBCA* + tantalum + Lipiodol), silk suture, polyvinyl alcohol, "cocktails."
16. Repeat neurologic examination.
17. Repeat steps 8–15.

Postoperative
1. Sheath and heparinization until next morning, intensive care unit until next evening.
2. Consider calcium channel blockers and beta blocker.

* NBCA = *N*-butyl-2-cyanoacrylate.

important nuances of interventional methods are best learned through one-on-one instruction.

Superselective angiography and superselective Wada testing are extremely useful in limiting postembolization neurologic deficit even in small AVMs (32,33). They are particularly useful in patients who have had a previous stroke or embolization. Mean pressure measurements within the feeding arteries give useful information regarding the effectiveness of embolization. Pressure recordings can give information regarding such different occurrences as kinks in the catheter, hemodynamic changes during embolization, or risks of bleeding (34). The author's preference for embolic agents is acrylate: NBCA because it is permanent, controllable, gives excellent penetration, allows deep penetration into the nidus, can be placed through a tiny catheter, and sets up a reactive scarring (35). The polymerization time can be altered by adding iodized oil (Lipiodol) or glacial acetic acid (36). The addition of over 50 percent Lipiodol may lead to absorption of the adhesive (37). Silk has been preferred by some, but this enthusiasm is not shared by all (38). Other agents, such as cocktails of PVA, Avatine, and 30 percent ethanol, can induce changes similar to acrylates (39). PVA and coils can also be used and are preferred by some (40,41). Balloons can be helpful in some situations with large fistulas (42). More on agents can be found in the section on materials. Superselective amobarbital or sodium methohexital and lidocaine injections are used for provocative testing during brain embolotherapy and appear to be both sensitive and specific in avoiding embolization of important areas of the brain (43).

REFERENCES

1. McCormick WF: The pathology of vascular ("arteriovenous") malformations. J Neurosurg 1966;24:807–816.
2. McCormick W, Nofzinger J: "Cryptic" vascular malformations of the central nervous system. J Neurosurg 1966;24:865–870.
3. Perret G, Nishioka H: Report on the Cooperative Study of Intracranial Aneurysms and Subarachnoid Hemorrhage VI. J Neurosurg 1966;25:467–490.
4. Pile-Spellman J, Baker KF, Liszczak TM, et al: High flow angiopathy: Cerebral blood vessel changes in experimental chronic arteriovenous fistula. Am J Neuradial 1986;7:811–815.
5. Kader A, Young WL, Pile-Spellman J, et al: The influence of hemodynamic and anatomic factors on hemorrhage from cerebral arteriovenous malformations. Neurosurgery 1994;34:801–807.
6. Horton J, Chambers W, Lyons S, et al: Pregnancy and the risk of hemorrhage from cerebral arteriovenous malformations. Neurosurgery 1990;27:867–873.
7. Graft C, Perret G, Torner J: Bleeding from cerebral arteriovenous malformations as part of their natural history. J Neurosurg 1983; 58:331–337.
8. Crawford P, West C, Chadwick D, Shaw M: Arteriovenous malformations of the brain: Natural history in unruptured aneurysms. J Neurol Neurosurg Psychiatry 1986;49:1–10.
9. Parkinson D, Pachers G: Arteriovenous malformations: Summary of 100 consecutive supratentorial cases. J Neurosurg 1980;53:285–293.
10. Spetzler RF, Martin NA: A proposed grading system for arteriovenous malformations. J Neurosurg 1986;65:476–483.
11. Hamilton MG, Spetzler RF: The prospective application of a grading system for arteriovenous malformations. Neurosurgery 1994;34: 2–6.
12. Lunsford LD, Kondziolka D, Flickinger JC, et al: Stereotactic radiosurgery for arteriovenous malformations of the brain. Neurosurg 1991;75:512–524.
13. Young WL, Pile-Spellman J, Prohovnik I, Kader A, Stein BM: Evidence for adaptive autoregulatory displacement in hypotensive cortical territories adjacent to arteriovenous malformations. Columbia University AVM Study Project. Neurosurgery 1994;34:601–610.
14. Petty GW, Massaro AR, Tatemichi TK, et al: Transcranial Doppler ultrasonographic changes after treatment for arteriovenous malformations. Stroke 1990;21:260–266.
15. Zentner J, Schumacher M, Bien S: Motor evoked potentials during interventional neuroradiology. Neuroradiology 1988;30:252–255.
16. Grzyska U, Westphal M, Zanella F, et al: A joint protocol for the neurosurgical and neuroradiologic treatment of cerebral arteriovenous malformations: Indications, technique, and results in 76 cases. Surg Neurol 1993;40:476–484.
17. Stein BM, Kader A: Intracranial arteriovenous malformations. Clin Neurosurg 1992;39:76–113.
18. Scoles J, Canter M, Turndorf H, Puig MM: Anesthesia for angioembolization of brain arteriovenous malformations: A retrospective assessment. Methods Find Exp Clin Pharmacol 1990;12:575–578.
19. Young WL, Pile-Spellman J: Anesthesia for interventional neuroradiology. Anesthesia 1994;80:427–456.
20. Willis D, Harbit MD: Transcatheter arterial embolization of cerebral arteriovenous malformations. J Neurosci Nurs 1990;22: 280–284.
21. Vinuela F, Dion JE, Duckwiler G, et al: Combined endovascular embolization and surgery in the management of cerebral arteriovenous malformations: Experience with 101 cases. J Neurosurg 1991; 75:856–864.
22. Hodes JE, Aymard A, Casasco A, Rufenacht D, Reizine D, Merland JJ: Embolization of arteriovenous malformations of the temporal lobe via the anterior choroidal artery. AJNR 1991;12:775–780.
23. Hurst RW, Hackney DB, Goldberg HI, Davis RA: Reversible arteriovenous malformation-induced venous hypertension as a cause of neurological deficits. Neurosurgery 1992;30:422–425.

24. Jafar JJ, Davis AJ, Berenstein A, Choi IS, Kupersmith MJ: The effect of embolization with *N*-butyl cyanoacrylate prior to surgical resection of cerebral arteriovenous malformations. J Neurosurg 1993;78: 60–69.
25. Guo WY, Wikholm G, Karlsson B, Lindquist C, Svendsen P, Ericson K: Combined embolization and gamma knife radiosurgery for cerebral arteriovenous malformations. Acta Radiol 1993;34: 600–606.
26. Jafar JJ, Rezai AR: Acute surgical management of intracranial arteriovenous malformations. Neurosurgery 1994;34:8–12.
27. Kashii S, Solomon SK, Moser FG, Tostanowski J, Burde RM: Progressive visual field defects in patients with intracranial arteriovenous malformations. Am J Ophthalmol 1990;109:556–562.
28. Lasjaunias P, Garcia-Monaco R, Rodesch G, et al: Vein of Galen malformation: Endovascular management of 43 cases. Childs Nervous System 1991;7:360–367.
29. Sugita M, Takahashi A, Ogawa A, Yoshimoto T: Improvement of cerebral blood flow and clinical symptoms associated with embolization of a large arteriovenous malformation: Case report. Neurosurgery 1993;33:748–751.
30. Spetzler RF, Martin NA, Carter LP, Flom RA, Raudzens PA, Wilkinson E: Surgical management of large AVM's by staged embolization and operative excision. J Neurosurg 1987;67:17–28.
31. Rodesch G, Lasjaunias P, TerBrugge K, Burrows P: Intracranial arteriovenous vascular lesions in children: Role of endovascular techniques apropos of 44 cases. Neurochirurgie 1988;34:293–303.
32. Vinuela F, Fox AJ, Debrun G, Pelz D: Preembolization superselective angiography: Role in the treatment of brain arteriovenous malformations with isobutyl-2 cyanoacrylate. AJNR 1984;5:765–769.
33. Willinsky R, TerBrugge K, Montanera W, Wallace C, Aggarwal S: Microarteriovenous malformations of the brain: Superselective angiography in diagnosis and treatment. AJNR 1992;13:325–330.
34. Handa T, Negoro M, Miyachi S, Sugita K: Evaluation of pressure changes in feeding arteries during embolization of intracerebral arteriovenous malformations. J Neurosurg 1993;79:383–389.
35. Klara PM, George ED, McDonnell DE, Pevsner PH: Morphological studies of human arteriovenous malformations: Effects of isobutyl 2-cyanoacrylate embolization. J Neurosurg 1985;63:421–425.
36. Pelz DM, Fox AJ, Vinuela F, Drake CC, Ferguson GG: Preoperative embolization of brain AVMs with isobutyl-2 cyanoacrylate. AJNR 1988;9:757–764.
37. Rao VR, Mandalam KR, Gupta AK, Kumar S, Joseph S: Dissolution of isobutyl 2-cyanoacrylate on long-term follow-up. AJNR 1989;10: 135–141.
38. Deveikis JP, Manz HJ, Luessenhop AJ, et al: A clinical and neuropathologic study of silk suture as an embolic agent for brain arteriovenous malformations. AJNR 1994;15:263–271.
39. Lylyk P, Vinuela F, Vinters HV, et al: Use of a new mixture for embolization of intracranial vascular malformations: Preliminary experimental experience. Neuroradiology 1990;32:304–310.
40. Schweitzer JS, Chang BS, Madsen P, et al: The pathology of arteriovenous malformations of the brain treated by embolotherapy: II. Results of embolization with multiple agents. Neuroradiology 1993; 35:468–474.
41. Nakstad PH, Bakke SJ, Hald JK: Embolization of intracranial arteriovenous malformations and fistulas with polyvinyl alcohol particles and platinum fibre coils. Neuroradiology 1992;34:348–351.
42. Halbach VV, Higashida RT, Yang P, Barnwell S, Wilson CB, Hieshima GB: Preoperative balloon occlusion of arteriovenous malformations. Neurosurgery 1988;22:301–308.
43. Purdy PD, Batjer HH, Risser RC, Samson D: Arteriovenous malformations of the brain: Choosing embolic materials to enhance safety and ease of excision. J Neurosurg 1992;77:217–222.

SUGGESTED READINGS

Han MH, Chang KH, Han DH, Yeon KM, Han MC: Preembolization functional evaluation in supratentorial cerebral arteriovenous malformations with superselective intraarterial injection of thiopental sodium solution. Acta Radiol 1994;35:212–216.

Hecht ST, Horton JA, Kerber CW: Hemodynamics of the central nervous system arteriovenous malformation nidus during particulate embolization: A computer model. Neuroradiology 1991;33:62–64.

Jungreis CA, Horton JA: Pressure changes in the arterial feeder to a cerebral AVM as a guide to monitoring therapeutic embolization. AJNR 1989;10:1057–1060.

Khayata MH, Zabramski JM, Johnson PC, Flom R: False aneurysm associated with rupture of an arteriovenous malformation—implications for treatment: Case report. Neurosurgery 1993;33:753–756.

Lanman TH, Martin NA, Vinters HV: The pathology of encephalic arteriovenous malformations treated by prior embolotherapy. Neuroradiology 1988;30:1–10.

Lasjaunias P, TerBrugge KG, Chiu MC: Coaxial balloon-catheter device for treatment of neonates and infants. Radiology 1986;159:269–271.

Norbash AM, Marks MP, Lane B: Correlation of pressure measurements with angiographic characteristics predisposing to hemorrhage and steal in cerebral arteriovenous malformations. AJNR 1994;15:809–813.

Perata HJ, Tomsick TA, Tew J Jr: Feeding artery pedicle aneurysms: Association with parenchymal hemorrhage and arteriovenous malformation in the brain. J Neurosurg 1994;80:631–634.

Peters KR, Quisling RG, Gilmore R, Mickle P, Kuperus JH: Intraarterial use of sodium methohexital for provocative testing during brain embolotherapy. AJNR 1993;14:171–174.

Purdy PD, Batjer HH, Samson D: Management of hemorrhagic complications from preoperative embolization of arteriovenous malformations. J Neurosurg 1991;74:205–211.

Purdy PD, Samson D, Batjer HH, Risser RC: Preoperative embolization of cerebral arteriovenous malformations with polyvinyl alcohol particles: Experience in 51 adults. AJNR 1990;11:501–510.

Rauch RA, Vinuela F, Dion J, et al: Preembolization functional evaluation in brain arteriovenous malformations: The ability of superselective Amytal test to predict neurologic dysfunction before embolization. AJNR 1992;13:309–314.

Rodesch G, Garcia-Monaco R, Lasjaunias P: False aneurysm associated with rupture of an arteriovenous malformation—implication for treatment: Case report (letter, comment). Neurosurgery 1994;34:769.

Taki W, Handa H, Yonekawa Y, et al: Detachable balloon catheter systems for embolization of cerebrovascular lesions. Neurol Med Chir 1981;21:709–719.

Wolpert SM, Barnett FJ, Prager RJ: Benefits of embolization without surgery for cerebral arteriovenous malformations. Am J Roentgenol 1982;138:99–102.

18.5 Dural Arteriovenous Malformations

Key Points

1. Dural AVMs appear to be acquired diseases initiated by venous sinus occlusion.
2. Reflux into the cerebral venous system puts patients at risk for bleeding and venous ischemia.
4. Venous hypertension causes symptomatic decreased cerebral blood flow.

5. Dural shunts developing in areas that are likely to drain into cortical veins (anterior falx) are much more likely to bleed than those that have many options to drain extracranially (cavernous).
6. Obliteration of the shunt with a permanent agent is needed to treat the AVM effectively when there is cortical venous drainage. Nonpermanent agents can be used when there is no cortical drainage, since these AVMs seem to obliterate themselves spontaneously and are at little risk for bleeding.
7. Care must be taken during embolization not to hurt the cranial nerves supplied by the arteries that supply both the fistula and the nerves in the dura, or to obliterate the venous outflow of the dural AVM and normal tissue.

Development

Dural arteriovenous malformations appear to be acquired lesions. There are three phases in their development (Fig. 18.24). Stage I: normally the heavily vascularized dura has a network of meningeal arteries. For whatever reasons, thrombosis of the sinus occurs (stage II). This leads to an increase in venous pressure. Increased venous pressure is thought to act as a stimulus for angiogenesis, as well as for relaxation of the arterioles. AV shunts that are present under normal conditions dilate, or they may develop in the recanalized clot (stage III). These shunts lead to an increase in the venous hypertension, and a positive feedback loop develops, causing a "growth" of the dural AVM.

What is the evidence for this theory? Angiographic demonstration of sigmoid (1 year) or transverse sinus occlusion (4 years) before the development of an AVM in the appropriate sinus in two patients prompted Houser et al. to postulate that dural sinus occlusion may precede the development of a dural AVM and that the pathogenesis may be partial recanalization of a thrombus (1). Arteriographic investigations of four patients who, after a head injury, developed dural arteriovenous fistulas led Chaudhary et al. to agree that these abnormal communications were acquired, with thrombosis or thrombophlebitis in the dural sinus or vein being the primary event in their formation (2). Others have reported the association of sinus occlusion with previous trauma and sometimes following surgery (3–5). The role of venous hypertension is less well established but has been postulated as the cause of dural AVMs (6,7). Relief of the venous hypertension by recanalization of an occluded sinus has in some instances led to obliteration of the AVM shunts. These results suggest that venous hypertension has a role in the development and maintenance of dural AVMs (8). More recently, dural AVMs have been created in rats using venous hypertension. Similar arguments have been advanced for cerebral AVMs (9). The dynamic nature of AVMs may explain changes sometimes seen with partial embolization; the altered hemodynamics cause the AVM to "shift" as both feeders and drainers become partially occluded (10).

Histologic studies showing the actual fistula (11) have convinced some that dural AVMs are acquired as a result of venous occlusion (12) and others that they are congenital (13). Persistent fetal venous system features occasionally seen in dural AVMs have led others to believe that they are developmental in origin (14–16).

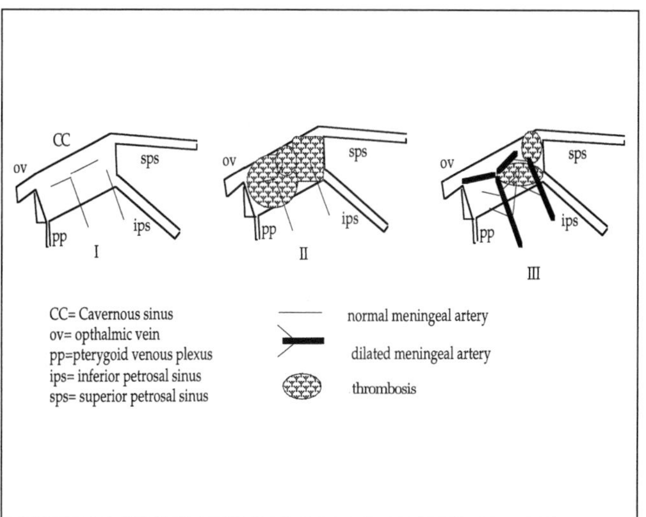

Figure 18.24. Dural arteriovenous malformations (AVMs). Dural AVMs develop in stages. As can be seen in this schematic of the cavernous sinus region, the dura is heavily vascularized by meningeal vessels (I). Thrombosis of the sinuses may develop for a variety of reasons (II). This thrombosis leads to an increase in venous pressure, which in turn acts as a stimulus for angiogenesis and relaxation of arterioles (III). AV shunts may dilate and develop in the recanalized clot.

Classification, Clinical Features, and Prognosis

Dural AVMs can be classified by location (Table 18.26), the amount of cortical venous drainage (ref), a angioarchitecture (17,18), or angiographic and clinical features (19) (Tables 18.27 and 18.29).

The natural history of dural AVMs is highly variable, depending on the location and amount of venous drainage. No doubt many dural AVMs are asymptomatic (20). Spontaneous occlusion is common in the cavernous sinus dural AVMs; it occurs at other locations as well but less commonly (21–24), and it can be related to angiography (25).

In adults, dural AVMs are usually single lesions (26). The greater the cortical venous drainage and venous stasis within the cortical system, the greater the chance for bleeding or neurologic impairment. In infants, children, and those with extensive venous occlusion, extremely extensive and multiple dural AVMs can be seen. These patients present with cerebral and cardiovascular hemodynamic problems: hydrocephalus, progressive neurologic dysfunction, and, in the younger patient, cardiac failure (Table 18.28) (27–30).

Dural AVMs involving the anterior falx, the anterior fossa, and the tentorial incisura, although uncommon, have

Table 18.26.
Location, Pathophysiology, Clinical Presentation, and Type of Treatment for Dural AVMs

Malformation	Frequency	Usual Presentation	Risks of bleeding	Usual Indications for Treatment	Therapeutic Options	Materials
Cavernous sinus dural AVMs	Very common	Proptosis, chemosis, exophthalmus, pain, glaucoma, central retinal vein occlusion, failing visual acuity	Very low	Cortical drainage, medically intractable glaucoma, failing vision	Trial of carotid compression, gentle arterial embolization, trans–superior ophthalmic vein, transfemoral petrosal vein	Transarterial embolization, transvenous cocktail embolization
Sigmoid sinus dural AVMs	Common	Bruit, headache	Low	Cortical drainage, incapacitating bruit or headache	Transarterial embolization, transvenous embolization, combined approach	NBCA, PVA-ethanol cocktail
Transverse sinus dural AVMs	Common	Bruit, headache, bleeding, progressive neurologic deficit	Low	Cortical drainage, headache, hemorrhage, neurologic deficit		NBCA, PVA-ethanol cocktail
Torcular AVMs	Rare	Bruit, headache, bleeding, progressive neurologic deficit	High	Cortical drainage, headache, hemorrhage, neurologic deficit	Transarterial embolization, transvenous embolization, combined approach	NBCA, PVA-ethanol cocktail
Incisural AVMs	Rare	Bleeding, impaired neurologic function	Very high	Cortical drainage, headache, hemorrhage, neurologic deficit	Transarterial embolization, radiosurgery	NBCA, PVA-ethanol cocktail
Sagittal sinus dural AVMs	Rare	Headache, bleeding, progressive neurologic deficit	High	Cortical drainage, headache, hemorrhage, neurologic deficit	Combined embolization and surgery	NBCA, PVA-ethanol cocktail, coils
Vein of Galen dural AVMs	Rare	Neonates: cardiac failures Infants: hydrocephalus Adults: seizures and bleeding	Low	High output failure, failure to thrive	Transarterial embolization, transvenous embolization	NBCA, coils
Anterior fossa dural AVMs	Rare	Bleeding	Very high	Presence should prompt immediate treatment	Surgery	NA

an aggressive course, and present with intracranial hemorrhage. Hemorrhage occurs even with those draining into the dural vein without the pial vein, possibly as a result of rupture of a venous aneurysm (31–35). Those presenting with venous drainage into the cervical region and presenting with myelopathy also have an aggressive course (36). Dural AVMs with aneurysmal dilatation and deep venous drainage warrant vigorous treatment (34) (Table 18.29).

Table 18.27.
Djindjian Classification of Dural AVMs

Total extracranial drainage
Intracranial reflux
Mixed intracranial-extracranial drainage
Total intracranial drainage
Intracranial stasis

Source: Djindjian R, Merland JJ, Theron J: Superselective arteriography of the external carotid artery. New York: Springer-Verlag, 1977.

Cerebral hemorrhage from cavernous (37) and even cervical spinal (36) dural AVMs can occur, but are very uncommon.

Pathophysiology

The importance of venous hypertension in the development of symptomatic ischemia and hemorrhage has been stressed by numerous authors (38–40). Demonstrations of this can be seen in clinical practice when reversible AVM-induced venous hypertension is linked with reversing the neurologic deficits (41). CT and MRI show an ischemic region mainly affecting the white matter, single photon emission computed tomography (SPECT) shows an in-

Table 18.28.
Hemorrhage Risk Factors for Dural AVMs

Aneurysms
Cortical drainage
Anterior falx or tentorial location

Table 18.29.
Classification of AVMs by Angioarchitecture and Hemodynamics

Angioarchitecture	
Nidus	Capillary/arterial
Fistula	Yes/no
Venous anomaly	Yes/no
Ectasia	Yes/no
Hemodynamics	
Flow	High/low
Arterial steal	Yes/no
Blush	Yes/no
Mass effect	Yes/no
Feeding vessel	Type
Compartment	Single/multiple

crease in blood volume and a decrease in cerebral blood flow, and angiography shows venous congestion. The brain edema that can be associated with these lesions is considered "hydrostatic." It is caused by an increased hydrostatic pressure in the capillary bed. Vascular permeability is not thought to be the cause. Venous hypotension causes expansion of the extracellular spaces by a protein-free plasma ultrafiltrate affecting both the gray and white matter. The neurologic deficit and the image changes are reversed with successful embolization (42). Similar findings in a dural AVM patient with dementia, leucoaraiosis, increased blood volume, and a reduced oxygen extraction fraction on a positron emission tomography (PET) scan have been reported (43). Prolonged transit time on contrast enhanced CT (CECT) caused by venous hypertension associated with dural AVMs has also been reported (44).

Intracranial aneurysms may be associated with dural AVMs, but the relationship is unknown (45–47).

Work-up

CLINICAL

Generally, dural AVM symptoms depend on the location and hence the drainage pattern (Fig. 18.25). The most common type, those of the cavernous sinus, present with proptosis, chemosis, and bruit. Those of the sigmoid and jugular region present with bruit and headache (Fig. 18.26), and those of the falx and incisura present with intracranial bleeds. Venous ischemia is seen in those with extensive venous occlusion and cortical venous drainage (40). Cardiac failure is seen in infants with large shunts. The symptoms can be quite variable and include increased intracranial pressure (48,49), papilledema (50,51), amaurosis fugax (52), prefrontal syndrome (53), subacute diencephalic angioencephalopathy (54), trigeminal neuralgia (55), painful oculomotor palsy (56,57), facial nerve palsy (58), pulsatile tinnitus (59–61), seizures and electroencephalographic changes (62), dementia with leucoaraiosis (43), progressive dysarthria (63), thalamic infarctions (64), central retinal vein occlusion and neovascularity (65), and superior ophthalmic vein thrombosis (66).

Dural thrombosis can be associated with recognizable hypercoagulable states. Although these are rare, they should be sought and treated (67). The classical Virchow triad is (a) *stasis*, (b) *abnormal blood*, and (c) *abnormal vessels*. A myriad of clinical conditions have been related to dural AVMs, including diabetes, pulmonary disease, hyper- and hypothyroidism, Behçet disease (68), protein S deficiency, protein C deficiency, pregnancy, glomus tumors, systemic lupus erythematosus, Wegener granulomatosis, non-Hodgkin lymphoma, trauma, dehydration, and increased intracranial pressure (Table 18.30).

A change in a patient's symptoms, such as resolution of proptosis or disappearance of a bruit, could paradoxically bode poorly, since it could represent increased venous drainage. Such "spontaneous cures" need to be confirmed by angiography.

RADIOLOGICAL

CT and MR angiography (MRA) are useful in identifying the fistula (69–71). Gadolinium MRI may be used (72). MRI and MRA are relatively insensitive to the cortical veins, feeding arteries, sinus occlusion, or fistula site associated with dural AVMs (69). MRI should not be counted on either to find the dural AVM or to follow the effects of treatment. MRI can be used effectively to follow the parenchymal changes seen from venous hypertension, since these will start to reverse within a few days after effective

Table 18.30.
Work-up of a Patient with a Dural AVM

Investigative goal	Studies	Criteria/Comment
Hypercoagulable states, Virchow triad, stasis, abnormal blood vessels, abnormal blood	Pulm function test, thyroid studies, fasting blood sugar, coagulation profile, protein C antigen or activity, VDRL, antiplatelet factor III activity, protein S antigen, liver function tests	The younger the patient, the more aggressive the hunt
Volume, location, extent	Angiogram	
Feeding arteries, draining veins, venous occlusion	Superselective angiogram	Flow rate, nidal aneurysm
Venous hypertension	MRI, T2 images	
Functional impairment	Complete and formal neurologic, ophthalmologic and psychological testing	

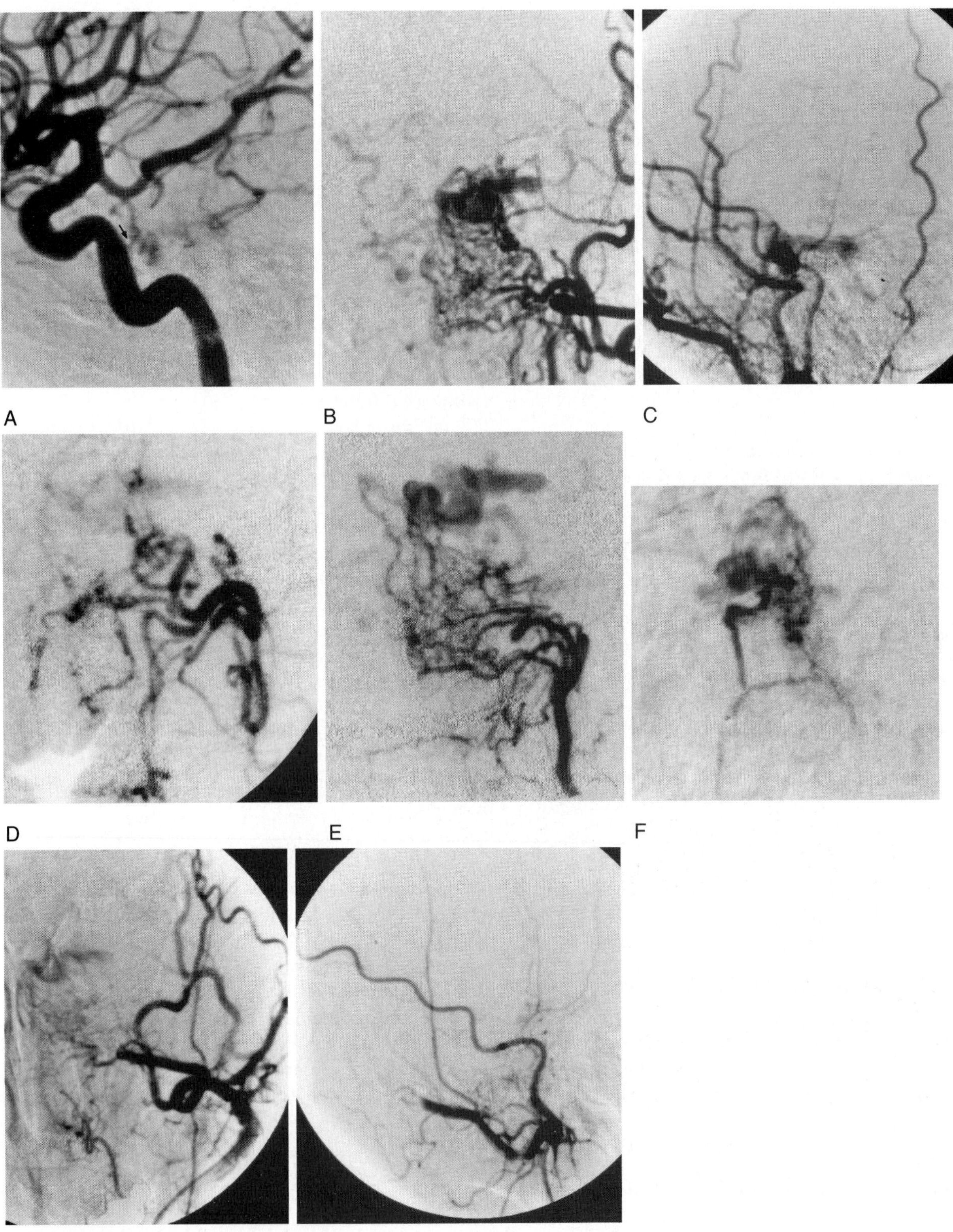

Figure 18.25. Left cavernous sinus dural AVM in a 48-year-old female presenting with left sixth-nerve palsy, headache, and dizziness. **A** to **C.** Angiograms. **A.** Left ICA angiogram showing meningeal branches off the C5 segment going to the left cavernous sinus (arrow). **B** and **C.** Anteroposterior and lateral views of the external carotid artery (ECA) showing branches off the left middle meningeal artery, the accessory meningeal artery, and the artery of the foramen rotundum, as well as clival branches off the left ascending pharyngeal artery to the left cavernous sinus. **D** to **F.** Superselective angiograms. **D.** Anteroposterior view of the distal left internal maxillary artery, showing the artery of the foramen rotundum going to the left cavernous sinus. **E.** View of the left ascending pharyngeal artery showing clival branches to the left cavernous sinus. **F.** Superselective left middle meningeal artery injection showing communication with the left cavernous sinus. Note the dilated cortical veins consistent with cortical venous hypertension, probably accounting for the patient's headaches and dizziness. **G** and **H.** Left ECA angiogram postembolization, anteroposterior and lateral views, showing occlusion of the AV shunting between the ECA branches and the left cavernous sinus. The ICA meningeal branches were not approached. The patient's symptoms resolved within a few weeks, including the left sixth-nerve palsy.

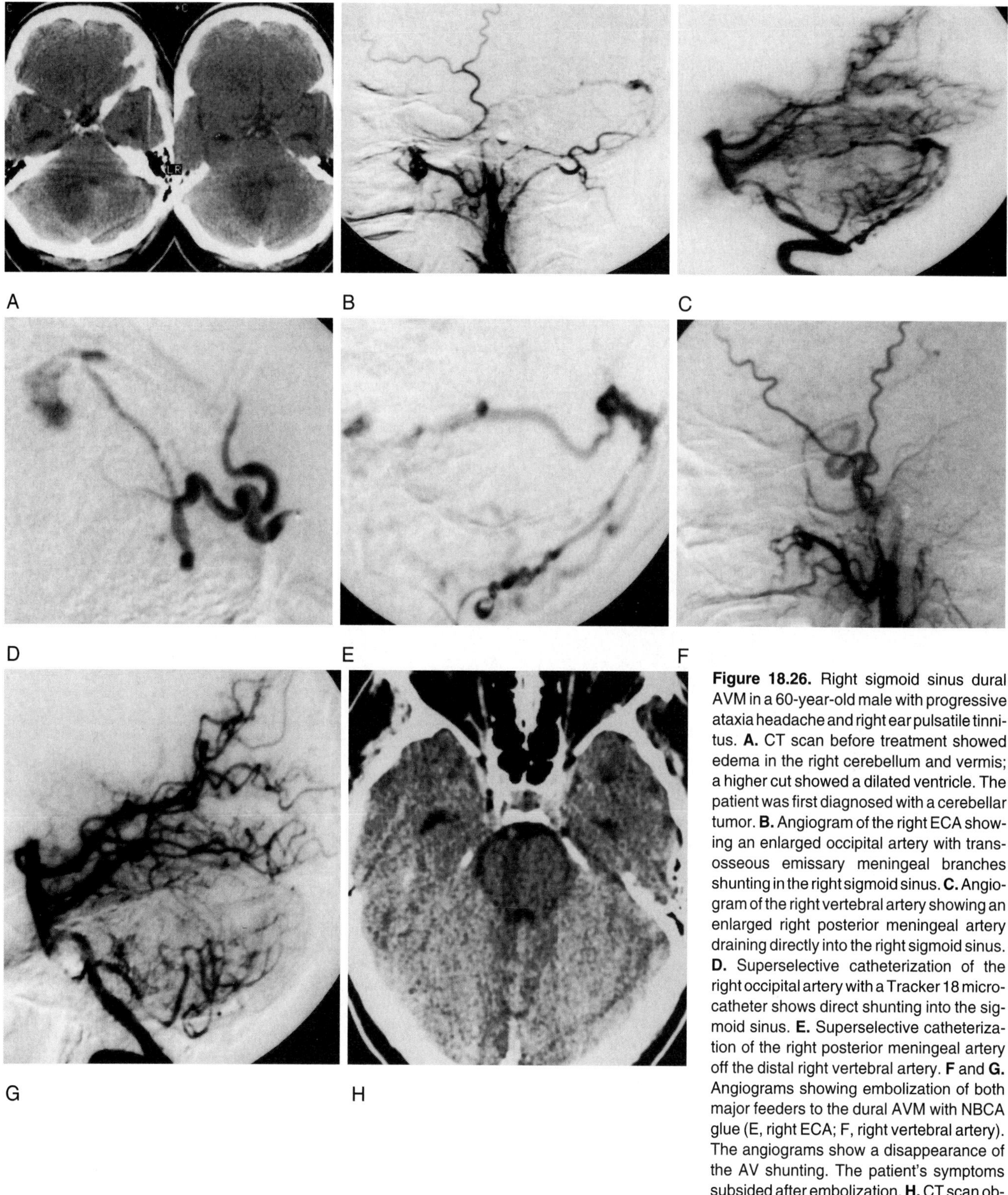

Figure 18.26. Right sigmoid sinus dural AVM in a 60-year-old male with progressive ataxia headache and right ear pulsatile tinnitus. **A.** CT scan before treatment showed edema in the right cerebellum and vermis; a higher cut showed a dilated ventricle. The patient was first diagnosed with a cerebellar tumor. **B.** Angiogram of the right ECA showing an enlarged occipital artery with transosseous emissary meningeal branches shunting in the right sigmoid sinus. **C.** Angiogram of the right vertebral artery showing an enlarged right posterior meningeal artery draining directly into the right sigmoid sinus. **D.** Superselective catheterization of the right occipital artery with a Tracker 18 microcatheter shows direct shunting into the sigmoid sinus. **E.** Superselective catheterization of the right posterior meningeal artery off the distal right vertebral artery. **F** and **G.** Angiograms showing embolization of both major feeders to the dural AVM with NBCA glue (E, right ECA; F, right vertebral artery). The angiograms show a disappearance of the AV shunting. The patient's symptoms subsided after embolization. **H.** CT scan obtained 4 weeks after endovascular treatment shows regression of the cerebellar edema.

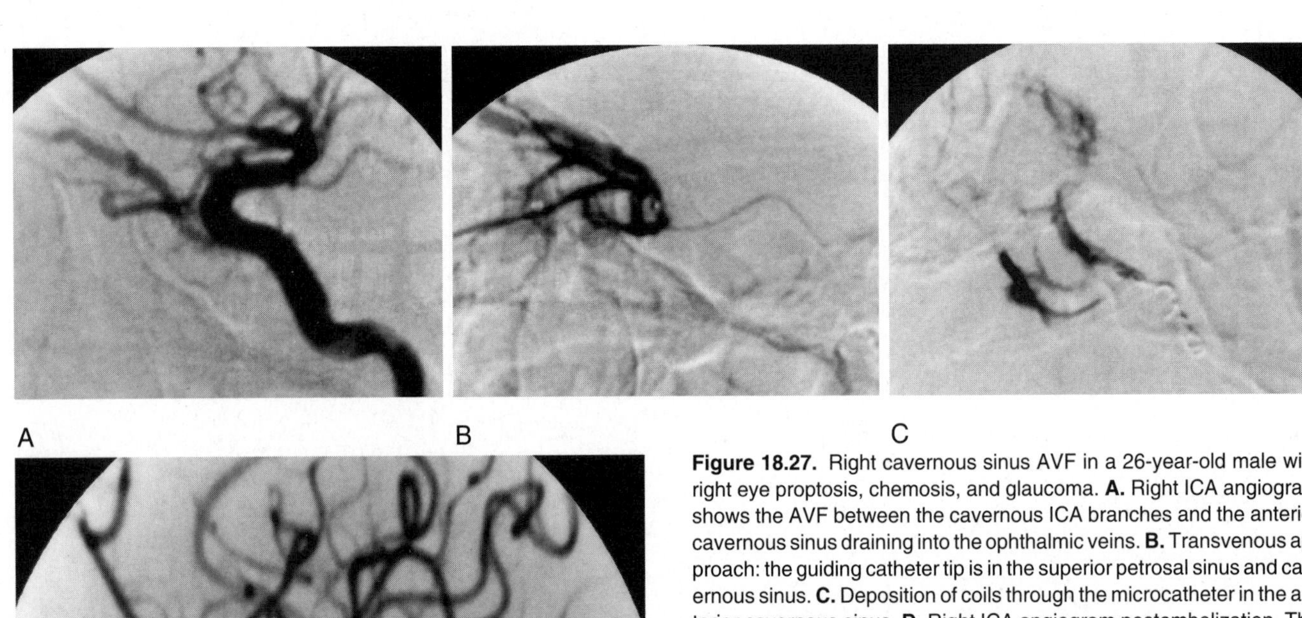

A B C

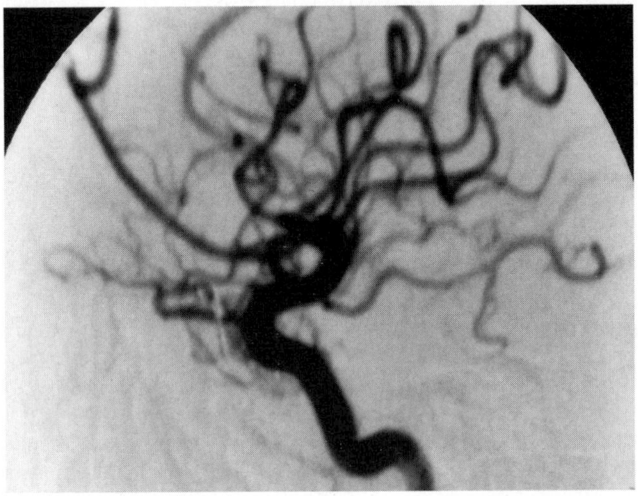

D

Figure 18.27. Right cavernous sinus AVF in a 26-year-old male with right eye proptosis, chemosis, and glaucoma. **A.** Right ICA angiogram shows the AVF between the cavernous ICA branches and the anterior cavernous sinus draining into the ophthalmic veins. **B.** Transvenous approach: the guiding catheter tip is in the superior petrosal sinus and cavernous sinus. **C.** Deposition of coils through the microcatheter in the anterior cavernous sinus. **D.** Right ICA angiogram postembolization. The AVF is not seen.

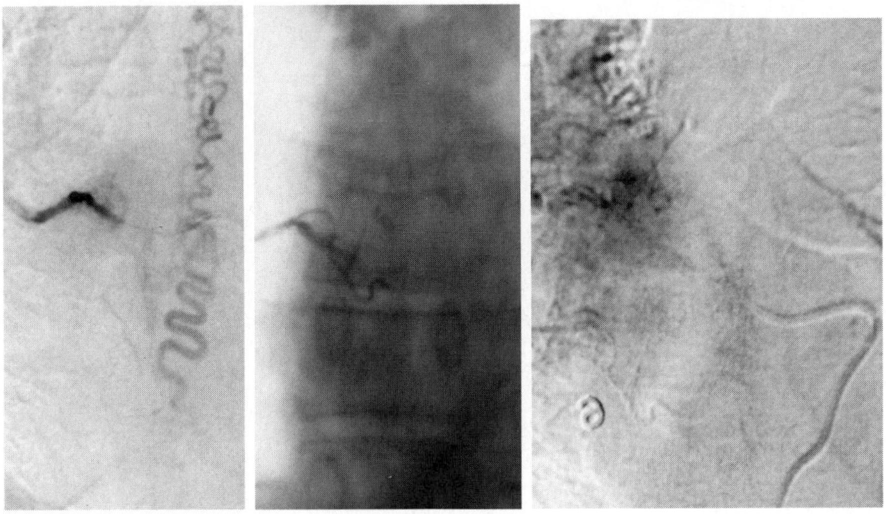

A B C

Figure 18.28. Thoracolumbar spinal AVM. **A.** Spinal angiogram, selective right T6 intercostal view, shows a fistula between the meningeal branches of the intercostal artery and the perimedullary venous plexus. **B.** Plain film of thoracic spine (detail). The cast of the opacified polymerizing material (acrylate glue) is seen in the proximal intercostal artery, its meningeal branches, and the proximal venous structures. **C.** Right T5 intercostal angiogram, late view. There is no filling of the venous system. The fistula is occluded.

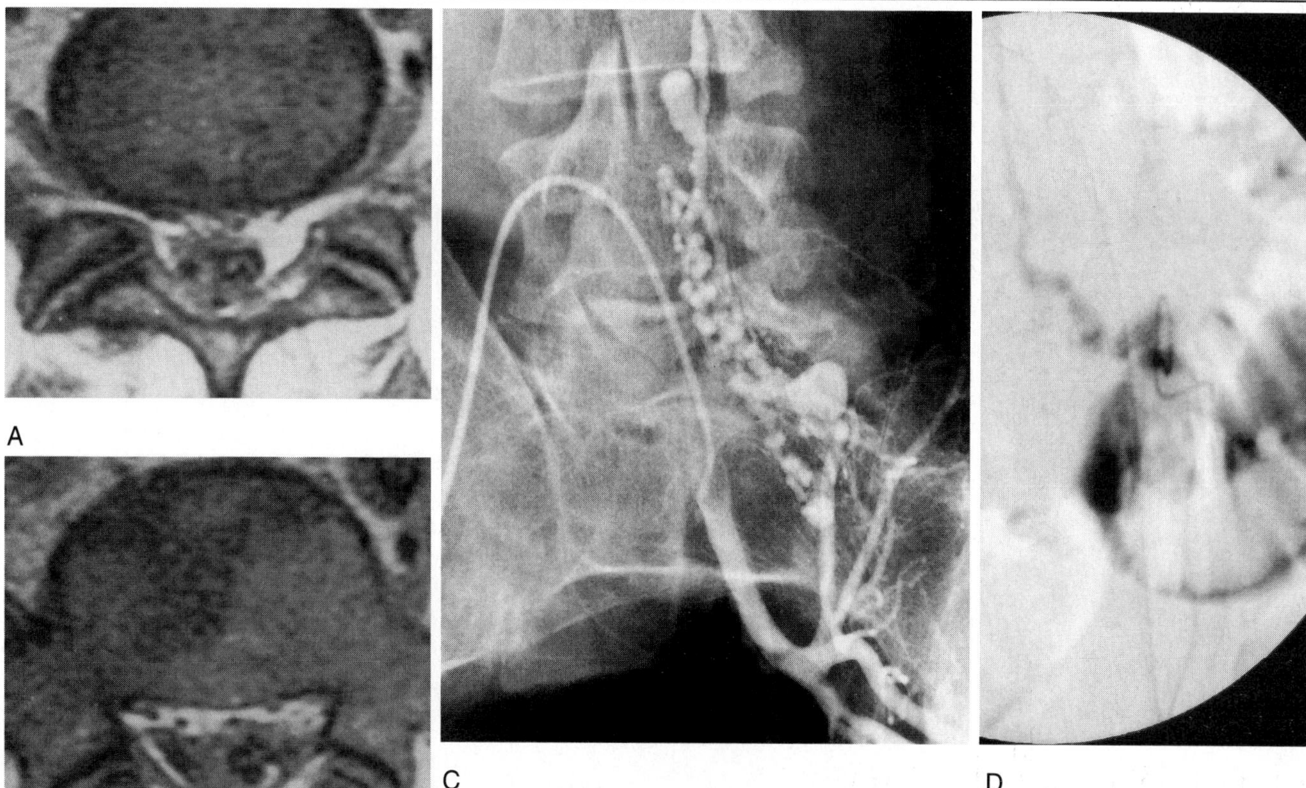

Figure 18.29. Spinal AVM-AVF in a 28-year-old male with pelvic pain and increasing difficulty walking. The left perimedullary AVM-AVF was at the conus level, was fed from the left hypogastric artery, and was draining into the perimedullary venous plexus. **A.** MR axial T1-weighted image at the L5 level. **B.** Axial T1-weighted image at the S1 level shows flow voids anterior to the spinal roots. **C.** Left hypogastric angiogram, oblique view, shows the AVM with a large AVF. The draining vein is midline. **D.** Superselective injection of the AVM feeder from Tracker 18 microcatheter. Embolization with coils was performed at this level.

embolization. Contrast-enhanced CT can also be used for this purpose; it demonstrates cortical enhancement (70) but is also not sensitive enough to find or follow dural AVMs.

The diagnostic angiogram remains the gold standard and should be performed in all cases when the diagnosis of dural AVM is being considered.

Management

GOALS AND INDICATIONS FOR TREATMENT

Obliteration of cortical venous drainage and venous hypertension is the goal of treatment. Treatment can be based on a classification of dural AVMs into four groups based on features and clinical and imaging findings:

Group 1. Anterior cavernous malformations with predominant superior ophthalmic vein drainage and symptoms and signs of carotid cavernous fistula

Group 2. Superior petrosal, transverse, and sigmoid sinus regions, presenting predominantly with bruit

Group 3. Basal sinuses and prominent cortical venous drainage, presenting with intracranial hemorrhage, headache, and impaired cortical function

Group 4. Infrequent manifestations

Group 1 and 2 patients are readily recognized and diagnosed. Group 3 and 4 patients are often misdiagnosed. Group 1 patients are the most amenable to transarterial embolization as well as to carotid compression and transvenous embolization. Group 3 patients carry a grave prognosis unless effectively treated (19).

ENDOVASCULAR STRATEGY

Obliteration of the fistula can be done with a permanent agent to cause obliteration of all the fistula or obliteration of all venous outflow. The first is best accomplished by staged acrylate embolization (Figs. 18.26; 18.28; 18.29); the second is done by transvenous embolization with coils (Fig. 18.27). In all cases care must be taken to avoid reflux of the material into normal veins that are carrying blood in a retrograde fashion, since this might well exacerbate symptoms (73). Staged treatment with both surgery and embolization is occasionally needed (74–77) (Fig. 18.30).

Strategies and tactics vary somewhat by location. Embolization for a cavernous dural fistula is usually straightforward and effective (46,78). Sigmoid sinus AVMs usually require multiple treatments. Superior sagittal sinus AVMs, because of their unique midline location, multiplicity of arterial feeders, and critical venous drainage of the superior

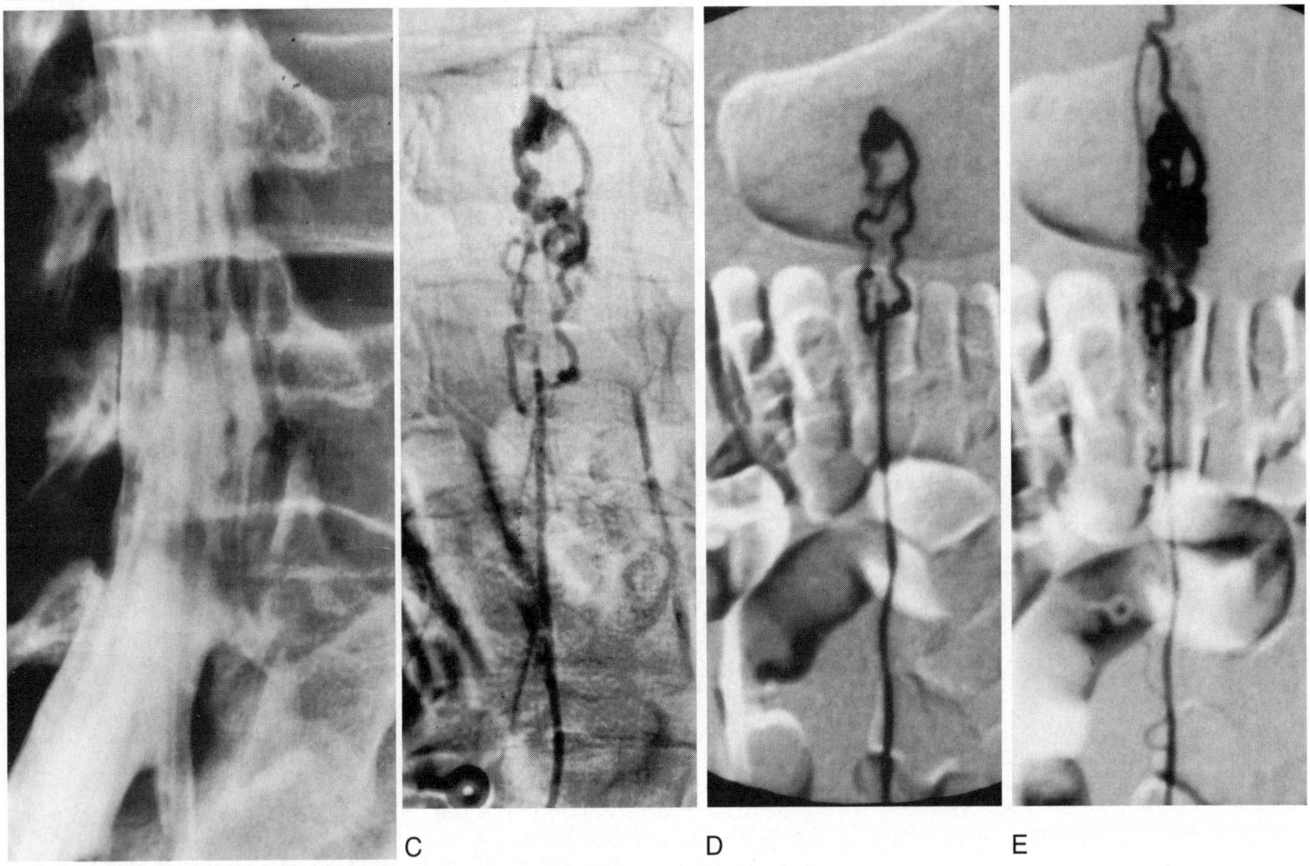

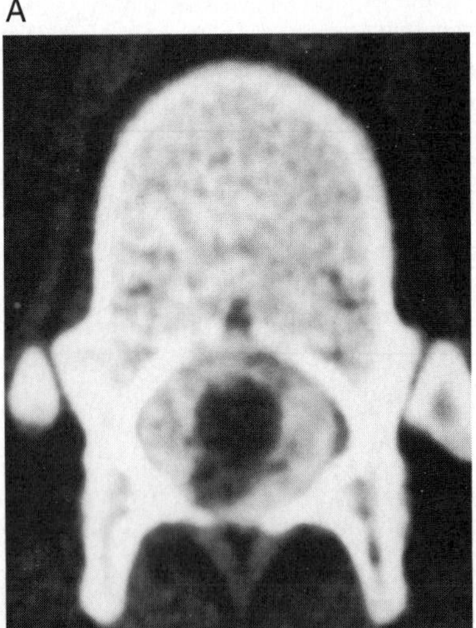

A B C D E

Figure 18.30. Spinal AVF (type 4; see Table 18.32) in a 25-year-old male with progressive left lower extremety paresis and numbness and diminished sphincter tone. **A.** Myelogram showing serpiginous vessels at L2-L3. **B.** Myelo-CT showing a mass behind the conus medullaris. **C** and **D.** Angiograms of the left hypogastric artery. **C.** Anteroposterior view shows the spinal AVM at the conus level. The anterior spinal artery off the left hypogastric artery gives off two posterior spinal arteries at the conus level feeding the AVM posterior to the conus. Drainage is via the large anterior spinal vein. **D** and **E.** Superselective anterior spinal artery angiograms. **D.** Early view. **E.** Late view showing the AVM nidus anatomy and the fistula exquisitely defined. The patient was treated with surgery and did well.

sagittal sinus, often require unusual and aggressive forms of therapy (79). The same can be said for tentorial AVMs (80). Anterior fossa dural AVMs require vigorous treatment, often surgical (25).

ENDOVASCULAR TACTICS

Particulate embolic treatment for dural AVMs has been in use for over 20 years (81). Since most cavernous dural AVMs will obliterate with incomplete embolization, and since polyvinyl alcohol (PVA) in this region can in many operators' hands be delivered safely, it may well be the agent of choice (82).

Permanent agents such as NBCA are needed in other locations. Care must be taken to avoid embolizing meningeal branches that feed cranial nerves. This can best be avoided by knowing the anatomy (see section on external

Table 18.31.
Treatment Guidelines for Dural AVMs

Preoperative
1. Evaluate goal of embolization and timing of treatment.
2. Anticonvulsant levels, complete blood count, coagulation profiles.

Operative
1. Monitoring ECG, O_2 saturation, baseline neurologic exam, blood pressure.
2. Mild anesthetic (see section on anesthetics this chapter).
3. Foley catheter, intravenous access (2).
4. 6.0F sheath.
5. Heparinization (ACT 2.5 × normal).
6. 5F guiding catheter in parent vessel.
7. Biplane angiogram.
8. Road map.
9. Navigate microcatheter (wire-directed) into fistula position.
10. Superselective angiogram through microcatheter.
11. Tailored neurologic examination.
12. Xylocaine 40 mg superselective angiograms.
13. Repeat neurologic examination.
15. Embolization: acrylate embolization (NBCA* + tantalum + Lipiodol), ethanol-PVA†-Avaline "cocktails."
16. Repeat neurologic examination.
17. Repeat steps 8–15.

Postoperative
1. If extensive venous occlusion: sheath and heparinization until next A.M., ICU until next P.M. If no venous occlusion: reverse heparin.
2. Consider calcium channel blockers and beta blocker.

* NBCA = *N*-butyl-2-cyanoacrylate.
† PVA = polyvinyl alcohol.

carotid artery anatomy), by practicing meticulous technique, and by using preembolization Xylocaine testing.

The author tends to use transvenous approaches if transarterial embolization has been ineffective. Transfemoral vein catheterization and insertion of coils or copper wires are often effective (83). The transophthalmic vein (84) approach is useful in treating cavernous sinus dural AVMs when the arterial approach and the transfemoral approach are unsuccessful. Combined surgery and embolization with sinus packing may also be needed (Tables 18.26 and 18.31).

OTHER TREATMENT OPTIONS

The Matas procedure (carotid compression) can be offered to all patients with cavernous AVMs who do not have either atherosclerosis of the bifurcation or cortical venous reflux. In patients with a single cortical venous drainage, interruption of this outflow can result in a cure and should strongly be considered (85). Radiosurgery (3000 cGy) can be effective for anterior fossa (86) and cavernous (87,88) dural AVMs and should be offered to patients who fail endovascular therapy.

The intellectually interesting procedure of opening up the venous occlusive disease with a venous bypass has been used to treat the venous hypertension, but there is little experience with this approach (89).

REFERENCES

1. Houser OW, Campbell JK, Campbell RJ, Sundt T Jr: Arteriovenous malformation affecting the transverse dural venous sinus—an acquired lesion. Mayo Clin Proc 1979;54:651–661.
2. Chaudhary MY, Sachdev VP, Cho SH, Weitzner I Jr, Puljic S, Huang YP: Dural arteriovenous malformation of the major venous sinuses: An acquired lesion. AJNR 1982;3:13–19.
3. Nabors MW, Azzam CJ, Albanna FJ, Gulya AJ, Davis DO, Kobrine AI: Delayed postoperative dural arteriovenous malformations: Report of two cases. J Neurosurg 1987;66:768–772.
4. Ugrinovski J, Vrcakovski M, Lozance K: Dural arteriovenous malformation secondary to meningioma removal. Br J Neurosurg 1989; 3:603–607.
5. Nakahara S, Katoh Y: A case of posttraumatic vascular abnormality similar to dural arteriovenous malformation. [Japanese]. No Shinkei Geka 1986;14:1371–1375.
6. Brainin M, Samec P: Venous hemodynamics of arteriovenous meningeal fistulas in the posterior cranial fossa. Neuroradiology 1983; 25:161–169.
7. Watanabe A, Takahara Y, Ibuchi Y, Mizukami K: Two cases of dural arteriovenous malformation occurring after intracranial surgery. Neuroradiology 1984;26:375–380.
8. Kutluk K, Schumacher M, Mironov A: The role of sinus thrombosis in occipital dural arteriovenous malformations: Development and spontaneous closure. Neurochir 1991;34:144–147.
9. Mullan S: Reflections upon the nature and management of intracranial and intraspinal vascular malformations and fistulae. J Neurosurg 1994;80:606–616.
10. Nakagawa H, Kubo S, Nakajima Y, Izumoto S, Fujita T: Shifting of dural arteriovenous malformation from the cavernous sinus to the sigmoid sinus to the transverse sinus after transvenous embolization: A case of left spontaneous carotid-cavernous sinus fistula. Surg Neurol 1992;37:30–38.
11. Nishijima M, Takaku A, Endo S, et al: Etiological evaluation of dural arteriovenous malformations of the lateral and sigmoid sinuses based on histopathological examinations. J Neurosurg 1992;76: 600–606.
12. Sakurai N, Koike Y, Hashizume Y, Takahashi A: Dural arteriovenous malformation and sinus thromboses in a patient with prostate cancer: An autopsy case. Internal Med 1992;31:1032–1037.
13. Sakaki S, Furuta S, Fujita M, Kohno K: Dural arteriovenous malformation of the transverse and sigmoid sinus with special reference to its pathological features. Br J Neurosurg 1991;5:87–92.
14. Vidyasagar C: Persistent embryonic veins in arteriovenous malformations of the posterior fossa. Acta Neurochir 1979;48:67–82.
15. Velut S: Embryology of the cerebral veins. Neurochir 1987;33: 258–263.
16. Vidyasagar C: Persistent embryonic veins in the arteriovenous malformations of the dura. Acta Neurochir 1979;48:199–216.
17. Houdart E, Gobin YP, Casasco A, Aymard A, Herbreteau D, Merland JJ: A proposed angiographic classification of intracranial arteriovenous fistulae and malformations. Neuroradiology 1993;35: 381–385.
18. Lasjaunias P, Manelfe C, Chiu M: Angiographic architecture of intracranial vascular malformations and fistulas: Pretherapeutic aspects. Neurosurg Rev 1986;9:253–263.
19. ApSimon HT, Ives FJ, Khangure MS: Cranial dural arteriovenous malformation and fistula: Radiological diagnosis and management. Review of thirty four patients. Australas Radiol 1993;37:2–25.
20. Aminoff MJ, Kendall BE: Asymptomatic dural vascular anomalies. Br J Radiol 1973;46:662–667.
21. Bitoh S, Sakaki S: Spontaneous cure of dural arteriovenous malformation in the posterior fossa. Surg Neurol 1979;12:111–114.
22. Endo S, Koshu K, Kodama N, Okada H: Spontaneous regression of a posterior fossa dural arteriovenous malformation (author's transl). No Shinkei Geka 1979;7:1001–1004.
23. Ito Y, Fukumura A, Seto H, Ikeda J, Matsukado Y, Kodama T: Internal carotid aneurysmal formation following spontaneous regression of the dural arteriovenous malformation in the posterior fossa: A case report. No Shinkei Geka 1985;13:1215–1220.

24. Kataoka K, Taneda M: Angiographic disappearance of multiple dural arteriovenous malformations: Case report. J Neurosurg 1984; 60:1275–1278.
25. Reul J, Thron A, Laborde G, Bruckmann H: Dural arteriovenous malformations at the base of the anterior cranial fossa: Report of nine cases. Neuroradiology 1993;35:388–393.
26. Kuwayama N, Takaku A, Nishijima M, Endo S, Hirao M: Multiple dural arteriovenous malformations: Report of two cases. J Neurosurg 1989;71:932–934.
27. Al-Mefty O, Jinkins JR, Fox JL: Extensive dural arteriovenous malformation: Case report. J Neurosurg 1986;65:417–420.
28. Albright AL, Latchaw RE, Price RA: Posterior dural arteriovenous malformations in infancy. Neurosurgery 1983;13:129–135.
29. Chan ST, Weeks RD: Dural arteriovenous malformation presenting as cardiac failure in a neonate. Acta Neurochir 1988;91:134–138.
30. Garcia-Monaco R, Rodesch G, TerBrugge K, Burrows P, Lasjaunias P: Multifocal dural arteriovenous shunts in children. Childs Nervous System 1991;7:425–431.
31. Agawa M, Kohno T, Sogabe K. Dural arteriovenous malformation in the falx with subarachnoid hemorrhage. No Shinkei Geka 1991; 19:841–845.
32. Dardenne GJ: Dural arteriovenous anomaly fed by ethmoidal arteries. Surg Neurol 1978;10:384–388.
33. Espinosa JA, Mohr G, Robert F: Dural arteriovenous malformations of the ethmoidal region: Report of two cases. Br J Neurosurg 1993; 7:431–435.
34. Awad IA, Little JR, Akarawi WP, Ahl J: Intracranial dural arteriovenous malformations: Factors predisposing to an aggressive neurological course. J Neurosurg 1990;72:839–850.
35. Hayashi T, Tokunaga T, Matsuo M: Dural arteriovenous malformation in the anterior fossa with subarachnoid hemorrhage. Kurume Med J 1986;33:187–191.
36. Morimoto T, Yoshida S, Basugi N: Dural arteriovenous malformation in the cervical spine presenting with subarachnoid hemorrhage: Case report. Neurosurgery 1992;31:118–120.
37. Harding AE, Kendall B, Leonard TJ, Johnson MH: Intracerebral hemorrhage complicating dural arteriovenous fistula: A report of two cases. J Neurol Neurosurg Psychiatry 1984;47:905–911.
38. Lasjaunias P, Chiu M, TerBrugge K, Tolia A, Hurth M, Bernstein M: Neurological manifestations of intracranial dural arteriovenous malformations. J Neurosurg 1986;64:724–730.
39. Malik GM, Pearce JE, Ausman JI, Mehta B: Dural arteriovenous malformations and intracranial hemorrhage. Neurosurgery 1984;15: 332–339.
40. Vinuela F, Fox AJ, Pelz DM, Drake CG: Unusual clinical manifestations of dural arteriovenous malformations. J Neurosurg 1986;64: 554–558.
41. Hurst RW, Hackney DB, Goldberg HI, Davis RA: Reversible arteriovenous malformation-induced venous hypertension as a cause of neurological deficits. Neurosurg 1992;30:422–425.
42. Kurata A, Miyasaka Y, Yoshida T, Kunii M: Venous ischemia caused by dural arteriovenous malformation: Case report. J Neurosurg 1994;80:552–555.
43. Nencini P, Inzitari D, Gibbs J, Mangiafico S: Dementia with leucoaraiosis and dural arteriovenous malformation: Clinical and PET case study. J Neurol Neurosurg Psychiatry 1993;56:929–931.
44. Kawaguchi T, Fujita S, Yamada H, Nishida Y, Mori E: Hemodynamics before and after the total removal of a dural arteriovenous malformation of the posterior fossa: Case report. Surg Neurol 1988; 30:457–461.
45. Kaech D, de Tribolet N, Lasjaunias P: Anterior inferior cerebellar artery aneurysm, carotid bifurcation aneurysm, and dural arteriovenous malformation of the tentorium in the same patient. Neurosurgery 1987;21:575–582.
46. Lasjaunias P, Halimi P, Lopez-Ibor L, Sichez JP, Hurth M, de Tribolet N: Endovascular treatment of pure spontaneous dural vascular malformations: Review of 23 cases studied and treated between May 1980 and October 1983. Neurochirurgie 1984;30:207–223.
47. Okada T, Matsuda M, Handa J: Association of cerebral aneurysm and dural arteriovenous malformation in the anterior cranial fossa: A case report. No Shinkei Geka 1988;16:903–906.
48. Lamas E, Lobato RD, Esperarza J, Escudero L: Dural posterior fossa AVM producing raised sagittal simus pressure: Case report. J Neurosurg 1977;46:804–810.
49. Tsugane R, Sato O, Watabe T: Non-communicating hydrocephalus caused by dural arteriovenous malformation. Surg Neurol 1979;12: 393–396.
50. Gelwan MJ, Choi IS, Berenstein A, Pile-Spellman JM, Kupersmith MJ: Dural arteriovenous malformations and papilledema. Neurosurgery 1988;22:1079–1084.
51. Rozot P, Berrod JP, Bracard S, Roy D, Vespignani H: Papilledema and dural fistula. J Fr Ophtalmol 1991;14:13–19.
52. Bogousslavsky J, Vinuela F, Barnett HJ, Drake CG: Amaurosis fugax as the presenting manifestation of dural arteriovenous malformation. Stroke 1985;16:891–893.
53. Cerqueira L, Coimbra J, Matos E, Reis FC, Beirao JC: Prefrontal syndrome as a manifestation of intracranial dural arterio-venous malformation. Acta Med Port 1992;5:503–505.
54. Nakada T, Kwee IL, Ellis WG, et al.: Subacute diencephalic necrosis and dural arteriovenous malformation. Neurosurgery 1985;17: 653–656.
55. Harders A, Gilsbach J, Hassler W: Dural AV malformation of the lateral and sigmoid sinuses as possible cause of trigeminal neuralgia: Case report. Acta Neurochir 1982;66:95–102.
56. Hawke SH, Mullie MA, Hoyt WF, Hallinan JM, Halmagyi GM: Painful oculomotor nerve palsy due to dural-cavernous sinus shunt. Arch Neurol 1989;46:1252–1255.
57. Nazarian SM, Janati A, Angtuaco EJ, Jay WM: Oculomotor palsy and papilledema with pial-dural arteriovenous malformation. J Clin Neuro Ophthalmol 1987;7:98–103.
58. Moster ML, Sergott RC, Grossman RI: Dural carotid-cavernous sinus vascular malformation with facial nerve paresis. Can J Ophthalmol 1988;23:27–29.
59. Hofmann E, Nadjmi M, Ratzka M, Schuknecht B: Pulse synchronous vascular tinnitus: Radiologic diagnosis and therapy. HNO 1987; 35:211–218.
60. Morrison GA: Pulsatile tinnitus and dural arteriovenous malformation. J Laryngol Otol 1989;103:1073–1075.
61. Sila CA, Furlan AJ, Little JR: Pulsatile tinnitus. Stroke 1987;18: 252–256.
62. Nazarian SM, Potts RE, Chesser MZ, Janati A: Frontal intermittent rhythmic delta activity (FIRDA) in pial-dural arteriovenous malformation. Clin Electroencephalogr 1987;18:227–232.
63. Ono S, Tamura E, Oishi M, Takasu T, Kido G: Chronic slowly progressive dysarthria due to posterior fossa dural arteriovenous malformation. Rinsho Shinkeigaku 1988;28:1–3.
64. Uchino A, Ohno M: Bilateral venous infarctions of the thalamus: A case report. Radiat Med 1987;5:34–35.
65. Barke RM, Yoshizumi MO, Hepler RS, Krauss HR, Jabour BA: Spontaneous dural carotid-cavernous fistula with central retinal vein occlusion and iris neovascularization. Ann Ophthalmol 1991;23: 11–17.
66. Sergott RC, Grossman RI, Savino PJ, Bosley TM, Schatz NJ: The syndrome of paradoxical worsening of dural-cavernous sinus arteriovenous malformations. Ophthalmology 1987;94:205–212.
67. Enevoldson TP, Russell RW: Cerebral venous thrombosis: New causes for an old syndrome? Q J Med 1990;77:1255–1275.
68. Imaizumi M, Nukada T, Yoneda S, Abe H: Behçet's disease with sinus thrombosis and arteriovenous malformation in brain. J Neurol 1980;222:215–218.
69. Chen JC, Tsuruda JS, Halbach VV: Suspected dural arteriovenous fistula: Results with screening MR angiography in seven patients. Radiology 1992;183:265–271.
70. Chiras J, Bories J, Leger JM, Gaston A, Launay M: CT scan of dural arteriovenous fistulas. Neuroradiology 1982;23:185–194.
71. Hirabuki N, Fujita N, Hashimoto T, et al: Follow-up MRI in dural arteriovenous malformations involving the cavernous sinus: Empha-

sis on detection of venous thrombosis. Neuroradiology 1992;34: 423–427.

72. Wang PY, Shen WC: Gadolinium-DTPA enhanced magnetic resonance imaging of dural sinus occlusion in dural arteriovenous malformation: A case report. Chung Hua i Hsueh Tsa Chih 1993;52: 403–407.
73. Hashimoto M, Yokota A, Matsuoka S, Tsukamoto Y, Higashi J: Central retinal vein occlusion after treatment of cavernous dural arteriovenous malformation. AJNR 1989;10:S30–31.
74. Andrews BT, Wilson CB: Staged treatment of arteriovenous malformations of the brain. Neurosurgery 1987;21:314–323.
75. Barnwell SL, Halbach VV, Higashida RT, Hieshima G, Wilson CB: Complex dural arteriovenous fistulas: Results of combined endovascular and neurosurgical treatment in 16 patients. J Neurosurg 1989; 71:352–358.
76. Mendelowitsch A, Gratzl O, Radu EW: Current therapeutic methods of dural arteriovenous malformation: Are there any alternatives? Two case reports of infratentorial AVM's. Neurosurg Rev 1989;12: 141–145.
77. Sundt T Jr, Nichols DA, Piepgras DG, Fode NC: Strategies, techniques, and approaches for dural arteriovenous malformations of the posterior dural sinuses. Clin Neurosurg 1991;37:155–170.
78. Halbach VV, Higashida RT, Hieshima GB, Hardin CW, Pribram H: Transvenous embolization of dural fistulas involving the cavernous sinus. AJNR 1989;10:377–383.
79. Halbach VV, Higashida RT, Hieshima GB, Rosenblum M, Cahan L: Treatment of dural arteriovenous malformations involving the superior sagittal sinus. AJNR 1988;9:337–343.
80. Picard L, Bracard S, Islak C, et al: Dural fistulae of the tentorium cerebelli: Radioanatomical, clinical and therapeutic considerations. J Neuroradiol 1990;17:161–181.
81. Kendall B: Percutaneous embolic occlusion of dural arterio-venous malformation. Br J Radiol 1973;46:520–523.
82. Nakstad PH, Bakke SJ, Hald JK: Embolization of intracranial arteriovenous malformations and fistulas with polyvinyl alcohol particles and platinum fibre coils. Neuroradiology 1992;34:348–351.
83. Takahashi A, Yoshimoto T, Kawakami K, Sugawara T, Suzuki J: Transvenous copper wire insertion for dural arteriovenous malformations of cavernous sinus. J Neurosurg 1989;70:751–754.
84. Teng MM, Guo WY, Huang CI, Wu CC, Chang T: Occlusion of arteriovenous malformations of the cavernous sinus via the superior ophthalmic vein. AJNR 1988;9:539–546.
85. Thompson BG, Doppman JL, Oldfield EH: Treatment of cranial dural arteriovenous fistulae by interruption of leptomeningeal venous drainage. J Neurosurg 1994;80:617–623.
86. Chandler H Jr, Friedman WA: Successful radiosurgical treatment of a dural arteriovenous malformation: Case report (review). Neurosurgery 1993;33:139–141.
87. Chen MN, Imaya H, Nakazawa S: Four cases of intracranial AVM successfully treated by radiation therapy. No Shinkei Geka 1990; 18:1161–1166.
88. Hidaka H, Terashima H, Tsukamoto Y, Nakata H, Matsuoka S: Radiotherapy of dural arteriovenous malformation in the cavernous sinus. Radiat Med 1989;7:160–164.
89. Niwa J, Ohtaki M, Morimoto S, Nakagawa T, Hashi K: Reconstruction of the venous outflow using a vein graft in dural arteriovenous malformation associated with sinus occlusion. No Shinkei Geka 1988;16:1273–1280.
90. Djindjian R, Merland JJ, Theron J: Superselective Arteriography of the External Carotid Artery. New York: Springer, 1977, pp 606–628.

18.6 Spinal Arteriovenous Malformations

Key Points

1. A high index of suspicion is needed to avoid missing the diagnosis in patients with unexplained myelopathy or radiculopathy.
2. Complete spinal angiography is indicated in these patients.
3. Spinal AVMs cause problems with venous hypertension (T2-bright) or bleeding (T1-bright).
4. Obliteration of the AVM is indicated in most cases.
5. Permanent agents such as acrylates are indicated if long-term patency is expected.

Spinal AVMs are a relatively rare vascular condition (1). Most patients who have the condition will become symptomatic (2). These conditions represent a heterogeneous group of diseases that differ by etiology, pathophysiology, and clinical presentation (2–4). Endovascular therapy is indicated in most patients (5).

Anatomy and Physiology

See the section on spinal angiography in Chapter 17. The blood supply to the spinal cord is metameric (6). Segmental arteries coming off the aorta or the vertebral, subclavian, or iliac arteries divide into a ventral or dorsal trunk to give supply to the spine, the paraspinal muscles, the dura, and the spinal cord. Longitudinal anastomotic arteries both short and long connect these "latitudinal" metameric branches. Veins are also metameric, with a predominance of the longitudinal components. The spinal vasculature has a number of peculiarities: (a) a single small vessel (the anterior spinal artery) feeds a long segment of the CNS; (b) the pressure of the tissue drained by the veins varies tremendously; and (c) the gray/white matter tissue distribution is lined up in an inside-outside fashion, opposite the cerebrum. These changes may under certain conditions make the cord more susceptible to watershed ischemia and venous hypertension.

Diagnosis

Spinal AVMs can most confidently be diagnosed or excluded by complete angiography. MRI is excellent for assessing edema and cord extension (7). CT myelography can usually identify the presence of a spinal AVM. Clinical suspicion should be high in any patient with unexplained SAH, myelopathy, or radiculopathy and should prompt angiography. There is often a significant time between the initial signs and symptoms and the diagnosis.

Table 18.32.
Types of Spinal AVMs

Characteristics	Dural AVF	Intramedullary AVM	Perimedullary AVF	Metameric AVM
Synoname	Type 1	Type 2 Juvenile, ?glomus	Type 4 ?Type 3 ?Glomus	Cobb syndrome
Presentation	Slowly progressive paraparesis, dorsal column	Acute onset, pain leading to quadriplegia	Slowly progressive paraparesis or acute-onset pain and paraplegia	Acute-onset pain leading to quadriplegia
Pathophysiology	Venous hypertension	Subarachnoid hemorrhage	Venous hypertension or subarachnoid hemorrhage	Mass effect or subarachnoid hemorrhage
Age	Elderly	Adolescents	Young adults	Young adults
Sex	M>>>F	M>F	M>F	?
MRI findings	Perimedullary flow voids, edematous cord	Intra- and perimedullary flow voids, old and new blood	Perimedullary flow voids, edematous cord, old and new blood	Perispinal, perimedullary, intramedullary flow voids, old and new blood
Feeding arteries	Radiculomedullary arteries, dural branch, usually one level	Usually anterior spinal artery axis with contributions from posterolateral branches	Dominance of either the anterior spinal axis or posterior lateral vessels with collateral augmentation to distal feeding vessels from nondominant vessel just proximal to fistula	
Draining veins	Intradural veins	Intradural veins	Intradural veins	Intra and extradural veins
Associated findings	Low flow; delayed draining of the anterior spinal artery territory: tissue staining	High flow	High flow; large venous or arterial aneurysm	High flow; osseous changes

Classification, Clinical Features, and Prognosis

Spinal AVMs can be divided by the location of the shunt (e.g., dural versus intradural) or by the size of the shunt (high flow versus low flow) (Table 18.32). Patients with spinal AVMs develop symptoms related to (a) venous hypertension (spinal dural fistula, or perimedullary AVFs), (b) aneurysm formation and rupture (perimedullary AVFs and intramedullary AVMs), and (c) mass effect (intramedullary AVM and metameric AVMs).

Dural AVFs are located within the nerve root and adjacent spinal dura, are supplied by the radicular-meningeal arteries, and drain into the dilated intradural medullary veins (8) (Fig. 18.28). The dural fistulas present almost exclusively with symptoms of venous hypertension (9). The venous hypertension is characterized by initial edema of the cord, with T2-bright areas in the conus region as well as slight swelling of the cord. The edematous areas usually enhance after gadalinum administration (see Chapter 16). Over time this increases to involve the lower thoracic cord. The upper and midthoracic cord are almost always spared. Over time there is atrophy of the cord. Clinically, a slowly progressive, distal to proximal myelopathy is seen, with bladder and bowel involvement. Dorsal column and lower motor neuron involvement is seen, more commonly in elderly males.

Intramedullary AVMs are located within the substance of the cord and are supplied by the anterior and posterior spinal arteries. They are associated with aneurysms on the feeding arteries and veins and tend to rupture, presenting plegia and pain. Rarely, they present as venous hypertension and mass effect, unless there is associated venous occlusion.

Perimedullary AVFs, located on the cord surface, are supplied by either the anterior or posterior spinal artery (3) (Fig. 18.30). They present with bleeds, mass effect, or venous hypertension.

Metameric AVMs are organized along the course of the dermatome and often are associated with cutaneous lesions. They are fed from both ventral and lateral divisions of the metameric vessels. Osseous involvement is common. They present bleeds, mass effect, or venous hypertension.

Management and Treatment

INDICATIONS FOR TREATMENT

Patients with spinal AVMs should be considered for prompt treatment. Endovascular obliteration of the fistula or nidus is usually possible. Intranidal aneurysms are highly likely to rupture and should be treated. Venous hypertension is progressive and often reversible and therefore needs to be treated urgently.

Surgical treatment is highly effective in patients with well-defined AVMs that are less than two vertebral bodies in length, are located posteriorly and medially, and are away from the anterior spinal artery (10). Embolization is helpful in patients with feeding from the dura and posterior lateral spine or dilated anterior spinal arteries, and vessels that end in the AVM or have good collaterals (5). Extensive AVMs and metameric AVMs are usually not amenable to total obliteration. Palliative embolization may be indicated for aneurysms (11) and venous hypertension in these cases. Radiation therapy is contraindicated.

Table 18.33.
Treatment Methods for Spinal AVMs

Preoperative
1. Baseline neurologic exam, cytometrics, electrophysiologic studies.
2. Discuss "wake-up call."
3. Diagnostic angiogram at separate sitting for intradural AVMs.

Operative
1. Sensory- and motor-evoked responses.
2. General anesthetic if evoked responses allow adequate intraoperative monitoring.
3. Cytometric setup if conus lesion.
4. Guiding catheter in parent vessel.
   Navigate small low-profile catheter into fistula.
   Angiogram.
   Superselective catheterization with microcatheter.
   Baseline neurologic exam/evoked responses.
   Amytal/Xylocaine angiogram.
   Embolize.
   Repeat catheterization, angiography testing, embolization as needed.

Postoperative
1. Keep heparinized × 24 h.
2. Close monitoring.
3. In occlusive venous disease (dural fistula, considered long term) anticoagulation with Coumadin.

WORK-UP

A high index of suspicion must be maintained in any patients with unexplained myelopathy (12). Myelogram-CT and MRI are relatively sensitive and specific, but if negative should be followed up with spinal angiography, since there are many false positives and negatives.

TREATMENT

Treatment must be done in a permanent fashion with a permanent agent or there will be recurrence (Fig. 18.28). Treatment methods are similar to other embolization procedures (Table 18.33).

Obliteration of aneurysms is indicated to prevent devastating bleeding or rebleeding. Usually perimedullary AVMs bleed in the subarachnoid space and intramedullary AVFs in the parenchyma, and dural AVFs do not bleed. They carry significant risk if they are on the anterior spinal arteries, since critically important vessels of passage may be involved. The central commissural artery, if obliterated, can lead to a devastating syndrome of a unilateral anterior spinal syndrome (13). Some have approached this problem with repeated embolizations with particulate agents such as PVA, with encouraging results (14) (Fig. 18.29).

Venous hypertension is effectively treated by obliteration of the shunt. Care must be taken to avoid obliteration of the venous drainage. Embolic agents passing into the venous outflow at the time of embolization can cause progressive antegrade thrombosis after the embolization. Relief of venous hypertension can lead to gratifying improvement over a few days. Usually the improvement takes weeks and continues for months. Failure to find improvement should prompt repeat angiography to exclude continued venous drainage. Surgery for recurrence after embolization is indicated. Progressive venous thrombosis in the face of obliteration of the AVF is cause for great concern, and vigorous anticoagulation with Coumadin is indicated. Progression of the disease in spite of angiographically full treatment is occasionally seen.

Mass effect can be seen and is usually related to aneurysms. It is challenging to treat because complications can result from obliteration of the vessels of passage or venous hypertension.

Results

Endovascular obliteration of dural arteriovenous fistulas (AVF) with acrylate is effective in most cases, as is surgery (15,16) (Fig. 18.28). Embolization with particulate agents is not indicated because the nidus will almost certainly recanalize. Adjuvant therapy prior to surgery is helpful for intramedullary AVMs.

REFERENCES

1. Djindjian R, Cophignon J, Theron J, Merland JJ, Houdart R: Embolization by superselective arteriography from the femoral route in neuroradiology: Review of 60 cases: 1. Technique, indications, complications. Neuroradiology 1973;6:20–26.
2. Hurth M, Houdart R, Djindjian R, Rey A, Djindjian M: Arteriovenous malformations of the spinal cord: Clinical, anatomical and therapeutic consideration—a series of 150 cases. Prog Neurol Surg 1978; 9:238–266.
3. Merland JJ, Riche MC, Chiras J: Intraspinal extramedullary arteriovenous fistulae draining into the medullary veins. J Neuroradiol 1980;7:271–320.
4. Riche MC, Reizine D, Melki JP, Merland JJ: Classification of spinal cord vascular malformations. Med Imag Radiat Oncol 1985;3: 17–24.
5. Merland JJ, Reizine D, Laurent A, et al: Embolization of spinal cord vascular lesions. In F Vinuela, VV Halbach, JE Dion (eds), Interventional Neuroradiology: Endovascular Therapy of the Central Nervous System. New York: Raven, 1992.
6. McCormick PC, Stein BM: Functional anatomy of the spinal cord and related structures. Neurosurg Clin N Am 1990;1:469–489.
7. Yoon SS, Silver AJ, Khandji AG, Pile-Spellman J, Chan S, Hilal SK: MR Imaging and Angiography of Spinal Cord Vascular Malformations. Radiographics (CD-ROM) 1995.
8. Kendall BE, Logue V: Spinal epidural angiomatous malformations draining into intrathecal veins. Neuroradiology 1977;13:181–189.
9. Hassler W, Thron A, Grote EH: Hemodynamics of spinal dural arteriovenous fistulas: An intraoperative study. J Neurosurg 1989; 70:360–370.
10. Yasargil MG, Symon L, Teddy PJ: Arteriovenous malformations of the spinal cord. Adv Tech Stand Neurosurg 1984;11:61–102.
11. Rodesch G, Lasjaunias P, Berenstein A: Embolization of spinal cord arteriovenous malformations. Riv Neuroradiol 1992;5:67–92.
12. Zervas NT, Pile-Spellman JM: Case records of the Massachusetts General Hospital. Weekly clinicopathological exercises. Case 12-1992. A 64-year-old woman with the abrupt onset of paraparesis after 10 months of increasing episodic leg weakness. N Engl J Med 1992;326:816–824.
13. Riche MC, Melki JP, Merland JJ: Embolization of spinal cord vascular malformations via the anterior spinal artery. AJNR 1983;4: 378–381.
14. Biondi A, Merland JJ, Reizine D, et al: Embolization with particles in thoracic intramedullary arteriovenous malformations: Long-term angiographic and clinical results. Radiology 1990;177:651–658.

15. Merland JJ, Assouline E, Ruffenacht D, Guimaraes N: Dural spinal arteriovenous fistulae draining into medullary veins: Clinical and radiological results of treatment (embolization and surgery) in 56 cases. Neuroradiology 1985/1986;

16. Mourier KL, Gelbert F, Rey A, et al: Spinal dural arteriovenous malformations with perimedullary drainage: Indications and results of surgery in 30 cases. Acta Neurochir 1989;100:136–141.

18.7 Aneurysms

Key Points

1. Treat aneurysms to eliminate the risk of bleeding or the presence of mass effect.
2. Permanent obliteration of the aneurysm with parent vessel sparing is the goal of aneurysm treatment.
3. Berry aneurysms can be considered *cold, hot, giant*, or *asymptomatic*. Nonberry aneurysms usually have a worse natural history than berry aneurysms.
4. The management outcome of hot aneurysms rests primarily on the Hunt and Hess grade (key factor level of consciousness); cold aneurysms on size and location. Rebleed, vasospasm, mass effect, and heart attacks account for most of the morbidity of aneurysmal subarachnoid bleeds.
5. Proper patient selection, meticulous procedural technique, fastidious postembolization management, and teamwork are essential to obtaining acceptable results in aneurysm patients.
6. Hunterian ligation (parent vessel occlusion) is highly effective and safe in properly selected patients.
7. Only patients with adequate cerebral *and* cardiopulmonary reserve are candidates for parent vessel occlusion.
8. Total permanent obliteration of an aneurysm with parent vessel sparing is difficult to obtain in large aneurysms (2.0 cm) with wide necks by either surgical or endovascular methods.
9. Endovascular coil obliteration of the aneurysm with vessel sparing alleviates the risk of acute bleeding, but with present methods it appears to be less effective in preventing the subsequent regrowth of the aneurysm.

Prevalence of Aneurysms and Incidence of Bleeds

The prevalence of aneurysms is related to the age of the population. Aneurysms are rarely found in autopsies of young patients but are common in elderly patients. The autopsy-derived prevalence of aneurysms varies considerably depending on the examiners' methodology, criteria, and results, but it appears that 2 to 5 percent of the population harbor aneurysms. This translates to over 400,000 people in the United States (1).

The incidence of bleeds from aneurysm is greatest in the sixth decade of life and is in the range of 12 per 100,000 people per year in North America. This brings the estimated number of patients in the United States to nearly 30,000 per year. The incidence throughout the world varies from 0.5 per 100,000 for Hong Kong Chinese to 15.7 for Finnish and 17.5 for Japanese. Besides age, smoking, atherosclerosis, diet, and genetic predisposition no doubt play a role.

The mortality and morbidity of aneurysm rupture remain high. Close to half of the patients will be dead within the first 3 months. More than half of the patients will have major disability, and only a third who leave the hospital will ever enjoy the quality of life they had before they bled. There does not appear to be any activity that promotes bleeding, with the exception of the second trimester of pregnancy.

Pathophysiology

The exact causes of aneurysms remain unclear, although it appears that the major ingredients have been identified. They include aging, flow stress (shear forces), and collagen abnormalities. The cause of rupture is not understood, nor are the factors that cause aneurysms to grow. Both growth and rupture appear to be related. Aneurysms can grow in a short time, and in the smaller aneurysms this is probably the natural history. Giant aneurysms may grow by different mechanisms. Hypertension has been associated with rerupture of an aneurysm in the acute state. Berry aneurysms make up the vast majority of aneurysms (Table 18.34).

The natural history of nonberry aneurysms is less well understood, but they appear to have a significantly higher risk of bleeding and management morbidity. *Aneurysms associated with AVMs* can be classified as (a) distal intralesion, (b) proximal, or (c) remote. Proximal aneurysms appear to regress with effective treatment of the AVMs. Aneurysms on the feeding pedicle appear to be associated with a high rate of bleeding (2,3). Aneurysms may be caused by trauma to the elastic membrane by increased flow (4). *Infectious cerebral aneurysms* are uncommon, accounting for only 2.6 to 6 percent of all intracranial aneurysms according to autopsy studies. Arising from an intravascular or extravascular source of infection, the vast majority occur in the setting of bacterial endocarditis with an intravascular source of infection due to embolization of fragments of infected cardiac valve emboli. Infectious aneurysms are usually discovered after a devastating intracranial hemorrhage that carries a 60 to 90 percent mortality. Fungal infectious aneurysms, which carry an even graver prognosis, have become more common. A high index of suspicion and early diagnosis of infectious aneurysms prior to hemorrhage are important factors in reducing morbidity and mortality.

Table 18.34
Types of Aneurysms

Type	Factors	Associated Conditions	Comments
Berry	Media or elastic defects and/or degeneration, flow stresses, arteriosclerotic vascular disease	Ehlers-Danlos, familial, adult polycystic disease, coarctation of the aorta, AVMs, fibromuscular disease, agenesis of the carotid, arterial anomalies of the carotid	Occur at branching points of proximal intracranial cerebral arteries
Atherosclerotic	Medial degeneration or absence	Atherosclerosis and hypertension, corpus callosum lipoma	Usually occurs on the vertebrobasilar system
Trauma (dissections and penetrating)	Spontaneous dissection, cystic degeneration of media, penetration of the blood vessel, penetrating trauma		Vertebral site most common, young age, headache, antecedent trauma, usually fatal
Mycotic	Septic degeneration of media	Subacute bacterial endocarditis, cerebral infarctions	Treat infection, serial angiogram, treat if aneurysm grows
Tumor	Tumor invasion of media	Atrial myxoma	

Some lesions are effectively treated with antibiotics alone, but others require surgical intervention. Intracranial neoplastic aneurysms can result from metastatic tumor embolization of the cerebral vessels associated with cardiac myxoma and choriocarcinoma as well as bronchogenic carcinoma (5). Like mycotic aneurysms, carcinomatous aneurysms are small, multiple, located in the peripheral branches of the cerebral artery, and often rupture, obscuring the tumor (6). *Fusiform vertebral basilar aneurysms* tend to present with ischemic or mass symptoms; the former symptoms can often be effectively treated with anticoagulation. Postclipping *aneurysm residual necks* (and presumably postendovascular packing necks) may well increase over time and pose a risk of rebleeding (7).

Experimental aneurysms have been made in a variety of ways. In biological models, increased flow, hypertension, and abnormal collagen production have all been implicated. Models for endovascular therapy are increasingly important in the development of new embolic materials and methods (8–12). A useful *experimental canine giant aneurysm* can be produced by initially producing a fistula between the common carotid artery and the external jugular vein and 1 week later ligating the vein above and below the fistula to create a blind aneurysmal pouch (8).

Work-up

The work-up for a patient with an aneurysm is directed at answering key questions with near certainty (Table 18.35).

CLINICAL

Prompt treatment requires prompt diagnosis, which is not always made. Ten percent of patients do not seek medical attention with an SAH. Twenty-five percent have a diagnosis other than SAH made, which delays treatment by an average of 4 days. These delays are most common in the patients not injured by the initial bleed who would be more likely to benefit from early treatment. Small warning bleeds are not uncommon, nor are new cranial nerve findings, both of which probably represent a growth of the aneurysm.

After the diagnosis has been made, the clinical history and examination are directed at determining what has happened to the patient and what options are available for effective treatment. How badly the patient has already been hurt by the aneurysmal SAH can in large part be determined by the Hunt and Hess grade of the patient. The grade is determined by how much meningeal irritation there is and by the level of consciousness. The Hunt and Hess classification is simple and is most commonly used (Table 18.36). The International grading system is also useful and has the advantage of being a modification of the Glasgow coma scale, which is used routinely throughout the world for other clinical situations, such as trauma.

Initial grading may overestimate the severity of the disease in patients with hydrocephalus, fever, or metabolic derangement. Acute severe hydrocephalus treated effectively by a ventricular drain can often lead to a profound improvement in the patients' state and grade. This is most true for patients with large intraventricular bleeds.

RADIOLOGICAL

Initial CT will confirm the diagnosis of SAH, help prognosticate the probability of symptomatic vasospasm, evaluate for hydrocephalus, give some indication of where the bleeding aneurysm is, and offer an invaluable baseline. A blood clot thicker than 1 cm or in the vertical cisterns is associated with a high incidence of vasospasm. It is highly sensitive and usually specific.

Initial MRI/MRA may demonstrate the aneurysm and the source of bleeding. It is indicated in patients with large and giant aneurysms to help determine intraluminal clot, mass effect, and associated edema. It is indicated in all complex aneurysms.

Early angiogram guides treatment. Identification of the aneurysm's location, size, neck, geometry, and topology, as well as collateral circulation, other aneurysms, vasospasm,

Table 18.35.
Work-up Questions for Aneurysm

Question	Impact	Techniques	Comments
Has the patient bled?	If patient has bled, there is a high management morbidity.	CT positive 95% of the time. LP* positive for small bleed, but false-positive with traumatic tap.	Delayed presentations can require an LP* looking for xanthochromia.
Does the patient have an aneurysm?	If demonstrated after an SAH, usually the source of bleeding. If not demonstrable, repeat angiogram with cross compression of opposite carotid, as well as external carotid injection.	CECT can show aneurysms of 3.0 mm 87% of the time. MRI/MRA can show aneurysms of 5.0 mm > 85% of the time. Four-vessel angiogram is gold standard.	PICA, ACA, MCA† areas can be missed due to technique. Vasospasm or clot can hide aneurysms.
What aneurysm bled?	Treat aneurysm that will rebleed.	CT (MRI) shows area of blood. Angiogram shows large, irregular tit.	Exploration is indicated if unknown.
What is the anatomy of the aneurysm neck?	Small, noncalcified necks without perforators off the aneurysm are straightforward for surgical clipping.	CT shows calcification. Superselective angiography shows flow arrest.	Superselective angiogram usually not indicated.
What is the collateral flow?	Excellent collateral flow makes emergent vessel occlusion or temporary occlusion less risky.	Cross-compression angiography or transcranial Doppler, carotid ultrasound.	Can be dangerous in face of ruptured aneurysm.
Is there significant clot with mass effect?	Clot can be knocked off during surgery or endovascular procedure. Edematous brain can cause mass effect.	On CT/MRI, edema vs. infarct related to aneurysms can be difficult to tell apart.	Edema needs to be treated vigorously. Perianeurysm infarct bodes poorly.
Are there multiple aneurysms or other "surgical" problems?	Hematoma, AVMs, ASVD‡, stenosis, and multiple aneurysms may need to be treated.	Generally treat the symptomatic lesion first.	
Are there other medical problems?	Generally multiple system disease favors endovascular treatment.	Proactive intensive monitoring is indicated in patients with multiple disease.	Fluid shifts and pain can be significant in endovascular procedures if one is not vigilant.

* LP = Lumbar Puncture.
† PICA, ACA, MCA = Posterior/inferior cerebellar artery, arterior cerebral artery, middle cerebral artery.
‡ ASVD = arteriosclerotic vascular disease.

vascular malformations, stenosis, emboli, and mass effect, is important. A four-vessel selective angiogram in the hours following the SAH is indicated when early treatment can be considered. All views and maneuvers needed to answer the previously mentioned questions without excessive discomfort and contrast load are indicated. *The suspicious locations should be examined first.* If an aneurysm is not found in spite of a technically good angiogram, a delayed repeat angiogram should be performed that includes the external carotid and cervical spinal vessels to exclude spasm, aneurysm recanalization, or AVM of the dural or upper cervical cord (13,14,15,16).

Table 18.36.
Aneurysmal SAH Grades

Grade	Hunt and Hess
0	No SAH, intact
1	Asymptomatic with slight headache
1a	No acute meningeal/reaction, fixed focal deficit
2	Moderate headache, nuchal rigidity without neurologic deficit other than cranial nerve
3	Drowsy or confused or minor focal defect
4	Stupor, moderate focal deficit
5	Deep coma, decerebrate rigidity

Source: Hunt W. E., Hess R. M.: Surgical Risk as Related to Time of Intervention in the Repair of Intracranial Aneurysm. J. Neurosurgery 28:14–20, 1968.

LABORATORY

Laboratory work-up includes a complete blood count, electrolytes, and an ECG. Many of these patients are very sick, having suffered periods of metabolic and respiratory stress during the subarachnoid bleed.

Management

GOALS

The goal of treatment is to keep the aneurysm from bleeding or growing. This can be accomplished by isolating the neck from the blood flow or by thickening the effective aneurysm wall.

Methods are available that can be viewed as "thickening the aneurysm wall" endovascularly or by direct surgery, such as packing an aneurysm dome with balloons or coils or wrapping an aneurysm dome with muslin. Since there

Table 18.37.
Aneurysm Neck

	Morphological	Anatomical	Flow
Definition	Plane where contrast column intersects with contrast ellipsoid	Plane where media-rich vessels intersect media-absent area	Plane where inflow and outflow intersect column of laminar flowing blood
Forms of treatment	Endovascular packing	Clipping	Hunterian ligation

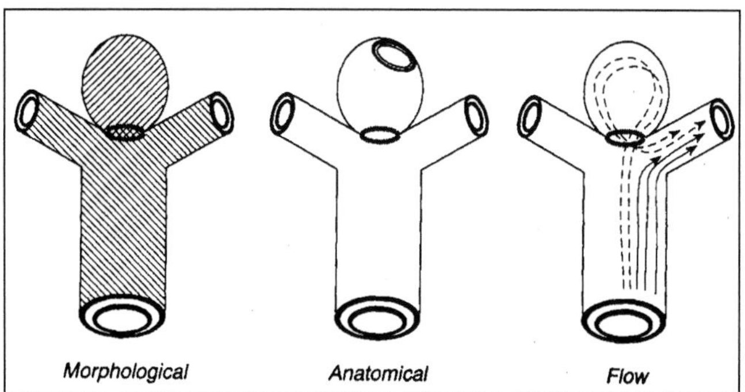

Figure 18.31. Aneurysm neck. The *morphological neck* is the plane where the contrast column intersects with the contrast ellipsoid. The *anatomical neck* is the plane where media-rich vessels intersect with the media-absent area. The *flow neck* is the plane where inflow and outflow columns intersect.

appears to be only a small difference in the bleeding rates of different aneurysm sizes, after aneurysms reach 7 to 10 mm, a partial reduction in the aneurysm size is unlikely to lead to a partial reduction in the bleeding rate.

Obliteration of the aneurysm neck is highly effective in keeping an aneurysm from rebleeding and should be considered the preferred approach. In discussions of the aneurysm "neck" there can be some ambiguity (Table 18.37 and Fig. 18.31). What is perceived by the angiographer, neurosurgeon, and surgical angiographer can in fact be different. The angiographer sees the "morphological neck," the surgeon the "anatomical neck," and the interventional angiographer the "flow neck." All types of aneurysms can be approached endovascularly. The long-term results have not been determined. If these results are as effective as they have initially appeared, all aneurysms presenting as SAH will have to be considered for endovascular treatment as well as for surgical treatment.

COMPLICATIONS OF THE DISEASE

Complications of the aneurysmal SAH include cerebral ischemia, hydrocephalus, electrolyte abnormalities, and myocardial infarction (17), as well as those complications related to decreased level of consciousness, such as aspiration pneumonia and pulmonary emboli (Table 18.38). Each possible complication must be identified, guarded against, and treated effectively if it develops. These associated conditions often alter the management options, making the less invasive approaches preferable.

Anticoagulants routinely used for embolizations in patients can have their own challenges. Minor surgical procedures such as lumbar punctures and central lines can be more difficult, and the procedures used prior to instituting anticoagulation or other methods must be carefully timed.

TREATMENT AND TIMING

Endovascular treatment of aneurysms has been used with varying indications, methods, and results. There are three distinctly different approaches: (a) parent vessel sparing, (b) parent vessel occlusion, and (c) adjuvant treatment (Table 18.39).

The timing of treatment can be a difficult decision. In patients who have bled, the high rebleed rate in the following days to weeks requires early decisions as to treatment. In addition, patients who develop vasospasm cannot be treated effectively with hypervolemic hypertension if the aneurysm has not been effectively obliterated. Aneurysms are often, therefore, divided into four types: (a) *hot*, having just bled, (b) *cold*, not having bled in the last 3 weeks, (c)

Table 18.38.
Disease Complications of Aneurysms

Aneurysmal SAH complications	Prophylaxis and treatment	Possible effect on endovascular treatment
Hydrocephalus	Baseline CT, elevated HOB*, ventricular drains if needed	
Electrolyte abnormalities	Baseline and q daily electrolyte and osmolality	
Myocardial ischemia	Baseline ECG	
Vasospasm	Early aneurysm obliteration, allowing safe hypervolemic hypertension; if fails, angioplasty	May require angioplasty
Aspirations		
Pulmonary emboli	Pneumatic boots, low-dose heparin after treatment	Heparinized patients can be treated endovascularly

* HOB = head of bed

Table 18.39.
Types of Endovascular Treatment

	Vessel sparing	Vessel sacrificing	Adjuvant treatment
Definition	The aneurysm neck and/or aneurysm is blocked with an endovascular device.	The parent vessel of the aneurysm (+/− the aneurysm mouth) is blocked with an aneurysm endovascular device.	Partial treatment of aneurysm dome in the acute stage. Temporary or permanent occlusion of a vessel as part of the planned treatment.
Also known as	Reconstructive; endovascular clipping.	Deconstructive; parent vessel occlusion; Hunterian ligation; trapping.	
Indications	Acute SAH	Giant "neckless" aneurysm	Difficult large aneurysms with acute SAH
Relative contraindications	Fresh trauma or dissection.	Hemodynamically ineffective collateral; impaired cerebral vascular reserve; acute SAH with vasospasm threatening; hemodynamically significant impaired cardiovascular reserve; vessel-sparing procedure considered.	
Materials	Coils, Balloons	Coils, Balloons	Coils, Balloons
Technical considerations	A definable neck is usually needed to be optimistic that the aneurysm can be obliterated and the parent vessel spared.	Test occlusion prior to occlusion. Revascularization prior to occlusion may be needed. Postocclusion anticoagulation. The vessels occluded are just below the aneurysm and the aneurysm is below the first major collateral.	Logistically demanding.
Results	Variably effective or of unknown effectiveness.	Highly effective. Safe if tolerated. Long-term increased risk of collateral failure by stenosis or aneurysm development not known.	In selected patients, the combined results can be quite satisfying.
Comments	Preferred treatment if effective.	May always have place in the treatment of giant aneurysms of the vertebral and proximal internal carotid artery in patients who present with mass effect.	Helpful in complex aneurysms.

giant, being larger than 2.5 cm, and (d) *asymptomatic*, being found on an examination instituted for nonaneurysm-related symptoms. Generally, uncomplicated hot aneurysms should be treated urgently, and giant and cold aneurysms are treated electively. Anatomically uncomplicated asymptomatic aneurysms smaller than 5 mm tend to be watched in the elderly and operated on in the young and middle-aged. Bifurcation aneurysms (anterior communicating artery, basilar artery) are far more likely to bleed than lateral wall aneurysms.

PARENT VESSEL OCCLUSION

Strategy

In properly selected patients, occlusion is safe, effective, and the preferred treatment. The parent vessel is occluded proximal to the aneurysm. For the occlusion to be effective and safe, the origin of the aneurysm must be below the first major, hemodynamically effective collateral. Since the cerebral vascular reserve has been reduced, at least temporarily, occlusion is contraindicated whenever the cardiovascular or cerebral vascular hemodynamic stability cannot be maintained. This includes patients with acute SAH in whom vasospasm can develop or in patients with acute myocardial infarctions who may develop hypotension or decreased effective cardiac output. If the aneurysm is large, direct aneurysm attack sometimes should be contemplated with caution and alternative solutions sought. In a large published series of 174 patients with giant aneurysms, 62 percent were found to be unclippable (12). Unruptured intracranial aneurysms ($n = 202$) treated with surgery obtained an excellent or good outcome in 100 percent of patients with aneurysms less than 10 mm in diameter, in 95 percent with aneurysms 11 to 25 mm, and in 79 percent with aneurysms greater than 25 mm. Except for giant basilar aneurysms, *size* (and not location) of the aneurysm was the key predictor of risk for surgical morbidity (18).

Traumatic or neoplastic pseudoaneurysms are treacherous. Proximal parent vessel occlusion is indicated when vigorous medical treatment is thought likely to fail. Early diagnosis and successful management of *traumatic carotid artery dissections* require a high index of clinical suspicion. The diagnostic study of choice is cerebral arteriography. Presenting signs and symptoms include Horner's syndrome, dysphasia, hemiparesis, obtundation, and monoparesis. In one study, patients detected early with mild neurologic deficits fared well with treatment, whereas those with profound neurologic deficits and delayed diagnoses had poor outcomes. *Aggressive nonsurgical treatment is advocated* with cerebral ischemia, including anticoagulation therapy for prevention of progressive thrombosis and arterial occlusion and/or distal arterial embolization with resultant cerebral ischemia. Direct surgical thromboendarterectomy is considered to carry high morbidity and mortality rates (19).

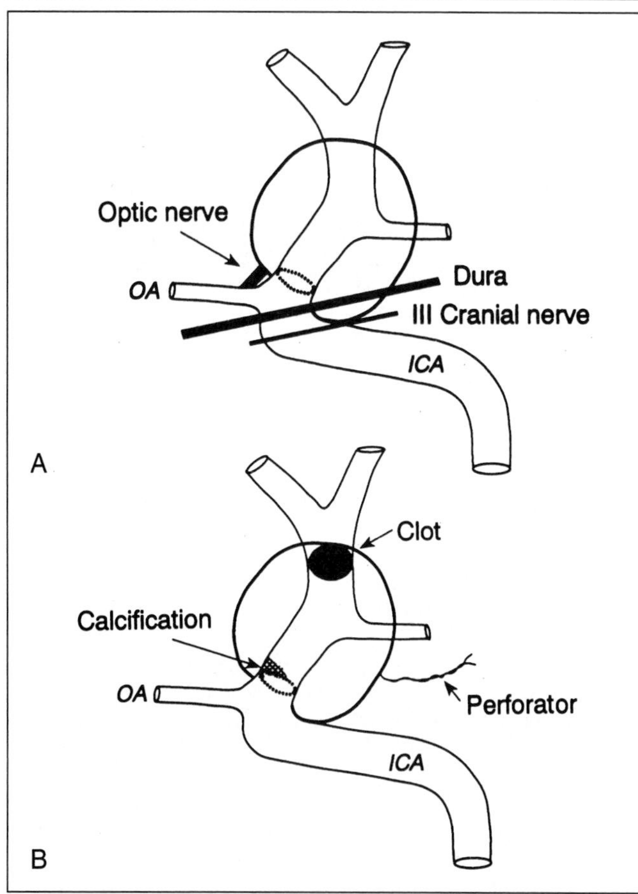

Figure 18.32. The close proximity of larger ophthalmic aneurysms (periclinoid) to the visual apparatus can exert a scissors effect on the optic chiasm causing a field cut or compressing the third nerve, causing diplopia. Uncommonly, a perforator arising from the dome or wall of the aneurysm also can make successful clipping more challenging. A clot within the aneurysm can rarely act as a source of emboli and can increase the risk of both direct surgery and endovascular treatment.

Certain aneurysm locations command additional caution. Some aneurysms, such as cavernous aneurysms, are difficult to reach surgically and tend to be best handled by the endovascular approach (Fig. 18.33). The close proximity of most ophthalmic aneurysms to the visual apparatus exerts a scissors effect on the optic chiasm, often causing a field cut or compressing the third nerve, causing diplopia (Fig. 18.32). Intra- and extradural extension, as with heavily calcified aneurysms, may make clipping impossible or may lead to intraoperative ruptures. The uncommon condition in which a perforator arises from the dome or wall of the aneurysm also can make successful clipping more challenging (Figs. 18.32 and 18.34). High or low basilar apex aneurysms, midbasilar aneurysms, and others can be challenging.

A clot within the aneurysm can rarely act as a source of emboli and can increase the risk of both direct surgery or endovascular treatment. Anticoagulation and parent vessel occlusion are sometimes needed in this uncommon condition. Some authors feel that the prognosis for unruptured aneurysms presenting with transient focal ischemia is good, regardless of therapy (20). This is also the author's impression. Four criteria have been suggested to determine whether embolization is likely: (a) clinical TIA or completed stroke, (b) arteriographic or surgical evidence of an aneurysm, (c) no other lesions that could produce a stroke, and (d) no recent evidence of SAH or vasospasm (21).

Preocclusion Tolerance Testing Cerebrovascular reserve can best be measured with balloon tolerance test occlusion of the vessel prior to occlusion under close neurologic, EEG, and physiologic monitoring. Provocative lowering of the blood pressure helps determine who are candidates for external carotid–internal carotid bypass prior to carotid occlusion and is useful in guiding postocclusion blood pressure guides. Data obtained from the test occlusion are only applicable for the same physiologic conditions (hematocrit, PaO_2, cardiac output) as those prevailing when the test was performed (Table 18.40). The author uses repeated meticulous neurologic examinations and xenon CBF measurements with provocative hypotension to determine occlusion safety. Postoperative management is guided by serial SPECT scans.

Patients with stump pressures below 55 mm Hg have a markedly increased risk of stroke, whereas those with a stump pressure over 70 mm Hg have a markedly decreased stroke rate (22). Patients can be divided into four groups based on XeCT-CBF mapping (23). XeCT-CBF mapping can be correlated with internal carotid artery stump pressures and clinical neurologic assessment during temporary internal carotid artery occlusion. It can also be divided into four groups, with patients becoming symptomatic below a CBF of 30 cc of blood/100 gm of brain/min (24) (Table 18.41). Temporary occlusion of the internal carotid artery with a balloon catheter (balloon Matas test) and simultaneous dynamic computerized tomography (DCT) scanning can be used to calculate the mean transit time (MTT) and the percentage of transit time (MTT of the occluded side × 100/MTT of the control side). The critical percent transit time value to cause symptomatic ischemia is reported to be 200 (25). Test occlusion has been reported to

Table 18.40.
Criteria for a Passing Test Occlusion

Normal neurologic examination
Adequate angiographic cross filling
CBF > 30 ml/min/dl
Stump pressure > 70% mBP
Asymmetric and bilateral decreased CBF*
Percent transit time (%TT) < 155
Normal EEG
MCA† velocity > 35

* CBF = cerebral blood flow.
† MCA = middle cerebral artery.

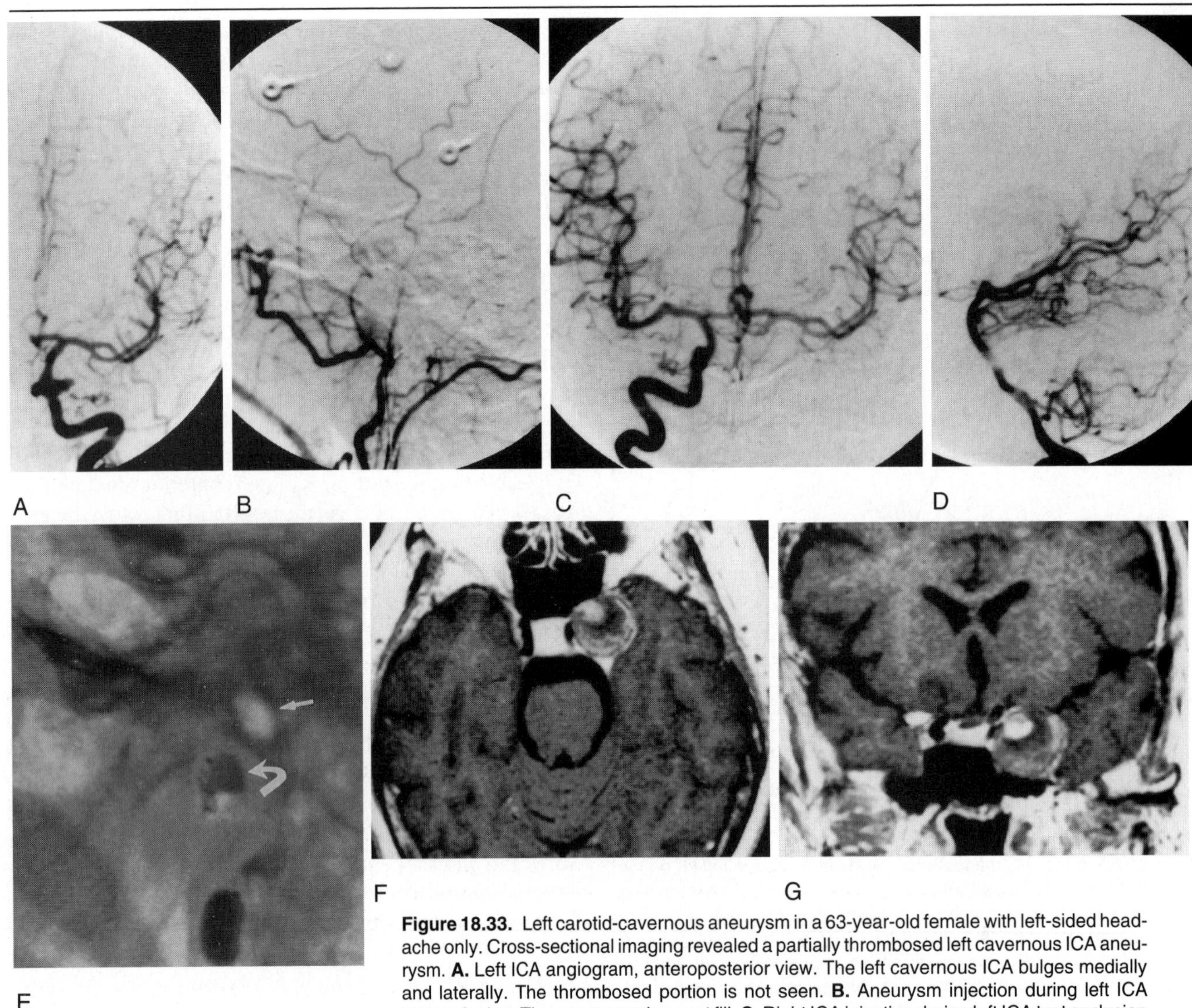

Figure 18.33. Left carotid-cavernous aneurysm in a 63-year-old female with left-sided headache only. Cross-sectional imaging revealed a partially thrombosed left cavernous ICA aneurysm. **A.** Left ICA angiogram, anteroposterior view. The left cavernous ICA bulges medially and laterally. The thrombosed portion is not seen. **B.** Aneurysm injection during left ICA test occlusion. The aneurysm does not fill. **C.** Right ICA injection during left ICA test occlusion shows excellent cross filling through the anterior circle of Willis. **D.** Left vertebral artery injection during test occlusion shows good collateral flow from both posterior communicating arteries. **E.** Plain film shows balloons in the left ICA after occlusion. The top balloon is beyond the aneurysm neck to ensure trapping (arrow). The second balloon from the top (curved arrow) is filled with a solidifying substance (silicone), which is radiolucent. Two other balloons are seen below. **F** and **G.** MRI 3 weeks after ICA occlusion shows a laminated thrombus in the aneurysm sac of different ages; the thrombus with bright signal corresponds to a recently occluded aneurysm lumen filled with intermediate-aged blood products (extracellular methemoglobin).

Table 18.41a.
CBF Classification of Carotid Occlusion

Group I	No significant change.
Group II	Symmetric decrease.
Group III	Asymmetric decrease, greater on the occluded side; very high risk for delayed neurologic injury due to a compromised CBF; should have arterial bypass grafts before carotid occlusion.
Group IV	Patients clinically failed to tolerate even brief carotid occlusion.

Source: SM Erba, JA Horton, RE Latchaw et al: AJNR 1988;9:533–538.

Table 18.41b.
Xe-CT-CBF Classification of Carotid Occlusion

	CT-CBF	Neurologic exam	*N*	Stump BP/BP
Group I	no Δ*	nl	40	86/128
Group II	$-\ \Delta$, >30	nl	50	86/130
Group III	<30	nl	13	
Group IV	<30	+ *!!!neur*	11	

Source: DL Steed, MW Webster, EJ DeVries, et al: J Vasc Surg 1990;11:38–43, with permission.

* Δ = change

† nl = normal

‡ +!!!neur = neurological symptoms

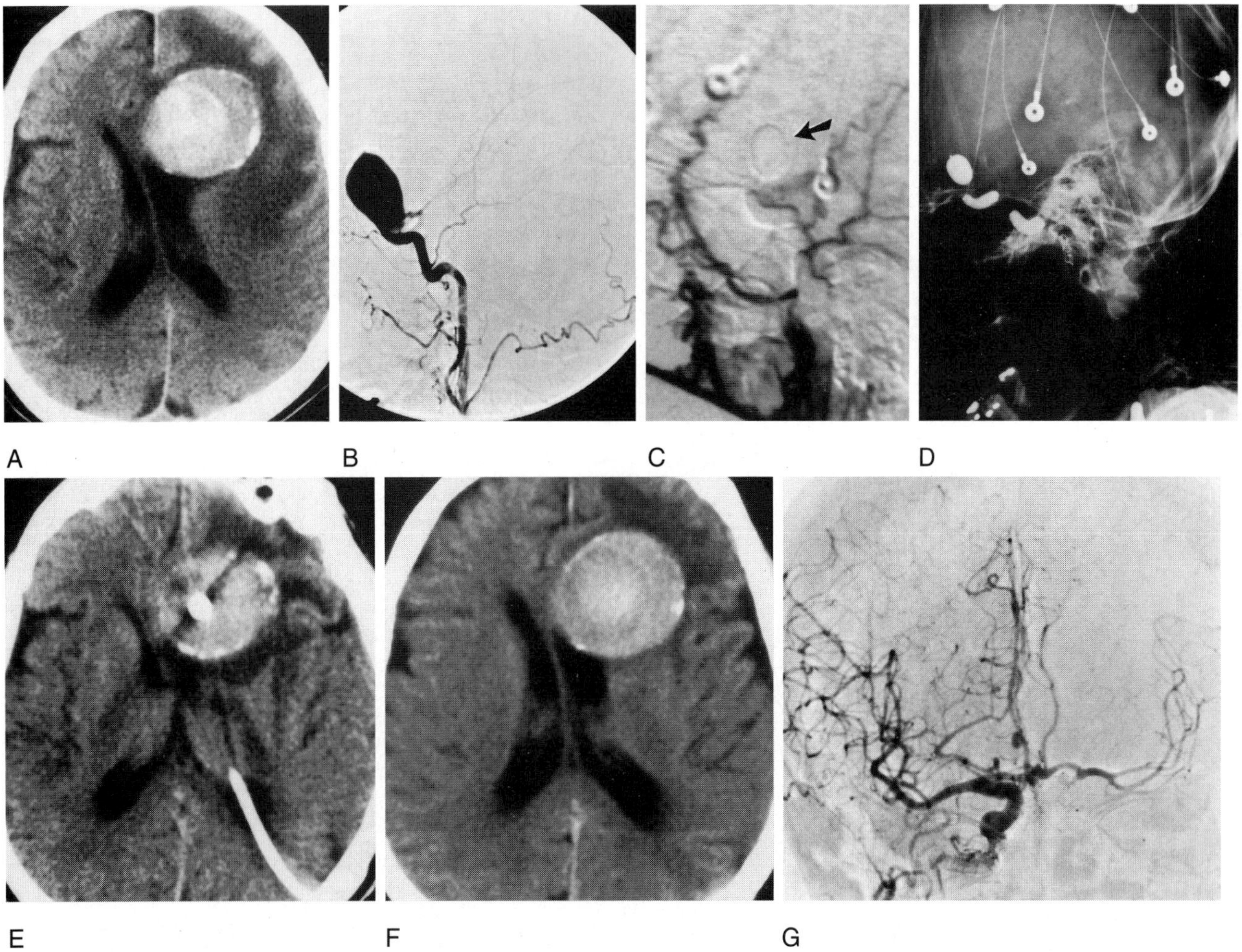

A B C D

E F G

Figure 18.34. Giant left carotid–ophthalmic aneurysm causing brain edema in a 68-year-old female with progressive onset of blindness in the right eye, headaches, and confusion. **A.** CT scan upon admission showed a giant calcified left carotid aneurysm with surrounding left frontal lobe edema and mass effect. **B.** Left ICA angiogram, lateral view, demonstrates the patent lumen of the giant aneurysm. **C.** Left ICA angiogram. The vessel was occluded with three balloons and coils; the top balloon is in the aneurysm neck (arrow). **D.** Plain film of neck showing balloons and coils. **E.** CT scan showing top balloons in aneurysm neck. There is significant perianeurysmal left frontal lobe edema. Note the left occipital ventricular drain to help control intracranial pressure. **F.** CT scan 2 weeks after treatment shows that the edema is much reduced. **G.** Right ICA angiogram 3 weeks after treatment shows excellent cross filling to the left hemisphere.

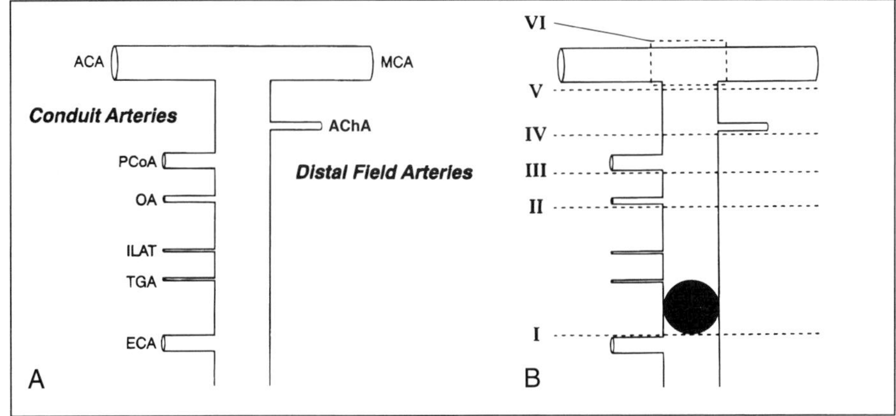

Figure 18.35. A. The vessels around an aneurysm can be grouped into *distal field vessels* and *conduit vessels*. The conduit vessels can have nutrient flow in either direction under nonpathologic conditions and can usually be counted on for collateral circulation. The distal field vessels are vessels that under normal conditions never have blood flowing in a retrograde fashion, and when this occurs it will almost always lead to ischemia. (ACA, anterior cerebral artery; MCA, middle cerebral artery; AChA, anterior choroidal artery; PCoA, posterior communicating artery; OA, ophthalmic artery; ILAT, inferior lateral trunk; TGA, trigeminal artery; ECA, external carotid artery.) **B.** The internal carotid can be schematized. Occlusion at I is highly effective for treating aneurysms below II, less effective for aneurysms above II, and ineffective for aneurysms above III. Similarly, occlusion at II is highly effective for treating aneurysms below III, less effective for aneurysms above IV, and ineffective for aneurysms at or above V.

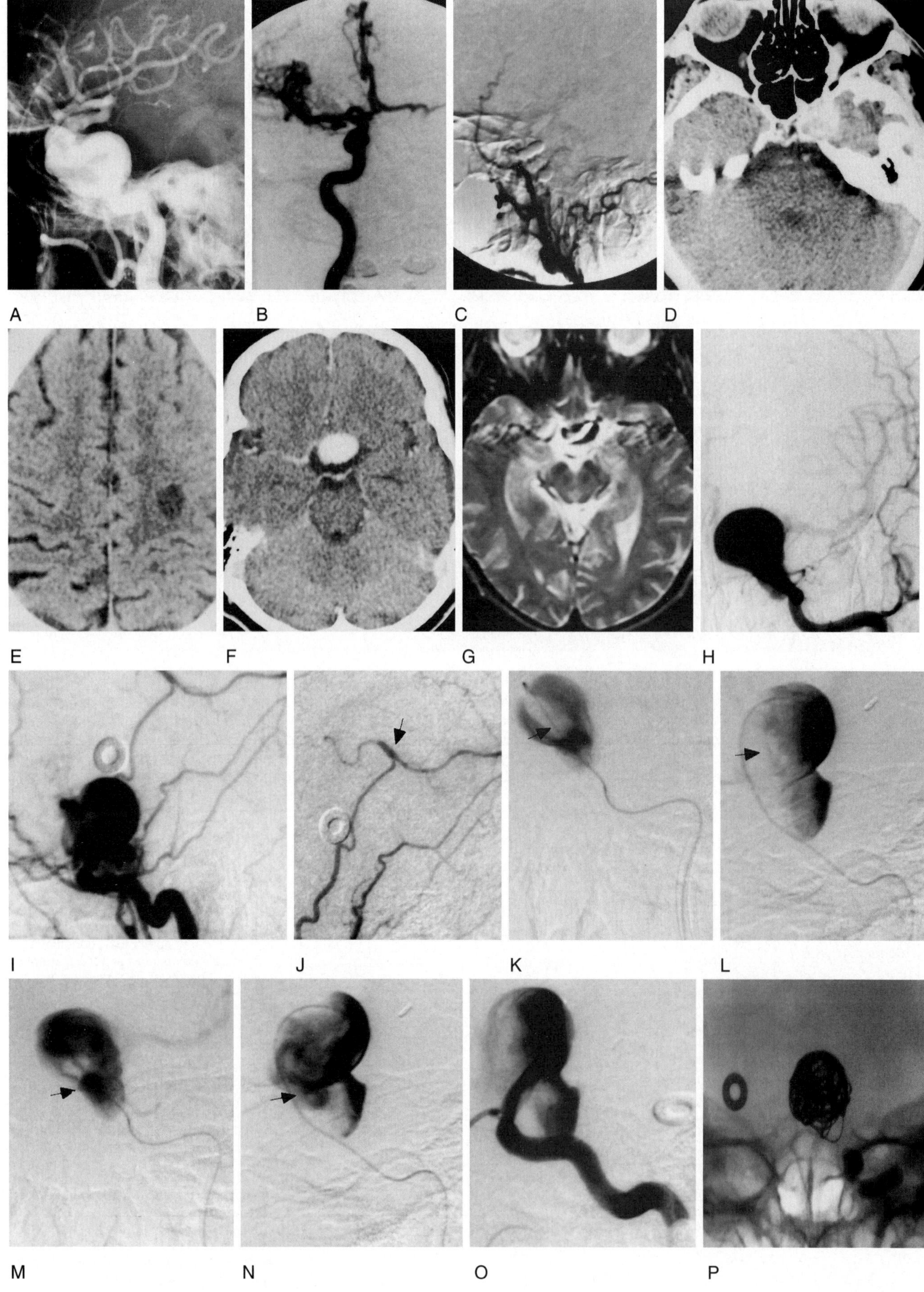
A
B
C
D
E
F
G
H
I
J
K
L
M
N
O
P

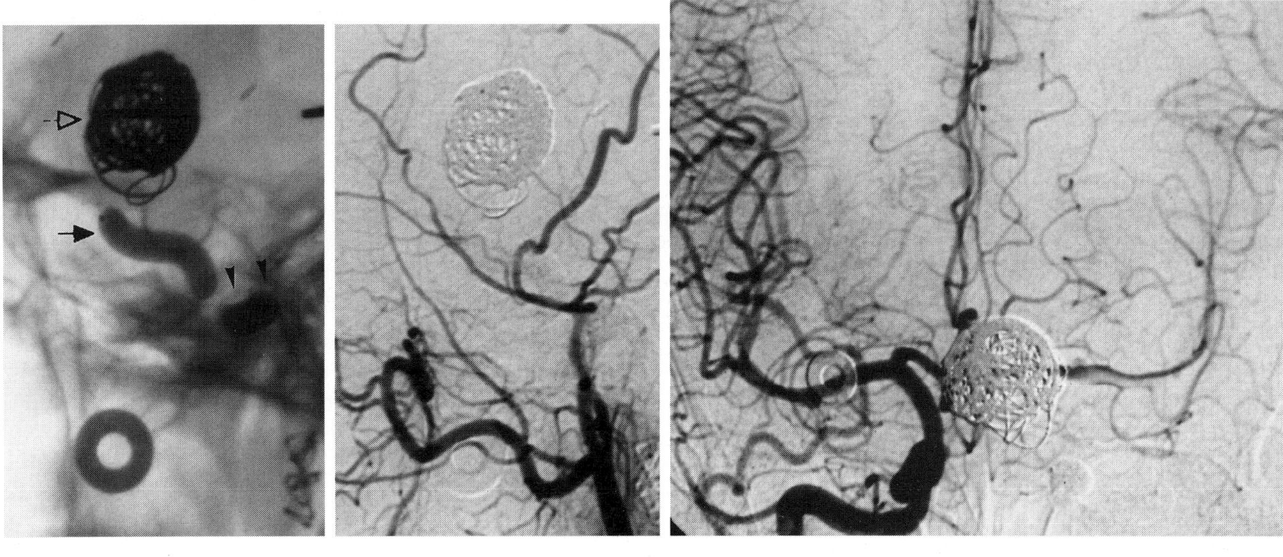

Figure 18.36. **A** to **E**. Giant left cavernous ICA aneurysm in a 67-year-old female with left sixth-nerve palsy and headaches. **A.** Left ICA angiogram shows a giant aneurysm of the left cavernous ICA. **B.** Left carotid artery test occlusion with right ICA angiogram shows good cross filling. The systolic blood pressure lowered to 90 mm Hg without symptoms. **C.** Aneurysm injection after left ICA balloon occlusion. **D** and **E.** CT scans 10 days after treatment. **D.** Scan showing intra-aneurysmal thrombosis. **E.** A higher cut demonstrates a small infarct in the left frontal lobe. The patient had transient Gertsmann syndrome attributed to loss of blood from groin hematoma. **F** to **S.** A second patient presented a giant supraclinoid carotid aneurysm treated with aneurysm coil filling followed by carotid occlusion. This patient was a 50-year-old female who had headaches and progressive loss of vision in the left eye. CECT scan (**F**) and MRI scan (**G**) show a giant carotid aneurysm that occupies most of the suprasellar cistern. **H** and **I.** Left carotid angiogram shows a giant aneurysm pointing superiorly and to the midline. The lateral view shows a patent EC-IC bypass, which was performed after the patient failed to tolerate test occlusion of the left carotid artery. **J.** Selective left external carotid artery injection shows the patent STA-MCA (angular branch) bypass (arrow). **K** and **L.** Superselective exploration of the aneurysm with a microcatheter (early view) shows the inflow neck (arrow). **M** and **N.** Superselective exploration of the aneurysm with a microcatheter (late view) shows the outflow neck (arrow). **O.** Balloon catheter in the petrous carotid artery to obtain flow arrest prior to coil packing of the aneurysm so as to avoid distal embolic migration from the aneurysm. **P** and **Q.** Plain films, anteroposterior and lateral views, showing the mesh of coils within the aneurysm (large arrow), the top balloon in the internal carotid artery across the ophthalmic artery to prevent aneurysm rupture (small arrow), and a second balloon immediately behind it (arrowheads). **R.** Control angiogram of the left common carotid artery showing IC bypass and no residual aneurysm. **S.** Control angiogram of the right internal carotid artery showing excellent cross filling through the anterior communicating artery with no aneurysm filling.

have a 1.7 percent complication rate but significant risk, including dissection and occlusion (23–25).

Obliterating Potential Collateral Flow Proximal ligation of the parent vessel can be carried out surgically or by endovascular means. To be most effective, occlusion should be *above the last conduit vessel and below the aneurysm.* Occlusion is generally well tolerated if the conduit vessels distal to the aneurysm are hemodynamically adequate for the distal fields. The stump may act as a source of emboli during the clotting process because it will fill up with clot up to the level of the next major collateral. Minor collaterals such as the inferolateral trunk are not adequate to keep the aneurysm open but may allow enough flow to wash out catastrophic clot distally and therefore should be occluded.

The vessels around an aneurysm can be grouped as distal field vessels and conduit vessels (Fig. 18.35). Aneurysms that cross the conduit vessel input can be most challenging and should be considered as requiring "trapping." Ophthalmic artery occlusion may be mandatory in cases of carotid-cavernous aneurysms when a low inserted ophthalmic artery is seen to supply the aneurysmal sac from external carotid injection during temporary occlusion of the internal carotid artery. The ophthalmic artery territory is immediately taken over by abundant external carotid artery collaterals, and vision is not at risk.

Burdens of Therapy Vessel occlusion diminishes a patient's cerebral vascular reserve, which is often balanced with the cardiovascular reserve. In patients who may soon have a decrease in either, vessel occlusion is contraindicated. This includes patients who may soon develop vasospasm or who have had recent myocardial infarction or intermittent congestive heart failure, chronic obstructive pulmonary disease (COPD), pneumonia, sepsis, or uncontrolled bleeding (Fig. 18.36).

The long-term effects of parent vessel occlusion are not known but can be relatively well tolerated in a majority of patients. Parent vessel occlusion must carry an increase risk of ischemia. Vessel occlusion without revascularization may be considered primarily in the age group between 60 and 75. In younger patients, bypass surgery prior to vessel occlusion is almost always indicated.

Tactics

Operative Methods and Materials Safe occlusion of the parent vessel has been done with a variety of agents (25). The author prefers a detachable balloon. The target occlusion site is determined, and all materials that will be used are prepared and tolerances checked. A balloon 20 to 30 percent larger than the target vessel is chosen. The author prefers to use a second nondetachable "shepherd balloon" via the second triaxial catheter system through the other groin. The nondetachable catheter is navigated to the lower edge of the target site.

Postocclusion Medical Care After occlusion, the patient is maintained in optimal hemodynamic conditions to avoid stressing an impaired cerebral vascular reserve. Bed rest, adequate hydration, high normal blood pressure, a hematocrit over 33, adequate oxygenation, and anticoagulation are maintained and monitored. Vigorous intensive care management is needed in those patients with either borderline cerebral or cardiovascular reserve. This includes close neurologic and cardiac monitoring. The postocclusion condition of these patients is similar to that of patients with SAH and vasospasm, and a similar patient management algorithm is applicable (Table 18.41). In postocclusion patients without neurologic deficit, the central venous pressure is kept at 8 to 10 cmH_2O, the pulmonary wedge pressure at 12 to 14 mm Hg, the cardiac index high, and the blood pressure normal. In postocclusion patients who are developing neurologic deficit, with a negative CT scan (blood or large infarction), there should be an increase in the blood pressure and pulmonary wedge pressure until the deficit is reversed or the cardiac index is high (26).

Serial brain SPECT scans are quite helpful in monitoring changes in cerebral vascular reserve. Return of normal cerebral vascular reserve can be documented with a normal acetazolamide (Diamox) challenge SPECT scan. The author intensively monitors and keeps patients at bed rest until SPECT is normal. Patients are anticoagulated and may not return to work or normal activity until the Diamox SPECT is normal. Anticoagulation is indicated until at least 2 months have passed and the Diamox SPECT documents no tissue with diminished cerebral vascular reserve.

After endovascular therapy, continuous short-term (2- to 4-month) anticoagulation is possible to reduce the risks of emboli and thrombosis. Patients to be anticoagulated for some period of time need guaiac stools, preoperatively; procedure a low, single stick, single wall arterial puncture, and the prothrombin time kept in the range of 13 to 15 sec to avoid catastrophic bleeding.

Results

Endovascular balloon occlusion of the internal carotid artery (ICA) as a treatment for large and giant aneurysms of the cervical, petrous, and cavernous portions is extremely effective (26–32). Parent vessel occlusion is highly effective in treating mass effect involving peridural structures and moderately effective if the mass effect is directly on the brain parenchyma (32,33) or the anterior visual pathway (34). Aneurysms involving the posterior communicating artery, the ophthalmic artery, and the ICA bifurcation can be treated, providing takedown of the collateral artery in most cases (Fig. 18.36).

In one study, results in patients who had embolization for aneurysms and symptoms related to mass effect could be classified into one of three groups: resolved (50 percent), improved (42 percent), and unchanged (7.7 percent). Patients with less wall calcification, shorter symptom duration, and total aneurysm occlusion tended to improve. Endosaccular embolization therapy can improve or alleviate presenting neurologic signs unrelated to hemorrhage or distal embolization in the majority of cases (33–37).

Eighty-seven patients with intracavernous aneurysms presenting with mass effect (79.3 percent), carotid-cavernous sinus fistula (9.2 percent), pseudoaneurysm (8.0 percent), or hemorrhage (3.4 percent) were treated with detachable silicone balloons filled with a permanent solidifying agent (2-hydroxyethyl methacrylate). Therapeutic occlusion of the ICA across or just proximal to the aneurysm neck (78.2 percent) or with preservation of the parent artery (22 percent) effected complete thrombosis, with partial or total alleviation of symptoms in all patients with therapeutic occlusion of the parent vessel. Patients with preservation of the parent artery had total exclusion (63 percent) and subtotal occlusion (37 percent), with clinical improvement in all cases. Complications included transient cerebral ischemia (8 percent) and strokes (5 percent). There were no deaths.

Balloon embolization for carotid-cavernous aneurysms showed success in 92 percent of patients presenting with progressive pain, ophthalmoplegia, or visual loss in which functional angiography under systemic heparinization using double-lumen balloon catheters to test tolerance to carotid occlusion was carried out. Twelve percent had unplanned deflation of the balloon necessitating reembolization, without serious permanent neurologic complications. All patients had complete resolution of pain, and 80 percent had improvement in the extraocular eye muscle and lid function. Balloon trapping of the carotid-cavernous artery, rather than placing the balloon directly into the aneurysm, was thought to result in involution of the aneurysm and decompression of the involved cranial nerves (35).

Long-term (17 to 112 months) follow-up study of inaccessible giant aneurysms ($n = 8$) of the internal carotid artery treated with ICA occlusion ($n = 3$) showed a gradual decrease of the size of the aneurysms on CT scan and improvement of signs in three out of three patients, whereas repeated Matas maneuver was effective in only one out of five patients (36).

In a report of giant posterior cerebral artery aneurysms ($n = 3$), clinically manifesting as cerebral ischemia, mass effect, and subarachnoid hemorrhage, all aneurysms were partially thrombosed, originated at the P2 segment, and possessed broad necks. Surgical neck clipping was difficult, but proximal occlusion of the parent artery was feasible. Aneurysm occlusion sparing the parent artery was attempted in all cases, but failed because the detachable balloon did not successfully block the aneurysmal neck. All patients tolerated test occlusion at the P2 segment, so the parent artery was occluded proximally with detachable balloons, leaving the important perforating arteries unaffected. Two transient ischemic attacks were associated with the procedure. When surgical treatment is unusually difficult, and proximal ligation or trapping is feasible, embolization with detachable balloons is an acceptable substitute (37).

Posterior inferior cerebellar artery aneurysms can be successfully treated by endovascular occlusion of the vertebral artery at the C1 level (Hunterian ligation).

Nonberry aneurysms can often be effectively treated with parent vessel occlusion. Intranidal aneurysms associated with AVMs are effectively treated with acrylate embolization (38). Parent vessel occlusion is effective in treating mycotic aneurysms (39), and acute traumatic pseudoaneurysms must be approached with extreme caution (40). Parent vessel occlusion is usually needed because direct surgical or endovascular repair is difficult. Hemorrhage, emboli, and thrombosis may complicate the disease course. Traumatic dissections require a high index of clinical suspicion (41). Presenting signs and symptoms for carotid dissections include Horner syndrome, dysphasia, hemiparesis, obtundation, and monoparesis. Patients detected early with mild neurologic deficits fare well with aggressive anticoagulant therapy treatment, whereas those with profound neurologic deficits and delayed diagnoses had poor outcomes (19). Chronic traumatic aneurysms, with their thicker wall and neoendothelial-lined pouch, can be approached with the expectation of good long-term results using either surgical or endovascular methods (42).

In summary, test occlusion is an essential part of management. Dramatic test occlusion failure, young patients, or aneurysms on the collateral vessels are situations that command preocclusion bypass surgery. Endovascular treatment is safe and effective if one avoids (a) aneurysm rupture during balloon inflation, (b) balloon rupture with distal migration of silicone, and (c) occlusion in the post-SAH vasospasm-prone period. In the postocclusion period, avoidance of hypotension and thromboembolic complications is essential. Neurologic intensive care is crucial. Mycotic aneurysms and acute traumatic aneurysms carry a high mortality.

PARENT VESSEL SPARING

Strategy

Vessel-sparing endovascular operations are physiologically gentler but also more demanding than nonvessel-sparing operations. Because they effectively treat acute aneurysms without decreasing cerebral vascular reserve, they are the preferred method in most patients (Fig. 18.37). The preferred method at this time is coil packing.

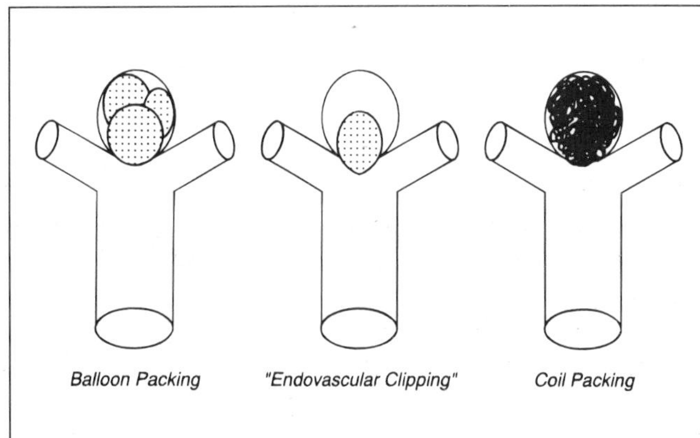

Figure 18.37. Endovascular aneurysm obliteration.

Endovascular navigation into an aneurysm was first demonstrated by Luessenhop in the late 1960s (43,44). Hilal in the late 1960s showed that endovascular methods could be used to produce thrombosis of an aneurysm (45,46). Serbinenko in the early 1970s showed that detachable balloons could be used effectively (47). Shcheglov and the Kiev group have effectively treated a large number of patients in the nonacute stage with "surgically respectable aneurysms" with detachable balloons (48). Hieshima and his group at San Francisco have effectively treated a large series of "nonsurgical" aneurysms using detachable balloons. Hilal in the late 1980s demonstrated that coils could be used to obliterate aneurysms.

A very important development has been the Guglielmi detachable coils. Guglielmi and the UCLA group have demonstrated that specially designed electrolytically detachable coils can be a highly effective way to treat aneurysms in patients in whom surgery is not an attractive option (49). Importantly, their results have been able to be shared by others using the same protocol. The complication rate appears relatively low and the effectiveness relatively high. This method is considered in any patients in whom excellent surgical results might be difficult to obtain. Methods are undergoing rapid development, and clinical trials are now under way to help assess the long-term results.

Tactics

Operative Methods and Materials Obliteration of the aneurysm can be done with coils, balloons, or even adhesives. Care must be taken to navigate gently. All force must be avoided. Any sign of headache usually signals stretching of the vessels and is to be avoided. Catheter manipulation, if associated with nausea, vomiting, or neurologic change, usually represents vessel damage (50). The dome of the

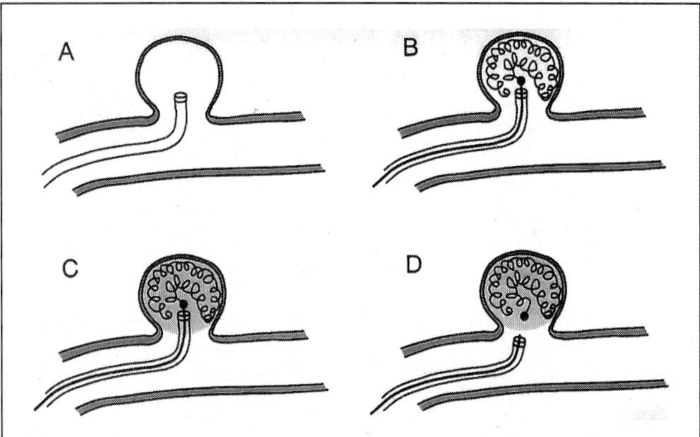

Figure 18.38. Endovascular technique for aneurysm treatment with detachable coils. **A.** The top of a microcatheter is positioned within the aneurysm. **B.** The platinum coil is deposited into the aneurysm through the microcatheter. The black dot represents the solder between the platinum coil and the stainless steel delivery wire. **C.** After applying a positive direct electric current to the proximal end of the delivery wire (not shown), the negatively charged blood elements become attracted to the positively charged platinum, thus eliciting thrombus formation. **D.** After 4 to 12 minutes, the current has also dissolved by electrolysis the uninsulated stainless steel proximal to the solder. The platinum coil is therefore detached in the aneurysm. (Reprinted with permission from: Guglielmi G, Endovascular treatment of intracranial aneurysms, in Neuroimaging Clinics of North America, F. Vinuela, J. Dion, and G. Duckwiler, Editors. 1992, W. B. Saunders Company: Philadelphia. p. 269–278.)

aneurysm can be packed, or the neck of the aneurysm can be occluded (Table 18.42) (Fig. 18.38).

The standard of care for the endovascular treatment of aneurysms today is vessel sparing with GDC coils. A microcatheter is navigated into the aneurysm, and the coil is navigated into the vessel (Figs. 18.38 and 18.39). (See also Figs. 18.7 to 18.9.)

Table 18.42.
GDC Technique for Aneurysms

Preoperative
1. Evaluate goal of embolization and timing of treatment.
2. Calcium channel blockers 12 h prior, anxiolytics on call.
3. Anticonvulsant levels, CBC, coagulation profiles.

Operative
1. Monitoring, ECG, O_2 saturation, baseline neurologic exam, BP.
2. Consider general anesthesia (see section on anesthetics).
3. Foley catheter, intravenous access (3a) consider CVP* or PA† line.
4. 7.5F sheath in femoral artery.
5. Heparinization (ACT 2.5 × normal).
6. 7F guiding catheter in parent vessel in neck, can also use a Tracker 38 to navigate intracranially.
7. Biplane angiogram with sizing markers anteroposterior and right/left.
8. Road map.
9. Navigate microcatheter with double marker into aneurysm dome.
10. Gentle superselective angiogram through microcatheter.
11. Pick coil size so as to fill the aneurysm.
12. Gently advance coils into aneurysm.
13. Stop when wire marker is at catheter marker.
14. Repeat angiogram.
15. Detach coil electrolytically by connecting the proximal wire to the positive pole and the negative wire to the skin electrode.
16. Repeat steps 12–15 until aneurysm is fully packed. A range of coils can be needed to pack the aneurysm fully.

Postoperative
1. Sheath and heparinization until next A.M., intensive care unit until next P.M.
2. Consider calcium channel blockers and beta blockers.

* CVP = central venous pressure
† PA = pulmonary artery pressure

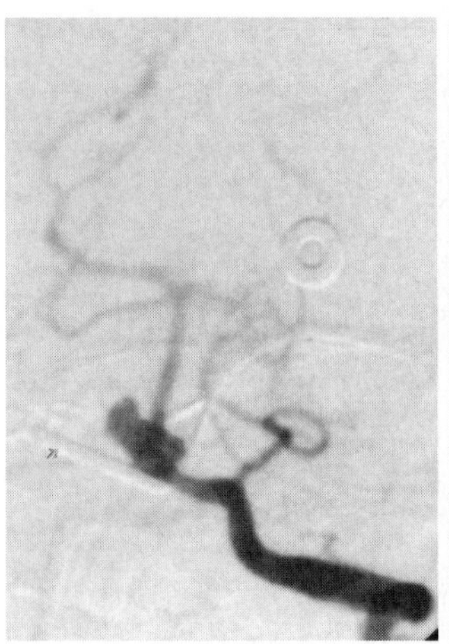
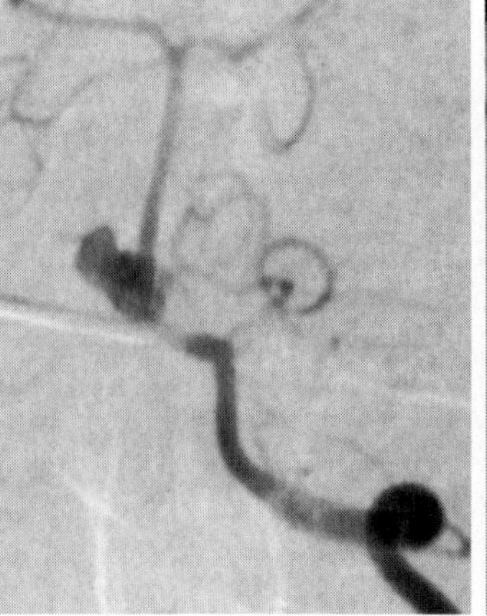
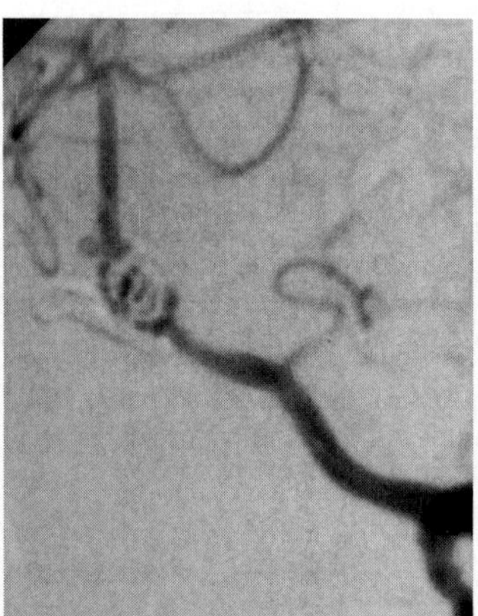
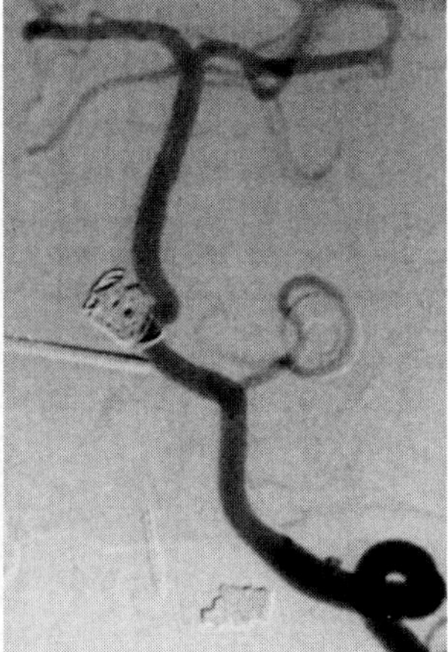

A B C D

Figure 18.39. GDC coil embolization of vertebrobasilar junction aneurysm. **A.** Left vertebral angiogram shows the left vertebrobasilar junction aneurysm. A surgical clip (arrow) is seen across the right vertebrobasilar junction. **B.** Left vertebral angiogram, slightly oblique view, shows the aneurysm. **C.** Superselective catheterization of the aneurysm with a microcatheter during intraaneurysmal GDC coil delivery. **D.** Control angiogram at 2 months shows no residual aneurysm.

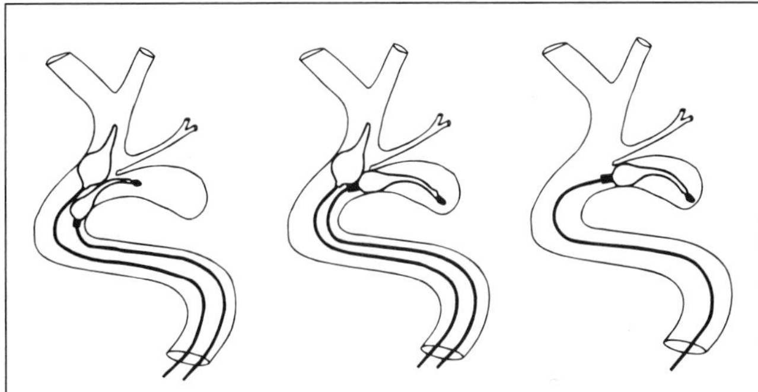

Figure 18.40. The Shcheglov balloon is a very soft balloon. The balloon has a small heavy tip. The balloon is trained by repeatedly inflating the balloon while holding part of it giving the balloon a tendency to turn and bend as it is inflated. The proper balloon is picked so that it can be placed across the neck and blown up, with the tip gently curved in the aneurysm sac abutting the distal wall. Two balloon catheters are introduced via the carotid artery. The first balloon is a non-detachable,"shepherd balloon" and is used to explore the aneurysm, guide the working detachable balloon into the aneurysm, brace the detachable balloon during deflation, and occlude the parent vessel if there is inadvertent rupture during manipulation. After the balloon is navigated into the aneurysm, a trial obliteration with contrast in the aneurysm is performed. The contrast is removed and replaced with silicone. The contrast in the catheter cannot be removed and remains in the balloon with the radiolucent bouyant silicone acting as a plug across the neck. Slight tension on the balloon can be placed to help contour the balloon as the silicone dries. The shepherd balloon may also be placed proximal to the aneurysm to help the detachable balloon pass into the aneurysm.

Shcheglov balloons and other balloons are highly effective in some operators' hands (Fig. 18.40). Initial balloon obliteration of the aneurysm is followed by scarring, particularly with the latex balloons (Figs. 18.41 and 18.42).

The Shcheglov balloon is a very soft latex balloon with a small, heavy tip. The balloon is trained by repeatedly inflating it while holding part of it, thus giving it a tendency to turn and bend as it is inflated. The proper balloon is picked so that the balloon can be placed across the neck and blown up with the tip gently curved in the aneurysm sac abutting the distal wall. Two balloon catheters are introduced via a carotid artery. The first balloon is a nondetachable "shepherd balloon" and is used to explore the aneurysm, guide the working detachable balloon into the aneurysm, brace the detachable balloon during deflation, and occlude the parent vessel if there is inadvertent rupture during manipulation. After the balloon is navigated into the aneurysm, a trial obliteration with contrast can be carried out (51).

The contrast is removed and replaced with silicone. The contrast in the catheter cannot be removed and remains in the balloon with the radiolucent buoyant silicone acting as a plug across the neck. Slight tension on the balloon can be placed to help contour the balloon as the silicone dries. The shepherd balloon may also be placed proximal to the aneurysm to help the detachable balloon pass it into the aneurysm (Fig. 18.40). The balloon sets up a significant amount of scarring (Fig. 18.41).

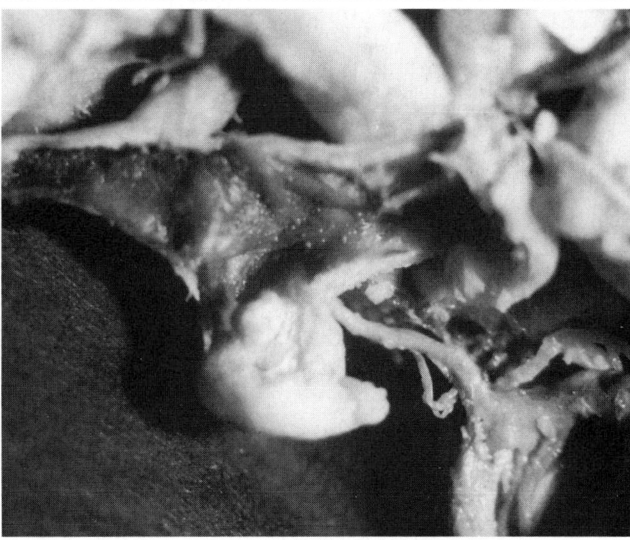

Figure 18.41. Autopsy photograph of a middle cerebral artery aneurysm of a patient who died from unrelated causes. The aneurysm that had been successfully treated by Dr. Shcheglov is replaced with scar.

A number of materials have been used to occlude aneurysms and spare parent vessels. They include (a) latex and silicone balloons, (b) platinum and steel coils, (c) stents, (d) polymers (53–55), and (e) thrombin (52). It should be noted that polymers are also used to fill the balloons so that over time the balloon does not deflate (Fig. 18.43).

Postoperative Management Patients who have undergone endovascular occlusion of aneurysms are treated by the author's service with close monitoring, low normal blood pressure, and a short course of mild anticoagulants. Embolic complications have happened in spite of this treatment, usually related to unmet goals regarding management. Untreated aneurysms may well rebleed.

Managing Complications Complications during treatment need to be handled immediately. Parent vessel occlusion, thrombolysis, rupture site obliteration, and surgical correction are all desperate options that must be instituted swiftly and expertly to be of benefit (52,56).

Perioperative Management Although endovascular methods are generally considered to have significantly less associated trauma than direct surgical approaches, there is still significant physiologic disruption that must be considered in very ill patients (Table 18.43).

Results

The results from vessel-sparing procedures can be excellent (Table 18.44). The results are complex and need to be stratified as to (a) time since bleeding, that is, cold versus hot and grade, (b) size, and (c) location. Comparison of treatment options must be made within each class. Endovascular techniques have until the very recent past been offered only

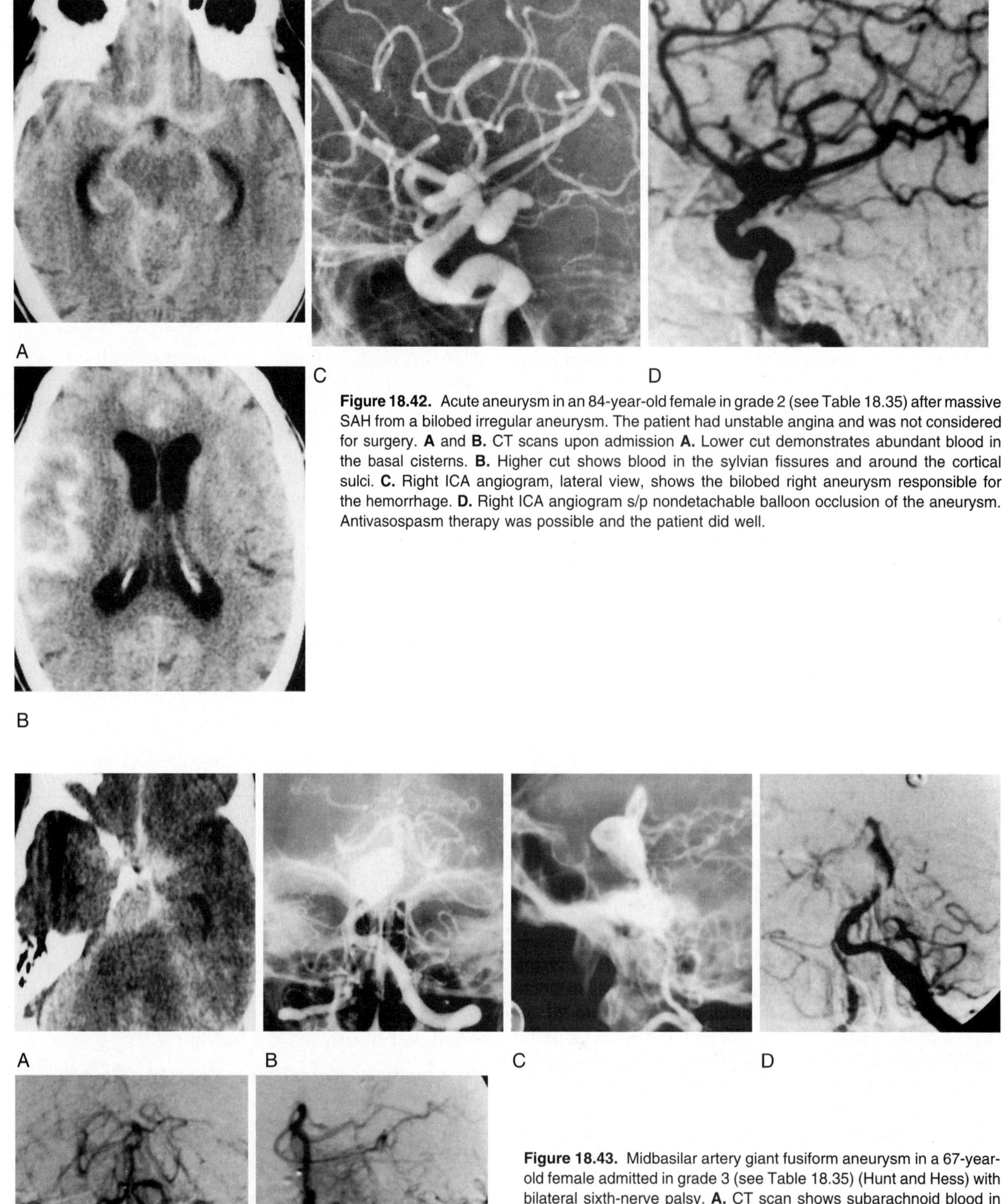

Figure 18.42. Acute aneurysm in an 84-year-old female in grade 2 (see Table 18.35) after massive SAH from a bilobed irregular aneurysm. The patient had unstable angina and was not considered for surgery. **A** and **B.** CT scans upon admission **A.** Lower cut demonstrates abundant blood in the basal cisterns. **B.** Higher cut shows blood in the sylvian fissures and around the cortical sulci. **C.** Right ICA angiogram, lateral view, shows the bilobed right aneurysm responsible for the hemorrhage. **D.** Right ICA angiogram s/p nondetachable balloon occlusion of the aneurysm. Antivasospasm therapy was possible and the patient did well.

Figure 18.43. Midbasilar artery giant fusiform aneurysm in a 67-year-old female admitted in grade 3 (see Table 18.35) (Hunt and Hess) with bilateral sixth-nerve palsy. **A.** CT scan shows subarachnoid blood in the suprasellar, interhemispheric, and interpeduncular cisterns. Prepontine mass effect is evident. **B** and **C.** Left vertebral artery angiogram shows a giant midbasilar fusiform aneurysm. **D.** Left vertebral artery angiogram during inflation of nondetachable balloon in the basilar artery **E** and **F.** Left vertebral artery posttreatment angiogram shows successful exclusion with preservation of the basilar artery. Anticoagulation and intensive care were crucial in obtaining this result. The patient fully recovered.

Table 18.43.
Perioperative Considerations for Aneurysms

Agent/Event	Magnitude	Comments
Blood loss	40–1500 ml	Large-bore arterial catheters, manipulation through O-rings, frequent blood sampling, and hematoma with heparinization all make large blood losses possible.
Fluid shifts	500–2500 ml	Three to five pressurized arterial and venous catheter lines make inadvertent fluid delivery possible. The osmotic diuretic effect of contrast can cause dehydration.
Contrast load	100–600 ml	Repeated injections required for safe navigation.
Vessel trauma	5–8F, dissections and occlusions	Stiff, straight, large-bore catheters in relatively small, curved, soft vessels account for the microscopic and macroscopic vessel disruption that can be seen and must always be presumed to be present.
Anesthesia	MAC*, GA†, GA† with wake-up	Difficulty in close visual monitoring of patient, cumbersomeness of x-ray equipment, distance of angiosuite from remaining ORs, shifts in BP and LOC‡ required by the procedure, and lack of understanding by collateral staff as to the nature and difficulty of the task may add to the possible trauma of anesthesia.
Pain	Mild discomfort to moderately severe pain	Vascular access, back discomfort, anxiety and claustrophobia, cold, and being restrained are all associated with pain and discomfort.
Time	1–8 h	

* MAC = monitored anesthesia care
† GA = general anesthesia
‡ LOC = level of consciousness

to that class of patients for whom surgical management is unfavorable.

ADJUVANT OR TEAM TREATMENT

Strategy and Results

Adjuvant endovascular treatment for aneurysms includes a variety of methods that have been developing as the endovascular and surgical teams work more closely in patient selection and treatment. A great variety of methods could be classified under this "team treatment." In difficult management cases, some type of adjuvant treatment can often be helpful:

1. Intraoperative angiogram
2. Aneurysmography
3. Temporary intraoperative occlusion
4. Test occlusion
5. Temporary endovascular trapping
6. Superficial-temporal artery-middle cerebral artery bypass → endovascular occlusion
7. Transaneurysm embolization
8. Acute endovascular aneurysm dome obliteration with delayed surgical aneurysm neck clipping
9. Back-up for a failed alternative treatment
10. Angioplasty for vasospasm prior to treatment

These different twists can be quite helpful in technically challenging large and giant aneurysms in difficult locations.

An intraoperative angiogram is useful to confirm clip placement in difficult aneurysms such as periclinoid or high basilar tip aneurysms. It is not without risk, and there is a significant learning curve (Table 18.45) (57–58).

Aneurysmography, or an angiogram within the dome of the aneurysm, is useful and, although routinely done before coil treatment, can be useful in large aneurysms that may

Table 18.44.
Results of Aneurysm Vessel Sparing

Method	Human/ animal	Parent vessel sparing	Delayed regrowth	M/M*	*N*	In use	Comments
Acrylate/polymer injection	H/A	80%	?	High	<10	–	
Electrolytic thrombosis	H	High	High	?	1	–	
Laser	A	90%	Low	?	<20	–	Very encouraging, no human trials
Serbinenko balloon	H	?	?	High	<20	–	
Shcheglov balloon	H	93%	?15%	5%	<20	+/–	
Rütenacht latex balloon	H/A	>90%	>10%			+/–	
Debrun latex balloon	H	?		High		–	
Nondetachable balloons	H	>99%	>10%	Moderate	<20	–	
ITC silicone balloon	H/A		?	5%		–	
Hilal coil	H/A		?	Moderate		+/–	
GDC coil	H/A		>15%	Low		+ + + +	
MDC coils	H/A					+	
Stents	A	High	?	?	?	–	

* M/M = morbidity and mortality

Table 18.45.
Adjuvant Tactics for Aneurysms: Intraoperative Angiography and/or Embolization

	Considerations	Comments
Staff	Neurointerventional staff and team, operating surgeon and team, attending anesthesiologist and team.	Communication is essential.
Equipment	Radiolucent OR table, radiolucent head holder, portable angio unit with DSA*, radiolucent anesthetic tubes, leads, and support.	The equipment must all be compatible and tested. Possible problems must be understood by everyone involved in the case.
Method	Sheath, heparinization, triaxial system to conduit vessel target, balloon placement, confirmation with repeated deflations and inflations under fluoroscopy, setup for clipping of aneurysm, balloon inflation, aneurysm clipping, balloon deflation and hemostasis, control angiogram of neck.	
Special considerations	Patients undergoing aneurysm surgery tend to be relatively hypercoagulable, dehydrated, and hypotensive in comparison to patients undergoing routine endovascular procedures.	These conditions can and often do lead to spasm and possible dissection. Heparinization after aneurysm dissection with hemostasis and sheath placement is essential.

* DSA = digital subtraction angiogram

have perforators incorporated into the dome (15). The aneurysm neck can occasionally be seen to better advantage by contrast injection distal to temporary balloon occlusion, or by injecting collateral with proximal temporary occlusion (59).

Temporary intraoperative occlusion or trapping performed during surgical approaches to the aneurysm may be indicated in those situations where proximal control of the parent vessel is difficult or ineffective, such as carotico-ophthalmic (31,34) or low-lying basilar tip aneurysms (60). Temporary occlusion of the proximal parent vessel with a microballoon performed under full heparinization after the operative dissection, but before clip placement, has been useful. This can be done instead of cardiac arrest or proximal carotid cutdown. Decompression of the aneurysm by aspiration may also be helpful.

Test occlusion is an essential part of treatment and has been discussed in the preceding section. Superficial temporal artery–middle cerebral artery bypass followed by endovascular occlusion is the standard of care for giant symptomatic cavernous aneurysms. It is also highly effective for giant unresectable paraclinoid aneurysms (see Fig. 18.34).

Transaneurysm embolization is best reserved for thick-walled extradural aneurysms. An entirely different set of materials and methods needs to be developed to allow this to be done with any degree of safety on a routine basis.

Acute endovacular aneurysm dome obliteration with delayed surgical aneurysm neck clipping is sometimes helpful (61). Clipping is not always possible after partial treatment by coils and can in some instances be treacherous. Partial coil treatment may be a source for emboli, and partial coil treatment may make surgery dangerous.

Occasionally, failed endovascular therapy can be saved by direct surgery, and vice versa (61–63). In traumatic disruptions and mycotic aneurysms, direct surgical care and endovascular therapy have been combined.

Occasionally, angioplasty for vasospasm must be done that vasospasm protects from rebleeding may not be true, but it is probably advisable to correct both if doing either endovascularly (64,65).

Tactics

Logistically challenging, adjuvant therapy often requires the simultaneous involvement of both operative and endovascular teams and excellent communication. These challenges are not a significant impediment if dealt with individually with all involved (Table 18.45).

Future Trends

Both endovascular and direct surgical results will improve over time. This will increase the indications for treatment. Poor-grade patients after a SAH continue to have a dismal outlook in spite of increasing sophistication of treatment. Giant clot-filled aneurysms with mass effect and fusiform aneurysms also are somewhat recalcitrant to treatment. Smaller asymptomatic aneurysms also present a challenge, since benefit to the patient can only be offered by highly effective and highly safe treatment. Interestingly, as the diagnostic tests increase in sensitivity and the therapeutic intervention decreases in burden, screening for aneurysms may become of value to the patient. In a recent study, 400 volunteers underwent angiography, and 20 of the 26 showing an aneurysm underwent surgery for elective clipping of their aneurysm without significant morbidity or mortality (1). In an environment that is increasingly outcome-driven and transparent, meeting these challenges will be like "learning to play the violin in public."

REFERENCES

1. Nakagawa T, Hashi K: The incidence and treatment of asymptomatic, unruptured cerebral aneurysms. J Neurosurg 1994;80:217–223.
2. Perata HJ, Tomsick TA, Tew J Jr: Feeding artery pedicle aneurysms: Association with parenchymal hemorrhage and arteriovenous malformation in the brain. J Neurosurg 1994;80:631–634.

3. Lasjaunias P, Piske R, TerBrugge K, Willinsky R: Cerebral arteriovenous malformations (C. AVM) and associated arterial aneurysms (AA): Analysis of 101 C. AVM cases, with 37 AA in 23 patients (review). Acta Neurochir 1988;91:29–36.
4. Ohno K, Tone O, Inaba Y, Terasaki T: Coexistent congenital arteriovenous malformation and aneurysms. (author's transl). No Shinkei Geka 1981;9:1187–1191.
5. Seigle JM, Caputy AJ, Manz HJ, Wheeler C, Fox JL: Multiple oncotic intracranial aneurysms and cardiac metastasis from choriocarcinoma: Case report and review of the literature. Neurosurgery 1987;20:39–42.
6. Ho KL: Neoplastic aneurysm and intracranial hemorrhage. Cancer 1982;50:2935–2940.
7. Nayeem SA, Tada Y, Takagi A, Sato O, Miyata T, Idezuki Y: Carotid artery pseudoaneurysm following internal jugular vein cannulation. J Cardiovasc Surg 1990;31:182–183.
8. Varsos V, Heros RC, DeBrun G, Zervas NT: Construction of experimental "giant" aneurysms. Surg Neurol 1984;22:17–20.
9. Nishikawa M, Smith RD, Yonekawa Y: Experimental intracranial aneurysms. Surg Neurol 1977;7:241–244.
10. Kerber CW, Cromwell LD, Zanetti PH: Experimental carotid aneurysms: Part 2. Endovascular treatment with cyanoacrylate. Neurosurgery 1985;16:13–17.
11. O'Reilly GV, Forrest MD, Schoene WC, Clarke RH: Laser-induced thermal occlusion of berry aneurysms: Initial experimental results. Radiology 1989;171:471–474.
12. Kerber CW, Heilman CB: Flow in experimental berry aneurysms: Method and model. AJNR 1983;4:374–377.
13. Machida T, Hayashi N, Sasaki Y, et al: Posterior cranial fossa dural arteriovenous malformation with a varix mimicking a thrombosed aneurysm: Case report. Neuroradiology 1993;35:210–211.
14. Manacas R, Cerqueira L: Angiography in the diagnosis of cerebrovascular pathology: Current indications and controversies (review). Acta Med Port 1993;6:411–420.
15. Kurata A, Miyasaka Y, Yada K, Kan S: Aneurysmography for visualizing large aneurysms. Neurosurgery 1994;34:745–747.
16. Nagata I, Kikuchi H, Karasawa J, Mitsugi T, Naruo Y, Takamiya M: Digital subtraction angiography of the cerebral vessels by intraarterial injection. No Shinkei Geka 1984;12:1273–1278.
17. Matsumura H, Iwai F, Ichikizaki K: Ischemic myocardial disorder in acute phase subarachnoid hemorrhage: Clinical study of 52 patients. No Shinkei Geka 1991;19:349–357.
18. Solomon RA, Fink ME, Pile-Spellman J: Surgical management of unruptured intracranial aneurysms. J Neurosurg 1994;80:440–446.
19. Watridge CB, Muhlbauer MS, Lowery RD: Traumatic carotid artery dissection: Diagnosis and treatment. J Neurosurg 1989;71: 854–857.
20. Przelomski MM, Fisher M, Davidson RI, Jones HR, Marcus EM: Unruptured intracranial aneurysm and transient focal cerebral ischemia: A follow-up study. Neurology 1986;36:584–587.
21. Strother CM, Eldevik P, Kikuchi Y, Graves V, Partington C, Merlis A: Thrombus formation and structure and the evolution of mass effect in intracranial aneurysms treated by balloon embolization: Emphasis on MR findings. AJNR 1989;10:787–796.
22. Steed DL, Webster MW, DeVries EJ, et al: Clinical observations on the effect of carotid artery occlusion on cerebral blood flow mapped by xenon computed tomography and its correlation with carotid artery back pressure. J Vasc Surg 1990;11:38–43.
23. Terada T, Nishiguchi T, Hyotani G, et al: Assessment of risk of carotid occlusion with balloon Matas testing and dynamic computed tomography. Acta Neurochir 1990;103:122–127.
24. Russell EJ, Goldberg K, Oskin J, Darling C, Melen O: Ocular ischemic syndrome during carotid balloon occlusion testing. AJNR 1994;15:258–262.
25. Linskey ME, Sekhar LN, Hecht ST: Emergency embolectomy for embolic occlusion of the middle cerebral artery after internal carotid artery balloon test occlusion: Case report. J Neurosurg 1992;77: 134–138.
26. Taptas JN: The treatment of carotid-cavernous aneurysms with embolization of the cervical internal carotid: Apropos of 3 cases, including a case of bilateral carotid-cavernous aneurysm treated with muscular embolization. Rev Neurol 1971;124:277–290.
27. Taki W, Handa H, Yamagata S, et al: Balloon embolization of a giant aneurysm using a newly developed catheter. Surg Neurol 1979; 12:363–365.
28. Rand RW: Thrombogenic microballoon for cerebral aneurysms, arteriovenous malformations, and carotid cavernous fistula occlusion: Preliminary technical note. Surg Neurol 1991;35:403–407.
29. Medlock MD, Dulebohn SC, Elwood PW: Prophylactic hypervolemia without calcium channel blockers in early aneurysm surgery. Neurosurgery 1992;30:12–16.
30. Wholey MH, Kessler L, Boehnke M: A percutaneous balloon catheter technique for the treatment of intracranial aneurysms. Acta Radiol Diagn 1972;13:286–292.
31. Kessler LA, Wholey MH: Carotid artery occlusion in the management of selected giant intracranial aneurysms and carotid cavernous fistula: Percutaneous use of the balloon catheter. Cardiovasc Intervent Radiol 1981;4:187–192.
32. Higashida RT, Halbach VV, Dowd C, et al: Endovascular detachable balloon embolization therapy of cavernous carotid artery aneurysms: Results in 87 cases. J Neurosurg 1990;72:857–863.
33. Kondo S, Aoki T, Nagao S, Gi H, Matsunaga M, Fujita Y: A successful treatment of giant carotid artery aneurysm by a detachable balloon technic: A child case. No Shinkei Geka 1988;16:1299–1304.
34. Vargas ME, Kupersmith MJ, Setton A, Nelson K, Berenstein A: Endovascular treatment of giant aneurysms which cause visual loss. Ophthalmology 1994;101:1091–1098.
35. Kupersmith MJ, Berenstein A, Choi IS, Ransohoff J, Flamm ES: Percutaneous transvascular treatment of giant carotid aneurysms: Neuro-ophthalmologic findings. Neurology 1984;34:328–335.
36. Miyagi J, Shigemori M, Lee S, Tokunaga T, Watanabe M, Kuramoto S: Follow-up study of inaccessible giant aneurysms of the intracranial internal carotid artery. No Shinkei Geka 1987;15: 1257–1263.
37. Yamashita K, Taki W, Nishi S, et al: Treatment of unclippable giant posterior cerebral artery aneurysms with detachable balloons—report of three cases. Neurol Med Chir 1992;32:679–683.
38. Marks MP, Lane B, Steinberg GK, Snipes GJ: Intranidal aneurysms in cerebral arteriovenous malformations: Evaluation and endovascular treatment. Radiology 1992;183:355–360.
39. Khayata MH, Aymard A, Casasco A, Herbreteau D, Woimant F, Merland JJ: Selective endovascular techniques in the treatment of cerebral mycotic aneurysms: Report of three cases. J Neurosurg 1993;78:661–665.
40. Komiyama M, Yasui T, Yagura H, Fu Y, Nagata Y: Traumatic carotid-cavernous sinus fistula associated with an intradural pseudoaneurysm: A case report. Surg Neurol 1991;36:126–132.
41. Lazarev VA, Smirnov NA: Arterial aneurysms of the petrous portion of the carotid artery. Zhurnal Vopr Neirokhir 1982;2:9–12.
42. Sundt T Jr, Pearson BW, Piepgras DG, Houser OW, Mokri B: Surgical management of aneurysms of the distal extracranial internal carotid artery. J Neurosurg 1986;64:169–182.
43. Luessenhop AJ. Interventional neuroradiology: A neurosurgeon's perspective. AJNR 1990;11:625–629.
44. Luessenhop AJ, Spence WT: Artificial embolization of cerebral arteries. Report of use in a case of arteriovenous malformation. JAMA 1960;172:1153–1155.
45. Hilal SK, Michelsen WJ, Driller J, Leonard E: Magnetically guided devices for vascular exploration and treatment: Laboratory and clinical investigations. Radiology 1974;113:529–540.
46. Driller J, Hilal SK, Michelsen WJ, Sollish B, Katz L, Konig W Jr: Development and use of the POD catheter in the cerebral vascular system. Med Res Eng 1969;8:11–16.

47. Serbinenko FA: Fifteen years of endovascular neurosurgery. Seara Med Neurocir 1984;13:1–16.
48. Romodanov AP, Shcheglov VI: Intravascular occlusion of saccular aneurysms of the cerebral arteries by means of a detachable balloon catheter. In: Krayenbuhl H, ed. Advances and technical standards in neurosurgery. Zurich: Springer-Verlag, 1982;25–48
49. Guglielmi G, Vinuela F, Sepetka I, Macellari V: Electrothrombosis of saccular aneurysms via endovascular approach. Part 1: Electrochemical basis, technique, and experimental results. J Neurosurg 1991;75:1–7.
50. Martins IP, Baeta E, Paiva T, Campos J, Gomes L: Headaches during intracranial endovascular procedures: A possible model of vascular headache. Headache 1993;33:227–233.
51. Higashida RT, Hieshima GB, Halbach VV, et al: Intravascular detachable balloon embolization of intracranial aneurysms: Indications and techniques. Acta Radiol Suppl 1986;369:594–596.
52. Lapresle J, Lasjaunias P, Verret JM, Dhaene T: Giant aneurysm of the intracavernous carotid, complicated by subarachnoid haemorrhage: Emergency treatment by occlusive balloon and thrombosis in situ (author's transl). Nouv Presse Med 1979;8:3037–3040.
53. Terada T, Nakamura Y, Nakai K, et al: Embolization of arteriovenous malformations with peripheral aneurysms using ethylene vinyl alcohol copolymer: Report of three cases. J Neurosurg 1991;75: 655–660.
54. Iwata H, Hata Y, Matsuda T, Taki W, Yonekawa Y, Ikada Y: Solidifying liquid with novel initiation system for detachable balloon catheters. Biomaterials 1992;13:891–896.
55. Kinugasa K, Mandai S, Tsuchida S, et al: Cellulose acetate polymer thrombosis for the emergency treatment of aneurysms: Angiographic findings, clinical experience, and histopathological study. Neurosurgery 1994;34:694–701.
56. Hodes JE, Fox AJ, Pelz DM, Peerless SJ: Rupture of aneurysms following balloon embolization. J Neurosurg 1990;72:567–571.
57. Martin NA, Bentson J, Vinuela F, et al: Intraoperative digital subtraction angiography and the surgical treatment of intracranial aneurysms and vascular malformations. J Neurosurg 1990;73:526–533.
58. Molsen HP, Grawe A, Nisch G, Rost H, Siedschlag WD: Intraoperative angiography and embolization in intracranial AVM's and aneurysms. Neurosurg Rev 1992;15:285–288.
59. Mikabe T, Tomita S, Watanabe S, Oya S, Yuzurihara M, Mochida H: Identification of the proximal neck of giant paraclinoidal aneurysms: Technical note. J Neurosurg 1991;75:331–332.
60. Hieshima GB, Higashida RT, Wapenski J, Halbach VV, Cahan L, Bentson JR: Balloon embolization of a large distal basilar artery aneurysm: Case report. J Neurosurg 1986;65:413–416.
61. Kurokawa Y, Abiko S, Okamura T, Watanabe K: Direct surgery for giant aneurysm exhibiting progressive enlargement after intraaneurysmal balloon embolization. Surg Neurol 1992;38:19–25.
62. Nakahara I, Handa H, Nishikawa M, et al: Endovascular coil embolization of a recurrent giant internal carotid artery aneurysm via the posterior communicating artery after cervical carotid ligation: Case report. Surg Neurol 1992;38:57–62.
63. Ladouceur DL: Transcranial clipping of recurrent cerebral aneurysms after endovascular treatment. Stroke 1993;24:1087–1089.
64. Higashida RT, Halbach VV, Cahan LD, et al: Transluminal angioplasty for treatment of intracranial arterial vasospasm. J Neurosurg 1989;71:648–653.
65. Kaku Y, Yonekawa Y, Tsukahara T, Kazekawa K: Superselective intra-arterial infusion of papaverine for the treatment of cerebral vasospasm after subarachnoid hemorrhage. J Neurosurg 1992;77: 842–847.

SUGGESTED READING

Ishikawa S, Kajikawa H, Hibino H, Shima T, Miyazaki M: Massive epistaxis from intracranial extradural aneurysm of the internal carotid artery associated with head injury (author's transl). No Shinkei Geka 1976;4:953–961.

Meder JF, Gaston A, Merienne L, Godon-Hardy S, Fredy D: Traumatic aneurysms of the internal and external carotid arteries: One case and a review of the literature (review). J Neuroradiol 1992;19:248–255.

Nishimoto A, Kuyama H, Nagao S, Kinugasa K, Kunishio K: Artificial embolization with isobutyl-2-cyanoacrylate for the treatment of carotid-ophthalmic aneurysm. Surg Neurol 1987;28:46–50.

Samii M, Turel KE: Possibility of the excision of aneurysms in the vertebrobasilar system followed by end-to-end anastomosis for the maintenance of circulation. Neurol Res 1985;7:39–45.

Zubkov YN, Nikiforov BM, Shustin VA: Balloon catheter technique for dilatation of constricted cerebral arteries after aneurysmal SAH. Acta Neurochir 1984;70:65–79.

18.8 Vasospasm

Key Points

1. Vasospasm starts a few days after a subarachnoid hemorrhage and is usually over after 2 weeks.
2. Early surgical obliteration of the aneurysm with washing out of the cisterns and use of calcium channel blockers, hypervolemic hemodilution and hypertension have markedly decreased the incidence and severity of symptomatic vasospasm.
3. Suspect vasospasm if there is a decreased level of consciousness and new focal neurologic deficits, and transcranial Doppler shows high velocities (>200 cm/sec); CT helps rule out new hemorrhage or hydocephalus.
4. Angioplasty is effective in focal vasospasm. Take care not to rupture vessels.
5. Papaverine is effective in diffuse vasospasm. Take care not to elevate intracranial pressure (ICP).

Background

Over half of patients after subarachnoid hemorrhage (SAH) will develop radiographic vasospasm, and half of these will evidence symptoms of ischemia (1). One in seven patients with subarachnoid bleed will die or have a stroke due to vasospasm. Vasospasm is delayed for a few days after the initial bleed, and may develop as late as 17 days after the bleed (2). This delay has led to its other name of *delayed ischemic neurologic deficit* (DIND).

The pathologic changes in vasospasm involve all three layers of the blood vessel. Inflammatory changes of the adventitia, muscle necrosis, and corrugation of the internal elastic membrane are noted, as well as swelling of the endothelial cells (3). The exact cause of vasospasm is unclear, but it is related to the blood being in contact with the arteries in their cisternal portion. The amount and duration

Table 18.46.
Work-up of Patient with Possible Vasospasm

Question	Studies	Criteria
Rule out causes of neurologic deterioration (rebleed, hydrocephalus, hyponatremia)?	CT, intracranial pressure, electrolyte	
Rule in vasospasm?	Transcranial Doppler	>250 cm/sec
Rule in maximum medical treatment?	CBC, cerebral venous pressure, pulmonary wedge pressure	Depending on status of aneurysm

of the blood around the blood vessel all increase the chance of vasospasm (4).

Diagnosis

Cerebral vasospasm should be suspected in any post-SAH patient with a focal neurologic deficit that can be traced to a given arterial distribution, especially if this follows a decline in the level of consciousness. Ideally, a TCD (transcranial Doppler) examination is performed immediately to evaluate blood flow velocities in the insonated intracranial arteries. Normal flow velocities range between 50 and 100 cm/sec; moderate elevations will go up to 180 cm/sec. Flow velocities in the range of 250 cm/sec suggest severe vasospasm (Table 18.46).

Angiography has long been the sole method of confirmation for vasospasm. It should be said that angiographic vasospasm is more frequent (50 percent) than clinically symptomatic vasospasm (33 percent). Moreover, the severity of angiographic vasospasm does not necessarily correlate with that of the clinical deficit.

CT permits one to evaluate other possible causes for clinical deterioration following SAH, such as a rebleed or hydrocephalus. Before considering mechanical cerebral arterial dilatation, it is imperative to rule out an infarction or rebleed by CT.

Treatment

STANDARD THERAPY

A great number of agents have been tried to treat vasospasm (5).

A recently published article summarizes the current treatment guidelines with regard to limiting the possibility of vasospasm, and the effectiveness of its treatment after a subarachnoid hemorrhage (5). It appears that in patients who are treated within the first 3 days after aneurysm rupture, the standard therapy is early definitive clipping associated with mechanical clot removal, whenever practical, and instillation of fibrinolytic agents. Calcium channel blockers (nimodipine) are also given to the patients, and a normal fluid and electrolyte balance is maintained. As soon as a delayed ischemic deficit is suspected, hypervolemia and hypertension should be instituted. Should the clinical deterioration persist or become progressive despite maximum medical therapy, consideration should be given to intra-arterial vasodilators or balloon angioplasty. For patients who are seen more than 3 days after hemorrhage, the same therapeutic plan is recommended, unless the patient is already suffering from severe symptomatic vasospasm, in which case surgery is likely to be associated with a high mortality and morbidity. In these patients, intra-arterial vasodilators or balloon angioplasty may well be the best first line of treatment despite the presence of an unclipped aneurysm.

ENDOVASCULAR METHODS AND MATERIALS

Angioplasty or intra-arterial vasodilators are indicated when standard methods have failed and before irreversible ischemia has occurred (Table 18.47). Since endovascular methods are reserved for those patients in whom the less invasive and more routine care has been ineffective to stop the development of new neurologic deficits, care must be exercised to be certain that the cause of the clinical deterioration is vasospasm. Therefore, gentle yet reliable diagnotic methods must be used, such as TCD. The beginning of vasospasm can sometimes be difficult to determine exactly because the main sign is a decrease in the level of consciousness. The work-up for vasospasm is outlined in Table 18.46.

The methods can be broken down in a step-by-step way to include preoperative, operative and postoperative considerations (Table 18.47).

Table 18.47.
Operative Methods for Angioplasty of Vasospasm

Preoperative
1. Rule out rebleed, large infarct, hydrocephalus.
2. Rule in maximal medical treatment.
3. Aggressive early treatment.

Operative
1. Consider intubation.
2. Baseline angiogram with markers for measurement. Compare with pre-VSP angiogram to identify areas of small perforators and level of branching.
3. Heparin and moderate hypertension.
4. Guiding catheter in parent vessel.
   - Navigate small low-profile balloon catheter across narrowing.
   - Inflate balloon.
   - Deflate balloon.
   - Advance balloon.
   - Repeat inflation angiogram.
   - Repeat as needed.
5. Treat distal vasospasm with intra-arterial papaverine.
6. Monitor arterial blood pressure, cerebral venous pressure, intracranial pressure, cerebral perfusion pressure.
7. Titrate dose appropriately.

Postoperative
1. Baseline noninvasive studies.
2. Close neurologic intensive care monitoring.

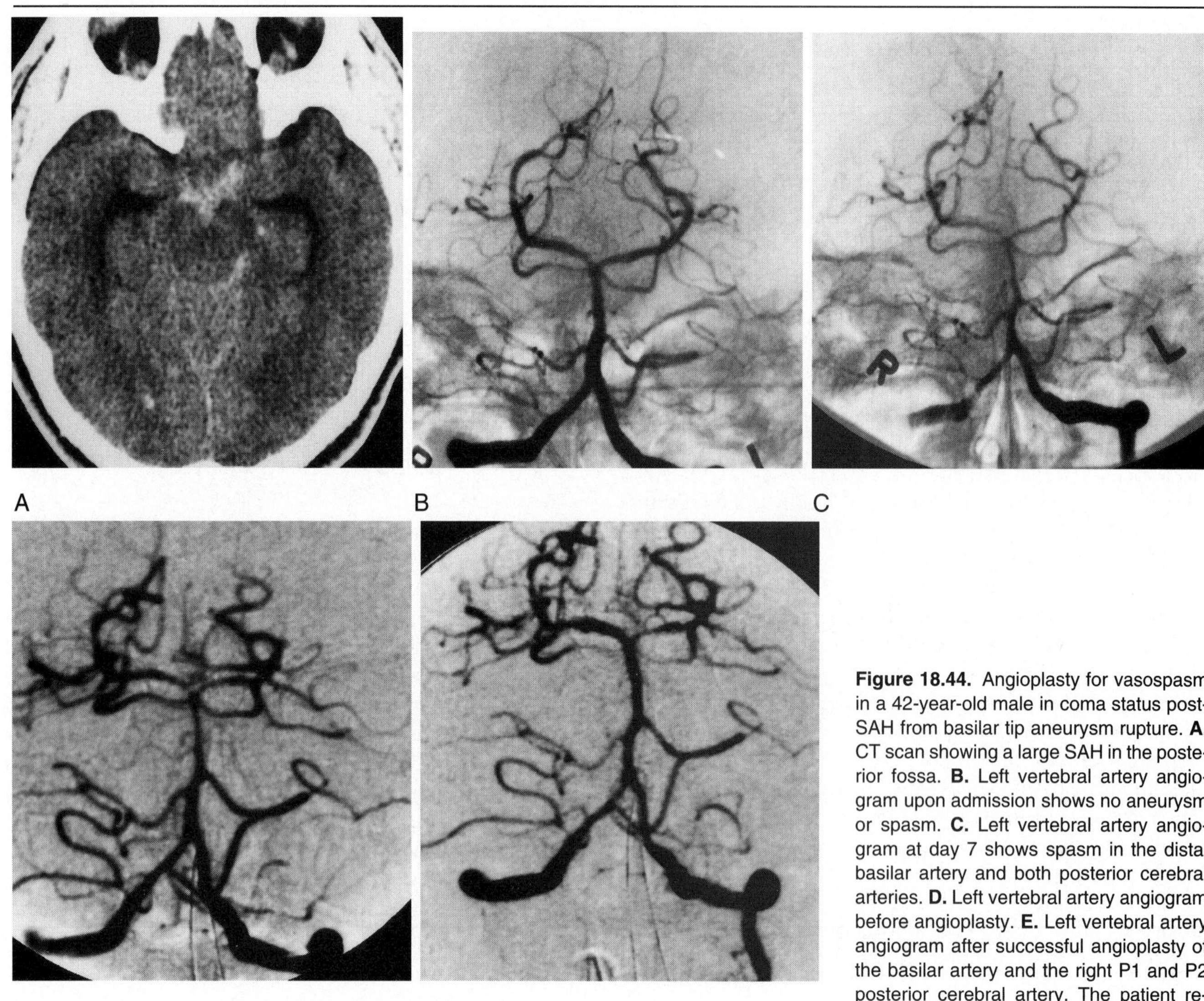

Figure 18.44. Angioplasty for vasospasm in a 42-year-old male in coma status post-SAH from basilar tip aneurysm rupture. **A.** CT scan showing a large SAH in the posterior fossa. **B.** Left vertebral artery angiogram upon admission shows no aneurysm or spasm. **C.** Left vertebral artery angiogram at day 7 shows spasm in the distal basilar artery and both posterior cerebral arteries. **D.** Left vertebral artery angiogram before angioplasty. **E.** Left vertebral artery angiogram after successful angioplasty of the basilar artery and the right P1 and P2 posterior cerebral artery. The patient recovered gradually to baseline.

Small-size latex balloons,* silicone balloons,† or polyethylene balloon systems‡ have all been effectively used for angioplasty of vasospasm. The balloon should not be more than 4 mm in diameter and should have a very soft profile. Navigation of the balloon past the bifurcation of the long circumferential arteries (M2, P2, A2) and overdistention of the vessel or perforator off the parent vessel can easily lead to catastrophic rupture (6).

A balloon that the author has found appropriate is the No. 15 Ingenor, which can be secured on a Tracker microcatheter with a commercial acrylate glue (iso-butyl-cyanoacrylate). The Stealth catheter‡ is also highly useful in the posterior circulation.

* Nycomed-Ingenor, Paris, France.

† ITC, San Francisco, Calif.

‡ Stealth Target, Target Therapeutics, San Jose, Calif.

MONITORING

Transcranial Doppler has a significant role in the management of patients undergoing interventional neuroradiologic treatment for intracranial vasospasm. Persistence of elevated TCD-obtained flow velocities after intracranial angioplasty suggests the need for repeat angiographic evaluation and possibly further therapy. In one study, intracranial angioplasty for clinically evident vasospasm after subarachnoid hemorrhage was performed in four patients (7). In two patients, transcranial Doppler flow velocities remained elevated despite initial anatomic correction of the vasospasm. Control angiography revealed new areas of involvement by vasospasm. Reangioplasty or papaverine infusion treatment of the new lesions resulted in decreased flow velocities and clinical improvement in all patients.

Brain SPECT (^{99m}Tc-HMPAO) after cerebral angioplasty can be seen to improve by visual interpretation rela-

Table 18.48.
Published Angioplasty Results

Study	Number of patients/lesions	% Improved angio/clinical	Complications: Dead/Major/Minor
Zubkov*	33/105	97%/?	?
Higashida†	13/36	100%/69%	0
Eskridge‡			

* Zubkov YN NB, Shustin VA: Acta Neurochir 1984;70:65–79, with permission.
† Higashida RT, Halback VV, Cahan LD, Brant-Zawczki M, Barnwel S, Dowel C, Hieshima GB: Transluminal angioplasty for the treatment of intracranial arterial vasospasm Jour Neurosurg 1989;71:648–653.

tive to an internal reference (cerebellum). In one study, manual, semiquantitative region of interest (ROI) analysis revealed improvement by 10.5 percent of regional cerebral blood flow (rCBF) in patients that improved clinically.

Endovascular Results

ANGIOPLASTY

Published results have been extremely encouraging, with 60 to 80 percent of patients showing improvement. The authors point to the need for early treatment and vigorous attempts to treat all vessels involved. The long-term follow-up of these patients has demonstrated angiographically normal vessels (8–12). The author has found the A1-anterior cerebral artery (ACA) difficult to gain access for geometric reasons. Angioplasty for vasospasm appears to be a relatively safe and effective procedure, though not without difficulty or risk (Fig. 18.44; Table 18.48). Overdilation can lead to rupture and dissection (Fig. 18.45).

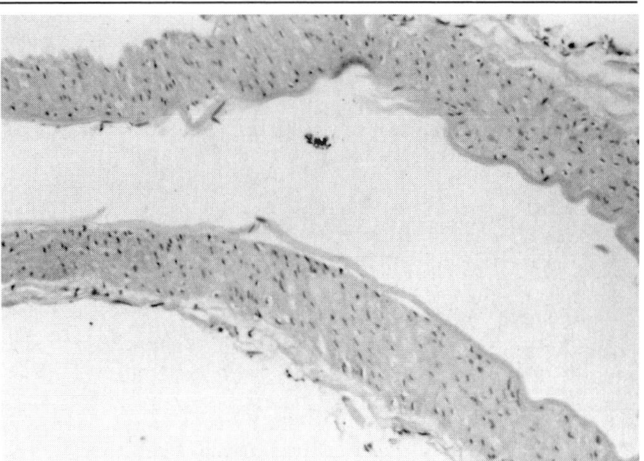

Figure 18.45. Dog basilar artery histology subjected to overdilation showing fracture of internal elastic membrane.

VASODILATORS

Papaverine is not without some problems. Clinically significant increase in intracranial pressure (ICP), blindness (13), and precipitation (14) have all been reported. It is suggested that if there is any possibility of increased ICP, that papaverine be titrated with monitoring of cerebral perfusion pressure. Blindness can be avoided by keeping the concentration low, less than 0.3 percent (Table 18.49). Nimodipine has been used intra-arterially via local injection with superselective technique with excellent results outside of the United States. It is not approved for intra-arterial use in the United States at this writing.

Future Directions

Diffuse vasospasm distal to the basal cisterns and vasospasm in the ACA distribution remain problematic. Pharmacologic prophylactic strategies are likely to have the greatest impact. Technical advances such as laser and advances in superselective pharmacology are promising. Angioplasty with "fluid bullets" has been reported by a Boston group using the anterior spinal artery in a canine subarachnoid hemorrhage model. Pulsed laser flashes from a 200μ tip created fluid waves that dissipated the vasospasm in front of the tip (15).

In summary, although we have seen in recent years significant progress in the understanding and the management of vasospasm, too many lives are still being claimed. Only generalized prophylaxis, a high level of suspicion, and an extremely aggressive attitude toward vasospasm can help create the hope that it may be eradicated in the future.

Table 18.49.
Results with Treatment of Vasospasm with Papaverine

Study	Number of patients	Outcome	Dose	Comments
Eskridge*	21	Papaverine caused increased ICP and decreased CPP#	300 mg/20 ml	Must watch ICP‡ if using papaverine
Mumaguchi†	14	17/19 better by angiography, 50% patients improved immediately, death none	150–600 mg	

* Eskridge JW, et al: Paper 175, ASNR meeting, 1994, with permission.
† Mumaguchi, T: Paper 176, ASNR meeting, 1994, with permission.
‡ ICP = intracranial pressure
# CPP = cerebral perfusion pressure

REFERENCES

1. Kassell NF, Sasaki T, Colohan AR, Nazar G: Cerebal vasospasms following aneurysmal hemorrhage [Review]. Stroke, 1985;16: 562–572.
2. Weir B, Grace M, Hansen J, Rothberg C: Time course of vasospasm in man. Journal of Neurosurgery 1978;48:173–178.
3. Sasaki T, Kassell NF, Yamashita M, et al: Barrier disruption in the major cerebral arteries following experimental subarachnoid hemorrhage. Journal of Neurosurgery 1985;63:433–440.
4. Fisher CM, Kistler JP, Davis JM: Relation of cerebral vasospasm to subarachnoid hemorrhage visualized by computerized tomographic scanning. Neurosurgery 1980;6:1–9.
5. Wilkins RH: Attempts at prevention or treatment of intracranial arterial spasm: an update. [Review]. Neurosurgery 1986;18: 808–825.
6. Linskey ME, Horton JA, Rao GR, Yonas H: Fatal rupture of the intracranial carotid artery during transluminal angioplasty for vasospasm induced by subarachnoid hemorrhage. Journal of Neurosurgery. 1991;74:985–990.
7. Hurst RW, Schnee C, Raps EC, Farber R, Flamm ES: Role of transcranial Doppler in neuroradiological treatment of intracranial vasospasm. Stroke 1993;24:299–303.
8. Weir B, MacDonald L: Cerebral vasospasm. [Review]. Clinical Neurosurgery 1993;40:40–55.
9. Zubkov YN, Nikiforov BM, Shustin VA: Balloon catheter technique for dilation of constricted cerebral arteries after aneurysmal SAH. Acta Neurochirurgica 1984;70:65–79.
10. Hieshima GB, Higashida RT, Wapenski J, Halbach VV, Cahan L, Bentson JR: Balloon embolization of a large distal basilar artery aneurysm. Case report. Journal of Neurosurgery 1986;65:413–416.
11. Eskridge JM, et al: ICP and Papaverine on vasospasm. Paper 176 presented at the American Society of Neuroradiology meeting, 1994.
12. Clouston JE, Numaguchi Y, Zoarski GH, Aldrich EF, Simard JM, Zitnay KM: Intraarterial papaverine infusion for cerebral vasospasm after subarachnoid hemorrhage. American Journal of Neuroradiology 1995;16:27–38.
13. Blindness and Papaverine. Paper 183 presented at the American Society of Neuroradiology meeting, 1994.
14. Dion J: In vivo incompatibilities of papaverine. Poster 42 presented at the American Society of Neuroradiology meeting, 1994.
15. Zervas NC: Angioplasty of SAH-induced VSP with pulsed dye laser. Paper 177 presented at the American Society of Neuroradiology meeting, 1994.

18.9 Hyperacute Intra-arterial Thrombolysis for Thromboembolic Stroke

John Pile-Spellman and Ichiro Nakara

Key Points

1. The role of acute endovascular treatment, if any, in acute stroke is unknown.
2. Thrombolysis is under vigorous investigation, and the initial work leads to the following four observations:
   a. Patient selection is critical.
      Rule out bleed, aneurysms, bleeding risk.
      Rule out completed infarction(>6 h).
   b. Restore bulk flow quickly and effectively.
   c. Thrombolytic agents found useful include urokinase, pro-urokinase, and tPA.
   d. Monitor patients closely.

Background

Interventional techniques can make the greatest contribution in the next 5 to 10 years in the area of thromboembolic stroke. This field is in its infancy. The information offered here is a guide to help direct the study and exploration of this field, and is only a suggestion of how one can proceed.

Strokes affect approximately 375,000 Americans each year. Strokes kill one-third of these patients and disable an additional one-third. Stroke ranks as the third leading cause of death in the United States. Eighty percent of these strokes are caused by embolism or thrombosis. Despite tremendous efforts, there has been little progress in the treatment or outcome of patients with stroke the last 25 years.

The brain's sensitivity to ischemia and/or reperfusion is the problem. Reduction of the cerebral blood flow (CBF) below 10 ml/100 g/min causes irreversible neuronal damage within 6 to 8 min due to disintegration of the membrane following failure of energy-dependent ionic transport (1). Between about 10 and 18 ml/100 g/min of CBF, electrical dysfunction without neuronal death may occur. However, sustained ischemia could cause irreversible damage even in this range of CBF. In focal ischemia, there may be a perifocal ischemic tissue that is in dysfunction but not dead ("penumbra"), surrounding the core of infarct according to the collateral circulation (1) (Fig. 18.46). Functional recovery is possible by restoration of CBF within 4 to 6 h, depending on the severity of the ischemia (1–3). Occlusive lesions are found angiographically in 90 percent of these stroke patients (4). From these observations, clearly early "hyperacute" revascularization is needed to avoid ischemic damage (5,6).

Thromboembolic stroke is a serious condition, with 20 percent of the patients dying in the first month after the stroke (7). Long-term outcome carries significant morbidity for the surviving patients, with almost two-thirds having decreased vocational and social function, half having peripheral motor weakness, one-third having a markedly decreased activity of daily living, and one-sixth being institutionalized (8). Progression of stroke after admission to the hospital may be as high as 40 percent (7). Methods of curtailing the progression of the deficit in stroke patients have been, as one author states, "woefully inadequate."

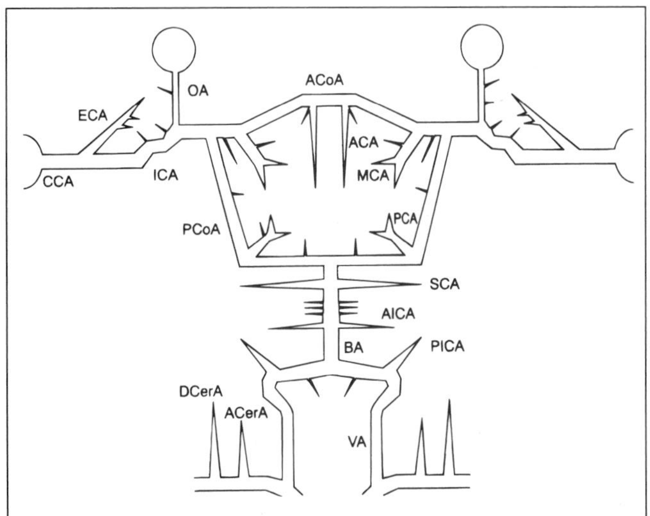

Figure 18.46. Pull-out projection of cerebral blood vessels. By drawing the circle of Willis around the brain, and the long circumferentials (anterior, middle, and posterior cerebral arteries) as spokes off this rim, a map can be made that helps delineate the areas of angiographic watershed. We have found this useful in cases of occlusive and embolic disease.

Current customary therapies for thromboembolic strokes rest on management of potential complications and attempts to reverse and stabilize neurologic impairment. Improvement in outcome for these patients has rested primarily on management of complications. A great variety of therapeutic maneuvers have been tried. A review of measures to reverse and stabilize neurologic impairment is beyond the scope of this book. Until recently a therapeutic nihilism based on effective treatment was common.

Clinical studies beginning in the late 1950s showed that delayed revascularization not only failed to treat cerebral ischemia but also caused hemorrhagic complications leading to neurologic deterioration. Failure of these patients to improve is not unexpected, since few if any had revascularization within 4 to 6 h. Sporadic case reports of "hyperacute" revascularization have, on the contrary, been encouraging. By the late 1970s revascularization for stroke was considered relatively contraindicated (9–14). Thrombolytic therapy for arterial thrombus has been reported in almost all organs (15–17). Regional perfusion in the arteries of the extremities, the superior mesenteric artery, the hepatic artery, and the renal arteries has had successful results. The higher reperfusion rate of regional intra-arterial (IA) infusion (approximately 70 to 80 percent) over systemic intravenous (IV) infusion (approximately 40 percent) has justified its use. The problem is the lack of large controlled studies on the long-term clinical benefits of this approach as against conventional treatment or systemic IV administration. Thrombolysis in coronary artery occlusion is well documented in many articles and reviews (15–21). Reperfusion rates range between 35 and 95 percent for various doses and durations of treatment. Approximately 50 to 70 percent of these patients have beneficial cardiac functions. Meanwhile, intracoronary infusion with angiographic confirmation of reperfusion with advanced imaging techniques showed a definitely improved reperfusion rate among 50 to 90 percent. Intravenous use of urokinase (UK) and streptokinase (SK) has seemed to provide clinical benefits in patients with pulmonary embolism (15–17). Because of its specific effects on circulation and pathophysiology, prolonged IV infusion even up to 72 h is preferred. The reperfusion rate is 80 to 90 percent.

Early cerebral revascularization using hyperacute IV thrombolytic therapy with tissue plasminogen activator (tPA) is not encouraging for serious major cerebral vessel occlusions (22–26), but has been encouraging in relatively mild branch occlusions (25).

On the other hand, in the early 1980s coronary artery IA infusion of UK or SK for acute myocardial infarction was demonstrated to be highly effective (15–21). These results motivated some to begin IA administration of such thrombolytic agents to the occluded cerebral vessels (5,6,27–32). Regionally delivered thrombolytics recanalize approximately 45 percent of occluded vessels. Technical advances have allowed for the routine catheterization of intracranial vessels. Using superselective microcatheters, revascularization of cerebral vessels has been possible in approximately 95 percent of patients (33–36). The demonstrated benefits of hyperacute local infusion of thrombolytic agents made swift and effective clot lysis possible without the need to keep patients systematically thrombolytic after demonstrated revascularization.

Hemorrhagic complication with clinically significant deterioration occurs in 5 to 10 percent of patients with thromboembolic stroke (37). Prompt thrombolytic therapy prevents an increased hemorrhagic rate (5,6,27–30,32,34–36).

Intra-arterial thrombolysis is not the established or customary care for stroke patients, but there is increasing evidence that it is highly effective in patients with severe stroke. Some consider IA thrombolysis the best possible treatment. Questions remain, even for the convinced, concerning patient selection, methodology, reperfusion injury,

Table 18.50.
Intra-arterial Thrombolytic Therapy for Acute Stroke: Types of Studies

Investigator	*N*	Agent	Infusion	Onset-Tx**
Carotid				
del Zoppo*	20	UK/SK	Regional/Local	7.6 h
Mori†	22	UK	Regional	4.5 h
Theron‡	9	SK	Local	6.4 h
Vertebrobasilar				
Hacke§	43	UK	Regional/Local	<24 h
Zeumer‖	7	UK	Local	4–48 h

* GJ del Zoppo, et al: Stroke 1988;19:307–313, with permission.
† E Mori, et al: Stroke 1989;19:802–812, with permission.
‡ J Theron, et al: AJNR 1989;10:753–765, with permission.
§ W Hacke, et al: Stroke 1988;19:1216–1222, with permission.
‖ H Zeumer, et al: Neuroradiology 1989;31:336–340, with permission.
** Onset-Tx = onset from ictus to time of treatment.

Table 18.51.
Intra-arterial Thrombolytic Therapy for Acute Stroke: Result of Studies

Investigator	N	Recanalization	Favorable outcome	Mortality	Hemorrhagic infarction
Carotid					
del Zoppo*	20	18 (90%)	12 (60%) R: 12, U: 0	3 (15%) R: 2, U: 1	4 (20%) R: 4, U: 0
Mori†	22	10 (45%)	10 (45%) R: 8, U: 2	3 (14%) R: 0, U: 3	4 (18%) R: 1, U: 3
Theron‡	9	8 (89%)	6 (67%) R: 6, U: 0	1 (11%) R: 1, U: 0	3 (33%) R: 3, U: 0
Vertebrobasilar					
Hacke§	43	19 (44%)	10 (24%) R: 10, U: 0	30 (70%) R: 6, U: 24	4 (9%) R: 2, U: 2
Zeumer‖	7	7 (100%)	4 (57%) R: 4, U: 0	2 (22%) R: 2, U: 0	1 (14%) R: 1, U: 0

Note: R = recanalized, U = unrecanalized.
* GJ del Zoppo, et al: Stroke 1988;19:307–313, with permission.
† E Mori, et al: Stroke 1989;19:802–812, with permission.
‡ J Theron, et al: AJNR 1989;10:753–765, with permission.
§ W Hacke, et al: Stroke 1988;19:1216–1222, with permission.
‖ H Zeumer, et al: Neuroradiology 1989;31:336–340, with permission.

and comparison with the natural course (5,6). The success of coronary artery infusion of thrombolytic agents for acute myocardial infarction motivated cerebral IA use in the 1980s (31,35,36). Acceptable results with cerebral IA thrombolytic therapy have been reported (Tables 18.50 to 18.53) (5,6,27–30,32,33,38).

CAROTID ARTERY TERRITORY

In the pilot study reported by del Zoppo et al. (28), 20 patients with angiographically demonstrated acute occlusion in the carotid territory were treated with IA thrombolytic therapy in two institutes. The dosage and rate of thrombolytic agents were rather variable (UK: 40,000 to 300,000 U/1 to 4 h; SK 6,000 to 7,000 U/0.5 to 2 h or 250,000 U/1 h). In some cases, concomitant heparinization and hemodilution therapy was used. Treatment was started within 8 h. Recanalization was achieved in 18/20 patients (90 percent; complete: 15, partial: 3). Favorable improvement was observed in 12/20, all of which were in the recanalized group. Hemorrhagic transformations were demonstrated in 4 (20 percent) of the recanalized patients with no clinical deterioration. In all of these cases with hemorrhage, anticoagulant was administered immediately after the treatment. Three patients died (recanalized: 2, unrecanalized: 1). One patient death was unrelated to the hemorrhagic transformation.

Table 18.52.
Intra-arterial Thrombolytic Therapy for Acute Stroke: Analysis of Results in Relation to Recanalization

Therapy	N	Favorable outcome	Mortality	Hemorrhagic infarction
Carotid	51	28 (55%)*	7 (14%)	11 (22%)
Recanalized	36	26 (72%)	3 (8%)	8 (22%)
Unrecanalized	15	2 (13%)	4 (27%)	3 (20%)
Vertebrobasilar	50	14 (28%)†	32 (64%)†	5 (10%)
Recanalized	26	14 (54%)	8 (31%)	3 (12%)
Unrecanalized	24	0 (0%)	24 (100%)	2 (8%)
Total	101	42 (42%)†	39 (39%)†	16 (16%)
Recanalized	62	40 (65%)	11 (18%)	11 (18%)
Unrecanalized	39	2 (5%)	28 (72%)	5 (13%)

* $p < 0.005$.
† $p < 0.001$:chi.

Table 18.53.
Intra-arterial Thrombolytic Therapy for Acute Stroke: Analysis of Results in Relation to Hemorrhagic Infarction

Therapy	N	Favorable outcome	Mortality
Carotid	51	28 (55%)	7 (14%)
Hemorrhaged	11	6 (55%)	3 (27%)
Nonhemorrhaged	40	22 (55%)	4 (10%)
Vertebrobasilar	50	14 (28%)	32 (64%)
Hemorrhaged	5	1 (20%)	4 (80%)
Nonhemorrhaged	45	13 (29%)	28 (62%)
Total	101	42 (42%)	39 (39%)
Hemorrhaged	16	7 (44%)	7 (44%)
Nonhemorrhaged	85	35 (41%)	32 (38%)

Mori et al. (30) reported 22 patients with acute middle cerebral artery occlusion treated with intra-arterial UK infusion (180,000 to 320,000 U/0.5 h) started after 0.83 to 12 h (mean 4.5 h) from onset. Recanalization occurred in 10/22 cases (45 percent; complete: 4, partial with sufficient flow: 4, partial with restricted flow: 4). Improved neurologic outcome and decreased volume of infarction were demonstrated in the recanalized group versus the unrecanalized group (recanalized: 8/10, 80 percent, versus unrecanalized: 4/12, 33 percent). Hemorrhage was observed in 4 cases (18 percent; recanalized: 1, unrecanalized: 3). Three patients died in the unrecanalized group for causes unrelated to hemorrhage. Rapid amelioration of symptoms was noticed in patients with successful recanalization.

Theron et al. (32) also tried intra-arterial SK (50,000 to 150,000 U) infusion in 12 patients with carotid territory occlusion. In 9 patients without combined surgical intervention, 8 patients (89 percent) achieved recanalization, and in 6 of these a favorable outcome (66 percent) was observed. Hemorrhage was observed in 3 cases (33 percent) in the lenticulostriate artery territory after recanalization. One patient died in relation to hemorrhage. The author suggested that the risk of basal ganglia hemorrhage is high if treatment is delayed (more than 6 h) in patients with lenticulostriate artery involvement.

VERTEBROBASILAR ARTERY TERRITORY

After the encouraging results in the carotid artery territory, IA infusion of thrombolytic agents was extended to use with acute vertebrobasilar occlusion by German investigators (30,35,39). Hacke et al. (29) treated 43 patients with vertebrobasilar occlusion presenting with acute (8/43) or progressive (35/43) neurologic deterioration; 100,000 U UK/h for up to 4 h (10,000 U/h for 12 to 24 h in some initial cases) was administered intra-arterially into the clotted vertebrobasilar arteries. Treatment was begun within 24 h after the onset of the stroke in most patients. Results were compared with 22 patients treated by conventional therapy (antiplatelet drugs or anticoagulant) retrospectively. Recanalization was obtained in 19/43 (44 percent) patients, with favorable outcomes in 10 patients and death in 6 patients. In contrast, poor clinical outcome with high mortality was evident in 24/43 patients without recanalization (favorable outcome: 0, death: 24), and in all of the 22 patients who received the conventional therapy (favorable outcome: 3, death: 19). Hemorrhage occurred in 4 patients (9 percent; recanalized: 2, unrecanalized: 2), with 2 deaths following acute deterioration in the treated group. Three of 4 patients who hemorrhaged had been treated with prolonged low-dose infusion concomitant with heparinization. The authors concluded that successful thrombolysis of vertebrobasilar occlusion could offer beneficial clinical outcome in life-threatening brainstem strokes.

Recently, Zeumer et al. (34) reviewed the study just described and reported on 7 new patients treated by superselective IA infusion under the revised protocol. On the basis of their experiences, they recommended high doses with shorter duration of treatment. Patients received up to 500,000 U of UK in 1 h and 250,000 U in the next hour through a microcatheter navigated close to or into the clot. Recanalization was obtained in all cases (100 percent), with recovery in 4/7 (58 percent), a locked-in state in 1/7 (14 percent), and death in 2/7 (29 percent). Heparinization was started after partial thromboplastin time was shown to be twice or less than the normal value. A small intracerebellar hemorrhage was observed in 1 patient (14 percent) under heparinization without clinical deterioration. The authors emphasized the progressive course of acute vertebrobasilar stroke leading to coma, decerebration, and finally death, and indicated that treatment should be determined not by time limit but by careful neurologic examinations combined with angiographic findings. Furthermore, it was suggested that high-dose local administration with short duration using a superselective catheterization technique would decrease the risk of hemorrhage and work more effectively on recanalization (see Tables 18.50 to 18.53).

In summary, recanalization has been achieved in 62/101 cases (61 percent) in these studies, which consisted of 36/51 cases (71 percent) in carotid artery territory and 26/50 (52 percent) in vertebrobasilar artery territory. Favorable outcome has been shown in 42/101 cases (42 percent; *carotid:* 28/51, 55 percent, versus *vertebrobasilar:* 14/50, 28 percent). The number of dead patients was 39/101 (39 percent; *carotid:* 7/51, 14 percent, versus *vertebrobasilar:* 32/50, 64 percent). Hemorrhagic infarction occurred in 14/101 (14 percent; *carotid:* 9/51, 18 percent, versus *vertebrobasilar:* 5/50, 10 percent). The outcomes, deaths, and hemorrhages are summarized in relation to recanalization in Table 18.53.

From these results, it appears that the recanalized group shows a better clinical outcome than the unrecanalized group in carotid territory ($p < 0.005$, chi square test), in vertebrobasilar territory ($p < 0.001$), and in both territories combined ($p < 0.001$), whereas there is no correlation between recanalization and the occurrence of hemorrhagic infarction. In addition, the number of deaths has been significantly decreased in the recanalized group in vertebrobasilar territory ($p < 0.001$), and in both territories combined ($p < 0.001$). On the other hand, no correlation was demonstrated between hemorrhagic infarction and outcomes or deaths in carotid, vertebrobasilar, or both territories (see Table 18.53). In addition to these published data, several challenges in superselective IA thrombolytic therapy have been tried with encouraging notices in the United States, Germany, Japan, France, and some other countries.

RECENT RESULTS WITH tPA IN ACUTE STROKES

Tissue plasminogen activator (tPA) is a fibrin-specific endogenous plasminogen activator that is made by modern DNA recombinant technique. As described in text preceding, tPA predominantly acts on fibrin-bound plasminogen activated by fibrin, causing less systemic fibrinolytic and anticoagulant effects with sufficient thrombolytic potency. tPA has already been used widely in thrombolysis for acute myocardial infarction, with great efficacy and safety. However, high-dose administration of tPA also can cause hemorrhagic complications, including intracranial hemorrhage, as observed rarely in acute myocardial infarction. Therefore, the risk of hemorrhagic infarction must be taken into account, as with exogenous plasminogen activators like UK or SK (15–17,23,24,40).

Many authors in the past few years have reported the efficacy of tPA in experimental stroke following successful results in its application for acute myocardial ischemia and infarction. Intravenous infusion of tPA has been employed mostly in rabbit acute stroke models after 0 to 4 h from onset, with 0.6 to 2.0 mg/kg given over 30 to 120 min (41–48). tPA was efficient in decreasing the size of infarction and in improving neurologic deficits, cerebral blood flow (CBF), or EEG results. In most of these reports, secondary hemorrhages were not observed in up to 24 h of the follow-up period, though some authors disclosed a 25 to 30 percent chance of secondary hemorrhage with rather high doses (3 to 5 mg/kg over 30 min) of tPA with a longer follow-up period (1 to 8 days). Recently, Lyden et al. (49) demonstrated that thrombolysis was achieved with high probability without increasing risk of hemorrhage even with 10 mg/kg over 30 min beginning 90 min after the onset in tPA. In contrast, SK infusion (30,000 U/kg) with the same time course regimen caused significant increase in the risk of hemorrhage, although the efficacy of thrombolysis was the same as with tPA. Philips et al. (50) compared the effects of a new type of tPA (Fb-Fb-CF, a catalytic fragment of the tPA molecule with a longer half-life) with SK in IV infusion after 3 h from the onset, in which they found the superior effect of tPA in restoring CBF.

In terms of intra-arterial infusion, Benes et al. (51) reported a study comparing tPA (1 mg in bolus and 1 mg/kg/h over 2 h) with UK (25,000 U in bolus and 25,000 U/kg/h over 2 h) started after 30 min from the onset. Both agents reduced the number of emboli and the size of infarction with no hemorrhage, but only tPA decreased the incidence of infarction. In addition, Kawakami et al. (52) observed that small-dose tPA achieved better clot lysis compared with UK in IA injection of a canine common carotid artery thrombosis model.

Concerning hemorrhagic infarction, del Zoppo et al. (53) demonstrated in an experimental 3-h middle cerebral artery occlusion baboon model (treated 30 min after reperfusion with 0.3 to 10 mg/kg over 60 min) that most of the hemorrhages associated with tPA infusion were no different in type (petechial) or frequency than the control (saline infusion) group. However, in a rabbit ligation/hypotension model treated with tPA 24 h after ischemia, gross hemorrhage was observed in 75 percent (3/4), suggesting that early treatment is essential with tPA as well as with other exogenous thrombolytic agents (54).

Clinical dose-range trials using IV-tPA in acute thrombotic and thromboembolic stroke have been started (22–24,26,32,55). Del Zoppo et al. (tPA acute stroke study group) (26) found that recanalization occurred in 22/57 (39 percent) patients (18 partial; 4 complete) treated within 8 h with various doses, and hemorrhagic infarcts occurred in 23/57 (40 percent) not associated with clinical deterioration or recanalization. Most of them were petechial in type; parenchymatous hemorrhage occurred in 4/57 (7 percent), with 3 deaths (3/57; 5 percent). On the other hand, Brott et al. (NINCDS tPA study, NIH-sponsored) (23) treated 74 patients who received IV-tPA (0.35 to 0.85 mg/kg,) within 90 min of onset. Early neurologic improvement (within 6 h of tPA infusion) was observed in 29 patients (39 percent), and hemorrhagic infarction occurred in 2 patients (3 percent). Recent reports, including these studies, indicate the possible benefits of IV-tPA treatment for acute stroke, though further case-controlled study focused on the benefits in neurologic outcome remains to be performed.

Table 18.54.
Result of IV-tPA Study (tPA Acute Stroke Study Group)

104/139 (75%) received IV tPA therapy	
94/104 included	
Recanalization	33/94 (35%)
Partial	29/94 (31%)
Complete	4/94 (4%)
Hemorrhagic infarction (HI; petechial hemorrhage)	23/104 (22%)
Clinical improvement in 17/23	
Parenchymatous hemorrhage (PI)	10/104 (9.6%)
Deterioration in 6/10	

* Source: Stroke 1991;22:153.

A recently published abstract of the final report on the IV-tPA study (tPA acute stroke study group) gave the results shown in (Table 18.54) (25). Recanalization was noted mostly in distal (branch) occlusions. A relationship between dose and recanalization was not achieved. Hemorrhagic infarction (HI) and parenchymal hemorrhage (PH) were not associated with dose or recanalization, but were significantly associated with initiation of treatment after 6.0 h. The effect of the treatment on clinical outcome has not been reported yet. From this result, early IV administration seems not to increase the risk of hemorrhage. However, frequency of recanalization is not so high as recent IA studies.

Experiences in arterial infusion of tPA are still rather limited. Henze et al. (56) reported complete clot lysis in acute basilar artery occlusion with intra-arterial tPA injection of the proximal left vertebral artery (15 mg in bolus, followed by continuous infusion of 50 mg over 30 min and 35 mg over the next 60 min; total dose 100 mg; 1.5 mg/kg). The patient, who was comatose and decerebrated initially, recovered up to mild deficits without any hemorrhagic complications. Buteux et al. (57) treated acute bilateral posterior cerebral artery occlusion successfully with local IA-tPA infusion (20 mg in bolus and 50 mg continuously over 4 h). In addition, a recent work of Takahashi et al. (58) showed 100 percent recanalization in 15 patients (9 complete; 6 partial) of acute middle cerebral artery occlusion utilizing IA-tPA infusion (1.2 to 9.6 mg) combined with superselective catheterization within 6 h (mean 3.2 h). Eight out of 15 (53 percent) improved immediately, and excellent or good outcome was observed in 9 out of 15 (60 percent) without any intracranial hemorrhage and systemic hemorrhagic tendency. These promising results, accompanied by the experimental findings previously described, justify further well-designed study in IA-tPA infusion for acute stroke.

THROMBOLYSIS AND THROMBOLYTIC AGENTS

Much of the information that follows repeats information found in the Materials section. Its new importance to neuroradiology justifies such repetitions.

In arterial thrombosis and its extension, many factors, such as endothelial injury, platelet aggregation, thrombin generation, and stasis, are involved in variable degrees. Platelets adhere and aggregate to the surface of the damaged endothelium, which is normally thrombus resistant. Activation of the platelet membrane via platelet surface receptors induces catalytic processes in the platelets, which promotes further aggregation of platelets, vasoconstriction, and activation of the intrinsic coagulation pathway. Platelet membrane phospholipids react with factors VIII and V, which promote activation and conversion of factor X to Xa, and prothrombin II to thrombin IIa, respectively. The platelet membrane provides efficient reaction sites through receptors for several clotting factors, and the positive feedback mechanism accelerates thrombin generation on the platelet surface. Cleavage of fibrinogen mediated by thrombin produces the fibrin-platelet network that is necessary to stabilize the thrombus (5,6,15–17,40).

Dissolution of the thrombus is mediated by fibrinolysis within the thrombus (thrombolysis). Degradation of fibrin is catalyzed by plasmin activated from plasminogen. Normally, the fibrinolytic system exists in circulating blood as plasminogen, the precursor of plasmin, and has no enzyme activity. The formation of plasmin is promoted by the appearance of plasminogen activator, which is neutralized instantly in normal circulating blood by alpha$_2$-antiplasmin, a plasmin inhibitor. A systemic fibrinolytic state is achieved by excessive production of plasmin over plasmin inhibitor following activation of plasminogen due to administration of large doses of exogenous plasminogen activator such as UK and SK. In the thrombus, plasminogen is bound with fibrin and platelets, where it is activated by plasminogen activator derived from vessel walls (tPA). Fibrin binding to plasminogen interferes with the reaction of alpha$_2$-antiplasmin. This causes the localized release of plasmin, as well as in situ fibrinolysis in the thrombus without the effect of alpha$_2$-antiplasmin. Fibrinolysis is also regulated by some other modulators, including plasminogen activator inhibitor. It is secreted from the endothelium, rapidly binds to plasminogen activator, and attenuates its activity. It is also neutralized by fibrin binding to plasminogen in the thrombus (5,6,15–17,40).

Exogenous plasminogen activators, such as UK, SK, or acylated plasminogen-streptokinase activator complex (APSAC), have been used in thrombolytic therapy. Different mechanisms are involved in the activation of plasminogen to plasmin in circulating blood with these agents. UK, which is a serine protease produced from human urine or fetal renal cell culture, directly activates plasminogen. In contrast, SK, which is derived from culture of beta-hemolytic streptococcus, has no direct effect on plasminogen. SK combines with plasminogen to form a plasminogen-streptokinase complex, which activates circulating plasminogen to plasmin. Free plasmin in the circulating blood activated by these agents degrades fibrin and fibrinogen, causing fibrinolysis. These exogenous agents also inactivate prothrombin II and factors V and VIII, thereby inhibiting systemic coagulation. Also, fibrin degradation products (FDPs) act as potent anticoagulants. Thus large doses of these agents could cause a prolonged systemic anticoagulant state. SK is less expensive than UK, and mass production is easy. However, the half-life of SK is longer (18 to 83 min) than that of UK (11 to 18 min), and it has more side effects, such as fever or allergy, than UK because of its immunogenetic property. Its activity may be unstable in patients with a myocardial infarction.

In patients with MI treated with UK or SK, the risk of hemorrhagic complication varies between 23 and 47 percent (40). The most common one is oozing around the punctured site, easily controlled by local pressure. In approximately 5 percent, blood transfusion or surgical repair of the vessel is required. Hematuria, hematemesis, hemoptysis, GI bleeding, or retroperitoneal bleeding occurs in about 14 percent. Intracranial hemorrhage occurs in up to 1.7 percent (15–17,40,59).

In assessing the efficacy and safety of thrombolytic therapy in acute stroke, spontaneous recanalization and hemorrhagic infarction in the natural course must be taken into consideration. Spontaneous recanalization of the occluded vessel secondary to intrinsic thrombolysis is known to occur, especially in embolic stroke (40,60). The probability of spontaneous recanalization in embolic stroke has been reported as 40 to 59 percent. In one report (61), 38 out of 52 (73 percent) patients were angiographically positive for emboli within 2 days of stroke, whereas 8 out of 29 (28 percent) performed after the second day showed emboli. The incidence of recanalization in thromboembolic occlusion is unknown, though it seems to be less than with embolic stroke. Spontaneous recanalization does not seem to be completed within a short period (that is, hours), as is expected in thrombolytic therapy (5,6).

Secondary hemorrhage is sometimes known to occur after cerebral infarction (hemorrhagic infarction; HI). It is related to increased permeability through ischemic endothelium, reopening of the occluded vessel due to the spontaneous recanalization or migration of the embolus, development of the collateral circulation, or rupture of the vessel secondary to necrosis (37,40,62–64). The secondary hemorrhage varies in size and pattern from a few scattered petechiae within an ischemic or infarcted tissue without mass effect (hemorrhagic transformation) to massive intracerebral hematoma (5,6). The occurrence is influenced by various factors, such as the etiology of the vessel occlusion (thrombus versus embolus), the size of the infarction, the age of the patient, the patient's medical condition (hypertension, coagulopathy, etc.), or concomitant treatment (e.g., thrombolytic therapy, anticoagulant therapy)

(5,6,40). The reported incidence of HI has been influenced by the type of study. In the pathologic examination, the frequency of HI has been reported as about 30 percent (18 to 42 percent; 51 to 71 percent in embolic stroke and 2 to 21 percent in nonembolic stroke) (40,62). The clinically or radiologically detectable evidence would be less, and one study showed that HI was observed in 5 percent within 24 h and in 20 percent within 2 weeks after the onset in CT examination (62,65). In the most recent series, the incidence of HI demonstrated on CT scan has been presumed to be 10 percent or less in occlusive stroke without anticoagulant (66). HI usually occurs within the first 2 weeks, beginning 24 to 48 h after onset (64). Significant deterioration associated with HI has been reported in 11 to 15 percent, most of which are massive intracerebral hematomas occurring within 48 h from onset (37). Since the severity of HI has been known to be influenced by thrombolytic or anticoagulant drugs, it is important to minimize the incidence of intracerebral hematoma with clinical deterioration in the processing of the protocol for intra-arterial thrombolytic therapy (ITT) (5,6).

Methods and Materials

LOGISTICAL GROUNDWORK

Because these patients must be treated quickly, sufficient understanding by all medical staff, including doctors, technologists, and nurses, is necessary to carry out this project successfully (67,68). Informational meetings with the emergency ward, neurology, and neuroradiology staff and residents are needed.

PATIENT SELECTION

In patients who are having a serious acute thromboembolic stroke, hyperacute revascularization may offer significant benefit. Differentiation of an acute stroke from a transient ischemic attack (TIA), which is defined as up to 24 h, can be difficult. However, in an extensive study on TIAs, the median duration was 14 min (69), and dense hemiplegia, global aphasia, or forced eye deviation were hardly detected (70). A trained neurologist can almost always differentiate a TIA from an acute stroke. This will be based on history, physical examination, CT, and, when indicated, additional tests such as transcranial Doppler (TCD) or EEG. MR diffusion imaging with echoplanar techniques allows for early differentiation of a stroke that is likely to progress to cerebral infarction, and if expeditiously obtained may be useful (see Chapters 2 and 10). Ongoing studies at the Massachusetts General Hospital with diffusion-weighted imaging (DWI) carried out routinely in all patients indicate that it is possible reliably to differentiate TIAs from ischemic infarction because DWI is negative to TIAs.

Only patients in whom revascularization can be completed in the hyperacute period should be offered treatment. In acute ICA territory stroke, the interval between onset and the expected completion of the treatment should not be longer than 4 to 6 h from the standpoint of hemorrhagic infarction, reperfusion injury, and reversibility of the neuronal tissue (5,6,27,28,30,32). Treatment in progressive stroke characterized as vertebrobasilar stroke can be delayed up to 24 h because of its specific pathophysiology (29,34).

Patients with conditions that would markedly enhance the risk of thrombolytic therapy should be excluded, including those with cerebral hemorrhage, recent surgery, and other conditions, as described in text following.

WORK-UP

1. Standardized neurologic examinations (Glasgow or NIH stroke) should be repeatedly given and documented. Additional tests, such as TCD (68), EEG, and blood tests are often useful.
2. An initial CT scan to exclude cerebral hemorrhage and recent infarction, MR diffusion and perfusion imaging, (follow-up CT or MRI scan to examine the progress of infarction and to rule out hemorrhagic transformation at appropriate intervals are indicated).
3. Blood tests, including of the coagulation system, are monitored to estimate systemic fibrinolytic and anticoagulant activity.
4. An initial and control angiogram prior to thrombolysis is indicated.

TECHNIQUE

1. Because localized infusion of thrombolytic agents close to or into the clot enhances the possibility of recanalization (33,34), superselective catheterization should be employed using interventional neuroradiologic technique whenever possible. When this is not possible without delay, regional infusion (common carotid, internal carotid, etc.) should be considered.
2. UK, tPA, and proUK are appropriate thrombolytic agents. SK has a longer half-life and may not be appropriate.
3. UK is available, and many workers have experience with it. High doses of short duration are thought to be desirable to achieve earlier recanalization (34). The maximum dose should be less than 1,000,000 to 1,250,000 U for fear of the anticoagulant effect of UK (30). The duration of treatment has been reported as up to 1 to 2 h in recent successful studies. Continuous infusion with a higher initial dose is also needed because of the short half-life of UK (11 to 18 min) (15–17,40).
4. Anticoagulant agents following thrombolytic treatment might increase the risk of hemorrhagic complications; however, they may help prevent reocclusion in the atherosclerotic vessel, incomplete recanalization, or new emboli in patients with persistent atrial fibrillation. Low-dose heparin appears to be an appropriate compromise. Therefore, low-dose heparinization after thrombolytic therapy under strict monitoring and controlling of PTT at one-and-a-half to twice normal value (5,6) should be considered. If there is no recanalization, heparinization is unlikely to help and is likely to contribute to bleeding.

Table 18.55.
Modified TIMI Scale: Definitions of Perfusion

Grade 0 (no perfusion):
There is no antegrade flow beyond the point of occlusion.
Grade 1 (penetration without perfusion):
The contrast material passes beyond the area of obstruction but "hangs up" and fails to opacify the entire vascular bed distal to the obstruction for the duration of the angiographic filming sequence.
Grade 2 (partial perfusion):
The contrast material passes across the obstruction. However, the rate of entry of contrast material into the vessel distal to the obstruction or its rate of clearance from the distal bed (or both) is perceptibly slower than its entry into or clearance from comparable areas not perfused by the previously occluded vessel, e.g., the opposite cerebral artery or the vascular bed proximal to the obstruction.
Grade 3 (complete perfusion):
Antegrade flow into the bed distal to the obstruction occurs as promptly as antegrade flow into the bed proximal to the obstruction, and clearance from an uninvolved bed in the same vessel or the opposite artery.

Source: N Engl J Med 1985;312:932–936, with permission.

Inclusion and exclusion criteria are under development. The following are offered as a guideline.

Inclusion Criteria:

1. Acute or progressive neurologic deficits exist consistent with acute occlusive cerebrovascular disease.
2. Angiographically demonstrated arterial occlusion with grade 0 and grade 1 perfusion (TIMI perfusion grade [20]), which are appropriate to the neurologic deficits (see Table 18.55).
3. The interval between the onset and the expected completion of ITT is within 6 h in carotid territory and 24 h in vertebrobasilar territory.

Exclusion Criteria:

1. CT scan shows recent cerebral infarction corresponding to the neurologic deficits or shows intracranial hemorrhage.
2. The patient has an AVM, an aneurysm, arterial dissection, vasculitis, or intracranial tumor.
3. The patient has minimal neurologic deficits, is in deep coma, or is already severely disabled by the previous neurologic disorder.
4. The patient has a known allergic reaction to contrast material or thrombolytic agents.
5. The patient has one or more of the following:
   - An uncompensated coagulopathy or anticoagulant therapy compromising coagulation activity
   - An unstable cardiopulmonary condition, uncontrolled hypertension, severe hepatic disorder, or renal disorder
   - Another serious medical condition, such as cancer, severe congenital disorder, severe malnutrition, or severe infection
6. The patient has a history of one or more of the following:
   - A hemorrhagic insult, including intracranial hemorrhage, GI bleeding, hematuria, or hemoptysis, within 3 months
   - A major surgery or major trauma within 1 month
   - A vascular occlusive disease, including cerebral infarction, myocardial infarction, or other visceral or peripheral arterial occlusion, within 1 month
7. The patient is in pregnancy or its possibility, lactation, or parturition within 1 month.

Catheterization

Angiography can be done by the transfemoral approach with a sheath introducer using a conventional 5.5F angiographic catheter with digital subtraction angiography (DSA). After the angiographic study, a microcatheter is positioned into or over the clot. Any available microcatheters can be used. However, flow-guided catheterization is usually difficult in arterial occlusions, and wire-guided catheterization utilizing a superselective infusion catheter and steerable guidewire (e.g., Tracker-18)* is usually employed through a coaxial 5.5F guiding catheter. The position of the tip of the catheter can be advanced with a short interruption of drug administration, if necessary. The sheath introduced is left in place after the procedure with continuous infusion of flush solution and is removed on the next day (24 h after treatment).

Dose and Rate of Thrombolytic Agent

The optimal dose and rate of thrombolytic agents are not known, and the following is offered for consideration. Continuous infusion of thrombolytic agents is started with an initially high concentration. UK is administered in pulses at an overall rate of 7500 U/kg in the first 8 min, followed by 7500 U/kg in the subsequent 16 min (7500 U/kg in 10 ml of saline). Infusion is discontinued when grade 3 reperfusion (complete reperfusion) is acquired, or stopped after 90 min. (Figure 18.47a).

Concomitant Treatment

The status of additional anticoagulant therapy is unclear and in the past has been withheld as far as possible after thrombolysis. However, low-dose heparin administered under controlling PTT at one-and-a-half to twice normal value after thrombolytic therapy may well be useful. Conventional treatments such as hypervolemic therapy, hemodilution therapy, hyperosmolar agents for brain swelling, vasodilators for microcirculation, pharmacologic cell protection drugs or antiplatelet drugs, and anticoagulants should be administered as needed.

POSTHROMBOLYSIS MONITORING

After intra-arterial thrombolysis, patients need to be admitted to the neurology intensive care unit, where their vital signs and physical and neurologic status can be continuously monitored. Neurologic examination, CT scan, laboratory tests, and TCD should be performed as needed. Neurologic examination should be carried out more frequently, depending on the patient's condition. CT scan

* Target, Temecula, Calif.

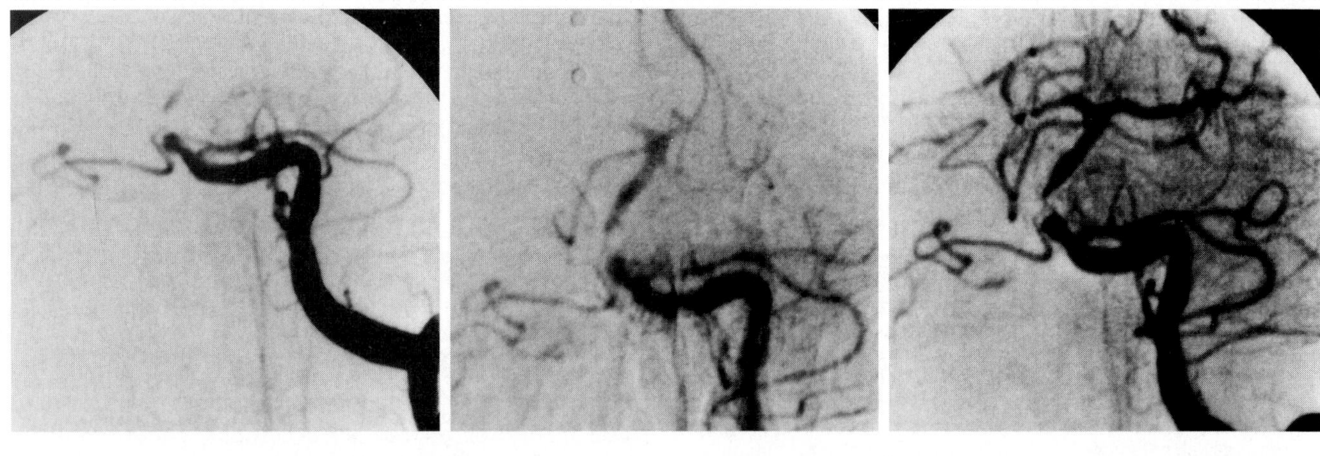

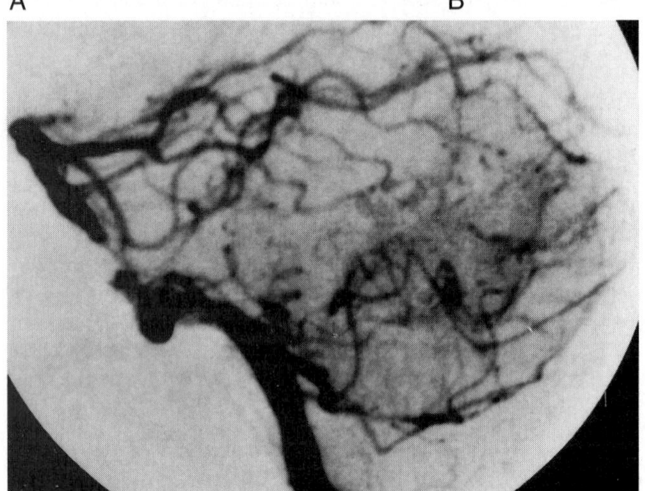

Figure 18.47. Acute basilar artery (BA) thrombolysis in a 69-year-old male. **A.** Left vertebral artery angiogram, anteroposterior view, shows total BA occlusion. **B.** Left vertebral artery angiogram, anteroposterior view, before thrombolysis shows progressive BA opening. **C** and **D.** Left vertebral artery angiogram after thrombolysis (C, anteroposterior view; D, lateral view). The patient received a total of 900,000 IU of UK in situ. The view shows the patency of the distal BA and branches. Note the residual area of tight stenosis in the proximal BA.

and TCD should be performed if unexpected deterioration occurs. Emergency angiography may be considered when these results suggest reocclusion.

Standard neurologic examinations are essential, since the patient's status is quite dynamic and trends are essential to follow. Evaluation of deficits using the modified NIH stroke scale (71,72) (Table 18.56) or the Glasgow coma scale at baseline (prethrombolysis, immediately, and 12 h after thrombolysis) as well as daily is needed to follow these patients. Clinical outcome should also be evaluated by the Barthel index (Table 18.57) at 6 months after treatment.

TCD can be beneficial in bedside evaluation of the patency of the occluded or recanalized vessel (68), obtained as a baseline, at the end of thrombolysis, and repeated daily. Noncontrast CT scan at baseline, 1 week, and 1 month after the onset to assess the progress of cerebral infarction and to rule out hemorrhagic transformation is indicated. CT scan is indicated if the patient deteriorates. Laboratory tests including coagulation parameters should be carried out to estimate systemic fibrinolytic and anticoagulant activities at baseline, immediately, and 12 h after in any group treated by ITT. The items to be monitored are the same as those in the preentry initial examination.

All patients should have an ECG and cardiac enzymes to rule out acute myocardial infarction as well as ectopy. Most patients will require a cardiac echo to look for the source of the emboli and to assess wall motion. These tests should be done early, since optimal cardiac function is essential.

POSTTHROMBOLYSIS MANAGEMENT

It is beyond the scope of this book to do any more than suggest some of the challenges in caring for these patients. Excellent textbooks in the care of neurologic and nonneurologic intensive care are available.

Acute stroke patients are usually very ill, usually with multisystem disease. Concomitant cardiovascular disease is the rule, and acute myocardial ischemia or infarction is frequently seen. Most of these patients are older and have significant risk factors for arteriosclerotic vascular disease. Also increasing significantly are other age-related conditions, such as diabetes, chronic obstructive pulmonary dis-

Table 18.56.
Neurologic Stroke Scale (modified from NIH Stroke Scale)

Domain	Score	Description
Level of consciousness[*1]	0	Alert
	1	Drowsy
	2	Stuporous
	3	Coma
consciousness questions[t2]	0	Answers both correctly
	1	Answers one correctly
	2	Answers both incorrectly
consciousness commands[*3]	0	Obeys both correctly
	1	Obeys one correctly
	2	Obeys both incorrectly
Best gaze[*4]	0	Normal
	1	Partial gaze palsy
	2	Forced deviation
Best visual field[*5]	0	No visual loss
	1	Partial hemianopia
	2	Complete hemianopia
	3	Bilateral hemianopia
Facial palsy	0	Normal
	1	Minor
	2	Partial
	3	Complete
Best motor arm[*6]	0	No drift
	1	Drift
	2	Can't resist gravity
	3	No effort against gravity
	4	No movement
Opposite arm[*6] (brainstem stroke)	0	No drift
	1	Drift
	2	Can't resist gravity
	3	No effort against gravity
	4	No movement
Best motor leg[*7]	0	No drift
	1	Drift
	2	Can't resist gravity
	3	No effort against gravity
	4	No movement
Opposite leg[*7]	0	No drift
	1	Drift
	2	Can't resist gravity
	3	No effort against gravity
	4	No movement
Limb ataxia[*8]	0	Absent
	1	Present in either upper or lower
	2	Present in both upper and lower
Sensory[*9]	0	Normal
	1	Partial loss
	2	Dense loss
Neglect[*10]	0	None
	1	Partial
	2	Complete
Dysarthria[*11]	0	Normal articulation
	1	Mild to moderate dysarthria
	2	Near unintelligible or worse
Best language[*12]	0	No aphasia
	1	Mild to moderate aphasia
	2	Severe aphasia
	3	Mute

Sources: T Brott, et al: Stroke 1989;20:864–870; and LB Goldstein, C Bertels, JN Davis: Arch Neurol 1989;46:660–662.

*1 0: alert, keenly responsive. 1: drowsy, but arousable by minor stimulation to obey, answer, or respond. 2: requires repeated stimulation to attend, or lethargic or obtund requiring strong or painful stimulation to make movements (not stereotyped). 3: responds only with reflex motor or autonomic effects, or totally unresponsive, flaccid, reflexless.

*2 The patient is asked the month and his or her age; only the initial answer is graded. 0: answers both correctly. 1: answers one correctly. 2: answers both incorrectly or unable to speak.

*3 The patient is instructed to open or close his or her hand or eyes; only initial responses are graded; credit is given if an unequivocal attempt is made but not completed. 0: obeys both correctly. 1: obeys one correctly. 2: incorrect.

*4 0: normal. 1: partial gaze palsy; score is given when gaze is abnormal in one or both eyes, but when forced deviation or total gaze paresis is not present. 2: forced deviation or total gaze paresis not overcome by the oculocephalic maneuver.

*5 Test for hemianopia using moving fingers on confrontation with both of patient's eyes open; double simultaneous stimulation is also performed; use visual threat where level of consciousness or comprehension limits testing, but score 1 only if clear-cut asymmetry is found; complete hemianopia [score 2] is recorded for dense loss extending to within 5 to 10 degrees of fixation. 0: no visual loss. 1: partial hemianopia. 2: complete hemianopia.

*6 Patient is examined with arms outstretched at 90 degrees if sitting, or at 45 degrees if supine; request full effort for 10 sec; if consciousness or comprehension is abnormal, cue the patient by actively lifting his or her arms into position as request for effort is orally given. 0: limb holds for 90 degrees for full 10 sec. 1: limb holds 90 degrees but drifts before full 10 sec. 2: limb cannot hold 90-degree position for full 10 sec, but there is some effort against gravity. 3: limb falls, no effort against gravity, but there is some movement. 4: no movement.

*7 While supine, patient is asked to maintain weaker leg at 30 degrees for 5 sec; if consciousness or comprehension is abnormal, cue the patient by actively lifting the leg into position as the request for effort is orally given. 0: leg holds 30-degree position for 5-sec period. 1: leg falls to intermediate position by the end of the 5-sec period. 2: leg falls to bed by 5 sec, but there is some effort against gravity. 3: leg falls to bed immediately with no effort against gravity. 4: no movement.

*8 Finger-to-nose and heel-to-shin tests are performed; ataxia is scored only if clearly out of proportion to weakness; limb ataxia would be "absent" in the hemiplegic, not untestable. 0: absent. 1: ataxia is present in one limb. 2: ataxia is present in two limbs.

*9 Test with pin; when consciousness or comprehension is abnormal, score sensory normal unless deficit is clearly recognized (e.g., by clear-cut grimace asymmetry, withdrawal asymmetry); only hemisensory losses are counted as abnormal. 0: normal, no sensory loss. 1: mild to moderate; patient feels pinprick is less sharp or is dull on the affected side; or there is a loss of superficial pain with pinprick but patient is aware of being touched. 2: severe-to-total sensation loss; the patient is not aware of being touched.

*10 0: no neglect. 1: visual, tactile, or auditory hemi-inattention. 2: profound hemi-inattention to more than one modality.

*11 0: normal. 1: mild to moderate; patient slurs at least some words, and, at worst, can be understood with some difficulty. 2: patient's speech is so slurred as to be unintelligible (in absence of, or out of proportion to, any dysphasia).

*12 The patient is asked naming and reading; comprehension is judged from responses to all of the commands in the preceding general neurologic examination: 0: normal. 1: mild to moderate, as follows: naming errors, word-finding errors, paraphasias, and/or impairment of comprehension or expression disability. 2: severe: fully developed Broca or Wernicke aphasia (or variant). 3: mute or global aphasia.

Table 18.57.
Barthel Index

Index item	Score weight	Description
1. Feeding	10	Independent (able to apply any necessary device, feeds in reasonable time)
	5	Needs help (e.g., for cutting)
2. Bathing	5	Performs without assistance
3. Personal toilet (grooming)	5	Washes face, combs hair, brushes teeth, shaves (manages plug if electric razor)
4. Dressing	10	Independent (ties shoes, fastens fasteners, applies braces)
	5	Needs help (at least half of task within reasonable time)
5. Bowel control	10	No accidents (able to use enema or suppository, if needed)
	5	Occasional accidents (or needs help with enema or suppository)
6. Bladder control	10	No accidents (able to care for collecting device if used)
	5	Occasional accidents (or needs help with device)
7. Toilet transfers	10	Independent (with toilet or bedpan; handles clothes, wipes, flushes, or cleans pan)
	5	Needs help (for balance, handling clothes or toilet paper)
8. Chair/bed transfers	15	Independent (including locks of wheelchair and lifting footrests)
	10	Minimum assistance (or supervision)
	5	Able to sit but needs maximum assistance to transfer
9. Ambulations	15	Independent for 50 yards (may use assistive devices, except for rolling walker)
	10	With help for 50 yards
	5	Wheelchair for 50 yards (only if unable to walk)
10. Stair climbing	10	Independent (may use assistive devices)
	5	Needs help (or supervision)

Sources: RJ Adams, FT Nichols, WO Thompson, in Clinical Trial Methodology in Stroke, London: Baillere Tindal, 1989, pp 54–74; and FI Mahoney and DW Barthel: Md State Med 1965;14:61–65.

ease, obesity, and a history of smoking. Age also brings a decreased physiologic reserve and recuperative potential. In treating the stroke patient in the hyperacute setting, it is best to assume that all of these concomitant conditions are present and exclude them by tests. Finesse and gentleness in treatment is needed.

Cardiac function will often need to be optimized. Early in the course, relative hypertension with hypervolemia may be useful, whereas a few hours later, relative hypovolemic hypotension may be indicated.

Pulmonary function is equally critical, since retained P_{CO_2} or falling P_{O_2} can compromise the ischemic brain significantly by increasing intracranial pressure and thus tissue pressure or by decreasing the O_2 being delivered to the tissue.

Even a low-grade fever significantly decreases the brain's ability to withstand ischemia and needs to be treated vigorously.

Future Trends

Studies of acute revascularization in stroke patients will in the near future help delineate its role in treatment. A greater understanding of the "therapeutic window" will lead to better patient selection and enlarging of that window.

REFERENCES

1. Astrup J, Siesjö BK, Symon L: Thresholds in cerebral ischemia: The ischemic penumbra. Stroke 1981;12:723–725.
2. Crowell RM, Olsson Y, Klatzo I, Ommaya A: Temporary occlusion of the middle cerebral artery in the monkey. Stroke 1970;1:439–448.
3. Jones TH, Morawetz RB, Crowell RM, et al: Thresholds of focal cerebral ischemia in awake monkeys. J Neurosurg 1981;54:773–782.
4. Solis OJ, Roberson GR, Taveras JM, Mohr J, Pessin M: Cerebral angiography in acute cerebral infarction. Rev Interam Radiol 1977; 2:19–25.
5. del Zoppo GJ, Zeumer H, Harker LA: Thrombolytic therapy in stroke: Possibilities and hazards. Stroke 1986;17:595–607.
6. del Zoppo GJ: Thrombolytic therapy in cerebrovascular disease. Stroke 1988;19:1174–1179.
7. Toole JF: Cerebrovascular Disorders, ed 4. New York: Raven, 1990, p 293.
8. Greham GE: The rehabilitation of the stroke survivor. In HM Barnett, JP Mohr, BM Stein, FM Yatsu (eds), Stroke: Pathophysiology, Diagnosis, and Management. New York: Churchill Livingstone, 1986, pp 1259–1274.
9. Abe T, Kazawa M, Naito I: Clinical evaluation for efficacy of tissue culture urokinase (TCUK) on cerebral thrombosis by means of multicenter double blind study. Blood Vessels 1981;12:321–341.
10. Abe T, Kazawa M, Naito I: Clinical effect of urokinase (60,000 units/day) on cerebral infarction: Comparative study by means of multicenter double blind test. Blood Vessels 1981;12:342–358.
11. Fletcher AP, Alkjaersig N, Lewis M, et al: A pilot study of urokinase therapy in cerebral infarction. Stroke 1976;7:135–142.
12. Hanaway J, Torack R, Fletcher AP, Landau WM: Intracranial bleeding associated with urokinase therapy for acute ischemic hemispheral stroke. Stroke 1976;7:143–146.
13. Herndon RM, Nelson JN, Johnson JF, Meyer JS: Thrombolytic treatment in cerebrovascular thrombosis. In RL MacMillan, JF Mustard (eds), Anticoagulants and Fibrinolysis. Philadelphia: Lea and Febiger, 1961, pp 154–164.
14. Meyer JS, Gilroy J, Barnhart ME, Johnson JF: Therapeutic thrombolysis in cerebral thromboembolism: Randomized evaluation of intravenous streptokinase. In CH Millikan, RG Siekert, JP Whisnant (eds), Cerebral Vascular Diseases, Fourth Princeton Conference. New York: Grune and Stratton, 1965, pp 200–213.
15. Marder VJ, Bell WR: Fibrinolytic therapy. In RW Colman, J Hirsh, VJ Marder, EW Salzman (eds), Hemostasis and Thrombosis. Philadelphia: Lippincott, 1987, pp 1393–1437.
16. Marder VJ, Sherry S: Thrombolytic therapy: Current status (first of two parts). N Engl J Med 1988;318:1512–1520.
17. Marder VJ, Sherry S: Thrombolytic therapy: Current status (second of two parts). N Engl J Med 1988;318:1585–1595.

18. Garabedian HD, Gold HK, Leinbach RC, Yasuda T, Johns JA, Collen D: Dose-dependent thrombolysis, pharmacokinetics and hemostatic effects of recombinant human tissue-type plasminogen activator for coronary thrombosis. Am J Cardiol 1986;58:673–679.
19. NIH Consensus Conference: Thrombolytic therapy in treatment. Br Med J 1980;280:1585–1587.
20. TIMI Study Group: The thrombolysis in myocardial infarction (TIMI) trial. N Engl J Med 1985;312:932–936.
21. Yasuda T, Gold HK. Acute myocardial infarction and thrombolytic therapy. Thromb Res 1990;10 (suppl):73–79.
22. Brott T, Haley EC, Levy DE, et al: Investigational use of tPA for stroke. Ann Emerg Med 1988;17:1202–1205.
23. Brott T, Haley EC, Levy D, et al: Safety and potential efficacy of tissue plasminogen activator (tPA) for stroke. Stroke 1990;21:181.
24. del Zoppo GJ: Investigational use of tPA in acute stroke. Ann Emerg Med 1988;17:1196–1201.
25. The rt-PA/Acute stroke study group: An open safety/efficacy trial of rt-PA in acute thromboembolic stroke: Final report. Stroke 1991; 22:153.
26. The tPA-acute stroke study group: An open multicenter study of the safety and efficacy of various doses of rt-PA in patients with acute stroke: Preliminary results. Stroke 1990;21:181.
27. del Zoppo GJ, Copeland BR, Waltz TA, Zyroff J, Plow EF, Harker LA: The beneficial effect of intracarotid urokinase on acute stroke in a baboon model. Stroke 1986;17:638–643.
28. del Zoppo GJ, Ferbert A, Otis S, et al: Local intra-arterial fibrinolytic therapy in acute carotid territory stroke: Pilot study. Stroke 1988;19:307–313.
29. Hacke W, Zeumer H, Ferbert A, Brückmann H, del Zoppo GJ: Intra-arterial thrombolytic therapy improves outcome in patients with acute vertebrobasilar occlusive disease. Stroke 1988;19: 1216–1222.
30. Mori E, Tabuchi M, Yoshida T, Yamadori A: Intracarotid urokinase with thromboembolic occlusion of the middle cerebral artery. Stroke 1989;19:802–812.
31. Nenci GG, Gresele P, Taramelli M, Agnelli G, Signotini E: Thrombolytic therapy for thromboembolism of vertebrobasilar artery. Angiology 1983;34:561–571.
32. Theron J, Courtheoux P, Casasco A, et al: Local intraarterial fibrinolysis in the carotid territory. AJNR 1989;10:753–765.
33. Jungreis CA, Wechsler LR, Horton JA: Intracranial thrombolysis via a catheter embedded in the clot. Stroke 1989;20:1578–1580.
34. Zeumer H, Freitag HJ, Grzyska U, Neunzig HP: Local intraarterial fibrinolysis in acute vertebrobasilar occlusion: Technical developments and recent results. Neuroradiology 1989;31:336–340.
35. Zeumer H, Hacke W, Ringelstein EB: Local intraarterial thrombolysis in vertebrobasilar thromboembolic disease. AJNR 1983;4: 401–404.
36. Zeumer H, Hundgen R, Ferbert A, Ringelstein EB: Local intraarterial fibrinolytic therapy in inaccessible internal carotid occlusion. Neuroradiology 1984;26:315–317.
37. Hornig CR, Dorndorf W, Agnoli AL: Hemorrhagic cerebral infarction: A prospective study. Stroke 1986;17:179–185.
38. Tsai F, Shah D, Matovich V, Alfieri K: Intra-arterial therapy for acute cerebral infarction and progressive stroke. Proc ASNR 1988; 26:288.
39. Maiza D, Theron J, Pelouze GA, et al: Local fibrinolytic therapy in ischemic carotid pathology. Ann Vasc Surg 1988;2:205–214.
40. Sloan MA: Thrombosis and stroke: Past and future. Arch Neurol 1987;44:748–768.
41. Bednar MM, McAuliffe T, Raymond S, Gross CE: Tissue plasminogen activator reduces brain injury in a rabbit model of thromboembolic stroke. Stroke 1990;21:1705–1709.
42. Chehrazi BB, Seibert JA, Kissel P, Hein L, Brock JM: Evaluation of recombinant tissue plasminogen activator in embolic stroke. Neurosurgery 1989;24:355–360.
43. Kissel P, Chehrazi B, Seibert JA, Wagner FC Jr: Digital angiographic quantification of blood flow dynamics in embolic stroke treated with tissue–type plasminogen activator. J Neurosurg 1987; 67:399–405.
44. Lyden PD, Zivin JA, Clark WA, et al: Tissue plasminogen activator–mediated thrombolysis of cerebral emboli and its effect on hemorrhagic infarction in rabbits. Neurology 1989;39:703–708.
45. Papadopoulos SM, Chandler WF, Salamat MS, Topol EJ, Sackellares JC: Recombinant human tissue-type plasminogen activator therapy in acute thromboembolic stroke. J Neurosurg 1987;67: 394–398.
46. Penar PL, Greer CA: The effect of intravenous tissue-type plasminogen activator in a rat model of embolic cerebral ischemia. Yale J Biol Med 1987;60:233–243.
47. Phillips DA, Davis MA, Fisher M: Selective embolization and clot dissolution with tPA in the internal carotid artery circulation of the rabbit. AJNR 1988;9:899–902.
48. Zivin JA, Lyden PD, DeGirolami U, et al: Tissue plasminogen activator: Reduction of neurologic damage after experimental embolic stroke. Arch Neurol 1988;45:387–391.
49. Lyden PD, Madden KP, Clark WA, Sasses KC, Zivin JA: Incidence of cerebral hemorrhage after antifibrinolytic treatment for embolic stroke in rabbits. Stroke 1990;21:1589–1593.
50. Phillips DA, Fisher M, Davis MA, Smith TW, Pang RHL: Delayed treatment with a t-PA analogue and streptokinase in a rabbit embolic stroke model. Stroke 1990;21:602–605.
51. Benes V, Zabramski JM, Boston M, Puca A, Apetzler RF: Effect of intra-arterial antifibrinolytic agents on autologous arterial emboli in the cerebral circulation of rabbits. Stroke 1990;21:1594–1599.
52. Kawakami K, Takahashi A, Yoshimoto T: An experimental study of local fibrinolysis using tissue plasminogen activator and urokinase in a canine common carotid thrombus model. No To Shinkei 1990; 42:193–201.
53. del Zoppo GJ, Copeland BR, Anderchek K, Hacke W, Koziol JA: Hemorrhagic transformation following tissue plasminogen activator in experimental cerebral infarction. Stroke 1990;21:596–601.
54. Slivka A, Pulsinelli W: Hemorrhagic complications of thrombolytic therapy in experimental stroke. Stroke 1987;18:1148–1156.
55. Wildemann B, Hutschenreuter M, Krieger D, Hacke W, von Kummer R: Infusion of recombinant tissue plasminogen activator for treatment of basilar artery occlusion. Stroke 1990;21:1513–1514.
56. Henze T, Boeer A, Tebbe U, Romatowski J: Lysis of basilar artery occlusion with tissue plasminogen activator. Lancet 1987;2:1391.
57. Buteux G, Jubault V, Suisse A, Courtheoux P: Local recombinant tissue plasminogen activator to clear cerebral artery thrombosis developing soon after surgery. Lancet 1988;2:1143–1144.
58. Takahashi A, Sugawara K, Mizoi K, Yoshimoto T, Fujimori K, So K: Superselective local thrombolysis for acute MCA embolism utilizing tPA. Abstracts of Sixth Annual Meeting of Japanese Society for Intravascular Neurosurgery Paper II, 29, 1990.
59. Aldrich MS, Sherman SA, Greenberg HS: Cerebrovascular complications of streptokinase infusion. JAMA 1985;253:1777–1779.
60. Dalal PM, Shah PM, Sheth SL, Deshpande CK: Cerebral embolism: Angiographic observation on spontaneous clot lysis. Lancet 1965; 1:61–64.
61. Mohr JP, Caplan LR, Melski JW, et al: The Harvard Cooperative Stroke Registry: A prospective registry. Neurology 1978;28: 754–762.
62. Hart RG, Easton JD: Hemorrhagic infarcts. Stroke 1986;17: 586–589.
63. Okada Y, Yamaguchi T, Minematsu K, et al: Hemorrhagic transformation in cerebral embolism. Stroke 1989;20:598–603.
64. Ott BR, Zamani A, Kleefield J, Funkenstein HH: The clinical spectrum of hemorrhagic infarction. Stroke 1986;4:630–637.
65. Lodder J: CT-detected hemorrhagic infarction: Relation with size of the infarct, and the presence of midline shift. Acta Neurol Scand 1984;70:329–335.

66. Fisher M, Zito JL, Siva A, DeGirolami U: Hemorrhagic infarction: A clinical and CT study. Stroke 1984;15:192.
67. Barsan WG, Brott TG, Olinger CP, Adams HP Jr, Haley EC Jr, Levy DE: Identification and entry of the patient with acute cerebral infarction. Ann Emerg Med 1988;17:1192–1195.
68. Fieschi C, Argentino C, Lenzi GL, Sacchetti ML, Toni D, Bozzao L: Clinical and instrumental evaluation of patients with ischemic stroke within the first six hours. J Neurol Sci 1989;91:311–322.
69. Dyken ML, Conneally PM, Haerer AF, et al: Cooperative study of hospital frequency and character of transient ischemic attacks: I. Background, organization, and clinical survey. JAMA 1977;237: 882–886.
70. Price TR, Gotshall RA, Poskanzer DC, et al: Cooperative study of hospital frequency and character of transient ischemic attacks: VI. Patients examined during an attack. JAMA 1977;238:2512–2515.
71. Brott T, Adams HP Jr, Olinger CP, et al: Measurements of acute cerebral infarction: A clinical examination scale. Stroke 1989;20: 864–870.
72. Goldstein LB, Bertels C, Davis JN: Interrater reliability of the NIH stroke scale. Arch Neurol 1989;46:660–662.

SELECTED READINGS

Adams RJ, Nichols FT, Thompson WO: Neurological assessment in acute stroke issues in the use of rating scales. In WK Amery, MG Boursser, FC Rose (eds), Clinical Trial Methodology in Stroke. London: Baillere Tindal, 1989, pp 54–74.

Bartlett RH, Roloff DW, Cornell RG, Andrews AF, Dillon PW, Zwischenberger JB: Extracorporeal circulation in neonatal respiratory failure: A prospective randomized study. Pediatrics 1985;76:479–487.

Berenstein A, Choi IS, Kuppersmith M, Flam E, Kricheff II, Madrid M: Complications of endovascular embolization in 182 patients with cerebral AVMs. Proc ASNR 27:57, 1989.

Earnst F IV, Forbes G, Sandok BA, et al: Complications of cerebral angiography: Prospective assessment of risk. AJR 1984;142:247–253.

Hacke W (ed): Neurocritical Care. Berlin: Springer, 1994.

Hankey GJ, Warlow CP, Sellar RJ: Cerebral angiographic risk in mild cerebrovascular disease. Stroke 1990;21:209–222.

Mahoney FI, Barthel DW: Functional evaluation. The Barthel Index. Md State Med 1965;14:61–65.

Ropper AH (ed): Neurological and Neurosurgical Intensive Care, ed 3. New York: Raven Press, 1993.

Wei LJ, Durham S: The randomized play-the-winner rule in medical trial. J Am Stat Assoc 1978;73:840–843.

Zelen M: Play the winner rule and the controlled clinical trial. J Am Stat Assoc 1969;64:131–146.

Zelen M: A new design for randomized clinical trials. N Engl J Med 1979; 300:1242–1245.

18.10 Brachiocephalic Angioplasty

Key Points

1. Stenotic disease of brachiocephalic vessel origin is effectively and safely treated by angioplasty.
2. Stenotic disease of the low to mid-cervical internal carotid bulb is well treated by surgery. Angioplasty should be considered for patients for whom surgical risks are thought excessive.
3. Stenotic disease of the high cervical and intracranial internal carotid and vertebral arteries can be effectively treated with angioplasty.
4. Techniques for angioplasty are undergoing changes.

Stroke is the third leading cause of death in the United States. It is estimated that there are over 2 million survivors of strokes in the United States and that each year over 150,000 people die from strokes. At least two-fifths of these strokes are caused by atherothrombotic events, and a large number are unclassifiable. The incidence is related to age, increasing from about 2/1000 at age 50 to nearly 18/1000 at age 80.

Treatment indications and options for stenotic disease of the great vessels are changing. Prophylactic surgical endarterectomy for carotid arteries narrowed by more than 70 percent by (ASVD) significantly decreases the stroke rate in patients. Prophylactic angioplasty for cerebral vascular disease is an uncharted territory. The experience with angioplasty in the peripheral vascular bed has shown that it can keep blood vessels open in more than 85 percent of patients for over 3 years and that it has a very low complication rate. Angioplasty has been performed for vessels of any size, from the aorta to the popliteals, on systemic and pulmonary arteries as well as on systemic veins, on native vessels and on operated vessels, and in the angiography suite as well as in the operating room. Although results vary, there is every indication that it is a well-tolerated procedure (1–11).

Between the islands of data is the uncharted territory of the role of angioplasty for stroke prophylaxis. Acute cerebral resuscitation by cerebral revascularization lies well past these islands of knowledge and has been a frustrating goal, fostering therapeutic nihilism even in the optimistic. However, our understanding of the pathophysiology of cerebral ischemia has increased tremendously. Dynamic imaging (CT, MRI/MRA, US/TCD, SPECT/PET) has allowed increased understanding of the disease processes not possible until recently. Optimism is indicated. Treatment of carefully selected patients in well-controlled studies will hopefully make possible successful intervention and greater understanding of the expanding role of interventional neuroradiology in the treatment of stenotic and occlusive disease. Specific indications for specific diseases with specific interventions and specific limitations will need to be delineated.

Background

Angioplasty of the brachiocephalic arteries is a viable therapeutic option. Concerns regarding distal emboli continue but can be minimized with proper patient selection and technical advances (see contraindications in text following).

The rate of restenosis appears to be higher than that of direct surgical approaches, and this limitation is under vigorous study.

CAROTID ANGIOPLASTY

Although carotid disease is far more common than brachiocephalic disease, endovascular methods have been slow to develop because surgery is an excellent therapy, with a high success rate and a low complication burden. In spite of this, preliminary experience with angioplasty of the carotid artery has been very encouraging (12). When data are pooled from reported cases, it appears that technical success (90 to 98 percent) and a low complication rate (2 to 5 percent) make it comparable to direct surgical methods. Angioplasty for the carotid artery may in the near future be reserved for restenosis, inflammatory disease, hemodynamically unstable patients, and patients with strokes in evolution.

Carotid angioplasty has been effective for difficult situations such as stroke in evolution and recurrent stenosis (Fig. 18.48). Progressive strokes in the middle cerebral artery territory can also be treated even if they require percutaneous transluminal angioplasty (PTA) of multiple brachiocephalic

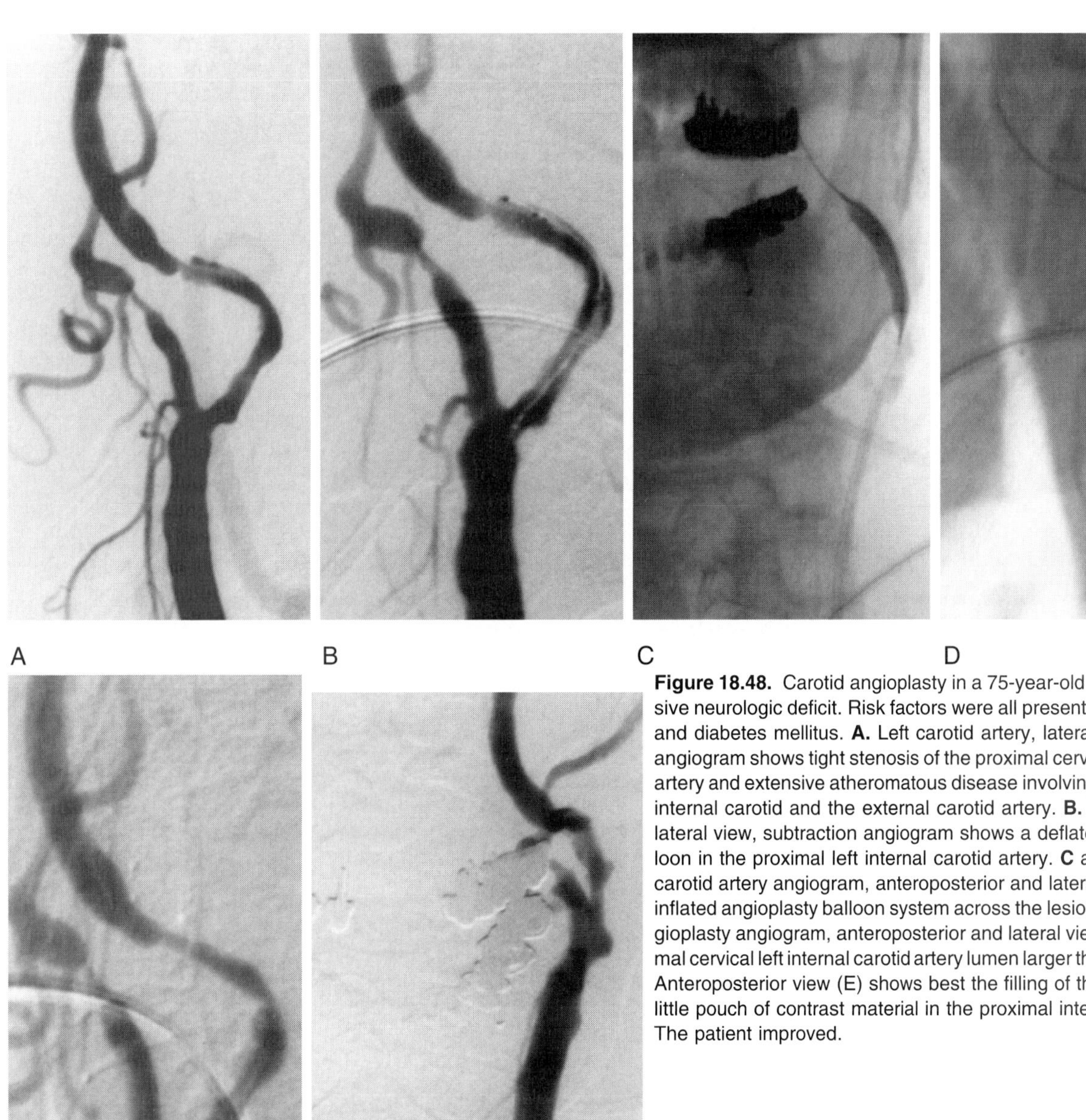

Figure 18.48. Carotid angioplasty in a 75-year-old male with progressive neurologic deficit. Risk factors were all present: age, tobacco use, and diabetes mellitus. **A.** Left carotid artery, lateral view, subtraction angiogram shows tight stenosis of the proximal cervical internal carotid artery and extensive atheromatous disease involving both the proximal internal carotid and the external carotid artery. **B.** Left carotid artery, lateral view, subtraction angiogram shows a deflated angioplasty balloon in the proximal left internal carotid artery. **C** and **D.** Left internal carotid artery angiogram, anteroposterior and lateral views, shows an inflated angioplasty balloon system across the lesion. **E** and **F.** Postangioplasty angiogram, anteroposterior and lateral views, shows a proximal cervical left internal carotid artery lumen larger than preangioplasty. Anteroposterior view (E) shows best the filling of the intimal tear as a little pouch of contrast material in the proximal internal carotid artery. The patient improved.

Table 18.58.
Carotid Angioplasty Experience

Study	*N:* att/pt/l*	Patency t† = 0	Patency at time	Complications: Dead/Major/Minor	Cerebral protection	Comments
Kerber	1/1	1	?	0/0	No	Common carotid
Mullan	1/1	1	?	0/0	No	Internal carotid
Tsai	34/27/29	?	?	0/0/0	No	Carotid
Becker	?/?/165	85%		3.6%	No	
Kachel	?/?/37	92.5%	?	4%	No	
Theron	?/?/123	?	?	(9%→→0%)	No→Yes	

Kerber CW, Cromwell LD, Loehden OL: Catheter dilatation of proximal stenosis during distal bifurcation endarterectomy. AJNR 1980;1:348–349.
Mullan S, Duda EE, Patro NAS: Some examples of balloon technology in neurosurgery. J Neurosurg 52:321–329, 1980.
Tsai FY, Higashida RT, Matovich V, et al: Seven year's experience with PTA of carotid artery. Neuroradiology 33(suppl):397–398, 1991.
Becker GJ, Katzen BT, Dake MD: Noncoronary angioplasty. Radiology 170:921–940, 1989.
Kachel R, Endert G, Basche S, Grossman, Glaser F: Percutaneous transluminal angioplasty (dilatation) of carotid, vertebral and innominate artery stenoses. Cardiovasc Intervent Radiol 1987;10:142–146.
Theron J: Angioplasty of brachiocephalic vessel. In Vinuela F, Halbark VV, Jaryl ED, (eds), Interventional Neuroradiology: Endovascular therapy of the CNS, Chap 13. New York: Raven Press, 1992:167–180.
* att/pt/l = attempted angioplasty/number of patients/lesions treated
† t = time

vessels: in these patients surgery and general anesthesia would probably be very risky (13). Angioplasty and thrombolysis can be used together, for example, to treat underlying stenosis or distal emboli. Total thrombotic occlusion of the cervical internal carotid artery with distal embolic occlusion of the ipsilateral middle cerebral artery can be treated with intra-arterial fibrinolysis and balloon angioplasty. Endovascular treatment for a totally occluded internal carotid artery is indicated in the very early stage when there is no thrombus or a short thrombus that can be evacuated (14). Angioplasty of recurrent stenosis after endarterectomy has been reported to be effective though not without some difficulty (15). In one series, 7 patients with hemodynamic transient ischemic attacks and decreased cerebral vascular reserve were successfully treated with PTA (Table 18.58) (16).

BRACHIOCEPHALIC/SUBCLAVIAN/ VERTEBRAL ANGIOPLASTY

Arguably, angioplasty appears to be the treatment of choice for inflammatory and atherosclerotic stenoses of the main trunks arising from the aortic arch (Table 18.59). Stenoses of the origin of the vertebral artery are not often ulcerated and may also be treated by angioplasty as long as the stenosis has been recognized as the cause of vertebral insufficiency symptoms, particularly when they are recognized early by Doppler examination (12). Angioplasty is suitable for management of a selected group of patients with nonocclusive vertebral artery lesions leaving some degree of antegrade flow, in whom a subclavian steal phenomenon is evident in the initial angiogram, thus putting them at high risk of cerebral embolization during angioplasty (17).

In another series of 46 patients with *subclavian artery stenosis* and brachial or cerebral symptoms, PTA was reported to be successful in 83 percent (18). The complications that were observed were residual stenosis ($n = 2$) and thrombotic material on the arterial wall ($n = 5$); the patients were treated with self-expandable stents. Residual stenoses were considered by the authors to have been successfully treated with stents. There were no cerebral or brachial complications. During a mean follow-up of 33

Table 18.59.
Noncarotid Brachiocephalic Experience

Study	*N:* att/pt/l*	Patency t† = 0	Patency at time	Complications: Dead/Major/Minor	Cerebral protection	Comments
Becker	?/?/258	92%	?	?/1/4	?	pooled
Kachel	?/?/75	92%		9%	No	
Theron	?/?/144	95%				
Higashida	?/?/42	93%		7%	No	Vertebrobasilar

Tsai FY, Higashida RT, Matovich V, et al: Seven year's experience with PTA of carotid artery. Neuroradiology 33(suppl):397–398, 1991.
Becker GJ, Katzen BT, Dake MD: Noncoronary angioplasty. Radiology 170:921–940, 1989.
Kachel R, Endert G, Basche S, Grossman, Glaser F: Percutaneous transluminal angioplasty (dilatation) of carotid, vertebral and innominate artery stenoses. Cardiovasc Intervent Radiol 1987;10:142–146.
Theron J: Angioplasty of brachiocephalic vessel. In Vinuela F, Halbark VV, Jaryl ED, (eds), Interventional Neuroradiology: Endovascular therapy of the CNS, Chap 13. New York: Raven Press, 1992:167–180.
* att/pt/l = attempted angioplasty/number of patients/lesions treated
† t = time

months, occlusion recurred after 3 months in one patient and recurrent stenosis in five (18).

Studies have confirmed the satisfactory efficacy of subclavian angioplasty and its low complication rate. Thus it seems legitimate to suggest angioplasty as the first-line treatment of stenosis of the subclavian artery and to reserve surgery for failures or contraindications to the technique. A retrospective study concerning 30 attempted angioplasties in 30 patients with tight stenoses of the subclavian artery showed 23 patients to have symptoms and 7 to be asymptomatic (19). There were 2 technical failures related to impossibility of balloon catheter passage through the stenosis. In the immediate postoperative period, 2 complications were observed in the form of obstruction at the arterial puncture site, with no long-term functional consequences. Clinical evaluation after a mean follow-up of 32.5 months showed that 25 out of 28 patients (89.2 percent) with a good primary result were improved from a clinical and/or blood pressure standpoint (19). These results are similar to other reported results showing success rates of 89 percent and clinical improvement of 94 percent for brachial ischemia and 72 percent for neurologic symptoms, with no major complications, 8.6 percent minor complications, and a reported restenosis rate of 6 percent in 2.5 years (20).

Not all series have reported such excellent results, particularly if they include patients with complete occlusions and high-risk patients. In a study by Sharma et al. (17), percutaneous transluminal angioplasty in subclavian (4 stenoses, 3 occlusions) and innominate (2 stenoses) artery obstructions was successful in 4 out of 6 stenoses (2 subclavian and both innominate arteries) but in none of the 3 occlusions. Three of the 4 subclavian artery stenoses were located proximal to the vertebral artery origin, and antegrade vertebral flow without subclavian steal was present in 2 of these lesions. Three patients had complications during the procedure: 2 developed symptoms and signs of cerebral embolization (both had shown antegrade vertebral flow and no evidence of subclavian steal in the initial angiogram), and one developed angina pectoris. The follow-up period ranged from 4 to 18 months (mean 10.8 months), and no restenosis was detected (17).

Hemodynamically significant stenoses (>70 percent) involving the posterior cerebral circulation and affecting the vertebral or basilar artery have been successfully treated by PTA techniques in a growing number of series. In one series of 42 patients (21), the proximal vertebral artery was involved in 34 cases, the distal vertebral artery in 5, and the basilar artery in 3. The success rate was 98 percent. Three (7.1 percent) permanent complications occurred, consisting of stroke in 2 cases and vessel rupture in 1. There were 4 (9.5 percent) transient complications (<30 mins): 2 cases of vessel spasm and 2 of cerebral ischemia. Clinical follow-up examination demonstrated improvement of symptoms in 39 cases (92.9 percent). Radiographic follow-up studies demonstrated 3 cases (7.1 percent) of restenosis involving the proximal vertebral artery; 2 were treated by repeat angioplasty without complication, and the third is being followed clinically while the patient remains asymptomatic. In patients with significant atherosclerotic stenosis involving the vertebral or basilar artery territories, transluminal angioplasty may be of significant benefit in alleviating symptoms and improving blood flow to the posterior cerebral circulation (Fig. 18.49) (21).

The *relative efficacy* of brachiocephalic angioplasty in preventing strokes associated with symptomatic brachiocephalic stenosis has yet to be determined and will take clinical trials.

The *relative indications and contraindications* for offering angioplasty have also yet to be determined. Extreme caution is advised in those patients with the following:

1. Lesions 3 cm in length, highly ulcerated, or occluded
2. Large stroke within last week with area of infarction on CT or MRI greater than 2.5 cm in diameter

Methods and Materials

The appropriate *work-up* for patients requiring supra-aortic vessel angioplasty has yet to be determined. The work-up must clearly answer a number of questions. The long-term implementation of angioplasty will be determined by the outcome. Physicians involved in this procedure would do a service to medicine and themselves if they collected data, with outcome adjusted for case mix (Table 18.60) (22).

METHODS

The methods can be broken down into a step-by-step way to include preoperative, operative, and postoperative considerations (Table 18.61).

Cerebral Protection and Monitoring

The procedure can be performed without vascular protection or with proximal or distal vascular protection. The need for distal protection from emboli has been considered by many to be critical, and special triple coaxial catheter systems for carotid angioplasty with cerebral protection have been designed (23). Protective mechanisms can apply to proximal or distal protection. The author does not routinely use them. A "seesaw balloon technique" has also been developed that is thought to help prevent cerebral embolization with debris from the dilated internal carotid artery stenosis (24). An occlusive balloon in the internal carotid artery for cerebral protection during PTA of atherosclerotic symptomatic stenosis of the brachiocephalic artery can also be used (25).

Anticoagulation

Anticoagulation, including heparin and antiplatelets agents, is crucial. The *amount of heparin* administered varies greatly, and complications may result from both excessive and insufficient anticoagulation. Determination of the

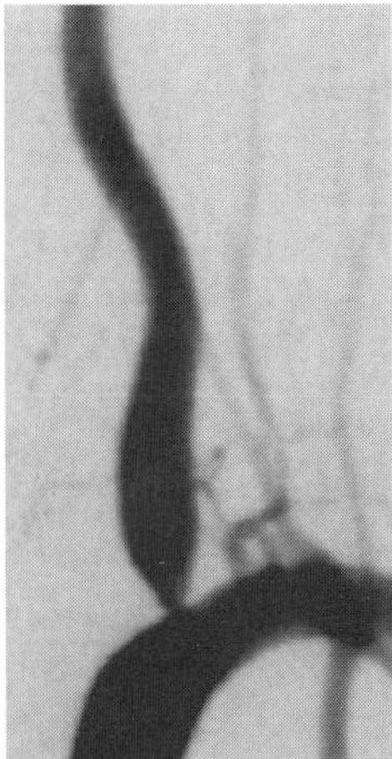

A

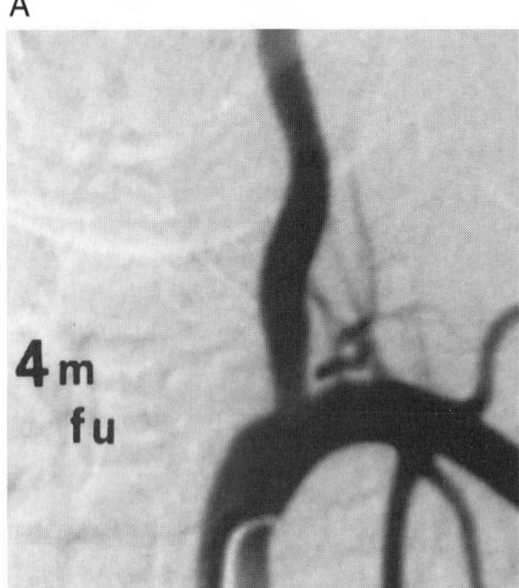

E

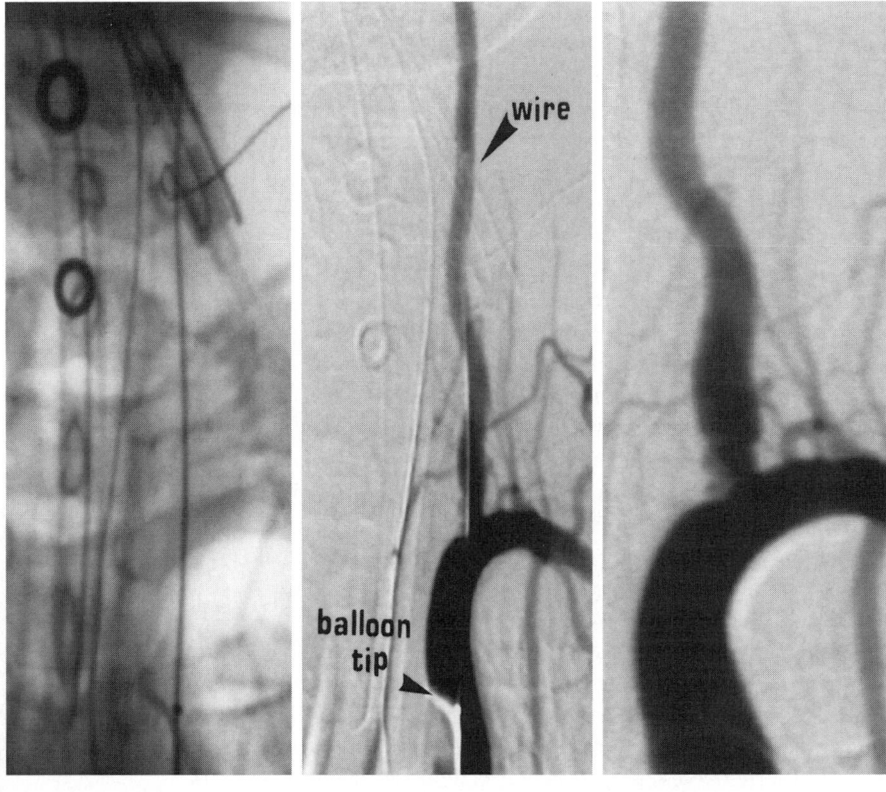

B C D

Figure 18.49. Vertebral angioplasty in a 65-year-old female with vertebrobasilar insufficiency. There was an occluded right vertebral artery and a tight left vertebral artery ostium stenosis. **A.** Left subclavian artery angiogram, subtraction view, shows tight stenosis of the ostium of the left vertebral artery. **B.** Nonsubtracted view shows a guide wire across the left vertebral artery stenosis. **C.** Angioplasty system being passed through the left vertebral artery. The balloon is in the proximal subclavian artery and is advanced through the guide wire in the left vertebral artery. **D.** Immediate postangioplasty result shows that the proximal left vertebral artery is widely patent. A filling defect is seen that corresponds to subintimal atheromatous material. **E.** Four-month follow-up shows that the left vertebral artery ostium has remained patent; there has been interval remodeling of the vessel, with a smoother appearance. The patient was asymptomatic.

Table 18.60.
Pretreatment Work-up

Question	Studies	Criteria
Identify the offending lesion.	History, physical Cerebral MRI MRA, US, transcranial Doppler Scintigraphic platelets study Angiogram	Transient ischemic attack or stroke in vascular territory of lesion that has hemodynamic changes. Clot formation.
Assess the severity and extent of associated vascular pathology.	See above	History of ischemic events in other territory, coronary artery disease, peripheral vascular disease, hypertension, DM, smoking history.
Assess cerebral vascular reserve.	Provocative (acetazolamide) SPECT	20% reduction in CBF with provocative test or baseline hypoperfusion.
Assess associated morbidity.	See above ECG, thallium stress test	
Assess the effectiveness and risk of all treatment alternatives.	ASA* class Sundt† grade SCIRS‡ grade	The longer and tighter, the more irregular the lesion, the more difficult the angioplasty.

* American Society of Anesthesia
† Sundt Risk Factor Grade
‡ SCIRS = Standards of Practice Committee of the Society of Cardiovascular and Interventional Radiology. Guidelines for percutaneous transluminal angioplasty. Radiology, 1990;177:619–626.

Table 18.61.
Angioplasty Treatment Methods

Preoperative	1. Patient selection.
	2. Cardiovascular evaluation and optimization.
	3. Pretreatment with aspirin, heparin, and calcium channel blockers, ? steroids.
	4. In questions of intraluminal thrombus, 1 week of heparin.
Operative	1. Baseline angiogram with markers for measurement.
	2. Consider intubation.
	3. Heparin and moderate hypertension.
	4. Consider initial thrombolysis.
	5a. NO EMBOLIC CEREBRAL PROTECTION
	Cross lesion with wire.
	Follow with small low-profile catheter.
	Exchange for stiff exchange wire.
	Exchange for angioplasty catheter.
	Remove wire.
	Inflate angioplasty balloon while perfusing distally with oxygenated blood.
	Aspirate distally while deflating balloon.
	Replace wire.
	Exchange for diagnostic catheter.
	Angiogram.
	Repeat as needed.
	5b. DISTAL EMBOLIC CEREBRAL PROTECTION
	Guiding catheter in immediately proximal vessel/Occlusive and angioplasty catheter at level of stenosis.
	Inflate occlusive balloon.
	Inflate angioplasty balloon.
	Remove angioplasty balloon and aspirate debri from guiding catheter.
	Deflate occlusion balloon.
	Angiogram.
	5c. PROXIMAL EMBOLIC CEREBRAL PROTECTION
	Guiding catheter in parent vessel proximal to intracranial and extracranial feeder.
	Occlusive balloon in parent vessel.
	Angioplasty catheter at level of stenosis.
	Inflate occlusive balloon.
	Remove angioplasty balloon and aspirate debri from guiding catheter.
	Deflate occlusion balloon.
	Angiogram.
	6. Retreat spasm with nitroglycerine or verapamil.
	7. Consider reangioplasty, thrombolysis, or stent placement if result suboptimal.
Postoperative	1. Close monitoring in ICU for 10 to 24 h.
	2. Adequate hydration.
	3. Anticoagulation (heparin changing to Coumadin).
	4. Control of risk factors for atherosclerotic vascular disease.

anticoagulant response to heparin in patients undergoing angioplasty by means of the activated clotting time (ACT) shows a linear relationship between heparin dose and ACT ($p = .0001$), but the slope of this relationship varies from patient to patient ($r^2 = .232$). Use of the ACT is a convenient and reproducible means of monitoring heparin administration and may increase safety and efficacy during peripheral angioplasty (26). Platelet-rich thrombus formation is a complication of arterial wall deep injury by balloon angioplasty that may lead to acute arterial occlusion and may contribute to restenosis. This mural thrombosis cannot usually be identified by angiography. Aspirin, although helpful, may not be enough, and other antithrombotic therapy using thrombin inhibition appears to be needed (27).

Hyperperfusion syndrome, a rare complication following revascularization for severe cerebrovascular occlusive disease, has been reported in a case with milder manifestations of this syndrome in the form of unilateral headache following balloon angioplasty of the brachiocephalic arteries. The author has also seen it. It is important to recognize this phenomenon so that one can treat it and avoid the more severe consequences (28).

MATERIALS

Catheters

Low-profile, high-pressure, highly trackable balloons are needed. The authors use a Utrathin ST Balloon Catheter by Meditech (Watertown, MA). For intracranial navigation, only the Stealth dilatation catheter* can be navigated intracranially in our hands around the carotid siphon or a tortuous distal vertebral.

Thrombolytic Agents

Urokinase (UK) thrombolysis can be needed prior to angioplasty. Pretreatment of all lesions with UK may be considered, and if there is any suggestion in our minds that part of the angiographic stenosis is due to a thrombus, we treat with 100 to 250,000 IU UK IA prior to angioplasty. At present we do not use the pulse-spray method. In the peripheral system some authors feel that *pulse-spray pharmacomechanical thrombolysis* markedly increases the efficiency and acceptability of thrombolysis: dialysis grafts usually require only 20 to 35 min for thrombolysis; bypass grafts or native arteries, 60 to 150 min (29).

Future Trends

STENTS, ATHERECTOMY DEVICES, LASERS, AND DRUGS

Stents may well prove to be extremely useful. They help with dissections, and covered stents help with emboli. They will no doubt revolutionize endovascular treatment. The *Palmaz balloon-expandable vascular stent* and its effect on the results of PTA were assessed in a prospective study of the peripheral system with excellent results: technical success was achieved in the placement of 34 of 35 stents (97 percent), with improved angiographic and hemodynamic results in 74 percent (30). The Strecker flexible stent also shows some promise (31).

The use of *atherectomy catheters* in the peripheral arterial system is under investigation but currently has limited application because of frequent early thromboembolic complications and poor late patency rates. If atherectomy became routine, it would permit the examination of the excised tissue and might provide insight into the efficacy of vascular interventions and the phenomenon of postintervention restenosis (32).

The integration of fluorescent guidance with *pulsed dye laser ablation* is feasible, but additional refinements are necessary to increase safety and efficacy (excimer laser) (33). Although satisfactory immediate results have been achieved by excimer laser angioplasty, intermediate follow-up studies have revealed a restenosis rate in the same range as with balloon angioplasty (34).

Some authors believe that angioscopy permits one to identify the nature of treated lesions and to predict possible complications, which are usually underrated by angiography (35). However, it is unlikely that this will find wide usage in interventional neuroradiology.

Various modes of *thermal energy used adjunctively* during balloon angioplasty have demonstrated the potential to enhance the results of acute lumen dilatation in animal studies (36). Ultrasound energy applied to normal and atherosclerotic human vessel segments obtained at autopsy has shown some promise as an adjunctive modality to balloon angioplasty (37).

DRUG DELIVERY

Still more in the future, and still more promising, are drugs for the prevention of restenosis, such as *Angiopeptin* (38) and *Carvedilol* (39).

Local intramural delivery of therapeutic agents during balloon angioplasty has been proposed as an adjunctive technique for preventing early intracoronary thrombosis and late restenosis. In vitro agent delivery has been successful with a depth of penetration of horseradish peroxidase related to both balloon pressure and duration of inflation. Hydrogel-coated balloons can deliver biologically active agents to the vessel wall without gross tissue disruption and may provide an atraumatic method for the local delivery of therapeutic agents during balloon angioplasty (40). The potent, irreversible thrombin inhibitor *D*-Phe-L-Pro-L-Arginyl chloromethyl ketone (PPACK) has been used to inhibit thrombus formation in chronic porcine arteriovenous shunts. The PPACK is delivered locally with a hydrogel-coated angioplasty balloon without alteration of bleeding parameters (41). Even direct *arterial gene transfer* has been achieved using double-balloon catheters and perforated balloons, or more simply with naked genetic material from a thin coat of hydrogel polymer applied to a standard angioplasty balloon. The idea of gene transfer without liposomes or viral vectors using DNA applied to a standard angioplasty catheter balloon coated with hydrogel is breathtaking (42).

REFERENCES

1. Mehan VK, Meier B: Interventional cardiology: State of the art (review). Presse Med 1994;23:339–344.
2. Lorenzi G, Domanin M, Constantini A: PTA and laser assisted PTA combined with simultaneous surgical revascularization. J Cardiovasc Surg 1991;32:456–462.
3. Pimentel Filho WA, Ascer E, Buchler JR, et al: Anatomical limitations for the performance of angioplasty in coronary multivessel disease. Arquivos Brasileiros de Cardiologia 1992;58:1–4.
4. Gasparini D, Camerini E: Renal angioplasty in the treatment of renovascular hypertension: A comparison of results and the authors' own experience. Radiol Med (Torino) 1992;83:91–96.
5. Hijazi ZM, Fahey JT, Kleinman CS, Hellenbrand WE: Balloon angioplasty for recurrent coarctation of aorta: Immediate and long-term results. Circulation 1991;84:1150–1156.
6. Plouin PF, Jeunemaitre X, Chatellier G, Julien J, Raynaud A: Value and limits of renal artery examination in the aged. Nephrologie 1990;11:297–299.
7. Ramsay LE, Waller PC: Blood pressure response to percutaneous transluminal angioplasty for renovascular hypertension: An overview of published series. BMJ 1990;300:569–572.
8. Wisselink W, Money SR, Becker MO, et al: Comparison of operative reconstruction and percutaneous balloon dilatation for central venous obstruction. Am J Surg 1993;166:200–204.
9. Gentles TL, Lock JE, Perry SB: High pressure balloon angioplasty for branch pulmonary artery stenosis: Early experience. J Am Coll Cardiol 1993;22:867–872.
10. Machleder HI: Evaluation of a new treatment strategy for Paget-Schroetter syndrome: Spontaneous thrombosis of the axillary-subclavian vein. J Vasc Surg 1993;17:305–315.
11. Shoenfeld R, Hermans H, Novick A, et al: Stenting of proximal venous obstructions to maintain hemodialysis access. J Vasc Surg 1994;19:532–538.
12. Theron J, Courtheoux P, Alachkar F, Maiza D: Intravascular technics of cerebral revascularization. J Mal Vasc 1990;15:245–256.
13. Inomori S, Fujino H, Yamataki A, Abe H, Takada H: Percutaneous transluminal angioplasty for multiple brachiocephalic artery stenosis: Case report. No Shinkei Geka 1990;18:295–299.
14. Komiyama M, Nishio A, Nishijima Y: Endovascular treatment of acute thrombotic occlusion of the cervical internal carotid artery associated with embolic occlusion of the middle cerebral artery: Case report. Neurosurgery 1994;34:359–363.
15. Bergeon P, Rudondy P, Benichou H, et al: Transluminal angioplasty for recurrent stenosis after carotid endarterectomy: Prognostic factors and indications. Int Angiol 1993;12:256–259.
16. Brown MM, Butler P, Gibbs J, Swash M, Waterston J: Feasibility of percutaneous transluminal angioplasty for carotid artery stenosis. J Neurol Neurosurg Psychiatry 1990;53:238–243.
17. Sharma S, Kaul U, Rajani M: Identifying high-risk patients for percutaneous transluminal angioplasty of subclavian and innominate arteries. Acta Radiol 1991;32:381–385.
18. Mathias KD, Luth I, Haarmann P: Percutaneous transluminal angioplasty of proximal subclavian artery occlusions. Cardiovasc Intervent Radiol 1993;16:214–218.
19. Trinca M, Millaire A, Marache P, Jabinet JL, Sergeant O, Ducloux G: Angioplasty of the subclavian arteries: Immediate and mid-term results (review). Ann Cardiol Angeiol (Paris) 1993;42:127–132.
20. Tesdal IK, Jaschke W, Haueisen H, et al: Percutaneous transluminal angioplasty (PTA) of the arteries of the arm in brachial and cerebral ischemia. Rofo Fortschr Geb Rontgenstr Neuen Bildgeb Verfahr 1991;155:363–369.
21. Higashida RT, Tsai FY, Halbach VV, et al: Transluminal angioplasty for atherosclerotic disease of the vertebral and basilar arteries. J Neurosurg 1993;78:192–198.
22. Hunink MG, Wong JB: Meta-analysis of failure-time data with adjustment for covariates. Med Decis Making 1994;14:59–70.
23. Theron J, Courtheoux P, Alachkar F, Bouvard G, Maiza D: New triple coaxial catheter system for carotid angioplasty with cerebral protection. AJNR 1990;11:869–874.
24. Kinoshita A, Itoh M, Takemoto O: Percutaneous transluminal angioplasty of internal carotid artery: A preliminary report of seesaw balloon technique. Neurol Res 1993;15:356–358.
25. Gobin Y, Hassani R, Batellier J, Casasco A, Aymard A, Merland JJ: Transluminal angioplasty of the brachiocephalic artery with cerebral protection. J Mal Vasc 1991;16:188–190.
26. Sharma S, Kaul U, Misra N, Rajani M: Percutaneous supra-aortic angioplasty in a high risk coronary patient. Clin Radiol 1990;42: 57–59.

27. Lam JY, Chesebro JH, Steele PM, et al: Antithrombotic therapy for deep arterial injury by angioplasty: Efficacy of common platelet inhibition compared with thrombin inhibition in pigs. Circulation 1991;84:814–820.
28. Mandalam KR, Rao VR, Neelakandhan KS, Kumar S, Unnikrishnan M, Mukhopadhyay S: Hyperperfusion syndrome following balloon angioplasty and bypass surgery of aortic arch vessels: A report of 3 cases. Cardiovasc Intervent Radiol 1992;15:108–112.
29. Bookstein JJ, Valji K: Pulse-spray pharmacomechanical thrombolysis. Cardiovasc Intervent Radiol 1992;15:228–233.
30. Bonn J, Gardiner G Jr, Shapiro MJ, Sullivan KL, Levin DC: Palmaz vascular stent: Initial clinical experience. Radiology 1990;174: 741–745.
31. Kuhn FP, Kutkuhn B, Torsello G, Modder U: Renal artery stenosis: Preliminary results of treatment with the Strecker stent. Radiology 1991;180:367–372.
32. Johnson DE, Hinohara T, Selmon MR, Braden LJ, Simpson JB: Primary peripheral arterial stenoses and restenoses excised by transluminal atherectomy: A histopathologic study. J Am Coll Cardiol 1990;15:419–425.
33. Douek PC, Leon MB, Geschwind H, et al: Occlusive peripheral vascular disease: A multicenter trial of fluorescence-guided, pulsed dye laser-assisted balloon angioplasty. Radiology 1991;180: 127–133.
34. Werner G, Buchwald A, Unterberg C, Voth E, Kreuzer H, Wiegand V: Excimer laser angioplasty in coronary artery disease. Eur Heart J 1991;12:24–29.
35. Foucart H, Carlier C, Baudrillard JC, Joffre F, Cecile JP: Femoral angioplasty: Long-term results (review). J Mal Vasc 1990;15: 229–233.
36. Fram DB, Gillam LD, Aretz TA, et al: Low pressure radiofrequency balloon angioplasty: Evaluation in porcine peripheral arteries. J Am Coll Cardiol 1993;21:1512–1521.
37. Weber W, Strunk H, Schild H, Steffen W, Stahr P, Erbel R: Percutaneous ultrasonic angioplasty: Initial results of an in-vitro study on normal and atherosclerotic human vessel segments. Ann Acad Med Singapore 1993;22:696–700.
38. Howell MH, Adams MM, Wolfe MS, Foegh ML, Ramwell PW: Angiopeptin inhibition of myointimal hyperplasia after balloon angioplasty of large arteries in hypercholesterolaemic rabbits. Clin Sci 1993;85:183–188.
39. Ohlstein EH, Douglas SA, Sung CP, et al: Carvedilol, a cardiovascular drug, prevents vascular smooth muscle cell proliferation, migration, and neointimal formation following vascular injury. Proc Natl Acad Sci USA 1993;90:6189–6193.
40. Fram DB, Aretz T, Azrin MA, et al: Localized intramural drug delivery during balloon angioplasty using hydrogel-coated balloons and pressure-augmented diffusion. J Am Coll Cardiol 1994;23: 1570–1577.
41. Nunes GL, Hanson SR, King S, Sahatjian RA, Scott NA: Local delivery of a synthetic antithrombin with a hydrogel-coated angioplasty balloon catheter inhibits platelet-dependent thrombosis. J Am Coll Cardiol 1994;23:1578–1583.
42. Riessen R, Rahimizadeh H, Blessing E, Takeshita S, Barry JJ, Isner JM: Arterial gene transfer using pure DNA applied directly to a hydrogel-coated angioplasty balloon. Hum Gene Ther 1993;4: 749–758.

18.11 Craniofacial Pathology

Lotfi Hacein-Bey and John Pile-Spellman

Key Points

1. Cranial-facial hemangiomas are:

- very common tumors of childhood
- grow → regress
- seldom need embolization.

2. Cranial-facial arteriovenous malformations are:

- congenital lesions, high flow lesions
- relentlessly progressive → deformity, ischemia, bleeding
- challenging, requiring embolization and surgery
- bleeding is a hyperacute emergency.

3. Cranial-facial arteriovenous fistulae usually are:

- posttraumatic
- symptomatic
- treatment beneficial/occlusion fistula site

4. Cranial-facial venous malformations are:

- congenital, slowly progressive venous dilations
- cosmetic deforming, episodically painful and swollen, functionally impairing
- responsive to transcutaneous ethanol sclerotherapy.

5. Cranial-facial tumors are:

- sometimes hypervascular (paragangliomas, juvenile angiofibromas, meningiloma, hypervascular metastases)
- helped by adjuvant particle embolization
- to be embolized with cognizance and respect of the dangerous anastomoses.

6. Cranial-facial bleeding is:

- well handled by embolization
- identified by superselective angiograms in trauma, tumor, but not epistaxis
- challenging in multiple trauma cases
- to be embolized with cognizance and respect of the anastomoses.

Vascular Anomalies

The vast and complex spectrum of vascular anomalies has been described in the literature with a wealth of details. Confusing terminologies combining attributes such as *cav-*

Assistant Professor of Radiology, Department of Interventional Neuroradiology, Columbia University College of Physicians & Surgeons, New York, New York.

ernous, *racemose*, *cirsoid*, *varicose*, and *pulsatile* with words like *hemangioma*, *angioma*, *hemolymphangioma*, and *cavernoma* have greatly contributed to blurring physicans' understanding of vascular lesions. Yet a simple and logical classification of vascular anomalies is conceivable and has been established by Mulliken and coworkers (1–4). It is based on histologic characteristics, cellular turnover pattern, clinical history, and physical findings. In this text we will refer to this classification, which distinguishes *hemangiomas* from *vascular malformations*, and further separates the latter according to their rheologic features (slow- versus high-flow lesions).

HEMANGIOMAS

Hemangiomas appear to be true neoplasms of endothelial cells that are present in infancy and exhibit a distorted cellular behavior. The typical hemangioma is a "cherry red spot" skin lesion that appears after birth, undergoes a proliferative phase, and grows before involuting spontaneously before age 5 (1–4). However, hemangiomas can be of any size and can be located anywhere. Large hemangiomas can have macroshunts and can be responsible for high-output cardiac failure (4,5). They can trap platelets and induce a thrombocytic coagulopathy (Kasabach-Merritt syndrome) (6) and serious bleeding. Depending on their location, hemangiomas can be a threat to function or even to life: orbital hemangiomas can cause blindness; cervicofacial hemangiomas involving the airway can cause asphyxiation.

The diagnosis of hemangiomas is clinical. In doubtful cases, cross-sectional imaging, especially MRI (4,7), shows a densely enhancing soft-tissue tumor. Angiography should be done only in atypical presentations, in which case it demonstrates a dense "parenchymal" staining in addition to possible macroshunts (3). It is only rarely necessary to establish the diagnosis histologically.

When treatment is warranted because of signs of aggressiveness, corticosteroids are the first choice, although the use of radiation therapy, cyclophosphamide, and other immunosuppressive agents has been reported. However, steroids have a 40 to 60 percent failure rate; intralesional corticosteroid injection is reported to have a beneficial effect in facial and orbital hemangiomas (8). A recent report credits interferon alpha-2a with a good angiogenic effect (5). Still, transarterial particulate embolization might represent the only palliative treatment option in aggressive hemangiomas with macroshunts and consumptive coagulopathy (9).

MALFORMATIONS

Vascular malformations demonstrate a normal endothelial cellular turnover, are lined by a normal "mature" endothelium, are always present at birth though often undetected, and grow commensurately with the child. They can be capillary, venous, arteriovenous, lympathic, or combined, depending on the stage at which a developmental aberration takes place. Furthermore, malformations can be distinguished as slow-flow or high-flow lesions (4).

Slow-Flow Vascular Malformations

Venous Malformations Venous malformations (VMs) often go undetected until they manifest during adolescence or early adulthood. They usually grow at the same pace as the child but can quickly enlarge due to thrombosis, trauma, or hormonal changes (4). Intralesional thrombosis is common and is responsible for episodic pain and swelling; calcified thrombi become phleboliths, which are quasi-pathognomonic on radiologic studies. CT shows best the phleboliths (Fig. 18.50*C*), although MRI, by virtue of its exquisite tissue resolution as well as its capability to separate fast from slow flow, is presently the best means of assessing these lesions that present as spontaneously bright on T2-weighted sequences (Fig. 18.50*A*), that do not have precise boundaries, that involve the surrounding anatomic compartments, and that often communicate with the normal venous system (7).

Arteriography is not very useful and involves some risk (3). Venography, or preferably an angiogram obtained from direct puncture of the malformation, helps identify a communication with normal veins and gives an estimate of the lesional volume before treatment.

Surgical excision of all but small VMs is unsatisfactory because of the diffuse and indistinct nature of the lesions; moreover, postoperative bleeding may occur, attributable to consumptive coagulopathy. Large craniofacial VMs are considered unresectable, especially if they extend to the airway (4). Sclerotherapy of VMs is an attractive treatment option, alone or in preparation for surgery. Several sclerosing agents are available. Mild agents, such as sodium tetradecyl sulfate, are commonly used (4). In Europe, Ethibloc, a mixture of corn protein and papaverine oil in a 60 percent alcohol suspension, is used with apparently good results (10,11). Cryoprecipitate admixtures are concentrated blood products that are rich in fibrinogen, factor VIII, and von Willebrand factor. Mixed with thrombin, they are highly thrombogenic and are currently used in surgery as tissue adhesives, as well as in hemophiliacs. Homologous cryoprecipitates obtained from the patient's blood have been used in VM sclerotherapy (12).

Absolute ethanol is the most potent of all sclerosing agents (10,13,14). It has been widely used to produce thrombosis and necrosis in neoplastic kidneys (13), and its use has been extended to vascular malformations (10,14). Slowly injected into a vascular space, ethanol instantly and irreversibly denatures blood proteins, red blood cells, and platelets, resulting in formation of a large thrombus and intense intimal necrosis (13,14); at first the lesion exhibits marked swelling. The long-term effect is marked fibrosis of the perivascular spaces, followed by shrinkage due to resorption by phagocytes (14). Extensive craniofacial VMs can be treated effectively with ethanol sclerotherapy, and when the airway is threatened, a tracheostomy tube is of great help while the VM undergoes massive swelling before shrinking. We have treated four such lesions either with sclerotherapy alone or in preparation for surgery with good results (Fig. 18.50).

Lymphatic Malformations Lymphatic anomalies are all present at birth, although they can go undetected for some time. The cervicofacial area is the most common site for lymphatic anomalies (4). The multiple possibilities in lymphatic channel size and morphology, depth of lesional extent, and degree of reactive surrounding fibrosis account for the various manifestations of lymphatic malformations. Cystic forms are common in the cervicofacial area, made either of large cysts or of multilocular microcystic lesions that are often labeled *cystic hygromas* or *lymphangiomas.* The cysts can experience hemorrhage, superinfection (cellulitis), or fibrosis.

The lesions are well shown by CT and MRI. MRI suggests best the various stages a cystic malformation may undergo, due to susceptibility artifacts.

Lymphatic malformations classically keep growing and can cause bony or soft-tissue deformity. Their preferred treatment is surgical excision (4). Sclerotherapy can be attempted, although recurrence is common, attributable to the multiplicity of lymphatic channels in communication with the lesion. If the lesion is combined and has a venous component, sclerotherapy is more likely to be partially effective.

Capillary Malformations Pure capillary malformations, also called *port-wine stains,* are easily diagnosed, and are at best accessible to laser therapy. It is important to recognize that these dermal lesions are often overly associated with vascular lesions (lymphatic, VMs, arteriovenous malformations); in this instance, the treatment is first aimed at managing the more concerning underlying lesion (4).

Combined Malformations Vascular malformations can be mixed and complex. More so than for simple lesions, ideal management of these lesions involving the craniofacial area

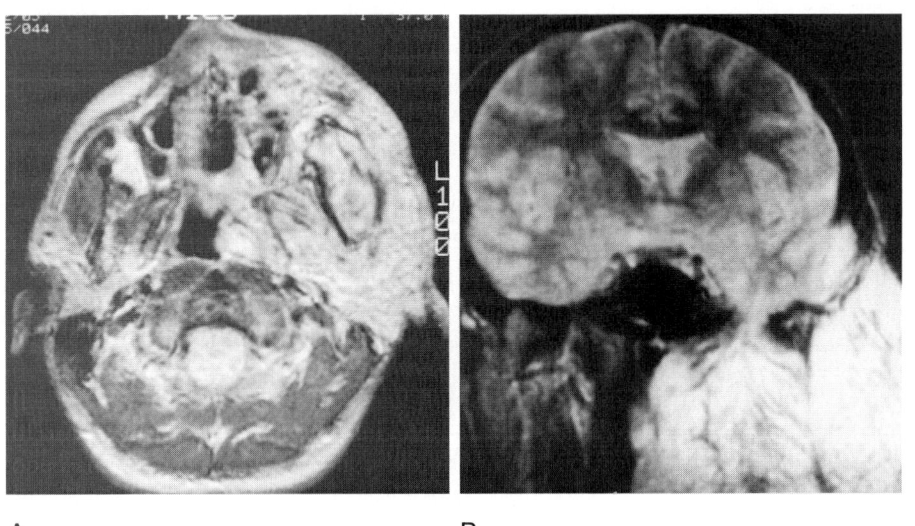

A B

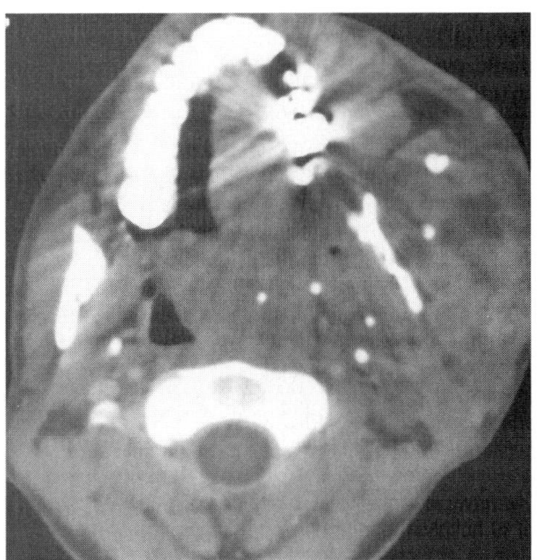

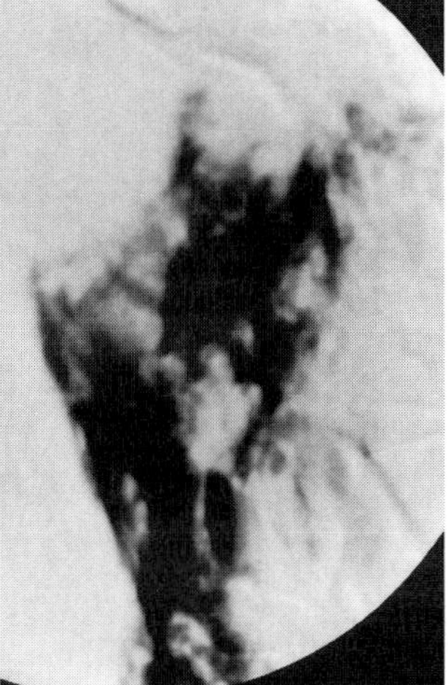

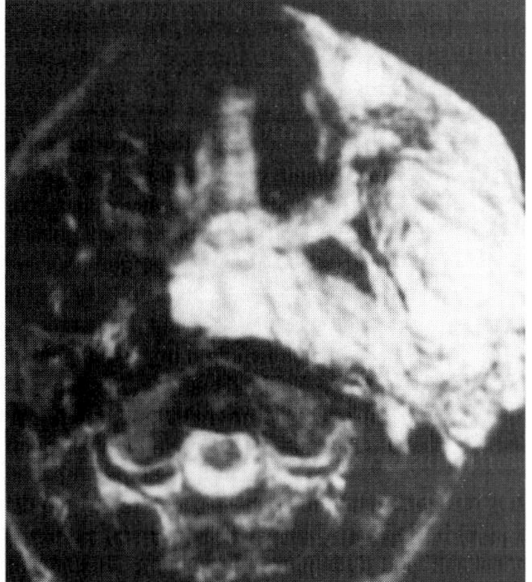

C D E

Figure 18.50. Massive craniofacial venous malformation in a 27-year-old male with sleep apnea, facial deformity, and pain. **A.** Axial T2-weighted MR image showing massive soft-tissue mass in left pharyngeal space extending to the airway. **B.** Coronal T2-weighted MR image showing the venous malformation extending from the infratemporal fossa and parotid space down to the paratracheal space and compromising the airway. **C.** Axial CT scan shows the presence of phleboliths within the lesion. **D.** Direct injection of left parapharyngeal component with 95 percent ethanol mixed with metrizamide under fluoroscopic control. Patient had a tracheostomy tube placed prior to procedure. **E.** Coronal T2-weighted MR image obtained after three sclerotherapy sessions. Airway patency improved, and the patient subsequently underwent further treatment.

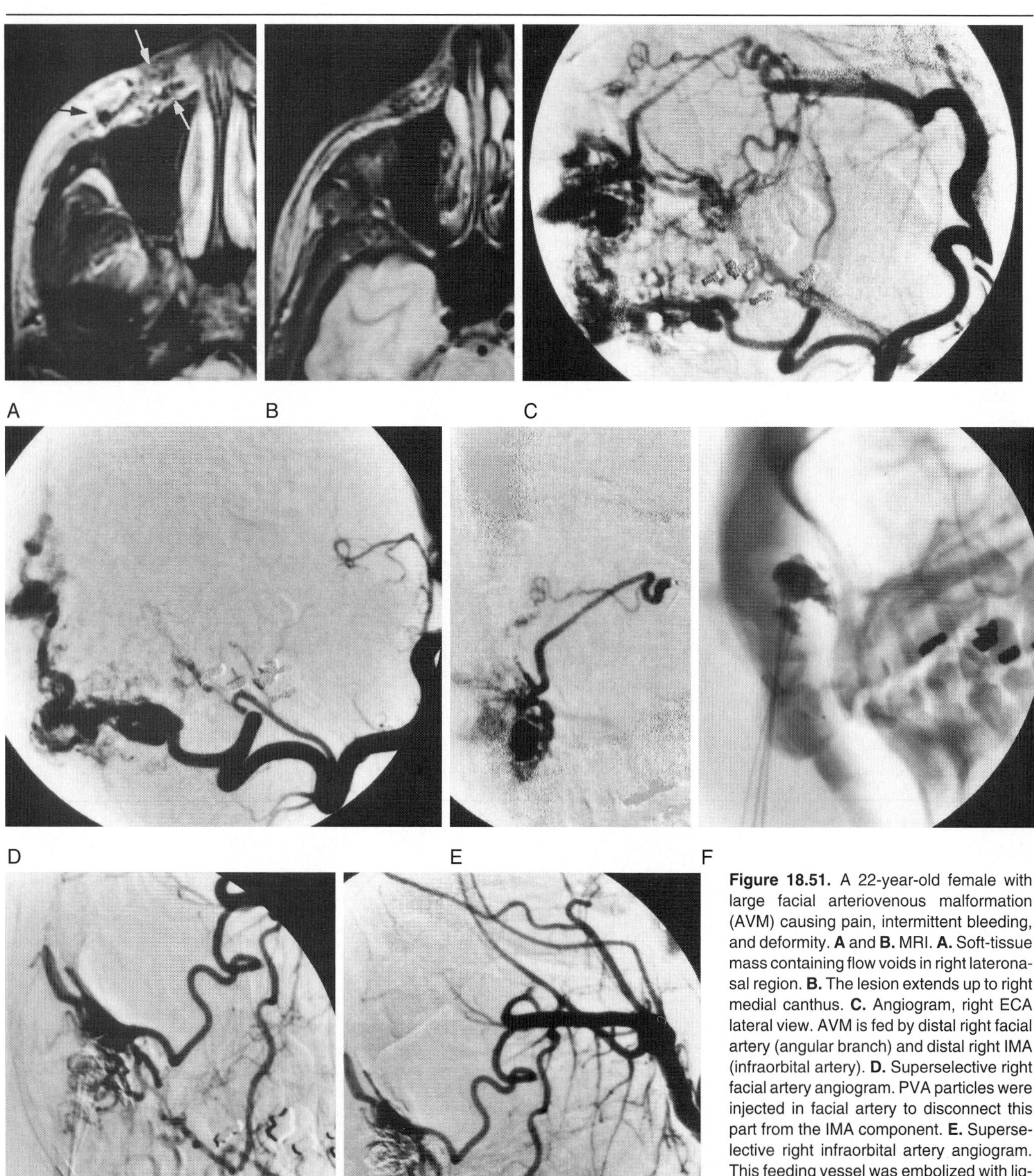

Figure 18.51. A 22-year-old female with large facial arteriovenous malformation (AVM) causing pain, intermittent bleeding, and deformity. **A** and **B.** MRI. **A.** Soft-tissue mass containing flow voids in right lateronasal region. **B.** The lesion extends up to right medial canthus. **C.** Angiogram, right ECA lateral view. AVM is fed by distal right facial artery (angular branch) and distal right IMA (infraorbital artery). **D.** Superselective right facial artery angiogram. PVA particles were injected in facial artery to disconnect this part from the IMA component. **E.** Superselective right infraorbital artery angiogram. This feeding vessel was embolized with liquid glue (NBCA) with good intranidal penetration. Plain film (**F**) and angiogram from right ECA injection. Direct transcutaneous injection of AVM nidus with NBCA glue under angiographic control. This gives more complete nidus obliteration and provides markers to the surgeon (glue is mixed with tantalum powder). **G** and **H.** Control right ECA angiogram. Glue cast is well seen in AVM. Satisfactory AVM obliteration. Patient is ready for surgery.

should involve a pluridisciplinary team of oral and plastic surgeons, interventional neuroradiologists, and anesthesiologists (4–15).

High-flow Vascular Malformations

Arteriovenous malformations (AVMs) and arteriovenous fistulae (AVFs) of the craniofacial region are uncommon. With the exception of rare traumatic fistulae, they are present at birth even though they might not be detected. Like other malformations, they keep growing with time. High-flow malformations have low-resistance shunts with (AVMs) or without (AVFs) intervening nidus, which makes them prone to recruit flow from surrounding vessels.

Arteriovenous Malformations Craniofacial AVMs are 20 times less common than their intracranial counterparts (4). Depending on their size and flow pattern, they can present with high-output cardiac failure or with less dramatic signs such as deformity with or without bony involvement, pain, a constant whooshing sound that can cause sleep deprivation, epistaxis, or a chronic consumptive coagulopathy. The diagnosis is strongly suggested at physical examination: palpation discloses an elevated temperature and a thrill; auscultation reveals a bruit.

CT with intravenous contrast enhancement shows the vascular mass within the soft tissues of the face as well as bony involvement or deformity when present. MRI (Fig. 18.51) reveals the presence of flow voids suggestive of a high-flow vascular lesion with hyperintense T2 signal. Doppler examination measures the arterial peak velocities within the lesion. Angiography is the gold standard in AVMs (Fig. 18.51*C* and *D*), showing the dilated arterial feeders, preferential flow to the shunt areas, size and morphology of the nidus, and the early draining veins, and giving an idea of potential collateral arterial supply.

The treatment of choice is surgical excision, which is greatly facilitated by preoperative embolization (4). Lack of effectiveness and even dangers of proximal feeding vessel ligation are never overemphasized. Decision to treat must be made thoughtfully, since incomplete treatment may result in AVM activation and rapid expansion. Carefully planned preoperative embolization markedly reduces intraoperative blood loss and permits precise and complete AVM excision, leading to optimal cosmetic result. Embolization can be carried out with flow-guided particles (Fig. 18.51*E*) or liquid agents (Fig. 18.51*F* and *G*). When liquid NBCA glue is used, it is best to mix it with tantalum oxide, which does not result in skin discoloration and yet provides a marker for the surgeon. Extreme attention to external carotid artery (ECA) to internal carotid artery (ICA) anastomoses is mandatory. More so than in other areas of the body, immediate collateral flow recruitment occurs after partial embolization in the craniofacial area (4); therefore, incomplete or poorly planned embolization may be more detrimental than helpful.

Arteriovenous Fistulae Most AVFs are congenital; they are nothing but AVMs that lack a nidus between a dilated artery and its venous drainage, and they are thought to occur at the same developmental stage as AVMs. However, traumatic AVFs can occur at any age, and once the shunt is established, they continue to grow and recruit more collateral flow (Fig. 18.52*B* to *D*).

AVFs present clinically as AVMs, and sometimes cross-sectional imaging can establish the diagnosis, showing a high-flow vascular shunt without soft-tissue mass. MR angiography is particularly useful, especially when using the

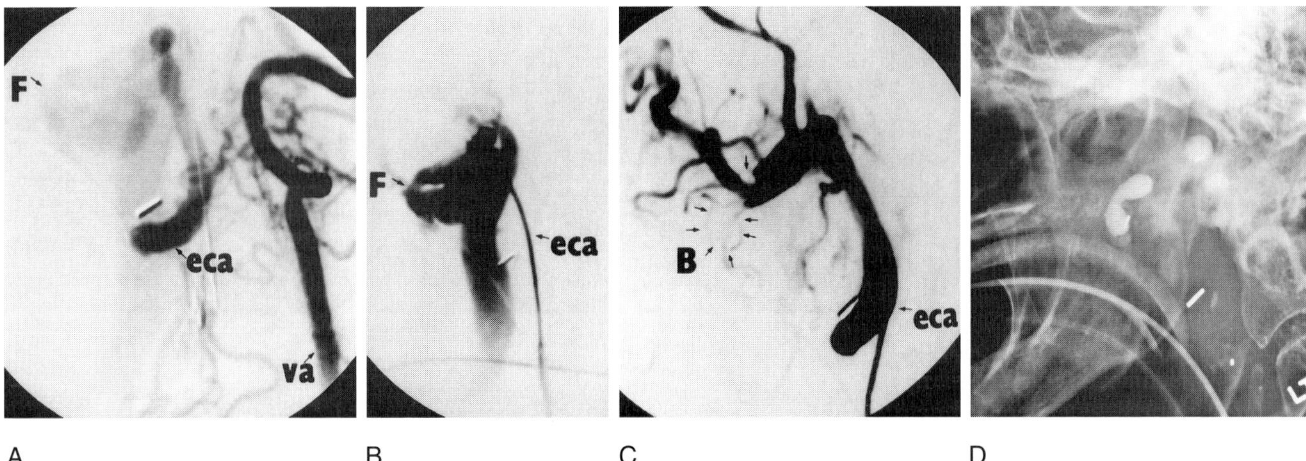

Figure 18.52. Facial arteriovenous fistula (AVF) in a 70-year-old female with epistaxis and left-sided facial bruit. The patient had left ECA clipping for fistula. **A.** Left vertebral artery angiogram showing reconstitution of left ECA via collaterals. **B.** Angiogram from direct puncture of left ECA shows direct fistula between proximal IMA and external carotid vein. **C.** Occlusion of fistula with detachable balloon. **D.** Plain film showing balloon in fistula; note shape of balloon corresponding to fistula configuration.

phase-contrast technique that permits encoding of any flow velocity. Nevertheless, as for AVMs, the diagnosis is confirmed at angiography, which shows the dilated artery communicating directly with a massively distended vein (Fig. 18.52*B*); the fistula itself often shows the typical pattern of prefistulous arterial dilatation followed by stenosis and again dilatation on the venous side (Fig. 18.52*D*). Again, as for AVMs, the myth of proximal ligation should be fought against.

TUMORS

Tumors originate from a specific group of cells and usually expand centrifugally, invading or displacing the surrounding tissues. The preferred treatment for most tumors is surgical excision whenever possible. Preoperative tumor evaluation must answer the following questions: Where does the tumor originate? Where does the tumor grow, and what is the extent of invasion? Where does it get its vascular supply? Furthermore, in cases where preoperative embolization is desired, these questions arise: How safe is embolization? Is proximal feeding artery occlusion a satisfactory option prior to surgery? The following concepts are helpful in obtaining as good a result as possible in a stepwise fashion (Table 18.62).

Compartments and Invasion

Cross-sectional imaging usually suffices to determine the location of a tumor and its precise relation to adjacent structures. MRI, with its inherent multiplanar capability and high tissue resolution, provides precise anatomic data; the presence of intratumoral flow voids reflects the hypervascular nature of certain tumors; the use of intravenous gadolinium furthermore permits differentiating tumor margins from surrounding edema. CT is still superior in determining bony involvement and erosion and the presence of calcifications (16–18). Angiography definitely establishes the hypervascular nature of a tumor. Superselective angiography allows recognition of vascular compartments within a tumor. Two types of lesions can be recognized (16,19,20).

In *monocompartmental tumors* the entire tumor is opacified from injection of each of its feeding arteries. This has a direct therapeutic consequence: a satisfactory "single-vessel embolization" can be performed, providing the feeding artery to be embolized has been selected with care; postembolization selective angiogram of the other feeders will confirm lack of tumor opacification. Monocompartmental tumors may grow as such, or may become multicompartmented as surrounding tissues are invaded.

In *multicompartmental tumors* injection of each of the feeding arteries will result in opacification of a specific compartment, hemodynamically independent from others. If embolization is planned, each pedicle must be selected and embolized as distally as possible. Components of multicompartmental tumors may grow at a different pace; also, additional compartments may be recruited over time. These factors will have a direct impact on staging and prognosis.

Some tumors with angiogenic capabilities, such as juvenile nasopharyngeal angiofibromas, can promote formation of new vascular channels (5,6).

Vascular Pedicles

The concept of arterial pedicles to tumors has an impact on preoperative angiographic staging as well as embolization technique. Although the arterial supply to a lesion usually can be predicted from its anatomic location, surprises may be seen; as a rule, satisfactory angiographic evaluation includes superselective catheterization of each potential feeder to demonstrate the territory involved and the relative contribution of each pedicle; peripheral vessels that do not supply the tumor must be studied because their territories will constitute the boundaries of the lesion (16).

Vessels theoretically unrelated to a specific tumor will be major or even exclusive feeders: for example, the occipital artery can be the only source of supply to a posterior fossa meningioma by means of transosseous feeders through emissary channels. Therefore, angiographic evaluation of potential contributors routing via skull base foramina or channels is necessary.

Another important point about vascular pedicles is that cranial nerves are supplied by arteries that also feed the surrounding soft tissues. Severe deficits can be observed

Table 18.62.
Work-up of a Patient with Tumor/Bleeding Prior to/During Embolization

Tumor/Bleeding site	Studies	Criteria/Comment
Biology, volume, location, extent, scope	Biopsy, MRI, CT	Aggressive vs quiescent Large vs small Critical vs redundant Multiple vs single system
Plan/other therapeutic options	Consults/collaboration	Coordination of sequential treatments
Angioarchitecture, collateral flow	Angiogram, TCD	High flow/low flow
Functional involvement	Superselective lidocaine testing Test occlusions	Clearest for superselective Wada testing
Baseline physical exam	Complete and formal neurologic and psychological testing	Progression deficits Limiting deficits

TCD = Transcranial Doppler

after excessive embolization of such arteries, more so with liquid agents than with particles that stop at the precapillary level (16,20,21).

Dangerous Anastomoses

Normal communications are present between vessels. Knowledge of these dangerous anastomoses is mandatory in order to avoid catastrophic complications. Depending on the type of communication, strokes or cranial nerve palsies can be inflicted on patients. Strokes result from passage of embolic material in the internal carotid, ophthalmic, or vertebrobasilar arterial systems, usually from the external carotid territory (16). Dangerous anastomoses involved in this type of complication include the following:

ECA to ICA: middle meningeal to cavernous ICA via the foramen spinosum; artery of the foramen rotundum to cavernous ICA; accessory meningeal to cavernous ICA via foramen ovale; ascending pharyngeal carotid and clival branches to cavernous ICA via the foramen lacerum; vidian artery to petrous ICA via the pterygoid (vidian) canal; ascending pharyngeal to internal maxillary via the pterygovaginal canal.

ECA to ophthalmic: middle meningeal via the superior orbital fissure or transosseous via sphenoid bone; anterior deep temporal via the inferior orbital fissure.

ECA to vertebral artery: ascending pharyngeal via musculospinal artery (C2–C3 levels) and odontoid arch system (C3 level); occipital artery at C1 and C2 levels.

Cranial nerve palsies are usually the consequence of vigorous liquid (cyanoacrylate glue) embolization of arteries feeding both soft tissues and unrecognized cranial nerve vasa vasorum. These vasa vasorum measure less than 150 μm, and particulate embolization (most particles are larger than 150 μm, with the exception of Gelfoam powder, rarely used) is unlikely to produce a permanent deficit (16). Arteries of concern include the following:

Superior pharyngeal branch of ascending pharyngeal artery: cranial nerves V and VI

Stylomastoid artery off posterior auricular artery or occipital artery: cranial nerve VII

Petrous branch of middle meningeal artery: cranial nerve VII

Inferior tympanic branch of ascending pharyngeal artery: cranial nerve VIII

Anterior tympanic artery off proximal internal maxillary artery: cranial nerve VIII

Neuromeningeal trunk of ascending pharyngeal artery: cranial nerves IX through XII

Knowledge of these potential anastomoses and constant attention are mandatory. In doubtful cases, a provocative test with lidocaine (cardiac 2 percent lidocaine is preferred to 1 percent lidocaine since it is not acid and is not mixed with an allergenic preservative) injected in the "dangerous" artery will induce a transient nerve deficit (22).

Still, embolization can be carried out in "dangerous vessels." "Flow control" can be obtained with the use of maneuvers such as balloon protection of a large vessel, proximal "disconnection" of a dangerous vessel with a piece of nonpermanent embolic material such as Gelfoam, or simply by advancing the catheter tip distal to dangerous branches (16,20,22).

Tumor Bed Versus Conduit Embolization

From all the preceding concepts, a decision as to the most appropriate embolization technique can be made (Table 18.63). Most desirable is deep embolic penetration within the tumor. Most tumors have capillary bed units that measure less than 200 μm; therefore, the use of small embolic particles is usually adequate. Further ischemia can be obtained with the use of proximal feeding artery occlusion with a nonpermanent agent, such as gelatin foam (Gelfoam).

However, some configurations will preclude such management: the presence of macroshunts within one or several tumoral compartments, unfavorable feeding artery anatomy with normal branches taking off too close to the tumor, and tumor location in anatomic areas making postembolization edema unforgiving, such as the spinal canal, are such examples.

Judgment must be made in every single circumstance as to what is safest in terms of technique and final result. The use of large embolic particles may be granted. "Conduit" arterial occlusion with a big piece of Gelfoam or a thrombogenic coil may sometimes be all the patient needs in preparation for surgery.

Table 18.63.
Cranial-Facial Technique

Preoperative	Evaluate goal of embolization and timing of treatment
	Coags, type and cross
	Hydrate patient properly
	Consider calcium channel blockers and anxiolytics on call
Operative	Monitoring, EKG, O_2 saturation baseline neurologic exam, blood pressure
	Mild anesthetic (see section on anesthesia)
	Foley catheter, intravenous access
	7.5-French femoral sheath
	Heparinization (ACT 2.5 $\times$ normal)
	7-French guiding catheter in parent vessel
	Biplane angiogram; identify pathology
	Road map
	Navigate microcatheter into tumor/bleeding position
	Superselective angiogram through microcatheter
	Tailored neurologic examination
	Lidocaine 40-mg superselective angiograms
	Repeat neurologic exam
	Embolization, silk suture, PVA, "cocktails"
	Repeat neurologic exam
	Repeat steps 8–15
Postoperative	Reverse heparinization
	Consider calcium channel blockers and beta blockers

ACT = activated clotting time.

TYPES OF NEOPLASMS

Juvenile Nasopharyngeal Angiofibroma

Juvenile nasopharyngeal angiofibromas (JNAs) occur in adolescent males. The presenting symptom is almost always nasal stuffiness; epistaxis may occur spontaneously or may result from biopsy; anosmia, nasal discharge, and deformity in large tumors can be seen. JNAs are benign tumors that originate from the fibrovascular stroma of the posterior nasal wall at the level of the sphenopalatine foramen. As JNAs grow, they extend into the pterygopalatine fossa, the nasopharynx, the infratemporal fossa, and even to the middle cranial fossa and the orbit through skull base foramina or areas of extreme bony thinning and destruction (17,23).

Preoperative evaluation is done with cross-sectional imaging. CT in the axial and coronal planes helps evaluate thinning and bowing of the nasal septum, maxillary sinus walls, and skull base. MRI, because of its excellent tissue resolution on T2-weighted images, shows well the extent of the tumor (Fig. 18.53 *A* and *B*). Contrast-enhanced MRI helps distinguish the boundaries of the tumor from mucus retention due to obstruction. Angiography is an essential part of the preoperative workup. The arterial supply to JAFs is primarily from distal internal maxillary artery branches, commonly the sphenopalatine, descending palatine, and posterior superior alveolar branches (Fig. 18.53 *C* and *D*). The ascending pharyngeal artery not infrequently supplies JNAs (Fig. 18.53 *E*). The distal facial artery can contribute indirectly via angular or alar arteries reaching the sphenopalatine region. Internal carotid artery branches are recruited in large tumors, most commonly the mandibular branch of the petrous ICA (Fig. 18.53 *F*), but also branches of the inferolateral trunk (artery of the foramen rotundum, accessory meningeal artery, and anastomotic branches to the middle meningeal artery), as well as ethmoidal branches of the ophthalmic artery can constitute ICA-to-ECA channels because of flow demand induced by tumor angiogenesis (16).

Surgical resection of JNAs is difficult because of abundant tumor vasculature; moreover, incomplete resection

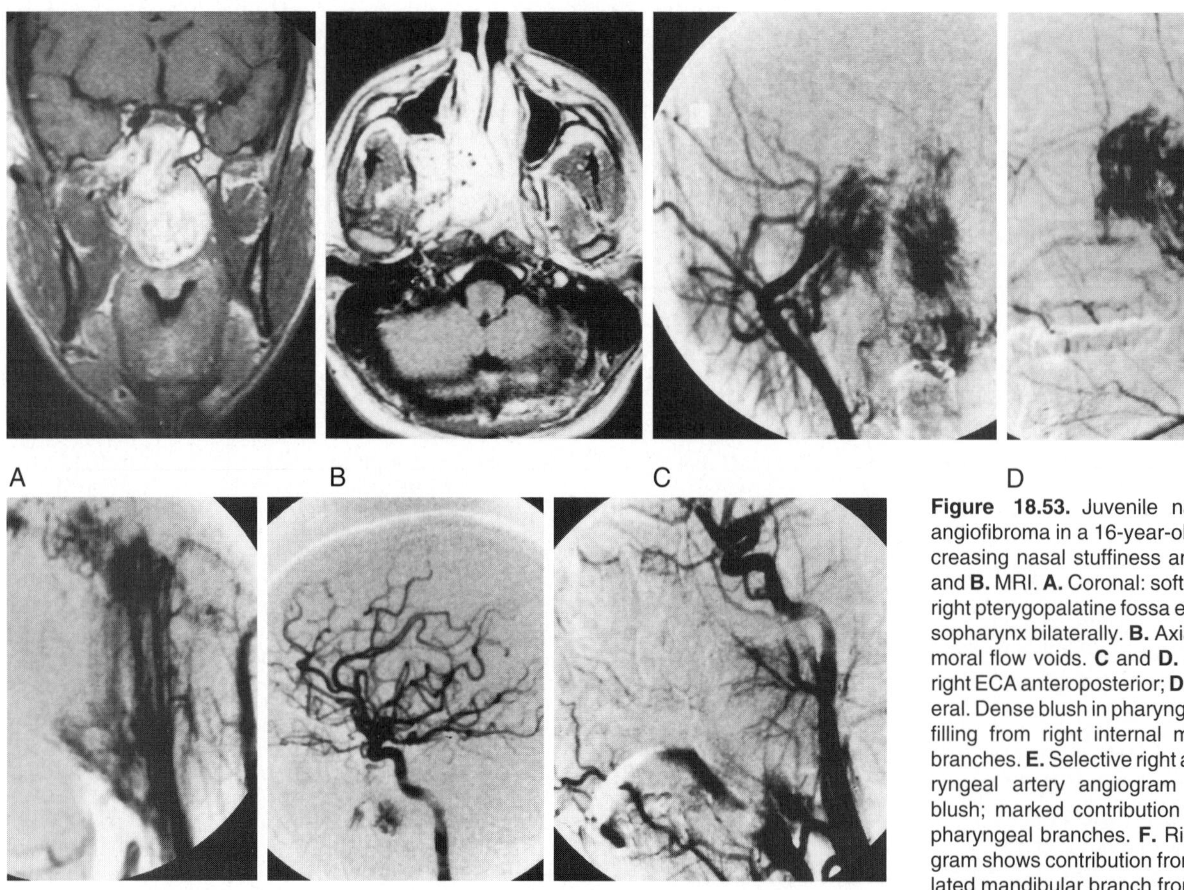

Figure 18.53. Juvenile nasopharyngeal angiofibroma in a 16-year-old male with increasing nasal stuffiness and epistaxis. **A** and **B.** MRI. **A.** Coronal: soft-tissue mass in right pterygopalatine fossa extending to nasopharynx bilaterally. **B.** Axial: note intratumoral flow voids. **C** and **D.** Angiogram. **C.** right ECA anteroposterior; **D.** Right ECA lateral. Dense blush in pharyngeal soft tissues filling from right internal maxillary artery branches. **E.** Selective right ascending pharyngeal artery angiogram shows dense blush; marked contribution to tumor from pharyngeal branches. **F.** Right ICA angiogram shows contribution from right ICA. Dilated mandibular branch from petrous segment of right ICA contributes to tumor vasculature; this vessel was not embolized. **G.** Postembolization right CCA angiogram. Right ECA angiogram no longer shows dense blush after satisfactory embolization of right IMA and ascending pharyngeal artery.

not infrequently results in tumor recurrence (17). Preoperative tumor embolization can greatly facilitate surgery. We routinely perform particulate embolization using polyvinyl alcohol (PVA) particles 150 to 250 μm in size for good tumor penetration and gelatin foam (Gelfoam) pledgets to induce further ischemia. Thrombogenic silk suture can also be used. In this fashion, distal internal maxillary artery and ascending pharyngeal artery branches feeding the tumor are embolized. As usual with the external carotid territory, very careful attention must be paid to potential collaterals with the intracranial or intraorbital circulation. Internal carotid artery branch embolization carries too high a risk and too little a benefit to be worthwhile. Embolization is stopped if collaterals are seen to open up. Dangerous collaterals include ascending pharyngeal-to-vertebral anastomoses (musculospinal artery at C3 and C2, odontoid arch system at C3), ascending pharyngeal-to-internal carotid anastomoses (lateral and medial clival branches), and internal maxillary-to-internal carotid collaterals (middle meningeal, artery of the foramen rotundum, accessory meningeal, vidian, anterior deep temporal arteries). Carefully performed, preoperative embolization of JNAs induces sufficient intratumoral thrombosis and necrosis to make surgery safer and easier; surgery usually is done 1 or 2 days following embolization to allow for maximum intratumoral thrombosis and ischemia.

Meningiomas

Meningiomas constitute about 15 percent of all brain tumors. They are commonly seen between the ages of 20 and 60, with a peak at age 45. Meningiomas are seen twice as frequently in women as in men, which may relate to the presence of estrogen and progesterone receptors within the tumor (18). Meningiomas arise from meningoendothelial cells, which are particularly concentrated in arachnoid villi; this explains why meningiomas are more likely to arise around dural sinuses. Meningiomas can be parasagittal and involve the convexity, the falx cerebri, the tentorium cerebelli, the skull base, the floor of the middle cranial fossa, and the tuberculum sellae; meningiomas are intraventricular in less than 2 percent of cases. The presenting symptoms depend upon tumor location: headaches, seizures, and progressive focal neurologic deficit should prompt clinical and radiologic evaluation. Some conditions predispose patients for developing a meningioma, including neurofibromatosis type 2 (NF2) or previous exposure to radiation therapy (18,23). Six histologic variants can be described: syncytial, fibroblastic, transitional, psammomatous, angioblastic, and sarcomatous. Hemangiopericytomas arise from meningoendothelial cells, are nonmalignant aggressive tumors, and may represent an angioblastic form of meningiomas.

CT and MRI usually establish the diagnosis showing an extra-axial tumor with a variable amount of vasogenic brain edema. CT clearly shows calcifications, common within the tumor, as well as hyperostosis adjacent to it. Gadolinium-enhanced MRI is very useful, as meningiomas enhance markedly (18). Angiography is an important part of the pretherapeutic work-up. The dilated feeding arteries to the tumor are displayed, usually originating from the middle meningeal artery (Fig. 18.54). Meningeal branches from the internal carotid system (marginal tentorial branch, an-

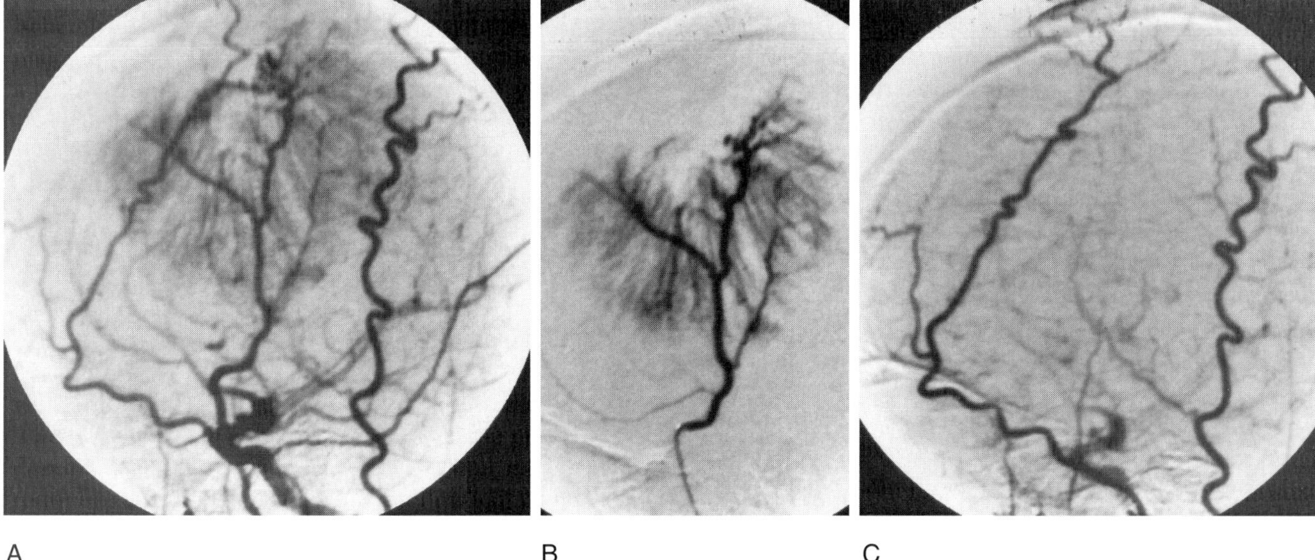

Figure 18.54. Right parasagittal meningioma in a 50-year-old female. **A.** Right ECA angiogram showing large middle meningeal artery feeding meningioma; tumor has typical "sunburst" appearance. **B.** Superselective angiogram of right MMA past point of potential anastomoses to ophthalmic or carotid arteries. The tumor was embolized with PVA particles and a pledget of Gelfoam. **C.** Control angiogram following embolization showing no residual tumor opacification.

terior falcine artery) or posterior circulation (posterior meningeal branch off the vertebral artery, meningeal branch off the posterior cerebral artery) can be recruited, and the surgeon needs that information, since deep, uncontrollable bleeding may occur from those branches. Large meningiomas will recruit pial branches at their periphery.

Hypervascular meningiomas have the typical "sunburst" appearance (Fig. 18.54) at the capillary phase of angiography. Perhaps most important, the venous phase tells whether the dural sinus adjacent to the tumor is patent; this information is crucial, since an occluded portion of a sinus can be resected by the surgeon, the rationale being that collateral transmedullary venous channels have had time to develop. If the sinus is still patent but engulfed, surgery to preserve the venous sinus, will be tedious and difficult.

Preoperative embolization of meningiomas can be routinely performed prior to surgery in most major institutions (16–20,22,23). Typical hypervascular convexity meningiomas usually necessitate only middle meningeal artery embolization (Fig. 18.54*B* and *C*). As usual, positioning of the microcatheter tip beyond the takeoff of critical potential anastomoses with the ophthalmic or carotid systems, and beyond the petrous branch which can supply the facial nerve or the geniculate ganglion, is the rule. Embolization with small (150 to 250 μm) PVA particles is preferred over the use of Gelfoam powder, which is less controllable. Excellent tumor bed obliteration can be obtained (Fig. 18.54*C*), along with occlusion of the feeding artery with a pledget of Gelfoam for maximum control. If the brain surrounding the tumor shows evidence of vasogenic edema, administration of corticosteroids and scheduling of surgery immediately after embolization are safest.

Paragangliomas

Paragangliomas are also called *chemodectomas* or *glomus tumors*. These locally infiltrative soft-tissue tumors derive from the neural crest and therefore can be found anywhere along the migration pathway of autonomic ganglionic cells. However, some sites are characteristic in the head and neck region. In the temporal bone, glomus jugulare and tympanicum tumors are the most frequent, followed by carotid body tumors at the carotid bifurcation. Glomus vagale tumors can be found anywhere in the neck along the course of the vagus nerve. The orbit, nasopharynx, and larynx are other possible sites for paragangliomas (20,24–27).

Paragangliomas can be multiple, bilateral, or malignant; they occur sporadically, although a familial form has been described that is transmitted in the autosomal dominant mode (27). Paragangliomas rarely can secrete catecholamines and serotonin, responsible for blood pressure swings, headaches, and agitation.

Paragangliomas manifest differently, depending on their location. Glomus tympanicum and jugulare tumors may present with otalgia, pulsatile tinnitus, conductive hearing loss, lower cranial involvement, or as a retrotympanic mass. Carotid body and glomus vagale tumors present as neck masses, with or without associated pain; lower cranial nerve dysfunction is less common than in paragangliomas of the temporal bone.

The diagnosis of typical paragangliomas is suggested by radiologic studies according to their anatomic location. Glomus tympanicum is seen in the middle ear abutting the cochlear promontory; glomus jugulare occupies the jugular foramen, which is usually eroded; carotid body paraganglioma is seen in the carotid bifurcation, which is usually splayed; glomus vagale has a less typical anatomic location and can be seen in the neck anywhere along the vagus nerve. CT, MRI, and ultrasound in the neck are useful. Dense tumoral enhancement and adjacent bony erosion, in addition to the highly suggestive anatomic location, are characteristic features. Once one tumor is diagnosed, screening for additional tumors should be performed. In secreting paragangliomas, blood and urine sampling for catecholamine or serotonin metabolites vanillylmandelic acid (VMA) or 5-hydroxyindoleacetic acid (5-HIAA) is of help; so can be 131I metaiodobenzoguanidine (MIBG) nuclear scanning.

Angiography is characteristic, showing the dilated feeding arteries and the dense and persistent tumoral blush; early venous shunting is not common; glomus jugulare tumors can be intravascular, within the vein. The arterial supply depends on tumor location, although the ascending pharyngeal artery is a ubiquitous feeder of paragangliomas. Glomus jugulare and tympanicum tumors are commonly supplied by the ascending pharyngeal artery, the posterior auricular artery, the stylomastoid artery, the occipital artery, as well as the caroticotympanic branch of the ICA; the anterior tympanic branch of the internal maxillary artery and the anteroinferior cerebellar artery (AICA) can be recruited. Carotid body tumors can derive their supply from the ascending pharyngeal, occipital, superior thyroidal, ascending cervical, and deep cervical arteries, depending on their size. The concept of vascular compartments applies particularly to paragangliomas, and monocompartmental forms are not uncommon (19,20).

The preferred treatment of paragangliomas is surgical excision. Radiation therapy used to be a popular form of treatment, but recurrences are frequent. Preoperative interventional management is important for several reasons. First of all, complete superselective angiography is necessary; since triggering of a hypertensive or hypotensive crisis can be disastrous, this is best done in the appropriate setting, that is, with the help of an anesthesiologist. Second, and perhaps most important in the management of carotid body tumors, a tolerance test occlusion of the ICA must be carried out (28,29) since the vessel wall may be invaded by the tumor, and subadventitial arterial dissection might result in uncontrollable ICA bleeding, necessitating ICA sacrifice (Fig. 18.55). Last, preoperative embolization of paragangliomas is presently regarded as a necessary step prior to surgery in major institutions (16,19,20,24–27),

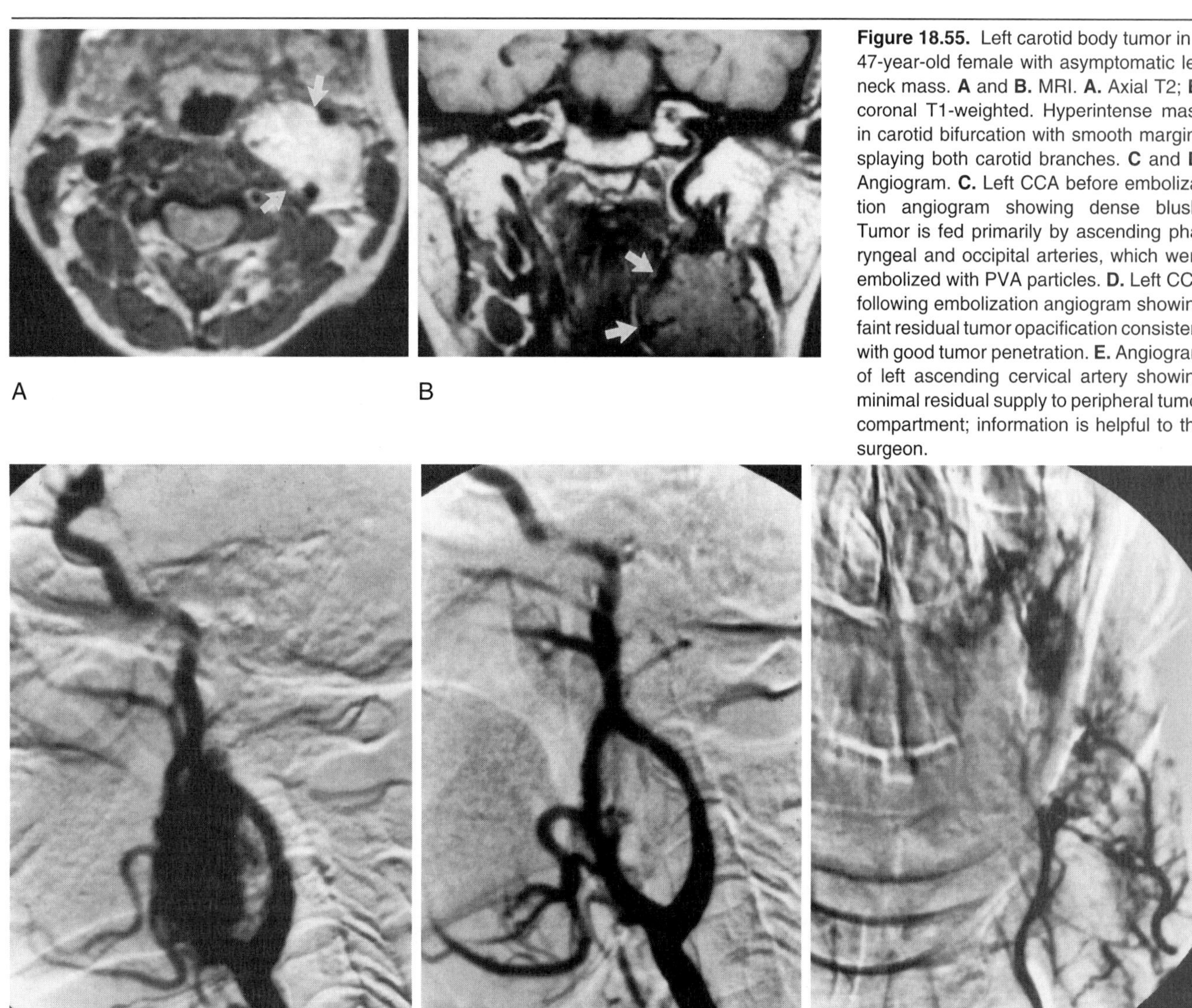

Figure 18.55. Left carotid body tumor in a 47-year-old female with asymptomatic left neck mass. **A** and **B.** MRI. **A.** Axial T2; **B.** coronal T1-weighted. Hyperintense mass in carotid bifurcation with smooth margins splaying both carotid branches. **C** and **D.** Angiogram. **C.** Left CCA before embolization angiogram showing dense blush. Tumor is fed primarily by ascending pharyngeal and occipital arteries, which were embolized with PVA particles. **D.** Left CCA following embolization angiogram showing faint residual tumor opacification consistent with good tumor penetration. **E.** Angiogram of left ascending cervical artery showing minimal residual supply to peripheral tumor compartment; information is helpful to the surgeon.

having been shown to reduce mortality, morbidity, and even length of hospital stay (20,24). The feeding vessels are catheterized as distally as possible, and particulate embolization is performed, usually with PVA particles 150 to 250 μm in size; larger particles may be needed to prevent reflux in anastomoses. Attention to branches supplying cranial nerves is the rule. Gelfoam pieces in the feeding artery trunk are a useful adjunct to promote further ischemia.

Other Tumors

Squamous cell carcinoma is the most common malignant tumor of the temporal bone. It is usually seen between the fifth and seventh decades following chronic ear infection. The tumor develops from the mucosa of the external auditory canal and spreads to the middle ear cavity. Otalgia and bloody ear drainage are early signs; later on, tumoral involvement of cranial nerves can result in facial palsy, tinnitus, dizziness, and hearing loss (30). CT and MRI show an irregular soft-tissue mass with bone destruction; CT can show sclerosis of the temporal bone; MRI shows an enhancing mass. The tumor is not hypervascular at angiography. When indicated, preoperative interventional management usually consists of tolerance test occlusion of the ipsilateral internal carotid artery and/or vertebral artery when strong suggestion of vessel wall invasion is present, or when surgery is not felt to be compatible with vessel sparing. Carotid or vertebral balloon occlusion can be performed in the standard way. Superselective injection of chemotherapeutic agents is currently under consideration.

Chordomas are slow-growing neoplasms that arise from notochord remnants. In the head and neck region, the most common site for chordomas is the clivus. The tumor is twice as common in males, and the peak incidence is between the third and seventh decades. Chordomas are median or slightly paramedian in location. There are two distinct subtypes, and their recognition bears prognostic implications: in the physaliphorous type, survival is around 4 years; in the chondroid type, it is around 16 years (31,32). CT shows a locally aggressive tumor with bone destruction and calcifications; bone sequestration is a feature of chordomas. MRI shows a mass that is hyperintense on T2-weighted sequences, iso- or hypointense on T1-weighted images, and enhances markedly (31,32). Chordomas are not hypervascular at angiography. Here, too, possible presurgical interventional management consists of tolerance test and/or permanent balloon occlusion of encased intracranial arteries.

Chondrosarcomas are rare in the skull. They usually arise at the petroclival junction, directly from bone, or from a preexisting exostosis. Chondrosarcomas are twice as frequent in females, and their peak incidence is between the fourth and sixth decades (31). They are slow growing, locally invasive, and extend to the cavernous sinus region, causing cranial nerve palsies. CT shows an osteolytic lesion associated with a soft-tissue mass that enhances. MRI shows best the extent of soft-tissue involvement and brainstem compression. Chondrosarcomas are not hypervascular at angiography, and again, when considered, preoperative interventional care consists of temporary tolerance test or permanent balloon occlusion of encased artery.

Trauma

PENETRATING INJURIES

Penetrating injuries of the head and neck are associated with an extremely high morbidity and mortality. Death occurs following exsanguination or cerebral ischemia. If the patient survives the initial hours, distal embolization of the arterial injury site is common. Particularly treacherous are injuries to the high neck, where surgical control of the high cervical or petrous internal carotid artery, the external carotid artery, or the vertebral artery is poor. Large veins may also be damaged, causing additional significant bleeding.

The patient is usually seen in a dramatic context of profuse bleeding from the nose, mouth, throat, or ear from a gunshot wound (Fig. 18.56). Less frequently, assault or accident results in blunt or sharp trauma to the neck. An expanding hematoma to the neck or nasopharynx can rapidly compromise airway patency. A neurologic deficit is frequently present, due to injury to the cranial nerves (33–37).

Angiography plays a crucial role in the diagnosis and management of such lesions. Direct contrast medium extravasation is rarely observed; the bleeding rate must be 2 ml per second or higher for extravasation to be noted. AVFs, pseudoaneurysms (Fig. 18.57), or total arterial occlusions do not pose a diagnostic problem. Intimal flaps (Fig. 18.58; 18.61) can be hard to demonstrate, and extreme attention must be given to irregularities of arterial wall contour. Vessel spasm can be seen in the form of smooth tapering, as can extrinsic compression from a hematoma (33–35).

Endovascular management of acute arterial hemorrhage in the head and neck can be rewarding (33–36). In cases of profuse hemorrhage, proper recognition of the bleeding source can have a dramatic impact on the patient's life. Figure 18.56 illustrates the case of a policeman who sustained a close-range gunshot wound to the head and neck while cleaning his loaded gun. He was bleeding profusely from the nose and mouth, and angiography, although demonstrating intracranial arterial spasm adjacent to multiple intracranial bullet fragments, did not show convincing evidence of internal carotid arterial injury. The bleeding source was identified as bilateral internal maxillary arteries, which were occluded with thrombogenic coils. Both internal carotid arteries were spared, and the patient eventually made a good recovery. Figure 18.57 illustrates an example of blunt trauma to the neck in a young man who was bleeding profusely from his mouth. Angiography showed the bleeding vessel to be the lingual artery. Coil embolization of this small vessel was successful in arresting the hemorrhage.

In cases when the ICA is recognized as the source of bleeding, the best treatment is detachable balloon occlusion. In imminent life-threatening situations, alternate techniques, such as the use of nondetachable balloon systems or detachable coils, are acceptable forms of management.

Management of head and neck trauma in the nonacute period is also sometimes best done by endovascular means. Figure 18.58 illustrates the case of a 19-year-old female who had been stabbed in the neck. Bleeding was not profuse, and an initial angiogram (not shown) disclosed complete left vertebral artery occlusion. A subsequent angiogram showed recanalization of the vessel, with an extensive and irregular intimal flap (Fig. 18.58*A* and *B*). The decision was made to occlude the vertebral artery in order to protect the patient from intracranial migration of emboli forming at the dissection site. Preservation of the distal vertebral artery through normal abundant collateral channels was confirmed (Fig. 18.58*E*), guaranteeing patency of crucial vessels such as the anterior spinal and posteroinferior cerebellar (PICA) arteries.

EPISTAXIS

Life-threatening epistaxis may result from trauma to the face. Although epistaxis is usually benign and self-containing, requiring nasal packing at the most, conditions other than trauma may result in uncontrollable epistaxis (16,38,39) (Fig. 18.62). Atrophic rhinitis, seen in the elderly and related to hypertension and arteriosclerosis, benign or malignant tumors of the nasopharynx (pyogenic granuloma, a rare fibrous tumor, is one such cause), true granulomatous disease (Wegener granulomatosis), arteriovenous malformations, and fistulae all can be responsible for nosebleeds that are difficult to control surgically.

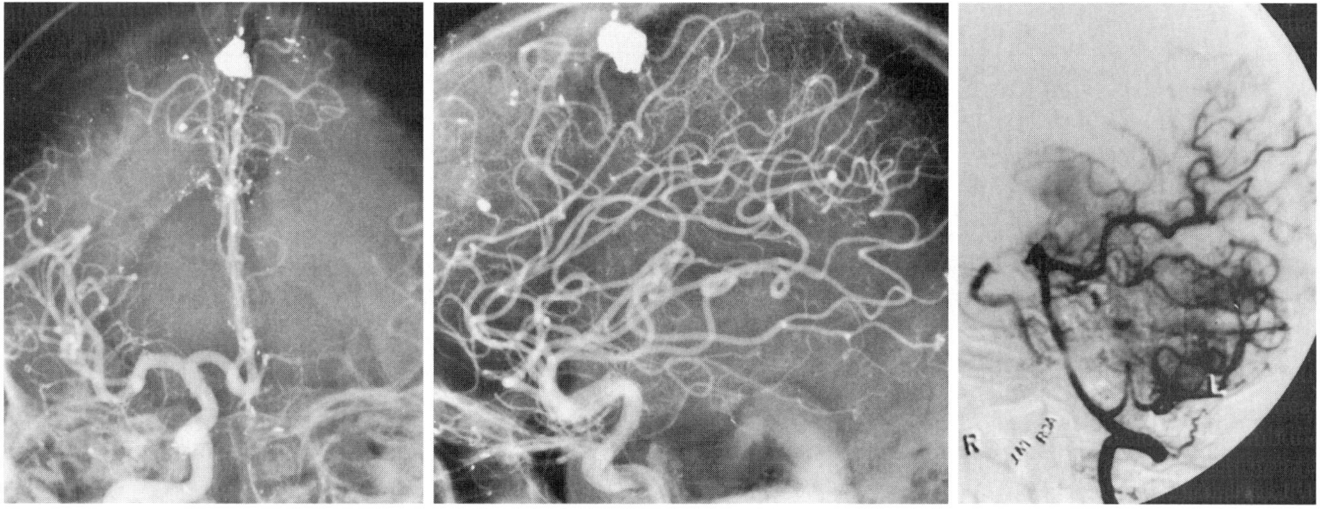

A B C

Figure 18.56. A 25-year-old unconscious policeman with profuse facial bleeding status post from a close-range gunshot wound to the head. **A.** Right ICA angiogram AP. Multiple metallic foreign bodies in the soft tissues of the face as well as within the skull cavity. Note localized vessel spasm contiguous to foreign bodies. No extravasation is noted from internal carotid artery; note mass effect from edema and hemorrhage. **B.** Right ICA angiogram lateral: orthogonal view confirming findings. The pericallosal artery is displaced downward. **C.** Left VA angiogram showing no injury to posterior circulation. The source of bleeding was bilateral internal maxillary arteries, which were proximally embolized with coils. Angiogram and embolization were performed within 30 minutes from trauma. Patient made a good recovery.

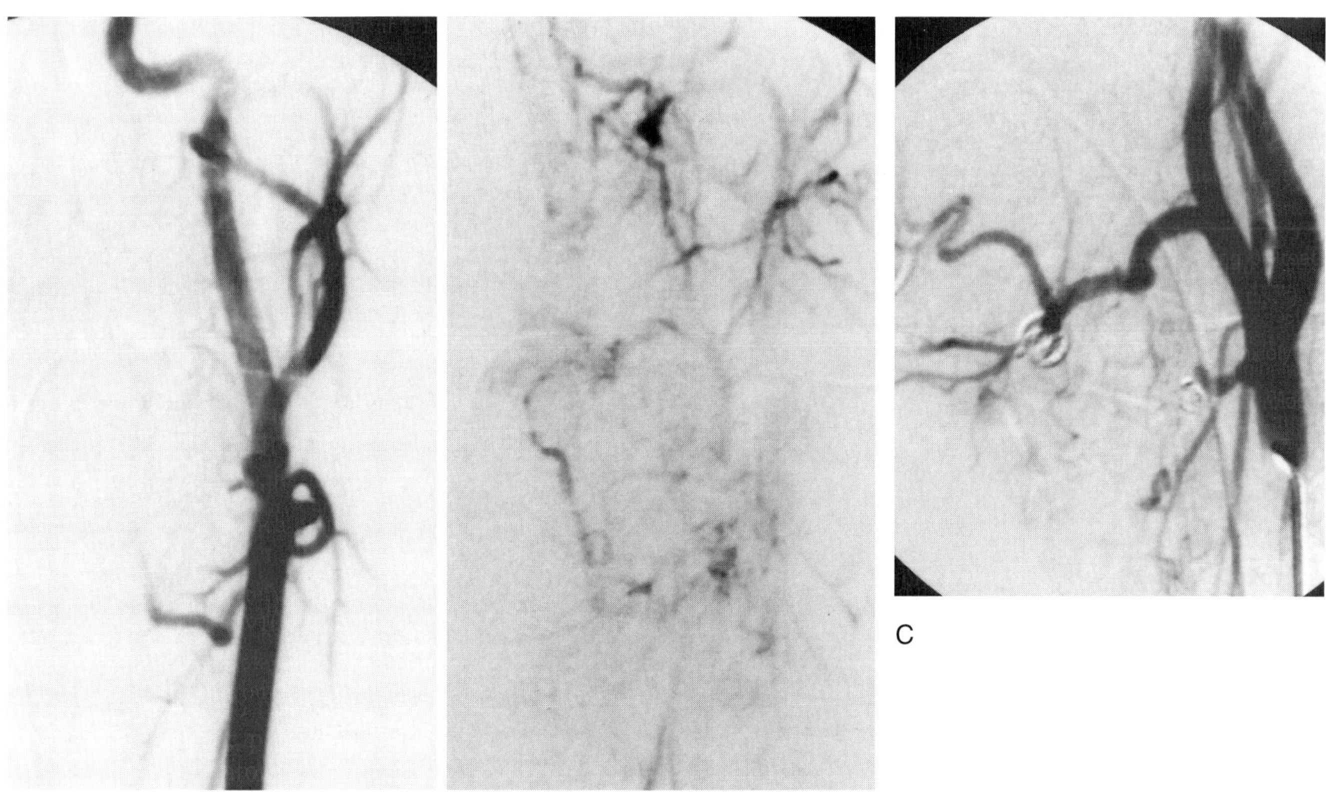

C

A B

Figure 18.57. Traumatic carotid blow-out in a 24-year-old male with oral bleeding status post neck trauma. **A** and **B.** Left CCA angiogram lateral view. **A.** Early phase; **B.** late phase. No contrast extravasation from or wall abnormality in ICA; bleeding is from lingual artery. Note slow initial filling and delayed emptying. **C.** Left CCA angiogram lateral view late phase following embolization of lingual artery with coils: cessation of bleeding.

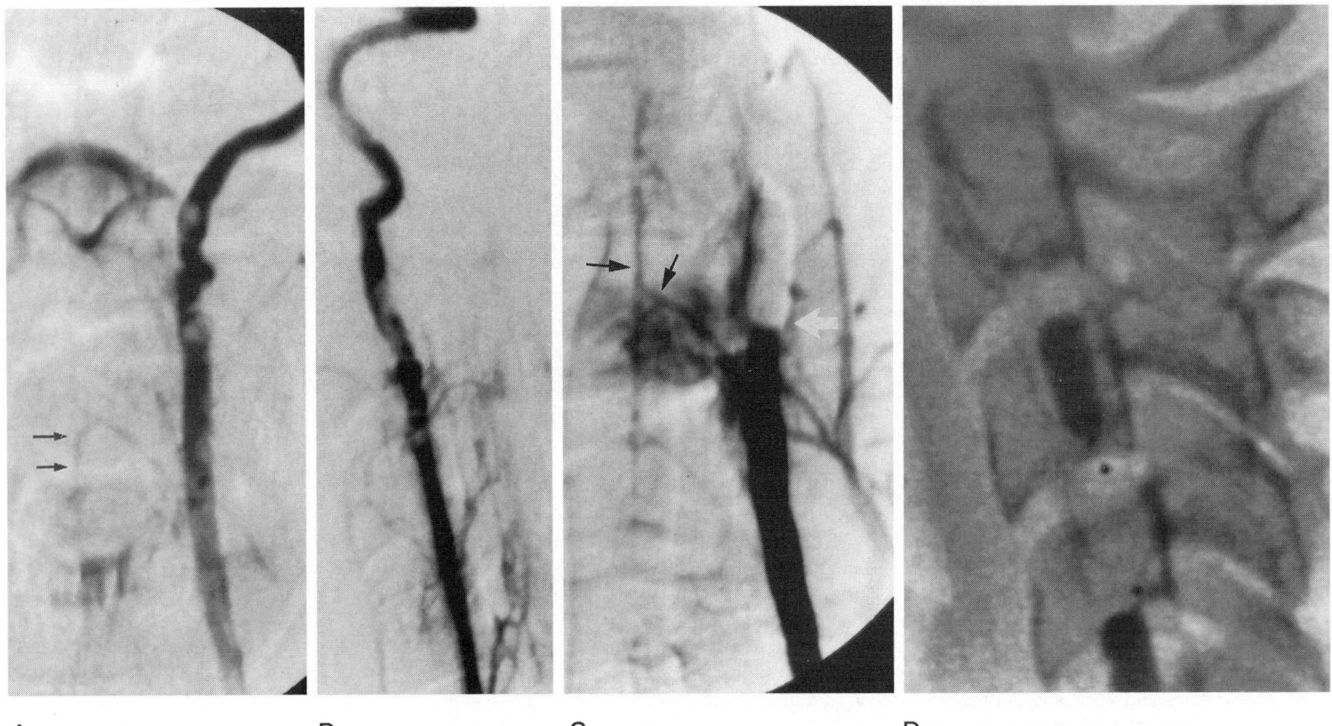

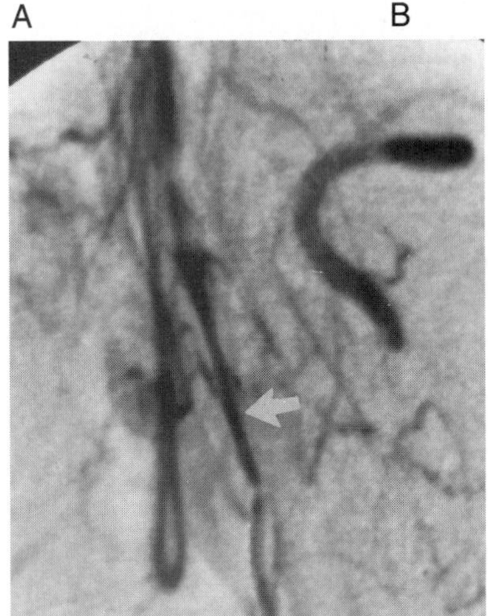

Figure 18.58. A 19-year-old female with traumatic left vertebral artery (VA) dissection status post penetrating injury. **A** and **B.** Left VA before treatment. A. anteroposterior; B. lateral. Left VA dissection seen at level of C3 vertebral body. Note anterior spinal artery well seen on AP at C5 (arrow). **C** and **D.** Left VA balloon occlusion. **C.** Left VA anteroposterior with balloon occluding distal vessel. Note anterior spinal artery filling from just below base of balloon (arrow). **D.** Plain film showing balloons in left VA following treatment. **E.** After treatment. Verification of patency of distal left VA: lateral view of left ascending pharyngeal artery injection (arrow) showing reconstitution of distal left VA from C3 anastomoses (odontoid arch system).

The usual therapeutic steps are, in a crescendo fashion, nasal packing with cotton, Gelfoam or balloon catheter, and surgical clipping of distal internal maxillary branches or of the external carotid artery trunk. Embolization is an accepted and very efficient form of epistaxis treatment, when cautiously performed and with careful attention to anatomy (21,38–40). The arterial supply to the nasopharynx is rich, and abundant anastomoses exist, some of which are unforgiving. Dangerous anastomoses are described earlier in this chapter; the potential risk is mostly to the eye, brain, and facial nerve. Embolization carried out for atrophic rhinitis (Fig. 18.59), tumors, or granulomas is most hazardous in inexperienced hands, since the use of particulate emboli is warranted for deep-tisue penetration. In cases of trauma with laceration of nasopharyngeal arteries, embolization with thrombogenic coils can suffice to arrest the bleeding, and carries less of a risk of distal migration in a normal vessel or an unsuspected anastomosis. One has to be aware of the possibility of a nasopharyngeal ulcer after vigorous embolization that usually heals spontaneously. Also, a low-grade fever can be observed.

Iatrogenic

Arterial trauma can result from medical intervention. Recognition of the problem may be the single most important step in managing the condition.

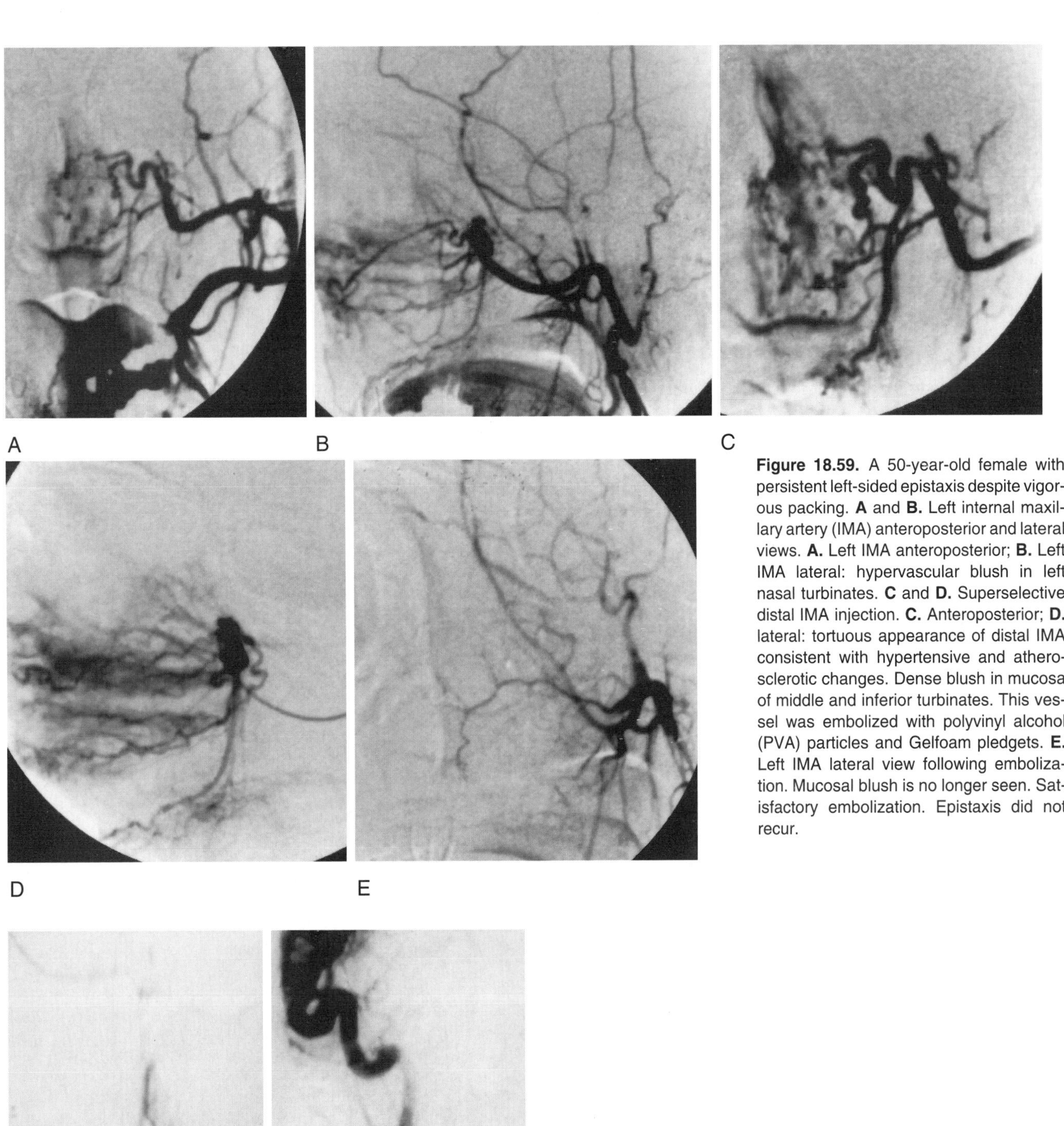

Figure 18.59. A 50-year-old female with persistent left-sided epistaxis despite vigorous packing. **A** and **B.** Left internal maxillary artery (IMA) anteroposterior and lateral views. **A.** Left IMA anteroposterior; **B.** Left IMA lateral: hypervascular blush in left nasal turbinates. **C** and **D.** Superselective distal IMA injection. **C.** Anteroposterior; **D.** lateral: tortuous appearance of distal IMA consistent with hypertensive and atherosclerotic changes. Dense blush in mucosa of middle and inferior turbinates. This vessel was embolized with polyvinyl alcohol (PVA) particles and Gelfoam pledgets. **E.** Left IMA lateral view following embolization. Mucosal blush is no longer seen. Satisfactory embolization. Epistaxis did not recur.

A B

Figure 18.60. Carotid blowout status post surgery and radiation. This 85-year-old male underwent status post radical neck dissection and radiation therapy for squamous cell carcinoma. **A.** Selective right superior thyroidal artery angiogram. Note irregular distal vessel at lower edge of film: source of bleed. Internal carotid artery was intact. **B.** Right CCA angiogram following embolization. No residual bleeding. Patient did not rebleed.

Endovascular

Vessel perforation can occur, either intracranially or in the neck, during an interventional procedure. Immediate recognition of this complication and prompt treatment will dramatically reduce morbidity. At all times during a procedure, there should be detachable balloons and liquid glue available to the interventional neuroradiologist. The adage "Fix what you broke" is most appropriate here, and the situation commands fast and skilled action.

Surgical

Occasionally, the interventional neuroradiologist may be called to the operating room to help manage profuse arterial bleeding resulting from inadvertent vessel laceration that is uncontrollable surgically. Such circumstances include difficult ear, nose, and throat surgery for tumors extending from the nasopharynx or the infratemporal fossa to the intracranial space and encasing the cavernous or petrous internal carotid artery, or surgery on the cervical spine resulting in vertebral artery laceration. In these instances, transfer of a hemodynamically unstable patient to the angiography suite might be too hazardous, and endovascular occlusion is best carried out in the operating room, under fluoroscopic control of a C-arm x-ray machine if at all possible.

Surgery can also be the cause of hemorrhage in patients with head and neck cancer who have sustained a radical neck dissection (41). However, surgery alone is rarely implicated: the association of surgery to radiation therapy, and less often to infection with fistula formation, more commonly predisposes to the so-called carotid blowouts (42).

Radiation

Total excision of head and neck tumors that surround and invade the carotid artery is not always possible at surgery; therefore, alternative forms of surgical management are considered, such as "peeling off" as much tumor as possible around the vessel, carotid ligation, and carotid reconstruction (usually with a saphenous vein graft) (43). Needless to say, in cases where the possibility of carotid artery sacrifice is considered, tolerance test occlusion of the vessel with recording of the patient's blood pressure gives invaluable information to the surgeon (28,43,44). We also believe that in situations where carotid sacrifice is granted, balloon occlusion is safer than abrupt intraoperative occlusion, allowing for postocclusion heparin therapy, and blood pressure control with vasopressors in the intensive care unit in a conscious patient to permit optimal intracranial collateral circulation buildup. Most of these patients receive radiation treatment.

Radiation injury to arterial walls has long been recognized as a cause of head and neck hemorrhage (41). Pulsatile flow in the carotid arteries, their branches, or the reconstruction graft after radiation does not encounter the usual elastic resistance. The vessel walls that have undergone microscopic radiation changes may be associated with small "sentinel" bleeds that precede catastrophic uncontrollable hemorrhage (41–43,45). The assumption that the internal carotid artery is the source of bleeding has not been verified in our experience (42). Careful angiographic technique and analysis disclose that in over half of the cases, occlusion of an external carotid branch (lingual, superior thyroidal, proximal facial artery) is sufficient to stop the bleeding (Fig. 18.60). Tolerance occlusion of the internal carotid artery in the same setting provides crucial information as to the safety of occluding the vessel, even at bedside if indicated as a lifesaving maneuver at a later time. Radiation injury seems to affect more medium-sized arteries than large trunks; a "sentinel" bleed should not necessarily mean that the internal or common carotid artery must be sacrificed.

REFERENCES

1. Mulliken JB, Glowacki J: Hemangiomas and vascular malformations: A classification based on endothelial characteristics. Plast Reconstr Surg 1982;69:412–420.
2. Glowacki J, Mulliken JB: Mast cells in hemangiomas and vascular malformations. Pediatrics 1982;70:48–51.
3. Burrows PE, Mulliken JB, Fellows KE: Childhood hemangiomas and vascular malformations: Angiographic differentiation. AJR 1983;141:483–488.
4. Mulliken JB: Vascular malformations of the head and neck. In JB Mulliken, AE Young (eds), Vascular Birthmarks: Hemangiomas and Malformations. Philadelphia: WB Saunders, 1988, pp 301–340.
5. Ezekowitz RAB, Mulliken JB, Folkman J: Interferon alpha-2a therapy for life-threatening hemangiomas of infancy. N Engl J Med 1992;326:1456–1463.
6. Kasabach HH, Merritt KK: Capillary hemangioma with extensive purpura: Report of a case. Am J Dis Child 1940;59:1063–1070.
7. Huston J III, Forbes GS, Ruefenacht DA, et al: Magnetic resonance imaging of facial vascular anomalies. Mayo Clin Proc 1992;67:739–747.
8. Sloan GM, Reinish JP, Nichter LS, et al: Intra-lesional corticosteroid therapy for infantile hemangiomas. Plast Reconstr Surg 1989;83:459–467.
9. Stanley P, Gomperts E, Woolley MM: Kasabach-Merritt syndrome treated by therapeutic embolization with polyvinyl-alcohol. Am J Pediatr Hematol Oncol 1986;8:308–311.
10. Riche MC, Merland JJ: Embolization of vascular malformations. In JB Mulliken, AE Young (eds), Vascular Birthmarks: Hemangiomas and Malformations. Philadelphia: WB Saunders, 1988.
11. Riche MC, Hadjean E, Tran-Ba-Huy P, Merland JJ: The treatment of capillary-venous malformations using a new fibrosing agent. Plast Reconstr Surg 1983;71:607–614.
12. Luedke MD, Pile-Spellman JMD, Huggins CE, et al: Cryoprecipitate admixtures: In vitro testing as an embolic agent. ASNR abstract. AJNR 1988;9:1030.
13. Ellman BA, Parkhill BJ, Carry TS, et al: Ablation of renal tumors with absolute ethanol: A new technique. Radiology 1981;141:619–626.
14. Berenstein A: Ethanol injection in venous malformations. In P Lasjaunias, A Berenstein (eds), Surgical Neuroangiography. Vol. 2: Endovascular Treatment of Craniofacial Lesions. Berlin: Springer, 1987.
15. Lasjaunias P, Berenstein A: Surgical Neuroangiography. Vol 2: Endovascular Treatment of Craniofacial Lesions. Berlin: Springer, 1987.
16. Lasjaunias P, Berenstein A: Surgical Neuroangiography. Vol. 1: Functional Anatomy of Craniofacial Arteries. Berlin: Springer, 1987.
17. Davis KR: Embolization of epistaxis and juvenile nasopharyngeal angiofibromas. AJNR 1986;7:953–962.

18. Elster AD, Challa VR, Gilbert TH, et al: Meningiomas: MR and histopathologic features. Radiology 1989;170:857–862.
19. Moret J, Delvert G, Lasjaunias P: Vascular architecture of tympanicojugular glomus tumors: Its application regarding therapeutic angiography. J Neuroradiol 1982;9:237–260.
20. Valavanis A: Preoperative embolization of the head and neck: Indications, patient selection, goals and precautions. AJNR 1986;7:943–952.
21. De Vries N, Vershuis RG, Valk G, et al: Facial nerve paralysis following embolization for severe epistaxis. J Laryngol Otol 1986;100:207–210.
22. Horton JA, Kerber CW: Lidocaine injection into the external carotid artery branches: Provocative test to preserve cranial nerve function in therapeutic embolization. AJNR 1986;7:105–108.
23. Vinuela F, Halbach VV, Dion JE: Interventional Neuroradiology: Endovascular Therapy of the Central Nervous System. New York: Raven Press, 1992.
24. Lacour P, Doyon D, Manelfe C, et al: Treatment of chemodectomas by arterial embolization. J Neuroradiol 1975;2:275–287.
25. Borges LF, Heros RC, Debrun GM: Carotid body tumors managed with preoperative embolization: Report of two cases. J Neurosurg 1983;59:867–870.
26. Spector GJ, Sobol S, Thawley SE, et al: Glomus jugulare tumors of the temporal bone: Patterns of invasion of the temporal bone. Laryngoscope 1979;89:1628–1639.
27. Ward PH, Liu C, Vinuela F, et al: Embolization: An adjunctive measure for removal of carotid body tumors. Laryngoscope 1988;98:1287–1291.
28. Mount LA, Taveras JM: Arteriographic demonstration of the collateral circulation of the cerebral hemispheres. Arch Neurol Psychiatry 1957;78:235–253.
29. Serbinenko FA: Balloon catheterization and occlusion of major cerebral vessels. J Neurosurg 1974;41:125–145.
30. Friedman DP, Rao VM: MR and CT of squamous cell carcinoma of the middle ear and mastoid complex. AJNR 1991;12:872–874.
31. Oot RF, Melville GE, New PFJ, et al: The role of MR and CT in evaluating clival chordomas and chondrosarcomas. AJNR 1988;9:715–723.
32. Sze G, Vichanco LS, Brant-Zawadski MN, et al: Chordomas: MR imaging. Radiology 1988;166:187–191.
33. Panetta T, Sclafani SJA, Goldstein AS, et al: Percutaneous transcatheter embolization for arterial trauma. J Vasc Surg 1985;2:54–64.
34. Sclafani SJA, Panetta T, Goldstein AS, et al: The management of arterial injuries caused by penetration of zone III of the neck. Trauma 1985;25:871–881.
35. Sclafani SJA, Becker JA: The arteriographic diagnosis and management of presacral hemorrhage. AJR 1982;138:123–126.
36. Khoo CTK, Molyneux AJ, Rayment R, et al: The control of carotid arterial hemorrhage in head and neck surgery by balloon catheter tamponade and detachable balloon embolisation. Br J Plast Surg 1986;39:72–75.
37. Mehringer CM, Hieshima GB, Grinnell VS, et al: Therapeutic embolization for vascular trauma of the head and neck. AJNR 1983;4:137–142.
38. Lasjaunias P, Marsot-Dupuch K, Doyon D: The radio-anatomical basis of arterial embolization for epistaxis. J Neuroradiol 1979;6:45–53.
39. Merland JJ, Melki JP, Chiras J, et al: Place of embolization in the treatment of severe epistaxis. Laryngoscope 1980;90:1694–1704.
40. Vitek JJ: Idiopathic intractable epistaxis: Endovascular therapy. Radiology 1991;181:113–116.
41. Heller KS, Strong EW: Carotid arterial hemorrhage after radical head and neck surgery. Am J Surg 1979;138:607–610.
42. Pile-Spellman J, Sanchez R, Chin J, et al: Carotid artery blow-outs: Importance of external carotid artery sources and endovascular treatment. ASNR abstract. 28th Annual Meeting of the ASNR, March 19–23, 1990.
43. Olcott C, Fee WE, Enzmann DR, et al: Planned approach to the management of malignant invasion of the carotid artery. Am J Surg 1981;142:123–127.
44. Moore OS, Karlan M, Sigler L: Factors influencing the safety of carotid ligation. Am J Surg 1969;142:123–127.
45. McReady RA, Hyde GL, Bivins BA, et al: Radiation induced arterial injuries. Surgery 1983;93:306–312.

18.12 Endovascular Management of Injuries to the Extracranial Carotid and Vertebral Arteries

E. Sander Connolly, Jr.* and John Pile-Spellman

Key Points

1. Traumatic injuries to the cervical carotid and vertebral arteries may result in transection, laceration, occlusion, dissection, false aneurysm, and arteriovenous fistula.
2. Trauma may be closed or penetrating, iatrogenic or accidental, may present acutely or subacutely, and is often overlooked in severe multisystem injury.
3. Early panangiography is indicated in all but the acutely exsanguinating patient; it provides critical information about the injury, gives information about general cerebrovascular physiology, lessens bleeding, decreases the incidence of iatrogenic injury by subsequent surgery, and can serve as the initial step in therapeutic embolization.
4. Ongoing bleeding is controlled proximally, with neurologic assessment to determine tolerance to vessel occlusion.
5. When endovascular occlusion is not tolerated, when symptoms are progressive and flow related, or when the ease of repair makes salvage of the parent vessel attractive, operative revascularization is warranted.
6. Dissection is generally treated with anticoagulation; thrombosis or occlusion is usually treated with balloons and anticoagulation; pseudoaneurysms and fistulas are usually treated with coils and microballoons, respectively.
7. Vessel patency is often achieved with endovascular and medical management alone.

Traumatic injuries to the cervical carotid and vertebral arteries may result in transection, laceration, occlusion, dissection, false aneurysm, and arteriovenous fistula. Trauma may be closed or penetrating, iatrogenic or accidental, and

* Neurological Surgery staff member, Columbia Presbyterian Medical Center, New York, N.Y.

may present acutely or subacutely. In spinal and severe multisystem trauma, injury can easily be misdiagnosed. Better understanding of the underlying pathophysiology of these lesions, together with recent advances in angiographic and endovascular techniques, should lead both to better patient selection and to more successful management.

GENERAL MANAGEMENT PRINCIPLES

Panangiography

Taken as a group there are very few patients who, having suffered penetrating or nonpenetrating cervical trauma, cannot endure panangiography in an institution prepared to administer it quickly and at short notice. Patients suffering exsanguinating hemorrhage may represent a rare exception. But even in cases where aggressive packing and intubation are necessary for immediate control, angiography can, with minimal added delay, allow exact identification of bleeding points and provide invaluable data regarding associated occlusions, collateral vascular supply, as well as general circulatory physiology. Contrast transit times give information about cerebral blood flow, and test occlusions may be performed on awake patients. Associated lesions such as subdural and epidural hematomas can be diagnosed, and access to the arch is rarely complicated or time-consuming in this younger population. Moreover, patients actively bleeding are generally coagulopathic and require no additional heparin to perform the procedure. Venous and arterial access at the groin has often already been obtained. In short, preoperative angiography is almost always warranted. It saves time, lessens bleeding, decreases the risk of associated iatrogenic lesions created by vascular clamps, and can often serve as the initial necessary step toward therapeutic embolization (1,2).

When ongoing hemorrhage is not a concern, this is even more true, yet there still exist situations in which angiography is unwisely omitted. Cases include those in which external signs of cervical trauma are mild and neurologic symptoms are either absent, subtle, or obscured by associated head or spinal cord injury. In the case of head and neck trauma with suspected intracranial injury, negative CT scans should at least be accompanied by cervical and transcranial Doppler studies and should probably lead one to angiography in any case. Duplex ultrasound followed by angiography should also be offered to patients with certain high-risk cervical fractures and to neurologically intact patients with highly suggestive symptomatology (i.e., bruit, partial Horner syndrome, basilar TIAs).

Embolization

Once angiography has been performed, embolization may be of either therapeutic or further diagnostic use and may be accomplished without delay (3,4). The decision whether to embolize, and if so how, depends on several factors. Most important is the pathology. Ongoing bleeding as detected by contrast extravasation should be immediately controlled by acquiring proximal control of the vessel with either the catheter itself or a detachable balloon (5). When the transected or lacerated vessel is the carotid or the vertebral artery itself, this, in essence, constitutes a test occlusion. All other extracranial branches of these vessels may be taken without deficit. In cases where the test occlusion is tolerated or sacrifice is known to be safe, permanent occlusion can be obtained using either metal coils or detachable balloons.

In cases that require patency of the damaged vessel, proximal control can be left in place temporarily, greatly simplifying the ensuing operative approach and reconstruction. This, of course, presumes accessibility to an able surgical staff and lesions not impossibly located. In the latter case, endovascular stents may offer another option. In any case, once bleeding has been controlled, consideration must be immediately given to anticoagulation, for it is at this point that the patient becomes hypercoagulable.

For cases in which angiography discloses nonhemorrhagic lesions such as dissections, thromboses, fistulas, or pseudoaneurysms, endovascular management is quite varied and will be discussed in detail in the text following. Generally, however, in dissection, therapy is delayed until an aggressive course of anticoagulation has failed. Thromboses or dissections leading to complete occlusion, if being tolerated, are usually permanently occluded with balloons, followed by anticoagulation. Acute fistulas and pseudoaneurysms may also be treated with balloons and coils, respectively. Parent vessel patency rates, which are quite good for both, are discussed in greater detail in text following.

Surgery

Although once the mainstay of treatment, surgery's role in the management of cervical vascular injuries remains critical, albeit less dominant. And while there are still cases of massive hemorrhage that require split-second exploration, surgery is now most often employed for the reconstruction of vessels whose endovascular occlusion cannot be tolerated and for the rerouting of flow in cases of flow-related deficits. In short, open surgery is employed when the likelihood of its success and the need of the vessel are both judged to be great. Several approaches have been developed for each cervical section of the carotid and vertebral arteries, but their discussion is beyond the scope of this text. Like any other endovascular procedure, adequate proximal and distal control is of paramount importance. Also important is ready access to vascular substitutes should primary repair prove impossible. Most surgeons prefer autologous saphenous vein, for its increased patency as well as its decreased risk for infection. Most also prefer intraoperative heparinization without reversal when possible and routinely monitor intraoperative EEG. When possible, neuroprotective anesthetics, hypothermia, and calcium channel blockers are also employed.

Specific Clinical Management

NONPENETRATING CAROTID INJURIES

Nonpenetrating trauma to the carotid artery may be the result of a direct blow but is more commonly secondary to stretching, tearing, or compression (6,7). All etiologies taken together, nonpenetrating carotid trauma is, however, rare (8,9). Rarity, and the fact that only a few patients will demonstrate external signs of direct cervical injury, make it necessary to have a high index of suspicion when examining patients who develop, either subacutely or in a delayed fashion, an unexplained mono- or hemiparesis or change in mental status, especially after MVAs or falls (10,11). Despite the common finding of a normal head computed tomography (CT), but, in part, because of the actual coexistence of head injury and other multisystem trauma, the unprepared clinician often attributes carotid symptoms to head injury or shock, with disastrous consequences (12). Better understanding of the various pathologic states that result from thrombosis, dissection, false aneurysm formation, and fistula formation will undoubtedly provide for earlier and more effective management.

Thrombosis

While nonpenetrating cervical trauma leading to carotid thrombosis is a rare event, approximately 15 percent of all cases of carotid thrombosis have associated histories of craniocervical trauma (13). Presentation of traumatic carotid thrombosis most commonly consists of a progressive focal deficit with delay in onset ranging from 1 to 24 h (14). Most patients have been hospitalized with the diagnosis of closed head injury (11). Half will have evidence of neck trauma as well (15).

Doppler ultrasonography is gaining popularity as a screening test, but, if negative, angiography should still be considered in any patient with a focal neurologic deficit and a negative CT scan. Magnetic resonance angiography (MRA) is also of potential benefit in more stable patients but is probably not sensitive enough to replace angiography, especially in high-risk patients such as those with progressive vascular distribution edema on serial CT scans (16,17). At angiography the majority will demonstrate occlusion, but high-grade stenosis or intraluminal thrombus with partial occlusion can also be seen. The vast majority of lesions occur between the bifurcation and the skull base (18).

Classification of thrombotic lesions focuses on etiology, with type I injuries occurring secondary to direct trauma to older atherosclerotic vessels resulting in intimal and medial damage. Type II, III, and IV injuries also involve intimal and medial damage but occur in the following less frequent settings: stretching of a hyperextended axially rotated artery against the transverse processes of C2 or C3, childhood intraoral trauma, and fracture of the skull base (14). In each of these an intimal flap is raised, leading to initiation of local thrombus, which quickly propagates to total occlusion. Delayed symptomatology is felt to be due to embolism from the thrombotic occlusion, and therefore, flow independent (19).

Traditional management of these lesions, whether medical or surgical, has unfortunately been associated with an approximately 33 percent mortality rate. Furthermore, only about 25 percent of patients escape permanent neurologic deficit. Medical management consists of full and aggressive anticoagulation with heparin (20). Surgical options, although less attractive, have included arteriotomy with thrombus removal using Fogarty catheters followed by intimal flap repair and arterial resection with interposition reversed saphenous vein graft repair (21). Comparison of the two approaches as analyzed by surgeons has favored surgery, but invalidating biases exist (22).

More recently, an initial nonsurgical trial of anticoagulation in good-grade patients has yielded good results in 87 percent (10). Nonetheless, even in patients with good surgical results, postoperative angiograms often show occluded vessels (10). Furthermore, anticoagulation appears safe in multiply traumatized victims (12). We therefore reserve procedural intervention in good-grade patients for those with progressive symptoms on full anticoagulation. We evaluate this subset with repeat angiography and transcranial Doppler to determine the degree of collateral flow. Operative revascularization is offered to those with poor or questionable flow, and endovascular proximal and distal balloon occlusion provides a simple and effective alternative to the traditional stumpectomy. Postoperative anticoagulation is vital in avoiding thrombus propagation from either the balloon or the suture line. Poor-grade patients are more controversial, having been shown to do better with surgery (50 percent good outcome) than with medical treatment alone (18 percent) (10). For patients with total occlusion, we feel that endovascular balloon occlusion with heparinization has been just as effective, allowing edematous areas to recover without subjecting them to the extremes of anesthetic hypoperfusion and revascularized hyperperfusion. Patients with high-grade stenosis are generally spared endovascular therapies until such time that they can be evaluated by test occlusion.

Dissection

Carotid dissection, although infrequently spontaneous or secondary to intrinsic arterial pathology, is most frequently traumatic in origin (23,24). Common etiologies include hyperextension with lateral rotation, chiropractic manipulation, attempted strangulation, and cerebral angiography (25–27). These insults may be either minor or severe, unilateral or bilateral, and the patient may present with either delayed or acute focal symptoms. An incomplete Horner syndrome, headache, facial pain, carotidynia, bruit, or some combination thereof is suggestive (28,29). Case-control analysis has shown significantly increased incidence in those with coexistent facial fractures and head injury (30).

Ultrasound, both cervical and transcranial, has been used acutely to screen patients, but angiography remains definitive (30,31). Diagnostic findings at angiography, in decreasing order of frequency, include pouch formation, luminal stenosis as manifested by the "string sign," tapering to near occlusion, "double lumen sign" with intimal flap, distal branch occlusion, and slow ICA-to-MCA flow (29). Follow-up angiography has shown that posttraumatic dissections are associated with a threefold increased likelihood of progressing to occlusion than are spontaneous dissections (29). Most commonly, the plane is subintimal, causing thromboembolic symptoms, but occasionally, and less commonly in the carotid than the vertebral artery, the dissection can be subadventitial, thus predisposing to subarachnoid hemorrhage (24).

Treatment is usually anticoagulation with intravenous heparin for 10 to 14 days, then sodium warfarin for an additional 3 to 4 months. With this approach there is a small risk of hematoma extension and intracranial hemorrhage, but the vast majority of lesions have healed by the time of repeat angiography at 6 weeks (24). An alternative approach with antiplatelet agents has been suggested for those not experiencing ischemic symptoms (29). If thromboembolic symptoms persist despite anticoagulation or if hemorrhagic complications develop, endovascular or surgical intervention is necessary. Resection and grafting and extracranial-to-intracranial (EC-IC) bypass followed by carotid ligation (29,32) have been described, but a balloon trapping procedure in those tolerating test occlusion is an acceptable alternative in those with good collaterals. Simple flap repair by direct tacking of the intima is rarely possible, but Fogarty catheter placement can be effective (33). Overall, these patients do quite well, with approximately 75 percent returning to normal and 15 percent demonstrating only minor deficits (29,34). Occasionally surgery is necessary prior to medical trial in the rare patient who presents with acute deterioration secondary to low flow, unresponsive to endovascular dilation.

False Aneurysm Formation

Although more commonly the result of penetrating trauma, the formation of false aneurysms due to rupture of the vessel wall with containment by laminated thrombus may occur in the setting of blunt trauma, especially in concert with distal dissections, and therefore will be discussed here. Unlike aneurysms secondary to penetrating trauma, which tend to occur on the common carotid, blunt traumatic aneurysms most commonly arise from the high internal carotid adjacent to the styloid process, which may play a role in their genesis (35,36). Presentation may include neurologic symptoms secondary to embolization or local symptoms of a pulsatile neck mass (37,38). Demonstration on angiography may be difficult secondary to poor filling (39). Conservative therapy has long been felt to be unsafe, with recent studies supporting operative evaluation for any symptomatic lesion (12,40–42).

Surgical therapy may consist of either carotid ligation, with or without EC-IC bypass, excision with or without reversed saphenous vein reconstruction, or, very rarely, clipping (38,43). Intraoperative monitoring of EEG and xenon washout monitoring are especially useful in determining which patients should undergo EC-IC bypass procedures as intraoperative shunting is often impossible in this location. Flow-related rather than exposure-related operative decision making owes much to recent technical improvements in the operative approach (38). These methods have decreased the perioperative stroke rate from the 30 percent associated with unselected ligation of the internal carotid artery to less than 5 percent. Some of this improvement may also be related to more aggressive perioperative heparinization of ICA ligation cases in addition to nonreversal of heparin in bypass and reconstruction cases.

Alternatively, false aneurysms can be treated at angiography, endovascularly. Test occlusion of the parent vessel provides as good or better information about physiologic reserve, and techniques are available for both preserving and sacrificing the main trunk. In those who do not tolerate the occlusion, detachable platinum coils can be positioned through the neck of the pseudoaneurysm, thus thrombosing it. In those with permissive vasculature, additional proximal occlusion with detachable balloons provides additional protection. Anticoagulation is necessary but poses few risks. Such an approach is exceptionally attractive in institutions not accustomed to approaching very high carotid pathology and/or performing bypass procedures.

PENETRATING CAROTID INJURIES

Penetrating injuries of the carotid artery are nearly 10 times as common as those caused by nonpenetrating trauma and occur in about 10 percent of cases of penetrating cervical trauma (44,45). Gunshot wounds are the most common etiology, followed by knife wounds (8,12,45). The most common injury is tangential or partial laceration of the common carotid artery, with total transection less frequent but not uncommon (46). Still less common are fistulas, usually involving the internal jugular vein, and false aneurysms.

Partial Laceration and Total Transection

Penetrating cervical trauma resulting in either laceration or transection of the carotid artery most often causes symptoms related either to hemorrhage (local hematoma, shock, etc.) or to cerebral ischemia. Hemorrhage can result in tracheal compromise, and initial management with intubation is generally recommended. Ischemic symptoms occur in about a third of patients and are felt to be more commonly embolic, but as many as a third of patients cannot tolerate common carotid occlusion, leading to the belief that, at least in some, symptoms may be in part flow related. Some flow-related symptomatology may also be the result of simultaneous injury to other major neck arteries, which occurs in 10 percent of cases. Also necessary for optimal management of these patients is the understanding that an additional 10 percent will have tracheal and laryngeal injuries, and nearly a third will have coexistent internal jugular vein injuries (9).

Management has traditionally included plain C-spine films and chest x-ray to rule out hemothorax, pneumothorax, and vertebral body lesions leading to instability. The decision to proceed to angiography is undisputed for Zone I and III lesions, namely, those below the sternal notch and those above the lower mandible, where vascular injury is felt to be particularly common. Others have maintained that all Zone II injuries should also be studied prior to exploration if time permits (47). In all but the most acute cases preoperative esophagram is also usually indicated (48,49).

At angiography, lacerations and transections show themselves as abnormal cutoffs with or without extravasation of contrast, depending on whether spontaneous thrombosis has occurred. For noncritical vessels, permanent occlusion of either thrombosed or actively bleeding vessels is best accomplished with a nonabsorbable embolic material. Such materials have a wide range of advantages, but most important prevent delayed recanalization and future hemorrhage.

Each has its own specific advantages, but, in short, barium-impregnated silicone microspheres are useful in slowing flow prior to definitive embolization, and detachable balloons are helpful in medium-sized vessels to proximally complete a distal occlusion begun with thrombogenic platinum coils. The incidence of unintentional coil migration is lower when balloons are used simultaneously. We have also developed a coaxial catheter system for the delivery of coils with no incidence of migration in 22 patients. For larger vessels, the extremely expandable polyvinyl alcohol foam sponge is particularly useful. Newer glues are generally more difficult to manipulate and polymerize rapidly, making them unforgiving and probably not indicated in this setting.

In cases where the damaged vessel is thought to be critical, due to failed test occlusion, poor collaterals, or attendant symptoms, placement of deflated silicone balloons may aid immediate surgical intervention by providing temporary occlusion during periods of brisk bleeding not controlled by compression. Surgical mortality remains about 20 percent in such cases, with most of the deaths occurring in those presenting either in coma or severely neurologically compromised (12,45). Seventy percent of survivors, however, returned to work.

FISTULA FORMATION

Traumatic carotid arteriovenous fistulas are encountered frequently (i.e., carotid-cavernous), but cervical carotid-jugular fistulas are decidedly rare (50,51). It has been the experience of those recently treating these lesions that a combined surgical and endovascular approach is advisable. Theoretically, direct balloon occlusion of the fistula could, in itself, be successful, but the increasing diameter of the jugular vein and the high-flow shunt make balloon migration and pulmonary embolism a real hazard. Transarterial balloon trapping of the fistula should therefore be the treatment of choice. This, however, is often difficult secondary to increasing stenosis of the distal ICA, which may again predispose to balloon migration. Transvenous approaches are of little additional help unless flow can be reduced by prior distal and proximal internal carotid occlusion. The safest order in which to proceed is therefore as follows: (a) endovascular ICA test occlusion; (b) STA-MCA bypass with surgical clip occlusion of the high cervical ICA (note: below the ophthalmic to reduce retrograde filling); (c) endovascular balloon occlusion of the ICA just above the bifurcation; and (d) transvenous placement of the distal ICA balloon. Patients not tolerant of balloon test occlusion are candidates for direct surgical ligation of the fistula. This, however, can be very difficult, as many of these are wide-necked, and disastrous complications can ensue if large rents develop unexpectedly in either the carotid, the -jugular, or both. See under "Arteriovenous Fistulas," Chapter 18.

Vertebral Artery Injuries

Injury to the extracranial vertebral artery, like injury to the carotid, can occur in the setting of both mild and severe, nonpenetrating or penetrating trauma. Once thought to be a rare sequela of trauma, frequent angiography has shown vertebral artery injury to represent one-fifth of all traumatic cervical vascular injuries (52). Several anatomic factors contribute to the spectrum and sequelae of injuries seen. Most important, perhaps, is the fact that most vertebral arteries can be occluded without neurologic sequelae, despite their role in supplying the upper spinal chord and medulla. Vertebral arteries that solely supply the basilar trunk or those ending in the posterior inferior cerebellar artery represent uncommon exceptions. Other important anatomic factors include the artery's bony encasement, which makes it very vulnerable in cases of cervical fracture, and extreme cervical spondylosis. The artery's horizontal course along the arch of the atlas also exposes it to compression in extended rotation.

Penetrating injuries of the vertebral artery are more common than nonpenetrating injuries, and because of the good collateral flow, symptoms are generally related to hemorrhage with few neurologic sequelae. Nonetheless, associated trauma to the brachial plexus, the spinal chord, and other cervical vasculature can often complicate this presentation. This is in contrast to nonpenetrating injuries, which have the propensity for developing ischemic complications of posterior circulation thromboembolism. Treatment is therefore quite different, with anticoagulants for cases of ischemia, and ligation, preferably via balloon embolization, for cases of persistent hemorrhage. More complicated surgical approaches are generally reserved for those rare cases of recurrent embolization, despite medical management, and for cases in which vertebral sacrifice cannot be tolerated.

PENETRATING VERTEBRAL ARTERY INJURIES

Penetrating wounds to the vertebral artery are almost always the result of gunshot or stab wounds and are frequently associated with other cervical soft-tissue and vascular trauma (53,54). Interestingly, as many as three-quarters of these injuries occur in patients with no clinical findings specifically implicating the vertebral artery other than a penetrating wound or stable hematoma (55). Injury most commonly results in unilateral **thrombosis,** but **fistula** formation and stenosis are not uncommon (53,55). Injury is equally distributed by location: Zone I (clavicle to C6), Zone II (C2 to C6), Zone III (occiput to C2). Only a quarter of all injuries are associated with major neurologic deficits, and only rarely is the deficit referable to the vertebral artery injury. Furthermore, while overall mortality is still a notable 17 percent, it is due entirely to direct central nervous system injury and is independent of both vertebral artery injury and attendant local injury secondary to cervical fracture, carotid injury, or pharyngoesophageal injury. This view is debated, however, with some groups finding arterial injury responsible for as much as 80 percent of mortality. Direct exploration of these wounds, often without the aid of preoperative angiography, has been supplanted by the aggressive use of early (<4 h of admission) aortic arch and four-vessel angiography. Management is largely related to the underlying pathology.

OCCLUSION OR STENOSIS

Occlusion or stenosis of the vessel can result from either intimal flap–associated thrombus or dissection with luminal compromise (Figs. 18.58 and 18.61) (56). In those with a patent contralateral vertebral and an ipsilateral vertebral not ending in posterior inferior cerebellar artery, asymptomatic occlusion or stenosis can usually be treated conservatively with or without antiplatelet or anticoagulant therapy. Symptomatic patients with contralateral vertebral atrophy (8 percent) or contralateral termination in PICA (2.5 percent) may, however, represent good candidates for revascularization (see operative approaches in text following).

In addition, those with persistent embolic symptoms despite medical management may benefit from either therapeutic detachable balloon occlusion or direct operative occlusion (see operative opproaches in text following). For short-segment dissections and intimal flaps, a single balloon, placed as proximal to the pathology as possible, is usually sufficient, but long-segment dissections may reconstitute themselves with distal flow and require balloon trapping (57). Distal balloon placement can be achieved either by directly traversing the injured segment with special guide wires or via the contralateral vertebral artery. Endovascular therapy offers the advantage of immediate and aggressive postprocedure anticoagulation, which is so important.

ARTERIOVENOUS FISTULA

Vertebral arteriovenous fistulas are rare but are most commonly secondary to penetrating trauma. They occur mostly in Zones I and II, and, when traumatic, are associated with transection of the vertebral artery half of the time. Symptoms usually consist of only neck pain or bruit, but massive hemorrhage and progressive neurologic deficit secondary to steal or venous hypertension are not uncommon. Transvascular techniques have been the treatment of choice in recent years and are associated with closure of the fistula in nearly all cases and preservation of the vertebral artery in half (66 percent without associated transection, 33 percent with transection) (58). Morbidity with these procedures is very low, and they rarely, if ever, are associated with the massive blood loss seen with past direct surgical approaches, which necessarily traversed the dense vertebral venous plexus (53,59). Silicone or latex balloons are most commonly employed in the obliteration of these fistulas and are placed via coaxial catheter systems under mild heparinization if not contraindicated. When distal access is difficult, as in cases associated with transection, either gentle advancement with guide wires or use of the contralateral vertebral artery may be employed. In any case, distal occlusion and occlusion of the fistula should always precede proximal occlusion in cases where patency is not a concern so as to avoid increased retrograde filling, collateral filling, and/or steal. Furthermore, staged procedures may be necessary, especially with large, long-standing lesions, which may show signs of reversible deterioration on inflation of the occluding balloon.

PSEUDOANEURYSM

Pseudoaneurysms most often present after penetrating trauma but also can be seen in blunt trauma (Fig. 18.62). They are most commonly associated with bruit, neck mass, and cranial nerve deficit. Pseudoaneurysms are best treated with test occlusion followed by percutaneous transcatheter coil or balloon occlusion of the proximal and distal vertebral artery. The decision to treat these lesions is based on their ability to cause future permanent neurologic disability even while some will spontaneously regress. In cases where the pathology arises from a dominant vertebral artery within the bony canal (C2–C6), staged placement of electrolytically detachable platinum coils can, in certain cases, successfully occlude pseudoaneurysms without migration of embolic material through the thrombus wall and with preservation of the parent vessel (57). The low morbidity of this endovascular approach, combined with the fact that several communications with the dense vertebral venous

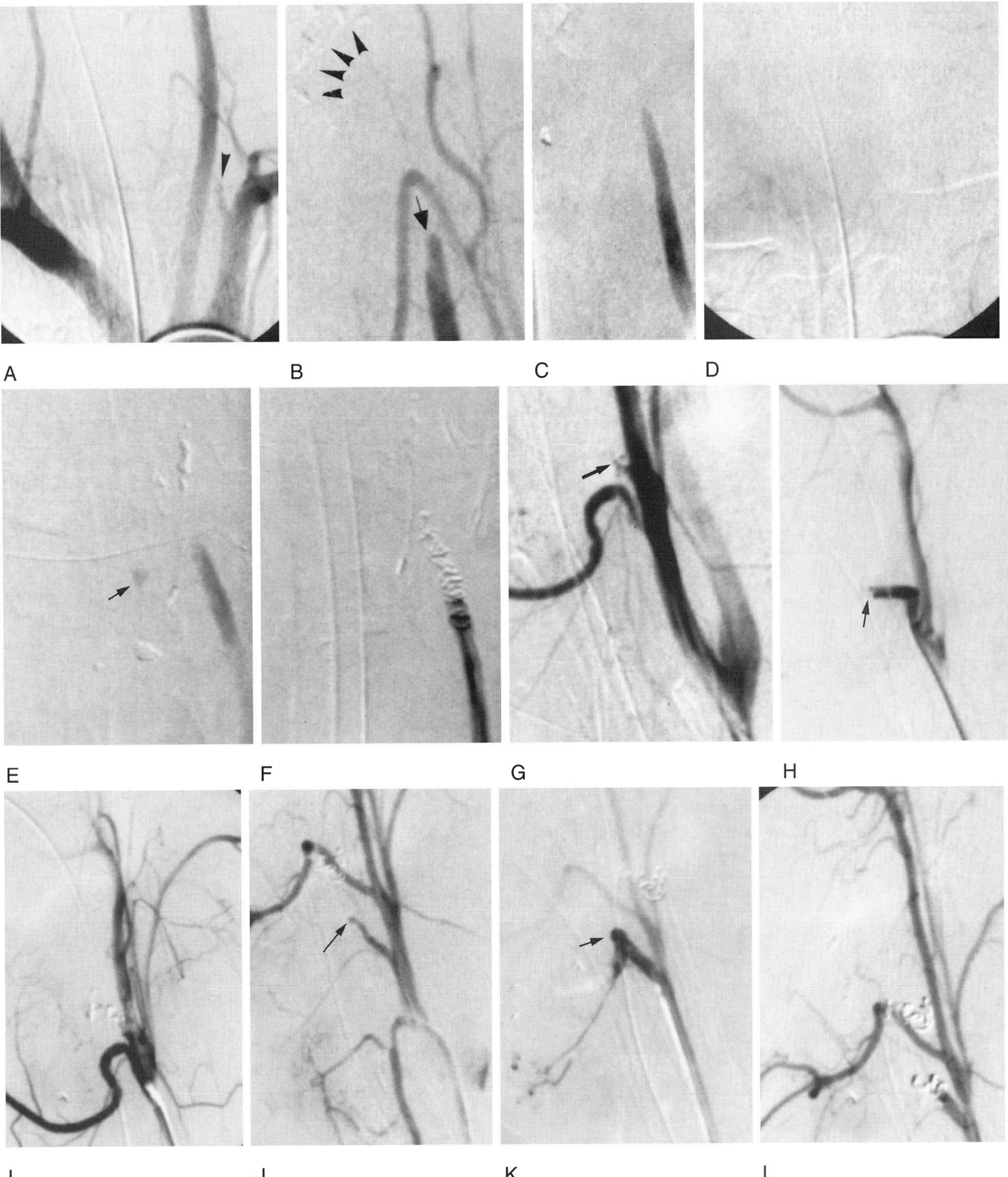

Figure 18.61. Multiple arterial occlusions. Young gunfighter who sustained multiple gunshot wounds to his neck and face. After an initial angiogram, he underwent surgical exploration with subsequent angiogram and embolization. There was a vertebral occlusion, with subsequent bleeding. Note that bleeding can occur in delayed fashion and from a vessel that initially seems "occluded." **A.** Initial arch angiogram showing cutoff of the left vertebral artery (arrow). **B.** Left subclavian artery angiogram showing occlusion of the proximal vertebral artery (arrow) and attempted collaterals (arrowheads). Late (**C**) and very late (**D**) films of the left subclavian artery without evidence of extravasation. **E.** Follow-up anteroposterior subclavian angiogram 6 h after the initial angiogram with extravasation noted projecting over the spinal canal (arrow). **F.** Left vertebral artery angiogram following occlusion of the vertebral artery. External carotid injection. **G.** Left lateral common carotid artery injection with stump of facial artery with bullet fragment (arrow). **H.** Selective catheterization of the facial artery showing cutoff of the vessel (arrow). **I.** Postcoil occlusion of the facial artery. **J.** Right lateral common carotid artery angiogram. Note cutoff of lingual artery (arrow). **K.** Superselective catheterization of lingual artery, with cutoff and pooling of contrast. **L.** Right lateral external carotid status following occlusion of lingual artery.

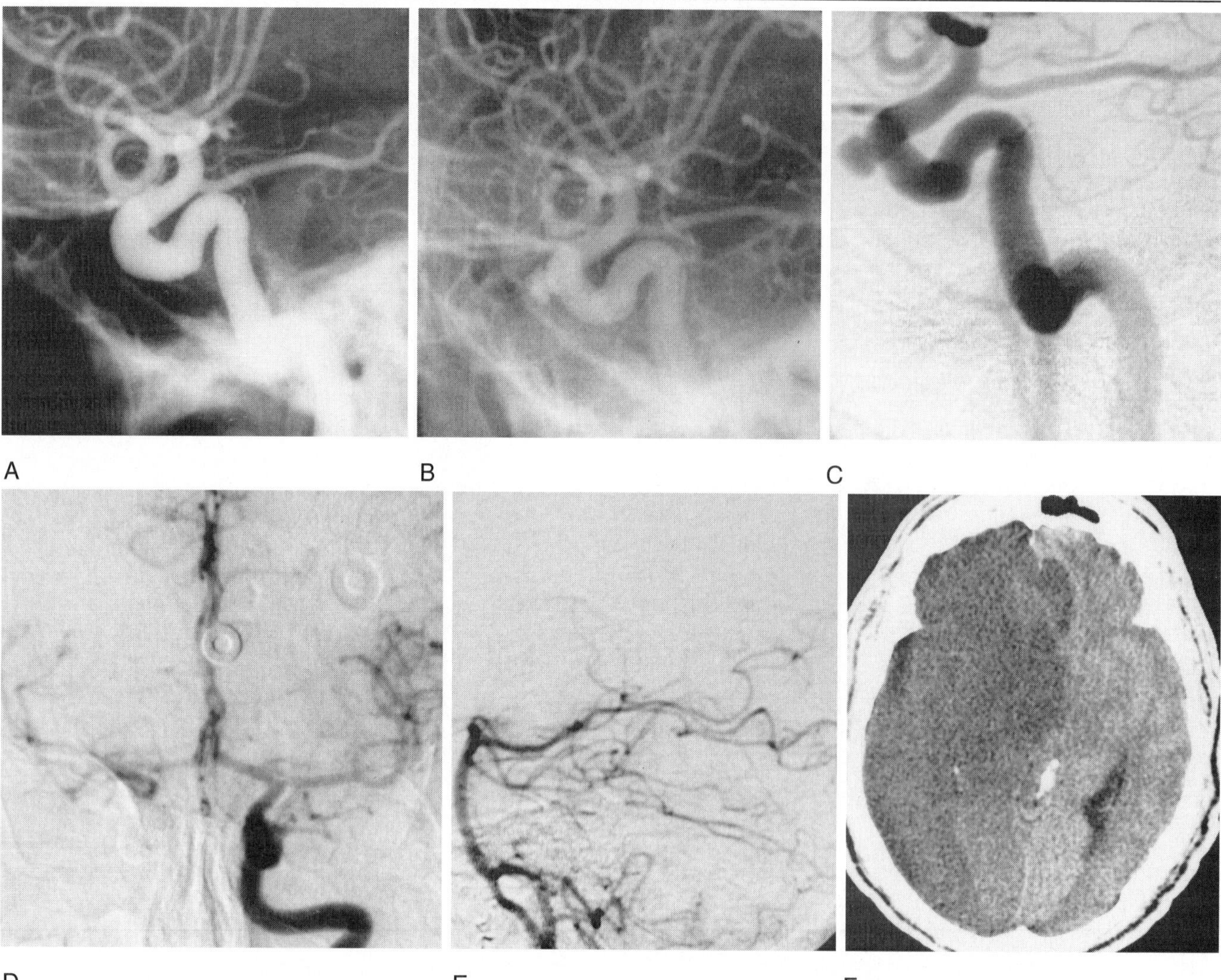

Figure 18.62. Pseudoaneurysm, posttraumatic, of carotid siphon. Brisk arterial bleeding (ca. 5 L) was encountered during abdominal surgery of this man. The patient was initially treated with packing, but when he rebled, repeat angiogram was done. A third angiogram was performed that showed that the aneurysm had grown, and the patient was treated with carotid occlusion. Following occlusion the patient developed a massive GI bleed, became hypotensive, developed a massive stroke, and died. **A.** Initial right lateral carotid angiogram without clear evidence of pseudoaneurysm. **B.** Angiogram done 12 days later, with pseudoaneurysm clearly seen projecting anteriorly from the anterior cavernous carotid. **C.** Angiogram done two days later, with interval growth of the pseudoaneurysm; carotid occlusion was carried out. **D.** Left anteroposterior internal carotid injection with cross-filling. **E.** Left lateral vertebral artery revealed atretic posterior communicating arteries. There was carotid origin of the right posterior cerebral artery as shown in A. **F.** CT showing massive hemispheric stroke developing after hypotension secondary to massive GI bleed.

plexus may exist in cases of associated fistula, has led groups to abandon a direct surgical approach for most of these lesions (53). For pseudoaneurysms of Zones I and III, however, several groups have maintained that the traditional surgical approach with either proximal ligation or trapping not only is safe and efficacious but can be intraoperatively modified to allow for arterial preservation in cases where vertebral sacrifice cannot be tolerated (60). Vertebral preservation techniques via primary vascular oversewing, interposed vein, or arterialized bypass can also be employed in the usual setting of vertebral expendability if the anatomy and the patient's condition are favorable (60).

ONGOING BLEEDING

Ongoing bleeding due to vessel transection is probably underdiagnosed. Bleeding can often be internal and delayed. When misdiagnosed on preoperative angiogram, occlusion is the most common errant reading. Management of this condition, when correctly recognized, is safest with proximal and distal endovascular occlusion after test occlusion. The greatest difficulties in delivering this form of embolotherapy involve distal control, but failure to achieve it has been associated with rebleeding (55). Guide wires can be used to traverse the level of injury in Zones I and II but are useless in situations of proximal thrombosis and in Zone

III. Distal control in these settings has been obtained using detachable balloons delivered from the contralateral vertebral artery, but this requires considerable expertise and in some institutions can only be approached surgically (61). For those who fail test occlusion, who suffer flow-related symptoms, or in whom distal control cannot be achieved endovascularly, operative exploration for either ligation or revascularization may be indicated (54,55,62–64).

Nonpenetrating Vertebral Artery Injuries

Nonpenetrating trauma to the cervical vertebral artery generally results from the extreme lateral rotation seen with events such as chiropractic manipulation, wrestling, or football tackling. It most frequently affects the vertebral artery at C1-2 (Zone III), and may occur in those with normal vertebrae, but it is often associated with underlying osteoarthritic spurring (65). Fracture/dislocations of the cervical spine, including the dens but especially between C2 and C6 (Zone II) with subluxations >1 cm, and fracture of the lateral masses or foramen transversarium are particularly associated with injury to the vertebral artery.

In fact, recent prospective angiographic studies suggest that 46 to 75 percent of patients with injuries involving the facet or the foramen transversarium between C2 and C6 will have angiographic evidence of vertebral injury (66,67). In the 26 patients prospectively identified by Willis, none, however, suffered any neurologic sequelae. This is in agreement with the other authors' findings that only 5 percent of cervical facet fractures developed vertebrobasilar insufficiency (0.75 percent of all cervical fractures). Subpopulations do, however, exist with greater incidences of symptomatic vertebral injury and include the rare facet injury coexistent with lateral dislocation (vertebrobasilar ischemia 60 percent) (68). For these patients, angiography should be performed prior to cervical reduction, but for others at lesser risk, duplex ultrasound and MRA may represent more reasonable screening methods (69,70). The latter is easily obtained in the setting of the routine conventional MRI evaluation for disc and soft-tissue pathology.

Blunt trauma secondary to fracture/dislocation or lesser trauma is similar in that the mechanism, whether stretching or direct trauma, appears to result in the same initial pathologic substrate—intimal injury. This, in turn, can precipitate thrombotic or dissecting stenosis or occlusion with or without embolization (71). Pseudoaneurysms can form and may either bleed or serve as a source for emboli. Fistulas and pronounced spasm may also develop. As with most vertebral pathology, collateral flow allows many lesions to remain either asymptomatic or symptomatic secondary to embolism alone (23).

These embolic symptoms and asymptomatic dissections are generally treated with anticoagulation, whereas the rare case of flow-related symptoms may be treated with either interposition vein graft or occipital-to-PICA bypass. Antiplatelet agents may initially be substituted for heparin in appropriate cases if severe head trauma coexists. When symptoms are positional, reduction of external compression can be accomplished through either removal of osteophytes or cervical fusion (72). When symptoms exist in the setting of persisting subluxation, reduction should be achieved despite case reports of occasional worsening. Fistulas and pseudoaneurysms are most often treated by intravascular balloon obliteration, as outlined earlier, as are embolic symptoms resistant to medical management (52, 73).

REFERENCES

1. Belkin M, Dunton R, Crombie HD Jr, Lowe R: Preoperative percutaneous intraluminal balloon catheter control of major arterial hemorrhage. J Trauma 1988;28:548–550.
2. Scalea TM, Sclafani SJA: Angiographically placed balloons for arterial control: A description of a technique. J Trauma 1991;31: 1671–1677.
3. McNeese S, Finck E, Yellin AE: Definitive treatment of selected vascular injuries and post-traumatic arteriovenous fistulas by arteriographic embolization. Am J Surg 1980;140:252–259.
4. Mehringer CM, Hieshima GB, Grinnell VS, et al: Therapeutic embolization for vascular trauma of the head and neck. AJNR 1983;4: 137–142.
5. Hieshima GB, Mehringer CM, Grinnell VS, Hasso AN, Siegel NH, Pribram HF: Emergency occlusive techniques. Surg Neurol 1978; 9:293–302.
6. Batzdorf U, Bentson JR, Machleder HI: Blunt trauma to the high cervical carotid artery. Neurosurgery 1979;5:195–201.
7. Chandler WF: Trauma to the carotid artery and other cervical vessels. In Julian R. Youmans (ed), Neurological Surgery, ed 3, vol 4. Philadelphia: WB Saunders, 1985, pp 2367–2377.
8. Fry RE, Fry WJ: Extracranial carotid artery injuries. Surgery 1980; 88:581–587.
9. Rubio PA, Ruel JG, Beall AC, et al: Acute carotid artery injury: 25 years' experience. J Trauma 1974;14:967–973.
10. Li MS, Smith BM, Espinosa J, Brown RA, Richardson P, Ford R: Nonpenetrating trauma to the carotid artery: Seven cases and a literature review. J Trauma 1994;36:265–272.
11. Yamada S, Kindt GW, Youmans JR: Carotid artery occlusion due to nonpenetrating injury. J Trauma 1967;7:333–344.
12. Fabian TC, George SM, Croce MA, Mangiante EC, Voeller GR, Kudsk KA: Carotid artery trauma: Management based on mechanism of injury. J Trauma 1990;30:953–961.
13. Garg AG, Gordon DS, Taylor AR, et al: Internal carotid artery thrombosis secondary to closed cranio-cervical trauma. Br J Surg 1968;55:4–9.
14. Fleming JFR, Petrie D: Traumatic thrombosis of the internal carotid artery with delayed hemiplegia. Can J Surg 1968;11:166–175.
15. Olfson RA, Christoferson LA: The syndrome of carotid occlusion following minor craniocerebral trauma. J Neurosurg 1970;33: 636–639.
16. French BN, Cobb CA, Dublin AB: Cranial computed tomography in the diagnosis of symptomatic indirect trauma in the carotid artery. Surg Neurol 1981;15:256–267.
17. Zuber M, Meary E, Meder J-F, Mas J-L: Magnetic resonance imaging and dynamic CT scan in cervical artery dissections. Stroke 1994; 25:576–581.
18. Zilkha A: Traumatic occlusion of the internal carotid artery. Radiology 1970;97:543–548.
19. Loar CR, Chadduck WM, Nugent GR: Traumatic occlusion of the middle cerebral artery: Case report. J Neurosurg 1973;39:753–756.
20. Towne JP, Neis ND, Smith JW: Thrombosis of the internal carotid artery following blunt cervical trauma. Arch Surg 1972;104: 565–568.
21. Crissey MM, Bernstein EF: Delayed presentation of carotid intimal tear following blunt craniocervical trauma. Surgery 1974;75: 543–549.

22. Krajewski LP, Hertzer NR: Blunt carotid artery trauma: Report of two cases and review of the literature. Ann Surg 1980;191:341–346.
23. Davis JM, Zimmerman RA: Injury of the carotid and vertebral arteries. Neuroradiology 1983;25:55–69.
24. Friedman WA, Day AV, Quisling RG, et al: Cervical carotid dissecting aneurysms. Neurosurgery 1980;7:207–214.
25. Biller J, Hingtgen WL, Adams HP, et al: Cervicocephalic arterial dissections: A ten-year experience. Arch Neurol 1986;43:1234.
26. Stringer WL, Kelly DL Jr: Traumatic dissection of the extracranial internal carotid artery. Neurosurgery 1980;6:123–130.
27. Zelenock GB, Kazmers A, Whitehouse WM Jr, et al: Extracranial internal carotid artery dissection: Noniatrogenic traumatic lesions. Arch Surg 1982;11:425–432.
28. Anson JA, Crowell RM: Cervicocranial arterial dissection. Neurosurgery 1991;29:89–96.
29. Mokri B, Piepgras DG, Houser OW: Traumatic dissections of the extracranial internal carotid artery. J Neurosurg 1988;68:189–197.
30. Davis JW, Holbrook TL, Hoyt DB, Mackersie RC, Field TO Jr, Shackford SR: Blunt carotid artery dissection: Incidence, associated injuries, screening, and treatment. J Trauma 1990;30:1514–1517.
31. Hennerici M, Steinke W, Rautenberg W: High-resistance Doppler flow pattern in extracranial carotid dissection. Arch Neurol 1989; 46:670–672.
32. Bergquist BJ, Boone SC, Whaley RA: Traumatic dissection on the internal carotid artery treated by ECIC anastomoses. Stroke 1981; 12:73–76.
33. Ojemann RG, Fisher CM, Rich JC: Spontaneous dissecting aneurysm of the internal carotid artery. Stroke 1972;3:434–440.
34. Hart RG, Easton JD: Dissections of cervical and cerebral arteries. Neurol Clin North Am 1983;1:255.
35. Deysine M, Adiga R, Wilder JR: Traumatic false aneurysm of the cervical internal carotid artery. Surgery 1969;66:1004–1007.
36. McCollum CH, Wheeler WG, Noon GP, et al: Aneurysms of the extracranial carotid artery: Twenty-one years' experience. Am J Surg 1979;137:196–200.
37. Rittenhouse EA, Radke HM, Sumner DS: Carotid artery aneurysm. Arch Surg 1972;105:786–789.
38. Sundt TM, Pearson BW, Piepgras DG, Houser OW, Mokri B: Surgical management of aneurysms of the distal extracranial internal carotid artery. J Neurosurg 1986;64:169–182.
39. Sullivan HG, Vines FS, Becker DP: Sequelae of indirect carotid injury. Radiology 1973;109:91–98.
40. Mokri B, Piepgras DG, Sundt TM Jr, et al: Extracranial internal carotid artery aneurysms. Mayo Clin Proc 1982;57:310–321.
41. Teal JS, Bergeron RT, Rumbaugh CL, et al: Aneurysms of the cervical portion of the internal carotid artery associated with nonpenetrating neck trauma. Radiology 1972;105:353–358.
42. Weaver FA, Yellin AE, Wagner WH, et al: The role of arterial reconstruction in penetrating carotid injuries. Arch Surg 1988;123: 1106–1111.
43. Fein JM, Flamm E: Planned intracranial revascularization before proximal ligation for traumatic aneurysm. Neurosurgery 1979;5: 254–255.
44. Calcaterra TC, Holt CP: Carotid artery injuries. Laryngoscope 1972;82:321–329.
45. Unger SW, Tucker WS, Mrdeza MA, et al: Carotid artery trauma. Surgery 1980;87:477–487.
46. Thal ER, Snyder WH, Hays RJ, et al: Management of carotid artery injuries. Surgery 1974;76:955–962.
47. McCormick TM, Burch BH: Routine angiogram for evaluation of neck and extremity injuries. Trauma 1979;19:384–387.
48. Flynn TC: Comment on Fabian TC, et al: Carotid artery trauma: Management based on mechanism of injury. J Trauma 1990;30: 961–962.
49. Panetta T, Sclafani SJA, Goldstein AS, Phillips TF: Percutaneous transcatheter embolization for arterial trauma. J Vasc Surg 1985;2: 54–64.
50. Morawetz RB, McDowell HA, Richardson JV: Obliteration of an internal carotid-internal jugular fistula using a prolo catheter. Surg Neurol 1978;10:276–278.
51. Niijima KH, Yonekawa Y, Taki W: A detachable balloon procedure for a traumatic internal carotid–internal jugular fistula: Report of a case. Neurosurgery 1990;27:809–812.
52. Ben-Menachem Y, Fields WS, Cadavid G, Gomez LS, Anderson EC, Fisher RG: Vertebral artery trauma: Transcatheter embolization. AJNR 1987;8:501–507.
53. Golueke P, Sclafani S, Phillips T, Goldstein AM, Scalea T, Duncan A: Vertebral artery injury: Diagnosis and management. J Trauma 1987;27:856–865.
54. Meier DE, Brink BE, Fry WJ: Vertebral artery trauma. Arch Surg 1981;116:236–239.
55. Reid JDS, Weiglet JA: Forty-three cases of vertebral artery trauma. J Trauma 1988;28:1007–1012.
56. Mas JL, Bousser MG, Hasboun D, et al: Extracranial vertebral artery dissections: A review of 13 cases. Stroke 1987;18:1037–1047.
57. Halbach VV, Higashida RT, Dowd CF, et al: Endovascular treatment of vertebral artery dissections and pseudoaneurysms. J Neurosurg 1993;79:183–191.
58. Halbach VV, Higashida RT, Hieshima GB: Treatment of vertebral arteriovenous fistulas. Am J Neuroradiol 1987;8:1121–1128.
59. Roper PR, Guinto FC, Wolma FJ: Posttraumatic vertebral artery aneurysm and arteriovenous fistula: A case report. Surgery 1984;96: 556–559.
60. de los Reyes RA, Moser FG, Sachs DP, Boehm FH: Direct repair of an extracranial vertebral artery pseudoaneurysm: Case report and review of the literature. Neurosurgery 1990;26:528–533.
61. Miller RE, Hieshima GB, Giannotta SL, et al: Acute traumatic vertebral arteriovenus fistula: Balloon occlusion with the use of a contralateral approach. Neurosurgery 1984;14:225.
62. Berguer R: Distal vertebral artery bypass: Technique, the "occipital connection," and potential uses. J Vasc Surg 1985;2:621–626.
63. Edwards WH, Mulherin JL: The surgical approach to significant stenosis of vertebral and subclavian arteries. Surgery 1980;87:20–28.
64. Miyamoto S, Kikuchi H, Nagata I, et al: Saphenous vein graft to the distal vertebral artery between C-1 and C-2 using a lateral-anterior approach. Technical note. J Neurosurg 1992;77:812–815.
65. Schneider RC, Gosch HH, Taren JA, et al: Blood vessel trauma following head and neck injuries. Clin Neurosurg 1972;19:312–354.
66. Louw JA, Mafoyane NA, Small B, Neser CP: Occlusion of the vertebral artery in cervical spine dislocations. J Bone Joint Surg Br 1990; 72:679–681.
67. Willis BK, Greiner F, Orrison WW, Benzel EC: The incidence of vertebral artery injury after midcervical spine fracture or subluxation. Neurosurgery 1994;34:435–442.
68. Parent AD, Harkey HL, Touchstone DA, Smith EE, Smith RR: Lateral cervical spine dislocation and vertebral artery injury. Neurosurgery 1992;31:501–509.
69. Meisner M, Paun M, Johansen K: Duplex scanning for arterial trauma. Am J Surg 1991;161:552–555.
70. Quint DJ, Spickler EM: Magnetic resonance demonstration of vertebral artery dissection. J Neurosurg 1990;72:964–967.
71. Hugenholtz H, Pokrupa R, Montpetit VJA, et al: Spontaneous dissecting aneurysm of the extracranial vertebral artery. Neurosurgery 1982;10:96–100.
72. Yang PJ, Latack JT, Gabrielsen TO, et al: Rotational vertebral artery occlusion at C1–C2. Am J Neuroradiol 1985;6:98–100.
73. Debrun G, Legre J, Kadsbarian M, Tapias PL, Caron JP: Endovascular occlusion of vertebral fistulae by detachable balloons with conservation of vertebral blood flow. Radiology 1979;130:141–147.

SUGGESTED READINGS

Bradley EL: Management of penetrating carotid injuries: An alternative approach. J Trauma 1973;13:248–255.

Brown MF, Graham JM, Feliciano DV, et al: Carotid artery injuries. Am J Surg 1982;144:748–753.

Ledgerwood AM, Mullins RJ, Lucas CE: Primary repair versus ligation for carotid artery injuries. Arch Surg 1980;115:488–493.

ACKNOWLEDGMENTS

Dr. Pile-Spellman is grateful to his many teachers, including Alex Berenstein, MD; Robert Crowell, MD; Ken Davis, MD; Gerard Debrun, MD; Roberto Heros, MD; J. P. Mohr, MD; Josephine Moore, PhD; Victor Shcheglov, MD; Bennett Stein, MD; Juan Taveras, MD; and William L. Young, MD.

He appreciates the continued support of all of his associates at the Neurological Institute in New York at Columbia Presbyterian Medical Center and hopes that this chapter may be of use to young colleagues in neuroradiology and neurosurgery.

Index

D